D1064583

Fifth Edition

JOSEPHSON'S

# Clinical Cardiac Electrophysiology

## Techniques and Interpretations


Mark E. Josephson, MD

*Herman C. Dana Professor of Medicine*
*Harvard Medical School*

*Chief of the Cardiovascular Division*
*Beth Israel Deaconess Medical Center*

*Director, Harvard-Thorndike Electrophysiology Institute and Arrhythmia Service*
*Beth Israel Deaconess Medical Center, Boston, Massachusetts*



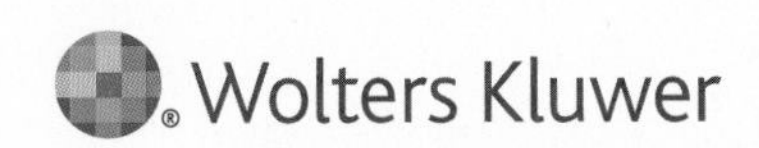


Philadelphia • Baltimore • New York • London
Buenos Aires • Hong Kong • Sydney • Tokyo

*Acquisitions Editor:* Julie Goolsby
*Product Development Editor:* Andrea Vosburgh
*Marketing Manager:* Stephanie Kindlick
*Production Project Manager:* David Saltzberg
*Design Coordinator:* Steven Druding
*Manufacturing Coordinator:* Beth Welsh
*Prepress Vendor:* Aptara, Inc.

5th edition


351 West Camden Street
Baltimore, MD 21201

Two Commerce Square/2001 Market Street
Philadelphia, PA 19103



9 8 7 6 5 4 3 2 1

Printed in China

**Library of Congress Cataloging-in-Publication Data**

Josephson, Mark E., author.
[Clinical cardiac electrophysiology]
Josephson's clinical cardiac electrophysiology : techniques and interpretations / Mark E. Josephson. – Fifth edition.
p. ; cm.
Previously published as: Clinical cardiac electrophysiology / Mark E. Josephson.
Includes bibliographical references and index.
ISBN 978-1-4511-8741-0
I. Title.
[DNLM: 1. Electrophysiologic Techniques, Cardiac–methods. 2. Arrhythmias, Cardiac–diagnosis. 3. Arrhythmias, Cardiac–therapy. 4. Heart Conduction System–physiopathology. WG 141.5.F9]
RC683.5.E5
616.1'207547–dc23

2015018611



LWW.com

CCS0815

*This book is dedicated to my family—Sylvie, Elan, Sydney, Rachel, Todd, Stephanie, Jesse, and particularly, to my wife Joan—for their love, support, and understanding. Joan, you have been the wind beneath my wings.*

FOREWORD

# Historical Perspectives

The study of the heart as an electrical organ has fascinated physiologists and physicians for nearly a century and a half. Matteucci[1] studied electrical current in pigeon hearts, and Kölliker and Müller[2] studies discrete electrical activity in association with each cardiac contraction in the frog. Study of the human electrocardiogram awaited the discoveries of Waller[3] and, most important, Einthoven,[4] whose use and development of the string galvanometer permitted the standardization and widespread use of that instrument. Almost simultaneously, anatomists and pathologists were tracing the atrioventricular (A-V) conduction system. Many of the pathways, both normal and abnormal, still bear the names of the men who described them. This group of men included His,[5] who discovered the muscle bundle joining the atrial and ventricular septae that is known as the common A-V bundle or the bundle of His.

During the first half of the 20th century clinical electrocardiography gained widespread acceptance, and, in feats of deductive reasoning, numerous electrocardiographers contributed to the understanding of how the cardiac impulse in man is generated and conducted. Those researchers were, however, limited to observation of atrial (P wave) and ventricular (QRS complex) depolarizations and their relationships to one another made at a relatively slow recording speed (25 mm/s) during spontaneous rhythms. Nevertheless, combining those carefully made observations of the anatomists and the concepts developed in the physiology laboratory, these researchers accurately described, or at least hypothesized, many of the important concepts of modern electrophysiology. These included such concepts as slow conduction, concealed conduction, A-V block, and the general area of arrhythmogenesis, including abnormal impulse formation and reentry. Some of this history was reviewed by the late Langendorf.[6] Even the mechanism of pre-excitation and circus movement tachycardia were accurately described and diagrammed by Wolferth and Wood from the University of Pennsylvania in 1933.[7] The diagrams in that manuscript are as accurate today as they were hypothetical in 1933. Much of what has followed the innovative work of investigators in the first half of the century has confirmed the brilliance of their investigations.

In the 1940s and 1950s, when cardiac catheterization was emerging, it became increasingly apparent that luminal catheters could be placed intravascularly by a variety of routes and safely passed to almost any region of the heart, where they could remain for a substantial period of time. Alanis et al. recorded the His bundle potential in an isolated perfused animal heart,[8] and Kottmeier et al. recorded the His bundle potential in man during open heart surgery.[9] Giraud et al. were the first to record electrical activity from the His bundle by a catheter;[10] however, it was the report of Scherlag et al.,[11] detailing the electrode catheter techniques in dogs and humans, to reproducibly record His bundle electrogram, which paved the way for the extraordinary investigations that have occurred over the past two and a half decades.

At about the time Scherlag et al.[11] were detailing the catheter technique of recording His bundle activity, Durrer et al. in Amsterdam and Coumel and his associates in Paris independently developed the technique of programmed electrical stimulation of the heart in 1967.[12,13] This began the first decade of clinical cardiac electrophysiology. Although the early years of intracardiac recording in man were dominated by descriptive work exploring the presence and timing of His bundle activation (and that of a few other intracardiac sites) in a variety of spontaneously occurring physiologic and pathologic states, a quantum leap occurred when the technique of programmed stimulation was combined with intracardiac recordings by Wellens.[14] Use of these techniques subsequently furthered our understanding of the functional component of the A-V specialized conducting system, including the refractory periods of the atrium, A-V node, His bundle, Purkinje system, and ventricles and enables us to assess the effects of pharmacologic agents on these parameters, to induce and terminate a variety of tachyarrhythmias, and, in a major way, has led to a greater understanding of the electrophysiology of the human heart. Shortly thereafter, enthusiasm and inquisitiveness led to placement of an increasing number of catheters for recording and stimulation to different locations with the heart, first in the atria and thereafter in the ventricle. This first led to development of endocardial catheter mapping techniques to define the location of bypass tracts and the mechanisms of supraventricular tachyarrhythmias.[15,16]

Beginning in the mid-1970s, Josephson and his colleagues at the University of Pennsylvania were the first to use vigorous, systematic, multisite programmed stimulation in the study of sustained ventricular tachycardia (VT) resulting from myocardial infarction, which allowed induction of VT in more than 90% of the patients in whom this rhythm occurred spontaneously.[17–19] Subsequent investigators sought to establish a better understanding of the methodology used in the electrophysiology study to induce arrhythmias. Several studies validated the sensitivity and specificity of programmed stimulation for induction of uniform tachycardias, and the nonspecificity of polymorphic arrhythmias induced with vigorous programmed stimulation was recognized.[19,20]

In the same time period, Josephson et al.[21–23] developed the technique of endocardial catheter mapping of VT, which for the first time demonstrated the safety and significance of placing catheters in the left ventricle. This led to the recognition of the subendocardial origin of the majority of ventricular tachyarrhythmias, associated with coronary artery disease and the development of subendocardial resection as a therapeutic cure for this arrhythmia.[24]

For the next decade, electrophysiologic studies continued to better understand the mechanisms of arrhythmias in man by comparing the response to programmed stimulation in man in the response to in vitro and in vivo studies of abnormal automaticity, triggered activity caused by delayed and early afterdepolarizations, and anatomical functional reentry. These studies, which used programmed stimulation, endocardial catheter mapping, and response of tachycardias to stimulation and drugs, have all suggested that most sustained paroxysmal tachycardias were due to reentry. The reentrant substrate could be functional or fixed or combinations of both. In particular, the use of entrainment and resetting during atrial flutter and VT were important techniques used to confirm the reentrant nature of these arrhythmias.[25–30] Resetting and entrainment with fusion became phenomena that were diagnostic of reentrant excitation. Cassidy et al.[31] using left ventricular endocardial mapping during sinus rhythm, for the first time described an electrophysiologic correlate of the pathophysiologic substrate of VT in coronary artery disease—a low-amplitude fragmented electrograms of long duration and late potentials.[31,32] Fenoglio, Wit, Josephson, and their colleagues from the University of Pennsylvania documented for the first time that these arrhythmogenic areas were associated with viable muscle fibers separated by and imbedded in scar tissue from the infarction.[33] They demonstrated that the quality and quantity of abnormal electrograms (and, hence, the pathophysiologic substrate) differed for sustained monomorphic VT, nonsustained VT, and ventricular fibrillation in patients with prior infarction and cardiomyopathy. Experimental studies by Gardner et al.[34] demonstrated that these fractionated electrograms resulted from poorly coupled fibers that were viable and maintained normal action potential characteristics but that exhibited salutatory conduction and caused by nonuniform anisotropy. Further exploration of contributing factors (triggers), such as the influence of the autonomic nervous system or ischemia, will be necessary to further enhance our understanding of the genesis of the arrhythmias. This initial decade or so of electrophysiology could be likened to an era of discovery.

Subsequently, and overlapping somewhat with the era of discovery, was the development of the concept and use of programmed stimulation as a tool for developing therapy for arrhythmias. The ability to reproducibly initiate and terminate arrhythmias led to the development of serial drug testing to assess antiarrhythmic efficacy.[35] The ability of an antiarrhythmic drug to prevent initiation of a tachycardia that we reliably initiated in the control state appeared to predict freedom from the arrhythmia in the 2- to 3-year follow-up. This was seen in many nonrandomized clinical trials from laboratories in the early 1980.

The persistent inducibility of an arrhythmia universally predicted an outcome that was worse than that in patients in whom tachycardias were made noninducible. The natural history of recurrences of ventricular tachyarrhythmias (or other arrhythmias for that matter) and the changing substrate for arrhythmias were recognized potential imitations of drug testing. It was recognized very early that programmed stimulation was not useful in selecting drugs to treat ventricular tachyarrhythmias in patients without coronary artery disease (i.e., cardiomyopathy).[36] Despite the fact that all studies showed that patients with spontaneous VT whose arrhythmias were rendered noninducible by antiarrhythmic agents far better than patients with persistently inducible arrhythmias, the inability to accurately predict freedom from recurrence led to abandonment of programmed stimulation as a modality to select antiarrhythmic agents. The ESVEM study,[37] although plagued by limitations in protocol and patient selection, put the nail in the coffin for programmed stimulation as a method of selecting antiarrhythmic therapy of arrhythmias.

With the known limitation of EP-guided therapy to predict outcomes uniformly and correctly, as well as the potentially lethal proarrhythmic effect of antiarrhythmic agents demonstrated in the CAST study,[38] the desire for nonpharmacologic approaches to therapy grew. Surgery had already become a gold standard therapy for Wolff–Parkinson–White syndrome, and innovative surgical procedures for VT had grown from our understanding of the pathophysiologic substrate of VT and coronary disease and the mapping of VT from the Pennsylvania group. However, surgery was considered a rather drastic procedure for patients with a relatively benign disorder (supraventricular tachycardia and the Wolff–Parkinson–White syndrome), and although successful for VT for coronary artery disease, was associated with a high operative mortality. These limitations have led to two major areas of nonpharmacologic therapy that have dominated the last 25 years; implantable antitachycardia/defibrillator devices and catheter ablation. These techniques were the natural evolution of our knowledge of arrhythmia mechanisms (e.g., the ability to initiate and terminate the reentrant arrhythmias by pacing and electrical conversion) and the refinement of catheter mapping techniques and the success of surgery used with these techniques.

It was Mirowski who initially demonstrated that an implantable defibrillator could convert VT or ventricular fibrillation to sinus rhythm regardless of underlying pathophysiologic substrate and prevent sudden cardiac death.[39] The initial devices were implanted epicardially via thoracotomy have been replaced by small devices with active cans and prevenous leads that are implanted pectorally similar to a pacemaker. Current devices may have single chamber, dual chamber, and biventricular pacing capability. The antitachycardia pacing modalities which evolve from clinical EP studies are widely employed and effective in terminating monomorphic gradient from VT particularly those with rates. With several major trials showing a statistical benefit of ICDs in reducing sudden death, there has been a widespread, logarithmic increase in the use of the device. I have removed the chapter on implantable devices from this edition because there are multiple texts on the topic and the electrophysiologic basis for their use is in the text.

The major thrust of the last 25 years has been the development and the use of catheterization techniques to manage cardiac arrhythmias. The concept of using a catheter to deliver energy as an antitachycardia therapeutic modality came from Dr. Melvin Scheinman[40] who was the first to demonstrate the ability to ablate the A-V junction via a catheter to control a ventricular rate in atrial fibrillation. Subsequently, the energy sources changed from a defibrillator to radiofrequency energy which is the standard at this point in time. Nonetheless, additional energy sources such as cryothermal energy, focused ultrasound, and laser energy are all currently being evaluated as modalities to be delivered by a catheter to treat arrhythmias. At the present time focal ablation using radiofrequency is the treatment of choice for all supraventricular tachyarrhythmias, including A-V nodal reentry, circus movement tachycardias using concealed or manifested accessory pathways, incessant automatic atrial tachycardia, isthmus-dependent atrial flutter as well as other macroreentrant atrial tachycardias, and VTs in both normal hearts and those associated with prior infarction.[41–55] In addition, ablation has become the treatment of choice for VPC-induced cardiomyopathy. Most exciting has been the development of the potential for ablation use in the treatment of atrial fibrillation. While the initial studies suggested that isolating the pulmonary veins to prevent the pulmonary vein foci from initiating and maintaining atrial fibrillation[56–59] have been used successful in paroxysmal atrial fibrillation, how best to treat persistent and chronic atrial fibrillation still remains unclear. We still do not understand the basic mechanisms of maintenance of atrial fibrillation, so it is not surprising that we don't know how to "fix" it. While isolations with radiofrequency energy have a reasonable acute success for paroxysmal atrial fibrillation reconnections are common and recurrences frequent, particularly if monitoring is done continuously. There has been an interest in using a variety of other lesion sets to treat persistent atrial fibrillation, but none have proved successful, and many times additional atrial tachycardias are a consequence of additional linear lesions. Most recently new high-resolution mapping systems and phase mapping using a new technology have been introduced in an attempt to improve success and understand the underpinnings of the arrhythmia.

In order to reduce stroke cool-tip radiofrequency catheters have been deployed to decrease the coagulant information resulting from noncooled-tip catheters to decrease the incidence of stroke, which remains a potential complication of this ablation. There is an interest in developing new methods to decrease strokes by use of left atrial occlusion devices one of which has just been FDA approved. How wide spread the use of these devices will be is unclear, but they are certainly reasonable for patients who can't take anticoagulation and do not wish to undergo a left atrial appendagectomy. New anticoagulants have been developed which will likely replace Coumadin.

One major concept I believe that is critical is that we need to understand the mechanism of arrhythmias before we try to "cure" them with ablation. This was easily done for supraventricular arrhythmias. The ability to accurately define reentrant circuits causing VT and even the underlying mechanism of atrial fibrillation needs further work. Although much has been accomplished, much work still remains. We must not let technology lead the way. We electrophysiologists must maintain our interest in understanding the mechanisms of arrhythmias to that we can devise nonpharmacologic or even pharmacologic approaches that would be more effective and safe to manage these arrhythmias. New molecular approaches may be forthcoming in the near future. The world of molecular biology has seen the recognition of ion channelopathies such as long QT syndrome, Brugada syndrome, idiopathic ventricular fibrillation, and catecholaminergic polymorphic VT. Early understanding of these disorders has led to potential ablative therapy, particularly in the Brugada syndrome, and the reintroduction of old fashioned drugs like quinidine and programmed stimulation to treat the short QT syndrome, Brugada syndrome, and idiopathic ventricular fibrillation.[60–62] Cardiovascular genomics will play an important role in risk stratification of arrhythmias in the future and new fields of proteomics and metabolomics will be essential if we are to develop specifically targeted molecules to treat arrhythmias.

The past 45 years have seen a rapid evolution of electrophysiology, from one of understanding the simple mechanisms to one of developing therapeutic interventions. The future will require us to go back to the past and continue to understand more complex underlying mechanisms so that our therapeutic modalities will be more successful and safe.

## REFERENCES


1. Matteucci C. Sur le courant électrique de la grenouille: second mémoire sur l'electricité animale, fasout suite à celui sur to torpille. *Ann Chim Phys* 1842;6:301.
2. Kölliker A, Müller H. Nachweis der negativen Schuankung des Muskelstroms am náturlich sich contrahirenden Muskel. *Verh Phys Med Ges* 1858; 6:528–533.
3. Waiter AD. A demonstration on man of electromotive changes accompanying the heart's beat. *J Physiol* 1887;8:229–234.
4. Einthoven W. Un noveau galvanométre. *Arch n se ex not* 1901;6:625.
5. His W. Die ThŠtigkeit des embryonalen Herzens and deren Bedeu-tung fŸr de Lehre yon der Herzbewegung helm Erwachsenen. *Arb Med Kiln (Leipzig)* 1893;14.
6. Langendorf R. How everything started in clinical electrophysiology. In: Brugada P, Wellens HJJ, eds. *Cardiac arrhythmias: where do we go from here? Mount Kisco*. NY: Futura Publishing Company, 1987:715–722.
7. Wolferth CC, Wood FC. The mechanism of production of short PR intervals and prolonged QRS complexes in patients with presumably undamaged hearts: hypothesis of an accessory pathway of auricolo-ventricular conduction (Bundle of Kent). *Am Heart J* 1933;8:297–311.
8. Alanis J, Gonzales H, Lopez E. Electrical activity of the bundle of His. *J Physiol* 1958;142:127–140.
9. Kottmeier PK, Fishbone H, Stuckey JH, et al. Electrode identification of the conducting system during open-heart surgery. *Surg Forum* 1959;9: 202.
10. Giraud G, Puech P, Letour H, et al. Variations de potentiel liŽes a l'activitŽ du system de conduction auriculoventriculaire chez l'homme (enregistrement electrocardiographique endocavitaire). *Arch Mat* 1960;53:757–776.
11. Scherlag BJ, Lau SH, Helfant RA, et al. Catheter technique for recording His bundle stimulation and recording in the intact dog. *J Appl Physiology* 1968;25:425.
12. Durrer D, Schoo L, Schuilenburg RM, et al. The role of premature beats in the initiation and termination of supraventricular tachycardias in the WPW syndrome. *Circulation* 1967;36:644.

13. Coumel P, Cabrol C, Fabiato A, et al. Tachycardiamente par rythme rŽciproque. *Arch Mat Coeur* 1967;60:1830–1864.
14. Wellens HJJ. *Electrical stimulation of the heart in the study and treatment of tachycardias*. Leiden: Stenfert Kroese, 1971.
15 Josephson ME, Scharf L, Kastor JA, et al. Atrial endocardial activation in man. Electrode catheter techniques for endocardial mapping. *Am J Cardiol* 1977;39:972–981.
16. Josephson ME. Paroxysmal supraventricular tachycardia: an electrophysiologic approach. *Am J Cardiol* 1978;41:1123–1126.
17. Josephson ME, Horowitz LN, Farshidi A, et al. Recurrent sustained ventricular tachycardia. 1. Mechanisms. *Circulation* 1978;57:431–440.
18. Michelson EL, Spielman SR, Greenspan AM, et al. Electrophysiologic study of the left ventricle - Indications and safety. *Chest* 1979;*75*:592–596.
19. VandePol CJ, Farshidi A, Spielman SR, et al. Incidence and clinical significance of tachycardia. *Am J Cardiol* 1980;45:725–731.
20. Brugada P, Greene M, Abdollah H, et al. Significance of ventricular arrhythmias initiated by programmed ventricular stimulation: the importance of the type of ventricular arrhythmia induced and the number of premature stimuli required. *Circulation* 1984;69:87–92.
21. Josephson ME, Horowitz LN, Farshidi A, et al. Recurrent sustained ventricular tachycardia. 2. Endocardial mapping. *Circulation* 1978;57:440–447.
22. Josephson ME, Horowitz LN, Farshidi A, et al. Recurrent sustained ventricular tachycardia. 4. Pleomorphism. Circulation 1979;59:459–468.
23. Josephson ME, Horowitz LN, Farshidi A. Continuous local electrical activity: a mechanism of recurrent ventricular tachycardia. *Circulation* 1978; 57:659–665.
24. Josephson ME, Harken AH, Horowitz LN: Endocardial excision - A new surgical technique for the treatment of ventricular tachycardia. *Circulation* 1979;60:1430–1439.
25. Waldo AL, MacLean WAH, Karp RB, et al. Entrainment and interruption of atrial flutter with atrial pacing: studies in man following open heart surgery. *Circulation* 1977;56:737–745.
26. Okamura K, Henthorn RW, Epstein AE, et al. Further observation of transient entrainment: importance of pacing site and properties of the components of the reentry circuit. *Circulation* 1985;72:1293–1307.
27. Almendral JM, Rosenthal ME, Stamato NJ, et al. Analysis of the resetting phenomenon in sustained uniform ventricular tachycardia: incidence and relation to termination. *J Am Coll Cardiol* 1986;8:294–300.
28. Almendral JM, Stamato NJ, Rosenthal ME, et al. Resetting response patterns during sustained ventricular tachycardia: relationship to the excitable gap. *Circulation* 1986;74:722–730.
29. Almendral JM, Gottlieb CD, Rosenthal ME, et al. Entrainment of ventricular tachycardia: explanation for surface electrocardiographic phenomena by analysis of electrograms recorded within the tachycardia circuit. *Circulation* 1988;77:569–580.
30. Rosenthal ME, Stamato NJ, Almendral JM, et al. Resetting of ventricular tachycardia with electrocardiographic fusion: incidence and significance. *Circulation* 1988;77:581–588.
31. Cassidy DM, Vassallo JA, Buxton AE, et al. Catheter mapping during sinus rhythm: relation of local electrogram duration to ventricular tachycardia cycle length. *Am J Cardiol* 1985;55:713–716.
32. Cassidy DM, Vassallo JA, Miller JM, et al. Endocardial catheter mapping in patients in sinus rhythm: relationship to underlying heart disease and ventricular arrhythmias. *Circulation* 1986;73:645–652.
33. Fenoglio JJ, Pham TD, Harken AH, et al. Recurrent sustained ventricular tachycardia: structure and ultra-structure of subendocardial regions in which tachycardia originates. *Circulation* 1983;68:518–533.
34. Gardner PI, Ursell PC, Fenoglio JJ Jr, et al. Electrophysiologic and anatomic basis for fractionated electrograms recorded from healed myocardial infarcts. *Circulation* 1985;72:596–611.
35. Horowitz LN, Josephson ME, Farshidi A, et al. Recurrent sustained ventricular tachycardia. 3. Role of the electrophysiologic study in selection of antiarrhythmic regimens. *Circulation* 1976;58:986–997.
36. Poll DS, Marchlinski FE, Buxton AE, et al. Sustained ventricular tachycardia in patients with idiopathic dilated cardiomyopathy: electrophysiologic testing and lack of response to antiarrhythmic drug therapy. *Circulation* 1984;70:451–456.
37. Mason JW. A comparison of seven antiarrhythmic drugs in patients with ventricular tachyarrhythmias. Electrophysiologic Study versus Electrocardiographic Monitoring Investigators. *N Engl J Med* 1993;329:452–458.
38. Cardiac Investigators. Preliminary report: effect of encainide and flecainide on mortality in a randomized trial of arrhythmia suppression after myocardial infarction. The Cardiac Arrhythmia Suppression Trial (CAST) Investigators. *N Engl J Med* 1989;321:406–412.
39. Mirowski M, Reid PR, Mower MM, et al. Termination of malignant ventricular arrhythmias with an implanted automatic defibrillator in human beings. *N Engl J Med* 1980;303:322.
40. Scheinmann MM, Laks MM, DiMarco J, et al. Current role of catheter ablative procedures in patients with cardiac arrhythmias. A report for health professionals from the Subcommittee on Electrocardiography and Electrophysiology, American Heart Association. *Circulation* 1991;83: 2146–2153.
41. Haissaguerre M, Dartigues JP, Warin JP, et al. Electrogram patterns predictive of successful catheter ablation of accessory pathways. Value of unipolar recording mode. *Circulation* 1991;84:188–202.
42. Jackman WM, Wang X, Friday KJ, et al. Catheter ablation of accessory atrioventricular pathways (Wolff-Parkinson-White syndrome) by radiofrequency current. *N Engl J Med* 1991;324:1605–1611.
43. Scheinman MM, Huang S. The 1998 NASPE prospective catheter ablation registry. *Pacing Clin Electrophysiol* 2000;6:1020–1028.
44. Nakagawa H, Lazzara R, Khastgir T, et al. Role of the tricuspid annulus and the eustachian valve/ridge on atrial flutter: relevance to catheter ablation of the septal isthmus and a new technique for rapid identification of ablation success. *Circulation* 1996;94:407–424.
45. Poty H, Saoudi N, Nair M, et al. Radiofrequency catheter ablation of atrial flutter: further insights into the various types of isthmus block: application to ablation during sinus rhythm. *Circulation* 1996;94:3204–3213.
46. Schwartzman D, Callans DJ, Gottlieb CD, et al. Conduction block in the inferior vena caval-tricuspid valve isthmus: association with outcome of radiofrequency ablation of type I atrial flutter. *Am Coll Cardiol* 1996;28: 1519–1531.
47. Cosio FG, Arribas F, Lopez-Gil M, et al. Radiofrequency ablation of atrial flutter. *J Cardiovasc Electrophysiol* 1996;7:60–70.
48. Stevenson WG, Khan H, Sager P, et al. Identification of reentry circuit sites during catheter mapping and radiofrequency ablation of ventricular tachycardia late after myocardial infarction. *Circulation* 1993;88:1647–1670.
49. Morady F, Harvey M, Kalbfleisch SJ, et al. Radiofrequency catheter ablation of ventricular tachycardia in patients with coronary artery disease. *Circulation* 1993;87:363–372.
50. Stevenson WG, Friedman PL, Kocovic D, et al. Radiofrequency catheter ablation of ventricular tachycardia after myocardial infarction. *Circulation* 1998;98:308–314.
51. El Shalakany A, Hadjis T, Papageorgiou P, et al. Entrainment mapping criteria for the prediction of termination of ventricular tachycardia by single radiofrequency lesion in patients with coronary artery disease. *Circulation* 1999;99:2283–2289.
52. Marchlinski FE, Callans DJ, Gottlieb CD, et al. Linear ablation lesions for control of unmappable ventricular tachycardia in patients with ischemic and non-ischemic cardiomyopathy. *Circulation* 2000;101:1288–1296.
53. Callans DJ, Menz V, Schwartzman D, et al. Repetitive monomorphic tachycardia from the left ventricular outflow tract: electrocardiographic patterns consistent with a left ventricular site of origin. *J Am Coll Cardiol* 1997;29:1023–1027.
54. Coggins DL, Lee RJ, Sweeney J, et al. Radiofrequency catheter ablation as a cure for idiopathic tachycardia of both left and right ventricular origin. *J Am Coll Cardiol* 1994;23:1333–1341.
55. Varma N, Josephson ME. Therapy of idiopathic ventricular tachycardia. *J Cardiovasc Electrophysiol* 1997;8:104–116.
56. Haissaguerre M, Jais P, Shah DC, et al. Spontaneous initiation of atrial fibrillation by ectopic beats originating in the pulmonary veins. *N Engl J Med* 1998;339:659–666.
57. Haissaguerre M, Jais P, Shah DC, et al. Catheter ablation of chronic atrial fibrillation targeting the reinitiating triggers. *J Cardiovasc Electrophysiol* 2000;11:2–10.
58. Haissaguerre M, Jais P, Shah DC, et al. Electrophysiological end point for catheter ablation of atrial fibrillation initiated from multiple pulmonary venous foci. *Circulation* 2000;101:1409–1417.
59. Chen SA, Hsieh MH, Tai CT, et al. Initiation of atrial fibrillation by ectopic beats originating from the pulmonary veins: electrophysiological characteristics, pharmacological responses, and effects of radiofrequency ablation. *Circulation* 1999;100:1879–1886.
60. Belhassen B, Glick A, Viskin S. Efficacy of quinidine in high-risk patients with Brugada syndrome. *Circulation* 2004;110:1731–1737.
61. Belhassen B. Is quinidine the ideal drug for brugada syndrome? *Heart* 2012;9:2001–2002.
62. Belhassen B, Glick A, Viskin S. Excellent long-term reproducibility of the electrophysiologic efficacy of quinidine in patients with idiopathic ventricular fibrillation and Brugada syndrome. *Pacing Clin Electrophysiol* 2009;32:294–301.

# PREFACE

The past 45 years have witnessed the birth, growth, and evolution of clinical electrophysiology, from a field whose initial goals were the understanding of arrhythmia mechanisms to one of significant therapeutic impact. The development and refinement of implantable devices and, in particular, catheter ablation have made nonpharmacologic therapy a treatment of choice for most arrhythmias encountered in clinical practice. Unfortunately, these new therapeutic tools have captured the imagination of young electrophysiologists to such an extent that terms such as *ablationist*, *defibrillationist*, or *implanter* are used to describe their practice. Their zest for the application of such therapeutic modalities has been associated with a decrease in the emphasis of understanding the mechanisms, clinical implications, and limitations of the therapeutic interventions used to treat arrhythmias. Such behavior is often associated with a lack of, or limited, critical thought that is essential to the development of a new therapeutic concept. There should be the development of a hypothesis, questioning the rationale of the hypothesis, and the testing the hypothesis prior to widespread application of the therapeutic strategy.

The purpose of this book is to provide the budding electrophysiologist with an *electrophysiologic* approach to arrhythmias, which is predicated on the hypothesis that a better understanding of the mechanisms of arrhythmias will lead to more successful and rationally chosen therapy. As such, this book will stress the methodology required to define the mechanism and site of origin of arrhythmias so that safe and effective therapy can be chosen. The techniques suggested to address these issues and specific therapeutic interventions employed represent a personal view, one that is based on experience and, not infrequently, on intuition.

MARK E. JOSEPHSON, MD

# ACKNOWLEDGMENTS

I would like to thank the current and recently graduated electrophysiology fellows and faculty at the Beth Israel Deaconess Medical Center, without whose help in the performance of electrophysiologic studies this book could not have been written. Additional thanks to the technical staff of the electrophysiology laboratory, especially Belinda Morse, whose skills and constant supervision made our laboratory function efficiently and safely for our patients. Special thanks Anuj Basil, a budding electrophysiology fellow, for reviewing Chapter 12. I am greatly indebted to David Callans, who reviewed, updated, and edited Chapter 13 on catheter ablation of arrhythmias. This was an enormous amount of work without which the chapter would have been incomplete. I am eternally grateful to Eileen Eckstein for her superb photographic skills and guardianship of my original graphics, and to Angelika Boyce and Susan Haviland, my administrative assistants during the writing of each edition, for protecting me from distractions. Finally, this book could never have been completed without the encouragement, support, and tolerance of my wife Joan.

# CONTENTS

CHAPTER 1

# Electrophysiologic Investigation: Technical Aspects

## PERSONNEL

The most important aspects for the performance of safe and valuable electrophysiologic studies are the presence and participation of dedicated personnel. The minimum personnel requirements for such studies include at least one physician, one or two nurses (two nurses for complex ablations requiring conscious sedation), a technician with radiation expertise, an anesthesiologist on standby, and an engineer on the premises to repair equipment. With the widespread use of catheter ablation, appropriate facilities and technical support are even more critical.[1,2] The most important person involved in such studies is the physician responsible for the performance and interpretation of these studies. This person should have been fully trained in clinical cardiac electrophysiology in an approved electrophysiology training program. The guidelines for training in clinical cardiac electrophysiology have undergone remarkable changes as interventional electrophysiology has assumed a more important role. The current training guidelines for competency in cardiac electrophysiology have been developed by the American College of Cardiology and the American Heart Association, and the American College of Physicians-American Society of Internal Medicine in collaboration with the Heart Rhythm Society (formerly, the North American Society for Pacing and Electrophysiology).[3,4] Based on these recommendations, criteria for certification in the subspecialty of clinical cardiac electrophysiology have been established by the American Board of Internal Medicine. Certifying exams are now given twice a year. Recertification is required every 10 years. The clinical electrophysiologist should have electrophysiology in general and arrhythmias in particular as his or her primary commitment. As such, they should have spent a minimum of 1 year, preferably 2 years, of training in an active electrophysiology laboratory and have met criteria for certification. The widespread practice of device implantation by electrophysiologists will certainly make a combined pacing and electrophysiology program mandatory for implanters. This should be a 2-year program. Recently, with the development of resynchronization therapy for heart failure, there has been an interest in developing a program to train heart failure physicians to implant devices in their patients. At the least this should be a program of 1 year, and in my opinion, should include training in basic electrophysiology. Such programs are currently available in a few centers. Sufficient training is necessary for credentialing, which will be extremely important for practice and reimbursement in the future.

One or, preferably, two nurses and a technician are the bare minimum support for simple EP studies and devices. Complex ablations (AF, VT, etc.) should be supported by two nurses and a technician. This is critical for safety, particularly with use of conscious sedation or anesthesia in patients in whom there is risk of life-threatening complications. These nurse–technicians must be familiar with all the equipment used in the laboratory and must be well trained and experienced in the area of cardiopulmonary resuscitation. We use two or three dedicated nurses and a technician in each of our electrophysiology laboratories. Their responsibilities range from monitoring hemodynamics and rhythms, using the defibrillator/cardioverter when necessary, and delivering antiarrhythmic medications and conscious sedation (nurses), to collecting and measuring data online during the study. They are also trained to treat any complications that could possibly arise during the study. An important but often unstressed role is the relationship of the nurse and the patient. The nurse is the main liaison between the patient and physician during the study—both verbally, communicating symptoms, and physically, obtaining physiologic data about the patient's clinical status. The nurse–technician may also play an invaluable role in carrying out laboratory-based research. It is essential that the electrophysiologist and nurse–technician function as a team, with full knowledge of the purpose and potential complications of each study being ensured at the outset of the study. A radiation technologist should also be available to assure proper equipment function and monitor radiation dose received by patients and laboratory personnel.

An anesthesiologist and probably a cardiac surgeon should be available on call in the event that life-threatening arrhythmias or complications requiring intubation, ventilation, thoracotomy, and potential surgery should arise. This is important in patients undergoing stimulation and mapping studies for malignant ventricular arrhythmias and, in particular, catheter ablation techniques (see Chapter 14). In addition, an anesthesiologist or nurse-anesthetist usually provides anesthesia support for ICD implantation and/or testing. We use anesthesia for all our atrial fibrillation ablations, and for ablative procedures in patients with fragile hemodynamics to enable us to maintain smooth hemodynamic control during the procedure. Anesthesia is also extremely useful in elderly patients because of the frequent paradoxical response to standard sedation. Although conscious sedation is usually given by laboratory staff, in the substantial minority of laboratories, anesthesia (e.g., propofol) is given by the laboratory staff (nurse or physician) and not by an anesthesiologist.

A biomedical engineer and/or technician should be available to the laboratory to maintain equipment so that it is properly functioning and electrically safe. It cannot be stated too strongly that electrophysiologic studies must be done by personnel who are properly trained in and who are dedicated to the diagnosis and management of arrhythmias. This opinion is shared by the appropriate associations of internal medicine and cardiology.[1–4] Finally a radiation technologist should be available to assure that excessive radiation is not delivered to the patient or electrophysiology team.

## EQUIPMENT

The appropriate selection of tools is of major importance to the clinical electrophysiologist. Although expensive and elaborate equipment cannot substitute for an experienced and careful operator, the use of inadequate equipment may prevent the maximal amount of data from being collected, and it may be hazardous to the patient. To some degree, the type of data collected determines what equipment is required. If the only data to be collected involve atrioventricular (A-V) conduction intervals (an extremely rare situation), this can be determined with a single catheter and a simple ECG-type amplifier and recorder, which are available in most cardiology units. However, a complete evaluation of most supraventricular arrhythmias, which may require activation mapping, necessarily involves the use of multiple catheters and several recording channels as well as a programmable stimulator. Thus, an appropriately equipped laboratory should provide all the equipment necessary for the most detailed study. In the most optimal of situations, a room should be dedicated for electrophysiologic studies. This is not always possible, and in many institutions, the electrophysiologic studies are carried out in the cardiac hemodynamic–angiographic catheterization laboratory. A volume of more than 100 cases per year probably requires a dedicated laboratory. The room should have air-filtering equivalent to a surgical operating room, if it is used for ICD and pacemaker implantation. This is the current practice in more than 90% of centers and is likely to be the universal practice in the future. It is important that the electrophysiology laboratory have appropriate radiographic equipment. The laboratory must have an image intensifier that is equipped for at least fluoroscopy, and, in certain instances, is capable of cine-fluoroscopy if the laboratory is also used for coronary angiography. To reduce radiation exposure, pulsed fluoroscopy or other radiation reduction adaptations are required. This has become critical in the ablation era, when radiation exposure can be prolonged and risk of malignancy increased. Currently the best systems are pulsed and digitally based, which reduces the radiation risk and allow for easy storage of acquired data. The equipment must be capable of obtaining views in multiple planes. Newer systems which markedly reduce radiation exposure enable the electrophysiologist to move catheters at a distance or in the absence of the fluoroscopic system. Examples of such systems are the Stereotaxis magnetic guided catheter positioning system and Hanson robotic system. The Stereotaxis system is available at this time; it is expensive and requires special catheters, which add to the expense. The Hanson system is currently not approved in the US, but is likely to be within the year. It is less expensive but all catheters can be used. These systems are of most value for complex ablations (e.g., atrial fibrillation or untolerated ventricular tachycardia), but seem excessive for most procedures. Other navigation systems are also being developed with the goal of reproducible three-dimensional navigation and reduction of fluoroscopy time and exposure. Currently, state-of-the-art equipment for the gamut of electrophysiologic studies includes permanent radiographic equipment of the C-arm, U-arm, or biplane varieties. It is critical that dosimetry to the patient is monitored. Guidelines for total dosage delivered during a single procedure are needed to prevent radiation-induced injury should be mandated.

### Electrode Catheters

A variety of catheters is currently available with at least two ring electrodes that can be used for bipolar stimulation and/or recording. The catheter construction may be of the woven Dacron variety or of the newer extruded synthetic materials such as polyurethane. As a general all-purpose catheter, we prefer the woven Dacron catheters (Bard Electrophysiology, Billerica, MA) because of their greater durability and physical properties. These catheters come with a variable number of electrodes, electrode spacing, and curves to provide a range of options for different purposes (Fig. 1-1). Although they have superior torque characteristics, their greatest advantage is that they are stiff enough to maintain a shape and yet they soften at body temperature so that they are not too stiff for forming loops and bends in the vascular system to adapt a variety of uses. The catheters made of synthetic materials cannot be manipulated and change shapes within the body, so they are less desirable. Many companies make catheters for specific uses such as coronary sinus cannulation, His bundle recording, etc., but in most cases I believe this is both costly and unnecessary. The advantages of the synthetic catheters are that they are cheaper and can be made smaller (2 to 3 French) than the woven Dacron types. Currently, most electrode catheters are size 3 to size 8 French. The smaller sizes are used in children. In adult patients, sizes 5 to 7 French catheters are routinely used. Other diagnostic catheters have a deflectable tip (Fig. 1-2). These are useful to reach and record from specific sites (e.g., coronary sinus, crista terminalis, tricuspid valve). In most instances the standard woven Dacron catheters suffice, and they are significantly cheaper. Although special catheters

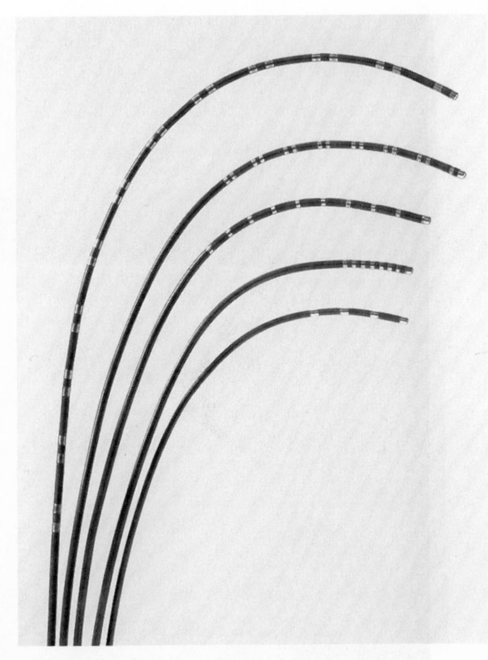

**FIGURE 1-1** *Electrode catheters routinely used.* Woven Dacron catheters with varying number of electrodes and interelectrode distances.

are useful for specific indications described below, standard catheters can be used for most standard pacing and stimulation protocols. We save our hospital thousands of dollars by using standard woven Dacron catheters for all but the ablation catheter. Skilled catheterizers rarely require steerable catheters for positioning, the cost of which is often >$500 in excess of standard catheters.

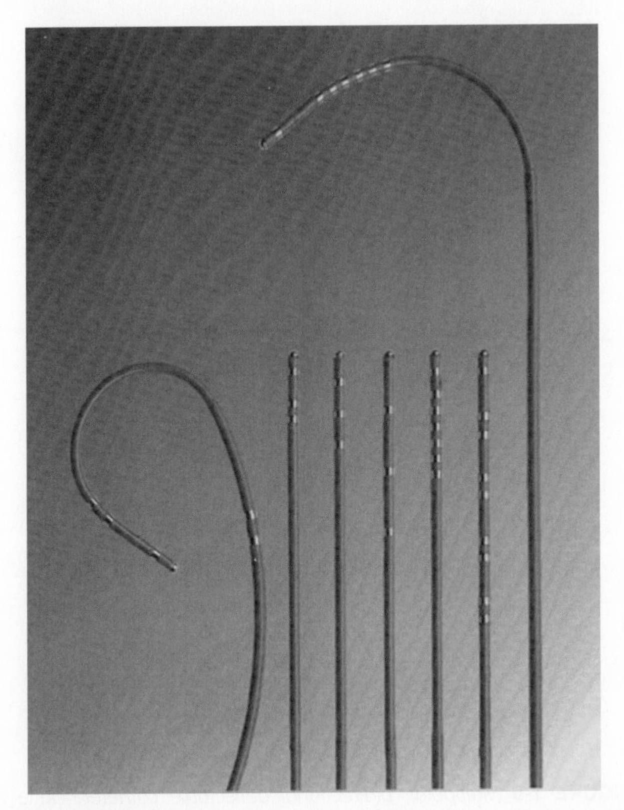

**FIGURE 1-2** *Electrode catheter with deflectable tips.* Different types of catheters with deflectable tips. These are primarily made of extruded plastic.

Electrode catheters have been designed for special uses. Catheters with an end hole and a lumen for pressure measurements may be useful in: (a) electrophysiologic hemodynamic diagnostic studies for Ebstein's anomaly; (b) validation of a His bundle potential by recording that potential and the right atrial pressure simultaneously (see Chapter 2); (c) the occasional instance when it may be desirable to pass the catheter over a long guidewire or transseptal needle; and (d) electrophysiologic studies that are part of a more general diagnostic study and/or for which blood sampling from a specific site (e.g., the coronary sinus) or angiography in addition to pacing is desirable. Special catheters have also been designed to record a sinus node electrogram, although we believe that such electrograms can be obtained using standard catheters (see Chapter 3). Other catheters have been specially designed to facilitate recording of the His bundle potential using the antecubital approach, which occasionally may be useful when the standard femoral route is contraindicated. This catheter has a deflectable tip that permits it to be formed into a pronounced J-shape once it has been passed into the right atrium.

In the last decade the evolution of ablation techniques for a variety of arrhythmias necessitated the development of catheters that enhance the ability to map as well as to safely deliver radiofrequency energy. Mapping catheters fall into two general categories: (a) deflectable catheters to facilitate positioning for mapping and delivering ablative energy and (b) catheters with multiple poles (8 to 64) that allow for simultaneous acquisition of multiple activation points. The former category includes a variety of ablation catheters as well as catheters to record and pace from specific regions (e.g., coronary sinus, tricuspid annulus, slow pathway [see Chapter 8], crista terminalis [see Chapter 9]). Some ablation catheters have a cooled tip, one through which saline is infused to allow for enhanced tissue heating without superficial charring (Biosense Webster and St Jude) or internal cooling (Chili; Boston Scientific) (Fig. 1-3). Ablation catheters deliver RF energy through tips that are typically 3.5 to 5 mm in length but may be as long as 10 mm. Catheters that are capable of producing linear radiofrequency lesions are being developed to treat atrial fibrillation by compartmentalizing the atria, but currently the ability of these catheters to produce transmural linear lesions that have clinical benefit and are safe is not proven. Catheters that deliver microwave, laser, cryothermal, or pulsed-ultrasound energy to destroy tissue are currently under active investigation. The cryothermal catheters have recently been approved by the FDA for A-V nodal modification for A-V nodal tachycardia (see Chapter 14) but are also being evaluated for other uses, that is, atrial fibrillation. For this latter use a cryoballoon catheter has been developed (Arctic; Medtronic [Fig. 1-4]). In the second category are included standard catheters with up to 24 poles that can be deflected to map large and/or specific areas of the atrium (e.g., coronary sinus, tricuspid annulus, etc.) (Fig. 1-5). Of particular note are catheters shaped in the

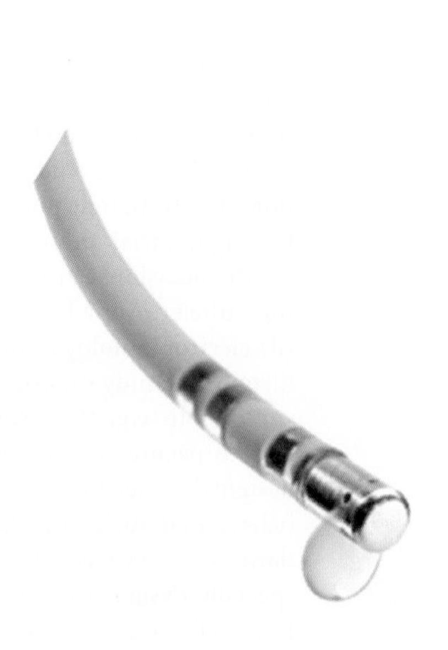

FIGURE 1-3 *Cool tip ablation catheter.* Saline spray through the catheter tip is used to maintain "low" tip temperature to prevent charring while at the same time increasing lesion size. See text for discussion.

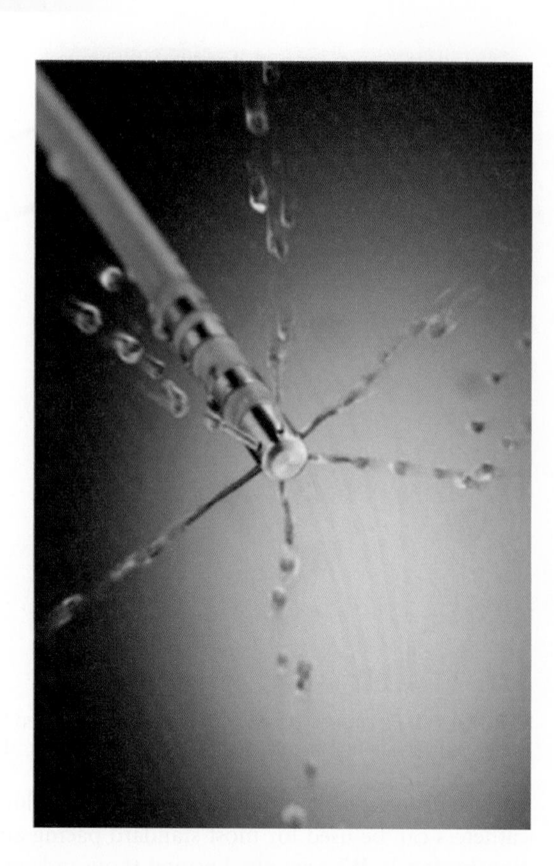

form of a "halo" to record from around the tricuspid ring (Fig. 1-6), or a lasso catheter on a deflectable shaft to record from 10 to 20 electrodes in the pulmonary vein/ostia, (Biosense Webster and St Jude) (Fig. 1-7) and basket catheters (Fig. 1-8), which have up to 64 poles or prongs that spring open and which are used to acquire simultaneous data

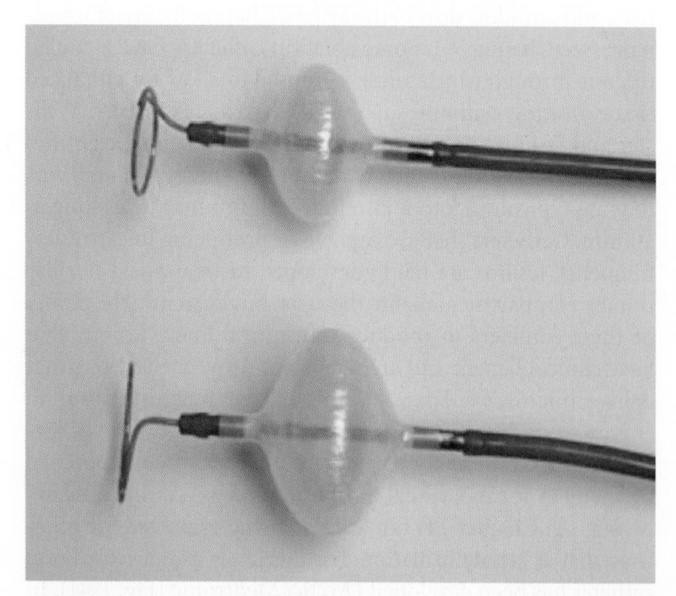

FIGURE 1-4 *Cryoballoon catheter for pulmonary vein isolation.* Two sizes of balloon catheters (24 and 28 cm) are available to deliver cryothermal lesions to the pulmonary vein ostia. A flexible lasso insets thru a lumen to identify the osyia and record pulmonary vein potentials. See Chapter 14 for further discussion.

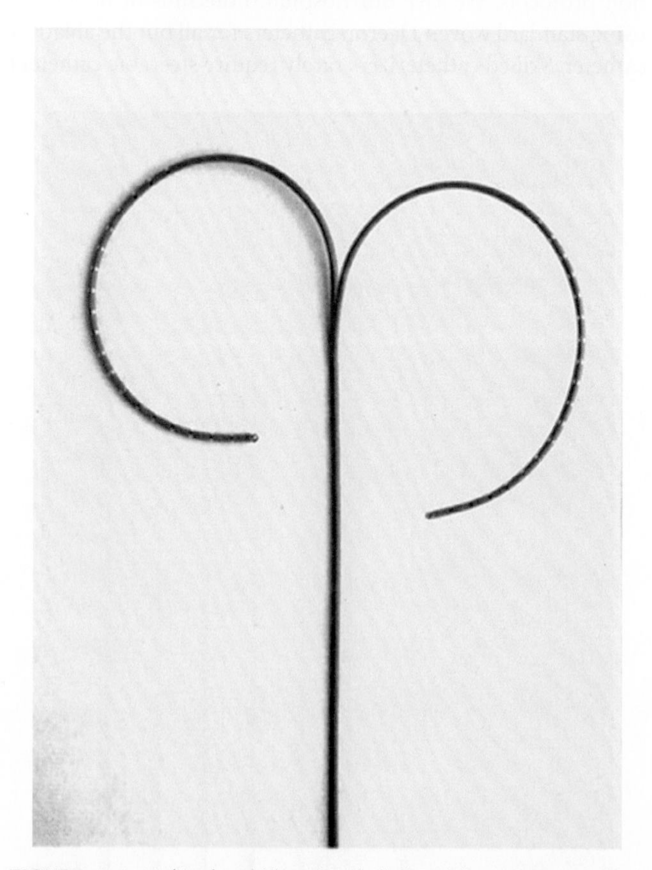

FIGURE 1-5 *Multipolar, bidirectional deflectable catheter.* Deflectable catheters with 10 to 24 poles that have bidirectional curves are useful for recording from the entire coronary sinus or the anterolateral right atrium along the tricuspid annulus.

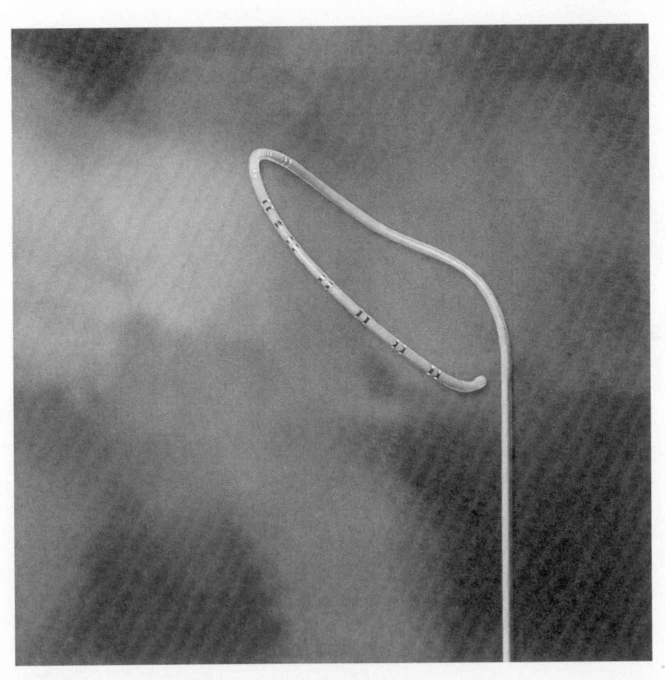

**FIGURE 1-6** *Multipolar deflectable catheter for recording around the tricuspid annulus.* While standard 10 to 20 pole woven Dacron or deflectable catheters can be used to record along the anterolateral tricuspid annulus, a "halo" catheter has been specifically designed to record around the tricuspid annulus.

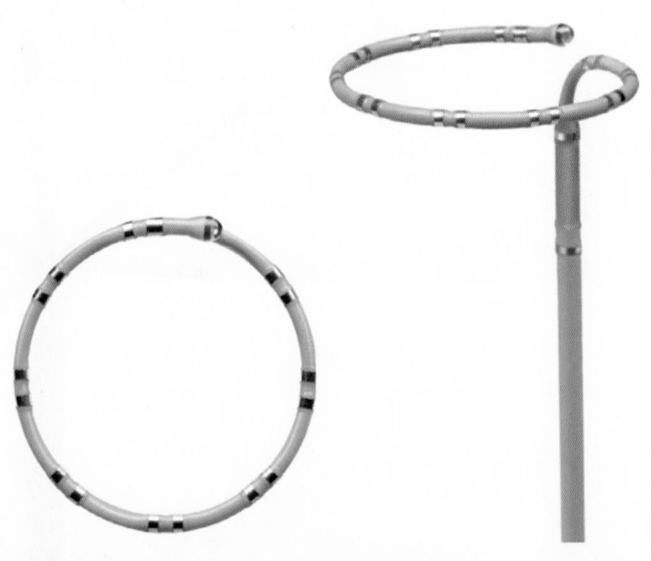

**FIGURE 1-7** *Lasso catheter.* This lasso catheter is used to record from and pace inside the pulmonary vein ostia before and after pulmonary vein isolation procedures (see Chapter 14). The catheter can also be used to create an "anatomic" shell of a chamber as well as to acquire multiple simultaneous activation times.

from within a given cardiac chamber. A PentaRay catheter (Fig. 1-9) is available from Biosense Webster which has five flexible splines with 4 electrodes on each spline allowing on to acquire 20 sites of activation. The 2-mm interelectrode distance allows for high-density mapping. The floppiness of

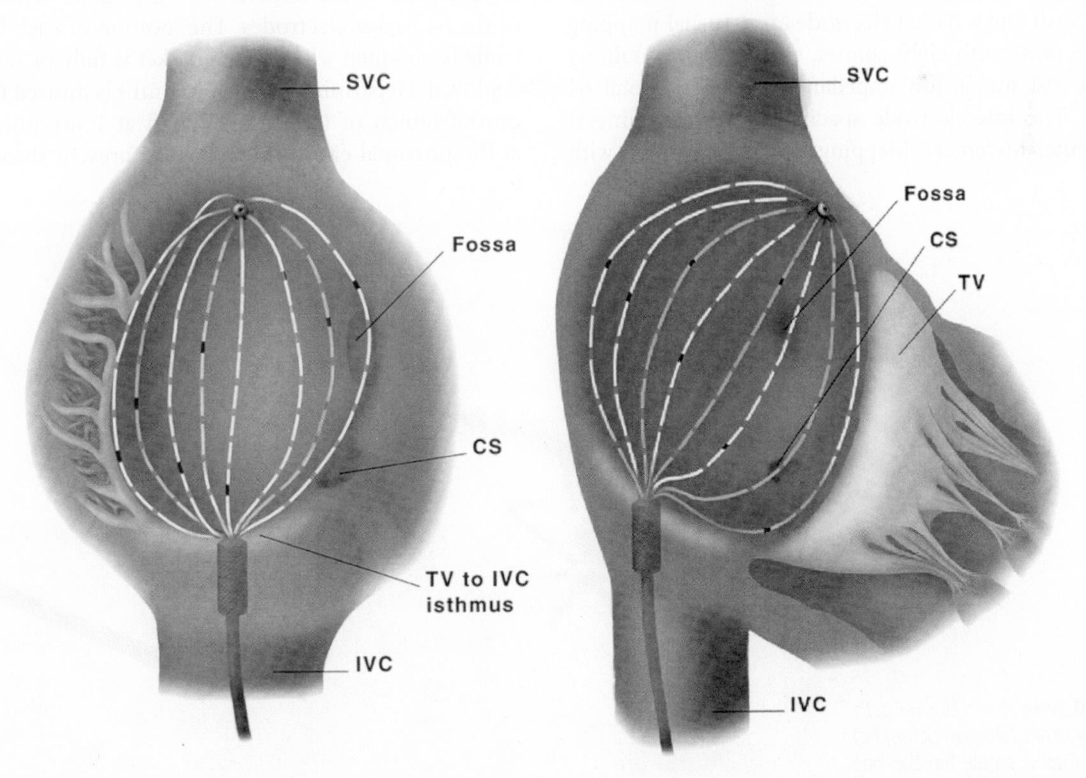


**FIGURE 1-8** *Basket catheter.* A 64-pole retractable "basket" catheter with 8 splines is useful for simultaneous multisite data acquisition for an entire chamber. The schema demonstrates the catheter position in the right atrium when used for the diagnosis and treatment of atrial tachyarrhythmias.

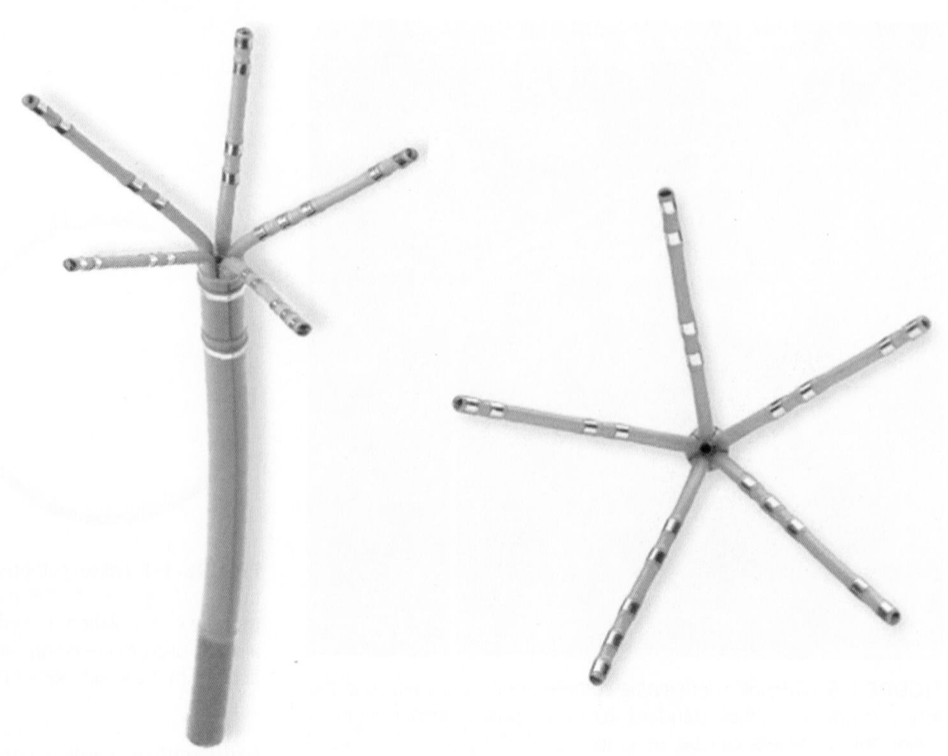

**FIGURE 1-9** *PentaRay mapping catheter*. This flexible, 20 pole catheter on 5 splines allows for high-density activation mapping.

the splines sometimes makes for variable contact in misinterpretation of data. More recently Rhythmia Medical (Boston Scientific) has developed a 64 pole roving catheter (Fig. 1-10). This mapping (minibasket) catheter has an 8 F bidirectional deflectable shaft and a basket electrode array (usual mapping diameter 18 mm) with eight splines, each spline containing eight small (0.4 $mm^2$), low-impedance electrodes (total 64 electrodes). The interelectrode spacing along the spline is 2.5 mm (center-to-center). Mapping can be performed with the basket in variable degrees of deployment (diameter ranging 3 to 22 mm). The location of each of the 64 electrodes is identified by a combination of a magnetic sensor in the distal region of the catheter and impedance sensing on each of the 64 basket electrodes. The location of each basket electrode is obtained whether the basket is fully or only partially deployed. Heparinized saline (1 U/mL) is infused through the central lumen of the catheter shaft at 1 mL/min, emerging at the proximal end of the basket to prevent thrombus. This

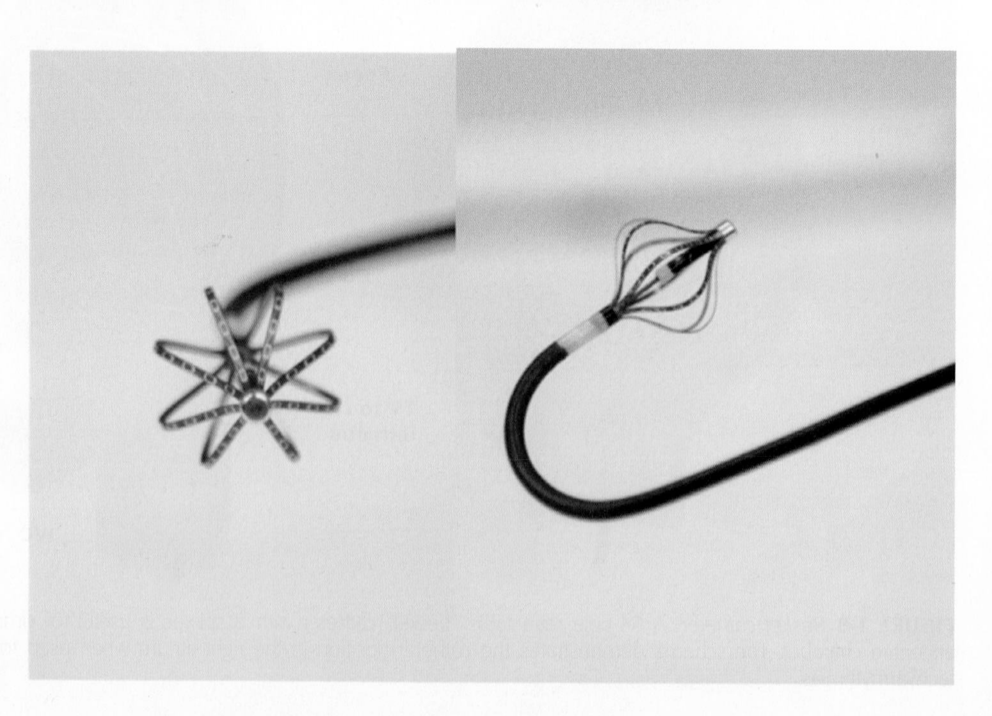

**FIGURE 1-10** *New micro basket catheter from Rhythmia (Boston Scientific)*. This catheter has a small, flexible basket with 64 poles on 8 splines using small (0.4 mm) low impedance electrodes. It also has bidirectional steering.

catheter has a magnetic sensor and with its respiratory gating in the accompanying mapping system provides the most accurate high-density mapping currently available. The magnetic locating system is similar to Carto, Biosense Webster (see below).

Another catheter that has the characteristics and appearance of a standard ablation catheter that has a magnetic sensor within the shaft near the tip is made by Biosense, Webster (see Fig. 1-3). Together with a reference sensor, it can be used to precisely map the position of the catheter in three dimensions. This Biosense electrical and anatomic mapping system is composed of the reference and catheter sensor, an external, ultra-low magnetic field emitter, and the processing unit.[5] The amplitude, frequency, and phase of the sensed magnetic fields contain information required to solve the algebraic equations yielding the precise location in three dimensions (x, y, and z axes) and orientation (roll, yaw, pitch) of the catheter tip sensor. A unipolar or bipolar electrogram can be recorded simultaneously with the position in space. An electrical anatomic map can, therefore, be generated. This provides precise (~1 mm) accuracy and allows one to move the catheter back to any desirable position, a particularly important feature in mapping. In addition, the catheter may be moved in the absence of fluoroscopy, thereby saving unnecessary radiation exposure. The catheter, because of its ability to map the virtual anatomy, can display the cardiac dimensions, volume, and ejection fraction. New enhancements include respiratory gating, assessment of catheter stability prior to ablation, and measurement of contact force to optimize the ablation lesion. This is similar to the Rhythmia Medical mapping system which records from 64 poles in unipolar and bipolar modes yielding the highest accuracy, but which requires a separate ablation catheter.

Another new mapping methodology, with its own catheter, is Ensite noncontact endocardial mapping system. An intracavitary multielectrode probe (Fig. 1-11) is introduced retrogradely, transseptally, or pervenously into the desired chamber and endocardial electrograms are reconstructed using inverse solution methods.[6] Endocardial potentials and activations sequences are reconstructed from intracavitary probe signals by a mathematical process called the "inverse solution." Beat-to-beat activation sequences of the entire chamber are generated. It represents both the inverse solution for 64 poles from which several thousand signals are interpolated in space. Whether this technique offers enough spatial resolution to be used to guide precise ablation in large, and/or diseased hearts, requires validation.

The number and spacing of ring electrodes on standard, contact mapping catheters may vary. Specially designed catheters with many electrodes (up to 24), an unusual sequence of electrodes, or unusual positioning of bipolar pairs may be useful for specific indications. For routine pacing or recording, a single pair of electrodes is sufficient; simultaneous recording and stimulation require two pairs; and studies requiring detailed evaluation of activation patterns or pacing from multiple sites may require several additional pairs. It is important to realize that while multiple poles can gather

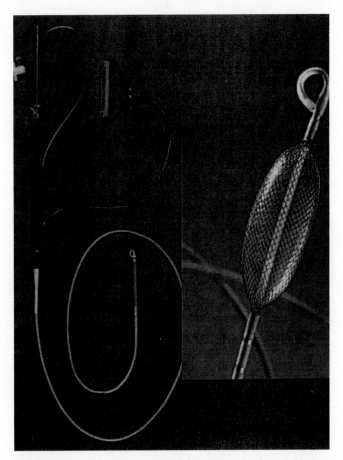

**FIGURE 1-11** *The EnSite noncontact mapping probe.* Mathematically derived electrograms from more than 3,000 sites can be generated from this olive-like probe (see Chapter 14).

simultaneous and accurate data, only the distal pole of an intracavitarily placed electrode will have consistent contact with the wall; thus, electrograms from the proximal electrodes may yield unreliable data. In general, a quadripolar catheter suffices for recording and stimulation of standard sites in the right atrium, right ventricle, and for recording a His bundle electrogram. We routinely use the Bard Electrophysiology multipurpose quadripolar catheter with a 5-mm interelectrode distance for recording and stimulation of the atrium and ventricle as well as for recording His bundle.

The interelectrode distances may range from 1 to 10 mm or more. In studies requiring precise timing of local electrical activity, tighter interelectrode distances are theoretically advantageous. We have evaluated activation times comparing 5- and 10-mm interelectrode distance on the same catheter and have found they do not differ significantly. It is unclear how much different the electrogram timing is using 1- to 2-mm apart electrodes. In my experience, the "local activation time" is similar in normal tissue. The width and amplitude of the electrogram and sometimes additional components of a multicomponent electrogram are more frequently seen with interelectrode distances of ≥5 mm and may be absent when very narrow interelectrode distances are used. This is not surprising since most of the local information recorded is from

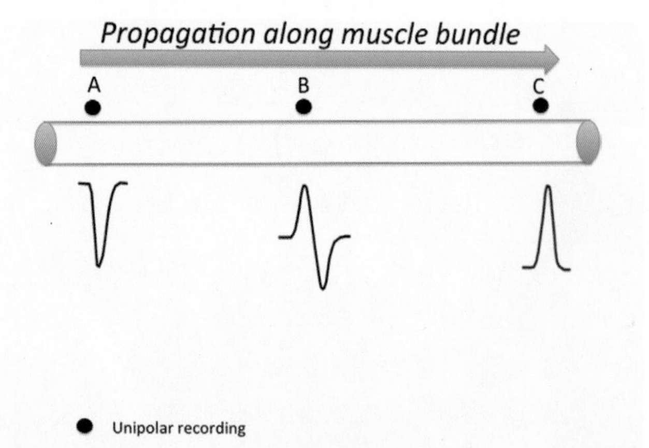


**FIGURE 1-12** *Unipolar recordings.* The unipolar recording identifies local activity by the most rapid negative (intrinsicoid) deflection.

the tip electrode. If careful attention is paid to principles of measurement, an accurate assessment of local activation time on a bipolar recording can be obtained with electrodes that are 5 or 10 mm apart. As stated above, we routinely use catheters with a 2-mm or 5-mm interelectrode distance for most general purposes. Very narrow interelectrode distances (less than or equal to 1 mm) may, however, be useful in understanding multicomponent electrograms. In similar fashion, orthogonal electrodes may provide particularly advantageous information regarding the presence of bypass tract potentials. In certain circumstances, unipolar, unfiltered, or filtered recordings are used since they provide the most accurate information regarding local activation time as well as directional information (Fig. 1-12). The peak negative deflection of the unfiltered bipolar signal corresponds to the intrinsicoid deflection of the unfiltered unipolar signal (Fig. 1-13). The filtered unipolar signal times with the most rapid dV/dT of the unfiltered signal and is the best approximate of local activation. Using simultaneous unipolar and bipolar recordings allows one to determine

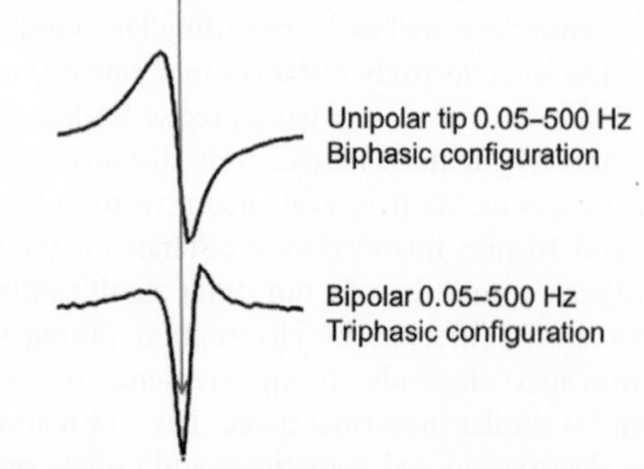


**FIGURE 1-13** *Relationship of unfiltered unipolar and unfiltered bipolar signals.*

which component of a multicomponent signal is local and what the sequence of activation is (Fig. 1-14).[7] To facilitate recording unipolar potentials without electrical interference, catheters have been developed with a fourth or fifth pole, 20 to 50 cm from the tip. This very proximal pole can be used as an indifferent electrode, and unipolar unfiltered recordings can be obtained without electrical interference. We have found this method to be more consistently free of artifact than unipolar signals generated using a Wilson central terminal. If handled with care, electrode catheters, specifically the woven Dacron types without a lumen, may be resterilized and reused almost indefinitely. However, there is much disagreement about the policy of reuse of catheters. Whereas, many of the early electrophysiologists have used the woven Dacron catheters multiple times without infection, there has been some concern in some laboratories about resterilization. While sterilization using ethylene oxide may leave deposits, particularly in extruded catheters, other forms of sterilization are safe. Contrarily, all catheters with lumens must be discarded after a single use. If catheters are reused prior to sterilization, they should be checked to assess electrical continuity. This can be done with a simple application of an ohmmeter to the distal ring and the corresponding proximal connectors. Currently the FDA has proposed strict guidelines for the resterilization of catheters. As a consequence, most institutions now send out their catheters to companies with approved resterilization facilities or, more commonly, have gone to single use.

## Laboratory Organization

As stated previously, a dedicated electrophysiologic laboratory and equipment dedicated to that laboratory are preferred. Use of stimulation and recording equipment in such a laboratory is schematically depicted in Figure 1-15. The equipment may be permanently installed in an area set apart for electrophysiologic work, or it may be part of a general catheterization laboratory such that it is installed in a standard rack mount that includes the hemodynamic monitoring amplifiers. In most laboratories, a stimulator and a computer system that modifies all input signals and stores them on optical disk are used. Some centers still use older systems, such as the E for M electronics DR 8, 12, or 16, in which signals are conditioned and visualized on an oscilloscope and printed out on a strip chart recorder. Such data may also be separately saved on tape for subsequent review. These systems, some of which may be more than 20 years old, are no longer commercially available, but work well. The recent development of computerized recording systems with optical disks has obviated the need for a tape recorder or VCR for clinical studies and has made storage of data much easier. However, current proprietary software limits the ability to analyze data acquired on computers with different software. Conversely, research data stored on a VCR tape recorder can be more widely used. In the near future, several manufacturers of recording equipment will allow storage of individual cases on CDs. Currently this is possible on the Bard system. This may allow analysis "off-site,"

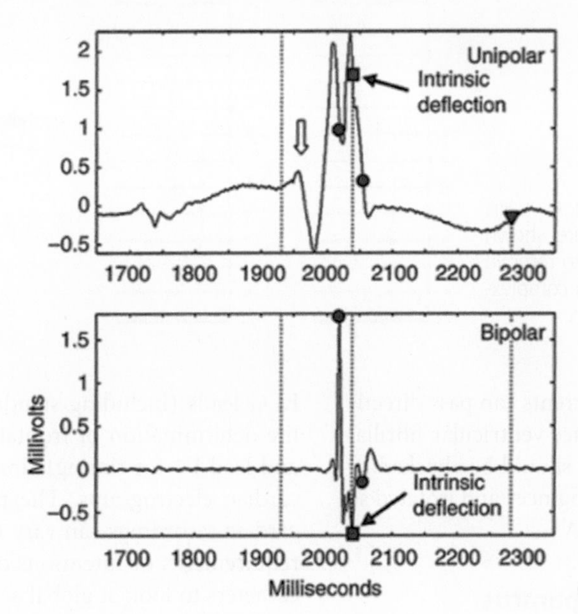


**FIGURE 1-14** *Usefulness of unipolar recordings to identify the local activation in a multicomponent bipolar signal.*

although tools for measurements are not readily available on standard laptops. There are several computerized recording systems available; the most commonly used are Marquette (formerly Prucka) and Bard (see below). The quality of the signal in each of the systems varies because of the way they are processed and filtered. I believe the Bard system currently provides purer signals the Marquette but it is less user-friendly. Further refinement should improve both systems. Filtering the signal can remove or add components to the signal which are not the pure signal. Even a notch filter (60 Hz) can introduce artifactual complexity to the signal (Fig. 1-16).[7]

While computers are superb for storing data, they cannot automatically "mark" events of interest. Such events are frequently missed by the electrophysiologist and, in my opinion, a direct writer is still the best method for recording the data as they are obtained (see following discussion). It is likely in time that computer systems will become more universally useable and all data can be saved, marked, and reviewed. This, in my opinion, in no way eliminates the advantage of having a hard copy of the data on a strip chart for subsequent analysis and review. I personally believe that the strip chart recorders are infinitely better for education. No events are missed and many individuals can analyze and discuss data together. The limitation of strip chart recorders is difficult data storage and the fact that most centers are paperless.

A fixed cinefluoroscopic C-arm or a biplane unit is preferred to any portable unit because it always has superior image intensification and has the ability to reduce radiation by pulsing the fluoroscopy. All equipment must be appropriately grounded, and other aspects of electrical safety must be

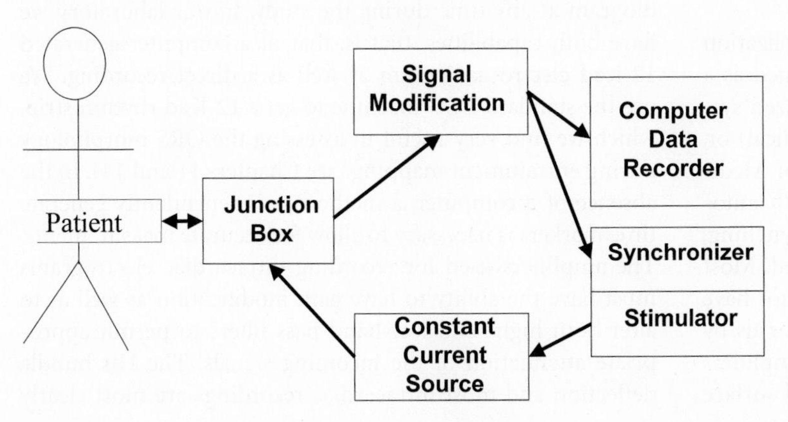


**FIGURE 1-15** *Schema of laboratory setup for data acquisition, processing, and analysis.*

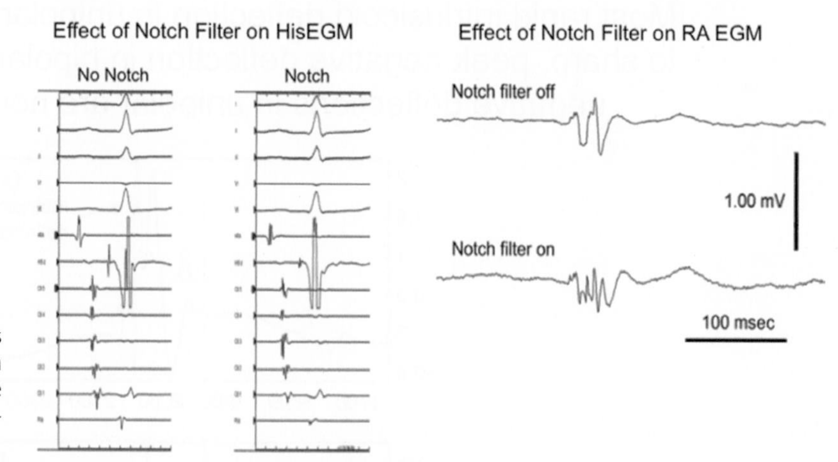


**FIGURE 1-16** *Effect of notch filter on signals.* A His bundle electrogram and right atrial (RA) are shown with and without the use of notch filtering to remove 60 cycle interference. Notice the increase in complexity of the electrogram with the notch filter on.

ensured because even small leakage currents can pass directly to the patient and potentially can induce ventricular fibrillation. All electrophysiologic equipment should be checked by a technical specialist or a biomedical engineer and isolated so leakage current remains less than 10 mA.

## Recording and Stimulation Apparatus

### *Junction Box*

The junction box, which consists of pairs of numbered multiple pole switches matched to each recording and stimulation channel, permits the ready selection of any pair of electrodes for stimulation or recording. Maximum flexibility should be ensured. This can be done by incorporating the capability of recording unipolar and bipolar signals from the same electrodes simultaneously on multiple amplifiers. Most of the current computerized systems fail in flexibility. Such systems have a limited number of groups of amplifiers and do not allow for the capability of older systems, which allowed one to record unipolar and bipolar signals from the same electrodes, even when numbering more than 20. Current computer junction boxes come in banks of 8 or 16 and thus, at best, could record only that number of signals.

### *Recording Apparatus*

The signal processor (filters and amplifiers), visualization screen, and recording apparatus are often incorporated as a single unit. This may be in the form of a computerized system (e.g., Prucka [now Marquette], Bard, or EP Medical) or, as mentioned earlier, an old-fashioned Electronics for Medicine VR or DR 16. Custom-designed amplifiers with automatic gain control, variable filter settings, bank switching, or common calibration signals, etc., can also be used. Most of the newer systems are computer-driven and do not have such capabilities as the system originally designed for us by Bloom, Inc. (Reading, PA). For any system 8 to 14 amplifiers should be available to process a minimum of 3 to 4 surface ECG leads (including standard and/or augmented leads for the determination of frontal plane axis and P-wave polarity, and lead V1 for timing) simultaneously with multiple intracardiac electrograms. The number of amplifiers for intracardiac recordings can vary from 3 to 128, depending on the requirements or intentions of the study. Studies using basket catheters to look at global activation might require 64 amplifiers while a simple atrial electrogram may suffice if the only thing desired is to document the atrial activity during a wide complex tachycardia. I believe an electrophysiology laboratory should have maximum capabilities to allow for both such simple studies and more complex ones. Intracardiac recordings should always be displayed simultaneously with at least 3 or 4 ECG leads to ensure accurate timing, axis determination, and P-wave/QRS duration and morphology. The ECG leads should at least be the equivalent of X, Y, and Z leads. Ideally, 12 simultaneous ECG leads should be able to be recorded, but this is not mandatory. Most computers allow several "pages" to be stored. One of these pages is always a 12-lead electrocardiogram. The advantage of computers is that you can always have a 12-lead electrocardiogram simultaneously recorded during a study when the electrophysiologist is observing the intracardiac channels. In the absence of a computer system, a 12-lead electrocardiogram should also be simultaneously attached to the patient. This allows recording of a 12-lead electrocardiogram at any time during the study. In our laboratory we have both capabilities, that is, that of a computer-generated 12-lead electrocardiogram as well as a direct recording. We use the standard ECG machine to get a 12-lead rhythm strip, which we find very useful in assessing the QRS morphology during entrainment mapping (see Chapters 11 and 14). In the absence of a computer, a method to independently generate time markers is necessary to allow for accurate measurements. The amplifiers used for recording intracardiac electrograms must have the ability to have gain modification as well as to alter both high- and low-band pass filters to permit appropriate attenuation of the incoming signals. The His bundle deflection and most intracardiac recordings are most clearly

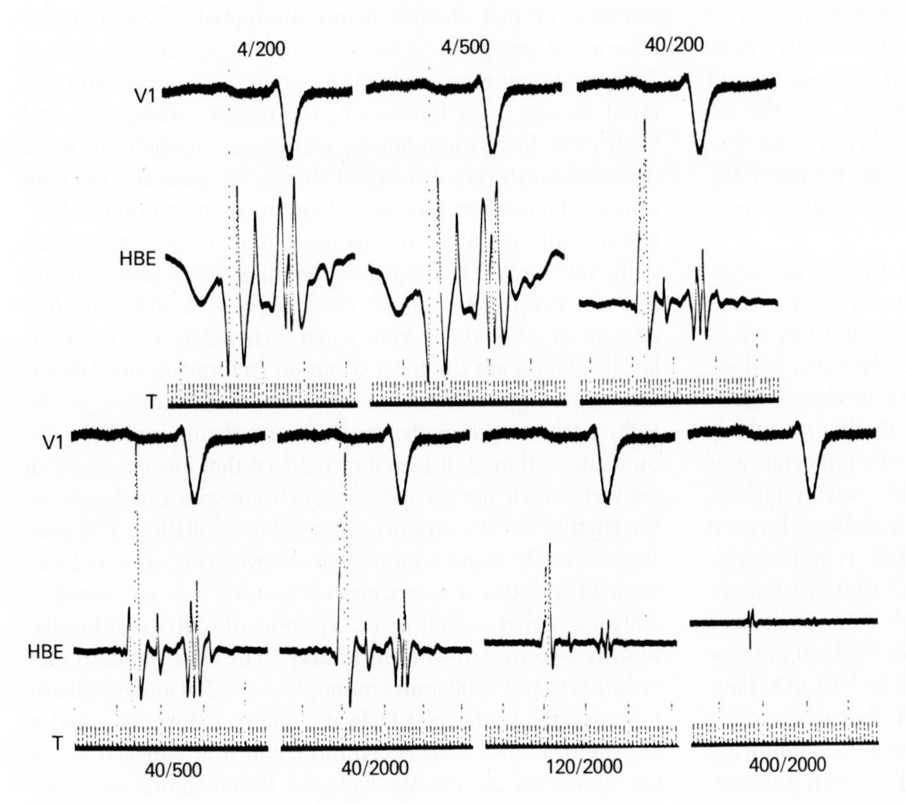


**FIGURE 1-17** *Effect of filtering frequency on the His bundle electrogram.* From **top** to **bottom** in each of the seven panels: a standard lead V1, a recording from a catheter in the position to record the His bundle electrograms, and time lines at 10 and 100 msec. Note that the clearest recording of the His bundle electrogram occurs with a filtering of signals below 40 Hz and above 500 Hz.

destined when the signal is filtered between 30 or 40 Hz (high pass) and 400 or 500 Hz (low pass) (Fig. 1-17). The capability of simultaneously acquiring open (0.05–0.5 to 500 Hz) and variably closed filters is imperative to use both unipolar and bipolar recordings. This is critical for selecting a site for ablation that requires demonstration that the ablation tip electrode is also the source of the target signal to be ablated.

The recording apparatus, or direct writer, is preferable if one desires to see a continuous printout of what is going on during the study. Most current computerized systems, however, only allow snapshots of selected windows. Obviously this can result in missing some important data. If one does have a direct writer, it should be able to record at paper speeds of up to 200 mm/s. While continuously recording information has significant advantages, particularly for the education of fellows, storage of the paper and limited ability to note phenomenon on line have led to the use of computers for data acquisition and storage. Such computerized systems, as noted above, store amplified signals on a variety of pages. These data can be evaluated on- or off-line and can be measured at a distant computer terminal. This specifically means that in order for people to perform their measurements, there needs to be a downtime of the laboratory or a separate slave terminal that can be used just for analysis at a site distant from the catheterization lab. As stated earlier, computerized systems have the limitation of only saving that which the physician requests; much data are missed as a consequence. The ability to store an entire case on a CD will make home evaluation of cases possible.

### *Stimulator*

A programmable stimulator is necessary to obtain data beyond measurement of basal conduction intervals and activation times. Although a simple temporary pacemaker may suffice for incremental pacing for assessment of A-V and ventriculoatrial (V-A) conduction capabilities and/or sinus node recovery times, a more complex programmable stimulator is required for the bulk of electrophysiologic studies. An appropriate unit should have: (a) a constant current source; (b) minimal current leakage (less than 10 μA); (c) the ability to pace at a wide range of cycle lengths (10 to 2,000 msec) from at least two simultaneous sites; (d) the ability to introduce multiple (preferably a minimum of three) extrastimuli with programming accuracy of 1 msec; and (e) the ability to synchronize the stimulator to appropriate electrograms during intrinsic or paced rhythms. The stimulator should be capable of a variable dropout or delay between stimulation sequences so that the phenomena that are induced can be observed. Other capabilities, including A-V sequential pacing, synchronized burst pacing, and the ability to introduce multiple sequential drive cycle lengths, can be incorporated for research protocols. We have found that the custom-designed unit manufactured by Bloom-Fischer, Inc. (Denver, CO) fulfills all the standard requirements and can be modified for a wide range of research purposes. I believe that the range of devices currently available from Bloom-Fischer and their predecessors can more than adequately satisfy the needs of any electrophysiologist. Many of the Bloom stimulators built more than 20 years ago are still functional. Many stimulators are incorporated into the lab systems and are computer based. I believe they are less flexible than the Bloom stimulator and do not have the capability to respond with multiple modalities of stimulation during a tachycardia.

The stimulator should also be able to deliver variable currents that can be accurately controlled. The range of current strengths that could be delivered should range from 0.1 to 10 mA, although greater currents may be incorporated in these devices for specialized reasons. The ability to change pulse widths is also useful. The standard Bloom-Fischer stimulator has pulse width ranges of 0.1 to 10 msec. The importance of a variable constant current source cannot be overemphasized. The results of programmed stimulation may be influenced by the delivered current (usually measured as milliamps); hence, the current delivered to the catheter tip must remain constant despite any changes in resistance. For consistency and safety, stimulation has generally been carried out at twice the diastolic threshold. Higher currents, 5 and 10 mA, have been used in some laboratories to reach shorter coupling intervals or to obtain strength interval curves (see following discussion). The safety of using increased current, however, particularly with multiple extrastimuli, has not been established. Observations in our laboratory and recent studies elsewhere[8] suggest that the use of currents of 10 mA with multiple extrastimuli can result in a high incidence of ventricular fibrillation that has no clinical significance.

### *Cardioverter/Defibrillator*

A functioning cardioverter/defibrillator should be available at the patient's side throughout all electrophysiologic studies. This is particularly true during electrophysiologic studies with patients who have malignant ventricular arrhythmias because cardioversion and/or defibrillation is necessary during at least one study in 25% to 50% of such patients. A wide variety of cardioverter/defibrillators are available and have similar capabilities as far as delivered energy, although they vary in the waveform by which the energy is delivered. There is currently a move toward biphasic waveforms because of the enhanced defibrillation efficacy when compared to monophasic waveforms. We have recently switched to PhysioControl-Medtronic biphasic devices. Other biphasic systems are also available. We routinely employ disposable defibrillation pads which are connected via an adaptor to the cardioverter/defibrillator. The ECG is recorded through the pads as a modified bipolar lead during cardioversion. Use of these pads has led to a marked improvement in tolerance and anxiety of the patients for cardioversion/defibrillation because the nurse–technician need not hover over the patient with paddles.

The success and/or complications of cardioversion/defibrillation depend on the rhythm requiring conversion, the duration of that rhythm before attempted conversion, the amount of energy used, and the underlying cardiac disease. The most common arrhythmias requiring conversion are atrial flutter, atrial fibrillation, ventricular tachycardia, and ventricular fibrillation. Since patients are anesthetized or are unconscious during delivery of shocks, we generally use high output to maximize success and minimize induction of fibrillation. Although atrial fibrillation often can be cardioverted with 100 joules, it frequently requires ≥200 joules. Thus, it is our practice to convert atrial fibrillation with an initial attempt at ≥200 joules. Ventricular tachycardia and ventricular fibrillation are the most common rhythms in our laboratory requiring cardioversion. The rate and duration of the tachycardia as well as the presence of ischemia influence the outcome. Although it is well recognized that low energies can convert ventricular tachycardia, such energies can accelerate the rhythm and/or produce ventricular fibrillation. In a prospective study using a monophasic waveform, we noted that 41 of 44 episodes of ventricular tachycardia were converted by 200 joules, whereas only 6 of 13 episodes of ventricular fibrillation were converted with this energy.[9] Thus our standard procedure is to use ≥300 joules monophasic or 200 joules biphasic for sustained ventricular tachyarrhythmias. Burning noted at the site of the R2 pads is common, and it is assuaged by the use of steroid creams. We have not found significant elevations of myocardial-specific creatine phosphokinase (CPK) although repeated episodes of high-energy cardioversion have resulted in a release of muscle CPK from the chest wall.[9] A variety of bradyarrhythmias and tachyarrhythmias as well as ST-segment changes can be noted postcardioversion. ST elevation and/or depression are seen in 60% of conversions and usually resolve within 15 minutes. The development of bradycardia appears most common with multiple cardioversions for arrhythmia termination in patients with inferior infarction.[5] Ventricular arrhythmias, when induced, are usually short-lived. Similar findings have been observed by Waldecker et al.[10] The high incidence of bradyarrhythmia, particularly in those patients with prior inferior infarction or those on negative chronotropic agents (e.g., blockers or amiodarone), suggests the necessity of having the capability for pacemaker support postconversion. It is necessary in certain patients.

## CARDIAC CATHETERIZATION TECHNIQUE

Intracardiac positioning of electrode catheters requires access to the vascular tree, usually on the venous side but occasionally on the arterial side as well. The technical approach is dictated by (a) the venous and arterial anatomy and the accessibility of the veins and arteries and (b) the desired ultimate location of the electrodes (Table 1-1). In the great majority of cases, the percutaneous modified Seldinger technique is the preferred method of access in either the upper or lower extremity. The percutaneous approach is fast, relatively painless, allows for

TABLE 1-1 Catheter Approach for Electrophysiologic Study

| Electrogram | Technique | Entry Site |
|---|---|---|
| RA | – | Any vein |
| HBE | Standard | FV (R > L) |
| | Torque-cont. | MBV (L > R) |
| | Figure-of-6 | MBV |
| | Left-sided | Any artery |
| CS | – | MBV (L > R) |
| LA | CS | MBV (L > R) |
| | Retrograde | Any artery |
| | RVOT | Any artery |
| | PFO (TS) | RFV |
| RV | – | Any vein |
| LV | Retrograde | Any artery |
| | TS | RFV |

A, artery; CS, coronary sinus; FV, femoral vein; HBE, His bundle electrogram; LA, left atrium; LV, left ventricle; MBV, median basilic vein; PFO, patent foramen ovate; RA, right atrium; RV, right ventricle; RVOT, right ventricular outflow tract; TS, transseptal; V, vein.

prompt catheter exchange, and most important, often allows the vein to heal over a period of days. After healing, the vein can often be used again for further studies. Direct vascular exposure by cut down is only occasionally necessary in the upper extremity, and it is rarely, if ever, warranted in the lower extremity. Specific premedication is generally not required: If it is considered necessary because the patient is extremely anxious, diazepam or one of its congeners is used. Diazepam has not been demonstrated to have any electrophysiologic effects.[11] We prefer the short-acting medazolan (Versed) for sedation in our laboratory.

## Femoral Vein Approach

Either femoral vein may be used, but catheter passage from the right femoral vein is usually easier, primarily because most catheterizers are right-handed and laboratories are set up for right-handed catheterization. The major contraindication in the right-femoral vein approach is acute and/or recurrent iliofemoral thrombophlebitis. Severe peripheral vascular disease or the inability to palpate the femoral artery, which is the major landmark, is relative contraindication. The appropriate groin is shaved, prepared with an antiseptic solution, and draped. The femoral artery is located by placing one's fingertips between the groin crease inferiorly and the line of the inguinal ligament superiorly, which extends from the anterior superior iliac spine to the symphysis pubis; the femoral vein lies parallel and within 2 cm medial to the area just described. A small amount of local anesthetic (e.g., a 1% to 2% solution of lidocaine hydrochloride or its equivalent) is infiltrated into the area, and a small stab wound is made in the skin with a No. 11 blade. A small, straight clamp or curved hemostat is used to make a plane into the subcutaneous tissues. A 2¾-in, 18-gauge, thin-walled Cournand needle or an 18-gauge Cook needle is briskly advanced through the stab wound until the vein or pelvic bone is encountered. The patient may complain of some pain if the pelvic bone is encountered. Additional lidocaine may be infiltrated into the periosteum through the needle. A syringe half-filled with flush solution is then attached to the hub of the needle, and the needle and syringe are slowly withdrawn, with the operator's left hand steadying the needle and his right hand withdrawing gently on the syringe. When the femoral vein is entered, a free flow of blood into the syringe is apparent. While the operator holds the needle steady with his left hand, he removes the syringe and inserts a short, flexible tip-fixed core (straight or "floppy J"), Teflon-coated stainless steel guidewire. The wire should meet no resistance to advancement. If it does, the wire should be removed, the syringe reattached, and the needle again slowly withdrawn until a free flow of blood is reestablished. The wire should then be reintroduced. Often, depressing the needle hub (making it more parallel to the vein) and using gentle traction result in a better intraluminal position for the needle tip and facilitate passage of the wire. If the wire still cannot be passed easily, the needle should be withdrawn, and the area should be held for approximately 5 minutes. After hemostasis is achieved, a fresh attempt may be made.

Once the wire is comfortably in the vein, the needle can be removed and pressure can be applied above the puncture site with the third, fourth, and fifth fingers of the operator's right hand while his thumb and index finger control the wire. The appropriate-sized dilator and sheath combination is slipped over the wire; and, with approximately 1 cm of wire protruding from the distal end of the dilator, the entire unit is passed with a twisting motion into the femoral vein. The wire and dilator are removed, and the sheath is ready for introduction of the catheter. We often insert two sheaths into one or both femoral veins. The insertion of the second sheath is facilitated by the use of the first as a guide. The Cournand needle or Cook needle should puncture the vein approximately 1 cm cephalad or caudal to the initial site. At least one of the sheaths should have a side arm for delivery of medications into a central vein. Frequently, we use a sheath with a side arm in each femoral vein for administration of drugs and removal of blood samples for plasma levels. Recently sheaths through which multiple catheters can pass have become available. Many are so large that multiple sticks are preferable from a hemostasis standpoint. Newer, 8 French, multicatheter sheaths will be more widely used as 3 to 4 French catheters become available.

Heparinization is used in all studies that are expected to last more than 1 hour. During venous studies, a bolus of 2,500 U of heparin is administered followed by 1,000 U/h, and for arterial sticks and direct left atrial access via transseptal puncture a bolus of 5,000–7,500 U of heparin is used followed by 1,000 to 2,000 U/h. The activated clotting time (ACT) is checked every 15 to 30 minutes and heparin dosage is adjusted to maintain an ACT, $t \geq 250$ seconds.

### *Inadvertent Puncture of the Femoral Artery*

Directing the needle too laterally (especially at the groin crease, where the artery and vein lie very close together) may result in puncture of the femoral artery. This complication may be handled in several ways: (1) The needle may be withdrawn and pressure put on the site for a minimum of 5 minutes before venous puncture is reattempted. (Closure of the puncture is important because persistent arterial oozing in a subsequent successful venous puncture can lead to the formation of a chronic arteriovenous fistula.); (2) the short guidewire may be passed into the artery and then replaced with an 18-gauge, thin-walled 6-in Teflon catheter, which can be used to monitor systemic arterial pressure continuously, a procedure that may be desirable in a patient with organic heart disease; (3) or a dilator-sheath assembly may be introduced as if it were the femoral vein, and a catheter may be then passed retrogradely for recording in the aortic root, left ventricle, or left atrium. When there is a doubt, option No. 2 is preferred because the small Teflon catheter is the least traumatic and it can be easily removed or replaced by a guidewire and dilator-sheath assembly should the need arise.

## Upper Extremity Approach

Catheter insertion from the upper extremity is useful if (a) one or both femoral veins or arteries are inaccessible or unsuitable, (b) many catheters are to be inserted, or (c) catheter passage will be facilitated (e.g., to the coronary sinus). The percutaneous technique is identical to that used for the femoral vein. A tourniquet is applied, and ample-sized superficial veins that course medially are identified for use. Lateral veins are avoided because they tend to join the cephalic vein system, which enters the axillary vein at a right angle that perhaps could not be negotiated with the catheter. However, lateral veins can be used successfully in approximately 50% to 75% of patients. If a superficial vein cannot be identified or entered percutaneously, a standard venous cut down can be used. The median basilic vein is generally superficial to the brachial artery pulsation, and the brachial vein lies deep in the vascular sheath alongside the artery. Some investigators prefer the subclavian or jugular approach, but I believe the arm approach is safer. Inadvertent pneumothorax or carotid artery puncture are known complications of subclavian jugular approaches, respectively. Use of left subclavian or brachial vein should be avoided if pacemaker or ICD implantation is being considered. The choice depends on the skill and experience of the operator. Percutaneous brachial artery puncture or brachial artery cut down are rarely used, but may be helpful when left ventricular access is required and the patient has significant abdominal aortic or femoral disease-limiting access. While transseptal catheterization is an alternative option, left ventricular access may be impossible in the presence of a mechanical mitral valve.

The order in which specific catheters are inserted is usually not crucially important. In a patient with left bundle branch block, the first catheter inserted should be passed quickly to the right ventricular apex for pacing because manipulation in the region of the A-V junction can precipitate traumatic right bundle branch block and thus complete heart block.

## Right Atrium

The right atrium can be easily entered from any venous site, although maintenance of good endocardial contact may be difficult when the catheter is passed from the left arm. The most common site for stimulation and recording is the high posterolateral wall at the junction of the superior vena cava (SVC) in the region of the sinus node or in the right atrial appendage. If one is primarily interested in assessing the intraaerial conduction times during sinus rhythm, the SVC–atrial junction is the site depolarized earliest in approximately 50% of patients; in the other 50% of patients, the mid-posterolateral right atrium (some 2 to 3 cm inferior to this site) is depolarized somewhat earlier.[12] Other identifiable and reproducible sites in the right atrium are the inferior vena cava (IVC) at the right atrial junction, the os of the coronary sinus, the atrial septum at the limbus of the fossa ovalis, the atrial appendage, and the A-V junction at the tricuspid valve. Further detailed mapping is difficult and less reproducible for single point mapping the absence of a localizing system (Biosense, Webster). Multipolar catheters or "basket" catheters may provide simultaneous data acquisition from multiple sites. However, the anatomic localization of these sites is variable from patient to patient.

## Left Atrium

Left atrial recording and stimulation are more difficult. The left atrium may be approached directly across the atrial septum through an atrial septal defect or patent foramen ovale or, in patients without those natural routes, by transseptal needle puncture.[13] All these routes are best approached from the right femoral vein. The left atrium may also be approached directly by retrograde catheterization from the left ventricle across the mitral valve.[14] Direct left atrial approaches are mandatory for ablation of left atrial or pulmonary vein foci or isolation of the pulmonary veins (see Chapter 14). Most often, however, for routine diagnostic purposes initial assessment of left atrial activation is approached indirectly by recording from the coronary sinus. This is most easily accomplished from the internal jugular, subclavian, or brachial vein in the antecubital fossa (particularly from the left arm) because the valve of the coronary sinus, which may cover the os, is oriented anterosuperiorly, and a direct approach from the leg is somewhat more difficult, although safer than the jugular or subclavian approaches, since pneumothorax or carotid artery injury cannot occur. Nevertheless, we routinely

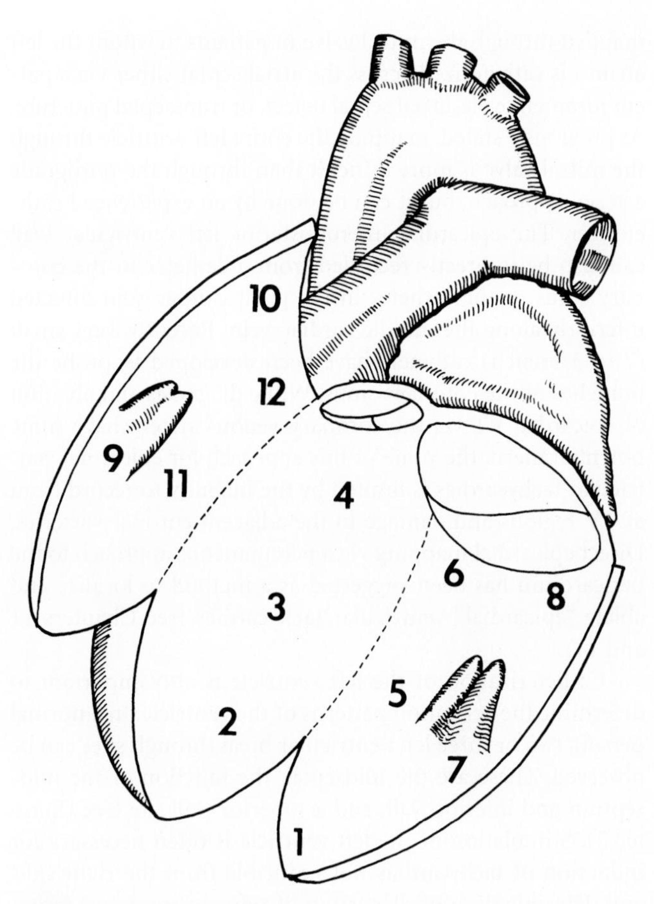


**FIGURE 1-18** *Schema of left ventricular endocardium.* The left ventricle is opened showing the septum (2, 3, 4), anterolateral free wall (7, 9, 11), superior and posterobasal wall (10, 12), and inferior surface (5, 6, 1, 8). Site 1 is the apex.

cannulate the coronary sinus with a standard woven Dacron decapolar catheter from the femoral approach nearly 90% of the time. Any difficulty may at times be circumvented by formation of a loop in the atrium or by using steerable catheters (Fig. 1-18). Steerable catheters cost 50% to 500% more than the woven Dacron catheter, so we use it only if the woven Dacron catheter cannot be positioned in the coronary sinus. The os of the coronary sinus lies posteriorly, and its intubation may be confirmed by: (a) advancement of the catheter to the left heart border, where it will curve toward the left shoulder in the left anterior oblique (LAO) position; (b) posterior position in the right anterior oblique (RAO) or lateral view, which can be seen as posterior to the A-V sulcus, which usually is visualized as a translucent area; (c) recording simultaneous atrial and ventricular electrograms with the atrial electrogram in the later part of the P wave; and (d) withdrawal of very desaturated blood (less than 30% saturated) through a luminal catheter.

Potentials from the anterior left atrium may be recorded from a catheter in the main pulmonary artery,[15] and potentials from the posterior left atrium may be recorded from the esophagus.[16] Left atrial pacing, however, is often impractical or impossible from these sites because of the high currents required. Nonetheless, transesophageal pacing has been used, particularly in the pediatric population, in the past to assess antiarrhythmic efficacy in patients with the Wolff–Parkinson–White syndrome (see Chapter 10).

## Right Ventricle

All sites in the right ventricle are accessible from any venous site. The apex is the most easily identified and reproducible anatomic site for stimulation and recording. The entire right side of the intraventricular septum is readily accessible from outflow tract to apex. However, basal sites near the tricuspid ring (inflow tract) and the anterior free wall are accessible but are more difficult to obtain. Deflectable tip catheters, with or without guiding sheaths, may be useful in this instance.

## Left Ventricle

Direct catheterization of the left ventricle has not been a routine part of most electrophysiologic studies because either the retrograde arterial approach or transseptal approach is required. However, complete evaluation of patients with preexcitation syndromes, and particularly recurrent ventricular arrhythmias, often requires access to the left ventricle for both stimulation and recording. This is particularly important for understanding the pathophysiology and ablation of ventricular tachycardia. Obviously, mapping the site of origin or critical components of a reentrant circuit of the tachycardia or determining whether an anatomic substrate for ventricular arrhythmias is present requires access to the entire left ventricle. We have not hesitated to use the femoral or even brachial approach when indicated. A transseptal approach may be necessary if there is no arterial access due to peripheral vascular disease, amputation, etc. Some prefer this approach for left-sided accessory pathways. The transseptal approach may be useful for ventricular tachycardias rising on the septum, but it is more difficult to maneuver to other left ventricular sites than when the retrograde arterial approach is used. As noted previously, systemic heparinization is mandatory during this procedure. Mapping has become routine in evaluating ventricular tachycardias in humans, especially those associated with coronary artery disease. A schema of the mapping sites of both the left and right ventricle is shown in Figure 1-19. The entire left ventricle is readily approachable with the retrograde arterial approach while the transseptal approach is particularly good for left ventricular septal tachycardias.

Multiple plane fluoroscopy is mandatory to ensure accurate knowledge of the catheter position. Electroanatomic mapping with the Biosense Carto system or the recently approved Rhythmia Medical System (Boston Scientific) provides the ability to accurately localize catheter position in three dimensions without fluoroscopy. This allows one to return to areas of interest. The system also provides activation and voltage analysis, making it ideal for ablation of stable rhythms. The Ensite system (Navix processing) can give activation mapping in 3-dimensions, similar to Carto and Rhythmia Medical, but requires two steps. The chamber must initially be created

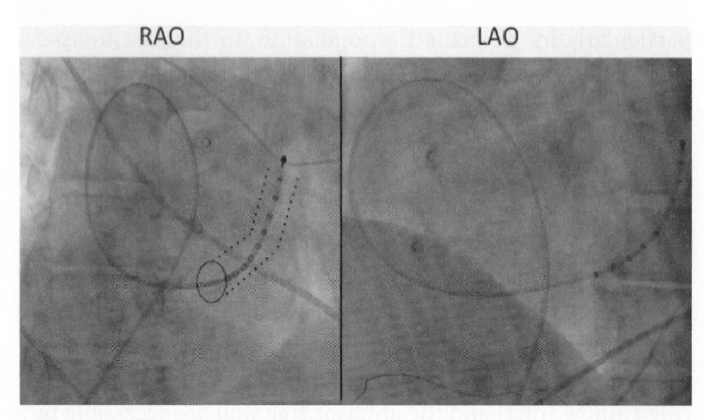


**FIGURE 1-19** *Cannulation of the coronary sinus by looping the catheter in the right atrium.* In this RAO view cannulation of the CS was achieved by looping the catheter in the RA (*red arrows*). Dashed lines outline body of coronary sinus.

by contact mapping, following which point to point contact mapping is repeated. In my experience, the Navix activation maps are similar to Carto or Rhythmia Medical, but not as accurate. Rhythmia Medical provides the most accurate maps of stable tachycardias. Voltage mapping correlating with scar has only been validated using Carto. Another localizing system, which can be used with multiple catheters, but which has only localizing (no activation maps), is also available (LocaLisa, Medtronic, Inc.).

Regardless of the navigating system one uses, we believe that the activation time should be assessed using bipolar electrograms with ≤5 mm interelectrode distance, in which the tip electrode, which is the only one guaranteed to be in contact with the ventricular myocardium, is included as one of the bipolar pair. Unipolar unfiltered recordings, which may provide important information regarding direction of activation, are less useful in mapping hearts scarred by infarction because often no rapid intrinsicoid deflection is seen due to the large size of the far field and/or cavity potential which swamp local unipolar signal because the amplitudes are restricted by the recording apparatus. However, filtering the unipolar signals will remove the far field signal, allowing one to assess local activation. The negative peak deflection of the filtered unipolar (30 to 500 Hz) signal corresponds to the maximum dV/dT of the unfiltered signal, thereby identifying local activation (see Fig. 1-13).[7] Unipolar recordings allow one to assess whether the tip or second pole is responsible for the early components of the bipolar electrogram. Unipolar (unfiltered and/or filtered) recordings are particularly useful in normal hearts or in evaluating atrial and ventricular electrograms in the Wolff–Parkinson–White syndrome or focal tachycardias. Recordings from proximal electrodes of a quadripolar catheter do not provide reliable information in general because the electrodes are not in contact with the muscle. They can, at best, be used as an indirect measure of the distal electrodes during entrainment mapping of ventricular tachycardia (see Chapters 11 and 14). In the left ventricle, electrograms may be recorded from Purkinje fibers, particularly along the septum. As noted above, the left ventricle may also be entered and mapped through the mitral valve in patients in whom the left atrium is catheterized across the atrial septal either via a patent foramen ovale, atrial septal defect, or transseptal puncture. As previously stated, mapping the entire left ventricle through the mitral valve is more difficult than through the retrograde arterial approach, but it can be done by an experienced catheterizer. The epicardial inferoposterior left ventricular wall can also be indirectly recorded from a catheter in the coronary sinus or the catheter in the great cardiac vein directed inferiorly along the middle cardiac vein. Recently, very small (2 to 3 French) catheters have been developed to probe the branches of the coronary sinus. While diagnosis and ablation of epicardial VT via the coronary venous system have some potential merit, the value of this approach for epicardial ventricular tachycardias is limited by the inability to record from all LV regions and damage to the adjacent coronary arteries. Direct epicardial mapping via a percutaneous approach to the pericardium has been suggested as a method to localize and ablate "epicardial" ventricular tachycardias (see Chapters 11 and 14).[17]

Catheterization of the left ventricle is also important to determine the activation patterns of the ventricle. In a normal person, two or three left ventricular breakthrough sites can be observed. These are the midseptal, the junction of the midseptum and inferior wall, and a superior wall site (see Chapter 2). Stimulation of the left ventricle is often necessary for induction of tachycardias not inducible from the right side, and determination of dispersion of refractoriness and recovery times requires left ventricular mapping and stimulation. These will be discussed further in Chapter 2.

## His Bundle Electrogram

The recording of a stable His bundle electrogram is best accomplished by the passage of a size 6 or size 7 French tripolar or quadripolar catheter from a femoral vein; however, almost any electrode catheter can be used. Tightly spaced octapolar or decapolar catheters are often used if activation of the triangle of Koch is being analyzed (see Chapter 8). The catheter is passed into the right atrium and across the tricuspid valve until it is clearly in the right ventricle. The catheter is then withdrawn across the tricuspid orifice with fluoroscopic monitoring. A slight clockwise torque helps to keep the electrodes in contact with the septum until a His bundle potential is recorded. It is often advantageous to attempt to record the His bundle potential between several lead pairs during this maneuver (e.g., using a quadripolar catheter–the distal and second pole, the second and third pole, and the third and fourth pole as individual pairs).

Initially, a large ventricular potential can be observed, and as the catheter is withdrawn, a narrow spike representing a right bundle branch potential may appear just before (less than 30 msec before) the ventricular electrogram. When the catheter is further withdrawn, an atrial potential appears and becomes larger. Where atrial and ventricular potentials are approximately equal in size, a biphasic or triphasic deflection

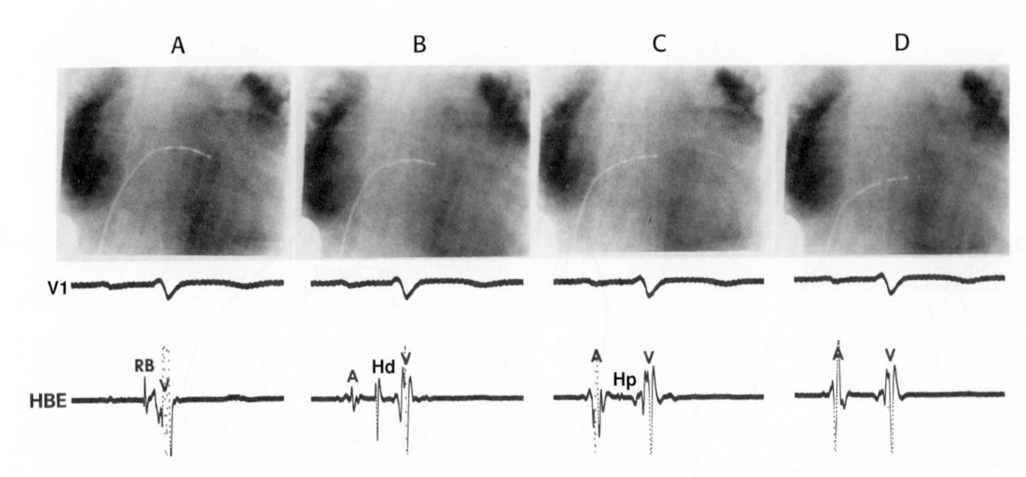


**FIGURE 1-20** *Method of recording the His bundle electrogram.* The ECG lead V1 and the electrogram recorded from the catheter used for His bundle recording (HBE) are displayed with roentgenograms to demonstrate how the catheter should be positioned for optimal recording. The catheter is slowly withdrawn from ventricle to atrium in panels **(A)** to **(D)**. Hd, distal His bundle potential; HP, proximal His bundle potential; RB, right bundle branch potential; V, ventricle. See text for explanation.

appears between them, representing the His bundle electrogram (Fig. 1-20). The most proximal pair of electrodes displaying the His bundle electrograms should be chosen; it cannot be overemphasized that a large atrial electrogram should accompany the recording of the proximal His bundle potential. The initial portion of the His bundle originates in the membranous atrial septum, and recordings that do not display a prominent atrial electrogram may be recording more distal His bundle or bundle branch potentials and therefore miss important intra-His bundle disease. The use of a standard Bard Electrophysiology Josephson quadripolar multipolar catheter for His bundle recording allows recording of three simultaneous bipolar pairs that can help evaluate intra-His conduction (Fig. 1-21). Distal and proximal His potentials can often be recorded and intra-His conduction evaluated. A 2-mm decapolar catheter can occasionally be used to record from the proximal His bundle to the right bundle branch. (This point and methods of validating the His bundle electrogram are discussed further in Chapter 2.) Should the first pass prove unsuccessful in locating a His bundle potential, the catheter should be passed again to the right ventricle and withdrawn with a slightly different rotation so as to explore a different portion of the tricuspid ring. The orientation of the tricuspid ring may not be normal (i.e., perpendicular to the frontal plane) in some patients, especially those with congenital heart disease, and more prolonged exploration may be required. If after several attempts a His bundle electrogram cannot be obtained, the catheter should be withdrawn and reshaped, or it should be exchanged for a catheter with a deflectable tip. Once the catheter is in place, stable recording can usually be obtained for several hours with no further manipulation. Occasionally, continued torque on the catheter shaft is required to obtain a stable recording. This can be accomplished by making a loop in the catheter shaft remaining outside the body, torquing it as necessary, and placing one or two towels on it to hold it; it is rarely necessary for the operator to hold the catheter continuously during the procedure. When the approach just described is used, satisfactory tracing can be obtained in less than 10 minutes in more than 95% of patients.

Both the upper extremity approach and the retrograde arterial approach can be used for recording the His bundle electrogram when the femoral vein cannot be used. The femoral veins should be avoided in the presence of (a) known or suspected femoral vein or IVC interruption or thrombosis, (b) active lower extremity thrombophlebitis or postphlebitic syndrome, (c) infection in the groin, (d) bilateral lower extremity amputation, (e) severe peripheral vascular diseases when the landmark of the femoral artery is not readily palpable, or (f) extreme obesity.

The natural course of a catheter passed from the upper extremity generally does not permit the recording of a His

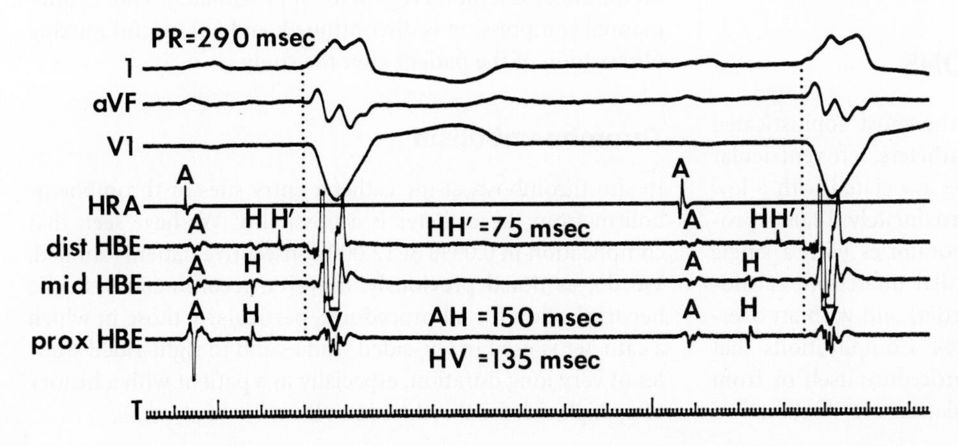


**FIGURE 1-21** *Use of quadripolar catheter to study intra-His conduction.* The quadripolar catheter allows for recording three bipolar signals (distal, mid, and proximal) from which His bundle electrograms can be recorded. Marked intra-His delays (HH′ = 75 msec) can be recognized using these catheters. A, atrium; HBE, His bundle electrogram; HRA, high-right atrium.

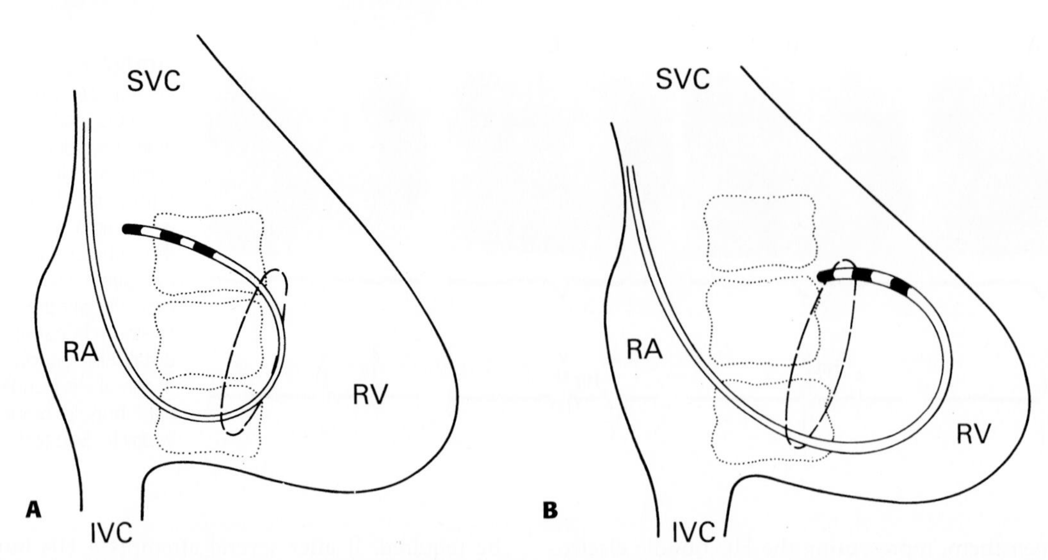


**FIGURE 1-22** *Upper extremity approach for recording His bundle electrograms. Schematic drawing in anteroposterior view.* The catheter is looped in the right atrium (RA), with the tip directed at the lateral wall **(A)** and then gently withdrawn **(B)**. The dotted circle represents tricuspid minutes. IVC, inferior vena cava; SVC, superior vena cava.

bundle electrogram, because the catheter does not lie across the superior margin of the tricuspid annulus. Two techniques are available to overcome this difficulty. One technique involves the use of a deflectable catheter with a torque control knob that allows the distal tip to be altered from a straight to a J-shaped configuration once it has been passed to the heart. The tip is then "hooked" across the tricuspid annulus to obtain a His bundle recording. The second technique and its variations are performed with a standard electrode catheter (Fig. 1-22). Rather than the catheter's being passed with the tip leading, a wide loop is formed in the right atrium with a "figure-of-6," with the catheter tip pointing toward the lateral right atrial wall. The catheter is then gently withdrawn so that the loop opens in the right ventricle with the tip resting in a position to record the His bundle electrogram. Recordings obtained in this fashion are comparable to those obtained by the standard femoral route (Fig. 1-23). As an alternative to any venous route, the His bundle electrogram may be recorded by a retrograde arterial catheter passed through the noncoronary (posterior) sinus of Valsalva, just above the aortic valve or just below the valve along the intraventricular septum (Fig. 1-24).

## RISKS AND COMPLICATIONS

In electrophysiologic studies, even the most sophisticated ones requiring the use of multiple catheters, left ventricular mapping and cardioversion should be associated with a low morbidity. We have performed approximately 12,000 procedures in our electrophysiology laboratories with a single death (a women with acute myocardial infarction, cardiogenic shock, and ventricular tachycardia) and with an overall complication rate of less than 2%. Complications that may arise from the catheterization procedure itself or from the consequences of electrical stimulation are discussed in the following sections. In general, the complication rates are higher in elderly patients and those undergoing catheter ablation than in patients less than 20-years old undergoing diagnostic procedures alone. Complications in diagnostic studies were approximately 1% and in ablation studies were approximately 2.5% and, in are higher for ablative procedures for atrial fibrillation (see Chapter 14). The increased complications of procedures in which RF ablation has been part of the procedure are consistent with recent observations in the US and abroad.[18–22]

### Significant Hemorrhage

Significant hemorrhage is occasionally seen, particularly, hemorrhage from the femoral site. The danger of hemorrhage is greater when the femoral artery is used, particularly in the obese patient. The danger can be minimized by: (a) maintaining firm manual pressure on puncture sites for 10 to 20 minutes after the catheters are withdrawn; (b) having the patient rest in bed with minimal motion of the legs for 12 to 24 hours after the study; (c) having a 5-pound sandbag placed on the affected femoral region for approximately 4 hours after manual compression is discontinued; and (d) careful nursing observation of the patient after the study.

### Thromboembolism

In situ thrombosis at the catheter entry sites or thromboembolism from the catheter is a possibility. We have seen that complication in 0.05% of 12,000 consecutive patients studied. We do, as noted previously, however, recommend systemic heparinization for all procedures, particularly those in which a catheter is used in left-sided studies and in right-sided studies of very long duration, especially in a patient with a history of or high risk for thromboembolism.

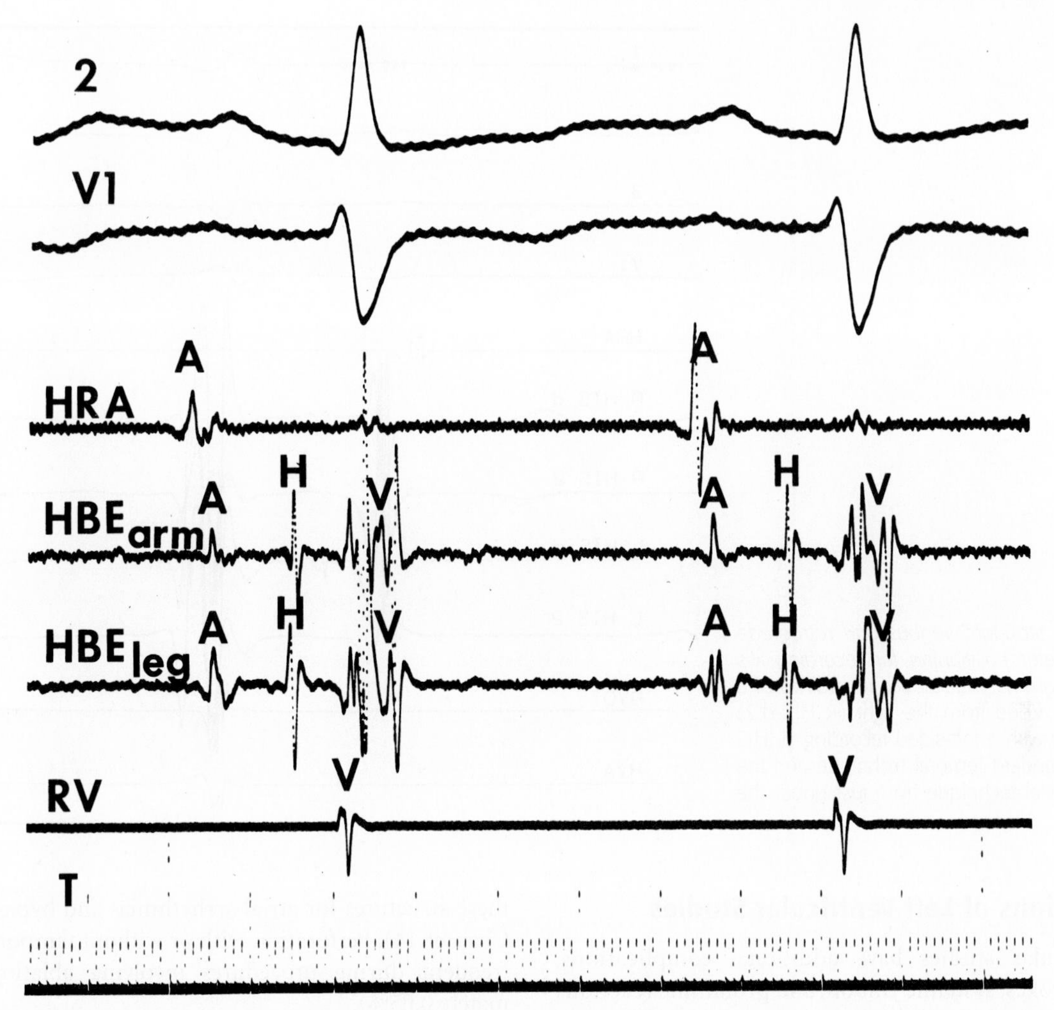


**FIGURE 1-23** *Simultaneous recording of the His bundle electrogram from catheters advanced from the upper and lower extremities.* From **top** to **bottom**: standard leads 2 and V1, a high-right atrial (HRA) electrogram; His bundle electrograms (HBE) obtained from the arm by the figure-of-6 technique and from the leg by the standard femoral technique, right ventricular-potential, and time lines at 10 and 100 msec. Note that the electrograms obtained from the His bundle catheters placed from the upper and lower extremities are nearly identical.

## Phlebitis

Significant deep vein phlebitis, either sterile or septic, has not been a serious problem in our practice (it has occurred in 0.03% of 12,000). We do not routinely use antibiotics prophylactically, although in certain selected patients (e.g., those with prosthetic heart valves) such treatment may be reasonable.

## Arrhythmias

Arrhythmias induced during electrophysiologic stimulation are common; indeed, induction of spontaneous arrhythmias is often the purpose of the study. A wide variety of reentrant tachycardias may be induced by atrial and/or ventricular stimulation; these often can be terminated by stimulation as well. (The significance of these arrhythmias, especially in regard to ventricular stimulation, is discussed in subsequent chapters.) Atrial fibrillation is particularly common with the introduction of early atrial premature depolarizations or rapid atrial pacing, more commonly from the right atrium than the left atrium. It is usually transient, lasting a few seconds to several minutes. If the fibrillation is well tolerated hemodynamically, no active therapy need be undertaken; the catheter may be left in place and the study continued when the patient's sinus rhythm has returned to normal. However, if the arrhythmia is poorly tolerated, especially if the ventricular response is very rapid (as it sometimes is in patients with A-V bypass tracts), IV pharmacologic therapy with a Class III agent (ibutilide or dofetilide) or electrical cardioversion is mandatory. The risk of ventricular fibrillation can be minimized by stimulating the ventricle at twice the threshold using pulse widths of ≤2 msec. A functioning defibrillator is absolutely mandatory. We also have a switch box that allows defibrillation between RV electrode and disposable pad on the chest wall. This can be lifesaving when external DC shocks fail. Such junction boxes are now commercially available.

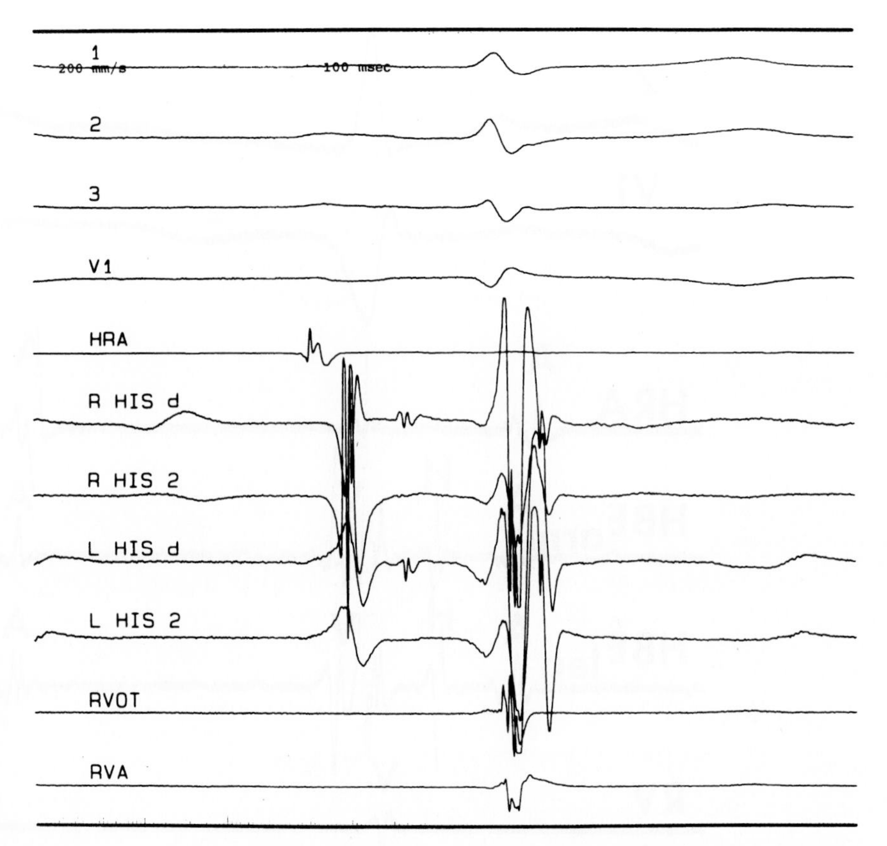


**FIGURE 1-24** *Standard venous and retrograde left-heart catheter positioning for recording His bundle electrograms.* Intracardiac recordings of a His bundle recorded from the right (R HIS d,2) simultaneously with a left-sided recording (L HIS d,2) via the standard femoral technique and the retrograde arterial technique from just under the aortic valve.

## Complications of Left Ventricular Studies

Left ventricular studies have additional complications, including strokes, systemic emboli, and protamine reactions during reversal of heparinization. These are standard complications of any left heart catheterization. Loss of pulse and arterial fistulas may also occur, but with care and attention, the total complication rate should be less than 1%. DiMarco et al.[18] have published their complications in 1,062 cardiac electrophysiologic procedures. No death occurred in their series due to intravascular catheterization, including thromboembolism, local or systemic infections, and pneumothorax. All their patients recovered without long-term sequelae.

## Tamponade

Perforation of the ventricle or atrium resulting in tamponade is a possibility and has occurred clinically in <0.1% undergoing diagnostic studies. The incidence is highest during AF ablation (0.75% in our lab and as high as 1.9% in other labs [Behassen abstract]) primarily because of the need for transseptal puncture and high anticoagulation (ACT 275 to 375 seconds). All required pericardiocentesis; one required an intraoperative repair of a torn coronary sinus. The right ventricle is more likely to perforate than the left ventricle because it is thinner. Perforation of the atrium or coronary sinus is more likely to occur as the result of ablation procedures in these structures for atrial arrhythmias and bypass tracts (see Chapter 14). Perforation with or without tamponade is more frequent during procedures involving ablation (approximately 0.05%).

The safety of electrophysiologic studies has been confirmed in other laboratories and in published reviews of this type.[17,18]

# ARTIFACTS

Otherwise ideal recordings can be rendered less than ideal or at least difficult to interpret by artifacts. Sixty-cycle interference from line currents should be eliminated by proper grounding of equipment and by shielding and suspension of wires and cables. Turning off fluoroscopic equipment (including the x-ray generator) once the catheters are in place may further improve the tracings. Use of notch filters can rid the signal of 60-cycle interference but will alter the electrogram size and shape (see Fig. 1-16).[7] Likewise, firm contact of standard ECG leads (which should be applied after the skin is slightly abraded) is imperative. Tremor in the patient can be dealt with by reassurance and by maintaining a quiet, warm laboratory; when necessary, small doses of an intravenous benzodiazepam may be necessary. Occasionally, the recording of extraneous electrical events, especially repolarization, can confound the interpretation of some tracings (Fig. 1-25).

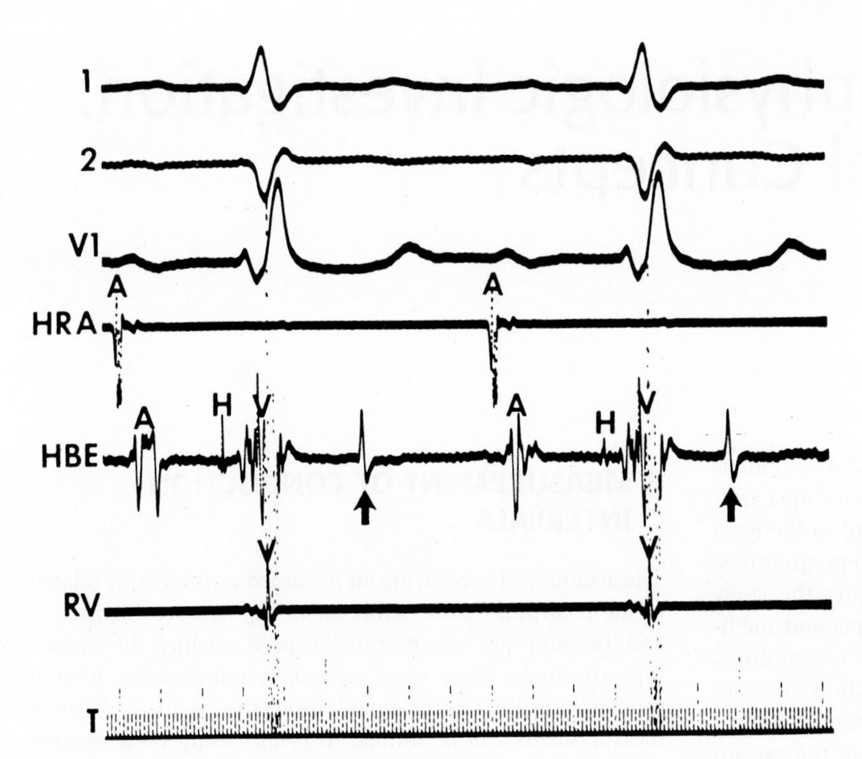


**FIGURE 1-25** *Repolarization artifacts*. From **top** to **bottom**: standard leads 1, 2, and V1, high-right atrial, His bundle, and right ventricular electrograms, and time lines at 10 msec and 100 msec. In the His bundle electrogram tracing, the sharp spike that occurs in the middle of electrical diastole could lead to confusion. It probably represents local repolarization (T-wave) activity or motion artifact.

## ■ REFERENCES


1. Fisher JD, Cain ME, Ferdinand KC, et al. Catheter ablation for cardiac arrhythmias: clinical applications, personnel and facilities. American College of Cardiology Cardiovascular Technology Assessment Committee. *J Am Coll Cardiol.* 1994;24:828–833.
2. Zipes DP, DiMarco JP, Gillette PC, et al. Guidelines for clinical intracardiac electrophysiological and catheter ablation procedures. A report of the American College of Cardiology/American Heart Association Task Force on Practice Guidelines (Committee on Clinical Intracardiac Electrophysiologic and Catheter Ablation Procedures), developed in collaboration with the North American Society of Pacing and Electrophysiology. *J Am Coll Cardiol.* 1995;26:555–573.
3. Josephson ME, Maloney JD, Barold SS, et al. Guidelines for training in adult cardiovascular medicine. Core Cardiology Training Symposium (COCATS). Task Force 6: training in specialized electrophysiology, cardiac pacing and arrhythmia management. *J Am Coll Cardiol.* 1995;25:23–26.
4. Tracy CM, Akhtar M, DiMarco JP, et al. American College of Cardiology/American Heart Association clinical competence statement on invasive electrophysiology studies, catheter ablation, and cardioversion. A report of the American College of Cardiology/American Heart Association/American College of Physicians–American Society of Internal Medicine Task Force on clinical competence. *J Am Coll Cardiol.* 2000;36:1725–1736.
5. Shpun S, Gepstein L, Hayam G, et al. Guidance of radiofrequency endocardial ablation with real-time three-dimensional magnetic navigation system. *Circulation.* 1997;96:2016–2021.
6. Khoury DS, Taccardi B, Lux RL, et al. Reconstruction of endocardial potentials and activation sequences from intracavitary probe measurements. Localization of pacing sites and effects of myocardial structure. *Circulation.* 1995;91:845–863.
7. de Bakker JM, Wittkampf FH. The pathophysiologic basis of fractionated and complex electrograms and the impact of recording techniques on their detection and interpretation. *Circ Arrhythm Electrophysiol.* 2010;3:204–213.
8. DiCarlo LA Jr., Morady F, Schwartz AB, et al. Clinical significance of ventricular fibrillation-flutter induced by ventricular programmed stimulation. *Am Heart J.* 1985;109:959–963.
9. Eysmann SB, Marchlinski FE, Buxton AE, et al. Electrocardiographic changes after cardioversion of ventricular arrhythmias. *Circulation.* 1986;73:73–81.
10. Waldecker B, Brugada P, Zehender M, et al. Dysrhythmias after direct-current cardioversion. *Am J Cardiol.* 1986;57:120–123.
11. Ruskin JN, Caracta AR, Batsford W, et al. Electrophysiologic effects of diazepam in man. *Clin Res.* 1974;22:302A.
12. Josephson ME, Scharf DL, Kastor JA, et al. Atrial endocardial activation in man. Electrode catheter technique of endocardial mapping. *Am J Cardiol.* 1977;39:972–981.
13. Ross J Jr. Considerations regarding the technique for transseptal left heart catheterization. *Circulation.* 1966;34:391–399.
14. Shirey EK, Sones FM Jr. Retrograde transaortic and mitral valve catheterization. Physiologic and morphologic evaluation of aortic and mitral valve lesions. *Am J Cardiol.* 1966;18:745–753.
15. Amat-y-Leon F, Deedwania P, Miller RH, et al. A new approach for indirect recording of anterior left atrial activation in man. *Am Heart J.* 1977;93:408–410.
16. Puech P. The P wave: correlation of surface and intra-atrial electrograms. *Cardiovasc Clin.* 1974;6:43–68.
17. Narula OS. *Advances in clinical electrophysiology: contributions of His bundle recordings.* New York: Grune & Stratton, 1973.
18. Dimarco JP, Garan H, Ruskin JN. Complications in patients undergoing cardiac electrophysiologic procedures. *Ann Intern Med.* 1982;97:490–493.
19. Horowitz LN. Safety of electrophysiologic studies. *Circulation.* 1986;73:II28–II31.
20. Chen SA, Chiang CE, Tai CT, et al. Complications of diagnostic electrophysiologic studies and radiofrequency catheter ablation in patients with tachyarrhythmias: an eight-year survey of 3,966 consecutive procedures in a tertiary referral center. *Am J Cardiol.* 1996;77:41–46.
21. Hindricks G. The Multicentre European Radiofrequency Survey (MERFS): complications of radiofrequency catheter ablation of arrhythmias. The Multicentre European Radiofrequency Survey (MERFS) investigators of the Working Group on Arrhythmias of the European Society of Cardiology. *Eur Heart J.* 1993;14:1644–1653.
22. Scheinman MM, Huang S. The 1998 NASPE prospective catheter ablation registry. *Pacing Clin Electrophysiol.* 2000;23:1020–1028.

CHAPTER

# 2 Electrophysiologic Investigation: General Concepts

The electrophysiologic study should consist of a systematic analysis of dysrhythmias by recording and measuring a variety of electrophysiologic events with the patient in the basal state and by evaluating the patient's response to programmed electrical stimulation. To perform and interpret the study correctly, one must understand certain concepts and methods, including the different types of electrogram recordings, measurement of atrioventricular (A-V) conduction intervals, activation mapping, and response to programmed electrical stimulation. Knowledge of the significance of the various responses, particularly to aggressive stimulation protocols, is mandatory before employing such responses to make clinical judgments. Although each electrophysiologic study should be tailored to answer a specific question for the individual patient, understanding the spontaneous electrophysiologic events and responses to programmed stimulation is necessary to make sound conclusions.

## ELECTROGRAM RECORDINGS

As discussed in Chapter 1, electrograms can be recorded as unfiltered or filtered unipolar signal or bipolar signals. Unipolar signals provide precise activation and give directional information. When unfiltered, significant far field activity is recorded that can make it difficult to see small local unipolar signals without increasing the size of the signal so much it swamps the amplifier. Respiratory drift is another problem. Filtering the unipolar signal gives precise localization and removes far field activity but often results in a very small signal, particularly in infarcted tissue. A bipolar signal approximates the timing recorded by the filtered unipolar signal, particularly with narrow interelectrode distances (≤2 mm) and removes far field signals, but does not give the directional information of the unfiltered unipolar signal. For ablation, particularly for the WPW syndrome and idiopathic VPCs/VT (see Chapter 14), it is important to record both simultaneously to assure the earliest components of the bipolar signal are derived from the distal pole, which is used for ablation, and not the proximal pole. Use of notch filters can add artifactual complexity to the signal and should not be used routinely. If there is severe 60-Hz interference, eliminating such noise is preferable.

## MEASUREMENT OF CONDUCTION INTERVALS

The accuracy of measuring an intracardiac interval is related to the recording mode (unipolar or bipolar; see Chapter 1) and the computer screen or paper speed at which the recordings are made. Since most electrophysiologists use filtered bipolar recordings as the default mode the discussion of such measurements will be limited to results using these recordings. The range of speeds generally used is 100 to 400 mm/sec. The accuracy of measurements made at 100 mm/sec is approximately ±5 msec, and the accuracy of measurements made at 400 mm/sec is increased to ±1 msec. To evaluate sinus node function, for which one is dealing with larger intervals (i.e., hundreds of milliseconds), a recording speed of 100 mm/sec is adequate. Routine refractory period studies require slightly faster speeds (150 to 200 mm/sec), especially if the effects of pharmacologic and/or physiologic maneuvers are being evaluated. For detailed mapping of endocardial activation, paper speeds of ≥200 mm/sec or more should be used.

### His Bundle Electrogram

The His bundle electrogram is the most widely used intracardiac recording to assess A-V conduction because more than 90% of A-V conduction defects can be defined within the His bundle electrogram.[1–6] Before measuring the conduction intervals, however, one must validate the His bundle deflection because all measurements are based on the premise that depolarization of the His bundle is being recorded. As noted in Chapter 1, using a 5- to 10-mm bipolar recording, the His bundle deflection appears as a rapid biphasic or triphasic spike, 15 to 25 msec in duration, interposed between local atrial and ventricular electrograms. To evaluate intra-His bundle conduction delays, one must be sure that the spike represents activation of the most proximal His bundle and not the distal His bundle or the right bundle branch (RBB) potential. Validation of the His bundle potential can be accomplished by several methods, described below.

## Assessment of "H"-V Interval

The interval from the apparent His bundle deflection to the onset of ventricular depolarization should be no less than 35 msec in adults. Intraoperative measurements of the H-V interval have demonstrated that, in the absence of pre-excitation, the time from depolarization of the proximal His bundle to the onset of ventricular depolarization ranges from 35 to 55 msec.[7,8] Furthermore, the RBB deflection invariably occurs 30 msec or less before ventricular activation. Thus, during sinus rhythm an apparent His deflection with an H-V interval of less than 30 msec either reflects recording of a bundle branch potential or the presence of pre-excitation.

## Establishing Relationship of the His Bundle Deflection to other Electrograms: Role of Catheter Position

Because, anatomically, the proximal portion of the His bundle begins on the atrial side of the tricuspid valve, the most proximal His bundle deflection is that associated with the largest atrial electrogram. Thus, even if a large His bundle deflection is recorded in association with a small atrial electrogram, the catheter must be withdrawn to obtain a His bundle deflection associated with a larger atrial electrogram. This maneuver can on occasion markedly affect the measured H-V interval and can elucidate otherwise inapparent intra-His blocks (Fig. 2-1).[9] Thus, when a multipolar (≥3) electrode catheter is used, it is often helpful to simultaneously record from the proximal and distal pair of electrodes to ensure that the His bundle deflection present in the distal pair of electrodes is the most proximal His bundle deflection. Use of a quadripolar catheter with a 5-mm interelectrode distance has facilitated recording proximal and distal His deflections without catheter manipulation, enabling one to record three bipolar electrograms over a 1.5 cm distance. Use of more closely spaced electrodes (1 to 2 mm) does not add a more accurate recording of the proximal His potential, since a His potential can be recorded up to 8 mm from the tip. However, use of a decapolar catheter with 1- to 2-mm interelectrode distance can record proximal, mid, and distal recordings of the His bundle as well as the RBB potential. Occasionally a "His bundle" spike can be recorded more posteriorly in the triangle of Koch. Abnormal sites of His bundle recordings may be noted in congenital heart disease, that is, septum primum atrial septal defect. Another method to validate a proximal His bundle deflection is to record pressure simultaneously with a luminal electrode catheter. The proximal His bundle deflection is the His bundle electrogram recorded with simultaneous atrial pressure. Atrial pacing may be necessary to distinguish a true His deflection from a multicomponent atrial electrogram. If the deflection is a true His deflection, the A-H should increase as the paced atrial rate increases.

## Simultaneous Left-sided and Right-sided Recordings

As noted in Chapter 1, a His bundle deflection can be recorded in the aorta from the junction of the noncoronary and right coronary cusp or from just inside the ventricle under the aortic valve. Because these sites are at the level of the central fibrous body, the proximal penetrating portion of the His bundle is recorded and can be used to time the His bundle deflection recorded via the standard venous route. Simultaneous left-sided and right-sided depolarization is being recorded. An example of this technique is demonstrated in Figure 2-2, in which the standard His bundle deflection by the venous route is recorded simultaneously with the His bundle deflection obtained from the noncoronary cusp in the left-sided His bundle recording. Advancement of the left-sided catheter into the left ventricle often results in the recording of a left bundle

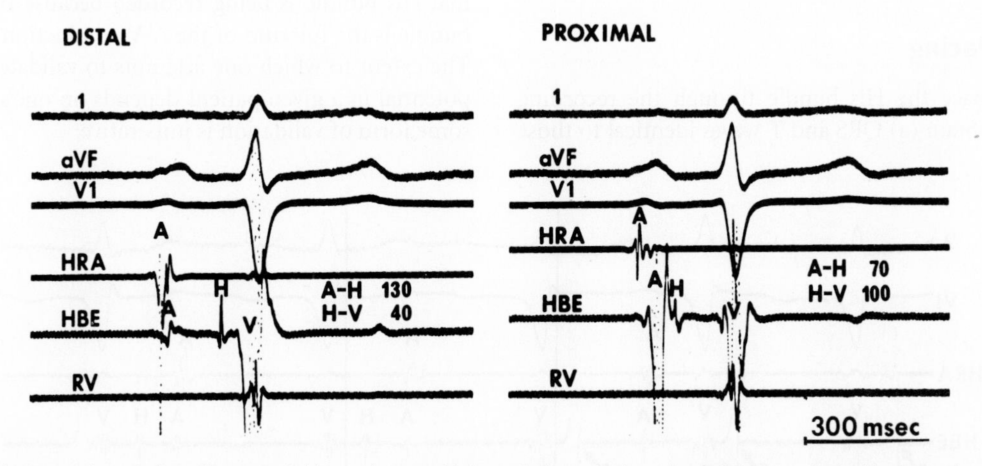


**FIGURE 2-1** *Validation of the His bundle potential by catheter withdrawal.* The panel on the **left** is recorded with the catheter in a distal position, that is, with the tip in the right ventricle. A small atrial electrogram and an apparently sharp His bundle deflection with an H-V interval of 40 msec are seen. However, when the catheter is withdrawn to a more proximal position **(right panel)** so that a large atrial electrogram is present, a His bundle deflection with an H-V of 100 msec is present. Had the distal recording been accepted at face value, a clinically important conduction defect would have been overlooked. Complete intra-His block subsequently developed. 1, aVF, and V1 are ECG leads. HBE, His bundle electrogram; HRA, high-right atrium; RV, right ventricle.

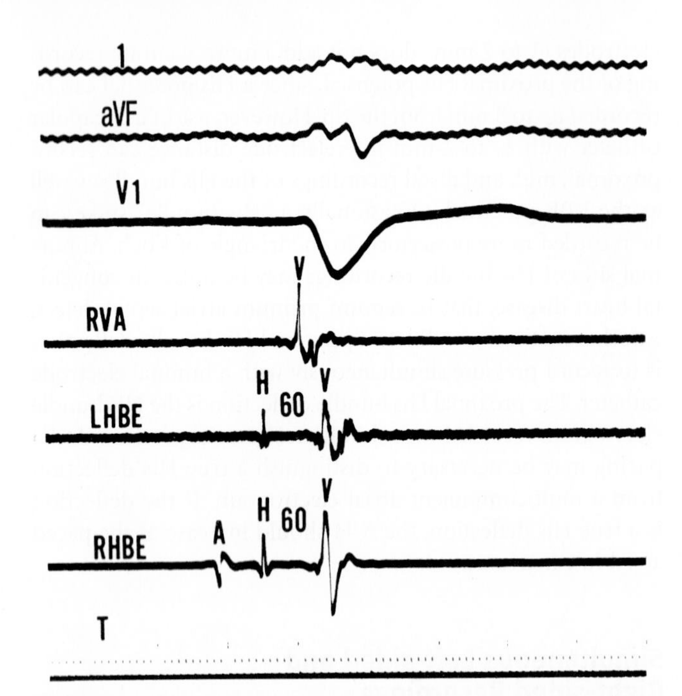


**FIGURE 2-2** *Validation of the His bundle potential by simultaneous right- and left-sided recordings.* ECG leads 1, aVF, and V1 are displayed with right-sided (RHBE) and left-sided (LHBE-from the aorta in the noncoronary cusp) His bundle electrograms and an electrogram from the right ventricular apex (RVA). The H-V intervals are identical.

branch (LBB) potential; therefore, care must be exercised in using a left-sided potential for timing. Thus, recording from the noncoronary cusp is preferred because only a true His bundle deflection can be recorded from this site. Because the LBBs and RBBs are depolarized virtually simultaneously,[10] the LBB potential can be used to distinguish a true His bundle potential from an RBB potential; earlier inscription of the venous His bundle deflection suggests that it is a valid His bundle potential.

## His Bundle Pacing

The ability to pace the His bundle through the recording electrodes and obtain (a) QRS and T waves identical to those during sinus rhythm in multiple leads and (b) a stimulus-to-V interval identical to the H-V interval measured during sinus rhythm perhaps provides the strongest criteria validating the His bundle potential.[11–15] Although the stimulus-to-V criterion is frequently met, multiple-surface ECG lead recordings are needed to ensure that no changes in the QRS or T waves appear during His bundle pacing. Sometimes simultaneous atrial pacing can distort the QRS, making it difficult to ensure true His bundle pacing. Although continuous His bundle pacing is difficult, the demonstration of His bundle pacing for two or three consecutive beats may suffice for validation (Fig. 2-3). Occasionally, one can pace the His reliably over a wide range of cycle lengths (Fig. 2-4). This allows one to obtain a 12-lead ECG to ensure His bundle pacing.

The major criticism of this technique is the inconsistency with which His bundle pacing can be accomplished, especially at low current output (mA).[16–18] Higher mA may result in nonselective His bundle pacing, particularly if a catheter with an interelectrode distance of 1 cm is used. In experienced hands, however, His bundle pacing can usually be accomplished safely at relatively low mA (i.e., 1.5 to 4 mA). The use of more closely spaced electrodes and the reversal of current polarity, i.e., anodal stimulation, may facilitate the pacing of the His bundle.[19] Because intraoperative pacing of the distal His bundle usually results in ventricular pacing (in 94% of patients) over a wide range of mA, one might record a true His bundle (distal) deflection but be incapable of selectively pacing the His bundle. His bundle pacing can frequently be performed from the proximal His bundle. Pacing from that site provides the strongest evidence that a true His bundle deflection has been recorded. The failure to selectively pace a His bundle, however, does not necessarily imply that the deflection recorded is a bundle branch potential.

In summary, measurement of conduction intervals within the His bundle electrogram requires validation that the proximal His bundle is being recorded because the proximal His bundle is the fulcrum of the A-V conduction system (AVCS). The extent to which one attempts to validate the His bundle potential in a given patient depends on one's experience, but some form of validation is imperative.

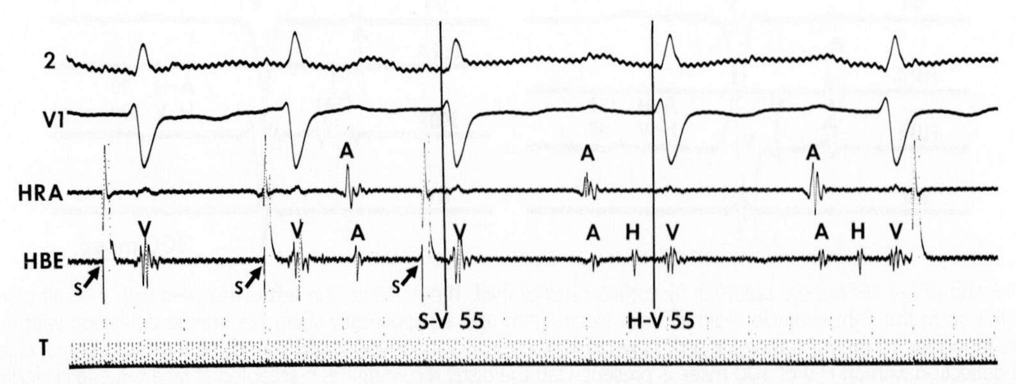


**FIGURE 2-3** *Validation of the His bundle potential by His bundle pacing.* The first three complexes are the result of His bundle pacing at a cycle length of 400 msec. The QRS complexes during pacing are identical to the sinus beats and the stimulus-to-V (S-V) interval equals the H-V interval.

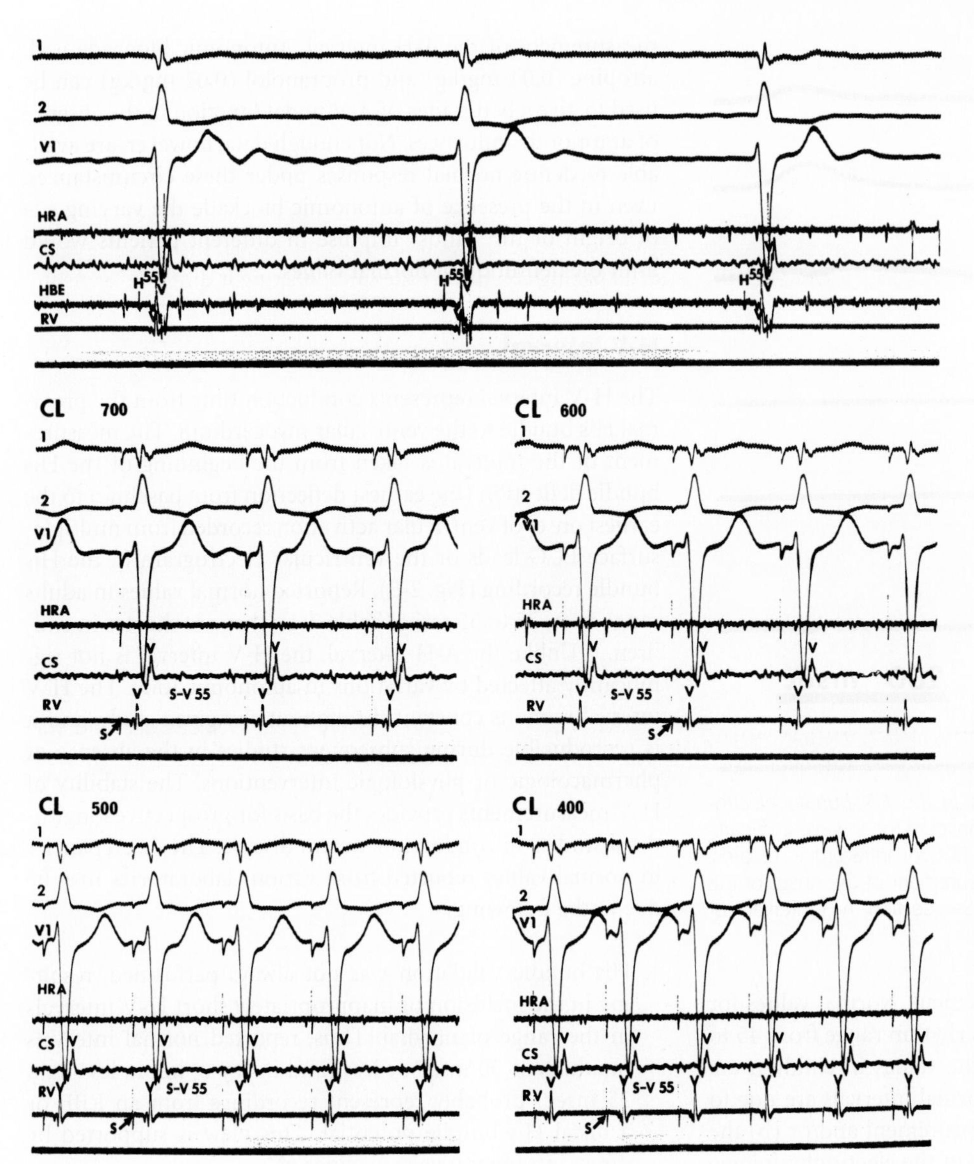


**FIGURE 2-4** *His bundle pacing at multiple cycle lengths.* All panels are arranged from top to bottom as leads 1, 2, V1, high-right atrium (HRA), coronary sinus (CS), His bundle electrogram (HBE), and right ventricular (RV) electrograms. Atrial fibrillation and complete A-V block are present in the top panel. The QRS is normal, and the H-V interval is 55-msec His bundle pacing performed at cycle lengths of 700, 600, 500, and 400 msec. The stimulus-to-V interval remains constant at 55 msec, and the QRS remains identical to that during A-V block. CL, cycle length.

## A-H Interval

The A-H interval represents conduction time from the low-right atrium at the interatrial septum through the A-V node to the His bundle. Thus, the A-H interval is at best only an approximation of A-V nodal conduction time. The measurement should therefore be taken from the earliest reproducible rapid deflection of the atrial electrogram in the His bundle recording to the onset of the His deflection defined by the earliest reproducible deflection from baseline (Fig. 2-5). This is not the activation time at the site (see Chapter 1). Because the exact point in time within the atrial electrogram when the impulse encounters the A-V node is not known, and the atrial component of the HBE often has multiple components, the most important criterion for measurement is reproducibility. One must make these measurements at the same gain because the first visible rapid deflection of the atrial electrogram may differ, depending on the gain. Furthermore, the A-H interval can be markedly affected by the patient's autonomic state. The interval may vary 20 to 50 msec during a single study merely because of a change in the patient's sympathetic and/or parasympathetic tone.[20] Thus, it is important to realize that one should not consider that the absolute value of the A-H interval represents a definitive assessment of A-V nodal function; extranodal influences may make an A-H interval short (when sympathetic tone is enhanced) or long (when vagal tone is enhanced) in the absence of any abnormality of A-V nodal function. Moreover, some investigators have demonstrated that the A-H interval may vary according to the site of the atrial pacemaker.[21,22] This is commonly observed when atrial activation is initiated in the left atrium or near the os of the coronary sinus. In both instances, the impulses may either enter the A-V node at a different site that bypasses part of the A-V node, or they may just enter the A-V node earlier with respect to the atrial deflection in the His bundle electrogram. Both mechanisms can give rise to a "shorter" A-H interval than during sinus rhythm but one could not tell whether A-V nodal conduction was the same or shorter than that during

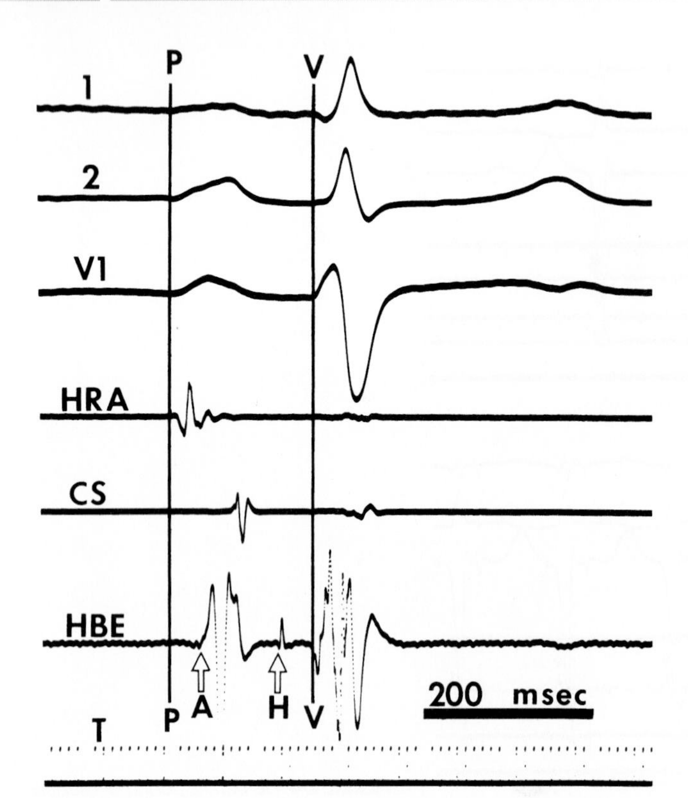


**FIGURE 2-5** *Method of measurement in the His bundle electrogram.* The *vertical black lines* mark the onset of the P wave and earliest ventricular activation in the surface ECG or intracardiac records. The *open arrows* show the site of measurement of the onset of the low atrial and His bundle electrograms. See section "A-H interval" for discussion. CS, coronary sinus.

sinus rhythm by this single measurement. Normal values for A-H intervals in adults during sinus rhythm range from 45 to 140 msec (Table 2-1)[1–6,9,14,18,23–28]; the values in children are lower.[7,8,29] Variations in reported normal intervals are due to differences in (a) the method of measurement and/or (b) the basal state of the patient at the time of the electrophysiologic study. The response of the A-H interval to pacing or drugs (e.g., atropine) often provides more meaningful information about the functional state of the A-V node than an isolated measurement of the A-H interval. Autonomic blockade with atropine (0.04 mg/kg) and propranolol (0.02 mg/kg) can be used to give a better idea of A-V nodal function in the absence of autonomic influences. Not enough data, however, are available to define normal responses under these circumstances. Even in the presence of autonomic blockade the varying site of origin of the "sinus" impulse in different patients would limit the definition of normal values.

## H-V Interval

The H-V interval represents conduction time from the proximal His bundle to the ventricular myocardium. The measurement of the interval is taken from the beginning of the His bundle deflection (the earliest deflection from baseline) to the earliest onset of ventricular activation recorded from multiple-surface ECG leads or the ventricular electrogram in the His bundle recording (Fig. 2-5). Reported normal values in adults range from 25 to 55 msec (Table 2-1); they are shorter in children.[7,8] Unlike the A-H interval, the H-V interval is not significantly affected by variations in autonomic tone. The H-V interval remains constant throughout any given study, and it is reproducible during subsequent studies in the absence of pharmacologic or physiologic interventions. The stability of H-V measurements provides the basis for prospective longitudinal studies in conduction system disease. The discrepancies in normal values reported from various laboratories may be due to the following:

1. His bundle validation was not always performed, resulting in the inclusion of inappropriately short H-V intervals in the range of normal. Thus, reported normal intervals in adults of 30 msec or less (and in my opinion, less than 35 msec) probably represent recordings from an RBB or a distal His bundle potential. This view is supported by direct intraoperative recordings.[7,8]
2. The peak or first high-frequency component of the His bundle deflection was taken as the onset of His bundle depolarization. Since the width of the His bundle potential

TABLE 2-1 Normal Conduction Intervals in Adults

| Laboratory | P-A | A-H | H-V | H |
|---|---|---|---|---|
| Narula et al.[2,5] | 25–60 | 50–120 | 35–45 | 25 |
| Damato et al.[1,3,18,28] | 24–45 | 60–140 | 30–55 | 10–15 |
| Castellanos et al.[6] | 20–50 | 50–120 | 25–55 | — |
| Schuilenburg[23,24] | 85–150 | 35–55 | — | — |
| Puech et al.[4,14] | 30–55 | 45–100 | 35–55 | — |
| Bekheit et al.[25,26] | 10–50 | 50–125 | 35–45 | 15–25 |
| Rosen[27] | 9–45 | 54–130 | 31–55 | — |
| Author | 60–125 | 35–55 | 10–25 | — |

has been demonstrated to correlate with intra-His conduction time,[30] the onset of His bundle activation should be taken as the initial movement, slow or fast, from baseline. Exclusion of initial low amplitude and/or slow components in H-V measurements may yield a short H-V interval. This is of particular importance in the presence of intra-His conduction defects, when improper measurements can result in the failure to identify a clinically significant conduction disturbance.

3. Multiple ECG leads were not used in conjunction with the intracardiac ventricular electrogram in the His bundle tracing to delineate the earliest ventricular activity, and thus, falsely long H-V intervals were produced. This situation is most likely to occur when a single standard ECG lead is used to analyze earliest ventricular activation, as graphically demonstrated in Figure 2-5, in which the H-V interval shown would be falsely lengthened by 20 msec if the onset of ventricular activation were taken as the onset of the R wave in the lead 2 surface electrogram. If only one ECG channel is available, a V1 or V2 lead should be used because the earliest ventricular activity is usually recorded in one of these leads in the presence of a narrow QRS.[31] Data from our laboratory have shown that ventricular activation can, and often does, occur before the onset of the QRS. This is particularly true when infarction of the septum and/or intraventricular conduction defects are present. Thus, even if V1 is used, the H-V interval can be falsely long (Fig. 2-6). New values for normal are probably not necessary, but the significance of a long H-V must be interpreted in light of these findings (see Chapter 4).

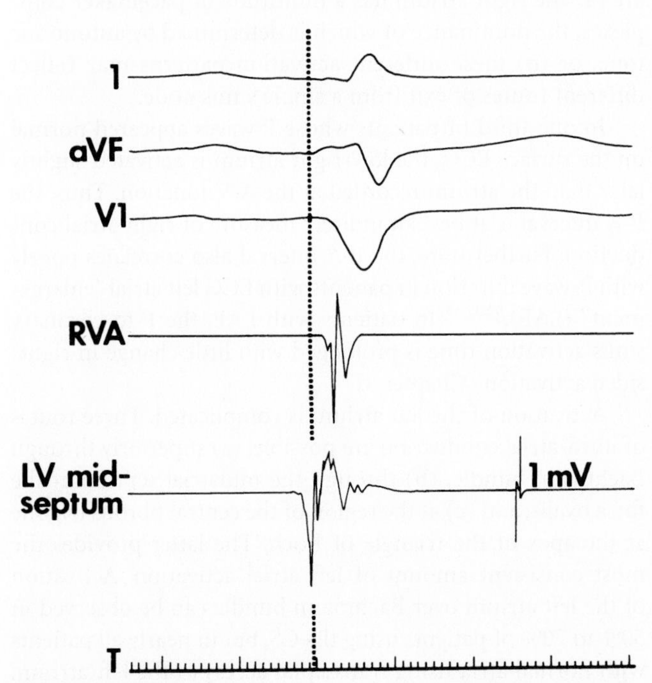


**FIGURE 2-6** *Presystolic electrogram at the left ventricular septum.* Leads 1, aVF, and V1 are shown with electrograms from the right ventricular apex (RVA) and left ventricular (LV) midseptum. An electrogram recorded at the midleft ventricular septum precedes the onset of the QRS by 20 msec. The recognition that presystolic activity exists may play a role in determining the risk of A-V block in patients with conduction disturbances (see Chapter 5).

## Intra-atrial Conduction

The normal sequence of atrial activation and intra-atrial conduction times has not been extensively studied. Many investigators have used the P-A interval (from the onset of the P wave to the onset of atrial activation in the His bundle electrogram) as a measure of intra-atrial conduction (Table 2-1).[1–6,9,14,18,23–28] Several factors, however, render the P-A interval an unsuitable measure of intra-atrial conduction:

1. The onset of endocardial activation may precede the P wave (Fig. 2-7).[32]
2. A more distal position of the His bundle catheter can result in a longer P-A interval.[33]
3. There is no a priori reason that the P-A interval should be a measure of intra-atrial conduction. At best, the P-A interval may reflect intra–right-atrial conduction, but studies have demonstrated that even this assumption is not universally true.[32]

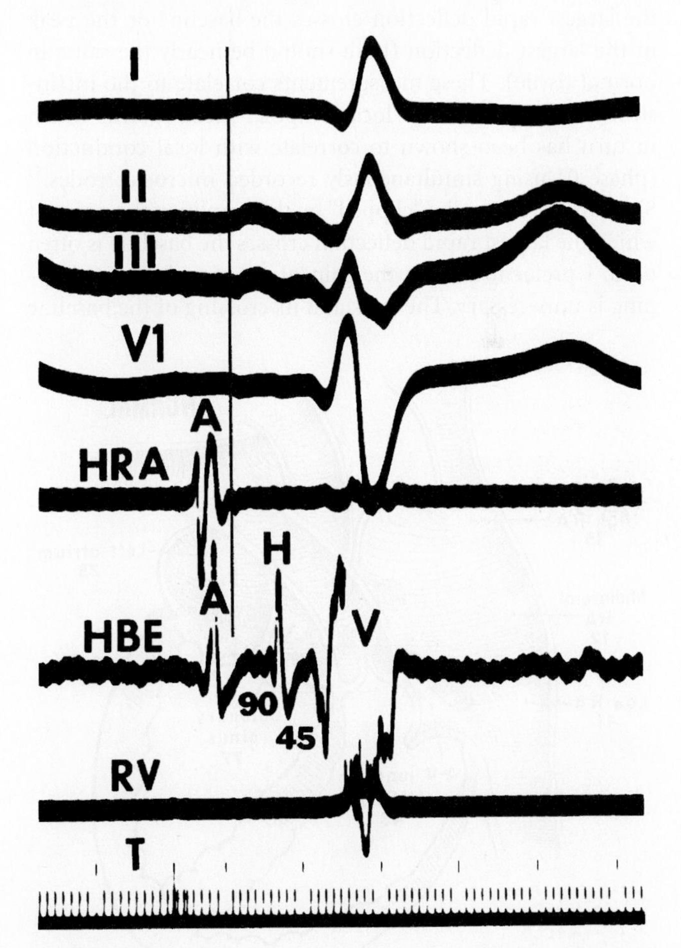


**FIGURE 2-7** *Limitations of the P-A interval.* Atrial activation as recorded in the high-right atrium (HRA) and His bundle electrograms (HBE) precedes the P wave by 40 and 30 msec, respectively, in this patient with dextroversion.

4. The onset of atrial activation appears to vary depending on the rate. In sinus tachycardia, the P waves in the inferior leads appear more upright and the onset of atrial activation is most often recorded high in the right atrium. During relatively slow rates, 50 to 60, the P waves become flat in these leads and the earliest onset of atrial activation is often recorded at the midlateral atrial sites.

To assess atrial conduction more accurately, we have used endocardial mapping of the atria in our laboratory for several years. A general assessment of intra-atrial conduction can be made using catheter recordings obtained from the high- and low-right atrium at the junctions with the venae cavae, midlateral right atrium, A-V junction (in the His bundle electrogram), proximal, mid- and distal coronary sinus, and/or left atrium. The normal activation times at those sites are shown in Figure 2-8. Detailed mapping of the left atrium requires a transseptal approach or use of a patent foramen ovale. Although the retrograde approach can be used, it is far more difficult to reproducibly map the entire left atrium. Entry to the pulmonary veins by the transseptal approach is readily achievable. When mapping is performed, conduction times should be determined using the point at which the largest rapid deflection crosses the baseline or the peak of the largest deflection (both should be nearly the same in normal tissue). These measurements correlate to the intrinsicoid deflection of the local unipolar electrogram, which in turn has been shown to correlate with local conduction (phase 0) using simultaneously recorded microelectrodes.[34] Since the peak may be "clipped" by the amplifier, the point at which the largest rapid deflection crosses the baseline is often used. I prefer to reduce the gain of the signal so that clipping is unnecessary. The peak and its crossing of the baseline are then easy to measure and are more accurate. This differs from the technique of measuring the onset of the His bundle deflection, in which the onset of depolarization of the entire His bundle rather than local activation is desired. Although close (1- to 2-mm) bipolar electrodes record local activity most discriminately, we have obtained comparable data using catheters with a standard (0.5- and/or 1-cm) interelectrode distance. How to best measure activation times of a multicomponent atrial electrogram has not been established. In my opinion, all rapid deflections can be considered relatively local activations (i.e., within a few millimeters). Unipolar signals can help determine the component which is closest to any recording electrode (see Chapter 1). Such electrograms may be caused by a specific anatomic substrate producing nonuniform anisotropy leading to asynchronous activation in the region from which the electrogram is recorded (see Chapter 11). As such, fragmented electrograms are a manifestation of nonuniform anisotropy. A normal atrial endocardial map is shown in Figure 2-9.

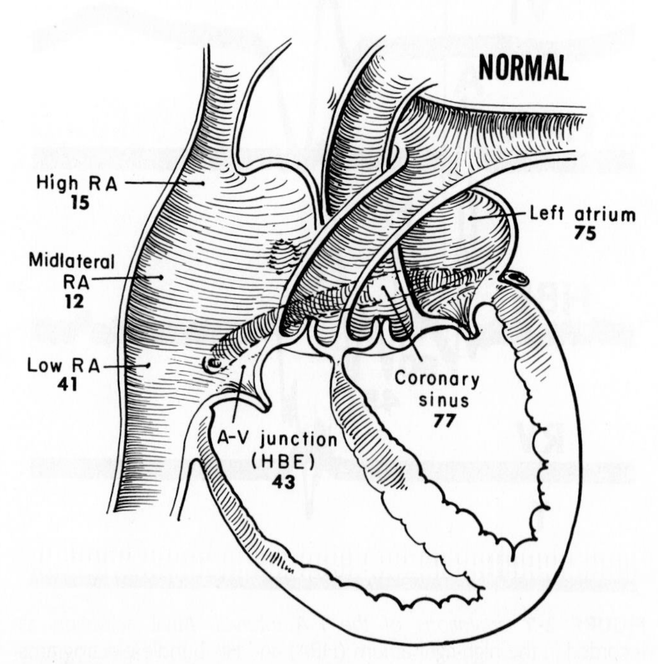


**FIGURE 2-8** *Atrial endocardial mapping sites and mean activation times in normal persons.*

Our data have shown that normal atrial activation can begin in either the high or the midlateral right atrium, spread from there to the low atrium and A-V junction, and then spread to the left atrium. As noted previously, in our experience, earlier activation of the high-right atrium is more likely to occur at faster rates (i.e., more than 100 beats per minute [bpm]), and early activation of the midright atrium is more common at rates less than 60 bpm. The mechanism of these findings is uncertain. Two possibilities exist, which are (a) the right atrium has a multitude of pacemaker complexes, the dominance of which is determined by autonomic tone, or (b) these different activation patterns may reflect different routes of exit from a single sinus node.

In one-third of patients whose P waves appeared normal on the surface ECG, the low-right atrium is activated slightly later than the atrium recorded at the A-V junction. Thus, the P-A interval is at best an indirect measure of right atrial conduction. Furthermore, the P-A interval also correlates poorly with P-wave duration in patients with ECG left atrial "enlargement" (LAE).[32,33,35] In patients with LAE, the P-to-coronary sinus activation time is prolonged with little change in right-sided activation (Chapter 4).[36]

Activation of the left atrium is complicated. Three routes of intra-atrial conduction are possible: (a) superiorly through Bachmann bundle, (b) through the midatrial septum at the fossa ovalis, and (c) at the region of the central fibrous trigone at the apex of the triangle of Koch. The latter provides the most consistent amount of left atrial activation. Activation of the left atrium over Bachmann bundle can be observed in 50% to 70% of patients using the CS, but in nearly all patients with normal atria using transseptal access to the left atrium. It can be demonstrated by distal (superior and lateral) coronary sinus activation preceding midcoronary sinus activation but following proximal (os) coronary sinus activation (Fig. 2-10). The Carto system allows for accurate display of right and left atrial activation, since one can record several hundred sites in both atria. A detailed map of both atria using

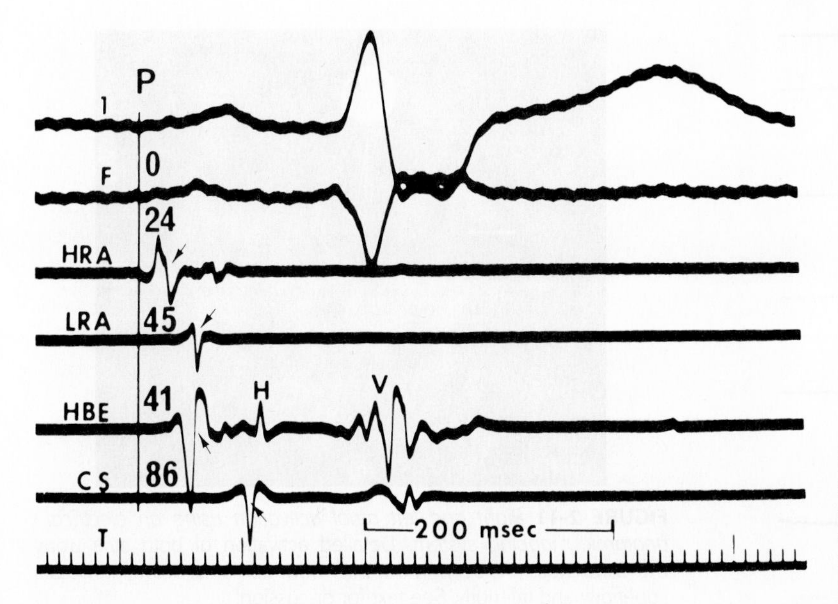


**FIGURE 2-9** *Map of normal antegrade atrial activation.* Activation times are determined by the first rapid deflection as it crosses the baseline (*arrows*). The onset of the P wave is the reference. CS, coronary sinus; HBE, his bundle electrogram; HRA, high-right atrium; LRA, low-right atrium.

this technology is shown in Figure 2-11. Left-to-right atrial activation during distal coronary sinus pacing rarely appears to use Bachmann bundle but primarily crosses at the fossa and low septum. This is particularly true when the recording from the "HRA" is from a catheter in the right atrial appendage, which, not unexpectedly, fails to demonstrate early high-right atrial activation in response to such pacing. If the superior septum is carefully mapped during distal CS pacing, an early breakthrough is usually seen, suggesting propagation over Bachmann Bundle.

Information about the antegrade and retrograde atrial activation sequences is critical to the accurate diagnosis of supraventricular arrhythmias (Chapter 8).[32,37–40] Normal retrograde activation proceeds over the A-V node. Early observations using His bundle, coronary sinus, and high-right atrial recordings using quadripolar catheters suggested that retrograde atrial activation in response to ventricular premature beats or His bundle rhythms normally begins at the A-V junction, with apparent simultaneous radial spread to the right and left atria.[32,41] Thus, the earliest retrograde atrial depolarization is recorded in the His bundle electrogram, then in the adjacent right atrium and coronary sinus, and finally, in the high-right and high-left atria (Fig. 2-12). Recently more detailed atrial mapping during ventricular pacing has demonstrated a complex pattern (see Chapter 8). Basically, at long-paced cycle lengths or coupling intervals atrial activation along a close-spaced (2-mm) decapolar catheter recording a His deflection at the tip is earliest. Secondary breakthrough sites in the coronary sinus catheter and/or posterior triangle of Koch occur in ~50% of patients (Fig. 2-13). The early left atrial breakthrough probably reflects activation over the left atrial extension of the A-V node. At shorter coupling intervals, particularly during pacing-induced Wenckebach cycles, retrograde activation changes and earliest activation is typically found at the posterior triangle of Koch, the os of the coronary sinus, or within the coronary sinus itself (Fig. 2-14).

## Intraventricular Conduction

Intracardiac analysis of intraventricular conduction has not been a routine procedure in most electrophysiologic laboratories. We, however, believe both right and left ventricular mapping are useful in analyzing intraventricular conduction defects, dispersion of ventricular activation and recovery of excitability, and localizing the site of origin of ventricular tachycardias. Specific areas in which left and/or right ventricular mapping has been particularly useful are (a) the finding of presystolic electrical activity on the left ventricular septum causing a "pseudo" H-V prolongation; (b) the finding of abnormal dispersion of activation, refractoriness, and total recovery (sum of local activation and refractoriness) in arrhythmogenic conditions; (c) to distinguish between proximal and distal RBB block; (d) to distinguish LBB block from left ventricular intraventricular conduction defects; (e) to define the site of origin of ventricular tachycardia; (f) to localize the ventricular site of pre-excitation; (g) to evaluate the degree of inter- and intraventricular dysynchrony as a predictor of resynchronization therapy and optimal LV lead placement, and (h) to define a pathophysiologic substrate of arrhythmogenesis that may help to distinguish patients predisposed to lethal arrhythmias.[42–49]

Although recording electrograms from the right ventricular apex has been used during the past 40 years to distinguish proximal from distal RBB block,[44,50,51] the potential role for right ventricular mapping to distinguish tachycardias related to arrhythmogenic right ventricular dysplasia (fractionated electrograms on the free wall of the right ventricle) from right ventricular outflow tract tachycardias that arise on the free wall or "septal" side of the outflow tract in patients without ventricular disease has been recognized (see Chapter 11). In the presence of a normal QRS, the normal activation times from the onset of ventricular depolarization to the electrogram recorded from the catheter placed near the

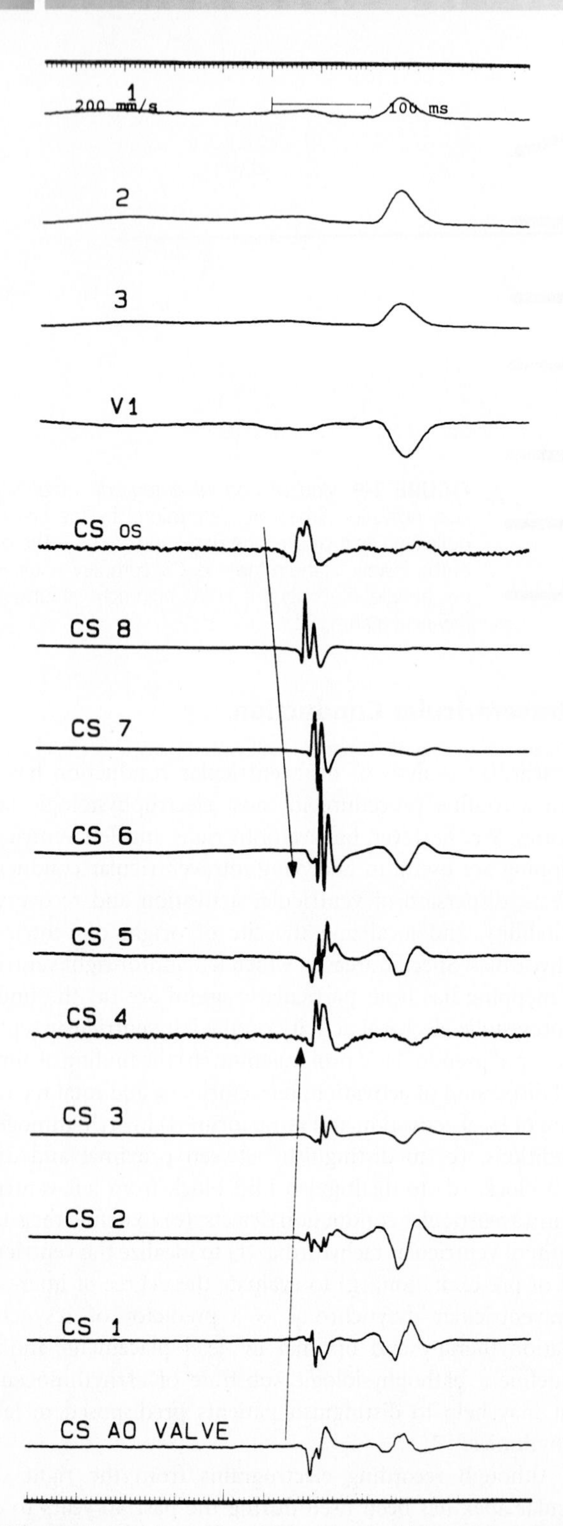


**FIGURE 2-10** *Evidence of multiple routes of left atrial activation.* Leads 1, 2, 3, and V1 are shown with electrograms from the HRA, His bundle, and left atrium from the coronary sinus (CS). The distal CS (CS 1) is located anteriorly, CS 3 is lateral, and CS os is ~1 cm inside the ostium of the CS. Note the CS is activated earlier than the lateral CS, but the proximal CS is activated even earlier. This suggests left atrial activation occurs over both Bachmann bundle and the low atrial septum. See text for discussion.

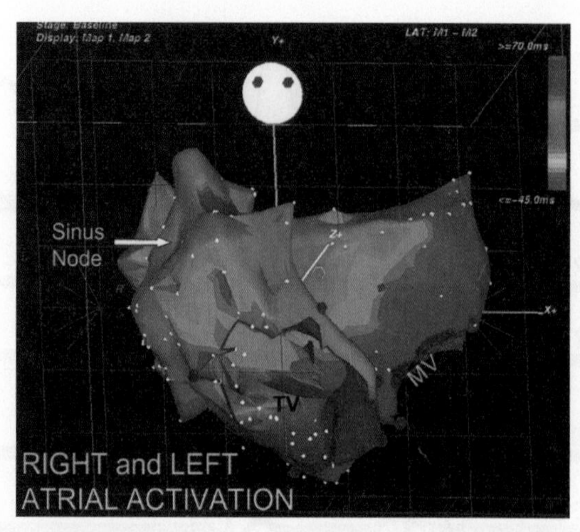


**FIGURE 2-11** *Right and left atrial activation using an electrical–anatomic mapping system.* Detailed activation of both atria using the Carto system is seen in the LAO view. Left atrial activation occurs superiorly and inferiorly. See text for discussion.

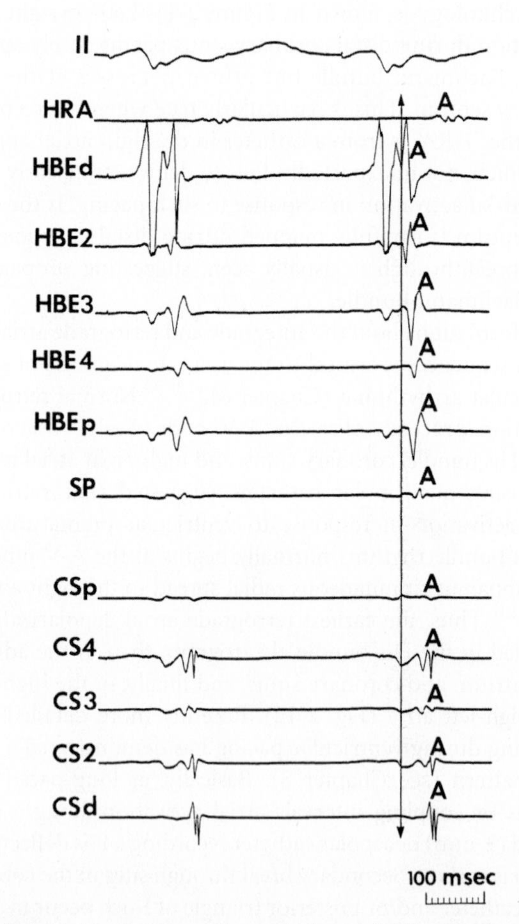


**FIGURE 2-12** *Focal pattern of retrograde atrial activation.* Retrograde atrial activation is recorded during ventricular pacing. Multiple recordings along the tendon of Todaro are made with a decapolar catheter (2-mm interelectrode distance), posterior triangle of Koch (SP), and left atrium via a decapolar catheter in the coronary sinus. Earliest activation is seen in the distal poles of the HBE with subsequent spread to the SP and CS. See text.

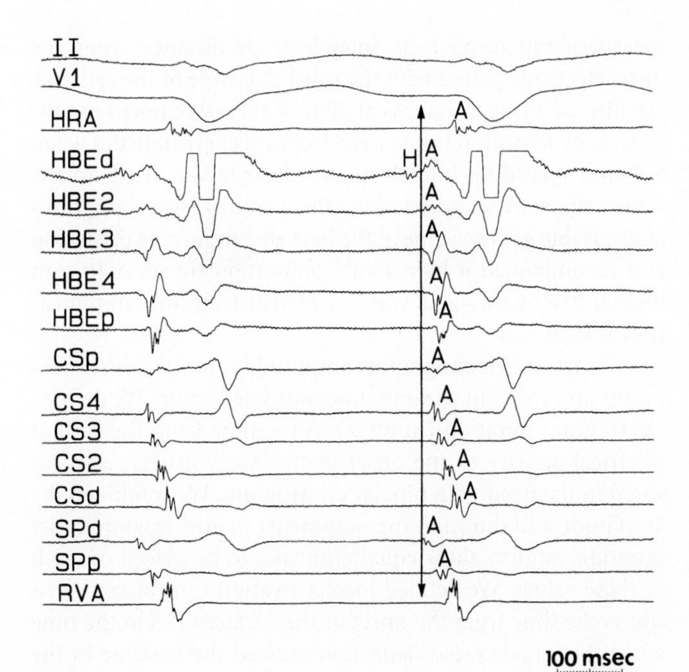


**FIGURE 2-13** *Complex pattern of retrograde atrial activation in response to a ventricular premature depolarization.* Retrograde atrial activation is recorded during ventricular pacing. Multiple recordings along the tendon of Todaro are made with a decapolar catheter (2-mm interelectrode distance), posterior triangle of Koch (SP), and left atrium via a decapolar catheter in the coronary sinus. Note early breakthroughs occur in the His bundle recording and secondarily in the CS (or SP). See text.

right ventricular apex range from 5 to 30 msec.[50,51] The RV free wall at the insertion of the moderator band into the anterior papillary muscle (apical third of the RV free wall) is typically the earliest site of RV activation and precedes the apical septum by 5 to 15 msec. This is dependent on if there is continuation of the RBB toward the apical septum (<25%) or the apical septum is activated from Purkinje fibers coming off the RBB in the moderator band (see Chapter 5). Differences in this timing relate to catheter placement more toward right ventricular apex or more toward the free wall at the base of insertion of the papillary muscle or after the takeoff of the moderator band. In addition, most investigators record from the proximal poles of a quadripolar catheter. Multiple levels of block in the right-sided conduction system can be assessed.[44] Patients with proximal RBB block (long V to RV apex activation time) and long H-V intervals found postoperatively after repair of tetralogy of Fallot may be at high risk for heart block and subsequent sudden cardiac death caused by ventricular arrhythmias. Use of simultaneous recordings from a multipolar catheter positioned along the RBB can facilitate determining the site of RBB block/delay or establish whether a tachycardia mechanism requires the RBB (e.g., bundle branch reentry).

We have actively pursued detailed evaluation of endocardial activation of the left ventricle during sinus rhythm in our laboratory.[42,43,45,48,49] We believed it was imperative to establish normal electrogram characteristics as well as activation patterns and recovery times to evaluate conduction defects related to the specialized conducting system or myocardial infarction or electrophysiologic abnormalities associated with a propensity to ventricular arrhythmias. We performed characterization of electrograms, both qualitatively and quantitatively, and particularly, activation patterns in 15 patients with no evidence of cardiac disease. In all cases, we performed left ventricular mapping using a Josephson quadripolar catheter (0.5-cm interelectrode distance). We inserted the catheter percutaneously into the femoral artery and advanced it to the left ventricle under fluoroscopic guidance. We inserted one to two quadripolar catheters percutaneously in the right femoral vein and advanced to the right ventricular apex and

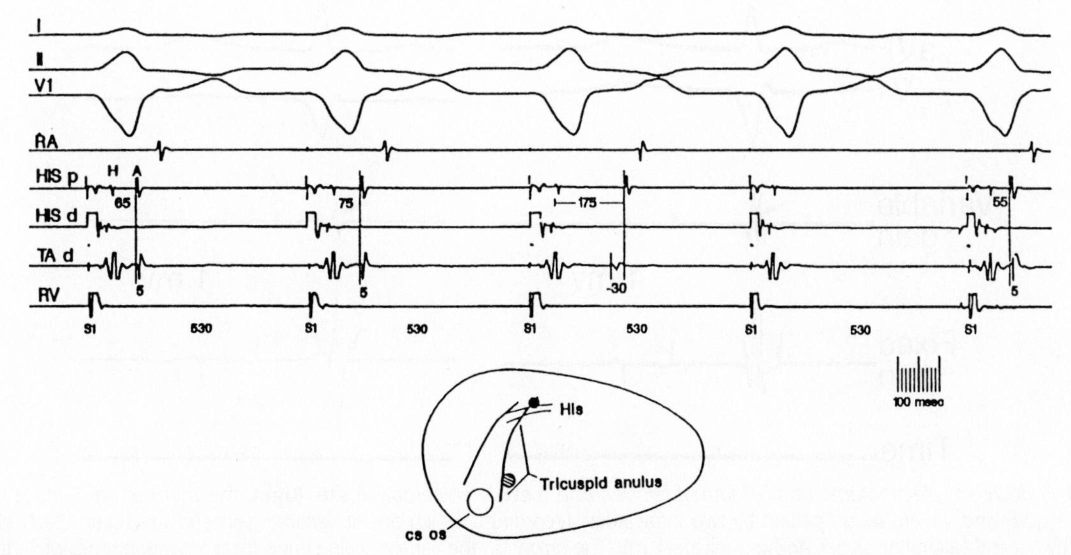


**FIGURE 2-14** *Change in retrograde atrial activation during ventricular pacing.* Leads I, II, and V1 are shown with electrograms from the high-right atrium (RA), proximal (p) and distal (d) HIS, and distal tricuspid annulus TA d (schematically show below), and RV. During ventricular pacing at 530 msec, earliest activation is at the HIS p with TA d following almost simultaneously (5 msec). The third paced complex shows a more marked delay in activation at the HIS p than the TA d so that the TA d now precedes the HIS p by 30 msec.

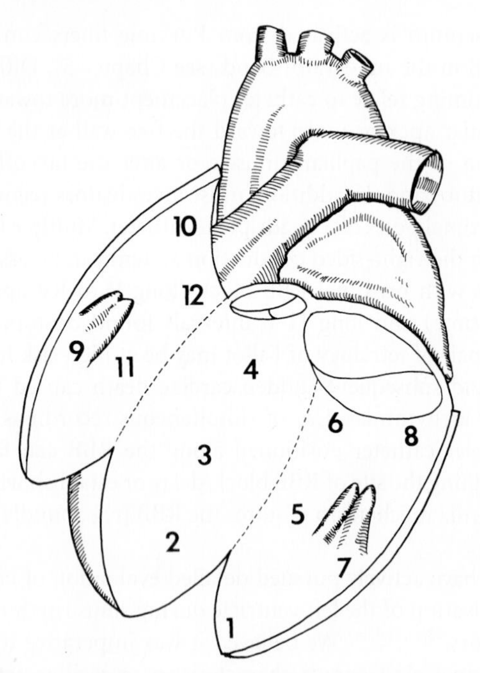


**FIGURE 2-15** *Schema of left ventricular endocardial mapping sites.* (Modified from Josephson ME, Horowitz LN, Spielman SR, et al. The role of catheter mapping in the preoperative evaluation of ventricular tachycardia. *Am J Cardiol* 1982;49:207.)

outflow tract as reference electrodes. We used the left ventricular mapping schema representing 12 segmental areas of the left ventricle (Fig. 2-15). We recorded 10 to 22 electrograms in each patient with the catheter sites verified by multiplane fluoroscopy. We ensured stability by recording from each site for a minimum of 5 to 30 seconds. We made all electrogram measurements using 1-cm interelectrode distance, using the distal electrode paired with the third electrode of the catheter. We filtered all electrograms at 30 to 500 Hz. We noted no difference in activation time or electrogram characteristics when a 5-mm recording interelectrode distance was used on the same catheter. We also recorded the intracardiac electrograms at a variable gain to achieve the best electrographic definition and accompanied it by a 1-mV calibration signal. A 10-mm bipolar fixed-gain signal was recorded at 1-cm/mV amplification at each site.

We defined electrographic amplitude (in mV) as the maximum upward to maximum downward deflection. We defined electrogram duration (in msec) as the time from the earliest electrical activity to the onset of the decay artifact as measured in the fixed-gain bipolar electrogram. We combined the amplitude and duration measurements to give an amplitude/duration ratio to allow equal emphasis to be placed on each of these values. We defined local activation time at any given site as the time from the onset of the surface QRS to the time when the largest rapid deflection crossed the baseline in the 10-mm variable-gain electrogram. Examples of these techniques are shown in Figure 2-16.

We defined normal electrogram amplitude and duration as those within 95% confidence limits for all electrograms for those measurements. We defined electrograms as basal (sites 4, 6, 8, 10, and 12) or nonbasal (sites 1, 2, 3, 5, 7, 9, and 11). Newer technologies for mapping (e.g., Carto System, Biosense, Inc.) require new standards for normals since different electrode size, interelectrode distance, and configuration (unipolar vs. bipolar) as well as different filtering are used. The Biosense Webster system can measure absolute unipolar

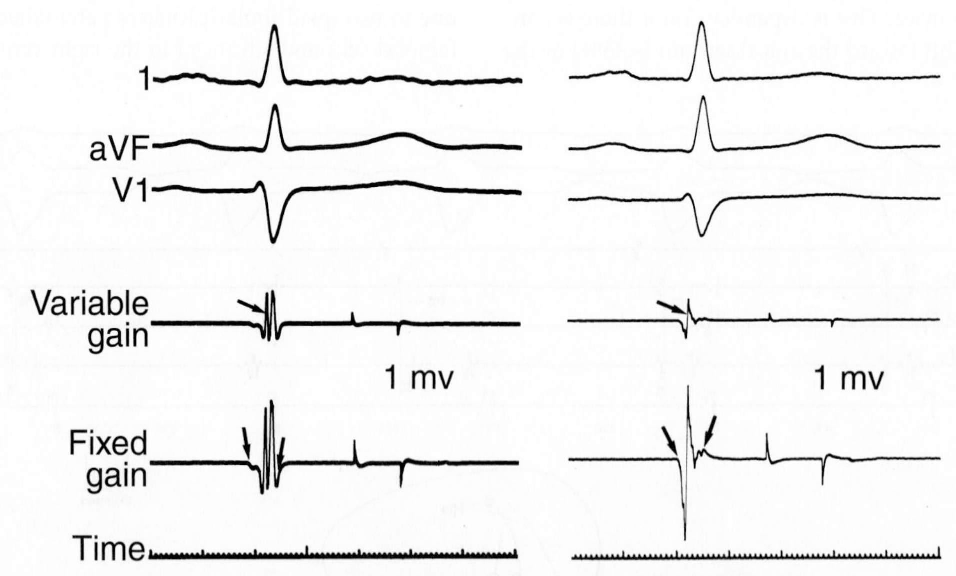


**FIGURE 2-16** *Endocardial electrograms from a normal left ventricle.* **Left**, a posterobasal site. **Right**, the midseptum. Surface electrocardiographic leads 1, aVF, and V1 are accompanied by two intracardiac recordings, which are of variable gain and fixed gain. Each electrogram is accompanied by a 1-mV calibration signal. *Arrows* indicate 1 mV. The *arrow* on the variable gain shows local activation time, while the *arrows* on the fixed-gain electrograms show onset and offset of local electrical activity. Note that the *arrows* marking the offset show the artifact produced by the decay of the amplified filtered signal. This is also seen on the 1-mV calibration signals. Time line is marked at the bottom of the figure. (From Cassidy DM, Vassallo JA, Marchlinski FE, et al. Endocardial mapping in humans in sinus rhythm with normal left ventricles: activation patterns and characteristics of electrograms. *Circulation* 1984;70:37–42.)

or bipolar voltage and automatically chooses an activation time which can be adjusted by the operator. In early versions it was possible to create off-line late potential and electrogram duration maps. This will probably be reintroduced in newer models. Integration with laboratory systems is possible, and has already been accomplished in the Prucka system. With the Carto system, which uses a 4-mm tip and 2-mm interelectrode distance, the Penn group[52,53] found normal bipolar LV electrograms to have an mean amplitude of 1.62 mV and the RV an amplitude of 1.47 mV. These signals were filtered at 30 to 150 Hz. We have noted similar values of ~1.5 mV in the LV and 1.40 mV in the RV, with higher values in the LV in the presence of LVH. Callans et al.[54] defined scar in an porcine model of infarction of ~0.5 mV using both echo and pathology. Similar values in humans have been proposed by Marchlinski et al.[52] using nuclear scan as a correlate. We have found dense transmural scar to have amplitudes of <0.1 mV in our initial mapping studies,[49] and similar values using Carto with MRI defined scar as a correlate. These findings are critical for substrate mapping (see Chapter 14). The Penn group[55,56] has suggested that unipolar recordings may be useful in detecting subepicardial or intramural disease. Normal LV values are >8.3 mV; lower values are said to represent loss of cells and fibrosis/scar. They even suggest it might be able to distinguish nonreversible cardiomyopathy.[55,56] I believe this requires validation. We have seen patients, particularly those with hypertrophy, have extensive scar detected by diffuse delayed gadolinium enhancement on MRI but who have normal bipolar and unipolar recordings. The degree of filtering effects recordings. Filtered bipolar recordings are a reflection of rapid conduction, while unfiltered (0.05 to 500 Hz) recordings reflect volume of tissue and direction of propagation. Hence they measure different things.

Any time catheters with different sized electrodes are used, new normal values need to be established. It is important to recognize the fact that our initial studies used both amplitude and duration to define electrograms. This requires a fixed gain at which the electrograms are recorded, something newer technology currently does not have available.

## DESCRIPTION OF ELECTROGRAMS

In our initial studies we obtained 156 electrograms (both variable and fixed gain) in 10 patients for quantitative analysis of characteristics of amplitude and duration. The use of mean values for multiple electrograms recorded from the same defined site left 112 electrograms for analysis. We obtained 215 electrograms (variable gain only) in 15 patients for analysis of left ventricular endocardial activation time. When only 1 electrogram per site was used, 169 electrograms were analyzed for activation time. We found no significant difference in activation times or electrographic characteristics when analyzing the total number of electrograms or the per-site mean average of electrograms. We have therefore reported our results using the per-site mean average.

### Descriptive Characteristics

Electrograms from normal left ventricles had rapid deflections and distinct components. We recorded low-amplitude slow activity of only a few milliseconds' (range, 2 to 15 msec) duration at the beginning of all electrograms. We observed no split, fractionated, or late electrograms (e.g., after the QRS) (see Chapter 11).[48,49]

### Quantitative Characteristics

Results of the quantitative analysis of normal electrographic characteristics are listed in Table 2-1. Mean electrographic amplitude was 6.7 ± 3.4 mV, and 95% of the electrograms were of an amplitude of 3 mV or greater. Mean electrogram duration was 54 ± 13 msec; 95% of the electrograms were of 70 msec or less duration. Mean electrogram/duration ratio was 0.133 ± 0.073 mV/sec, and the ratio for 95% of the electrograms was 0.045 mV/msec or greater. Quantitative descriptions of all electrograms recorded are listed in Tables 2-2 and 2-3 Basal electrograms tended to be of lower amplitude (6.5 vs. 6.9 mV; $p$ = NS), of greater duration (60 vs. 50 msec; $p <$ 0.001), and to have a lower amplitude/duration ratio (0.166 vs. 0.144 mV/msec; $p < 0.05$) (Table 2-2). As noted earlier normal RV and LV voltage have been determined using the Navistar (Biosense Webster) 4-mm tip catheter. No other catheters have been used to obtain normal values. As such, normal values for voltage need to be determined when other tip size or interelectrode distance is used.

### Left Ventricular Endocardial Activation

Left ventricular endocardial activation began at 0 to 15 msec (mean, 6 msec) after the onset of the QRS. Left ventricular endocardial activation was completed at 29 to 52 msec (mean, 43 msec). The duration of left ventricular endocardial activation ranged from 28 to 50 msec (mean 36). This comprised 41% of the total surface QRS complex (mean QRS duration, 87 msec; range, 80 to 100 msec). An analog map is shown in Figure 2-17.

We observed a definite pattern of left ventricular endocardial activation, although some patient-to-patient variability existed. The midseptum and the inferior wall adjacent to the midseptum was the earliest area of left ventricular endocardial activation, while the superior-basal aspect of the free wall was a third endocardial breakthrough site. Sometimes the earliest septal and inferior sites were close to one another, but in the majority (10/15, 67%) earliest sites of endocardial breakthrough were nonadjacent. Activation then appeared to spread radially from these breakthrough sites, so that the apex was activated relatively late, whereas the base at the inferior-posterior wall was consistently the last area to be activated. Analog records of ventricular activation are shown in Figure 2-17.

Using our mapping techniques (5-mm bipolar recordings filtered at 30 to 500 Hz), we were able to discern a distinct third endocardial breakthrough site, in the vast majority of patients analogous to that noted by Durrer et al.[57] The inability to see

**TABLE 2-2 Summary of Electrogram Characteristics in Normal Left Ventricles**

| Characteristics | All Sites | Basal Sites | Nonbasal Sites | p Value |
|---|---|---|---|---|
| Amplitude (mV) | — | — | — | — |
| Mean ± SD | 6.7 ± 3.4 | 6.5 ± 3.2 | 6.9 ± 3.5 | NS |
| 95% ≥3.0 | — | — | — | — |
| Range 1.5–21 | — | — | — | — |
| Duration (msec) | — | — | — | — |
| Mean ± SD | 54 ± 13 | 60 ± 14 | 50 ± 11 | <0.001 |
| 95% ≤70 | — | — | — | — |
| Range 18–82 | — | — | — | — |
| Amplitude/duration ratio (mV/msec) | — | — | — | — |
| Mean | 0.133 ± 0.073 | 0.116 ± 0.070 | 0.144 ± 0.074 | <0.05 |
| 95% ≥0.046 | — | — | — | — |
| Range 0.031–438 | — | — | — | — |
| Number of electrograms | 112 | 45 | 67 | — |

this universally was most likely due to the limitation of defining discrete activation sites, particularly at the midseptum and adjacent inferior wall using nonsteerable catheters. Using the Carto system (Biosense, Inc.) we have been more consistently able to define separate septal and inferior wall breakthrough sites comparable to those described by Durrer et al.[57]

Our data had limitations. One was the use of a 1-cm interelectrode distance for recording our electrograms. We compared 5- and 10-mm interelectrode distances and found no difference in activation times. Thus, the use of a 5-mm interelectrode distance would not change the data. However, tighter (i.e., 1- to 2-mm) bipolar pairs might alter the results. Certainly, use of a 1-mm interelectrode distance between poles, each of which, having a small surface area, has demonstrated electrograms of different duration. However, local activation appears similar using the largest rapid deflection for measurement. A negative feature of using such tight electrodes is that reproducible placement at the same recording site is more difficult. Whether or not 1-mm recordings will provide more clinically useful information is not yet established. As noted above, use of different catheters and recording techniques will necessitate establishing new "normal" values for each technique. For the last decade we have used the electrical–anatomic mapping system (Carto System, Biosense,

**TABLE 2-3 Electrogram Amplitude and Duration Characteristics in Normal Left Ventricles by Left Ventricular Site[a] Number**

| Patient | 1 A/D | 2 A/D | 3 A/D | 4 A/D | 5 A/D | 6 A/D | 7 A/D | 8 A/D | 9 A/D | 10 A/D | 11 A/D | 12 A/D |
|---|---|---|---|---|---|---|---|---|---|---|---|---|
| 1 | 6.7/45 | 4.8/50 | 5.4/62 | 3.1/69 | 6.5/62 | 3.7/72 | 7.0/60 | .0/70 | 4.2/52 | 3.2/70 | 6.0/50 | 6.2/56 |
| 2 | 8.5/60 | 9.0/55 | 7.3/56 | — | 7.8/55 | 7.5/50 | 11.2/50 | 7.5/52 | 3.2/60 | 8.5/60 | 4.5/52 | 8.5/48 |
| 3 | 21/48 | 5.6/48 | 4.5/57 | 3.3/62 | 9.3/53 | 4.4/62 | 7.0/46 | 2.0/48 | 4.8/56 | 3.0/63 | — | — |
| 4 | 4.8/47 | 4.7/48 | 6.0/40 | — | 5.1/40 | 4.8/48 | 9.7/40 | 9.3/46 | 5.4/18 | 11.5/62 | 5.2/40 | 8.2/40 |
| 5 | 3.3/48 | 10/40 | 2/25 | 6.3/42 | 6.2/26 | 8.0/22 | 3.3/26 | 9/43 | 7/30 | 10.6/46 | 3/58 | 6/28 |
| 6 | 6.8/46 | 8.5/50 | 5.3/52 | — | 7.8/52 | 5.2/70 | 3.9/33 | 7.1/59 | — | 3.4/76 | 4.8/53 | 6.2/68 |
| 7 | 11.2/58 | 5.4/65 | 4.4/60 | 3.8/69 | 2.9/55 | 7.2/79 | 6.4/65 | 11.5/80 | 17.5/62 | 7.8/56 | 4.5/70 | 3.6/58 |
| 8 | 2.7/37 | 8.5/40 | 1.6/51 | 3.4/56 | 5.2/47 | 3.0/49 | 4.5/46 | 4.5/59 | 5.0/64 | 2.8/58 | 4.7/21 | 1.5/46 |
| 9 | 9.2/55 | 6.7/57 | 14.5/60 | 5.0/75 | 15.1/53 | 6.0/82 | 7.8/45 | .0/78 | 8.5/60 | 14.5/75 | 8.8/50 | — |
| 10 | 13/50 | 6.6/50 | 4.4/54 | 6.4/70 | — | 11.4/75 | 9.3/46 | 5.0/70 | 10.0/60 | 15.5/70 | 6.5/49 | 8.5/67 |

[a]Sites correspond to those in Figure 2-15.

A, amplitude in millivolts; D, duration in milliseconds; —, no electrogram recorded.

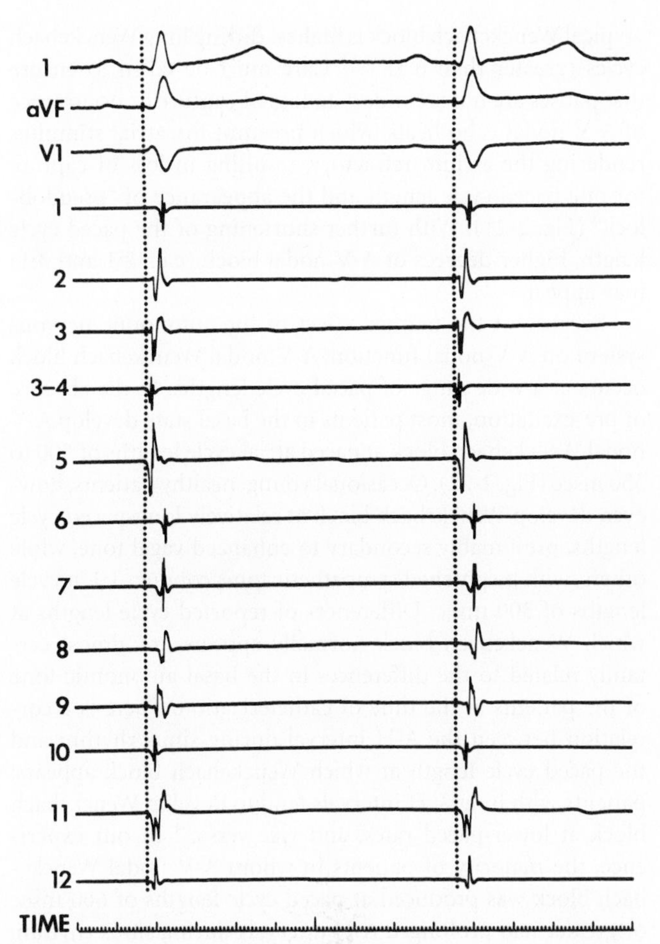


**FIGURE 2-17** *Analog record and isochronic map of ventricular endocardial activation for a normal patient.* On the right are analog recordings of 1, aVF, V1, and electrograms from left ventricular endocardial sites. Note that the electrograms recorded from the left endocardial sites are rapid, with activation complete in the first half of the QRS complex. Notice there are probably three breakthrough sites, one at the midseptum at site 3–4; one at the inferior wall, site 5; and one at the anterosuperior wall, site 11–12. See text for further discussion.

Inc.) and have been able to routinely acquire 100 to 200 activation points in the left ventricle (Fig. 2-18) which are also spatially depicted and stored in three dimensions. The data were similar to our original findings but could distinguish in greater detail breakthrough sites and conduction abnormalities. The "normal" standards are available for this system (see preceding paragraphs), although this is more relevant to evaluation of electrogram amplitude, width, and configuration, not activation.

## PROGRAMMED STIMULATION

Incremental pacing and the introduction of programmed single or multiple extrastimuli during sinus or paced rhythms are the tools of dynamic electrophysiology. The normal heart responds in a predictable fashion to those perturbations, which may be used to achieve the following:

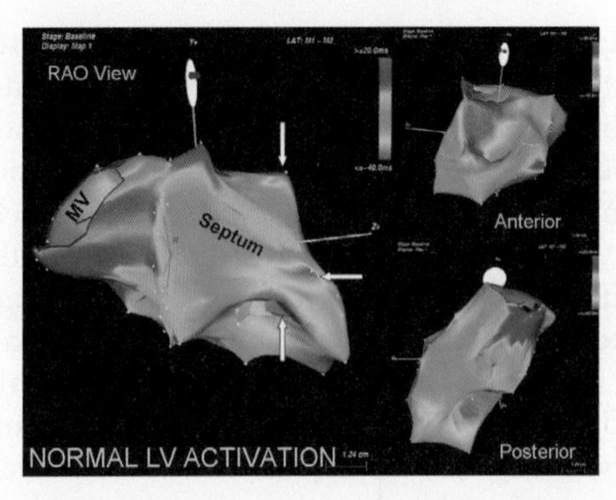


**FIGURE 2-18** *Electrical–anatomic map of normal left ventricular activation.*

1. Characterize the physiologic properties of the AVCS, atria, and ventricles.
2. Induce and analyze mechanisms of arrhythmias.
3. Evaluate both the effects of drug and electrical interventions on the function of the AVCS, atria, and ventricles and their efficacy in the treatment of arrhythmias.

Like hemodynamic catheterizations, electrophysiologic studies must be tailored to the individual patient.

Stimulation is usually carried out with the use of an isolated constant current source that delivers a rectangular impulse at a current strength that is twice-diastolic threshold. We chose this current strength because of its reproducibility and safety. Some investigators advocate the use of stimuli delivered at 5 and 10 mA, but the safety of this current strength, particularly when used with multiple extrastimuli, remains to be determined. This will be discussed subsequently in this chapter in the section entitled Safety of Ventricular Stimulation. Regardless of what current strength is used, the stimulation system must allow the precise determination of the current strength delivered. The amount of current used is crucial in evaluating sensitivity and specificity of induction of arrhythmias and, in particular, in evaluating pharmacologic effects and therapy. Threshold, the lowest current required for consistent capture, is determined in late diastole, and must be redetermined after the administration of any drug to assess the effect of that drug on excitability.

Because the threshold can be influenced by the paced cycle length, one should determine threshold at each paced cycle length used. One must also ascertain that stimulation is carried out at twice-diastolic threshold both before and after drug intervention to distinguish changes in diastolic excitability (threshold) from changes in refractoriness.

### Incremental Pacing

Atrial pacing provides a method of analyzing the functional properties of the AVCS. Pacing from different atrial sites may result in different patterns of A-V conduction.[21,22,58] Thus, pacing should be performed from the same site if the effects of drugs and/or physiologic interventions are to be studied.

Atrial pacing should always be synchronized because alteration of the coupling interval of the first beat of a drive can affect subsequent A-V conduction. Atrial pacing is most commonly performed from the high-right atrium in the region of the sinus node. It is begun at a cycle length just below that of sinus rhythm with progressive shortening of the cycle length, in 10- to 50-msec decrements, to a minimum of 250 msec and/or cycle length at which A-V Wenckebach occurs. Zhang et al.[59] have compared ramp pacing, which is a gradual decrease in cycle length after several paced complexes at each cycle length, to the stepwise decremental atrial pacing technique and found both to be comparable. The use of the ramp technique might shorten the study if the cycle length of A-V nodal Wenckebach is all that is required. We prefer decremental pacing in our laboratory because it also allows assessment of sinus node recovery times at each drive cycle length (see Chapter 3). We maintain each paced cycle length for 15 to 60 seconds to ensure stability of conduction intervals. This is necessary to overcome two factors that significantly influence the development of a steady state. First is a phenomenon that has been termed accommodation by Lehmann et al.[60] They have found that during decremental pacing, if the coupling interval at the first beat of the drive is not synchronized, one can observe an increasing, decreasing, or stable A-H pattern for several cycles. Lehmann et al.[60] noted this when shifting from one drive cycle length to another without a pause. When the second cycle length was begun asynchronously and the coupling interval of the first beat of the new cycle length was significantly less than that of the second drive cycle length, the initial A-H intervals are longer than during steady state A-H. Oscillations of the A-H interval, which dampen to a steady level, or A-V nodal Wenckebach can occur under these circumstances. If the coupling interval of the first beat of the train is longer than the cycle length of the train, then the first A-H interval will be shorter and then gradually lengthen to reach a steady state level. If the coupling interval of the first beat is approximately the same as the cycle length of the train, there will be rapid attainment of the steady state A-H interval. These patterns of A-V nodal accommodation can be avoided by synchronized atrial pacing.

A second problem that cannot be readily resolved is the influence of autonomic tone on A-V conduction. Depending on the patient's autonomic status, rapid pacing can produce variations in A-V nodal conduction. The effect of paced cycle length and P-R interval on hemodynamics can produce reflexes that alter A-V nodal conduction. A stable interval is usually achieved after 15 to 30 seconds.

The normal response to atrial pacing is for the A-H interval to gradually lengthen as the cycle length is decreased until A-V nodal block (Wenckebach type) appears (Fig. 2-19). Infranodal conduction (H-V interval) remains unaffected (Fig. 2-20).[1–6] Wenckebach block is frequently "atypical" in that the A-H interval does not gradually prolong in decreasing increments. The A-H interval may remain almost unchanged for several beats before block, and/or it may show its greatest increment on the last conducted beat. The incidence of atypical Wenckebach block is highest during long Wenckebach cycles (greater than 6:5).[61–63] Care must be taken to ensure that pauses are not secondary to loss of capture or occurrence of A-V nodal echo beats, which preempt the atrial stimulus, rendering the atrium refractory, resulting in loss of capture for one paced cycle length and the appearance of "pseudoblock" (Fig. 2-21). With further shortening of the paced cycle length, higher degrees of A-V nodal block (e.g., 2:1 and 3:1) may appear.

Because of the marked effect of the autonomic nervous system on A-V nodal function, A-V nodal Wenckebach block occurs at a wide range of paced cycle lengths. In the absence of pre-excitation, most patients in the basal state develop A-V nodal Wenckebach block at paced atrial cycle lengths of 500 to 350 msec (Fig. 2-22). Occasional young, healthy patients, however, develop Wenckebach block at relatively long-paced cycle lengths, presumably secondary to enhanced vagal tone, while others, with heightened sympathetic tone, conduct 1:1 at cycle lengths of 300 msec. Differences of reported cycle lengths at which Wenckebach block normally appears are almost certainly related to the differences in the basal autonomic tone of the patients at the time of catheterization. There is a correlation between the A-H interval during sinus rhythm and the paced cycle length at which Wenckebach block appears; patients with long A-H intervals tend to develop Wenckebach block at lower-paced rates, and vice versa.[64] In our experience, the majority of patients in whom A-V nodal Wenckebach block was produced at paced cycle lengths of 600 msec or greater had prolonged A-H intervals during sinus rhythm. In the absence of drugs, this tends to occur in older patients or in young athletic patients with high vagal tone. In some young athletes Wenckebach block may be seen during sinus rhythm at rest.

At very short cycle lengths (350 msec or less), infra-His block may occasionally be noted in patients with normal resting H-V and QRS intervals (Fig. 2-23).[65] Infra-His block occurs when the refractory period of the His–Purkinje system exceeds the paced atrial cycle length. Although some investigators consider infra-His block abnormal at any paced cycle length,[21,25] it can clearly be a normal response at very short cycle lengths. This is a particularly common phenomenon, because if pacing is begun during sinus rhythm, the first or second complex (depending on the coupling interval from the last sinus complex to the first paced complex) acts as a long-short sequence. The long preceding cycle will prolong the His–Purkinje refractoriness; thus, the next impulse will block. The His–Purkinje system may also show accommodation following the initiation of a drive of atrial pacing in an analogous way to the A-V node.[66] In this instance, however, one may see block initially in the His–Purkinje system followed by decreasing H-V intervals before resumption of 1:1 conduction at a fixed H-V interval. Occasionally persistent two-to-one block occurs as a self-perpetuating phenomenon. Repeating the atrial pacing at log cycle lengths with gradual reduction of the paced cycle length will show normal one-to-one conduction up to A-V nodal Wenckebach; thereby demonstrating the

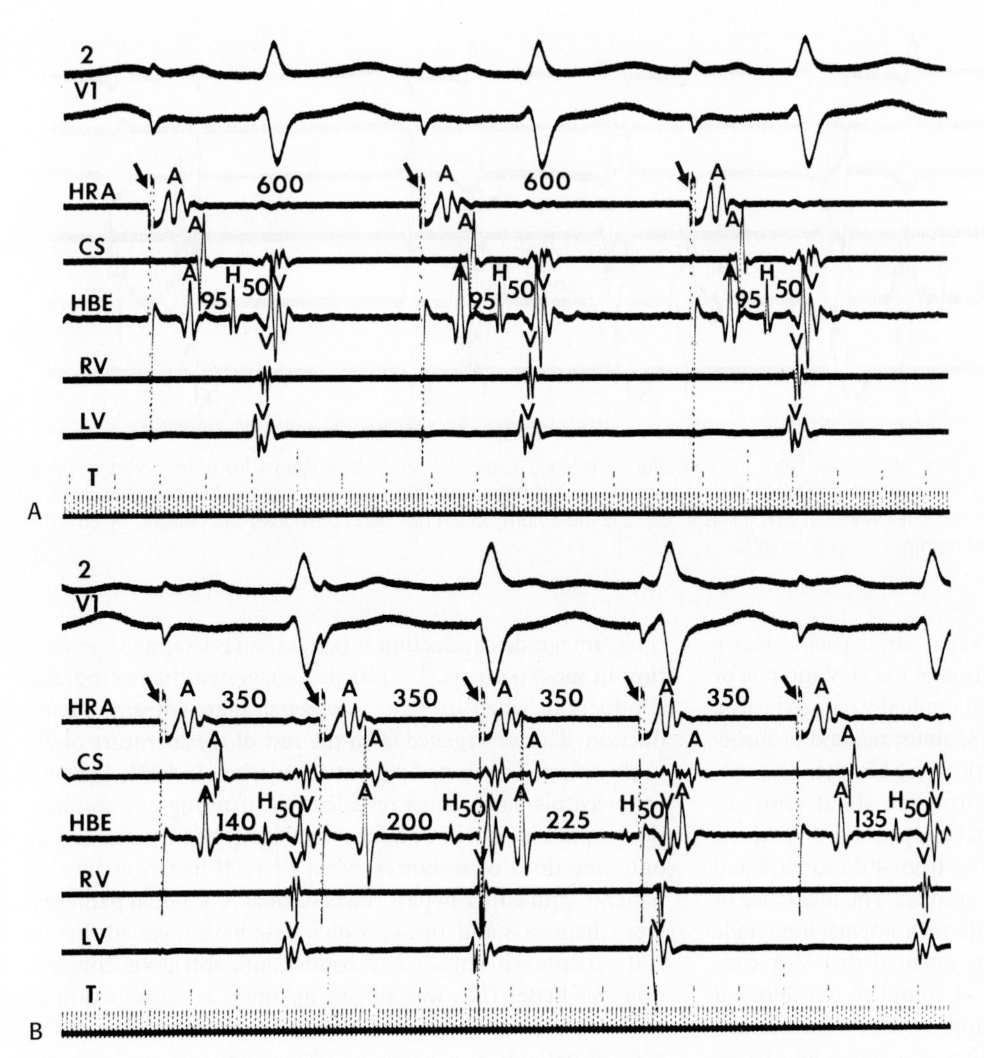


**FIGURE 2-19** *Normal response to incremental atrial pacing.* **A:** At a paced cycle length of 600 msec, the A-H is 95 msec and the H-V is 50 msec. Shortening the cycle length to 350 msec **(B)** results in A-V nodal Wenckebach block; that is, progressive A-H prolongation (140, 200, 225 msec) terminating in block of the P wave in the A-V node (no His bundle deflection after the fourth paced beat). No changes are noted in atrial, right (RV), or left (LV) activation time.

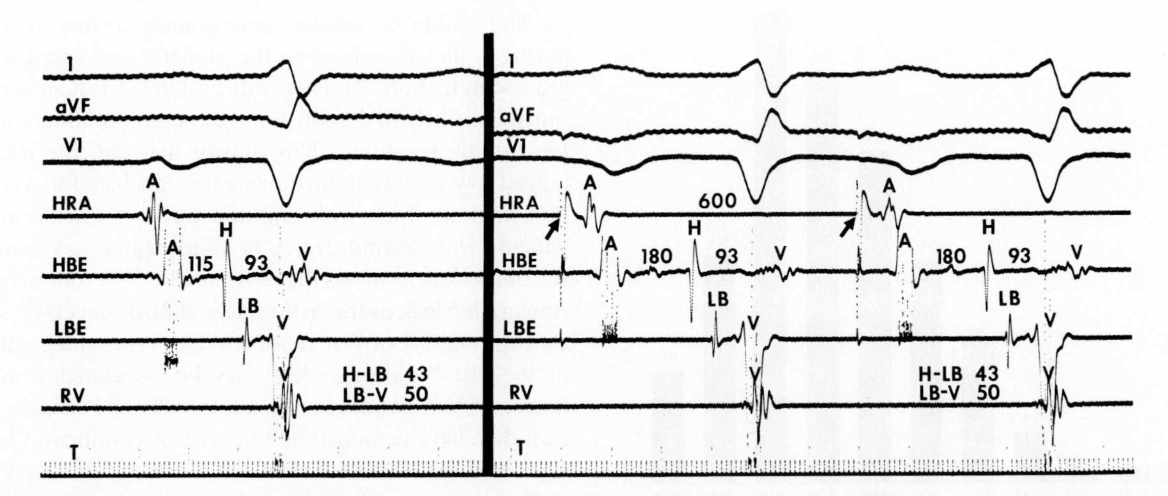


**FIGURE 2-20** *Effect of atrial pacing on the various components of the A-V conduction system.* On the **left** is a sinus beat. The A-H and H-V intervals are 115 and 93 msec, respectively. A left bundle branch electrogram (LBE) allows division of the H-V interval into an H-LB interval (43 msec) and an LB-V of 50 msec. Atrial pacing at a cycle length of 600 msec **(right panel)** produces prolongation of A-V nodal conduction (increase A-H to 180 msec) while infranodal conduction is unaffected (H-V, H-LB, and LB-V remain constant).

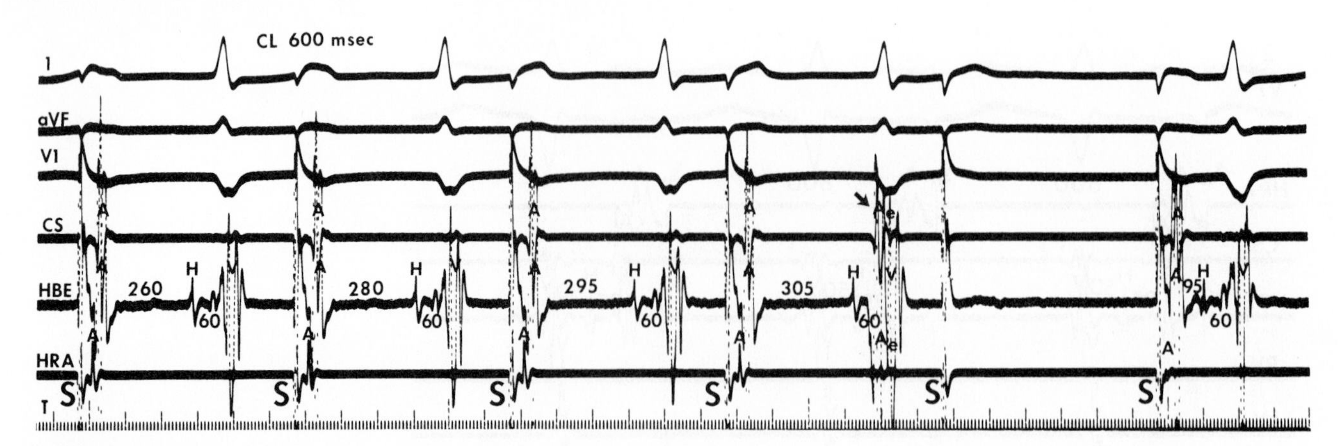


**FIGURE 2-21** *"Pseudoblock" owing to failure of capture.* From top to bottom are leads 1, aVF, V1, and electrograms from the coronary sinus (CS), His bundle electrogram (HBE), and high-right atrium (HRA). Pacing from the HRA is begun, and apparent block of the fast-paced impulse is not due to block in the A-V node. The stimulus is delivered, which fails to capture the atrium, which has been previously depolarized by an atrial echo (Ae, *arrow*) that is due to A-V nodal reentry. CL, cycle length.

production of infra-His block by rapid atrial pacing was a physiologic phenomenon. Prolongation of the H-V interval or infra-His block, however, produced at gradually reduced paced cycle lengths of 400 msec or more are abnormal and probably signify impaired infranodal conduction (see Chapter 5).

Ventricular pacing provides information about ventriculoatrial (V-A) conduction. The exact proportion of patients demonstrating V-A conduction varies from 40% to 90% and depends on the patient population studied. The incidence of V-A conduction is higher in patients with normal antegrade conduction, although it is well documented that V-A conduction can occur in the presence of complete A-V block if block is localized to the His–Purkinje system.[67–70] Although most studies have demonstrated that at comparable paced rates, antegrade conduction is better than retrograde conduction in most patients.[70–72] Narula[73] suggested that retrograde conduction, when present, was better than antegrade conduction. This divergence from the rest of the literature obviously reflected a selected patient population. In 1981, Akhtar[74] reviewed his data, which revealed that if retrograde conduction is present, it will be better than antegrade conduction in only one-third of instances. Most of such instances involve patients with either bypass tracts or dual A-V nodal pathways (see Chapters 8 and 10). Our own data have revealed that in 750 patients with intact A-V conduction, antegrade conduction was better (i.e., was able to maintain 1:1 conduction at shorter-paced cycle lengths) than retrograde conduction in 62% of patients, was worse in 18% of patients, and was the same in 20% of patients. These data, which exclude patients with bypass tracts, are comparable to those of Akhtar who only considered patients with intact retrograde conduction.[74]

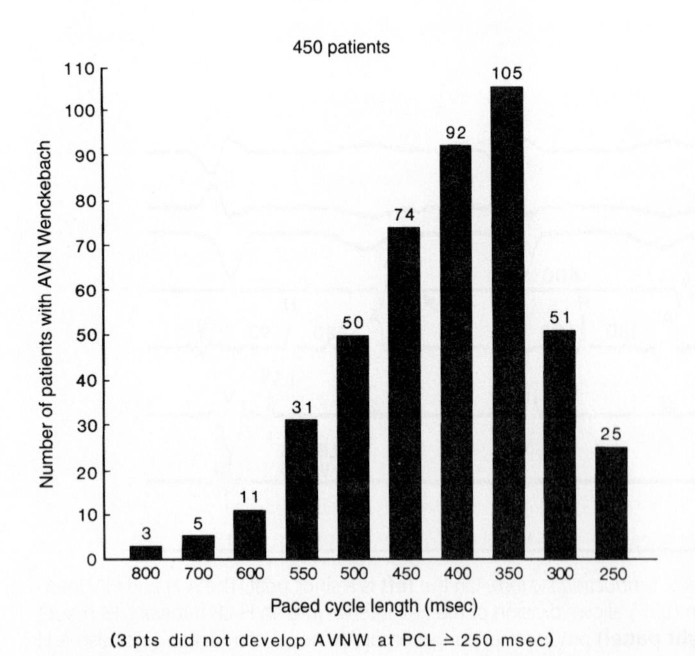


**FIGURE 2-22** *Paced cycle lengths producing A-V nodal Wenckebach block (AVNW).*

The ability to conduct retrogradely during ventricular pacing is directly related to the presence and speed of antegrade conduction. Patients with prolonged P-R intervals are much less likely to demonstrate retrograde conduction.[70–72,74] His bundle recordings have shown that patients with prolonged A-V nodal conduction are less capable of V-A conduction than are those with infranodal delay.[70] Furthermore, in patients with second-degree or third-degree A-V block, the site of block determines the capability for V-A conduction.[70,74] Antegrade block in the A-V node is almost universally associated with failure of V-A conduction, whereas antegrade block in the His–Purkinje system may be associated with some degree of V-A conduction in up to 40% of instances.[70] Our own data have demonstrated intact V-A conduction in 42 of 172 (29%) patients with infra-His block and in only 4 of 173 (1.7%) patients with A-V nodal block. Thus, A-V nodal conduction appears to be the major determinant of retrograde conduction during ventricular pacing.

Ventricular pacing is usually carried out from the right ventricular apex. No difference in capability of V-A conduction

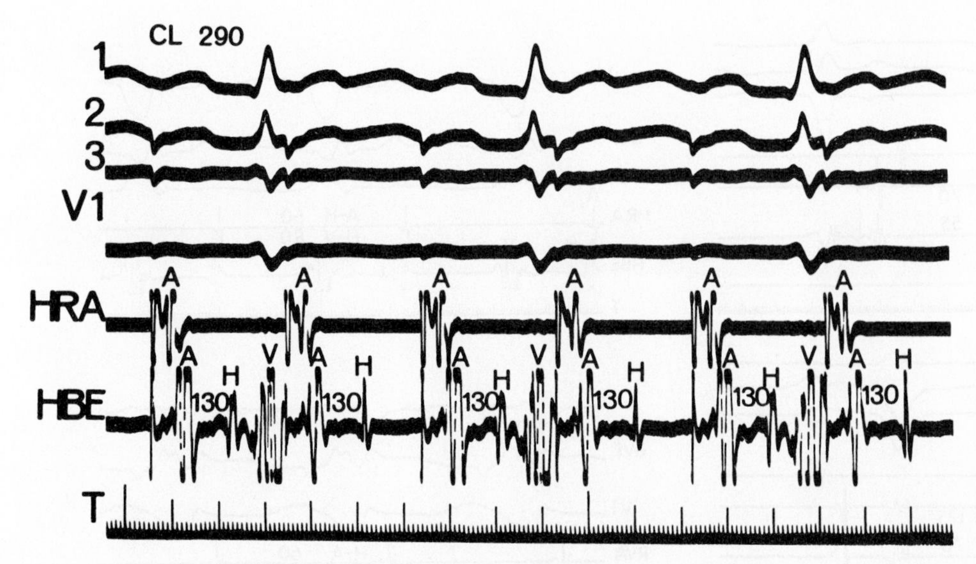


**FIGURE 2-23** *Functional 2:1 infranodal block.* Atrial pacing at a cycle length (CL) of 290 msec results in 2:1 block below the His bundle despite the normal QRS complex and basal H-V interval of 40 msec. This response occurred because the effective refractory period of the His–Purkinje system was 350 msec, which is longer than the paced cycle length.

has been demonstrated between right ventricular apical pacing and pacing from the right ventricular outflow tract or left ventricle in patients with normal A-V and intraventricular conduction. As with atrial pacing, ventricular pacing is begun at a cycle length just below the sinus cycle length. The paced cycle length is gradually reduced until a cycle length of 300 msec is reached. Further shortening of the ventricular-paced cycle length may also be used, particularly in studies assessing rapid retrograde conduction in patients with supraventricular arrhythmias (see Chapter 8) or during stimulation studies to initiate ventricular arrhythmias (see Chapter 11). During ventricular pacing, a retrograde His deflection can be seen in the His bundle electrogram in the majority of cases. If careful attention is paid to obtaining the His deflection (this may require multiple readjustments), particularly using a narrow bipolar pair at relatively low gain settings, a His deflection may be observed nearly 85% of the time in patients with a normal QRS complex during sinus rhythm. We have used the Bard Electrophysiology Josephson quadripolar catheter for obtaining distal and proximal His deflections (Chapter 1). Using this catheter, we observed a retrograde His potential in 86 of 100 consecutive patients in whom we attempted to record it. Ventricular pacing at the base of the heart opposite the A-V junction (Para-Hisian pacing) facilitates recording a retrograde His deflection, particularly when the His bundle recording is made with a narrow bipolar signal (i.e., 2 mm). This allows the ventricle to be activated much earlier relative to His bundle activation, because the ventricular impulse must propagate from the base to the apex before it engages the RBB and subsequently conduct to the His bundle. Retrograde His deflections are much less often seen in the presence of ipsilateral bundle branch block. In all instances, V-H (or stimulus-H) interval exceeds the anterograde H-V by the time it takes for the stimulated impulse to reach the ipsilateral bundle branch. In patients with normal QRS complexes and normal H-V intervals, a retrograde His deflection usually can be seen before inscription of the ventricular electrogram in the His bundle recording site during right ventricular apex stimulation (Fig. 2-24). In contrast, when ipsilateral bundle branch block is observed, particularly with prolonged H-V intervals, a retrograde His is less commonly seen, and when it is seen, it is usually inscribed after the QRS when pacing is carried out in the ipsilateral ventricle. This is most commonly observed in patients with RBB block during right ventricular pacing (Fig. 2-24), but can be seen during LV stimulation or spontaneous LV impulse formation in patients with LBBB.

The normal response to ventricular pacing is a gradual prolongation of V-A conduction as the ventricular-paced cycle length is decreased. Retrograde (V-A) Wenckebach-type block and higher degrees of V-A block appear at shorter cycle lengths (Fig. 2-25). Although Wenckebach-type block usually signifies retrograde delay in the A-V node, it is only when a retrograde His deflection is present that retrograde V-A Wenckebach and higher degrees of block can be documented to be localized to the A-V node (Fig. 2-25C). Occasionally, retrograde (V-A) Wenckebach cycles are terminated by an early beat with a normal QRS morphology and a relatively short A-H interval (Fig. 2-26). This extra beat is termed a ventricular echo and is not infrequent during retrograde Wenckebach cycles.[74–76] Such echoes may be seen in at least 25% to 30% of patients if care is taken to evaluate V-A conduction at small increments of paced rates. Ventricular echoes of this type are due to reentry secondary to a longitudinally dissociated A-V node and require a critical degree of V-A conduction delay for their appearance. Patients with a dual A-V nodal pathway manifesting this type of retrograde Wenckebach and reentry are generally not prone to develop clinical supraventricular tachycardia that is due to A-V nodal reentry (see Chapter 8).

Because a retrograde His bundle deflection may not always be observed in patients during ventricular pacing, in the presence of V-A block, localization of the site of block in such patients must be inferred from the effects of the ventricular-paced beat on conduction of spontaneous or

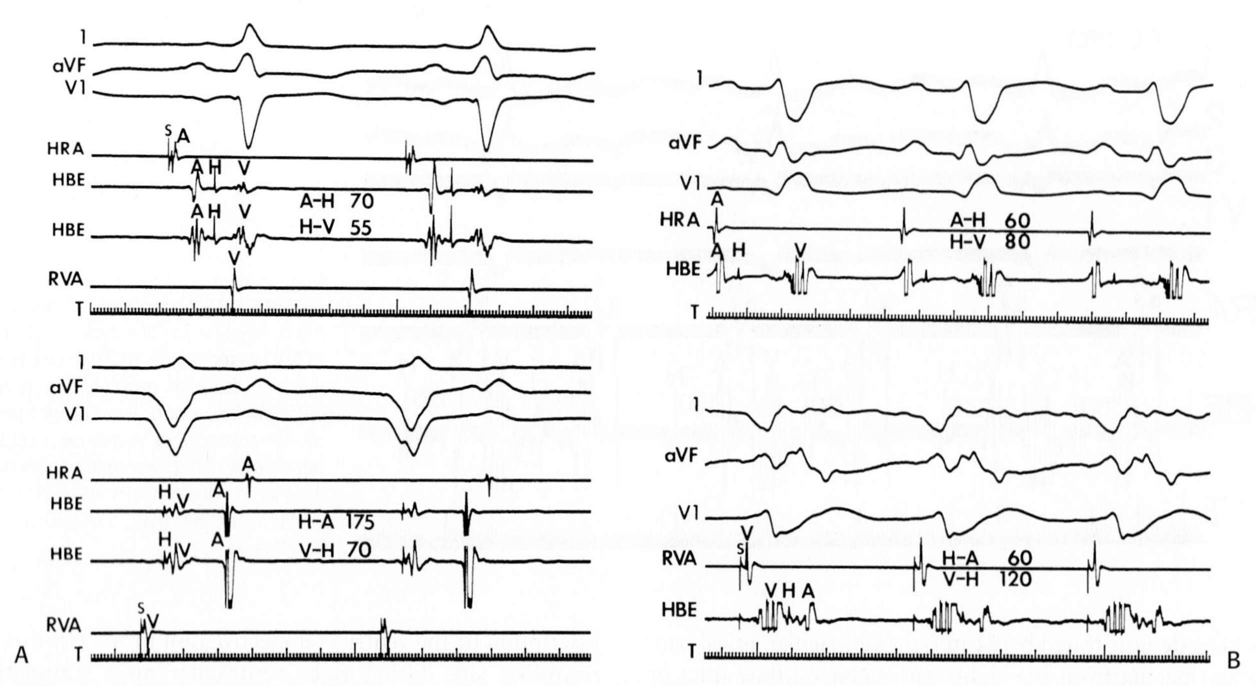


**FIGURE 2-24** *Relationship of antegrade H-V interval to V-H interval during ventricular pacing.* All four panels are organized as leads 1, aVF, V1, high-right atrium (HRA), two His bundle electrograms (HBE), and the right ventricular apical (RVA) electrogram. **A:** On the **top**, atrial pacing at a cycle length of 700 is associated with an H-V interval of 55 msec with a normal QRS. On the **bottom,** ventricular pacing at the same cycle length is associated with the V-H interval of 70 msec. The retrograde His can be seen to occur before the local V in the HBE. **B:** During sinus rhythm at a cycle length of 550 msec, the right bundle branch block is present with an H-V interval of 80 msec. On the **bottom**, right ventricular pacing is shown from the RVA along with a single HBE. The paced cycle length is just faster than the sinus cycle length. A retrograde H can be seen to follow the paced QRS complex, with a V-H interval of 120 msec. T, time line.

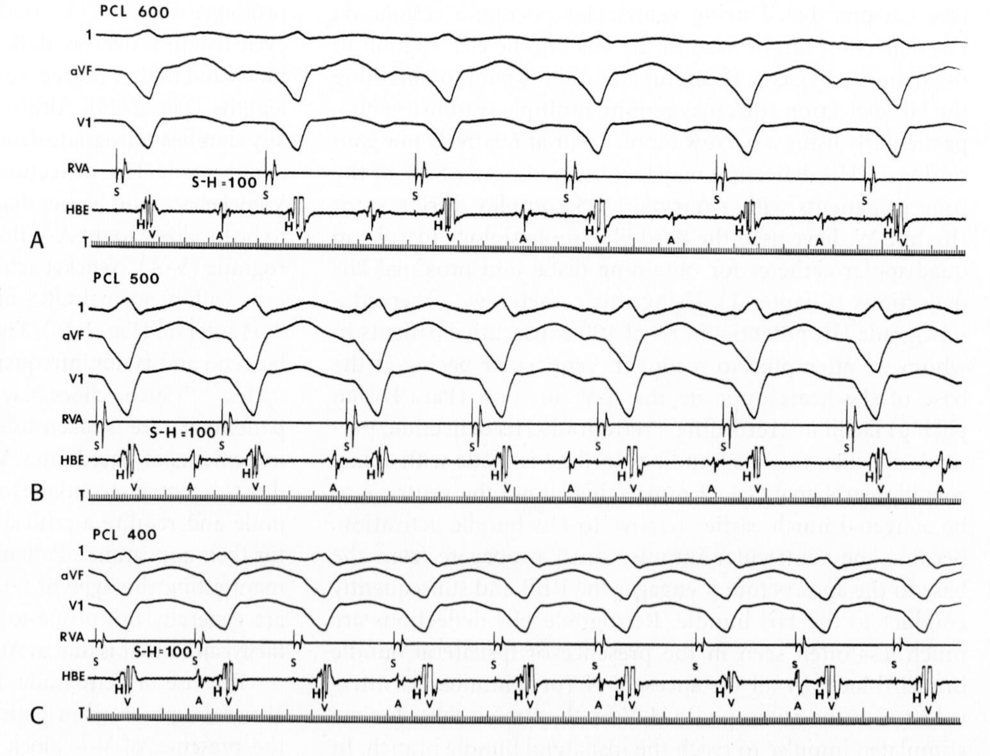


**FIGURE 2-25** *Ventricular pacing resulting in retrograde A-V nodal Wenckebach block.* **A:** During right ventricular pacing at a paced cycle length (PCL) of 600 msec, 1:1 V-A conduction is present. **B:** As the PCL is shortened to 500 msec, 3:2 retrograde Wenckebach block appears. **C:** As the PCLs decrease to 400 msec, 2:1 V-A block occurs. The presence of a retrograde His deflection allowed the site of block to be localized to the A-V node. Note that the S-H interval remains constant at the three PCLs.

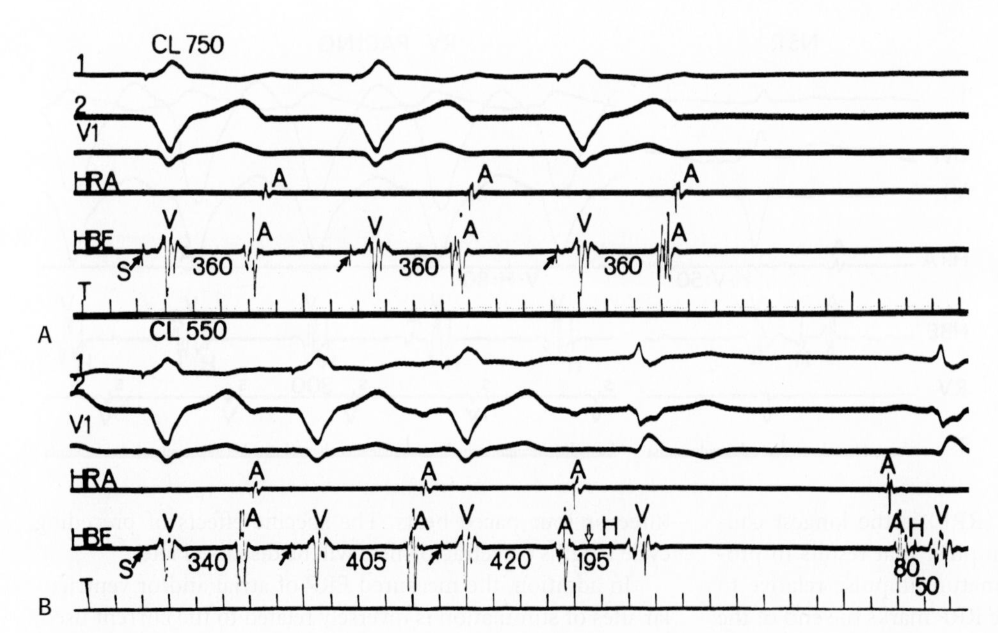


**FIGURE 2-26** *Retrograde Wenckebach cycle terminated by an echo beat.* **A:** Prolonged retrograde conduction (S-A, 360 msec) is noted in response to a ventricular-paced cycle length (CL) of 750 msec. **B:** As the CL is shortened to 550 msec, progressive delay in retrograde conduction results. After the third paced ventricular complex, pacing is terminated (*open arrow*) and a return beat appears that has the same configuration as the subsequent sinus beat. See text for further discussion.

stimulated atrial depolarizations. Thus, one localizes the site of delay by analyzing the level of concealed retrograde conduction. If the A-H interval of the spontaneous or induced atrial depolarization is independent of the time relationship of ventricular-paced beats, then by inference, the site of retrograde block is infranodal in the His–Purkinje system. On the other hand, variations in the A-H intervals that depend on the coupling interval of the atrial complex to the ventricular-paced beat, or failure of the atrial impulse to depolarize the His bundle, suggest retrograde penetration and block within the A-V node (Fig. 2-27). Another method of evaluating the site of retrograde block in the absence of a recorded retrograde His potential is to note the effects of drugs, such as atropine or isoproterenol, which affect only A-V nodal conduction, on V-A conduction. Improvement of conduction following administration of these drugs suggests that the site of block is in the A-V node. Using narrow bipolar electrograms to obtain retrograde His potentials, particularly with right ventricular para-Hisian pacing, and pharmacologic manipulations when these are not observed, it is possible to localize the site of block during ventricular pacing at cycle lengths of 300 msec or more to the A-V node in more than 95% of patients with normal QRS complexes in sinus rhythm.

In contrast to the development of the V-A Wenckebach, if one can record a retrograde His deflection, it is possible to demonstrate that V-H conduction remains relatively intact at rapid rates despite the development of retrograde block within the A-V node (Fig. 2-28).

## Refractory Periods

The refractoriness of a cardiac tissue can be defined by the response of that tissue to the introduction of premature stimuli. In clinical electrophysiology, refractoriness is generally expressed in terms of three measurements: relative, effective, and functional. The definitions differ slightly from comparable terms used in cellular electrophysiology.

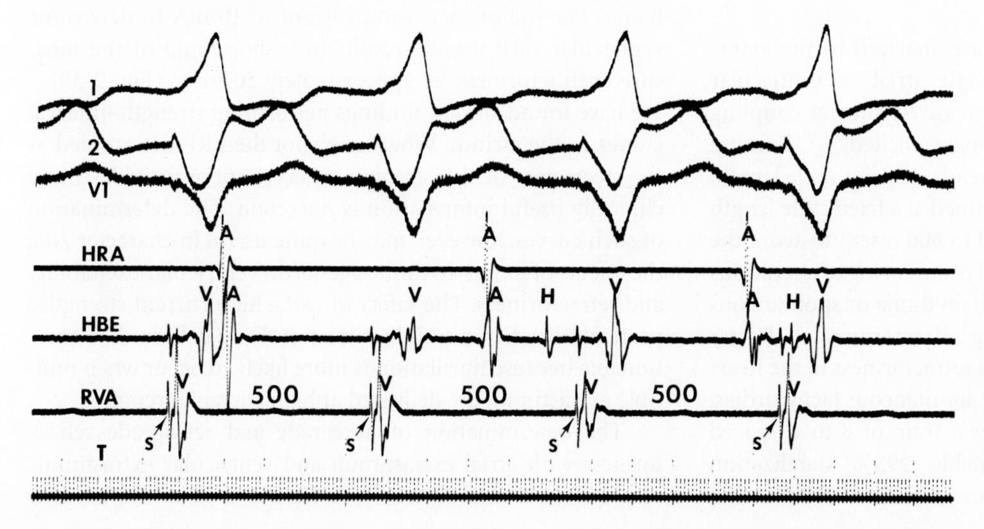


**FIGURE 2-27** *Diagnosis of site of retrograde block by inference.* During ventricular pacing (S, *arrow*) from the right ventricular apex (RVA), A-V dissociation is present. Despite the presence of a visible retrograde His deflection the site of block is shown to be the A-V node because antegrade A-V nodal conduction (A-H) depends on the relationship of the sinus beats A to the ventricular complexes. See text for further discussion.

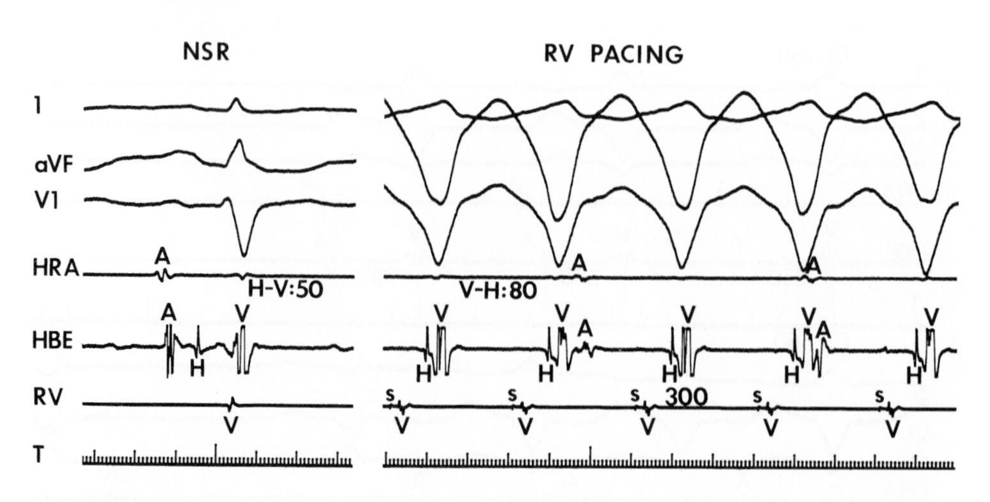


**FIGURE 2-28** *Stability of retrograde His conduction during rapid ventricular pacing.* Leads 1, aVF, V1 are shown with the high-right atrium (HRA), His bundle electrogram (HBE), and right ventricular (RV) electrograms. The H-V in sinus rhythm (NSR) is 50 msec, and the V-H during RV pacing at all cycle lengths was 80 msec. On the right, during RV pacing at a cycle length of 300 msec, the retrograde His conduction time is 80 msec and is constant during complete V-A dissociation.

1. The relative refractory period (RRP) is the longest coupling interval of a premature impulse that results in prolonged conduction of the premature impulse relative to that of the basic drive. Thus, the RRP marks the end of the full recovery period, the zone during which conduction of the premature and basic drive impulses is identical.
2. The effective refractory period (ERP) of a cardiac tissue is the longest coupling interval between the basic drive and the premature impulse that fails to propagate through that tissue. It therefore must be measured proximal to the refractory tissue.
3. The functional refractory period (FRP) of a cardiac tissue is the minimum interval between two consecutively conducted impulses through that tissue. Because the FRP is a measure of output from a tissue, it is described by measuring points distal to that tissue. It follows that determination of the ERP of a tissue requires that the FRP of more proximal tissues be less than the ERP of the distal tissue; for example, the ERP of the His–Purkinje system can be determined only if it exceeds the FRP of the A-V node.

The concepts of refractory period measurements can be applied to each component of the AVCS, and they can be schematically depicted by plotting the input against the output of any component of the AVCS. The definitions of antegrade and retrograde refractory periods of the components of the AVCS are given in Table 2-4.

In humans, refractory periods are analyzed by the extrastimulus technique, whereby a single atrial or ventricular extrastimulus is introduced at progressively shorter coupling intervals until a response is no longer elicited.[77–80] Because refractoriness of cardiac tissues depends on prior cycle length, refractory periods should be determined at a fixed cycle length within the physiologic range (1,000 to 600 msec) to avoid the changes in refractoriness that would occur owing to alterations in cycle length secondary to sinus arrhythmia or spontaneous premature complexes. Determining refractoriness at shorter cycle lengths may be useful to assess refractoriness in the heart at rates comparable to those during spontaneous tachycardias. The extrastimulus is delivered after a train of 8 to 10 paced complexes to allow time for reasonable (≥95%) stabilization of refractoriness, which is usually accomplished after the first three or four paced beats. The specific effects of preceding cycle lengths on refractoriness will be discussed later.

In addition, the measured ERP of atrial and/or ventricular sites of stimulation is inversely related to the current used; that is, the measured ERP will decrease when higher stimulus strengths are used. In most electrophysiologic laboratories, stimulus strength has been arbitrarily standardized as being delivered at twice-diastolic threshold. Some standardization of stimulus strength is necessary if one wishes to compare atrial and/or ventricular refractoriness before and after an intervention. Although use of current at twice-diastolic threshold gives reproducible and clinically relevant information, and has a low incidence of nonclinical arrhythmia induction, the use of higher currents has been suggested.[81] Certainly, a more detailed method of assessing refractoriness, or more appropriately, ventricular or atrial excitability, would be to define the strength–interval curves at these sites. This would entail determining the ERP at increasing current strengths from threshold to approximately 10 mA. An example of a strength–interval curve to determine ventricular refractoriness is shown in Figure 2-29. Note there is a gradual shortening of measured ventricular refractoriness as the current is increased until the point is reached where the refractory period stays relatively constant despite increasing current strengths. The steep portion of the strength–interval curve defines the ERP of that tissue. The use of increasing current to 10 mA to determine ventricular ERP usually results in a shortening of the measured refractoriness by approximately 30 msec (Fig. 2-30).[81] We have found similar findings performing strength–interval curves in the atrium. Whether or not the ERP determined as the steep part of the strength–interval curve provides more clinically useful information is uncertain. The determination of such curves, however, may be quite useful in characterizing the effects of antiarrhythmic agents on ventricular excitability and refractoriness. The safety of using high current strengths, particularly when multiple extrastimuli are delivered, is questionable because fibrillation is more likely to occur when multiple extrastimuli are delivered at high current strengths.

The determination of antegrade and retrograde refractoriness with atrial extrastimuli and ventricular extrastimuli, respectively, is demonstrated in Figures 2-31 and 2-32. It is

TABLE 2-4 Definition of Terms

S1, A1, H1, V1: stimulus artifact, atrial, His bundle, and ventricular electrograms of basic drive
S2, A2, H2, V2: stimulus artifact, atrial, His bundle, and ventricular electrograms of premature beat

**Antegrade Refractory Periods**

Effective refractory period (ERP) of the atrium: the longest S1-S2 interval that fails to result in atrial depolarization
ERP of the A-V node: the longest A1-A2 interval measured in the His bundle electrogram that fails to propagate to the His bundle
ERP of the His–Purkinje system (HPS): the longest H1-H2 interval that fails to result in ventricular depolarization
ERP of the atrioventricular conduction system (AVCS): the longest S1-S2 interval that fails to result in ventricular depolarization
Functional refractory period (FRP) of the atrium: the shortest A1-A2 interval in response to any S1-S2 interval
FRP of the A-V node: the shortest H1-H2 interval in response to any A1-A2 interval
FRP of the HPS: the shortest V1-V2 interval in response to any H1-H2 interval
FRP of the AVCS: the shortest V1-V2 interval in response to any S1-S2 interval
Relative refractory period (RRP) of the atrium: the longest S1-S2 interval at which the S2-A2 interval exceeds the S1-A1 interval (latency)
RRP of the A-V node: the longest A1-A2 interval at which the A2-H2 interval exceeds the A1-H1 interval
RRP of the HPS: the longest H1-H2 interval at which the H2-V2 interval exceeds the H1-V1 interval or results in an aberrant QRS complex

**Retrograde Refractory Periods**

ERP of the ventricle: the longest S1-S2 interval that fails to evoke a ventricular response
ERP of the HPS: the longest S1-S2 or V1-V2 interval at which S2 or V2 blocks below the bundle of His. This measurement can be made only if H2 is recorded before the occurrence of retrograde block
ERP of the A-V node: the longest S1-H2 or H1-H2 interval at which H2 fails to propagate to the atrium
ERP of the ventriculoatrial conduction system (VACS): the longest S1-S2 interval that fails to propagate to the atrium
FRP of the ventricle: the shortest V1-V2 interval as measured on the surface
ECG or local ventricular electrogram in response to any S1-S2 interval
FRP of the HPS: the shortest S1-H2 or H1-H2 interval in response to any V1-V2 interval
FRP of the AVN: the shortest A1-A2 interval in response to any H1-H2 interval
FRP of VACS: the shortest A1-A2 interval in response to any S1-S2 interval
RRP of the ventricle: the longest S1-S2 interval at which the S2-V2 interval exceeds the S1-V1 interval. The V is measured from the surface ECG or a local electrogram at the site of ventricular stimulation
RRP of VACS: the longest S1-S2 interval at which the S2-A2 interval exceeds the S1-A1 interval

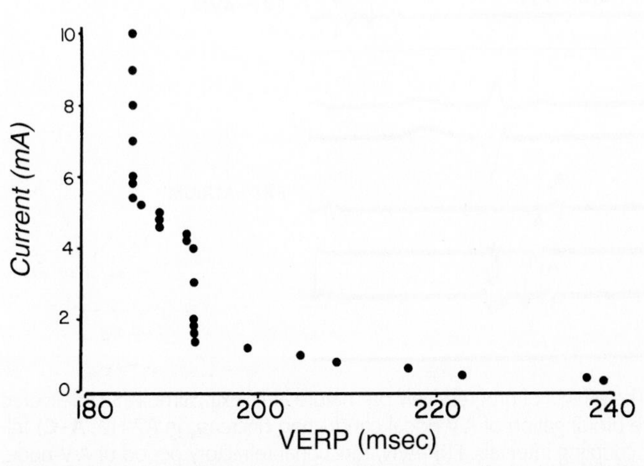


**FIGURE 2-29** *Typical curve relating current strength and ventricular refractoriness.* The ventricular effective refractory period (VERP) at a given current strength (abscissa) is plotted against the current strength of the stimuli (ordinate). At diastolic threshold, 0.35 mA, the ventricular effective refraction period is 238 msec. With increases in stimulus current, there is a decrease in the measured VERP until it becomes fixed at 185 msec, despite further increases in current from 5 to 10 mA. (From Greenspan AM, Camardo JS, Horowitz LN, et al. Human ventricular refractoriness: effects of increasing current. *Am J Cardiol* 1981;47:244.)

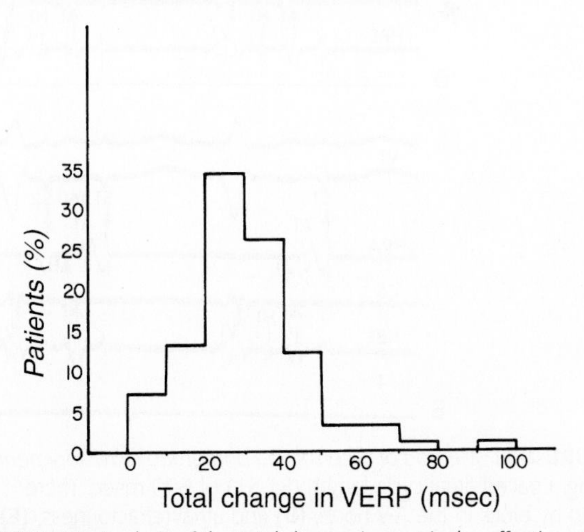


**FIGURE 2-30** *Analysis of the total change in ventricular effective refractory period (VERP) with increasing current.* The total change in VERP with increasing current from threshold to 10 mA (abscissa) is plotted against the percentage of patients demonstrating such a total change. In three patients (7%) with a high diastolic threshold, the total change in VERP was less than 10 msec; in 72% of the patients the total change with increasing current was between 20 and 40 msec. (From Greenspan AM, Camardo JS, Horowitz LN, et al. Human ventricular refractoriness: effects of increasing current. *Am J Cardiol* 1981;47:244.)

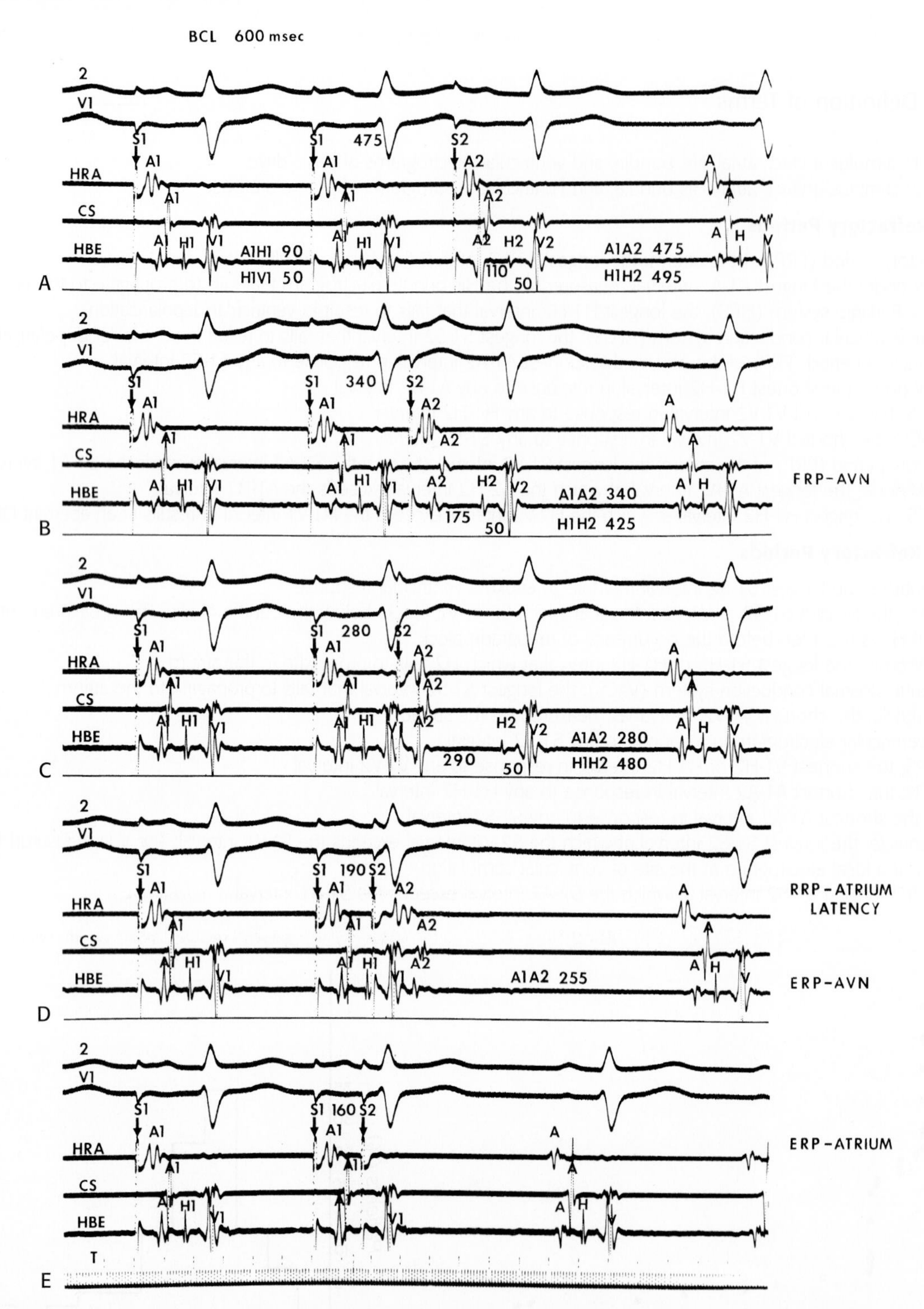


**FIGURE 2-31** *Method of determining antegrade refractory periods.* **A–E:** The effects of progressively premature atrial extrastimuli (S2) delivered during a paced atrial cycle length (S1-S1) of 600 msec. There is progressive prolongation of A-V nodal conduction (increase in A2-H2; **A–C**) followed by block in the A-V node, **(D)** and atrial refractoriness, **(E)** at shorter coupling intervals. FRP-AVN, functional refractory period of A-V node; RRP, relative refractory period; ERP, effective refractory period; S, stimulus artifact. See Table 2-4 for definitions and text for further discussion.

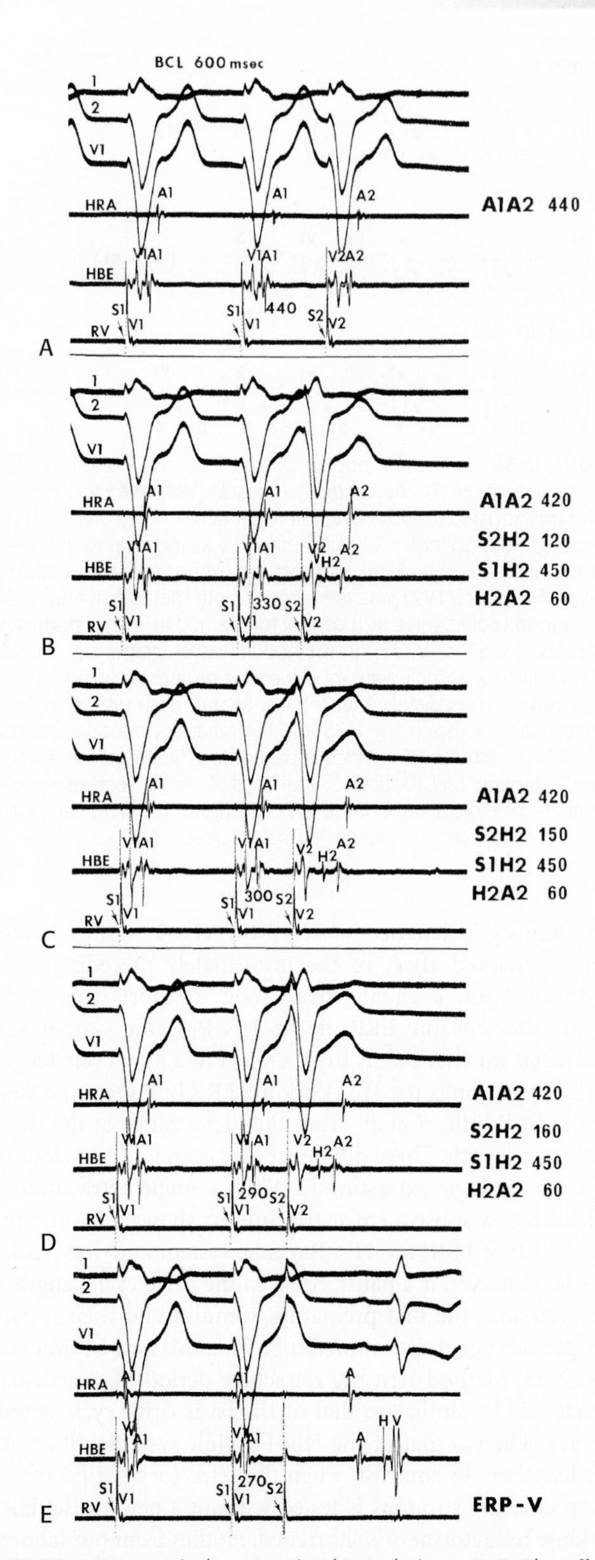


**FIGURE 2-32** *Ventricular extrastimulus technique.* **A–E:** The effects of progressively premature right ventricular (RV) extrastimuli (S2) at a basic cycle length (BCL; S1-S1) of 600 msec are shown. At long coupling intervals, **(A)** there is no retrograde delay. **B–D:** Conduction delay appears in the His–Purkinje system (S2-H2 prolongation). At a very short coupling interval (S1-S2 = 270 msec), the effective refractory period of the ventricle (ERP-V) is reached. See Table 2-4 for definitions and text for discussion.

extremely important that measurements in refractory periods be taken at specific sites; measurements of atrial and ventricular refractory periods are taken at the site of stimulation, and measurements of A-V nodal refractory periods and His–Purkinje refractory periods are taken from the His bundle electrogram.

## *Cycle Length Responsiveness of Refractory Periods*

Determinations of refractoriness should be performed at multiple drive cycle lengths to assess the effect of cycle length on the refractory periods. There are expected physiologic responses to alterations in drive cycle lengths. Normally, atrial, His–Purkinje, and ventricular refractory periods are directly related to the basic drive cycle length; that is, the ERP tends to decrease with decreasing drive cycle lengths.[82,83] This phenomenon is most marked in the His–Purkinje system (Fig. 2-33). Of note the refractory period of the RBB, which is longer than the LBB during sinus rhythm, tends to shorten more than the LBB explaining the increased prevalence of RBBB aberration at long cycle lengths and LBBB aberration at short cycle lengths. The A-V node, in contrast, behaves in an opposite fashion; the ERP increases with decreasing cycle lengths.[21,82,83] The explanation for the behavior of A-V nodal tissue has been

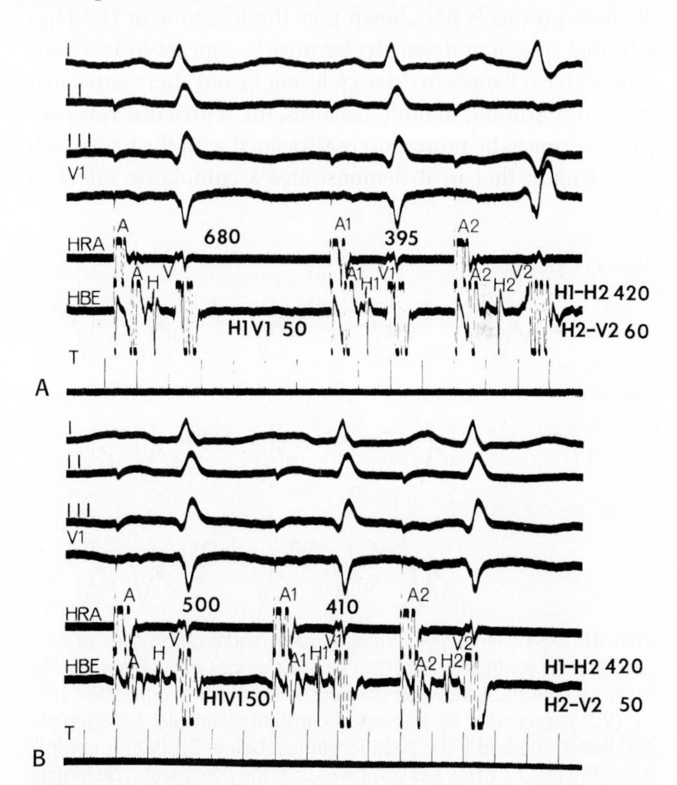


**FIGURE 2-33** *Effect of cycle length on His–Purkinje refractoriness.* **A:** The basic paced cycle length is 680 msec, and the H-V is 50 msec. An atrial premature stimulus (A2), delivered at a coupling interval (Al-A2) of 395 msec, conducts with an Hl-H2 interval of 420 msec, resulting in the development of right bundle branch block and H2-V2 prolongation to 60 msec. **B:** At a shorter cycle length of 500 msec, a premature atrial impulse with an identical H1-H2 of 420 msec is conducted without aberration or H2-V2 prolongation. Thus, the relative refractory period of the His–Purkinje system is shortened as the paced cycle length decreases.

suggested by Simson et al.[84] to be due to a fatigue phenomenon that most likely results because A-V nodal refractoriness (unlike His–Purkinje refractoriness) is time dependent and exceeds its action potential duration (APD). On the other hand, the response of the FRP of the A-V node to changes in cycle length is variable but tends to decrease with decreasing cycle lengths. This paradox occurs because the FRP is not a true measure of refractoriness encountered by the premature atrial impulse (A2). It is significantly determined by the A-V nodal conduction time of the basic drive beat (Al-Hl); the longer the Al-Hl, the shorter the calculated FRP at any A2-H2 interval (FRP = Hl-H2 = [Al-A2 + A2-H2] − [Al-H1]).

Although the basic drive cycle length affects the refractory periods in this predicted way, abrupt changes in the cycle length may alter refractoriness differently. The effect of abrupt changes in drive cycle length and/or the effect of premature impulses on subsequent refractoriness of His–Purkinje and ventricular tissue has recently been studied.[65–90] Specific ventricular pacing protocols have been used to assess the role of abrupt changes in drive cycle length (Fig. 2-34) and of postextrasystolic pauses during a constant drive cycle length (Fig. 2-35) on subsequent retrograde His–Purkinje refractoriness and ventricular myocardial refractoriness.[66,86] Use of these protocols has shown that the behavior of the His–Purkinje system and ventricular muscle appears to be divergent both to changes in drive cycle length and after ventricular premature stimuli. In both instances, the ventricular refractoriness seems to be more closely associated with the basic drive cycle length; that is, it demonstrates a cumulative effect of

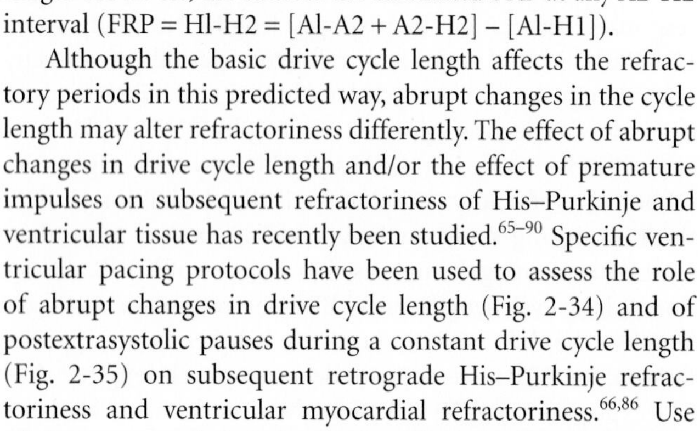

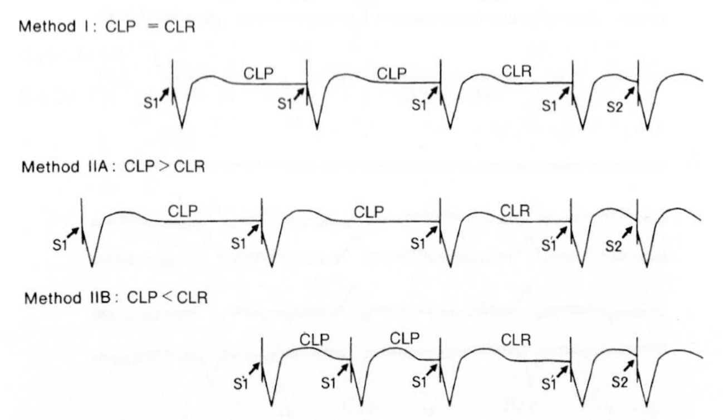


**FIGURE 2-34** *Stimulation protocols to evaluate differences of His–Purkinje and ventricular refractoriness to changes in cycle length.* The essential difference between methods I and II is that in method I the S2 (V2) is preceded by a series of constant ventricular cycle lengths and that in method II the cycle length just before S2 (V2) is abruptly altered (S1S1′ or V1V1′) as compared with the preceding cycle lengths (S1 S1 or V1 V1). In all methods the reference cycle lengths (CLR) are the ventricular cycle length to which S2 (V2) is coupled, whereas the cycle lengths preceding the CLR are designated as CLP. Note that CLR is identical for all methods, whereas CLP is equal to CLR during method I, where cycle length is constant; CLP is greater than CLR during method IIA, where cycle length is abruptly decreased; CLP is less than CLR during method IIB, where cycle length is abruptly increased. (From Denker S, Lehmann MH, Mahmud R, et al. Divergence between refractoriness of His–Purkinje system and ventricular muscle with abrupt changes in cycle length. *Circulation* 1963;68:1212.)

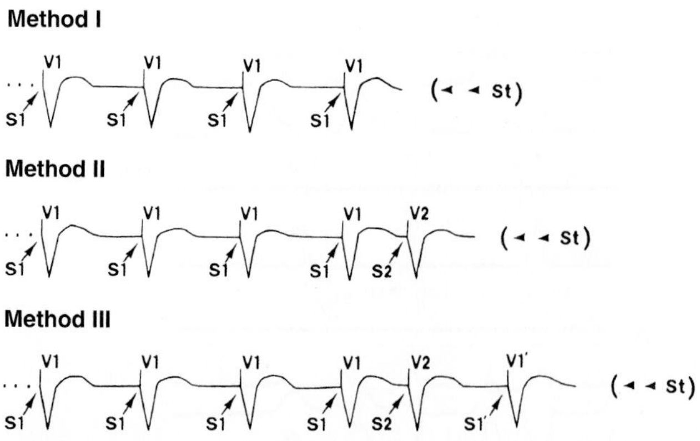

Method I

Method II

Method III

**FIGURE 2-35** *Ventricular pacing protocol used to analyze His–Purkinje system (HPS) and ventricular muscle (VM) refractory periods during an extrasystole–postextrasystole sequence.* The constant basic cycle length (S1 S1 or V1 V1) of method I was identical to that used with methods II and III. Note also that the extrasystolic beat coupling interval (S1 S2 or V1V2) was the same in both methods II and III. So that method I could serve as a control for method III, the postextrasystolic pause (S2S1′ or V2V1′) in method III was programmed to equal S1S1. Ventricular stimuli were introduced at progressively closer coupling intervals immediately after the last beat of each pacing method to determine corresponding HPS and VM refractory periods. See text for details. S, stimulus; V, ventricular-paced beat; St, premature stimuli. (From Lehmann MH, Denker S, Mahmud R, et al. Postextrasystolic alterations in refractoriness of the His–Purkinje system and ventricular myocardium in man. *Circulation* 1984;69:1096.)

preceding cycle lengths, whereas the His–Purkinje system shows a marked effect of the immediately preceding cycle length(s). Thus, a change from long to short drive cycle lengths shortens the ERP of the His–Purkinje system and ventricular muscle; a shift from a short to a long cycle length markedly prolongs the His–Purkinje ERP but alters the ventricular ERP little, if at all, from that determined at the short drive cycle length. These differences are even more obvious in response to single extrastimuli. When a single extrastimulus is delivered, a subsequent extrastimulus shows a shortening of the ERP of both the His–Purkinje system and ventricular muscle. However, if a pause equal to the drive cycle length is delivered after the first premature stimulus and then refractory periods again determined following this new S1' interval (Fig. 2-35, Method III), the refractory period of ventricular muscle will be similar to that of the basic drive cycle length (S1-S1), whereas that of the His–Purkinje system will markedly lengthen. In contrast, when the refractory period of the first premature stimulus is tested without a new pause, His–Purkinje refractoriness is shortened. Studies from our laboratory have shown that the ability of a premature stimulus to shorten the ventricular ERP is related to the coupling interval of the extrastimulus.[87–89] Shortening of the ERP primarily occurs at short coupling intervals beginning from 50 to 100 msec above the ERP determined during the basic drive cycle length. This effect on refractoriness was linearly related to the drive cycle length such that premature stimuli at comparable coupling intervals delivered at 400 msec would produce a shorter ERP than those associated with 600 msec.

This marked effect of the preceding cycle length, either in exaggerated abbreviation or prolongation of refractoriness, may explain what were previously felt to be paradoxical responses in conduction during long, short-long, or long-short sequences during antegrade or retrograde conduction. These findings may also explain some of the variability of initiation of tachycardias depending on preceding cycle lengths. The mechanism of these abnormalities has not been well worked out but appears related to the diastolic interval between action potentials of premature and drive beats (Fig. 2-36). As can be seen in Figure 2-36, although the drive cycle length affects the action potential during that drive, the diastolic interval (the interval from the end of the action potential to the beginning of the next action potential) can be markedly affected by short-long, or long-short intervals, which can affect the refractory period of the subsequent complex. The role of the diastolic interval on ventricular refractoriness has been studied by Vassallo et al.[87–89] in our laboratory. In this study, we evaluated the effect of one and two extrastimuli on subsequent ventricular refractoriness using a protocol that kept the coupling interval of the first and second stimulus equal (S1-S2 = S2-S3). Because a single premature stimulus (S2) can shorten ventricular refractoriness, as measured by S3, keeping S1-S2 and S2-S3 equal would directly assess the effect of the diastolic interval on refractoriness. Using this method, we clearly showed that the refractory period following one extrastimulus (S2) was shorter than a refractory period following two extrastimuli (S2, S3) delivered at the same coupling intervals. This was probably related to an increase in the diastolic interval preceding S3 (Fig. 2-37). This finding implies that the diastolic interval is probably the key determinant in alterations in refractoriness in response to sudden changes in cycle length and suggests that the His–Purkinje system and ventricular muscle differ more quantitatively than qualitatively.

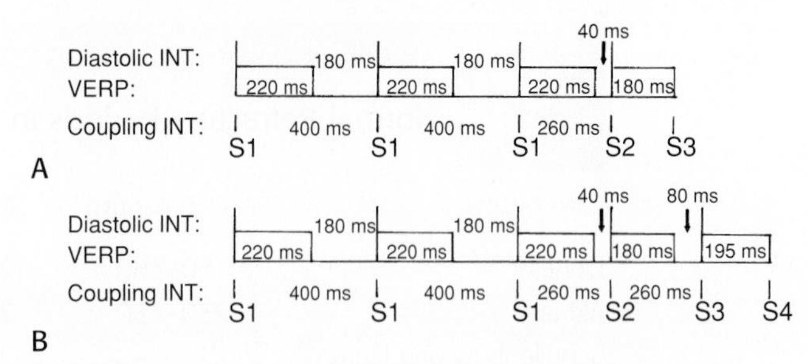


**FIGURE 2-37** *Diagrammatic representation of the influence of preceding diastolic interval and preceding refractory period on shortening of subsequent refractory period in one patient.* During a paced cycle length of 400 msec, refractoriness was determined to be 220 msec. **A:** Double extrastimuli (S2 and S3) are delivered with an S1-S2 coupling interval equal to 260 msec (diastolic interval of 40 msec). This results in shortening the refractory period of S2 to 180 msec compared to the drive cycle length. **B:** Double ventricular extrastimuli at the same coupling intervals (260 msec) are delivered and a third extrastimulus (S4) is introduced to determine ventricular effective refractory period (VERP) of S3. Refractoriness of S3 now depends on previous diastolic interval (80 msec), as well as a refractory period of S2 (which is shorter than the refractory period of S1). This results in a refractory period of S3 at an S1-S2 = S2-S3 of 260 msec that is 195 msec. This compares to a refractory period of 220 msec during the drive and a ventricular refractory period of S2 of 180 msec. (From Vassallo JA, Marchlinski FE, Cassidy DM, et al. Shortening of ventricular refractorines with extrastimuli: Role of the degree of prematurity and number of extrastimuli. *J Electrophysiol* 1988;2:227.)

Because the diastolic interval influences the response of both His–Purkinje system and ventricular refractoriness to single extrastimuli, what is the cause of the "quantitative" differences? The difference in APD between ventricular muscle and His–Purkinje system and the more pronounced effect of drive cycle length on the duration of the action potential of the His–Purkinje system probably cause the apparent differences in the

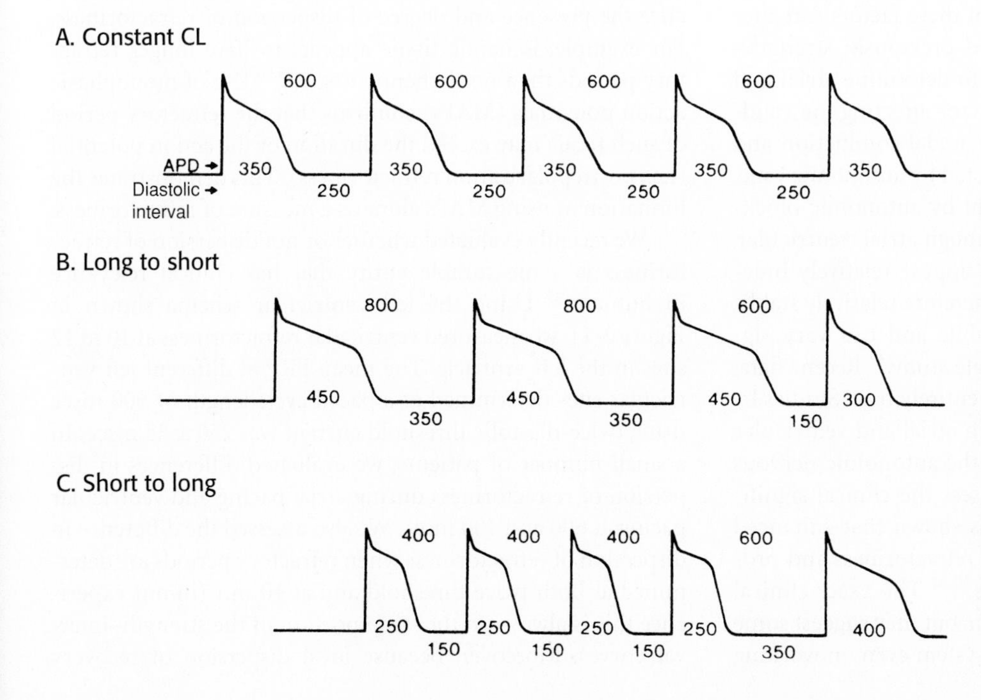


**FIGURE 2-36** *The schema depicts the action potential duration (APD) and the diastolic intervals during a pacing protocol.* **A–C:** The stimulus-to-stimulus intervals (in milliseconds) are shown along the top of action potentials. The values of APD and diastolic intervals are only a rough approximation and were derived from the actual values of relative refractory period-His–Purkinje system (RRP-HPS) obtained during studies. (From Akhtar M, Denker ST, Lehmann MH, et al. Effects of sudden cycle length alteration on refractoriness of human His–Purkinje system and ventricular myocardium. In: Zipes DP, Jalife J, eds. *Cardiac electrophysiology and arrhythmias*. Orlando, FL: Grune & Stratton, 1985:399.)

TABLE 2-5 Normal Refractory Periods in Adults

| Laboratory | ERP Atrium | ERP AVN | FRP AVN | ERP HPS | ERP V |
|---|---|---|---|---|---|
| Denes[83] | 150–360 | 250–365 | 350–495 | – | – |
| Akhtar[71] | 230–330 | 280–430 | 320–680 | 340–430 | 190–290 |
| Schuilenburg and Durrer[23] | – | 230–390 | 330–500 | – | – |
| Author | 170–300 | 230–425 | 330–525 | 330–450 | 170–290 |

[a]Only includes patients with normal A-H and H-V. Studies performed at twice threshold.
AVN, A-V node; ERP, effective refractory period; FRP, functional refractory period; HPS, His–Purkinje system.

effect of premature stimuli on the diastolic interval and subsequent refractoriness between these two tissues. Demonstration of the effects of the diastolic interval on refractoriness of ventricular muscle requires short coupling intervals. In 1987 Marchlinski[88] demonstrated that very short drive cycle lengths and coupling intervals produce oscillations of ventricular refractoriness analogous to that shown for the His–Purkinje system. Thus, the diastolic interval appears to be the major determinant of the refractory period following extrastimuli in both structures. Differences in the basic action potentials of ventricular muscle and His–Purkinje fibers are responsible for the apparent differences in their response to changes in cycle length and premature stimulation.

A wide range of normal values has been reported for refractory periods (Table 2-5).[23,71,83] The major difficulty with interpreting these "normal" values is that they represent pooled data of refractory periods at different cycle lengths. The data would be more meaningful if they were all obtained at comparable cycle lengths using the same stimulus strength and pulse width. In these different laboratories, stimulus strengths vary from twice threshold to 5 mA, and pulse widths vary from 1 to 2 msec; both of these factors can alter the so-called normal value. As noted previously, strength–interval curves may be the best way to determine atrial and ventricular refractoriness. Another factor affecting the validity of such "normal" data is that A-V nodal conduction and refractoriness are both markedly affected by autonomic tone, an impossible factor to control except by autonomic blockade, which is not done routinely. Although atrial, ventricular, and His–Purkinje refractory periods appear relatively independent of autonomic tone and are therefore relatively stable, A-V nodal refractory periods are labile and can vary significantly during the course of a single study.[20] Recent data, however, suggest that even this is not entirely true. Studies by Prystowsky et al.[91,92] suggest that both atrial and ventricular refractory periods are influenced by the autonomic nervous system. Although it is difficult to assess the clinical significance of his findings, Prystowsky has shown that enhanced parasympathetic tone shortens atrial refractoriness and prolongs right ventricular refractoriness.[91,92] The exact clinical relevance of these findings is uncertain, but they suggest some influence of the autonomic nervous system even on working muscle. Thus, the values listed in Table 2-5 should serve only as approximate guidelines. The effect of drive cycle length on ventricular refractoriness in any given patient may represent a means of discriminating between abnormal and normal refractoriness when the absolute value of a single refractory period determination is borderline. For example, if the ERP of the His–Purkinje system is 450 msec at a basic cycle length of 1,000 msec, failure of the ERP to decrease when the basic drive cycle length is shortened confirms an abnormal response, whereas a marked decrease suggests that the initial value was at the upper limits of normal because of the slow intrinsic rate.

### *Dispersion of Refractoriness*

Dispersion of ventricular refractory periods has been suggested as an indicator of an arrhythmogenic substrate based on animal experiments.[93–96] As noted, differences in refractory periods depend on how they were determined, related to both stimulus strength and drive cycle length.[97,98] The types of tissue in which the refractory period is measured also influence the presence and degree of dispersion of refractoriness. For example, ischemic tissue appears to have longer refractory periods than nonischemic tissue.[95,96] Use of monophasic action potentials (MAPs) confirms that the refractory period of such tissue may exceed the duration of the action potential (i.e., postrepolarization refractoriness). This demonstrates the limitation of using MAPs alone as a measure of refractoriness.

We recently evaluated whether or not dispersion of refractoriness is a measurable entity that has clinical relevance in humans.[43] Using the left ventricular schema shown in Figure 2-11, we measured ventricular refractoriness at 10 to 12 sites in the left ventricle. The mean ERP at different left ventricular sites determined at a paced cycle length of 600 msec using twice-diastolic threshold current was 250 ± 38 msec. In a small number of patients, we evaluated differences in dispersion of refractoriness during atrial pacing and ventricular pacing at 600 and 400 msec. We also assessed the difference in dispersion of refractoriness when refractory periods are determined at both twice threshold and at 10 mA (in our experience this is always on the steep portion of the strength–interval curve). Moreover, because local dispersion of recovery may be more important than dispersion of refractory period measurements per se, intraventricular activation must also be considered. Thus, we evaluated both dispersion of refractoriness and dispersion of recovery (local activation plus local refractoriness) at each site. In seven patients without heart disease, the normal dispersion of the left ventricular ERP was 40 ± 14 msec, and dispersion of the total recovery time was 52 ± 14 msec using a twice-diastolic threshold current strength and 600-msec drive cycle lengths from the left ventricle. In five patients, we studied the effect of drive cycle length on dispersion of refractoriness. At a paced cycle length of 600 msec, the dispersion of refractoriness was 66 ± 41 msec, and it was similar at a paced cycle length of 400 msec at 65 ± 45 msec. Total dispersion of recovery was 89 ± 40 msec at a paced cycle length of 600 and 88 ± 38 msec at a paced cycle length of 400 msec. Of note, the maximum dispersion at any two adjacent sites of refractoriness was 33 ± 12 msec, and for total recovery it was 41 ± 15 msec.

Thus, in our studies,[43] cycle lengths from 600 to 400 msec did not alter dispersion of refractoriness, as seen in experimental studies.[93–97] We also compared dispersion of refractoriness at both twice-diastolic threshold and at 10 mA in selected normal patients. In these patients we found no significant difference in dispersion of refractoriness. The dispersion of refractoriness was 62 msec at twice threshold and 50 msec at 10 mA, and the total recovery was 79 msec at twice threshold and 68 msec at 10 mA. Neither of these reached statistical significance. A limitation of these preliminary data is that in these patients, dispersion measurement methods were mixed, some having twice threshold and 10 mA performed at sinus rhythm and some during a different ventricular-paced cycle length.

Luck et al.[98] evaluated bradycardia on dispersion of ventricular refractoriness using only three right ventricular sites in 16 patients with severe bradycardia. They found that patients with bradycardia had significantly longer right ventricular ERPs than normals, but they found a comparable dispersion of refractoriness among these three right ventricular sites (43 ± 38 msec vs. 37 ± 12 msec). Pacing at rates of 120 bpm tended to shorten the refractoriness of both groups as well as the dispersion of refractoriness in both groups, but the ERP at this paced cycle length of the group with spontaneous bradycardia remained longer than the ERP in those patients with normal sinus rhythm. The difference between this study and our data[43] probably relates to the fact that we could not compare very slow rates with faster rates and only studied rates of 100 and 150 bpm in detail. Moreover, the effect of chronic bradycardia and subsequent ventricular enlargement may play an important role in refractory period measurements. The fact that only right ventricular sites were evaluated by Luck et al.[98] limits their conclusions.

Other workers have looked at the effect of site of pacing on refractoriness, considering, for example, whether atrial pacing differed from ventricular pacing. Friehling et al.[99] showed longer ERPs and greater dispersion of ERP from three right ventricular sites determined during atrial pacing when compared to refractoriness determined by pacing and stimulating the right ventricular site. In contrast, when we compared dispersion of refractoriness and recovery from multiple left ventricular sites measured during atrial pacing and ventricular pacing at the stimulation site in five patients, we found no significant difference in dispersion of refractory periods of total recovery times. The difference between these results is unclear, although the small number of pacing sites in the study by Friehling et al.,[99] the difference between right and left ventricular stimulation, and the small number of patients in both studies limit the interpretation of the data. Our data on normal left ventricular dispersion of refractoriness and total recovery time serve as a reference for evaluating the role of dispersion refractoriness and/or recovery in arrhythmogenesis. The use of MAPs may provide useful information about dispersion of refractoriness that is independent of stimulation.[100] This technique uses a contact electrode to basically record an injury potential. The signals recorded are quite comparable to intracellular microelectrode recording, and if properly done are stable for a few hours. The APD corresponds to the ERP in normal tissue, but in diseased tissue the ERP exceeds the ERP. Thus, the value of this technique in abnormal tissue or in the presence of Na channel blockers is uncertain. The demonstration that drugs produce an ERP that exceeds the APD may be useful, but this would be demonstrated by ERP prolongation by stimulation techniques alone. The limited ability to readily map all areas of the left ventricle with current MAP catheters may further limit the utility of this technique.

### *Patterns of Response to Atrial Extrastimuli*

Several patterns of response to programmed atrial extrastimuli are characterized by differing sites of conduction delay and block and the coupling intervals at which they occur.[68,69] The most common pattern (Type I) is seen when the atrial impulse encounters progressively greater delay in the A-V node without any change in infranodal conduction (Fig. 2-31). Block eventually occurs in the A-V node or the atrium itself. With the Type II response, delay is noted initially in the A-V node, but at shorter coupling intervals, progressive delay in the His–Purkinje system appears. Block usually occurs first in the A-V node, but it may occur in the atrium and occasionally in the His–Purkinje system (modified Type II). With the Type III response (which is least common), initial slowing occurs in the A-V node, but at critical coupling intervals, sudden and marked prolongation of conduction occurs in the His–Purkinje system. The His–Purkinje system is invariably the first site of block with this pattern. Although it has been stated that any prolongation of His–Purkinje conduction is an abnormal response, it is not. The only requirement for such prolongation to occur is that the FRP of the A-V node be less than the RRP of the His–Purkinje system. Previous studies demonstrated that 15% to 60% of normal patients can show some prolongation of the H-V interval in response to atrial extrastimuli.[79,80] Infranodal delay or block is more likely to occur at longer basic drive cycle lengths because His–Purkinje refractoriness frequently exceeds the FRP of the A-V node at slower rates. Thus, block below the His bundle in response to an atrial extrastimulus delivered during sinus rhythm may be a normal response.

The pattern of conduction (Type I, II, or III) is not fixed in any patient. Pharmacologic interventions (e.g., atropine, isoproterenol, or antiarrhythmic agents) or changes in cycle length can alter the refractory period relationships between different tissues so that one type of response may be switched to another. Atropine, for example, shortens the FRP of the A-V node and allows the impulse to reach the His–Purkinje system during its relative and effective refractory periods. As a result, a Type I pattern could be changed to a Type II or III pattern.[101]

These patterns of A-V conduction can best be expressed by plotting refractory curves relating the coupling intervals of the premature atrial impulse (A1-A2) to the responses in the A-V node and the His–Purkinje system. The curves may be drawn in two ways: (a) by plotting A1-A2 versus H1-H2 and V1-V, which gives the functional input–output relationship between the basic drive beat and the premature beat, and (b) by plotting the actual conduction times of the premature beat through the A-V node (A2-H2) and His–Purkinje system (H1-V2) versus the A1-A2 intervals. Both methods are useful: The former provides an assessment of the FRP of the AVCS, whereas the latter allows one to actually determine the conduction times through the various components of the AVCS. We use both types of curves, but we feel that the latter curve (A1-A2 vs. A2-H2 and H2-V2) allows a purer evaluation of the response to A2 because, unlike the former curve, the results are not affected by conduction of the basic drive beat. This becomes particularly important when the effects of drugs or cycle length on the conduction of premature atrial impulses are being evaluated.

### *Type I Response*

Type I response (Fig. 2-38) is characterized by an initial decrease in the H1-H2 and V1-V2 intervals as the coupling interval of the premature atrial impulse (A1-A2) decreases. During this limited decrease, A-V nodal conduction (A2-H2) and His–Purkinje conduction (H2-V2) are unchanged from the basic drive so that the curve moves along the line of identity. The RRP of the A-V node is encountered at the A1-A2, at which H1-H2 and V1-V2 move off the line of identity. The H1-H2 and V1-V2 curves remain identical, localizing the delay to the A-V node, as shown in the right-hand panel as an increase in the A2-H2 interval without any change in the H2-V2. The curve continues to descend at a decreasing slope as further A-V nodal delay is encountered. At a critical Al-A2 interval, the delay in the A-V node becomes so great that the H1-H2 and V1-V2 intervals begin to increase. The minimum H1-H2 and V1-V2 attained define the FRP of the A-V node and entire AVCS. The increase in H1-H2 and V1-V2 continues until the impulse is blocked within the A-V node or until atrial refractoriness is reached. A-V nodal conduction (A2-H2) usually is prolonged two to three times control values before A-V nodal block. The analog records of a typical Type I response are shown in Figure 2-26.

### *Type II Response*

At longer A1-A2 intervals, the Type II response (Fig. 2-39) is similar to the Type I response in that the H1-H2 and V1-V2 intervals fall along the line of identity as A2-H2 and H2-V2

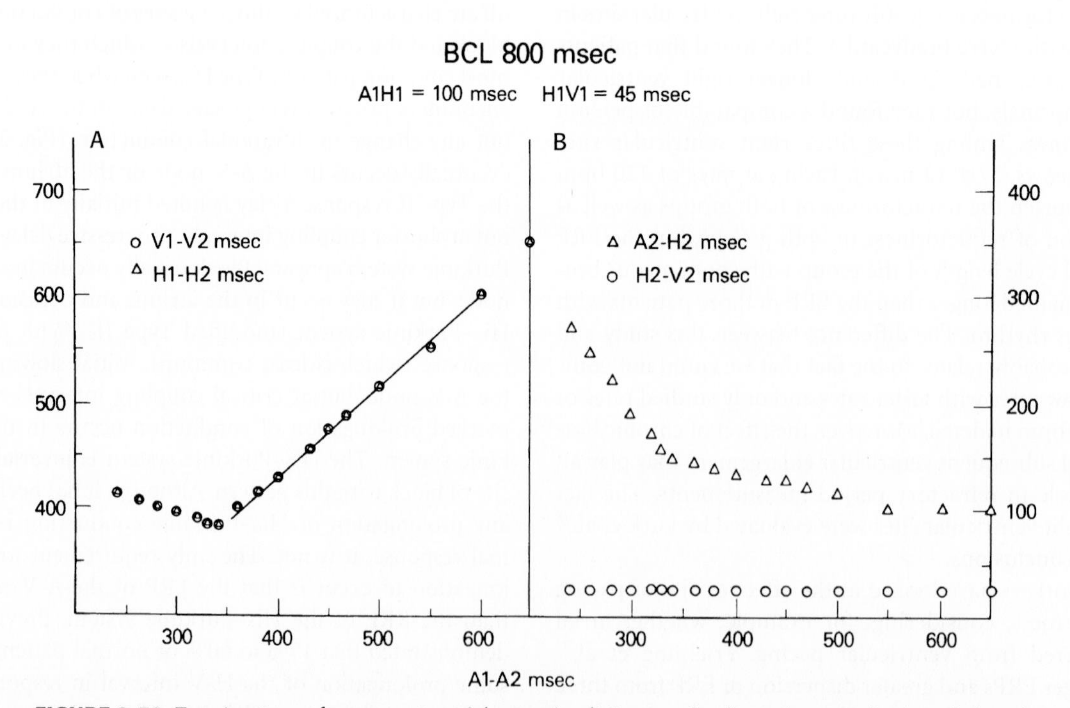


**FIGURE 2-38** *Type I pattern of response to atrial extrastimuli.* See text for discussion. BCL, basic cycle length.

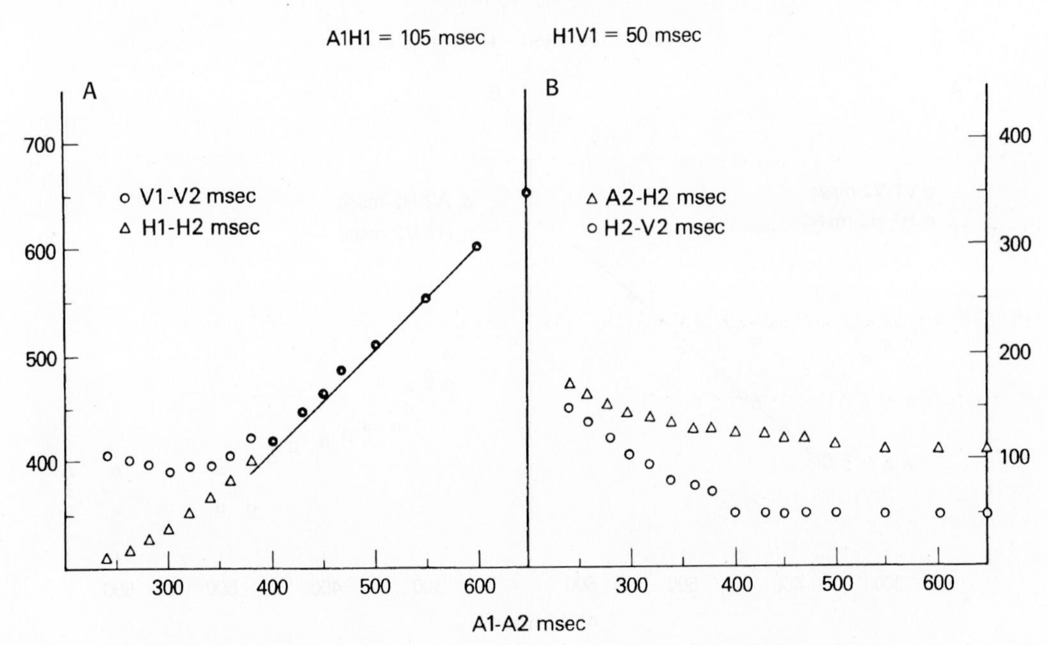


**FIGURE 2-39** *Type II pattern of response to atrial extrastimuli.* See text for discussion.

remain stable. At closer coupling intervals, in addition to an increase in the A2-H2 interval, H2-V2 becomes prolonged as the RRP of the His–Purkinje system is encountered. This prolongation results in divergence of the H1-H2 and V1-V2 curves. If the increment in H2-V2 approximates the decrement in A1-A2, V1-V2 assumes a relatively fixed value, producing a horizontal limb. Aberration is the rule as His–Purkinje conduction delay is encountered. Further shortening of A1-A2 results in block in either the A-V node or the His–Purkinje system; or in some instances, the ERP of the atrium is reached first. Thus, in the Type II response, the His–Purkinje system determines the FRP of the entire AVCS, whereas the ERP of the AVCS may be determined at any level. The total increase in A-V nodal conduction delay in the Type II is less than twofold, and no ascending limb appears on the H1-H2 curve.

### *Type III Response*

The Type III response (Fig. 2-40) is the least common response to atrial extrastimuli. At longer coupling intervals, conduction is unchanged and the curve decreases along the line of identity. Shortening of A1-A2 results in a gradual increase in A-V nodal conduction. Further shortening, however, produces a sudden jump in the H2-V2 interval, resulting in a break in the V1-V2 curve, which subsequently descends until, at a critical Al-A2 interval, the impulse usually blocks within the A-V node or His–Purkinje system. Aberrant conduction invariably accompanies beats with prolonged His–Purkinje conduction times. The FRP of the His–Purkinje system occurs just before the marked jump in H2-V2. The FRP of the AVCS in the Type III pattern is determined by the His–Purkinje system, but the ERP can be determined at any level. As in the Type II response, A-V nodal delay is not great, and no ascending limb of the H1-H2 curve appears.

## The Atrium as a Limiting Factor in A-V Conduction

The ERP of the atrium is not infrequently encountered earlier than that of the A-V node, particularly when (a) the basic drive is relatively slow, a situation that tends to lengthen atrial refractoriness and shorten A-V nodal refractoriness, or (b) the patient is agitated, and his heightened sympathetic tone shortens A-V nodal refractoriness. In our experience with 450 patients, the A-V node was the first site of block in 355 patients (57%), the ERP of the atrium was longest in 150 patients (33%), and the His–Purkinje system was the first site of block in 45 patients (10%). The figures are similar to those of Akhtar et al.[71] (45%, 40%, 15%, respectively) but differ somewhat from those of Wit et al.[80] who found the ERP of the atrium to be the longest in only 15% of patients, whereas the A-V node was longest in 70% of patients, and the His–Purkinje system was longest in 15% of patients. Again, autonomic tone at the time of catheterization can markedly affect the percentage of patients whose A-V nodes have the longest refractory periods during antegrade stimulation. The cycle lengths at which these refractory period measurements were made were highly variable, and inconsistent use of sedation, I believe, explains the disparate results.

### *Patterns of Response to Ventricular Extrastimuli*

Retrograde conduction has been less well characterized than antegrade conduction. The use of the ventricular extrastimulus

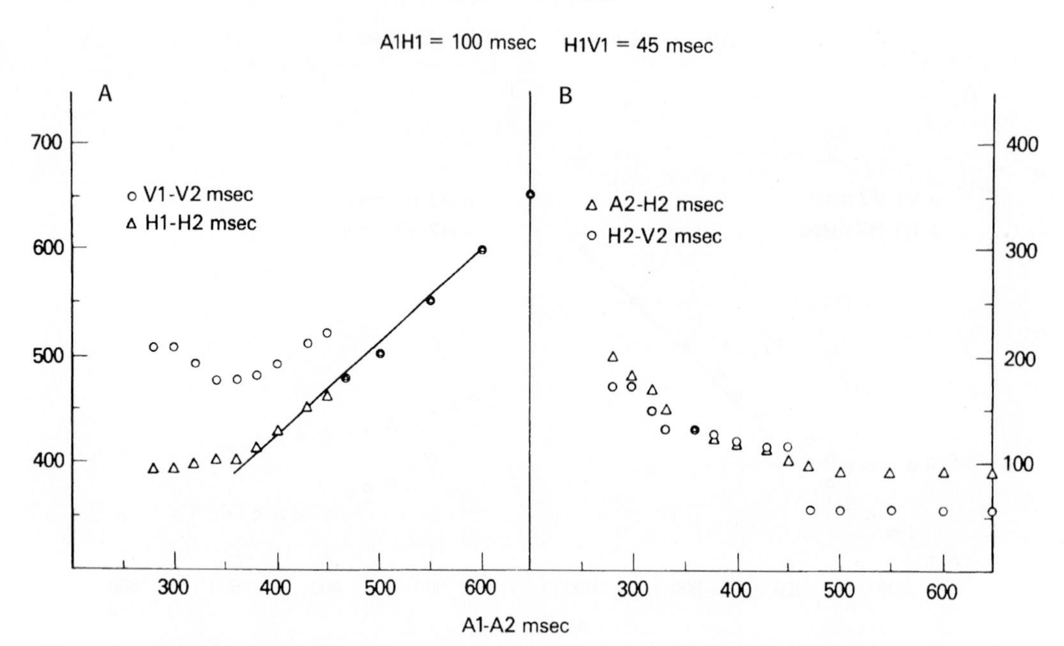


**FIGURE 2-40** *Type III pattern of response to atrial extrastimuli.* See text for discussion.

technique provides a method of systematically evaluating patterns of V-A conduction.[69–72,74,102] The technique is analogous to that used in antegrade studies and involves the introduction of progressively premature ventricular extrastimuli after every eighth to tenth beat of a basic paced ventricular rhythm until ventricular refractoriness is reached (Fig. 2-32). In patients with A-V dissociation, we employ simultaneous atrial and ventricular pacing during the basic drive to prevent supraventricular captures from altering refractoriness by producing sudden changes in cycle length. Moreover, potential changes in hemodynamics related with A-V dissociation may also affect the reproducibility of refractory period studies. Thus, attention should be given to ensuring a constant 1:1 relationship between ventricular pacing and atrial activation. We have found differences in measured refractoriness based on volume changes. Refractory periods measured during A-V pacing (P-R 150 to 200 msec) were 12.1 msec longer than during simultaneous A and V pacing at cycle lengths <600 msec but not at cycle lengths >800 msec. Similar stimulation methods must be used, therefore, when drug effects or other interventions are to be compared.

Definitions of retrograde refractoriness are given in Table 2-4. Although the functional properties of conduction and refractoriness follow principles similar to those of antegrade studies, the most common site of retrograde delay and block is in the His–Purkinje system.[70,71,74,102,103] Retrograde conduction to the His bundle is commonly seen even during A-V dissociation owing to nodoatrial block or during atrial fibrillation (Fig. 2-41).

Detailed assessment of retrograde conduction was limited in the past by the fact that the His bundle deflection was not uniformly observed during the basic drive, thus making the cases reported relatively selected. More recently, using bipolar electrodes with a 5-mm interelectrode distance and being extremely careful, we have been able to record retrograde His deflections during the ventricular-paced drive in up to 85% of our patients. A second limiting factor is that during ventricular extrastimuli the His deflection can be buried within the ventricular electrogram over a wide range of ventricular coupling intervals, therefore making measurements of ventricle to His bundle conduction times impossible in these circumstances. Using even narrower interelectrode distances (e.g., 2 mm) and pacing the para-Hisian right ventricle facilitate observation of His potentials since the His is recorded after the local ventricular electrogram (Fig. 2-42). This technique, although not widely used, offers the best method of evaluating retrograde His–Purkinje conduction during programmed ventricular stimulation.

Since a retrograde His potential may not be observed even at close coupling intervals in approximately 15% to 20% of patients using standard techniques (pacing the right ventricular apex), evaluation of His–Purkinje and consequently A-V nodal conduction is at best incomplete. Furthermore, in the absence of a recorded His bundle deflection during ventricular pacing (H1), the FRP of the His–Purkinje system (theoretically, the shortest H1-H2 at any coupling interval) must be approximated by the S1-H2 (S1 being the stimulus artifact of the basic drive cycle length). The rationale for choosing S1-H2 is the observation in animals and in occasional patients that over a wide range of ventricular-paced rates, S1-H1 remains constant (Figs. 2-25 and 2-28)[71,74,102] so that S1-H2 approximates H1-H2 but exceeds it by a fixed amount, the S1-H1 interval. The typical response shown in Figures 2-43 and 2-44 may be graphically displayed by plotting S1-S2 versus

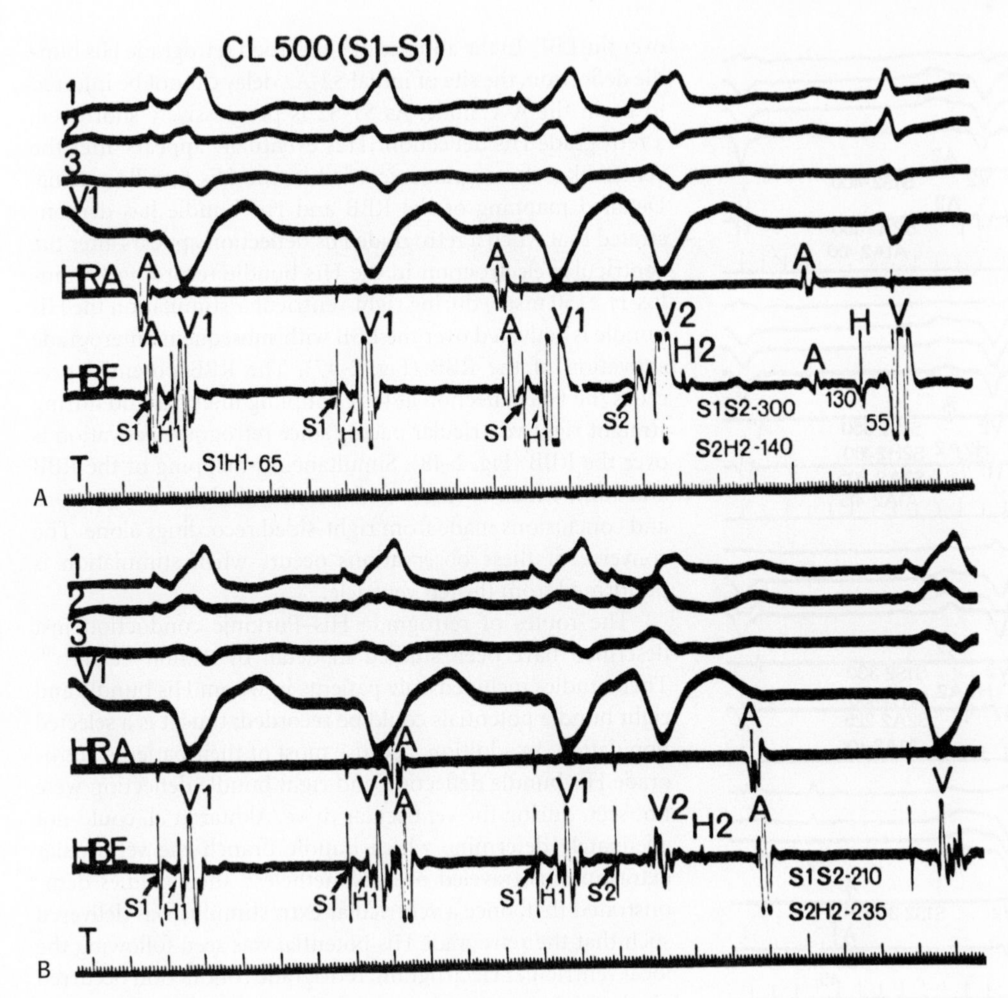


**FIGURE 2-41** *Retrograde conduction to the His bundle during A-V dissociation.* The right ventricle is being paced at a cycle length (CL; S1-S1) of 500 msec. A-V dissociation is present with block in the A-V node. A retrograde His bundle deflection (H1) is noted in the paced beats. As the ventricular extrastimuli are delivered at progressively premature coupling intervals (S1-S2), progressive delay in retrograde His–Purkinje conduction (S2-H2) is noted **(A, B)**. S, stimulus artifact.

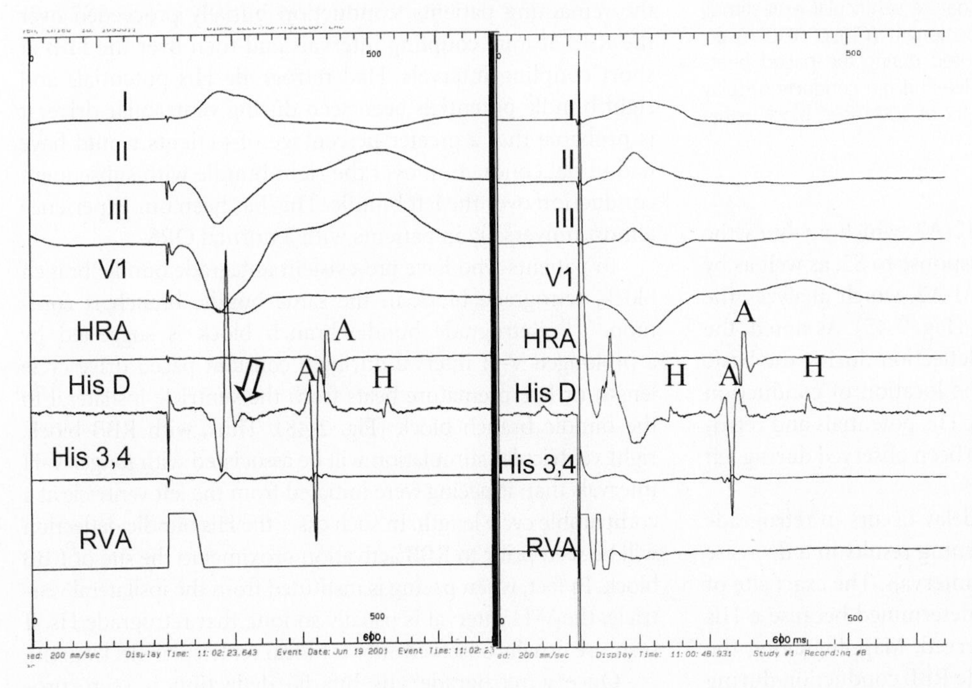


**FIGURE 2-42** *Para-Hisian ventricular pacing to identify retrograde His potential.* Both panels show response to UPC. In each case UPC is followed by an A-V nodal echo which blocks below the His. On the **left**, during RV apical pacing the retrograde His cannot be clearly distinguished from local ventricular electrogram (*open arrow*). On the **right**, during para-Hisian pacing, a retrograde His is clearly seen prior to the echo beat. See text for discussion.

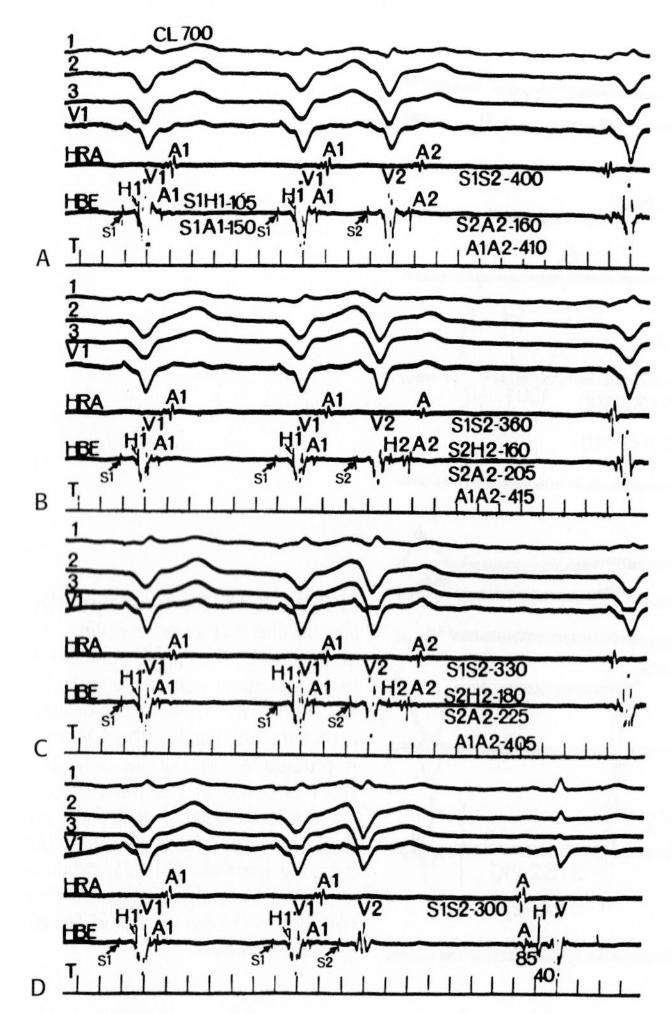


**FIGURE 2-43** *Block within the His–Purkinje system during ventricular stimulation.* **A–D:** Progressively premature ventricular extrastimuli (S2) are delivered during a paced cycle length (CL) of 700 msec. A retrograde His bundle potential is noted during the paced beats (S1-H1). **B–C:** Progressive retrograde His–Purkinje conduction delay appears as S1-S2 shortens. **D:** At an S1-S2 of 300 msec, block within the His–Purkinje system occurs.

the resulting S2-H2, S2-A2, and H2-A2, which analyzes the specific pattern of conduction in response to S2, as well as by plotting S1-S2 versus S1-H2 and Al-A2, which analyzes the FRP of the V-A conducting system (Fig. 2-45). As noted, the ability to record a retrograde His deflection during the basic drive greatly facilitates analyzing the location of conduction delays and block. Similar retrograde His potentials and retrograde V-A conduction patterns have been observed during left ventricular stimulation (Fig. 2-46).

At long coupling intervals, no delay occurs in retrograde conduction (S2-A2). Further shortening results in a decrease in A1-A2 and an increase in S2-A2 intervals. The exact site of this initial delay cannot always be determined because a His bundle deflection may not be observed. Mapping along the RBB shows initial delay in retrograde RBB conduction during right ventricular stimulation. At a critical coupling interval, block in the RBB occurs and retrograde conduction proceeds over the LBB. In the absence of a recorded retrograde His bundle deflection, the site of initial S2-A2 delay cannot be inferred to be in the A-V node. As S1-S2 is progressively shortened, a retrograde His deflection (H2) eventually appears after the ventricular electrogram recorded in the His bundle tracing. Detailed mapping of the RBB and His bundle has demonstrated that when a retrograde His deflection appears after the ventricular electrogram in the His bundle recording (stimulus-H ≥150 msec) during right ventricular stimulation the His bundle is activated over the LBB with subsequent anterograde activation of the RBB (Fig. 2-47). The RBB potential precedes the His deflection at long coupling intervals and during straight right ventricular pacing since retrograde activation is over the RBB (Fig. 2-48). Simultaneous mapping of the RBB and LBB, which is rarely done, confirms these observations and conclusions made from right-sided recordings alone. The converse of these observations occurs when stimulation is performed from the left ventricle.

The routes of retrograde His–Purkinje conduction just described have been studied in detail by Akhtar et al.[74,104] Their studies included only patients in whom His bundle and right bundle potentials could be recorded; thus it is a selected population. In addition, because most of their patients' retrograde His bundle deflection and right bundle deflection were not seen during the ventricular drive, Akhtar et al. could not adequately determine which bundle branch the ventricular extrastimulus traveled over. Nonetheless, their studies demonstrated that, once a ventricular extrastimulus was delivered such that the retrograde His potential was seen following the local ventricular electrogram, retrograde conduction occurred via the LBB system in the majority of instances (67%). In only 12.5% conduction proceeded over the RBB system, while in the remaining patients, conduction initially proceeded over the RBB at long coupling intervals and then over the LBB at short coupling intervals. Had retrograde His potentials and right bundle potentials been seen during ventricular drive, it is probable that a greater percentage of patients would have had initial conduction over the right bundle with subsequent conduction over the left bundle. This has been our experience almost universally in patients with a normal QRS.

In patients who have pre-existent antegrade bundle branch block, retrograde block in the same bundle branch is common.[74,104] Retrograde bundle branch block is suggested by a prolonged V-H interval during a constant paced drive cycle length or late premature beats from the ventricle ipsilateral to the bundle branch block (Fig. 2-48). Thus, with RBB block, right ventricular stimulation will be associated with longer V-H intervals than if pacing were initiated from the left ventricle at a comparable cycle length. In such cases the His bundle deflection will be seen prior to RBB activation proximal to the site of RBB block. In fact, when pacing is instituted from the ipsilateral ventricle, the V-H interval is usually so long that retrograde Hs, if seen, are usually observed after the local ventricular electrogram.

Once a retrograde His bundle deflection is seen, progressive prolongation of His–Purkinje conduction (S2-H2) occurs as the S1-S2 interval decreases. The degree of S2-H2

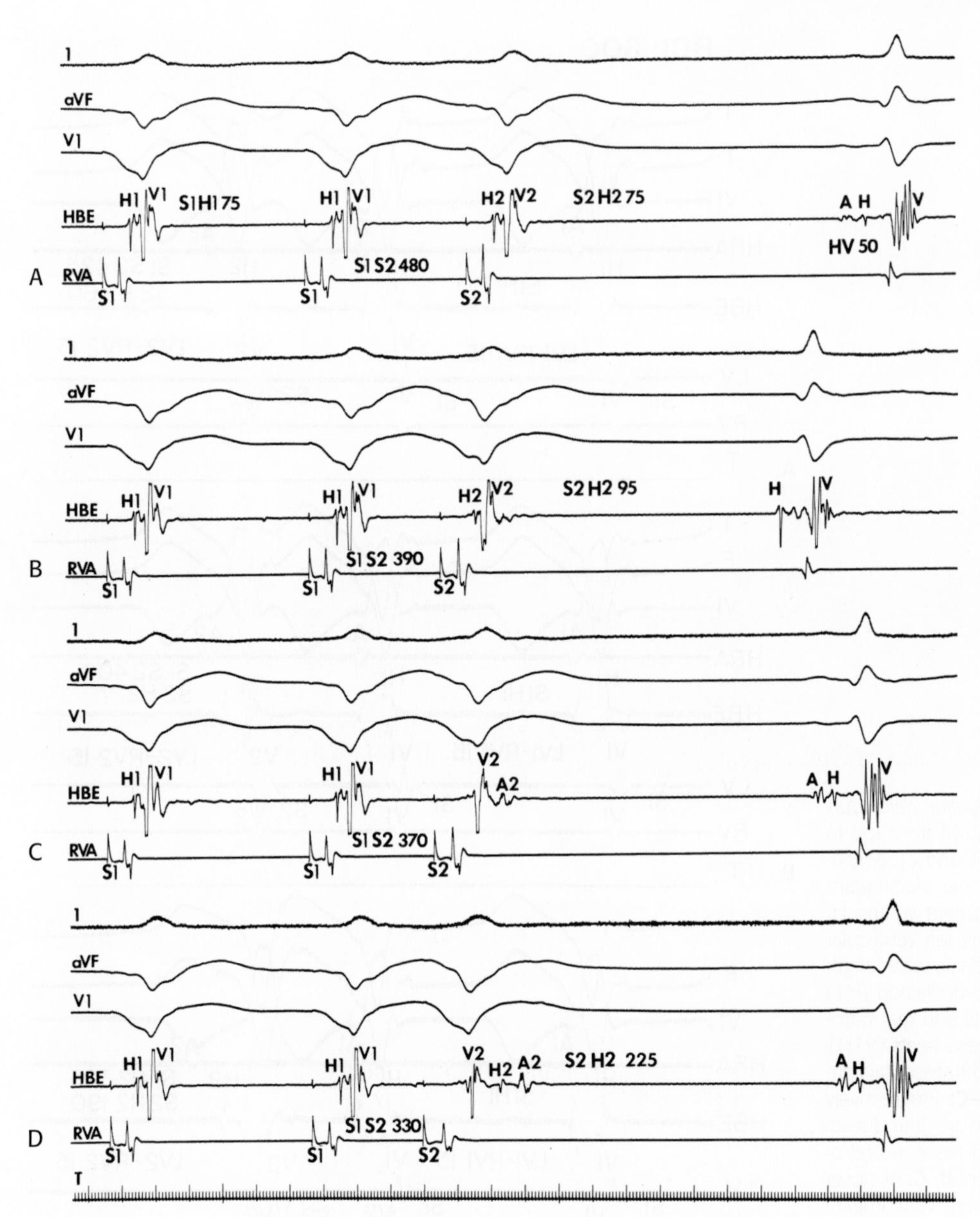


**FIGURE 2-44** *Use of retrograde His to demonstrate site of delay during retrograde stimulation.* All panels are arranged as leads 1, aVF, V1, His bundle electrogram (HBE), and right ventricular apex (RVA). **A–D:** Progressively premature ventricular extrastimuli (S1 S2) are introduced. The retrograde His deflection as seen on the drive beat (S1H1 = 15 msec) allows one to assess the sites of delay during progressively premature S1 S2. See text for discussion.

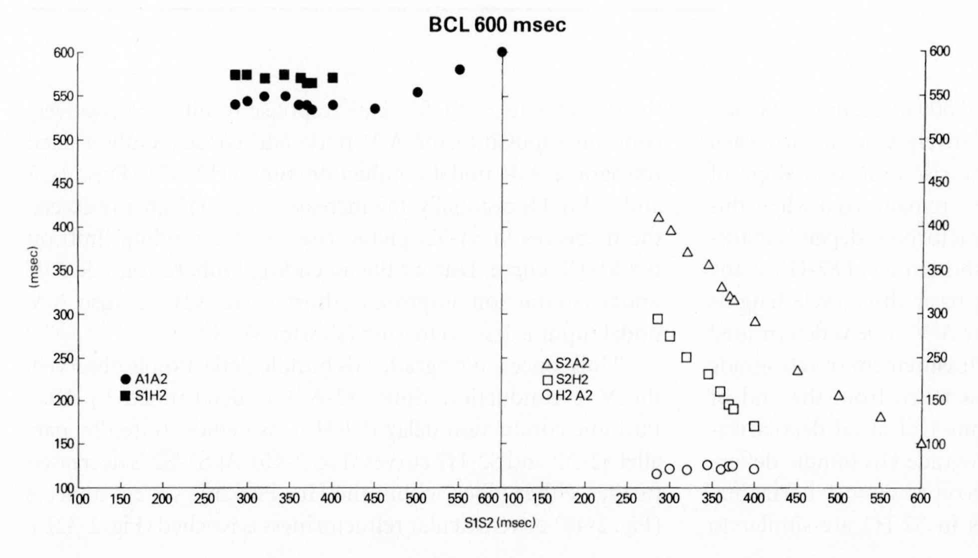


**FIGURE 2-45** *Normal pattern of retrograde conduction in response to ventricular extrastimuli.* See text for discussion.

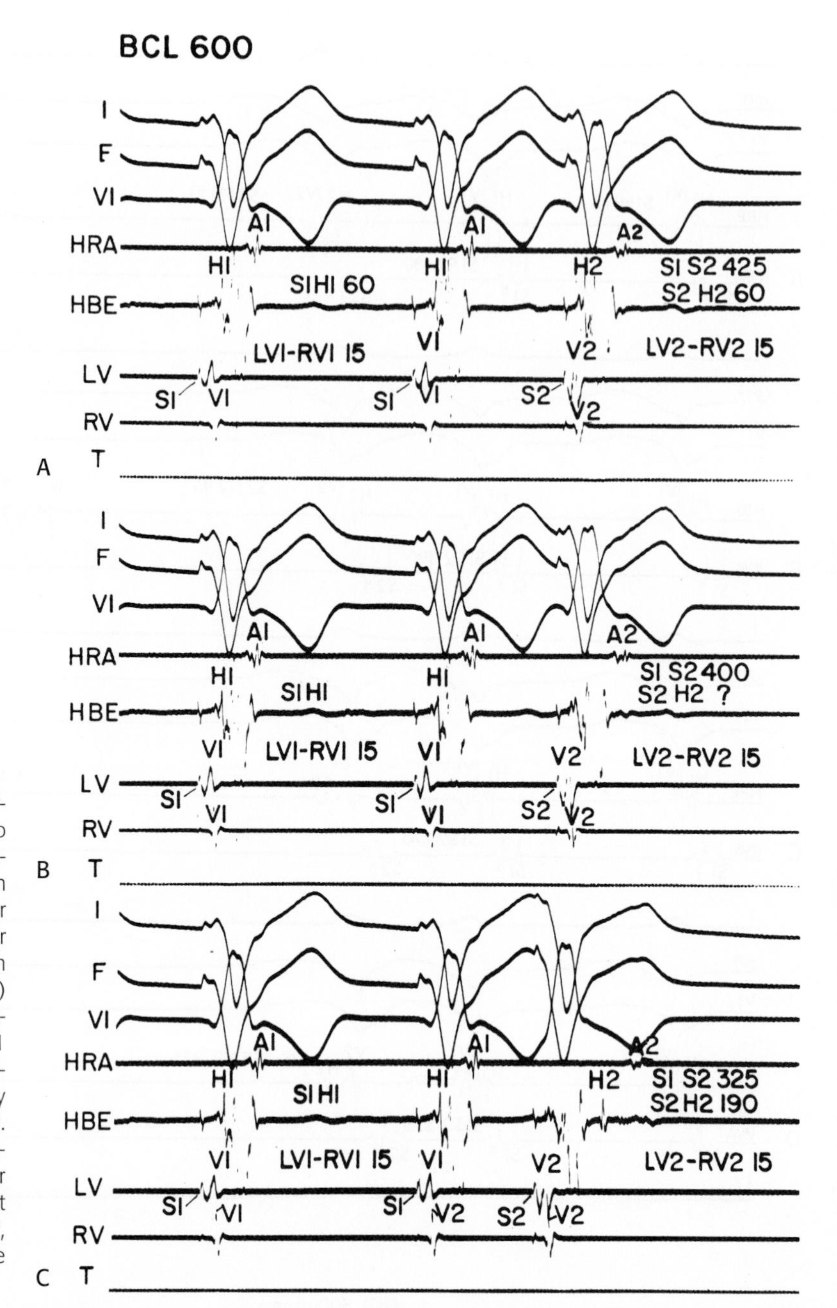


**FIGURE 2-46** *Site of His–Purkinje conduction delay during premature stimulation.* **A–C:** Organized from top to bottom as follows: surface leads I, avF (F), and V1, a high-right atrial electrogram (HRA), His bundle electrogram (HBE), left ventricular electrogram (LV), right ventricular electrogram (RV), and time lines (T). The left ventricular electrogram is being paced (S1S1) at a basic cycle length of 600 msec. Note that a retrograde His deflection (H1) can be seen during the basic drive beats and that retrograde His–Purkinje conduction during these beats (S1H1 = 60 msec) exceeds local ventricular and transseptal conduction time (LV1-RV1 = 15 msec). **A–C:** Progressively premature ventricular extrastimuli (S2) are introduced. **A:** At a coupling interval (S1 S2) of 425 msec, no retrograde His–Purkinje delay (S2 H2) is seen. **B, C:** At closer coupling intervals, S2 H2 prolongs without concomitant local ventricular conduction delay. (From Josephson ME, Kastor JA. His–Purkinje conduction during retrograde stress. *J Clin Invest* 1978;61:171.)

prolongation varies, but it can exceed 300 msec. In most cases, the increase in S2-H2 remains relatively constant for each 10-msec decrement in S1-S2, giving rise to a fixed slope of S2-H2/S1-S2. The S1-H2 and A1-A2 remain fixed when this occurs (Fig. 2-45). His–Purkinje refractoriness depends markedly on the cycle length; consistent shortening of S2-H2 at any given S1-S2 is noted at decreasing basic drive cycle lengths (S1-S1).[102] Retrograde input into the A-V node is determined by measuring the S1-H2 interval. Measurement of retrograde A-V nodal conduction time is best taken from the end of the His bundle deflection to the onset of atrial depolarization. In most instances, once a retrograde His bundle deflection appears, the S1-H2 curve becomes almost horizontal (Fig. 2-45) because the increments in S2-H2 are similar to the decrements in S1-S2. This response results in a relatively constant input into the A-V node and consequently a fixed retrograde A-V nodal conduction time (H2-A2) (Figs. 2-32 and 2-45). Occasionally, the increases in S2-H2 greatly exceed the decreases in S1-S2, giving rise to an ascending limb on the S1-H2 curve. During the ascending limb, retrograde A-V nodal conduction improves (shorter H2-A2) because A-V nodal input is less premature (shorter S1-H2).

Thus, once a retrograde His bundle deflection is observed, the V-A conduction time (S2-A2) is determined by His–Purkinje conduction delay (S2-H2), as demonstrated by parallel S2-A2 and S2-H2 curves (Fig. 2-45). As S1-S2 is decreased further, either block within the His–Purkinje system appears (Fig. 2-48) or ventricular refractoriness is reached (Fig. 2-32E).

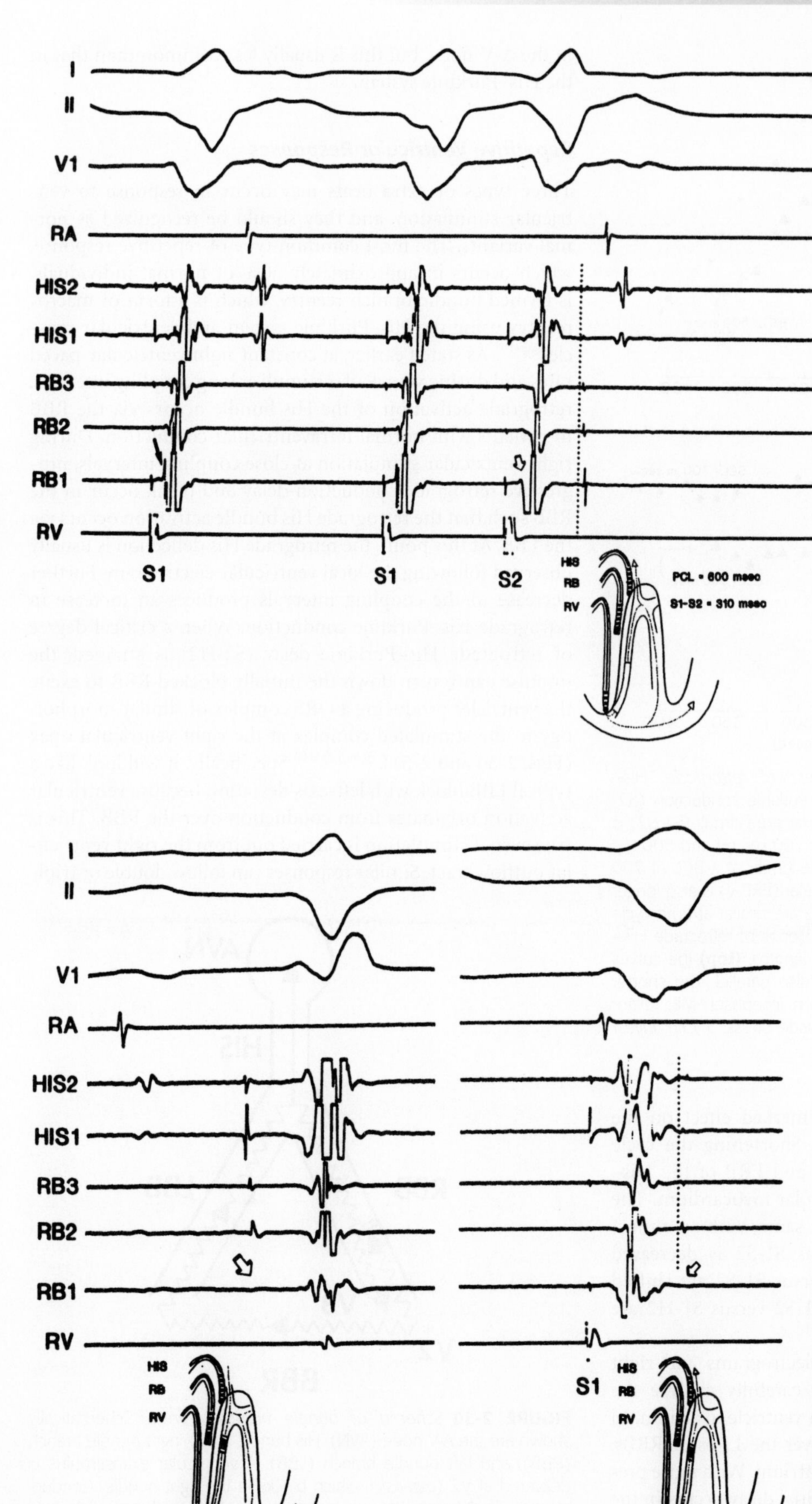


**FIGURE 2-47** *Retrograde conduction during ventricular pacing and early coupled ventricular extrastimuli.* Leads I, II, V1 are shown with electrograms from the right atrium (RA), proximal (HIS2) and distal (HIS1) His bundle, distal, mid, and proximal right bundle (RB1, RB2, RB3 respectively), and right ventricle (RV). Schema is below. During RV pacing (S1) RB1 is activated early with retrograde spread to the HIS. Following a ventricular extrastimulus (S2) activation is reversed, going from His to RB. See text for discussion.

**FIGURE 2-48** *Retrograde conduction in the presence of ipsilateral bundle branch block.* This figure is organized the same as Figure 2-47. Schemas are shown below. On the **left** activation during sinus rhythm with right bundle branch block (RBBB) is present. The *open arrow* demonstrates the site of RBBB. During ventricular pacing **(right panel)** retrograde conduction proceeds over the left bundle branch to activate the His bundle with subsequent engagement and block in the RB (*open arrow*).

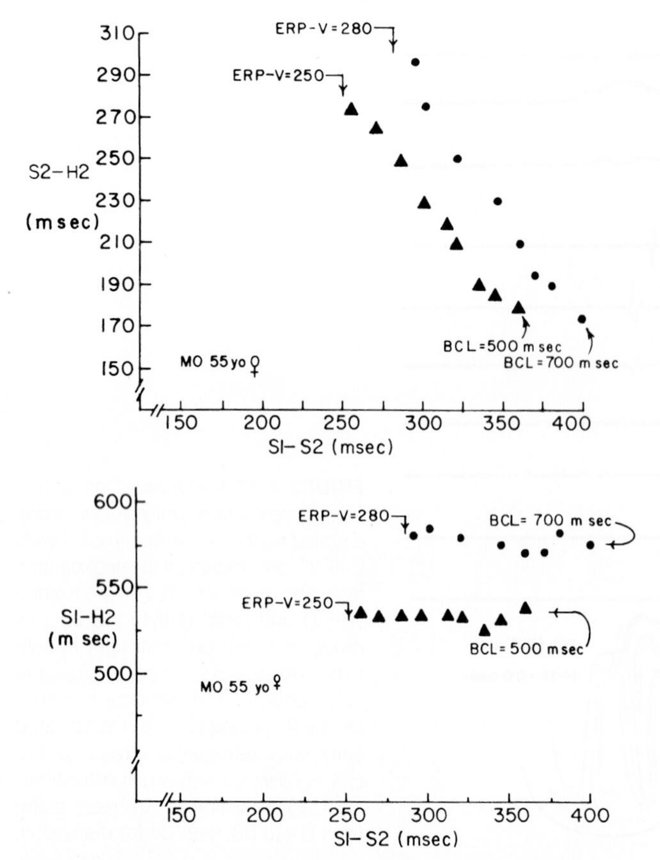


**FIGURE 2-49** *Cycle length responsiveness of retrograde.* His–Purkinje conduction delay. Retrograde His–Purkinje conduction (S2-H2) in response to variably coupled ventricular extrastimuli (S1 S2) is compared at two basic cycle lengths (BCL): 700 ms (•) and 500 ms (▲). At every S1 S2, the resultant S2 H2 is longer at a BCL of 700 msec. The effective refractory period-ventricular (ERP-V) is also longer at a BCL of 700 msec. The slopes of S2-H2 are similar at both cycle lengths in parallel curves. Inasmuch as the slopes of retrograde His–Purkinje delay are parallel at different cycle lengths, **(top)** the curves of resultant minimal outputs (S1-H2) are also parallel. The shorter the BCL, the less the minimal output. (From Josephson ME, Kastor JA. His–Purkinje conduction during retrograde stress. *J Clin Invest* 1978;61:171.)

Cycle length, as expected, has a marked effect on the response to ventricular extrastimuli. Shortening the cycle length decreases both the functional and ERP of the His–Purkinje system as well as the ventricular myocardium. The general pattern, however, remains the same, with an almost linear increase in S2-H2 intervals as S1-S2 is decreased (Fig. 2-49). The curves for S2-H2 versus S1-S2 are shifted to the left, and the curves relating S1-S2 versus S1-H2 are shifted down.

In summary, using His bundle electrograms and right bundle deflections, it is possible to carefully analyze the sequence of retrograde activation from ventricle to atrium. In most patients, conduction proceeds over the LBBs or RRBs, then to the His bundle, A-V node, and atrium. With more premature ventricular extrastimuli, the initial delay occurs in the His–Purkinje system. When block first occurs, it is also most likely in the His–Purkinje system. Delay and block can occur in the A-V node, but this is usually less common than that in the His–Purkinje system.

### *Repetitive Ventricular Responses*

Three types of extra beats may occur in response to ventricular stimulation, and they should be recognized as normal variants. The most common type of repetitive response, which occurs in approximately 50% of normal individuals, is termed bundle branch reentry, which is a form of macroreentry using the His–Purkinje system and ventricular muscle.[105–107] As stated earlier, at constant right ventricular-paced rates and during ventricular stimuli at long coupling intervals, retrograde activation of the His bundle occurs via the RBB in patients with normal intraventricular conduction. During right ventricular stimulation at close coupling intervals, progressive retrograde conduction delay and block occur in the RBB such that the retrograde His bundle activation occurs via the LBB. At this point, the retrograde His deflection is usually observed following the local ventricular electrogram. Further decrease in the coupling intervals produces an increase in retrograde His–Purkinje conduction. When a critical degree of retrograde His–Purkinje delay (S2-H2) is attained, the impulse can return down the initially blocked RBB to excite the ventricles producing a QRS complex of similar morphology to the stimulated complex at the right ventricular apex (Figs. 2-50 and 2-51).[70,96,105–110] Specifically, it will look like a typical LBB block with left-axis deviation because ventricular activation originates from conduction over the RBB. This is true even if stimulation is carried out from the right ventricular outflow tract. Similar responses can follow double or triple

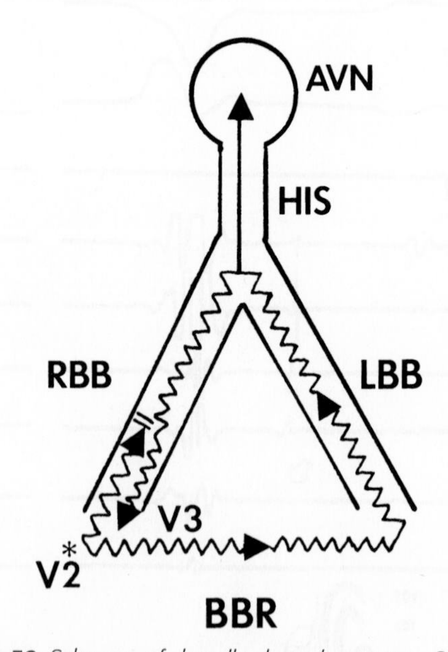


**FIGURE 2-50** *Schema of bundle branch reentry.* Schematically shown are the A-V node (AVN), His bundle (HIS), right bundle branch (RBB), and left bundle branch (LBB). A ventricular extrastimulus is delivered at V2 (*asterisk*), which blocks in the right bundle. Conduction proceeds across the ventricles, up the LBB, and if enough time is elapsed, the RBB has time to recover and the impulse to conduct through the RBB to produce V3. See text for discussion.

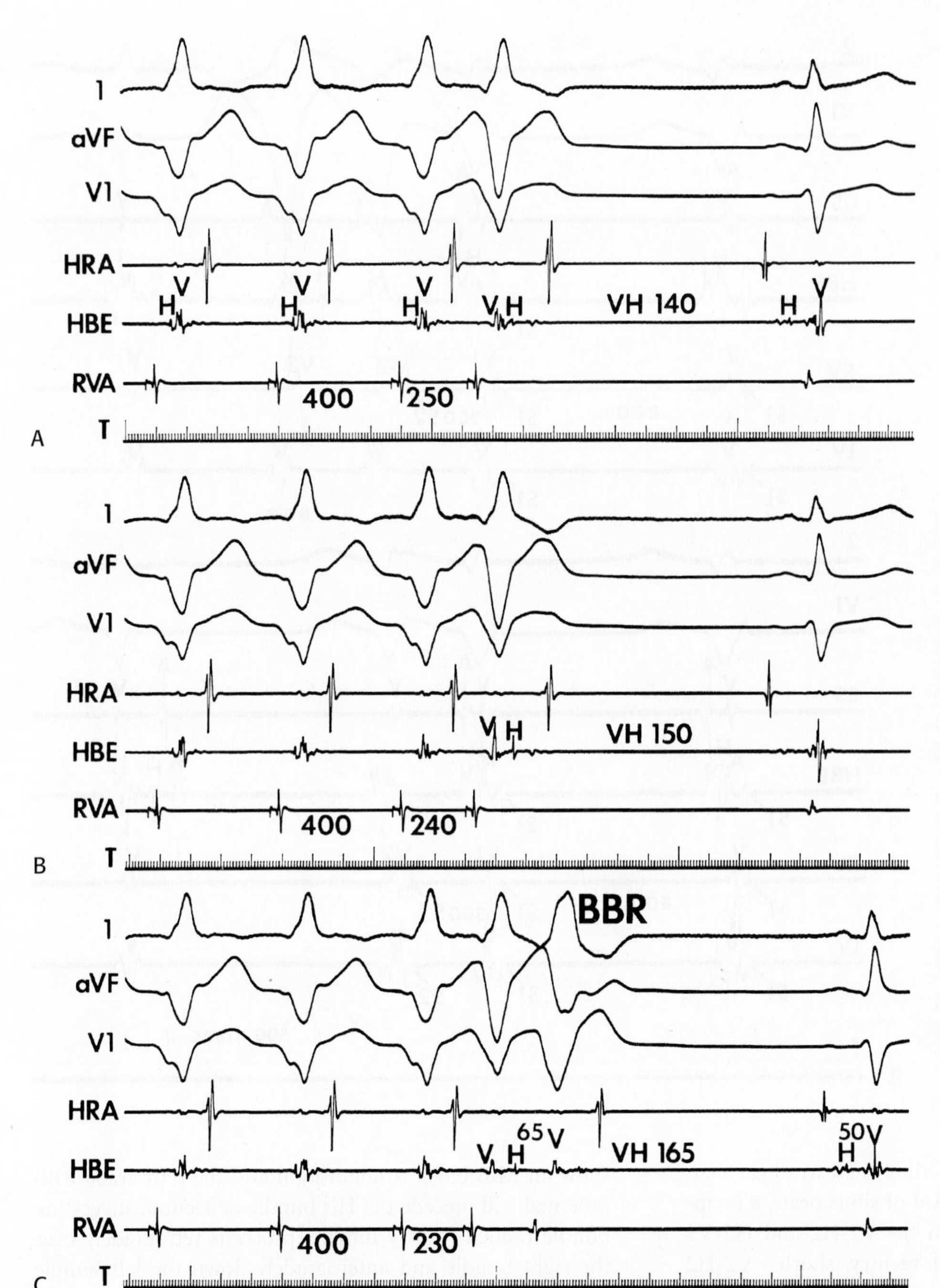


**FIGURE 2-51** *Demonstration of bundle branch reentry.* **A–C:** Organized as 1, aVF, V1, and electrograms from the high-right atrium (HRA), His bundle (HBE), and right ventricular apex (RVA). At a basic drive of 400 msec, progressively premature extrastimuli are delivered. A retrograde H can be seen during the drive beats. **A:** At a premature ventricular coupling interval of 250 msec, retrograde His–Purkinje delay is manifested by prolongation of the V-H to 140 msec. **B:** The V-H increases to 150 msec. **C:** At a coupling interval of 230 msec, the retrograde His–Purkinje delay reaches 165 msec and is followed by a bundle branch reentrant (BBR) complex. The H-V interval during this complex is 165 msec (15 msec greater than during sinus rhythm). Note that the QRS of the BBR has a left bundle branch block left-axis deviation. See text for discussion.

extrastimuli. Retrograde atrial activation, if present, follows the His deflection, and the H-V interval usually approximates that during antegrade conduction. However the H-V interval may be shorter or greater than the H-V interval during antegrade conduction. The H-V interval depends on (a) the site of His bundle recording relative to the turnaround point (Fig. 2-50). If the His bundle is recorded proximal to the turnaround, it will be recorded after the impulse has begun to travel down the RBB giving rise to a shorter H-V interval than in sinus rhythm. It will be shorter by twice the time it takes the impulse to reach the His recording site from the turnaround site, assuming antegrade conduction remains unaltered; (b) antegrade conduction down the RBB. If conduction down the RBB is slowed, the H-V interval can be prolonged. The H-V interval of the bundle branch reentrant beat, therefore, reflects the interplay of these factors.

Electrophysiologic features that suggest that this extra beat is in fact due to bundle branch reentry follow:

1. The extra response is always preceded by a retrograde His deflection and is abolished when retrograde block below the His bundle recording site is achieved, a phenomenon that may occur with simultaneous right and left ventricular stimulation (Fig. 2-52). Moreover, pre-excitation of the His bundle to produce block below the His bundle also prevents the repetitive response (Fig. 2-53).

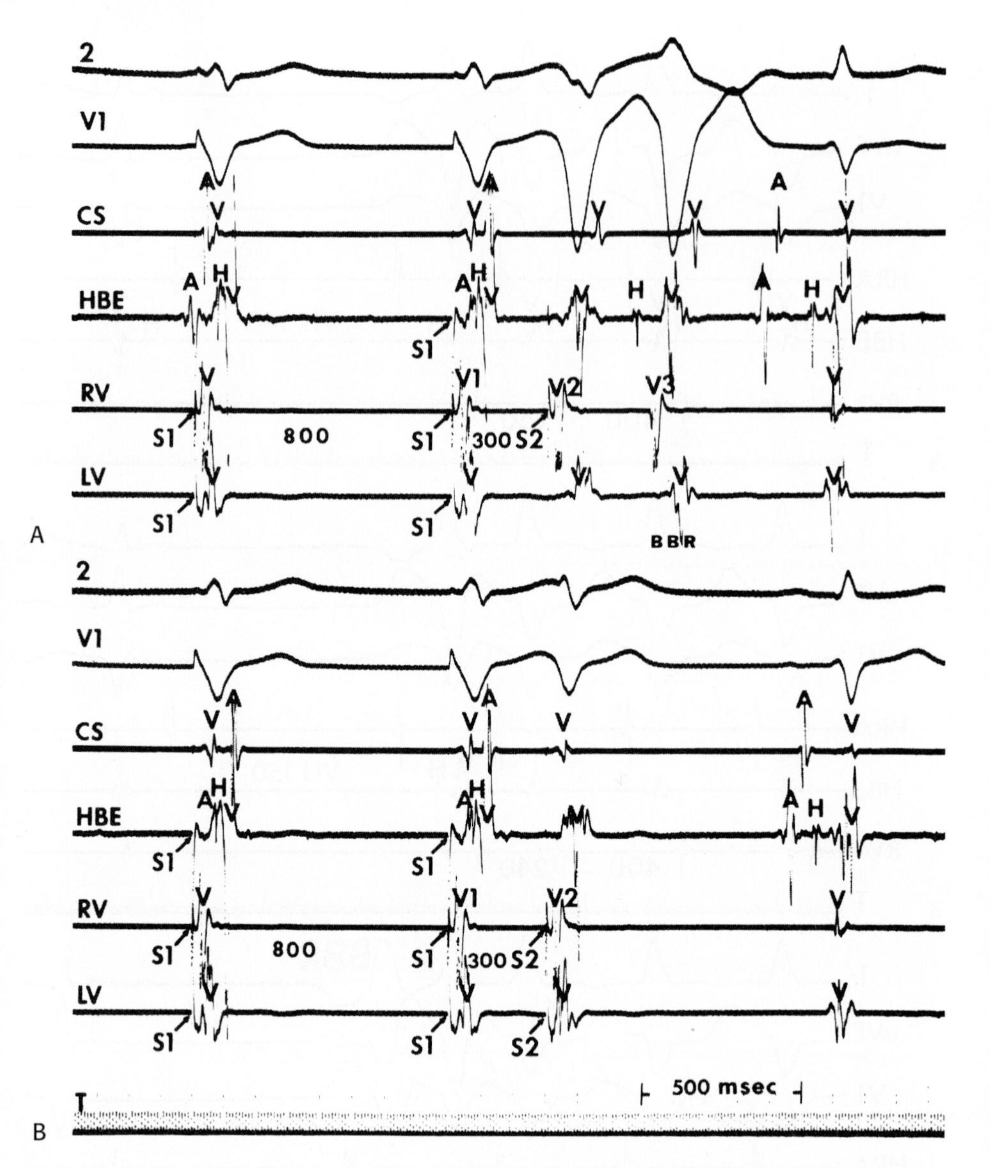


**FIGURE 2-52** *Prevention of bundle branch reentry by simultaneous right and left ventricular stimulation.* From top to bottom are ECG leads 2 and V1, and electrograms from the coronary sinus (CS), His bundle (HBE), right ventricle (RV), and left ventricle (LV). **A:** A right ventricular premature stimulus (S2) is delivered at a coupling interval of 300 msec during ventricular pacing (S1-S1) at a cycle length of 800 msec, resulting in bundle branch reentry (BBR), as previously described. **B:** Simultaneous right and left ventricular stimulation at the same coupling intervals as in **(A)** failed to induce BBR. Simultaneous stimulation of the opposite ventricle renders the retrograde limb of the BBR pathway (LV conduction system) refractory, thereby abolishing reentry. (From Farshidi A, Michelson EL, Greenspan AM, et al. Repetitive responses to ventricular extrastimuli: incidence, mechanism, and significance. *Am Heart J* 1980;100:59.)

2. Although the H-V interval preceding the extra beat usually approximates the H-V interval of sinus beats, a reciprocal relationship exists between the V2-H2 and H2-V3 intervals. Thus, at the onset of reentry, shorter V2-H2 intervals are associated with longer H2-V3 intervals. Progressive shortening of the coupling intervals results in longer V2-H2 intervals, which are then followed by shorter H2-V3 intervals. The H2-V3 interval reflects recovery of the RBB-Purkinje-muscle junction following initial block in that area.
3. This macroreentrant phenomenon during right ventricular stimulation is uncommon in patients with a pre-existing complete RBB block on the surface ECG.[105]
4. During bundle branch reentrant complexes produced by right ventricular stimulation with a LBB block configuration, the retrograde His bundle deflection (H2) precedes that of antegrade right bundle potential (RB2), which further supports activation of the His system via the left bundle (Fig. 2-54). In rare instances, the repetitive response will show an RBB block configuration and the retrograde RBB potential will precede the His bundle deflection, suggesting bundle branch reentry initially proceeds retrogradely over the right bundle and anterogradely down the left bundle (Fig. 2-55). Bundle branch reentry with an RBB block configuration is the rule during left ventricular stimulation. These types of repetitive responses can be noted during atrial fibrillation or in the absence of A-V conduction (Fig. 2-56).

In patients with normal hearts, bundle branch reentry is rarely sustained and usually is self-terminating in one or two complexes. The most common reason for failure to sustain bundle branch reentry is a retrograde block in the LBB system. Rarely, conduction will proceed retrogradely to the His bundle, and block will then occur in the RBB (Fig. 2-57). Sustained bundle branch reentry is rarely observed in patients with a normal QRS; however, it is not an uncommon phenomenon in patients with pre-existing conduction defects, producing a form of ventricular tachycardia (see

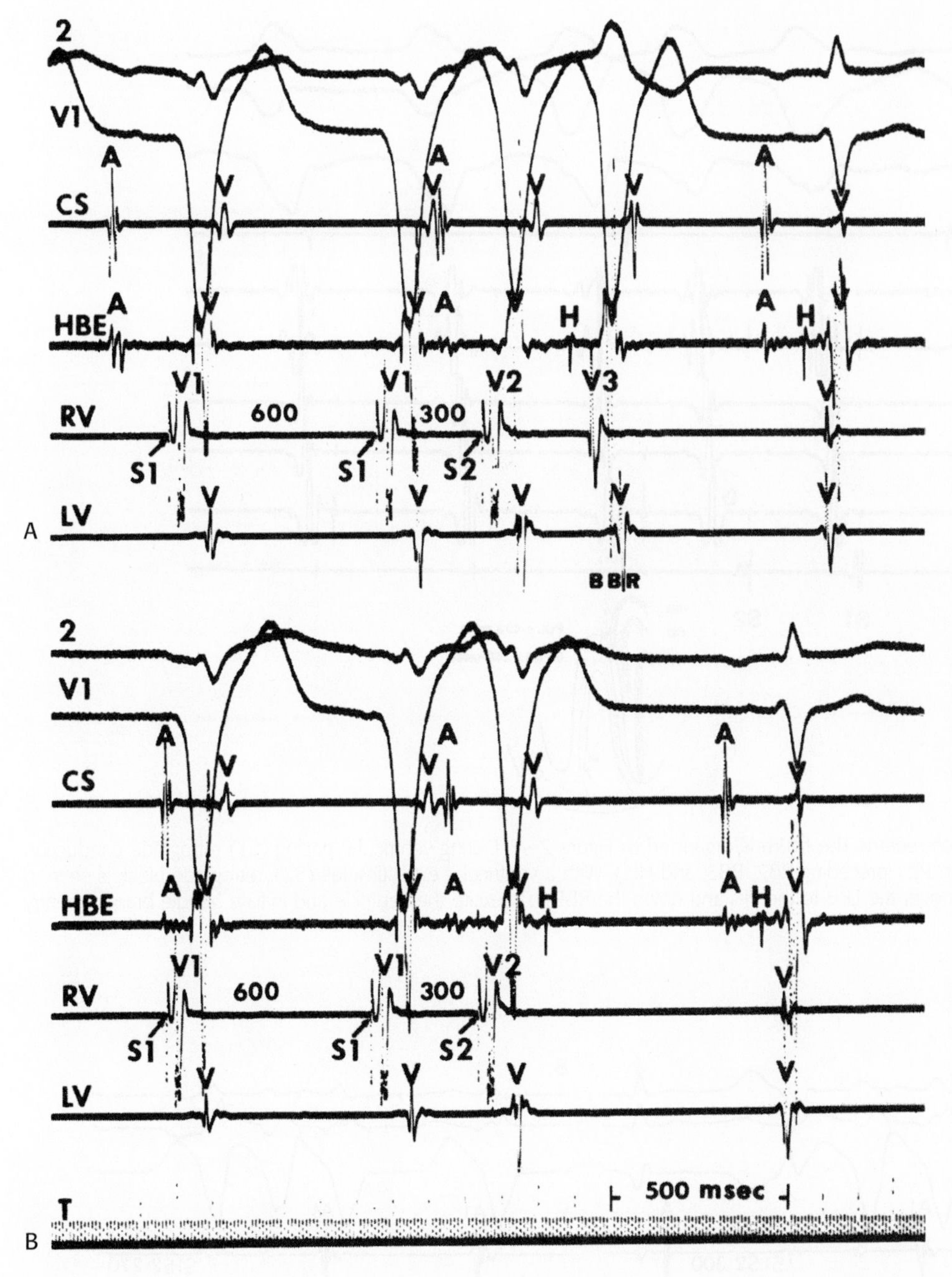


**FIGURE 2-53** *Abolition of bundle branch reentry by pre-excitation of the His bundle.* The panels are organized from top to bottom as ECG leads 2 and V1, and coronary sinus (CS), His bundle (HBE), right ventricular (RV), and left ventricular (LV) electrograms. **A:** A premature RV stimulus (S2) at a coupling interval of 300 msec results in bundle branch reentry (BBR). **B:** S2 is again delivered at a coupling interval of 300 msec, but no BBR occurs. BBR is prevented by a spontaneous sinus complex preceding V2, which conducts through the A-V node to pre-excite the His bundle by 50 msec, thereby rendering it refractory to retrograde activation. The supraventricular impulse blocks below the His bundle and no ventricular response occurs. (From Farshidi A, Michelson EL, Greenspan AM, et al. Repetitive responses to ventricular extrastimuli: incidence, mechanism, and significance. *Am Heart J* 1980;100:59.)

Chapter 11).[105] Nonsustained bundle branch reentry occurs in patients with and without heart disease and is unrelated to the presence of spontaneous arrhythmias. The only factor influencing the ability to demonstrate bundle branch reentry is the presence of antegrade bundle branch block during sinus rhythm. Farshidi et al.[106] from our laboratory showed that only 2 of 35 patients with RBB block and 1 of 17 patients with LBB block demonstrated bundle branch reentry during ventricular stimulation. A variant of bundle branch reentry is intrafascicular reentry. This universally occurs in patients with pre-existent complete RBB block and either left anterior or posterior fascicular "block" on the ECG (Fig. 2-58). The fascicular "block" is usually due to very slow conduction. Ventricular extrastimuli can conduct up the slowly conducting fascicle and down the "good" fascicle, giving rise to an extra beat that looks almost identical to the sinus complex. Atrial premature beats can also produce such repetitive responses by causing transient block in the slowly conducting fascicle. Conduction proceeds over the "good" fascicle and can return up the blocked fascicle if it has recovered. This often results in sustained reentry, producing a hemodynamically untolerated ventricular tachycardia. Since the turnaround point is always a distance below the His bundle, the H-V interval is always less than the H-V interval during sinus rhythm by at least 25 msec (Fig. 2-59). In addition, if recorded, an LBB potential will precede the His potential (Fig. 2-59).

In normal patients, the second most common repetitive response to single ventricular extrastimuli is a ventricular

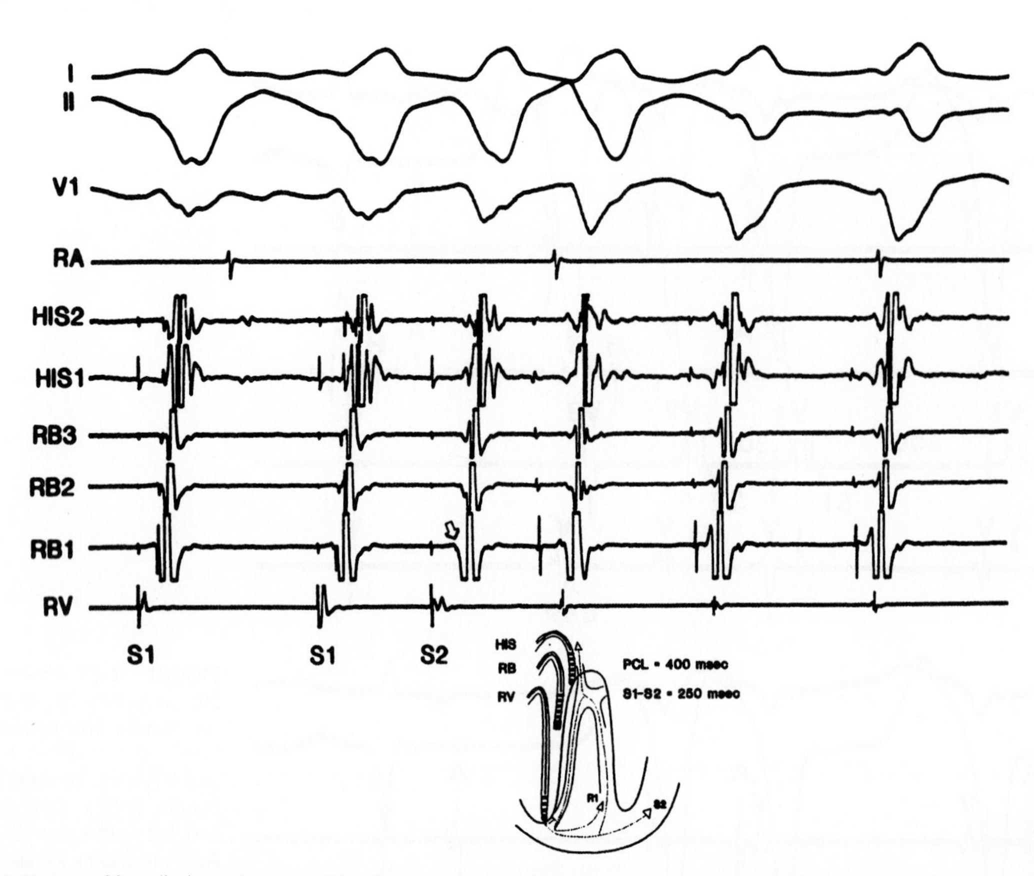


**FIGURE 2-54** *Initiation of bundle branch reentry.* The figure is organized as Figure 2-47. During ventricular pacing (S1) retrograde conduction goes over the RBB (note spike of RBB in RB1 preceding RB2, RB3, and HIS). With a ventricular extrastimulus (S2), retrograde block is seen in the RBB (*open arrow*), conduction goes over the LBB to the His and down the RBB to reexcite the ventricle and initiate bundle branch reentry (see schema below).

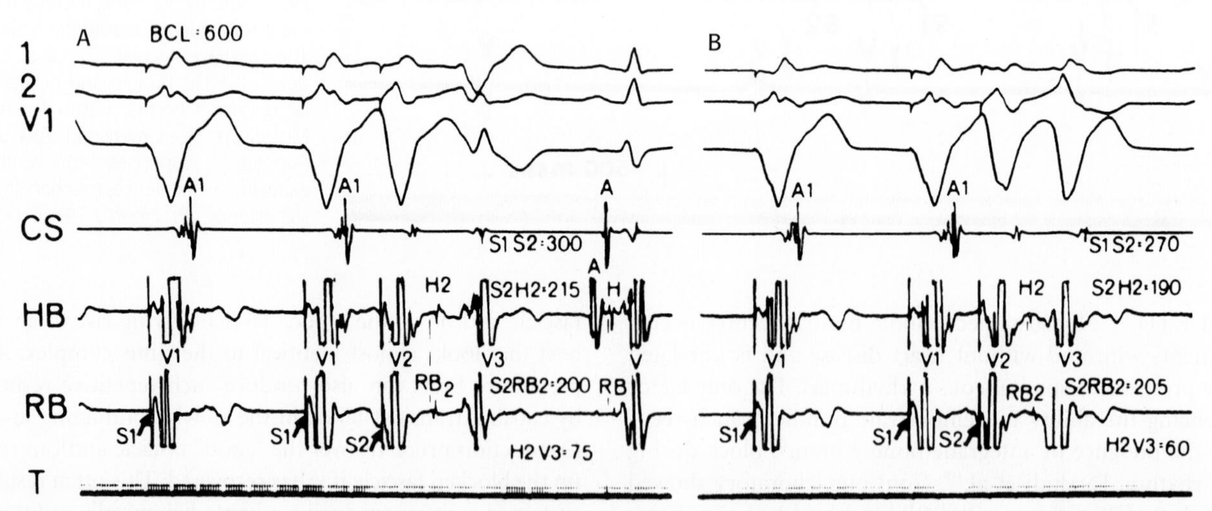


**FIGURE 2-55** *Bundle branch reentry showing both a right bundle branch block and left bundle branch block pattern.* Trading is arranged from top to bottom as leads 1, 2, and V1, along with electrograms from the coronary sinus (CS), His bundle (HB), and right bundle (RB). **A:** A right ventricular extrastimulus is delivered in which conduction proceeds up the right bundle and then returns to the ventricle over the left bundle branch system giving rise to a right bundle branch block configuration. Note right bundle potential precedes the His bundle potential following S2. **B:** At closer coupling intervals, typical bundle branch reentry occurs with the extrastimulus blocking in the right bundle, going retrogradely up the left bundle to return to the ventricles over the right bundle. In this instance note that H2 precedes RB2. (From Akhtar M, Denker S, Lehmann MH, et al. Macro-reentry within the His–Purkinje system. *PACE* 1983;6:1010.)

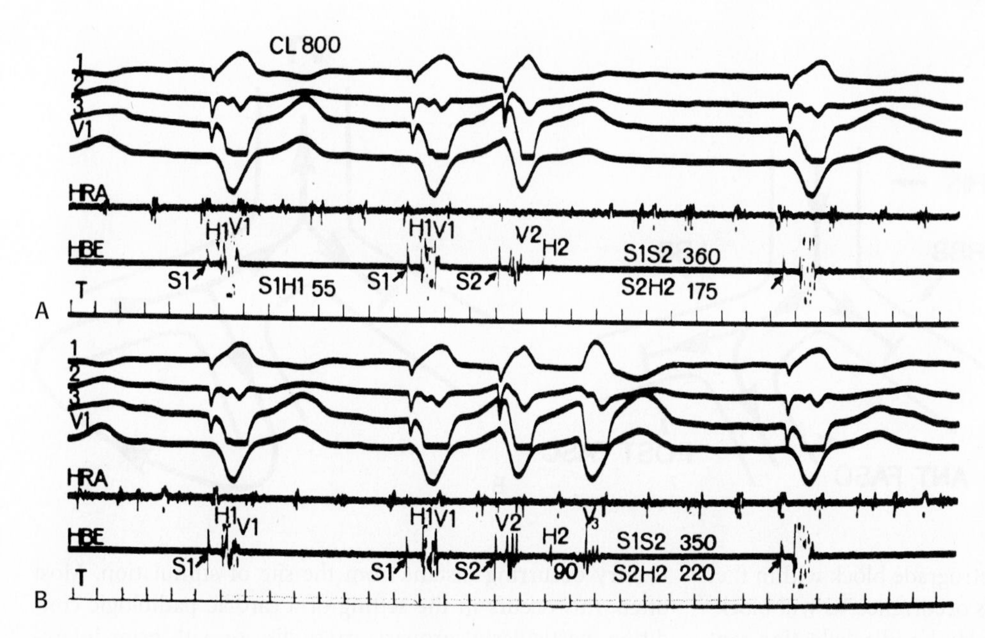


**FIGURE 2-56** *Presence of bundle branch reentry during atrial fibrillation.* **A, B:** Premature ventricular extrastimuli delivered during atrial fibrillation result in critical S2-H2 prolongation and bundle branch reentry. The production of this type of echo does not depend on A-V nodal participation.

echo that is due to reentry within the A-V node.[70,72,74,108–110] This phenomenon, which occurs in approximately 15% of patients, is identical to that occurring during ventricular pacing (Fig. 2-26). In fact, if such repetitive responses are noted in response to ventricular extrastimuli, they can invariably be produced by ventricular pacing, during which they are more commonly observed. This type of echo appears when a critical degree of retrograde A-V nodal delay is achieved. In most instances a critical degree of A-V nodal delay is achieved before the appearance of a retrograde His deflection beyond the local ventricular electrogram. If one can see the retrograde His deflection during the ventricular drive, one can occasionally note a retrograde His deflection during the ventricular extrastimulus and can measure the retrograde H2-A2 interval (Fig. 2-60). At a critical H2-A2 or, in some instances when the His deflection cannot be seen, V2-A2 interval, an extra beat with a normal antegrade QRS morphology results (Fig. 2-60). Atrial activity also precedes the His deflection before the extra QRS complex. This phenomenon may occur at long or short coupling intervals and depends only on the degree of retrograde

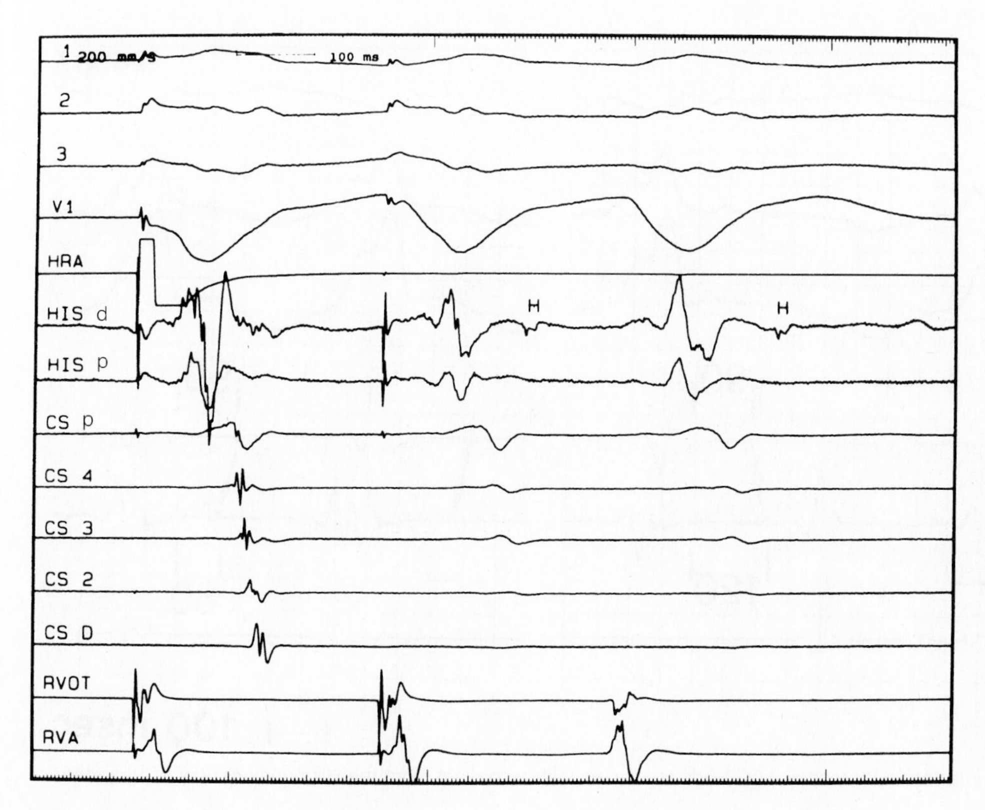


**FIGURE 2-57** *Termination of bundle branch reentry by antegrade block in the RBB.* ECG leads 1, 2, 3, and V1 are shown with electrograms from the high-right atrium (HRA), proximal and distal His bundle (HIS p, HIS d), proximal to distal coronary sinus (CS), right ventricular outflow tract and apex (RVOT, RVA). A ventricular extrastimulus from the RVA at 310 msec initiates bundle branch reentry, which does not sustain because of antegrade block in the RRB (below His).

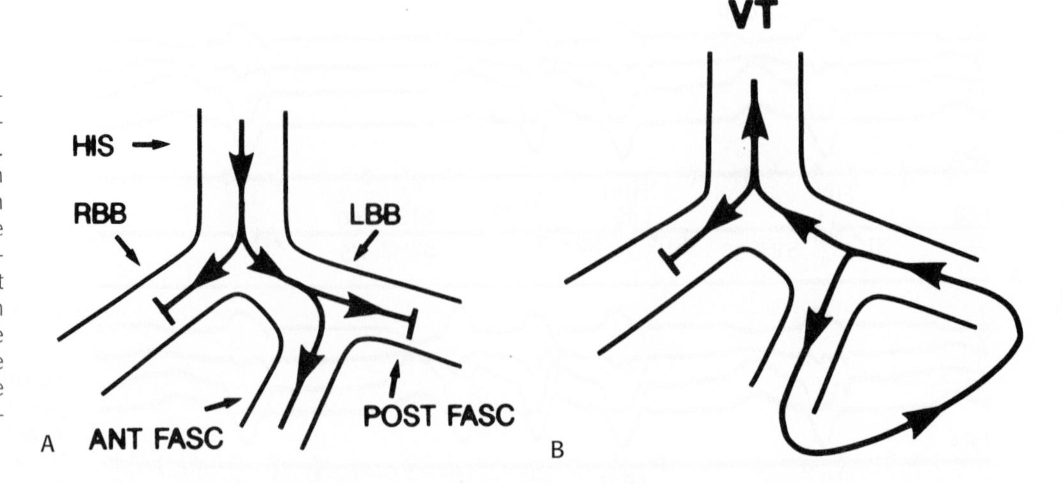


**FIGURE 2-58** *Schema of intrafascicular reentry.* Activation during sinus rhythm is shown in **(A)**. Intrafascicular reentry is shown in **(B)**. The impulse conducts down the anterior fascicle and up the posterior fascicle to form a sub-Hisian circuit. This is in contrast to bundle branch reentry, which uses the RBB as the retrograde limb that turns around at the distal His to conduct down one or both fascicles. See text for discussion.

A-V nodal delay. The presence of retrograde block within the His–Purkinje system will prevent its occurrence, as will block within the A-V node. If a retrograde His bundle deflection can be seen throughout the zone of intervals, one can frequently see a reciprocal relationship between the H2-A2 interval and the A2-H3 interval (compare Fig. 2-60A and C). This supports the fact that this echo is due to reentry within the A-V node. These patients therefore have dual A-V nodal pathways. The ventricular echo is produced by retrograde conduction up the slow pathway and antegrade conduction down the fast pathway (see Chapter 8).

The third type of repetitive ventricular response that can be observed consists of those that are due to intraventricular reentry occurring distant from the site of stimulation. Most often, this occurs in the setting of a cardiac pathologic condition, particularly coronary artery disease with prior infarction. These repetitive responses usually occur at short coupling intervals and may have any morphology, but are more often RBB block than LBB block in patients with prior myocardial infarction. In normal patients using single ventricular extrastimuli at twice threshold, repetitive responses occur less than 15% of the time and up to 24% with double extrastimuli. This is in marked contrast to patients with prior ventricular tachycardia and fibrillation and cardiac disease, in whom repetitive intraventricular reentry occurs in 70% to 75% of instances in response to single or double extrastimuli. The

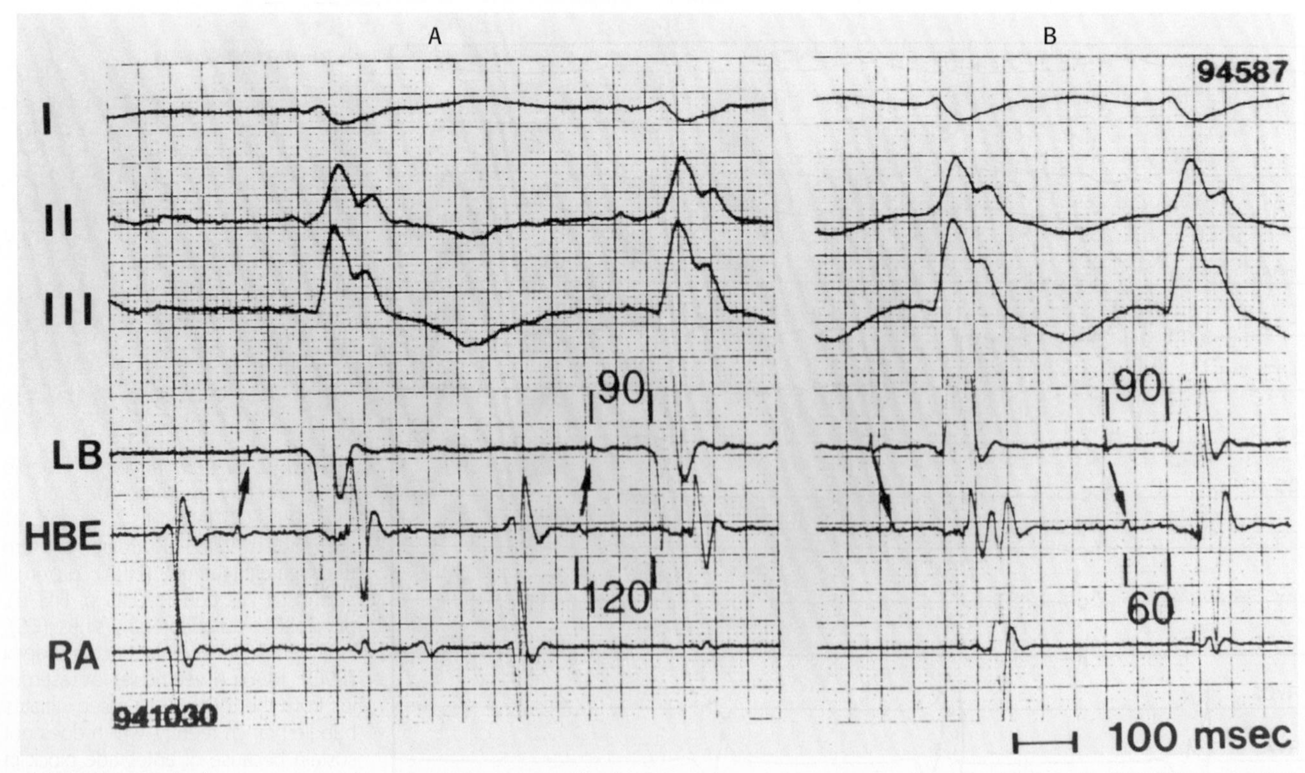


**FIGURE 2-59** *Analog recordings of intrafascicular reentry.* ECG leads are shown with recordings from the His bundle (HBE), LBB, and RV.

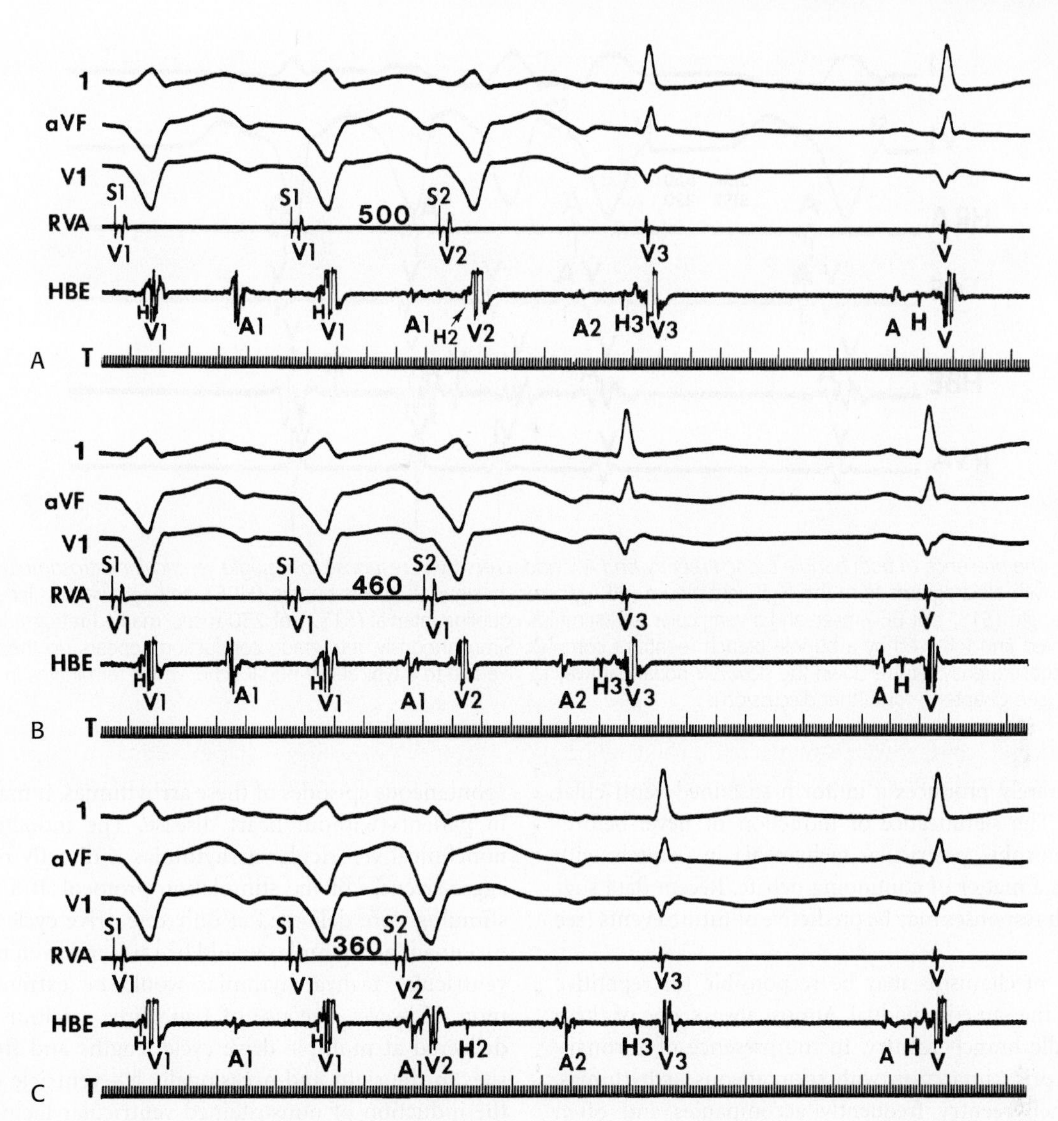


**FIGURE 2-60** *Repetitive responses that are due to A-V nodal reentry.* **A–C:** Leads 1, aVF, V1, and electrograms from the right ventricular apex (RVA) and His bundle (HBE). The basic drive cycle length is 600 msec when progressively premature ventricular extrastimuli (S2) are delivered. Note the presence of a retrograde His deflection on the basic drive complexes. **A:** An S2 delivered at 500 msec results in retrograde H-A delay (compare H2-A2, H1-A1) and an A-V nodal echo (H3-V3). **B:** As S1-S2 is shortened to 460 msec, the retrograde His becomes lost in V2. H2-A2 must have been similar to that in panel **(A)**, because A2-A3 in **(A)** and **(B)** are comparable. **C:** When S1-S2 is shortened to 360 msec, however, marked delay occurs in V2-H2. This results in more time for A-V nodal recovery so that H2-A2 decreases. As H2-A2 decreases, the incidence of fast pathway shortens, and the A2-H3 increases. The reciprocal relationship between H2-A2 and A2-H3 can therefore be seen because of the ability to note a retrograde His deflection.

incidence of repetitive responses increases when increasing number of stimuli, increasing number of drive cycle lengths, and increasing number of stimulation sites are used. When these responses last for several beats, they are frequently polymorphic, and in occasional instances they may even degenerate into ventricular fibrillation. In patients without prior clinical arrhythmias, such responses have not been found to have clinical significance.[106,111–114] The repetitive intraventricular reentrant responses that one observes are usually nonsustained (1 to 30 complexes) and typically polymorphic. As noted, in occasional instances polymorphic tachycardias may degenerate to ventricular fibrillation. These should be considered "normal" responses and should not be treated in patients with normal hearts and no clinical ventricular arrhythmias. This is in contrast to the induction of sustained monomorphic tachycardia by routine or even aggressive stimulation techniques, which in my opinion remains highly specific, occurring only in those populations of patients who have had sustained monomorphic tachycardia; symptoms compatible with this arrhythmia (e.g., syncope); and/or a substrate known to produce this arrhythmia, that is, recent myocardial infarction or old infarction, particularly with aneurysm. In the latter two instances, one may occasionally induce a uniform tachycardia that has not been seen before the electrophysiologic study. The clinical significance of these tachycardias remains to be evaluated by long-term follow-up. However, it can be stated in general that in the absence of spontaneous ventricular arrhythmias, and of acute infarction or a large ventricular aneurysm, ventricular

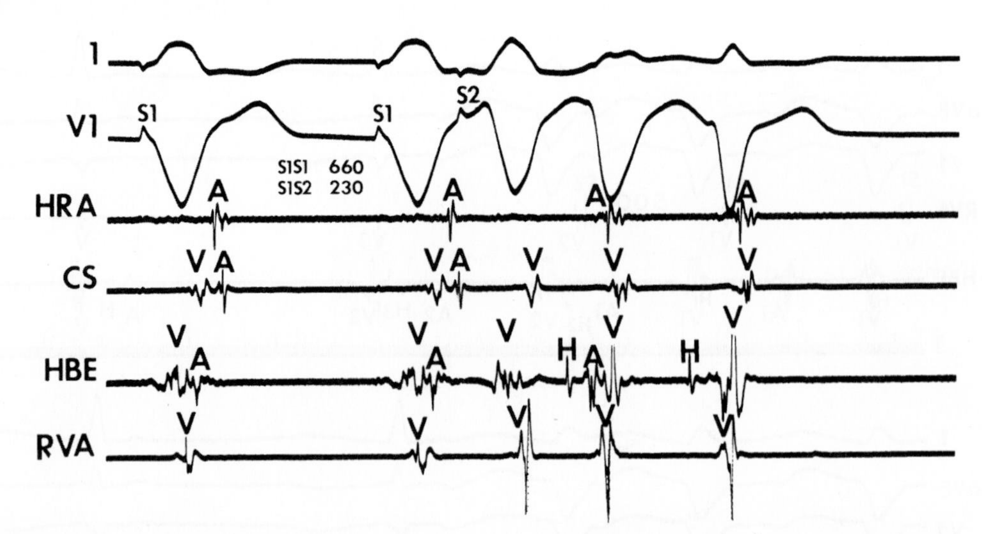


**FIGURE 2-61** *The presence of both bundle branch reentry and A-V nodal reentry in response to a single ventricular extrastimulus.* Leads 1 and V1 are shown with electrograms from the high-right atrium (HRA), coronary sinus (CS), His bundle (HBE), and right ventricular apex (RVA). At a drive cycle length (S1S1) of 660 msec and a ventricular extrastimulus coupling interval (S1S2) of 230 msec, marked retrograde His–Purkinje delay is observed and followed by a bundle branch reentrant complex. Simultaneously, retrograde conduction appears up the fast A-V nodal pathway and subsequently returns down the slow A-V nodal pathway to give rise to a typical A-V nodal echo, which terminates in the antegrade slow pathway (see Chapter 8 for further discussion).

stimulation rarely produces a uniform sustained ventricular tachycardia. The significance of induction of never-before-seen monomorphic ventricular tachycardia in patients with a substrate is a matter of continuing debate. Recent data suggest that such responses may be predictive of future events (see Chapter 11).

Multiple mechanisms may be responsible for repetitive responses in the same individual. Almost always, one of these will be bundle branch reentry. In the presence of coronary disease and prior infarction with spontaneous arrhythmias, bundle branch reentry frequently accompanies and often introduces intraventricular reentrant responses. Less commonly but also observed are the presence of bundle branch reentry and A-V nodal reentry, an example of which is shown in Figure 2-61. In this figure two repetitive responses are produced in response to an extrastimulus delivered from the right ventricular apex. The first is associated with V-H prolongation and has a configuration similar to that of pacing. The second has a normal QRS complex and is due to typical A-V nodal reentry with retrograde conduction during the bundle branch reentrant complex up the fast pathway, which subsequently conducts antegradely down the slow pathway to produce the second ventricular echo that is due to A-V nodal reentry. The responses terminate by block in the A-V node. Induction of A-V nodal reentry by ventricular stimulation is most common by this mechanism (see Chapter 8).

### *Safety of Ventricular Stimulation*

In more than 10,000 patients undergoing ventricular stimulation, I have observed that the induction of clinically irrelevant malignant ventricular arrhythmias, including ventricular fibrillation, can occur in patients who have not had spontaneous episodes of these arrhythmias. It may even occur in patients without heart disease. The induction of these nonclinical ventricular arrhythmias is directly related to the aggressiveness of the stimulation protocol. If a single extrastimulus were delivered at only one drive cycle length, such malignant arrhythmias would be rare, and even nonsustained ventricular tachyarrhythmias would be extremely uncommon. However, the use of two, three, or four extrastimuli delivered at multiple drive cycle lengths and from multiple sites in the right and occasionally left ventricle can result in the induction of nonsustained ventricular tachyarrhythmias (or ventricular fibrillation) in 40% to 50% of patients.[111,112] As a consequence, we have curtailed our stimulation protocol, limiting it to two extrastimuli, when patients without a clinical history compatible with malignant ventricular arrhythmias are studied. Where the induction of a lethal arrhythmia may have a clinical counterpart, more aggressive stimulation protocols will be used (see Chapter 11). It is important to note that the use of increased current may also produce nonclinical, and potentially lethal, arrhythmias. As a result, we continue to do our stimulation at twice threshold with 1-msec pulse width. In my opinion, pulses greater than 2 msec have not been shown to be safe. We currently use high current strengths in two circumstances. The first is when we are determining strength–interval curves. In this instance, we use high current strengths only with a single extrastimulus. Even this has led to sustained ventricular arrhythmias in one patient who had not had a similar arrhythmia spontaneously. We also use high current to overcome drug-induced prolongation of refractoriness to assess the presence and mechanism of effective antiarrhythmic therapy (see Chapter 13). We have observed an increased incidence of nonclinical arrhythmias using this protocol with up to three extrastimuli. Thus, it is apparent that great care must be used during ventricular stimulation, particularly when more than two extrastimuli are delivered. The entire electrophysiologic team, physicians and technicians, should be aware of the potential induction of lethal sustained arrhythmias when aggressive stimulation protocols are used.

## Comparison of Antegrade and Retrograde Conduction

Available data suggest that antegrade conduction is better than retrograde conduction in the majority of patients.[69–71] However, exact comparisons of antegrade and retrograde within different segments of the A-V conducting system cannot be made because of the inherent limitations of current techniques. Most obvious is the inability to record a His bundle deflection during ventricular stimulation. In its absence, the exact site of conduction delay or block cannot be ascertained; that is, one cannot distinguish retrograde His–Purkinje from A-V nodal delay. Furthermore, the exact retrograde input to the A-V node (H1-H2) cannot be determined. We overcome this problem by using narrower bipolar recording electrodes. Retrograde His deflections can now be recorded in the vast majority of patients with normal QRS complexes. Even when a His bundle deflection is recorded, exact comparisons of antegrade and retrograde A-V nodal conduction cannot be made, because it is not possible to determine the exact point at which an antegrade atrial impulse enters the A-V node. The A-H interval is only an approximation of A-V nodal conduction time; it is a measurement with a recognizable output time (the onset of the His bundle deflection) but no finite input. Retrograde measurement of A-V nodal conduction may be more accurate because the time of input can be defined by the end of the His bundle deflection and because the output is readily defined by the earliest onset of atrial activity.

In an analogous fashion, one cannot determine the site at which the ventricular stimulus enters the His–Purkinje system. During right ventricular stimulation, the site of entry certainly differs from the site of exit during antegrade conduction (i.e., the left ventricular endocardium). Furthermore, the measurement of retrograde His–Purkinje conduction includes an unknown and variable amount of time for the impulse to travel from the site of ventricular excitation to a site of entry into the His–Purkinje system. Finally, it is uncertain whether or not the same areas within the His–Purkinje system are stressed by antegrade and retrograde stimulation; that is, the actual site of antegrade and retrograde conduction delay and/or block may differ. Those factors invariably result in V-H intervals that are longer than H-V intervals at comparable cycle lengths and that preclude direct comparison of antegrade and retrograde His–Purkinje conduction times.

From a practical standpoint, prediction of the patterns of retrograde conduction from antegrade conduction patterns is not always possible. The response to incremental pacing at two cycle lengths may differ because of the opposite effects of cycle length on A-V nodal and His–Purkinje refractoriness. During incremental atrial and/or ventricular pacing, the A-V node is normally the site of conduction delay and block because progressive shorter cycle lengths produce progressive increases in A-V nodal refractoriness. In response to extrastimuli, however, any site may be associated with conduction delay or block. Although these sites may be markedly influenced by the drive cycle length, most commonly, delay or block occurs in the A-V node in response to atrial extrastimuli and in the His–Purkinje system during ventricular stimulation.

## ■ REFERENCES


1. Damato AN, Lau SH, Helfant R, et al. A study of heart block in man using His bundle recordings. *Circulation* 1969;39:297–305.
2. Narula OS, Cohen LS, Samet P, et al. Localization of A-V conduction defects in man by recording of the His bundle electrogram. *Am J Cardiol* 1970;25:228–237.
3. Damato AN, Lau SH. Clinical value of the electrogram of the conduction system. *Prog Cardiovasc Dis* 1970;13:119–140.
4. Puech P, Grolleau R. Les blocs auriculoventriculaires. Classification basée sur Fenregistrement de l'activité du tissue de conduction. *Coeur Med Interne* 1971;10:615.
5. Narula OS, Scherlag BJ, Samet P, et al. Atrioventricular block. Localization and classification by His bundle recordings. *Am J Med* 1971;50:146–165.
6. Castellanos A Jr., Castillo CA, Agha AS. Symposium on electrophysiologic correlates of clinical arrhythmias. 3. Contribution of His bundle recordings to the understanding of clinical arrhythmias. *Am J Cardiol* 1971;28:499–508.
7. Kupersmith J, Krongrad E, Waldo AL. Conduction intervals and conduction velocity in the human cardiac conduction system. Studies during open-heart surgery. *Circulation* 1973;47:776–785.
8. Kupersmith J. Electrophysiologic mapping during open heart surgery. *Prog Cardiovasc Dis* 1976;19:167–202.
9. Schuilenburg RM, Durrer D. Problems in the recognition of conduction disturbances in the His bundle. *Circulation* 1975;51:68–74.
10. Rosen KM, Rahimtoola SH, Sinno MZ, et al. Bundle branch and ventricular activation in man: a study using catheter recordings of left and right bundle branch potentials. *Circulation* 1971;43:193–203.
11. Narula OS, Scherlag BJ, Samet P. Pervenous pacing of the specialized conducting system in man. His bundle and A-V nodal stimulation. *Circulation* 1970;41:77–87.
12. Narula OS, Samet P. Pervenous pacing of the A-V junction in man. *Fed Proc* 1969;28:269.
13. Scherlac BJ, Samet P, Helfant RH. His bundle electrogram. A critical appraisal of its uses and limitations. *Circulation* 1972;46:601–613.
14. Puech P, Latour H, Grolleau R, et al. [Electric activity of atrioventricular conduction tissue in intracavitary electrocardiography. I. Identification]. *Arch Mal Coeur Vaiss* 1970;63:500–520.
15. Kupersmith J, Krongrad E, Bowman FO Jr, et al. Pacing the human cardiac conduction system during open-heart surgery. *Circulation* 1974;50:499–506.
16. Rosen KM, Heller R, Ehsani A, et al. Localization of site of traumatic heart block with His bundle recordings: electrophysiologic observations regarding the nature of "split" H potentials. *Am J Cardiol* 1972;30:412–417.
17. Haft JI. The His bundle electrogram. *Circulation* 1973;47:897–911.
18. Damato A, Schnitzler RN, Lau SH, eds. *Recent advances in the bundle of His electrograms* Philadelphia, PA: Lea & Febiger, 1973.
19. Williams DO, Scherlag BJ, Hope RR, et al. Selective versus non-selective His bundle pacing. *Cardiovasc Res* 1976;10:91–100.
20. Reddy CP, Damato AN, Akhtar M, et al. Time dependent changes in the functional properties of the atrioventricular conduction system in man. *Circulation* 1975;52:1012–1022.
21. Batsford WP, Akhtar M, Caracta AR, et al. Effect of atrial stimulation site on the electrophysiological properties of the atrioventricular node in man. *Circulation* 1974;50:283–292.
22. Leon FY, Denes P, Wu D, et al. Effects of atrial pacing site on atrial and atrioventricular nodal function. *Br Heart J* 1975;37:576–582.

23. Schuilenburg RM, Durrer D. Conduction disturbances located within the His bundle. *Circulation* 1972;45:612–628.
24. Schuilenburg RM. Evaluation of atrio-ventricular conduction by intracardiac electrocardiography and stimulation. *Heart Bull* 1974;5:11.
25. Bekheit S, Murtagh JG, Morton P, et al. Measurements of sinus impulse conduction from electrogram of bundle of His. *Br Heart J* 1971;33:612.
26. Bekheit S, Murtagh JG, Morton P, et al. Studies of heart block with His bundle electrograms. *Br Heart J* 1972;34:717–734.
27. Rosen KM. Evaluation of cardiac conduction in the cardiac catheterization laboratory. *Am J Cardiol* 1972;30:701–703.
28. Gallagher JJ, Damato AN, eds. *Technique of recording His bundle activity in man* Philadelphia, PA: Lea & Febiger, 1974.
29. Bekheit S, Morton P, Murtagh JG, et al. Comparison of sinoventricular conduction in children and adults using bundle of His electrograms. *Br Heart J* 1973;35:507–515.
30. Varghese PJ, Elizari MV, Lau SH, et al. His bundle electrograms of dog. Correlation with intracellular recordings. *Circulation* 1973;48:753–760.
31. Danzig MD, Robertson TL, Webber LS, et al. Earlier onset of QRS in anterior precordial ECG leads: precision of time interval measurements. *Circulation* 1976;54:447–451.
32. Josephson ME, Scharf DL, Kastor JA, et al. Atrial endocardial activation in man. Electrode catheter technique of endocardial mapping. *Am J Cardiol* 1977;39:972–981.
33. Wyndham CR, Shantha N, Dhingra RC, et al. P-A interval: lack of clinical, electrocardiographic and electrophysiologic correlations. *Chest* 1975;68:533–537.
34. Hoffman BF, Cranefield PF. *Electrophysiology of the heart.* Mount Kisco, NY: Futura Publishing Company, 1976.
35. Bekheit S, Murtagh G, Morton P, et al. His bundle electrogram in P mitrale. *Br Heart J* 1972;34:1057–1061.
36. Josephson ME, Kastor JA, Morganroth J. Electrocardiographic left atrial enlargement. Electrophysiologic, echocardiographic and hemodynamic correlates. *Am J Cardiol* 1977;39:967–971.
37. Josephson ME, Kastor JA. Supraventricular tachycardia: mechanisms and management. *Ann Intern Med* 1977;87:346–358.
38. Barold SS, Fracp MB, Coumel P. Mechanisms of atrioventricular junctional tachycardia. Role of reentry and concealed accessory bypass tracts. *Am J Cardiol* 1977;39:97–106.
39. Gallagher JJ, Gilbert M, Svenson RH, et al. Wolff-Parkinson-White syndrome. The problem, evaluation, and surgical correction. *Circulation* 1975;51:767–785.
40. Wellens HJ, Durrer D. The role of an accessory atrioventricular pathway in reciprocal tachycardia. Observations in patients with and without the Wolff-Parkinson-White syndrome. *Circulation* 1975;52:58–72.
41. Amat-y-Leon F, Dhingra RC, Wu D, et al. Catheter mapping of retrograde atrial activation. Observations during ventricular pacing and AV nodal re-entrant paroxysmal tachycardia. *Br Heart J* 1976;38:355–362.
42. Cassidy DM, Vassallo JA, Marchlinski FE, et al. Endocardial mapping in humans in sinus rhythm with normal left ventricles: activation patterns and characteristics of electrograms. *Circulation* 1984;70:37–42.
43. Vassallo JA, Cassidy DM, Kindwall KE, et al. Nonuniform recovery of excitability in the left ventricle. *Circulation* 1988;78:1365–1372.
44. Horowitz LN, Alexander JA, Edmunds LH Jr. Postoperative right bundle branch block: identification of three levels of block. *Circulation* 1980; 62:319–328.
45. Vassallo JA, Cassidy DM, Marchlinski FE, et al. Endocardial activation of left bundle branch block. *Circulation* 1984;69:914–923.
46. Josephson ME, Horowitz LN, Farshidi A, et al. Recurrent sustained ventricular tachycardia. 2. Endocardial mapping. *Circulation* 1978;57:440–447.
47. Josephson ME, Horowitz LN, Spielman SR, et al. Role of catheter mapping in the preoperative evaluation of ventricular tachycardia. *Am J Cardiol* 1982;49:207–220.
48. Cassidy DM, Vassallo JA, Buxton AE, et al. The value of catheter mapping during sinus rhythm to localize site of origin of ventricular tachycardia. *Circulation* 1984;69:1103–1110.
49. Cassidy DM, Vassallo JA, Miller JM, et al. Endocardial catheter mapping in patients in sinus rhythm: relationship to underlying heart disease and ventricular arrhythmias. *Circulation* 1986;73:645–652.
50. Sung RJ, Tamer DM, Garcia OL, et al. Analysis of surgically-induced right bundle branch block pattern using intracardiac recording techniques. *Circulation* 1976;54:442–446.
51. Kastor JA, Goldreyer BN, Moore EN, et al. Intraventricular conduction in man studied with an endocardial electrode catheter mapping technique. Patients with normal QRS and right bundle branch block. *Circulation* 1975;51:786–796.
52. Marchlinski FE Callans DJ, Gottlieb CD, et al. Linear ablation lesions for control of unmappable ventricular tachycardia in patients with ischemic and nonischemic cardiomyopathy. *Circulation* 2000;101:1288–1296.
53. Garcia FC, Bazan V, Zado ES, et al. Epicardial substrate and outcome with epicardial ablation of ventricular tachycardia in arrhythmogenic right ventricular cardiomyopathy/dysplasia. *Circulation* 2009;120:366–375.
54. Callans DJ, Ren JF, Michele J, et al. Electroanatomic left ventricular mapping in the porcine model of healed anterior myocardial infarction. Correlation with intracardiac echocardiography and pathological analysis. *Circulation* 1999;100:1744–1750.
55. Polin GM, Haqqani H, Tzou W, et al. Endocardial unipolar voltage mapping to identify epicardial substrate in arrhythmogenic right ventricular cardiomyopathy/dysplasia. *Heart Rhythm* 2011;8:76–83.
56. Hutchinson MD, Gerstenfeld EP, Desjardins B, et al. Endocardial unipolar voltage mapping to detect epicardial ventricular tachycardia substrate in patients with nonischemic left ventricular cardiomyopathy. *Circ Arrhythm Electrophysiol* 2011;4:49–55.
57. Durrer D, van Dam RT, Freud GE, et al. Total excitation of the isolated human heart. *Circulation* 1970;41:899–912.
58. Aranda J, Castellanos A, Moleiro F, et al. Effects of the pacing site on A-H conduction and refractoriness in patients with short P-R intervals. *Circulation* 1976;53:33–39.
59. Zhang X, Fisher JD, Kim SG, et al. Comparison of ramp and stepwise incremental pacing in assessment of antegrade and retrograde conduction. *Pacing Clin Electrophysiol* 1986;9:42–52.
60. Lehmann MH, Denker S, Mahmud R, et al. Patterns of human atrioventricular nodal accommodation to a sudden acceleration of atrial rate. *Am J Cardiol* 1984;53:71–76.
61. Castillo C, Maytin O, Castellanos A Jr. His bundle recordings in atypical A-V nodal Wenckebach block during cardiac pacing. *Am J Cardiol* 1971;27:570–576.
62. Dressier W, Swiller SL. Atypical Wenckebach periods with dropped atrial beats. *Am J Cardiol* 1958;2:575.
63. Denes P, Levy L, Pick A, et al. The incidence of typical and atypical A-V Wenckebach periodicity. *Am Heart J* 1975;89:26–31.
64. Bissett JK, Kane JJ, De Soyza N, et al. Electrophysiological significance of rapid atrial pacing as a test of atrioventricular conduction. *Cardiovasc Res* 1975;9:593–599.
65. Damato AN, Varghese PJ, Caracta AR, et al. Functional 2:1 A-V block within the His-Purkinje system. Simulation of type II second-degree A-V block. *Circulation* 1973;47:534–542.
66. Lehmann MH, Denker S, Mahmud R, et al. Postextrasystolic alterations in refractoriness of the His-Purkinje system and ventricular myocardium in man. *Circulation* 1984;69:1096–1102.
67. Castillo C, Samet P. Retrograde conduction in complete heart block. *Br Heart J* 1967;29:553–558.
68. Gupta PK, Haft JI. Retrograde ventriculoatrial conduction in complete heart block: studies with His bundle electrography. *Am J Cardiol* 1972;30:408–411.
69. Takeshita A, Tanaka S, Nakamura M. Study of retrograde conduction in complete heart block using His bundle recordings. *Br Heart J* 1974; 36:462–467.
70. Schuilenburg RM, ed. *Patterns of V-A conduction in the human heart in the presence of normal and abnormal A-V conduction.* Phildelphia, PA: Lea & Febiger, 1976.
71. Akhtar M, Damato AN, Batsford WP, et al. A comparative analysis of antegrade and retrograde conduction patterns in man. *Circulation* 1975; 52:766–778.
72. Goldreyer BN, Bigger JT Jr. Ventriculo-atrial conduction in man. *Circulation* 1970;41:935–946.
73. Narula OS. Retrograde pre-excitation. Comparison of antegrade and retrograde conduction intervals in man. *Circulation* 1974;50:1129–1143.
74. Akhtar M. Retrograde conduction in man. *Pacing Clin Electrophysiol* 1981;4:548–562.
75. Gallagher JJ, Damato AN, Varghese PJ, et al. Manifest and concealed reentry: a mechanism of A-V nodal Wenckebach in man. *Circulation* 1973;47:752–757.
76. Damato AN, Lau SH, Bobb GA. Studies on ventriculo-atrial conduction and the reentry phenomenon. *Circulation* 1970;41:423–435.
77. Krayer O, Mandoki JJ, Mendez C, et al. Studies on veratrum alkaloids. XVI. The action of epinephrine and of veratramine on the functional

refractory period of the auriculo-ventricular transmission in the heart-lung preparation of the dog. *J Pharmacol Exp Ther* 1951;103: 412–419.
78. Moe GK, Preston JB, Burlington H. Physiologic evidence for a dual A-V transmission system. *Circ Res* 1956;4:357–375.
79. Damato AN, Lau SH, Patton RD, et al. A study of atrioventricular conduction in man using premature atrial stimulation and His bundle recordings. *Circulation* 1969;40:61–69.
80. Wit AL, Weiss MB, Berkowitz WD, et al. Patterns of atrioventricular conduction in the human heart. *Circ Res* 1970;27:345–359.
81. Greenspan AM, Camardo JS, Horowitz LN, et al. Human ventricular refractoriness: effects of increasing current. *Am J Cardiol* 1981;47:244–250.
82. Cagin NA, Kunstadt D, Wolfish P, et al. The influence of heart rate on the refractory period of the atrium and A-V conducting system. *Am Heart J* 1973;85:358.
83. Denes P, Wu D, Dhingra R, et al. The effects of cycle length on cardiac refractory periods in man. *Circulation* 1974;49:32–41.
84. Simson MB, Spear JF, Moore EN. Electrophysiologic studies on atrioventricular nodal Wenckebach cycles. *Am J Cardiol* 1978;41:244–258.
85. Denker S, Shenasa M, Gilbert CJ, et al. Effects of abrupt changes in cycle length on refractoriness of the His-Purkinje system in man. *Circulation* 1983;67:60–68.
86. Denker S, Lehmann MH, Mahmud R, et al. Divergence between refractoriness of His-Purkinje system and ventricular muscle with abrupt changes in cycle length. *Circulation* 1983;68:1212–1221.
87. Cain ME, Martin TC, Marchlinski FE, et al. Changes in ventricular refractoriness after an extrastimulus: effects of prematurity, cycle length and procainamide. *Am J Cardiol* 1983;52:996–1001.
88. Marchlinski FE. Characterization of oscillations in ventricular refractoriness in man after an abrupt increment in heart rate. *Circulation* 1987;75:550–556.
89. Vassallo JA, Marchlinski FE, Cassidy DM, et al. Shortening of ventricular refractoriness with extrastimuli: role of the degree of prematurity and number of extrastimuli. *J Electrophysiol* 1988;2:227–236.
90. Akhtar M, Denker ST, Lehmann MH, et al., eds. *Effects of sudden cycle length alteration on refractoriness of human His-Purkinje system and ventricular myocardium.* Orlando, FL: Grune & Stratton, 1985.
91. Prystowsky EN, Jackman WM, Rinkenberger RL, et al. Effect of autonomic blockade on ventricular refractoriness and atrioventricular nodal conduction in humans. Evidence supporting a direct cholinergic action on ventricular muscle refractoriness. *Circ Res* 1981;49:511–518.
92. Prystowsky EN, Naccarelli GV, Jackman WM, et al. Enhanced parasympathetic tone shortens atrial refractoriness in man. *Am J Cardiol* 1983;51:96–100.
93. Han J, Moe GK. Nonuniform Recovery of Excitability in Ventricular Muscle. *Circ Res* 1964;14:44–60.
94. Kuo CS, Atarashi H, Reddy CP, et al. Dispersion of ventricular repolarization and arrhythmia: study of two consecutive ventricular premature complexes. *Circulation* 1985;72:370–376.
95. Burgess MJ, Coyle J. Effects of premature depolarization on refractoriness of ischemic canine myocardium. *J Electrocardiol* 1982;15:335–344.
96. Rozanski GJ, Jalife J, Moe GK. Determinants of postrepolarization refractoriness in depressed mammalian ventricular muscle. *Circ Res* 1984;55: 486–496.
97. Millar CK, Kralios FA, Lux RL. Correlation between refractory periods and activation-recovery intervals from electrograms: effects of rate and adrenergic interventions. *Circulation* 1985;72:1372–1379.
98. Luck JC, Minor ST, Mann DE, et al. Effect of bradycardia on dispersion of ventricular refractoriness. *Am J Cardiol* 1985;55:1009–1014.
99. Friehling TD, Kowey PR, Shechter JA, et al. Effect of site of pacing on dispersion of refractoriness. *Am J Cardiol* 1985;55:1339–1343.
100. Franz MR. Long-term recording of monophasic action potentials from human endocardium. *Am J Cardiol* 1983;51:1629–1634.
101. Akhtar M, Damato AN, Batsford WP, et al. Unmasking and conversion of gap phenomenon in the human heart. *Circulation* 1974;49:624–630.
102. Josephson ME, Kastor JA. His-Purkinje conduction during retrograde stress. *J Clin Invest* 1978;61:171–177.
103. Akhtar M, Damato AN, Caracta AR, et al. The gap phenomena during retrograde conduction in man. *Circulation* 1974;49:811–817.
104. Akhtar M, Gilbert CJ, Wolf FG, et al. Retrograde conduction in the His-Purkinje system. Analysis of the routes of impulse propagation using His and right bundle branch recordings. *Circulation* 1979;59:1252–1265.
105. Akhtar M, Denker S, Lehmann MH, et al. Macro-reentry within the His Purkinje system. *Pacing Clin Electrophysiol* 1983;6:1010–1028.
106. Farshidi A, Michelson EL, Greenspan AM, et al. Repetitive responses to ventricular extrastimuli: incidence, mechanism, and significance. *Am Heart J* 1980;100:59–68.
107. Roy D, Brugada P, Bar FW, et al. Repetitive responses to ventricular extrastimuli: incidence and significance in patients without organic heart disease. *Eur Heart J* 1983;4:79–85.
108. Schuilenburg RM, Durrer D. Ventricular echo beats in the human heart elicited by induced ventricular premature beats. *Circulation* 1969; 40:337–347.
109. Akhtar M, Damato AN, Ruskin JN, et al. Characteristics and coexistence of two forms of ventricular echo phenomena. *Am Heart J* 1976;92:174–182.
110. Castillo C, Castellanos A Jr. Retrograde activation of the His bundle in the human heart. *Am J Cardiol* 1971;27:264–271.
111. Brugada P, Green M, Abdollah H, et al. Significance of ventricular arrhythmias initiated by programmed ventricular stimulation: the importance of the type of ventricular arrhythmia induced and the number of premature stimuli required. *Circulation* 1984;69:87–92.
112. Brugada P, Abdollah H, Heddle B, et al. Results of a ventricular stimulation protocol using a maximum of 4 premature stimuli in patients without documented or suspected ventricular arrhythmias. *Am J Cardiol* 1983;52:1214–1218.
113. Breithardt G, Abendroth RR, Borggrefe M, et al. Prevalence and clinical significance of the repetitive ventricular response during sinus rhythm in coronary disease patients. *Am Heart J* 1984;107:229–236.
114. Morady F, Shapiro W, Shen E, et al. Programmed ventricular stimulation in patients without spontaneous ventricular tachycardia. *Am Heart J* 1984;107:875–882.

CHAPTER

# 3 Sinus Node Function

Disorders of sinus node function are an important cause of cardiac syncope. Approximately 50% of permanent pacemakers implanted at our own and other institutions are for the specific treatment of bradyarrhythmias, caused by sinus node dysfunction. This number is increasing as the number of elderly people in our population rises. This has been associated with an increase in symptomatic disorders of sinus node dysfunction, particularly the bradycardia–tachycardia syndrome. Clinical disorders of sinus node dysfunction can be characterized as abnormalities of automaticity or conduction, or both. Automaticity refers to the ability of pacemaker cells within the sinus node to undergo spontaneous depolarization and generate impulses at a rate faster than other latent cardiac pacemakers. Once generated, the impulses must be conducted through and out of the sinus node to depolarize the atrium. Delay or failure of conduction can occur within the sinus node itself or at the sinoatrial junction in the perinodal tissue. The methods by which sinus node automaticity and conduction are evaluated include ECG monitoring, atrial stimulation techniques, and direct recording of the sinus node. The assessment of the influence of autonomic tone on these parameters can provide additional information concerning inherent sinus node function.

## ELECTROCARDIOGRAPHIC FEATURES OF SINUS NODE DYSFUNCTION

Because no method is currently available to directly record sinus node activity from the body surface in humans, noninvasive evaluation of sinus node automaticity and conduction must be made by indirect methods. Therefore, we attempt to assess sinus function electrographically by analyzing the frequency and pattern of atrial depolarization, that is, P-wave morphology, frequency, and regularity.

### Sinus Bradycardia

When persistent and unexplained, sinus bradycardia (a rate less than 60 beats per minute [bpm]) is said to reflect impaired sinus automaticity. The value of 60 bpm, an arbitrary one, is extremely nonspecific, and it has led to the misclassification of many normal persons as abnormal. Kirk and Kvorning analyzed the ECGs of 482 consecutive patients admitted to the general medicine service; their results suggested that a rate of less than 60 bpm would classify one-third of all men and one-fifth of all women as abnormal.[1] A study that involved 24-hour Holter monitoring of 50 healthy medical students revealed that all the students had sinus bradycardia at some time during the 24-hour period and 26% of the students had significant sinus bradycardia (a rate less than 40 bpm) during the day.[2] Because autonomic tone plays such an important role in determining the sinus rate, we believe that an isolated heart rate of less than 60 bpm should not be considered abnormal, particularly in asymptomatic people, unless it is persistent, inappropriate for physiologic circumstances, and cannot be explained by other factors. Sinus bradycardia usually results in dizziness, fatigue, mental status changes, and dyspnea on exertion if chronotropic insufficiency is marked.

### Sinoatrial Block and Sinus Arrest

Both sinus arrest and exit block are definite manifestations of sinus node dysfunction. Although sinoatrial block is a conduction disturbance, it remained unsettled whether sinus arrest actually reflects impaired or absent sinus automaticity or varying degrees of sinus exit block. Recently, use of direct recordings of the sinus node has allowed one to ascertain the cause of such pauses (see later section in this chapter entitled Sinus Node Electrogram). Symptoms are uncommon unless pauses are marked. When this happens, syncope can occur.

### Bradycardia–tachycardia Syndrome

In our own experience and the experience of others, the bradycardia–tachycardia syndrome is the most frequently encountered form of symptomatic sinus node dysfunction, and it is associated with the highest incidence of syncope.[3] The syncope is generally associated with the marked pauses following the cessation of paroxysmal supraventricular tachyarrhythmias that occur in the setting of sinus bradycardia (primarily atrial fibrillation). Of importance is the recognition that a prolonged asystolic period occurring in the setting of any form of sinus node dysfunction also implies impaired function of lower (nonsinus) pacemakers. The drugs used to prevent atrial fibrillation or control its rate are often responsible for the symptomatic bradycardias following cessation of the arrhythmia, and hence, the need for pacemakers. Syncope is much rarer in patients with isolated sinus bradycardia. When these patients are symptomatic, it is usually fatigue or dyspnea on exertion. Syncope in patients with isolated sinus bradycardia is usually neurocardiac. Autonomic reflex abnormalities consistent with neurocardiac syncope (see below) are usually present when syncope occurs in patients with isolated sinus bradycardia.[4]

## ELECTROCARDIOGRAPHIC MONITORING OF PATIENTS SUSPECTED OF HAVING SINUS NODE DYSFUNCTION

If a random ECG in a patient with episodic symptoms is normal, prolonged (24-hour) ECG monitoring is the next step in evaluating sinus node function. Unfortunately, most episodes of syncope or dizziness are paroxysmal and unpredictable, and even 24-hour monitoring may fail to include a symptomatic episode. The use of event recorders has improved our ability to correlate symptoms with sinus node dysfunction. In cases with infrequent episodes of syncope, an implantable event recorder is now available. It must be interrogated as a pacemaker currently, but in the near future, it will have automatic detection. Although asymptomatic sinus bradycardia may be noted frequently, its significance remains uncertain. The appropriateness of the sinus rate relative to the physiologic circumstances under which it occurs is critical in deciding whether there is an abnormality of sinus automaticity.

The frequency and clinical significance of sinus pauses have been studied.[4,5] Sinus pauses greater than or equal to 2 seconds were found in 84 (2.6%) of 3,259 consecutive 24-hour Holter monitor studies.[4] The pauses ranged from 2 to 15 seconds. The length of pause correlated poorly with symptoms and did not predict death. Most pauses were asymptomatic, whereas in the remainder, pauses could have produced symptoms. Pacemakers did not benefit asymptomatic people and failed to prevent dizziness, presyncope, and syncope in one-third of the patients in whom such symptoms were felt to be secondary to the pauses. In a second study of 6,470 Holters, 0.3% had sinus pauses greater than or equal to 3 seconds.[5] Only one patient was symptomatic during a pause. All patients did well without a pacemaker. Other studies have demonstrated pauses >2 seconds in 11% normals and in one-third of trained athletes.[6–8] Despite the limitations of retrospective studies, these data suggest that although rare, sinus pauses equal to or greater than 3 seconds, particularly when asymptomatic, need not be treated. As noted above, syncope in such instances is more likely neurocardiac in origin (Alboni). However, demonstration of symptomatic unexplained sinus bradycardia, long asystolic periods following paroxysmal tachyarrhythmias, sinus exit block, or sinus arrest is diagnostic of sinus dysfunction and may obviate the need for further diagnostic evaluation. Furthermore, 24-hour monitoring and/or event recorders can exclude sinus node dysfunction, atrioventricular (A-V) block, or cardiac arrhythmias as causes of syncope by demonstrating sinus rhythm during an attack.

## ASSESSMENT OF AUTONOMIC TONE

The response of the sinus node, including heart rate and heart rate variability, to changes in autonomic tone should be assessed in all patients suspected of having sinus node dysfunction. The assessment can be made pharmacologically by evaluating the response of the sinus node to atropine, isoproterenol, and propranolol. The effects of "pharmacologic denervation" can be evaluated after the concurrent administration of atropine and propranolol. The response to carotid sinus massage may be diagnostically useful in patients with syncope that is due to carotid sinus hypersensitivity in which there is a heightened response to vagal stimuli. Exercise testing offers another method of assessing sinus node response to enhanced sympathetic tone.[9]

Atropine (1 to 3 mg) is the most widely used agent to assess parasympathetic tone. The normal response is an acceleration of heart rate to greater than 90 bpm and an increase over the control rate of 20% to 50%.[10–17] Most patients with symptomatic sinus node dysfunction exhibit a blunted response to atropine.[11,13,17,18] Failure to increase the sinus rate to above the predicted intrinsic heart rate (IHR, see following discussion) following 0.04% mg/kg of atropine is diagnostic of impaired sinus node automaticity. In our experience, patients with asymptomatic isolated sinus bradycardia commonly show a normal or sometimes exaggerated chronotropic response.

Isoproterenol (1 to 3 mg/min) produces sinus acceleration of at least 25% in normal people.[10–12,17,19] An impaired response to isoproterenol correlates well with a blunted heart rate response to exercise observed in some patients with sinus node dysfunction.[9] The response of some patients with suspected sinus node dysfunction to isoproterenol is occasionally normal or even exaggerated. Such responses are not unexpected because the chronotropic responses to exercise in those patients are usually normal. This exaggerated response may represent a form of denervation hypersensitivity, with basal bradycardia that is due to a low resting sympathetic tone in contrast to a primary lack of responsiveness to sympathetic stimulation.

Propranolol has not been extensively studied in patients with the sick sinus syndrome. In normal persons, propranolol (0.1 mg/kg, up to 10 mg) produces a 12% to 22.5% increase in sinus cycle length.[20–22] A similar (17.4%) increase in sinus cycle length has been noted in a study of 10 patients with symptomatic sinus node disease.[17] Thus, the chronotropic response to propranolol is usually no different in patients with and those without sinus node dysfunction, suggesting that sympathetic tone and/or responsiveness is intact in most patients with sinus node dysfunction at rest.

Pharmacologic denervation using atropine (0.4 mg/kg) and propranolol (0.2 mg/kg) has been used to determine an IHR.[23–25] Tonken et al.[26] have suggested that lower doses

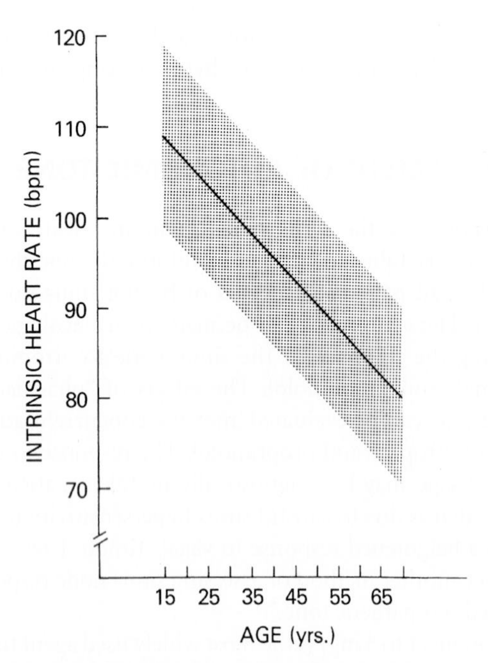


**FIGURE 3-1** *Relationship of intrinsic heart rate to age.* The stippled area delineates the normal range ±2 SD of intrinsic heart rate at different ages. (From Jose AD. Effect of combined sympathetic and parasympathetic blockade on heart rate and cardiac function in man. *Am J Cardiol* 1966;18:476.)

(0.03 mg/kg of atropine and 0.15 mg/kg of propranolol) are sufficient. The effects of this autonomic blockade peak after 5 minutes and are usually stable for 30 minutes. The IHR is age-dependent in persons 15- to 70-years old, and it can be defined by the regression equation: IHR = 117.2 − (0.57 × age) bpm (Fig. 3-1). Thus, the normal response to autonomic blockade usually results in an increase in heart rate. Because a depressed IHR correlates well with other abnormalities of sinus node function, the determination of the IHR in patients with isolated sinus bradycardia may more accurately identify patients who truly have sinus node dysfunction from those who have enhanced parasympathetic tone.[27]

This is evident from observations that tests of sinus node function are more often positive in patients with abnormal IHR. The IHR correlates well with the rate of the denervated sinus node of transplanted hearts.[28] Following autonomic blockade, the sinus cycle length is stable and allows for more reproducible results when electrophysiologic perturbations are employed (see following discussion). The response to atropine alone may provide as much information and obviate the need for propranolol. Failure of the sinus rate to accelerate above the predicted IHR is diagnostic of abnormal sinus automaticity.

Carotid sinus pressure (CSP) with ECG monitoring occasionally reveals patients in whom paroxysmal dizziness and/or syncope is due to a hypersensitive carotid sinus (see later section in this chapter entitled Vagal Hypersensitivity Syndromes). Pauses in excess of 3 seconds in response to 5 seconds of CSP are said to be abnormal and may be responsible for such symptoms. Similar pauses, however, may be observed in asymptomatic elderly people. We have observed ≥3 second pauses in 40% of asymptomatic patients ≥70-years old. Wellens (personal communication) has a similar experience. Thus, the use of CSP may give false-positive results. Only if pauses are long and produced symptoms identical to those occurring spontaneously should therapy be based on this isolated finding. Even then, all other potential causes of syncope should be ruled out. Other tests of autonomic reflexes include baroreceptor reflexes, valsalva maneuver, and, most commonly, the upright tilt test (see below).

Exercise testing using a Bruce or modified protocol has demonstrated that many patients with sinus node dysfunction have a blunted response to exercise when compared to controls at comparable oxygen consumption, but significant overlap exists. A chronotropic assessment protocol that focuses on intermediate workloads (3 to 5 METs) is more appropriate since symptomatic individuals have their symptoms at such activity. Even so, I believe too much overlap exists to rely on heart rate alone. Symptoms must be related to the inadequate heart rate.

## ELECTROPHYSIOLOGIC EVALUATION OF SINUS NODE FUNCTION

The evaluation of sinus node function should include the assessment of sinus automaticity and sinoatrial conduction as well as the effects of physiologic and pharmacologic interventions on these properties. Unfortunately, most methods used for these tests provide only indirect and impure analysis of sinus node automaticity and conduction. Notwithstanding, because of their widespread use, a description of these electrophysiologic tests follows. It is imperative that one understands the limitations of these tests if they are to be used to help make clinical decisions. The tests used to evaluate sinus node function have been recently evaluated by Benditt et al.

### Sinoatrial Conduction Time

The response of the sinus node to induced atrial premature depolarizations (APDs) has been used as an indirect method to evaluate sinoatrial conduction.[17,29–34] This method of evaluation involves the introduction of progressively premature APDs (A2) after every eighth to tenth beat of a stable sinus rhythm (A1-A1) and measurement of the first (A2-A3) and second (A3-A4) return cycles. Measurement A3-A4 allows one to assess the presence of depression of automaticity, which may be responsible for a variable component of the first return cycle. Four zones of response to APDs have been identified (Fig. 3-2). They can be best demonstrated by plotting the coupling interval of the APD (A1-A2) versus the return cycle (A2-A3) (Fig. 3-3). Many investigators prefer to normalize those values by dividing them by the spontaneous sinus cycle length (A1-A1) and deriving a percentage.

Zone I is the range of A1-A2 intervals at which the return cycle (A2-A3) is fully compensatory, that is, A1-A2 + A2-A3

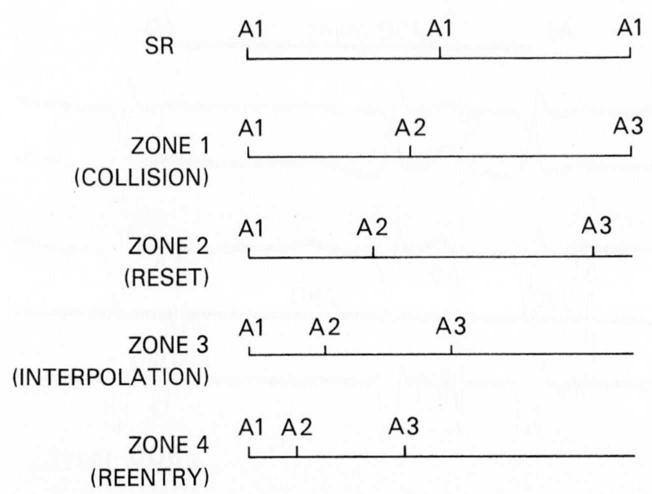


**FIGURE 3-2** *Response of the sinus node to atrial premature depolarizations (APDs).* Four zones of response are seen. A1-A1 is the spontaneous sinus cycle length. In zone 1 an APD (A2) delivered late in the cardiac cycle does not affect the sinus node, as manifested by the next sinus beats (A3) occurring on time. In zone II, a more premature A2 results in resetting of the sinus node so that A3 occurs early although A2-A3 is greater than A1-A1 owing to conduction time between the atrium and sinus node. In zone III, A2 results in a return cycle (A3) that is early. Since A2-A3 is less than A1-A1, that is, A2 is interpolated. In zone IV, A2 results in an even earlier return cycle, so that A1-A2 + A2-A3 < A1-A1 is consistent with sinus node reentry. See text for discussion.

(A1-A3) = 2 (A1-A1) (Fig. 3-4A). Zone I usually occurs in response to APDs falling in the last 20% to 30% of the spontaneous cycle length. Zone I is variously referred to as the zone of collision, interference, or nonreset because the mechanism of the response is a collision of the spontaneous sinus impulse with the stimulated atrial impulse (A2). Because the sinus pacemaker is therefore unaffected by A2, the subsequent sinus beat occurs "on time."

Zone II is the range of A1-A2 intervals at which reset of the sinus pacemaker occurs, resulting in an A2-A3 that exceeds the basic sinus cycle. However, the sum of A1-A2 and A2-A3 (A1-A3) is less than 2 (A1-A1); that is, it is less than compensatory (Fig. 3-4B). Zone II is a zone of long duration, typically occupying 40% to 50% of the cardiac cycle. In most patients, the pause (A2-A3) remains constant throughout zone II, producing a plateau in the curve. The plateau results because A2 penetrates the sinus node and resets the pacemaker without changing pacemaker automaticity. Because the duration of the return cycle (A2-A3) depends on conduction time into and out of the sinus node and sinus automaticity, the difference between A2-A3 and A1-A1 has been taken as an estimate of total sinoatrial conduction time. Conventionally, it has been assumed that conduction into and out of the sinus node is equal, resulting in the calculation of sinoatrial conduction time (SACT) as A2-A3-A1-A/-2 (Fig. 3-5).[25] Data suggest,

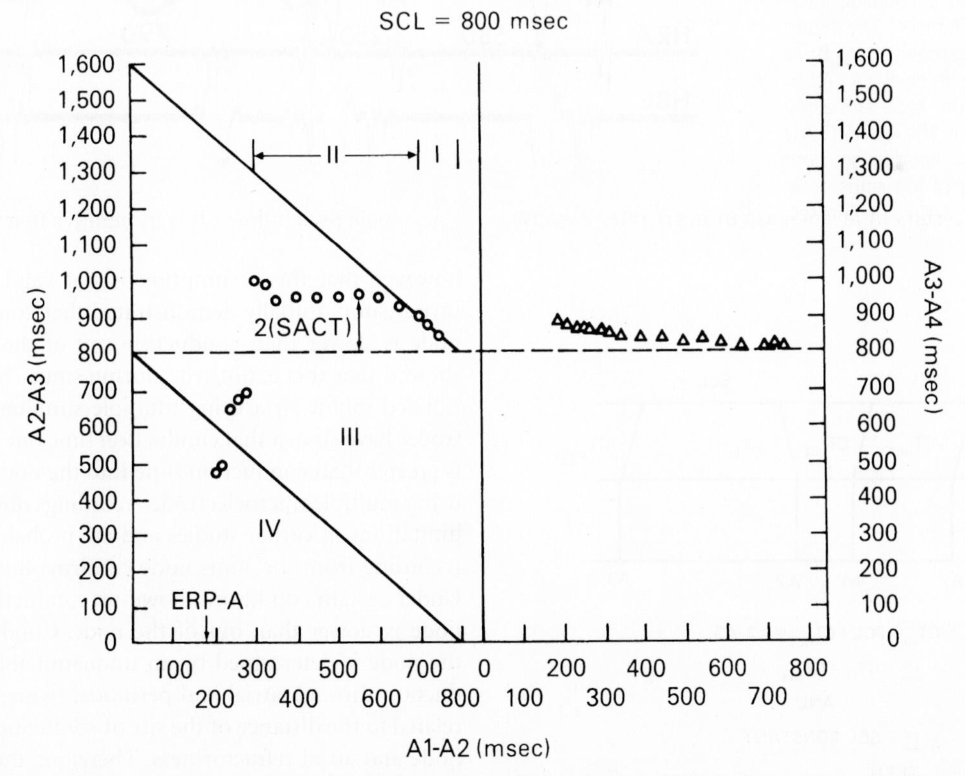


**FIGURE 3-3** *Graphic display of sinus node response to atrial premature depolarizations (APDs).* The spontaneous sinus cycle length (SCL) is 800 msec. The coupling intervals of the APD (A1-A2) are plotted on the abscissa, and the first return cycles (A2-A3, open circles) and the second return cycles (A3-A4, open triangles) are plotted on the ordinate. The upper and lower diagonal lines represent the lines of full compensatory pause (A1-A3 = 2[A1-A1]) and complete interpolation (A1-A3 = A1-A1), respectively. The horizontal dashed line is the SCL. In zone I, the responses fall along the line of compensatory pauses. In zone II they move off the line of compensatory pauses and produce a plateau in the curve. The difference between the A2-A3 of the plateau and the SCL is presumed to represent conduction time into and out of the sinus node. One-half of this difference is therefore taken as the sinoatrial conduction time (SACT). In zone III the return cycles lie between the line of complete interpolation and the SCL, and in zone IV the return cycles fall below the line of interpolation. ERP-A, atrial effective refractory period. See text for further discussion.

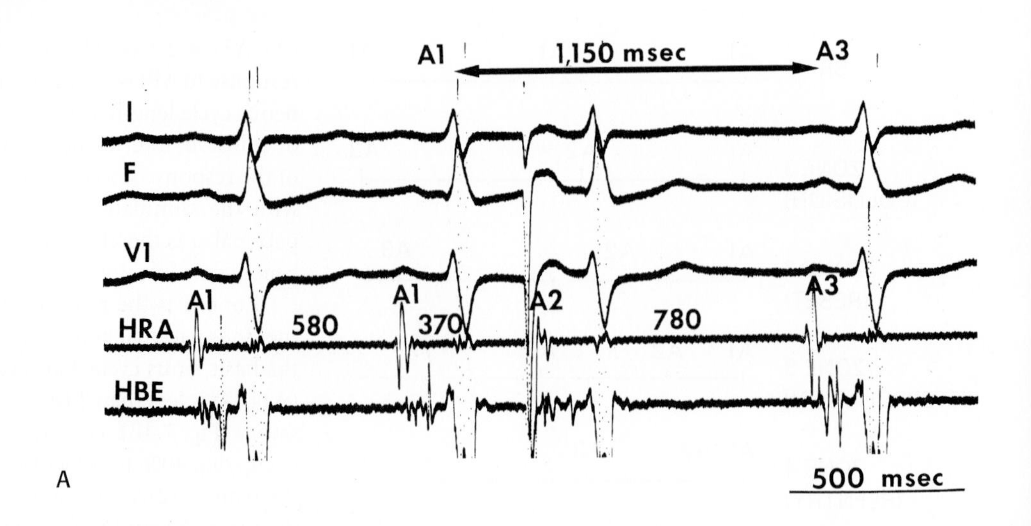


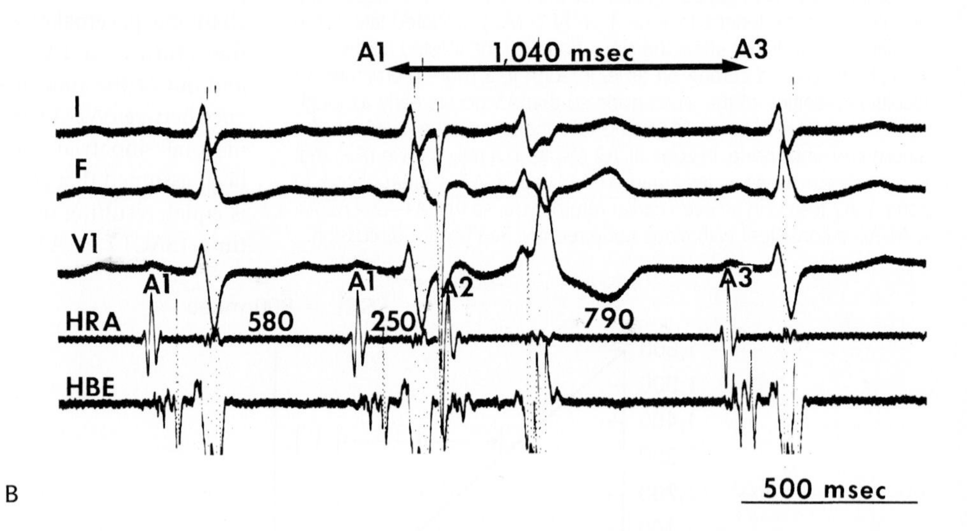


**FIGURE 3-4** *Analog records of zones I and II.* From **top** to **bottom**: ECG leads I and V1, and intracardiac electrograms from the high-right atrium in the area of the sinus node (HRA) and at the His bundle recording sight (HBE). The sinus cycle (A1-A1) is 580 msec. **A:** An APD (A2) is delivered at a coupling interval (A1-A2) of 370 msec. The return cycle (A3) is fully compensatory. **B:** At a shorter coupling interval (A1-A2 = 250 msec), the return cycle falls along the plateau of zone II. The A2-A3 (790) – A1-A1 (580) = conduction time of A2 into and out of the sinus node (210 msec); that is, SACT = 105 msec.

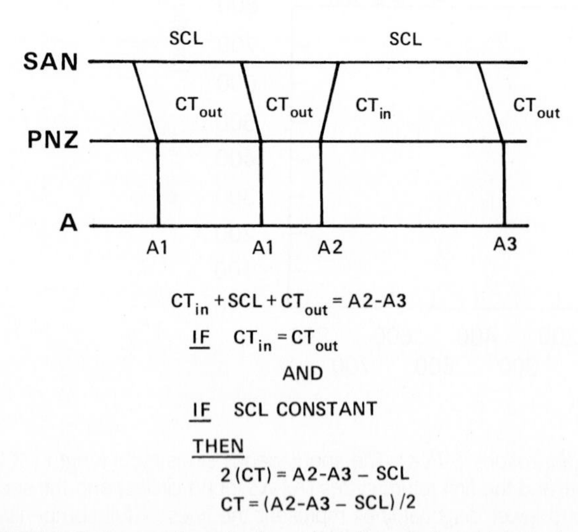


**FIGURE 3-5** *Assumptions in the calculation of sinoatrial conduction time.* SCL, sinus cycle length; SAN, sinoatrial node; PNZ, perinodal zone; A, atrium; CT, conduction time; A1-A1, SCL; A2, atrial premature depolarization; A3, sinus return cycle. See text for further discussion.

however, that this assumption is not valid. Although some investigators initially demonstrated that conduction into the node is slower than conduction out of the node, later data showed that this is not true during sinus rhythm. Studies in isolated rabbit atria using multiple simultaneous microelectrodes have shown that conduction time out of the sinus node is greater than conduction time into the node.[35–38] These data using multiple microelectrode recordings obviate many of the limitations of earlier studies and are probably correct. Direct recording from the sinus node confirms this (see following). Under certain conditions, however, conduction time into the node is slower than out of the node. Conduction time into the node is determined by an unquantifiable extent by conduction through atrial and perinodal tissue, which in turn is related to the distance of the site of stimulation from the sinus node and atrial refractoriness. Therefore, the site of stimulation is critical. The farther the site of stimulation from the sinus pacemaker site, the greater the overestimation of SACT. In addition, the more premature an APD, the more likely it will encroach on perinodal and/or refractoriness, which will slow conduction into the node. Early APDs commonly cause pacemaker shift to a peripheral latent pacemaker, which can

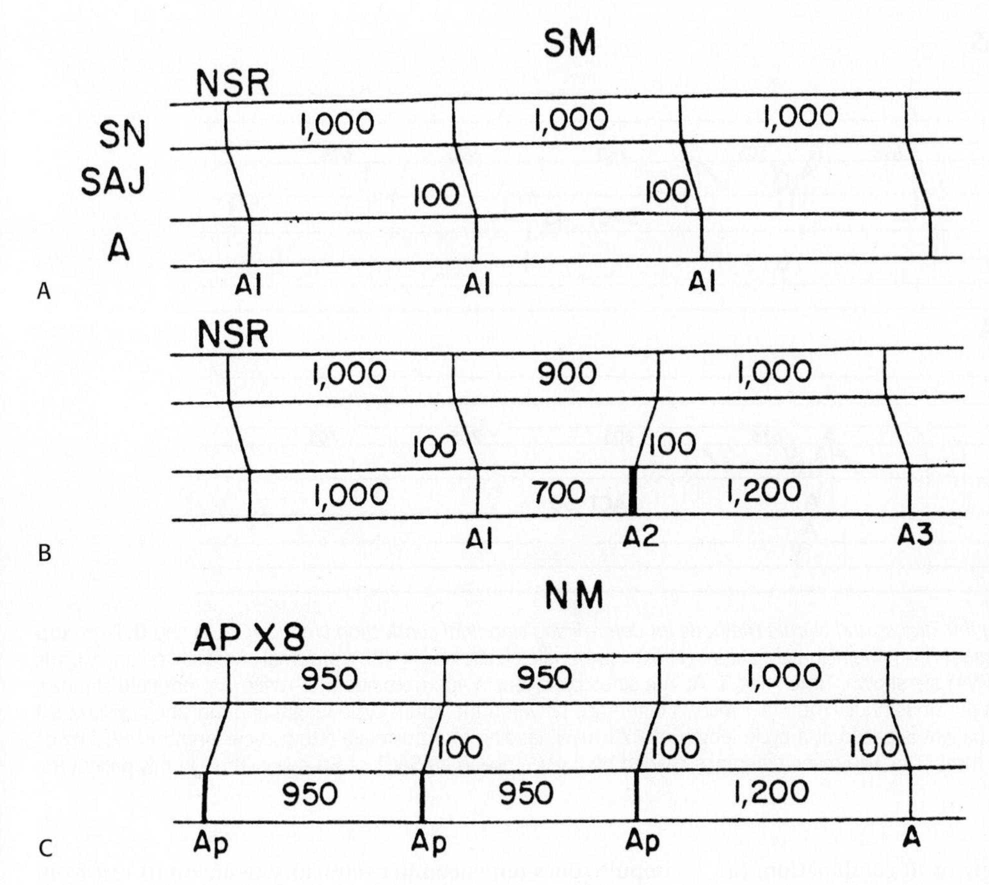


**FIGURE 3-6** *Schematic of Strauss method and Narula method for determining sinoatrial conduction time.* **A and B:** The Strauss method (SM). **C:** The Narula method. Each panel shows the sinus node (SN), sinoatrial junction (SAJ), and atrium (A). **A:** Sinus rhythm (NSR) is shown with A1-A1 equal in the sinus rate. **B:** An extrastimulus (A2) is delivered at 700 msec. It takes approximately 100 msec to read the sinus node, which gives rise to A3. The conduction into and out of the sinus node is assumed to be 100 msec, giving an A2-A3 of 1,200 msec. **C:** Atrial pacing (AP) for eight beats at a cycle length of 950 msec is performed with the sixth, seventh, and eighth paced complexes (Ap) shown. The last Ap takes 100 msec to get to the sinus node, resets the sinus node, leading to the subsequent atrial impulse. The SACT 100 msec also is depicted as an Ap-A interval of 1,200 msec.

excite the atrium earlier because of its proximity to that tissue; hence, conduction out of the node appears more rapid.[36,38–41] Despite these limitations, for practical purposes the SACT is a reasonable estimate of functional SACT, providing that stimulation is performed as close as possible to the sinus node and the measurement is taken when a true plateau is present in zone II. We usually take the measurement in the first third of zone II responses. In our laboratory, where patients range from 12 to 98 years of age, the normal SACT ranges from 45 to 125 msec.

The SACT appears to be independent of spontaneous cycle length,[34,42] although one report has shown an inverse relationship.[43] Marked sinus arrhythmia invalidates the calculation of SACT by APDS, because it is impossible to know whether the return cycle is as a result of spontaneous oscillation or a result of the induced APD. In the presence of mild sinus arrhythmia, this limitation may be partially overcome by performing multiple tests at each coupling interval. Still, the presence of even small degrees of sinus arrhythmia may produce errors in the measurement of SACT.

In an attempt to eliminate the effects of sinus arrhythmia, two other methods have been employed. Narula et al.[44] proposed that brief (eight-beat) periods of atrial pacing at rates just above sinus should be used instead of atrial extrastimuli delivered during sinus rhythm. The difference between the postpacing pause and the sinus cycle length would equal the SACT. The Strauss[17] and Narula methods[44] are schematically compared in Figure 3-6. Preliminary data from Breithardt and Seipel[45] comparing the two methods demonstrate that they are not always equivalent. Other studies show a reasonable correlation.[46–48] Reasons for differences may relate to the paced cycle length used for the Narula method. Inoue et al.[48] found that the correlation is best if pacing is performed 100 msec less than the sinus cycle length. If pacing is performed within 50 msec of the sinus cycle length, sinus acceleration occurs.[49] Thus, the postpacing sinus cycle length should be used as the control cycle length to compute the SACT if the Narula method is used. Other problems with both techniques include depression of automaticity, pacemaker shifts, sinus entrance block, and shortening of sinus action potential leasing to earlier onset of phase 4, each of which can give misleading results. We have found both techniques to give fairly comparable results in normal persons, particularly (but not necessarily) when cycle lengths of at least 50 msec less than sinus are used (Fig. 3-7). A second method for circumventing sinus arrhythmia is the use of atrial extrastimuli during atrial pacing. Kirkorian et al.[50] showed a close correlation of this method and the Strauss method. Further studies are required to corroborate these findings. Most studies using normal persons have shown that atropine with or without propranolol shortens the SACT unrelated to its effect on heart rate.[18,42,51–54]

In an occasional patient in response to progressively premature APDs, A2-A3 either continuously increases or increases after a brief plateau phase (in either instance, the pause remains less than compensatory). The progressive increase in A2-A3 during this zone may be due to any

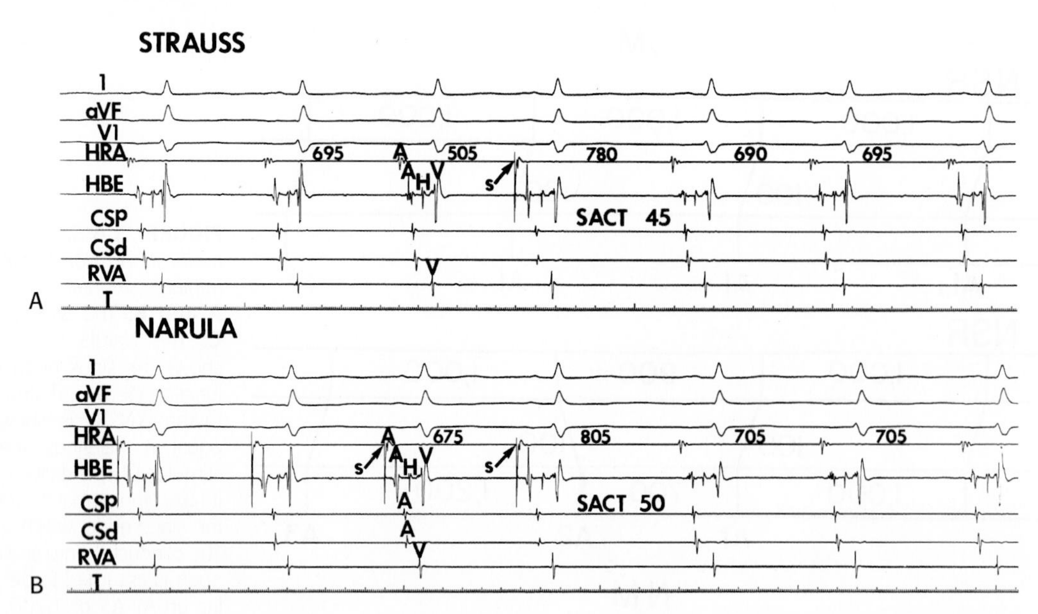


**FIGURE 3-7** *Analog records comparing the Strauss and Narula methods for determining sinoatrial conduction time (SACT).* **A** and **B:** From **top** to **bottom**, leads 1, aVF, and V1, electrograms from the high-right atrium (HRA), His bundle electrogram (HBE), proximal and distal coronary sinus (CSp, CSd), and right ventricular apex (RVA) are shown. Time lines, T. **A:** The sinus cycle length approximates 695 msec. A premature stimulus (*arrows*) delivered at 505 msec resents the sinus node. The SACT reveals difference between the return cycle length and the sinus cycle of 90 msec divided by 2 = 45. **B:** The same patient is paced at a cycle length of 675 msec leading to a postdrive return cycle length of 805 msec followed by a sinus cycle length of 705 msec. The 100 msec difference divided by 2 gives rise to an SACT of 50 msec. Thus, in this patient the two methods are comparable. T, time line.

of the following factors, either singly or in combination: (a) suppression of sinus pacemaker automaticity, (b) shift to a slower latent pacemaker, or (c) increase in conduction time into the sinus node that is due to A2 encountering perinodal tissue refractoriness. Thus, we recommend that the earliest third of zone II be used to measure the SACT because it is less likely to introduce errors that are due to any of those three factors. Analysis of postreturn cycles (A3-A4) may provide insight into changes in automaticity or pacemaker shift.[41,55] An A3-A4 greater than A1-A1 suggests depression of automaticity; in this instance, SACT calculated from A2-A3 yields an overestimation of the true SACT. Correction or exclusion of SACT using A2-A3 in the presence of an A3-A4 greater than A1-A1 is necessary. In this case, using A3-A4 as the basic sinus cycle length to which A2-A3 is compared will help correct a falsely prolonged SACT if A2-A3 were related to the prior sinus cycle length (A1-A1).

Zones III and IV are ranges of A1-A2 at which the A2-A3 shortens to less than A1-A1. Two types of early responses are found in these zones. The responses in zone III are termed complete and incomplete interpolation, and they include those in which A2-A3 is less than A1-A1 and A1-A3 is less than 2 (A1-A1) (see Fig. 3-3). The coupling interval at which incomplete interpolation is first observed defines the refractory period of the perinodal tissue. Some investigators refer to this as the sinus node refractory period. In this instance, A3 represents delay of A1 exiting the sinus node, which has not been affected. The A1-A2 at which complete interpolation is observed probably defines the effective refractory period of the most peripheral of the perinodal tissue, because the sinus impulse does not encounter refractory tissue on its exit from the sinus node. In this instance, A1-A2 + A2-A3 = A1-A1, and sinus node entrance block is said to exist. In our laboratory, zone II responses can be seen in 15% of patients using the Strauss method. This has ranged from 13% to 46%.[30,50,56] In two studies using atrial pacing and premature stimuli to evaluate SACT and "sinus node refractoriness," zone III responses were observed in 65% and 85%.[50,57] They also demonstrated an increase in sinus node refractoriness at decreasing paced cycle lengths. Increased perinodal refractoriness may have been responsible for their high incidence of zone III responses. Kerr and Strauss.[57] found the refractory period of the sinoatrial node to be 325 ± 39 msec at a paced cycle length of 600 msec in normals and 522 ± 20 msec at the same cycle length in patients with sinus node dysfunction. Autonomic blockade shortens the refractory period. More work is necessary to establish the utility of these measurements.

A second type of early response, which defines zone IV is due to sinus node reentry. This response by definition occurs when A1-A2 + A2-A3 is less than A1-A1 (Fig. 3-8) and the atrial activation sequence and P-wave morphology are identical to sinus. Dhingra et al.[30] found sinus node reentry in 11% of patients. In our laboratory, the incidence of this finding is similar (10%).

A wide range of "normal" values of SACT has been reported (Table 3-1). This, in large part, reflects the inherent limitations of these indirect methods. Even after autonomic blockade, the range of "normals" reflects the previously described fallibility of the assumptions of indirect measurements as well as the variability of pacing site relative to the site of sinus impulse formation.

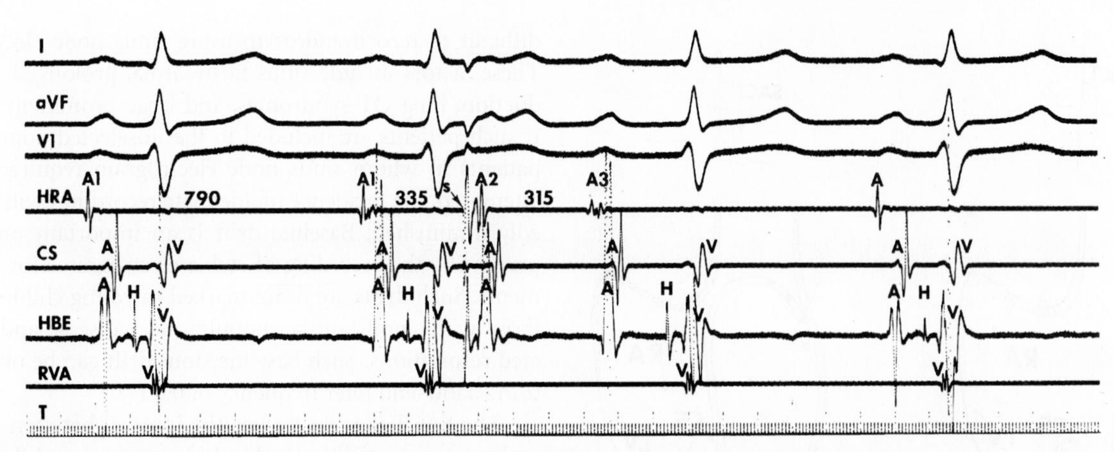


**FIGURE 3-8** *Sinus node echo in response to atrial premature depolarization (APD).* ECG leads 1, aVF, and V1 are displayed with electrograms from the high-right atrium (HRA), coronary sinus (CS), His bundle (HBE), and right ventricular apex (RVA). An APD (A2) is introduced at a coupling interval of 335 msec. There is an early return beat (A3), with an atrial activation sequence and P-wave morphology identical to that of sinus rhythm. Since the A1-A3 (650 msec) is less than the spontaneous sinus cycle length (790 msec), A3 is probably due to reentry in the region of the sinus node.

## Sinus Node Electrogram

In view of the limitations of indirect methods to assess sinoatrial conduction and the assumptions that are necessarily required to derive the SACT, a method of directly recording a sinus node electrogram was developed by Cramer et al.,[58] who identified extracellular potential changes associated with directly recorded electrical activity of the sinus pacemaker in isolated rabbit atria. Further work using endocardial recordings from the intact canine heart confirmed the ability to record diastolic phase 4 slope, followed by slow upstroke culminating in a rapid atrial electrogram.[59] Subsequently, several investigators developed techniques to record electrograms from human subjects with and without sinus node dysfunction.[46,60–62] To record sinus node electrograms, one can use catheters with 0.5- to 1.5-cm interelectrode distances. Two techniques have been employed; in one the catheter is positioned at the junction of the superior vena cava and right atrium in the region of the sinus node, and the other – which appears more reliable and from which more stable recordings can be obtained – requires that the catheter be looped in the right atrium with firm contact at the region of the superior vena cava and atrial junction (Fig. 3-9). This latter method, which produces firm contact against the atrial wall, produces an atrial injury potential simultaneously with the recording of the sinus node electrogram. The reported frequency for obtaining node electrograms ranges considerably, from 40% to 90%. Those studies using methods similar to the second method report higher success rates. In addition, filter settings play a prominent role in the ability to record stable electrograms that are not obscured by marked baseline drift. Use of low end (high-pass filters) of less than 0.1 Hz (0.01 to 0.05 Hz) is associated with marked baseline drift and difficulty in interpretation of the recordings. Use of low-end filter settings of 1 Hz or more produces diminution or loss of the sinus node electrogram. Thus, the low-end filter used should be between 0.1 and 0.6 Hz. The high-end or low-pass filter frequency can be set at 20 or 50 Hz, the latter being more commonly employed. The signal then must be gained using a range of 50 to 100 μV/cm. Using these techniques, which are time consuming, a stable sinus node electrogram without significant baseline shift can be recorded. However, in my opinion, the frequency and ease with which this recording can be made have been exaggerated. We obtained stable sinus node electrograms in only 50% of an unselected population of patients. It has been recognized that factors that produce encroachment of the T and U wave on the P wave make it

**TABLE 3-1 Normal Upper Limits for Sinoatrial Conduction Time (SACT[a], msec)**

| Investigators | Method | SACTa + r SACTa |
|---|---|---|
| Luderitz et al.[126] | PAS | ≥200[a] |
| Scheinman et al.[127] | PAS | ≥206[a] |
| Alboni et al.[124] | PAS | ≥214[a] |
| Jordan et al.[27] | PAS | ≥226[a] |
| Breithardt et al.[126] | PAS | ≥240[a] |
| Engel et al.[127] | PAS | ≥260[a] |
| Dhingra et al.[128] | PAS | ≥304[a] |
| Crook et al.[66] | PAS | ≥344[a] |
| Yabek and Jarmakani[128] | – | ≥210[b] |
| Kugler et al.[129] | – | ≥200[b] |
| Reiffel et al.[132] | SN electrogram | ≥120[a] |
| Juillard et al.[86] | SN electrogram | ≥137[a] |
| Bethge et al.[130] | SN electrogram | ≥107[a] |
| Gomes et al.[135] | SN electrogram | ≥112[a] |

[a]Based on the mean +2 SD.
[b]Measurement in children.
SACT, Sinoatrial conduction time; SACTa + r total SACT, A2-A3 minus A1-A1; SACTa, SACT in antegrade direction; PAS, premature atrial stimulation technique; SN electrogram, direct electrogram recording technique.

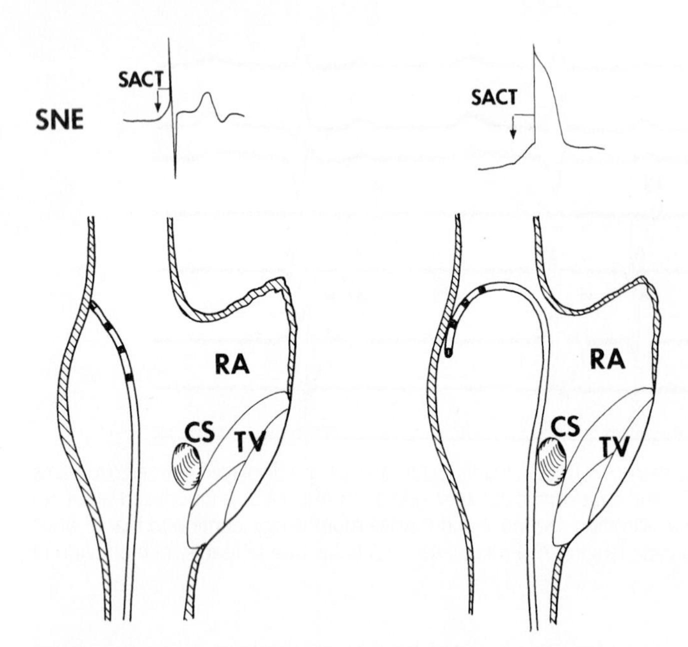


**FIGURE 3-9** *Schema of methods for obtaining sinus node electrograms.* The right atrium is depicted with a catheter in the region of the sinus node. Tricuspid valve (TV), coronary sinus (CS), and right atrial appendage (RA) are shown. In the **left** panel, where the catheter is merely positioned with the tip touching the region of the sinus node, one gets a sinus node electrogram (SNE) and calculated sinoatrial conduction time (SACT), as shown in the **upper left**. On the **right**, a second method of obtaining the sinus node electrogram is shown with a catheter-looped positioning of the recording electrodes at the sinus node area. The pressure caused by the looped catheter produces more of a monophase type of signal with a calculated SACT, as shown in the upper right.

difficult to record and/or measure sinus node electrograms. These factors include sinus tachycardia, prolonged A-V conduction, long QT syndromes, and large prominent U waves. If such patients are included in the unselected population of patients in whom sinus node electrogram requirements are attempted, the incidence of adequate recordings will be markedly diminished. Baseline drift is an important problem in preventing the recording of stable electrograms for measurements. Such drifts are more marked in young children and in those with significant cardiopulmonary disease and exaggerated respirations. Such baseline sinus drift can be obviated by using a low-end filter frequency of 0.6 Hz.

The SACT is measured as the interval between the pacemaker prepotential on the local electrogram and the onset of the rapid atrial deflection (Fig. 3-10). When SACT is normal, a smooth upstroke slope merges into the atrial electrogram (see Fig. 3-10). When sinoatrial conduction is slowed, an increasing amount of the sinus node potential becomes visible before the rapid atrial deflection is inscribed. Sinoatrial block is said to occur when the entire sinus node electrogram is seen in the absence of a propagated response to the atrium. These patterns are schematized in Figure 3-11. Validation of sinus node electrograms has included (a) the ability to record in only a local area,[46,61,62] (b) loss of the upstroke potential during overdrive atrial pacing,[46,63] and (c) the persistence of sinus node electrograms (with or without prior prolongation) following CSP, following induced pauses, or during pauses following overdrive suppression.[46,64,65] This latter finding in fact both defines and validates the concept of sinoatrial exit block. Another aspect of the sinus node electrogram that has been evaluated is the total time of diastolic depolarization.[63]

The major values of this technique have been: (a) to improve our understanding of physiologic phenomena related

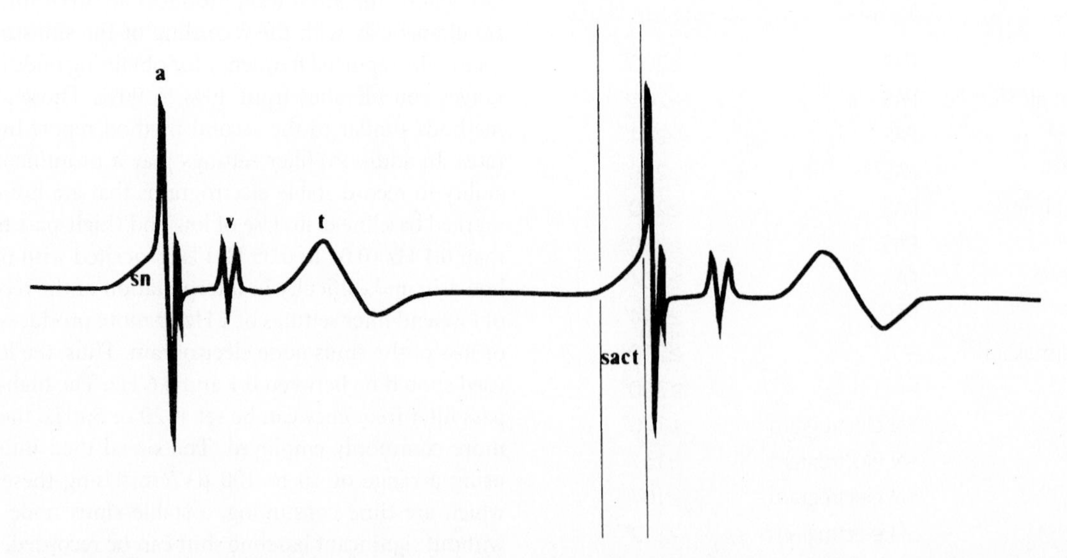


**FIGURE 3-10** *Schematic illustration showing the direct measurement of sinoatrial conduction time (SACT).* A schematic copy of a sinus node electrogram (SNE) is shown. On the SNE, high-right atrial depolarization (a), ventricular depolarization (v), the T wave (t), and the sinus node potential (sn) are identified. In the second beat, reference lines are drawn through the point at which the SN potential first becomes evident and the point at which atrial activation begins. The SACT is the interval between these two reference lines. (From Reiffel JA, Gang E, Gliklich J, et al. The human sinus node electrogram: a transvenous catheter technique and a comparison of directly measured and indirectly estimated sinoatrial conduction time in adults. *Circ* 1980;62:1324.)

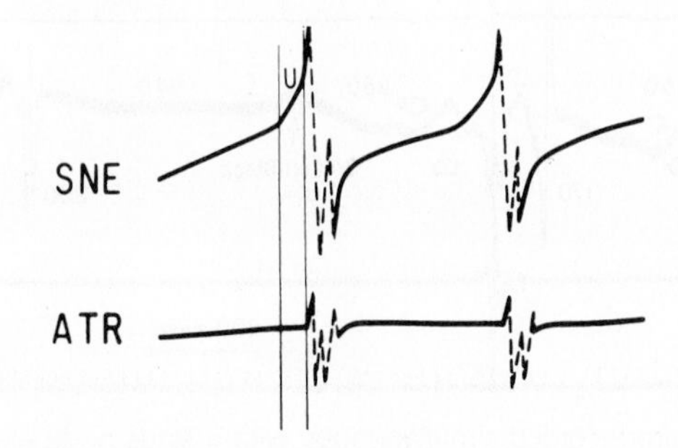


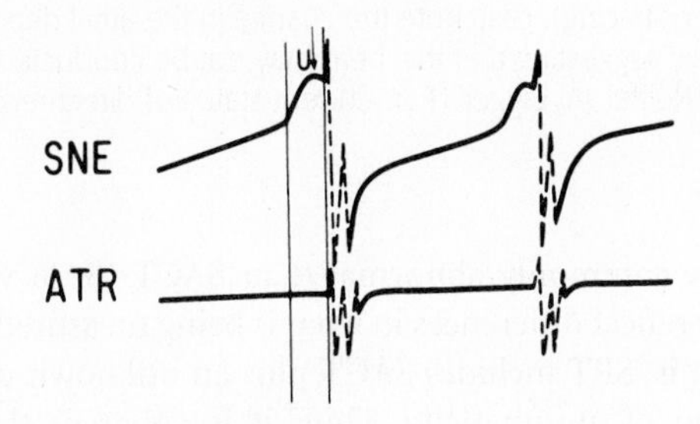


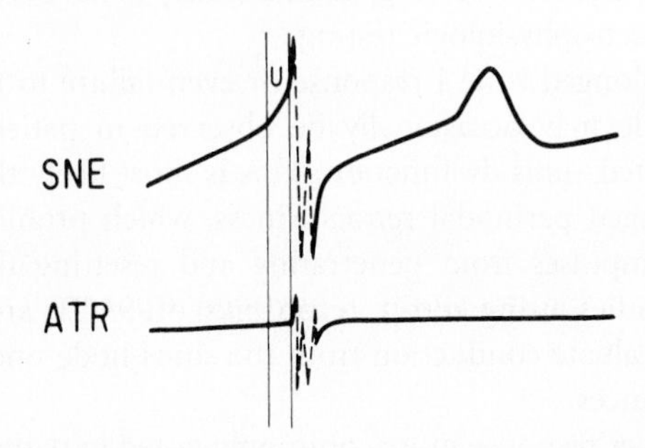


**FIGURE 3-11** *Schematic illustration of sinus node and atrial activity.* Three panels showing various sinoatrial activity are depicted. Normal sinoatrial conduction is shown on top. After the upstroke slope, atrial activation is recorded on the sinus node electrogram (SNE) and reference high-right atrial electrogram (ATR). The thin vertical lines delineate the sinoatrial conduction time (SACT), which is measured from the onset of the upstroke slope to the onset of atrial activity in the ATR. In the middle, first-degree sinoatrial block is shown. The SACT is prolonged; that is, the distance between onset of the upstroke slope in the SNE and atrial activation is prolonged. Note that the upstroke slope on the SNE rises to a peak (*arrow*) and then rolls off before atrial activation. The delay in sinoatrial conduction permits more of the contour of the sinus node potential to be inscribed on the SNE before it becomes obscured by atrial activation. On the bottom is shown second-degree sinoatrial block. The second sinus node depolarization is visualized but is not followed by atrial activation. (Adapted from Reiffel JA, Gang E, Gliklich J, et al. The human sinus node electrogram: a transvenous catheter technique and a comparison of directly measured and indirectly estimated sinoatrial conduction time in adults. *Circ* 1980;62:1324.)

to sinus node function and (b) to allow us to understand the values and limitations of indirect measurements of SACT and sinus node recovery time (SRT). As previously mentioned, the development of pauses during sinus rhythm has either been called sinus arrest or sinus exit block, depending on whether the next sinus impulse or impulse is a multiple of the basic sinus cycle length. The use of sinus node electrograms has shown us that in most instances sinoatrial block is present because persistence of the sinus node electrogram at similar or slightly slower rates has been observed (Fig. 3-12). This can also be seen following carotid sinus massage (see Vagal Hypersensitivity Syndromes later in this chapter). The use of the sinus node electrogram has demonstrated the limitation of the use of overdrive pacing as a means to evaluate sinus node automaticity. The pauses that follow overdrive suppression, particularly the long pauses associated with sinus node dysfunction, have in almost all instances been shown to have some component of sinus node exit block (complete or partial) with or without impaired sinus automaticity (see Sinus Node Recovery Time, later in this chapter).[46,64]

Several studies have been undertaken to compare the SACT measured by indirect methods (both the Strauss.[17] and Narula method[44]) with the directly recorded SACT. These studies have shown a good correlation between indirect and direct methods in patients without and with sinus node dysfunction.[46,61,62,65] In addition, the patterns and degree of inaccuracy associated with indirectly measured SACT have been reported by Reiffel et al.[55] A lengthened postreturn cycle (A3-A4) with respect to the basic sinus cycle suggests suppression of automaticity and an overestimation of SACT when the indirect methods are used. In this instance, use of A3-A4 as the "new" sinus cycle can correct for the overestimation. In the presence of sinoatrial entrance block, indirect methods cannot measure sinoatrial conduction. Finally, the effect of early APDs or sinoatrial conduction during zone III responses (i.e., complete and incomplete interpolation) can only be determined by direct recordings.

Recent data have also shown that sinoatrial conduction is directly related to the sinus cycle length, and this relationship persists during periods of vagal tone. This helped resolve the question of what the effect of sinus cycle length of SACT was, a problem previously unresolved by indirect methods.

Limited studies have been conducted of patients with sinus node dysfunction in whom both indirect and direct methods have been compared. The study by Gomes et al.[46] is the most detailed and shows a good correlation between directly measured SACT and that as made by the indirect techniques. However, in individual instances there were some discrepancies. It is of interest, however, that the range of normal values of directly recorded SACT was 60 to 112 msec in the study by Gomes et al.[46] and 46 to 116 msec in the initial study by Reiffel et al.[61] These are remarkably similar to the values previously reported using indirect techniques (Table 3-2). This suggests that differences in autonomic tone make this measurement inherently variable. No data are available in an age-matched, control population analyzing sinus node electrograms after autonomic blockade.

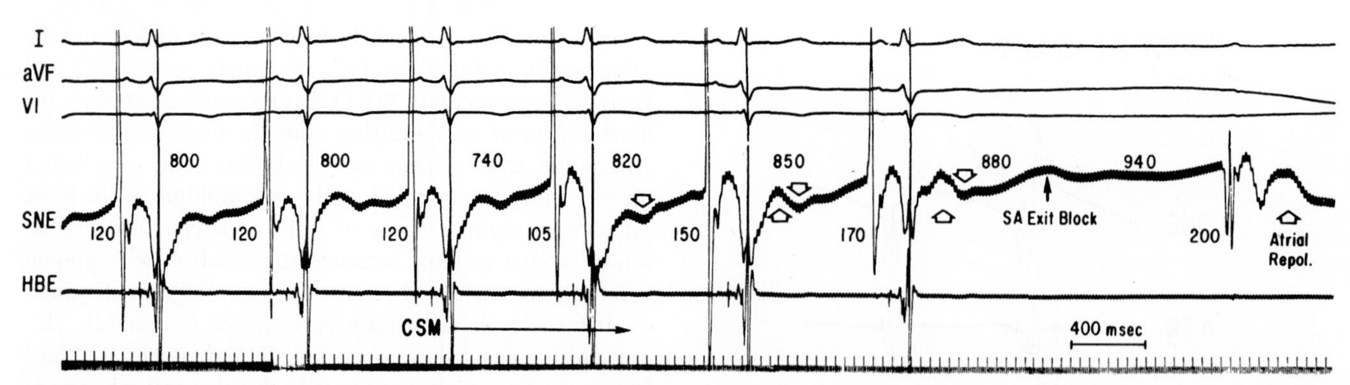


**FIGURE 3-12** *The response to carotid sinus massage.* ECG leads I, aVF, and V1 are recorded simultaneously with a sinus node electrogram (SNE) and a His bundle electrogram (HBE). The onset of carotid sinus massage as well as the presence of a blocked sinus node depolarization (labeled S-A exit block) and A-V nodal block of the following atrial depolarization (right-hand end of tracing) during carotid sinus massage. Note also the presence of the atrial repolarization waves (upward heavy *arrows*) and minimal manifestation of ventricular T waves (heavy downward *arrows*). T-wave activity is absent following the blocked atrial depolarization (right end of tracing). Last, note the change in the atrial depolarization configuration and slight change in the P wave in lead aVF of the blocked atrial complex, suggesting that this beat may not be conducted from the sinus node (an ectopic complex) or is using a different route out of the node. (From Reiffel JA, Bigger JT Jr. Current status of direct recordings of the sinus node electrogram in man. *PACE* 1983;6:1143.)

## Sinoatrial Conduction Time in Patients with Sick Sinus Syndrome

We and others have found the SACT to be an insensitive indicator of sinus node dysfunction,[14,25,27,62] because it has been prolonged in only 40% of our patients with clinical findings of sinus node dysfunction. Like SRT, SACT is least likely to be abnormal in patients with isolated sinus bradycardia.[17,34] In patients with sinus exit block and/or the bradycardia–tachycardia syndrome, the SACT is more frequently abnormal, positive responses being noted in as many as 78% of those patients.[34] In a comparison of SACT and SRT in patients with sinus pauses, Strauss et al.[33] found that corrected SRT was more commonly abnormal than SACT (80% vs. 53%). This may reflect differences in what is being measured by both tests; that is, SRT includes SACT plus an unknown degree of depression of automaticity. Thus, it is apparent that those patients with evidence of sinus node dysfunction undergoing ECG long-term monitoring are most likely to have abnormalities by electrophysiologic testing.

A prolonged zone I response or even failure to reset the sinus node may occasionally be observed in patients with documented sinus dysfunction. This is most likely the result of prolonged perinodal refractoriness, which prohibits premature impulses from penetrating and resetting the sinus node. Studies using direct recordings of SACT are necessary to evaluate conduction from the sinus node under such circumstances.

Another response more commonly noted in patients with clinical sinus dysfunction is the progressive lengthening of A1-A3, resulting in either abbreviation or abolition of the plateau portion of the curve.[66,67] Combined abnormalities of sinus automaticity and sinoatrial conduction are probably responsible for this phenomenon, the clinical significance of which is unknown.

Atropine shortens the SACT in most patients with sinus node dysfunction, occasionally to normal values.[42,51–53,68] Dhingra et al., however, noted a variable response with a decrease in 56% of patients and an increase in return cycles in 44% of patients with sick sinus syndrome.[18] The increase probably results from improvement in retrograde conduction into the sinoatrial node, resulting in depression of automaticity.

**TABLE 3-2 Diagnostic Evaluation of Sinus Node Function**

| |
|---|
| Electrocardiographic monitoring |
| Exercise testing |
| Autonomic testing |
| Clinical electrophysiologic testing<br>Response to rapid atrial pacing<br>Maximum sinus node recovery time (SNRTmax) and maximum corrected sinus node recovery time (CSNRTmax) |
| Secondary pauses |
| Total recovery time |
| Estimated sinoatrial conduction time (SACT)<br>Atrial extrastimulus technique<br>Constant atrial pacing technique<br>Direct sinus node electrogram recording<br>Duration of sinus node depolarization (SNDd) |
| Estimated sinus node refractory period (SNERP) |
| Observed intrinsic heart rate (IHR) |

## Sinus Node Recovery Time

Suppression of pacemaker activity by driving the heart at a faster rate was first noted by Gaskell.[68] The mechanism of overdrive suppression of the sinus node remains unclear; factors that appear to be involved include the release of acetylcholine, the efflux of potassium from cells during rapid atrial pacing, activation of electronic sodium pump, and altered calcium exchange across the membrane.[69–72] The degree of prolongation of postdrive cycles in excess of control cycle lengths has been assumed to reflect a degree of depression in sinus node automaticity. The SRT, however, is a more complex event, and many factors besides automaticity are involved. They include (a) proximity of the stimulation site to the sinus node, (b) local concentrations of acetylcholine and norepinephrine, and (c) conduction time into and out of the sinus node. In particular, sinoatrial conduction can significantly affect the SRT. Because conduction time to and from the atrial stimulation site and the sinus node can be as much as 250 msec, it may be a major component of the SRT. Moreover, sinus node entrance block during rapid atrial pacing may lead to a shortening of the SRT, whereas sinus node exit block after cessation of rapid atrial pacing may result in a marked prolongation of the SRT. Despite these reservations, the SRT is probably the best and most widely used test of sinus node automaticity, and perhaps of overall function.[10,13,33,34,43–76]

Performance of SRT requires stimulation of the right atrium near the sinus node at progressively shorter cycle lengths, starting at cycle lengths just below sinus. It is imperative that at least 1 minute be allowed between paced cycle lengths to ensure full recovery of the sinus node. High- and low-atrial electrograms are usually simultaneously recorded to enable one to determine whether escape beats at the termination of pacing originate from the sinus node. Confirmation of the sinus node as the origin of the escape beats depends on demonstration of a similar P-wave morphology and atrial activation sequence to that observed during sinus rhythm before atrial pacing. Changes in P-wave morphology and/or atrial activation sequence suggest a shift of pacemaker. Such shifts represent a limitation to all indirect methods of assessing sinus node function.

Several intervals have been used as a measure of the recovery time. They include (a) maximum SRT (SRT = the longest pause from the last paced atrial depolarization to the first sinus return cycle at any paced cycle length), (b) corrected SRT (CSRT = SRT – sinus cycle length), (c) SRT/sinus cycle length, and (d) total recovery time (TRT = time to return to basic sinus cycle length). In addition, the presence of junctional escapes and sudden unexpected pauses during the recovery period should be noted. Because resting sinus cycle length has a major influence on the SRT, we believe some form of adjustment for the sinus cycle length should be made. Normal values used in several laboratories for SRT are listed in Table 3-3. The marked differences in reported "normal" values probably reflect differences in patient populations with respect to autonomic tone and structural cardiac disease as well as to differences in methodology. Our normal values are CSRT less than 550 msec, SRT/NSR × 100% less than 150%, and TRT less than 5 seconds (usually by the fourth to sixth recovery beat).

Although we initially used the regression equation derived for SRT that takes into consideration the basic sinus cycle length as suggested by Mandel et al.,[10] use of a CSRT is simpler and takes into account the basic sinus cycle length. Using Mandel's[10] regression equation, the value of the first sinus cycle following termination of pacing is considered prolonged if it exceeds a value equal to 1.3 (mean spontaneous cycle length) + 101 msec, a value derived by plotting the maximum first

**TABLE 3-3 Normal Values (msec) for Maximum Sinus Node Recovery Time (SNRTmax) and Maximum Corrected Sinus Node Recovery Time (CSNRTmax)**

| Investigators | SNRTmax[a] | CSNRTmax[a] |
|---|---|---|
| Mandel et al.[136] | ≤1,207 | – |
| Breithardt et al.[126] | ≤1,475 | – |
| Benditt et al.[77] | ≤1.61 (SCL) for SCL < 800 msec | – |
| Narula et al.[138] | ≤1.83 (SCL) for SCL > 800 msec | ≤525 |
| Kulbertus et al.[74] | – | ≤533 |
| Gupta et al.[85] | ≤1,500 | ≤472 |
| Alboni et al.[124] | – | ≤354 |
| Engel et al.[127] | – | ≤533 |
| El Said et al.[131] | ≤1,250 | ≤250[b] |
| Yabek and Jarmakani[128] | – | ≤273[b] |
| Kugler et al.[129] | – | ≤275[b] |

[a]Where possible, values are mean +2 SD.
[b]Measurements in children.
SCL, Baseline sinus cycle length.

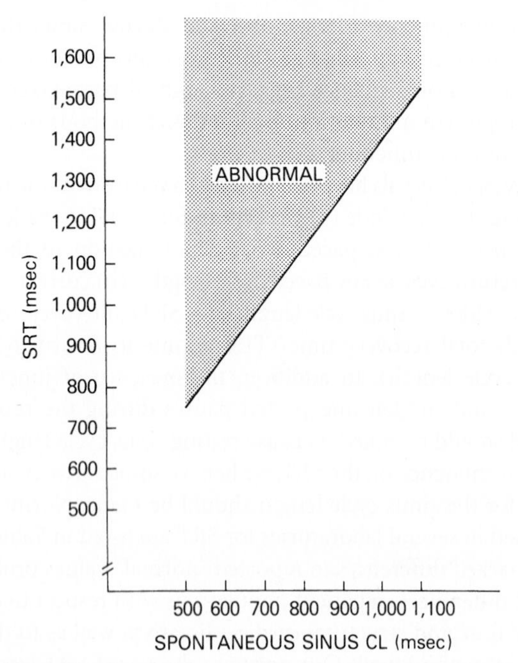


**FIGURE 3-13** *Relationship of maximum sinus node recovery time to spontaneous sinus cycle length.* At any spontaneous sinus cycle length, the normal sinus node recovery time (SRT) ± 2 SD should fall to the right of the stippled area. (From Mandel W, Hayakawa H, Allen HN, et al. Evaluation of sinoatrial node function in many by overdrive suppression. *Circ* 1971;44:59.)

escape cycle length against the control spontaneous cycle length (Fig. 3-13).[10] A normal response is shown in Figure 3-14. The basic sinus cycle length is 720 msec (upper panel). The maximum SRT occurred following a paced atrial cycle length of 400 msec (bottom panel). The calculated values are SRT 1,120 msec; CSRT, 400 msec; percentage of SRT over sinus cycle length, 156%; and TRT, 2.5 seconds. Note that despite normal values of SRT, CSRT, and TRT, the percentage of SRT over sinus cycle length is slightly prolonged. This prolongation may occur when the spontaneous sinus cycle length is less than 800 msec and thus should not be used in such circumstances.

Because the SRT has been shown to be proportional to the control sinus cycle length, in my opinion the CSRT is the most useful of the measurements just discussed. It may be normal in the presence of a prolonged SRT, particularly in the presence of a long basic sinus cycle length. For example, if the basic sinus cycle length is 1,200 msec, and the maximum SRT is 1,600 msec, some laboratories would consider it an abnormal response (see Table 3-1). However, the CSRT of 400 msec is well within normal limits. Thus, when sinus node recovery from overdrive suppression is evaluated, some consideration must be given to the basic sinus cycle length.

Normally, there is gradual warm-up (shortening of cycle length) following the cessation of overdrive pacing until the control sinus length is achieved (see Fig. 3-14). Usually, the control sinus length is achieved in four to six beats, giving a TRT of less than 5 seconds. It is not unusual to find oscillation of recovery cycle lengths before full recovery, but the pattern of oscillation of sinus cycle length shortening should fall within the limits described by Benditt et al.[77] (Fig. 3-15). A greater frequency of oscillation occurs at higher-paced rates.[10,42,54,74,76,77] Heddle, et al.[76] recently developed a nonlinear mathematical model to predict the pattern of overdrive recovery and to evaluate the effects of pacing on both sinoatrial conduction time and automaticity. This sophisticated technique is, however, limited by (a) effects of change in autonomic tone that are due to the hemodynamic consequences of pacing; (b) changes in P-wave morphology suggesting a change in pacemaker location and/or exit; (c) sinoatrial entrance block; and (d) secondary pauses. These are also limitations common to all methods analyzing the response to overdrive suppression. Although the utility of such an algorithm needs to be established, the CSRT and pattern of resumption to a stable sinus cycle length certainly are a measure of the effect of overdrive pacing on both sinoatrial conduction and automaticity.

Sudden and marked secondary pauses occurring during sinus recovery are abnormal and in most instances reflect changes in sinoatrial conduction; however, a change in automaticity with or without pacemaker shift is also possible. Because these secondary pauses represent abnormalities of sinus function and because they occur more frequently following rapid pacing, atrial pacing should be carried out at rates up to 200 bpm. Use of the sinus node electrogram has

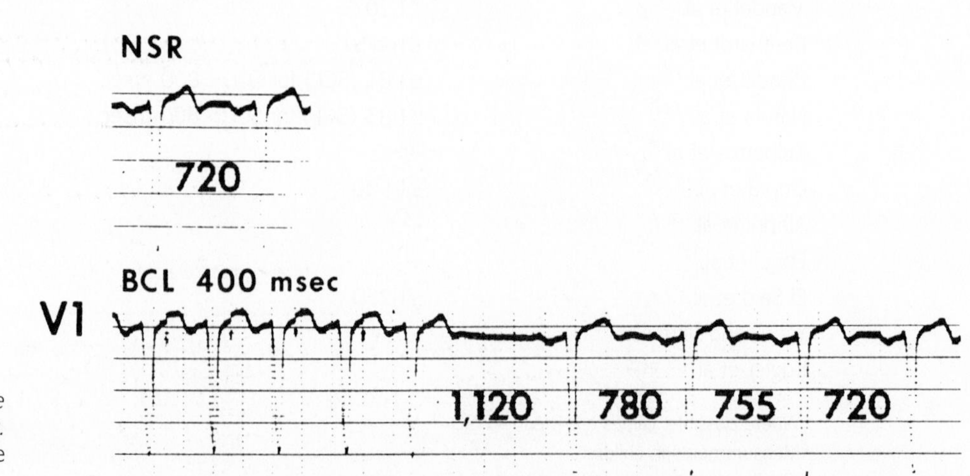


**FIGURE 3-14** *Normal sinus node response (NSR) to rapid atrial pacing.* See text for details. BCL, basic cycle length.

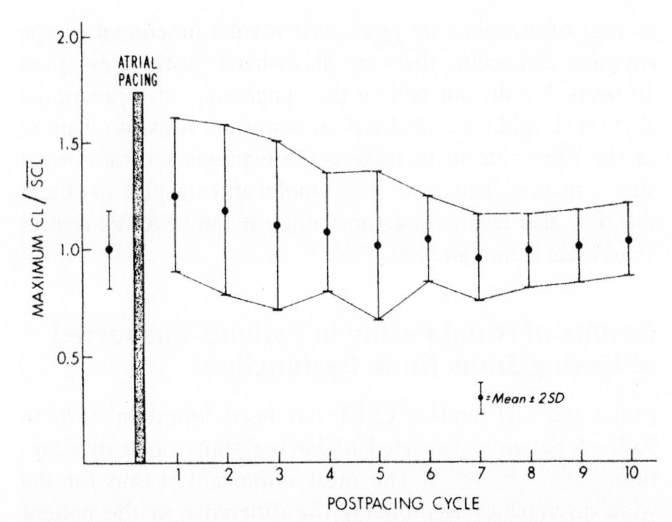


**FIGURE 3-15** *The limits of the normal recovery response for the first 10 postpacing cycles in patients with mean sinus cycle length greater than 800 msec.* The normal limits ± 2 SD of postpacing recovery cycles are determined by dividing the maximum recovery time for each postreturn cycle by the mean spontaneous sinus cycle length (SCL). The normalized mean value (1.0) and the 2 SD bars for variation in spontaneous cycle length are shown to the left of the vertical bar. Note that the gradual return toward SCL is usually completed by the fifth or sixth postpacing cycle. Marked pauses falling outside the 2 SD limits during the second to tenth return cycles suggest an abnormality of sinus node function. (From Benditt DG, Strauss HC, Scheinman MM, et al. Analysis of secondary pauses following termination of rapid atrial pacing in man. *Circ* 1976;54:436.)

helped resolve this issue. Several investigators have demonstrated sinoatrial exit block of variable duration to be the primary mechanism of prolonged pauses with a lesser component of depression of automaticity (Fig. 3-16).[46,62,64] Both may, and often do, coexist. This can clearly be demonstrated by persistence of sinus node electrograms during pauses. These studies suggest that in normal situations the CSRT is always a composite of sinoatrial conduction time and sinus automaticity. If the mean CSRT is 320 msec and SACT is 85 msec, and we assume a time into the sinus node of 60 msec, it is quite apparent that almost half of the measured CSRT is a reflection of sinoatrial conduction and atriosinus conduction and not of sinus node automaticity. It is impossible to predict to what extent sinoatrial conduction and depression of automaticity contribute to the pauses noted in any individual, and only through the use of sinus node electrograms can this be adequately assessed. Similar persistence of sinus node electrograms during pauses following CSP suggests sinus exit block as the mechanism of these pauses (see Vagal Hypersensitivity Syndromes, following).[46,62,64]

The normal sinus node is suppressed by as little as 15 seconds of atrial pacing at rates greater than sinus. Increase in the duration of pacing to 30, 60, 120, 180, or 300 msec has not been shown to alter the maximum SRT in normal patients.[10,73] The SRT is proportional to the paced rate (and inversely proportional to paced cycle length) up to heart rates of 130 to 150 bpm, at which point shortening of the return cycle is commonly noted (Fig. 3-17).[10] The mechanisms for the shortening may include (a) hemodynamic factors with reflex acceleration of the sinus rate in response to hypotension, (b) local release of catecholamines, and (c) entrance block of some of the paced atrial beats into the sinus node. In 1986 Nalos et al.[78] demonstrated that autonomic blockade abolishes reflex acceleration of the sinus node in response to pacing-induced hypotension. Following autonomic blockade, the CSRT increases as the paced cycle length is decreased.

Gang et al.[79] and Engel et al.[80] have demonstrated a good relationship between the pause following such rapid pacing

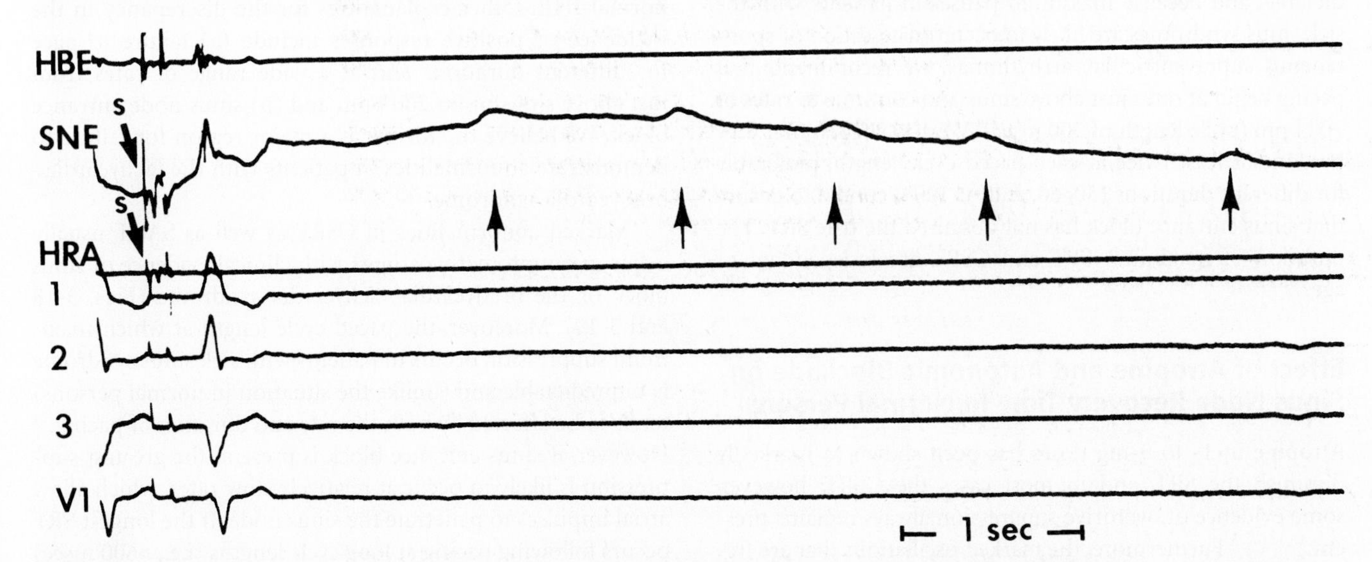


**FIGURE 3-16** *Effects of overdrive pacing on sinoatrial conduction and automaticity.* From **top** to **bottom** are shown the His bundle electrogram (HBE), sinus node electrogram (SNE), high-right atrial electrogram (HRA), and surface leads 1, 2, 3, and V1. Following the last stimulated complex of overdrive pacing (s, *arrow*), a long pause ensues. Five sinus node electrograms can be seen, the first four of which demonstrate progressive shortening of the intrasinus node electrogram cycle length followed by a pause. This suggests complete sinoatrial block as well as intrasinus Wenckebach-type block. (Adapted from Asseman P, Berzin B, Desry D, et al. Persistent sinus nodal electrograms during abnormally prolonged postpacing atrial pauses in sick sinus syndrome in humans: sinoatrial block vs. overdrive suppression. *Circ* 1983;68:33.)

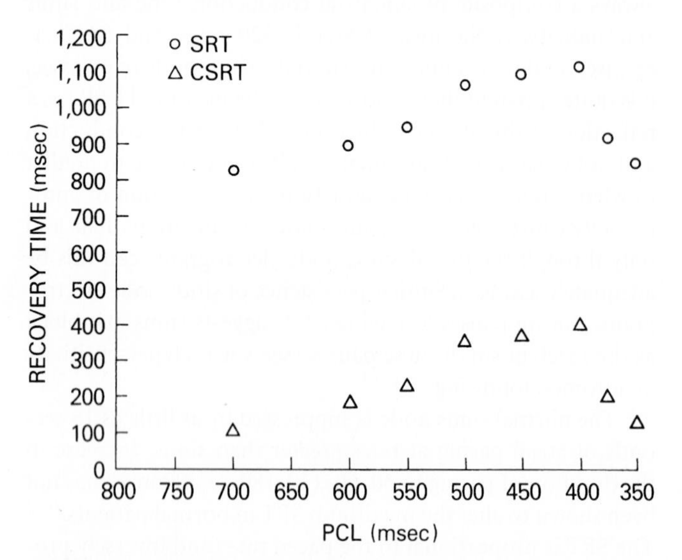


**FIGURE 3-17** *Typical relationship of sinus node recovery time (SRT) to paced cycle length in a normal person.* The paced cycle length (PCL) (abscissa) is plotted against recovery time (ordinate). SRT is shown by the open circles, and corrected sinus node recovery time (CSRT) is shown by the open triangles. There is a progressive increase in SRT and CSRT at shorter PCL, reaching a peak at a PCL of 400 msec. Further shortening of the PCL results in a decrease in recovery time. See text.

and spontaneous pauses following termination of tachycardias in patients with the tachycardia–bradycardia syndrome. Studies in our laboratory do not show a precise relationship between the duration of laboratory-produced and spontaneous pauses following cessation of tachycardias. However, because the rate at which the maximum SRT occurs is unpredictable, and because maximum pauses in patients with the sick sinus syndromes are likely to occur on cessation of spontaneous supraventricular arrhythmias, we recommend that pacing begin at rates just above sinus and continue to rates of 200 bpm (cycle length of 300 msec). We also suggest that they be done at least twice at each paced cycle length, preferably for different durations (30, 60, and/or 120 seconds) to ensure that sinus entrance block has not obscured the true SRT. The duration of maximum SRT and CSRT are independent of age.[10,12,34,74,75]

## Effect of Atropine and Autonomic Blockade on Sinus Node Recovery Time in Normal Persons

Atropine in 1- to 3-mg doses has been shown to markedly diminish the SRT, and in most cases the CSRT; however, some evidence of overdrive suppression always remains present.[10,42,67,73] Furthermore, the marked oscillations that are frequently noted following rapid-paced rates are abolished by atropine.[10,74,75] Atropine occasionally results in the appearance of junctional escapes before sinus escape in normal patients. This phenomenon occurs most frequently in healthy young men with borderline slow heart rates in whom lower doses (1 mg) of atropine are given. When such junctional escape rhythms do occur, they are short-lived, lasting less than 10 beats. We do not believe the appearance of a junctional rhythm should be considered an abnormal response. Failure of the sinus rate to increase is the expression of abnormal sinus function. The use of propranolol and atropine to obtain the IHR also results in a shortening of the CSRT as well as sinus cycle length and SACT.[27,51,52]

## Results of Atrial Pacing in Patients Suspected of Having Sinus Node Dysfunction

Prolonged SRT and/or CSRT has been found in 35% to 93% of patients suspected of having sinus node dysfunction.[11,13,17,33,34,73,75,81–85] The most important reason for the wide discrepancy is probably the difference in the patient populations studied. Those investigations that included a higher number of patients with isolated sinus bradycardia, particularly if asymptomatic, have the lowest incidence of positive responses.[34,73,85] In fact, Breithardt demonstrated no significant differences of CSRT between patients with asymptomatic sinus bradycardia and normal patients.[34] His data further suggest that isolated sinus bradycardia in most cases does not imply clinically significant sinus node dysfunction. Jordan et al., however, have demonstrated that if SRT is adjusted for the effects of autonomic tone, two groups of responses are observed.[27] Those patients with abnormal IHR have abnormal SRT, whereas those with normal IHR have normal SRT. These data have been supported in several other studies.[86] Thus, differences in basal autonomic tone may explain some discrepancies in SRT. In 1983 Alboni et al.[52] confirmed these findings and demonstrated a higher reproducibility following autonomic blockade in those with normal IHR. Other explanations for the discrepancy in the incidence of positive responses include (a) failure to pace for different durations and at a wide range of rates from just above sinus up to 200 bpm and (b) sinus node entrance block. We believe the former is a major reason for failure to demonstrate abnormalities in patients with the tachycardia–bradycardia syndrome.

Marked abnormalities in CSRT as well as SACT usually occur in symptomatic patients with clinical evidence of sinus block or the bradycardia–tachycardia syndrome (Figs. 3-18 and 3-19). Moreover, the paced cycle length at which maximum suppression occurs in patients with sick sinus syndrome is unpredictable and (unlike the situation in normal persons) tends to be affected by both the rate and duration of pacing.[24] However, if sinus entrance block is present, the greatest suppression is likely to occur at relatively slow rates, which allow atrial impulses to penetrate the sinus node. If the longest SRT occurs following pacing at long cycle lengths (i.e., >600 msec) a normal value may reflect the presence of sinus entrance block. In such cases the abnormal SRT is an unreliable assessment of sinus node function. The fact that the paced cycle length producing the longest SRT exceeds 600 msec is in itself a marker of sinus node dysfunction and correlates with

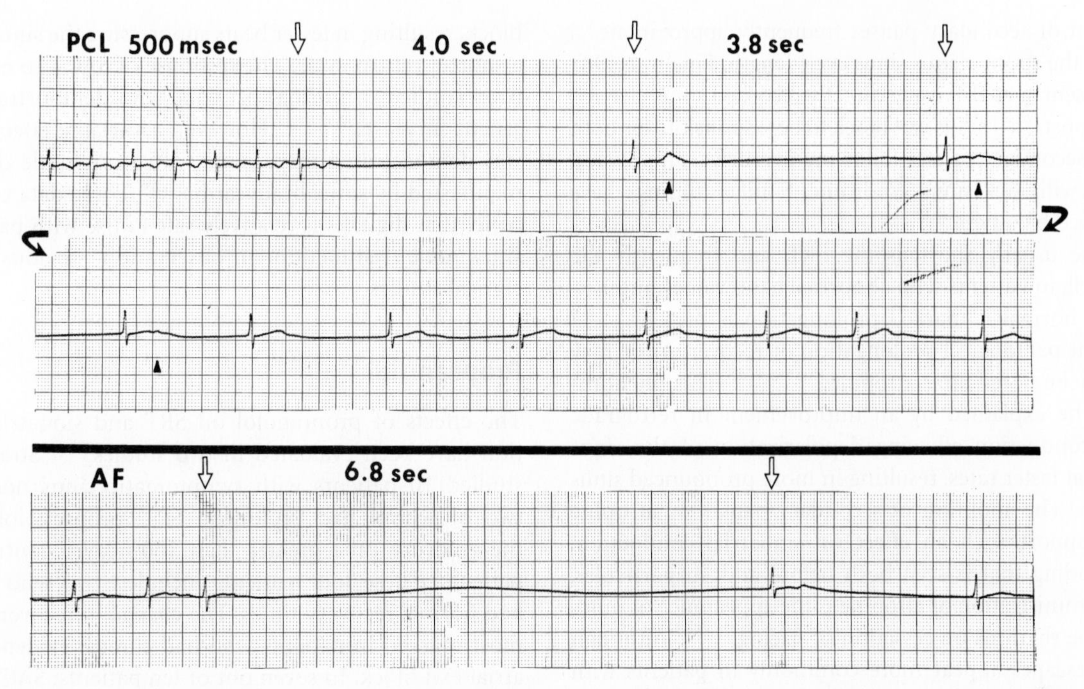


**FIGURE 3-18** *Abnormal sinus node recovery time in a patient with bradycardia–tachycardia syndrome.* In the **top** panel, cessation of atrial pacing at 500 msec results in a 4-second pause with a junctional escape and another 3.8 seconds elapse before the next escape, followed by more escapes. Small *arrowheads* mark sinus P waves that have recovered more slowly than the junction. The findings demonstrate impaired junctional as well as sinus node function. In the **bottom** panel, termination of spontaneous atrial fibrillation in the same patient is followed by similar pauses.

prolonged sinus node refractory and/or prolonged zone I during extrastimulation evaluation of SACT. The most abnormal responses (i.e., the longest SRT) occur in patients with spontaneous sinoatrial exit block or the bradycardia–tachycardia syndrome.[34] Use of sinus node electrogram shows sinus activity during these pauses, indicating a primary abnormality of sinoatrial conduction (see Fig. 3-17). The longest SRT that we have recorded is 23 seconds—in a patient who manifested the bradycardia–tachycardia syndrome.

Prolongation TRT and marked secondary pauses are other manifestations of impaired sinus node conduction and to a lesser extent, automaticity. Marked secondary pauses may occasionally occur in the absence of prolonged SRT; in those instances, sinoatrial block is the mechanism. This observation was substantiated in a study that demonstrated 69% of patients with secondary pauses had clinical evidence of sinoatrial exit block and, conversely, 92% of patients with sinoatrial exit block demonstrated marked secondary pauses.[77] Furthermore,

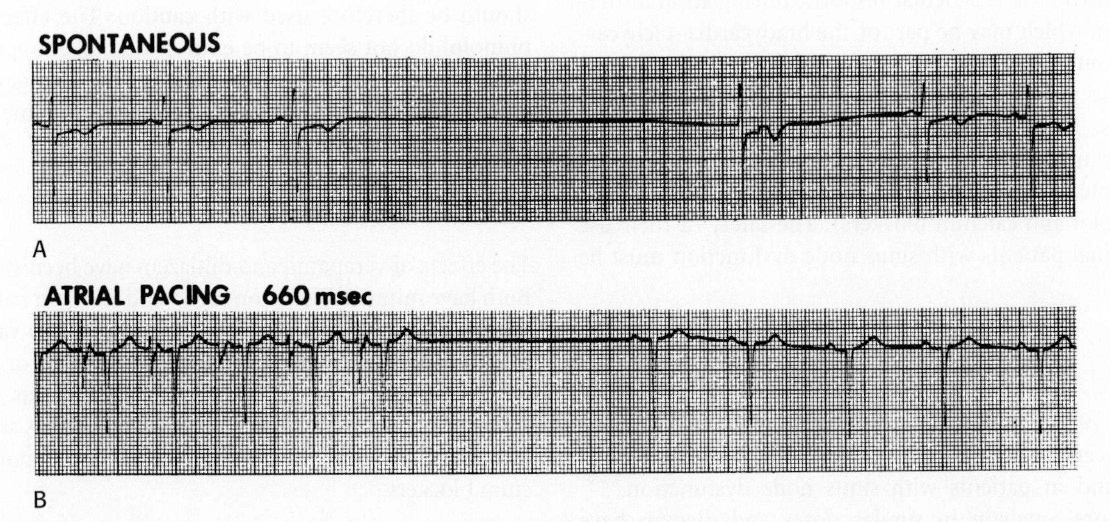


**FIGURE 3-19** *Relationships of overdrive pacing into sinoatrial exit block.* **A:** Following three sinus complexes a sudden pause occurs with an intersinus P-wave interval of approximately 5 seconds. The return of this P wave actually follows the first junctional escape complex. **B:** Atrial overdrive pacing at a cycle length of 660 msec also demonstrates a long pause of approximately 3 seconds. The pauses in **A** are slightly more than four sinus cycles, and the pauses in **B** are approximately three sinus cycles. In both cases, sinoatrial exit block appears to be the mechanism.

the duration of secondary pauses frequently approximates a multiple of the spontaneous sinus cycle length. Finally, a 1983 study by Asseman et al.[64] using directly recorded sinus electrograms demonstrated sinus exit block to be responsible for both initial and secondary pauses following overdrive suppression in patients with sick sinus syndrome. Similar findings have been observed by others.[46,62]

Atropine usually shortens the SRT, and frequently the CSRT as well, in patients with abnormal basal values but usually not to normal if marked prolongation is present.[11,72,74] A significant paradoxical prolongation of recovery time may occasionally be noted after atropine.[75,81,85,87,88] This phenomenon may be explained by an improvement in retrograde sinoatrial conduction allowing depolarization of the sinus pacemaker at faster rates, resulting in more pronounced sinus suppression. The abolition of secondary pauses by atropine tends to support such an effect on sinoatrial conduction. Another finding that is seen both before and, in particular, after the administration of atropine is the appearance of junctional escape rhythms on cessation of pacing.[73,75,85] Although junctional escapes appear more commonly in patients with clinical sinus node dysfunction than in normal persons, the frequency of this finding is further increased by atropine, and in one series, it was seen in 14 of 21 patients.[75] Whether this represents a paradoxical response of the sinus node to atropine and "normal" response of the A-V junction has not been established.

## EFFECT OF DRUGS ON SINUS NODE RECOVERY TIME AND SINOATRIAL CONDUCTION TIME

Digitalis, propranolol, and calcium blockers are commonly used to control the ventricular response during atrial flutter-fibrillation, which may be part of the bradycardia–tachycardia syndrome. Type I antiarrhythmic agents and amiodarone are used to prevent the occurrence of these atrial tachyarrhythmias. Furthermore, these drugs are extremely useful in the management of coexisting cardiac dysfunction, for example, congestive heart failure (digoxin) and angina (propranolol and calcium blockers). The safety of their use in individual patients with sinus node dysfunction must be evaluated.

### Digoxin

Ouabain (0.01 mg/kg) has been demonstrated to have no significant effect on resting heart rate in both normal persons and in patients with sinus node dysfunction.[85–91] Furthermore, ouabain in similar doses and digoxin have been demonstrated to shorten the SRT and/or CSRT in some patients with clinical sinus node dysfunction.[90–94] Shortening of the SRT in this situation may be due to an increase in perinodal refractoriness, which creates sinoatrial entrance block, resulting in fewer beats suppressing the sinus node and a shorter return cycle. The response of SACT to ouabain has been studied in normal patients, who demonstrated a consistent increase.[90,92,94,95] However, a variable effect on SACT was demonstrated in patients with sinus node dysfunction manifested by sinus bradycardia.[92,96] These data confirm the belief that digitalis is relatively safe to use with patients with sinus node dysfunction, an observation previously made in clinical studies.[97]

### Propranolol

The effects of propranolol on SRT and sinoatrial conduction have been evaluated in two studies.[22,98] Strauss et al.[97] studied 10 patients with symptomatic sinus node disease, two of whom had prolonged SRT; propranolol increased the recovery time greater than 160% over control in four patients. These four patients included two who previously had normal recovery times. The change in recovery time was most marked in patients who had clinical evidence of sinoatrial exit block. In seven out of ten patients, SACT could be calculated; it was abnormal in four patients and normal in three patients. Propranolol increased the SACT in six of seven patients. Because propranolol can increase perinodal refractoriness and therefore can prolong conduction into the sinus node as well as decrease the automaticity of the sinus node, the mechanism of SACT prolongation following its administration is unknown. Narula et al.[22] showed a significant increase in CSRT and SACT in patients with sinus dysfunction while no significant effect was observed in normals. No studies using direct recordings of SACT have been performed to clarify the mechanism of propranolol's effect on SACT and CSRT. Clearly, however, in some patients who manifest sinus node dysfunction, propranolol can markedly exacerbate the bradyarrhythmias associated with the syndrome, and it should be therefore used with caution. The effects of propranolol do not seem to be entirely due to unopposed vagal tone, because atropine cannot abolish the changes in SNRT and SACT produced by the drug, although some improvement may be noted.[22,98]

### Calcium Blockers

The effects of verapamil and diltiazem have been studied.[99,100] Both have minimal effects on SACT and CSRT in patients with no sinus dysfunction. The sinus rate response is variable but usually has little effect (less than 10% increase or decrease). Systematic studies of calcium blockers in patients with sinus dysfunction are not available. Many observations suggest that worsening of sinus function is the expected response to calcium blockers.

### Antiarrhythmic Agents

A variety of studies has shown that procainamide, quinidine, lidocaine, mexiletine, and amiodarone can adversely affect sinus node function in patients with evidence of sinus node dysfunction.[101–104] Severe sinus bradycardia and sinus pauses are the most common problems encountered. In my opinion, amiodarone is the worst offender and has even caused severe sinus dysfunction in patients without a prior history or laboratory evidence of sinus dysfunction. In general, the other drugs have minimal effects on sinus node dysfunction in normal persons. The increasing use of amiodarone has led to an increased requirement for pacemakers in patients with paroxysmal atrial fibrillation.

## VAGAL HYPERSENSITIVITY (NEUROCIRCULATORY) SYNDROMES

Vagal hypersensitive syndromes are probably the most important cause of noncardiac syncope in patients, particularly those without cardiac disease. The clinical history is the single most important diagnostic tool for these disorders. Failure to use the history has led to widespread use of costly neurologic and cardiac workups. In younger patients, vasovagal and vasodepressive syncope are by far the most common cause of syncope. This disorder results from an imbalance of autonomic reflexes in response to a variety of stimuli causing bradycardia and/or vasodilatation, and severe hypotension.

In normal patients, assumption of the upright position results in venous pooling, and a decrease in ventricular filling and cardiac output. A slight drop in systolic blood pressure, a rise in diastolic blood pressure, and an increase in heart rate and inotropy occur. These responses are due to compensatory baroreceptor reflexes. In patients with vasovagal or vasodepressor syncope in whom the trigger seems to be prolonged standing, post-exercising, or volume depletion, the compensatory increased inotropy is believed to activate left ventricular mechanoreceptors leading to a pronounced Bezold–Jarisch reflex, resulting in bradycardia and hypotension owing to vasodilatation.[105–110] Although the heart rate may begin to decrease first, the peak drop in blood pressure occurs prior to the peak drop in heart rate.[106,108,111,112] The vasodepressor component usually dominates the syndrome, but in occasional patients, prolonged asystolic periods due to either sinus arrest or exit block or A-V block may produce a near cardiac arrest.[113,114] Flammang et al. suggest that ATP (or adenosine) may be used to predict patients at risk for this type of response. Patients with pauses greater than 10 seconds following ATP are most likely to benefit from a pacemaker. While atropine may relieve the bradycardia component,[111,112] it does not significantly affect the hypotensive component. This suggests that the vasodilation is not mediated by enhanced parasympathetic tone. On the other hand, beta blockers or other negative inotropic agents (e.g., disopyramide) can reverse the hypotension.[111,112,115,116] Although these findings support a counter-compensatory mechanoreceptor reflex (Bezold–Jarisch reflex) as the mechanism of the vasovagal episode in hypovolemic triggered events, I am not convinced this mechanism is always responsible for this syndrome, particularly when it occurs in adults with organic heart disease or when other triggers are present. We have seen several patients in whom this syndrome has developed following cardiac transplant. This observation suggests an alternative mechanism, that is, failure of alpha receptor responsiveness, failure of activation and/or responsiveness of the renin-angiotensin system, or stimulation of serotonin receptors.

These observations have led to the widespread use of tilt testing to evaluate patients with unexplained syncope.[111–121] Such patients are tilted at 40° to 80° for 10 to 40 minutes. We use 60° tilt for 30 minutes, which reproduces the syndrome in 65% to 80% of patients within 30 minutes. The higher the degree of tilt, the shorter the duration of time prior to symptoms.[112,118–121] The use of isoproterenol in small boluses or short infusions increases the sensitivity of the tilt test,[111] but in my opinion, may give rise to false-positive results. It is certainly no surprise that beta blockers prevent the syndrome in patients requiring isoproterenol to achieve positive tilt test. Chen et al. have demonstrated reasonable reproducibility of such tests, potentially allowing for drug evaluation.[120] To date, however, no randomized controlled studies have demonstrated predictable responses to drugs. In our laboratory, we found the test to be useful primarily in young patients with cardiac disease who have a high likelihood of this cause of syncope but in whom a clinical history is not suggestive. Moreover, in patients with organic heart disease, and unexplained syncope, the outcome of patients with positive and negative tilt tests is similar. This has led to skepticism of the use of this technique in such patients. In these patients we believe that a full electrophysiologic study should be performed. Tachyarrhythmias are a very important cause of syncope in these patients, regardless of whether or not the tilt test is positive. Electrophysiologic assessment of sinus node function in patients with vasovagal or vasodepressor syncope has been invariably normal in our experience. This is not surprising since there are many triggers; for example, pain, abdominal distension, deglutination, micturition, which are totally different from the triggers induced by a tilt test. The tilt test may be useful to characterize the autonomic response to assuming the upright position and can be useful in diagnosing diabetic neuropathy and a variety of dysautonomic syndromes.

Another expression of vagal hypersensitivity is the so-called carotid sinus hypersensitivity syndrome, in which syncope may primarily be sinus inhibitory, although a vasodepressor component may also occur. Sinus node function as measured by direct and/or indirect SACT or sinus node response to overdrive pacing (CSRT) has generally been normal.[122–124] When abnormal, they can be normalized by atropine. The consistent findings in such patients are prolonged, usually right-sided, pauses following CSP (Fig. 3-20). Use of directly recorded sinus electrograms has shown that CSP usually produces a prolongation of sinoatrial conduction eventuating in sinoatrial block of one or more sinus impulses (see Fig. 3-12).[46,61–64,125] Slowing of sinus automaticity may also be present. Pacing, anticholinergic drugs, and

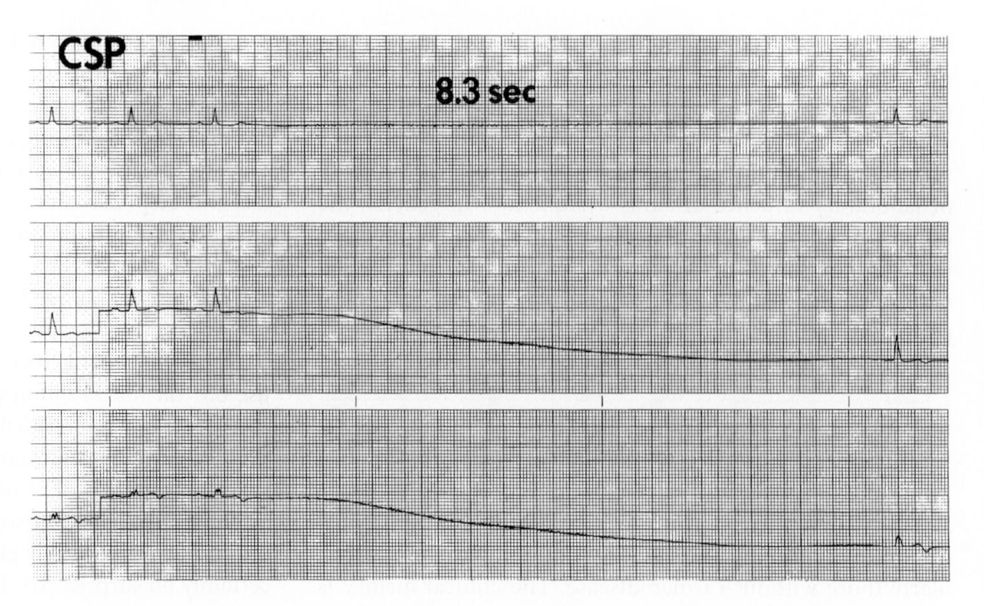


**FIGURE 3-20** *Effect of carotid sinus pressure on a patient with carotid sinus syncope.* Leads 1, 2, and 3 are displayed as carotid sinus pressure (CSP) is applied. An 8.3 second pause results. Near-syncope developed, linking the clinical episodes. See text for discussion.

theophylline have all been reported to be effective for the cardioinhibitory features of this. The vasodepressor component is difficult to treat, and pacemaker therapy with or without pharmacologic manipulation has been less than satisfactory. Moreover, the high incidence of spontaneous remission of this syncope makes assessment of the actual benefit of these therapies difficult.

Another less frequently observed phenomenon is paroxysmal "sinus arrest," which is usually preceded by a slowing of heart rate and occurs in people with normal sinus node function. We have seen 15 patients with pauses ranging from 6 to 55 seconds (Fig. 3-21). These episodes could happen during the day or night but invariably during inactivity. Three of these patients were sleeping; the others were either presyncopal or had true syncope. A vagal stimulus such as nausea or vomiting was present in 50% of our patients. The absence of any escape pacemaker for such extended pauses is remarkable. On electrophysiologic testing, all patients have had normal SACT and CSRT. None had directly recorded sinus electrograms during an episode, so the exact mechanism of these pauses remains unknown. Seven had exaggerated responses to CSP (4 to 10 seconds), which in each case was abolished by atropine. Pacemakers have relieved symptoms in the 12 symptomatic patients. The natural history and mechanism of this disorder require investigation, but they may represent a variant of vasovagal syncope,[113,114] although nocturnal episodes may be related to sleep apnea disorders.

## THERAPEUTIC IMPLICATIONS

The ECG patterns of sinus node dysfunction do not always correlate with the symptoms. A variety of interventions may be necessary to evaluate more carefully the presence and degree of abnormalities of sinus node automaticity and/or sinoatrial conduction. The use of invasive electrophysiologic studies has been decreasing as clinicians have recognized their limitations and the importance of the clinical history. Nevertheless, these studies have provided important information about normal and abnormal sinus node function. When the response to drugs and electrical stimulation is taken into consideration, overall function of the sinus node and perinodal tissue seems to be most severely disturbed in patients with spontaneous sinoatrial exit block or the bradycardia–tachycardia syndrome. Most of these patients, however, are symptomatic, and on clinical and ECG evidence alone, they can be correctly classified as having sinus node dysfunction. In such cases, electrophysiologic testing is not necessary to make a diagnosis of sinus node dysfunction. More difficult problems are presented by the patients who have isolated sinus bradycardia but symptoms compatible with sinus node dysfunction. Many of these people have neurocardiac symptoms and have normal electrophysiologic sinus node function studies. A good history could avoid EP studies in many of these patients. It may be important to test sinus node function in those patients with truly unclear causes of symptoms to avoid the unnecessary implantation of a cardiac pacemaker. Perhaps the most useful measures of their overall sinus node function are a combination of the responses to atropine and exercise and SNRT, particularly the CSRT. A marked prolongation of the CSRT and an absent or blunted response to atropine and exercise suggest impaired sinus node function. As noted previously, evaluation of CSRT following pharmacologic denervation may increase the sensitivity of the test.[27] If abnormal results are correlated with symptoms, pacemaker implantation may be considered. The same is true of patients in whom CSP produces pauses of greater than 3 seconds, because the specificity of this response is unknown, particularly in elderly patients. More than 50% of patients over 65 have pauses >3 seconds, which have no clinical significance. The significance of an isolated prolongation of sinus node conduction time is unclear in the absence of

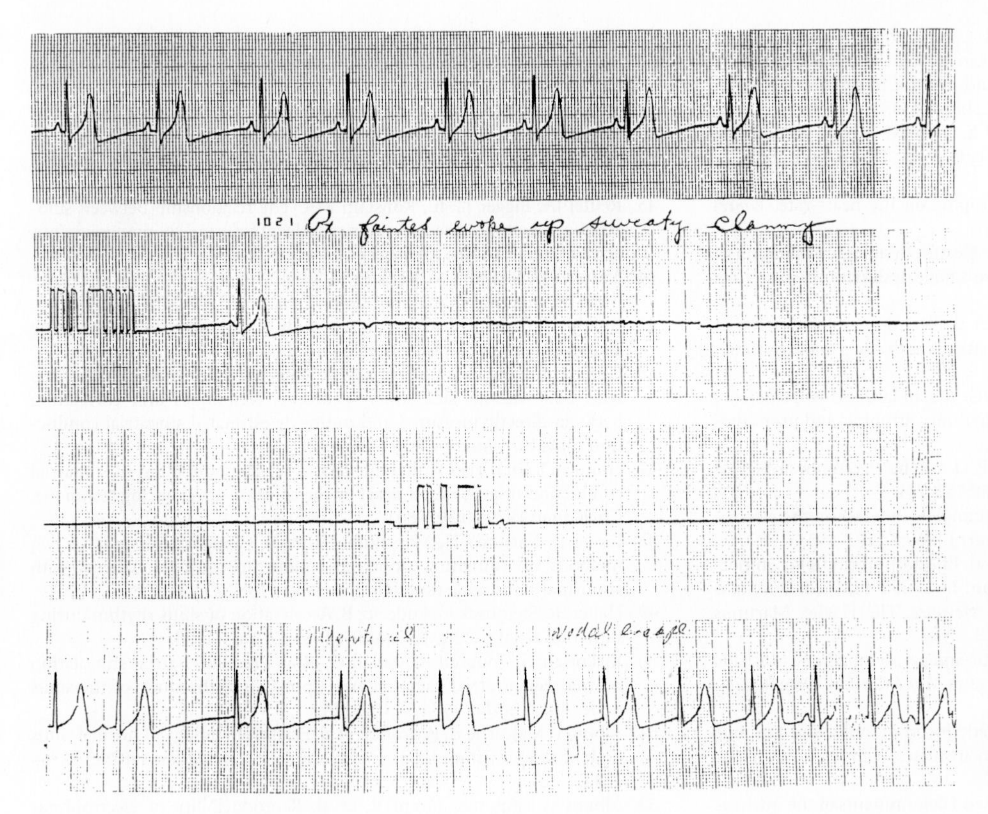


**FIGURE 3-21** *Paroxysmal sinus arrest.* This is a rhythm strip from a patient who developed paroxysmal sinus arrest. One can see slight slowing of the sinus cycle before a prolonged episode of asystole that lasted 20 seconds. The patient had no cardiac disease. See text for discussion.

clinically evident and symptomatic sinoatrial exit block. Thus, the presence of symptoms must be correlated with electrophysiologic findings for the results of these studies to be translated into clinically meaningful decisions.

When considering implantation of a permanent pacemaker, we recommend evaluating A-V nodal and infranodal conduction (Chapter 4) because a significant number of patients with sinus node dysfunction have abnormalities of A-V conduction.[13,34,126] Impaired A-V conduction may preclude the use of an atrial pacemaker when it might be advantageous hemodynamically. Currently, multiprogrammable dual-chambered pacemakers with rate responsive (physiologic) are recommended for patients with sinus node dysfunction. Patients with atrial tachyarrhythmias, particularly atrial fibrillation, may require VVIR or DDDR pacemakers with mode-switching capabilities. Patients with good ventriculoatrial conduction might develop a pacemaker tachycardia syndrome if only ventricular pacing is used.

Knowledge of the effects of potentially therapeutic drugs on sinus node function is of major clinical importance. Propranolol and calcium blockers, which may be desirable to treat angina in a patient who has sinus node dysfunction, may be shown to cause severe symptomatic bradyarrhythmias that require a pacemaker. Also, the safety of drugs such as digitalis and antiarrhythmic agents should be assessed in each patient before use. If these drugs are needed in the treatment of heart failure, arrhythmias, or angina but are shown in the laboratory to produce significant bradyarrhythmias, a pacemaker may be necessary if no other therapy is available.

## REFERENCES


1. Kirk JE, Kvorning SA. Sinus bradycardia; a clinical study of 515 consecutive cases. *Acta Med Scand Suppl* 1952;266:625–652.
2. Brodsky M, Wu D, Denes P, et al. Arrhythmias documented by 24 hour continuous electrocardiographic monitoring in 50 male medical students without apparent heart disease. *Am J Cardiol* 1977;39:390–395.
3. Short DS. The syndrome of alternating bradycardia and tachycardia. *Br Heart J* 1954;16:208–214.
4. Mazuz M, Friedman HS. Significance of prolonged electrocardiographic pauses in sinoatrial disease: sick sinus syndrome. *Am J Cardiol* 1983;52:485–489.
5. Hilgard J, Ezri MD, Denes P. Significance of ventricular pauses of three seconds or more detected on twenty-four-hour Holter recordings. *Am J Cardiol* 1985;55:1005–1008.
6. Johansson BW. Long-term ECG in ambulatory clinical practice. Analysis and 2-year follow-up of 100 patients studied with a portable ECG tape recorder. *Eur J Cardiol* 1977;5:39–48.
7. Lekieffre J, Libersa C, Caron J, et al. Electrocardiographic aspects of sinus node dysfunction. Use of the Holter electrocardiographic recording. In: Levy S, Scheinman MM, eds. *Cardiac arrhythmias. From diagnosis to therapy.* Mount Kisco, NY: Futura, 1984:73–86.
8. Grodman RS, Capone RJ, Most AS. Arrhythmia surveillance by transtelephonic monitoring: comparison with Holter monitoring in symptomatic ambulatory patients. *Am Heart J* 1979;98:459–464.
9. Holden W, McAnulty JH, Rahimtoola SH. Characterisation of heart rate response to exercise in the sick sinus syndrome. *Br Heart J* 1978;40:923–930.
10. Mandel W, Hayakawa H, Danzig R, et al. Evaluation of sino-atrial node function in man by overdrive suppression. *Circulation* 1971;44:59–66.
11. Mandel WJ, Hayakawa H, Allen HN, et al. Assessment of sinus node function in patients with the sick sinus syndrome. *Circulation* 1972;46:761–769.
12. Mandel WJ, Laks MM, Obayashi K. Sinus node function; evaluation in patients with and without sinus node disease. *Arch Intern Med* 1975;135:388–394.

13. Rosen KM, Loeb HS, Sinno MZ, et al. Cardiac conduction in patients with symptomatic sinus node disease. *Circulation* 1971;43:836–844.
14. Craig FN. Effects of atropine, work and heat on heart rate and sweat production in man. *J Appl Physiol* 1952;4:826–833.
15. Eckberg DL, Drabinsky M, Braunwald E. Defective cardiac parasympathetic control in patients with heart disease. *N Engl J Med* 1971;285:877–883.
16. Morton HJ, Thomas ET. Effect of atropine on the heart-rate. *Lancet* 1958;2:1313–1315.
17. Strauss HC, Bigger JT, Saroff AL, et al. Electrophysiologic evaluation of sinus node function in patients with sinus node dysfunction. *Circulation* 1976;53:763–776.
18. Dhingra RC, Amat YLF, Wyndham C, et al. Electrophysiologic effects of atropine on sinus node and atrium in patients with sinus nodal dysfunction. *Am J Cardiol* 1976;38:848–855.
19. Cleaveland CR, Rangno RE, Shand DG. A standardized isoproterenol sensitivity test. The effects of sinus arrhythmia, atropine, and propranolol. *Arch Intern Med* 1972;130:47–52.
20. Seides SF, Josephson ME, Batsford WP, et al. The electrophysiology of propranolol in man. *Am Heart J* 1974;88:733–741.
21. Stern S, Eisenberg S. The effect of propranolol (Inderal) on the electrocardiogram of normal subjects. *Am Heart J* 1969;77:192–195.
22. Narula OS, Vasquez M, Shantha N, et al. Effect of propranolol on normal and abnormal sinus node function. In: Bonke FIM, ed. *The sinus node: structure, function, and clinical relevance.* The Hague: Martinus Nijhoff Medical Division, 1978:112–128.
23. Jose AD. Effect of combined sympathetic and parasympathetic blockade on heart rate and cardiac function in man. *Am J Cardiol* 1966;18:476–478.
24. Jose AD, Taylor RR. Autonomic blockade by propranolol and atropine to study intrinsic myocardial function in man. *J Clin Invest* 1969;48: 2019–2031.
25. Jose AD, Collison D. The normal range and determinants of the intrinsic heart rate in man. *Cardiovasc Res* 1970;4:160–167.
26. Tonkin AM, Heddle WF. Electrophysiological testing of sinus node function. *Pacing Clin Electrophysiol* 1984;7:735–748.
27. Jordan JL, Yamaguchi I, Mandel WJ. Studies on the mechanism of sinus node dysfunction in the sick sinus syndrome. *Circulation* 1978;57: 217–223.
28. Mason JW. Overdrive suppression in the transplanted heart: effect of the autonomic nervous system on human sinus node recovery. *Circulation* 1980;62:688–696.
29. Strauss HC, Saroff AL, Bigger JT Jr, et al. Premature atrial stimulation as a key to the understanding of sinoatrial conduction in man. Presentation of data and critical review of the literature. *Circulation* 1973;47: 86–93.
30. Dhingra RC, Wyndham C, Amat YL, et al. Sinus nodal responses to atrial extrastimuli in patients without apparent sinus node disease. *Am J Cardiol* 1975;36:445–452.
31. Masini G, Dianda R, Graziina A. Analysis of sino-atrial conduction in man using premature atrial stimulation. *Cardiovasc Res* 1975;9: 498–508.
32. Breithardt G, Seipel L. The effect of premature atrial depolarization on sinus node automaticity in man. *Circulation* 1976;53:920–925.
33. Strauss HC, Scheinman MM, LaBarre A, et al. Programmed atrial stimulation and rapid atrial pacing in patients with sinus pauses and sinoatrial exit block. In: Bonke FIM, ed. *The sinus node: structure, function, and clinical relevance.* The Hague: Martinus Nijhoff Medical Division, 1978:56–64.
34. Breithardt G, Seipel L, Loogen F. Sinus node recovery time and calculated sinoatrial conduction time in normal subjects and patients with sinus node dysfunction. *Circulation* 1977;56:43–50.
35. Miller HC, Strauss HC. Measurement of sinoatrial conduction time by premature atrial stimulation in the rabbit. *Circ Res* 1974;35:935–947.
36. Strauss HC, Bigger JT Jr. Electrophysiological properties of the rabbit sinoatrial perinodal fibers. *Circ Res* 1972;31:490–506.
37. Steinbeck G, Allessie MA, Bonke FI, et al. Sinus node response to premature atrial stimulation in the rabbit studied with multiple microelectrode impalements. *Circ Res* 1978;43:695–704.
38. Bleeker WK, Mackaay AJ, Masson-Pevet M, et al. Asymmetry of the sino-atrial conduction in the rabbit heart. *J Mol Cell Cardiol* 1982;14: 633–643.
39. Bonke FI, Bouman LN, van Rijn HE. Change of cardiac rhythm in the rabbit after an atrial premature beat. *Circ Res* 1969;24:533–544.
40. Bonke FI, Bouman LN, Schopman FJ. Effect of an early atrial premature beat on activity of the sinoatrial node and atrial rhythm in the rabbit. *Circ Res* 1971;29:704–715.
41. Steinbeck G, Luderitz B. Sinoatrial pacemaker shift following atrial stimulation in man. *Circulation* 1977;56:402–409.
42. Steinbeck G, Luderitz B. Comparative study of sinoatrial conduction time and sinus node recovery time. *Br Heart J* 1975;37:956–962.
43. Reiffel JA, Bigger JT Jr., Konstam MA. The relationship between sinoatrial conduction time and sinus cycle length during spontaneous sinus arrhythmia in adults. *Circulation* 1974;50:924–934.
44. Narula OS, Shantha N, Vasquez M, et al. A new method for measurement of sinoatrial conduction time. *Circulation* 1978;58:706–714.
45. Breithardt G, Seipel L. Comparative study of two methods of estimating sinoatrial conduction time in man. *Am J Cardiol* 1978;42:965–972.
46. Gomes JA, Kang PS, El-Sherif N. The sinus node electrogram in patients with and without sick sinus syndrome: techniques and correlation between directly measured and indirectly estimated sinoatrial conduction time. *Circulation* 1982;66:864–873.
47. Grant AO, Kirkorian G, Benditt DG, et al. The estimation of sinoatrial conduction time in rabbit heart by the constant atrial pacing technique. *Circulation* 1979;60:597–604.
48. Inoue D, Katsume H, Matsukubo H, et al. Comparative study of two methods of estimating sinoatrial conduction time in patients with abnormal sinus node function. *Jpn Heart J* 1982;23:25–38.
49. Haberl R, Steinbeck G, Luderitz B. Acceleration of sinus rhythm during slow-rate atrial pacing. *Circulation* 1983;67:1368–1373.
50. Kirkorian G, Touboul P, Atallah G, et al. Premature atrial stimulation during regular atrial pacing: a new approach to the study of the sinus node. *Am J Cardiol* 1984;54:109–114.
51. Alboni P, Malcarne C, Pedroni P, et al. Electrophysiology of normal sinus node with and without autonomic blockade. *Circulation* 1982;65:1236–1242.
52. Alboni P, Filippi L, Pirani R, et al. Reproducibility of electrophysiological parameters of sinus node following autonomic blockade. *Int J Cardiol* 1983;4:431–442.
53. Breithardt G, Seipel L, Both A, et al. The effect of atropine on calculated sinoatrial conduction time in man. *Eur J Cardiol* 1976;4:49–57.
54. Bissett JK, de Soyza N, Kane JJ, et al. Improved sinus node sensing after atropine. *Am Heart J* 1976;91:752–756.
55. Reiffel JA, Gang E, Livelli F, et al. Indirectly estimated sinoatrial conduction time by the atrial premature stimulus technique: patterns of error and the degree of associated inaccuracy as assessed by direct sinus node electrography. *Am Heart J* 1983;106:459–463.
56. Goldreyer BN, Damato AN. Sinoatrial-node entrance block. *Circulation* 1971;44:789–802.
57. Kerr CR, Strauss HC. The measurement of sinus node refractoriness in man. *Circulation* 1983;68:1231–1237.
58. Cramer M, Siegal M, Bigger JT Jr., et al. Characteristics of extracellular potentials recorded from the sinoatrial pacemaker of the rabbit. *Circ Res* 1977;41:292–300.
59. Cramer M, Hariman RJ, Boxer R, et al. Electrograms from the canine sinoatrial pacemaker recorded in vitro and in situ. *Am J Cardiol* 1978;42: 939–946.
60. Hariman RJ, Krongrad E, Boxer RA, et al. Method for recording electrical activity of the sinoatrial node and automatic atrial foci during cardiac catheterization in human subjects. *Am J Cardiol* 1980;45:775–781.
61. Reiffel JA, Gang E, Gliklich J, et al. The human sinus node electrogram: a transvenous catheter technique and a comparison of directly measured and indirectly estimated sinoatrial conduction time in adults. *Circulation* 1980;62:1324–1334.
62. Reiffel JA, Bigger JT Jr. Current status of direct recordings of the sinus node electrogram in man. *Pacing Clin Electrophysiol* 1983;6:1143–1150.
63. Sharma AD, Klein GJ. Comparative quantitative electrophysiologic effects of adenosine triphosphate on the sinus node and atrioventricular node. *Am J Cardiol* 1988;61:330–335.
64. Asseman P, Berzin B, Desry D, et al. Persistent sinus nodal electrograms during abnormally prolonged postpacing atrial pauses in sick sinus syndrome in humans: sinoatrial block vs overdrive suppression. *Circulation* 1983;68:33–41.
65. Rakovec P, Jakopin J, Rode P, et al. Clinical comparison of indirectly and directly determined sinoatrial conduction time. *Am Heart J* 1981;102: 292–294.

66. Crook B, Kitson D, McComish M, et al. Indirect measurement of sinoatrial conduction time in patients with sinoatrial disease and in controls. *Br Heart J* 1977;39:771–777.
67. Breithardt G, Seipel L. Influence of drugs on the relationship between sinus node recovery time and calculated sinoatrial conduction time in man. *Basic Res Cardiol* 1978;73:68–76.
68. Gaskell WH. On the innervation of the heart with special reference to the heart of tortoise. *J Physiol* 1884;4:43–132.
69. Lange G. Action of driving stimuli from intrinsic and extrinsic sources on in situ cardiac pacemaker tissues. *Circ Res* 1965;17:449–459.
70. Lu HH, Lange G, Brooks CM. Factors controlling pacemaker action in cells of the sinoatrial node. *Circ Res* 1965;17:460–471.
71. Vassalle M. The relationship among cardiac pacemakers. Overdrive suppression. *Circ Res* 1977;41:269–277.
72. Kodama I, Goto J, Ando S, et al. Effects of rapid stimulation on the transmembrane action potentials of rabbit sinus node pacemaker cells. *Circ Res* 1980;46:90–99.
73. Narula OS, Samet P, Javier RP. Significance of the sinus-node recovery time. *Circulation* 1972;45:140–158.
74. Kulbertus HE, Leval-Rutten F, Mary L, et al. Sinus node recovery time in the elderly. *Br Heart J* 1975;37:420–425.
75. Delius W, Wirtzfeld A. The significance of the sinus node recovery time in the sick sinus syndrome. In: Luderitz B, ed. *Cardiac pacing, diagnostic and therapeutic tools.* Berlin, NY: Springer-Verlag, 1976:25–32.
76. Heddle WF, Dorveaux LD, Tonkin AM. Use of rapid atrial pacing to assess sinus node function. *Clin Prog Electrophysiol Pacing* 1985;3:299.
77. Benditt DG, Strauss HC, Scheinman MM, et al. Analysis of secondary pauses following termination of rapid atrial pacing in man. *Circulation* 1976;54:436–441.
78. Nalos PC, Deng Z, Rosenthal ME, et al. Hemodynamic influences on sinus node recovery time: effects of autonomic blockade. *J Am Coll Cardiol* 1986;7:1079–1086.
79. Gang ES, Reiffel JA, Livelli FD Jr., et al. Sinus node recovery times following the spontaneous termination of supraventricular tachycardia and following atrial overdrive pacing: a comparison. *Am Heart J* 1983;105:210–215.
80. Engel TR, Luck JC, Leddy CL, et al. Diagnostic implications of atrial vulnerability. *Pacing Clin Electrophysiol* 1979;2:208–214.
81. Reiffel JA, Bigger JT, Giardina EG. "Paradoxical" prolongation of sinus nodal recovery time after atropine in the sick sinus syndrome. *Am J Cardiol* 1975;36:98–104.
82. Lien WP, Lee YS, Chang FZ, et al. Electrophysiologic manifestations in so-called "sick sinus syndrome". *Jpn Circ J* 1978;42:195–206.
83. Reiffel JA, Bigger JT Jr., Cramer M, et al. Ability of Holter electrocardiographic recording and atrial stimulation to detect sinus nodal dysfunction in symptomatic and asymptomatic patients with sinus bradycardia. *Am J Cardiol* 1977;40:189–194.
84. Dhingra RC, Deedwania PC, Cummings JM, et al. Electrophysiologic effects of lidocaine on sinus node and atrium in patients with and without sinoatrial dysfunction. *Circulation* 1978;57:448–454.
85. Gupta PK, Lichstein E, Chadda KD, et al. Appraisal of sinus nodal recovery time in patients with sick sinus syndrome. *Am J Cardiol* 1974;34:265–270.
86. Juillard A, Guillerm F, Chuong HV, et al. Sinus node electrogram recording in 59 patients. Comparison with simultaneous estimation of sinoatrial conduction using premature atrial stimulation. *Br Heart J* 1983;50:75–84.
87. Bashour T, Hemb R, Strauss HC, et al. Letter: an unusual effect of atropine on overdrive suppression. *Circulation* 1973;48:911–913.
88. Dhingra RC, Amat YLF, Wyndham C, et al. The electrophysiological effects of ouabain on sinus node and atrium in man. *J Clin Invest* 1975;56:555–562.
89. Ticzon AR, Strauss HC, Gallagher JJ, et al. Sinus nodal function in the intact dog heart evaluated by premature atrial stimulation and atrial pacing. *Am J Cardiol* 1975;35:492–503.
90. Engel TR, Schaal SF. Digitalis in the sick sinus syndrome. The effects of digitalis on sinoatrial automaticity and atrioventricular conduction. *Circulation* 1973;48:1201–1207.
91. Reiffel JA, Bigger JT Jr., Cramer M. Effects of digoxin on sinus nodal function before and after vagal blockade in patients with sinus nodal dysfunction: a clue to the mechanisms of the action of digitalis on the sinus node. *Am J Cardiol* 1979;43:983–989.
92. Vera Z, Miller RR, McMillin D, et al. Effects of digitalis on sinus nodal function in patients with sick sinus syndrome. *Am J Cardiol* 1978;41:318–323.
93. Gomes JA, Kang PS, El-Sherif N. Effects of digitalis on the human sick sinus node after pharmacologic autonomic blockade. *Am J Cardiol* 1981;48:783–788.
94. Bond RC, Engel TR, Schaal SF. The effect of digitalis on sinoatrial conduction in man. *Circ* 1973; 48:147.
95. Reiffel JA, Bigger JT, Giardina EG. The effect of digoxin on sinus node automaticity and sinoatrial conduction. (Abstract). *J Clin Invest* 1974;53:64.
96. Rubenstein JJ, Schulman CL, Yurchak PM, et al. Clinical spectrum of the sick sinus syndrome. *Circulation* 1972;46:5–13.
97. Strauss HC, Gilbert M, Svenson RH, et al. Electrophysiologic effects of propranolol on sinus node function in patients with sinus node dysfunction. *Circulation* 1976;54:452–459.
98. Mitchell LB, Jutzy KR, Lewis SJ, et al. Intracardiac electrophysiologic study of intravenous diltiazem and combined diltiazem-digoxin in patients. *Am Heart J* 1982;103:57–66.
99. Kawai C, Konishi T, Matsuyama E, et al. Comparative effects of three calcium antagonists, diltiazem, verapamil and nifedipine, on the sinoatrial and atrioventricular nodes. Experimental and clinical studies. *Circulation* 1981;63:1035–1042.
100. Goldberg D, Reiffel JA, Davis JC, et al. Electrophysiologic effects of procainamide on sinus function in patients with and without sinus node disease. *Am Heart J* 1982;103:75–79.
101. Vera Z, Awan NA, Mason DT. Assessment of oral quinidine effects on sinus node function in sick sinus syndrome patients. *Am Heart J* 1982;103:80–84.
102. Strauss HC, Scheinman MM, Labarre A, et al. Review of the significance of drugs in the sick sinus syndrome. In: Bonke FIM, ed. *The sinus node: structure, function, and clinical relevance.* The Hague: Martinus Nijhoff Medical Division, 1978:103–111.
103. Reiffel JA. Drugs to avoid in patients with sinus node dysfunction. *Drug Ther* 1982;6:99.
104. Glick G, Yu PN. Hemodynamic changes during spontaneous vasovagal reactions. *Am J Med* 1963;34:42–51.
105. Epstein SE, Stampfer M, Beiser GD. Role of the capacitance and resistance vessels in vasovagal syncope. *Circulation* 1968;37:524–533.
106. Fitzpatrick A, Theodorakis G, Travill C, et al. Incidence of malignant vasovagal syndrome in 332 syncope patients: results of cardiac pacing. (Abstract). *Br Heart J* 1989;61:97.
107. Mark AL. The Bezold-Jarisch reflex revisited: clinical implications of inhibitory reflexes originating in the heart. *J Am Coll Cardiol* 1983;1:90–102.
108. Thoren P. Vagal depressor reflexes elicited by left ventricular C-fibers during myocardial ischemia in cats. In: Schwartz PJ, Brown AM, Maliani A, et al., eds. *Neural mechanisms in cardiac arrhythmias.* New York, NY: Raven Press, 1978:179–190.
109. Abboud FM. Ventricular syncope: is the heart a sensory organ? *N Engl J Med* 1989;320:390–392.
110. Waxman MB, Yao L, Cameron DA, et al. Isoproterenol induction of vasodepressor-type reaction in vasodepressor-prone persons. *Am J Cardiol* 1989;63:58–65.
111. Chen MY, Goldenberg IF, Milstein S, et al. Cardiac electrophysiologic and hemodynamic correlates of neurally mediated syncope. *Am J Cardiol* 1989;63:66–72.
112. Maloney JD, Jaeger FJ, Fouad-Tarazi FM, et al. Malignant vasovagal syncope: prolonged asystole provoked by head-up tilt. Case report and review of diagnosis, pathophysiology, and therapy. *Cleve Clin J Med* 1988;55:542–548.
113. Milstein S, Buetikofer J, Lesser J, et al. Cardiac asystole: a manifestation of neurally mediated hypotension-bradycardia. *J Am Coll Cardiol* 1989;14:1626–1632.
114. Goldenberg IF, Almquist A, Dunbar DN, et al. Prevention of neurally-mediated syncope by selective beta-1 adrenoreceptor blockade. (Abstract). *Circ* 1987;76(Suppl IV):IV-133.
115. Milstein S, Buetikofer J, Lesser J, et al. Disopyramide reversal of induced hypotension-bradycardia in neurally-mediated syncope. (Abstract). *Circ* 1987; 76(Suppl IV):IV-175.
116. Kenny RA, Ingram A, Bayliss J, et al. Head-up tilt: a useful test for investigating unexplained syncope. *Lancet* 1986;1:1352–1355.
117. Sutton R, Vardas P, Williams S, et al. Value of tilt-testing in unexplained syncope. (Abstract). *PACE* 1988;11:829.

118. Fitzpatrick A, Robinson S, Bower M, et al. Vasovagal syndrome: importance of tilt-testing methodology. (Abstract). *PACE* 1987;11: 829.
119. Chen XO, Milstein S, Dunnigan A, et al. Reproducibility of upright-tilt testing for eliciting neurally-mediated syncope. (Abstract). *Circ* 1988;78(Suppl):239.
120. Fitzpatrick A, Sutton R. Tilting towards a diagnosis in recurrent unexplained syncope. *Lancet* 1989;1:658–660.
121. Schneller SJ, Harthorne JW. Carotid sinus hypersensitivity. *Clin Prog Electrophysiol Pacing* 1985;3:389.
122. Stryjer D, Friedensohn A, Schlesinger Z. Electrophysiological studies in screening of the "mixed type" of carotid sinus syncope. In: Feruglio FA, ed. *Cardiac pacing, electrophysiology and pacemaker technology.* Padova: Piccin Medical Books, 1982:523–527.
123. Almquist A, Gornick C, Benson W Jr., et al. Carotid sinus hypersensitivity: evaluation of the vasodepressor component. *Circulation* 1985; 71:927–936.
124. Gang ES, Oseran DS, Mandel WJ, et al. Sinus node electrogram in patients with the hypersensitive carotid sinus syndrome. *J Am Coll Cardiol* 1985;5:1484–1490.
125. Narula OS. Atrioventricular conduction defects in patients with sinus bradycardia. Analysis by His bundle recordings. *Circulation* 1971;44:1096–1110.
126. Luderitz B, Steinbeck G, Naumann d'Alnoncourt C, et al. Relevance of diagnostic atrial stimulation for pacemaker treatment in sinoatrial disease. In: Bonke FIM, ed. *The sinus node: structure, function and clinical relevance.* The Hague: Martinus Nijhoff, 1978:77–88.
127. Scheinman MM, Strauss HC, Abbott JA, et al. Electrophysiologic testing in patients with sinus pauses and/or sinoatrial exit block. *Eur J Cardiol* 1978;8:51–60.
128. Yabek SM, Jarmakani JM. Sinus node dysfunction in children, adolescents, and young adults. *Pediatrics* 1978;61:593–598.
129. Kugler JD, Gillette PC, Mullins CE, et al. Sinoatrial conduction in children: an index of sinoatrial node function. *Circulation* 1979;59:1266–1276.
130. Bethge C, Gebhardt-Seehausen U, Mullges W. The human sinus nodal electrogram: techniques and clinical results of intra-atrial recordings in patients with and without sick sinus syndrome. *Am Heart J* 1986; 112:1074–1082.
131. El-Said GM, Gillette PC, Mullins CE, et al. Significance of pacemaker recovery time after the Mustard operation for transposition of the great arteries. *Am J Cardiol* 1976;38:448–451.

CHAPTER

# 4 Atrioventricular Conduction

The usefulness of intracardiac recording and stimulation techniques in humans was first realized during its application to patients with disorders of atrioventricular (A-V) conduction. Electrophysiologic study allowed confirmation and further elucidation of the underlying mechanisms and site of block suspected indirectly by surface ECG. The A-V block has been traditionally classified by criteria combining implications about anatomic site, mechanism, and prognosis. Analysis of A-V conduction from the surface ECG is confined to (a) the duration and shape of the P wave, (b) the duration and pattern of alternation of the P-R interval, (c) the QRS morphology and the duration of either conducted beats or escape rhythms, and (d) the rate of escape rhythms (if present). Because intracardiac studies can provide much of this information directly, a classification of A-V block that is applicable to the A-V conduction system as a whole or to any of its components is preferred (Table 4-1). Thus, in our laboratory, we prefer to consider first-degree, second-degree, and third-degree A-V block as prolonged conduction, intermittent conduction, and no conduction, respectively, because it more accurately defines the underlying physiology. For example, in the presence of first-degree block, impulse transmission (output/input) is 1:1 (hence the inappropriateness of the term block), although conduction through the whole A-V conduction system, or any of its parts, is prolonged; in the presence of second-degree block, impulse transmission is less than 1:1; and in the presence of third-degree block, no impulse transmission occurs.

Second-degree block is further subdivided into Types I and II. Type I second-degree block, to which the eponym Wenckebach block is often applied, is characterized by progressive prolongation in A-V conduction time preceding the nonconducted time in the conducted beat following the blocked impulse. In contrast, Type II second-degree block, to which the eponym Mobitz Type II is often applied, is characterized by sudden failure of conduction without alteration of conduction time of conducted beats either preceding or following the nonconducted one.

El-Sherif et al.[1] have described a canine model in which ligation of the anterior septal artery produced an apparent Type II second-degree block in the His bundle. However, careful measurement of intra-His conduction times with stable plunge wire electrodes revealed minimal (1- to 2-msec) increments before the blocked beat, a range that usually falls within the error of measurement of the recording techniques commonly used in humans. Furthermore, a temporal continuum between apparent Type II block and obvious Type I block in the His–Purkinje system has been demonstrated in these canine animals by Simson et al.[2] in our laboratory as well as in a few patients with acute myocardial infarction. Thus, the subdivision of second-degree A-V block into two distinct types may not be sound from a mechanistic viewpoint. Nevertheless, from a practical viewpoint it is worth noting that intermittent conduction (second-degree A-V block) associated with no (or undetectable) preceding increment is a behavior characteristic of the His–Purkinje system. Therefore, we shall continue to use the designations Type I block and Type II block as clinically descriptive terms. In the presence of 2:1 or higher-grade intermittent conduction, classification into Type I or II is not possible and is really a category unto itself. Therefore, block greater than second-degree A-V block includes 2:1 A-V block, high-degree A-V block (≥2 consecutive blocked P waves of intermittent conduction), and complete A-V block with evidence.

Theoretically, abnormalities of A-V conduction may result from conduction disturbances in any region of the heart, although certain patterns of block can be localized to specific sites (Table 4-2). Nevertheless, considerable overlap is seen, and the identification of the site of block on the basis of the surface ECG alone may not be possible. In the case of a prolonged P-R interval, intracardiac measurements may show normal intracardiac conduction (e.g., P-Atrioventricular junction [P-AVJ] atrium = 50, A-H = 125, H-V = 55). The chance of one's developing complete heart block, and its clinical significance, depends on the site of block. Hence, precise localization of a conduction disturbance may aid the clinician in planning the therapeutic approach.

Two questions must be addressed when deciding which patients should be referred for evaluation of A-V conduction disturbances: (a) When is the surface ECG likely to be misleading? (b) When does the localization of a conduction disturbance per se provide therapeutically important information independent of the patient's symptoms, surface ECG, and so on? Because of the lack of complete data, these questions are often answered on subjective rather than objective grounds; nevertheless, the following paragraphs present

**TABLE 4-1 Atrioventricular Block**

| Degree | Conduction |
|---|---|
| First degree | Prolonged conduction |
| Second degree | Intermittent conduction<br>Type I progressive prolongation<br>Type II sudden failure |
| Two-to-one | Two-to-one |
| High degree | Two consecutive from conducted P-waves with intermittent conduction |
| Third degree | No conduction |

information that may provide some guidelines for the use of intracardiac studies in defining A-V block.

## ATRIUM

An impulse originating in the sinus node must traverse the right atrium to reach the A-V node. Although there are no anatomic data supporting the presence of specific internodal tracts (anterior, middle, or posterior) that facilitate internodal conduction,[3] preferential pathways of atrial conduction exist, but they appear to be related to the spatial and geometric arrangement of atrial fibers rather than to specialized "tracts."

Because the sinus impulse can propagate directly through all types of atrial muscle as well as through these proposed preferred pathways, high-grade or complete heart block that is due to atrial disease in humans is virtually unknown. Of interest is the fact that a majority of dogs develop complete A-V block and a junctional rhythm if all three internodal tracts (found in dogs) are sectioned. On the other hand, prolonged A-V conduction (first-degree block) that is due to atrial conduction delay is not uncommon in humans. The ECG pattern of left atrial enlargement (a P wave ≥120 msec in duration with posteriorly and leftward directed terminal forces) is produced by delayed or prolonged left atrial activation rather than left atrial enlargement or hypertrophy in the absence of conduction delay.[4] A correlation between left atrial size and ECG left atrial enlargement is best seen in rheumatic and primary myocardial disease and rather poorly seen in coronary artery disease.[4] In all instances, however, delayed activation to the lateral left atrium is present. Therefore, so-called electrocardiographic "left atrial enlargement" is better thought of as an interatrial conduction delay (IACD).

The assessment of intra-atrial conduction demands the reproducible and accurate timing of local electrocardiograms from specific anatomic sites in the atria.[5] While high-density mapping may be useful to ascertain local atrial defects, fewer points are needed to demonstrate the cause of P-wave abnormalities (in a general way). For the reasons given in Chapter 2, simple measurement of the P-A interval is inadequate for the assessment of intra-atrial conduction. At a minimum, atrial electrograms from the high-right atrium (HRA) in the region of the sinus node, the A-V junction at the His bundle recording site, and the posterior lateral and even anterior left atrium recorded from various positions in the coronary sinus are required. Recordings from other sites along the lateral right atrial wall are easily obtained, whereas recordings from other sites in the left atrium are more difficult to obtain unless an atrial septal defect (ASD) or a patent foramen ovale is present, or a transseptal catheterization or retrograde approach is performed. These latter two procedures are not really justified unless a left atrial tachycardia is suspected. For accuracy and consistency, the principles of measurement described in Chapter 2 must be followed strictly. Accuracy is further enhanced by the use of rapid recording speeds (200 mm/sec or greater). A single catheter may be used to map more than one location as long as the rhythm (usually sinus) remains constant, and a reproducible reference electrogram is chosen (e.g., an intracardiac atrial electrogram and/or P wave in the surface ECG). Normal atrial activation using standard sites is shown in Figure 4-1. The mean activation time in a group of 24 patients with normal P waves and the mean values in a group of 15 patients with electrocardiographic left atrial enlargement are shown in Figure 4-2A,B, respectively. Obviously detailed atrial activation mapping using the Carto electroanatomic system is most accurate and is necessary for ablation of left atrial tachyarrhythmias. Normal activation is shown in Figure 4-3 in which activation of the left atrium occurs over Bachmann bundle, with additional conduits through the interatrial septum and coronary sinus (and potentially via interatrial bridges). In contrast, Figure 4-4 shows an atrial activation using standard catheter positions in a patient with a P wave that meets the standard ECG criteria for left atrial enlargement. In this patient, delayed activation of the left atrium (P to coronary sinus) and normal intra-right atrium conduction are shown by the atrial map. Biatrial conduction delay in standard catheter positions is shown in Figure 4-5.

Intra-atrial delay involving only the right atrium is far less common, but it is seen in the presence of congenital heart disease, particularly the endocardial cushion defects[6] and Ebstein anomaly of the tricuspid valve.[7] In approximately 20% of

**TABLE 4-2 Sites of Atrioventricular Block**

| | First Degree | Second Degree | | Third Degree |
|---|---|---|---|---|
| | | Type I | Type II | |
| Atrium | C | N | N | N |
| AVN | C | C | N | C |
| Intra-His | C | U | C | C |
| Infra-His | C | U | C | C |

AVN, atrioventricular node; C, common; N, virtually never; U, uncommon.

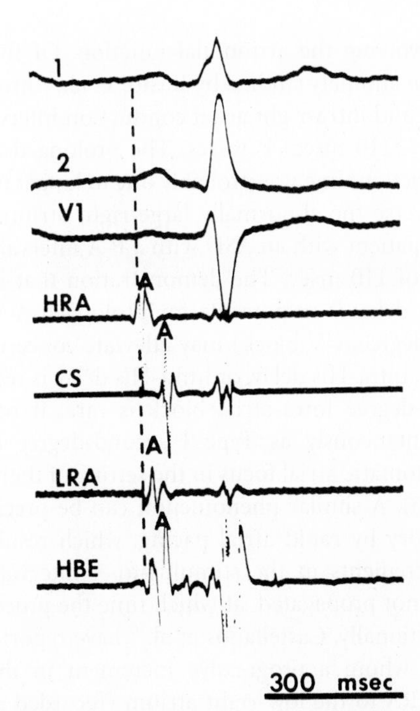


**FIGURE 4-1** *Normal sequence and timing of atrial endocardial activation.* Electrograms from the high-right atrium (HRA), coronary sinus (CS), low lateral right atrium (LRA), and His bundle area (HBE) are shown. The *vertical line* marks the reference point for measurement and is the earliest evidence of atrial electrical activity. Activation times in msec are HRA = 2, CS = 60, LRA = 28, and A in HBE = 25.

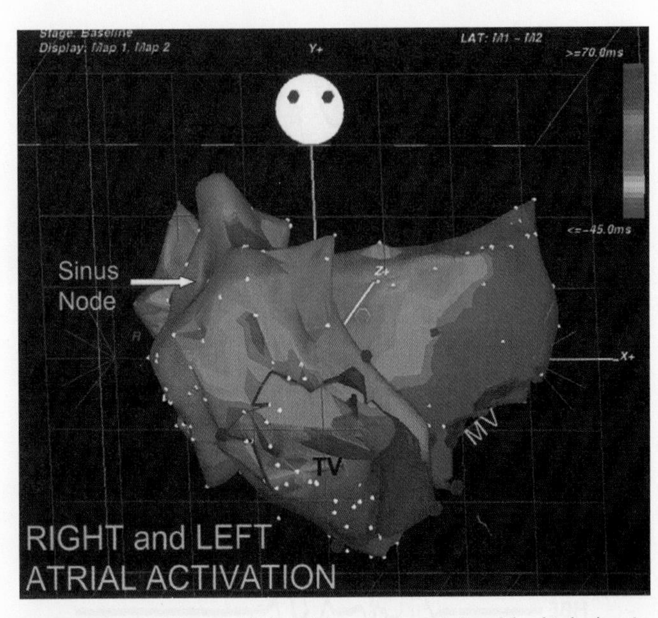


**FIGURE 4-3** *Right and left atrial activation defined by high-density electroanatomic mapping.* See section "Atrium."

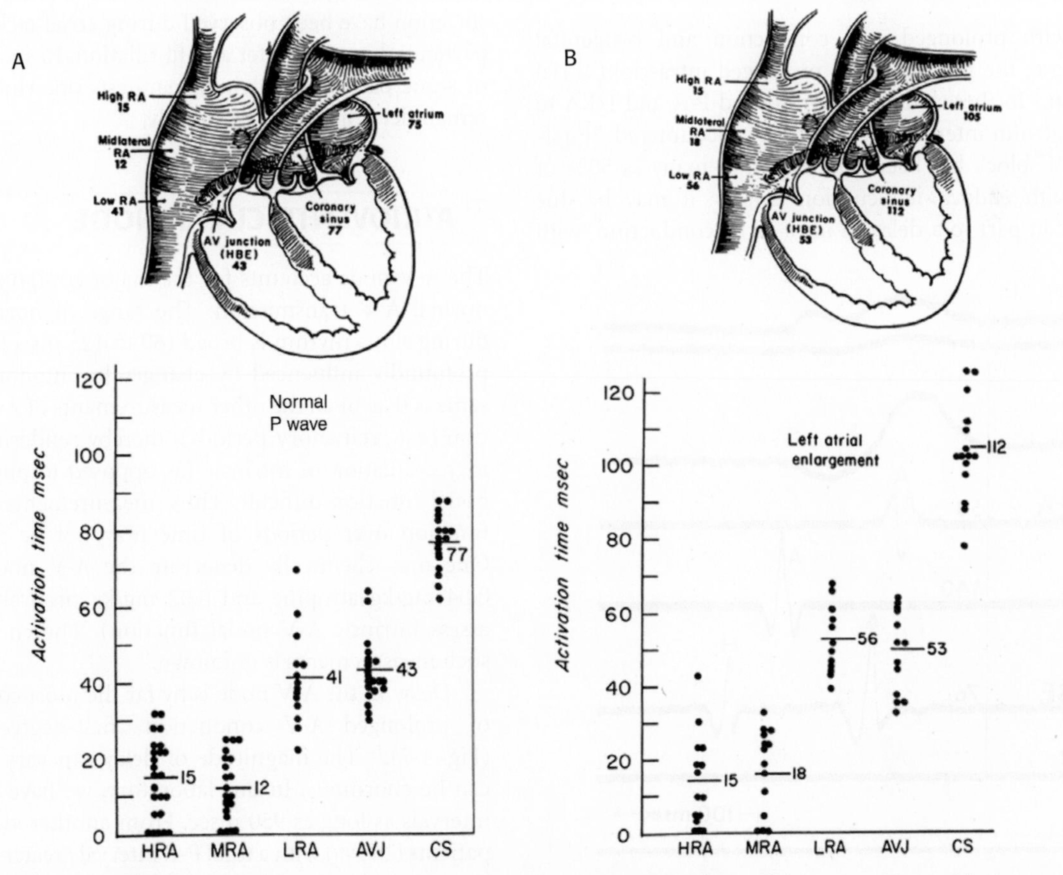


**FIGURE 4-2** *Atrial activation times in 24 patients with normal P waves on the surface ECG* **(A)** *and from 15 patients with electrocardiographic "left atrial enlargement"* **(B)**. Activation times are plotted from various standard sites in the atria, with mean activation time shown with a bar and number. AVJ, atrioventricular junction; MRA, midright atrium.

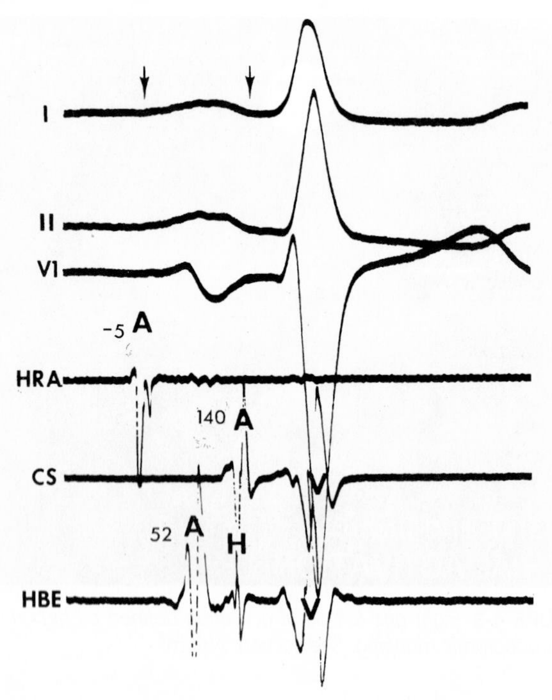


**FIGURE 4-4** *Atrial activation sequence in a patient with a broad P wave with posteriorly directed terminal forces-so-called left atrial enlargement.* Note the prolonged coronary sinus (CS) activation time (140 msec) in the face of a normal right atrial conduction time (P-A measured at HBE recording site = 52 msec) consistent with an interatrial and/or intra-left atrial conduction delay.

patients with prolonged A-V conduction and congenital heart disease, the mechanism is prolonged intra-right atrial conduction.[8] In these situations, prolonged P-A and HRA to low-right atrium intervals are frequently encountered. "First-degree A-V" block has been reported in as many as 50% of patients with endocardial cushion defects; it may be due entirely or in part to a delay in intra-atrial conduction, with

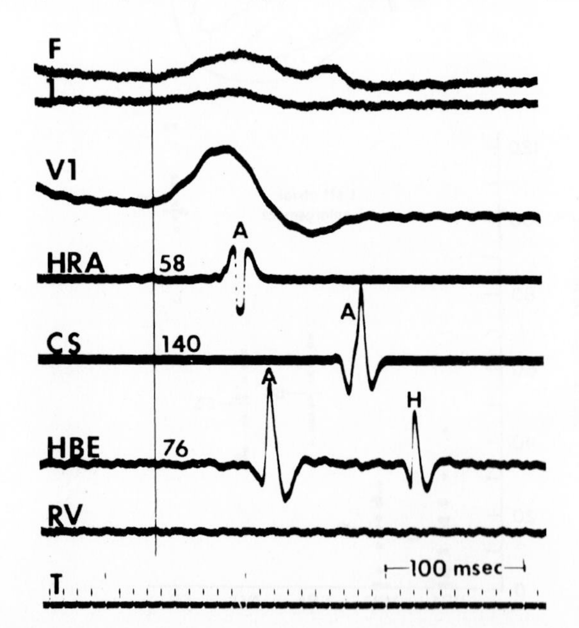


**FIGURE 4-5** *Biatrial conduction delay.* A single P wave is shown. Note the delayed activation of all atrial electrograms. T, time line.

a defect involving the atrionodal junction. Of five patients with Ebstein anomaly studied by Kastor et al.,[7] three had prolonged P-A and intra-right atrial conduction intervals and all had broad (≥110 msec) P waves. The prolonged intra-right atrial conduction time was probably due to longer time necessary to traverse the abnormally large right atrium. We have also seen a patient with an ASD with a P-A interval measured at the AVJ of 110 msec. The demonstration that intra-atrial conduction delay is responsible for prolonged A-V conduction (first-degree A-V block) may alleviate concern that A-V nodal delay, intra-His delay, or infra-His delay is responsible.

Second-degree intra-atrial block is rare. It occasionally occurs spontaneously as Type I second-degree exit block from an automatic atrial focus in the setting of digitalis toxicity (Fig. 4-6). A similar phenomenon can be precipitated in the laboratory by rapid atrial pacing, which results in progressive increments in the stimulus-to-A interval until the stimulus is not propagated, at which time the process repeats itself.[9] Additionally, Castellanos et al.[10] have reported on two patients in whom a progressive increment in the interval from the HRA to the low-right atrium (recorded at the A-V junction) occurred until the beat was dropped. Such types of intra-atrial delays appear to be substrates for intra-atrial reentry (Chapters 8, 9).

Type II second-degree block and complete heart block do not occur as manifestations of atrial conduction disease in humans during sinus rhythm. Interatrial and intra-atrial dissociation have been observed during atrial tachyarrhythmias, particularly atrial flutter and fibrillation. In such instances, all or some part of the atrium manifests one rhythm while the remainder is activated differently.

## ATRIOVENTRICULAR NODE

The A-V node accounts for the major component of time in normal A-V transmission. The range of normal A-H time during sinus rhythm is broad (60 to 125 msec), and it can be profoundly influenced by changes in autonomic tone. The same is true of all the other measurements of A-V nodal function (e.g., refractory periods), thereby rendering the laboratory evaluation of intrinsic (as opposed to physiologic) A-V nodal function difficult. Thus, measurements of A-V nodal function over periods of time may not be reproducible.[11] One may chemically denervate the A-V nodal node (i.e., 0.04 mg/kg atropine and 0.02 mg/kg propranolol to better assess intrinsic A-V nodal function). The clinical utility of such measurements is unknown.

Delay in the A-V node is by far the most common source of prolonged A-V conduction (first-degree A-V block) (Fig. 4-7).[12] The magnitude of delay can vary greatly, but it can be enormous. In our laboratory, we have observed A-H intervals as long as 950 msec. From another viewpoint, most patients (≥95%) with a total P-R interval greater than 300 msec have some degree of A-V nodal delay. It is worth reemphasizing that A-V conduction can vary greatly with changes in the

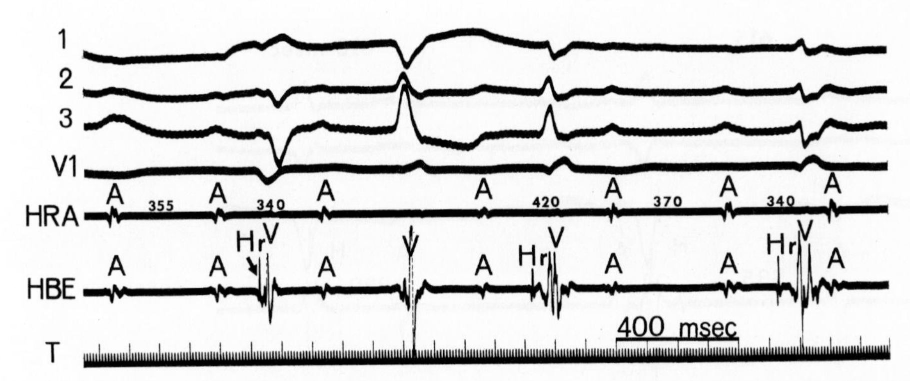


**FIGURE 4-6** *Automatic atrial tachycardia with exit Wenckebach block.* Atrial tachycardia with regularly irregular (i.e., group beating) atrial activity associated with complete heart block is present in a patient with digitalis intoxication (serum digoxin level = 3.8 ng/mL). Note the progressively decreasing A-A intervals followed by a pause and then resumption of the pattern. Hr are retrograde His bundle potentials associated with fascicular depolarizations (Chapter 7), another manifestation of digitalis intoxication.

patient's clinical state (i.e., influence of autonomic nervous system) and in response to pacing-induced changes in heart rate in a characteristic fashion (Chapter 3), with a prolongation in conduction time and refractoriness at increasing paced heart rates. On the other hand, clinical states with heightened sympathetic tone are accompanied by decreased A-V nodal and conduction time and refractoriness at any paced rate.

Second-degree block that is due to intermittent failure of conduction through the A-V node is very common in a wide variety of circumstances. The A-V node is the site of most Type I second-degree blocks. Type I second-degree block may be a manifestation of a pathologic process, or it may be a physiologic response within normal limits. This type of block may occur in the setting of any acquired or congenital disease of the A-V node, especially inferior wall myocardial infarction. It can also be precipitated by drugs such as digitalis, beta blockers, calcium channel blockers, or amiodarone. In addition, it may be seen in the young, healthy heart at rest in the presence of high levels of resting vagal tone, a state that is particularly common in well-trained endurance athletes. Furthermore, Type I second-degree block can be precipitated in almost all subjects by incremental atrial pacing (Chapter 2) and in an analogous fashion may be seen during atrial tachycardia.

The easily recognized typical Wenckebach periodicity (Fig. 4-8), with a gradual prolongation of each succeeding conduction interval with decreasing increments, may be relatively uncommon in clinical practice. More often, Wenckebach periodicity is atypical.[13] It is not uncommon to observe (a) the A-H interval stabilize for several beats, especially during long Wenckebach cycles (11 to 10, etc.); (b) the greatest increment occurs with the second beat after the pause; and (c) very little incremental conduction delay after a large initial "jump" (dual A-V nodal pathways present, see below and in Chapter 8, A-V nodal reentry), or only a relatively small overall increment in A-H associated with a modest decrease in A-H following the pause (Fig. 4-9). This latter phenomenon is often seen associated with an increased vagal tone. As shown in Figure 4-9, this usually is accompanied by slowing of the sinus rate. Typical Wenckebach periodicity is more frequently observed during pacing-induced second-degree A-V block (Fig. 4-10). In patients with dual A-V nodal pathways, Wenckebach cycles are almost always atypical. The greatest jump in A-H occurs when block in the fast pathway occurs, whichever complex this may be. In patients with A-V nodal reentry, Wenckebach cycles may be terminated by A-V nodal echoes or the development of supraventricular tachycardia (Chapter 8). These should really not be called Wenckebach cycles because there is no blocked paced impulse.

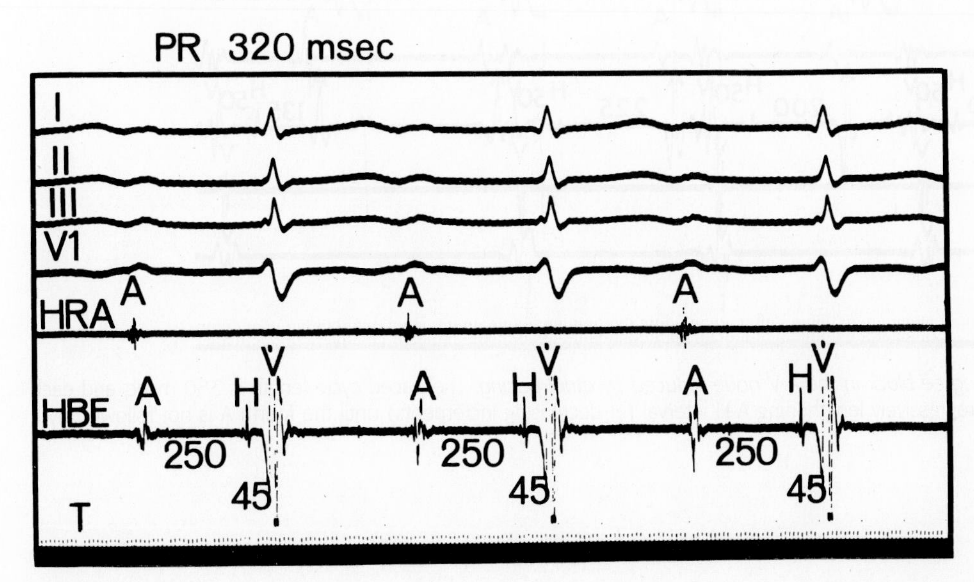


**FIGURE 4-7** *First-degree block (prolonged conduction) confined to the A-V node.* The A-H interval is prolonged to 250 msec. The H-V interval is 45 msec (normal).

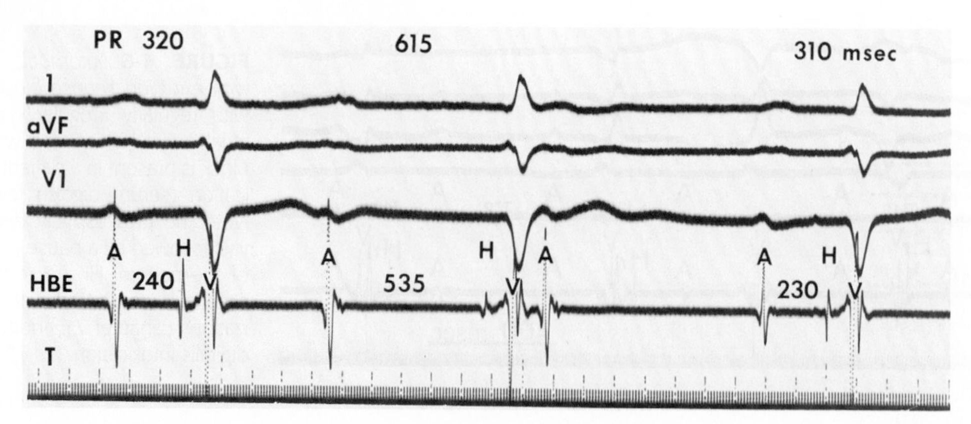


**FIGURE 4-8** *Typical spontaneous Type I second-degree block (intermittent conduction) in the A-V node.* Progressive prolongation of the A-H (and P-R) intervals occurs until the third atrial deflection A is not followed by a His bundle or a ventricular depolarization.

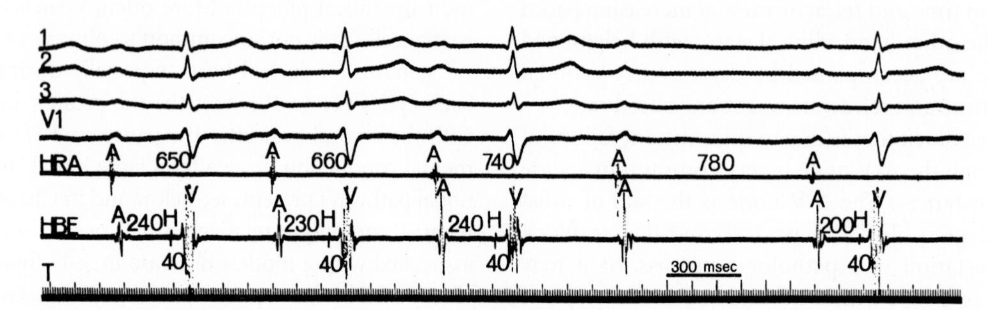


**FIGURE 4-9** *Spontaneous atypical Type I second-degree block in the atrioventricular node due to heightened vagal tone.* Note that there is little alteration in the A-H interval before the fourth A not conducting. The true nature of the arrhythmia, however, is revealed by the first conducted A after the pause, which is associated with substantial shortening of the A-H interval to 200 msec. The analysis or mechanism is clarified by the associated sinus slowing.

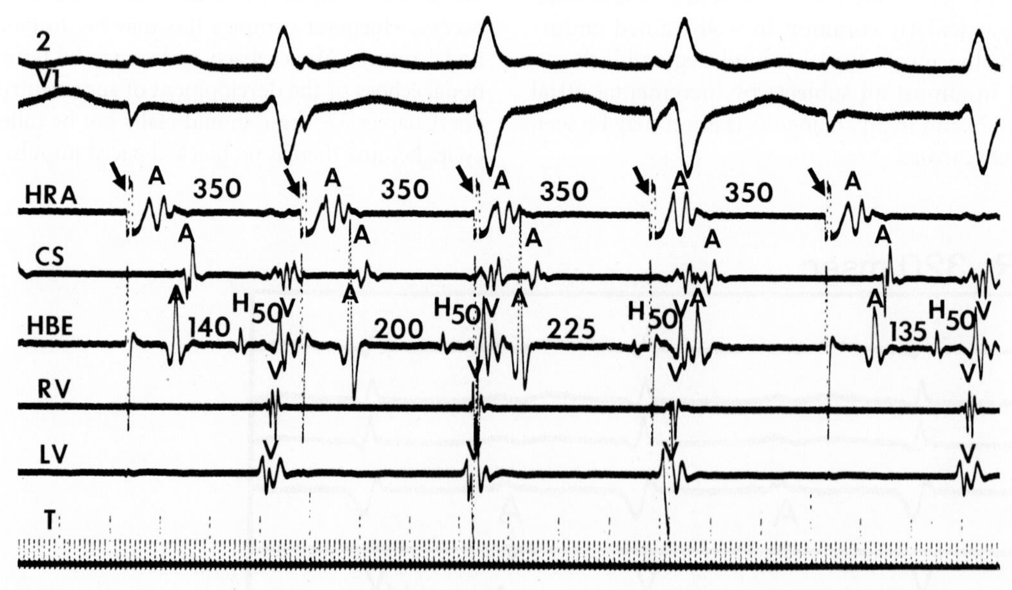


**FIGURE 4-10** *"Typical" Type I second-degree block in the A-V node induced by atrial pacing.* The paced cycle length is 350 msec, and each atrial depolarization A is followed by a progressively lengthening A-H interval (at decreasing increments) until the fourth A is not followed by a His bundle deflection.

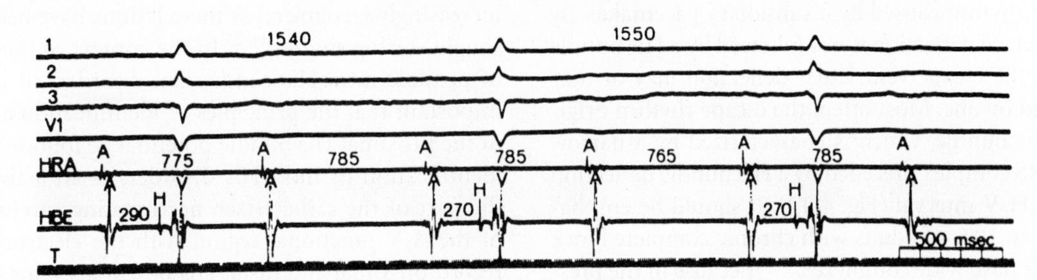


**FIGURE 4-11** *Spontaneous high-grade (2:1) block in the atrioventricular (A-V) node.* Alternative atrial depolarization A is not followed by either a His bundle or a ventricular depolarization. On the basis of the surface ECG, the finding of 2:1 A-V block with a narrow QRS complex is compatible with either an A-V node or an intra-His site of block. The intracardiac records localize the site of block to the A-V node.

Type II second-degree A-V block occurring in the A-V node has been reported,[14] but in each case, either the block could have been localized to a more likely site (usually the His bundle rather than the A-V node) or the block probably was atypical Type I, as suggested by a decrease in the A-H interval of the beat following the blocked impulse. One of the more common situations in which "apparent" Type II A-V nodal block can be seen is during heightened vagal tone during sleep. A clue to this phenomenon is associated sinus slowing (Fig. 4-9). Another rare cause of apparent Type II block with normal QRS complexes is concealed His bundle extrasystoles.[15] In my opinion, true Type II second-degree block occurring in the A-V node has never been adequately documented.

Second-degree A-V block in the A-V node can often be partially or completely reversed by altering autonomic tone. Hence, exercise (or other measures to increase sympathetic tone) or the administration of atropine (to decrease vagal tone) may produce reversion to 1:1 conduction. However, occasionally in the presence of structural damage (e.g., congenital heart block or inferior myocardial infarction), these measures may be ineffectual. In such cases spontaneous progression to third-degree block (complete A-V block) may occur. More than likely, in most instances, failure of conduction to improve following atropine or isoproterenol suggests block is probably high in the His bundle. In general, Type I second-degree A-V nodal block is usually well tolerated from a hemodynamic standpoint, and it seldom if ever merits pacemaker therapy on symptomatic grounds. Prophylactic therapy is discussed later in this chapter.

Two-to-one block in the A-V node (Fig. 4-11) is less common than Mobitz I block. It is often associated with organic disease of the A-V node (e.g., Lyme disease), myocardial infarction, s/p mitral valve or other cardiac (particularly congenital heart) surgery, or drug toxicity. Since the impaired function of the A-V node is present, the A-H, and hence, P-R, of the conducted beats is almost always prolonged. Two-to-one block with P-R ≤160 msec should suggest an intra- or infra-His site of block. Improvement of conduction by atropine, beta agonists, or exercise suggests an A-V nodal site of block. However, as stated above, if structure disease of the A-V node is present, improvement of A-V node conduction under these conditions may be small or inapparent.

Third-degree (complete) heart block occurring in the A-V node is relatively common. Most cases of congenital complete heart block are localized to the A-V node (Fig. 4-12),[16] as are most cases of transient complete heart block seen in acute inferior wall myocardial infarction.[17] This is also the site of block in digitalis intoxication or when block is produced by beta blockers and/or calcium blockers. Intracardiac

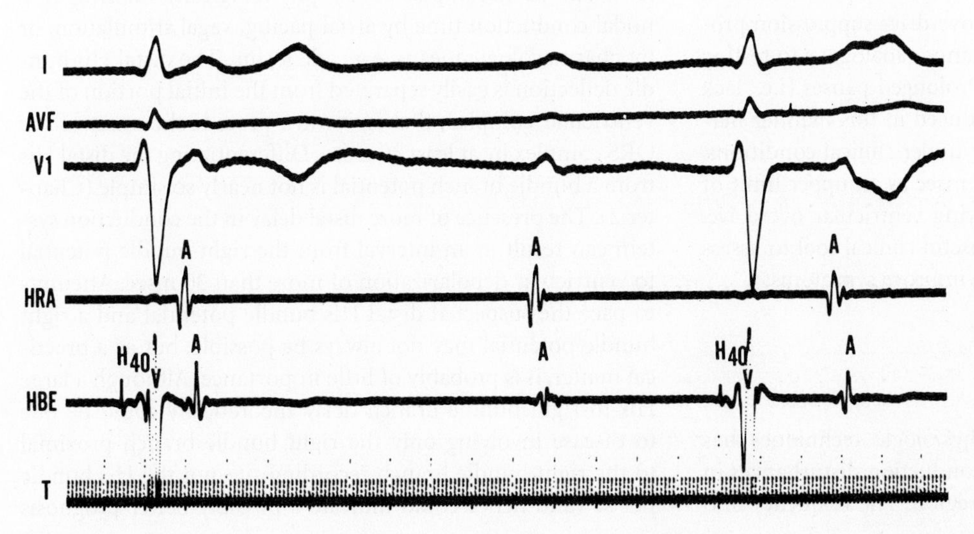


**FIGURE 4-12** *Congenital complete heart block in the A-V node.* All atrial impulses fail to conduct through the A-V node. Each junctional escape QRS complex is preceded by a His bundle deflection (H) with a normal H-V interval (40 msec). This patient's record is of a young man, 17 years old, who is asymptomatic.

recordings reveal atrial deflections that are dissociated from the ventricular rhythm caused by a subsidiary pacemaker. By definition, the atrial deflection is not followed by a His bundle deflection, but the escape ventricular deflection may or may not be preceded by one. Most often, the escape rhythm originates in the His bundle, which is characterized by a narrow ("normal") QRS complex preceded by a His bundle deflection with a normal H-V interval (Fig. 4-12). It should be emphasized that 20% to 50% of adults with chronic complete block in the A-V node have wide complexes.[18,19] Because in the presence of wide QRS complexes, many physicians assume block below His and implant pacemakers in asymptomatic people, such a finding, particularly in asymptomatic or minimally symptomatic patients, may be an indication for electrophysiologic study since A-V nodal block may be reversible.

His bundle escape rhythms typically have a rate of 45 to 60 beats per minute (bpm), and they are variably responsive to alterations in autonomic tone or manipulation of the autonomic nervous system by pharmacologic agents (e.g., atropine, isoproterenol) or exercise. Occasionally, the escape rhythm has a normal QRS complex but is not preceded by a His bundle deflection. This instance probably reflects a failure to record the His bundle deflection. Use of closely spaced electrodes and careful mapping may locate a His bundle potential, which may be in an unusual position. Occasionally the escape focus may originate more distally (i.e., in the fascicles or distal Purkinje fibers), producing a wide QRS complex. These distal rhythms are either preceded by a retrograde His bundle deflection or no deflection at all (Chapter 2). They are slower and unresponsive to atropine. Because of the wealth of potential subsidiary pacemakers with adequate rates, syncope is a rare presenting symptom in patients with third-degree block localized to the A-V node. In fact, many patients with congenital complete heart block are asymptomatic for many years. It is only when aging produces chronotropic insufficiency of the His rhythm that patients become symptomatic, usually with exertional fatigue. They are often referred for evaluation because of bradycardia detected on a routine examination. In rare circumstances, the His bundle rhythm may be unstable, and syncope can occur. The stability of the His bundle escape rhythm can be assessed by noting the effects of overdrive suppression produced by ventricular pacing in a manner analogous to testing sinus node function (Chapter 3). Prolonged pauses (i.e., lack of His bundle escape rhythm) produced in this manner herald failure of the escape pacemaker under clinical conditions. Narula and Narula[20] proposed 200 msec as an upper limit of corrected "His escape time" following ventricular overdrive. The response to exercise is also a useful clinical tool to assess when a pacemaker may be useful to improve symptoms.

## HIS BUNDLE

The use of intracardiac electrophysiologic techniques has done more to identify and clarify conduction disturbances in the His bundle than in any other region. The frequency and importance of intra-His conduction disturbances have been increasingly recognized as these lesions have been specifically sought during studies.[19–23] In the context of the investigation of possible intra-His conduction disorders, it is particularly important that the principles of identification and validation of the proximal His bundle potential be followed strictly. The identification of intra-His disorders is an active process on the part of the catheterizer, necessitating careful exploration of the A-V junctional region with the electrode catheter to record proximal and distal His potentials. This must be used in conjunction with manipulation of autonomic tone.

Given a conduction velocity of 1.3 to 1.7 m/sec in the normal human His bundle,[24] depolarization of the entire structure should take no more than 25 to 30 msec. The His bundle deflection as measured with bipolar catheter electrodes (10 mm apart) corresponds to total conduction time through the His bundle. Hence, prolonged intra-His conduction ("first-degree block" in the His bundle) can be said to be present if the total duration of the His bundle deflection is >30 msec, particularly if the deflection is notched or fragmented. In contrast to A-V nodal conduction, the range of values of intra-His conduction is typically small. Therefore, significant delays of intra-His conduction are usually not reflected by a prolongation of the P-R interval on the surface ECG (Fig. 4-13). The ultimate expression of intra-His delay is a splitting of the potential into separate and distinct proximal and distal deflections. These deflections occasionally may be separated by an interval of as much as several hundred milliseconds (Fig. 4-14). The interval between proximal and distal His bundle electrograms may be isoelectric or have low-amplitude indistinct activity (Figs. 4-13 and 4-14), which presumably is due to very slow conduction and to poor coupling in the area of damaged tissue. In pure intra-His delay, the A-to-proximal-His (A-H) and the distal His-to-V (H′-V) intervals are normal. However, coexistent conduction defects in other parts of the conduction system are common.

Confirmation of the His bundle origin of each of the "split His" potentials is critical. Separation of the proximal His bundle deflection from the terminal portion of the atrial deflection can be accomplished by physiologically altering A-V nodal conduction time by atrial pacing, vagal stimulation, or by pharmacologic means, e.g., adenosine. The distal His bundle deflection is easily separated from the initial portion of the ventricular complex; that is, it must precede the onset of the QRS complex by at least 30 msec. Differentiating the distal His from a bundle branch potential is not nearly so simple (Chapter 2). The presence of more distal delay in the conduction system can result in an interval from the right bundle potential to ventricular depolarization of more than 30 msec. Attempts to pace the suspected distal His bundle potential and a right bundle potential may not always be possible, but as a practical matter, it is probably of little importance. Although a large His-to-right bundle branch delay theoretically could be due to disease involving only the right bundle branch proximal to the right bundle branch recording site-not the His bundle per se (and hence could indicate a possibly better prognosis

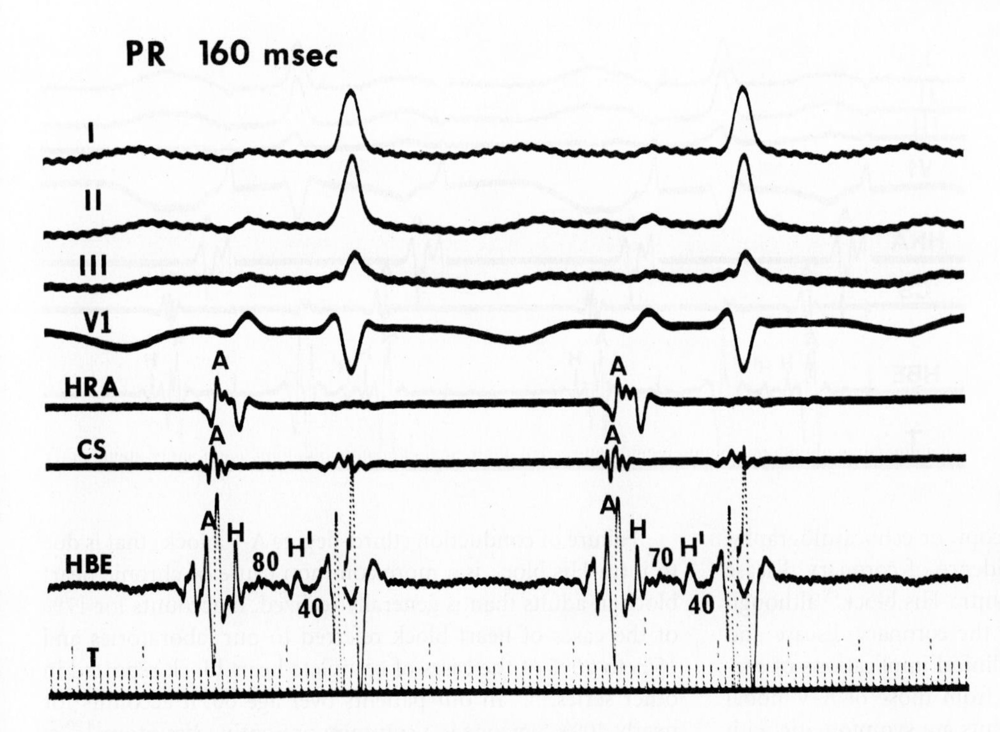


**FIGURE 4-13** *First-degree intra-His block.* Of interest is the low-amplitude electrical activity in the 70 to 80 msec between H and H′, as well as the width and direction of H′ itself in the markedly slow conduction through this region. Furthermore, the alteration in A-V conduction is well hidden in an overall P-R interval of 160 msec.

because the left bundle branch system is entirely intact)—it is very unlikely, especially with a normal QRS complex. In these cases, a main-stem His bundle lesion is almost certainly present. The prognosis in asymptomatic patients with prolonged intra-His conduction appears benign.

Second-degree intra-His block is defined by intermittent conduction between the proximal and distal His bundle potentials. Ideally, each atrial depolarization is followed by a proximal His bundle deflection with intermittent failure of conduction to the distal His bundle. Type I and Type II second-degree blocks are commonly seen as is 2:1 block (Figs. 4-15 and 4-16). In contrast to A-V nodal block, 2:1 block is more common than either Type I or II second-degree block. Because the conducted QRS complexes are narrow (in the absence of coexistent bundle branch block), block in the A-V node may be simulated if one fails to record the proximal His bundle deflection. Unfortunately failure to record split His deflections is more common than recording them. This probably accounts for some cases of Type II second-degree block that have been reported to occur in the A-V node. The presence of a narrow QRS with failure of conduction to improve with isoproterenol or atropine and paradoxically improve with carotid pressure suggests an intra-His lesion. On the other hand, failure to record the distal His bundle potential during second-degree A-V block can result in a mistaken diagnosis of infra-His block, especially in the presence of a wide QRS complex. Therefore, the techniques for validating the proximal and/or distal His bundle deflections given in Chapter 2 should be employed.

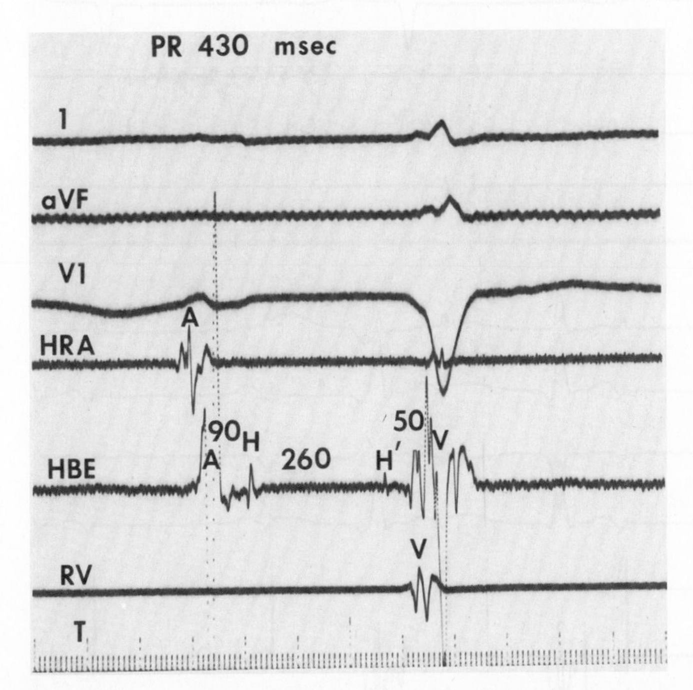


**FIGURE 4-14** *Marked first-degree block (prolonged conduction) confined to the His bundle.* Two distinct His bundle deflections (H and H′) are seen, separated by an isoelectric interval of 260 msec. Note that both the A-H (proximal) interval and the H′ (distal)-V interval are normal, indicative of normal A-V nodal and infra-His conduction times.

In contrast to A-V nodal block in two-to-one intra-His block, the P-R interval is usually normal in the absence of disease elsewhere in the conducting system. In fact, a normal P-R, particularly ≤160 msec during 2:1 block, is virtually diagnostic of intra-His block if the QRS is narrow. Moreover, atropine and exercise do not improve conduction, and may, in fact, worsen it. In contrast vagal maneuvers, which decrease the input into the His bundle (i.e., increase H-H), may actually improve conduction.

The clinical suspicion of intra-His disease should be heightened in the older (>60 years old) female patient, particularly in the presence of a calcified mitral valve annulus[25]

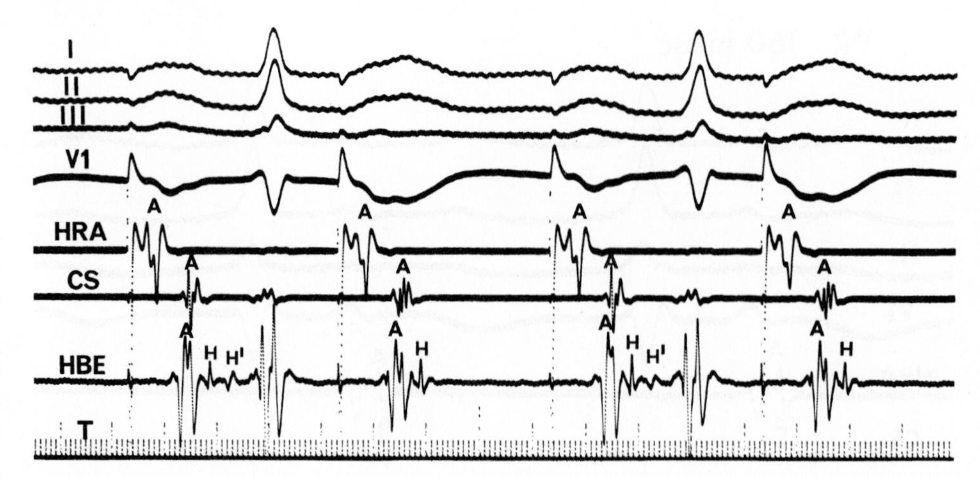


**FIGURE 4-15** *Second-degree block (intermittent conduction) in the middle of the His bundle induced by atrial pacing in the patient depicted in Figure 4-13.* Note that alternative A-H (proximal) complexes are not followed by H′ (distal)-V complexes with the impulse blocked within the His bundle distal to the H (proximal) recording site.

as identified by chest film, fluoroscopy, or echocardiography. We have also observed a high incidence of coronary disease in our patients with symptomatic intra-His block[23] although a cause and effect relationship of the coronary disease and intra-His block is uncertain. The clinical implications of second-degree intra-His block differ from those of A-V nodal block. Most commonly, these patients are symptomatic with recurrent syncope. Progression to high-grade or complete block may occur paroxysmally, with hemodynamic stability, depending on the emergence of a low junctional (distal His), fascicular, or idioventricular rhythm.

Failure of conduction (third-degree A-V block) that is due to intra-His block is a more common cause of chronic heart block in adults than is generally realized. It accounts for 17% of the cases of heart block referred to our laboratories and 15% to 20% of the cases of complete heart block reported in other series.[18,19] In our patients over age 60, it accounts for nearly 40%. Syncope is a common presenting symptom[18,20–22] because the escape pacemaker is at or distal to the low A-V junction with a slow rate (usually less than 45 bpm) and is unresponsive to autonomic interventions. One observes dissociation between the A-to-proximal-His complexes and

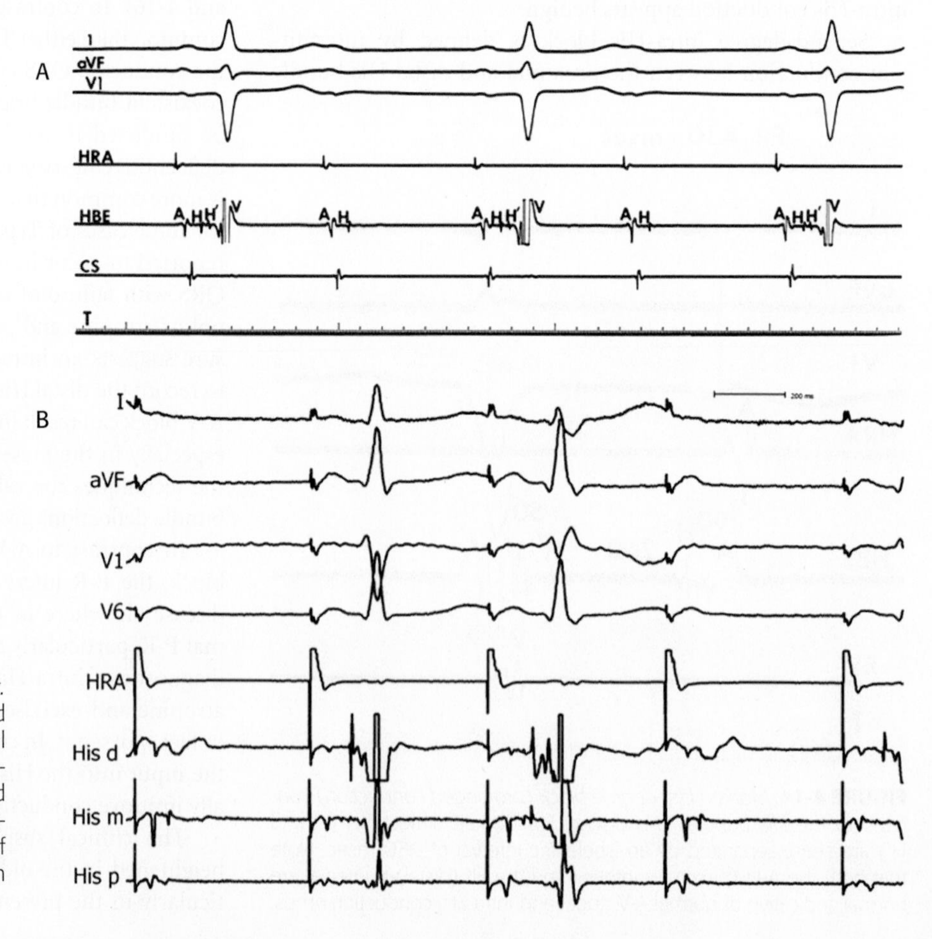


**FIGURE 4-16** *Two-to-one intra-His block.* **A:** Two-to-one block with a narrow QRS and normal P-R during sinus rhythm interval is shown. A split His (H-H′) is seen in conducted complexes, and block between H and H′ is noted in every other complex. **B:** Pacing-induced intra-His block at a cycle length of 500 msec is shown. The split His is best seen in the mid-His bipolar pair.

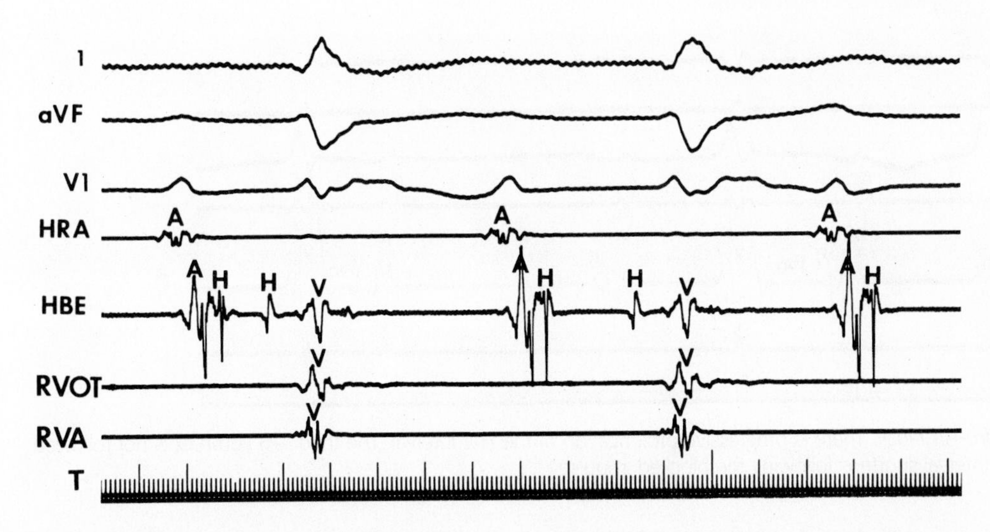


**FIGURE 4-17** *Complete heart block localized to the His bundle.* There is complete atrioverter dissociation. Each atrial complex is followed by a proximal His (H) bundle deflection with a fixed A-H interval, and each escape ventricular complex is preceded by a distal His bundle deflection with a normal H-V interval.

the escape distal His-to-V complexes (Fig. 4-17). Failure to record the distal His may simulate infra-His block in the presence of a wide QRS complex. If the escape rhythm is narrow (i.e., supraventricular morphology), even in the absence of a recorded distal His, one can assume an intra-His site of block. Because the escape rate is usually quite slow, these patients are almost always symptomatic with syncope or fatigue and shortness of breath. Because syncope may be related to an associated ventricular tachycardia, we believe symptomatic patients should be studied.

## INFRA-HIS CONDUCTION SYSTEM

The infra-His conduction system, which comprises the main bundle branches and fascicles, their ramifications, and the Purkinje network, is the source of most of the clinically important heart block in adults.[18] The His bundle is generally considered to trifurcate into the right bundle branch and the left bundle branch, which promptly fans out into an anterior (superior) fascicle and a posterior (inferior) fascicle. A fourth, septal fascicle[26] has been proposed to explain certain ECG patterns. However, because this fascicle probably contributes little to overall infra-His conduction, it is not discussed here. Although conduction disturbances can occur in each of the major fascicles, the integrity of overall A-V conduction can be maintained by a single functioning fascicle. Therefore, in this chapter the infra-His system is discussed as a single unit and the next chapter covers the implications of individual bundle branch and fascicular blocks.

As long as at least one fascicle conducts normally, the H-V interval, should not exceed 55 msec. It has been suggested, however, that the upper limit of normal may be 60 msec in the presence of complete left bundle branch block and an intact right bundle branch (Chapter 5). A prolonged H-V interval is almost always associated with an abnormal QRS complex because the impairment of infra-His conduction is not homogenous. In the absence of an abnormal QRS (i.e., presence of a normal QRS) complex, apparent infra-His delay or block should suggest intra-His delay or block with failure to record the distal His bundle potential.

The degree of infra-His conduction delay is variable. Most patients with infra-His delay have H-V intervals in the 60- to 100-msec range (Fig. 4-18). In occasional patients however, the H-V interval may exceed 100 msec (Fig. 4-19). This is most

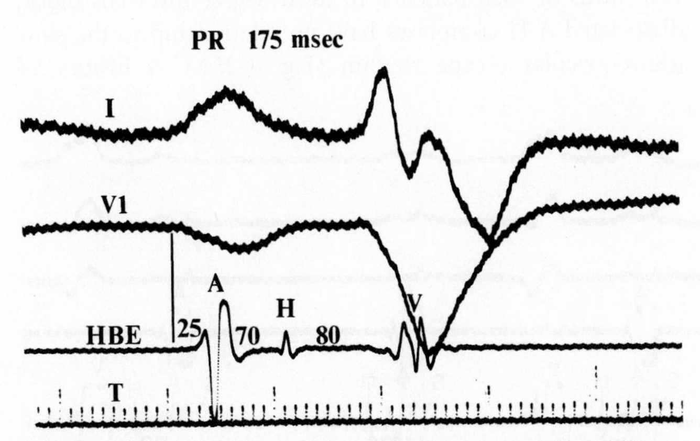


**FIGURE 4-18** *First-degree infra-His block (prolonged conduction) in a patient with an IVCD.* Note that the prolonged H-V interval of 80 msec is obscured in the overall P-R interval, which is normal at 175 msec.

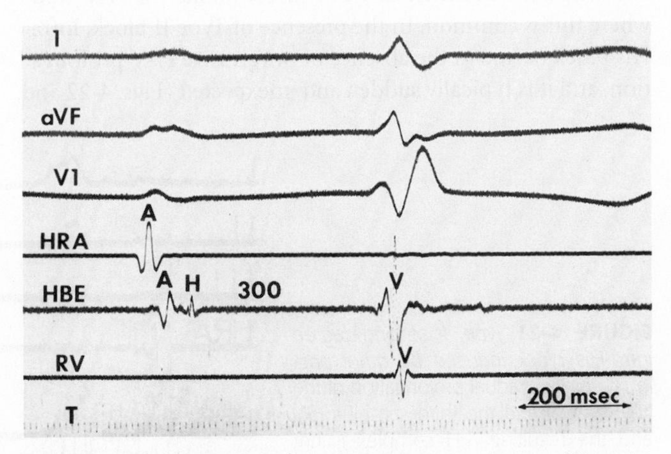


**FIGURE 4-19** *Markedly prolonged infra-His conduction delay.* The H-V interval is 300 msec, and it is largely responsible for P-R prolongation in this patient.

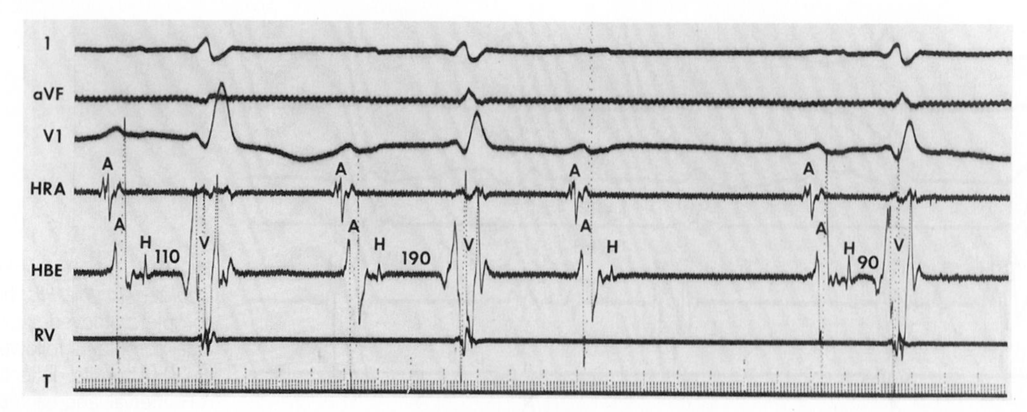


**FIGURE 4-20** *Type I second-degree infra-His block.* There is progressive prolongation of the H-V interval. The third A-H complex is not followed by a ventricular depolarization. The H-V interval shortens following the blocked impulse.

frequent in patients with alternating bundle branch block, in which case it is the rule (see Chapter 5). The longest H-V interval we have seen is 345 msec. Such marked infranodal delay is uncommon, and in our experience, it frequently progresses to high degrees of block.

H-V prolongation in the more usual ranges (60 to 100 msec) can exist without any or minimal prolongation of the P-R interval (Fig. 4-18) although, the longer the H-V interval, the less likely it is to "fit" into a P-R interval under 0.20 sec (in the absence of accelerated A-V nodal conduction). Similarly, a grossly prolonged H-V interval is unlikely in the presence of a P-R interval of 0.16 msec or less. Nevertheless, the P-R interval is an extraordinary poor predictor of the H-V interval because the H-V interval is usually significantly smaller than the A-H interval, which is the major component of the P-R interval.

Second-degree block with Type I or Type II characteristics can result from failure of infranodal conduction. In the presence of Type I block, a gradual prolongation of the H-V interval occurs until an A-H group is not followed by a ventricular depolarization (Figs. 4-20 and 4-21). This is much less common than Mobitz II, or two-to-one block. Although the H-V shows progressive prolongation, it is very rare for there to be a maximum increment of >100 msec, unlike the A-V node where this is common. In the presence of Type II block, infra-His block occurs in the absence of progressive H-V prolongation, and it is typically sudden and unexpected (Figs. 4-22 and 4-23). Not uncommonly, careful analysis reveals that block below the His is a rate-related phenomenon (Fig. 4-23). This can be demonstrated by pacing (Figs. 4-21 and 4-22). When it occurs spontaneously, it may be precipitated by a change in H-H of a few milliseconds (Figs. 4-20 and 4-21). Pacing-induced block below the His is considered an indication for a permanent pacemaker (see Chapter 5). Type II second-degree A-V block is more common than Type I when the site of block is below the His bundle.[18] Intermittent infra-His conduction is frequent in the presence of alternating bundle branch block (Chapter 5). In any case, second-degree infra-His block is indicative of impending high-grade or complete infra-His block with the attendant problem that hemodynamic survival depends on an idioventricular escape rhythm.

Two-to-one infra-His block is common (Fig. 4-24). Although the H-V is usually prolonged, the P-R interval is often normal. This may be a clue from the surface ECG that one is delaying with a His–Purkinje site of block. As with intra-His block, atropine and exercise failed to improve and may even have worsened conduction, while vagal maneuvers may actually improve conduction (Table 4-3).

Third-degree infra-His block is the most common cause of spontaneous chronic complete heart block in adults over 30 years old; in our laboratory it accounts for approximately two-thirds of such patients. In third-degree infra-His block, dissociated A-H complexes have no relationship to the slow idioventricular escape rhythm (Fig. 4-25A). A history of

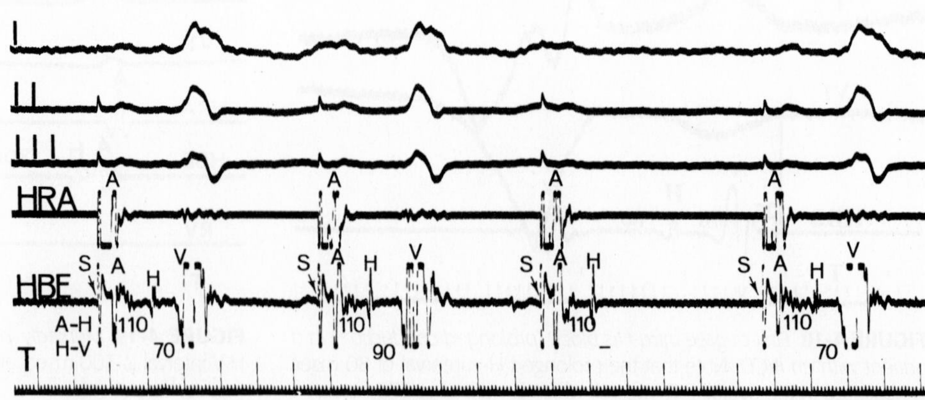


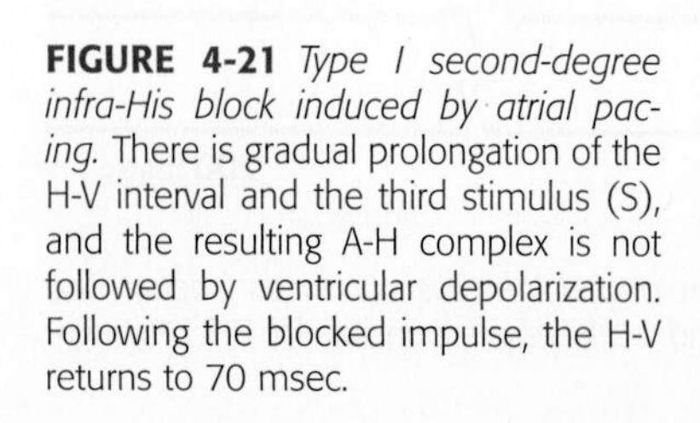

**FIGURE 4-21** *Type I second-degree infra-His block induced by atrial pacing.* There is gradual prolongation of the H-V interval and the third stimulus (S), and the resulting A-H complex is not followed by ventricular depolarization. Following the blocked impulse, the H-V returns to 70 msec.

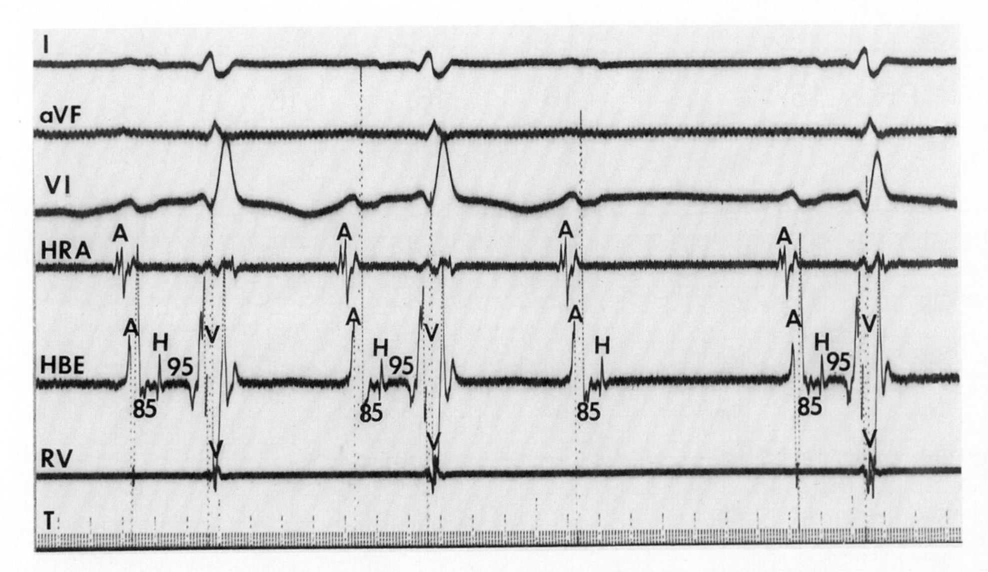


**FIGURE 4-22** *Spontaneous Type II second-degree infra-His block.* The A-H and H-V intervals remain constant during conducted impulses at 85 msec and 95 msec, respectively. The third A-H complex, however, is suddenly and unexpectedly not followed by a ventricular depolarization. The complex following the blocked impulse shows no alteration in the conduction intervals.

syncope (of "Adams–Stokes attacks") is the rule because the idioventricular escape rhythm is slow and often unreliable. In addition, this slow rhythm may precipitate Torsades de Pointes, which causes syncope. Of note, is that retrograde conduction may be present in 20% to 40% of patients with intra- or infra-His block (Figs. 4-25 and Table 4-4). The presence of one-to-one retrograde conduction during pacing (Fig. 4-25B) can produce a pacemaker syndrome.

## PAROXYSMAL A-V BLOCK

The sudden appearance of A-V block following a pause in HPS activation is called paroxysmal A-V block.[27] This disorder is rarely recognized and can be lethal because of unreliable escape rhythms. This pause may be produced by an APC (Fig. 4-26), VPC, CSP or other vagal maneuvers, His extrasystole, or posttachycardia sinus suppression. It may often be mistaken for a "benign" vagal episode, if the clinical situation suggests increased vagal tone; e.g., Valsalva. Electrocardiographic features suggesting *Paroxysmal A-V block* are failure to see significant P-R prolongation prior to block, sinus acceleration with failure to conduct, and sudden resumption of conduction following a VPC or junctional escape with a normal P-R interval. This is always a disorder of the HPS and is due to Phase 4 block in either the His bundle (baseline narrow QRS) or in the bundle branches (baseline wide QRS). Resumption of conduction requires an appropriately timed escape beat, premature beat (sinus or ectopic) relative to Phase 4 depolarization causing the block. Pacemakers are required in such cases.

## VALUE OF INTRACARDIAC STUDIES IN THE EVALUATION OF A-V CONDUCTION DISTURBANCES

Several specific points are discussed in this section to emphasize the value of intracardiac studies in the diagnosis and management of A-V conduction disturbances. (Points regarding patients with bundle branch block per se are discussed in Chapter 5.)

1. The ECG appearance of first- or second-degree block may not be due to a primary conduction disorder; rather, it may be due to junctional (His bundle) extrasystoles that are concealed (not conducted to the atria or ventricles) but render a portion of the conduction system refractory

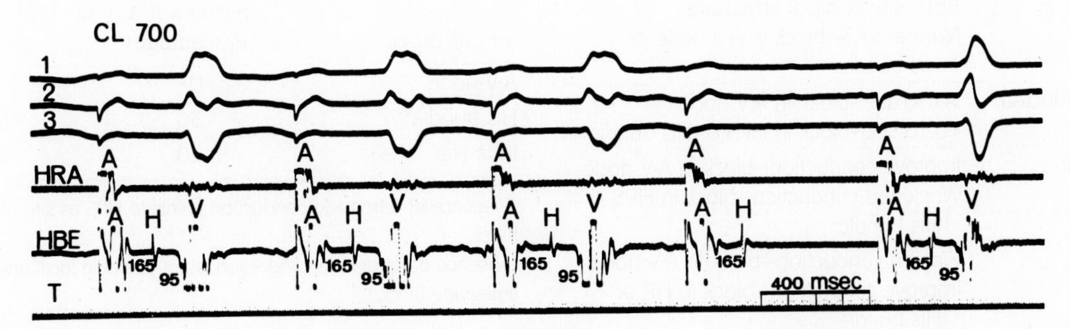


**FIGURE 4-23** *Type II second-degree infra-His block induced by atrial pacing.* The atrium is paced at a cycle length of 700 msec with stable conduction intervals. No ventricular depolarization follows the fourth paced atrial complex. Ventricular depolarization results from the fifth paced atrial complex and demonstrates no change in A-H or H-V intervals.

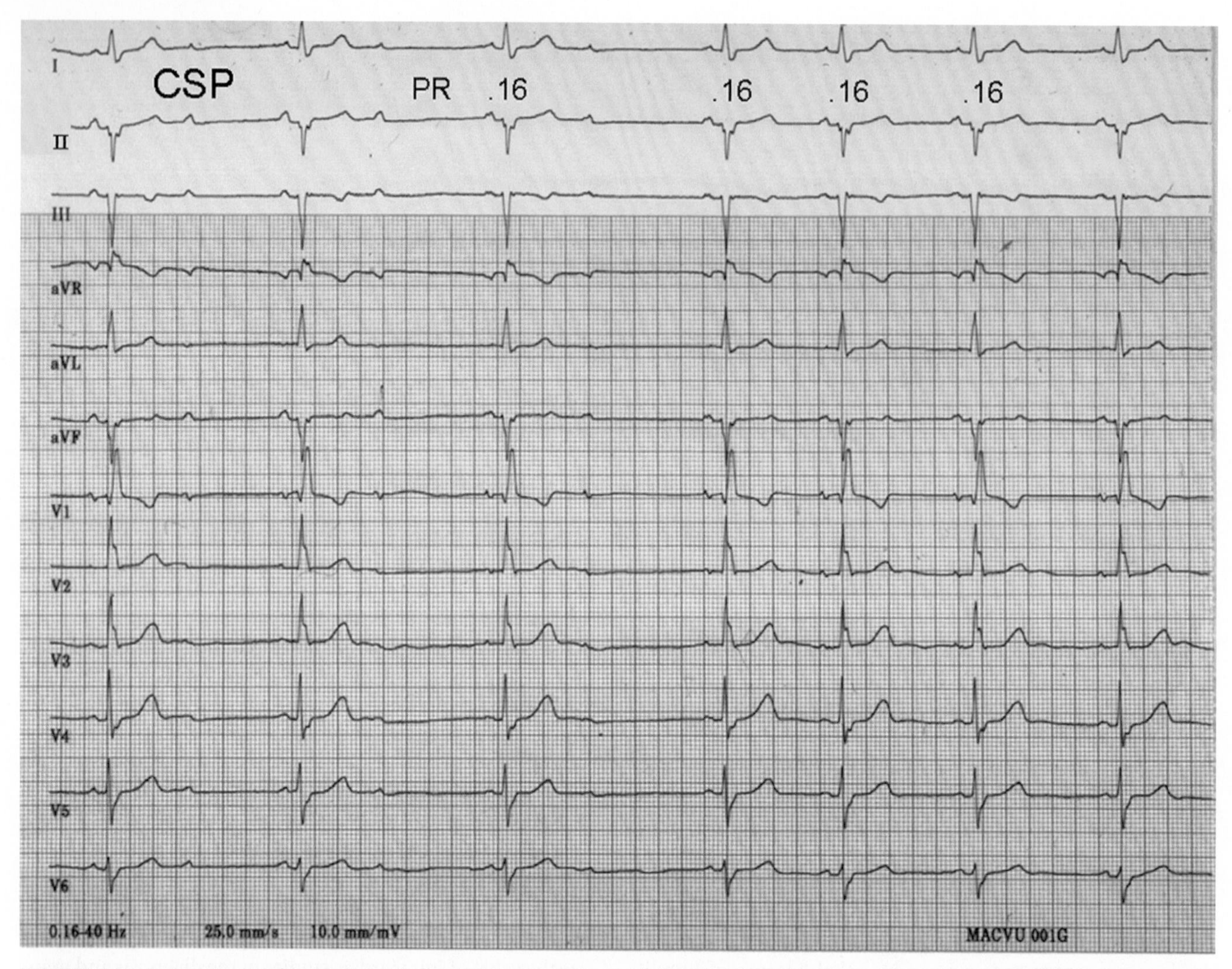


**FIGURE 4-24** *Two-to-one A-V block relieved by carotid sinus pressure.* Right bundle branch block with left anterior hemiblock and a P-R interval of 0.16 sec is presentment with two-to-one A-V block at a sinus rate of 70 bpm is present on the left. Carotid sinus pressure (CSP) is applied producing slowing of the sinus and one-to-one conduction, without a change in P-R or QRS. This is highly suggestive of block in the HPS.

### TABLE 4-3 Site of 2:1 A-V Block

| | |
|---|---|
| 1. QRS width | BBB—site of block anywhere<br>Normal QRS—block in A-V node or His bundle |
| 2. P-R of conducted P wave | >0.30 sec—block in A-V node<br><0.16 sec—block in HPS or His bundle |
| 3. Atropine or exercise | Improve conduction—block in A-V node<br>Worsened conduction—block in HPS or His bundle |
| 4. CSP | Worsen conduction—block in A-V node<br>Improve conduction—block in HP or His bundle |
| 5. Retrograde conduction | Present—block in HPS or His bundle<br>Absent—block may be anywhere |

### TABLE 4-4 Significance of Retrograde Conduction in the Presence of Antegrade Block

| Site of Block | Retrograde Conduction (Percentage) |
|---|---|
| A-V node | 0 |
| His bundle | 30 |
| Infra-His | 40 |

[a]Presence of retrograde conduction points to HPS as site of antegrade block.

[b]Absence of retrograde conduction is not useful in localizing the site of antegrade block.

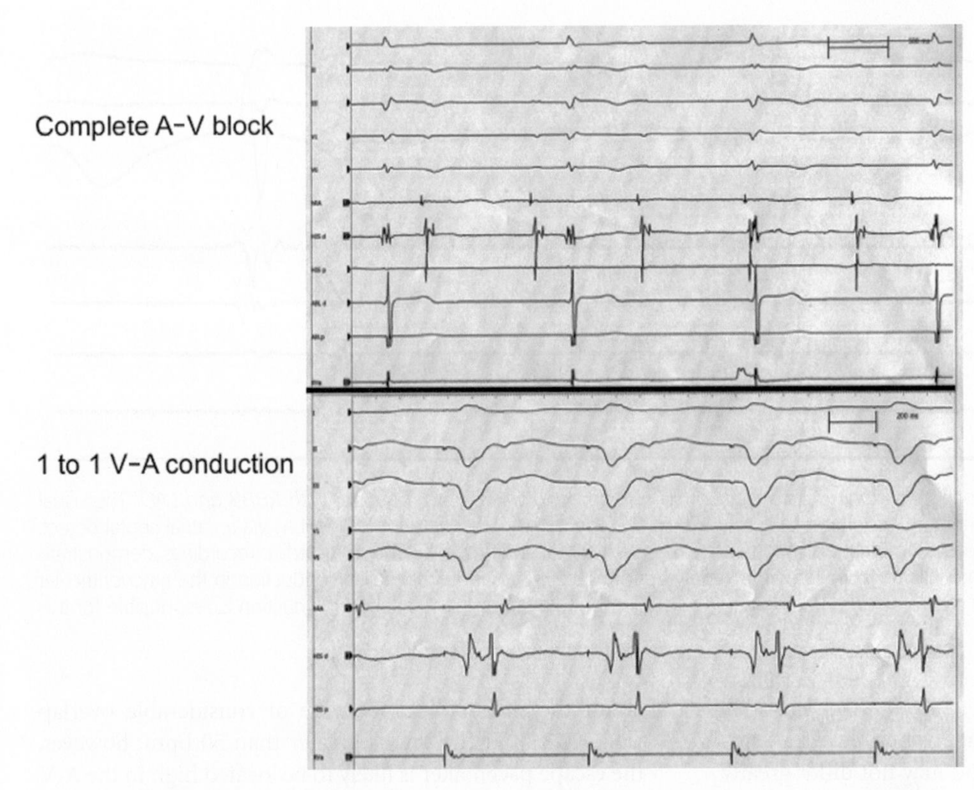


**FIGURE 4-25** *Antegrade infra-His block with intact retrograde conduction.* **Top:** Complete infra-His block with a ventricular escape of ≈ 1,450 msec is shown. **Bottom:** Ventricular pacing during complete antegrade A-V block demonstrates 1:1 V-A conduction. A retrograde His is seen following the ventricular electrogram during ventricular pacing because conduction proceeds up the left bundle branch. The patient had pre-existing RBBB during intact A-V conduction.

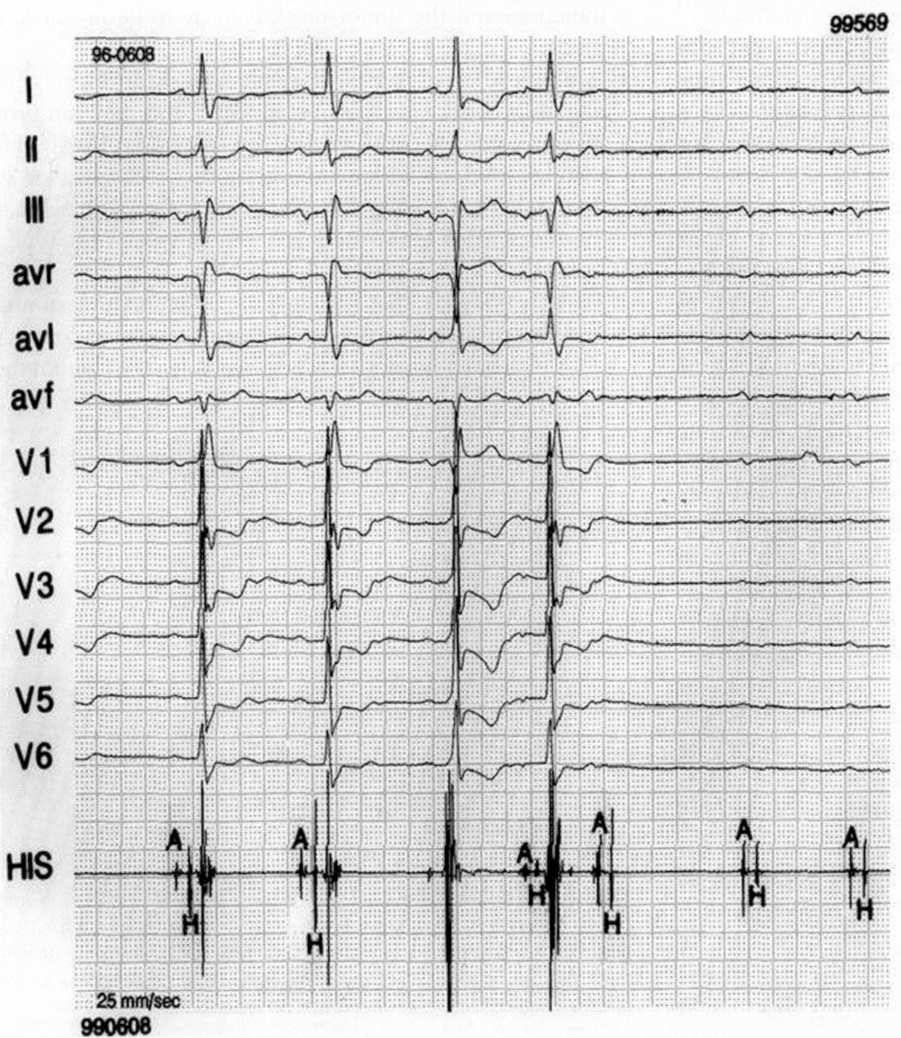


**FIGURE 4-26** *Paroxysmal A-V block.* Following three sinus beats two APCs are noted. The first, which is rather late, conducts rapidly through the A-V node and HPS. The second, earlier APC, blocks below the His. There is a sinus pause following the second APC resulting in a long H-H interval which then sets up Phase 4 block leading to complete A-V block. (Courtesy of Hein Wellens.)

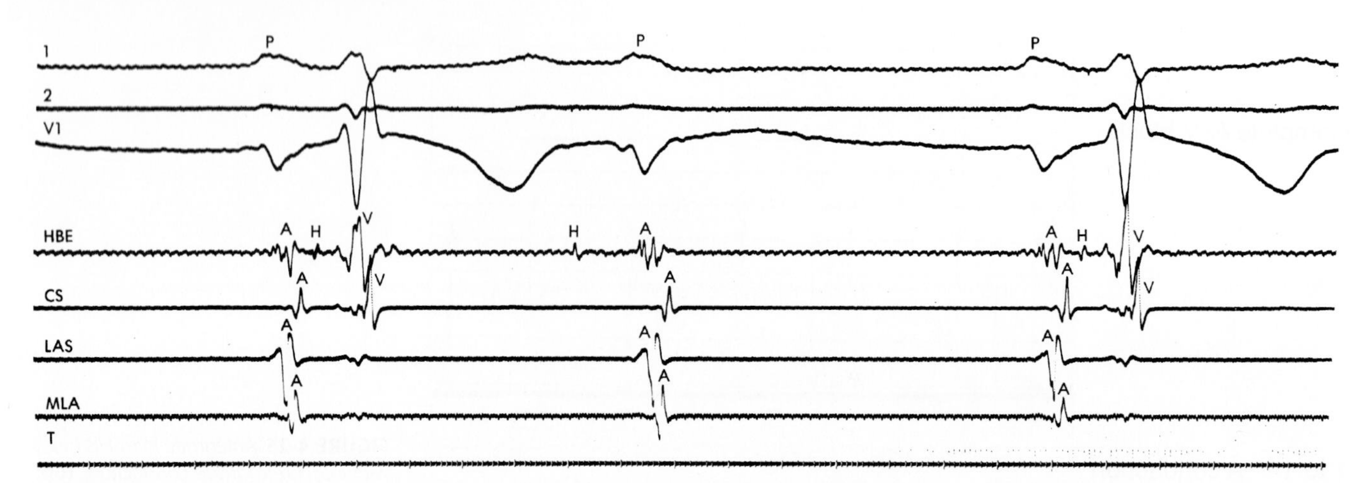


**FIGURE 4-27** *Pseudo-type II infra-His block secondary to a concealed His bundle depolarization in a patient with RBBB and LAD.* The usual electrograms are recorded, plus the left atrium at the intra-atrial septum (IAS) and the midleft atrial anterior wall (MLA) via an atrial septal defect. The "blocked" P wave in the surface leads has an atrial activation sequence identical to sinus rhythm. The intracardiac recordings demonstrate a junctional (His bundle) depolarization that fails to propagate antegradely but produces retrograde concealed conduction in the atrioventricular node, which is the cause of the blocked P wave. Increased automaticity in the His bundle rather than impaired conduction is responsible for this phenomenon. LAS, low atrial septum.

to propagation of a sinus beat (Fig. 4-27) (Chapter 7).[15] Although it has been suggested that His bundle extrasystoles reflect a diseased His bundle and may not differ greatly from His bundle block in their prognostic significance,[12] we believe that therapy should initially be directed at suppressing automaticity rather than at failing conduction. Although the observance of junctional premature depolarizations on the surface ECG suggests that concealed His bundle extrasystoles are responsible for the apparent A-V block, an intracardiac recording is the only method of positive identification.

2. Although 2:1 or higher degrees of block (e.g., 3:1 and 4:1) have traditionally been classified as Type II block, the site of those blocks cannot be reliably determined by the surface ECG. The observation of typical Type I block in the same patient, however, suggests that the site of block is the A-V node. Several clinical observations may point to the site of block (Table 4-4) that are based on known physiologic responses of the A-V node and diseased HPS to predictors that alter heart rate and autonomic tone. Because high-grade block can occur anywhere in the A-V conduction system, an intracardiac study is essential for accurate localization when the site of block cannot be really determined.
3. Data about the width of the QRS complex and the configuration of conducted beats and/or escape beats are of only limited value in localizing the site of block. Although a narrow QRS complex is most compatible with an A-V nodal or intra-His problem, and a wide QRS complex is most compatible with an infra-His problem, a wide QRS complex certainly may occur with A-V nodal or intra-His disease in the presence of coexistent bundle branch block. This is fairly common, occurring in 20% to 50% of such patients.[18,19]
4. In the presence of third-degree block, the rate of the escape pacemaker also provides only limited information about the site of block because of considerable overlap (Fig. 4-28).[18] If the rate is greater than 50 bpm, however, the escape pacemaker is likely to be located high in the A-V junction, and the site of block is likely to be in the A-V node.
5. Multiple levels of A-V block spontaneously or during pacing, may coexist in the same patient,[28] and they can produce a confusing ECG picture that is extraordinarily difficult to interpret without an intracardiac study (Figs. 4-29 and 4-30). Combined A-V nodal and infra-His block has been described as the mechanism in alternate-beat Type I block.[28]
6. Atrial pacing or the introduction of premature stimuli may precipitate latent prolongation or failure of conduction. The phenomenon may be physiologic (i.e., within the

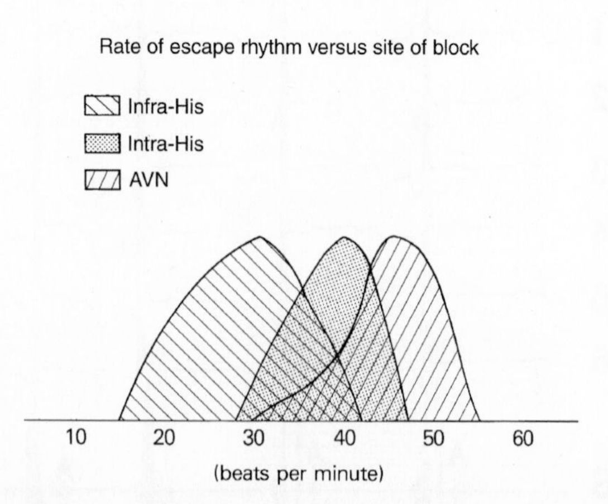


**FIGURE 4-28** *Relationship of site of complete A-V block to the rate of the escape rhythm.* Note that the range of rates in each site is rather broad although the means clearly differ. Only when the escape rhythm is very slow (<28 bpm) or relatively rapid (>50 bpm) can the rate be diagnostically useful information be deduced.

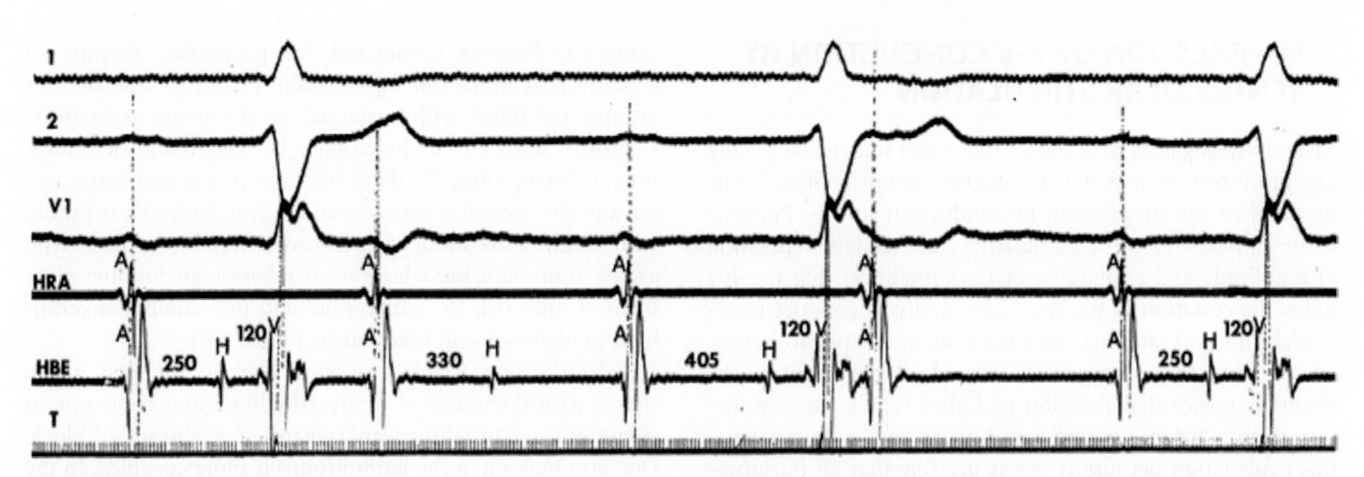


**FIGURE 4-29** *Spontaneous multiple levels of second-degree block in the same patient.* The rhythm is sinus, and there is a gradual prolongation of A-V nodal conduction (A-H interval) until the fourth atrial depolarization A is not followed by a His bundle deflection H or by ventricular depolarization V. Following the next (fifth) atrial depolarization, the A-H interval shortens to 250 msec; that is, typical Type I second-degree A-V nodal block occurs. Note that the H-V interval remains constant at 120 msec, except following the second atrial depolarization A, after which conduction fails following depolarization of the His bundle; that is, Type II second-degree infra-His block occurs.

range of the normal responses described in Chapter 2) or pathologic (Figs. 4-19 and 4-21; see also Chapter 5).

7. Presence of block may not be the sole cause of symptoms (see subsequent paragraphs on Therapeutic Considerations). This is particularly true in the presence of organic heart disease where ventricular tachycardia is the cause of syncope.
8. When a pacemaker is to be implanted for assumed or proven intra- or infra-His block, V-A conduction may be intact. This can lead to a pacemaker syndrome or pacemaker-mediated tachycardia. Recognition of these potential problems helps the physician choose the appropriate pacemaker and programming to prevent their occurrence.

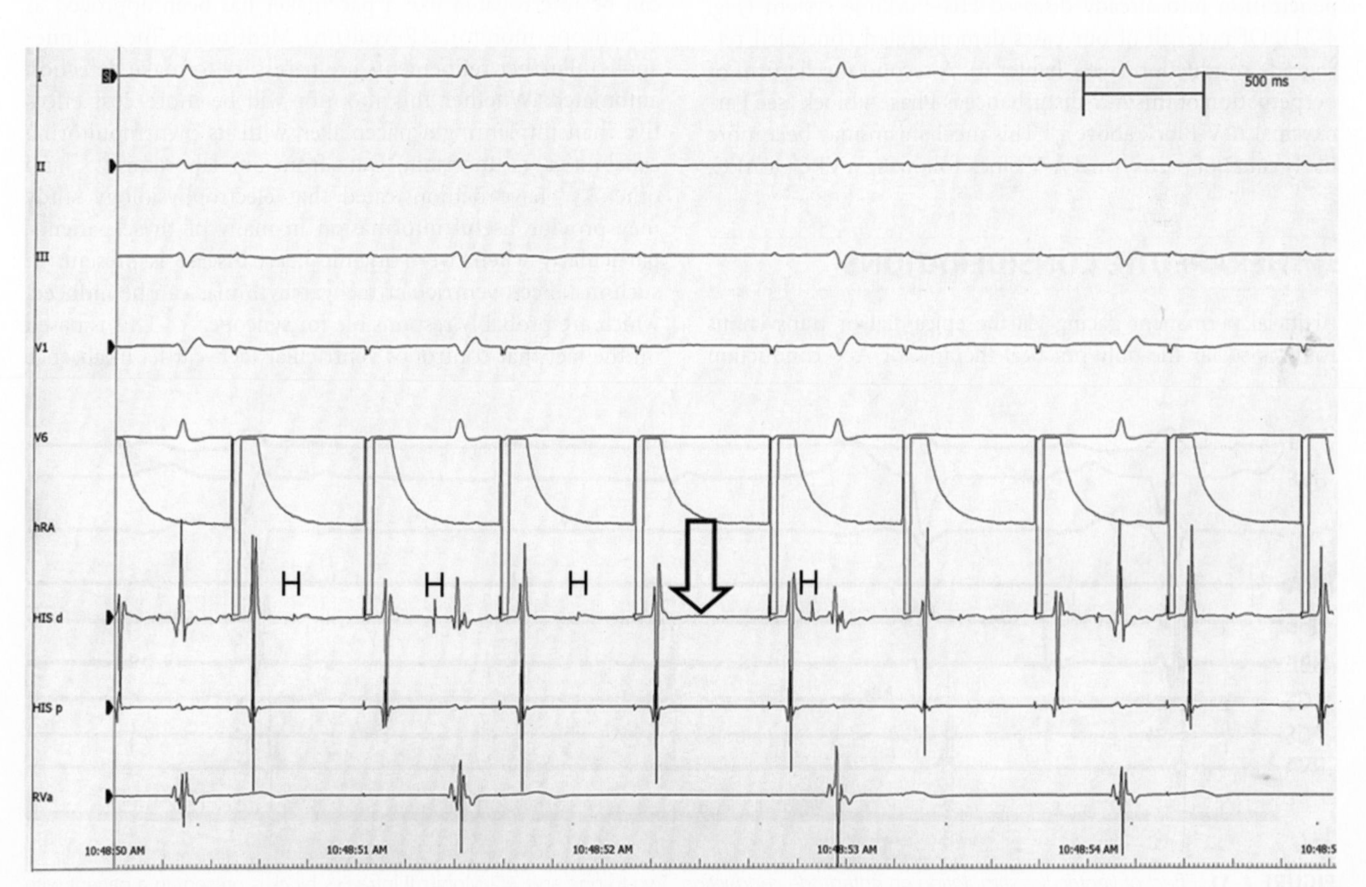


**FIGURE 4-30** *Pacing-induced multilevel block.* Atrial pacing process five-to-four A-V nodal Wenckebah (*open arrow*) and two-to-one block below the His H.

## SUPPRESSION OF A-V CONDUCTION BY VENTRICULAR STIMULATION

Several investigators have shown that rapid ventricular pacing can produce transient A-V conduction abnormalities.[29] The mechanism for suppression of conduction in His–Purkinje tissue appears to be a cumulative, rate-related depression of amplitude and excitability of Purkinje fibers that persists following cessation of pacing.[29] The ability to conduct retrogradely at rapid rates may be a requisite to this phenomenon. Most recent studies suggest that the block site might be the Purkinje–myocardial junction and that retrograde conduction to the Purkinje system is not necessary.[29] I do not favor this explanation because it seems unlikely that all Purkinje–myocardial junctions would be affected similarly and simultaneously. We have seen this phenomenon occasionally; it has always occurred in the presence of a pre-existent intraventricular and A-V conduction disturbance. Typically, we have seen this in the presence of bundle branch block and Mobitz II or 2:1 block. In such patients single ventricular premature depolarization or ventricular pacing can produce higher degree of heart block, which usually resolves in seconds. Wald and Waxman[30] have shown that both rate and duration can affect the duration of block. The ability of single ventricular premature depolarization as well as ventricular pacing to induce this phenomenon is more compatible with earlier reports of requiring penetration into already diseased His–Purkinje system (Fig. 4-31). Of note, all of our cases demonstrated concealed retrograde conduction (see Chapter 6). A second mechanism of perpetuation of this A-V disturbance is Phase 4 block (see Paroxysmal A-V Block above).[31] This mechanism may be a more likely cause of paroxysmal A-V block following a VPC or APC.

## THERAPEUTIC CONSIDERATIONS

Artificial permanent pacing via the epicardial or transvenous route is so far the only practical therapy for A-V conduction disorders. Patients considered for pacemaker therapy of a bradyarrhythmia can be generally placed in one of four groups: (a) those with sustained or documented bradyarrhythmia sufficient to precipitate hemodynamic deterioration and symptoms, (b) those with symptoms and suspected, but not documented paroxysmal bradyarrhythmia, (c) those with bradycardia-induced tachycardias, and (d) those who are asymptomatic but whose electrophysiologic findings place them at high risk for paroxysmal and potentially dangerous high-grade block and bradycardia (Table 4-5).

The decision to place a pacemaker in the first group (those with documented bradyarrhythmia and concomitant symptoms) is straightforward, regardless of the site of block. Decision making in the latter groups is more complex. In the second group (those with symptoms of a suspected bradyarrhythmic origin), one needs to weigh the chance of the symptomatology being cardiac against the evidence for an electrophysiologic substrate likely to cause paroxysmal block. Hence, the patient with paroxysmal syncope and no evidence of neurologic disease who has first-degree or second-degree intra-His or infra-His block appears to be a good candidate for a pacemaker despite the lack of direct correlation of bradyarrhytmia and the symptom. While the use of external event recorders may be useful in correlating symptoms with bradyarrhythmias, the relative infrequency of symptoms may make this impractical. Recently, an implantable loop recorder that can be interrogated like a pacemaker has been approved as a "syncope monitor" (Reveal(tm) Medtronics, Inc., Minneapolis). Further refinements are necessary to make detection automated. Whether this monitor will be more cost effective than implanting a pacemaker, with its own monitoring capabilities, is uncertain. Data from our laboratory[32,33] and others[34,35] have demonstrated that electrophysiology study may provide useful information in many of these patients, particularly when overt organic heart disease is present. In such instances, ventricular tachyarrhythmias can be induced, which are probably responsible for syncope.[33,35] This is based on the fact that control of ventricular tachycardia in absence

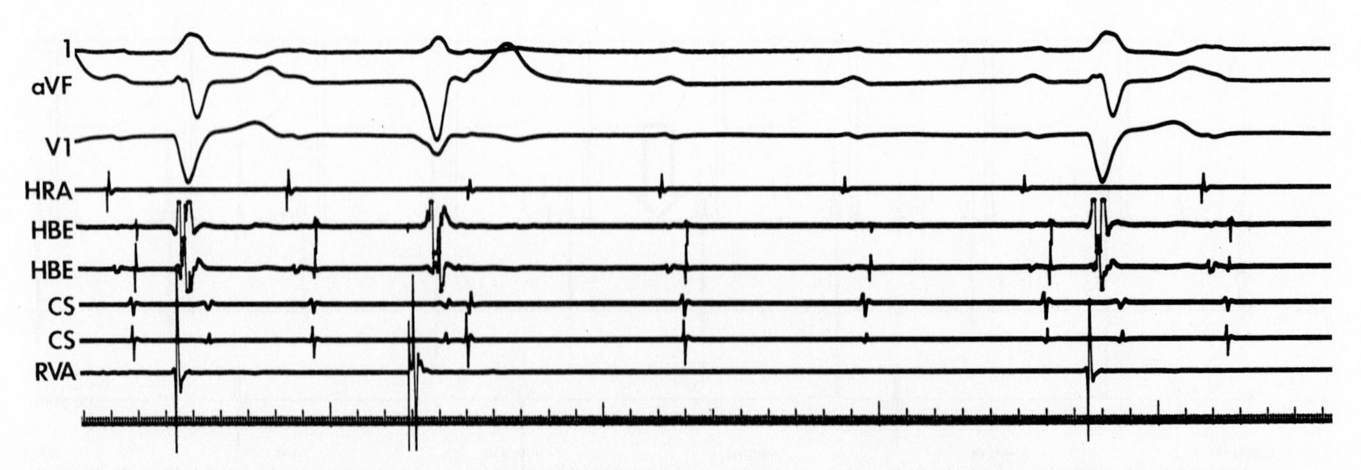


**FIGURE 4-31** *Effect of ventricular stimulation on antegrade conduction.* Two-to-one and 3:2 Mobitz II infra-His block is present in a patient with left bundle branch block and left anterior hemiblock. The H-V of conducted complexes was 140 to 150 msec. A ventricular premature complex (VPC) is introduced following the first blocked sinus beat. This VPC is associated with good retrograde conduction, which then produces a higher degree of antegrade infra-His block.

TABLE 4-5 Indications for Cardiac Pacing in Chronic Heart Block

| Degree | Intra-His or Infra-His | A-V Node |
|---|---|---|
| First degree (prolonged conduction) | Yes, with symptoms[a]<br>? without symptoms[a] | No[b] |
| Second degree (intermittent conduction) | Yes | Yes, with symptoms[a] |
| Third degree (no conduction) | Yes | Yes, with symptoms[a] |

[a]Symptoms must be of cardiac origin.
[b]Unless P-R is so long that the P wave occurs during the QRS and produces symptomatic Canon A waves or a "pacemaker syndrome."

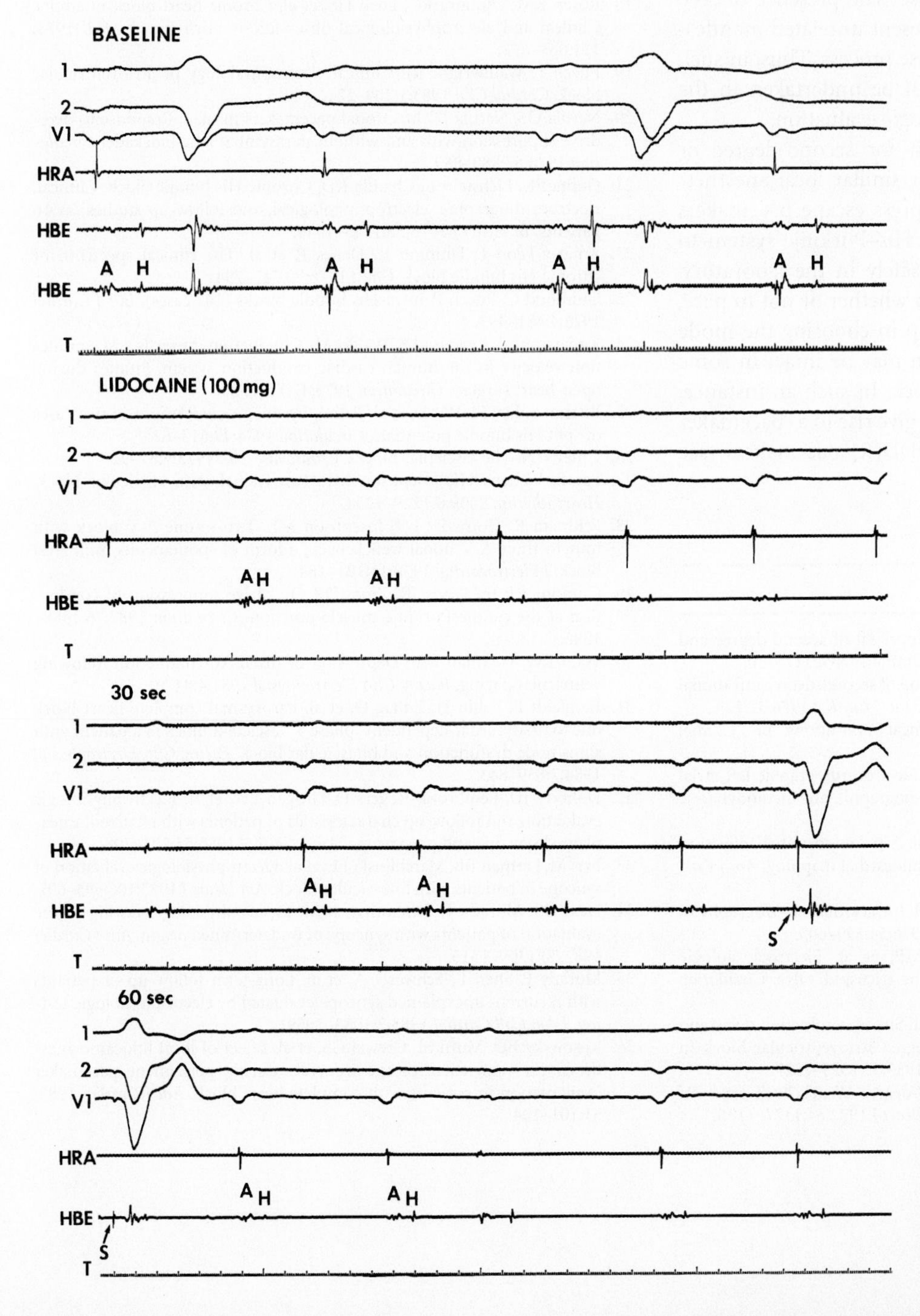


**FIGURE 4-32** *Depressant effects of lidocaine on diseased His–Purkinje tissue.* In the baseline state (**top panel**), 2:1 infra-His block is present. The conducted complexes show a left bundle branch block, left anterior hemiblock configuration, and have a markedly prolonged H-V interval of ≈ 120 msec. Lidocaine (100 mg) produced complete intra-His block with no escape for more than a minute.

of pacemaker relieves symptoms.[32] Many of these patients will still require pacemakers because antiarrhythmic agents required to suppress ventricular tachycardia increase third-degree A-V block. The decision to place a pacemaker in patients in the group of asymptomatic patients with alarming electrophysiologic findings is the most difficult and controversial one. In our experience, "first-degree" infra-His block with H-V intervals exceeding 100 msec, alternating bundle branch block with changing H-V intervals (see Chapter 5), as well as second- or third-degree intra-His or infra-His block, is so apt to result in severe paroxysmal symptoms that we recommend pacemaker therapy for all these patients, regardless of the absence of symptoms.

Full electrophysiologic studies are of value in patients with syncope (recurrent) and heart disease. The presence of A-V conduction defects may merely represent unrelated manifestations of the same or different disease process. Thus, in such cases, pacemaker therapy should not be undertaken in the absence of a complete electrophysiologic evaluation.

During pacemaker implantation for second-degree or third-degree A-V block, lidocaine or similar local anesthetics may increase A-V block and depress escape pacemakers (Fig. 4-32).[36] The sensitivity of the His–Purkinje system to lidocaine can be readily evaluated safely in the laboratory. In addition to aiding the decision on whether or not to pace, the electrophysiology study may help in choosing the mode of pacing. As noted, V-A conduction may be intact in some patients with complete infra-His block. In such an instance, ventricular pacing in the VVI(R) will give rise to a "pacemaker syndrome." Such patients require DDD(R) pacemakers (see Chapter 13).

## REFERENCES


1. El-Sherif N, Scherlag BJ, Lazzara R. An appraisal of second degree and paroxysmal atrioventricular block. *Eur J Cardiol* 1976;4:117–130.
2. Simson MB, Spear J, Moore EN. Comparison of second-degree infranodal with second-degree A-V block. (Abstract). *Am J Cardiol* 1976;37:173.
3. Sherf L. The atrial conduction system: clinical implications. *Am J Cardiol* 1976;37:814–817.
4. Josephson ME, Kastor JA, Morganroth J. Electrocardiographic left atrial enlargement. Electrophysiologic, echocardiographic and hemodynamic correlates. *Am J Cardiol* 1977;39:967–971.
5. Josephson ME, Scharf DL, Kastor JA, et al. Atrial endocardial activation in man. Electrode catheter technique of endocardial mapping. *Am J Cardiol* 1977;39:972–981.
6. Jacobsen JR, Gillette PC, Corbett BN, et al. Intracardiac electrography in endocardial cushion defects. *Circulation* 1976;54:599–603.
7. Kastor JA, Goldreyer BN, Josephson ME, et al. Electrophysiologic characteristics of Ebstein's anomaly of the tricuspid valve. *Circulation* 1975;52:987–995.
8. Sherron P, Torres-Arraut E, Tamer D, et al. Site of conduction delay and electrophysiologic significance of first-degree atrioventricular block in children with heart disease. *Am J Cardiol* 1985;55:1323–1327.
9. Narula OS, Runge M, Samet P. Second-degree Wenckebach type AV block due to block within the atrium. *Br Heart J* 1972;34:1127–1136.
10. Castellanos A Jr., Iyengar R, Agha AS, et al. Wenckebach phenomenon within the atria. *Br Heart J* 1972;34:1121–1126.
11. Reddy CP, Damato AN, Akhtar M, et al. Time dependent changes in the functional properties of the atrioventricular conduction system in man. *Circulation* 1975;52:1012–1022.
12. Narula OS, ed. *Current concepts of atrioventricular block.* Philadelphia, PA: FA Davis, 1975.
13. Denes P, Levy L, Pick A, et al. The incidence of typical and atypical A-V Wenckebach periodicity. *Am Heart J* 1975;89:26–31.
14. Rosen KM, Loeb HS, Gunnar RM, et al. Mobitz type II block without bundle-branch block. *Circulation* 1971;44:1111–1119.
15. Rosen KM, Rahimtoola SH, Gunnar RM. Pseudo A-V block secondary to premature nonpropagated His bundle depolarizations: documentation by His bundle electrocardiography. *Circulation* 1970;42:367–373.
16. Rosen KM, Rahimtoola SH, Gunnar RM, et al. Site of heart block as defined by His bundle recording. Pathologic correlations in three cases. *Circulation* 1972;45:965–987.
17. Rosen KM, Loeb HS, Chuquimia R, et al. Site of heart block in acute myocardial infarction. *Circulation* 1970;42:925–933.
18. Rosen KM, Dhingra RC, Loeb HS, et al. Chronic heart block in adults. Clinical and electrophysiological observations. *Arch Intern Med.* 1973;131:663–672.
19. Puech P, Wainwright RJ. Clinical electrophysiology of atrioventricular block. *Cardiol Clin* 1983;1:209–224.
20. Narula OS, Narula JT. Junctional pacemakers in man. Response to overdrive suppression with and without parasympathetic blockade. *Circulation* 1978;57:880–889.
21. Gupta PK, Lichstein E, Chadda KD. Chronic His bundle block. Clinical, electrocardiographic, electrophysiological, and follow-up studies on 16 patients. *Br Heart J* 1976;38:1343–1349.
22. Amat-y-Leon F, Dhingra R, Denes P, et al. The clinical spectrum of chronic His bundle block. *Chest* 1976;70:747–754.
23. Guimond C, Puech P. Intra-His bundle blocks (102 cases). *Eur J Cardiol* 1976;4:481–493.
24. Kupersmith J, Krongrad E, Waldo AL. Conduction intervals and conduction velocity in the human cardiac conduction system. Studies during open-heart surgery. *Circulation* 1973;47:776–785.
25. Bharati S, Lev M, Wu D, et al. Pathophysiologic correlations in two cases of split His bundle potentials. *Circulation* 1974;49:615–623.
26. Uhley HN. The fascicular blocks. *Cardiovasc Clin* 1973;5:87–97.
27. Lee S, Wellens HJ, Josephson ME. Paroxysmal atrioventricular block. *Heart Rhythm* 2009;6:1229–1234.
28. Feldman R, Horowitz LN, Josephson ME. Two-to-one A-V block with four-to-three A-V nodal wenckebach, a form of spontaneous multilevel block. *J Electrocardiol* 1978;11:181–184.
29. Gilmour RF Jr., Davis JR, Zipes DP. Overdrive suppression of conduction at the canine Purkinje-muscle junction. *Circulation* 1987;76:1388–1396.
30. Wald RW, Waxman MB. Depression of distal AV conduction following ventricular pacing. *Pacing Clin Electrophysiol* 1981;4:84–91.
31. Bergfeldt L, Vallin H, Edhag O, et al. Paroxysmal complete heart block due to bradycardia-dependent "phase 4" fascicular block in a patient with sinus node dysfunction and bifascicular block. *Pacing Clin Electrophysiol* 1984;7:839–843.
32. Doherty JU, Pembrook-Rogers D, Grogan EW, et al. Electrophysiologic evaluation and follow-up characteristics of patients with recurrent unexplained syncope and presyncope. *Am J Cardiol* 1985;55:703–708.
33. Ezri M, Lerman BB, Marchlinski FE, et al. Electrophysiologic evaluation of syncope in patients with bifascicular block. *Am Heart J* 1983;106:693–697.
34. Hess DS, Morady F, Scheinman MM. Electrophysiologic testing in the evaluation of patients with syncope of undetermined origin. *Am J Cardiol* 1982;50:1309–1315.
35. Morady F, Shen E, Schwartz A, et al. Long-term follow-up of patients with recurrent unexplained syncope evaluated by electrophysiologic testing. *J Am Coll Cardiol* 1983;2:1053–1059.
36. Kosowsky BD, Mufti SI, Grewal GS, et al. Effect of local lidocaine anesthesia on ventricular escape intervals during permanent pacemaker implantation in patients with complete heart block. *Am J Cardiol* 1983;51:101–104.

CHAPTER

# 5 Intraventricular Conduction Disturbances

Intraventricular conduction disturbances are the result of abnormal activation of the ventricles. Normal ventricular activation requires the synchronized participation of the distal components of the atrioventricular (A-V) conducting system, that is, the main bundle branches and their ramifications. In addition, abnormalities of local myocardial activation can further alter the specific pattern of activation in that ventricle. In the last chapter, I discussed the entire infra-His system as a unit as a site of prolonged, intermittent, or failed conduction. In this chapter, I address the consequences of impaired conduction in the individual fascicles. I will not detail the influences of pathologic processes, such as infarction, on ventricular activation. However, I will discuss the effects of infarction on the characteristic patterns of "bundle branch block."

Because it is often difficult, if not impossible, to measure conduction times and refractory periods directly from the individual fascicles via catheter, identification of specific conduction defects usually depends on recognition of an altered pattern of ventricular activation on the surface ECG. Measurement of activation times at different areas of the ventricles has been suggested as a means of indirectly assessing conduction properties of the right bundle branch (RBB) and the multiple divisions of the left bundle branch (LBB). This technique may be useful in evaluating conduction over the RBB, particularly if simultaneous measurements from the LBB are also obtained from the catheter and/or if the entire pattern of right ventricular activation is determined intraoperatively. It is possible because the anatomy of the RBB is generally uniform. In humans the RBB has its major route from the His bundle through the musculature of the ventricular septum. The septal band gives rise to the moderator band, which extends to the anterior papillary muscle at the apical third of the right ventricular free wall. Purkinje fibers extend from the moderator band to the remainder of the RV. In Tawara's text a branch from the RBB in the moderator band gives rise to Purkinje fibers that subsequently activate the septum (Fig. 5-1). In some patients there appears to be a small continuation of the RBB distal to the moderator band toward the apical septum, which is also supplied by extensions of the moderator band and Purkinje fibers. Mapping studies of the RBB by Durrer et al.[1] and Horowitz et al. showed that most individuals have the moderator band as the main source of right ventricular activation. Durrer et al.[1] also noted that one in four had relatively early activation of the right ventricular apical septum, but activation of the septum never occurred prior to activation of the right ventricular free wall.

However, there are many objections to its use in evaluating the LBB system. The major objection stems from the fact that the LBB does not divide into two discrete fascicles, but it divides into two or three broad fascicle, then rapidly fans out over the entire left ventricle. The size of the fascicles is highly variable as described by Tawara[2] more than 100 years ago (Figs. 5-2 and 5-3). Thus, a detailed assessment of infra-His conduction in humans can be made only intraoperatively, where direct mapping of the entire subendocardial conducting system can be performed. Use of mathematically derived electrograms from an intracoronary probe (Endocardial Solutions, Inc.) may provide assessment of His–Purkinje activation, particularly on the septum, but the use of this probe is complicated and expensive. Moreover, the value of data obtained from this probe has not been assessed. Therefore, for practical reasons, clinical evaluation has primarily involved observations of the surface ECG pattern and on the H-V interval. Recordings of potentials of the RBB and/or from the proximal and distal His bundle are of great help in determining sites of conduction delay or block associated with these specific electrocardiographic patterns and should be performed whenever possible.

Traditionally, in clinical electrocardiography, three major fascicles are considered to be operative in normal persons, even though a third fascicle of the LBB (septal fascicle) is usually responsible for the initiation of intraventricular septal depolarization (see Fig. 2-18).[3] Electrocardiographically the three major fascicles are (a) the RBB, which is an anatomically compact unit that travels as the extension of the His bundle after the origin of the LBB; (b) the anterior (superior) division of the left bundle branch block (LBBB); and (c) the posterior (inferior) division of the LBB. The LBB and its divisions are, unlike the RBB, diffuse structures that fan out just beyond their origin (some investigators have denied their distinct anatomic existence).[4,5] Nevertheless, specific patterns of altered ventricular activation as reflected in the QRS complex have been correlated experimentally, clinically, and anatomically with altered conduction in each of the fascicles. The contribution of the septal fascicle to the ECG is less well appreciated but is responsible for the initial left to right septal forces giving rise to a small r wave in lead V1 and a small q wave in lead I and/or aVL.

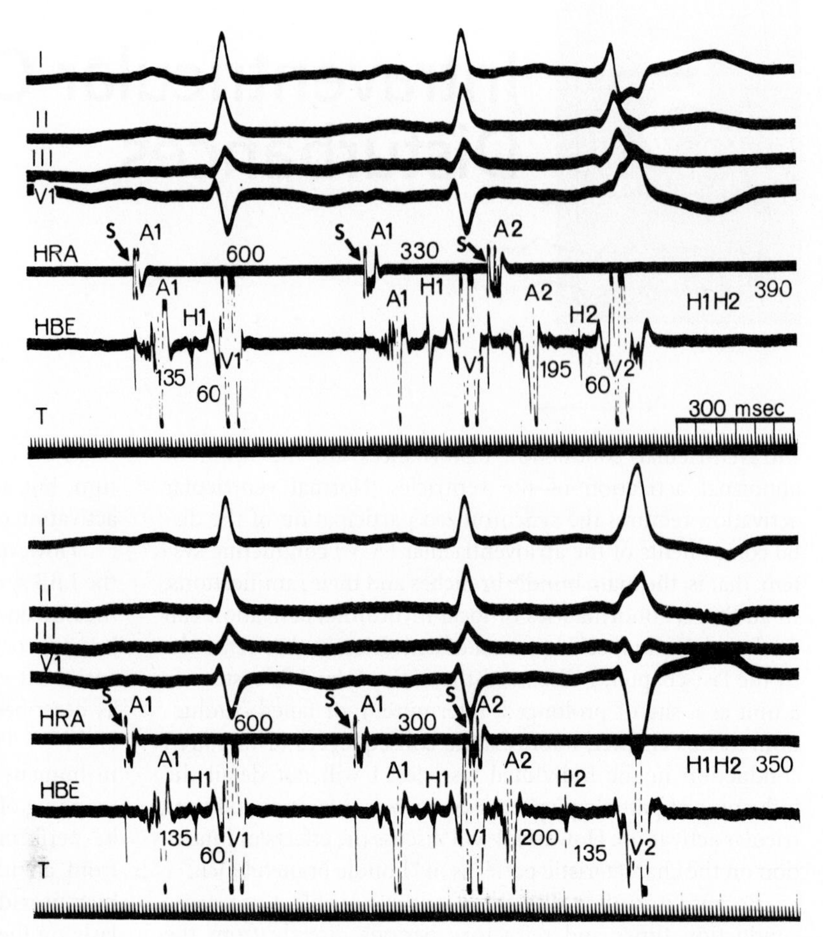


**FIGURE 5-1** *Incomplete nature of bundle branch block.* From **top** to **bottom** in each panel: surface ECG leads 1, 2, 3, and V1 high-right atrium (HRA), His bundle electrogram (HBE), and time lines (T) at 10 msec and 100 msec. In both panels, the basic atrial drive is at a cycle length of 600 msec. In the **top** panel, an atrial premature stimulus (A2) is introduced at a coupling interval of 330 msec. The resulting QRS complex is conducted in "complete" RBBB pattern. In the **bottom** panel, an atrial premature stimulus at a coupling interval of 300 msec results in a QRS complex conducted in an LBBB pattern.

## DEFINITIONS

1. Right bundle branch block (RBBB). QRS interval prolongation >120 msec with normal activation during the first half (approximately 60 msec) of the QRS complex, delayed intrinsicoid deflection in lead V1, and abnormal anterior and rightward forces during the terminal portion of the QRS complex.
2. Left bundle branch block. QRS interval prolongation >120 msec or (usually >140 msec) delayed intrinsicoid deflection in lead V6 (>0.075 seconds); absent Q waves and slurred broad R waves in leads I, aVL, and V6; rS or QS deflection in leads V1 and V2 (and often to V4); and an ST- and T-wave vector 180 degrees discordant to the QRS vector.
3. Left anterior hemiblock. QRS interval of 100 msec or shorter (unless complicated by bundle branch block, hypertrophy, etc.), with a frontal plane QRS axis to the left of −30 degrees with a counterclockwise loop, and initial activation in a rightward and inferior direction, with a small q wave in lead aVL and a small r wave in lead III, followed by leftward and superior forces with tall R waves in lead I and aVL and deep S waves in leads II, III, and aVF.

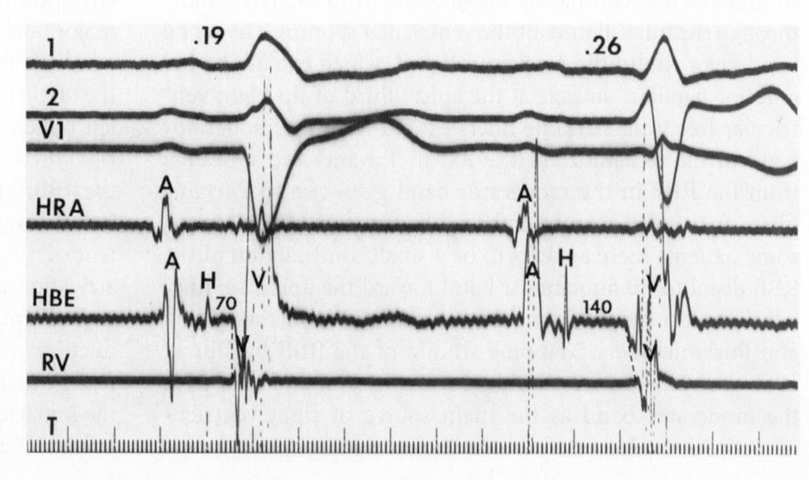


**FIGURE 5-2** *Alternating bundle branch block.* The first complex shows left bundle branch block and an H-V interval of 70 msec (with a corresponding P-R interval of 0.19 seconds). The second complex shows right bundle branch block with left anterior fascicular block and an H-V interval of 140 msec (with a corresponding P-R interval of 0.26 seconds). Note the relationship of the ventricular electrogram in the His bundle recording of the right ventricular apex electrogram (*dotted line*) during each conduction pattern.

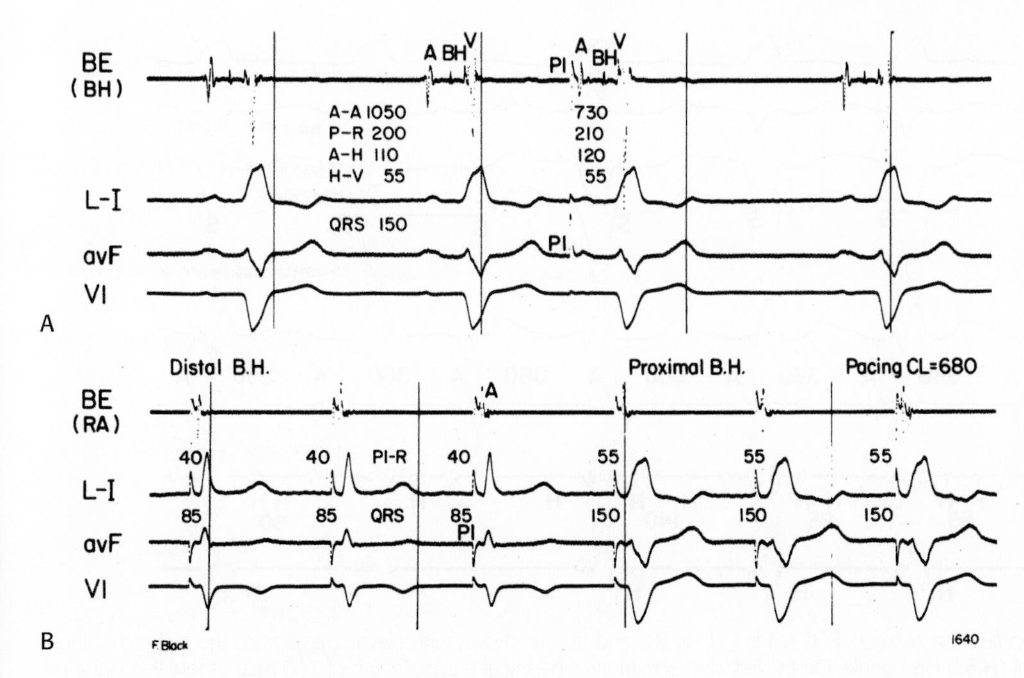


**FIGURE 5-3** *Normalization of left bundle branch block and left anterior fascicular block by distal His bundle (BH) stimulation.* **A:** Sinus rhythm with an H-V interval of 55 msec. **B:** QRS complex normalization for the first three beats during distal BH stimulation with a PI (pacing impulse)-R interval of 40 msec, which is 15 msec shorter than the basal H-V interval. The last three beats during proximal BH pacing demonstrate a QRS complex identical to those in panel A and a PI-R interval (55 msec) equivalent to the basal H-V interval. (From Narula OS. Longitudinal dissociation in the His bundle: bundle branch block due to asynchronous conduction within the His bundle in man. *Circulation* 1977;56:996.)

4. Left posterior hemiblock. Right ventricular hypertrophy, chronic lung disease, and extensive lateral wall myocardial infarction must be excluded. QRS interval of 100 msec or shorter (unless complicated by RBBB), a frontal plane QRS axis to the right of +110 degrees, with a clockwise loop, a small initial r wave in lead aVL, a small q wave in lead aVF, and a subsequently large terminal S wave in lead aVL and an R wave in aVF.
5. Intraventricular conduction defect (IVCD). QRS interval prolongation >120 msec with a pattern not conforming to LBBB or RBBB. An intraventricular conduction delay may be further classified as left or right ventricular, depending on the site of delayed intrinsicoid deflection and the direction of the terminal QRS forces.

Although the term bundle branch block is standard nomenclature, the pathophysiology of this electrocardiographic pattern should be thought of in terms of relative conduction delay (of varying degree and including failure of conduction) producing asynchronous ventricular activation without necessarily implying complete transmission failure. Thus, a typical bundle branch block appearance may be due to marked conduction delay in the bundle branch and not failure of conduction. The point is demonstrated by (a) varying degrees of "complete" bundle branch or fascicular block manifested by further axis shift or QRS widening either spontaneously or following premature extrastimuli[6] and (b) spontaneous or induced alternating "complete" bundle branch block (Figs. 5-1 and 5-2).[7] Obviously, in the latter instance, one could not have complete block in one bundle branch and then develop complete block in the other bundle branch without total failure of A-V conduction.

The marked H-V prolongation during LBBB in Figure 5-1 and during RBBB in Figure 5-2 reflects slowed conduction in the contralateral bundle branch to the one demonstrating "block" on the surface electrocardiogram. The difference in conduction time in the bundle branches allows the ventricles to be activated asynchronously, producing the typical QRS patterns of bundle branch block. Thus when alternating bundle branch "block" is observed, one assumes that the bundle branch block pattern associated with the long H-V is blocked, while the contralateral bundle is slowly conducting.

## SITE OF "BLOCK" OR CONDUCTION DELAY DURING BUNDLE BRANCH BLOCK

Interest in the site of block and/or conduction delay in the fascicles stems from the recognition that bifascicular block, especially RBBB with left anterior hemiblock, is the most common ECG pattern preceding the development of A-V block. Because these ECG patterns are common, we need to elucidate factors that can predict who will develop A-V block. Determining the site of bundle branch block is the first step in this process.

Despite the ECG-anatomic correlates that have been made, the exact site of block or conduction delay producing bundle branch block patterns is not certain in all cases. Longitudinal dissociation with asynchronous conduction in the His bundle may give rise to abnormal patterns of ventricular activation;[8] hence, the conduction problem may not necessarily lie in the individual bundle branch. This phenomenon has been substantiated in the case of both LBBB and left anterior hemiblock by normalization of the QRS complex, H-V interval, and ventricular activation times during His bundle stimulation (Fig. 5-3).[9,10] These findings suggest that fibers to the left and right ventricles are already predestined within the His bundle and that lesions in the His bundle may produce characteristic bundle branch block patterns. Moreover, it is not uncommon to observe intra-His disease (widened or split

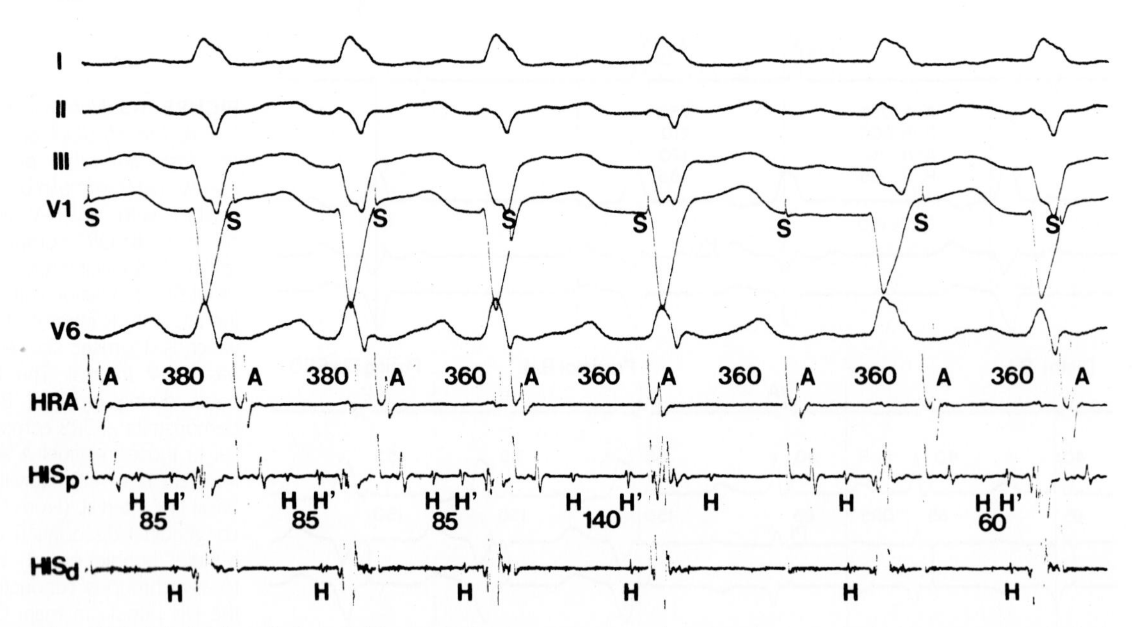


**FIGURE 5-4** *Site of block in left bundle branch block.* ECG leads I, II, III, V1, and V6 are shown with electrograms from the high-right atrium (HRA) and proximal (HISp) and distal (HISd) His bundle. On the left, during right atrial pacing at a cycle length of 380 msec, there is an intra-His conduction delay H-H′ of 85 msec but the H′-V is normal. With an abrupt to a paced cycle length of 360 msec, the H-H′ increases to 140 msec, then block occurs between the H and H′. Delay and block is therefore intra-His.

His potentials) accompanying bundle branch block, particularly LBBB.

The frequency with which conduction disturbances in the His bundle are responsible for the fascicular and bundle branch blocks is not known. The use of multipolar catheters to record distal, mid-, and proximal His bundle potentials or proximal right bundle and proximal His bundle potentials are of great use in delineating how frequently very proximal lesions result in a particular bundle branch block. It is theoretically appealing to postulate that such longitudinal dissociation in the His bundle causes the conduction abnormalities that ultimately result in complete A-V block in either the setting of acute anteroseptal infarction or sclerodegenerative diseases of the conducting system. The sudden simultaneous failure of conduction through all peripheral fascicles would appear much less likely than failure at a proximal site in the His bundle or at the truncal bifurcation. An example supporting this concept is shown in Figure 5-4, in which atrial pacing in a patient with LBBB and split His potentials produces progressive prolongation of conduction and ultimate block between the two His potentials, that is, in the His bundle.

The site of transient bundle branch block may differ from that of chronic or permanent bundle branch block. Studies in the clinical electrophysiology laboratory in which distal His bundle or proximal RBB recordings are used along with right and left ventricular endocardial mapping and/or intraoperative studies have both proved useful in better defining the sites of block in patients with either chronic or transient bundle branch block (i.e., aberration). Because the likelihood of developing complete A-V block may depend on the site of conduction or block in individual fascicles, obtaining such data is critical to predicting risk of A-V block. Failure to do so may explain variability of published data in predicting progression of bifascicular block to complete A-V block. (See section on predicting risk of heart block.) Results of activation studies during bundle branch block are described in the following paragraphs.

## Chronic Right Bundle Branch Block

Intraoperative studies have clearly shown that the electrocardiographic pattern of RBBB can result from lesions at different levels of the conducting system in the right ventricle.[11,12] These studies were performed during operative procedures for congenital heart disease, the most common of which was repair of tetralogy of Fallot. Endocardial mapping was performed from the His bundle along the length of the RBB, including the base of the moderator band, where it separated into the septal divisions, the anterior free wall, and the outflow tract. Epicardial mapping was also performed. The use of both endocardial and epicardial mapping clearly demonstrated three potential levels of block in the right ventricular conduction system that could lead to the electrocardiographic pattern of RBBB: (a) Proximal RBBB, (b) distal RBBB at the level of the moderator band, and (c) terminal RBBB involving the distal conducting system of the RBB or, more likely, the muscle itself.[12]

Proximal RBBB was the most common form noted after transatrial repair of tetralogy of Fallot,[11,12] and similar studies in adults suggest it is also the most common spontaneously occurring type of chronic RBBB.[13–15] In proximal RBBB, loss of the right bundle potential occurs where it is typically recorded (Fig. 5-5). Activation at these right ventricular septal sites is via transseptal spread from the left ventricle. This results in

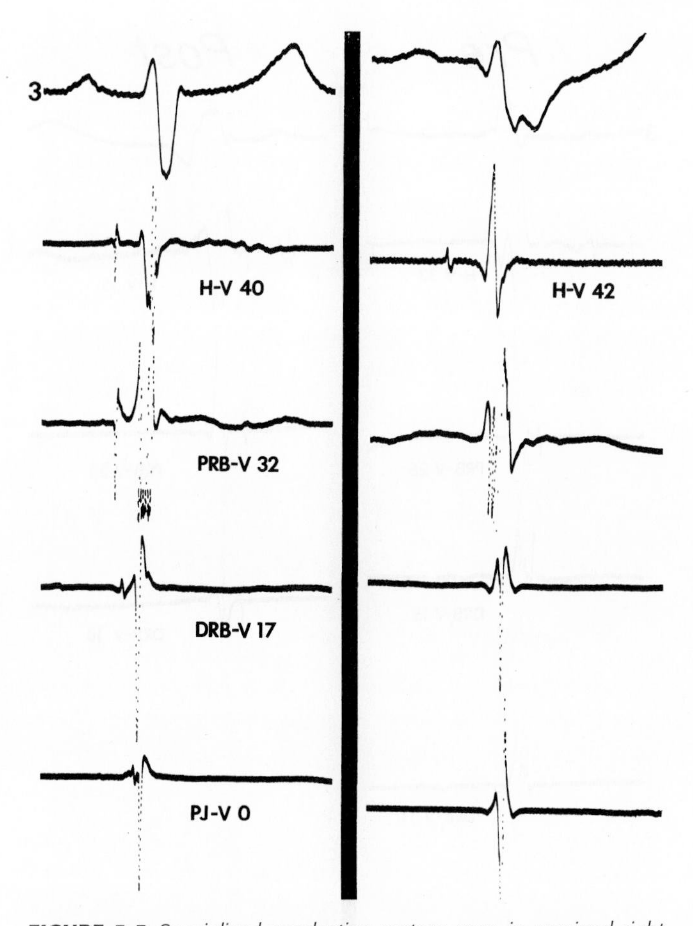


**FIGURE 5-5** *Specialized conduction system map in proximal right bundle branch block (RBBB).* ECG lead 3 is shown with electrograms recorded from the distal His bundle (H), proximal right bundle branch (PRB), distal right bundle branch (DRB), and anterior wall Purkinje fiber (PJ). Intervals (in milliseconds) measured from the conduction system electrograms to the onset of ventricular activation are shown. Before repair, sequential electrograms were recorded along the length of the right bundle branch. The ventricular septal electrograms recorded at each site occur early in the QRS complex. After repair, RBBB is present. A distal His bundle potential was recorded, but no other electrograms of the specialized conduction system could be recorded. The septal electrograms in the mid-RV and apical areas (PRB, DRB) are recorded later in the QRS. (From Horowitz LN, Alexander JA, Edmunds LH Jr. Postoperative right bundle branch block: identification of three levels of block. *Circulation* 1980;62:319.)

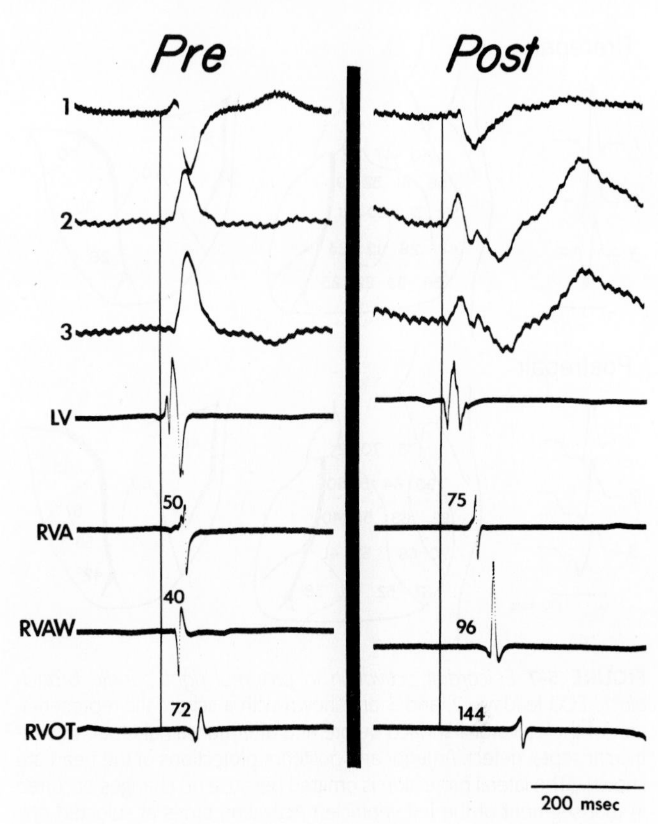


**FIGURE 5-6** *Selected epicardial electrograms in proximal right bundle branch block.* ECG leads 1, 2, and 3 are shown with a reference electrogram recorded in the left ventricle (LV) and mapping electrograms recorded at the right ventricular apex (RVA), right ventricular anterior wall (RVAW), and right ventricular outflow tract (RVOT) before and after transatrial repair of tetralogy of Fallot. The vertical lines indicate the onset of the QRS, and the numbers indicate time (in milliseconds) from the vertical line to the local electrogram. Before repair, the RVAW was the earliest site in the right ventricle. After repair, the earliest right ventricular site was the apex, which was activated 25 msec later than before repair. The latest ventricular epicardial activation occurred on the RVOT at 144 msec (cf. Fig. 5-7). (From Horowitz LN, Alexander JA, Edmunds LH Jr. Postoperative right bundle branch block: identification of three levels of block. *Circulation* 1980;62:319.)

delayed activation of the mid- and apical right ventricular septum, the right ventricular anterior wall at the insertion of the moderator band, and the right ventricular outflow tract (RVOT) (Fig. 5-6). Epicardial mapping in patients preoperatively and postoperatively shows a change from the normal right ventricular breakthrough at the midanterior wall with concentric spread thereafter, to a pattern showing no distinct right ventricular breakthrough but right ventricular activation occurs via transseptal spread following left ventricular activation. In Figure 5-7, this transseptal spread begins at the apex and then sequentially activates the midanterior wall and base of the heart. Left ventricular activation remains normal. In cases of proximal RBBB, the mid- and apical septa are activated at least 30 msec after the onset of the QRS.

In distal RBBB, activation of the His bundle and proximal RBB is normal. RBB potentials persist at the base of the moderator band and are absent at the midanterior wall, where the moderator band normally inserts (Fig. 5-8). This form of bundle branch block only occurred when the moderator band was cut during surgery. Thus, this form of RBBB is extremely rare as a spontaneous form of bundle branch block. In distal RBBB, the apical and midsepta are normally activated, but activation of the free wall at the level of the moderator band and subsequent activation of the RVOT is delayed (Figs. 5-9 and 5-10). Epicardial activation shows a small area of apical right ventricular activation that is the same as preoperatively. Activation at the midanterior wall, which was the site of epicardial breakthrough in the right ventricle preoperatively, was delayed, as was subsequent activation of the remaining right ventricle (Fig. 5-10).

Terminal RBBB was the second most common form of RBBB observed following either transatrial or transventricular

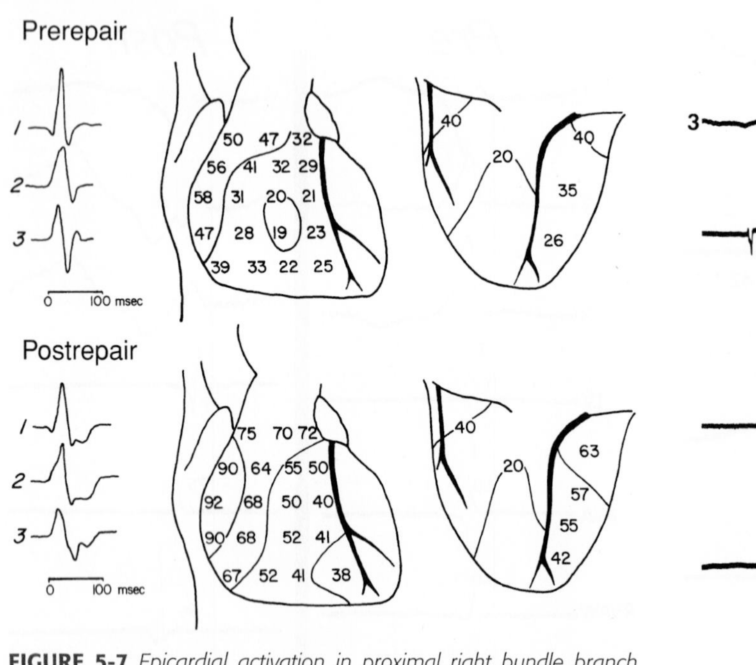


**FIGURE 5-7** *Epicardial activation in proximal right bundle branch block.* ECG leads 1, 2, and 3 are shown with a schematic representation of the epicardial surface before and after transatrial repair of ventricular septal defect. Anterior and posterior projections of the heart are shown. (The lateral projection is omitted because no changes occurred in that segment of the left ventricle.) Activation times at selected epicardial sites are shown with 20 msec, and the right ventricular activation pattern was normal. After repair, the QRS duration was 92 msec, and activation at all right ventricular sites was delayed. Right ventricular activation began along the anterior interventricular groove and spread radially to the base. (From Horowitz LN, Alexander JA, Edmunds LH Jr. Postoperative right bundle branch block: identification of three levels of block. *Circulation* 1980;62:319.)

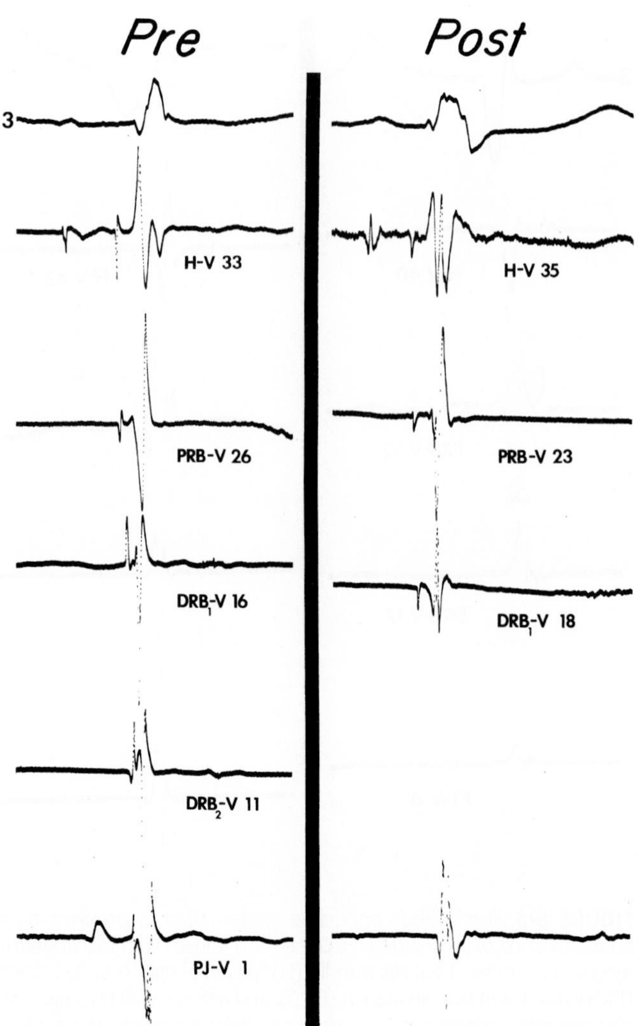


**FIGURE 5-8** *Specialized conduction system map in distal right bundle branch block.* ECG lead 3 is shown with electrograms recorded from the distal His bundle (H), proximal right bundle branch (PRB), two sites in the distal right bundle branch at the septal base of the moderator band (DRB1) and at the midportion of the moderator band (DRB2), and an anterior wall Purkinje fiber (PJ). Intervals (in milliseconds) measured from the conduction system electrograms to the onset of ventricular activation are shown. Sequential recordings along the course of the right bundle branch were obtained before the repair. After sectioning of the moderator band, conduction system recordings were obtained from PRB and DRB1. Electrograms recorded beyond this level showed no specialized conduction system potentials. The DRB2 electrogram recorded after repair is not shown because that area was resected. (From Horowitz LN, Alexander JA, Edmunds LH Jr. Postoperative right bundle branch block: identification of three levels of block. *Circulation* 1980;62:319.)

repair of tetralogy of Fallot. Activation along the specialized conducting system (i.e., His bundle branch and RBB) remains normal up to the Purkinje–myocardial junction (Fig. 5-11). In contrast to proximal and distal RBBB, activation of the midanterior wall is unchanged from normal, and only the RVOT shows delayed activation. Epicardial mapping demonstrates slowly inscribed isochrones from the infundibulum to the base of the heart (Figs. 5-12 and 5-13). Of note, terminal RBBB, which is probably due to interruption of the terminal Purkinje network and/or intramyocardial delay can have two quantitatively similar but qualitatively different patterns.[12]

During terminal bundle branch block produced by ventriculotomy, the latest activation is adjacent to the ventriculotomy scar. In contrast, when terminal bundle branch block is produced by transatrial resection, then the delayed activation appears as a smooth homogenous slow spread from the anterior infundibulum to the posterobasal aspects of the outflow tract. These data help resolve previously reported experimental work and clinical studies by a variety of authors.[16–21] Our findings were similar to those of Wyndham,[13] Wyndham et al.,[14] and Van Dam.[15]

Clinically, these findings[11–15] are relevant because terminal or distal bundle branch block, when accompanied by disorders of left ventricular conduction, may not indicate an increased risk of heart block. Such distal or terminal block has been seen in atrial septal defect, where conduction in the RBB is normal but stretching of terminal Purkinje fibers and/or muscle causes delayed activation of the RVOT.[19] I have also seen terminal bundle branch block in patients with cardiomyopathy and chronic lung disease. Finally, I have also seen this pattern in rare patients with right ventricular infarction associated with the development of an RBBB pattern. In this latter case the duration of the QRS does not exceed 120 msec. In my

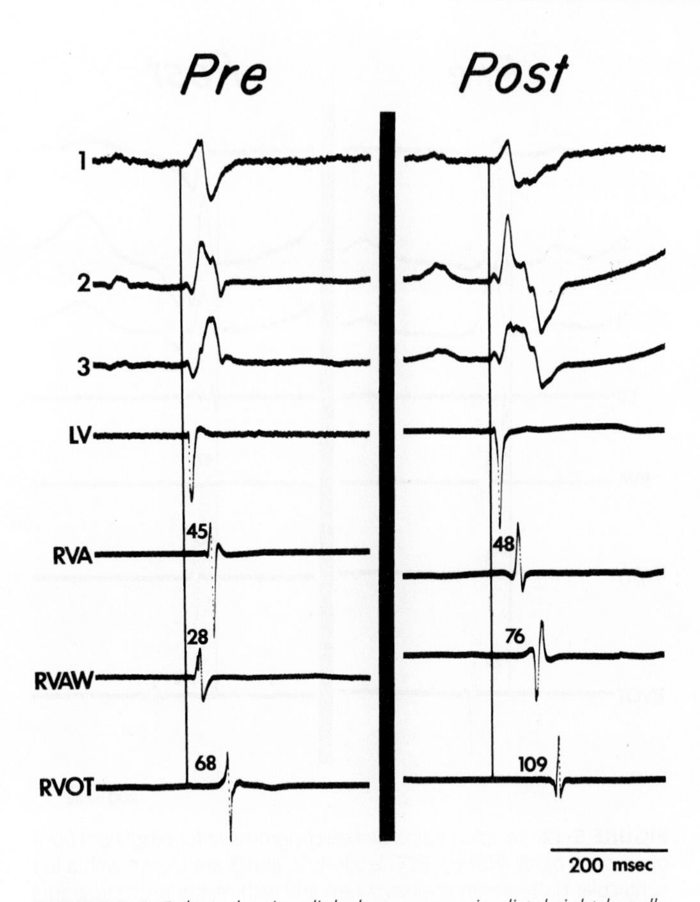


**FIGURE 5-9** *Selected epicardial electrograms in distal right bundle branch block.* ECG leads 1, 2, and 3 are shown with a reference electrogram recorded in the left ventricle (LV) and mapping electrograms recorded at the right ventricular apex (RVA), right ventricular anterior wall (RVAW), and right ventricle outflow tract (RVOT) before and after transatrial repair of tetralogy of Fallot. The vertical lines indicate the onset of the QRS, and numbers indicate time (in milliseconds) from the vertical line to the local electrograms. Before repair, the RVAW was the earliest right ventricular site. After repair, right bundle branch block (RBBB) was present, and the earliest activation was at the RVA. Despite the presence of RBBB, the RVA activation time after repair did not significantly differ from the value before repair. Activation of the RVAW and RVOT were delayed (cf. Fig. 5-10). (From Horowitz LN, Alexander JA, Edmunds LH Jr. Postoperative right bundle branch block: identification of three levels of block. *Circulation* 1980;62:319.)

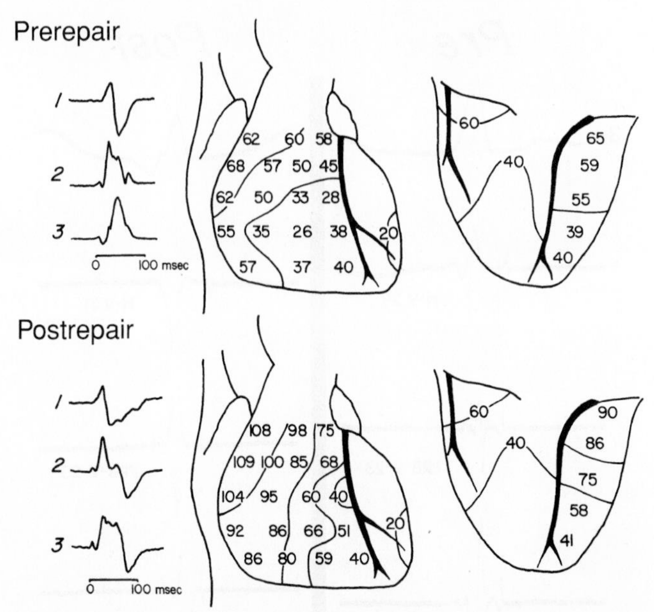


**FIGURE 5-10** *Epicardial activation in distal right branch block.* ECG leads 1, 2, and 3 are shown with a schematic representation of the epicardial surface before and after transatrial repair of tetralogy of Fallot. Anterior and posterior projections of the heart are shown. Activation times at selected epicardial sites are shown with 20-msec isochrones. Before repair, the right ventricular activation pattern was normal. After repair, the QRS duration increased and a terminal slurred S wave appeared. The earliest right ventricular activation occurred at the right ventricular apex and along the midanterior interventricular groove. Right ventricular apical activation times before and after repair were similar. Activation of the remainder of the right ventricle was delayed; left ventricular activation did not change. (From Horowitz LN, Alexander JA, Edmunds LH Jr. Postoperative right bundle branch block: identification of three levels of block. *Circulation* 1980;62:319.)

opinion, these data favor a delay in intramyocardial conduction as the primary cause of terminal conduction delay. Determination of either proximal or terminal bundle branch block can easily be made in the clinical electrophysiology laboratory by demonstrating normal activation time of the mid- and apical septa in the presence of RBBB. If RBBB is proximal, activation of the mid- and apical septa will be delayed, producing a V (onset of the QRS) to local RV activation time exceeding 30 msec.[22,23] If the RBBB is the rare distal type or, more commonly, the terminal RBBB, the local activation time at the mid- and apical septa will be normal (i.e., <30 msec), whereas that of the anterior wall (in the case of distal RBBB) and/or the outflow tract (either distal or terminal RBBB) will be delayed. Electroanatomic mapping allows one to display right and/or left ventricular activation during bundle branch block. An example of RBBB due to proximal RBBB and passive RV activation by transseptal spread from the left ventricle is shown in Figure 5-14.

## Left Bundle Branch Block

Far fewer data are available to evaluate the site of conduction abnormalities in LBBB. No human studies have traced conduction from the His bundle down the left bundle system, as done in RBBB.[11,12] Epicardial mapping data in a few patients with LBBB[13–15] demonstrate (a) that right ventricular activation is normal but occurs relatively earlier in the QRS; (b) that a discrete left ventricular breakthrough site is absent, in contrast to normal, in which two or three breakthrough sites may be observed; (c) that transseptal conduction is slow, as manifested by crowded isochrones in the interventricular sulcus with more rapid isochrones along the left ventricular free wall. In LBBB with normal axis, Wyndham[13] found that the latest left ventricular site activated was not the A-V sulcus, as it is with normal intraventricular conduction. These studies, however, not only were limited by the small number of patients but by the fact that the authors did not consider myocardial disease and did not adequately address the effect of axis deviation.

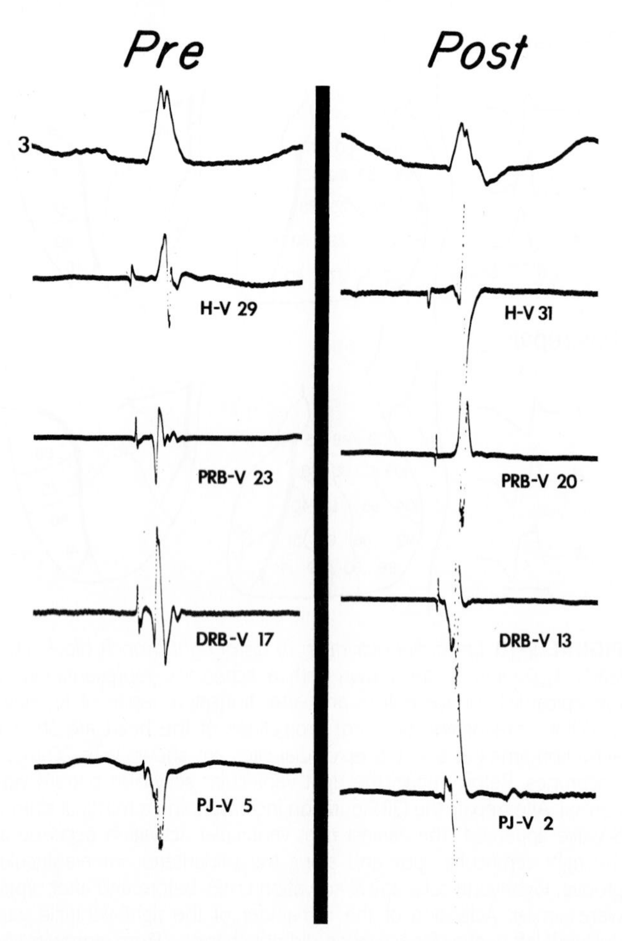


**FIGURE 5-11** *Specialized conduction system map in terminal right bundle branch block.* ECG lead 3 is shown with electrograms recorded from the distal His bundle (H), proximal right bundle branch (PRB), distal right bundle branch (DRB), and anterior wall Purkinje fiber (PJ) before and after transatrial repair of tetralogy of Fallot. Intervals (in milliseconds) measured from the conduction system electrograms to the onset of ventricular activation are shown. Sequential electrograms were recorded along the length of the right bundle branch before and after repair despite the presence of right bundle branch block after repair. (From Horowitz LN, Alexander JA, Edmunds LH Jr. Postoperative right bundle branch block: identification of three levels of block. *Circulation* 1980;62:319.)

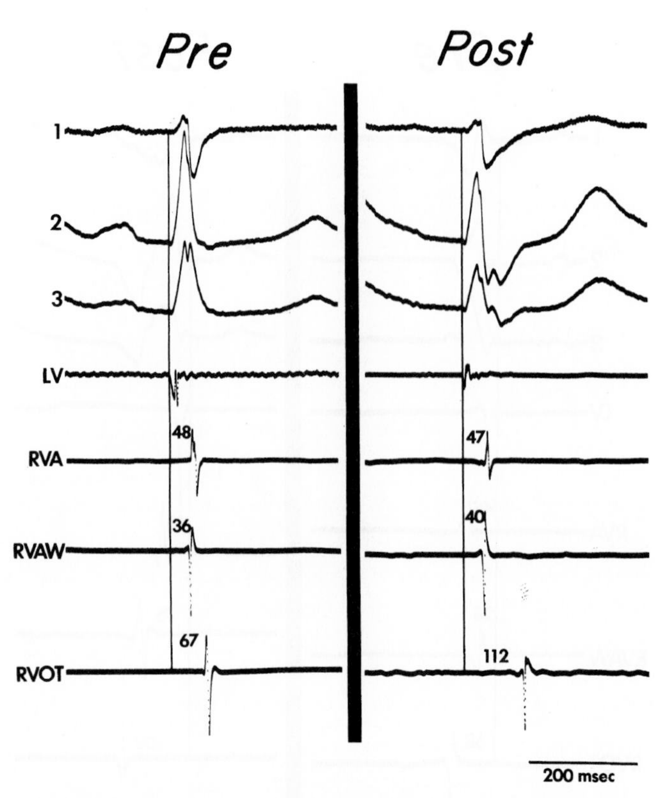


**FIGURE 5-12** *Selected epicardial electrograms in terminal right bundle branch block (RBBB).* ECG leads 1, 2, and 3 are shown with a left ventricular (LV) reference electrogram and with mapping electrograms recorded at the right ventricular apex (RVA), right ventricular anterior wall (RVAW), and right ventricular outflow tract (RVOT) before and after transatrial repair of tetralogy of Fallot. The vertical lines indicate the beginning of the QRS, and the numbers indicate time (in milliseconds) from the vertical line to the local electrograms. Before repair, right ventricular activation was earliest in the RVAW and latest in the RVOT, 67 msec after the onset of the QRS. After repair, RBBB was present and RVAW and RVA activation were not changed, but activation of the RVOT was delayed 45 msec (cf. Fig. 5-13). (From Horowitz LN, Alexander JA, Edmunds LH Jr. Postoperative right bundle branch block: identification of three levels of block. *Circulation* 1980;62:319.)

Furthermore, the extent to which intramural conduction delay contributed to QRS widening has never been assessed.

We therefore decided to evaluate endocardial activation during LBBB in a heterogenous group of patients, including four with no organic heart disease, six with congestive cardiomyopathy, and eight with coronary artery disease and previous infarction.[24] All but one patient had a QRS >140 msec. Only three patients had normal H-V times. Unfortunately, we did not record right bundle potentials or distal His potentials to localize the source of H-V prolongation (see the following discussion).

We performed catheter mapping studies, as described in Chapter 2. We recorded standard activation sites (Fig. 5-15) in the right and left ventricle in sinus rhythm with fixed and variable-gain electrograms using both a 1-cm and 5-mm interelectrode bipolar recording. There was no difference in activation times between them. We therefore defined local activation as the point on the 1-cm variable-gain electrogram at which the largest rapid deflection crossed the baseline. When a fractionated electrogram was present without a surface discrete deflection >1 mV in amplitude, we used the rapid deflection of highest amplitude as local activation time. In addition, we measured the onset and offset of local activation from the fixed-gain electrogram from the time the electrical signal reached 0.1 mV from baseline to the time of the amplifier decay signal (see Fig. 2-11). We defined transseptal conduction time as the difference between local activation time at the right ventricular septum (usually near the apex) and the earliest left ventricular activation time. We also evaluated the total left ventricular activation time, which was the difference in time from the earliest to the latest left ventricular endocardial activation. The average number of left ventricular sites mapped was 14 ± 3 per patient (range, 8 to 19). There was

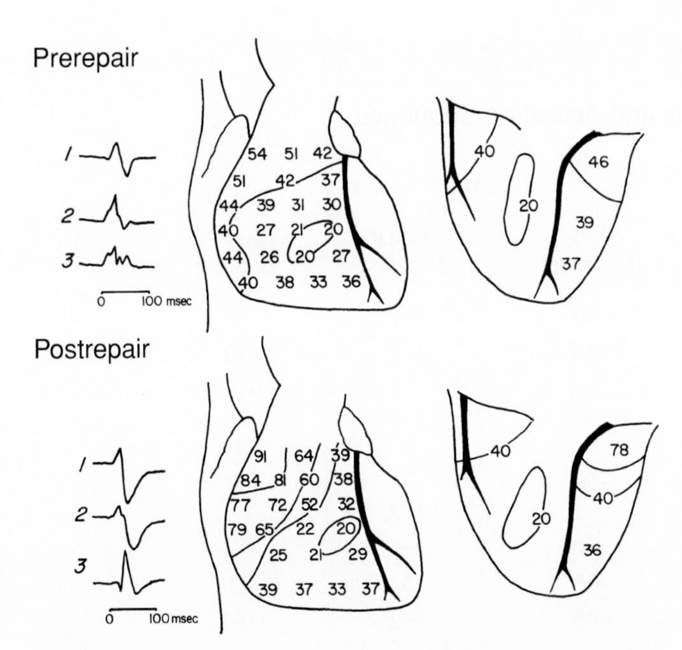


**FIGURE 5-13** *Epicardial activation in terminal right bundle branch block.* ECG leads 1, 2, and 3 are shown with a schematic representation of the epicardial surface before and after transatrial repair of tetralogy of Fallot. Anterior and posterior projections of the heart are shown. Activation times at selected epicardial sites are shown with 20-msec isochrones. Before repair, the right ventricular activation pattern was normal. After repair, right bundle branch block appeared, and outflow tract activation was delayed. Activation of the right ventricular anterior wall with a normal epicardial breakthrough site was unchanged after repair. (From Horowitz LN, Alexander JA, Edmunds LH Jr. Postoperative right bundle branch block: identification of three levels of block. *Circulation* 1980;62:319.)

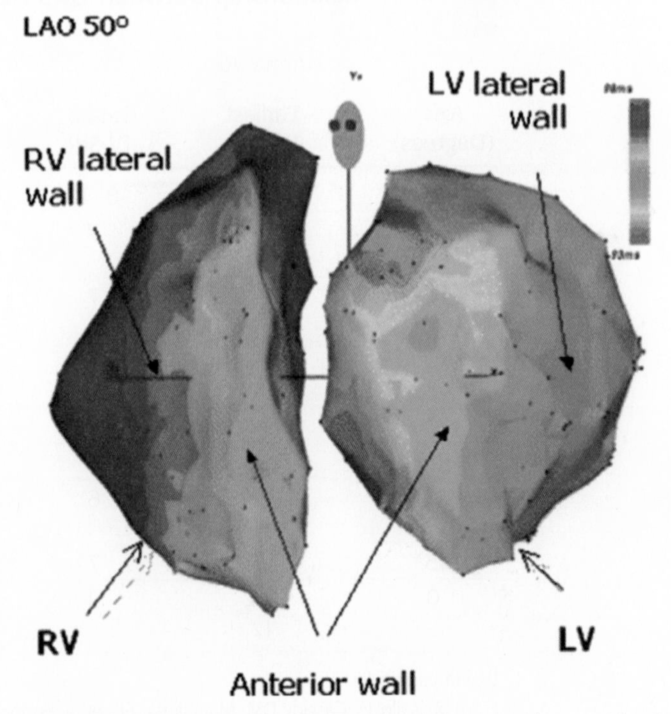


**FIGURE 5-14** *Electroanatomic mapping during complete, proximal RBBB.* The activation sequence of the RV and LV during RBBB is displayed with 10-msec colored isochrones (red early to blue/purple, late; see color bar). The LV is activated earliest with early breakthroughs on the anterior wall, septum, and inferior wall (not seen). Activation spreads transseptally to activate the RV sequentially.

no difference in a number of sites mapped among any of the three groups.

Twelve of 18 patients had only one site of a left ventricular endocardial breakthrough. In nine patients, this was in the middle third of the left ventricular septum, and in three patients, it was at the apical third of the septum. In the remaining six patients, we observed simultaneous early activation at two left ventricular sites; in two patients, two sites were on the septum (one in the middle third and one at the apical septum), and in one, the apical septum and superior basal free wall. In contrast to the studies of Wyndham,[13] we found that the latest site of left ventricular activation was frequently at the base of the heart in patients with normal axis, while it was more variable in those with left axis (Table 5-1).[24]

Left ventricular endocardial activation began a mean of 52 ± 17 msec after the onset of the surface QRS (Table 5-2). We observed no difference in any of the three groups. In the normal patients, left ventricular activation began 44 ± 13 msec after the QRS, in patients with cardiomyopathy, left activation began 58 ± 13 msec after the onset of the QRS, and in the patients with prior infarction, left ventricular septal activation began at 51 ± 20 msec after the QRS.

The earliest activity in local anteroseptal sites was similar in the normal and cardiomyopathic groups, at 23 ± 9 and 23 ± 19 msec. However, earliest activation recorded in the septum in

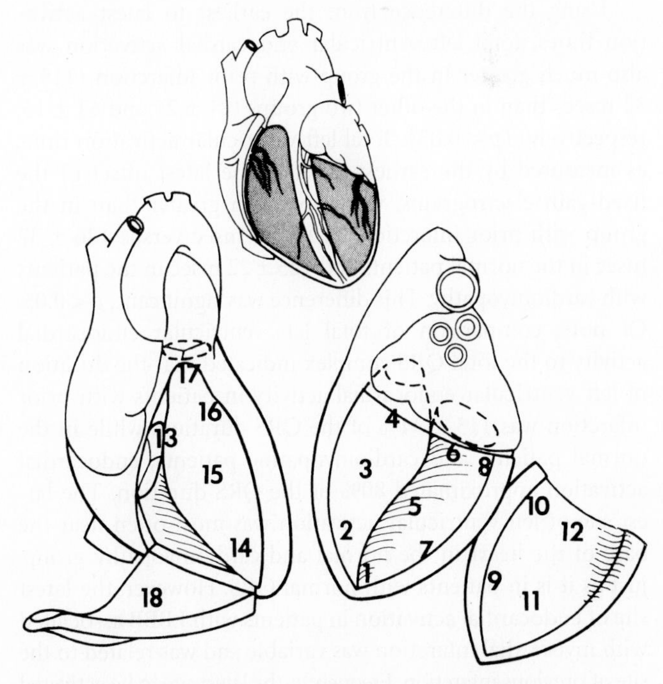


**FIGURE 5-15** *Schema of mapping sites in the right and left ventricles.* (From Josephson ME, Horowitz LN, Spielman SR, et al. Role of catheter mapping in the preoperative evaluation of ventricular tachycardia. *Am J Cardiol* 1982;49:207.)

TABLE 5-1 Relationship between QRS Axis and Activation Sequence

| Normal Axis | | | Left-Axis Deviation | | |
|---|---|---|---|---|---|
| Axis (Degrees) | Earliest LV Site | Latest LV Site | Axis (Degrees) | Earliest LV Site | Latest LV Site |
| +45 | 2–3 | 8–10 | −40 | 1–2 | 7 |
| +45 | 2–3<br>12 | 7 | −40 | 1–2 | 10 |
| +10 | 2<br>12 | 7 | −40 | 3–5 | 8 |
| −10 | 2–3 | 10 | −50 | 3<br>1–2 | 8 |
| +20 | 2–3 | 8 | −60 | 3–5 | 12 |
| +45 | 2–3 | 6 | −45 | 3 | 11 |
| +50 | 3<br>1–2 | 6 | −45 | 1–2 | 11–12 |
| +45 | 3 | 7 | −45 | 2–3 | 8 |
| 0 | 1–2<br>12 | 8 | −50 | 2–3<br>12 | 1 |

LV, left ventricular.
From Vassallo JA, Cassidy DM, Marchlinski FE, et al. Endocardial activation of left bundle branch block. *Circulation* 1984;69:914.

patients with prior anteroseptal infarction was only 11 ± 11 msec and was significantly shorter than that reported in the other groups ($p < 0.05$).

Using the difference from the earliest to latest activation times, total left ventricular endocardial activation was also much greater in the group with prior infarction (119 ± 32 msec) than in the other two groups (81 ± 26 and 61 ± 15, respectively) ($p < 0.05$). Total left ventricular activation time, as measured by the earliest onset to the latest offset of the fixed-gain electrograms, was also much greater than in the group with prior infarction: 219 ± 77 msec versus 126 ± 37 msec in the normal patients and 125 ± 22 msec in the patients with cardiomyopathy. This difference was significant, $p < 0.05$. Of note, comparison of total left ventricular endocardial activity to the total QRS complex indicated that the duration of left ventricular endocardial activity in patients with prior infarction was 113 ± 34% of the QRS duration, while in the normal patients and cardiomyopathic patients, endocardial activation approximated 80% of the QRS duration. The latest site of left ventricular activation was most often near the base of the heart in the normal and cardiomyopathy group, just as it is in patients with normal QRS. However, the latest site of endocardial activation in patients with LBBB associated with myocardial infarction was variable and was related to the site of previous infarction. Frequently, the latest site to be activated was within the site of prior infarction.

The interval between local activation at the right ventricular apex and the earliest rapid deflection noted in the left ventricle (i.e., transseptal activation) was similar in our groups of patients and averaged 33 msec. However, if one measured the interval between local activation at the right ventricular apex and the rapid deflection at the corresponding left ventricular site (site 2), it was longer, averaging 46 ± 50 msec; we noted no differences in any of the three groups. As noted earlier, when we used the fixed high-gain recording for earliest activation, the patients with prior anteroseptal infarction had the earliest activation recorded from onset of the QRS to the high-gain septal recording. We believe that this represents activation within the septum, which is thinner, and probably represents the right and medial part of the intraventricular septum. Patients with cardiomyopathy and normal hearts have thicker septa and therefore do not record right and intramural septal recordings from the endocardial surface of the left ventricle.

We performed right ventricular endocardial mapping in seven patients with LBBB.[24] One patient had a normal heart, three had cardiomyopathy, and three had prior infarctions. We mapped an average of six right ventricular sites. Right ventricular endocardial breakthrough occurred 8 ± 9 msec after the onset of the QRS and was usually at the midseptum. This corresponded with the initial 5% of the QRS complex. Activation then spread concentrically to the midanterior wall and the remainder of the septum, with latest activation at the RVOT. Total right ventricular endocardial activation using the beginning of the first to the last rapid deflection was completed in 36 ± 13 msec, which corresponded to the first 21 ± 7% of the surface QRS complex. We noted no difference in

TABLE 5-2 Results of Left Ventricular Mapping

| Patient Activation No. | Total LV QRS (msec) | LV Endocardial Breakthrough (msec) | Latest Endocardial Sites (msec) | Total LV Activation (msec) | Total LV Activation (% QRS) |
|---|---|---|---|---|---|
| Group 1 | | | | | |
| 1 | 160 | 26 | 105 | 79 | 49 |
| 2 | 160 | 58 | 115 | 57 | 36 |
| 3 | 150 | 52 | 170 | 118 | 77 |
| 4 | 155 | 38 | 108 | 70 | 45 |
| Group II | | | | | |
| 5 | 155 | 64 | 126 | 62 | 40 |
| 6 | 160 | 78 | 130 | 52 | 33 |
| 7 | 160 | 52 | 92 | 40 | 25 |
| 8 | 165 | 55 | 138 | 83 | 50 |
| 9 | 175 | 60 | 122 | 62 | 35 |
| 10 | 130 | 40 | 108 | 68 | 52 |
| Group III | | | | | |
| 11 | 185 | 32 | 160 | 128 | 69 |
| 12 | 200 | 53 | 196 | 143 | 72 |
| 13 | 190 | 70 | 15 | 80 | 42 |
| 14 | 180 | 28 | 152 | 124 | 69 |
| 15 | 215 | 50 | 230 | 180 | 84 |
| 16 | 195 | 89 | 183 | 94 | 48 |
| 17 | 170 | 42 | 134 | 92 | 54 |
| 18 | 195 | 45 | 158 | 113 | 58 |

LV, left ventricular.
From Vassallo JA, Cassidy DM, Marchlinski FE, et al. Endocardial activation of left bundle branch block. *Circulation* 1984;69:914.

right ventricular activation in any of the groups. When measurements were made using high-gain electrograms, earliest activity typically preceded the onset of the QRS and was at the midseptal site similar to using the rapid deflection.

Thus, although rapid delay of transseptal activation is common to all forms of LBBB, the type of heart disease markedly influences the subsequent pattern of left ventricular activation. Patients with prior and extensive infarction had the longer left ventricular activation times than those patients with no heart disease or cardiomyopathy. Of note, patients with cardiomyopathy and no heart disease had rapid left endocardial activation comparable to endocardial activation in patients with a normal QRS.

Examples of isochronic maps during LBBB in patients with normal left ventricular endocardial activation and cardiomyopathy are contrasted with that of a patient with delayed activation associated with anterior infarction in Figures 5-16 and 5-17. Analog recordings in comparable patients are shown in Figures 5-18 and 5-19. In patients with cardiomyopathy, left ventricular endocardial activation is rapid and smooth. In contrast, in patients with infarction, left ventricular endocardial activation is markedly delayed and associated with abnormal conduction, manifested by fractionated electrograms and narrowed isochrones. Higher density mapping (60 to 200 sites) using the Carto System (Biosense) has confirmed these data. Detailed mapping of LV activation has been part of the evaluation of resynchronization therapy. The area of latest activation is usually the posterolateral wall in patients with complete LBBB in the absence of infarction (Fig. 5-20), but may reside elsewhere in infarcted tissue in patients with old myocardial infarction. The fractionated electrograms and delayed activation form an arrhythmogenic substrate (see Chapters 11 and 13). Auricchio et al.[25] have described intraventricular block in the LV in LBBB of all etiologies using the EnSite system. We have not seen this using electroanatomic mapping. We believe that the multiple breakthroughs noted in many patients with LBBB (Tables 5-1 and 5-2) resulting in collision of wavefronts, as well as abnormal conduction in patients with infarction are responsible for the uniformly seen intra-LV block noted above. ESI, which really interpolates 64 noncontact activation points to produce several thousand "electrograms," may have yield artifacts in the interpolated format. Rodriguez et al.,[26] using electroanatomic mapping, confirms our data.

We believe that the heterogeneity of endocardial activation in patients with LBBB is a manifestation of the integrity of the distal specialized conducting system. Patients with

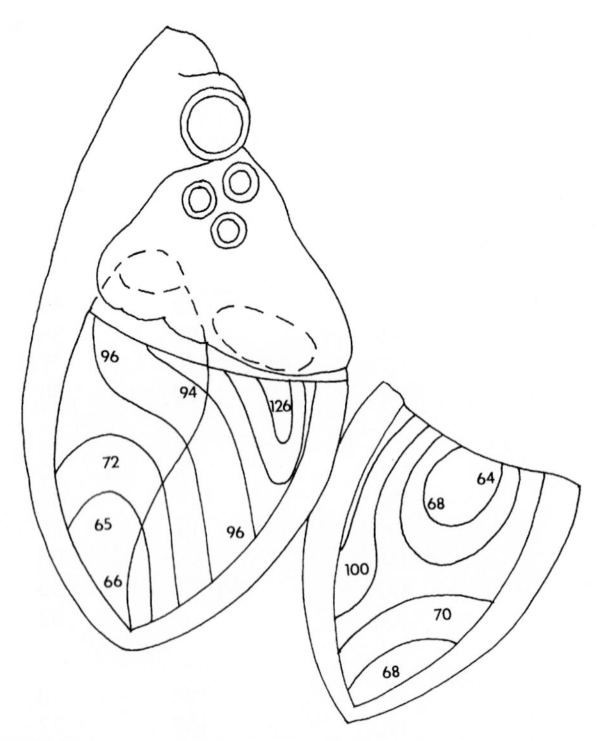


**FIGURE 5-16** *Isochronic map of left ventricular activation in a patient with a cardiomyopathy and two sites of left ventricular breakthrough.* Numbers represent local activation times, and lines represent 10-msec isochrones. Note early breakthrough at apical septum (site 2, 65 msec) and basal superior free wall (site 12, 64 msec). The isochrones are widely spaced, demonstrating a normal left ventricular endocardial activation. (From Vassallo JA, Cassidy DM, Marchlinski FE, et al. Endocardial activation of left bundle branch block. *Circulation* 1984;69:914.)

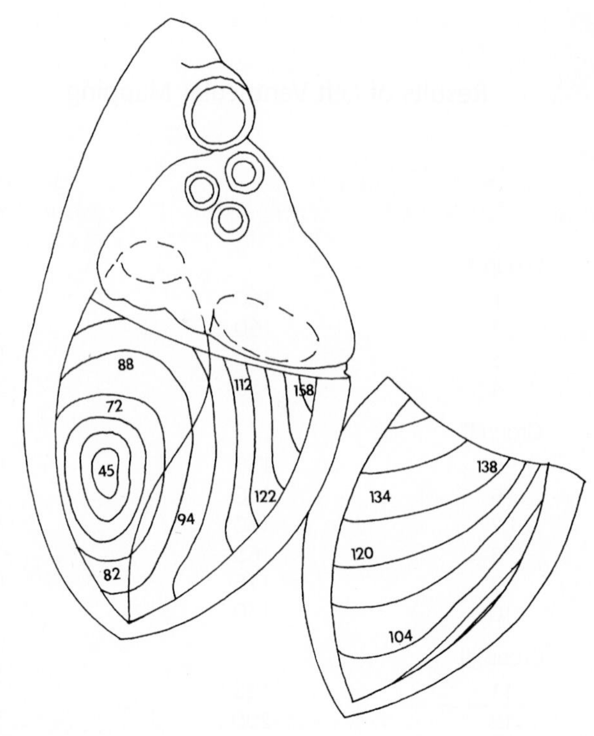


**FIGURE 5-17** *Isochronic map of left ventricular activation of a patient with coronary artery disease and one site of left ventricular breakthrough.* Numbers represent local activation times, and lines represent 10-msec isochrones. Earliest left ventricular breakthrough is at midseptum (site 3) 45 msec after the onset of the QRS. Note closely aligned isochrones and total endocardial activation, which is prolonged, ending 158 msec after the onset of the QRS. (From Vassallo JA, Cassidy DM, Marchlinski FE, et al. Endocardial activation of left bundle branch block. *Circulation* 1984;69:914.)

normal hearts and cardiomyopathies appear to have intact distal conducting system and, hence, early engagement and rapid spread through the rest of the intramural myocardium. In those patients with large anterior infarctions, the bulk of their distal specialized conducting system has been destroyed. As a consequence, their endocardial activation is via muscle-to-muscle conduction and thus is much slower. That hypothesis is strongly supported by our analysis of left ventricular endocardial maps in 40 patients during right ventricular pacing, which, we have shown, mimics LBBB.[27]

We compared patients with no heart disease, those with inferior infarction, and those with anterior infarction.[27] The data again demonstrated that left ventricular endocardial activation patterns and conduction times were markedly influenced by the site and extent of prior infarction. We always observed longer endocardial activation times in patients with large anterior infarctions. Left ventricular activation times in patients with inferior infarction were intermediate between those without heart disease and those with anterior infarction. We believe this may be due to a lower density of His–Purkinje fibers, which contribute less to activation of the basal inferior wall, which is normally activated late in the QRS. Thus, inferior infarction would have less of an effect on total endocardial activation.

Analog records and isochronic maps in a patient with no infarction and one with an anterior infarction are shown in Figures 5-21 to 5-23. They are remarkably similar to those comparable patterns recorded in spontaneous LBBB. Thus, the only common bond in patients with LBBB is a delay in transseptal activation.

The pattern in which the left ventricle is activated initially (i.e., site of breakthrough), as well as the remainder of left ventricular endocardial and transmural activation, depends critically on the nature of the underlying cardiac disease. Thus, the bizarreness of the QRS, that is, the greater QRS width, is more a reflection of left ventricular pathologic condition than of primary conduction disturbance. Our data[24,27] suggest that whenever the pattern of LBBB is present, regardless of variability of QRS patterns, a similar degree of "block" in the LBB is present in all groups of patients, at least as regards transseptal activation. This conclusion is at odds with others who suggest that left-axis deviation is required for "complete" LBBB.[28] Thus, the risks of A-V block associated with the appearance of LBBB should be similar in all groups of patients. However, the underlying cardiac disease is the major determinant of QRS width and morphology, left ventricular endocardial activation times, and overall mortality.

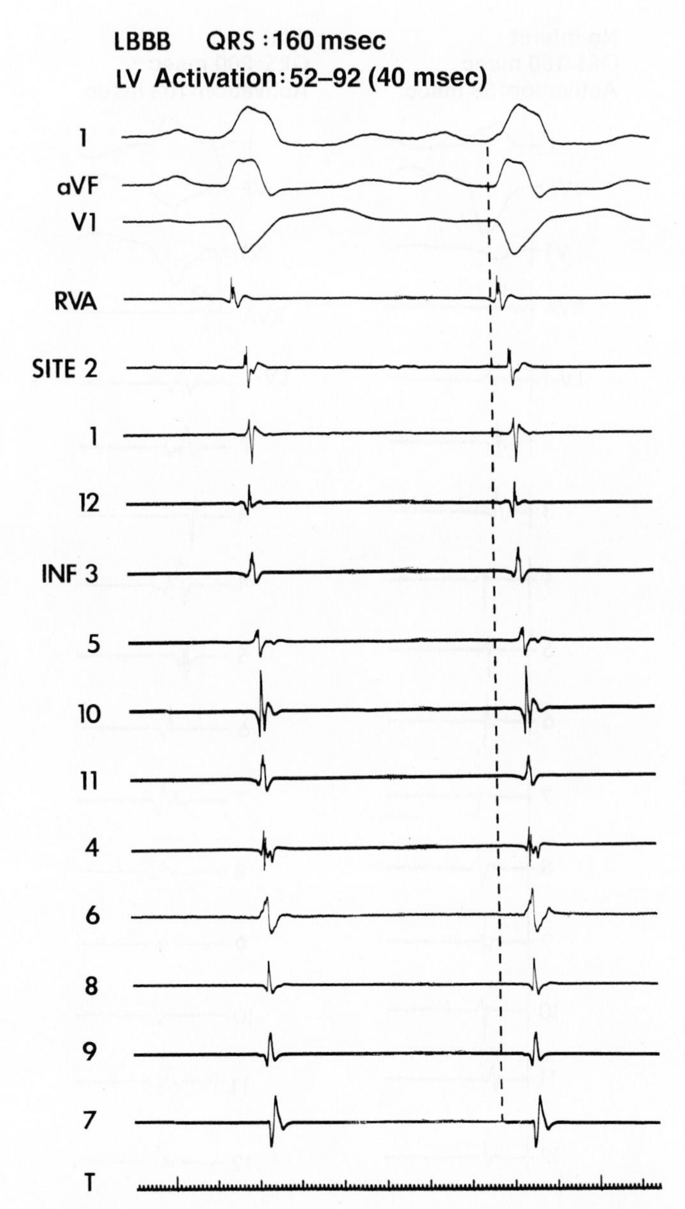


**FIGURE 5-18** *Analog map of patient with cardiomyopathy.* Surface leads 1, aVF, and V1 are displayed with local electrograms from the right ventricular apex (RVA) and designated left ventricular (LV) sites. The duration of total LV endocardial activation is 40 msec. (From Vassallo JA, Cassidy DM, Marchlinski FE, et al. Endocardial activation of left bundle branch block. *Circulation* 1984;69:914.)

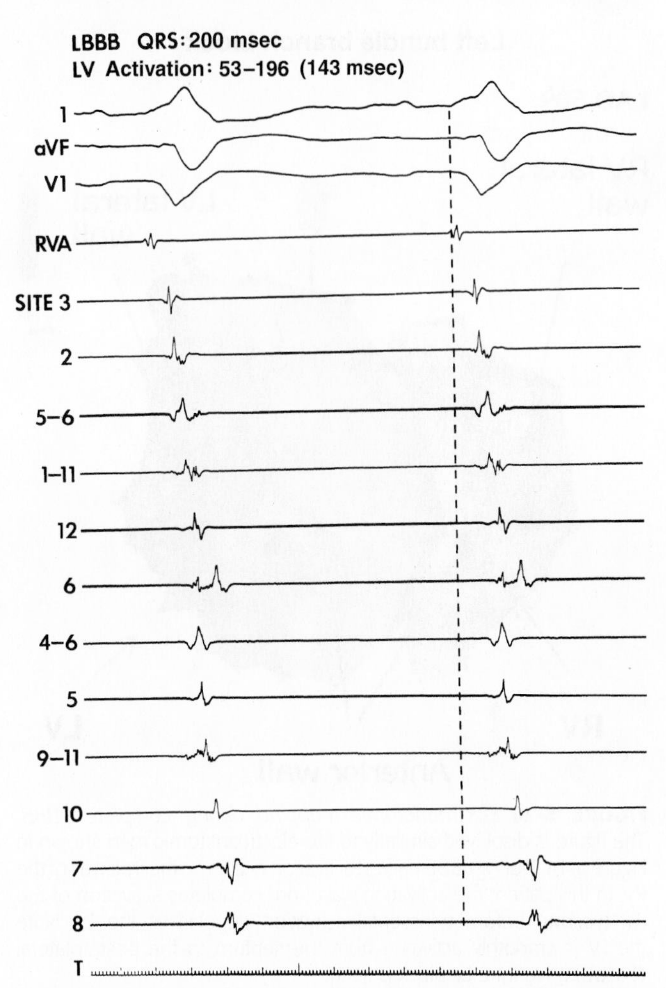


**FIGURE 5-19** *Analog map of a patient with coronary artery disease.* Surface leads 1, aVF, and V1 with local electrograms from the right ventricular apex (RVA) and designated left ventricular (LV) sites. The duration of total LV endocardial activation is 143 msec. (From Vassallo JA, Cassidy DM, Marchlinski FE, et al. Endocardial activation of left bundle branch block. *Circulation* 1984;69:914.)

## Transient Bundle Branch Block

Intermittent or transient bundle branch block (aberration) may have several mechanisms. These include (a) phase 3 block in which the initial aberrant complex is caused by encroachment on the refractory period (phase 3 of the action potential); (b) acceleration-dependent block in which at critical increasing rates (but well below the action potential duration) block occurs; (c) phase 4 or bradycardic-dependent block, which is due to a loss of resting membrane potential owing to disease and/or phase 4 depolarization; and (d) retrograde concealment in which retrograde penetration of a bundle branch renders it refractory to subsequent beats. Both acceleration-dependent and bradycardic-dependent block are manifestations of a diseased His–Purkinje system and should be thought of as abnormal. Phase 3 block, however, is physiologic.

These proposed mechanisms of aberration can occur anywhere in the specialized conducting system. Unlike chronic bundle branch block, the site of block during aberration can shift. The use of intracardiac recordings that contain proximal and distal His bundle recordings or proximal His bundle and proximal RBB recordings has been helpful in demonstrating this.[29]

Proximal RBBB has been defined by disappearance of a right bundle recording that was previously present. However, absence of a RBBB potential may represent block proximal to the right bundle potential, slow conduction proximal to the right bundle potential so that it is activated during the QRS, or such slow decremental conduction in the RBB that is not recordable as a "spike." Distal block in the RBB is said to exist when the proximal RBB recording remains present during intermittent bundle branch block.

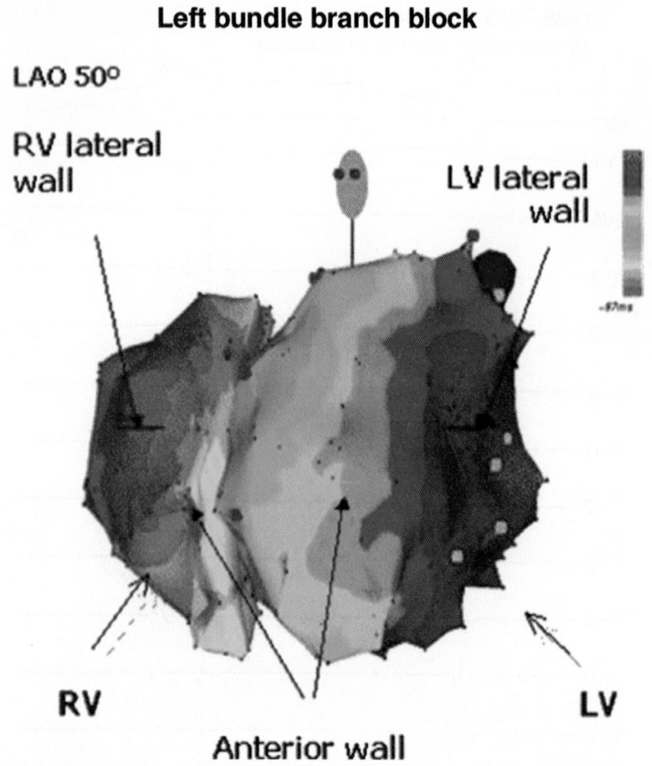

**Left bundle branch block**

LAO 50°

RV lateral wall

LV lateral wall

RV

LV

Anterior wall

**FIGURE 5-20** *Electroanatomic mapping during complete LBBB.* The figure is displayed similarly to the electroanatomic map shown in Figure 5-14. During LBBB earliest activation occurs on the free wall of the RV. In this patient the activation wavefront completes activation of the RV (*yellow*) before transseptal activation depolarizes the LV. Note the LV is smoothly activated from the septum to the posterolateral (base) LV. No intra-LV block is seen.

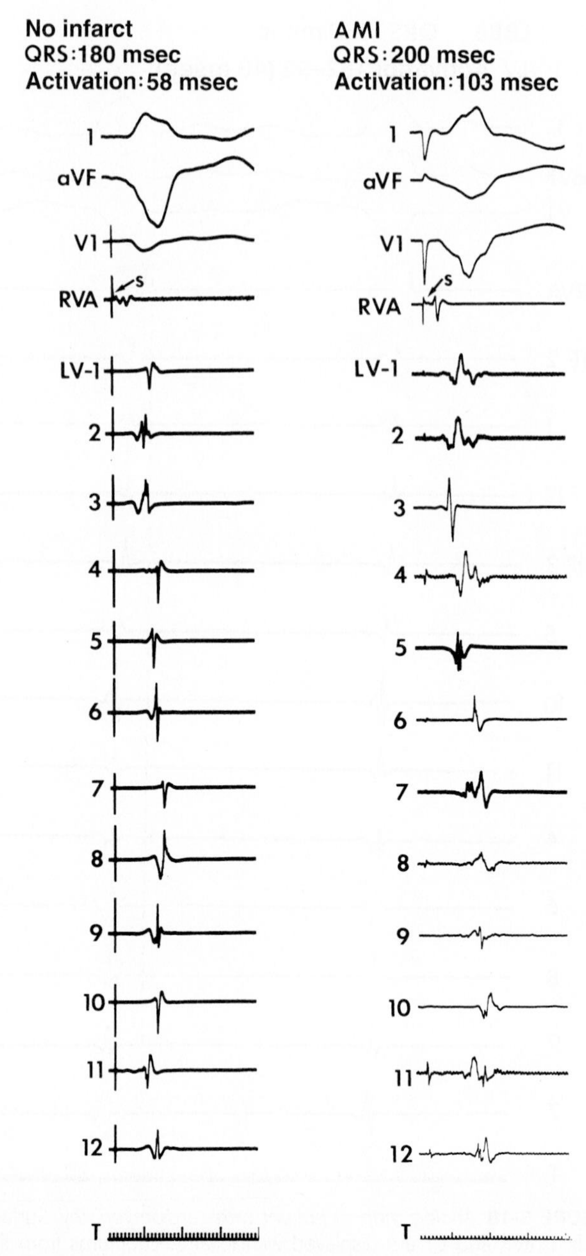


**FIGURE 5-21** *Analog map during right ventricular pacing.* Surface leads 1, aVF, and V1 are displayed with local electrograms from the right ventricular apex (RVA) and 12 designated left ventricular (LV) sites. Duration of LV endocardial activation is shorter in the group I patient without infarction (**left**) than in the group III patient with anterior myocardial infarction (AMI). (From Vassallo JA, Cassidy DM, Miller JM, et al. Left ventricular endocardial activation during right ventricular pacing: Effect of underlying heart disease. *J Am Coll Cardiol* 1986;7:1228.)

Most of the data suggest, however, that proximal block is responsible for at least the initial appearance of RBBB during phase 3 block. An observation that supports this concept is that during increasing "degrees" of RBBB in response to atrial premature stimuli, an increasing His to RBB potential is observed before the development of complete block, when absence of the right bundle recording is observed (Figs. 5-24 and 5-25).[30]

In addition to the absence of the proximal RBB potential, the time from the onset of QRS to the midseptal right ventricular recording site exceeds 30 msec, as noted previously, in chronic RBBB. Almost invariably, when right bundle block aberration occurs at long cycle lengths, the delay and block are proximal to the RBB recording. Distal delay (i.e., RBBB in the presence of a normal His to RBB potential recording) is rare but may occur at shorter cycle lengths (Fig. 5-26). Thus, there appears to be some cycle length dependency of the site of block, and shifts can occur. This is particularly so during rapid rhythms, whether paced or spontaneous, in which the initial site of block is almost always proximal with loss of a right bundle recording, but on subsequent complexes, the RBB potential may reappear, suggesting a shift from proximal to distal site of block.

Akhtar et al.[29] has clearly demonstrated a shift in the site of block during a rapid pacing producing 2:1 block below the His (Fig. 5-27). Although the initial site of block is below the His and above the recorded right bundle potential, on subsequent blocked atrial complexes, a right bundle potential reappears, suggesting that during trifascicular block the site of RBBB is distal to the right bundle recording. Persistence of RBBB during 1:1 conduction with a normal H-RB interval may be due to a shift to a distal site; however, I believe this

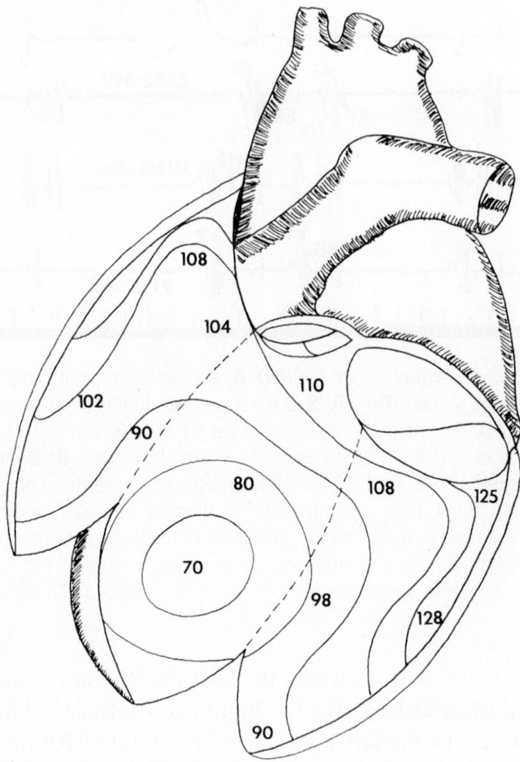


**FIGURE 5-22** *Isochronic map during right ventricular (RV) pacing in a group I patient: no infarct, QRS duration, 180 msec.* Left ventricular local activation times (in milliseconds) are indicated with 10-msec isochrones. Note one septal breakthrough site at 70 msec and complete activation in 58 msec. (From Vassallo JA, Cassidy DM, Miller JM, et al. Left ventricular endocardial activation during right ventricular pacing: effect of underlying heart disease. *J Am Coll Cardiol* 1986;7:1228.)

AMI RV PACE
QRS: 200 msec
Activation: 103 msec

168
128
142
122
100
65
128
155
85
84
140
94

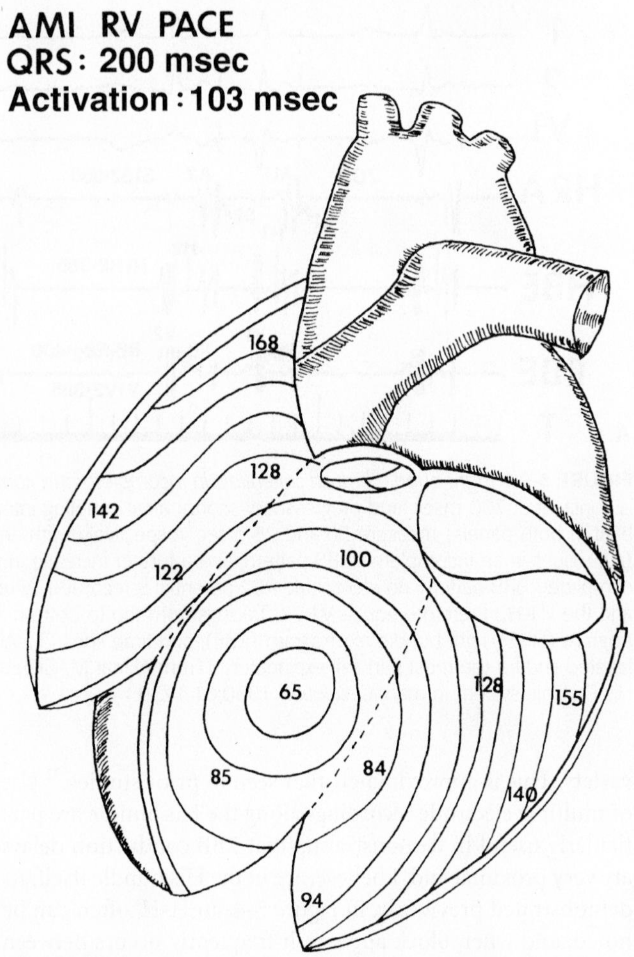

**FIGURE 5-23** *Isochronic map during right ventricular (RV) pacing in a group III patient: anterior myocardial infarction (AMI) QRS duration, 200 msec.* Local activation times are indicated with 10-msec isochrones. Note one septal breakthrough site at 65 msec and complete activation in 103 msec. (From Vassallo JA, Cassidy DM, Miller JM, et al. Left ventricular endocardial activation during right ventricular pacing: effect of underlying heart disease. *J Am Coll Cardiol* 1986;7:1228.)

more likely is due to retrograde concealed conduction with collision below the right bundle recording site (Fig. 5-27B).

The persistence of aberration at longer cycle lengths than that at which aberration was initially noted strongly favors retrograde concealment as the mechanism of persistent aberration. A shifting site of block should ultimately lead to resumption of normal conduction unless persistence of retrograde concealment is also present. Furthermore, in the presence of a shift, one would expect changing His-to-RB and RB-V intervals, because these intervals should change as the site of block changes. The sudden resumption of normal H-RB and RB-V times (Fig. 5-28) is more consistent, I believe, with retrograde concealment. The fact that ventricular premature complexes (VPCs) delivered during aberration can suddenly normalize conduction is further evidence that retrograde concealment is the responsible mechanism (see Chapter 6).[31]

Our experience is consistent with Akhtar's[29] in that the initial beat of long short-induced RBBB aberration almost always is proximal. The shift in site of block at short cycle lengths from proximal to distal may merely represent the difference in shortening of refractoriness at different levels in the RBB, which may be complicated by retrograde invasion of the right bundle following this development of RBBB. Chilson et al.[32] showed that the refractory period of the RBB shortens to a greater degree than that of the LBB system at increasing heart rates. This leads to the greater ability to demonstrate LBBB at short-drive cycle lengths and RBBB at long-drive cycle lengths. This is illustrated in Figure 5-27B where long H-H intervals precede RBBB and shorter H-H intervals are associated with LBBB. The shortening of RBB refractoriness at shorter-drive cycle lengths might also allow the impulse to penetrate distally to the proximal site of block noted at long drive cycle lengths. A graph showing this relationship is given in Figure 5-29.

Transient LBBB aberration is less common than RBBB. In our laboratory, at paced cycle lengths of 600 msec or longer, approximately 25% of phase 3 type aberration is of the LBBB

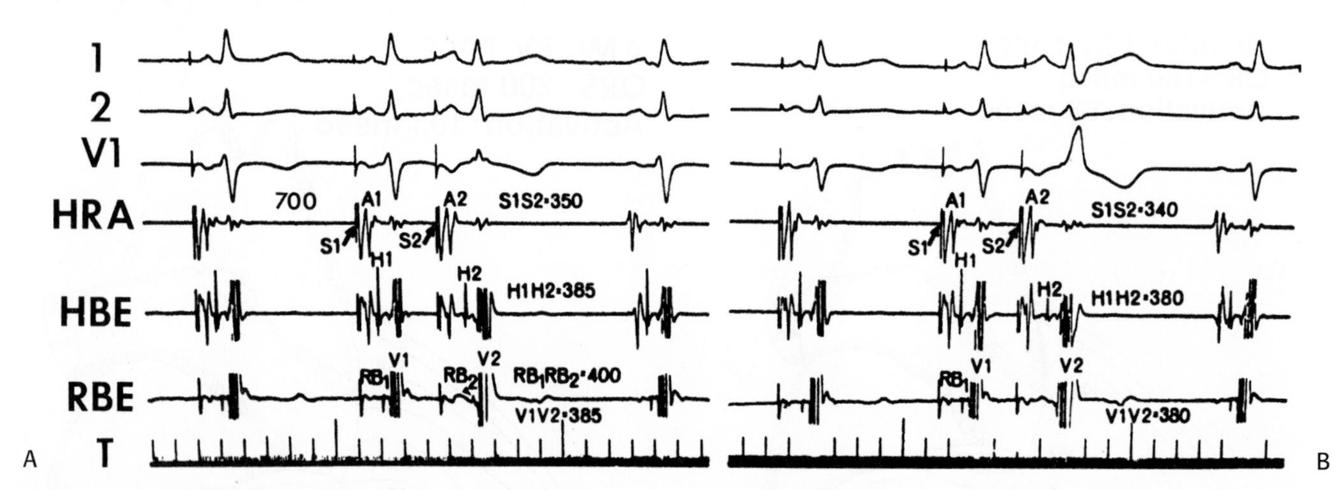


**FIGURE 5-24** *Right bundle branch potentials in incomplete and complete right bundle branch block (RBBB).* **A, B.** The basic atrial cycle length is constant at 700 msec, and progressively shorter atrial coupling intervals (A1-A2) are shown. The HV and RB-V interval during sinus beats (last beat in both panels) measure 50 and 25 msec, respectively, with an H-RB interval of 25 msec. Shortening in the S1-S2 interval to 350 msec, **(A)**, results in an incomplete RBBB pattern, and a further increase in the H2-RB2 occurs (RB1-RB2 exceeds H1-H2 by 15 msec). **B:** During the complete RBBB pattern, no identifiable RB2 potential is recorded. Although not labeled, H1-V1 and H2-V2 values measure the same in all panels, and the H1-H2 therefore equals V1-V2. Tracings from top to bottom are ECG leads I, II, V1, high-right atrial (HRA) electrogram, His bundle electrogram (HBE), right bundle electrogram (RBE), and time lines (T). All measurements are in milliseconds. Pertinent deflections and intervals are labeled and for the most part self-explanatory. (From Akhtar M, Gilbert C, Al-Nouri M, et al. Site of conduction delay during functional block in the His-Purkinje system in man. *Circulation* 1980;61:1239.)

variety. This is approximately that seen in prior studies.[32] Use of multiple electrode recordings along the His bundle are particularly useful in demonstrating that LBB conduction delays are very proximal and, I believe, are in the His bundle itself. As demonstrated previously, in Figure 5-4, an H-H' often can be noted, and when block appears, it frequently occurs between His spikes (Fig. 5-4). These data, along with prior data in chronic LBBB demonstrating normalization of the QRS by His bundle pacing, further support the His bundle origin of the conduction defect. Longitudinal dissociation in His bundle may cause individual fascicular block, which has been suggested by the observation that catheter manipulation in the His bundle region can produce left anterior hemiblock. Furthermore, if one records multiple His potentials, or even a His and proximal right bundle potential, the appearance of left anterior hemiblock in a patient with LBB is often associated with an intra-His conduction delay, or proximal His to proximal right bundle delay, as seen in Figure 5-30. In this figure, a leftward shift in axis is accompanied by H-V prolongation, which is caused by a 70-msec increment between proximal and distal His bundle recordings.

Regardless of axis deviation, the initiation of LBBB aberration by an atrial premature beat is almost always accompanied by an increase in H-V interval. In the majority (approximately 75%) of cases, multiple recordings from the His bundle or between the His and RBB show incremental delays within the His bundle or, when a RBB potential is measured, proximal to that RBB potential (Fig. 5-31).

In a smaller number of cases, the H-V interval is prolonged by 5 to 15 msec without a change in H-RB or H-RV, suggesting that the increase in H-V is due to a relative difference in ventricular activation over the LBB and RBB and is not due to conduction delay in the His bundle or contralateral bundle (Fig. 5-32). In the latter instances, the distal H-RB or distal H-RV would increase. These findings strongly suggest that the His bundle is probably longitudinally dissociated into fibers predestined to serve the right ventricle (RBB) and left ventricle (anterior and posterior fascicle). Distinguishing between the intra-His site and the truncal site just proximal to the division of the right and left bundle is impossible; however, I believe that in the majority of cases block at a very proximal site is responsible for both transient and permanent bundle branch block. In fact, when bifascicular block involving both bundle branches is observed, I believe it is only when the site of conduction delay and/or block is proximal that the risk of developing spontaneous heart block is increased. This is an important concept when one uses intracardiac recordings to predict risk of A-V conduction disturbances (see following discussion).

Bradycardia or phase 4 block almost always manifests a LBBB pattern. I have not yet seen a case of isolated bradycardia-dependent complete RBBB, although there is no particular reason why this should not occur. A possible explanation for this observation is that the left ventricular conducting system is more susceptible to ischemic damage and has a higher rate of spontaneous phase 4 depolarization than the right; therefore, it is more likely to be the site of bradycardia-dependent block. This may be one reason why some cases of bradycardia-dependent LBBB demonstrate an H-V interval no different from the normal H-V interval. That is, the His-to-RBB potential, or intra-His delay, is not the source of the conduction defect but that delay in

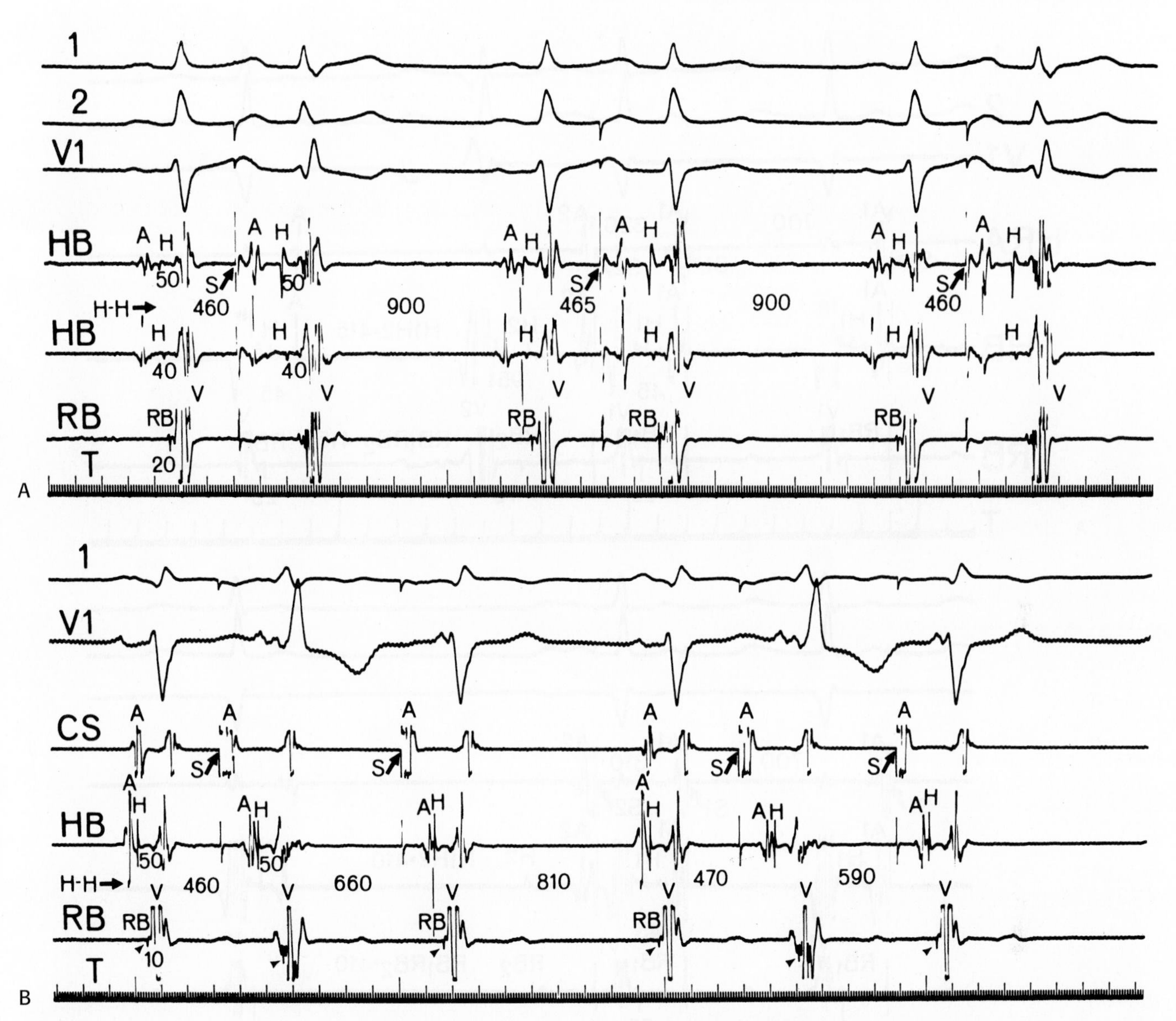


**FIGURE 5-25** *Disappearance of right bundle potential during right bundle branch block (RBBB) pattern in two patients.* **A:** Two recordings are from the His bundle (HB) region with HV intervals of 50 and 40 msec, respectively, and one is right bundle (RB) recording with an RB-V interval of 20 msec. With premature stimulation (S) at comparable atrial coupling intervals, the RB potential is not identifiable when the QRS complex shows an RBBB pattern (second and sixth beats) but is clearly recognizable when the QRS complex has a normal morphology (fourth beat). The HV interval measures the same for all beats. **B:** The HV and RB intervals are 40 and 10 msec, respectively. During premature atrial stimulation from the coronary sinus (CS, second and fifth beats), the QRS complex shows an RBBB pattern without concomitant change in the HV interval. The RB potential, however, disappears from its expected location and can be recognized within the local ventricular electrogram (*small arrows*), signifying a marked increase in H-RB interval after the atrial premature beats. All measurements are in milliseconds. (From Akhtar M, Gilbert C, Al-Nouri M, et al. Site of conduction delay during functional block in the His-Purkinje system in man. *Circulation* 1980;61:1239.)

the distal conducting system is responsible of bradycardia-dependent LBBB. Moreover, it has a higher rate of underlying automatically than the RBB system. An example of bradycardia-dependent LBBB is shown in Figure 5-33; a change from 1:1 conduction to 2:1 conduction with block in the A-V node resulted in a slower rate of engagement of the His–Purkinje system and the development of LBBB. Acceleration-dependent block in contrast is observed in both the RBBB and LBBB.

Clinically, both tachycardia or acceleration-dependent and bradycardia-dependent bundle branch blocks are often seen in the same patient with an intermediate range of cycle lengths and normal conduction. The range of normal conduction may be quite broad, with rapid pacing and/or prolonged carotid sinus pressure required to produce the extremes of cycle length that precipitate the bundle branch block.[28] In some cases, however, the range of cycle lengths resulting in normal conduction may be very narrow, and to some extent variable and affected

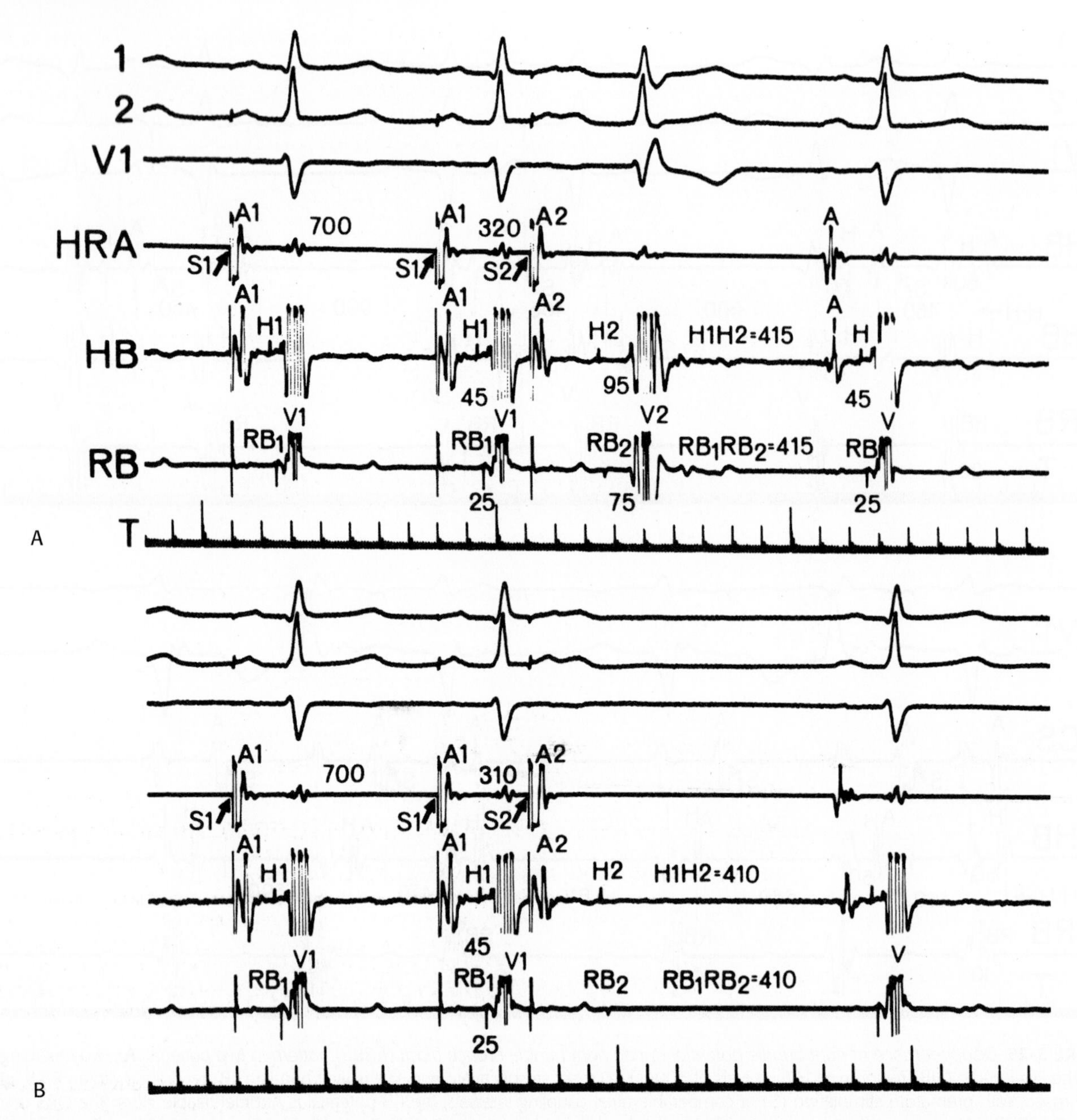


**FIGURE 5-26** *Distal block in the right bundle (RB) branch.* The basic atrial cycle length is 700 msec, and the H1-V1 and RB1-V1 measure 45 and 25 msec, respectively. **A:** The A1 conducts with a right bundle branch block (RBBB) pattern. **B:** A2 shows a block in the His–Purkinje system. In both panels, the H-RB interval is the same as sinus beats, and conduction delay and block are distal to the RB recording site. All measurements are in milliseconds. (From Akhtar M, Gilbert C, Al-Nouri M, et al. Site of conduction delay during functional block in the His-Purkinje system in man. *Circulation* 1980;61:1239.)

by drugs and other factors. However, the isolated appearance of bradycardia-dependent block is almost always associated with LBBB. The clinical implications of rate-dependent bundle branch block are not clear. Acceleration-dependent and bradycardia-dependent blocks usually occur in diseased tissue and, in the setting of infarction, usually an inferior infarction. The prognosis for such dependent blocks is purely related to the underlying cardiac disorder. On the other hand, phase 3 block is a physiologic normal response to encroachment on the refractory period of the bundle branch. Therefore, in and of itself, it should have no adverse prognostic implications.

## CLINICAL RELEVANCE OF INTRAVENTRICULAR CONDUCTION DISTURBANCES

The major interest in the study of IVCDs stems from early studies showing that bifascicular block, specifically RBBB with left-axis deviation, is the most common ECG pattern preceding complete heart block in adults.[33] Other forms of IVCD precede the bulk of the remaining instances of complete infra or infra-His heart block. Although the incidence

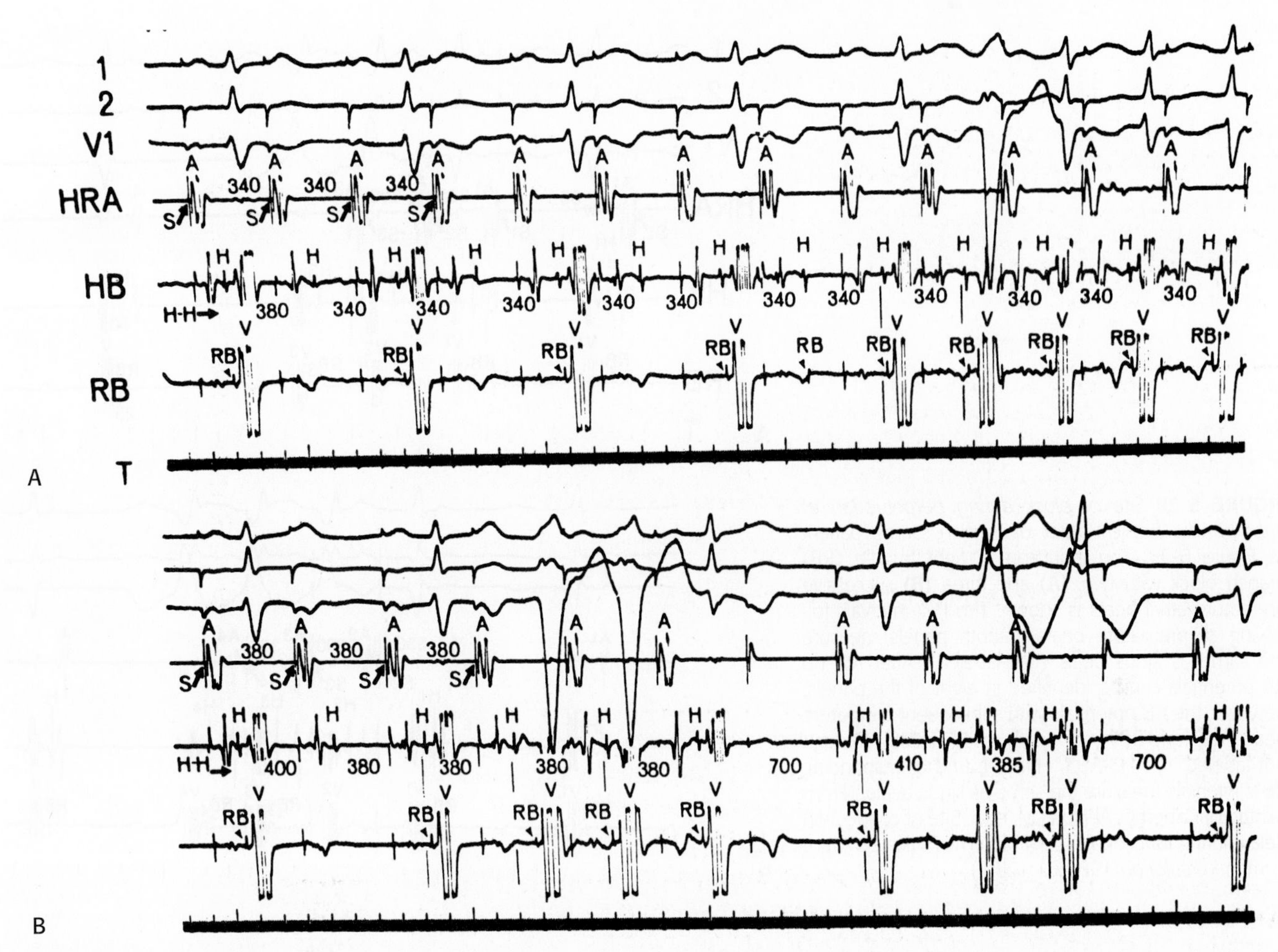


**FIGURE 5-27** *Migration of block in the right bundle (RB) branch during rapid pacing.* **A:** A period of stable function 2:1 atrioventricular block in the His–Purkinje system before resumption of 1:1 conduction. The second, fourth, and sixth impulses are followed by His (H) but no RB potentials. The eighth atrial impulse, however, is followed by both H and RB potentials, and the H-RB interval measures the same as sinus beats. The tenth atrial impulse conducts with a left bundle branch block (LBBB) pattern and is preceded by prolonged H-V and RB-V intervals and a normal H-RB interval. The association of delay distal to RB recording in association with LBBB at this moment is because the site of delay had already shifted from a proximal to a distal location (beyond the RB potential) before resumption of 1:1 conduction. Perpendiculars are drawn in appropriate places to show the timing of the H-RB activation. **B:** Atrial pacing at a constant cycle length of 380 msec and two missed atrial captures (seventh and eighth stimuli). The second atrial impulse is followed by H but no RB deflection, while the third atrial impulse conducts normally. The next two beats conduct with an LBBB pattern; the H-V and H-RB intervals preceding the first aberrant beat are prolonged but return to normal with the second aberrant beat. The RB-V interval preceding both beats with LBBB pattern measures the same as sinus beats (not labeled). During the first beat with an RBBB pattern (seventh QRS complex), the H-V interval is prolonged and no RB potential is recorded; however, the H-V and RB-V intervals preceding the second beat with RBBB measure the same as normal beats and are shown by perpendiculars. (From Akhtar M, Gilbert C, Al-Nouri M, et al. Site of conduction delay during functional block in the His-Purkinje system in man. *Circulation* 1980;61:1239.)

of progression of complete heart block varies from 2% to 6% a year, the method of patient selection markedly influences this.[34–38] The incidence in asymptomatic patient population studies is closer to 2%, while that in patients with neurologic symptoms, such as syncope, is closer to 6% a year. Unfortunately, these studies have not always localized the site of A-V block. When they have described it, however, they have noted that many instances of A-V block were, in fact, in the A-V node.[35] Many of these investigations also noted the high mortality associated with intraventricular conduction disturbances; however, this primarily reflects the underlying cardiac disease. Moreover, death was usually sudden and assumed to be due to ventricular tachyarrhythmias. The issue to be addressed in this chapter is the usefulness of intracardiac studies in identifying patients at risk for subsequent complete heart block among those with intraventricular conduction disturbances.

## Role of Electrophysiologic Studies in Predicting Risk of Heart Block

If one accepts the functional trifascicular or quadrifascicular nature of the His–Purkinje system, the evaluation of the patient with bundle branch block or fascicular block necessarily involves testing the integrity of the remaining "intact" fascicle. In the presence of bundle branch block, with or without

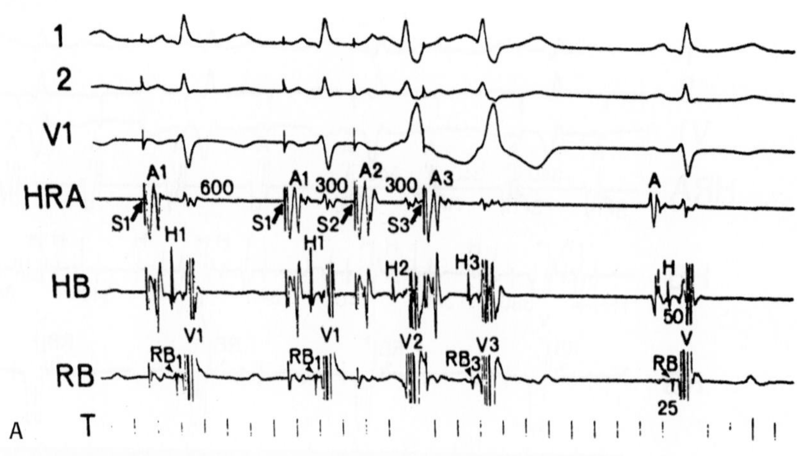


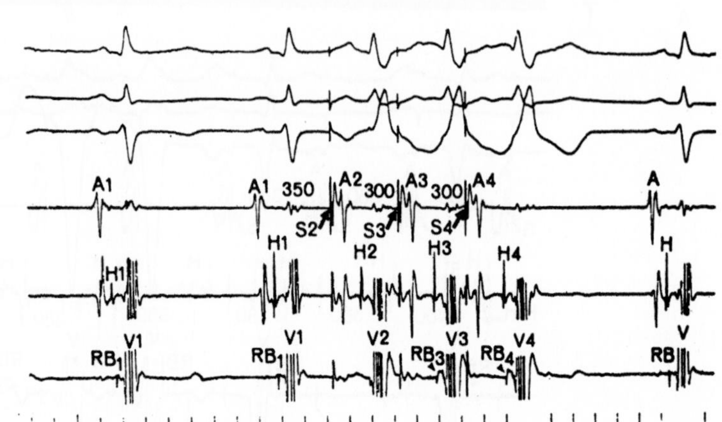


**FIGURE 5-28** *Site of block during perpetuation of right bundle branch block aberration.* Same patient as Figure 5-22. The induction of right bundle (RB) branch block with two, **(A)** and three **(B)** successive premature atrial beats is shown. The H-V intervals following all premature beats in both panels measure the same as sinus beats (not labeled). After A2, no RB potentials can be identified in eight of the panels; however, the RB potentials with subsequent premature beats (RB3 and RB4) are clearly recognizable. Although not labeled, the H3-RB3, H4-RB4, and corresponding RB-V intervals measure the same as sinus beats. (From Akhtar M, Gilbert C, Al-Nouri M, et al. Site of conduction delay during functional block in the His-Purkinje system in man. *Circulation* 1980;61:1239.)

additional fascicular block, the H-V interval should be normal as long as conduction is unimpaired in the remaining fascicle. This would be true even if the delays were within the His bundle that was longitudinally dissociated and the recorded His bundle potential was proximal to the site of the conduction disturbance. Even if the concept of a simple tri-/quadrifascicular system is naive, the patterns of bundle branch block at the very least are apparent markers for patients in whom His–Purkinje conduction may be jeopardized and in whom the degree of conduction "reserve" should be assessed. The simplest method of assessing His–Purkinje reserve is the measurement of basal H-V intervals (normal <55 msec).

**FIGURE 5-29** *Response of right bundle branch (RBB) and left bundle branch (LBB) to cycle length (CL).* Note that the refractory period of the RBB shortens to a greater degree than that of the LBB system at increasing heart rates.

As stressed previously, because the site of block or conduction delay may have important clinical significance, it is important to use multiple His bundle electrogram (proximal and distal) and/or the recording of a His bundle and proximal RBB potential to discern how proximal the site of the conduction disorder is. I believe that the more proximal the defect, the more likely the chance of progression to heart block. Although some investigators maintain that the earlier site of depolarization on the left side of the intraventricular septum via the LBB precedes activation of the RBB by 12 to 20 msec,[39] others have shown a nearly simultaneous activation on both sides of the septum.[1,40] We have seen differences of 5 to 15 msec with the development of LBBB in the absence of a change in H-RB or H-RV interval, suggesting that conduction time from the His bundle to the RV is longer than the His to LV (Fig. 5-31). Because of this finding, we believe that 60 to 70 msec may be a more appropriate upper limit of normal for the H-V interval in the presence of LBBB.

It has long been recognized that patients with second-degree or complete infra-His block have prolonged H-V

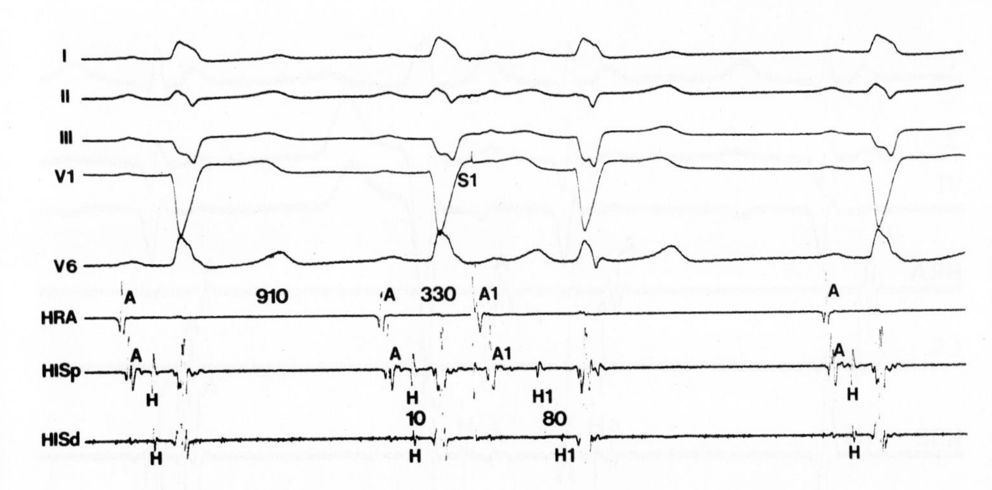


**FIGURE 5-30** *Longitudinal dissociation in the His bundle causing left anterior hemiblock.* (Same arrangement as in Fig. 5-4) Left bundle branch block with a 10-degree axis is shown. A premature atrial complex, A1, results in marked left-axis deviation and is associated with an increase between proximal (HISp) and distal (HISd) His deflections. No change of distal His-V occurs during the premature complex.

intervals during conducted complexes. Rarely, the H-V intervals have been normal, and two potential explanations may be invoked: (a) Measured "normal" H-V interval may not have been taken from the true proximal His bundle region, and no validation of His bundle proximity was performed; (b) within the range of normal H-V intervals (35 to 55 msec), an unsuspected change of perhaps 15 msec, resulting in an increase of the H-V interval from 40 to 55 msec, may have occurred before the development of the marked block. This may represent an extremely important alteration of infra-His conduction that may go undetected in the single study demonstrating an H-V interval within normal limits.

Because most patients developing complete infra-His block have prolonged H-V intervals, analysis of H-V interval was the factor initially evaluated as a predictor of subsequent heart block. Approximately 50% of patients with RBBB and left anterior hemiblock and 75% of patients with LBBB have prolonged H-V intervals.[6,40,41] Thus, it is obvious that this finding alone is nonspecific as a predictor of the development of high-grade heart block, because the incidence of heart block is low, yet the presence of prolonged H-V interval is great. Other criteria are therefore required to more adequately define the patient population at risk.

In the presence of RBBB and left anterior hemiblock or LBBB with or without left anterior hemiblock, the surface P-R interval does not appear to be of any value in selecting those patients with prolonged H-V intervals because (a) a normal P-R interval can easily "conceal" a significantly prolonged H-V interval (Fig. 5-34) and (b) a prolonged P-R interval can be the result of a prolonged A-H interval only (Fig. 5-35). Although it has been suggested that in the presence of LBBB, a P-R interval exceeding 0.22 seconds with a QRS duration of ≥0.14 seconds selects a group of patients who will have long H-V intervals,[42] we have not found this to be useful. In our experience and that of others,[40,41] most patients who have LBBB have prolonged H-V intervals, regardless of the length of the accompanying P-R interval. Conversely, a long P-R interval does not automatically mean a long H-V interval (Fig. 5-36). When the H-V interval is prolonged in LBBB, one frequently can observe a prolongation between the proximal

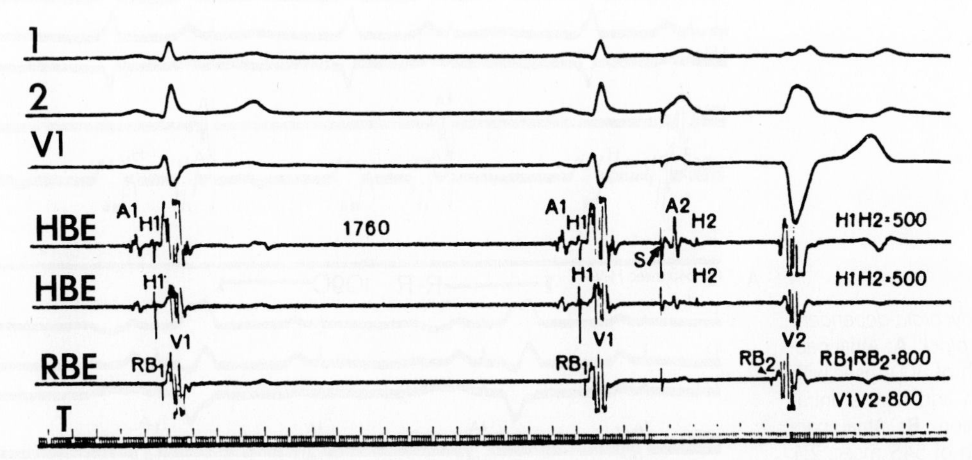


**FIGURE 5-31** *Site of conduction delay in left bundle branch block.* Two His bundle electrograms (HBE) and a right bundle electrogram (RBE) are shown. The H1-V1 and RV1-V1 are 40 and 20 msec, respectively. An atrial premature complex, A2, produces a marked increase in H2-RB2 interval (320 msec), which is associated with left bundle branch block aberration. Normal conduction beyond the RBE is evident by a persistent RB-V of 20 msec. This points to the His bundle as the location of the site of left bundle branch delay. T, time line. (From Akhtar M, Gilbert C, Al-Nouri M, et al. Site of conduction delay during functional block in the His-Purkinje system in man. *Circulation* 1980;61:1239.)

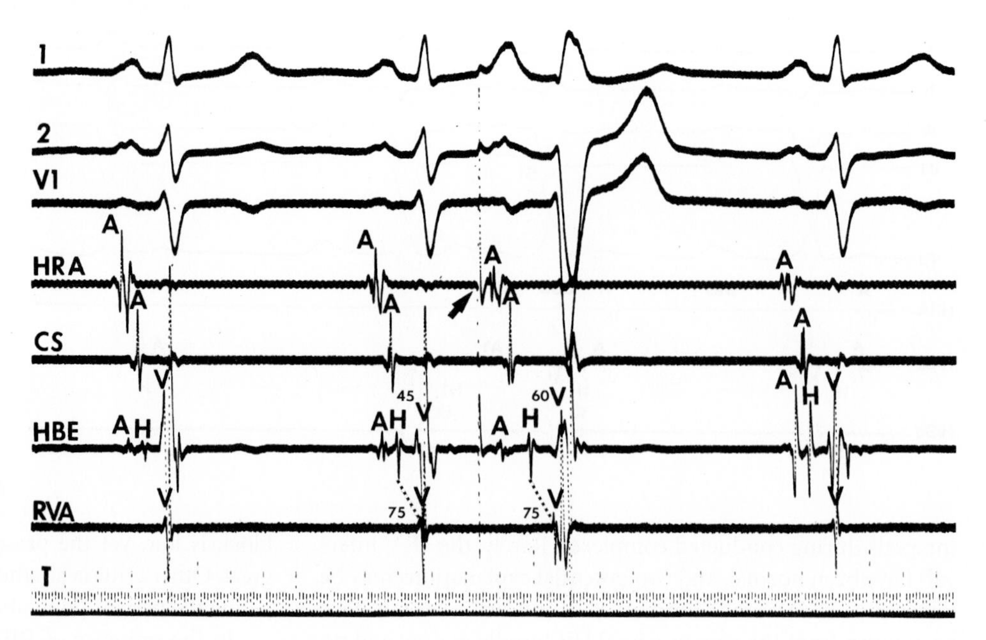


**FIGURE 5-32** *Effect of LBBB on the H-V interval.* During sinus rhythm (first two complexes) the H-V interval is 45 msec and the H-RV interval is 75 msec. An atrial extrastimulus (*arrow*) results in LBBB aberration and an increase in H-V to 60 msec. However, the H-RV remains the same. Thus despite the increase in H-V interval, the conduction down the right bundle branch is unaltered. Therefore, in the presence of LBBB, the H-V interval may be prolonged to 60 msec in the absence of trifascicular delay.

His deflection and the proximal RBB deflection or between the proximal and distal His deflections, suggesting that the increase in H-V interval is due to delay of conduction in the very proximal LBB or in fibers within the His bundle that are destined to form the LBB. In agreement with Dhingra et al.,[43] we have noted that patients with LBBB and left anterior hemiblock have longer H-V intervals (as well as longer A-H intervals) than those patients with normal axis, although there is considerable overlap. Such patients also appear to have a higher mortality and greater extent of cardiac disease.

Although a short P-R interval (i.e., ≤160 msec) makes a markedly prolonged H-V interval (i.e., ≥100 msec) unlikely, in a given patient, enhanced A-V nodal conduction may be present, in which case, a P-R interval of 160 msec could still be compatible with an H-V of 80 msec. Thus, predictions about conduction time of the intact fascicle or fibers predestined to become that fascicle cannot be made on the base of the P-R interval. Moreover, a P-R interval of >300 msec almost always means at least some abnormality, if not all, of A-V nodal conduction.

The specificity and sensitivity of a long H-V interval in predicting heart block has been a topic of continued controversy. Problems that have led to this controversy have, I believe, primarily been related to the nature of the patients enrolled in

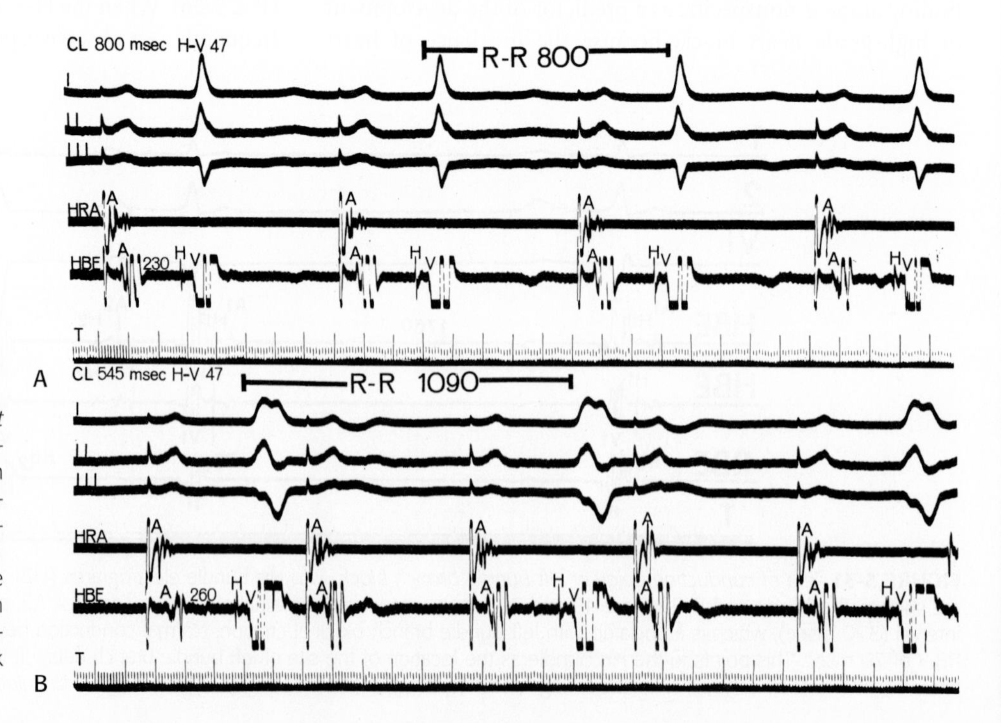


**FIGURE 5-33** *Bradycardia-dependent left bundle branch block.* **A:** Atrial pacing at a cycle length of 800 msec with 1:1 A-V conduction and normal intraventricular conduction. **B:** Atrial pacing at a cycle length of 545 msec, 2:1 block in the A-V node, and an effective cycle length in the His–Purkinje system of 1,090 msec. A widened QRS complex with a left bundle branch block configuration is evident.

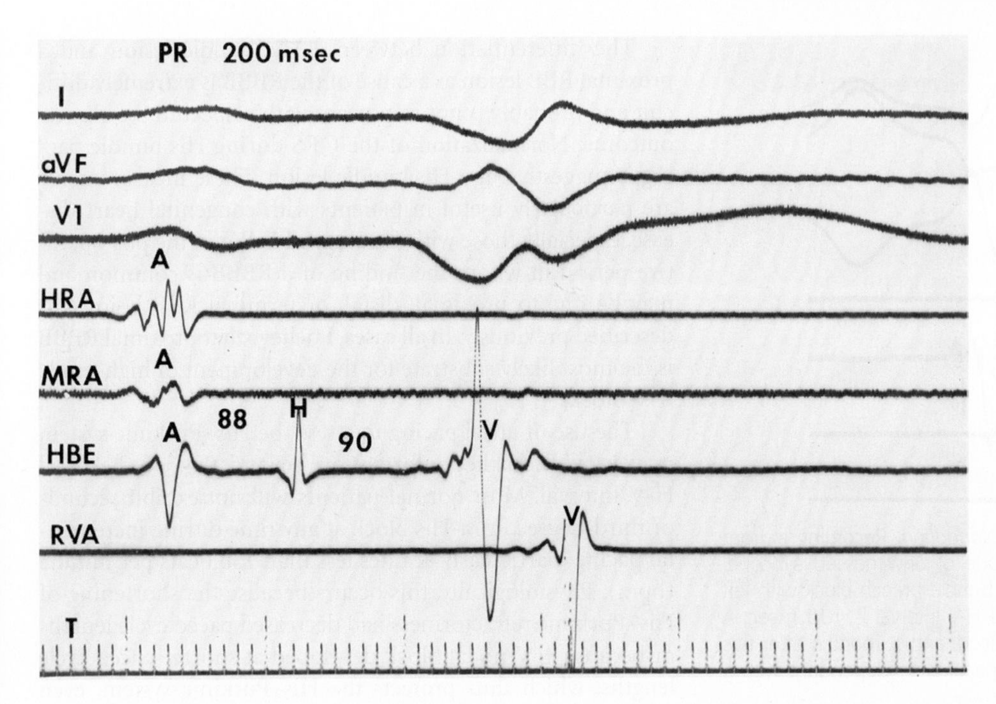


**FIGURE 5-34** *Markedly prolonged H-V interval in the presence of a normal overall P-R interval.* The P-R interval is at the upper limits of normal (200 msec), and the QRS complex is prolonged with a pattern of interventricular conduction defect of the LBBB type. The H-V interval is 90 msec.

the studies. Many of the differences can be resolved if one considers large asymptomatic population base studies and studies including patients with symptoms. Currently, three major studies in the United States, all prospective, have shown that prolonged H-V intervals exceeding 70 msec predict patients at higher risk of A-V block.[36–38] In two of the studies comparing symptomatic and asymptomatic patients, the symptomatic patients had a higher relative risk of block.[37,38] The risk of block, however, even in the high-risk group noted in many of the earlier studies (H-V of 80 msec or longer), only approaches at best 6% a year.[36–38] Thus, one cannot clinically use such data because of the low positive predictive value. It is, therefore, important to develop other criteria that will have a greater predictive accuracy.

We have noted that 50 of 72 patients who had H-V intervals ≥100 msec (Fig. 5-37) have developed second- or third-degree

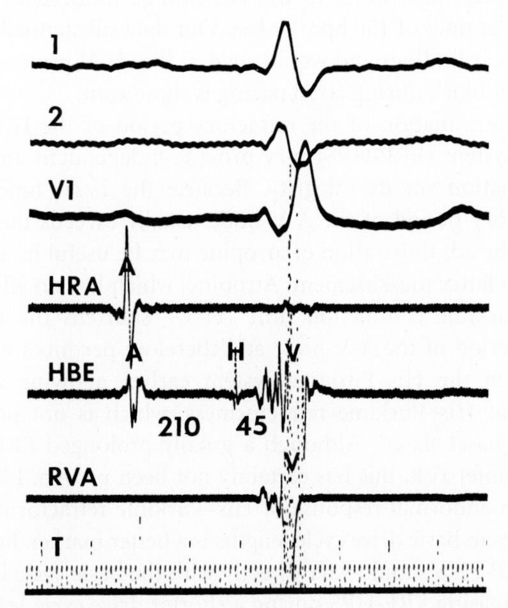


**FIGURE 5-35** *Prolonged P-R interval with a normal H-V interval.* The P-R interval is 290 msec, and the QRS complex is prolonged with a pattern of right bundle branch block and left anterior fascicular block. The H-V interval is normal at 45 msec, but the A-H interval is prolonged at 210 msec.

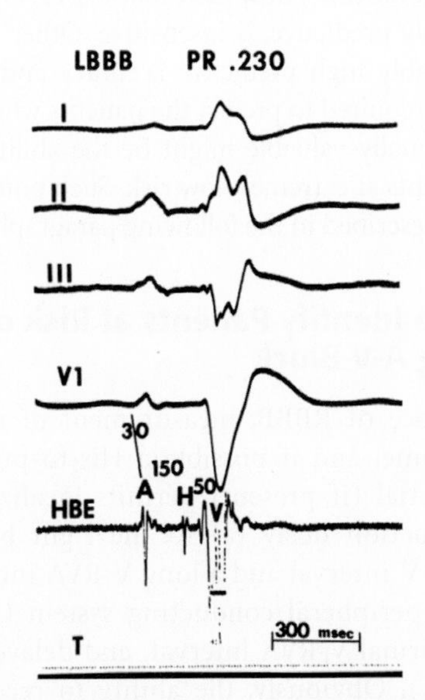


**FIGURE 5-36** *Normal H-V interval in left bundle branch despite P-R prolongation and marked QRS complex widening.* The P-R interval is 230 msec and QRS complex 210 msec yet the H-V interval is normal (50 msec). The P-R prolongation is due to A-V nodal delay (A-H interval = 150 msec).

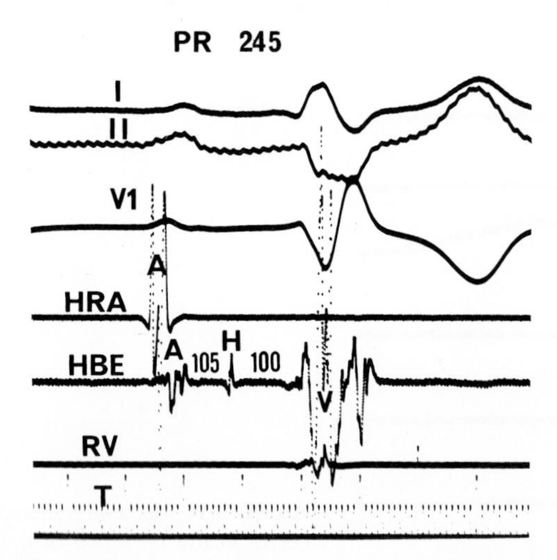


**FIGURE 5-37** *Marked H-V interval prolongation.* Recording is from a 62-year-old man with a single episode of unwitnessed syncope. The QRS complex is indicative of right bundle branch block with left anterior fascicular block. The measured H-V interval is 100 msec. A demand ventricular pacemaker was placed, and 5 months after this recording was made, the patient was pacemaker dependent with a 2:1 infra-His block.

infra-His block within a 24-month follow-up period. Only one-third of the patients had no symptoms before the study. Most of our patients (29/50) with H-V >100 msec have exhibited alternating bundle branch block (see below). A prospective study from Scheinman's laboratory[38] also found that an H-V interval exceeding 100 msec identified a subgroup of extremely high-risk patients. In his study, 25% of the patients having H-V intervals exceeding 100 msec developed heart block over a mean follow-up of 22 months. Unfortunately, H-V intervals in excess of 100 msec are uncommon (72/1,330 patients with bundle branch block). Thus, such marked H-V prolongation, although highly predictive, is insensitive. Other methods that are of reasonably high predictive accuracy and enhance the sensitivity are required to predict the patients who will develop A-V block. Equally valuable might be the ability to define a group of patients at extremely low risk. Such potentially useful methods are described in the following paragraphs.

## Methods to Identify Patients at Risk of Developing A-V Block

In the presence of RBBB, measurement of the H-V, the V-RV apex time, and if possible a His-to-proximal right bundle potential (if present) permits localization of the site of conduction delay (a) to the right bundle trunk (a normal H-V interval and a long V-RVA interval) or (b) to the more peripheral conducting system (normal H-V interval, a normal V-RVA interval, and delayed activation of the RVOT). Obviously, the ability to record multiple regions of the His bundle and/or His right bundle potential has been stressed before. I believe that the finding of a distal RBBB confers a low risk in the development of subsequent A-V block.

The differentiation between a His bundle lesion and a proximal RBB lesion as a cause of the RBBB is extremely difficult and probably is not important with respect to the clinical outcome. Normalization of the QRS during His bundle pacing is suggestive of a His bundle lesion. These measurements are particularly useful in patients with congenital heart disease, especially those with tetralogy of Fallot in the postoperative period in whom the finding of a RBBB is common and may be due to proximal, distal, or terminal RBB lesions, as described previously. In all cases, I believe that proximal RBBB is the most likely substrate for the development of high-grade A-V block.

The use of atrial pacing to stress the His–Purkinje system may provide further information beyond that of the basal H-V interval. Most normal patients will not exhibit second- or third-degree infra-His block at any time during incremental pacing, particularly at rates less than 150 beats per minute (bpm). Physiologically, this occurs because the shortening of His–Purkinje refractoriness had decreased paced cycle lengths or because A-V nodal block developed at shorter paced cycle lengths, which thus protects the His–Purkinje system, even H-V prolongation during atrial pacing at rates less than 150 bpm. Second- or third-degree block within the His–Purkinje system *in the absence of a changing A-H* interval at paced cycle lengths of 400 msec or greater is abnormal and suggests a high risk for A-V block (Figs. 5-38 and 5-39). One must be careful not to start pacing with a short coupling interval that can lead to the production of "pseudo A-V block" produced by initiating pacing producing a long short cycle. It is best to start pacing at a 100 msec less than sinus and gradually decrease the cycle length to avoid this situation. Dhingra et al.[44] showed a 50% progression to high-grade A-V block in patients who developed block distal to the His bundle induced by atrial pacing at rates of 150 bpm or less. Our data substantially support their findings and would suggest that H-V prolongation without block during atrial pacing is significant.

Determination of the refractory period of the His–Purkinje system (ERP-HPS) may provide independent ancillary information on its integrity. Because the basal functional refractory period of the A-V node usually exceeds the ERP-HPS, the administration of atropine may be useful in obtaining the latter measurement. Atropine, which has no effect on His–Purkinje conduction time (H-V), shortens the refractory period of the A-V node and therefore permits impulses to reach the His–Purkinje system earlier, allowing assessment of His–Purkinje refractoriness, which is not possible in the basal state.[45] Although a grossly prolonged ERP-HPS may confer risk, this has certainly not been proven. I believe that an abnormal response of His–Purkinje refractoriness to changes in basic drive cycle lengths is a better marker. Because the ERP-HPS should vary directly with the basic cycle length, an increasing ERP-HPS during a shorter drive cycle length is abnormal and indicates a markedly abnormal His–Purkinje system. In my opinion such a response is a better discriminator of abnormal His–Purkinje refractoriness than a prolonged refractory period during sinus rhythm. We have observed this

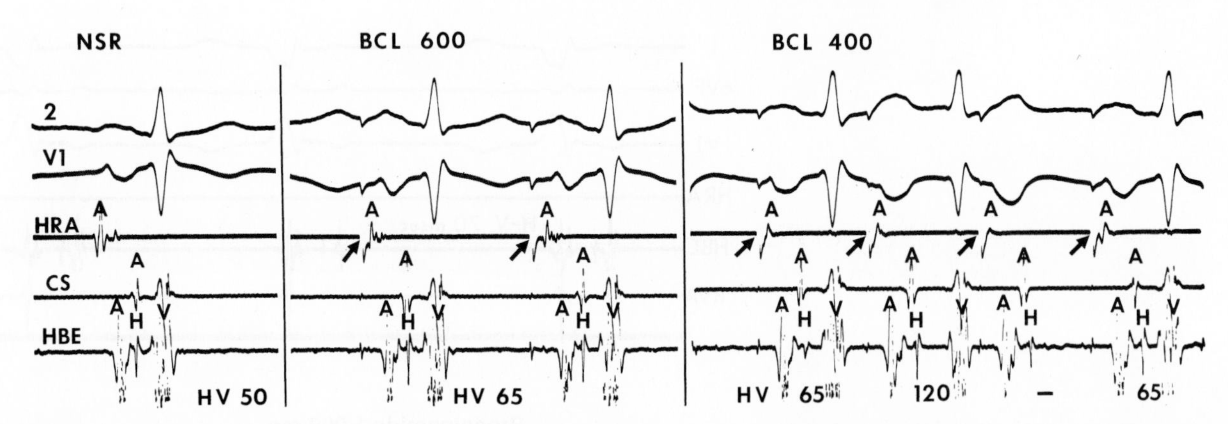


**FIGURE 5-38** *Unmasking of decreased infra-His conduction reserve by atrial pacing.* **Left panel** (during sinus rhythm), a right bundle branch block configuration is seen with a normal H-V interval of 50 msec. **Center panel**, atrial pacing (*arrows*) at a cycle length of 600 msec results in an increase in the H-V interval to 65 msec. **Right panel**, atrial pacing (*arrows*) at a cycle length of 400 msec precipitates infra-His type I second-degree block.

phenomenon when (a) the His–Purkinje system has been exposed to drugs with use-dependent sodium channel blocking effects (class IC), which can markedly prolong the H-V or (b) during recent infarction-related bifascicular block. It is therefore an insensitive marker, although it is usually associated with other findings confirming high risk of block.

The administration of pharmacologic agents known to impair His–Purkinje conduction (e.g., procainamide) may unmask extraordinary sensitivity to the usual therapeutic doses of the agent. Sensitivity to the drug may itself indicate poor His–Purkinje system reserve. Furthermore, because patients with bundle branch block often exhibit ventricular arrhythmias that warrant suppressive therapy (see following), the laboratory assessment of His–Purkinje system integrity following procainamide or similar agents may have practical implications. In normal persons as well as in most persons with moderately prolonged (55 to 80 msec) H-V intervals, procainamide typically produces a 10% to 20% increase in the H-V interval.[46,47] An increase of greater magnitude, including (a) doubling of the H-V interval, (b) a resultant H-V interval exceeding 100 msec, or (c) the precipitation of second- or third-degree infra-His block, all represent evidence of propensity for spontaneous infra-His block. Tonkin et al.[48] have reported that, in 5 of 12 patients with clinical features suggestive of A-V block, procainamide at a dose of 10 mg/kg intravenously produced intermittent second-degree or third-degree A-V block. Those authors documented progression to high degrees of spontaneous A-V block during a follow-up period of 1 year. Our experience in symptomatic patients with probable A-V block is similar. Neither Tonkin's nor our experience is necessarily applicable to patients with bundle branch block without symptoms; however, because such findings have been observed only in symptomatic patients and/or in those who progressed to A-V block, in our laboratory, we consider this a useful test. An example of a patient with bundle branch block in whom procainamide prolonged the H-V interval to 100 msec and in whom block below the His during atrial pacing was observed following procainamide is shown in Figures 5-40 and 5-41. This patient developed spontaneous heart block in a follow-up of less than 3 months.

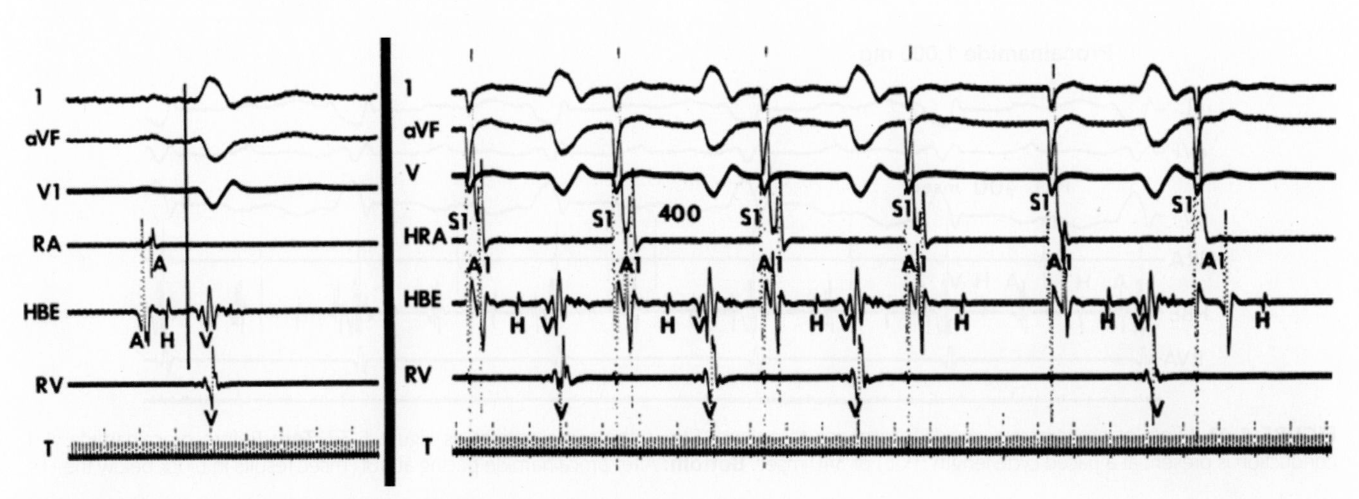


**FIGURE 5-39** *Mobitz II block below the His during atrial pacing.* **Left:** A sinus complex is shown on the left in a patient with right bundle branch block and left anterior hemiblock. **Right:** Atrial pacing at 400 msec results in Mobitz II block below the His. RA, right atrial electrogram; HBE, His bundle electrogram; RV, right ventricular electrogram; T, time line.

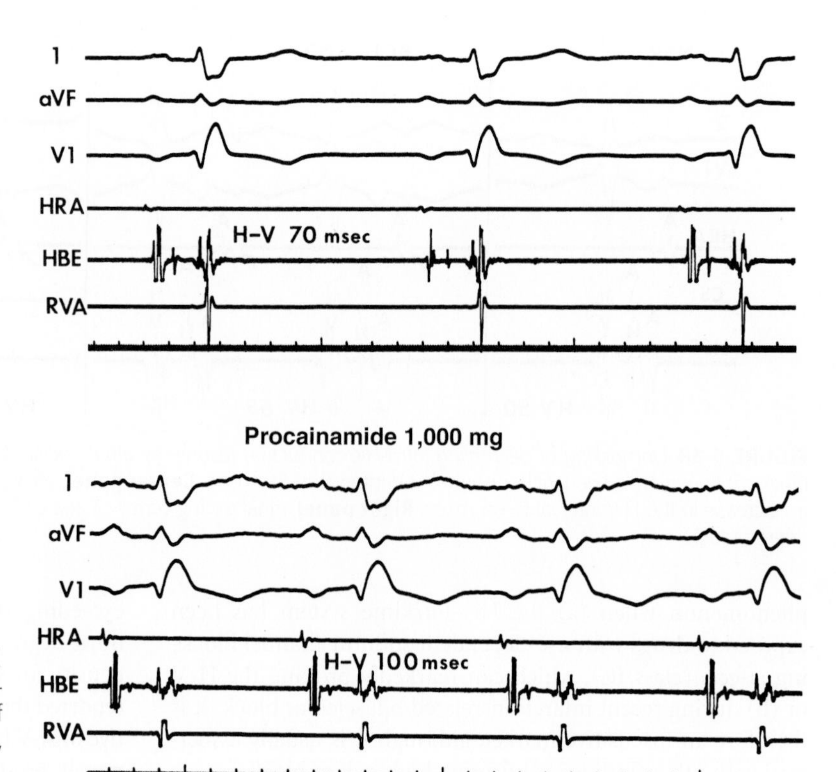


**FIGURE 5-40** *Effect of procainamide on H-V interval.* In the contra state (**top**) the patient manifests right bundle branch block and right-axis deviation with an H-V of 70 msec. After 1,000 mg of procainamide (**bottom**), the H-V markedly prolongs to 100 msec.

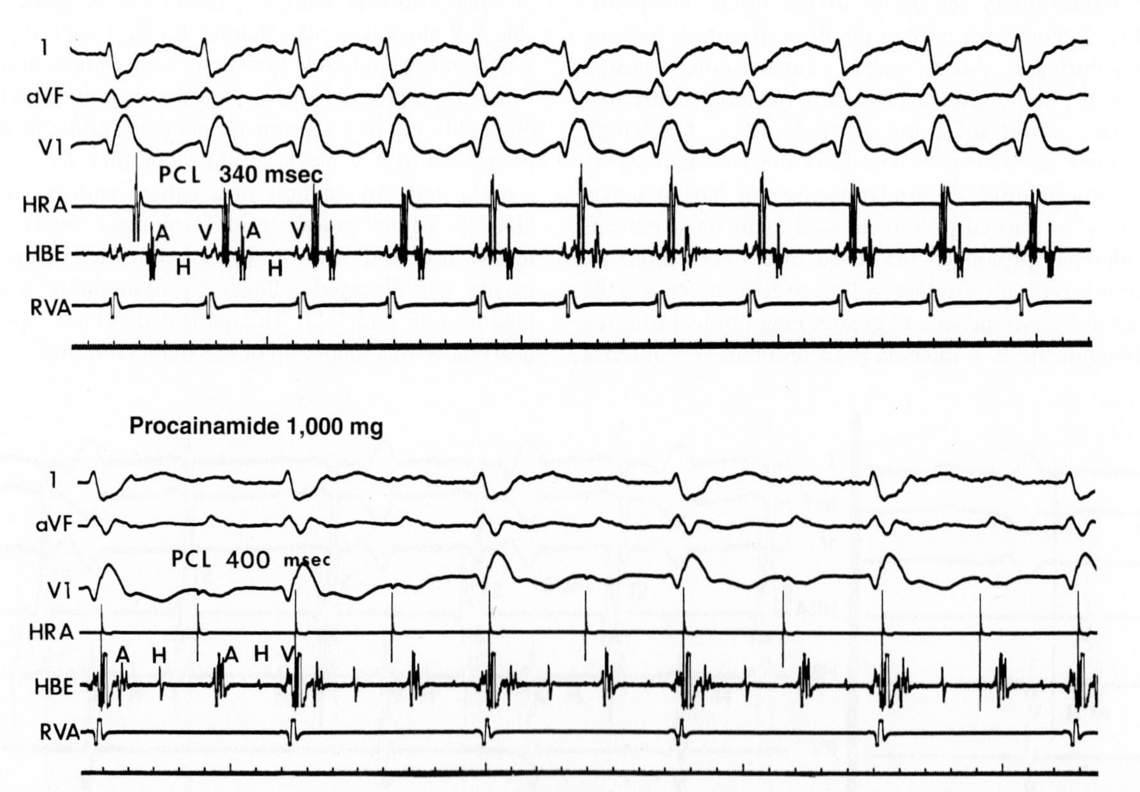


**FIGURE 5-41** *Effect of procainamide on H-V response to pacing.* This is the same patient as Figure 5-37. **Top:** Before procainamide, 1:1 conduction is present at a paced cycle length (PCL) of 340 msec. **Bottom:** After procainamide pacing at 400 msec results in block below the His.

Assessment of retrograde (V-H or ventriculoatrial [V-A]) conduction by ventricular stimulation has not been particularly useful as an indicator of antegrade His–Purkinje system reserve.[49] Different areas of the His–Purkinje system are tested during antegrade and ventricular stimulation. Many patients with RBBB or LBBB on their surface ECG have absent retrograde His–Purkinje system conduction during ventricular stimulation, and conversely, some patients with antegrade intermittent A-V block in the presence of bundle branch block have intact retrograde His–Purkinje system conduction. The sites of conduction delay and block probably differ antegradely and retrogradely. As noted, antegrade block in the RBB is usually proximal, whereas during ventricular stimulation, block usually occurs at the gate, which is at the His–Purkinje–myocardial junction. Thus, evaluation of the His–Purkinje system by retrograde stimulation is not useful for evaluating risk of A-V block.

## Alternating Bundle Branch Block

Besides active testing to assess His–Purkinje reserve, spontaneous alternating bundle branch block, particularly when associated with a change in P-R interval, represents the most ominous sign for progression to A-V block. Beat-to-beat alternation is the most ominous, whereas a change in bundle branch block noted on different days is somewhat less ominous. In either case, this finding portends the development of A-V block. This phenomenon implies instability of the His–Purkinje system and a disease process involving either both bundle branches, the His bundle, or main trunk. In most patients with diffuse His–Purkinje system disease, delay or block in one of the bundle branches consistently predominates and alternating bundle branch block is uncommon. The H-V interval in alternating bundle branch block is almost universally prolonged and typically varies with a change in bundle branch block. This group of patients has the highest incidence of H-V intervals exceeding 100 msec (Fig. 5-42). The infrequency with which this situation is seen makes it an insensitive predictor of patients at risk for developing heart block but it has a high predictive value. Twenty one of 29 patients manifesting alternating bundle branch block and changing, prolonged H-V intervals developed high-grade A-V block within weeks of documentation of this finding. Thus, despite its relative insensitivity, this finding is associated with the most predictable progression to complete heart block and mandates a pacemaker.

## Syncope and Sudden Death in Patients with Bundle Branch Block

Patients with bundle branch block have an unusually high incidence of cardiac disease and sudden death.[35–38,40,43,50] Most deaths have been sudden or due to heart failure. In these studies as well as those of our own, sudden death occurs with high frequency and does not seem to be related to the H-V interval. The highest incidence is among those patients with cardiac disease and with LBBB. Most sudden deaths are due to ventricular tachycardia and/or ventricular fibrillation. Moreover, permanent pacemaker implantation has relieved symptoms potentially due to heart block but never has been shown to prevent sudden death or alter mortality.[38,51] It is important to recognize that syncope, although perhaps resulting from intermittent heart block in these patients, may also be due to ventricular arrhythmias. Complete electrophysiologic studies, including programmed stimulation, are necessary in such patients because ventricular tachycardia will be found in one-third to one-half of patients.[52] Morady et al.[53] found a 50% incidence of ventricular tachycardia in patients with bundle branch block and syncope. Thus, tachyarrhythmias clearly are just as important a cause as bradyarrhythmias of both neurologic symptoms and sudden death. This suggests that complete studies need to be done to exclude a tachyarrhythmia cause of syncope because the therapies differ.

# THERAPEUTIC IMPLICATIONS

The electrophysiologic study should be used to obtain information that could predict which patients are at risk for syncope, heart block, or sudden death. Questions that the

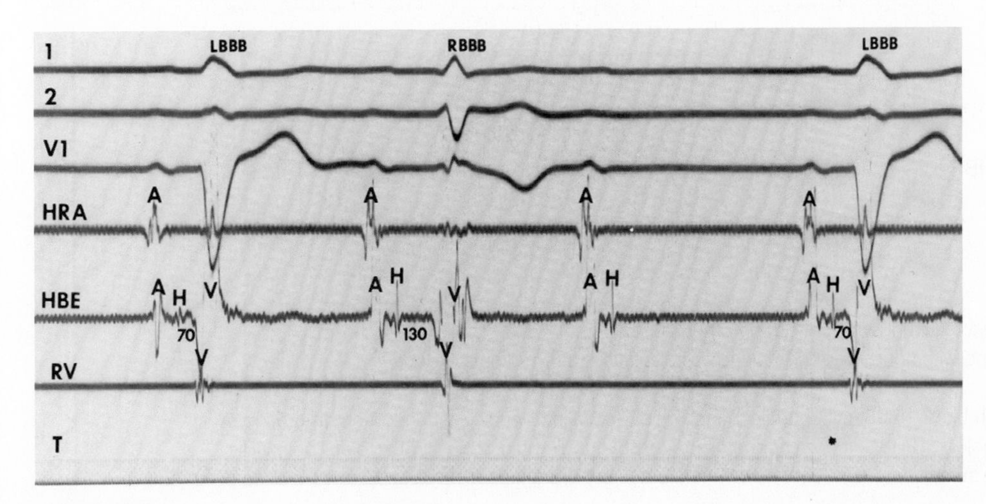


**FIGURE 5-42** *Development of intermittent A-V block during spontaneous alternating bundle branch block.* The first complex exhibits the ECG pattern of "complete" left bundle branch block (LBBB), and the second complex exhibits "complete" right bundle branch block (RBBB) with left anterior fascicular block. The third atrial depolarization (A) is followed by a His bundle deflection (H) but not ventricular depolarization. The fourth atrial complex conducts again with an LBBB pattern. HRA, high-right atrial electrogram; HBE, His bundle electrogram; RV, right ventricular electrogram; T, time line.

**TABLE 5-3 Intraventricular Conduction Disturbances: Assessment of HPS Reserve**

| Technique | Normal | Abnormal |
|---|---|---|
| Basal H-V | <55 msec[a] | >55 msec[a] |
| Atrial pacing | No BBH or BBH >150 bpm | BBH < 150 bpm[b] |
| Programmed APDs | ERP-HPS ≤ 450 msec and ≠ c_ Ø PCL | ERP-HPS ≥ 450 msec and ≠ c_ Ø PCL |
| Drug effect (e.g., PA) | H-V ≠ 15–20% | H-V ≠ 100% or >100 msec; second- or third-degree BBH |

[a]In the presence of left bundle branch block, normal = <60 msec.
[b]No change in A-V nodal conduction (i.e., stable act).
HPS, His–Purkinje system; BBH, block below His bundle; bpm, beats per minute; APD, atrial premature depolarization; ERP-HPS, effective refractory period of the His–Purkinje system; ≠, increase; Ø, decrease; PCL, paced cycle length; PA, procainamide.

electrophysiologic study should answer follow: (a) What prognostic indicators can be obtained for the development of A-V block or tachyarrhythmias? (b) Given a set of prognostic indicators, can the natural history be altered by the use of a pacemaker in the case of bradyarrhythmias and by drugs in the case of tachyarrhythmias? Although prolonged H-V intervals and poor prognosis associated with bundle branch block are related to myocardial dysfunction, heart failure, and ventricular fibrillation rather than to heart block, symptoms such as syncope are often related to heart block. When electrophysiologic studies demonstrate the likelihood of such, a pacemaker may be useful.

Pacemaker therapy clearly can help prevent syncope in patients among whom that event most likely was due to transient bradyarrhythmias, but it has not been shown to prevent sudden death or cardiac mortality.[35–38,50] The induction of ventricular tachycardia by programmed stimulation mandates therapy be directed toward the tachycardia (see Chapters 11 and 13 to 15). The use of antiarrhythmic agents to prevent tachyarrhythmias may in fact necessitate the implantation of a pacemaker if the antiarrhythmic agent produces a situation likely to be associated with the development of A-V block. The current policies in our laboratory are shown in Tables 5-3 and 5-4.

The methods of assessing His–Purkinje reserve are shown in Table 5-3. We generally use identification of abnormal responses to select patients at high risk for development of A-V block. These include H-V intervals ≥100 msec, block below the His or H-V prolongation at pacing cycle lengths ≥400 msec, refractory periods of the His–Purkinje system that are inversely related to paced cycle length, or block below the His or doubling of H-V intervals following procainamide in patients with neurologic symptoms compatible with bradyarrhythmias. Recommendations for pacemakers in such patients

**TABLE 5-4 Intraventricular Conduction Disturbances: Recommendations for Clinical Cardiac Pacing**

| | H-V | | |
|---|---|---|---|
| | ≤55 msec | 60–99 msec | ≥100 msec |
| LBBB, RBBB, IVCD | No[a] | Yes, with symptoms[b] | Yes |
| RBBB + LAHB or LPHB | No[a] | Yes, with symptoms[b] | Yes |
| Alternating BBB | ?[c] | Yes | Yes |
| BBH > 150 bpm | No[a] | Yes, with symptoms[c] | Yes |
| BBH < 150 bpm | Yes | Yes | Yes |

[a]Except with documented recurrent syncope with no other causes.
[b]Syncope or near-syncope with noncardiac and nontachycardia causes of symptoms excluded.
[c]Rarely occurs.
LBBB, left bundle branch block; RBBB, right bundle branch block; IVCD, intraventricular conduction disturbances; LAHB, left anterior hemiblock; LPHB, left posterior hemiblock; BBB, bundle branch block; BBH, block below His bundle; bpm, beats per minute.

is given in Table 5-4. In all such cases, it is important to recognize that tachyarrhythmias may be a cause of these symptoms and should be evaluated and treated when demonstrated. If antiarrhythmic agents are necessary to manage tachyarrhythmias, the effects of the antiarrhythmic agent on infra-His conduction must be assessed. The ideal therapy for patients at risk for both A-V block and ventricular tachycardias is an ICD with dual chamber pacing capability.

A pacemaker also may be implanted in the patient with recurrent neurologic symptoms and prolonged H-V intervals but without any of the abnormalities associated with markedly increased risk of developing A-V block when all other causes for symptoms have been excluded. It seems prudent in the presence of such symptoms and a long H-V interval to implant a pacemaker. Scheinman's study[38] demonstrated that prophylactic pacing does relieve neurologic symptoms in such patients. In patients without electrophysiologic risk factors implantible loop recorders (Reveal, Medtronic, Inc.) may provide diagnostic information that standard monitoring techniques are unlikely to yield.

In conclusion, patients with IVCDs appear to have a higher incidence of cardiac disease, overall cardiac mortality, sudden death, and development of A-V block. Electrophysiologic studies localizing the site of a block and abnormalities of the His–Purkinje system can be useful in determining who is likely to receive benefit from pacemaker therapy. Complete electrophysiologic studies are also necessary to establish whether syncope or other transient neurologic symptoms associated with bundle branch block are due to intermittent heart block or tachyarrhythmias, because the therapies for these disturbances are dissimilar.

## ■ REFERENCES


1. Durrer D, van Dam RT, Freud GE, et al. Total excitation of the isolated human heart. *Circulation* 1970;41:899–912.
2. Tawara S. Das Reizleitungssystem des Säugetierherzens (English: "The Conduction System of the Mammalian Heart"). Jena: Verlag von Gustav Fischer. 1906.
3. Uhley HN. The fascicular blocks. *Cardiovasc Clin* 1973;5:87–97.
4. Mossing G, James T, eds. *Anatomy and pathology of the conducting system.* New York, NY: Grune & Stratton, 1973.
5. Demoulin JC, Kulbertus HE. Histopathological examination of concept of left hemiblock. *Br Heart J* 1972;34:807–814.
6. Batsford WP, Akhtar M, Damato AN, et al. Electrophysiologic studies in asymptomatic patients with RBBB and LAH (Abstract). *Circulation* 1974; 50:214.
7. Wu D, Denes P, Dhingra R, et al. Bundle branch block. Demonstration of the incomplete nature of some "complete" bundle branch and fascicular blocks by the extrastimulus technique. *Am J Cardiol* 1974;33: 583–589.
8. Watt TB Jr, Pruitt RD. Focal lesions in the canine bundle of His. Their effect on ventricular excitation. *Circ Res* 1972;31:531–545.
9. Narula OS. Longitudinal dissociation in the His bundle. Bundle branch block due to asynchronous conduction within the His bundle in man. *Circulation* 1977;56:996–1006.
10. El-Sherif N, Amay YLF, Schonfield C, et al. Normalization of bundle branch block patterns by distal His bundle pacing. Clinical and experimental evidence of longitudinal dissociation in the pathologic his bundle. *Circulation* 1978;57:473–483.
11. Horowitz LN, Alexander JA, Edmunds LH Jr. Postoperative right bundle branch block: identification of three levels of block. *Circulation* 1980; 62:319–328.
12. Horowitz LN, Simson MB, Spear JF, et al. The mechanism of apparent right bundle branch block after transatrial repair of tetralogy of Fallot. *Circulation* 1979;59:1241–1252.
13. Wyndham CR. Epicardial activation in bundle branch block. *Pacing Clin Electrophysiol* 1983;6:1201–1209.
14. Wyndham C, Meeran M, Levitsky S, et al. Epicardial mapping in three patients with right bundle branch block (Abstract). *Circulation* 1976;54:2.
15. Van Dam RT, ed. *Ventricular activation in human and canine bundle branch block.* Philadelphia, PA: Lea & Febiger, 1976.
16. Gelband H, Waldo AL, Kaiser GA, et al. Etiology of right bundle-branch block in patients undergoing total correction of tetralogy of Fallot. *Circulation* 1971;44:1022–1033.
17. Krongrad E, Hefler SE, Bowman FO Jr, et al. Further observations on the etiology of the right bundle branch block pattern following right ventriculotomy. *Circulation* 1974;50:1105–1113.
18. Becker RA, Erickson RV, Scher AM. Ventricular excitation in experimental bundle-branch block. *Circ Res* 1957;5:5–10.
19. Moore EN, Hoffman BF, Patterson DF, et al. Electrocardiographic changes due to delayed activation of the wall of the right ventricle. *Am Heart J* 1964;68:347–361.
20. Uhley HN, Rivkin L. Electrocardiographic patterns following interruption of main and peripheral branches of the canine right bundle of His. *Am J Cardiol* 1961;7:810–816.
21. Amer NS, Stuckey JH, Hoffman BF, et al. Activation of the interventricular septal myocardium studied during cardiopulmonary bypass. *Am Heart J* 1960;59:224–237.
22. Sung RJ, Tamer DM, Garcia OL, et al. Analysis of surgically-induced right bundle branch block pattern using intracardiac recording techniques. *Circulation* 1976;54:442–446.
23. Kastor JA, Goldreyer BN, Moore EN, et al. Intraventricular conduction in man studied with an endocardial electrode catheter mapping technique. Patients with normal QRS and right bundle branch block. *Circulation* 1975;51:786–796.
24. Vassallo JA, Cassidy DM, Marchlinski FE, et al. Endocardial activation of left bundle branch block. *Circulation* 1984;69:914–923.
25. Auricchio A, Fantoni C, Regoli F, et al. Characterization of left ventricular activation in patients with heart failure and left bundle-branch block. *Circulation* 2004;109:1133–1139.
26. Rodriguez LM, Timmermans C, Nabar A, et al. Variable patterns of septal activation in patients with left bundle branch block and heart failure. *J Cardiovasc Electrophysiol* 2003;14:135–141.
27. Vassallo JA, Cassidy DM, Miller JM, et al. Left ventricular endocardial activation during right ventricular pacing: effect of underlying heart disease. *J Am Coll Cardiol* 1986;7:1228–1233.
28. Rosenbaum MB, Lazzari JO, Elizari MV, eds. *The role of phase 3 and phase 4 block in clinical electrocardiography.* Philadelphia, PA: Lea & Feiber, 1976.
29. Akhtar M, Gilbert C, Al-Nouri M, et al. Site of conduction delay during functional block in the His-Purkinje system in man. *Circulation* 1980; 61:1239–1248.
30. Flowers NC. Left bundle branch block: a continuously evolving concept. *J Am Coll Cardiol* 1987;9:684–697.
31. Wellens HJ, Ross DL, Farre J, et al., eds. *Function of bundle branch block during supraventricular tachycardia in man: observations on mechanisms and their incidence.* Orlando, FL: Grune & Stratton, Inc., 1985.
32. Chilson DA, Zipes DP, Heger JJ, et al. Functional bundle branch block: discordant response of right and left bundle branches to changes in heart rate. *Am J Cardiol* 1984;54:313–316.
33. Lasser RP, Haft JI, Friedberg CK. Relationship of right bundle-branch block and marked left axis deviation (with left parietal or peri-infarction block) to complete heart block and syncope. *Circulation* 1968;37:429–437.
34. Kulbertus HE. Reevaluation of the prognosis of patients with LAD–RBBB. *Am Heart J* 1976;92:665–667.
35. Dhingra RC, Wyndham C, Amat-y-Leon F, et al. Incidence and site of atrioventricular block in patients with chronic bifascicular block. *Circulation* 1979;59:238–246.
36. Dhingra RC, Palileo E, Strasberg B, et al. Significance of the HV interval in 517 patients with chronic bifascicular block. *Circulation* 1981;64:1265–1271.
37. McAnulty JH, Rahimtoola SH, Murphy E, et al. Natural history of "high-risk" bundle-branch block: final report of a prospective study. *N Engl J Med* 1982;307:137–143.
38. Scheinman MM, Peters RW, Suave MJ, et al. Value of the H-Q interval in patients with bundle branch block and the role of prophylactic permanent pacing. *Am J Cardiol* 1982;50:1316–1322.
39. Castellanos A Jr. H-V intervals in LBBB. *Circulation* 1973;47:1133–1134.

40. Narula OS, ed. *Interventricular conduction defects.* Philadelphia, PA: FA Davis, 1975.
41. Puech P, ed. *Atrioventricular block: the value of intracardiac recordings.* Philadelphia, PA: WB Saunders, 1975.
42. Rosen KM, Ehsani A, Rahimtoola SH. H-V intervals in left bundle-branch block. Clinical and electrocardiographic correlations. *Circulation* 1972;46:717–723.
43. Dhingra RC, Amat YLF, Wyndham C, et al. Significance of left axis deviation in patients with chronic left bundle branch block. *Am J Cardiol* 1978;42:551–556.
44. Dhingra RC, Wyndham C, Bauernfeind R, et al. Significance of block distal to the His bundle induced by atrial pacing in patients with chronic bifascicular block. *Circulation* 1979;60:1455–1464.
45. Akhtar M, Damato AN, Caracta AR, et al. Electrophysiologic effects of atropine on atrioventricular conduction studied by His bundle electrogram. *Am J Cardiol* 1974;33:333–343.
46. Josephson ME, Caracta AR, Ricciutti MA, et al. Electrophysiologic properties of procainamide in man. *Am J Cardiol* 1974;33:596–603.
47. Scheinman MM, Weiss AN, Shafton E, et al. Electrophysiologic effects of procaineamide in patients with intraventricular conduction delay. *Circulation* 1974;49:522–529.
48. Tonkin AM, Heddle WF, Tornos P. Intermittent atrioventricular block: procainamide administration as a provocative test. *Aust N Z J Med* 1978; 8:594–602.
49. Josephson ME, Kastor JA. His-Purkinje conduction during retrograde stress. *J Clin Invest* 1978;61:171–177.
50. Denes P, Dhingra RC, Wu D, et al. Sudden death in patients with chronic bifascicular block. *Arch Intern Med* 1977;137:1005–1010.
51. Peters RW, Scheinman MM, Modin C, et al. Prophylactic permanent pacemakers for patients with chronic bundle branch block. *Am J Med* 1979; 66:978–985.
52. Ezri M, Lerman BB, Marchlinski FE, et al. Electrophysiologic evaluation of syncope in patients with bifascicular block. *Am Heart J* 1983;106:693–697.
53. Morady F, Higgins J, Peters RW, et al. Electrophysiologic testing in bundle branch block and unexplained syncope. *Am J Cardiol* 1984;54:587–591.

CHAPTER 6

# Miscellaneous Phenomena Related to Atrioventricular Conduction

Concealed conduction, the gap phenomenon, and supernormality are physiologic events that may be considered to be variants of the normal response. These phenomena are responsible for many unusual or unexpected responses of atrioventricular (A-V) conduction. This chapter addresses these separate but interrelated phenomena of cardiac conduction.

## CONCEALED CONDUCTION

The definition of concealed conduction has been irrevocably altered by the availability of intracardiac electrophysiologic studies. The concept of concealed conduction, an explanation for the effects of incomplete penetration of an impulse into a portion of the A-V conduction system, was introduced (and then expanded on) by Langendorf[1,2] and by Katz and Pick.[3] The term was applied to unexpected phenomena observed on the surface ECG that were compatible with the effects of incompletely penetrating impulses that were not directly reflected on the surface ECG; hence the term concealed. Because intracardiac recordings can directly document the presence of these impulses during the electrophysiologic study, they are no longer truly concealed. Thus, specific consequences of incomplete penetration of impulses may be a less ambiguous term than concealed conduction of impulses to describe a variety of ECG findings.[4] Although the A-V node is the structure with which concealed conduction has been most often associated, this phenomenon can occur in any portion of the A-V conduction system. The manifestations of concealed conduction (i.e., the effects of incomplete penetration of an impulse) include (a) unexpected prolongation of conduction, (b) unexpected failure of propagation of an impulse, (c) unexpected facilitation of conduction by "peeling back" refractoriness, directly altering refractoriness, and/or summation,[4–6] and (d) unexpected pauses in the discharge of a spontaneous pacemaker. Excellent reviews of the ECG manifestations of concealed conduction are available.[7–11]

Concealed conduction may result from antegrade or retrograde penetration of an impulse into a given structure. The impulse producing concealment may originate anywhere in the heart – in the sinus node, an ectopic atrial site, the A-V junction, the fascicles, or the ventricles.[7] The most common site manifesting the effects of concealed conduction is the A-V node. The effects of retrograde concealment in the A-V node under different circumstances are shown in Figures 6-1 through 6-4. Impulses from any subnodal site can produce concealed conduction. The ability of ventricular premature complexes (VPCs) to produce concealment in the A-V node depends on intact retrograde His–Purkinje conduction. In Figure 6-4, similarly coupled VPCs, manifesting different patterns of retrograde His–Purkinje conduction, have totally different effects on A-V nodal conduction of the sinus complex that follows. The effect of His bundle, fascicular, or ventricular extrasystoles on subsequent A-V nodal conduction is inversely related to the coupling interval of the premature depolarization. In patients with dual A-V nodal pathways (see Chapter 8), VPCs, fascicular premature complexes, and His bundle complexes can shift conduction from the fast to the slow pathway. Slow pathway can be maintained by retrograde invasion into the fast pathway (see Chapter 8). Retrograde concealment at multiple levels of the A-V conduction system may also occur (Fig. 6-5). The levels of concealment depend on the relative timing of antegrade and retrograde impulses.

The most frequent clinical circumstances in which concealed conduction is operative are: (a) atrial fibrillation during which the irregular ventricular response is due to the varying depth of penetration of the numerous wavefronts bombarding the A-V node[8]; (b) prolongation of the P-R(A-H) interval or production of A-V nodal block by a premature depolarization of any origin; (c) reset of a junctional (His bundle) pacemaker by atrial or subjunctional premature depolarizations; and (d) perpetuation of aberrant conduction during tachyarrhythmias. In the latter circumstance, retrograde penetration of the blocked bundle branch subsequent to transeptal conduction perpetuates aberration.[12,13] This is the most common mechanism of perpetuation of aberration during supraventricular tachycardia observed in our laboratory (approximately 70% of cases). Wellens et al.[14] have found a similar incidence of retrograde concealment producing perpetuation of aberration.

Concealed His bundle depolarizations can produce many unusual patterns of conduction, including simulation of type II second-degree A-V block (see Chapters 4 and 7). His bundle depolarizations are frequently not recognized because they must conduct antegrade and/or retrograde to have any

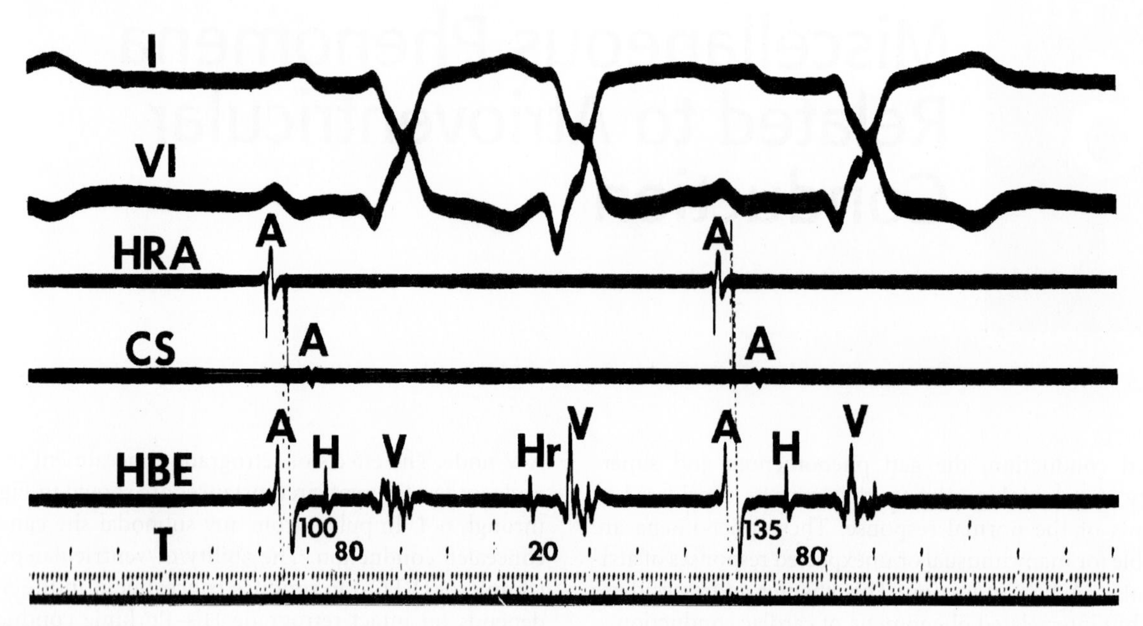


**FIGURE 6-1** *Retrograde concealed conduction by a fascicular extrasystole.* From **top** to **bottom**, tracings represent standard leads 1 and V1 and high-right atrium (HRA), coronary sinus (CS), and His bundle electrogram (HBE) and time lines (T) at 10 msec and 100 msec. The first beat is a conducted sinus beat, with an A-H = 100 msec, H-V = 80 msec, and a right bundle branch block configuration. The second beat is a fascicular extrasystole, with an "Hr-V" = 20 msec. Note that there is no manifest conduction above the atrioventricular (A-V) junction (i.e., no atrial electrogram). Note, however, in the next sinus beat that the A-H interval is prolonged to 135 msec, indicating that the retrograde wavefront from the preceding beat partially penetrated (concealed) in the A-V node, rendering it relatively refractory to the next sinus impulse. A, atrial deflection; H, His bundle deflection; Hr, retrograde His deflection; V, ventricular deflection.

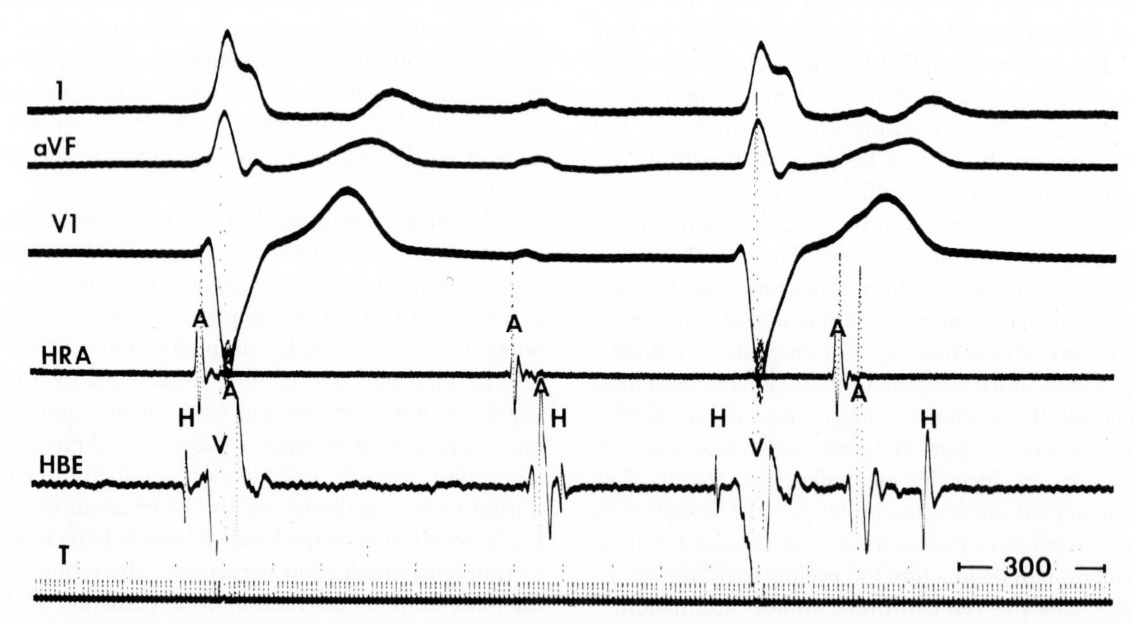


**FIGURE 6-2** *Retrograde concealed conduction by a junctional (His bundle) escape rhythm during intra-His complete heart block.* A-V dissociation is present, and there is no retrograde activation of the atria by the His bundle escape rhythm. There are three sinus depolarizations, as evidenced by early high-right atrial (HRA) activation. The first sinus impulse is blocked above the proximal His bundle (i.e., in the atrioventricular [A-V] node), the second conducts to the proximal His bundle with a short A-H interval, and it is then blocked; and the third conducts to the proximal His bundle with a longer A-H interval. The A-V nodal block in the first beat and the A-V nodal delay in the third beat are due to concealed retrograde conduction of the His bundle beats into the A-V node. Thus, despite antegrade intra-His block, the distal His bundle escape rhythm can conduct retrogradely and affect antegrade conduction (i.e., unidirectional antegrade block is present).

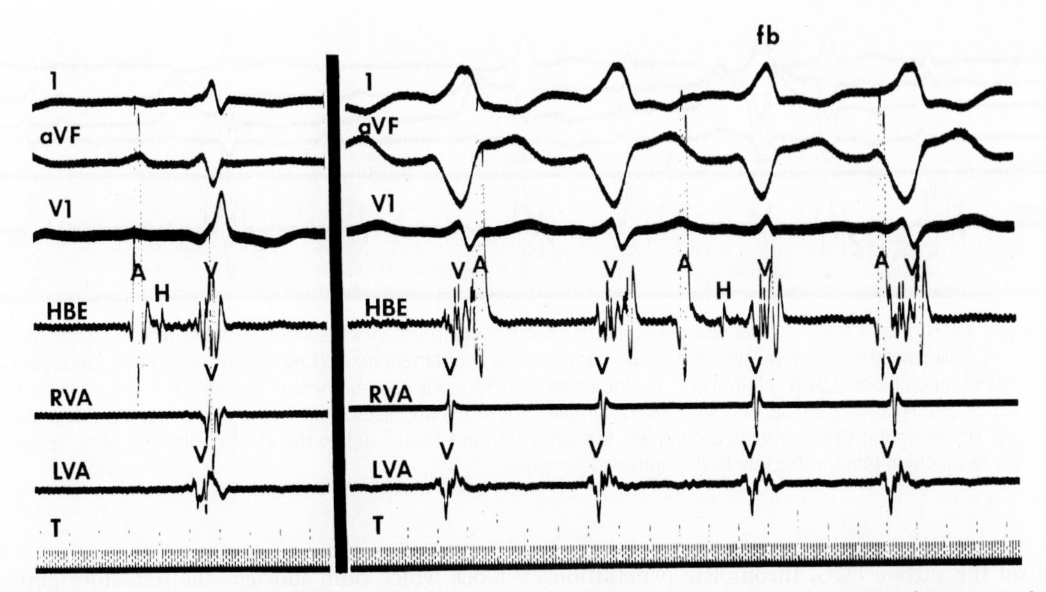


**FIGURE 6-3** *Retrograde concealed conduction during ventricular tachycardia.* The tracing is arranged from **top** to **bottom:** surface ECG leads 1, aVF, and V1, His bundle electrogram (HBE), right ventricular apex (RVA), left ventricular apex (LVA), and time lines (T) at 10 msec and 100 msec. The left panel represents sinus rhythm. The right panel represents ventricular tachycardia without manifest retrograde conduction. Retrograde His bundle or atrial deflections are not seen. There are three sinus complexes, as reflected by atrial deflections **(A)** in the HBE tracing. Only the second results in a propagated response with a His bundle deflection (H) and a slight alteration in the QRS complex characteristic of a fusion beat (fb). Block of the first and third sinus impulses in the atrioventricular (A-V) node results from retrograde concealed conduction of the ventricular beats into the A-V node, rendering it refractory.

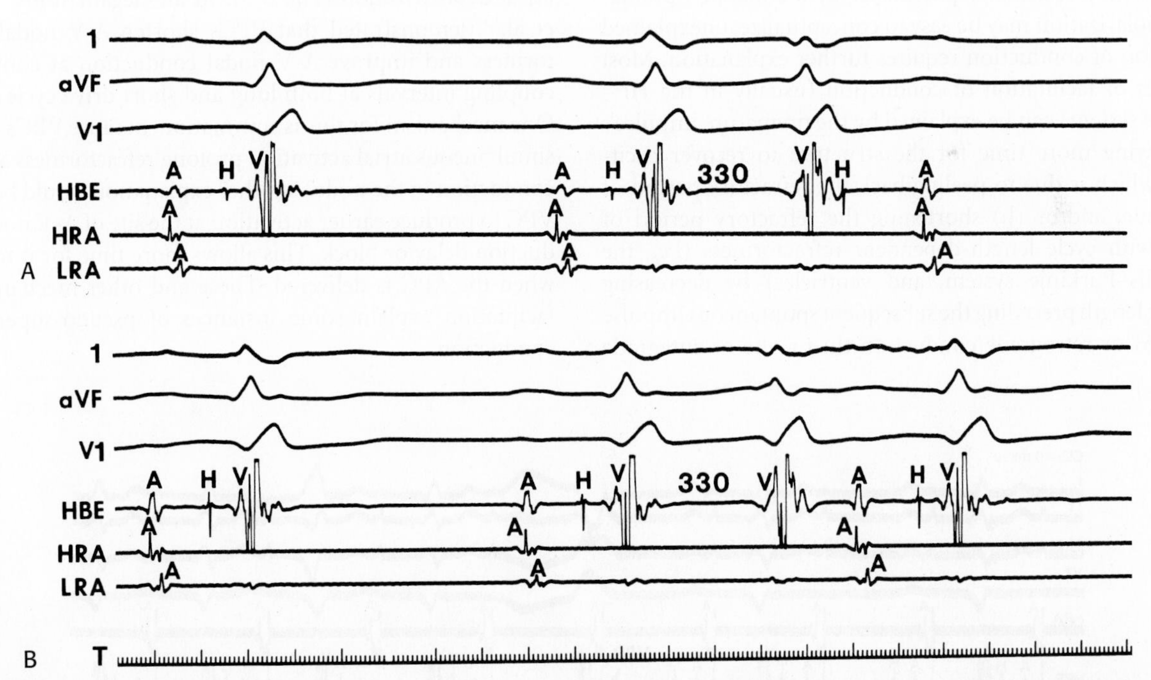


**FIGURE 6-4** *Concealed conduction by ventricular premature contractions (VPCs).* **A** and **B:** Leads 1, aVF, and V1 and electrograms from the His bundle (HBE), high-right atrium (HRA), and low-right atrium (LRA). Sinus rhythm is present in the first two complexes of each panel. **A:** A VPC is observed at a coupling interval of 330 msec with retrograde conduction through the His bundle to the atrioventricular (A-V) node. This results in concealed conduction so that the subsequent sinus complex is a block in the A-V node. **B:** A similarly coupled VPD fails to reach the His bundle so that no concealment in the A-V node is manifested and the sinus complex conducts with a normal HV and normal A-H. Thus, the ability to produce concealed conduction in the A-V node by VPC depends on the ability to penetrate the A-V node via the His–Purkinje system. T, time line.

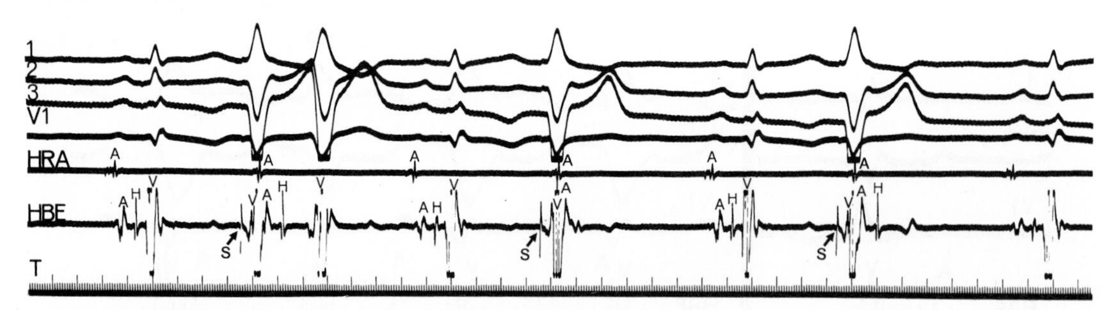


**FIGURE 6-5** *Multiple levels of concealed conduction during ventricular pacing.* The rhythm is sinus, with ventricular pacing at a cycle length of 1200 msec (S, *arrow*). Following the first stimulated ventricular complex, the spontaneously occurring sinus impulse is conducted with a long H-V interval and left bundle branch block (LBBB) aberration. This indicates asynchronous concealment into both left and right bundle branches (long H-V and LBBB morphology). Following the second stimulated complex, the sinus impulse blocks in the A-V node, indicating concealed conduction to that structure. Following the third stimulated complex, the sinus impulse blocks below the His bundle, indicating concealment into the His–Purkinje system, rendering it totally refractory to the antegrade impulse.

representation on the surface ECG. Incomplete penetration (concealment) of His bundle depolarizations in either direction, producing unexpected abnormalities of antegrade or retrograde conduction, may present a particularly difficult diagnostic problem.[9,10] The intracardiac study may be extremely useful in assessing the causes and sites of concealed conduction by making all the components of the A-V conduction system available for analysis.

Although interference with normal antegrade conduction or with a subsidiary pacemaker by a concealed premature depolarization may be easy to conceptualize, unexplained facilitation of conduction requires further explanation. Most examples of facilitation of conduction (usually in the His–Purkinje system) can be explained by the premature impulse's (a) allowing more time for the structure to recover excitability, which is due to peeling back the refractory period of that tissue, and/or (b) shortening the refractory period of tissues with cycle length-dependent refractoriness (i.e., the atria, His–Purkinje system, and ventricles) by decreasing the cycle length preceding the subsequent spontaneous impulse (Fig. 6-6) or retrograde conduction thru a site of antegrade block which both shortens the refractory period and allowing more time for recovery. Simultaneous shortening of refractoriness and providing more time to recover excitability is the most common mechanism. Abrupt normalization of aberration by a VPC (the finding of which proves retrograde concealment as the mechanism for perpetuation of aberration) is based on these principles (Figs. 6-7 and 6-8). Atrioventricular nodal conduction time and refractoriness may be shorted by VPCs delivered simultaneously with the prior atrial depolarization (Fig. 6-9). In an elegant study, Shenasa et al.[15] demonstrated that VPCs shorten A-V nodal refractoriness and improve A-V nodal conduction at comparable coupling intervals at both long and short drive cycle lengths. One mechanism for this is summation, because VPCs without simultaneous atrial activation prolong refractoriness and slow conduction in the node. Another explanation would be for the VPC to produce earlier activation at the site of A-V nodal conduction delay or block. This allows more time for it to record when the APC is delivered. These and other mechanisms of facilitation explain some instances of pseudo-supernormal conduction.

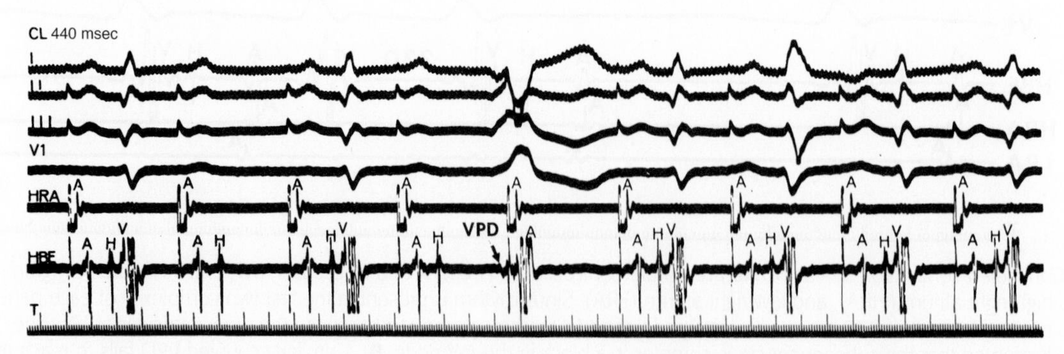


**FIGURE 6-6** *Facilitation of His–Purkinje conduction by a ventricular premature depolarization (VPD).* During atrial pacing at a cycle length of 440 msec, 2:1 block below the His bundle occurs. A VPD (*arrow*) is introduced just before the fifth atrial paced complex. Following the VPD, the P wave that should block in the 2:1 sequence conducts with the same A-H and H-V intervals as other conducted complexes. Facilitation of His–Purkinje conduction results because the VPD "peeled back" His–Purkinje refractoriness, allowing the atrial impulse to propagate through the previous site of block. See text for discussion. (From Gallagher JJ, Damato AN, Varghese PJ, et al. Alternative mechanisms of apparent supernormal atrioventricular conduction. *Am J Cardiol* 1973;31:362.)

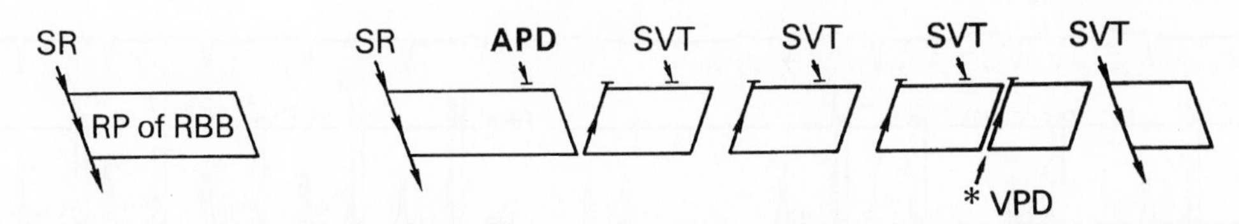


**FIGURE 6-7** *Mechanism of normalization of aberration during supraventricular tachycardia (SVT) by a ventricular premature depolarization (VPD).* Parallelograms represent the refractory period (RP) of the right bundle branch (RBB). During sinus rhythm (SR), an atrial premature depolarization (APD) initiates SVT with REB block because the APD occurred during the RP of the RBB. The RBB aberration persists, owing to continued retrograde concealment during the tachycardia. A VPD normalizes antegrade conduction by prematurely depolarizing the RBB, thereby "peeling back" its refractory period and allowing time for it to recover when engaged by the next impulse. In addition, the RP itself is shortened (decreased duration of parallelogram).

## GAP PHENOMENON

The term gap in A-V conduction was originally used by Moe et al.[16] to define a zone in the cardiac cycle during which premature atrial impulses failed to evoke ventricular responses, while atrial complexes of greater and lesser prematurity conducted to the ventricles. The gap phenomenon was attributed to functional differences of conduction and/or refractoriness in two or more regions of the conducting system. The physiologic basis of gap phenomenon in most instances

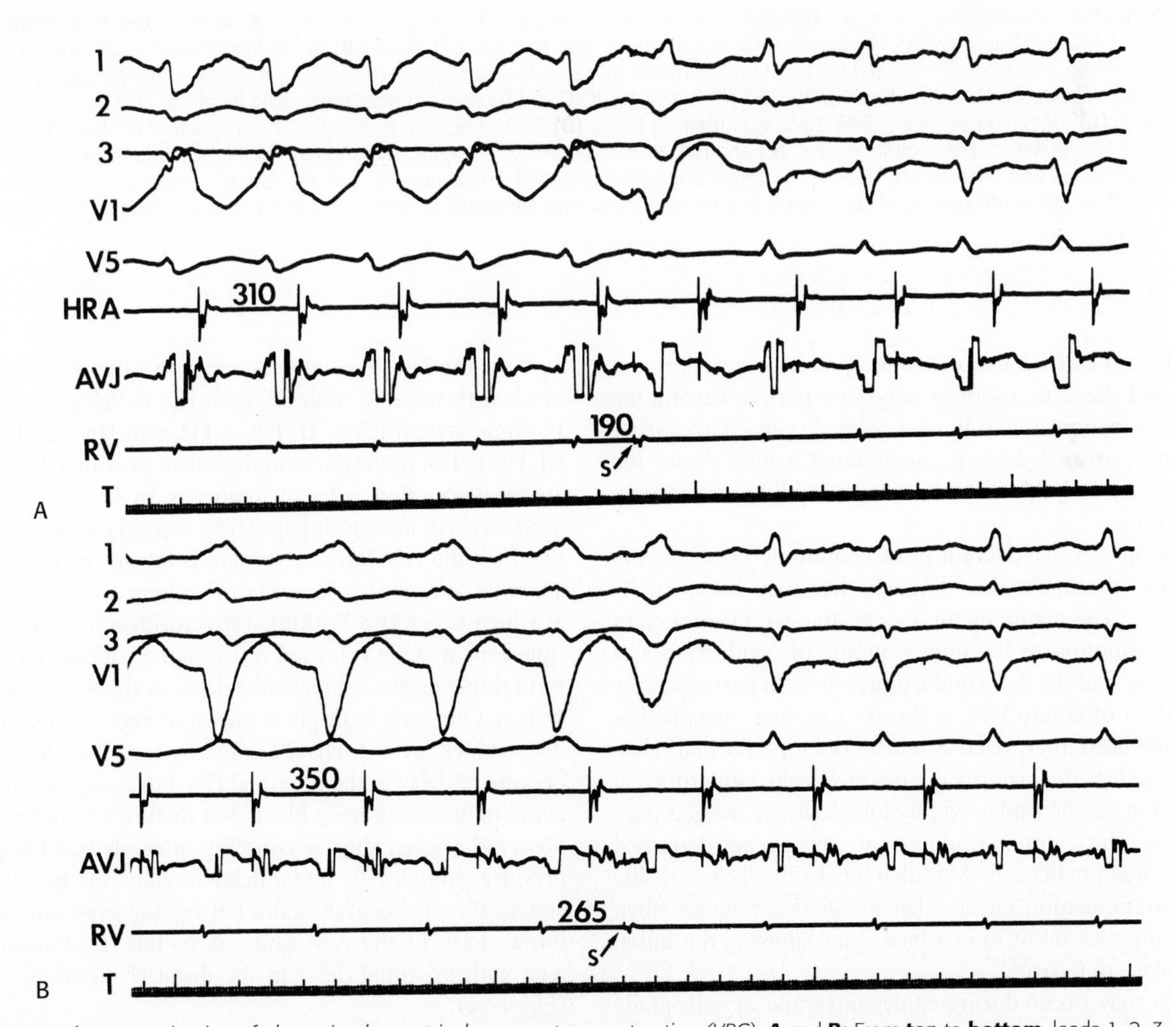


**FIGURE 6-8** *Abrupt termination of aberration by ventricular premature contraction (VPC).* **A** and **B:** From **top** to **bottom**, leads 1, 2, 3, V1, and V5, along with electrograms from the high-right atrium (HRA), atrioventricular junction (AVJ), and right ventricle (RV). **A:** Atrial pacing at a cycle length of 310 msec produces right bundle branch block aberration. A VPC (S, *arrow*) is introduced at a coupling interval of 190 msec, which immediately normalizes the QRS. **B:** Pacing at a longer cycle length of 350 msec produces left bundle branch block aberration. A premature VPC (S, *arrow*) is introduced at 265 msec, which abruptly normalizes the QRS as pacing is continued. In both instances, the VPC interrupted retrograde penetration of the blocked bundle branch as the cause of perpetuation of aberration. See text for discussion. T, time line.

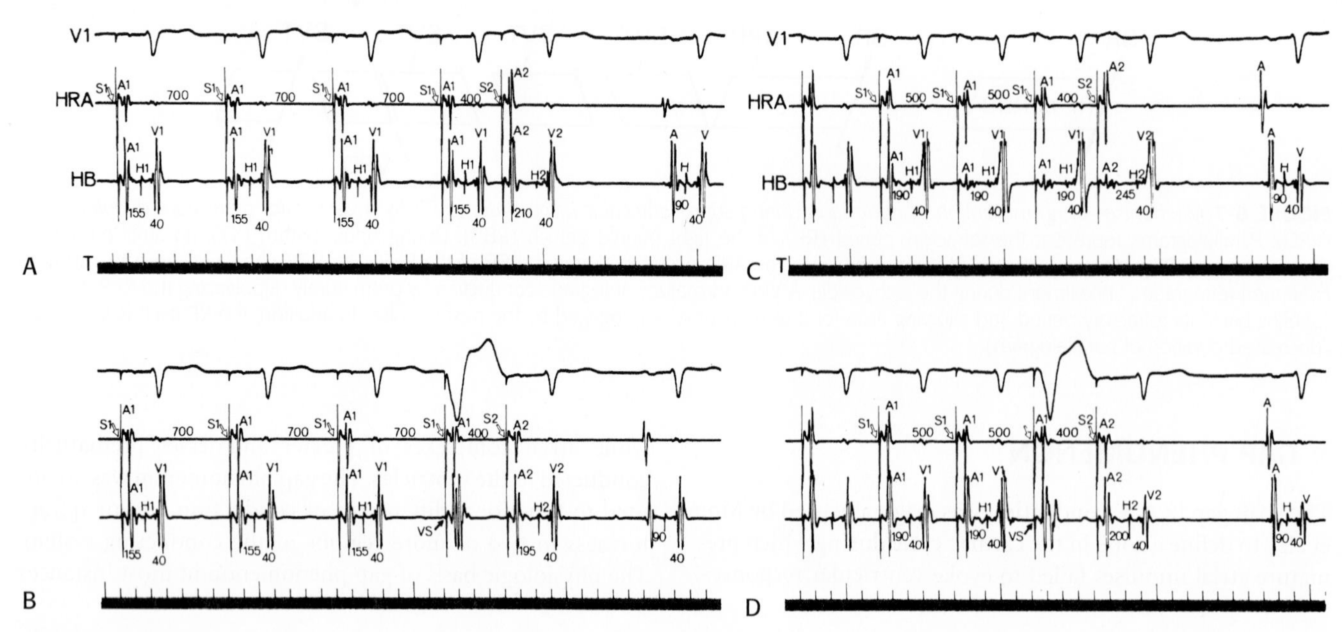


**FIGURE 6-9** *Effect of ventricular premature depolarization on atrioventricular (A-V) nodal conduction.* **A–D:** From **top** to **bottom** are surface ECG lead, high-right atrial (HRA), His bundle (HB) electrograms, and time line (T). **A** and **B:** At the longer basic cycle length (S1-S1) of 700 msec and an S1-S2 of 400 msec, **(A)** the S2-H2 is 210 msec with standard stimulation (method I). **B:** While with a preceding VPD simultaneous with the last paced beat (method II), the S21-H2 is 195 msec. **C** and **D:** At the shorter basic cycle length of 500 msec and an S1-S2 of 400 msec, **(C)** the S2-H2 interval is 245 msec with method I and, **(D)** 200 msec with method II. The magnitude of shortening in S2-H2 with method II is greater at shorter cycle lengths, **(C)** and **(D)**, than at longer cycle lengths, **(A)** and **(B)**. All measurements are in milliseconds; pertinent deflections and intervals are labeled. VS, ventricular beat introduced simultaneously with the last A1. (From Shenasa M, Denker S, Mahmud R, et al. Atrioventricular nodal conduction and refractoriness after intranodal collision from antegrade and retrograde impulses. *Circ* 1983;67:651.)

depended on a distal area with a long refractory period and a proximal site with a shorter refractory period. During the gap phenomenon, initial block occurs distally. With earlier impulses, proximal delay is encountered, which allows the distal site of early block to recover excitability and resume conduction.

Gaps in A-V conduction most commonly occur during programmed stimulation, although they may occur spontaneously.[17] The major significance of the gap phenomenon is its contribution to the understanding of conduction and refractoriness of the A-V conducting system. In particular, the resumption of conduction at shorter coupling intervals has frequently been interpreted as a form of "supernormal" conduction. In fact, the majority of cases of so-called supernormal conduction can be explained physiologically by the gap phenomenon. The common finding of all gaps already described has been that predicted by Moe; that block initially occurs distal to the stimulation site and that conduction resumes when earlier impulses result in proximal delay allowing the initial site of block to recover.[16]

Gaps may occur during either antegrade or retrograde stimulation. Any pair of structures in the A-V conduction system that have the appropriate physiologic relationship to one another can participate in gap phenomena. Six different types of antegrade gap and two types of retrograde gap have been described (Table 6-1).[18–20] In antegrade gap Types I, II, and III, the His–Purkinje system is the site of initial distal block with the A-V node (Type I, Fig. 6-10), proximal His–Purkinje system (Type II, Fig. 6-11), and His bundle (Type III, Fig. 6-12), respectively, as the site of proximal delay. These are, in descending order of frequency, by far the most common forms of antegrade gap. These three types, and all others in which the His–Purkinje system is the site of initial block, are most commonly observed during long drive cycle lengths, at which times His–Purkinje refractoriness is greatest. Multiple gaps may be recorded in the same patient. This is due to multiple levels of block and delay in the A-V conducting system. One such example is shown in Figure 6-13, in which distal block in the His–Purkinje system initially recovers because of delay in the proximal His–Purkinje system. Earlier coupling intervals again block, but dual A-V nodal pathways observed at even shorter coupling intervals (see Chapter 8) produce enough A-V nodal delay to allow the His–Purkinje system time to recover again. Retrograde gaps can manifest initial delay in the A-V node or in the His–Purkinje system, with proximal delay in the distal His–Purkinje system (Fig. 6-14).

Because the gap phenomenon depends on the relationship between the electrophysiologic properties of two sites, any interventions that alter these relationships (e.g., a change in cycle length or drug intervention) may eliminate or perpetuate the gap phenomenon and may also convert one type of

TABLE 6-1 Classification of Gap Phenomena in the Human Heart

| Type | Distal Site (Initial Block) | Proximal Site (Delay) |
|---|---|---|
| | **Antegrade** | |
| 1 | HPS | A-V node |
| 2 | HPS (distal) | HPS (proximal) |
| 3 | HPS | His bundle |
| 4 | HPS or A-V node | Atrium |
| 5 | A-V node (distal) | A-V node (proximal) |
| 6 | HPS | (?) True supernormality |
| | **Retrograde** | |
| 1 | A-V node | HPS |
| 2 | HPS (proximal) | HPS (distal) |

Adapted from Damato AN, Akhtar M, Ruskin J, et al. Gap phenomena: Antegrade and retrograde. In: Wellens HJJ, Lie KI, Janse MJ, eds. *The conduction system of the heart: Structure, function and clinical implications*. Philadelphia: Lea & Febiger, 1976:504.
A-V, atrioventricular; HPS, His–Purkinje system.

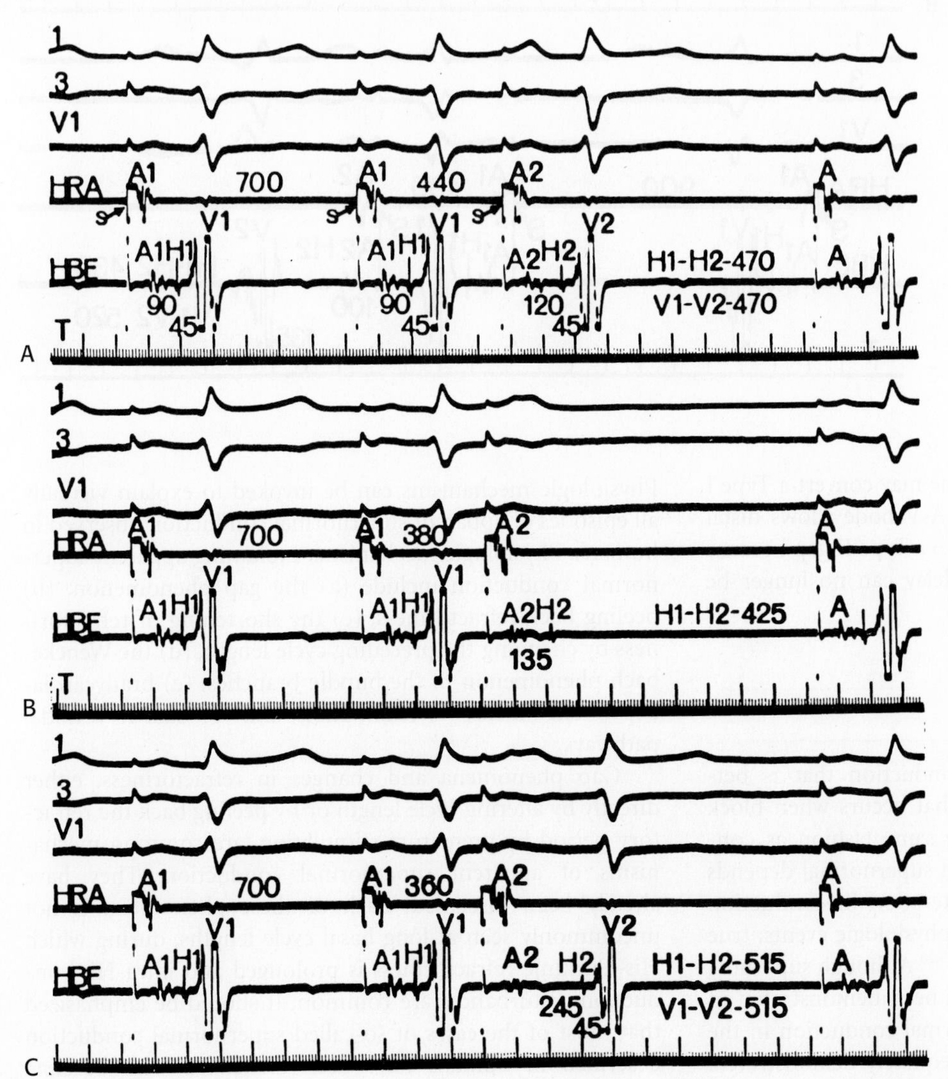


**FIGURE 6-10** *Type I gap in atrioventricular (A-V) conduction.* The basic atrial drive rate (A1-A1) in each panel is 700 msec, with the introduction of progressively premature atrial depolarization (A2). **A:** There is intact A-V conduction with a prolonged (120 msec) A2-H2 interval and an H1-H2 interval of 470 msec. **B:** Shortening A1-A2 to 380 msec results in an A2-H2 interval of 135 msec and an H1-H2 interval of 425 msec; the H1-H2 interval exceeds the effective refractory period (ERP) of the His–Purkinje system (HPS), and the atrial depolarization is blocked below the His bundle. **C:** Shortening A1-A2 to 380 msec results in a marked prolongation of the A2-H2 interval to 245 msec, and subsequent prolongation of the H1-H2 interval to 515 msec, which exceeds the ERP of the HPS, and A-V conduction resumes.

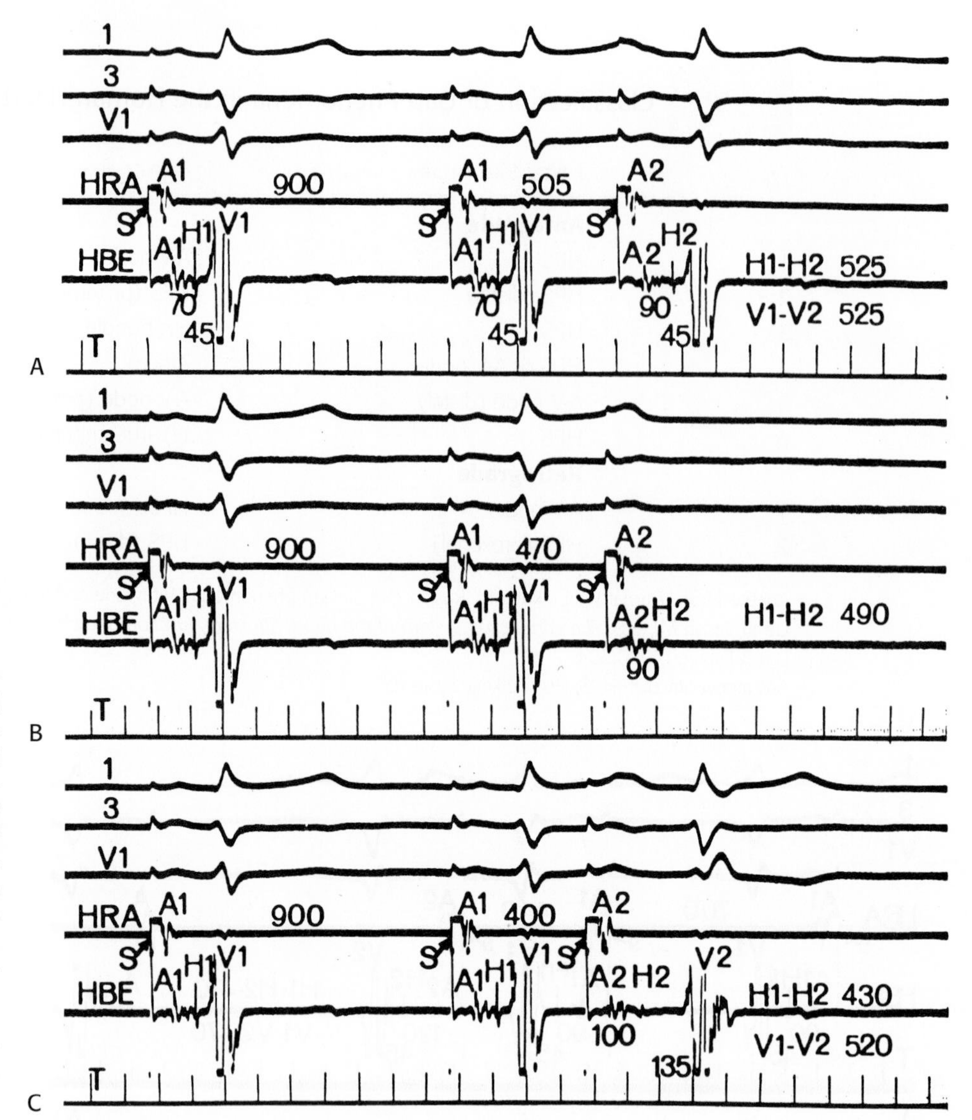


**FIGURE 6-11** *Type II gap in atrioventricular (A-V) conduction.* The basic atrial drive rate (A1-A1) is 900 msec. Progressively premature atrial extrastimuli (A2) are introduced. **A:** A-V conduction is intact. **B:** A2 is blocked below the His bundle as the H1-H2 interval of 490 msec exceeds the effective refractory period (ERP) of some portion of the HPS. **C:** Conduction resumes despite a still shorter A1-A2 (400 msec) and a shorter H1-H2 (430 msec). This resumption is postulated to be due to a delay in the proximal HPS, resulting in an H2-V2 interval of 135 msec, sufficient to allow the most refractory region (the "gate area") of the distal HPS to recover.

gap to another.[21] For example, atropine may convert a Type I gap, in which proximal delay in the A-V node allows distal recovery of the His–Purkinje system, to a Type II gap because the requisite degree of A-V nodal delay can no longer be achieved.[21]

## SUPERNORMALITY

Supernormal conduction implies conduction that is better than anticipated or conduction that occurs when block is expected.[22–24] Hence, in much the same fashion as concealed conduction, what is considered supernormal depends on what is anticipated. When an alteration in conduction can be explained in terms of known physiologic events, true supernormality need not be invoked.[25,26] Although supernormal conduction and excitability have been demonstrated in vitro,[23] the existence of true supernormal conduction in the intact human heart has not been adequately demonstrated. Physiologic mechanisms can be invoked to explain virtually all episodes of apparent supernormal conduction observed in humans. Physiologic mechanisms explaining apparent supernormal conduction include (a) the gap phenomenon, (b) peeling back refractoriness, (c) the shortening of refractoriness by changing the preceding cycle length, (d) the Wenckebach phenomenon in the bundle branches, (e) bradycardia-dependent blocks, (f) summation, and (g) dual A-V nodal pathways.

Gap phenomena and changes in refractoriness, either directly by altering cycle length or by peeling back the refractory period by premature stimulation, are common mechanisms of apparent supernormal conduction. They have already been discussed. Each of these phenomena is not uncommonly seen at long basal cycle lengths, during which His–Purkinje refractoriness is prolonged and infra-His conduction disturbances are common. It should be emphasized that most of the cases of so-called supernormal conduction described in humans have been associated with baseline

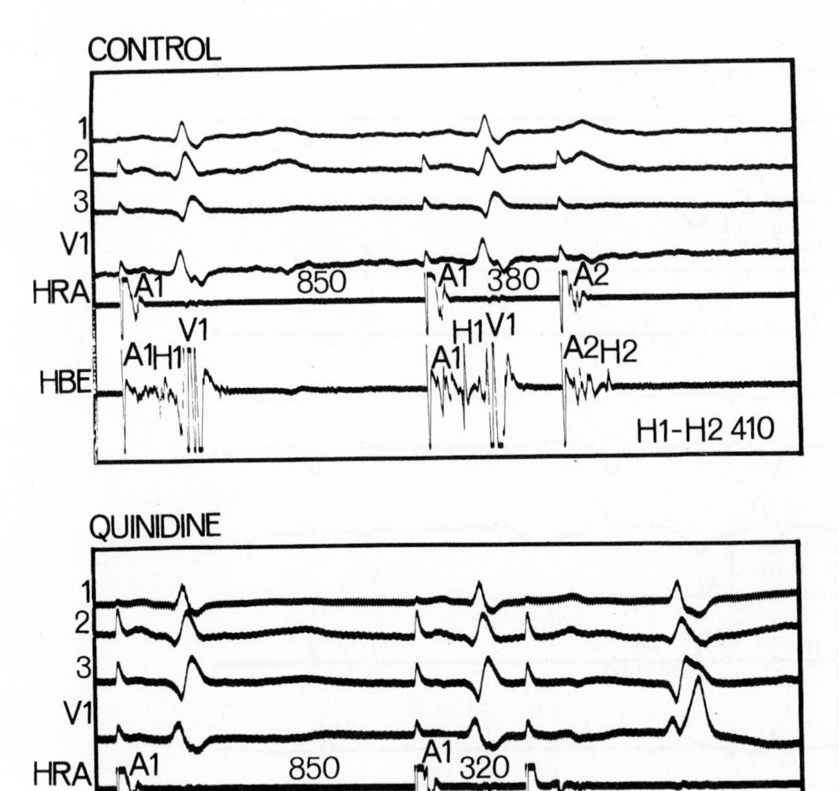


**FIGURE 6-12** *Type III gap in atrioventricular (A-V) conduction nduced by quinidine.* The basic atrial drive rate (A1-A1) in both panels is constant at 850 msec. A premature atrial stimulus (A2) introduced at a coupling interval (A1-A2) of 380 msec during the control period (**top** panel) results in an H1-H2 interval of 410 msec and block of the impulse in the HPS. One hour after the administration of quinidine gluconate, 800 mg intramuscularly (**bottom** panel), an identical H1-H2 interval (410 msec) A2 results in an intra-His delay (H2-H′) sufficient to allow the distal HPS to recover and conduct the beat to the ventricles. Note RBBB aberration in this conducted beat.

disturbances of A-V conduction. Therefore, the term supernormal has referred to improved conduction but not to conduction that is better than normal.[20]

The gap phenomenon and all its variants are probably the most common mechanisms of pseudo-supernormality (Figs. 6-10 through 6-14). An example of how marked delay in proximal His–Purkinje conduction allows an initial area of distal His–Purkinje block to recover excitability and to resume conduction is shown in Figure 6-15. Normalization of aberrant conduction with progressively premature APDs is associated with progressive intra-His delay (Fig. 6-16) or proximal His–Purkinje delay (Fig. 6-17), allowing recovery of the right bundle branch and left anterior division of the left bundle branch. Alternatively, Figure 6-17 may represent slowing of conduction in both the RBB and the left anterior fascicle in panel A; subsequently, further delay in the posterior fascicle, or more likely, the proximal LBB, produces equal delay in both the RBB and LBB so that the QRS "normalizes". As noted in Chapter 2, His–Purkinje refractoriness is cycle length dependent, and therefore aberration may not be manifested at identical coupling intervals if the preceding cycle length is shortened (see Fig. 2-17).

Type I (Wenckebach) second-degree block in the bundle branch system may result in either a progressive or a sudden normalization of aberration, with progressive delay being concealed in the surface ECG and with only the recovered cycle manifesting normal conduction (Fig. 6-18). Theoretically, any mechanism that removes retrograde invasion will normalize A-V conduction (see Fig. 6-7). Another cause of normalization of aberration is the appearance of a ventricular premature depolarization (VPD) from the "blocked" ventricle. This pattern, however, is rarely repetitive and/or reproducible. Although equal and sudden simultaneous delay in the opposite bundle branch could theoretically normalize the QRS, it would be associated with a prolonged H-V (and P-R) interval (see Fig. 6-16). Furthermore, further premature complexes would unlikely conduct with a normal QRS because it would require continuous equal slowing in both bundle branches.

Another form of pseudo-supernormal conduction is facilitation of A-V nodal conduction by a VPD (Fig. 6-19). Because A-V nodal refractoriness is inversely proportional to cycle length, facilitation of A-V nodal conduction by a VPD cannot implicitly be explained by alterations in refractoriness either directly or by peeling back. Such facilitation, which has been shown to require simultaneous atrial activation,[15] more likely results from summation, as suggested by Zipes et al.[6]

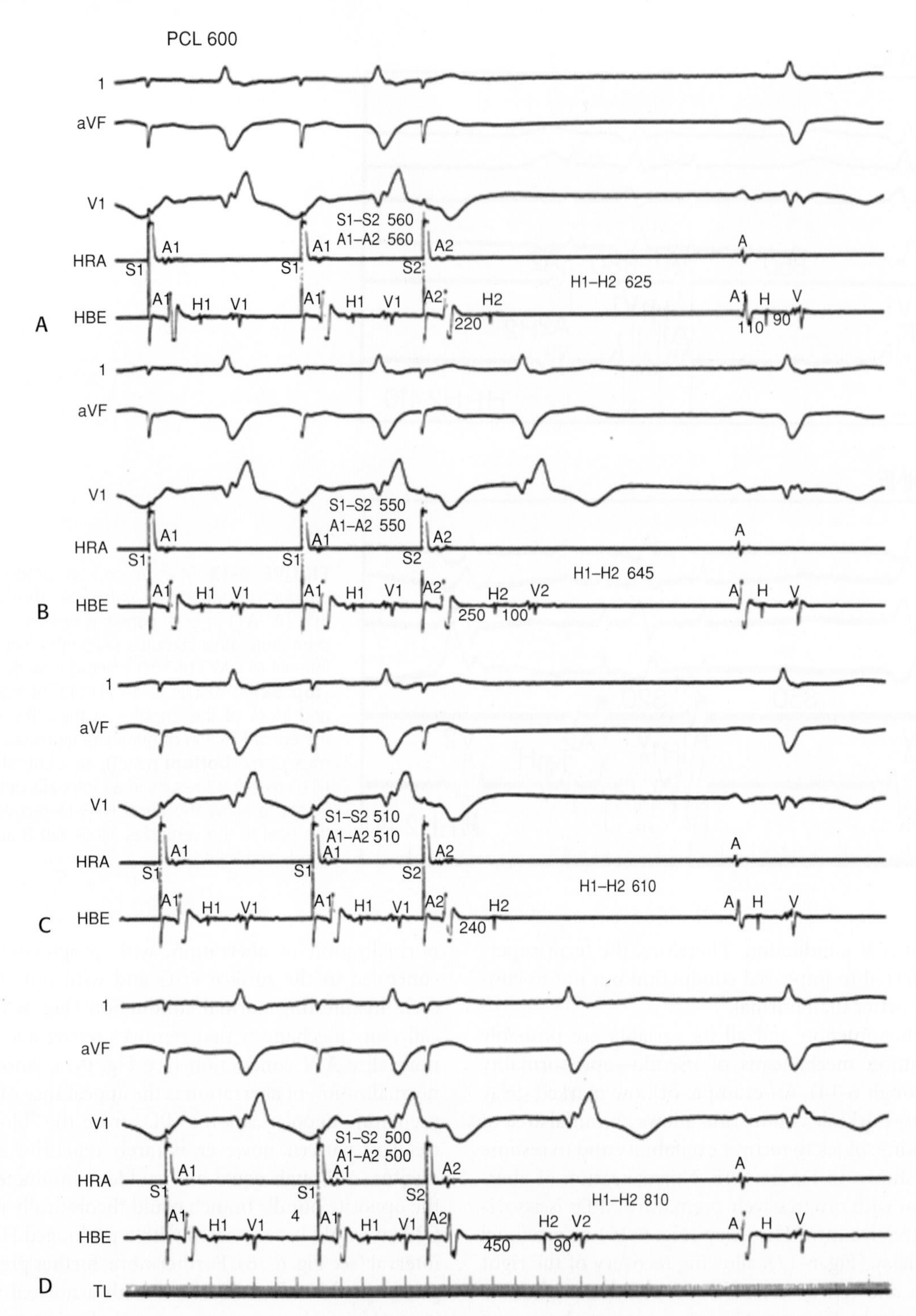


**FIGURE 6-13** *Multiple levels of conduction delay associated with gaps in the atrioventricular (A-V) conducting system.* **A** to **D:** From **top** to **bottom**, leads 1, aVF, and V1, and electrograms from the high-right atrium (HRA) and His bundle (HBE). In each panel, the atrium is paced at a constant paced cycle length (PCL) of 600 msec, and progressively premature atrial extrastimuli (A2) are delivered. **A:** A1A2 are 560 msec; A2 blocks below the His bundle. The effective refractory period (ERP) of the His–Purkinje system is defined as an H1–H2 of 625 msec. **B:** At a shorter coupled A2 delay in both the A-V node and proximal His–Purkinje system allow recovery of the initial site of block. **C:** At a shorter coupling interval, not enough delay is produced in the A-V node or proximal His–Purkinje system to allow conduction to occur. **D:** At a 10-msec shorter coupling interval, however, dual A-V nodal pathway producing a marked jump in the A2–H2 interval to 450 msec allows the initial site of block to recover. Thus, multiple levels of conduction delay and block are present, all of which contribute gap phenomena. See text for discussion. TL, time line.

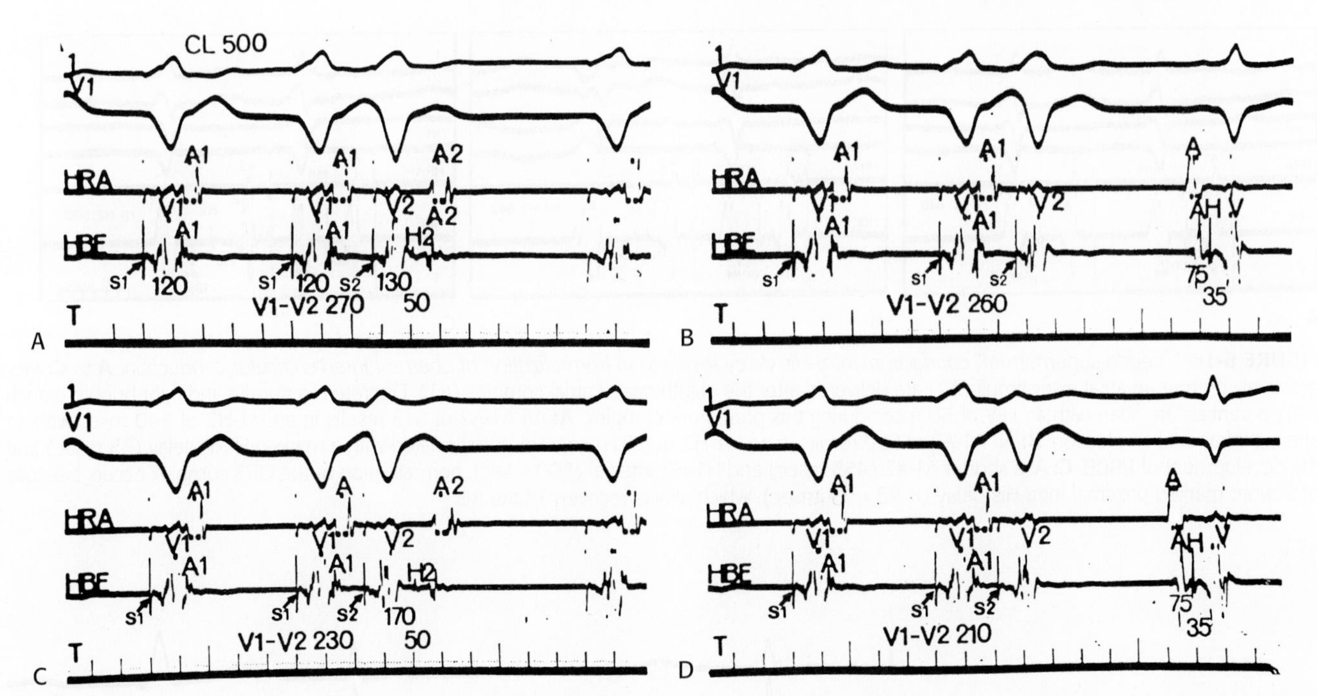


**FIGURE 6-14** *Type II retrograde gap in ventriculoatrial (V-A) conduction.* The ventricular drive rate is constant at 500 msec. Note the low-to-high sequence of atrial activation. **A:** V2 encounters retrograde conduction delay below the His bundle. The S2-H2 interval is 130 msec, and retrograde activation of the atria occurs. **B:** V2 blocks within the HPS and neither HZ nor AZ is seen. **C:** With further prematurity of V2, conduction resumes with a S2-H2 of 170 msec as V2 encounters delay before the site of initial block, allowing sufficient time for recovery. **D:** The effective refractory period of the site of delay is reached, and V-A conduction is again interrupted.

Another cause of pseudo-supernormal conduction is bradycardia-dependent bundle branch block with normalization of the QRS complexes at shorter cycle lengths or with APCs (Fig. 6-20). The physiologic explanation for phase 4 block is enhanced automaticity and/or partial depolarization of injured myocardial tissue. Propagation of supraventricular impulses is more difficult late in diastole because the impulses encounter partially depolarized tissue through which voltage-dependent conduction is not possible (Chapter 5).

Dual A-V nodal pathways can be manifested by intermittent long or short P-R intervals, depending on which pathway is used for antegrade conduction. Perpetuation of one pattern

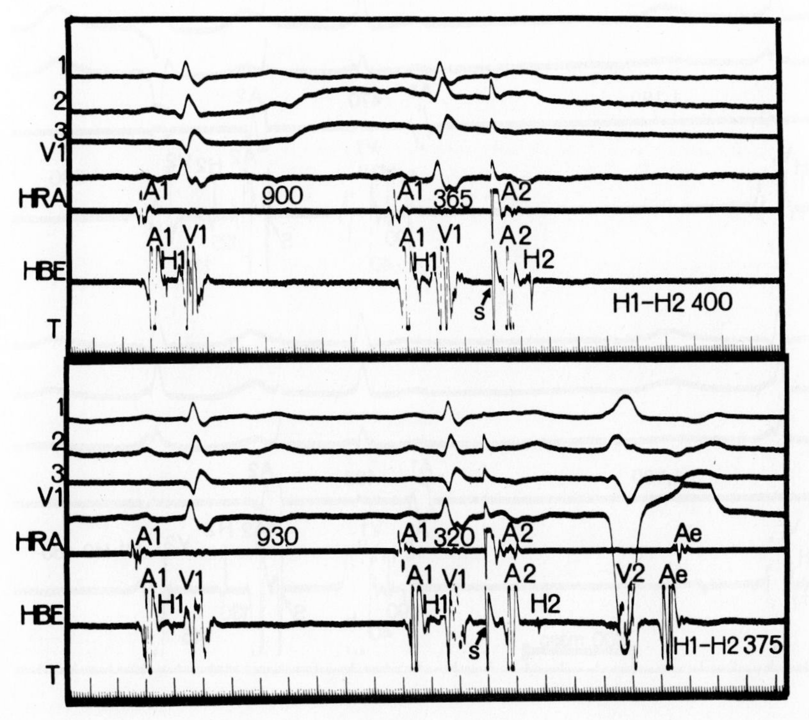


**FIGURE 6-15** *"Pseudo-supernormal" conduction that is due to Type II atrioventricular (A-V) gap.* In the **top** panel, an atrial extrastimulus (A2) that was introduced during sinus rhythm at a coupling interval (A1-A2) of 365 msec blocks below the His bundle deflection. In the **bottom** panel, an atrial extrastimulus (A2) that was introduced at a coupling interval of 320 msec is conducted despite a slightly longer preceding sinus cycle length that, if anything, would be expected to favor nonconduction. Note the strikingly long H2-V2 (235 msec), which has permitted the distal HPS to recover. The resultant beat is conducted with left bundle branch block, and it is followed by an atrial echo (Ae).

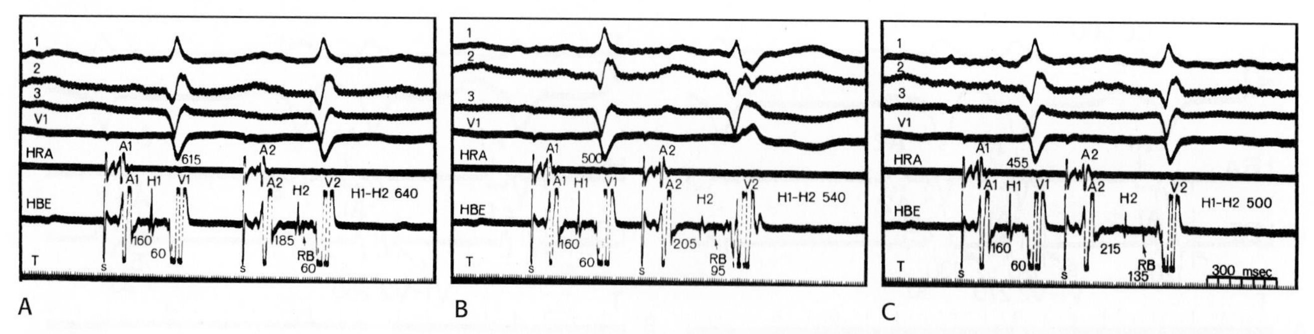


**FIGURE 6-16** *"Pseudo-supernormal" conduction; intra-His delay resulting in normalization of aberrant interventricular conduction.* **A** to **C:** Progressively premature atrial extrastimuli (A2) are delivered after the eighth paced atrial complex (A1). Discrete His bundle and right bundle branch (RB) potentials are seen with an H-V of 60 msec during this premature complex. **A:** An A1-A2 of 615 results in an H1-H2 of 640 msec without altering infranodal conduction. **B:** An A1-A2 of 500 results in an H1-H2 of 540 msec. This is associated with a marked H-RB delay (35 msec) and the development of RBBB. **C:** At a shorter A1-A2 (455 msec) and H1-H2 interval (500 msec), normalization of the QRS complex occurs because of a more marked proximal intra-His delay (H-RB = 75 msec), which allows recovery of the RB.

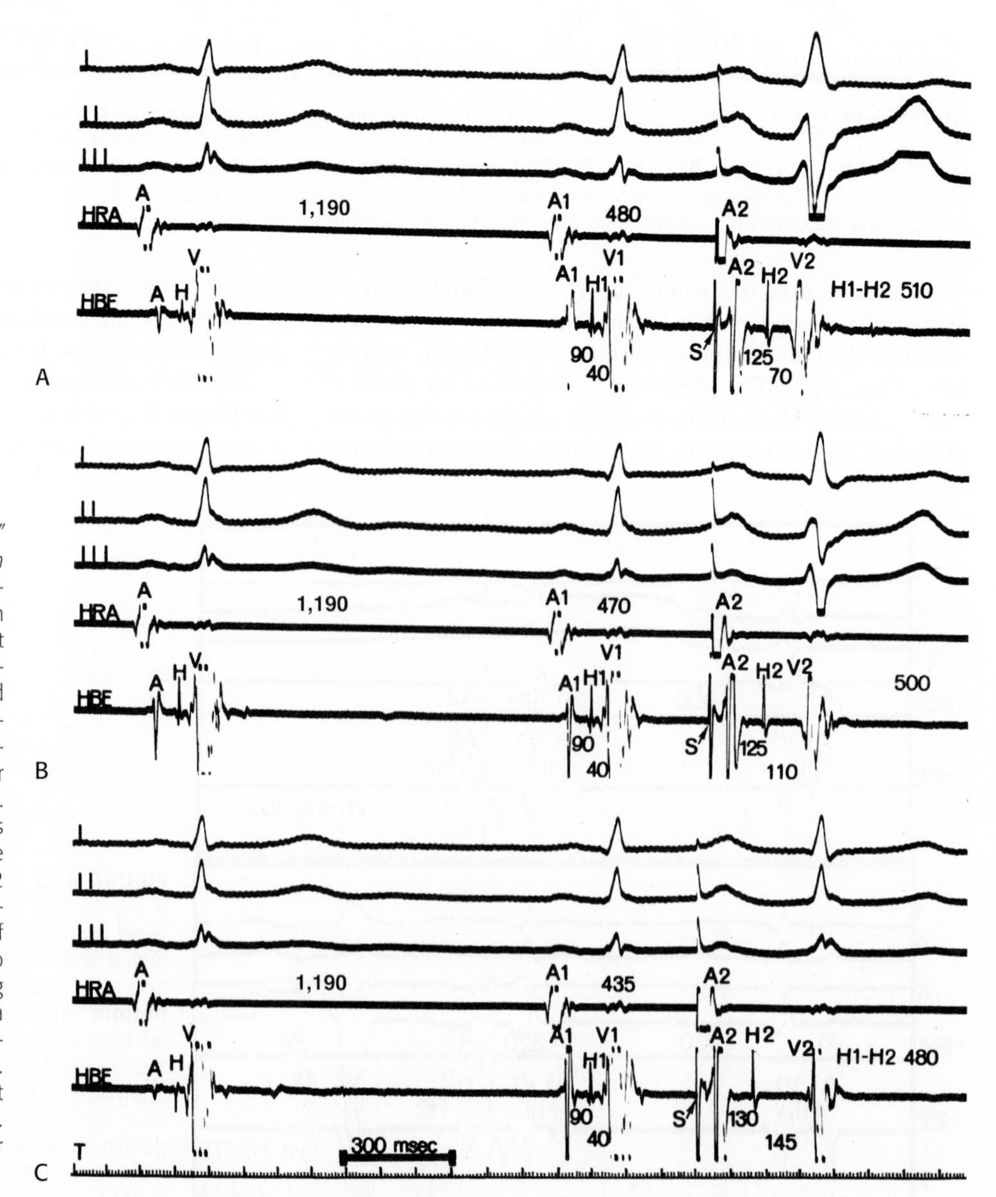


**FIGURE 6-17** *"Pseudo-supernormal" conduction; HPS delay resulting in normalization of aberrant interventricular conduction.* The basic rhythm in all panels is sinus, with a constant cycle length of 1,190 msec. A premature atrial stimulus (A2) is introduced at progressively shorter coupling intervals. **A:** The premature beat is conducted with a RBBB and left anterior hemiblock (axis 60 degrees) pattern. **B:** The conducted QRS complex is less aberrant. **C:** It is virtually identical to the sinus beats-despite decreasing H1-H2 intervals. However, the H2-V2 progressively increases, and normalization of the QRS complex can be attributed to proximal delay in the HPS, allowing progressive recovery of the distal area of delay and aberration. (From Gallagher JJ, Damato AN, Varghese PJ, et al. Alternative mechanisms of apparent supernormal atrioventricular conduction. *Am J Cardiol* 1973;31:362.) See text for discussion.

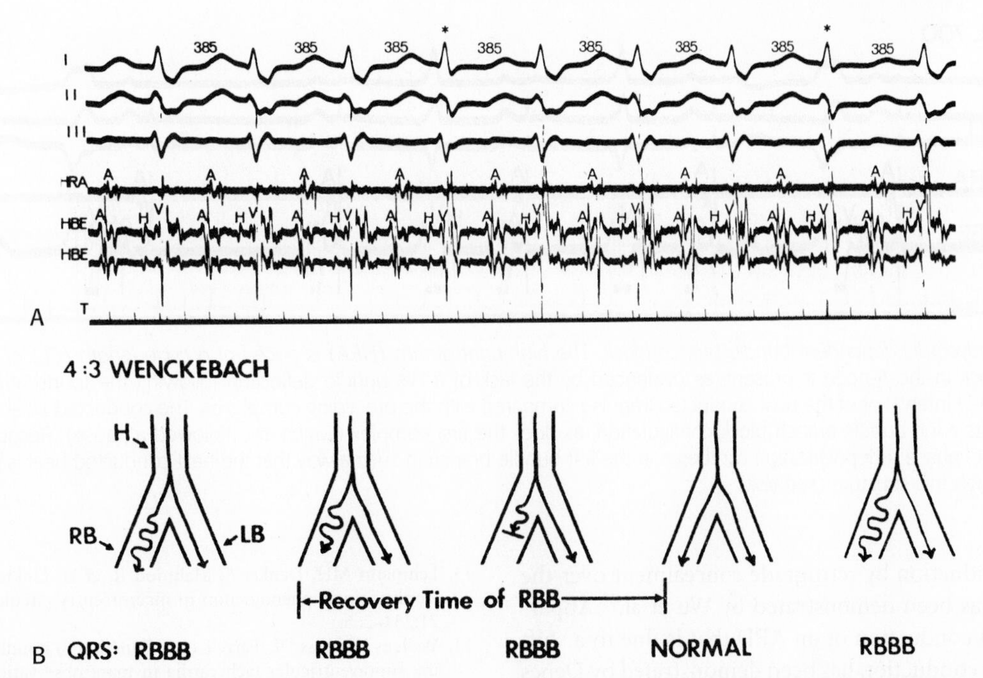


**FIGURE 6-18** *"Pseudo-supernormal" conduction that is due to Type I (Wenckebach) second-degree block in the right bundle branch (RBB).* **A:** Superventricular tachycardia with RBB block (RBBB) is shown at a cycle length of 385 msec. The fourth and eighth complexes (*asterisks*) manifest normal conduction. **B:** Repetitive normalization in this fashion can be explained by a Wenckebach-type block in the RBBB, which is schematically presented. In panel **(A)** the normal, constant H-V interval (45 msec) suggests normal conduction through the left bundle (LB) branches. Conduction through the RBB is progressively impaired because of some area of prolonged refractoriness. The first two impulses variably penetrate this area, while the third complex fails to engage the area. This effectively doubles the cycle length of the impulses that reach the critical area of delay, allowing time for recovery and subsequent normal conduction. (From Gallagher JJ, Damato AN, Varghese PJ, et al. Alternative mechanisms of apparent supernormal atrioventricular conduction. *Am J Cardiol* 1973;31:362.)

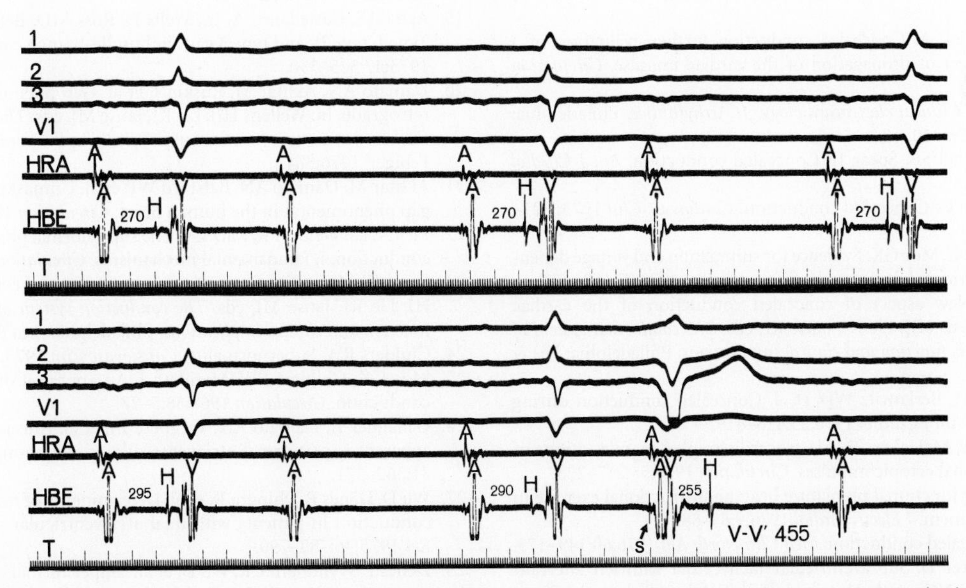


**FIGURE 6-19** *Facilitation of atrioventricular (A-V) modal conduction by a ventricular premature depolarization (VPD).* The basic rhythm is sinus with stable 2:1 block in the A-V node. The A-H interval on conducted beats ranges from 270 msec to 295 msec. A ventricular extrastimulus is introduced (S), and the sinus impulse that would have expected to block in the A-V node conducts through the node with an A-H interval of 255 msec. This probably results from summation of the blocked impulse and the retrogradely concealed VPD. See text for details.

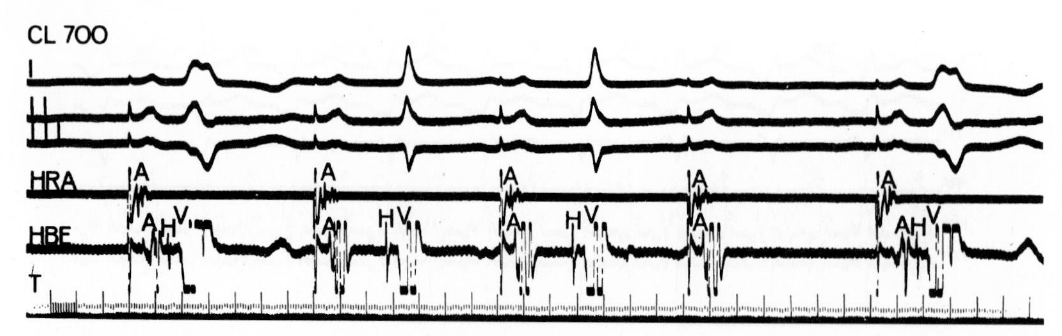


**FIGURE 6-20** *Bradycardia-dependent bundle branch block. The high-right atrium (HRA) is paced at a cycle length (CL) of 700 msec.* Type I second-degree block in the A-node is present, as evidenced by the lack of a His bundle deflection following the fourth atrial complex and a shortening of the A-H interval or of the next conducted impulse compared with the preceding complexes. The conducted atrial complex following the pause manifests a left bundle branch block configuration, as does the first complex (which also followed a pause). Because block is occurring in the A-V node, phase 4 depolarization can begin in the left bundle branch in such a way that the next conducted beat is propagated slowly (or not at all) through this structure (see text).

of antegrade conduction by retrograde concealment over the other pathway has been demonstrated by Wu et al.[27] Apparent supernormal conduction of an APD that is due to a shift from slow to fast conduction has been demonstrated by Denes et al.[28] We have seen spontaneous examples of junctional premature complexes and VPC shift fast to slow pathways and vice versa. The methods of evaluating dual A-V nodal pathways are described in Chapter 8.

## REFERENCES


1. Langendorf R. Concealed A-V conduction: the effect of blocked impulses on the formation and conduction of subsequent impulses. *Am Heart J* 1948;35:542.
2. Langendorf R, Pick A. Concealed conduction further evaluation of a fundamental aspect of propagation of the cardiac impulse. *Circulation* 1956;13:381–399.
3. Katz LN, Pick A. *Clinical electrocardiology. 1. Arrhythmias.* Philadelphia: Lea & Febiger, 1956:540.
4. Moore EN, Knoebel SB, Spear JF. Concealed conduction. *Am J Cardiol* 1971;28:406–413.
5. Knoebel SB, Fisch C. Concealed conduction. *Cardiovasc Clin* 1973;5:21–34.
6. Zipes DP, Mendez C, Moe GK. Evidence for summation and voltage dependency in rabbit atrioventricular nodal fibers. *Circ Res* 1973;32:170–177.
7. Langendorf R. New aspect of concealed conduction of the cardiac impulse. In: Wellens HJJ, Lie KI, Janse KI, eds. *The conduction system of the heart: structure, function and clinical implications.* Philadelphia: Lea & Febiger, 1976:410.
8. Cohen SI, Lau SH, Berkowitz WD, et al. Concealed conduction during atrial fibrillation. *Am J Cardiol* 1970;25:416–419.
9. Fisch C, Zipes DP, McHenry PL. Electrocardiographic manifestations of concealed junctional ectopic impulses. *Circulation* 1976;53:217–223.
10. Childers RW. The junctional premature beat: an instructional exercise in modes of concealment. *J Electrocardiol* 1976;9:85–88.
11. Childers R. Concealed conduction. *Med Clin North Am* 1976;60:149–173.
12. Wellens HJ, Durrer D. Supraventricular tachycardia with left aberrant conduction due to retrograde invasion into the left bundle branch. *Circulation* 1968;38:474–479.
13. Lehmann MH, Denker S, Mahmud R, et al. Linking: a dynamic electrophysiologic phenomenon in macroreentry circuits. *Circulation* 1985; 71:254–265.
14. Wellens HJ, Ross DL, Farre J, et al. Function of bundle branch block during supraventricular tachycardia in man: observations on mechanisms and their incidence. In: Zipes DP, Jalife J, eds. *Cardiac electrophysiology and arrhythmias.* Orlando: Grune and Stratton, Inc., 1985:435.
15. Shenasa M, Denker S, Mahmud R, et al. Atrioventricular nodal conduction and refractoriness after intranodal collision from antegrade and retrograde impulses. *Circulation* 1983;67:651–660.
16. Moe GK, Mendez C, Han J. Aberrant A-V impulse propagation in the dog heart: a study of functional bundle branch block. *Circ Res* 1965;16: 261–286.
17. Bonow RO, Josephson ME. Spontaneous gap phenomenon in atrioventricular conduction produced by His bundle extrasystoles. *J Electrocardiol* 1977;10:283–286.
18. Wu D, Denes P, Dhingra R, et al. Nature of the gap phenomenon in man. *Circ Res* 1974;34:682–692.
19. Agha AS, Castellanos A, Jr., Wells D, Ross MD, Befeler B, Myerburg RJ. Type I, type II, and type 3 gaps in bundle-branch conduction. *Circulation* 1973;47:325–330.
20. Damato AN, Akhtar M, Ruskin J, et al. Gap phenomena: antegrade and retrograde. In: Wellens HJJ, Lie KI, Janse MJ, eds. *The conduction system of the heart: structure, function and clinical implications.* Philadelphia: Lea & Febiger, 1976:504.
21. Akhtar M, Damato AN, Batsford WP, et al. Unmasking and conversion of gap phenomenon in the human heart. *Circulation* 1974;49:624–630.
22. Pick A, Langendorf R, Katz LN. The supernormal phase of atrioventricular conduction. I. Fundamental mechanisms. *Circulation* 1962;26:388–404.
23. Spear JP, Moore EN. Supernormal excitability and conduction. In: Wellens HJ, Lie KI, Janse MJ, eds. *The conduction system of the heart: structure, function and clinical implications.* Philadelphia: Lea & Febiger, 1976:111.
24. Childers RW. Supernormality. *Cardiovasc Clin* 1973;5:135–158.
25. Moe GK, Childers RW, Merideth J. An appraisal of "supernormal" A-V conduction. *Circulation* 1968;38:5–28.
26. Gallagher JJ, Damato AN, Varghese PJ, et al. Alternative mechanisms of apparent supernormal atrioventricular conduction. *Am J Cardiol* 1973; 31:362–371.
27. Wu D, Denes P, Dhingra R, et al. Determinants of fast- and slow-pathway conduction in patients with dual atrioventricular nodal pathways. *Circ Res* 1975;36:782–790.
28. Denes P, Wyndham CR, Wu D, et al. "Supernormal conduction" of a premature impulse utilizing the fast pathway in a patient with dual atrioventricular nodal pathways. *Circulation* 1975;51:811–814.

CHAPTER

# 7 Ectopic Rhythms and Premature Depolarizations

Ectopic depolarizations can arise from many areas of the heart, but the surface ECG is markedly limited in its ability to precisely define the origin of such ectopic activity. Although various ECG guidelines have been proposed to distinguish supraventricular depolarization from ventricular depolarizations, for example, none are foolproof. Nevertheless, knowledge of the origin of impulse formation has become critical in the current era of catheter ablation. Recording intracardiac electrograms is the most reliable method of defining the origin of ectopic activity. Such recordings have thus provided the most accurate method of localizing and characterizing ectopic activity and have made us aware of the many limitations of the surface ECG in the evaluation of these arrhythmias. More recently, Hariman et al.[1–4] have demonstrated that the use of high-gain specially filtered electrograms (0.1 to 25 to 50 Hz) can be used to detect automaticity in ectopic foci of the ventricle, atrium, and atrioventricular (A-V) junction (AVJ). The frequency with which such signals can be obtained has not yet been evaluated. However, it is logical that, analogous to sinus node electrograms, automaticity could be detected in very well-localized areas. Another potential method to localize and postulate mechanisms of arrhythmias is through the use of recording monophasic action potentials (MAPs) to record afterdepolarizations.[5–9] While many accept MAP recordings, much concern exists in my mind as to whether what is recorded is truly responsible for the arrhythmia it is being used to localize. In my opinion, further validation of these techniques demonstrating a causal relationship to arrhythmogenesis is needed before this technique is applied clinically.

## ATRIAL DEPOLARIZATIONS

The ability to assess atrial activity by standard ECG criteria is limited. Atrial anatomy, prior surgery, fibrosis, drugs, and atrial position in the thorax can influence propagation of atrial activity and, therefore, P-wave morphology. Thus, the predictive accuracy of P-wave morphology for sites of ectopic atrial impulses is limited in the presence of these factors. Although a P wave in the surface ECG is the manifestation of atrial activation, even the absence of P waves cannot be taken to exclude the presence of atrial activity. In an occasional patient, the surface ECG demonstrates the absence of P waves, a normal QRS complex, and a regular (Fig. 7-1) or an irregular rhythm (Fig. 7-2), suggesting either a junctional (His bundle) rhythm with atrial quiescence or atrial fibrillation. In such cases, atrial electrograms frequently can be recorded in either the left or right atrium, and in some cases they may be localized to a discrete site within one or both atria (Fig. 7-2).[10–12] This situation occurs not uncommonly in the setting of chronic heart disease (particularly rheumatic heart disease), with dilated diseased atria.[12] Moreover, in our experience, during so-called sinoventricular conduction that is due to hyperkalemia, atrial electrograms have always been recorded. Thus, because atrial activity may be present without representation on the ECG, intracardiac recordings may be the only method of assessing unexplained supraventricular rhythms.

Endocardial mapping of the atria is a tool with which the site of origin of atrial premature depolarizations (APDs) can be ascertained.[13] Because P-wave morphology on the surface ECG is determined by the patterns of interatrial and intra-atrial conduction, which can be markedly affected by disease and/or drugs, the ECG cannot always be used accurately before the site of origin of APDs.[11,14–16]

Figure 7-3 demonstrates an APD that originates in the left atrium. The pulmonary veins are an important source of APDs. Haissaguerre et al.[17,18] have shown that APDs originating in the pulmonary veins can initiate atrial fibrillation. Cure of atrial fibrillation can be accomplished by ablating such foci.[17,18] Other frequent sites of APDs and atrial tachycardias are the atrial appendages, crista terminalis, coronary sinus, ligament of Marshall, superior vena cava, and fibers around the mitral and tricuspid valve. The relative frequency of these sites, and their electrocardiographic features, in a large series of atrial tachycardias was recently reported by Kistler et al. (Fig. 7-4).[19] I believe the ECG is limited in precisely localizing the site of atrial foci not only because of limitations sited in preceding paragraphs, but because the entire P wave is frequently not discernible from the T wave. Because superiorly directed P waves can be observed with APDs that originate low in the right atrium, as well as in the left atrium or coronary sinus, intracardiac recording is the only method of localizing the origin of such P waves. Moreover, if P-wave morphologies of APDs appear similar to sinus P waves, the only method of differentiating those premature impulses from sinus arrhythmia or sinus node reentry (see Chapter 8) or ectopic impulses

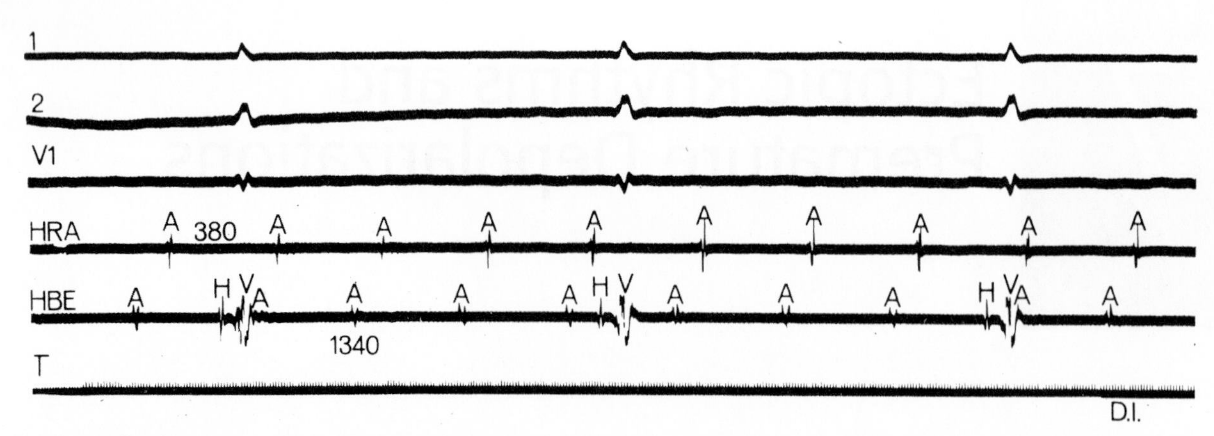


**FIGURE 7-1** *Atrial tachycardia in the absence of P waves on the surface QRS.* Leads 1, 2, and V1 are shown with electrograms from the high-right atrium (HRA), His bundle (HBE), and time lines (T). There is a dissociation of atrial activity and ventricular activity; thus, complete heart block is present. Simultaneously, a regular atrial rhythm at a cycle length of 380 msec is seen in the intracardiac recordings, yet there are no distinct P waves on the surface ECG. Hyperkalemia with so-called "sinoventricular rhythm" was assumed to be present in the patient.

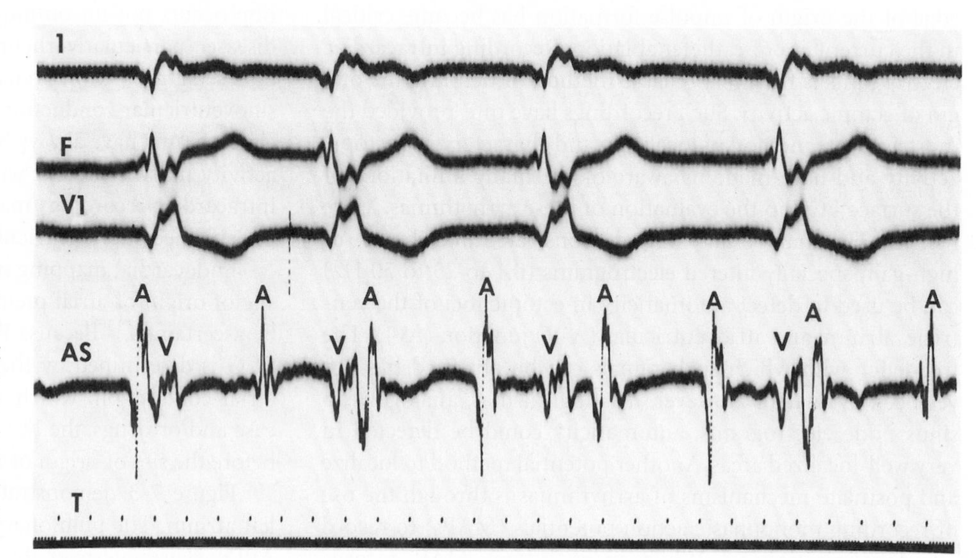


**FIGURE 7-2** *Atrial tachycardia with absence of P waves on the surface ECG.* ECG leads 1, F, and V1 are shown with an atrial electrogram recorded at the low atrial septum (AS). The surface ECG demonstrates an irregular rhythm and no P waves, suggesting atrial fibrillation. However, an intra-atrial electrogram from the AS revealed atrial tachycardia (A-A = 375 msec) with variable block. T, time line.

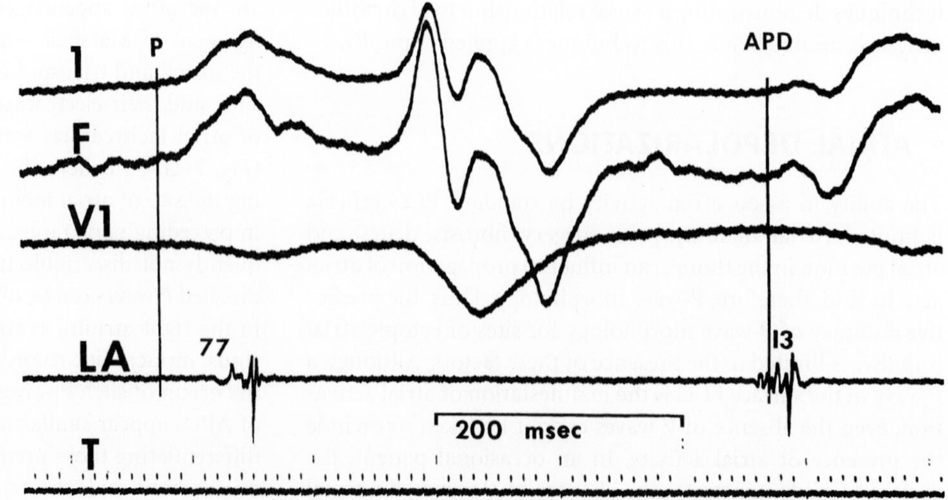


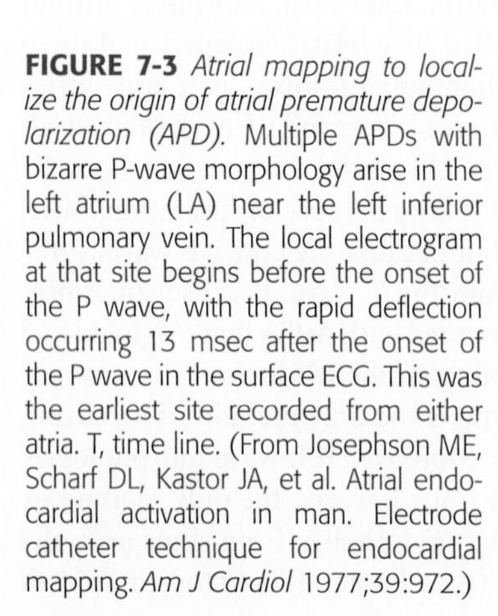

**FIGURE 7-3** *Atrial mapping to localize the origin of atrial premature depolarization (APD).* Multiple APDs with bizarre P-wave morphology arise in the left atrium (LA) near the left inferior pulmonary vein. The local electrogram at that site begins before the onset of the P wave, with the rapid deflection occurring 13 msec after the onset of the P wave in the surface ECG. This was the earliest site recorded from either atria. T, time line. (From Josephson ME, Scharf DL, Kastor JA, et al. Atrial endocardial activation in man. Electrode catheter technique for endocardial mapping. *Am J Cardiol* 1977;39:972.)

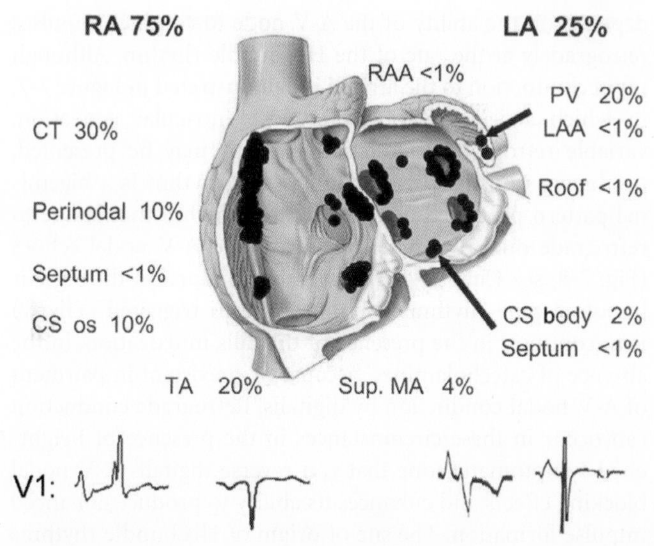


**FIGURE 7-4** *Sites of origin of atrial tachycardias.* The sites of mapped atrial tachycardias are shown on a schema of the heart. P waves characterizing these sites are possible, with limitations. (Modified from Kistler PM, Roberts-Thomson KC, Haqqani HM, et al. P-wave morphology in focal atrial tachycardia: development of an algorithm to predict the anatomic site of origin. *J Am Coll Cardiol* 2006;48:1010–1017.)

in the region of the sinus node is mapping the sequence of atrial activation of the early complexes. An atrial activation sequence different from that during sinus rhythm confirms the premature complexes as ectopic, despite a surface P-wave morphology similar to sinus. Automaticity (suggested by recording phase 4 activity) and triggered activity (suggested by recording delayed afterdepolarizations) have been postulated as the mechanism of APDs[2,3] based on experimental studies.[20–23] How valid these conclusions are and, if they are, how frequent such mechanisms are operative, remain speculative. Certainly many of the atrial tachycardias that are catecholamine sensitive are likely to be due to these mechanisms. The morphology of the electrogram at the site of origin, that is, fractionated, split, etc., does not determine the mechanism of the APD. It is only a reflection of propagation of the atrial impulse.

The site of origin of an atrial impulse can affect the P-R intervals.[24–26] Such an apparent alteration in A-V conduction (i.e., changing P-R interval) may result from a different input into the A-V node, either qualitatively or in relationship to the activation of the remainder of the atrium. An example of that phenomenon is depicted in Figure 7-5; different atrial rhythms are associated with different P-R intervals despite identical A-H intervals. This situation is a result of an earlier input into the A-V node relative to atrial activation during the rhythm shown on the left. Shorter A-H intervals than sinus are more often observed with ectopic atrial activation originating in the coronary sinus or inferoposterior left atrium (Fig. 7-6). The response of the A-V node to pacing and premature atrial stimulation from different sites suggests that in some instances atrial activation originating in the coronary sinus seems to bypass part of the node, leading to shorter A-V nodal conduction and Wenckebach cycles.

Finally, it is important to distinguish atrial echoes that are due to reentry in the sinus node, A-V node, or via a concealed A-V bypass tract from APDs. The relationship of these reentrant phenomena to conduction delay and the specific patterns of atrial activation associated with these echoes are discussed in Chapters 8 and 10.

## ■ JUNCTIONAL (HIS BUNDLE OR A-V NODAL) DEPOLARIZATIONS

His bundle depolarizations can be definitively recognized only by intracardiac recordings, especially if their manifestations are concealed. Junctional (most commonly, His bundle depolarizations) most frequently take the form of escape rhythms in the presence of sinus node dysfunction (Chapter 3) or A-V

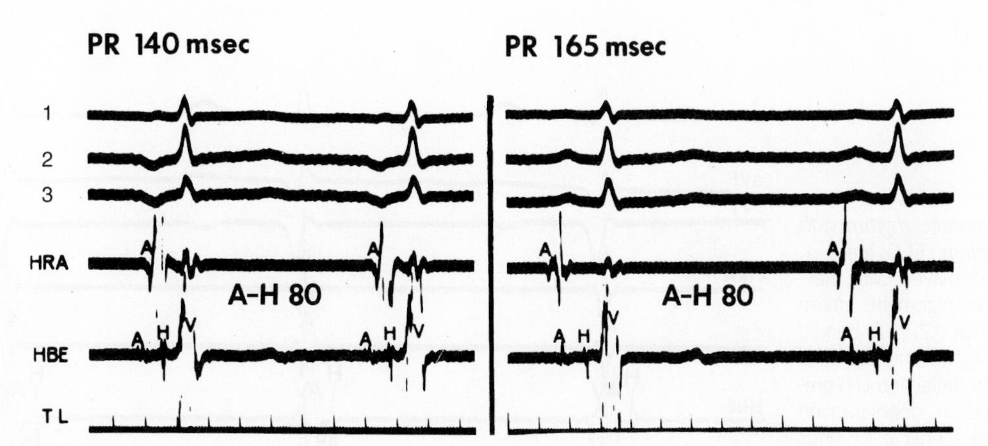


**FIGURE 7-5** *Different P-R intervals with identical A-H intervals, which is due to altered atrial activation and input into the atrioventricular (A-V) node.* ECG leads 1, 2, and 3 are shown with a high-right atrial (HRA) and a His bundle electrogram (HBE). The panel on the **left** was taken during a low-right atrial rhythm (A in HBE is earliest and precedes the onset of the surface P wave). The panel on the **right** was taken during sinus rhythm. Note that despite a difference in P-R intervals, A-V nodal conduction remains the same (A-H = 80 msec). TL, time line.

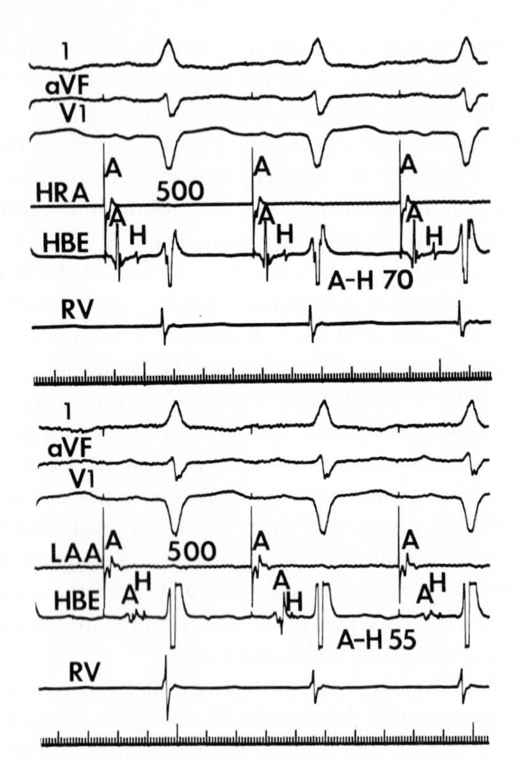


**FIGURE 7-6** *Effect of stimulation site on A-H interval.* The A-H intervals during pacing from the high-right atrium (HRA) and left atrial appendage (LAA) at a cycle length of 500 msec are shown. The A-H interval during left atrial pacing is shorter (55 msec) than that during HRA pacing (70 msec). This is likely due to left atrial input to the A-V node. HBE, His bundle electrogram; RV, right ventricle.

nodal block (Chapter 4). These escape rhythms usually have a QRS morphology identical to that during sinus rhythm. However, the hallmark of these rhythms is a His bundle deflection that precedes ventricular depolarization by a normal or greater than normal (in the case of bradycardia-dependent intra- or infra-His conduction disturbances) H-V interval (Fig. 7-7). In the latter instance (i.e., intra- or infra-His delay) the QRS usually is aberrant. Retrograde atrial activation may or may not accompany His bundle rhythms, and it depends on the ability of the A-V node to conduct impulses retrogradely at the rate of the His bundle rhythm. Although rapid conduction to the atrium is demonstrated in Figure 7-7, in which atrial activation precedes ventricular activation, variable retrograde conduction patterns may be presented, producing unusual rhythms. One such rhythm is a bigeminal pattern produced by a His bundle rhythm that is due to retrograde dual A-V nodal pathways and A-V nodal echoes (Fig. 7-8; see Chapter 8). Retrograde conduction during His bundle escape rhythms (or those due to triggered activity) is uncommon in the presence of digitalis intoxication, in the absence of catecholamines, because of coexistent impairment of A-V nodal conduction by digitalis. Retrograde conduction can occur in these circumstances in the presence of heightened symptomatic tone that can reverse digitalis A-V nodal blocking effects and enhances its ability to produce enhanced impulse formation. The site of origin of His bundle rhythms may differ. Hariman et al.,[1] using high-gain specially filtered unipolar signals, have detected phase 4 slope in such rhythms. He suggested that such junctional rhythms may arise in the node because overdrive suppression by atrial pacing did not depend on the impulse reaching the His bundle (i.e., during A-V nodal block) (Fig. 7-9).[1] However, electrotonic interactions within the node at the N-H region could alter the resulting escape rhythm. Theoretically, an automatic His bundle rhythm should demonstrate a greater degree of overdrive suppression than the A-V Node because it is lower in the hierarchy of "pacemaker" activity and it is sodium dependent. This should result in greater overdrive suppression than the calcium-dependent A-V node since overdrive suppression is based on the Na/K exchanger. The speed of retrograde conduction to the atrium has also been suggested as a means to help localize the site of the pacemaker, with a short retrograde conduction time suggesting an A-V nodal origin. This reasoning, however, is not valid, because retrograde conduction may be rapid (even more rapid than anterograde) if a "fast" A-V nodal pathway is used in the retrograde direction (see Chapter 8). Further proof of this is provided by the similarly short

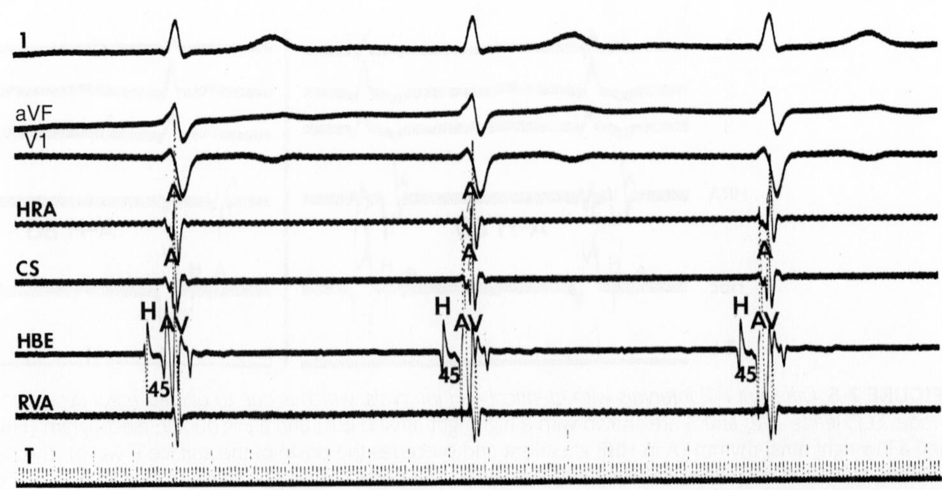


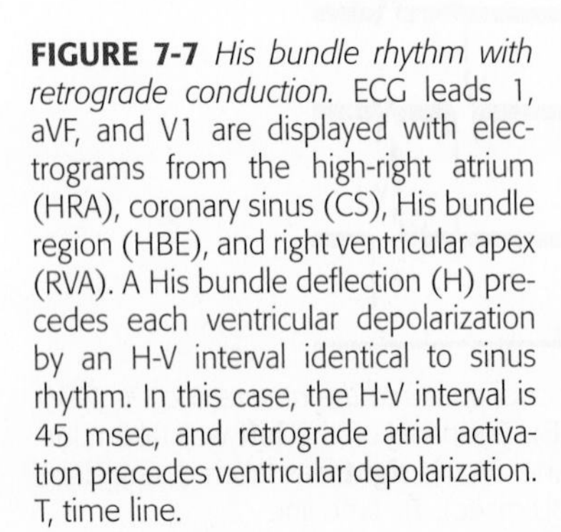
**FIGURE 7-7** *His bundle rhythm with retrograde conduction.* ECG leads 1, aVF, and V1 are displayed with electrograms from the high-right atrium (HRA), coronary sinus (CS), His bundle region (HBE), and right ventricular apex (RVA). A His bundle deflection (H) precedes each ventricular depolarization by an H-V interval identical to sinus rhythm. In this case, the H-V interval is 45 msec, and retrograde atrial activation precedes ventricular depolarization. T, time line.

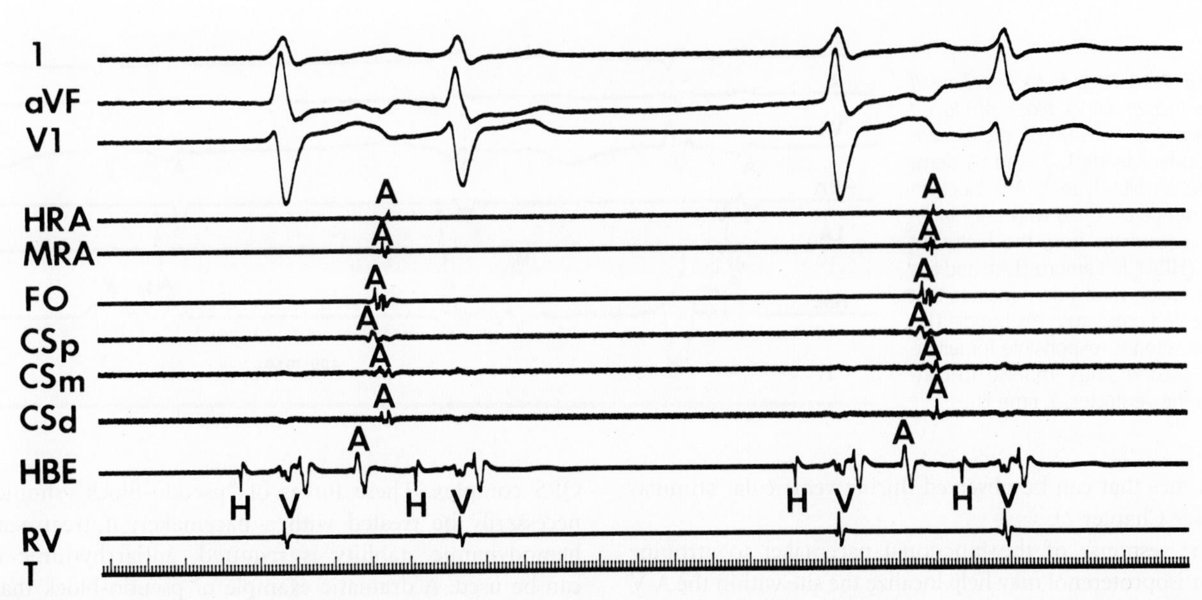


**FIGURE 7-8** *Junctional rhythm presenting as bigeminy owing to (A-V) nodal reentry.* Leads 1, aVF, and V1 are shown with electrograms from the high-right atrium (HRA), midright atrium (MRA), fossa ovalis (FO), and proximal, mid-, and distal coronary sinus (CSp, CSm, CSd) as well as His bundle electrogram (HBE), and right ventricular (RV) electrogram. The junctional rhythm is present. Each junctional escape beat is followed by retrograde conduction to the A-V node. Retrograde conduction is by way of the slow A-V nodal pathway, which allows reexcitation of the His bundle over the fast pathway. Thus, retrograde dual A-V nodal pathways with reentry in the presence of a junctional rhythm can give rise to a bigeminal rhythm. T, time line.

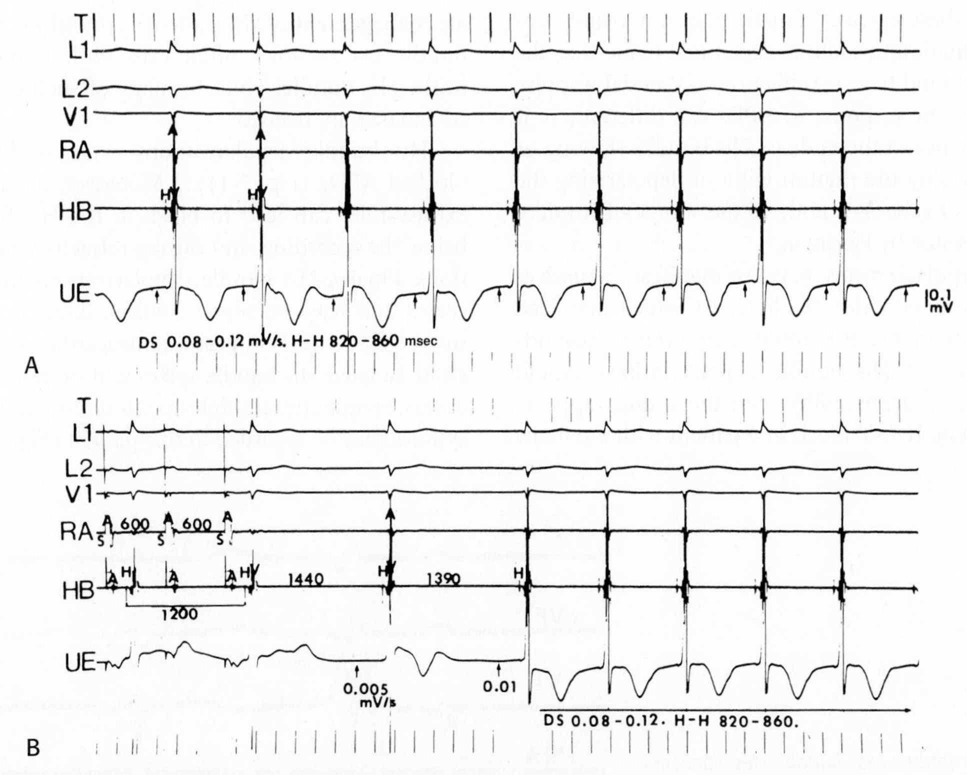


**FIGURE 7-9** *Effects of atrial pacing on the junctional rhythm and the junctional diastolic slope.* **A** and **B:** Tracings are arranged as follows: T, time lines; L1, L2, V1 = leads 1, 2, and V1 of the electrogram; RA, high-right atrial electrogram; HB, bipolar His bundle electrogram; and UE, unipolar electrogram of the His bundle. The *arrows* indicate junctional diastolic slopes (DS). A, H, and V are electrograms of the atria, the His bundle, and the ventricles. S, stimulus artifact. Voltage calibration is for UE. **A:** Control. **B:** Atrial pacing at 600-msec cycle length for 30 sec resulted in 2:1 conduction to the His bundle and the ventricles. After pacing, the junctional cycle length was prolonged from 820 to 860 msec in control to 1,440 msec, and the diastolic slope decreased from 0.08 to 0.12 mV/sec in control to 0.005 mV/sec. The junctional cycle length and the diastolic slope returned to control values after two beats. (From Hariman RJ, Gomes JAG, El-Sherif N. Recording of diastolic slope with catheters during junctional rhythms in humans. *Circulation* 1984;69:485–491.)

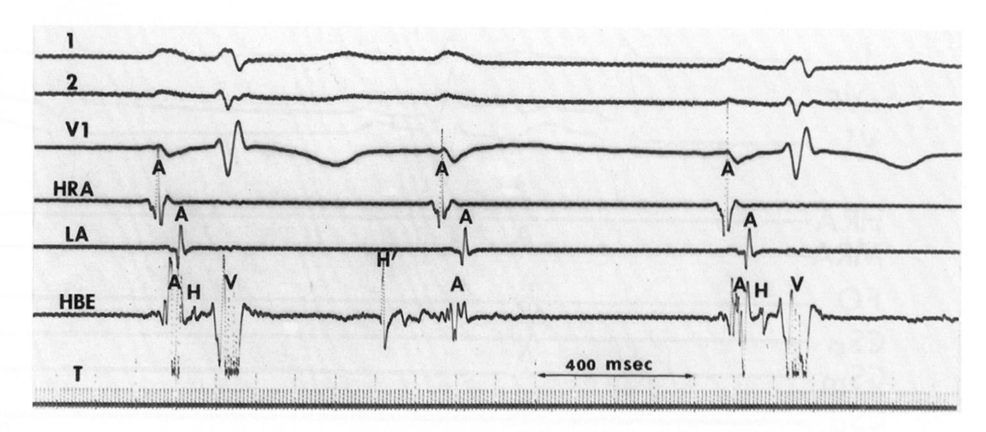


**FIGURE 7-10** *Pseudo-Mobitz Type II atrioventricular (A-V) block produced by concealed His bundle depolarizations.* Surface leads 1, 2, and V1 demonstrate Mobitz Type II A-V block in the presence of RBBB with LAH. Intracardiac recordings from the high-right atrium (HRA), left atrium (LA), and His bundle region (HBE) demonstrate that a concealed premature His bundle (H) depolarization is responsible for failure of the second sinus impulse to conduct to the ventricles. T, time lines.

H-A times that can be observed during ventricular stimulation (see Chapter 2).

The response of the junctional pacemaker to atropine and/or isoproterenol may help localize the site within the A-V junction from which the automatic focus arises.[27] A rapid response suggests a pacemaker in the proximal His bundle, N-H region of the node, or the node itself whereas a sluggish response suggests a more distal (or an impaired proximal) pacing focus. The use of calcium blockers, beta blockers, or adenosine may also be of value. A marked depression of automaticity suggests a nodal origin because it is the site most sensitive to these agents.[28] Finally lidocaine could suppress impulse formation in sodium-dependent tissue (i.e., the His bundle) but should have no effect on A-V nodal impulse formation. Finally, the response to APDs can differentiate if the impulse originates in the node or His bundle; slowing or transiently suppressing the rhythm without depolarizing the His Bundle points to the A-V node as the source of impulse formation as suggested by Hariman.[1]

His bundle depolarizations may also manifest themselves only by concealed conduction (Chapter 6), which may lead to sudden changes in the P-R interval or even to second-degree A-V block.[29–32] His bundle depolarizations should always be considered a possibility with the sudden appearance of Mobitz Type II A-V block in a patient with a narrow QRS complex. These forms of "pseudo-block" should not necessarily be treated with a pacemaker; if treatment for hemodynamic stability is required, antiarrhythmic drugs can be used. A dramatic example of pseudo-block that was successfully treated with quinidine is shown in Figure 7-10. This patient (described in Chapter 4), who had a right bundle branch block and left anterior hemiblock morphology, had experienced dizzy spells and had been referred for permanent implantation of a pacemaker. The electrophysiologic study revealed pseudo-block that was due to concealed His bundle depolarizations, a finding that was crucial to the appropriate management of the patient's condition. Nevertheless, His bundle extrasystoles often exist with impaired excitability in the His bundle. Thus, in many of such cases, drugs plus a pacemaker are needed.

His bundle depolarizations can also be manifested as blocked APDs (Fig. 7-11).[33] Moreover, the presence of such extrasystoles can lead to block in the His bundle (above or below the recording site) during refractory period determinations. Finally, His bundle depolarizations may be truly concealed and have no representation, direct or indirect, on the surface ECG. In this instance, intracardiac recordings demonstrate isolated His bundle spikes that do not affect subsequent events. Frequently, multiple manifestations of His bundle extrasystoles may be recorded in one patient (Fig. 7-12).[31] In such a

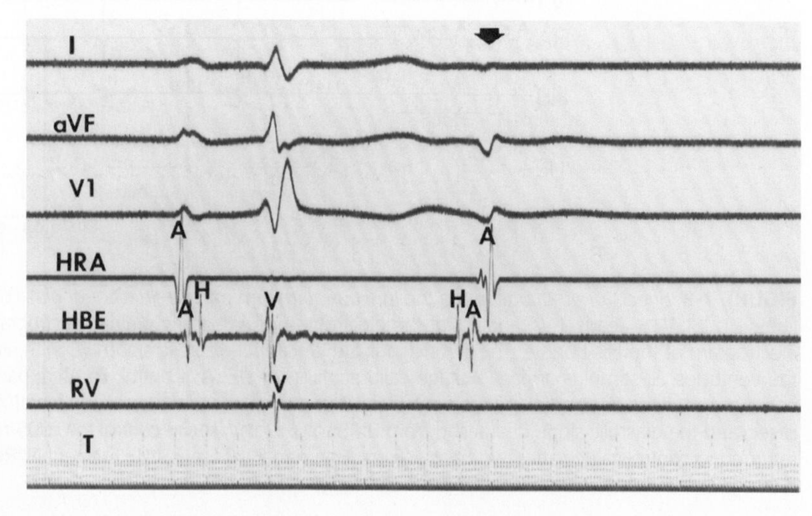


**FIGURE 7-11** *Premature His bundle depolarization manifested as a blocked atrial premature depolarization (APD).* In this patient, who has marked infranodal conduction delay (H-V = 330 msec), a premature His bundle depolarization blocks below the recorded His bundle deflection but is able to conduct retrogradely to the atrium, appearing as a blocked APD on the surface ECG (*arrow*). HBE, His bundle electrogram; HRA, high-right atrium; RV, right ventricle; T, time line.

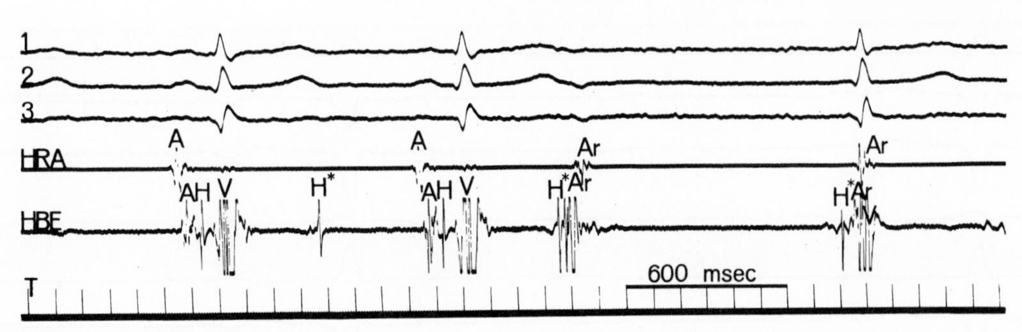


**FIGURE 7-12** *Multiple manifestations of His bundle depolarizations in the one patient.* Three His bundle depolarizations (H*) are recorded. The first H* has no manifestation on the surface ECG and appears as an isolated His spike without affecting subsequent atrioventricular conduction. The second H* blocks within the His–Purkinje system but conducts retrogradely to the atrium to be manifested as a blocked atrial premature depolarization. This resets the sinus node and allows the third H* to arise as an escape rhythm during the sinus pause.

patient, the presence of conducted His bundle extrasystoles on the ECG is an important clue to the diagnosis. Complex conduction problems including "gap" phenomena (see Chapter 6) may be observed with His extrasystoles (Fig. 7-13).[31] His extrasystoles can also produce unusual conduction patterns due to multilevel block (Fig. 7-14). The pattern of three-to-one block should suggest multilevel block, and in this case block in the more proximal structure (A-V node) was due to a His extrasystole. Junctional tachycardia can occur as a primary arrhythmia (usually in children-JET), secondary to digitalis intoxication, or in the setting of injury to the His bundle (i.e., valve surgery, abscess, sarcoidosis, etc.) (Fig. 7-15). Triggered activity due to

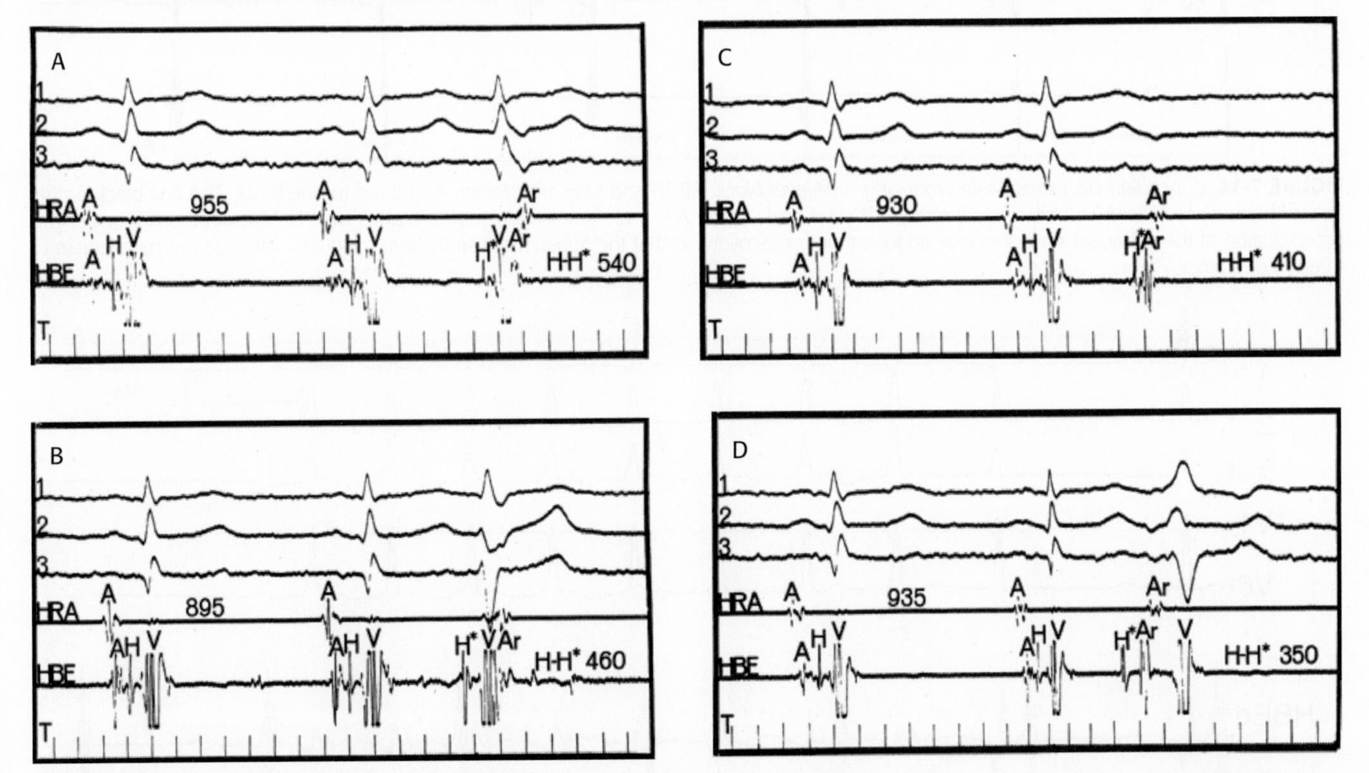


**FIGURE 7-13** *Conduction patterns of spontaneously occurring His extrasystoles.* **A–D:** Each panel shows the simultaneous recording from top to bottom of surface leads 1, 2, and 3, followed by high-right atrium (HRA) and His bundle electrogram (HBE) deflections. Time lines (T) on the bottom of each frame record 100 msec per large spike. The basic rhythm is sinus with similar cycle lengths (895 to 955 msec) in each frame. **A:** A His extrasystole (H*) with coupling interval (H-H*) of 540 msec, conducts antegrade with normal H*-V time (48 msec), as well as retrograde. Note the reversal of the intra-atrial conduction pattern of the retrograde atrial depolarization (Ar) in this and subsequent panels. **B:** A His extrasystole with a shorter coupling interval (H-H* = 460 msec) conducts to the ventricle with prolonged infranodal conduction (72 msec) and an RBBB pattern. Ar is clearly seen in the HRA and is partially buried within the ventricular depolarization in the HBE. **C:** Further prematurity of the His extrasystole (H-H* = 410 msec) causes block within the His–Purkinje system, and no ventricular depolarization occurs. **D:** With even greater prematurity (H-H* = 350 msec), infranodal conduction resumes, but with marked prolongation (H*-V = 172 msec) and the development of an LBBB pattern. (From Bonow RO, Josephson ME. Spontaneous gap phenomenon in atrioventricular conduction produced by His bundle extrasystoles. *J Electrocardiol* 1977;10:263.)

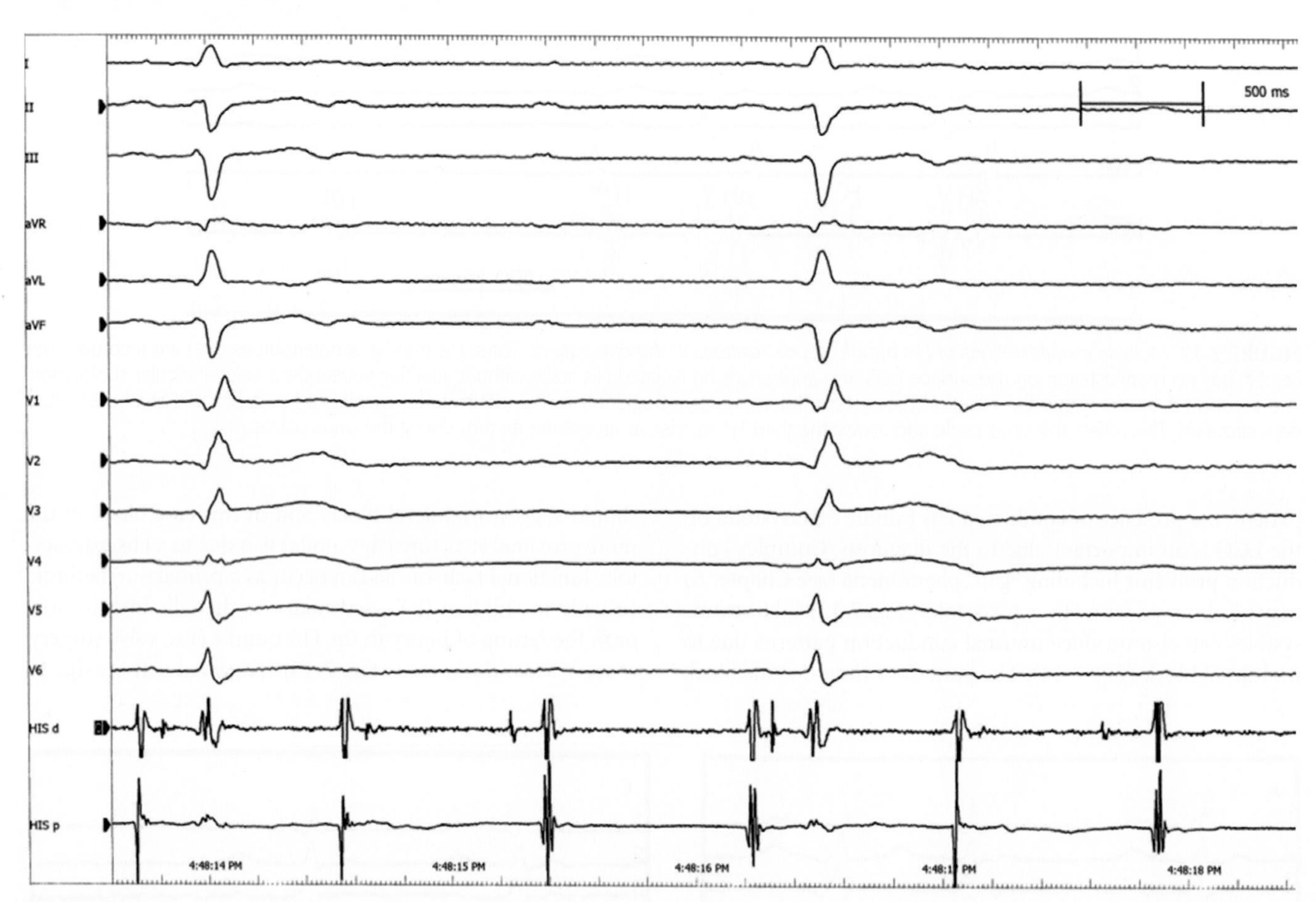


**FIGURE 7-14** *Concealed His extrasystole producing multilevel block.* RBBB and LAH are present with three-to-one block. The first block occurs below the recorded His. A His extrasystole retrogradely conceals in the A-V node resulting in the next sinus beat to block in the A-V node. The pre-excitation of the subnodal structures give enough time for recovery so that the subsequent sinus beat conducts. This was the mechanism of three-to-one block.

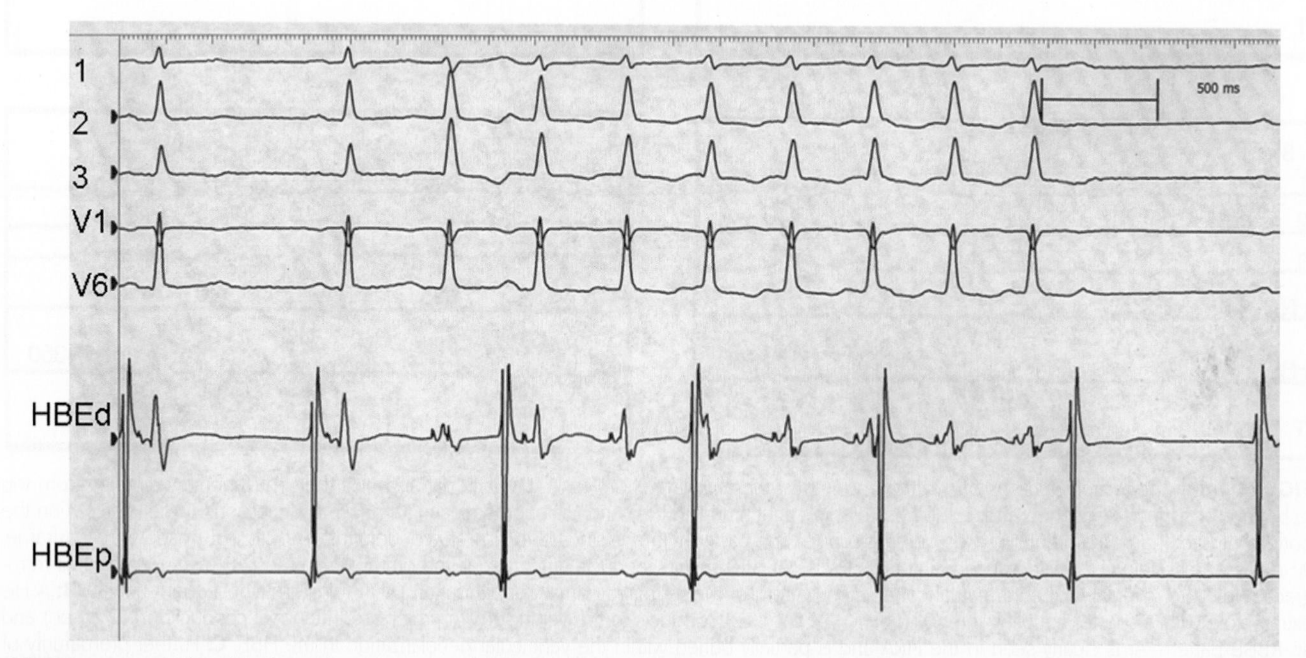


**FIGURE 7-15** *Junctional tachycardia postaortic valve replacement.* Following aortic valve replacement for aortic stenosis, incessant bursts of junctional tachycardia was observed. Note there is no retrograde conduction to the atrium, but there is concealed conduction in the A-V node. This rhythm was able to be reproducibly initiated by ventricular pacing and was catecholamine sensitive suggesting a triggered mechanism due to delayed afterdepolarizations.

delayed afterdepolarizations and abnormal automaticity are the mechanisms. The automatic rhythms are difficult to treat pharmacologically, and require large doses of antiarrhythmic agents, but on occasion must be ablated. We have encountered seven patients in the absence of digitalis, two of whom required ablation, in one of whom conduction was maintained. All of those due to triggered activity postsurgery disappeared after weeks on antiarrhythmic agents.

## FASCICULAR DEPOLARIZATIONS

Automatic or triggered foci in the fascicles of the proximal specialized conduction system can give rise to premature impulses or escape rhythms similar to those resulting from such foci in the His bundle.[34] These rhythms may be manifested by wide QRS morphologies, or they may produce concealed conduction analogous to His bundle depolarizations (Chapter 6). The diagnosis of fascicular rhythms relies on the ability to record His bundle deflections before or just within the ventricular electrogram. The recorded His bundle deflection results from retrograde His bundle depolarization, and its position relative to ventricular depolarization depends on the relative antegrade and retrograde conduction times from the site of impulse formation. If a His bundle spike appears before the QRS complex during a fascicular depolarization, by definition, it must have a shorter H-V interval than a sinus impulse (Fig. 7-16). If the His bundle is activated before ventricular activation, retrograde conduction of the impulse is faster than antegrade conduction. Most investigators have inferred that such a finding means that the origin of the impulse is closer to the His bundle than to the ventricles; however, their inference assumes that antegrade and retrograde conduction velocities are equal, an assumption that has not been validated in most cases.[35,36] It therefore only means retrograde conduction to the His bundle occurs earlier than antegrade conduction to the ventricles.

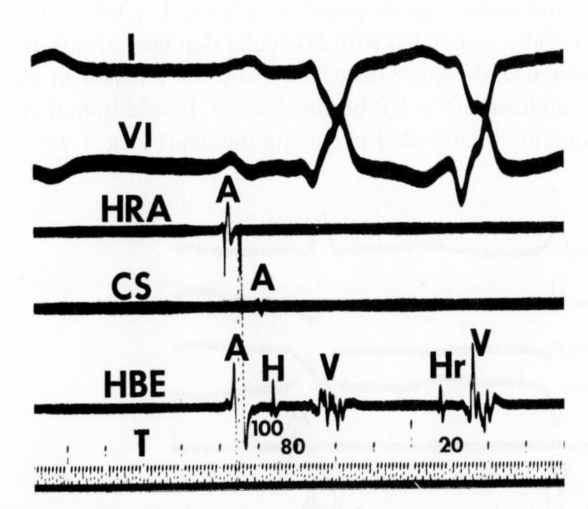


**FIGURE 7-16** *Premature fascicular depolarization with more rapid retrograde than antegrade conduction.* The sinus complex (first impulse) manifests a right bundle branch block pattern with right-axis deviation. The H-V of the sinus beats is 80 msec. A premature complex (second impulse) with a morphology very similar to that of sinus rhythm arises from the left anterior-superior fascicle. A retrograde His bundle deflection (H) appears 20 msec before ventricular depolarization. Thus, retrograde conduction from the site of impulse formation through the fascicles to the His bundle was faster than antegrade conduction to ventricular myocardium. This phenomenon results in a pattern of ventricular activation similar to that during sinus rhythm. CS, coronary sinus; HBE, His bundle electrogram; HRA, high-right atrium; T, time lines.

Retrograde His bundle deflections are seen in approximately 85% of patients during ventricular pacing when 5-mm interelectrode distances are used (see Chapter 2). Typically, the His deflection is recorded as a stimulus-to-retrograde His (S-H) interval that typically is 10 msec greater than the antegrade H-V interval. Use of para-Hisian pacing facilitates recording of a His bundle after the QRS. In my experience, ventricular stimulation from multiple sites in either ventricle has never resulted in an S-H interval less than the H-V interval (Chapter 2). An unquantifiable amount of time is required to reach the His–Purkinje system from the ventricular site of origin of a paced ventricular complex; the same would be true for spontaneous impulses arising from ventricular myocardial cells with abnormal automaticity and triggered activity. Thus, indirect evidence suggests that retrograde conduction to the His bundle is no faster than antegrade conduction. One therefore probably can safely assume that, in a normal heart, the impulse has a fascicular origin if the His bundle deflection occurs within 20 msec after the onset of ventricular activity. Certainly, the recording of a "retrograde" His potential before the QRS suggests an origin quite proximal in the fascicle. In general, fascicular rhythms or premature depolarizations that have short H-V intervals are narrower and show greater similarity to the sinus complex than do those with His bundle deflections inscribed just within the QRS complex (Fig. 7-17). Rhythms arising at the junction of the Purkinje fibers and ventricular myocardium, will have a His inscribed within the QRS and will look more like a VPD (Fig. 7-18). In cases where there is proximal conduction delay or block in the left bundle branch, a retrograde His will be buried in the QRS or seen after it due to retrograde conduction over the RBB (Fig. 7-19). Fascicular rhythms from all three fascicles theoretically can be observed. A right bundle branch block origin produces a left bundle branch block morphology, whereas origins from the anterior and posterior divisions of the left bundle branch produce a right bundle branch block. In my experience, however, I have never seen a right bundle branch extrasystole. This is consistent with the fact that the fascicles of the left bundle branch have a faster automatic rate, spontaneously and in response to a variety of perturbations, than the right bundle branch with right- or left-axis deviation, respectively.[34–36] While these comments regarding short H-V intervals signifying a fascicular origin are valid in normal hearts, occasionally a true ventricular extrasystole arising in a scarred ventricle can demonstrate a His deflection prior to the QRS (Chapter 11).

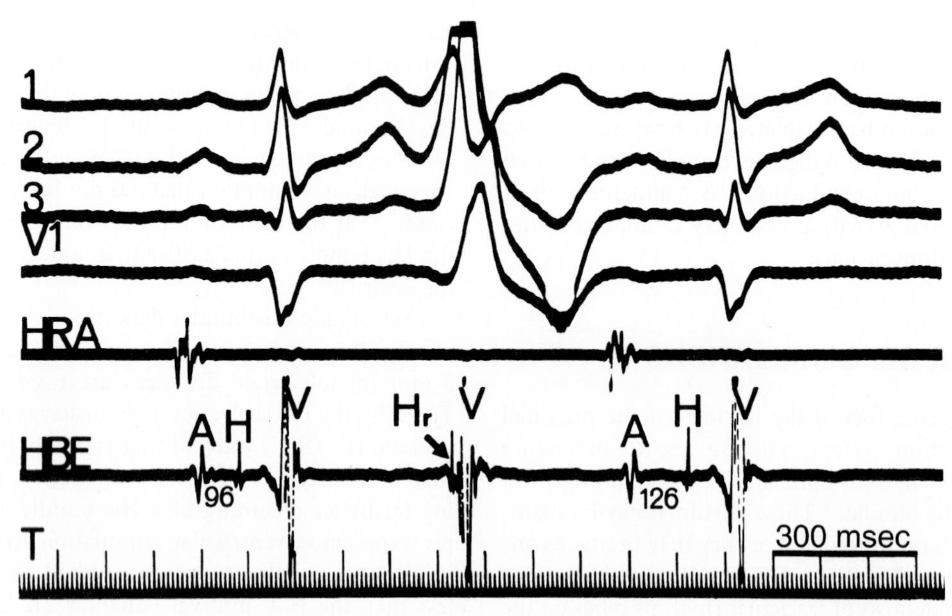


**FIGURE 7-17** *Purkinje depolarization with faster antegrade conduction to the ventricles than retrograde conduction to the His bundle.* The second complex is a Purkinje extrasystole with retrograde activation of the His bundle (Hr) occurring after the onset of the QRS complex by an interval just shorter than the H-V on the conducted complex. This phenomenon results in a wide, bizarre QRS complex because a great portion of the ventricles are depolarized by muscle-to-muscle activation before any ventricular depolarization can occur antegradely over the specialized conduction system. A minimum of 35 msec after His bundle depolarization is required for ventricular depolarization via the specialized conduction system to take place. This requirement suggests that the fascicular impulse arises distally and/or that the velocity of retrograde conduction over the fascicle is much slower than the velocity of antegrade conduction. HBE, His bundle electrogram; HRA, high-right atrium; T, time line.

The therapeutic implications of fascicular rhythms or fascicular premature depolarizations are not clear, although most physicians regard them as ventricular in origin and treat them as such. It has been suggested that in the setting of myocardial infarction, fascicular depolarizations associated with inferior infarction have a right bundle branch block and left-axis deviation morphology because they arise from the posterior-inferior fascicle of the left bundle branch. Those associated with anterior infarction arise from the anterior-superior fascicle and have a right bundle branch block with right-axis deviation pattern. Although those suggestions seem logical, proof is lacking. Digitalis intoxication is also associated with fascicular depolarizations. In our experience, these are invariably from the anterior or posterior division of the left bundle branch. In addition, they can frequently be initiated by pacing the heart (Fig. 7-19). This

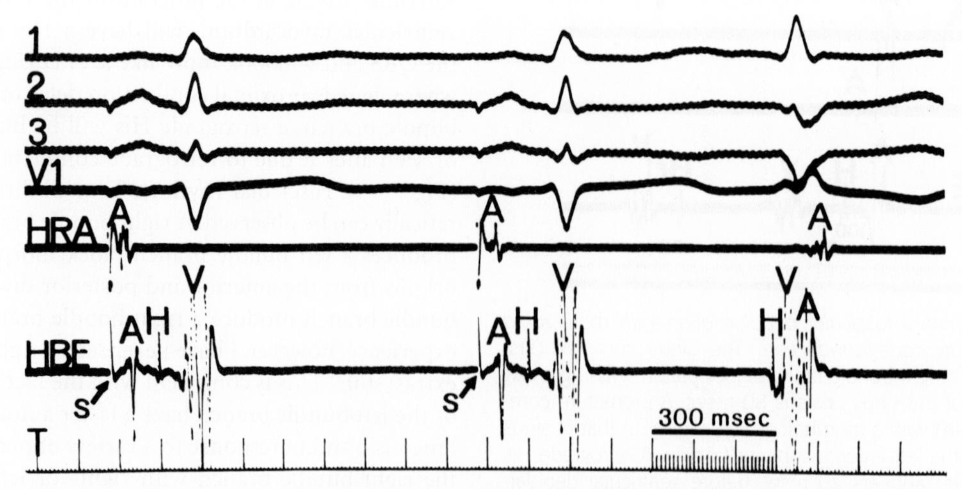


**FIGURE 7-18** *Fascicular extrasystole.* Leads 1, 2, 3, and V1 are shown with electrograms from the high-right atrium (HRA) and His bundle (HBE). During atrial pacing at 900 msec, spontaneous QRS complexes with a right bundle branch block, and left-axis deviation are induced. Each time this pattern was reproduced, a retrograde His bundle section was observed just at the onset of the QRS. The QRS width is 120 msec. This fascicular extrasystole was reproducibly initiated by atrial pacing suggesting triggered activity due to delayed afterdepolarizations as the mechanism of the fascicular complex. The presence of a His deflection prior to the onset of the QRS as well as the narrowness of the QRS suggests that the origin of the extrasystole is high in the fascicle. T, time line.

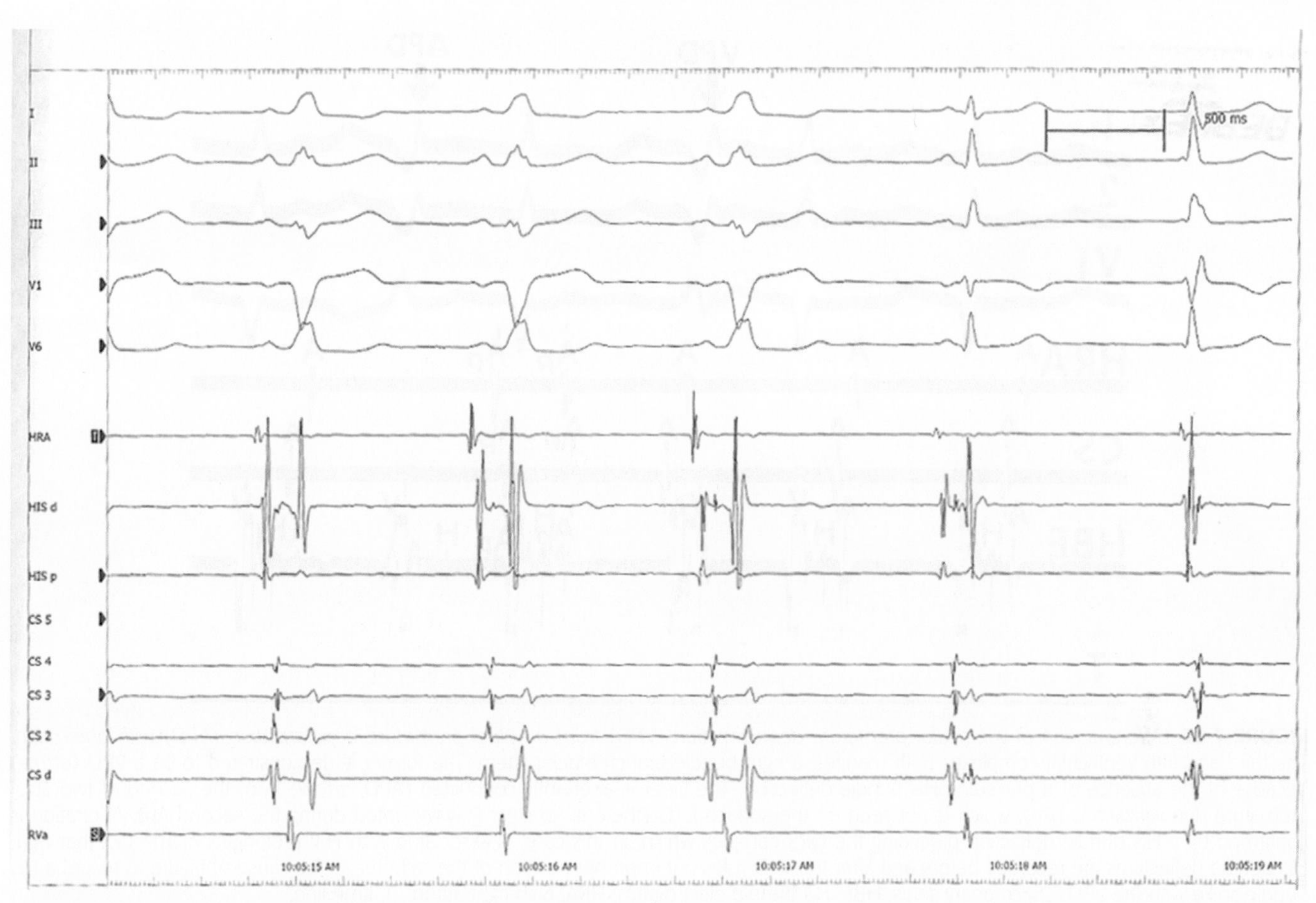


**FIGURE 7-19** *Pseudonormalization of an LBBB by a fascicular extrasystole.* LBBB is present on the first three complexes. A fascicular rhythm (below the site of LBBB) normalizes the QRS. Note a retrograde His does not precede the QRS due to the LBBB which prevented retrograde conduction over the LBBB to the His bundle. When observed on subsequent beats, the His followed the QRS because it was reached by trans-septal spread and retrograde activation over the RBB.

phenomenon is compatible with triggered activity that is due to delayed afterpotentials, the mechanism postulated for many digitalis-induced arrhythmias.[22,37,38] Such triggered fascicular rhythmias may be encountered in the absence of digitalis, and if incessant, may produce a tachycardia-mandated cardiomyopathy.[39]

## VENTRICULAR DEPOLARIZATIONS

The ECG criteria proposed to distinguish supraventricular depolarizations with aberrations from ventricular depolarizations are legion.[39,40] Despite the applicability of these criteria to large groups of patients, they may not be valid for a given person. Intracardiac recording is the most accurate diagnostic tool for evaluating the problem. His bundle recordings have demonstrated that bizarre QRS morphologies, A-V dissociation, and so on, may be encountered with supraventricular impulses as well as with impulses of ventricular origin.

By definition, a ventricular depolarization is one in which no His bundle deflection is seen before the QRS complex in the absence of pre-excitation (Chapter 10). The ventricular depolarization may be isolated (Fig. 7-20) or in runs such as an accelerated ventricular rhythm (Fig. 7-21)[41] or a sustained ventricular tachycardia (Chapter 11). Caution must be taken to ensure that the absence of a His bundle deflection is not due to poor placement of the catheter. From the appearance of a normal His bundle spike associated with the supraventricular complex immediately preceding or following the ventricular rhythm, it can be inferred that the catheter was placed correctly. Occasionally, His bundle spikes may be observed at the terminal portion of a premature ventricular complex. The relationship of ventricular activation to retrograde His bundle activation depends on the prematurity of the ventricular impulse (Chapter 2). The earlier the VPD, the longer the retrograde His–Purkinje conduction time.[42,43] In the presence of coronary artery disease with prior infarction, VPDs usually originate in areas of infarction characterized by abnormal fragmented electrograms (see Chapter 11; Fig. 7-22). Such VPDs may have a retrograde His deflection prior to the QRS (see Chapter 11). Such fragmented electrograms appear to be markers of a pathologic substrate that is potentially arrhythmogenic, and sustained ventricular rhythmias can occur as a consequence of reperfusion. These typically arise from the

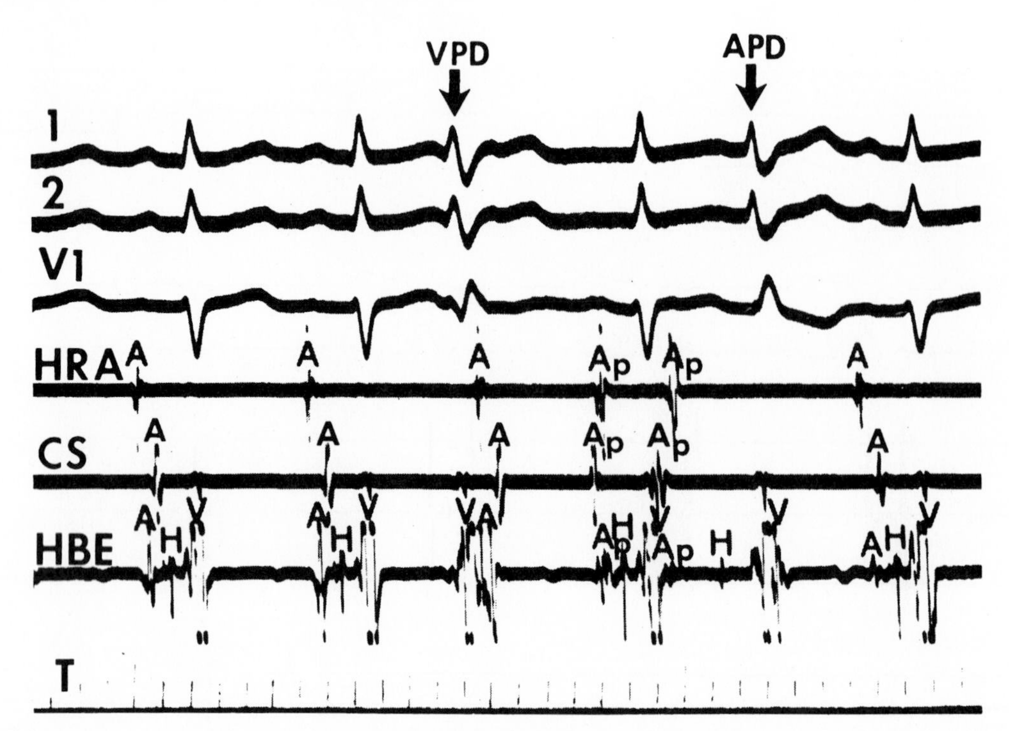


**FIGURE 7-20** *Differentiation of ventricular premature depolarization (VPD) from an atrial premature depolarization (APD) with aberration.* The third and fifth ventricular complexes both manifest a right bundle branch block pattern. The former is demonstrated to be a VPD (*arrow*) because of the absence of a preceding His bundle deflection. The latter is aberrantly conducted (APD, *arrow*) from the second of two atrial premature depolarizations (Ap), which is not seen on the surface ECG (there is no clear P wave noted during the second Ap). Aberration is confirmed by a His bundle deflection preceding the QRS complex which, in this case, is associated with H-V prolongation. The fact that clear His bundle deflections are recorded before and after the VPD rules out improper position of the catheter as the cause of failure to record a His bundle spike with the VPD. CS, coronary sinus; HBE, His bundle electrogram; HRA, high-right atrium; T, time line.

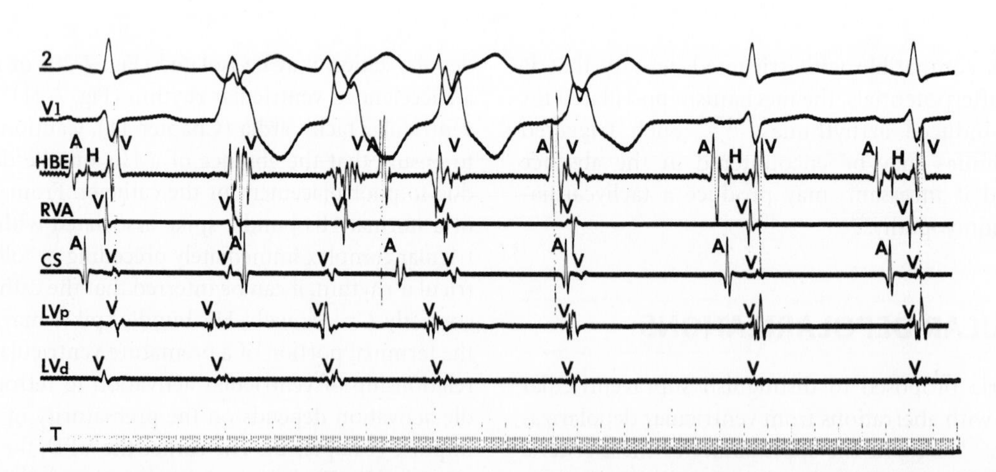


**FIGURE 7-21** *Accelerated idioventricular rhythm.* Leads 2 and V1 are shown with a His bundle electrogram (HBE) and electrograms from the right ventricular apex (RVA), coronary sinus (CS), and at the left ventricular apex from proximal (LVp) and distal (LVd) pairs of electrodes. After one sinus complex, four complexes of an accelerated ventricular rhythm with slightly irregular cycle length begin. No His bundle deflections are observed during the tachycardia, but they are clearly observed immediately before initiation and after termination. HBE, His bundle electrogram; T, time line.

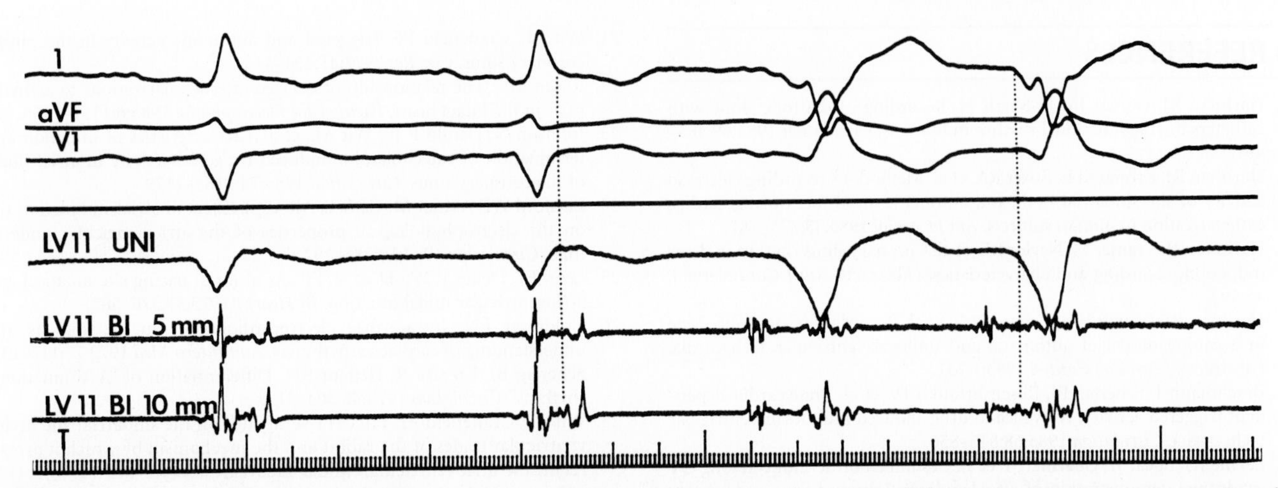


**FIGURE 7-22** *Premature ventricular complexes in a patient with prior infarction.* Leads 1, aVF, and V1 are shown with electrograms from left ventricle site 11 (LV11) (see Fig. 2-11). The top tracing is the unipolar (UNI) tracing, and the bottom two are bipolar (BI) with 5- and 10-mm interelectrode distances, respectively. During sinus rhythm, an anteroseptal infarction can be recognized. At the recording site, a split potential—the second component, inscribed well after the termination of the QRS—is observed (see Chapters 2 and 11). This electrogram denotes marked abnormalities of conduction associated with infarction. Two premature ventricular complexes are then observed originating from this site, with activity preceding the QRS by 90 msec. Note that during the premature complexes the electrogram is also split into two components. Close relationship of abnormalities of activation during sinus rhythm and sites of origin of ventricular complexes is discussed in Chapter 11. T, time line.

area of reperfusion and in my experience, signify successful reperfusion and have no negative clinical implications.

The ability to diagnose a ventricular origin using intracardiac recordings has important therapeutic implications, which are particularly evident in the setting of acute atrial fibrillation with a rapid ventricular response during which intravenous digitalization has begun. The appearance of rapid, bizarre QRS complexes may indicate digitalis intoxication if they are interpreted as VPDs. However, if they represent an aberrantly conducted ventricular impulse, they may suggest the need for further digitalization (Chapter 9). Once the diagnosis of a supraventricular complex with aberrancy is confirmed, the clinician can be sure that aggressive antiarrhythmic therapy is unnecessary. This confirmation may prevent iatrogenic disease, and it therefore may justify the performance of an electrophysiologic study. The appearance of premature depolarizations from multiple sites in the heart simultaneously is one of the signs of advanced digitalis intoxication (Fig. 7-23), which requires appropriate therapy.

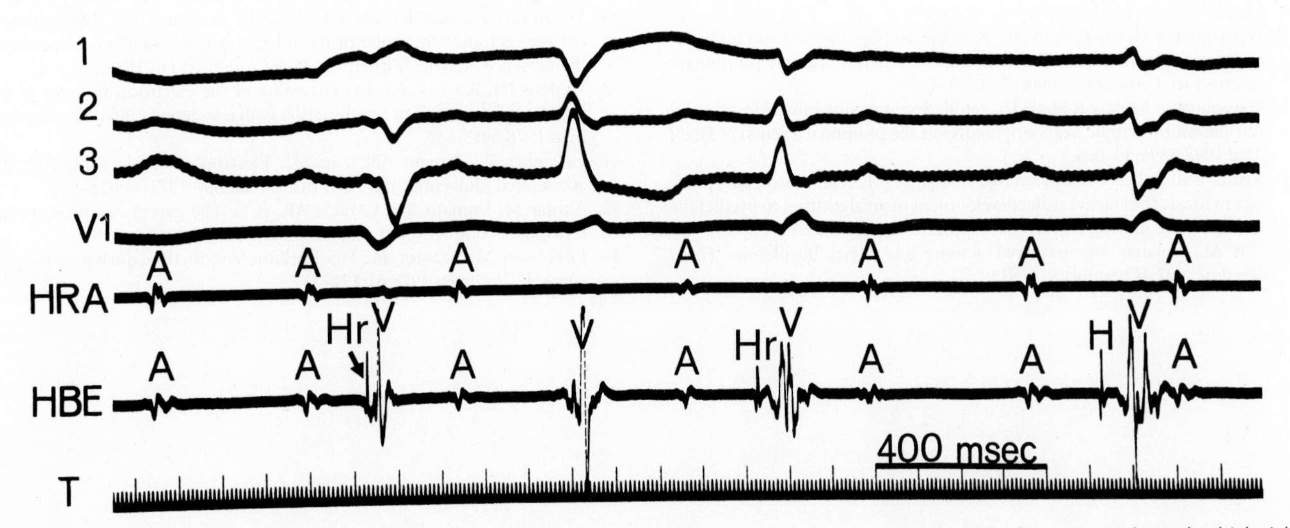


**FIGURE 7-23** *Premature complexes at multiple sites simultaneously.* Leads 1, 2, 3, and V1 are shown with electrograms from the high-right atrium (HRA) and His bundle (HBE). An atrial tachycardia is shown along with premature complexes from the right bundle branch (first wide complex), the ventricle (second wide complex), the anterior division of the left bundle branch. Prolonged A-V conduction is observed on the only wide complex that is conducted. The multiple levels of enhanced excitability should suggest digitalis intoxication. T, timeline.

## REFERENCES


1. Hariman RJ, Gomes JA, El-Sherif N. Recording of diastolic slope with catheters during junctional rhythm in humans. *Circulation* 1984;69:485–491.
2. Hariman RJ, Krongrad E, Boxer RA, et al. Method for recording electrical activity of the sinoatrial node and automatic atrial foci during cardiac catheterization in human subjects. *Am J Cardiol* 1980;45:775–781.
3. Hariman RJ, Cramer M, Naylor RE, et al. Coronary sinus rhythm in dogs: induction, recording and characteristics. (Abstract). *Am J Cardiol* 1980; 45:492.
4. Hariman RJ, Gough WB, Gomes JAG, et al. Recording of diastolic slope in a canine model of automatic and unifocal ventricular tachycardia. (Abstract). *J Am Coll Cardiol* 1983;1:731.
5. Brachmann J, Scherlag BJ, Rosenshtraukh LV, et al. Bradycardia-dependent triggered activity: relevance to drug-induced multiform ventricular tachycardia. *Circulation* 1983;68:846–856.
6. Levine JH, Spear JF, Guarnieri T, et al. Cesium chloride-induced long QT syndrome: demonstration of afterdepolarizations and triggered activity in vivo. *Circulation* 1985;72:1092–1103.
7. Gavrilescu S, Luca C. Right ventricular monophasic action potentials in patients with long QT syndrome. *Br Heart J* 1978;40:1014–1018.
8. Hariman RJ, Holtzman R, Gough WB, et al. In vivo demonstration of delayed afterdepolarizations as a cause of ventricular rhythms in 1-day-old infarction. (Abstract). *J Am Coll Cardiol* 1984;3:476.
9. Schechter E, Freeman CC, Lazzara R. Afterdepolarizations as a mechanism for the long QT syndrome: electrophysiologic studies of a case. *J Am Coll Cardiol* 1984;3:1556–1561.
10. Zipes DP, Dejoseph RL. Dissimilar atrial rhythms in man and dog. *Am J Cardiol* 1973;32:618–628.
11. Wu D, Denes P, Leon FA, et al. Limitation of the surface electrocardiogram in diagnosis of atrial arrhythmias. Further observations on dissimilar atrial rhythms. *Am J Cardiol* 1975;36:91–97.
12. Zipes DP, Gaum WE, Genetos BC, et al. Atrial tachycardia without P waves masquerading as an A-V junctional tachycardia. *Circulation* 1977; 55:253–260.
13. Josephson ME, Scharf DL, Kastor JA, et al. Atrial endocardial activation in man. Electrode catheter technique of endocardial mapping. *Am J Cardiol* 1977;39:972–981.
14. Waldo AL, Vitikainen KJ, Kaiser GA, et al. The P wave and P-R interval. Effects of the site of origin of atrial depolarization. *Circulation* 1970; 42:653–671.
15. MacLean WA, Karp RB, Kouchoukos NT, et al. P waves during ectopic atrial rhythms in man: a study utilizing atrial pacing with fixed electrodes. *Circulation* 1975;52:426–434.
16. Puech P. The P wave: correlation of surface and intra-atrial electrograms. *Cardiovasc Clin* 1974;6:43–68.
17. Haissaguerre M, Jais P, Shah DC, et al. Electrophysiological end point for catheter ablation of atrial fibrillation initiated from multiple pulmonary venous foci. *Circulation* 2000;101:1409–1417.
18. Haissaguerre M, Jais P, Shah DC, et al. Spontaneous initiation of atrial fibrillation by ectopic beats originating in the pulmonary veins. *N Engl J Med* 1998;339:659–666.
19. Kistler PM, Roberts-Thomson KC, Haqqani HM, et al. P-wave morphology in focal atrial tachycardia: development of an algorithm to predict the anatomic site of origin. *J Am Coll Cardiol* 2006;48:1010–1017.
20. Wit AL, Boyden PA. Triggered activity and atrial fibrillation. *Heart Rhythm* 2007;4(3 Suppl):S17–S23.
21. Wit AL, Cranefield PF. Triggered and automatic activity in the canine coronary sinus. *Circ Res* 1977;41:434–445.
22. Rosen MR. The relationship of delayed afterdepolarizations to arrhythmias in the intact heart. *Pacing Clin Electrophysiol* 1983;6:1151–1156.
23. Johnson N, Danilo P Jr., Wit AL, et al. Characteristics of initiation and termination of catecholamine-induced triggered activity in atrial fibers of the coronary sinus. *Circulation* 1986;74:1168–1179.
24. Batsford WP, Akhtar M, Caracta AR, et al. Effect of atrial stimulation site on the electrophysiological properties of the atrioventricular node in man. *Circulation* 1974;50:283–292.
25. Leon FY, Denes P, Wu D, et al. Effects of atrial pacing site on atrial and atrioventricular nodal function. *Br Heart J* 1975;37:576–582.
26. Goldreyer BN. Intracardiac electrocardiography in the analysis and understanding of cardiac arrhythmias. *Ann Intern Med* 1972;77:117–136.
27. Scherlag BJ, Lazzara R, Helfant RH. Differentiation of "A-V junctional rhythms". *Circulation* 1973;48:304–312.
28. Wit AL, Cranefield PF. Effect of verapamil on the sinoatrial and atrioventricular nodes of the rabbit and the mechanism by which it arrests reentrant atrioventricular nodal tachycardia. *Circ Res* 1974;35:413–425.
29. Rosen KM, Rahimtoola SH, Gunnar RM. Pseudo A-V block secondary to premature nonpropagated His bundle depolarizations: documentation by His bundle electrocardiography. *Circulation* 1970;42:367–373.
30. Damato AN, Lau SH, Bobb G. Cardiac arrhythmias simulated by concealed bundle of His extrasystoles in the dog. *Circ Res* 1971;28:316–322.
31. Bonow RO, Josephson ME. Spontaneous gap phenomenon in atrioventricular conduction produced by His bundle extrasystoles. *J Electrocardiol* 1977;10:283–286.
32. Dhurandhar RW, Valen FJ, Phillips J. Pseudo second degree atrioventricular block with bradycardia. Successful treatment with quinidine. *Br Heart J* 1976;38:1363–1366.
33. Cannom DS, Gallagher JJ, Goldreyer BN, et al. Concealed bundle of His extrasystoles simulating nonconducted atrial premature beats. *Am Heart J* 1972;83:777–779.
34. Castellanos A, Sung RJ, Mallon SM, et al. His bundle electrocardiography in manifest and concealed right bundle branch extrasystoles. *Am Heart J* 1977;94:307–315.
35. Massumi RA, Ertem GE, Vera Z. Aberrancy of junctional escape beats. Evidence for origin in the fascicles of the left bundle branch. *Am J Cardiol* 1972;29:351–359.
36. Massumi RA, Hilliard G, DeMaria A, et al. Paradoxic phenomenon of premature beats with narrow QRS in the presence of bundle-branch block. *Circulation* 1973;47:543–553.
37. Cranefield PF. Action potentials, afterpotentials, and arrhythmias. *Circ Res* 1977;41:415–423.
38. Moak JP, Rosen MR. Induction and termination of triggered activity by pacing in isolated canine Purkinje fibers. *Circulation* 1984;69:149–162.
39. Marriott HJL, Sandler IA. Criteria, old and new for differentiating between ectopic ventricular beats and aberrant ventricular conduction in the presence of atrial fibrillation. *Prog Cardiovasc Dis* 1966;9:18–28.
40. Wellens HJ, Bar FW, Lie KI. The value of the electrocardiogram in the differential diagnosis of a tachycardia with a widened QRS complex. *Am J Med* 1978;64:27–33.
41. Gallagher JJ, Damato AN, Lau SH. Electrophysiologic studies during accelerated idioventricular rhythms. *Circulation* 1971;44:671–677.
42. Akhtar M, Damato AN, Caracta AR, et al. The gap phenomena during retrograde conduction in man. *Circulation* 1974;49:811–817.
43. Josephson ME, Kastor JA. His-Purkinje conduction during retrograde stress. *J Clin Invest* 1978;61:171–177.

CHAPTER

# 8 Supraventricular Tachycardias

The development and refinement of the techniques of intracardiac recording and programmed stimulation, and our ability to compare these findings with experimental models, have resulted in a greater understanding of the physiologic mechanisms responsible for paroxysmal supraventricular tachycardias (SVTs). This has led to a more meaningful classification of these tachycardias. This chapter discusses analysis of SVT using these techniques.

## MECHANISMS OF SUPRAVENTRICULAR TACHYCARDIA

Our concepts of arrhythmogenic mechanisms have evolved over the past century. The two basic mechanisms responsible for SVT (and for that matter, all tachycardias) are enhanced impulse formation and abnormalities of conduction leading to reentry.[1,2] Enhanced impulse formation may be due to enhanced phase 4 automaticity in normal or abnormal cells (abnormal automaticity) or to triggered activity. Tachycardias that are due to enhanced automaticity, either normal or abnormal, can in general be neither predictively initiated nor terminated by electrical stimulation. Although experimental models suggest that annihilation of an automatic focus (not a tachycardia) is possible,[3] this is not predictable. The most common response of automatic rhythms to overdrive pacing is either overdrive suppression or no effect whatsoever.[1,2,4] Triggered rhythms that are due to delayed afterdepolarizations have been demonstrated in atrial and coronary sinus tissue under a variety of experimental conditions.[5–7] Observations in animal models and in vitro preparations have shown that electrical stimulation can induce tachycardias that are due to triggered activity secondary to delayed afterdepolarizations; however, the initiation of such arrhythmias is most consistently produced by overdrive pacing and is not associated with conduction delay and/or block. It is facilitated by catecholamines. Specific responses such as (a) a direct relationship between the coupling interval or paced cycle length initiating the rhythm and the interval to the onset of the rhythm and early cycle length of the rhythm and (b) overdrive acceleration are typical of such arrhythmias and distinguish them from reentrant arrhythmias (see following discussion).[4–7] The incidence of triggered activity as the mechanism of spontaneous paroxysmal SVTs is uncertain and, with the possible exception of digitalis-induced atrial tachycardias, is certainly uncommon.[8]

The second mechanism is reentry, which is an expression of abnormalities of impulse propagation.[1,2] These may be based on anatomic, functional, or a combination of anatomic and functional abnormalities, which provide the electrophysiologic inhomogeneity required for sustained reentry. The following three conditions are required for the initiation and maintenance of a reentrant rhythm: (a) at least two functionally (or anatomically) distinct potential pathways that join proximally and distally to form a closed circuit of conduction; (b) unidirectional block in one of these potential pathways; and (c) slow conduction down the unblocked pathway, allowing the previously blocked pathway time to recover excitability; that is, the conduction time along the alternative pathway must exceed the refractory period of the initially blocked pathway. If, and only if, conduction delay and refractoriness in both pathways are appropriate, a continuously circulating wavefront of electrical activity will ensue, resulting in a tachycardia. The sine qua non of a reentrant arrhythmia is the ability to reproducibly initiate the tachycardia by timed extrastimuli (particularly in association with evidence of conduction delay and block). Similarly, programmed stimulation can also reproducibly terminate the tachycardia. The mode of initiation and response to stimulation during a reentrant tachycardia differs from that of triggered activity. Timed extrastimuli are more effective than rapid pacing for initiation; there is no direct relationship of pacing cycle length or coupling of extrastimuli to the interval to the onset of the tachycardia or cycle length of the tachycardia; and resetting or entrainment of the tachycardia in the presence of fusion can be demonstrated.[1,2,4,7] The latter two phenomena are diagnostic of reentry.[9,10] In view of these responses to stimulation, the vast majority of paroxysmal SVTs appear to be reentrant.

## METHODS OF EVALUATION

Incremental pacing and programmed extrastimuli from both the atrium and ventricle may be used to initiate SVTs (see Chapter 2). After a tachycardia has been initiated, the stimulator is synchronized in, and triggered by, a suitable intracardiac

**TABLE 8-1 Electrophysiologic Evaluation of Supraventricular Tachycardia**

- Mode of initiation of the tachycardia
- Atrial activation sequence during the tachycardia
- Influence of bundle branch block on conduction and cycle length during the tachycardia
- Requirement of the atria and/or ventricles to initiate and sustain the tachycardia
- Effect of atrial and/or ventricular stimulation during the tachycardia
- Effects of drugs and/or physiologic maneuvers on the tachycardia

**TABLE 8-2 Mechanisms of SVT (2,789 Patients)**

| | |
|---|---|
| **AVNRT** | **1,433 (51%)** |
| Typical | 1,285 |
| Uncommon | 92 |
| Intermediate forms | 56 |
| **AVRT (CBT)** | **1,072 (38%)** |
| Fast conducting | 945 |
| Slow conducting | 127 |
| **Atrial Tachycardia** | **284 (11%)** |
| AAT | 191 |
| PAT | 65 |
| SNRT | 28 |

electrogram. One or more extrastimuli and overdrive pacing are then introduced to modify (reset, entrain, or terminate) the arrhythmia. The use of these techniques has demonstrated that most SVTs are due to reentry and that the general diagnostic category, SVT, is in reality composed of several different arrhythmias. Mechanisms and site of origin of SVT can be defined and classified by analysis of specific phenomena (Table 8-1) including the following:

1. The mode of initiation of the tachycardia, with particular attention to the site of conduction delay, which appears requisite for the development of the arrhythmia: to help distinguish reentry from triggered activity,[4,7] one should also analyze the relationship of the basic drive cycle length and the coupling interval of the extrastimulus that initiates the tachycardia to the onset of the tachycardia and the initial cycle length of the tachycardia.
2. The atrial activation sequence and relationship of the P wave to the QRS complex at the onset of and during the tachycardia.
3. The effect of bundle branch block, spontaneous or induced, on the cycle length and ventriculoatrial (V-A) conduction time during the tachycardia.
4. The requirement of atrial, His bundle, and/or ventricular participation in the initiation and maintenance of the tachycardia, that is, the effect of A-V dissociation or variable A-V or V-A conduction on the tachycardia.
5. The effect of atrial and/or ventricular stimulation during the tachycardia. Response to such stimulation allows one to assess the role of atrial, His bundle, and ventricular participation in the tachycardia and can be used to distinguish atrial tachycardia, A-V nodal tachycardia, and tachycardias using concealed accessory pathways from one another. Responses to extrastimuli can establish and quantitate the presence of an excitable gap within the reentrant circuit.[10–14]
6. The effects of drugs and/or physiologic maneuvers on the tachycardia. This allows one to characterize the properties of the tachycardia circuit as well as to establish which components of the heart are required to maintain the tachycardia.

The mechanisms and frequency of SVTs based on the results of such investigations and observations are listed in Table 8-2.

## SUPRAVENTRICULAR TACHYCARDIA RESULTING FROM ATRIOVENTRICULAR NODAL REENTRY

Supraventricular tachycardia due to A-V nodal reentry (AVNRT) is the most common form of SVT, accounting for approximately 50% of the cases.[15–18] This arrhythmia is more common in women and usually occurs before age 40, with a median age of onset of 28. However, this arrhythmia may be seen in children or the elderly. We have recently studied three nonagenarians with severely symptomatic AVNRT. The rates of AVNRT tachycardia vary widely. In our patient population, we have seen SVT rates ranging from 100 to 280 beats per minute (bpm) with a mean of approximately 170 bpm. Rates are slower in patients over 50 than in those under 50. Holter monitoring in such patients demonstrates atrial premature depolarizations (APDs) and isolated atrial echo beats between episodes.

The concept of AVNRT as a mechanism of SVT was first proposed by Mines[19] in 1913. Moe et al.[20] were the first to postulate that SVT could be produced by longitudinal dissociation of the A-V node (AVN) into two pathways in the AVN. They were also the first to demonstrate that atrial extrastimuli could actually initiate and terminate SVT in the rabbit.[21] Based on their experiments, these investigators postulated the presence of a dual A-V nodal transmission system with a slowly conducting alpha pathway with a short refractory period and a fast-conducting beta pathway with a longer refractory period. During sinus rhythm the impulse traverses the faster-conducting beta pathway to produce a single QRS complex (Fig. 8-1A). The impulse simultaneously conducts down the alpha pathway (slow), reaching

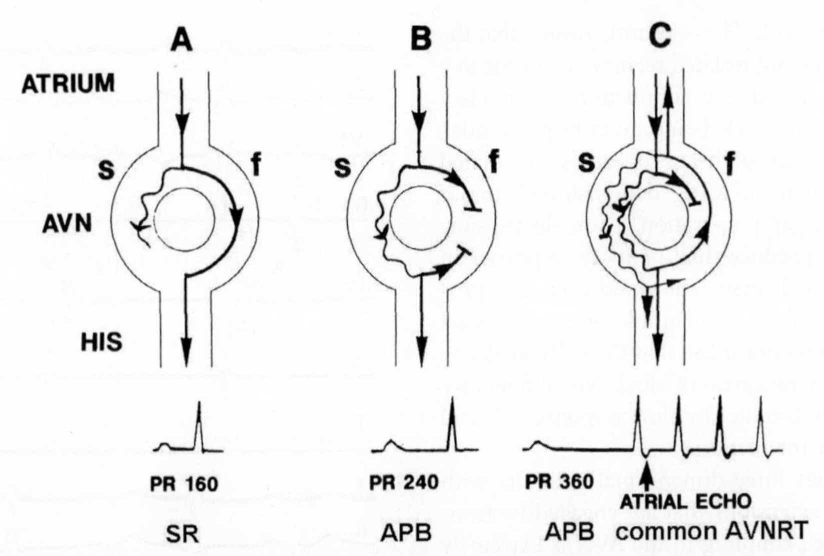


**FIGURE 8-1** *Mechanism of typical A-V nodal reentry.* The A-V node (AVN) is schematically drawn with fast and slow pathway. The beta pathway has fast conduction and long refractoriness, and the alpha pathway is slowly conducting with relatively shorter refractoriness. During sinus rhythm, the impulse traverses the faster-conducting beta pathway to produce a single QRS complex with a P-R interval of 160 msec **(A)**. The impulse simultaneously conducts down the alpha pathway (slow), reaching the lower part of the AVN or His bundle shortly after it has been depolarized and rendered refractory by the impulse that has conducted down the beta pathway. When an APD is delivered **(B)**, the impulse blocks in the beta pathway, because of its longer refractory period, and proceeds slowly down the alpha pathway. This leads to a prolonged P-R interval of 240 msec. If conduction down the alpha pathway is not slow enough to allow the previous refractory beta pathway time to recover reentry will occur. An earlier APD **(C)** also blocks in the beta pathway, but conducts more slowly down the alpha pathway (P-R of 360 msec). Because of the longer antegrade conduction time, the beta pathway has now had more time to recover excitability, and a sustained tachycardia results.

the lower part of the AVN or His bundle shortly after it has been depolarized and rendered refractory by the impulse that has conducted down the beta pathway. When an APD is delivered (Fig. 8-1B), the impulse blocks in the beta pathway, because of its longer refractory period, and proceeds slowly down the alpha pathway. This leads to a prolonged P-R interval. If conduction down the alpha pathway is slow enough to allow the previous refractory beta pathway time to recover, an atrial echo results. If, however, the alpha pathway does not itself recover excitability in time to permit subsequent antegrade conduction, only a single atrial echo results. An earlier APD (Fig. 8-1C) also blocks in the beta pathway, but conducts more slowly down the alpha pathway and arrives later to retrogradely excite the beta pathway, producing an echo. Because of the longer antegrade conduction time, the alpha pathway has now had more time to recover excitability, and a sustained tachycardia results. This schema depicts initiation of the most common form of A-V nodal reentrant tachycardia, typical AVNRT. Rarely, the beta pathway may have a shorter refractory period than the alpha pathway, and the tachycardia can be reversed, conducting antegradely down the fast pathway and retrogradely up the slow pathway to produce the uncommon variety of AVNRT (Fig. 8-2).[18,22–28] Women appear to have greater differences in the refractory periods of the fast and slow pathways, which may be why A-V nodal tachycardia is more common in women.

Recently, the concept of dual A-V nodal pathways causing longitudinal dissociation of the AVN permitting AVNRT has

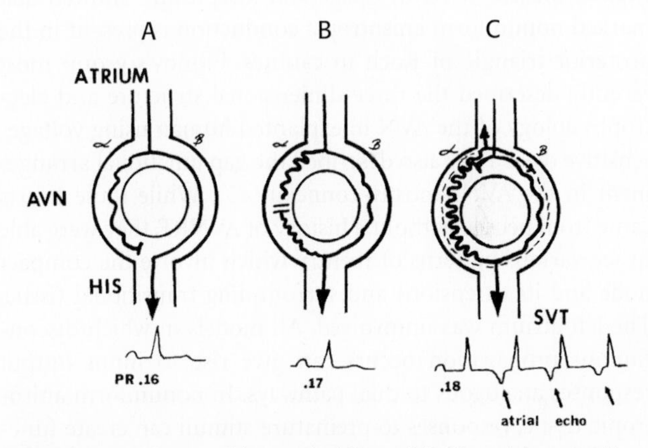


**FIGURE 8-2** *Schema of the atypical form of (A-V) nodal reentry.* Here, the A-V node (AVN) is schematically drawn, as in Figure 8-1, but here the beta pathway has fast conduction but a relatively shorter refractory period than the slowly conducting alpha pathway. **A:** In sinus rhythm, the impulse conducts over the fast pathway, giving rise to a normal P-R interval, as in Figure 8-1. **B:** However, in response to an APD, block now occurs in the slow pathway, but it is concealed because conduction proceeds over the fast pathway with minimal prolongation of the P-R interval. The impulse conducting over the fast pathway tries to return up the alpha pathway, but it has not recovered excitability, so no echo occurs. **C:** An even earlier APD blocks again in the slow pathway, which is not manifested on the surface ECG as the impulse proceeds over the fast pathway with slightly longer P-R prolongation. However, as the impulse reenters the slow-conducting alpha pathway, conduction through that pathway proceeds so slowly that the site of block has time to recover excitability and repetitive reentrance occurs, with the development of SVT. Note in this case that because retrograde activation occurs slowly over the alpha pathway, the P wave follows the QRS by a longer R-P interval. See text for further discussion.

been called into question. Jalife[29] has elegantly shown that the jump in conduction times and isolated reentry can occur in a nonhomogenous linear structure if conduction occurs electrotonically across an area of block. Using a sucrose gap model, he demonstrated classic dual-pathway responses in isolated Purkinje fibers. Antzelevitch and Moe[30] demonstrated similar responses in an ischemic gap preparation. Thus, electrotonic propagation clearly can produce dual-pathway responses in the absence of longitudinal dissociation and even can produce reflection of the impulse, a form of microreentry, at least for isolated beats. This does not mean that the AVN works by electrotonic conduction across areas of block. Nodal fibers are not inexcitable, and they conduct by slow responses[31,32] and not solely by electrotonic interaction.

The AVN is a complex three-dimensional structure with posterior and left atrial extensions that are engaged by transitional tissue. Cell-to-cell coupling in the AVN is extremely poor due to heterogenous connexins, both type and distribution, which is the main reason the node is so slowly conducting. In canines the posterior extension and transitional tissue in the posterior triangle of Koch are longitudinally arranged parallel to the tricuspid annulus with scant side-to-side connections. The anatomic characteristics create nonuniform anisotropic properties that could lead to saltatory conduction analogous to that shown by Spach et al.[33,34] in atrial tissue and recently by Dillon et al.[35] and Cardinal et al.[36] in ischemic ventricular muscle. Recently Spach and Josephson[37] showed that marked nonuniform anisotropic conduction is present in the posterior triangle of Koch in canines. Efimov's group most recently described the three-dimensional structure and electrophysiology of the AVN in explanted human using voltage-sensitive dyes. They also described the gap junctional arrangement in the AVN (mostly connexin 45). While these hearts came from people without a history of AVNRT, they were able to see various patterns of reentry which involve the compact node and its extensions and surrounding transitional tissue. The left atrium was uninvolved. All models in which discontinuous propagation occurs can give rise to input–output responses analogous to dual pathways. In nonuniform anisotropic tissue, responses to premature stimuli can create functional longitudinal dissociation and sustained reentry.[33–36] Dual pathways therefore could actually exist wholly secondary to nonuniform anisotropic conduction. Data in humans supporting the dual-pathway concept include the findings of two P-R or A-H intervals during sinus rhythm or at similar paced cycle lengths (Fig. 8-3);[38,39] the observation of double responses (1:2 conduction) either antegradely in response to atrial extrastimuli or retrogradely in response to ventricular extrastimuli; and the ability to preempt atrial echoes by ventricular extrastimuli delivered during slow-pathway conduction during SVT.[24,27,40–42] This latter phenomenon truly demonstrates two parallel pathways capable of conduction, because, if only a single pathway were present, the retrograde impulse from the ventricular extrastimulus would collide with the antegrade impulse and fail to reach the atrium. Thus, the concept of longitudinal dissociation of the AVN with dual

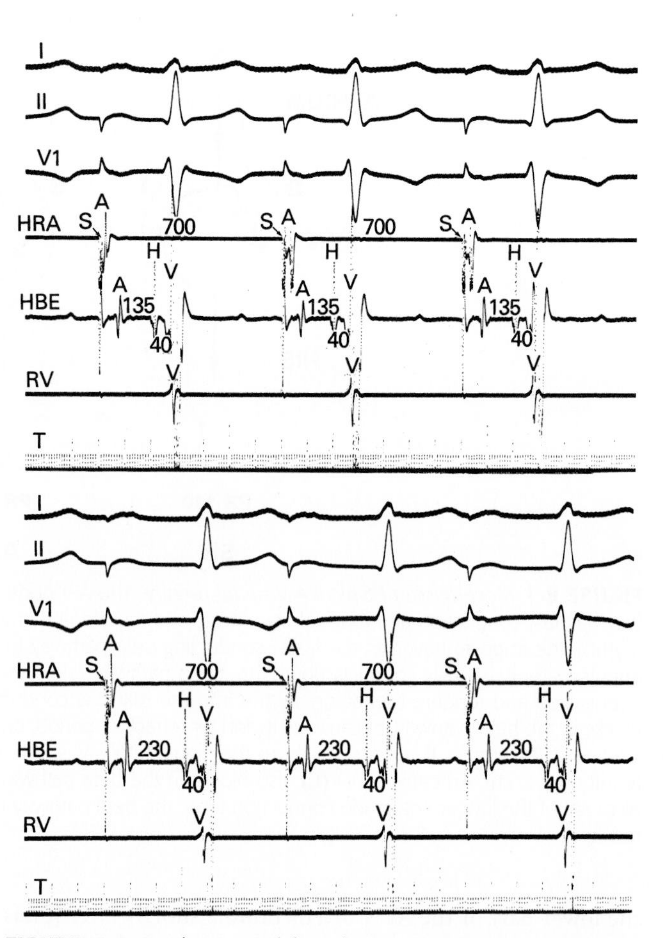


**FIGURE 8-3** *Dual A-V nodal pathways manifested by two P-R intervals that are comparable paced cycle lengths.* Both panels are arranged from top to bottom as leads I, II, $V_1$, and electrograms from the high-right atrium (HRA), His bundle electrogram (HBE), and right ventricle (RV), and time line (T). In the top and bottom panels, the atria are being paced at a cycle length of 700 msec. In the **top**, the A-H interval is 135 msec and is fixed and in the **bottom**, a totally different, markedly longer A-H interval (230 msec) is present. Two A-H intervals at the same paced cycle lengths suggest dual A-V nodal pathways.

A-V nodal pathways and the critical interrelationship of conduction and refractoriness in these two pathways best explain the mechanism of AVNRT.

While much of the literature implies that the fast and slow pathways are anatomically distinct structures, there is no anatomic evidence to support this concept. In fact analysis of the anatomy of the A-V nodal region of patients with and without AVNRT shows no differences and no evidence of specialized pathways.[43–45] Even the "slow pathway" potentials described by Jackman et al.[46] and Hassaguerre et al.[47] are nonspecific electrograms that can be recorded in all people in the posterior triangle of Koch.[48] The variations in retrograde activation in typical and uncommon forms of AVNRT support lack of anatomic pathways (see discussion of Atrial Activation During A-V Nodal Reentry later in this chapter). Therefore, I believe that it is most likely that electrophysiologic demonstration of dual A-V nodal pathways is a result of the influence of nonuniform anisotropy on propagation in the A-V junctional region.

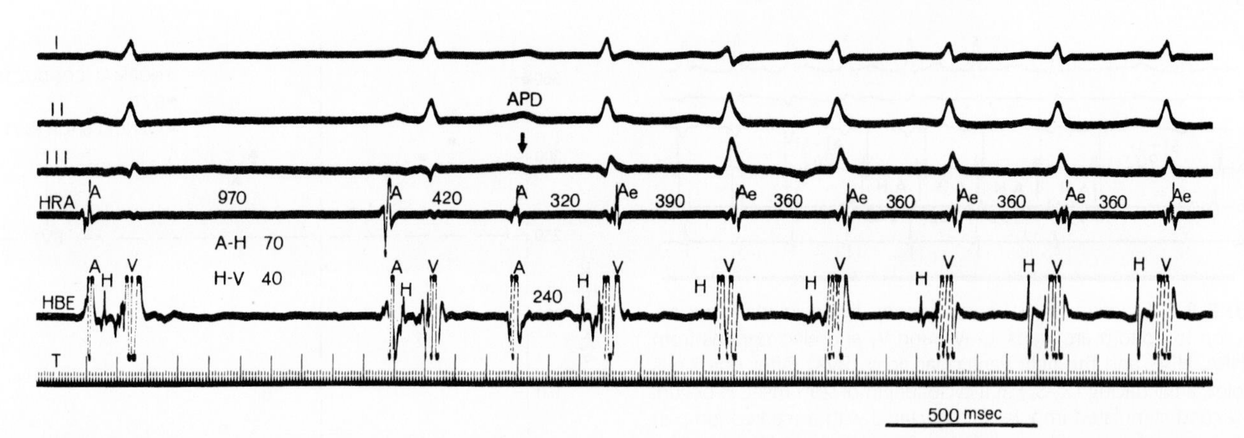


**FIGURE 8-4** *Spontaneous initiation of A-V nodal reentry.* Leads I, II, and III are displayed with an electrogram from the HRA and HBE. The A-H and H-V intervals during sinus rhythm are normal. Following two sinus complexes, spontaneous APD (*arrow*) occurs, initiating SVT. The initiating APD is associated with a markedly prolonged A-H interval (240 msec), and atrial activity during SVT occurs simultaneous with the QRS. T, time line.

## Mechanisms of Initiation of Atrioventricular Nodal Reentry

The spontaneous initiation of typical AVNRT is almost always by an APD that is associated with a long P-R and A-H interval leading to a tachycardia in which the atria and ventricles are activated nearly simultaneously (Fig. 8-4). Thus, in typical AVNRT, initiation is produced when an APD blocks in the fast pathway and conduction proceeds antegradely over the slow pathway and retrogradely over the fast pathway, as depicted in Figure 8-1. It is logical to assume that if spontaneous APDs were the most frequent method of initiation of AVNRT, then programmed atrial extrastimuli could simulate the spontaneous situation and induce the tachycardia. In nearly 100% of patients with a history of AVNRT their arrhythmia can be induced by programmed stimulation, most commonly by timed APDs introduced over a reproducible range of coupling intervals (Fig. 8-5).[15–18,27,43,49] In some instances, catecholamines and/or atropine are needed

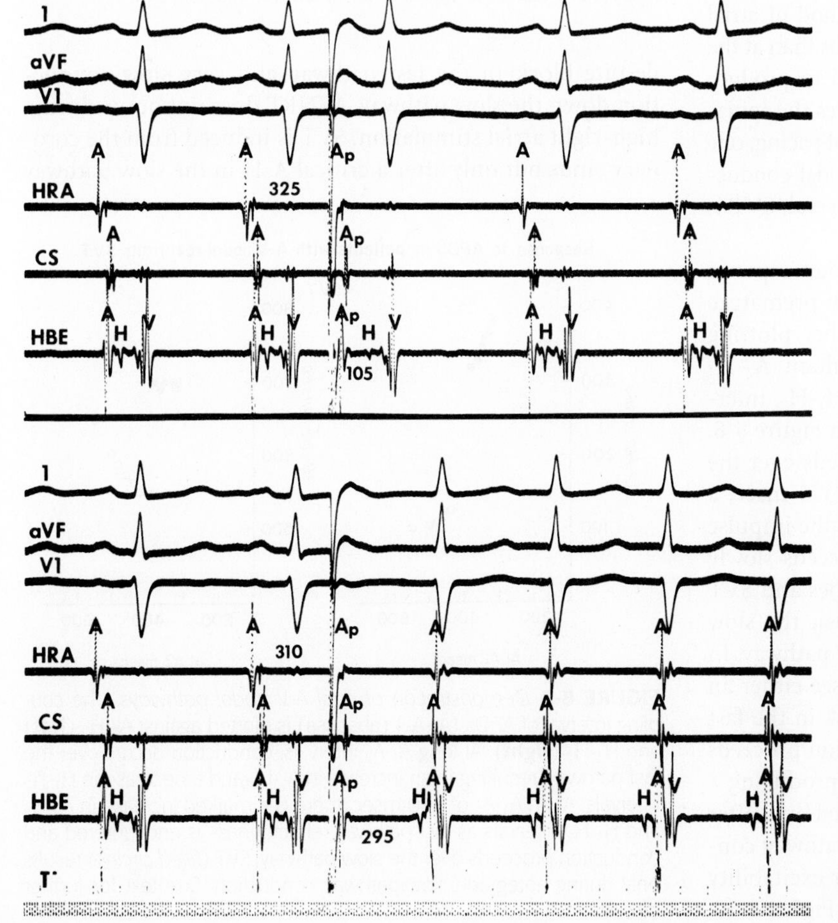


**FIGURE 8-5** *Initiation of (A-V) nodal reentrant SVT.* This and subsequent intracardiac recordings are similarly organized. From **top** to **bottom:** ECG leads 1, aVF, and $V_1$ and intracardiac recordings from the high-right atrium (HRA), coronary sinus (CS), A-V junction in the His bundle area (HBE), and time line (T). In the **top panel**, an atrial premature depolarization ($A_p$) delivered at a coupling interval of 325 msec is conducted with an A-H interval of 105 msec without inducing SVT. In the **lower panel**, at a slightly shorter coupling interval (310 msec), $A_p$ is conducted with a much larger A-H interval (295 msec) and initiates SVT. The sudden marked prolongation of the A-H interval is characteristic of a shift from fast to slow A-V nodal pathways. During SVT, retrograde atrial activation, which begins at the onset of the QRS complex, is earliest in the HBE, followed by HRA and CS. See text for further discussion.

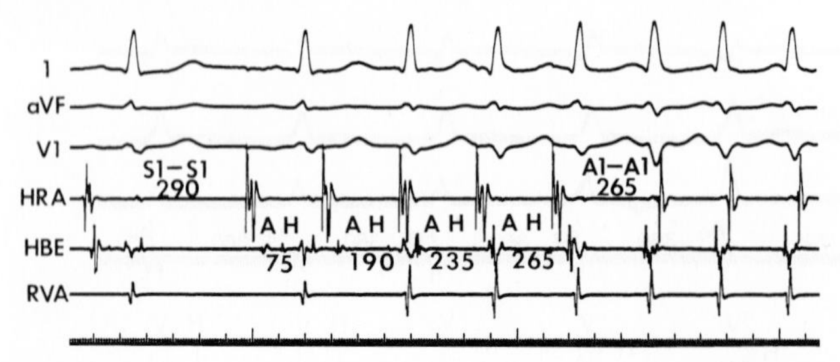


**FIGURE 8-6** *Initiation of A-V nodal reentry by rapid atrial pacing.* From top to bottom are leads 1, aVF, and $V_1$ and electrograms from the HRA, HBE, and the right ventricular apex (RVA). After one sinus complex, atrial pacing ($S_1$-$S_1$) at a cycle length of 290 msec is begun. The second stimulated impulse is associated with a marked jump in the A-H interval, and with progressive delays in the A-H interval on subsequent complexes, A-V nodal reentry is induced. Note that the A-V nodal reentrant tachycardia cycle length is 265 msec and the pacing cycle length at which Wenckebach-like activity was occurring in the A-V node was longer at 290 msec. See text for further discussion.

to facilitate induction. We have actually required stimulation during a 30-degree tilt to induce AVNRT in three patients. The zone of coupling intervals of atrial extrastimuli that induces A-V nodal echoes or sustained SVT (i.e., "echo or tachycardia zone") usually begins at coupling intervals associated with a marked prolongation of the P-R and A-H intervals. A-V nodal conduction delay (i.e., the increase in A-H interval), and not the coupling interval of the APD, is of prime importance in the genesis of A-V nodal reentrant SVT.[50] This can be demonstrated by initiation of AVNRT by using the alternative method of atrial pacing to produce A-H delays at longer cycle lengths than at the coupling intervals of single extrastimuli required to produce comparable A-H delays (Fig. 8-6). If one compares the initiation of SVT by atrial extrastimuli with that by atrial pacing, one can demonstrate that only after sufficient A-V nodal conduction delay is achieved, as reflected by the A-H interval, SVT is induced (Fig. 8-7).

Dual pathways are identified by a discontinuous response of A-V nodal conduction time to progressively premature APDs. Dual pathways can be identified by either plotting the $A_1$-$A_2$ coupling intervals against the resultant $A_2$-$H_2$ intervals or the $A_1$-$A_2$ intervals against the $H_1$-$H_2$ intervals. A typical dual-pathway curve is depicted in Figure 8-8. At longer coupling intervals, conduction proceeds over the fast (beta) pathway. At a coupling interval of 370 msec, a marked jump in the A-H interval is observed as the impulse blocks in the refractory beta pathway and proceeds slowly along the alpha pathway. Single A-V nodal echoes and SVT appear only during antegrade conduction down the slow pathway and retrograde conduction up the fast pathway. In approximately 25% of the cases, one does not see either an A-V nodal echo or SVT immediately after block in the fast pathway. In a smaller number of cases conduction proceeds down the fast pathway and the slow pathway producing a one-to-two response. An echo or SVT is observed only after a critical A-H interval is reached during slow-pathway conduction that allows the fast pathway to recover excitability and conduct retrogradely (Fig. 8-9). As seen in Figure 8-10,

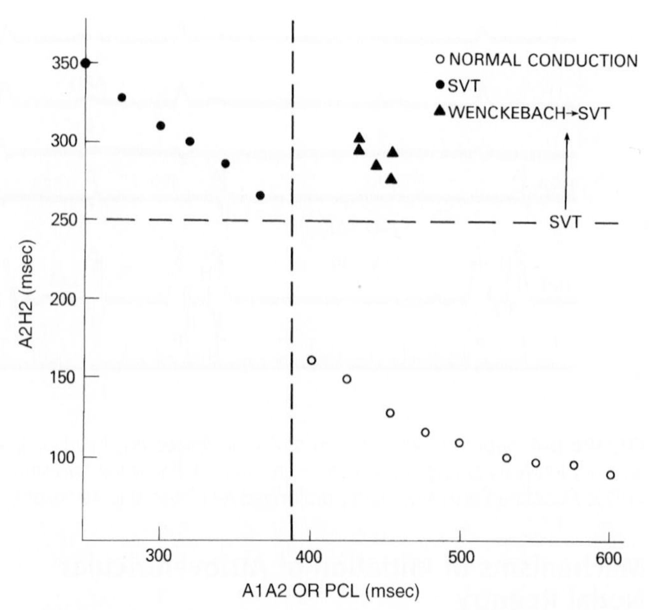


**FIGURE 8-7** *Primacy of (A-V) nodal conduction delay in the genesis of A-V nodal reentrant SVT.* The $A_1$-$A_2$ interval of stimulated APDs or paced cycle lengths (PCL) at which Wenckebach-induced SVT occurs (abscissa) is plotted against the resulting $A_2$-$H_2$ (ordinate). The *vertical dashed line* represents the $A_1$-$A_2$, below which SVT always results (*filled circles*). The *horizontal dashed line* represents the $A_2$-$H_2$ interval, above which SVT results (*filled circles* and *triangles*) only at $A_2$-$H_2$ intervals greater than 250 msec, independent of the coupling interval of the APD or PCL. Thus, A-V nodal delay ($A_2$-$H_2$), not the coupling interval or PCL, is the critical determinant for initiating SVT.

despite block in the fast pathway and very slow conduction down the slow pathway, AVNRT does not occur during high-right atrial stimulation. SVT is induced from the coronary sinus but only after a critical A-H in the slow pathway

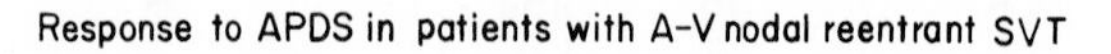

Response to APDS in patients with A-V nodal reentrant SVT


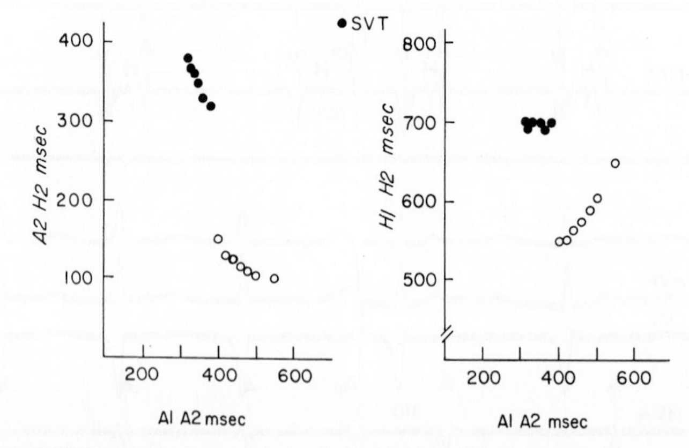


**FIGURE 8-8** *Demonstration of dual A-V nodal pathways.* The coupling interval of APDs ($A_1$-$A_2$) (abscissa) is plotted against $A_2$-$H_2$ (**left**) and $H_1$-$H_2$ (**right**). At long $A_1$-$A_2$ intervals, conduction occurs over the fast pathway, resulting in an increase in $A_2$-$H_2$ and a decrease in $H_1$-$H_2$ intervals. At an $A_1$-$A_2$ of 370 msec, there is a marked increase in $A_2$-$H_2$ and $H_1$-$H_2$ intervals as fast pathway refractoriness is encountered and conduction proceeds over the slow pathway. SVT (*filled circles*) results only during antegrade slow-pathway conduction. See text for further discussion.

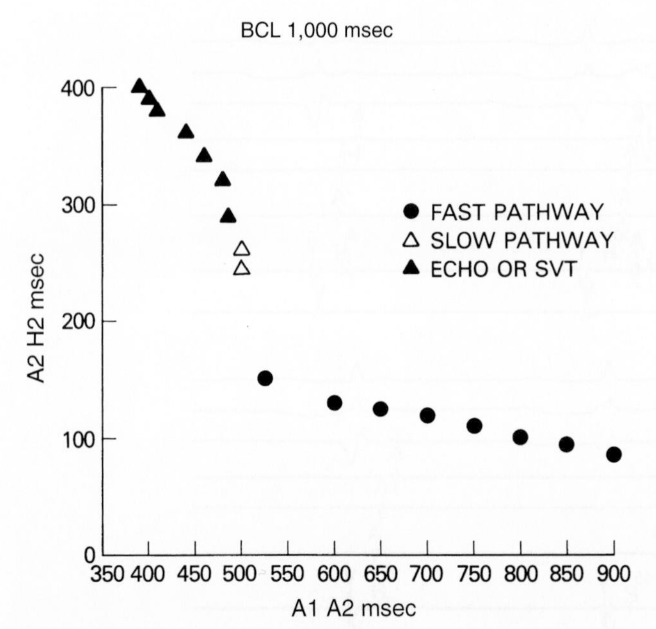


**FIGURE 8-9** *Requirement of critical A-H during slow-pathway conduction and initiation of SVT.* The coupling intervals of atrial extrastimuli ($A_1$-$A_2$) are shown on the *horizontal axis,* and resultant A-V nodal conduction times ($A_2$-$H_2$) are shown on the *vertical axis.* Block in the fast pathway occurs at an $A_1$-$A_2$ of 480 msec, but no SVT is induced. SVT is only induced when $A_2$-$H_2$ reaches 275 msec. See text for discussion. BCL, basic cycle length.

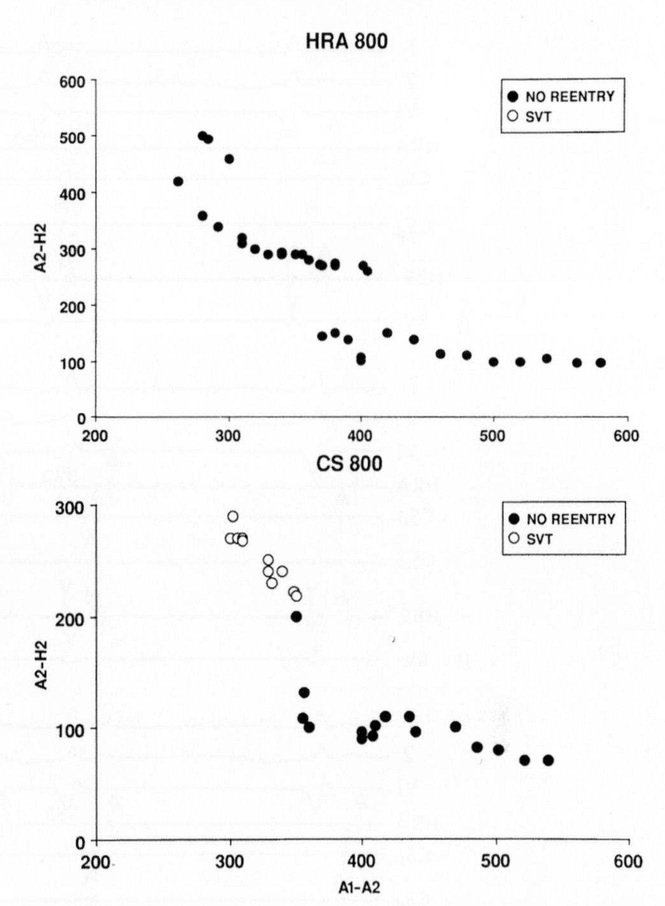


**FIGURE 8-10** *Comparison of stimulation from the high-right atrium and coronary sinus in a patient with SVT.* In both panels, the coupling interval of APDs is plotted on the *horizontal axis,* and the resultant $A_2$-$H_2$ interval is plotted on the *vertical axis.* **Top:** During high-right atrial stimulation, no reentry is observed, despite achieving coupling intervals of 270 msec and A-H intervals as long as 500 msec. Note the jump in A-H intervals, suggestive of dual pathways (see text), occurs at a coupling interval of 400 msec. **Bottom:** During coronary sinus stimulation, a jump in A-H intervals occurs at a shorter coupling interval of 350 msec. At coupling intervals from 290 to 340 msec, A-V nodal reentry is induced with the $A_2$-$H_2$ intervals at the time of induction ranging from 210 to 290 msec. See text for discussion.

is reached. Thus, relating these events to the proposed mechanism shown in Figure 8-1, one must conclude that typical nodal reentry is initiated by atrial stimulation producing block in the fast pathway with a jump to the slowly conducting pathway. Only when conduction is slow enough during slow-pathway conduction to allow recovery of the fast pathway does reentry occur.

By definition, in order to diagnose dual pathways in response to atrial extrastimuli, one must observe an increase of at least 50 msec in the A-H interval with a small (i.e., 10 msec) decrease in the coupling interval of the APD.[15,16,38,49] Although the jump is usually in the order of 70 to 100 msec, marked increases in the A-H of several hundred milliseconds can be observed (Fig. 8-11). As mentioned, dual pathways may also be manifested by different P-R or A-H intervals during sinus rhythm or at identical paced rates (Fig. 8-3). A sudden jump in the A-H during atrial pacing may also be a manifestation of dual A-V pathways. We use a similar beat-to-beat change in the A-H interval of 50 msec during atrial pacing as a marker for dual pathways. Baker et al.[51] suggested that another manifestation of dual A-V nodal pathways is the observation of atrial pacing-induced P-R interval exceeding the paced cycle length. This observation has been made only in patients with either overt dual pathways or AVNRT.

An uncommon manifestation of dual pathways is a double response to an atrial extrastimulus. In such an instance, an atrial extrastimulus can result in conduction down the fast pathway, and if conduction down the slow pathway is sufficiently prolonged, a second response to the ventricle can occur, which may be associated with an atrial echo or sustained AVNRT (Fig. 8-12). Occasionally, patients can exhibit spontaneous 1:2 conduction in sinus rhythm producing a nonreentrant tachycardia during sinus rhythm (Fig. 8-13). This situation requires slow enough conduction down the slow pathway that the HPS has time to recover to produce a second response. If conduction down the slow pathway is not long enough, block in the HPS will occur and the one-to-two response will be concealed (Fig. 8-14). Only a few such patients ever manifest spontaneous AVNRT, an example of which is shown in Figure 8-15. This reflects poor retrograde fast-pathway conduction and/or prolonged retrograde fast-pathway refractoriness, or both. In 11/12 cases I have studied AVNRT could be induced following isoproterenol and/or atropine (see **Pharmacologic and Physiologic Maneuvers** below).

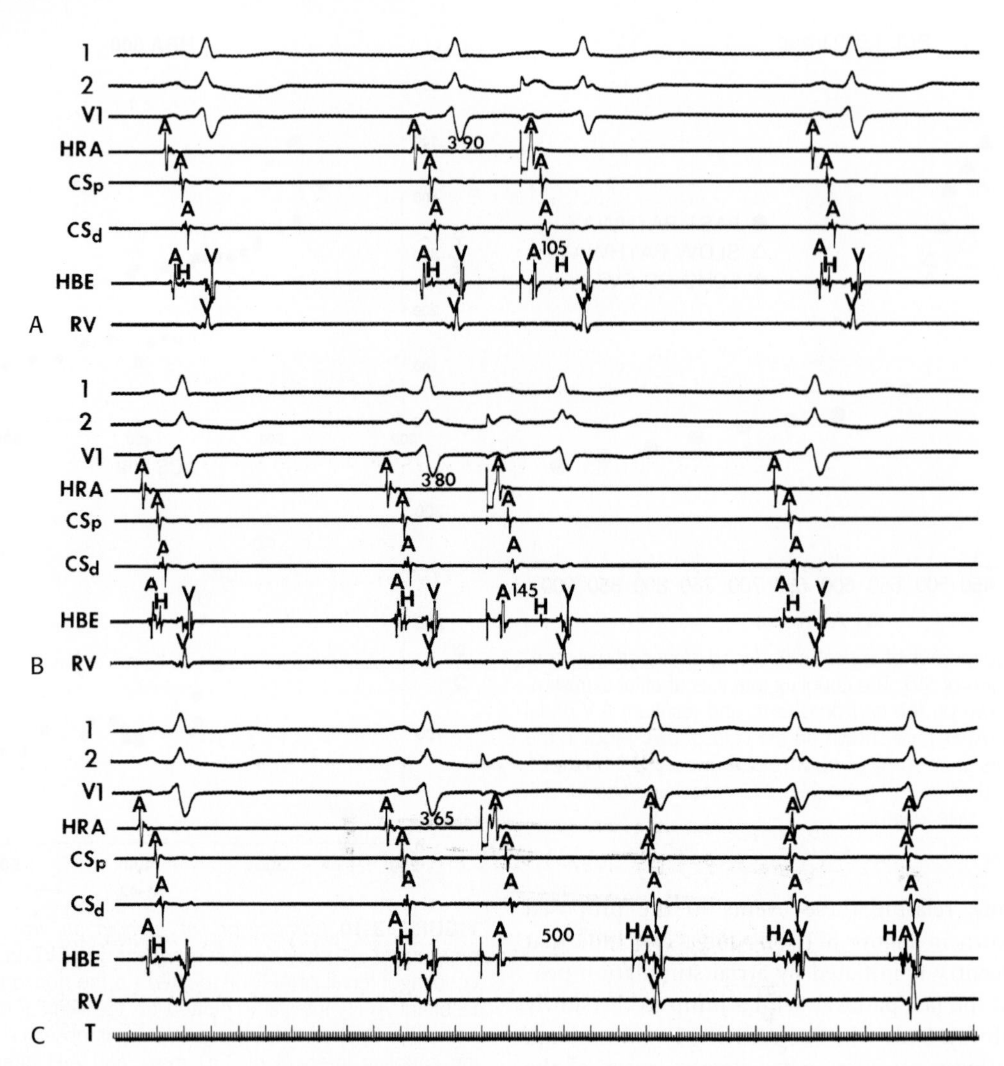


**FIGURE 8-11** *Magnitude of "critical A-H interval."* All three panels are arranged from top to bottom as leads 1, 2, and $V_1$, and electrograms from the HRA, proximal (p) and distal (d) CS ($CS_p$, $CS_d$), HBE, and RV. During sinus rhythm, APDs are delivered with increasing prematurity in all three panels. **A** and **B:** There is a minimal delay in A-H interval in response to the APD. **C:** With a small decrement in coupling interval of the APD there is a marked jump in A-H interval to 500 msec with the induction of A-V nodal reentry. In this case, not only was the jump in A-H intervals a remarkable 355 msec, but the critical A-H interval required for A-V nodal reentry was 500 msec. See text for discussion.

The site of stimulation can affect the ability to initiate dual pathways and induce AVNRT. Although Ross et al.[52] demonstrated that the site of stimulation may influence the A-H conduction times over the fast and slow pathways, they showed no significant alteration of refractoriness of these pathways or differences in the ease of induction of dual pathways or AVNRT. However, they noted variability of initiation from either site. Our experience differs slightly. We also have found that the conduction times over the fast and slow pathway may be different during high-right atrial and coronary sinus stimulation. The critical A-V nodal delay (i.e., A-H interval) required to initiate the tachycardia is different depending on the site of stimulation and is almost always shorter from the coronary sinus (Figs. 8-16 and 8-17).[53] Whether or not these differences are due to true shortening of A-V nodal conduction time because of differential input into the AVN—as suggested by Batsford et al.[54] and Aranda et al.[55]—or merely are due to apparent shortening of the A-H interval owing to the alteration of the relationship of the atrial electrogram in the His bundle recording and the true onset of A-V nodal depolarization is unclear. A shorter tachycardia cycle length associated with a shorter A-H at initiation would favor anisotropically based differences in conduction and refractoriness. Both of these mechanisms may play a role in individual patients.

In contrast to others, we have observed that dual A-V nodal pathways and reentry are easier to induce from the high-right atrium than from the coronary sinus, although in rare cases, induction of SVT can be accomplished only from the coronary sinus. The use of multiple drive cycle lengths, multiple extrastimuli, and rapid pacing make induction only by coronary sinus stimulation rare. Despite using these methods, we have observed induction of AVNRT by coronary sinus stimulation when high-right atrial stimulation failed in ~3% of cases in which we performed both high-right atrial and coronary sinus stimulation (Fig. 8-18). We agree with Ross et al.[52] that in most cases SVT can be induced with stimulation from both sites,

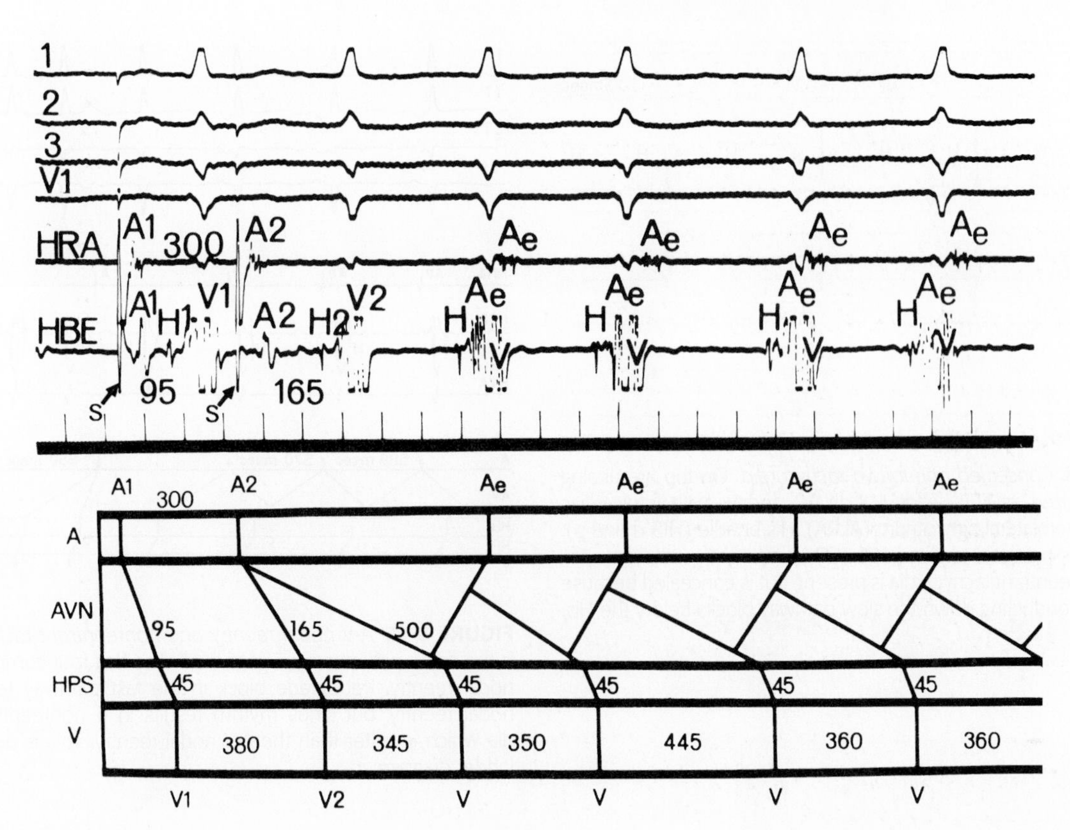


**FIGURE 8-12** *Induction of (A-V) nodal reentry with an APD resulting in two ventricular responses.* On **top** are the analog records organized as 1, 2, 3, and $V_1$, and electrograms from the HRA and HBE. On the **bottom** is an explanatory electrogram. As seen in the analog tracing, at a coupling interval of 300 msec $A_2$ results in two responses, one with an A-H interval of 165 msec and the other with an A-H interval of 500 msec. The second complex is followed by the initiation of SVT. An explanation is given in the ladder diagram below. In the ladder diagram the atrium **(A)**, A-V node (AVN), His–Purkinje system (HPS), and ventricle (V) are displayed. Last are the basic drive beats ($A_1$) and resultant $V_1$, displayed with A-H and H-V intervals of 95 and 45 msec, respectively. When the APD ($A_2$) is delivered, it initially conducts down a fast pathway with an A-H interval of 165 msec. The impulse also simultaneously conducts down the slow pathway with a markedly prolonged A-H interval of 500 msec. The impulse then returns up the fast pathway to initiate a run of A-V nodal reentry. Thus, one APD gave rise to two conducted responses over both the fast and slow pathway before initiation of SVT. See text for discussion.

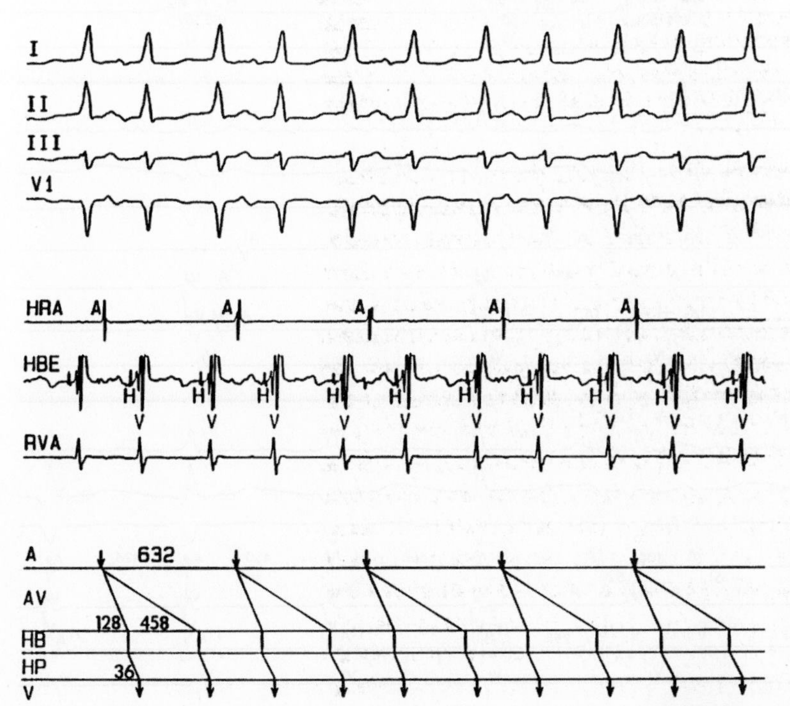


**FIGURE 8-13** *One-to-two tachycardia.* On **top** are analog records organized as ECG leads I, II, III, and $V_1$ with intracardiac recordings from HRA, HBE, and RVA. An explanatory ladder diagram is shown **below** with A, atrium, HB, His bundle, and V, ventricle. Sinus rhythm is present at a cycle length of 632 msec. Each sinus beat is conducted down both the fast and slow pathway, producing a double response, which results in a tachycardia of 316 msec.

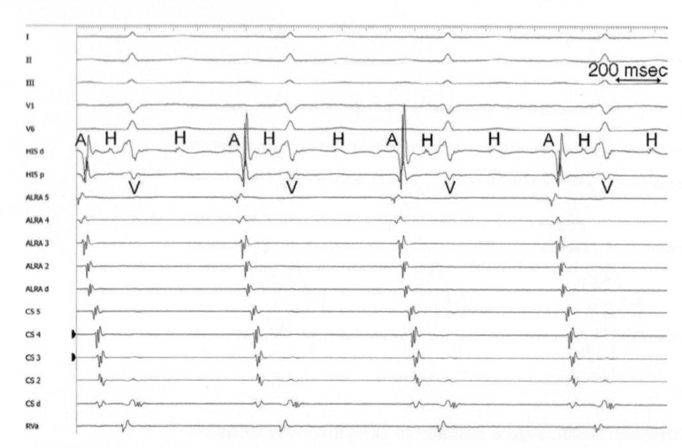


**FIGURE 8-14** *Concealed one-to-two tachycardia.* On top are analog records organized as ECG leads I, II, III, $V_1$, and $V_6$ with intracardiac recordings anterolateral right atrium (ALRA), His bundle (HIS d and p), coronary sinus proximal to distal ($CS_5$-$CS_1$) and right ventricular apex (RVA). A nonreentrant tachycardia is present, but is concealed because the impulse conducting down the slow pathway blocks below the His. See text.

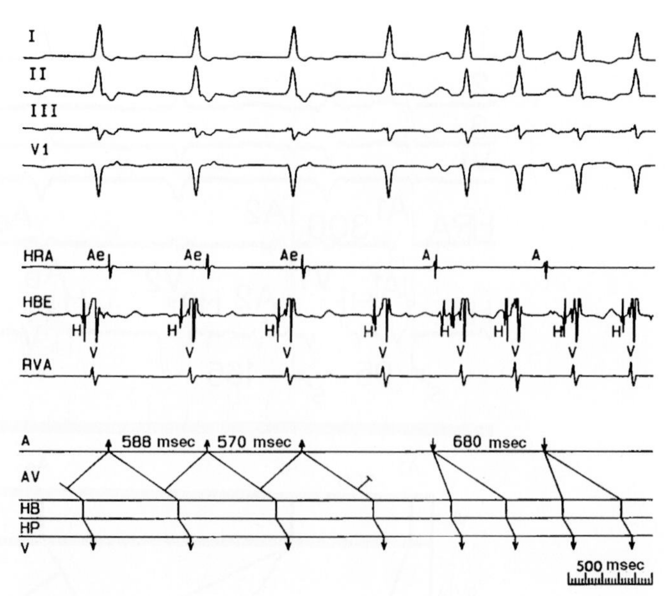


**FIGURE 8-15** *A-V nodal reentry and nonreentrant tachycardia.* This is the same patient as in Figure 8-13. The first four complexes are A-V nodal reentry. Retrograde block in the fast pathway terminates A-V nodal reentry, but sinus rhythm results in a nonreentrant tachycardia which is faster than the A-V nodal reentry. This is depicted in the ladder diagram.

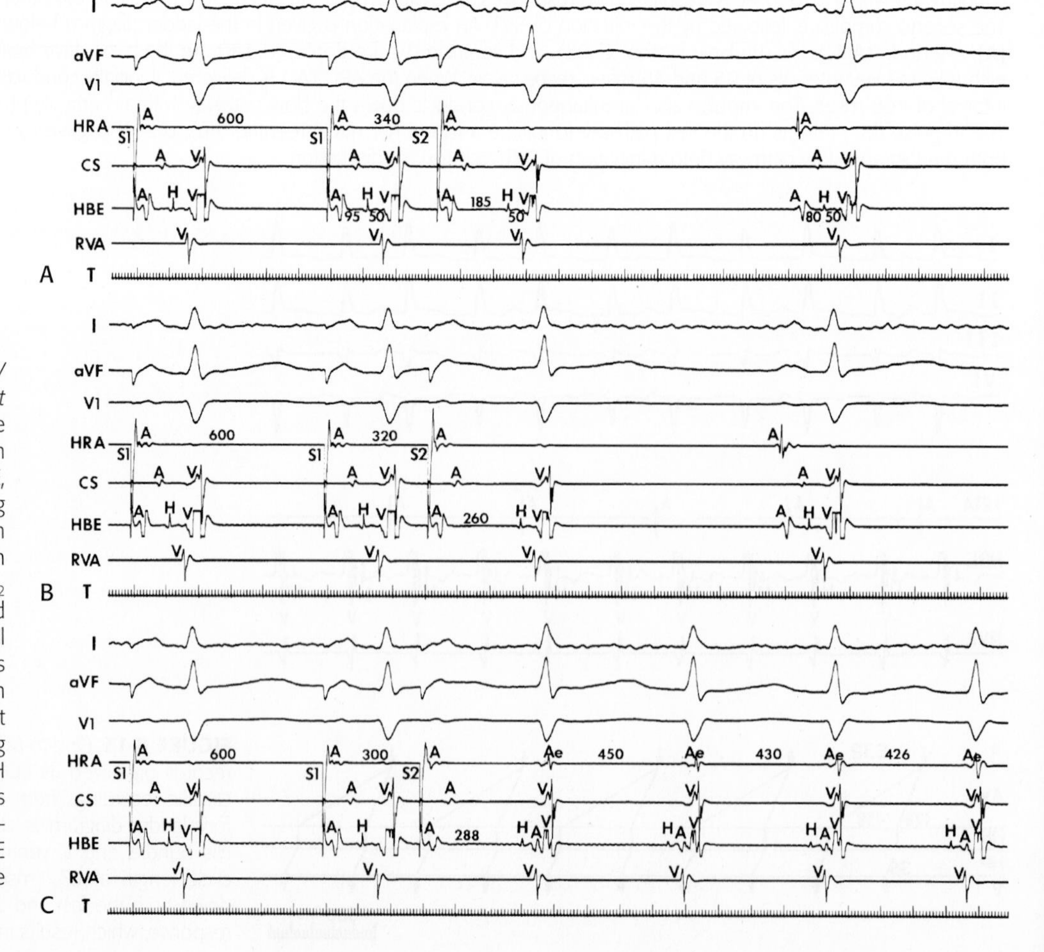


**FIGURE 8-16** *Initiation of A-V nodal reentry from the high-right atrium.* From top to bottom are leads 1, aVF, $V_1$, electrograms from the HRA, coronary sinus (CS), HBE, and RV apex. The HRA is being paced at a basic drive cycle length of 600 msec. The A-H interval on the basic drive is 95 msec. **A:** An $A_2$ delivered at 340 msec is associated with an A-H of 185 msec. **B:** A small decrement in coupling intervals is associated with a marked jump in the A-H interval to 260 msec but no echo occurs. **C:** At a coupling interval of 300 msec at a critical A-H of 288 msec, A-V nodal reentry is induced. The retrograde atrial activation sequence begins in the HBE with subsequent activation in the HRA and CS. T, time line.

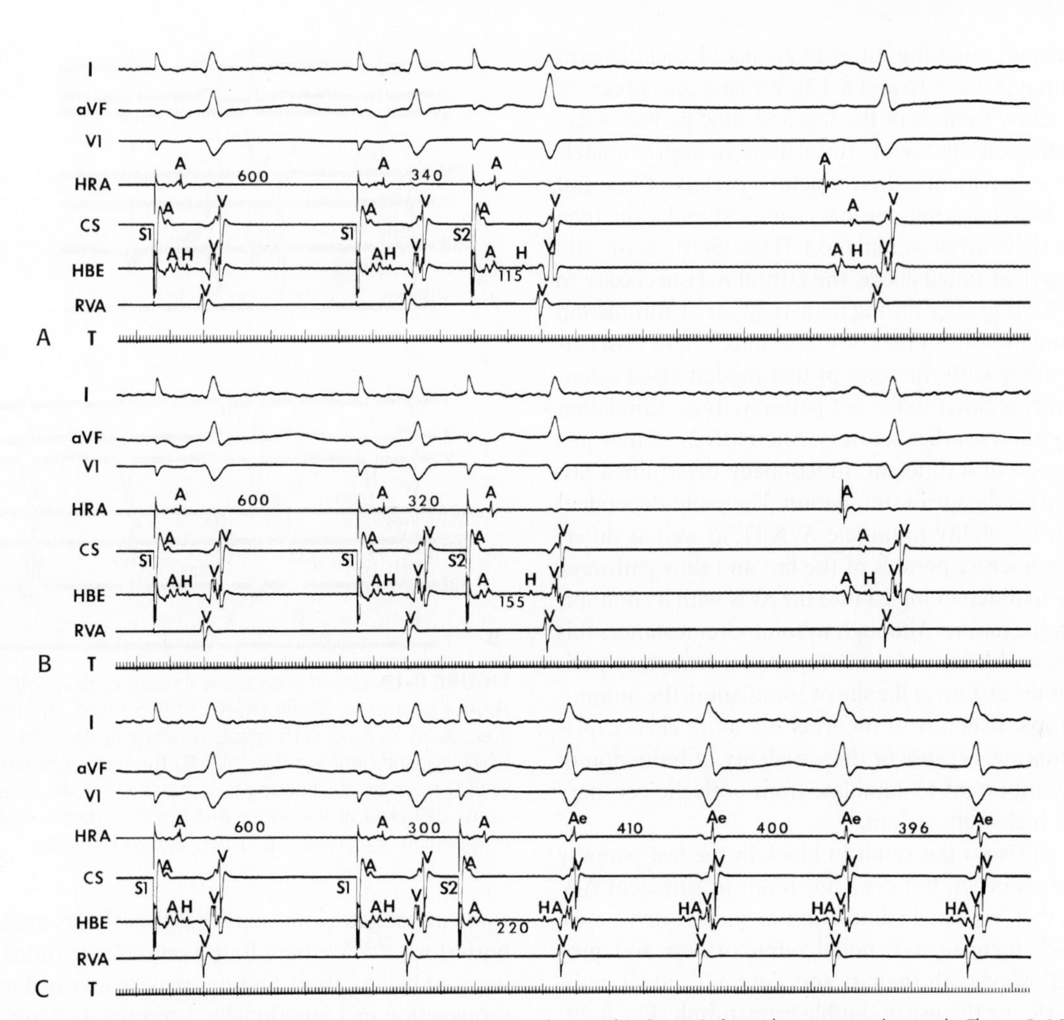


**FIGURE 8-17** *Induction of A-V nodal reentry by coronary sinus (CS) stimulation.* This figure is from the same patient as in Figure 8-16. In this figure, stimulation is carried out from the CS at a basic drive cycle length of 600 msec. **A:** At a coupling interval of 340 msec, the A-H is shorter than in Figure 8-16A during (HRA) stimulation. **B:** No jump in A-H intervals occurs at a coupling interval comparable to that in Figure 8-16B. **C:** Only at a coupling interval of 300 msec, a jump in the A-H interval occurs. However, here the A-H interval is only 220 msec, yet A-V nodal reentry is induced. Thus, despite the fact that a shorter coupling interval was required to initiate A-V nodal reentry from the CS, the critical A-H not only was shorter than the critical A-H in Figure 8-16C but was shorter than the A-H interval in **(B)** in which not even a single A-V nodal echo occurred. See text for discussion.

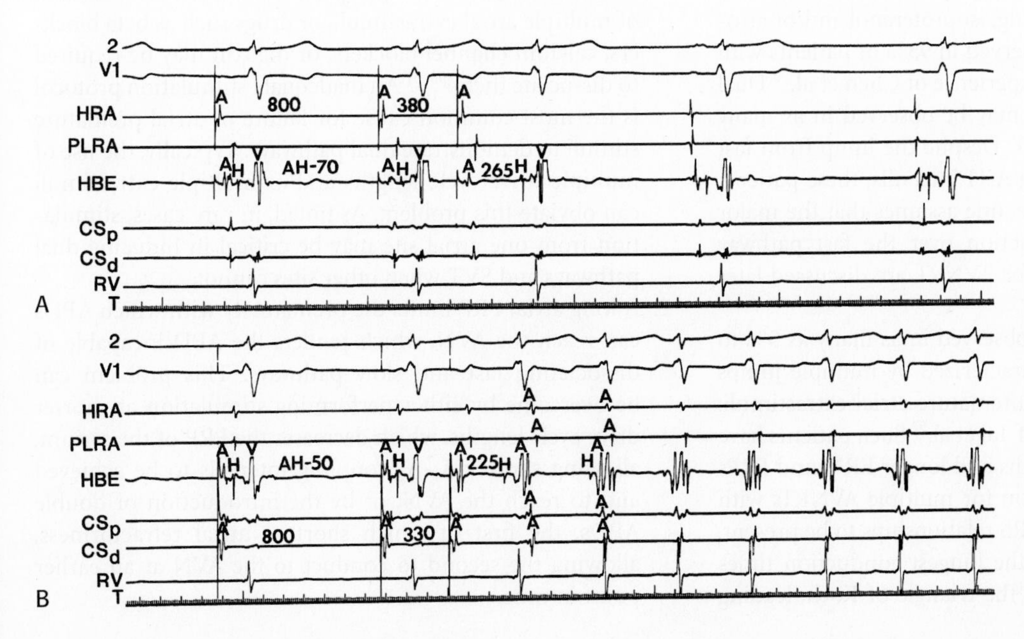


**FIGURE 8-18** *Induction of (A-V) nodal reentry by coronary sinus stimulation.* **A:** The closest-coupled HRA extrastimulus that conducts through the A-V node is associated with a long A-H (265 msec) but no echo. **B:** Stimulation from the CS allows achievement of closer coupling intervals, which initiate A-V nodal reentry despite an A-H interval that is shorter than that produced by HRA stimulation (225 msec). $CS_d$, distal CS; $CS_p$, proximal CS; PLRA, posterior low-right atrium.

although different coupling intervals or paced cycle lengths may be required (Figs. 8-16 and 8-17). We have also observed that the refractory periods of the fast and slow pathways can differ depending on the site of stimulation. In approximately one-third of our patients, the refractory period of the fast pathway is shorter during coronary sinus stimulation than during high-right atrial stimulation (Figs. 8-10, 8-16, and 8-17). Moreover, as noted above, the critical A-H necessary to initiate AVNRT is greater during high-right atrial stimulation than for stimulation from the coronary sinus.[53] This observation is compatible with the concept that the left atrial extension of the AVN is closer to the fast pathway, thus, stimulation from this site allows earlier recovery. Alternatively, it may just be an expression of a different, functionally determined fast pathway based on the site of stimulation. These site-dependent differences in the ability to initiate AVNRT, as well as differences in the refractory periods of the fast and slow pathways, are likely due to different inputs into the AVN with its nonuniform anisotropic nature. Although in some circumstances this may result from differences in the functional refractory periods (FRPs) of the atrium at the site of stimulation, the nonuniform anisotropic structure of the AVN is a more likely explanation. In any case, because of the variability of induction of AVNRT, it is important to stimulate from both the coronary sinus and the high-right atrium.

If single APDs do not result in block in the fast pathway or, if block does occur, but does not result in sufficient A-V nodal delay, then repeated stimulation at shorter drive cycle lengths, which increase A-V nodal refractoriness and prolong conduction of both the fast and slow A-V nodal pathways (Fig. 8-19), or the use of double extrastimuli (Fig. 8-20) or atrial pacing (Fig. 8-6) frequently produce the block and delay required to initiate SVT. Most patients (approximately 85%) with typical A-V nodal reentrant SVT exhibit dual A-V nodal pathways in response to single high-right atrial extrastimuli.[15,16,18,24,27,38] Using multiple drive cycle lengths and extrastimuli from both the high-right atrium and coronary sinus, as well as rapid atrial pacing, isoproterenol and/or atropine, dual pathways may be observed in 95% of patients with AVNRT. This is similar to the experience of Chen et al.[56] Dual pathways in response to APDs may be observed in as many as 25% of patients without SVT. Despite the jump from fast to slow pathway, with very long A-H intervals, these patients never have an atrial echo; hence, one assumes that the major limitation is retrograde conduction over the fast pathway (Fig. 8-21). The determinants for AVNRT are discussed later in this chapter.

Multiple pathways may be observed in as many as 5% to 10% of patients. These are characterized by multiple jumps of >50 msec with increasingly premature atrial extrastimuli. This is comparable to the data of Tai et al.[57] Such patients have AVNRTs with longer cycle lengths and longer ERPs and FRPs of the AVN. It is not uncommon for multiple AVNRTs with different cycle lengths and P–QRS relationships to be present. In general, the pathways with the longest conduction times are ablated more posteriorly in the triangle of Koch, leading

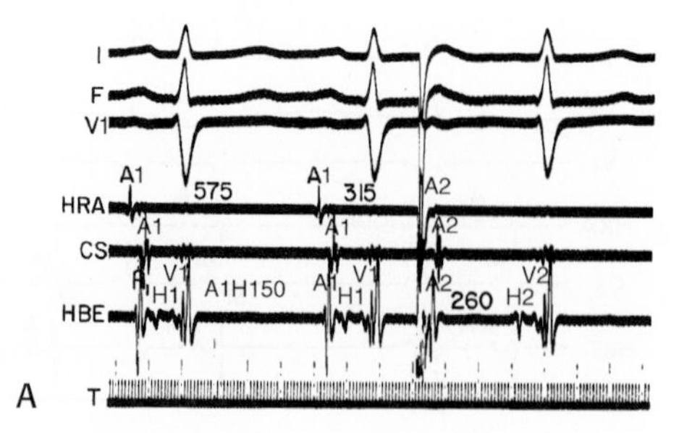


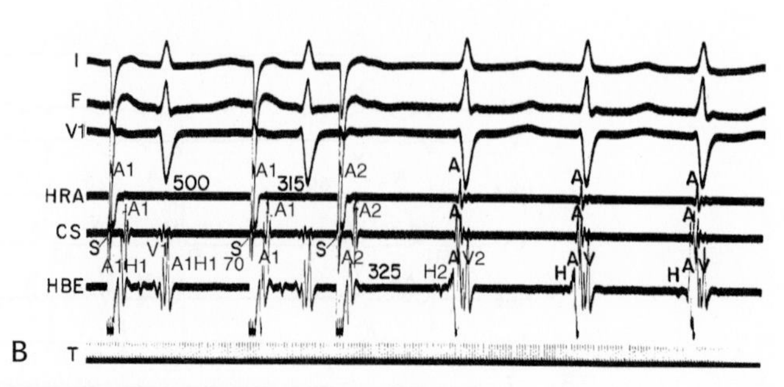


**FIGURE 8-19** *Use of a decrease in basic cycle length to initiate SVT.* **A:** At a basic cycle length ($A_1$-$A_1$) of 575 msec, an APD ($A_2$) is delivered at an $A_1$-$A_2$ of 315 msec, resulting in an $A_2$-$H_2$ of 260 msec, which is insufficient to initiate SVT. **B:** The basic cycle length is reduced to 500 msec by atrial pacing to increase A-V nodal refractoriness, and an $A_2$ delivered at the same $A_1$-$A_2$ of 315 msec results in a critical lengthening of $A_2$-$H_2$ to 325 msec, and SVT ensues.

some investigators to assert that these fibers are located more posteriorly.[56,57] We have found several exceptions to this finding, and believe these findings may be ascribed to anisotropic propagation in a functionally determined circuit.

Failure to demonstrate antegrade dual pathways in a patient with typical A-V nodal reentrant SVT in response to atrial extrastimuli is usually due to one of three factors:

1. The refractory periods of the alpha and beta pathways may be similar, and more rapid pacing rates, the introduction of multiple atrial extrastimuli, or drugs such as beta blockers, calcium channel blockers, or digoxin may be required to dissociate them.[58–61] An inadequate stimulation protocol is the most common cause for failure of atrial premature stimuli to demonstrate dual pathways. Typically, the use of multiple drive cycle lengths and/or multiple extrastimuli can obviate this problem. As noted, in rare cases, stimulation from one atrial site may be critical in inducing dual pathways and SVT when other sites cannot.
2. A long atrial FRP limits the prematurity with which APDs can reach the AVN, which renders the APD incapable of dissociating fast and slow pathways. This problem can be overcome by either performing stimulation at shorter drive cycle lengths, which decreases the FRP of the atrium, allowing shorter $A_1$-$A_2$ coupling intervals to be achieved and to reach the AVN; or by the introduction of double APDs, the first of which shortens atrial refractoriness, allowing the second to conduct to the AVN at an earlier point in time.

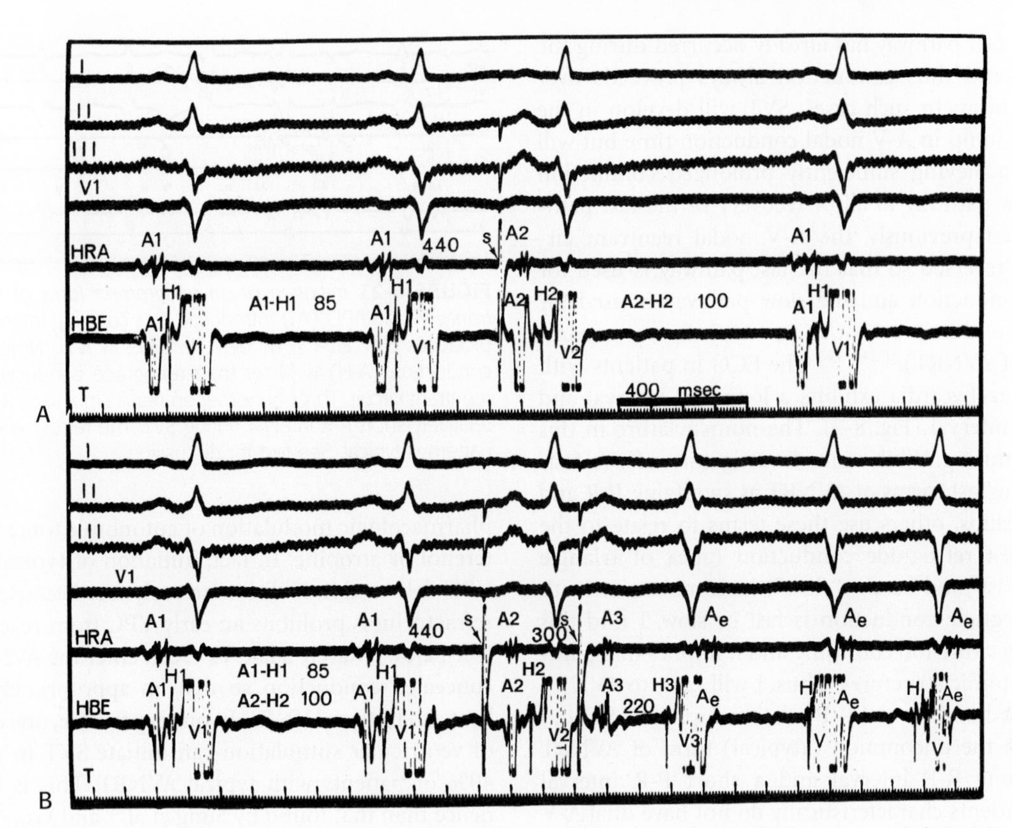


**FIGURE 8-20** *Use of APDs to initiate SVT.* **A:** An APD ($A_2$) delivered at a coupling interval ($A_1$-$A_2$) of 440 msec fails to initiate SVT. **B:** If $A_2$ is followed by a second APD ($A_3$), enough A-V nodal delay is produced ($A_3$-$H_3$ = 220 msec) to initiate SVT.

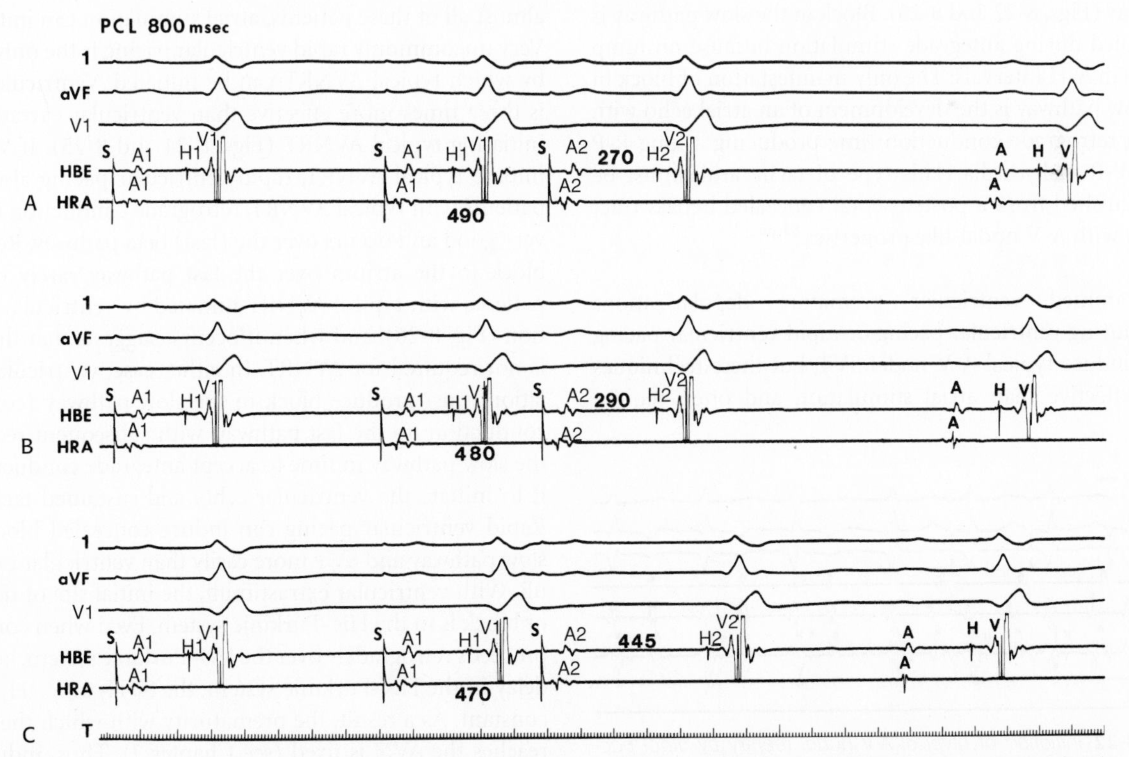


**FIGURE 8-21** *Demonstration of dual pathways with marked A-V nodal conduction delay in the balance of an A-V nodal echo.* **A, B**, and **C:** From top to bottom leads 1, aVF, and $V_1$ and electrograms from the HBE and HRA. In all three panels, stimulation is from the HRA. The basic paced cycle length (PCL) is at 800 msec. **A** and **B:** At 490- and 480-msec coupling intervals, the $A_2$-$H_2$ interval is prolonged to 290 msec without a jump. **C:** With a 10-msec decrement in $A_1$-$A_2$ intervals, however, there is a 155-msec increment in A-H intervals, diagnostic of dual pathways. Despite the marked delay in A-H intervals approximating the $A_1$-$A_2$ interval, no echo occurs. See text for discussion.

3. Block in the fast pathway has already occurred during the basal drive, and thus conduction always proceeds over the slow pathway. In such cases, SVT will develop in the absence of a jump in A-V nodal conduction time but will depend on achieving sufficiently prolonged conduction over the slow pathway to allow recovery of the fast pathway. As noted previously, the A-V nodal reentrant circuit may be reversed so that the fast pathway is used for antegrade conduction and the slow pathway is used for retrograde conduction (fast/slow, atypical, or uncommon form of AVNRT).[18,24–28,62] The ECG in patients with this type of tachycardia exhibits a long R-P interval and a short P-R interval (Fig. 8-2). The nomenclature in this matter is confusing. While many investigators refer to fast/slow and slow/fast forms of AVNRT as signifying P-R and R-P relationships, others use these terms to relate to the site of earliest retrograde conduction (apex of triangle of Koch = "fast" and base = "slow") in combination with whether antegrade conduction is fast or slow. I find this latter nomenclature too confusing and it implies that pathways are anatomic structures. Thus, I will refer to AVNRT subtypes based on P-R and R-P relationships. The ECG in patients with the uncommon (atypical) form of AVNRT exhibits a long R-P interval and a short P-R interval (Fig. 8-2). Patients characteristically do not have dual A-V nodal pathways in response to APDs or atrial pacing. The tachycardia is initiated with APDs or atrial pacing, producing modest increases of the A-H interval along the fast pathway (Figs. 8-22 and 8-23). Block in the slow pathway is concealed during antegrade stimulation because no jump occurs in A-H intervals. The only manifestation of block in the slow pathway is the development of an atrial echo with a long retrograde conduction time producing a long R-P short P-R tachycardia. This type of tachycardia must be distinguished from a posteroseptal concealed bypass tract (CBT) with A-V nodal-like properties.[63–66]

Programmed ventricular premature depolarizations (VPDs) during ventricular pacing or rapid ventricular pacing can also induce typical A-V nodal SVT, but these techniques are less effective than atrial stimulation and often require

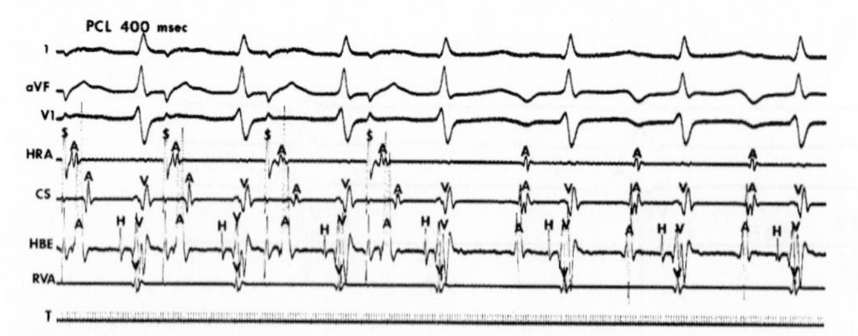


**FIGURE 8-22** *Initiation of atypical A-V nodal reentry by atrial pacing.* Leads 1, aVF, and $V_1$, and electrograms from the HRA, CS, HBE, and RVA are shown. Atrial pacing at a paced cycle length (PCL) of 400 msec results in a modest increase in the A-H interval. Following cessation of pacing, atypical A-V nodal reentry begins with a long R-P interval following the last paced complex. See text for discussion.

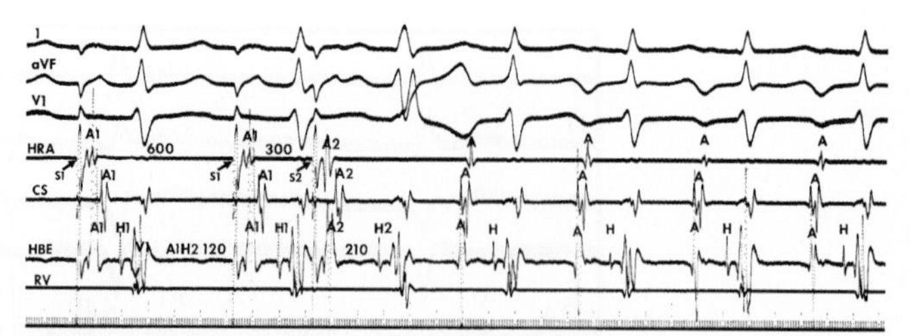


**FIGURE 8-23** *Initiation of an uncommon form of A-V nodal reentrant SVT.* An APD ($A_2$) introduced at a coupling interval of 300 msec produces SVT after a modest increase in A-H. Note that antegrade conduction (A-H) is faster than retrograde conduction (H-A) in the reentrant circuit. This phenomenon results in a long R-P interval and a relatively short P-R interval during SVT. The retrograde atrial activation pattern is typical. See text for discussion.

pharmacologic modulation of autonomic tone; that is, isoproterenol or atropine. In fact, initiation of typical AVNRT by a VPC delivered in NSR is extremely rare because His–Purkinje refractoriness prohibits an early VPC from reaching the AVN (see below). Rarely a late VPC can enter the AVN and produce concealed conduction so that an appropriately timed sinus beat can initiate AVNRT. In our experience, one or more forms of ventricular stimulation can initiate SVT in approximately 40% of patients with typical AVNRT. This is a higher incidence than that found by Sung et al.[26] and Wu,[24,66] who found ventricular stimulation–induced typical AVNRT in only 10% to 30% of patients. In contrast, atypical AVNRT is induced almost as frequently from the ventricle as from the atrium. In almost all of these patients, atrial stimulation can initiate SVT. Very uncommonly rapid ventricular pacing is the only method by which typical AVNRT can be initiated. Ventricular pacing is three times more effective than ventricular extrastimuli in initiating typical AVNRT (Figs. 8-24 and 8-25). If VPDs can initiate typical AVNRT, rapid ventricular pacing also can. In patients with typical AVNRT, retrograde conduction is usually very good and occurs over the (fast) beta pathway. Retrograde block to the atrium over the fast pathway rarely occurs in patients with typical AVNRT initiated by ventricular stimulation (Fig. 8-26), and when it occurs, suggests that the atrium is not required for AVNRT. In either case, ventricular stimulation must produce block in the slow pathway (concealed), conduction up the fast pathway, with subsequent recovery of the slow pathway in time to accept antegrade conduction over it to initiate the ventricular echo, and sustained tachycardia. Rapid ventricular pacing can induce concealed block in the slow pathway and SVT more easily than ventricular extrastimuli. With ventricular extrastimuli, the initial site of delay and/or block is in the His–Purkinje system. Even when conduction proceeds retrogradely over the His–Purkinje system, because of delay in the His–Purkinje system, the $S_1$-$H_2$ or $V_1$-$H_2$ remains constant. As a result, the prematurity with which the impulse reaches the AVN is fixed (see Chapter 2). Thus, induction of typical AVNRT by a single VPD during ventricular pacing only succeeds in approximately 10% of patients.

Specific reasons for failure to initiate typical AVNRT by VPDs include (a) block in the His–Purkinje system; (b) the

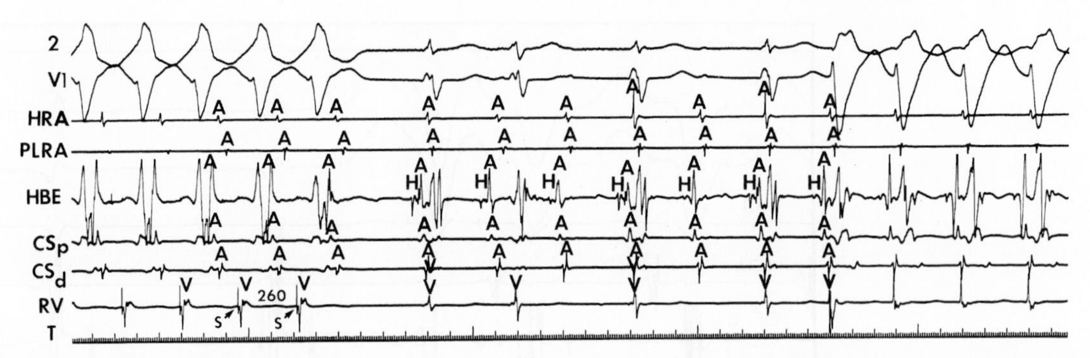


**FIGURE 8-24** *Initiation of typical AVNRT by ventricular pacing.* Leads 2 and $V_1$ are shown with electrograms from the (HRA), posterior low-right atrium (PLRA), HBE, proximal ($CS_p$) and distal ($CS_d$) coronary sinus, and RV. Ventricular pacing at 260 msec is shown on the left with 1:1 conduction up the fast pathway. On cessation of pacing following retrograde conduction up the fast pathway, conduction goes down the slow pathway, leading to typical A-V nodal reentry. Transient infra-His block is observed with resumption of 1:1 conduction with bundle branch block. See text for further discussion.

FRP of the His–Purkinje system exceeds the effective refractory period (ERP) of the slow pathway in the retrograde direction; (c) the ERP of the slow pathway is equal to that of the fast pathway in the retrograde direction; (d) the antegrade slow pathway ERP exceeds the ventricular-paced cycle length, therefore it cannot accept an input from the fast pathway at that cycle length; (e) following its engagement from the fast pathway, there is insufficient antegrade delay in the slow pathway to allow the fast pathway to recover; and (f) block in a lower final common pathway in the AVN (i.e., proximal to the slow and fast pathways in the retrograde direction), which thereby prohibits block in one of these pathways. Pacing at shorter drive cycle lengths may increase the percentage of patients in whom typical AVNRT can be induced by ventricular stimulation because of shortening the ERP and FRP of the His–Purkinje system.

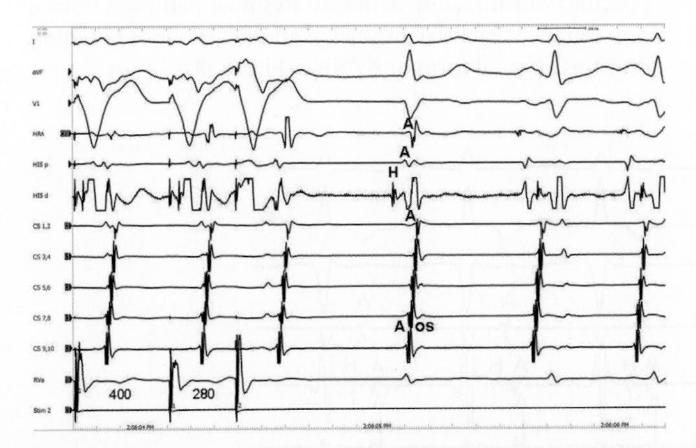


**FIGURE 8-25** *Initiation of typical A-V nodal reentry by a VPD.* Leads 1, aVF and $V_1$ are shown with electrograms from the HRA, proximal and distal HBE, proximal (9, 10) to distal (1, 2) CS, and RVA. The ventricles are paced at 400 msec, and a ventricular extrastimulus is delivered at 280 msec. This results in prolongation of the V-A. The relatively rapid retrograde conduction up the fast pathway is followed by antegrade conduction over the slow pathway, with a markedly prolonged A-H interval exceeding 400 msec and over the slow pathway to initiate A-V nodal reentry.

Many of the problems imposed by His–Purkinje refractoriness on induction of typical AVNRT by ventricular stimulation can be overcome by rapid ventricular pacing, during which the AVN is the primary site of delay. This explains why rapid pacing is more likely to longitudinally dissociate fast and slow pathways in the AVN than extrastimuli. The observation that ventricular pacing does not always induce typical A-V nodal SVT is explained in part by the occurrence of repetitive concealment, not block, in the slow pathway, rendering it incapable of antegrade conduction. Block cannot be distinguished from concealment in humans.

The specific mechanisms by which ventricular stimulation can induce A-V nodal reentrant SVT follows:

1. The most common method of inducing typical AVNRT depends on the retrograde refractory period of the alpha pathway exceeding that of the beta pathway. In this instance, VPDs or ventricular pacing induce typical AVNRT in the absence of the demonstration of retrograde dual pathways. Retrograde conduction proceeds up the fast pathway without prolonged retrograde conduction. Block in the slow pathway is not manifested (i.e., it is concealed) and is only inferred by initiation of the tachycardia. Thus, no critical V-A or H-A interval is required to induce the tachycardia. As mentioned, this is easier to achieve with ventricular pacing than ventricular extrastimuli. An example of the initiation of typical AVNRT by a VPD conducting up the fast pathway is shown in Figure 8-25. Initiation of a tachycardia by rapid ventricular pacing is shown in Figure 8-24.
2. Interpolated VPDs can result in the production of antegrade dual pathways; that is, retrograde concealed conduction can result in antegrade block in the fast beta pathway and allow slow conduction down the alpha pathway. This produces dual A-V nodal pathway physiology with induction of typical A-V nodal reentrant SVT. This is far less common than method 1.
3. If the retrograde refractory period of the fast pathway exceeds that of the slow pathway, VPDs or ventricular pacing can produce retrograde dual A-V nodal pathways. This

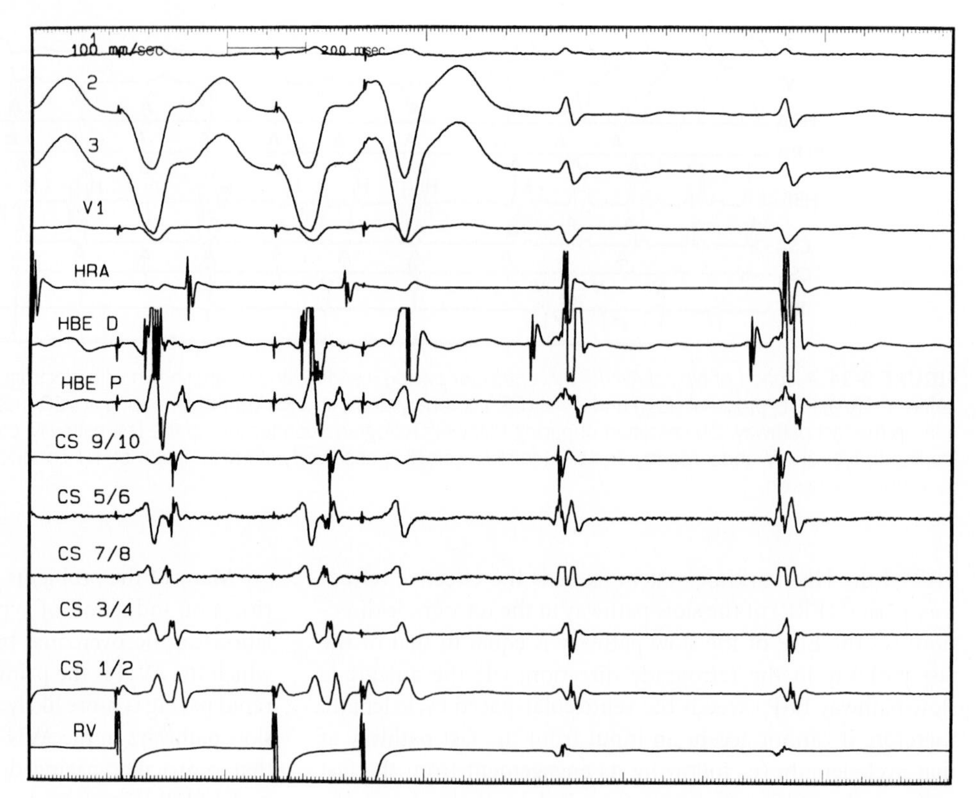


**FIGURE 8-26** *Induction of typical AVNRT by ventricular stimulation in the absence of atrial activation.* ECG leads 1, 2, 3, and $V_1$ are shown with recordings from the HRA, distal (d) and proximal (p) HBE, and five bilar pairs from the CS (electrode numbers shown), and RV. A premature ventricular depolarization is delivered at a coupling interval of 230 msec, which initiates typical AVNRT. Note that the VPD, which must go up the fast pathway, blocks to the atrium but still turns around to conduct antegradely down the slow pathway to initiate the tachycardia.

leads to the development of the uncommon type of A-V nodal SVT because initial block in the beta (fast) pathway results in a long retrograde conduction time up the alpha (slow) pathway, which is followed by antegrade conduction down the fast pathway. This is a common mechanism of induction of the atypical form of AVNRT in the laboratory. As noted, with atypical AVNRT, ventricular stimulation is equally as likely to initiate the rhythm as atrial stimulation. Occasionally, atypical AVNRT can be induced by ventricular extrastimuli demonstrating conduction over both the fast and slow pathways in response to the single ventricular extrastimulus (Fig. 8-27).[42] In Figure 8-27, conduction of $S_2$ occurs first over the fast, and then over the slow pathway. The H-A interval over the slow pathway at initiation of the tachycardia is much longer than the H-A interval during the tachycardia because of concealment into the slow pathway by the initial conduction over the fast pathway. This is analogous to initiation of AVNRT by atrial extrastimuli producing a one-to-two response (Fig. 8-12). Ventricular pacing, which readily demonstrates dual pathways during retrograde Wenckebach cycles, is another mode of initiation for this atypical form of AVNRT (Fig. 8-28).

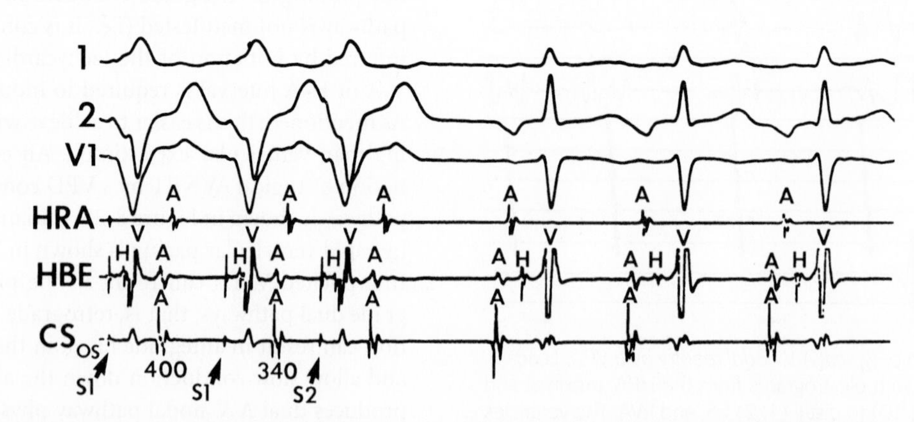


**FIGURE 8-27** *Induction of atypical A-V nodal reentry by ventricular stimulation.* Leads 1, 2, $V_1$ and electrograms from the HRA, HBE, and the os of the CS are shown. During a basic drive of 400 msec ($S_1$-$S_1$), a premature stimulus ($S_2$) is delivered at 340 msec. Retrograde His deflections can be seen on both the drive and premature complexes. With $S_2$, the impulse conducts retrogradely up the fast pathway with essentially no delay and also goes up the slow pathway with a markedly prolonged H-A interval to initiate the tachycardia as it returns down the fast pathway. Thus, one ventricular extrastimulus gave rise to two atrial responses, one over the fast pathway and one over the slow pathway, to initiate SVT. Note the $CS_{OS}$ is the earliest site of atrial activation. See text for discussion.

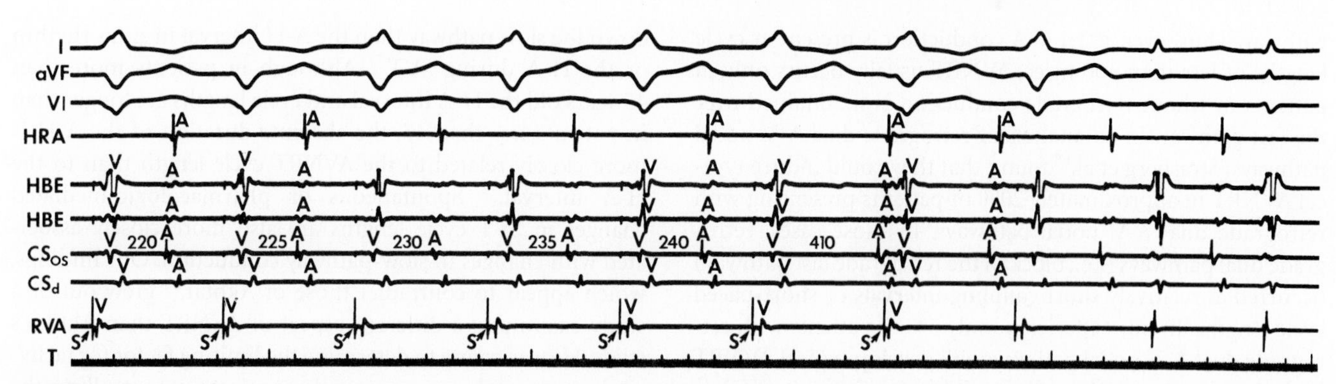


**FIGURE 8-28** *Initiation of atypical A-V nodal reentry by ventricular pacing.* Leads 1, aVF, and $V_1$ and electrograms from the RVA, HBE, os and distal pair of electrodes from the CS, and RVA are shown. Ventricular pacing is performed at a cycle length of 500 msec. There is progressive delay from A to V (see $CS_{os}$ tracing) until after the sixth stimulus. There is a jump in V-A intervals to 410 msec. When pacing is turned off, atypical A-V nodal reentry is present, having been initiated from the seventh stimulus. Therefore, the eighth stimulus is a fusion between the first beat of atypical A-V nodal reentry and ventricular pacing. Note the $CS_{os}$ is the earliest site of atrial activation.

## Determinants for the Induction of Atrioventricular Nodal Reentry

Some generalizations can be made regarding the determinants for developing typical AVNRT. Although dual A-V nodal pathways are required for AVNRT, they are insufficient. Many patients can demonstrate "dual pathways" but do not have spontaneous or inducible AVNRT. The most common finding in patients with dual A-V nodal pathways who do not develop SVT is the failure of the impulse to return up the fast pathway once antegrade conduction has proceeded over the slow pathway. There are four possible explanations for this phenomenon: (a) longitudinal dissociation of the AVN is not really present, but the pattern of conduction of "pseudo-dual" pathways is produced by electrotonic propagation across a nonhomogenous linear area in the AVN, as described previously[29]; (b) the APD that "blocks" in the fast pathway produces postdepolarization refractoriness (i.e., a manifestation of concealed conduction) resulting in the inability of the fast pathway to recover excitability in time to be reexcited; conduction down the slow pathway is insufficiently slow to allow the fast pathway to recover; (c) the fast pathway has a long retrograde refractory period, which renders it incapable of retrograde conduction despite slow antegrade conduction of the slow pathway; (d) there is no distal connection between the fast and slow pathways. Based on our data and that of others[67] the most common reason for failure to induce typical AVNRT in patients with antegrade dual pathways is that the fast pathway is incapable of rapid retrograde conduction.

This can be evaluated by using the maximum rates of 1:1 antegrade and retrograde conduction as indices of antegrade slow pathway refractoriness and retrograde fast pathway refractoriness. Denes et al.[67] first analyzed fast and slow pathway properties in detail and clearly showed that the ability to induce typical AVNRT required 1:1 V-A conduction. Absence of induction of typical AVNRT in patients with antegrade dual pathways was associated with either no V-A conduction or V-A Wenckebach at relatively long drive cycle lengths.[58] Most often, the ability to induce typical AVNRT requires the capability of one-to-one retrograde V-A conduction at paced ventricular cycle lengths of ≤400 msec.

Although retrograde fast-pathway characteristics determine if reentry can occur, slow-pathway conduction time determines when it will occur. Thus, the "critical A-H" concept depends on fast-pathway recovery at a given $A_2$-$H_2$ interval. When echoes do not occur as soon as the impulse blocks in the fast pathway and goes down the slow pathway, concealed conduction into the fast pathway by $A_2$ may be present, requiring a critical A-H for recovery. This can mimic a primary impairment of V-A fast-pathway conduction as the determinant of reentry. One can recognize the likely presence of concealment if the A-H interval not producing an echo exceeds the shortest cycle length of 1:1 retrograde conduction up the fast pathway.

Although an isolated A-V nodal echo can occur as long as V-A conduction is present, the ability to initiate sustained SVT also requires the capability of the slow pathway to sustain repetitive antegrade conduction. Denes et al.[67] found that sustained, typical AVNRT was initiated only if the slow pathway maintained 1:1 antegrade conduction at cycle lengths less than 350 msec. Patients who only had single A-V nodal echoes in response to APDs usually developed antegrade Wenckebach in the slow pathway at relatively long cycle lengths. Thus, the ability to initiate sustained SVT depends on the balance of a retrograde fast-pathway conduction and antegrade slow-pathway conduction.

Retrograde fast-pathway conduction appears to be the major determinant of the ability to initiate isolated A-V nodal echoes and/or sustained SVT. This is further supported by the fact that there is no difference in maximal A-H intervals during slow-pathway conduction in patients with and without echoes or SVT. The ability to initiate A-V nodal echoes by APDs thus depends primarily on the capability of V-A conduction over the fast pathway. This has been our experience almost universally. It is therefore obvious that patients with retrograde dual pathways will have a low incidence of sustained typical AVNRT, because the presence of dual pathways suggests relatively poor retrograde conduction over the fast pathway. Thus, even if 1:1 V-A conduction is present at cycle lengths of less than 400 msec, AVNRT usually occurs only in patients in whom retrograde conduction is maintained over the fast pathway. In an analysis of retrograde dual A-V nodal pathways, Strasberg et al.[68] found that they could induce typical AVNRT in approximately 20% of patients presenting with retrograde dual A-V nodal pathways. In those cases, retrograde dual pathways (i.e., block in the retrograde fast pathway) occurred at relatively short coupling intervals or short-paced cycle lengths. In our experience, only 5% of patients with retrograde dual A-V nodal pathways will develop typical AVNRT in the baseline state. We have found the use of atropine or isoproterenol, which shortens the retrograde refractory period of the fast pathway and improve retrograde fast-pathway conduction, increases the number of patients with retrograde dual pathways in the control state in whom sustained typical AVNRT can be induced by APDs to 20%. Others have found a slightly higher incidence.[67–70] In our patients, facilitation of induction of typical AVNRT depended on improving V-A conduction such that 1:1 V-A conduction over the fast pathway at cycle lengths of 425 msec or less was achieved in all patients in whom typical AVNRT could be induced. Thus, the markers that are predictive of a low likelihood of inducibility of typical AVNRT are (a) no V-A conduction, (b) V-A conduction worse than A-V conduction with retrograde Wenckebach at long cycle lengths (500 msec or more), and (c) retrograde dual pathways. Exceptions can occur if failure of V-A conduction results from retrograde block in the HPS or in a lower final common pathway in the AVN (see subsequent discussion). In the latter case, catecholamines and/or atropine can overcome the block. In addition, as noted earlier in the chapter (and to be discussed later) A-V nodal tachycardia can occur with block to the atrium; retrograde fast pathway is present but not manifested by atrial activation.

The A-H interval may be a useful marker in predicting the capability of rapid V-A conduction. In our experience, as well as that of Bauernfeind et al.,[71] the shorter the A-H interval, the better the V-A conduction. In fact, the shorter the A-H interval, the shorter the antegrade refractory period of the fast pathway, the shorter the cycle length at which block is produced in the fast pathway, and the shorter the cycle length at which 1:1 V-A conduction is maintained. In addition, although overlap existed, Bauernfeind et al.[71] found statistically significant relationships between retrograde H-A intervals and antegrade A-H intervals, shorter cycle lengths maintaining 1:1 V-A conduction and A-H interval, and a higher incidence of inducible SVT in patients with short A-H intervals and dual pathways than in those with longer A-H intervals and dual pathways.[64] These findings provide a potential explanation for the high incidence of SVT in patients with short P-R intervals giving rise to the so-called Lown–Ganong–Levine syndrome. It is of interest that Akhtar[18] also found that the shortest cycle length of typical A-V nodal SVT correlated best with the shortest cycle length of 1:1 V-A conduction, a finding that correlates with a short A-H interval. In contrast, we have found that the cycle length of SVT is more closely related to conduction down the slow pathway than the A-H interval in sinus rhythm or the H-A during SVT.[72] Although in patients more than 45 years old the H-A interval and cycle lengths are longer than in patients less than 45, the absolute duration of the A-H is more closely related to the AVNRT cycle length than to the H-A interval.[72] Spontaneous or pharmacologic-mediated changes in SVT cycle lengths are also more closely associated with changes in slow-pathway conduction. Our findings, which appear to contradict those of Akhtar,[18] grew out of a study examining a different aspect of AVNRT than Akhtar's study. He was trying to determine the limiting factor for tachycardia rate while we were analyzing factors controlling the tachycardia rate. Spontaneous termination of typical AVNRT can occur by either retrograde block in the fast pathway or antegrade block in the slow pathway. Although it is not always possible to predict which pathway will be the major limiting factor in maintaining AVNRT in an individual patient, a short P-R interval suggests that the fast pathway is unlikely to be the site of block. In addition, the direction (i.e., A-V or V-A) at which conduction fails at the longest cycle length provides a reasonable, but not absolute, marker for induction of spontaneous block.

Little data exist for the determinants of induction of atypical AVNRT because it is such an uncommon arrhythmia. It is our impression that retrograde slow-pathway conduction is the major determinant inducing this arrhythmia. Antegrade fast-pathway conduction is usually rapid enough and refractoriness is short enough to accept and conduct antegradely the impulse that has conducted retrogradely over the slow pathway. Thus, the development of atypical AVNRT by ventricular stimulation is determined primarily by the ability to demonstrate retrograde slow-pathway conduction, since the fast pathway almost always can return the impulse toward the ventricle. When the uncommon form of AVNRT is induced by atrial stimulation, the major determinant of retrograde slow-pathway conduction is insufficient antegrade concealment into the slow pathway so that retrograde conduction is possible.

## Atrial Activation Sequence and the P–QRS Relationship During Supraventricular Tachycardia

The sequence of retrograde atrial activation during typical A-V nodal reentrant tachycardia is more complex than previously believed. While early studies suggested that the initial site of retrograde atrial activation during typical AVNRT is recorded in the His bundle electrogram,[16,18,73–75] more detailed mapping using a decapolar catheter with 2-mm interelectrode distance to record the His bundle (distal pair) and electrograms along the tendon of Todaro, a deflectable quadripolar catheter (2-5-2–mm interelectrode distance) at the base of the triangle of Koch (area between the os of the coronary sinus and tricuspid annulus), and a decapolar catheter (5-mm interelectrode distance) in the coronary sinus with the proximal pair placed 1 to 2 cm inside the os

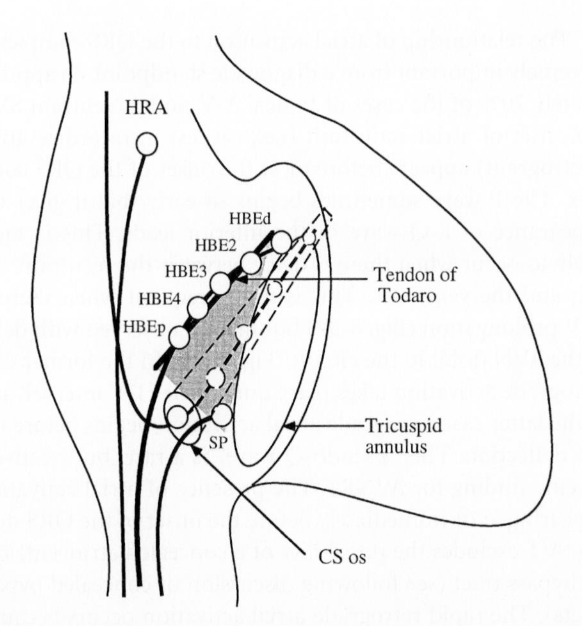


**FIGURE 8-29** *Schematic of recording sites relative to the triangle of Koch in the right anterior oblique view.* Five bipolar recordings along the tendon of Todaro are obtained from the His bundle catheter, five from the CS (proximal pole just inside the os). One or two recordings are also obtained at the posterior triangle of Koch at the "slow pathway" area.

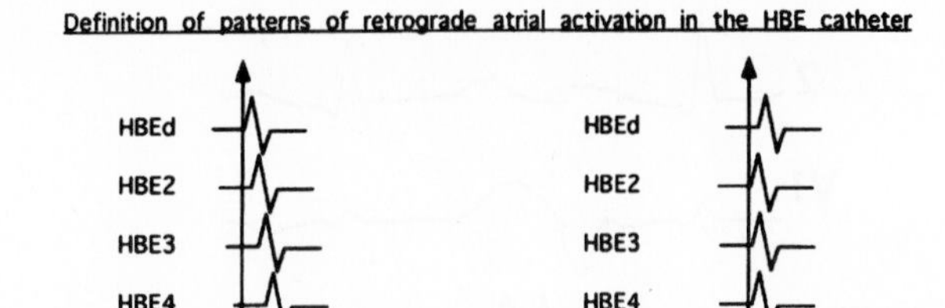


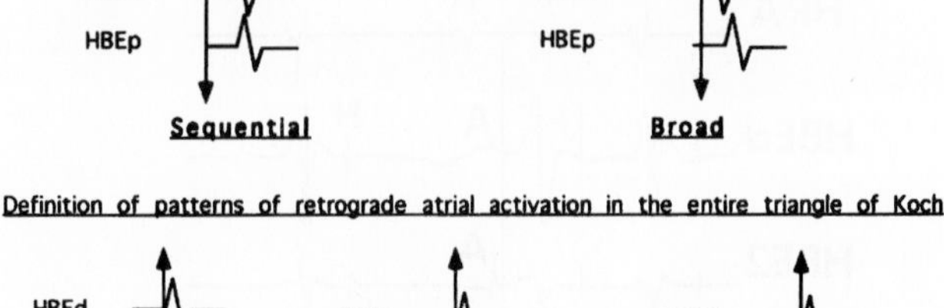


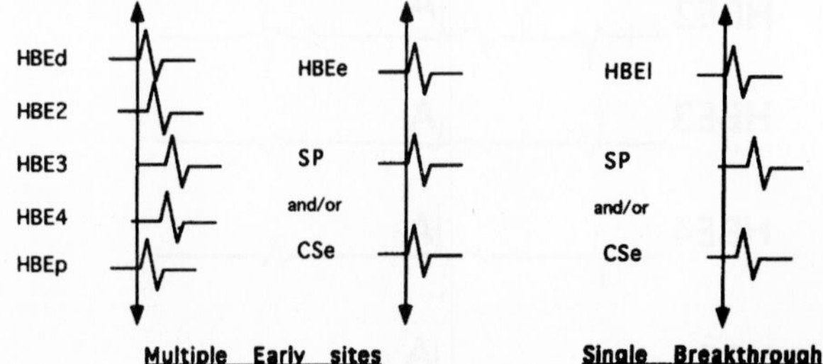


**FIGURE 8-30** *Patterns of retrograde atrial activation.* **Top:** Definition of patterns of activation along the His bundle catheter. Sequential is defined by spread away from a focal early site of activation. Broad is defined by simultaneous (within 5 msec) activation of three or more adjacent sites. **Bottom:** Definitions of activation of the entire triangle of Koch. Left and middle show multiple breakthrough patterns (two or more separate sites activated within 5 msec) or a single breakthrough (one early site at any location). See text for discussion. (From Anselme F, Fredericks J, Papageorgiou P, et al. Nonuniform anisotropy is responsible for age-related slowing of atrioventricular nodal reentrant tachycardia. *J Cardiovasc Electrophysiol* 1996;7:1145–5378.)

(Fig. 8-29).[76,77] of the triangle of Koch and coronary sinus shows marked heterogeneity in the pattern of activation.[76,77] Patterns were described along the tendon of Todaro as sequential or broad and throughout the triangle of Koch and coronary sinus as having single or multiple breakthrough sites (Fig. 8-30). Multiple breakthroughs were considered to be present when two or more activation times along the His bundle catheter within 5 msec of each other were separated by two later sites, or when one or more sites on the His bundle catheter and any other catheter (i.e., slow pathway or coronary sinus) occurred within 5 msec of each other. VPDs were introduced when necessary to accurately measure the atrial activation sequence. Examples of heterogenous atrial activation during AVNRT are shown in Figures 8-31 and 8-32 In nearly 50% of patients a secondary breakthrough in the coronary sinus was observed (Fig. 8-29); that is, an electrogram within the coronary sinus was bounded by sites with later electrograms.[78] Similar findings were observed, but not commented upon by McGuire et al.[79] Activation during AVNRT and ventricular pacing were discordant qualitatively and/or quantitatively in 60% of patients (Fig. 8-33). Similar heterogeneity was seen during atypical AVNRT although earliest activation tended to be at the base of the triangle of Koch or in the coronary sinus (Fig. 8-34).[76–78] Multiple breakthroughs, during detailed atrial mapping, are a useful discriminator of AVNRT from atrial tachycardia or circus movement tachycardia using a bypass tract. Although Jackman's group have described and depicted a number of large reentrant pathways involving the left atrium and coronary sinus, our mapping data have never found and do not support a macroreentrant circuit. The atrial activation pattern during AVNRT has important implications as to the role of the atrium in AVNRT (see discussion below). From these heterogenous activation patterns, the wave of atrial activation subsequently spreads cephalad and laterally to depolarize the remainder of the right and left atria. These findings suggest that retrograde activation during SVT spreads radially after leaving the AVN. Of note, studies by Ross et al.,[80] using intraoperative mapping, demonstrated a relationship of the earliest site of atrial activation to the retrograde H-A interval. In general, the shorter the H-A interval, the more likely the earliest atrial activation is recorded in the His bundle electrograms. As the H-A interval prolongs, the earliest activation moves closer to the base of the triangle of Koch or in the coronary sinus. Of importance is the recognition that identification of an "earliest" site of atrial activation does not mean that atrial activation is sequential from that site. As stated above, multiple breakthroughs are present in ~50% of patients. Recent experience using left atrial mapping in addition to detailed right atrial and coronary sinus mapping has confirmed the lack of sequential activation compatible with large reentrant circuits during AVNRT.

On the surface ECG the narrowest P waves are seen when atrial activation begins at the apex of the triangle of Koch. In our experience 7% of AVNRTs have earliest atrial activation

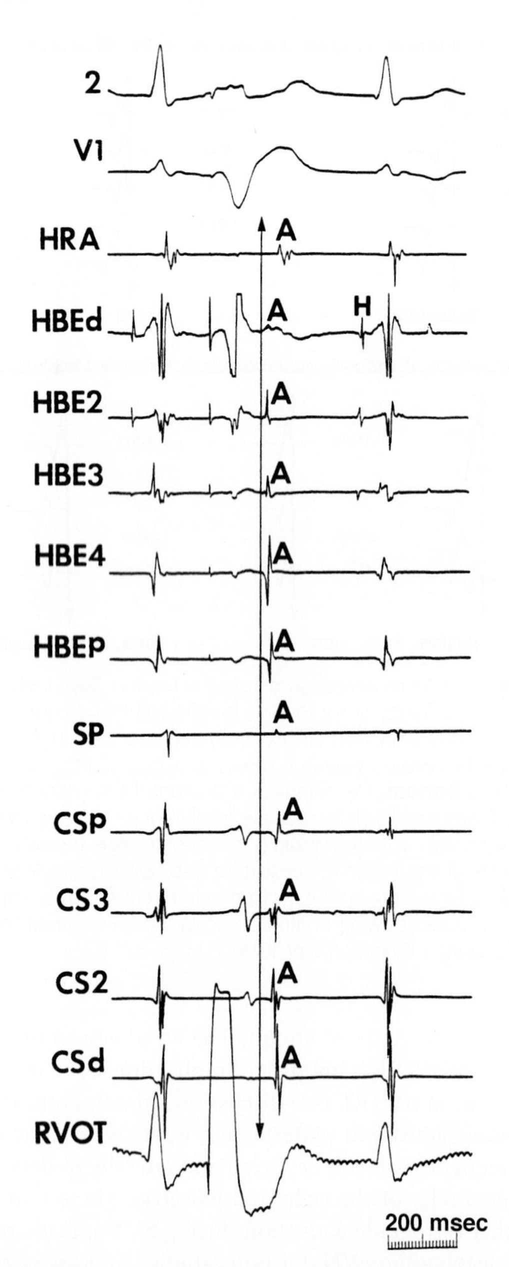


**FIGURE 8-31** *Example of single breakthrough with sequential activation.* Surface leads 2 and $V_1$ are shown with intracardiac electrograms from the HRA, HBE (five sites), slow pathway (SP), and proximal CS during AVNRT. A VPD delivered from the RVOT allows visualization of atrial activation. The earliest site is at the HBEd with sequential spread along the HBE recordings and later activation of the SP (slow pathway) and CSp. See text for discussion.

recorded in the coronary sinus, suggesting atrial activation via the left atrial extension of the AVN (Figs. 8-35 and 8-36) All of these patients were successfully ablated from the right side suggesting that the left atrial activation is an epiphenom. Others[81,82] have shown a high variability of the ***earliest site*** of activation in all varieties of AVNRT which further makes terms like fast-slow; slow-fast, or slow-slow dependent on the anatomic site of retrograde conduction and the R-P relationship, meaningless.

The relationship of atrial activation to the QRS complex is extremely important from a diagnostic standpoint. In approximately 70% of the cases of typical A-V nodal reentrant SVT, the onset of atrial activation (i.e., earliest intracardiac atrial electrogram) appears before or at the onset of the QRS complex. The P wave sometimes begins so early that it gives the appearance of a Q wave in the inferior leads. This is most likely to occur when there is delay between the reentrant circuit and the ventricles. This is most frequent when there is H-V prolongation (Fig. 8-37) but may be observed with delay in the AVN distal to the circuit (Fig. 8-38). In the former case retrograde activation takes place during the H-V interval, and in the latter case retrograde atrial activation begins before the His deflection. This "pseudo-Q wave" is a rare, but relatively specific finding for AVNRT. The presence of atrial activation appearing at or immediately before the onset of the QRS during SVT excludes the possibility of a concealed atrioventricular bypass tract (see following discussion of concealed bypass tracts). The rapid retrograde atrial activation occurs because, as discussed previously, the retrograde limb of the reentrant circuit is the fast beta pathway. In approximately 25% of the tachycardias, atrial activation begins just within the QRS. In 95% of patients, either no discrete P waves are noted on the surface electrocardiogram (40%), or the terminal part of the QRS is slightly distorted, possibly appearing as a "pseudo-S wave" in the inferior leads, a "pseudo-R'" in $V_1$, or a nonspecific terminal notching (57%). In the remaining patients, the P wave may be seen just after the end of the QRS. Intra-atrial conduction delays can alter the duration of atrial activation so that completion of atrial activation occurs slightly after termination of the QRS. In those patients in whom the P wave distorts the terminal QRS or appears at the end of the QRS, one must distinguish this tachycardia from the circus movement tachycardias using CBTs (see following discussion of concealed bypass tracts). Because completion of atrial activation arising in the midline usually requires at least 50 msec, the appearance of atrial activity as a terminal notch in the QRS, representing the end part of the P wave, suggests that atrial activation begins within the QRS and makes a bypass tract less likely. Sometimes, however, this is hard to distinguish from a bypass tract. In such cases atrial mapping as well as a variety of different responses to ventricular stimulation can help determine whether a bypass tract or atrial tachycardia is present (see following discussion of concealed bypass tracts and atrial tachycardia).

In patients who have the atypical form of AVNRT, the R-P interval is long because retrograde conduction proceeds over the slow pathway. Thus, the R-P/P-R ratio is greater than 1 (long R-P tachycardia). This pattern is extremely uncommon, representing perhaps only 5% of the instances of spontaneous sustained AVNRT in the absence of a prior ablation. The atypical form of AVNRT is often confused with an incessant form of tachycardia caused by a slowly conducting, concealed posteroseptal atrioventricular bypass tract[63–65] or an atrial tachycardia arising in the low intra-atrial septum. Atypical AVNRT is more often a paroxysmal arrhythmia, while atrial tachycardias

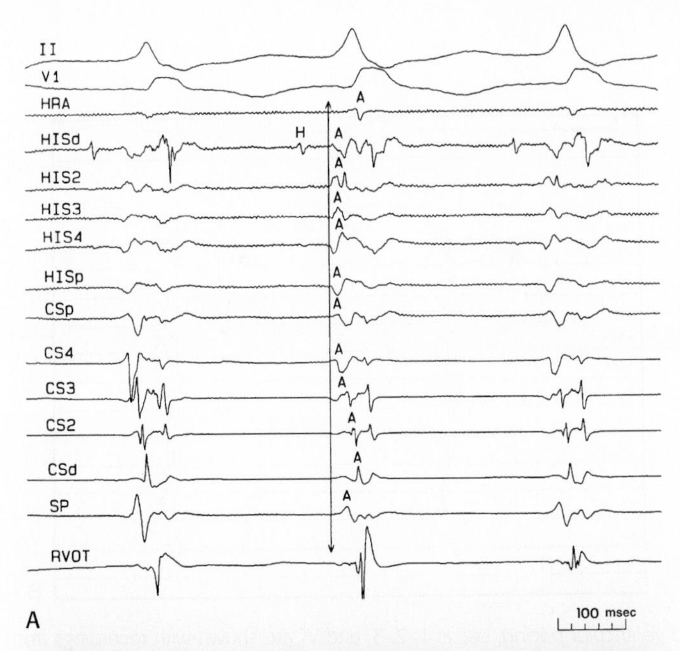


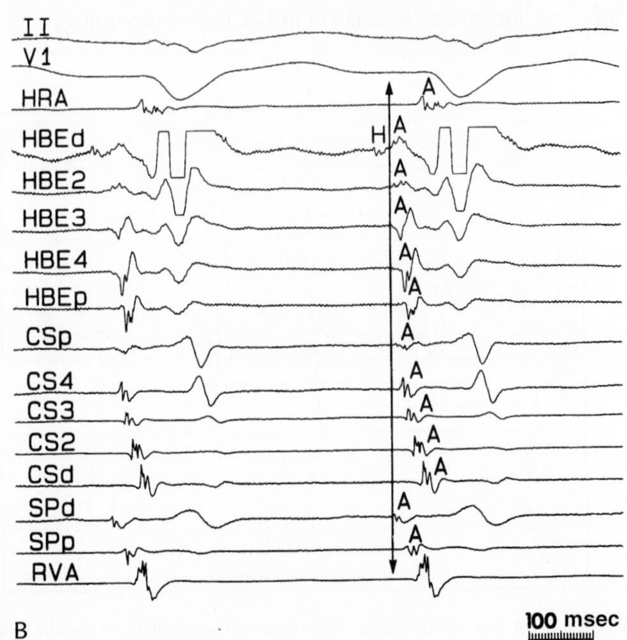


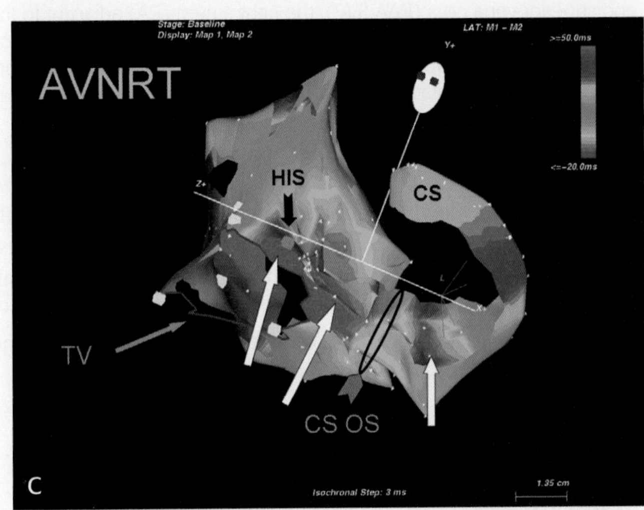


**FIGURE 8-32** *Examples of single and multiple breakthroughs of atrial activation during A-V nodal reentry.* **A:** Shows a single breakthrough with a broad wave of activation along the HBE. The figure is organized similar to Figure 8-31 with one additional SP recording and five CS recordings. Note that earliest activation occurs along the HBE, at which there is near simultaneous activation of all five poles (broad pattern), following which the rest of the triangle of Koch is activated. **B:** Shows an example of multiple breakthroughs and a broad wavefront of activation along the HBE. The figure is organized similar to the **left panel**. AVNRT with an LBBB is present. Atrial activation is easily seen because of the long H-V interval. Note that atrial activation begins simultaneously along the HBE (poles HBEd, 2, 3 are nearly simultaneous, i.e., broad pattern) and at the SPd. Thus the apex and base of the triangle of Koch demonstrate multiple breakthroughs. A Carto map showing multiple breakthroughs is shown in **C**. See text for further discussion.

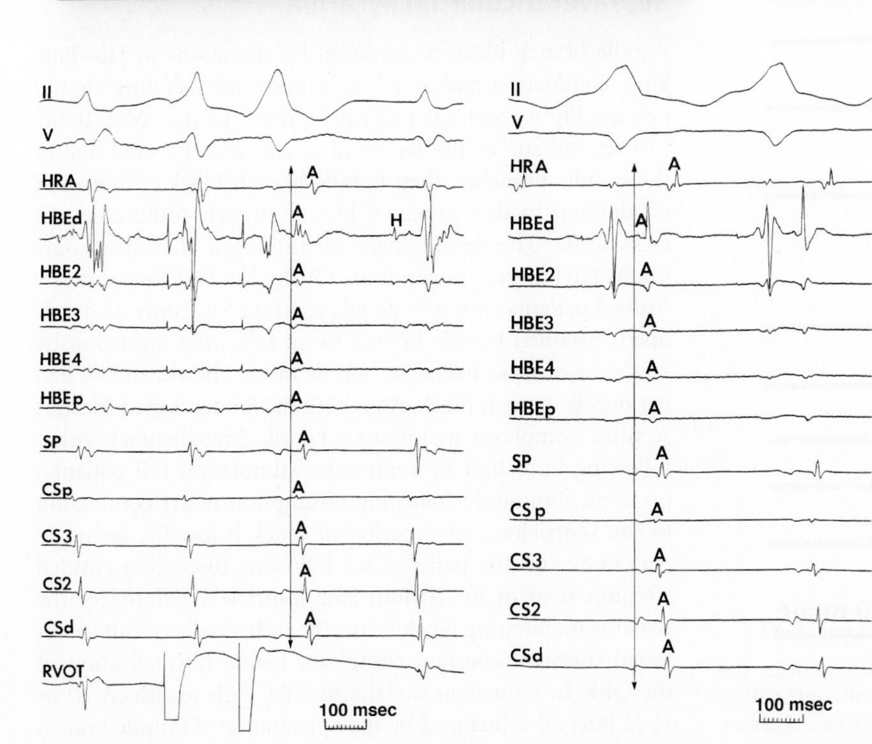


**FIGURE 8-33** *Discordant atrial activation between ventricular pacing and typical AVNRT.* The figure is organized as in Figure 8-29. On the **left** during typical AVNRT 2 VPDs expose atrial activation, which demonstrates a single breakthrough at the HBE with a broad pattern of HBE activation. During ventricular pacing on the right, atrial activation is single and sequential. The difference in activation is readily apparent. See text for discussion.

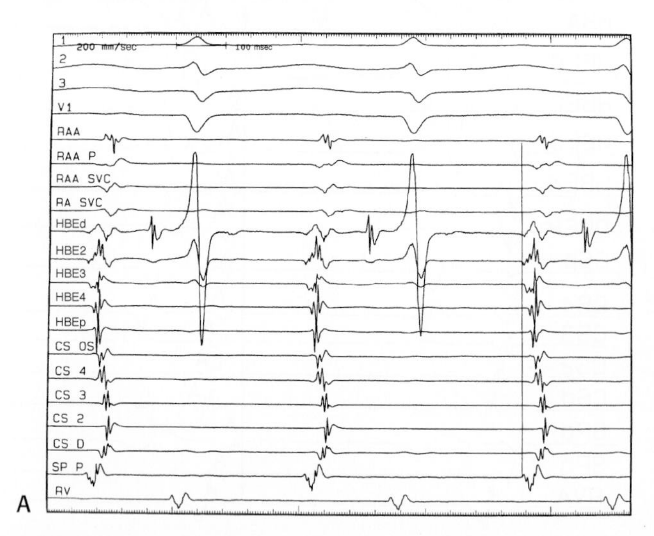


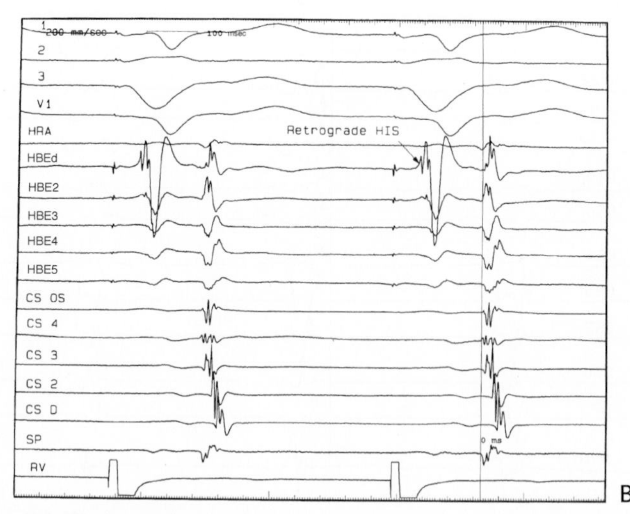


**FIGURE 8-34** *Discordant atrial activation between atypical AVNRT and ventricular pacing.* Leads 1, 2, 3, and $V_1$ are shown with recordings from the tip of the right atrial appendage (RAA), proximal RAA, junction of RAA, and superior vena cava (RAA SVC), the right atrium (RA) adjacent to the SVC, and standard recordings from the HBE, CS, and SP. **A:** During atypical AVNRT there are multiple breakthroughs with simultaneous activation of HBEd and HBE2 (focal, sequential) and the SP. **B:** During ventricular pacing multiple breakthroughs are present, but there is a broad wavefront along the HBE (HBEd–HBE4 nearly simultaneous). The SP and the CS os and CS4 are also simultaneously activated. See text for further discussion.

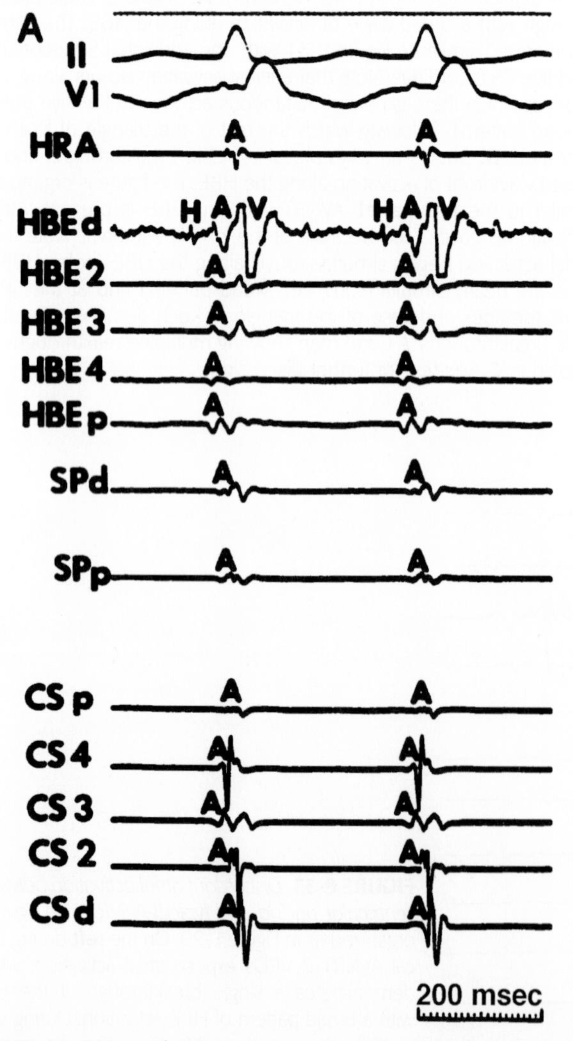


**FIGURE 8-35** *Typical AVNRT with earliest atrial activation in the CS.* This figure is organized similar to Figure 8-31. Typical AVNRT with a RBBB is present. Earliest atrial activation is noted at $CS_3$. See text for discussion.

or those using slowly conducting bypass tracts are frequently incessant and difficult to treat methods to distinguish these arrhythmias are discussed later in this chapter. The R-P intervals discussed above are in the absence of prior catheter ablation. We have noted a greater incidence of atypical R-P relationships and multiple tachycardias in patients postablation.

## Effect of Bundle Branch Block During Atrioventricular Nodal Reentrant Supraventricular Tachycardia

Bundle branch block is produced by alterations in His–Purkinje conduction and/or refractoriness and therefore should not modify a reentrant process localized to the AVN. If the turnaround site of the reentrant circuit incorporated one of the bundle branches, then bundle branch block or impaired conduction in that proximal bundle branch could alter the tachycardia. The development of prolonged aberration during AVNRT is very uncommon. Of the last 900 consecutively studied patients with A-V nodal reentrant SVT, only 43 developed sustained bundle branch block following induction by APDs; 25 of these had right bundle branch block, and 18 had left bundle branch block. An additional 85 developed ≥5 consecutive complexes manifesting bundle branch block either following induction by ventricular stimulation (19 patients) or, more commonly, following resumption of 1:1 conduction to the ventricles after a period of block below the tachycardia circuit (66/103 patients; see following discussion entitled "Requirement of the Atrium and Ventricle"). All 103 of the patients manifesting block below the tachycardia circuit manifested transient aberrant complexes before normalization of the QRS. In no patient was the AVNRT cycle length (A-A) or H-H interval influenced by the appearance of bundle branch

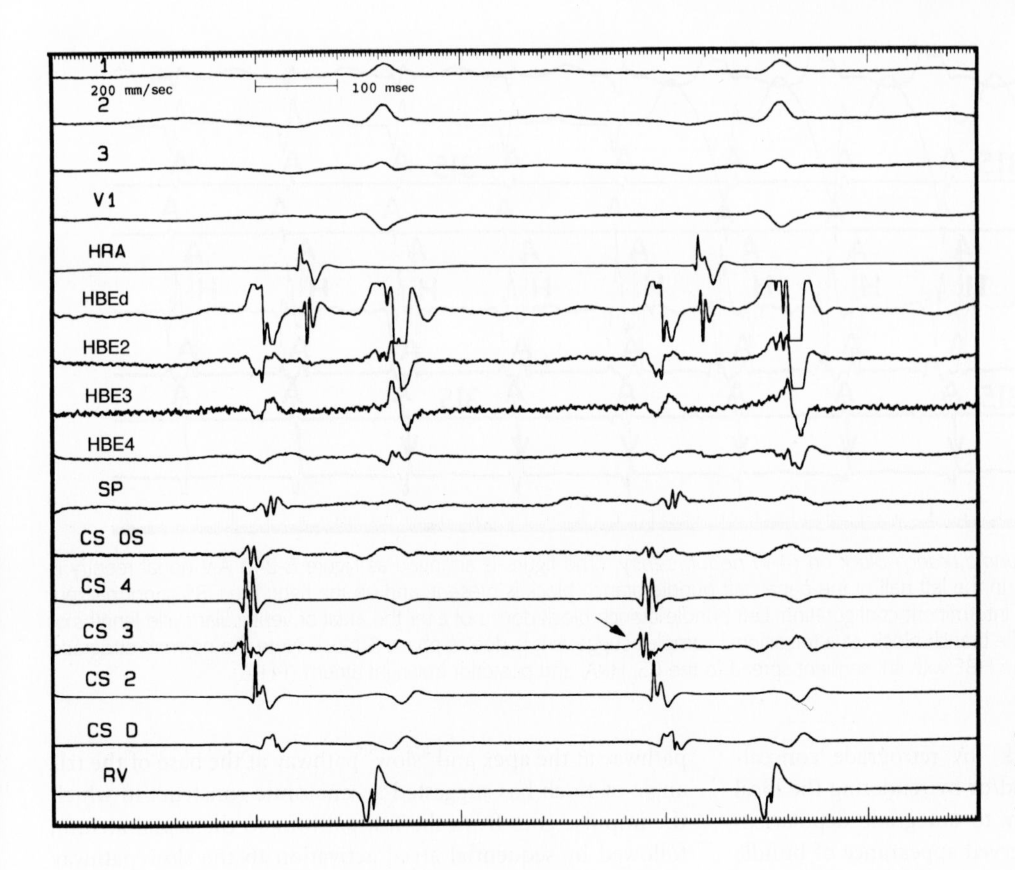


**FIGURE 8-36** *Atypical AVNRT with earliest atrial activation in the CS.* Atypical AVNRT is present. Earliest atrial activation occurs at CS 3 (*arrow*). See text for further discussion.

block. At the onset of bundle branch block, if the H-V interval is prolonged, an increase in the V-V interval equal to the increment in the H-V interval can occur; however, the following V-V time would be shortened by the same amount. During this transition, the A-A and H-H intervals generally remain constant, although if aberration occurs at the onset of the tachycardia, some oscillation of all electrograms can be observed, with some slight slowing prior to resumption of 1:1 conduction. Thus, it is safest to analyze the effects of bundle branch block after induction of the arrhythmia when the tachycardia is stabilized. During the tachycardia, the introduction of VPDs also may occasionally produce transient bundle branch block

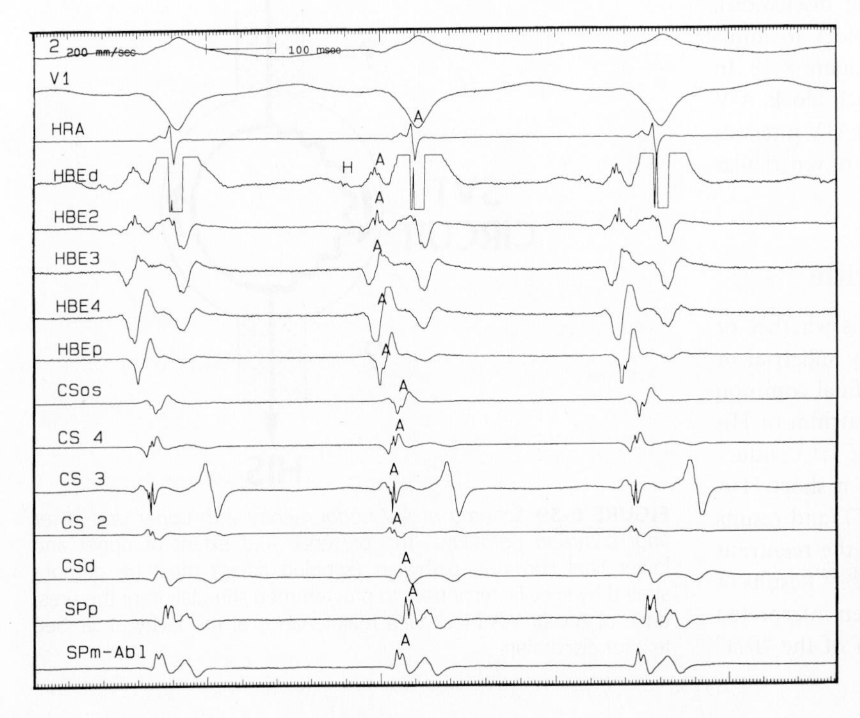


**FIGURE 8-37** *Atrial activation beginning prior to the QRS producing a pseudo-Q wave during typical AVNRT.* The figure is organized similar to Figure 8-31. Typical AVNRT with an LBBB is present. The H-V interval is prolonged (75 msec) so that atrial activation begins well before the QRS giving rise to a pseudo-Q wave in lead 2. See text for discussion.

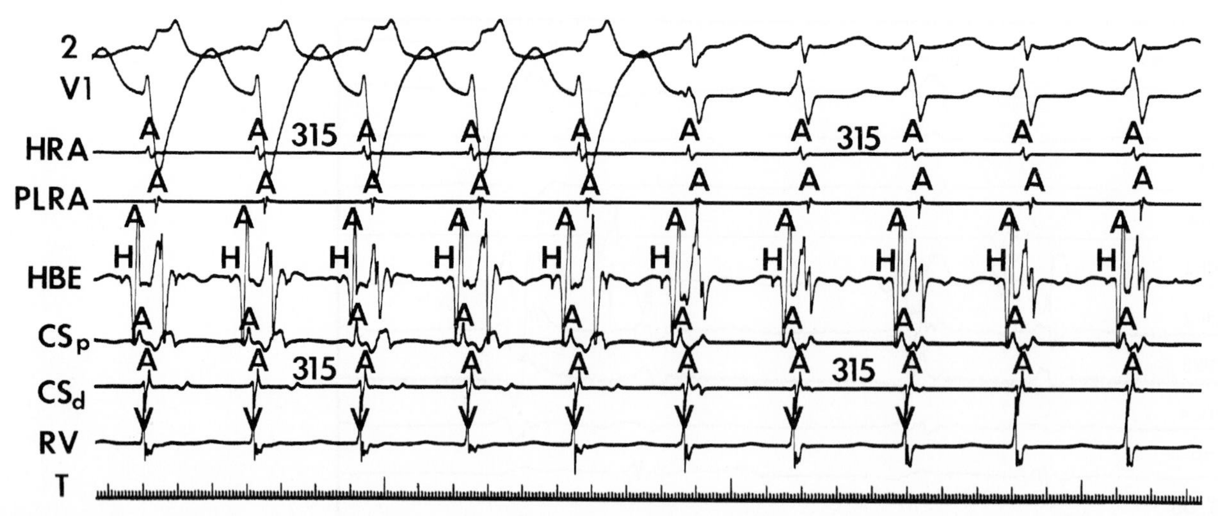


**FIGURE 8-38** *The lack of effect of bundle branch block on (A-V) nodal reentry.* (The figure is arranged as Figure 8-24.) A-V nodal reentry is present at a cycle length of 315 msec. In the left half of the panel, left bundle branch block is present, and on the right, the QRS is normalized. Between the transition is a complex of intermittent configuration. Left bundle branch block does not alter the atrial or ventricular cycle lengths of A-V nodal reentry. The loss of left bundle branch block via a transitional complex suggests it is due to phase 3 block. Note the normal retrograde activation sequence being earliest in the HBE with subsequent spread to the CS, HRA, and posterior low-right atrium (PLRA).

(usually left bundle branch block) by retrograde concealment into the bundle branches and/or by rendering the local ventricular myocardium refractory to antegrade depolarization. As in the spontaneously observed appearance of bundle branch block, no change in the A-A or H-H interval results. Whenever the H-V interval prolongs with the development of bundle branch block, the V-V interval also prolongs for one cycle, as mentioned. In this instance, however, because the circuit is not influenced, the A-A interval remains constant and the atrial electrogram, and even the P wave, can be seen before the QRS. The lack of influence of bundle branch block on A-V nodal reentrant SVT is in contrast to patients with SVTs incorporating free-wall bypass tracts (see following discussion). An example of the failure of bundle branch block to influence the tachycardia cycle length is shown in Figure 8-38. In this instance, after a period of left bundle branch block, A-V conduction normalizes. No change in the A-A or V-V intervals occurs during the stable portion of each pattern of ventricular activation.

## Requirement of the Atrium and Ventricle

One of the issues that remains controversial is whether or not the reentrant circuit in AVNRT is entirely subatrial or even intranodal, including "upper and lower" final common pathways, or whether some component of the atrium or His bundle is required (Fig. 8-39). The presence of 1:1 conduction at rapid rates with a short V-A interval, a short H-A interval that remains relatively fixed during SVT, and results of surgical interventions suggest to some that the reentrant circuit involves tissue above and below the AVN.[80,83] Results of catheter modification of the AVN have also been interpreted similarly (see Chapter 15). Successful ablation of the "fast" pathway at the apex and "slow" pathway at the base of the triangle of Koch has suggested an anatomic construct in which the impulse goes from the fast pathway to the septal atrium, followed by sequential atrial activation to the slow pathway through which the AVN is engaged. Pathologic specimens demonstrating radiofrequency-induced lesions not involving the compact node (no known extent of physiologic influences)

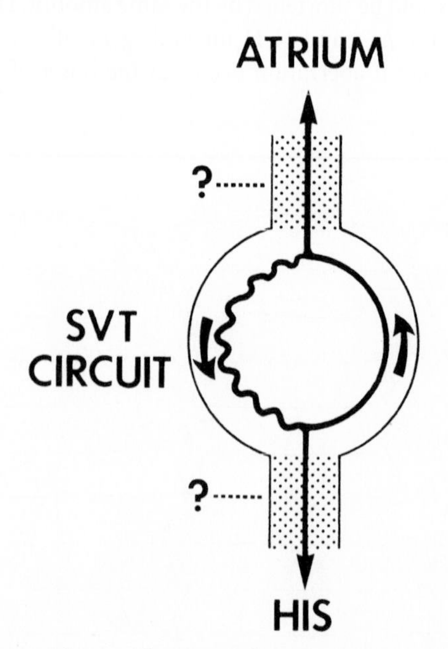


**FIGURE 8-39** *Schema of A-V nodal reentry with upper and lower final common pathways.* The presence and extent of upper and lower final common pathways (stippled areas) must be demonstrated by specific responses to programmed stimulation or the presence of A-V or V-A block with maintenance of the tachycardia. See text for discussion.

have been used to further support this construct. Still other investigators have taken the relative ease with which AVNRT can be reset from the base of the triangle of Koch as evidence of atrial participation in the circuit.[46] I believe all of these findings do not prove the requirement of the atrium, but only suggest that the circuit has dimension and/or has different inputs and outputs that are determined by the anisotropic nature of the compact node, its extensions, and the transitional fibers that can be more or less easily engaged depending on the site of stimulation.

I believe that the bulk of the evidence, both experimentally and clinically, suggests that, in most patients, AVNRT is a subatrial reentrant circuit based on the anisotropic properties of the AVN and transitional tissue.[41,77,78,84–92] As stated earlier, Efimov et al. using high-density voltage-sensitive dye mapped the AVN three dimensionally and found reentry was subatrial, involving the AVN +/– transitional cells. Cell-to-cell coupling in the AVN is extremely poor due to heterogenous connexins, both type and distribution (primarily connexin 45, with small amounts of connexin 40 near the His bundle) which is the main reason the node is so slowly conducting.

Clinical data, which come from observations during spontaneous SVT, at the time of induction of SVT, and response to stimulation during SVT are discussed in the following paragraphs and are summarized in Table 8-3. They include (a) initiation of AVNRT in the absence of an atrial echo; (b) maintenance of AVNRT in the presence of either a changing V-A relationship, 2:1 retrograde or V-A block and/or A-V dissociation; (c) depolarization of the atrium surrounding the AVN without influencing the tachycardia; (d) resetting AVNRT without atrial activation; (e) heterogenous atrial activation during AVNRT incompatible with atrial participation; and (f) atrial pacing and entrainment of AVNRT with a longer A-H than during the tachycardia entrainment suggesting that little if any of the atrium is required.

**TABLE 8-3 AVNRT: Evidence That the Atrium is not Necessary**

- Initiation of AVNRT in the absence of an atrial echo
- Maintenance of AVNRT in the presence of either a changing V-A relationship, 2:1 retrograde V-A block, or V-A dissociation
- Depolarization of the atria surrounding the A-V node without affecting the tachycardia
- Resetting the tachycardia by ventricular stimulation in the absence of atrial activation
- Heterogenous atrial activation during SVT which is incompatible with atrial participation
- Atrial pacing and entrainment at paced cycle length, comparable to the SVT cycle length producing a longer "A-H" interval than the A-H during SVT
- Atrial pacing produces A-V nodal Wenckebach at a cycle length SVT > cycle length

### *Requirement of the Atrium in AVNRT*

Initiation of AVNRT in the absence of atrial activation most frequently occurs during ventricular stimulation (Fig. 8-40). In virtually all of these cases the initial retrograde H (if seen) to antegrade H interval was longer than the subsequent H-H intervals, and the tachycardia cycle lengths were relatively long (i.e., >400 msec). As ventricular coupling intervals were decreased, the initial retrograde H (when observed) to antegrade H interval increased. While absence of atrial activation at the initiation of AVNRT is an uncommon observation, it will be missed if ventricular stimulation is not routinely performed. Rarely, retrograde block in the fast pathway can be observed at initiation of AVNRT by atrial stimulation or by induction during atrial flutter or fibrillation. The preceding findings were made only during *typical AVNRT.* The occurrence of the ventricular echoes during atrial fibrillation, a well-recognized phenomenon, suggests that the atrium is also not required for atypical AVNRT.

Retrograde block to the atrium during AVNRT is uncommon (96/1,798 of our cases) but has been reported.[78,85–88,90,93] In my experience it only occurs in typical AVNRT. AVNRT with 2:1 block to the atrium with resumption of 1:1 conduction and acceleration of the AVNRT following atropine is shown in Figure 8-41. Examples of AVNRT with both 2:1 block and Wenckebach to the atrium and AVNRT with A-V dissociation and intermittent capture are shown in Figure 8-42 (top and bottom, respectively). Adenosine-induced V-A block and A-V dissociation during AVNRT is shown in Figure 8-43. Whenever A-V dissociation occurs with apparent AVNRT, one must rule out the presence of a concealed nodofascicular or nodoventricular bypass tract as the retrograde limb. These extremely rare pathways are suggested by the influence of bundle branch block on the tachycardia cycle length or the ability to reset or terminate the SVT with ventricular extrastimuli or pacing delivered when the His bundle is refractory. An example of AVNRT with A-V dissociation unaffected by the appearance of RBBB is shown in Figure 8-44.

Two other related phenomena support lack of atrial requirement for AVNRT. First is the very common observation at the onset of AVNRT of changing V-A relationships with minimal or no change in tachycardia cycle length. This suggests that atrial activation is determined by the functional output to the atrium from the tachycardia, and not causally related to it. The finding of multiple tachycardias with identical retrograde atrial activation sequences and cycle lengths but different V-A relationships further supports the hypothesis that atrial activation is an epiphenomenon of AVNRT and is functionally determined by nodoatrial coupling and the anisotropic nature of the subatrial nodal structures (Fig. 8-45).

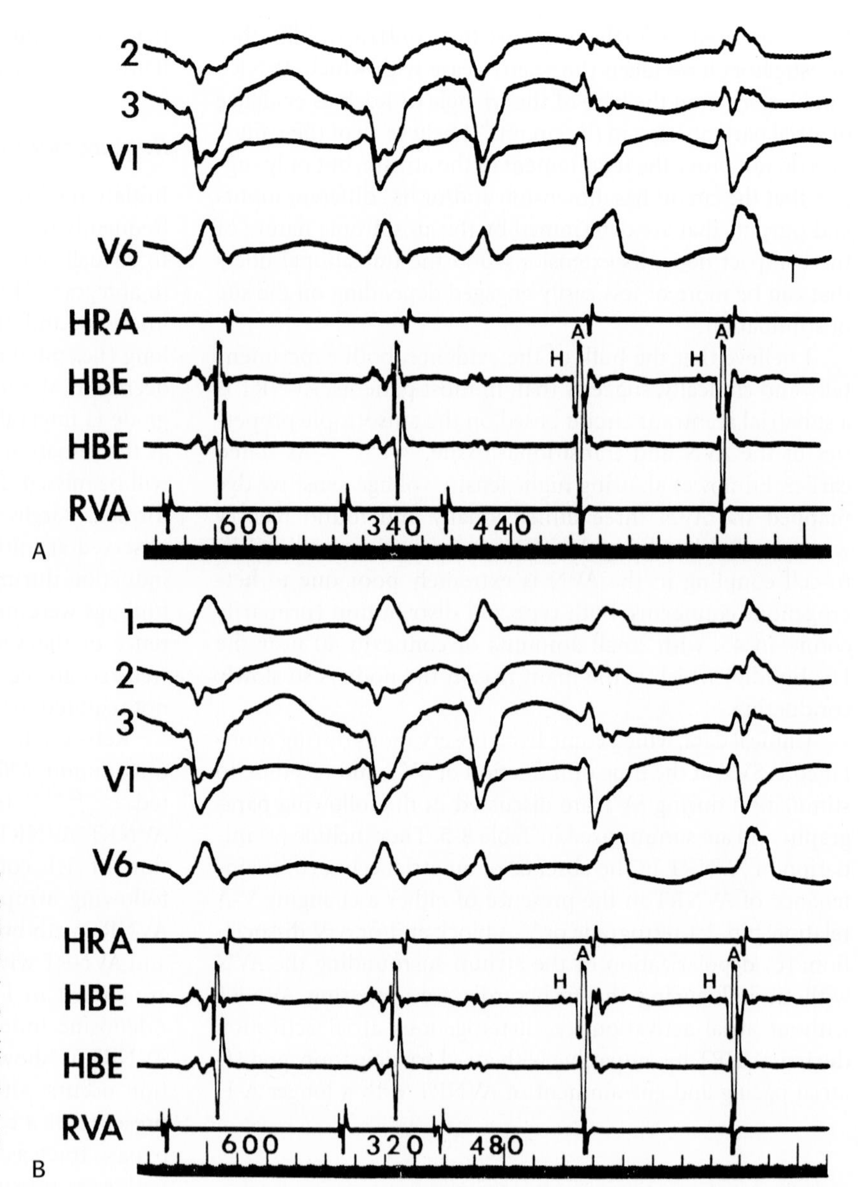


**FIGURE 8-40** *Initiation of AVNRT in the absence of atrial activation.* ECG leads 2, 3, $V_1$, and $V_6$ are shown with electrograms from the HRA, HBE, and RVA. In both panels VPDs are delivered during a paced cycle length of 600 msec. **A:** A VPD delivered at a coupling interval of 340 msec initiates AVNRT without depolarizing the atrium over the fast pathway. The AVNRT begins after an A-V delay of 440 msec. **B:** When a VPD is delivered at a coupling interval of 320 msec, AVNRT is induced without atrial activation but the first interval is increased to 480 msec. See text for discussion.

### *Responses to Stimulation During AVNRT—Role in Defining Atrial and Subnodal Participation*

During A-V nodal reentrant SVT, APDs can produce several responses (Fig. 8-46). Relatively late APDs fail to alter the cycle length of SVT; therefore, full compensatory pauses result (Fig. 8-45A) because of the inability of the atrial stimulus to depolarize the entire atria to reach the AVN or, if the atria are depolarized, failure to penetrate the reentrant circuit. The ability to depolarize the atria, specifically, the atrial tissue surrounding AVN (i.e., the atrium recorded at the His bundle electrogram and at the os and within the coronary sinus), without affecting the tachycardia provides evidence that the atria are not a necessary link in the reentrant circuit (Fig. 8-47). Demonstration of premature excitation of all the recordable atrial tissue around the AVN is imperative (i.e., the atrial electrograms at the os and within the CS, and the HBE), because these are the areas where earliest activity is recorded during mapping of SVT in the laboratory[24–26,77,78] or intraoperatively.[90] Because a noncompensatory pause may reflect delay in the slow pathway, which exactly compensates for the prematurity of the atrial extrastimulus (an unlikely but theoretically possible event), the investigation should attempt to demonstrate this response over a range of coupling intervals of ≥30 msec to ensure that the APD has not entered the node and fortuitously increased the A-H interval to produce a fully compensatory pause. If possible, stimulation should be performed from both the high-right atrium and os of the coronary sinus because stimulation at both those sites yields different A-H intervals, as mentioned earlier. If the same fully compensatory response occurs from stimulation at both sites, it is unlikely that compensatory A-H delay is responsible. This is clearly demonstrated in

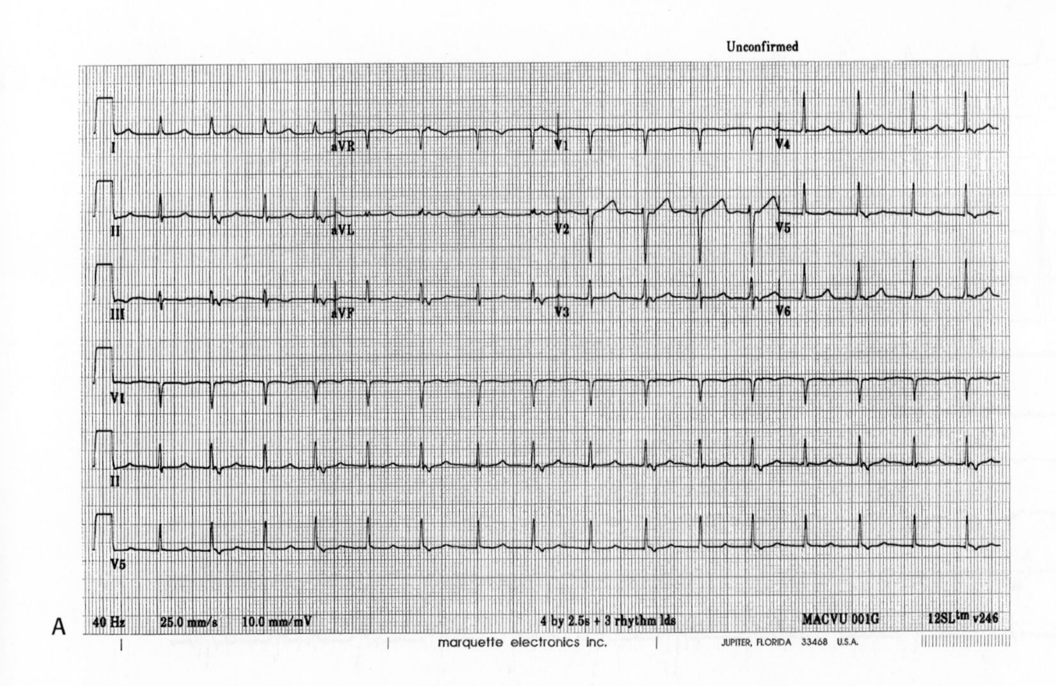


A

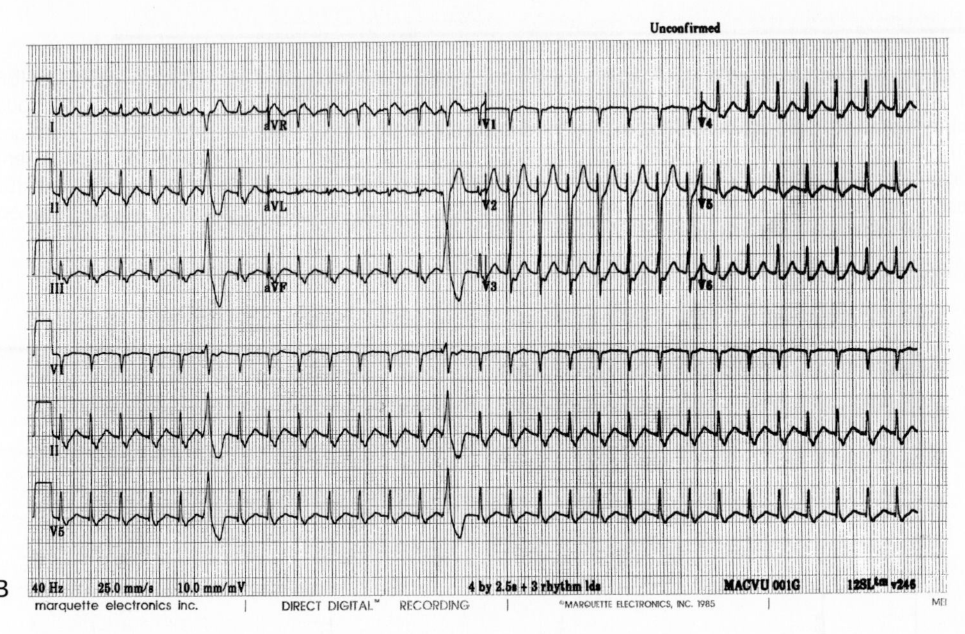


B

**FIGURE 8-41** *Typical AVNRT with two-to-one V-A block.* **A:** Typical AVNRT is present with 2:1 V-A block at a cycle length of 590 msec. Note the relatively long V-A interval of the complexes associated with atrial activity. **B:** Following atropine, the AVNRT speeds up to 360 msec and 1:1 conduction resumes with a shorter V-A interval. This can only be explained by retrograde V-A block localized to the A-V node. See text for discussion.

Figure 8-46. Simultaneous stimulation from the right atrium and coronary sinus can yield the same result (Fig. 8-48). The same phenomenon can occasionally be seen using double extrastimuli (Fig. 8-49), a situation that makes compensatory A-V nodal delays even more unlikely. The demonstration of this phenomenon may even be observed during atrial pacing or atrial fibrillation or flutter. This can be seen in Figure 8-50 in which the first two beats of AVNRT are unaffected by atrial flutter/fibrillation. The third QRS is advanced by ≈20 msec and AVNRT resumes without requiring an atrial echo (see prior discussion). It is important for the investigator to recognize that recordings from the os and within the coronary sinus as well as the His bundle electrogram are necessary to demonstrate local atrial capture around the AVN. The demonstration of a full compensatory pause after the introduction of an APD does not prove the atrium is unnecessary unless it can be shown that the atrial tissue surrounding the AVN is captured before it would have been depolarized by spontaneously occurring atrial echoes without altering the arrhythmia. Although, theoretically, a protected, nonrecordable bridge of atrial tissue could be involved in the circuit, entrance block to the area would be required to prevent its depolarization by APDs, and exit block would be required to prevent recording an atrial electrogram. Since the atria are normal in the vast majority of patients with AVNRT, and the APDs are delivered at intervals in excess of local atrial refractory periods, this is hardly conceivable.

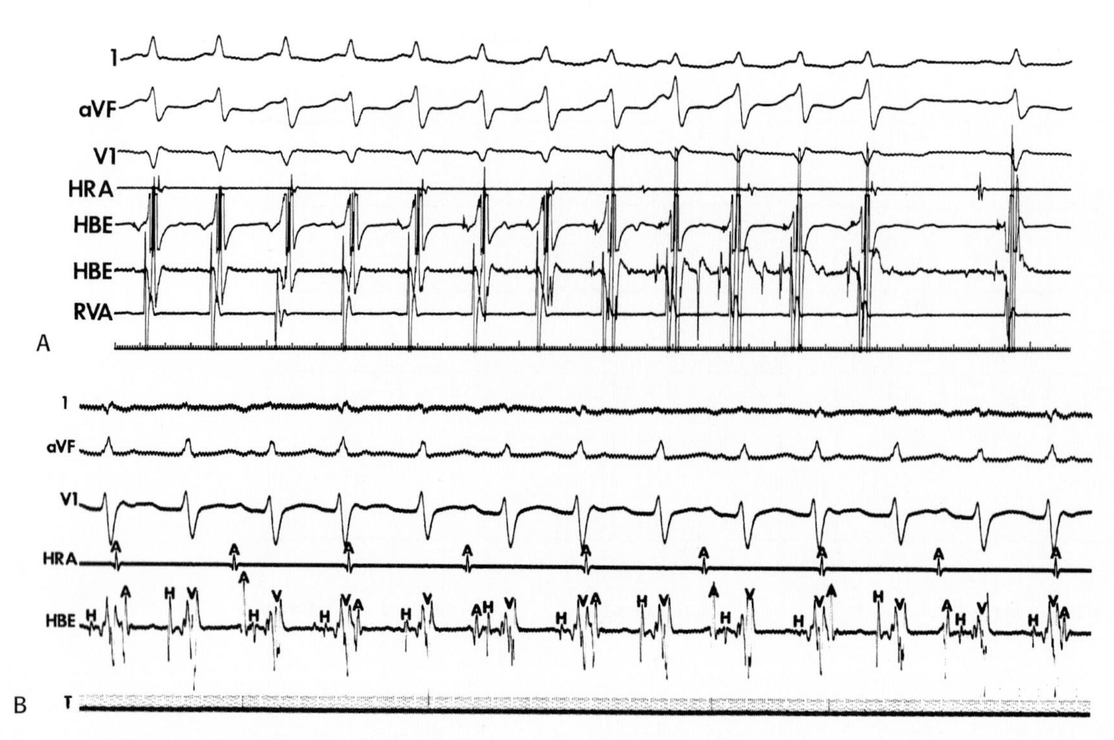


**FIGURE 8-42** *A-V nodal reentry with retrograde block to the atrium.* **A:** Leads 1, aVF, and $V_1$ are shown with electrograms from the HRA, HBE, and RVA. A-V nodal reentry is present, which eventually terminates (right-hand side of tracing). During the first seven complexes of A-V nodal reentry, 2:1 retrograde block to the atrium is present. On a subsequent complex, conduction suddenly appears with delay toward the atrium and then reverts back to 2:1 conduction. The lack of atrial requirement during the tachycardia suggests an upper final common pathway is present. See text for discussion. **B:** A-V dissociation during A-V nodal reentry. Leads 1, aVF, and $V_1$ are shown with electrograms from the HRA and HBE during A-V nodal reentry. A-V dissociation is present, and every other sinus complex penetrates the reentrant circuit, leading to an advancement of the subsequent QRS (QRS 1, 4, 7, 10, and 13). See text for discussion.

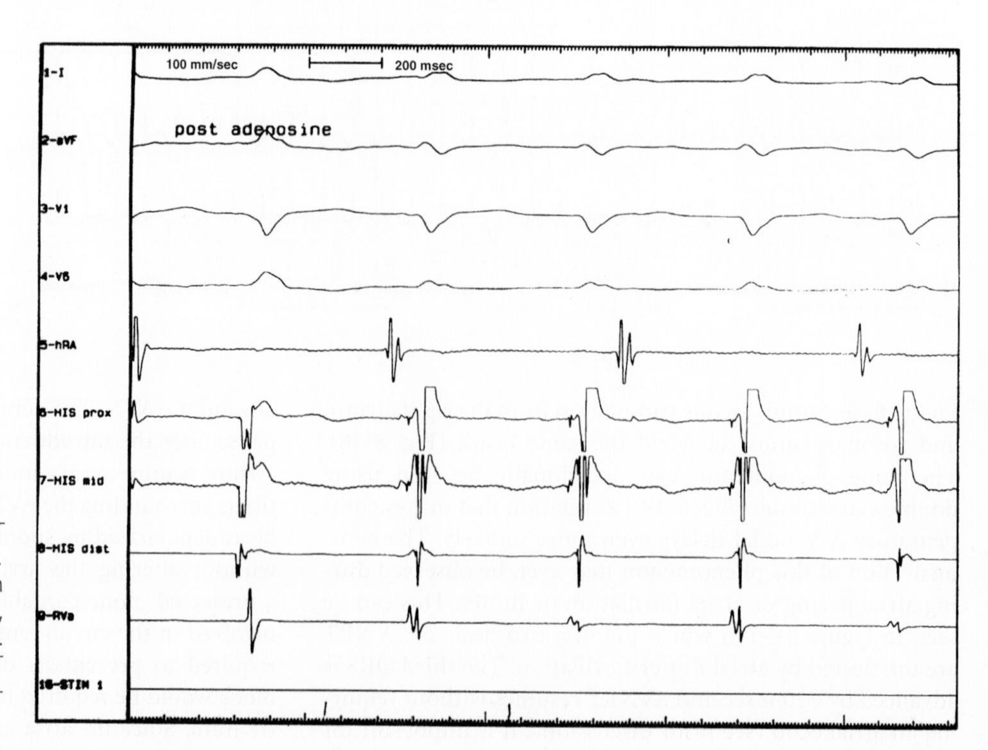


**FIGURE 8-43** *Persistence of AVNRT despite adenosine-induced V-A block.* Leads 1, aVF, $V_1$, and $V_6$ are shown with electrograms from the HRA proximal, mid, and distal His bundle, and RVA. Following 6 mg of adenosine AVNRT continues in the presence of A-V dissociation. See text for discussion.

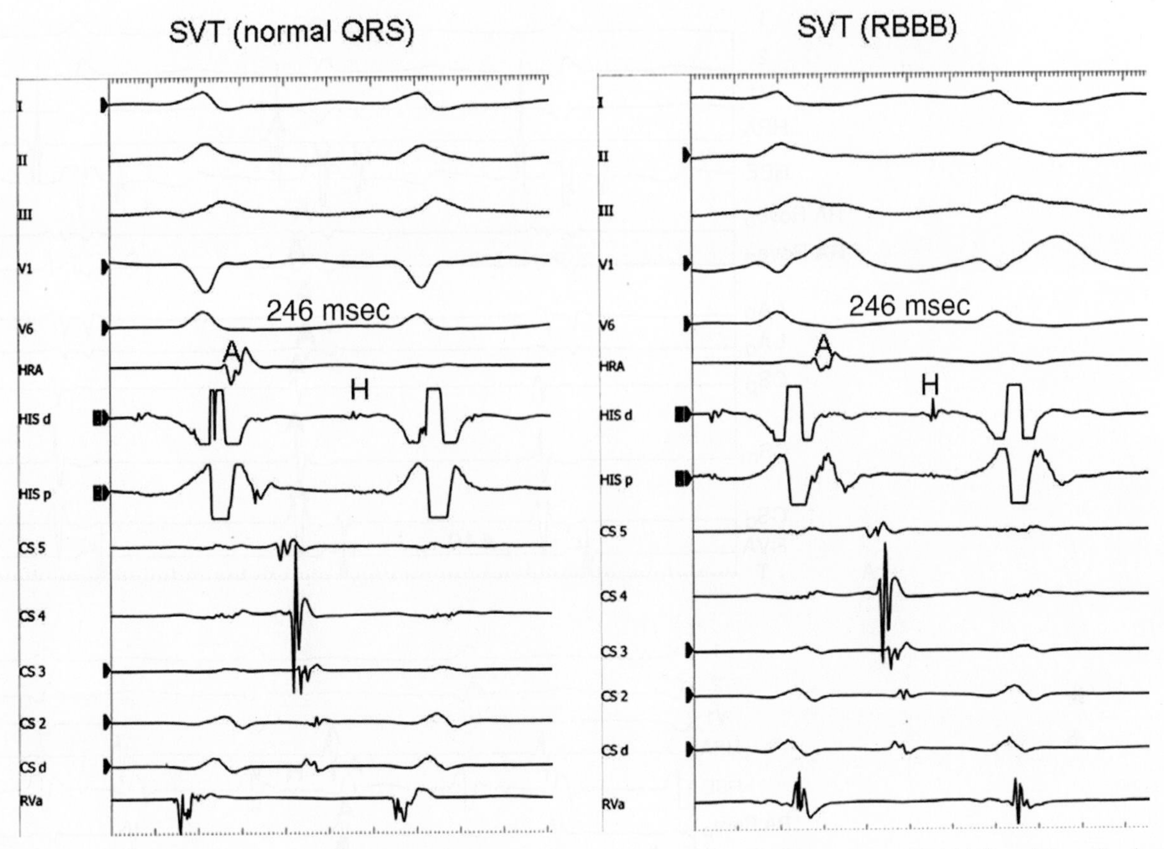


**FIGURE 8-44** *Failure of RBBB to influence A-V nodal tachycardia with A-V dissociation.* SVT is present with A-V dissociation. On the **left** the QRS is narrow and on the **right**, RBBB is present. The RBBB does not alter the tachycardia cycle length or H-V interval, excluding a concealed right-sided nodofascicular bypass tract. See text for discussion.

Another observation suggesting that the "upper common pathway" is located within the node (or at least, subatrial transitional zone) is the ability of an APD to retard the subsequent atrial echo without influencing the tachycardia (i.e., H-H interval). Hariman et al.[89] demonstrated that this phenomenon was most likely due to the APD producing concealed conduction into the AVN above the dual pathways so that, when the impulse returned up the fast pathway, the upper final common pathway had not recovered excitability completely, and retrograde nodal-atrial conduction was delayed.

Earlier APDs frequently penetrate the reentrant circuit and reset it (Fig. 8-46B). Depending on how slowly the APD is conducted down the antegrade limb of the reentrant circuit, less or greater than compensatory pauses can result. On occasion, an APD can produce such marked conduction delay in the slow pathway antegradely, or in a lower common pathway, that a greater than compensatory pause results. If an APD produces a long enough pause, spontaneous sinus P waves that depolarize the atrial tissue surrounding the AVN can occur (i.e., in the HBE and the os and/or within the coronary sinus), confirming a subatrial site of the reentrant circuit (Fig. 8-51). In addition, one or two atrial extrastimuli can produce delay in a lower final common pathway, which can be recognized by a shift in the relationship of the retrograde atrial activation and the His bundle deflection. Delay in the lower common pathway (see subsequent discussion) causes delay of the impulse reaching the His bundle without influencing the return to the atrium through the fast pathway. This results in atrial activation preceding the His deflection (Fig. 8-52) during the tachycardia instead of following the His bundle deflection, as it normally does. Continuous resetting of the A-V nodal reentrant tachycardia by atrial pacing can almost universally be achieved. Portillo et al.[87] also demonstrated that, although the tachycardia could be reset, rapid pacing could produce A-V dissociation and/or 2:1 nodoatrial block during the SVT, both of which further support a subatrial origin of the tachycardia.[87]

Finally, if the APD penetrates the circuit early enough, it will block antegradely in the slow pathway and usually collide with the circling wavefront in the beta pathway to terminate the arrhythmia (Fig. 8-53). If the rate of typical AVNRT is slow enough, and if the APD is appropriately timed, the presence of a wide and fully excitable gap (in the fast pathway) can be demonstrated by the ability of the APD to conduct down the fast pathway, capture the His bundle, and terminate the tachycardia before the wavefront in the slow pathway reaches the lower final common pathway. Thus, the last H and QRS are prematurely activated and advanced. This phenomenon is far more common in atypical AVNRT (Fig. 8-54). Here, the tachycardia is terminated by stimulation from either the high-right

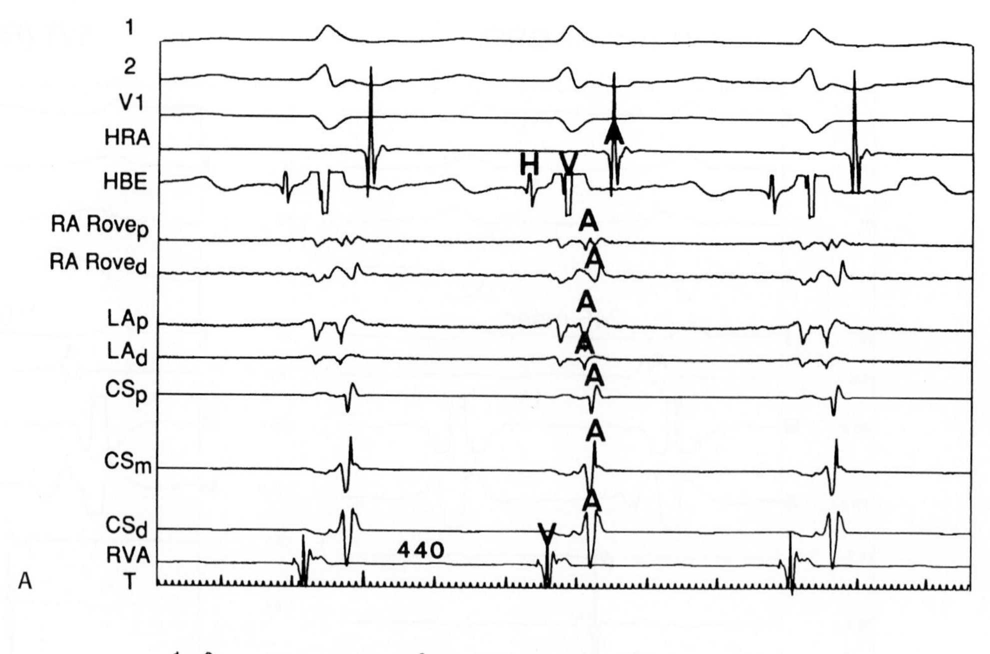


**FIGURE 8-45** *AVNRT with two different V-A intervals and the same cycle length.* ECG leads 1, 2, and $V_1$ are shown with electrograms from the HRA, HBE, distal (d) and proximal (p) right atrial (RA) rove, distal and proximal left atrium (LAd, LAp), CSp, CSm, CSd, and RVA. Two SVTs proven to be AVNRT have identical cycle lengths and atrial activation sequences. See text for discussion.

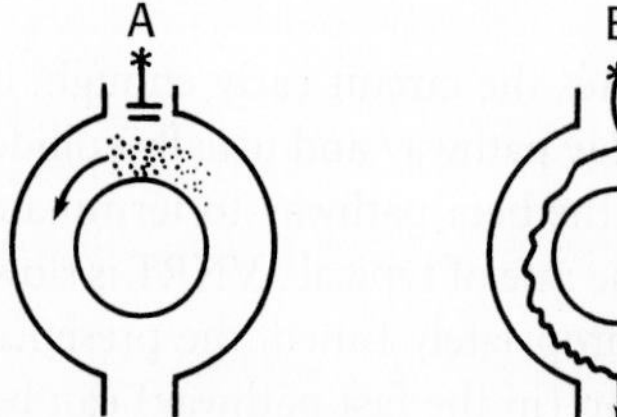


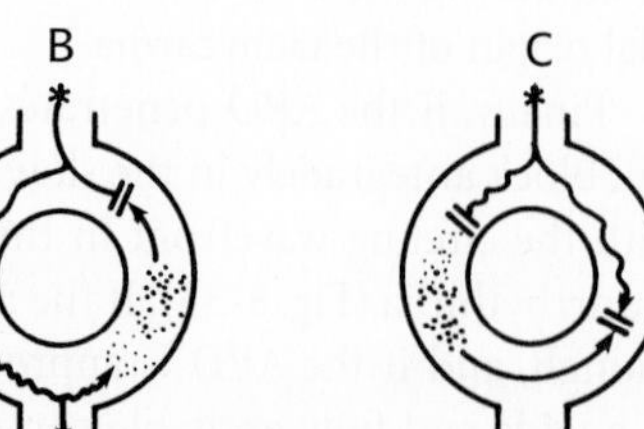


**FIGURE 8-46** *Response to APDs during SVT.* **A:** Late APDs find the reentrant circuit refractory and therefore cannot penetrate it, resulting in a full compensatory pause. **B:** Earlier APDs penetrate the reentrant circuit and conduct down the slow (alpha) pathway while colliding with a circulating wavefront in the fast (beta) pathway. This resets the SVT. **C:** Very early APDs encounter a refractory alpha pathway and collide with circulating wavefront in the beta pathway, terminating the arrhythmia. See text for further discussion.

atrium (Fig. 8-54A) or the coronary sinus (Fig. 8-54B), which conducts down the fast pathway during retrograde slow-pathway activation, and blocks retrogradely in the slow pathway. This is confirmed by termination of the SVT by an APD before the expected atrial echo that would have occurred over the slow pathway. The ability to conduct over the fast pathway during slow-pathway conduction and to terminate the tachycardia (whether typical or atypical AVNRT) suggests that an excitable gap exists in the reentrant circuit. (Further evidence of an excitable gap is described later in the discussion of the response to VPDs.)

The ability of an APD to terminate the arrhythmia depends on (a) the cycle length of the tachycardia, (b) the distance of the site of stimulation from the reentrant circuit, (c) the refractoriness of the intervening tissue, (d) the conduction velocity of the APD, and (e) an excitable gap in the reentrant circuit. A short SVT cycle length, a distant site of stimulation, a long atrial refractory period, a slowly conducting APD, and

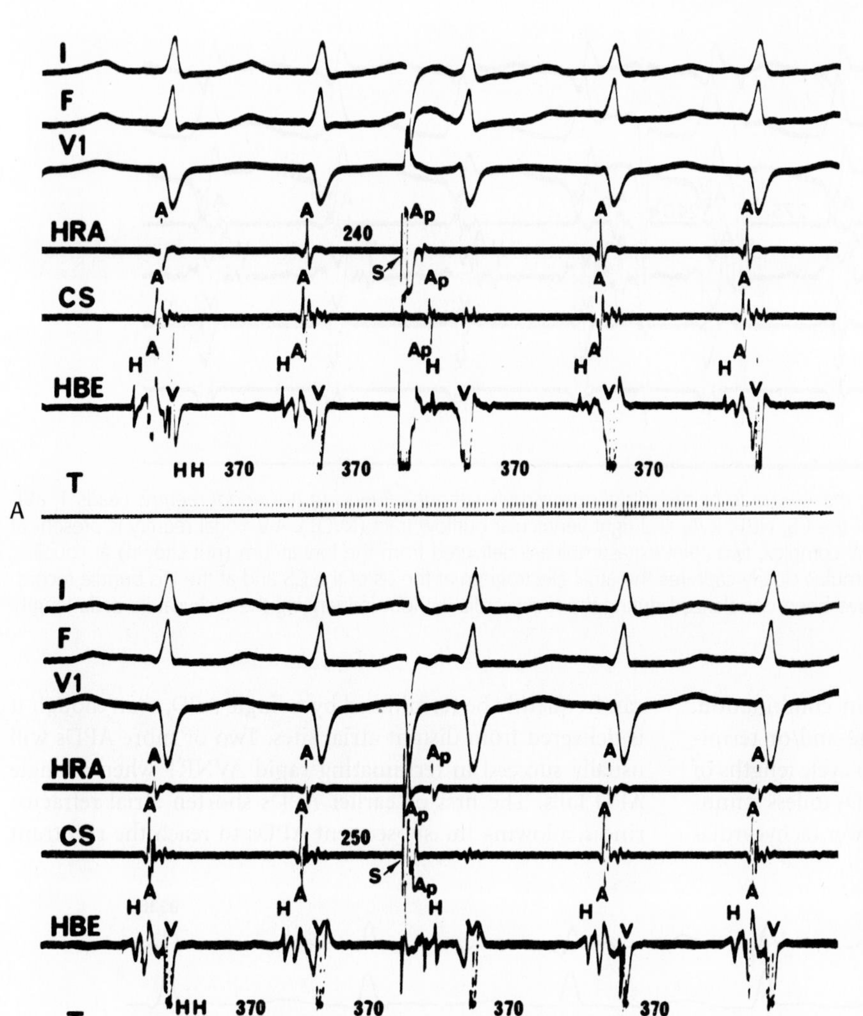


**FIGURE 8-47** *Lack of atrial requirement during A-V nodal reentrant SVT.* SVT is present at a cycle length of 370 msec. **A:** An APD ($A_p$) is introduced from the HRA, resulting in premature depolarization of the atrial recorded in the HRA, CS, and HBE by 130, 70, and 100 msec, respectively, without affecting the tachycardia. **B:** Similarly, an APD ($A_p$) is introduced from the proximal CS near the os, resulting in premature depolarization of the atria recorded in the HRA, CS, and HBE by 55, 120, and 60 msec, respectively, without affecting the tachycardia. See text for discussion. (From Josephson ME, Kastor JA. Paroxysmal supraventricular tachycardias: is the atrium a necessary link? *Circulation* 1976;54:430.)

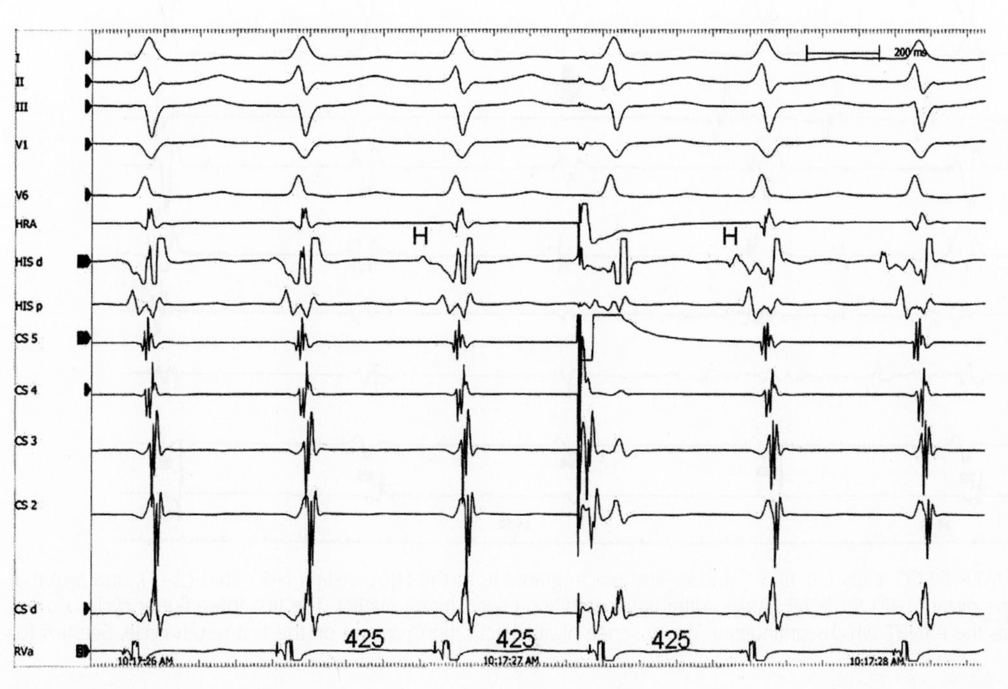


**FIGURE 8-48** *Simultaneous right and left atrial extrastimuli resulting in biatrial capture without affecting A-V nodal reentrant tachycardia.* The figure is organized similar to Figure 8-44. A-V nodal tachycardia is present at a cycle length of 425 msec. Simultaneous extrastimuli from HRA and proximal CS are delivered at 350 and 340 msec coupling intervals to their respective electrograms without affecting the tachycardia. See text for discussion.

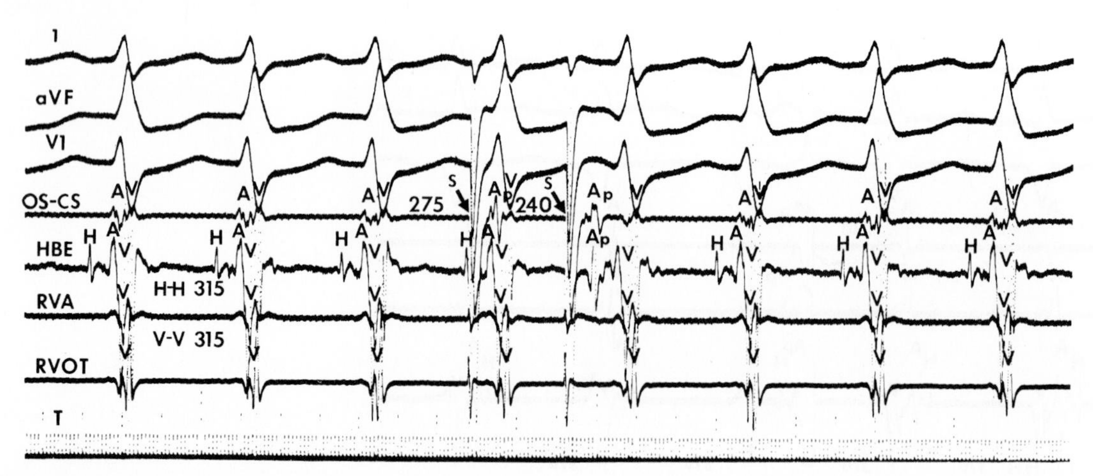


**FIGURE 8-49** *Capture of atrial tissue surrounding the A-V node by two atrial extrastimuli without influencing A-V nodal reentry.* Leads 1, aVF, and $V_1$ are shown with electrograms from the os of the CS, HBE, RVA, and right ventricular outflow tract (RVOT). A-V nodal reentry is present at a cycle length of 315 msec. Following the third QRS complex, two atrial extrastimuli are delivered from the low atrium (not shown) at coupling intervals of 275 and 240 msec. The second extrastimulus clearly captures the atrial electrogram at the os of the CS and at the His bundle recording nearly 15 msec before the time they would have been depolarized during the tachycardia without influencing the tachycardia cycle length. See text for discussion.

the absence of an excitable gap, singly or in combination, will result in failure of the APD to penetrate and/or terminate the SVT. In my experience, AVNRTs with cycle lengths of ≤325 msec are rarely terminated by single APDs unless stimulation is carried out adjacent to the AVN. Slower tachycardias can frequently be terminated by a single APD, even though it is delivered from distant atrial sites. Two or more APDs will usually succeed in terminating rapid AVNRT when a single APD fails. The first or earlier APDs shorten atrial refractoriness, allowing the subsequent APDs to reach the reentrant

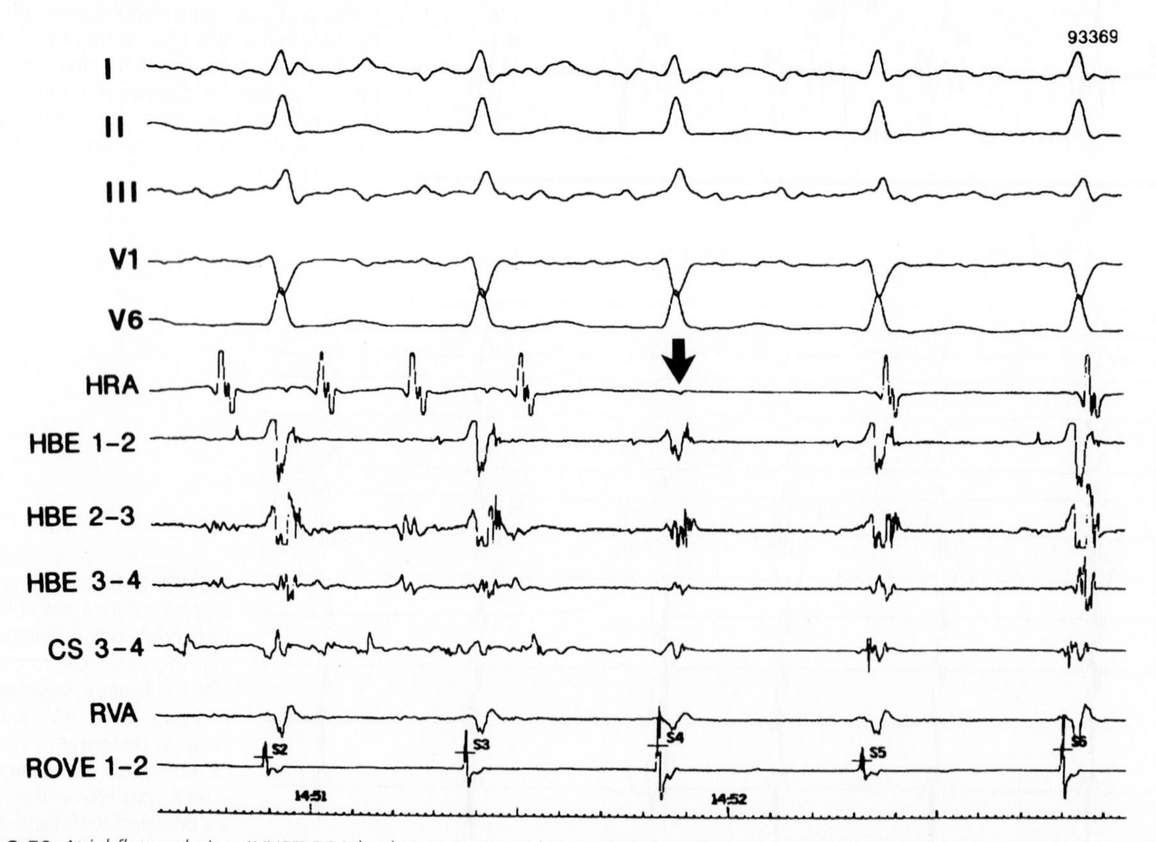


**FIGURE 8-50** *Atrial flutter during AVNRT.* ECG leads I, II, III, $V_1$, and $V_6$ and electrograms from the HRA, distal (1–2), mid (2–3), and proximal (3–4) HBE, mid (3–4) CS, RVA, and distal (1–2) RV ROVE. Atrial flutter is transiently present during AVNRT. The first three flutter cycles do not influence AVNRT but the fourth rests the AVNRT, which continues in the absence of atrial activation (*arrow*) on the first return cycle. See text for discussion.

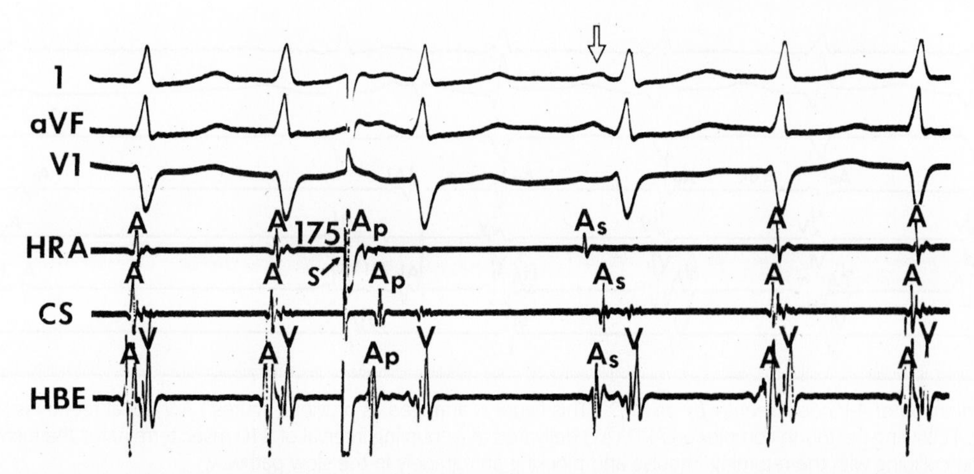


**FIGURE 8-51** *Production of A-V dissociation during A-V nodal reentrant SVT.* SVT is present at a cycle length of 370 msec. After the second QRS complex, an APD ($A_p$) is introduced at a coupling interval of 175 msec, which penetrates the reentrant circuit, producing a long pause. A spontaneous sinus P wave ($A_s$, *open arrow*) depolarizes all recorded atrial tissue before the time the spontaneous atrial echo would have occurred, resulting in A-V dissociation without terminating SVT. The HBE has moved slightly into the right atrium, and no His bundle deflections are recorded. (From Josephson ME, Scharf DL, Kastor JA, et al. Atrial endocardial activation in man. Electrode catheter technique for endocardial mapping. *Am J Cardiol* 1977;39:972–981.)

circuit at the critical time required for termination. This is also the mechanism by which rapid atrial pacing terminates arrhythmias.

In an analogous fashion to atrial stimulation, VPDs can produce similar responses.[94–96] The application of progressively premature VPDs during SVT can provide useful information regarding the presence of a lower common pathway. This depends critically on the ability to record a retrograde His potential and the capability of the VPD to reach the His bundle. As noted in Chapter 2, in approximately 85% of patients a

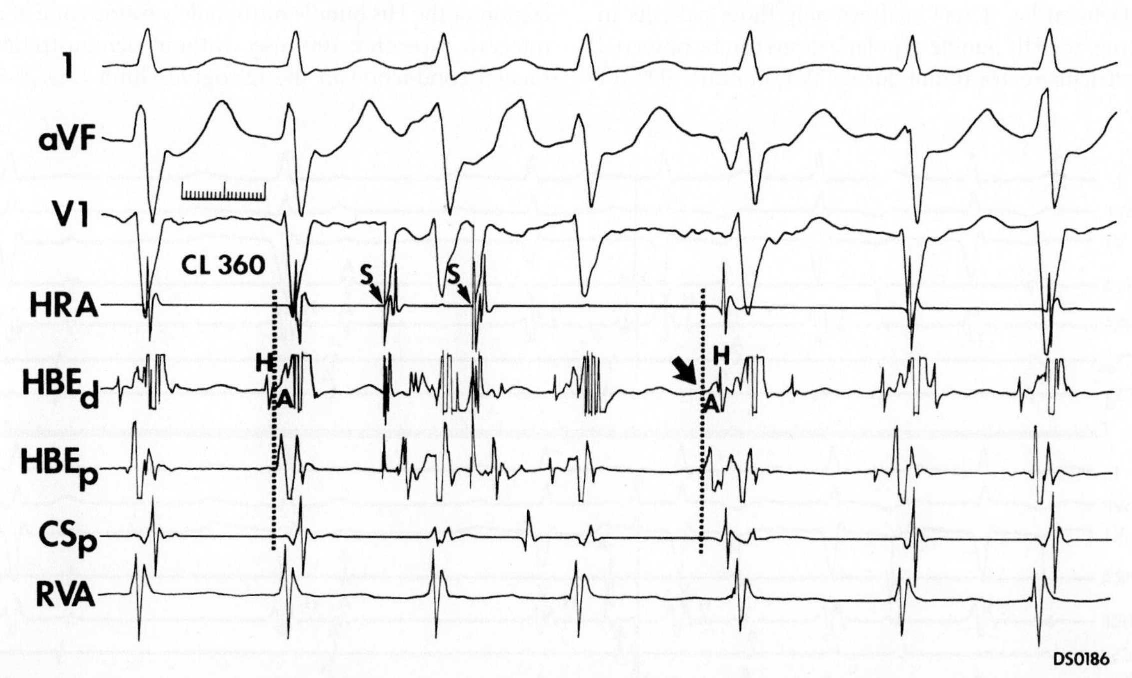


**FIGURE 8-52** *Atrial extrastimuli producing delay in the lower final common pathway during A-V nodal reentry.* Leads 1, aVF, and $V_1$ are shown with electrograms from the HRA, distal and proximal HBE, and the very proximal CS, and RVA. A-V nodal reentry with a cycle length of 360 msec is present. Note on the first two complexes retrograde atrial activation begins just before the onset of the QRS shown by the *dotted lines.* Two atrial extrastimuli are delivered, which influence the tachycardia. The second produces conduction delay in the lower final common pathway such that retrograde atrial activity now occurs before the inscription of the antegrade His bundle deflection, and an inverse P wave is seen before the onset of the QRS. The conduction delay, therefore, must be below the circuit in a lower final common pathway. See text for discussion. (From Miller JM, Rosenthal ME, Vassallo JA, et al. Atrioventricular nodal reentrant tachycardia: studies on upper and lower 'common pathways'. *Circulation* 1987;75:930–940.)

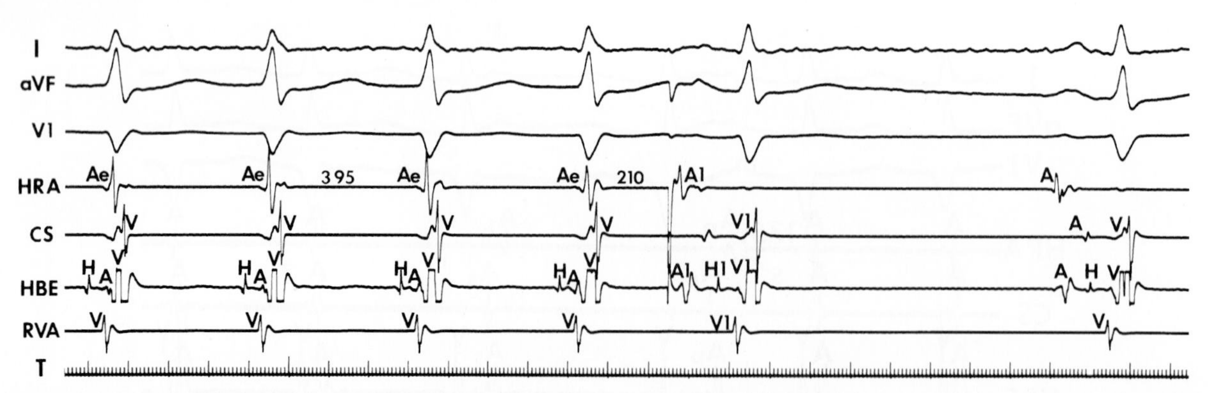


**FIGURE 8-53** *Termination of A-V nodal reentry by an APD.* (This figure is arranged as previous figures.) A-V nodal reentry is present at the cycle length of 395 msec. Following the fourth complex an APD ($A_1$) delivered at a coupling interval of 210 msec terminates the tachycardia by entering the fast pathway and colliding with the returning impulse and blocking antegradely in the slow pathway.

retrograde His deflection can be seen during ventricular pacing. The ability to reach the His bundle during a tachycardia by ventricular extrastimuli depends on the tachycardia cycle length, the local ventricular refractory period, the obligatory time required for the impulse to reach the bundle branches from the site of stimulation, and retrograde conduction time up the bundle branches to the His bundle. Thus, although VPDs can be introduced without any effect on AVNRT in all patients with A-V nodal reentrant SVT, the ability to document premature depolarization of the lower part of the AVN is limited to perhaps 60% of patients. This number can be augmented by using maneuvers or pharmacologic agents to slow the tachycardia. If one analyzes only those patients in whom retrograde His bundle depolarizations can be observed during ventricular extrastimuli during SVT, in nearly 90% of these patients the His bundle can be retrogradely captured prematurely by single (Fig. 8-55) and even double (Fig. 8-56) ventricular extrastimuli without affecting the tachycardia as manifested by a constant atrial cycle length.[96]

As with APDs, earlier VPDs can reset the tachycardia. This usually requires a very premature extrastimulus and/or a rather slow tachycardia (usually cycle lengths greater than 350 msec). Rosenthal et al.,[11] in our laboratory, demonstrated that if one can reset A-V nodal reentrant tachycardia by VPDs, the presence of an excitable gap can be demonstrated in the common form of AVNRT. During a slow typical A-V nodal reentrant tachycardia, he demonstrated premature depolarization of the His bundle retrogradely over a zone of coupling intervals exceeding 100 msec without demonstrating decremental conduction in the retrograde limb (Fig. 8-57). This

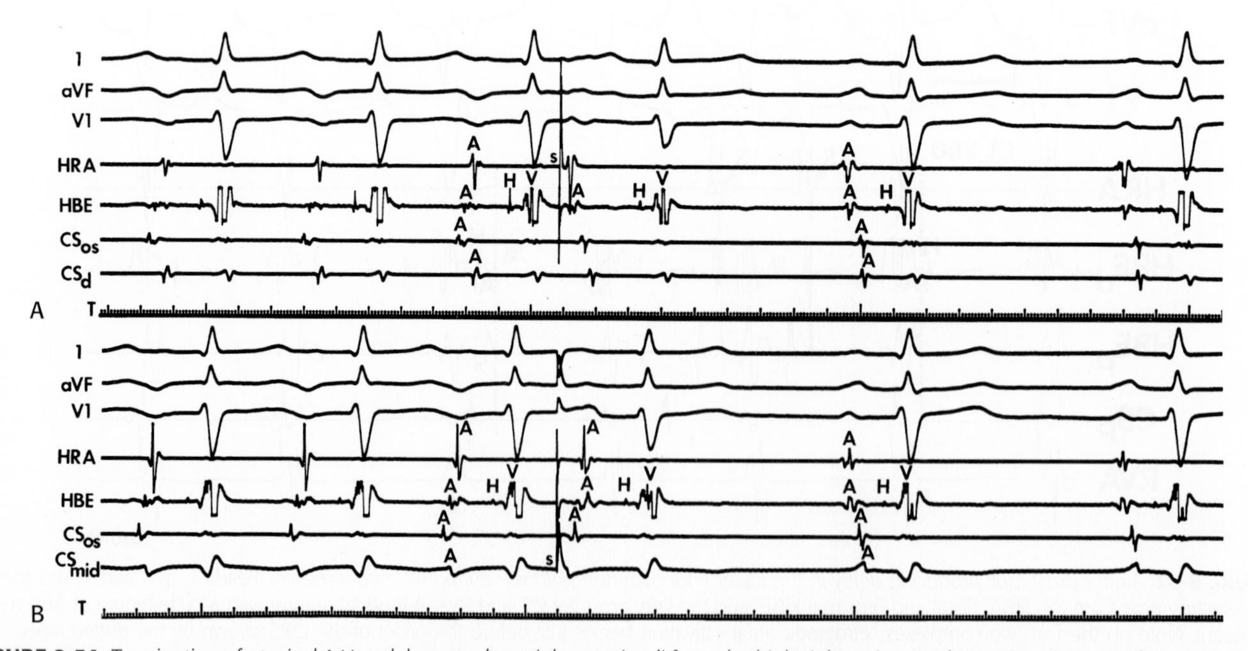


**FIGURE 8-54** *Termination of atypical A-V nodal reentry by atrial extrastimuli from the high-right atrium and coronary sinus.* Leads 1, aVF, and $V_1$ are shown with recordings from the HRA, HBE, CSos, CSmid, and time (T) lines. During atypical A-V nodal reentry, an atrial extrastimulus from the HRA **(A)** and the CS **(B)** terminate the tachycardia by conducting down the fast pathway during retrograde slow-pathway conduction, therefore preempting conduction over the slow pathway. The earlier impulse then blocks retrogradely in the slow pathway and the tachycardia terminates. See text for discussion.

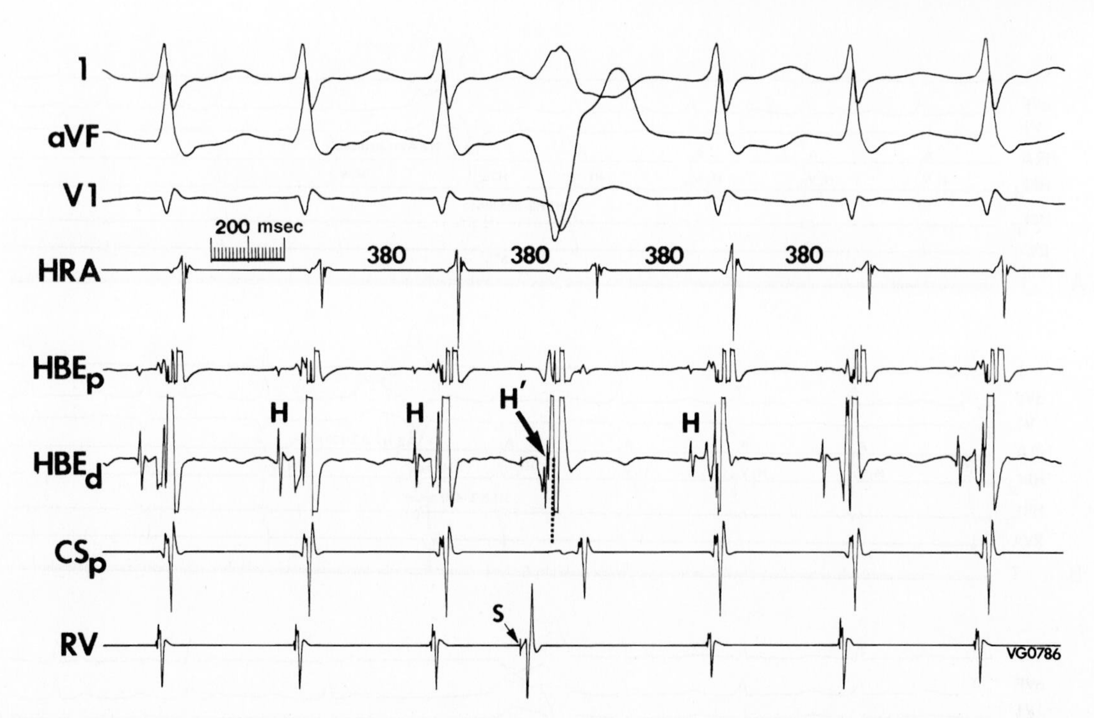


**FIGURE 8-55** *Retrograde capture of the His bundle by a ventricular extrastimulus without influencing the tachycardia.* (The figure is arranged identically to Figure 8-50.) Following three complexes of atrioventricular (A-V) nodal reentry at a cycle length of 380 msec, a ventricular extrastimulus is delivered and captures the His bundle retrogradely (H′, *arrow*) without influencing the tachycardia, as shown by a constant A-A interval. See text for discussion. (From Miller JM, Rosenthal ME, Vassallo JA, et al. Atrioventricular nodal reentrant tachycardia: studies on upper and lower 'common pathways'. *Circulation* 1987;75:930–940.)

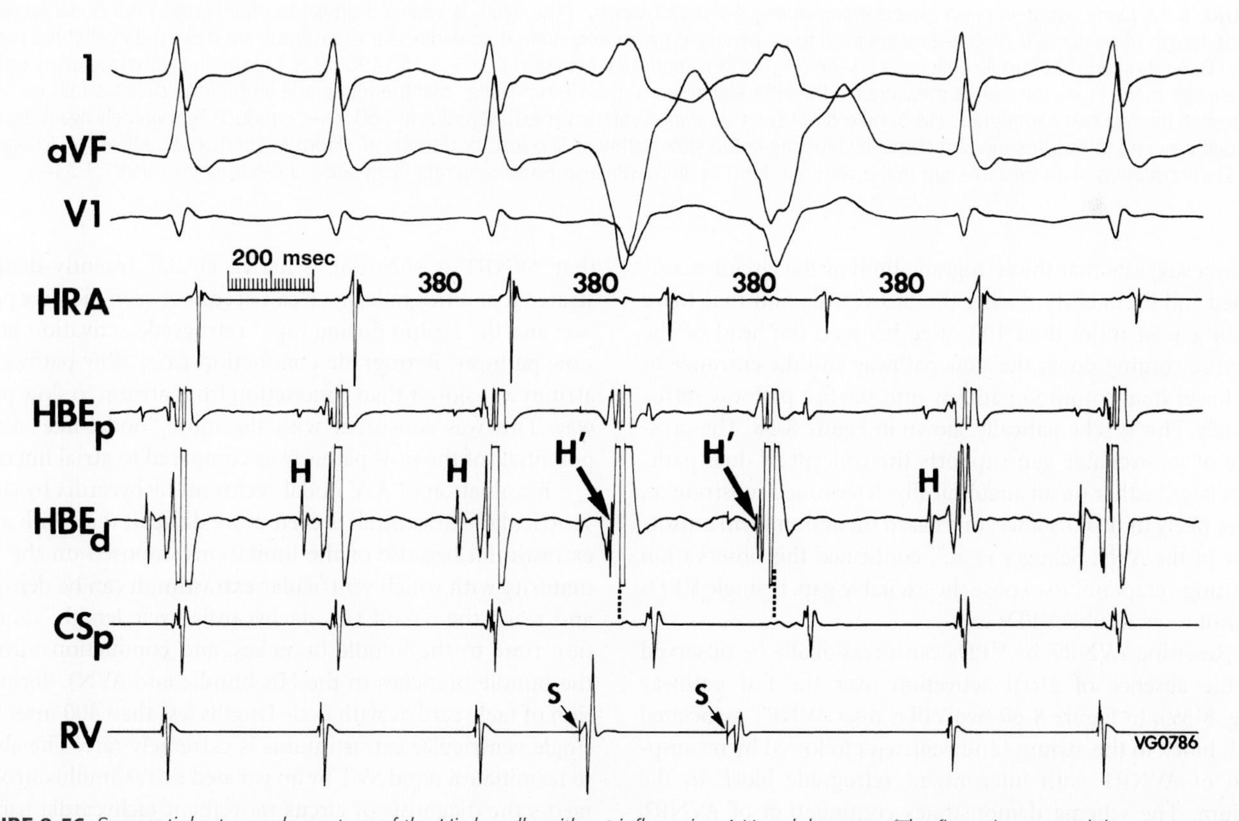


**FIGURE 8-56** *Sequential retrograde capture of the His bundle without influencing A-V nodal reentry.* (The figure is arranged the same as Figure 8-53.) Two ventricular extrastimuli capture the His bundle retrogradely (H′, *arrow*) without influencing the tachycardia. The *dotted lines* show where the His bundle would have been activated spontaneously during the tachycardia. See text for discussion. (From Miller JM, Rosenthal ME, Vassallo JA, et al. Atrioventricular nodal reentrant tachycardia: studies on upper and lower 'common pathways'. *Circulation* 1987;75:930–940.)

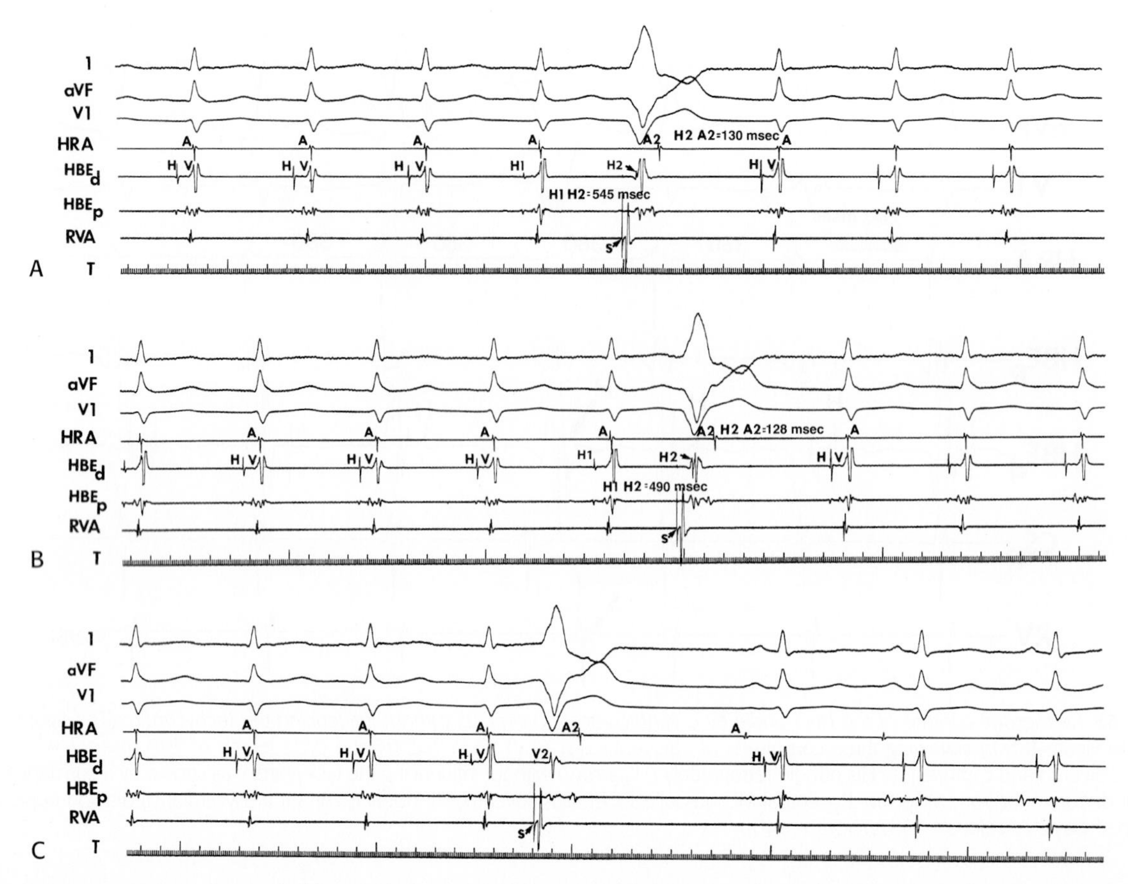


**FIGURE 8-57** *Demonstration of an excitable gap during A-V nodal reentry.* (The figure is arranged similar to prior figures.) A-V nodal reentry at a cycle length of nearly 600 msec is present in all three panels. Progressively premature ventricular extrastimuli are delivered in all three panels. **A** and **B:** A retrograde His bundle deflection is seen ($H_2$, *arrow*). Ventricular extrastimuli at 545 and 490 msec capture the His retrogradely without any change in the $H_2$-$A_2$ interval, as measured in the HRA electrogram. This demonstrates that the retrograde limb of the circuit is fully excitable. **C:** Despite the fact that a retrograde His bundle is not seen, an earlier ventricular extrastimulus at 260 msec conducts retrogradely again over the fast pathway and terminates the arrhythmia by blocking in the slow pathway. See text for discussion. (From Rosenthal ME, Miller JM, Josephson ME. Demonstration of an excitable gap in the common form of atrioventricular nodal reentrant tachycardia. *J Electrophysiol* 1987;1:334.)

finding suggests that the retrograde limb of the circuit maintained full excitability during the tachycardia and that there was a gap of more than 100 msec between the head of the impulse coming down the slow pathway and the entrance of the lower final common pathway into the fast pathway retrogradely. This is schematically shown in Figure 8-58. The presence of an excitable gap supports the concept of dual pathways based either on an anatomically determined substrate or, more likely in this instance, one based on nonuniform anisotropy in the AVN. Schuger et al.[94] confirmed this observation by using verapamil to expose the excitable gap. If single VPDs cannot reset, double VPDs can.

Resetting AVNRT by VPDs can occasionally be observed in the absence of atrial activation over the fast pathway (Fig. 8-59). In Figure 8-60 two VPDs reset AVNRT associated with block to the atrium (and ventricle) followed by resumption of AVNRT with intermittent retrograde block to the atrium. The schema demonstrates continuation of AVNRT with retrograde and antegrade block during the pause and intermittent block to the atrium following return of conduction to the ventricle. This finding also supports the concept that AVNRT is subatrial. Scherlag et al.[97] recently demonstrated that retrograde block can occur between the slow pathway and the atrium during rapid retrograde activation of the slow pathway. Retrograde conduction from slow pathway to atrium was slower than conduction from atrium to slow pathway. This was consistent with the more "nodal-like" action potentials of the slow pathway as compared to atrial fibers.

Termination of A-V nodal reentrant tachycardia by single ventricular extrastimuli is even more difficult than with atrial extrastimuli because of the limitations imposed on the prematurity with which ventricular extrastimuli can be delivered and reach the circuit (i.e., tachycardia cycle length, conduction time to the bundle branches, and conduction through the bundle branches to the His bundle and AVN). Termination of tachycardias with cycle lengths less than 400 msec by a single ventricular extrastimulus is extremely rare. The ability to terminate a rapid SVT by an isolated extrastimulus strongly favors the diagnosis of circus movement tachycardia using a CBT (see following discussion of concealed bypass tracts). Termination of AVNRT by a ventricular premature complex can occur either in the retrograde or antegrade limb. Usually,

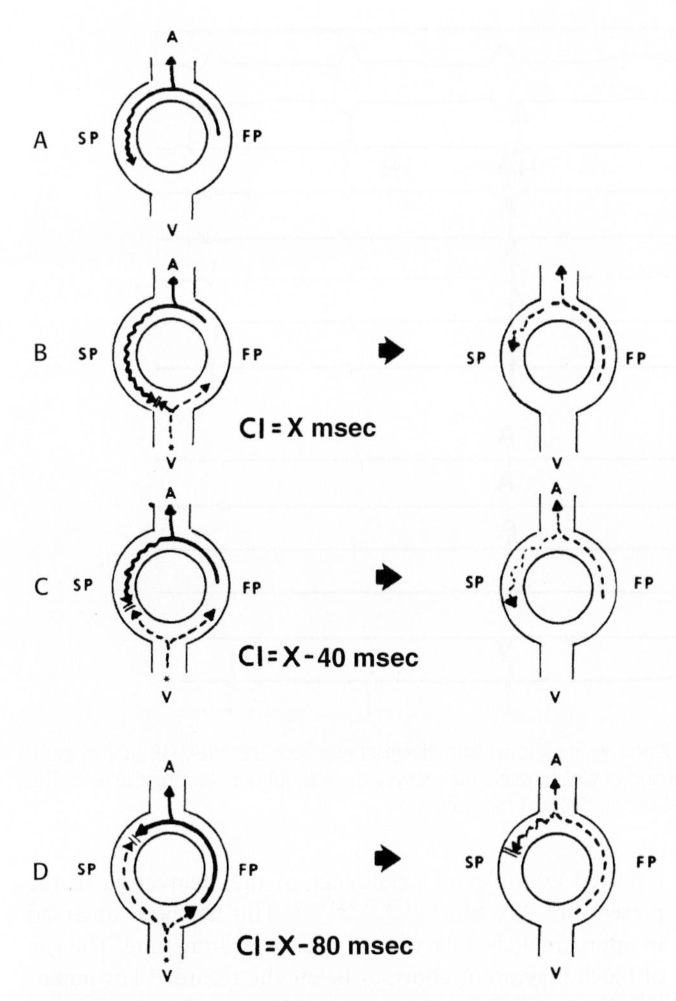


**FIGURE 8-58** *Schema of demonstration of excitable gap by ventricular extrastimuli.* **A, B, C,** and **D:** The tachycardia and effective premature stimuli delivered during the tachycardia over a range of 80 msec. See text for discussion. (From Rosenthal ME, Miller JM, Josephson ME. Demonstration of an excitable gap in the common form of atrioventricular nodal reentrant tachycardia. *J Electrophysiol* 1987;1:334.)

the slower the tachycardia, the more likely termination will be in the slow pathway. In contrast to isolated ventricular extrastimuli, rapid ventricular pacing can usually terminate even rapid tachycardias when single VPDs fail to do so. At longer-paced cycle lengths than those that terminate AVNRT, the AVNRT will be reset with a V-A-V response (see discussion later in this chapter regarding the use of overdrive ventricular pacing to distinguish AVNRT, AVRT, and AT).

To summarize, atrial and ventricular stimulation can terminate both typical and atypical AVNRT but are limited by several factors. When termination of typical AVNRT is by single APDs, more than 95% of the time this occurs with retrograde collision in the fast pathway and antegrade block in the slow pathway as shown in Figure 8-53. Occasionally, however, the APD can preempt slow-pathway conduction and go down the fast pathway while simultaneously blocking the slow pathway. In any event block in the slow pathway with either simultaneous collision in or capture of the fast pathway terminates the tachycardia. Similarly, in atypical AVNRT, APDs can terminate the tachycardia, but they do so almost universally by preempting conduction up the slow pathway. The APD conducts down the fast pathway, which produces block in the slow pathway retrogradely because of the earlier input into the slow pathway retrogradely by the earlier conducted impulse down the fast pathway. This is the typical mode of termination of a typical AVNRT by APDs, regardless of coupling interval or site of stimulation (Fig. 8-54).

Termination of AVNRT by single VPDs is more variable and is very uncommon if AVNRT has a cycle length of <320 msec. Although typical AVNRT can be terminated by a VPD, which usually conducts up the fast pathway and blocks on the return down the slow pathway, very early VPDs or multiple VPDs can, in fact, block in the fast pathway and collide with the impulse conduction down the slow pathway, terminating the arrhythmia. Thus, some variability in the site of termination exists. With atypical AVNRT, however, virtually 100% of the time the VPDs terminate the tachycardia by blocking the slow pathway retrogradely. These observations are for abrupt termination. Occasionally, however, delayed termination of A-V nodal reentrant tachycardia can occur following premature stimuli.[95] In this case, the effects of concealment in either of the two pathways can cause delayed block either antegradely in the slow pathway or retrogradely in the fast pathway during typical AVNRT. Thus, the site of termination is more variable when it does not occur abruptly.

### *Role of Atrial Activation Patterns in Evaluating the Role of the Atrium*

As noted earlier, during AVNRT retrograde atrial activation is heterogenous. The presence of multiple breakthroughs, particularly when activation at the slow pathway and/or in the coronary sinus was earlier than those sites on the proximal His bundle catheter, is incompatible with a macroreentrant circuit involving the atrium between the fast and slow pathways (Fig. 8-61A). Moreover, activation during AVNRT was discordant from that during ventricular pacing at comparable cycle lengths in half of our patients[77] (Fig. 8-61B). This further supports the functional nature of conduction and stresses the misconception of anatomically discrete pathways.

Loh et al.[98] performed high-density mapping (192 electrodes) of the triangle of Koch as well as of the left atrial septum during atypical A-V nodal echoes in canines and found no evidence of atrial activation that could be construed as participating in the reentrant circuit. They then made 1- to 3-mm deep incisions perpendicular to the tricuspid valve and the tendon of Todaro at the level of the coronary sinus os and at three more proximal levels closer to the compact node. These incisions, which separated the so-called fast and slow pathways, failed to prevent the A-V nodal echoes (Fig. 8-62). All these data suggest that the reentrant circuit involved in AVNRT has not been defined, but suggests it is subatrial perhaps related to the marked nonuniform anisotropy of the compact node and transitional nodal tissue around it.

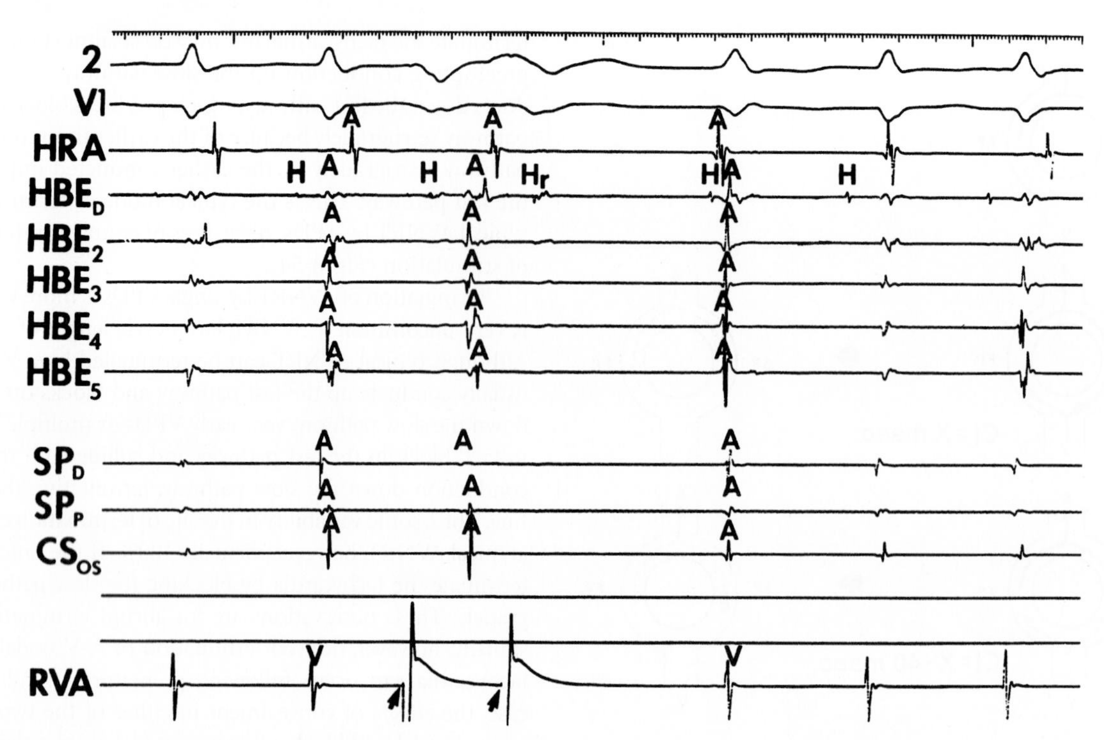


**FIGURE 8-59** *Resetting AVNRT without activating the atrium.* ECG leads 2 and $V_1$ are shown with electrograms from the HRA, HBE (slow pathway), CSos, and RVA. Two VPDs are delivered during typical AVNRT, the second of which resets the tachycardia without depolarizing the atria. The first VPD does not affect the tachycardia. These findings suggest a subatrial circuit. See text for discussion.

This is supported by the recent work of Efimov's group using optical mapping techniques in explanted human hearts, which has shown nonuniformities of connexins structure and function in a three-dimensional AVN/transitional zone structure in which reentry takes place.

## Requirement of Subnodal Structures in AVNRT

Many observations suggest that infranodal structures are not required to maintain AVNRT. There have been many reported examples of persistence of the tachycardia in the presence of A-V block.[18,28,85–88,99–104] This has been observed in approximately 13% of our patients at sometime. The site of block may occur above or below the recorded His potential, but most commonly occurs below the His in either a 2:1 or Wenckebach fashion at the onset of the tachycardia (Fig. 8-63). The observation of block below the His has no implication as to the site of turn around, since it is only seen at short H-H intervals as a manifestation of physiologic phase 3 block. Although A-V block has most commonly been

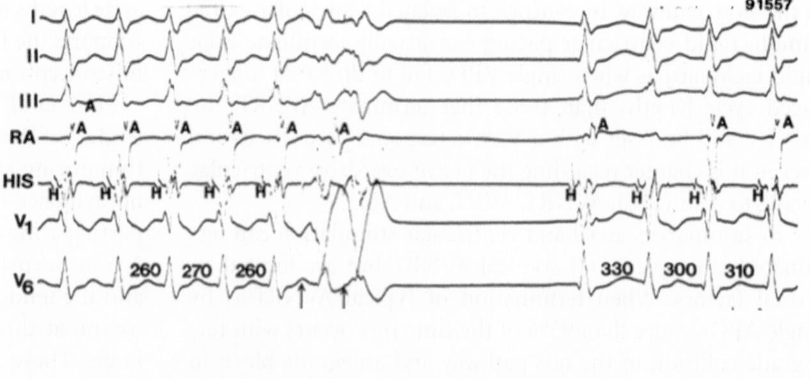


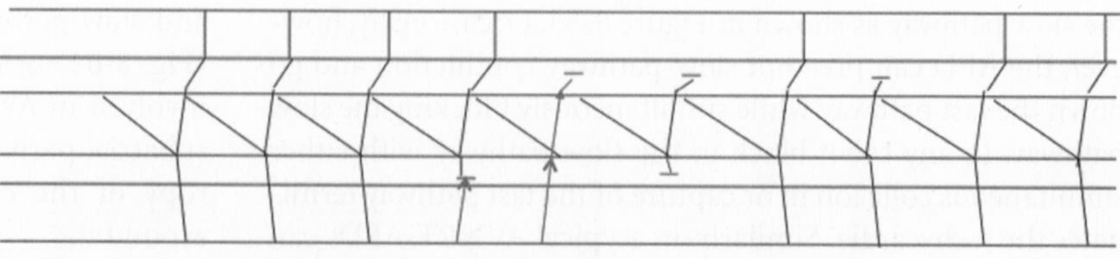

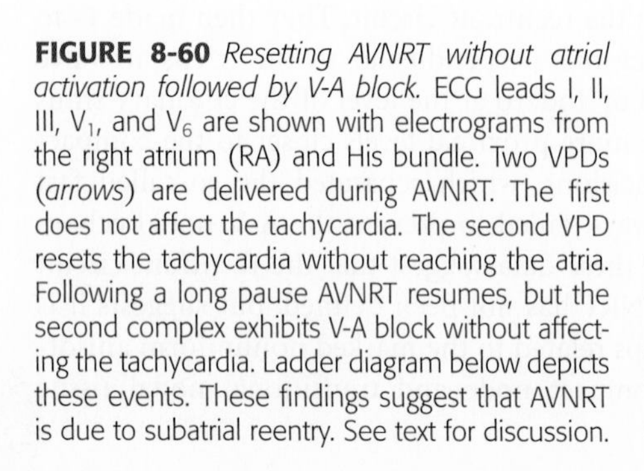

**FIGURE 8-60** *Resetting AVNRT without atrial activation followed by V-A block.* ECG leads I, II, III, $V_1$, and $V_6$ are shown with electrograms from the right atrium (RA) and His bundle. Two VPDs (*arrows*) are delivered during AVNRT. The first does not affect the tachycardia. The second VPD resets the tachycardia without reaching the atria. Following a long pause AVNRT resumes, but the second complex exhibits V-A block without affecting the tachycardia. Ladder diagram below depicts these events. These findings suggest that AVNRT is due to subatrial reentry. See text for discussion.

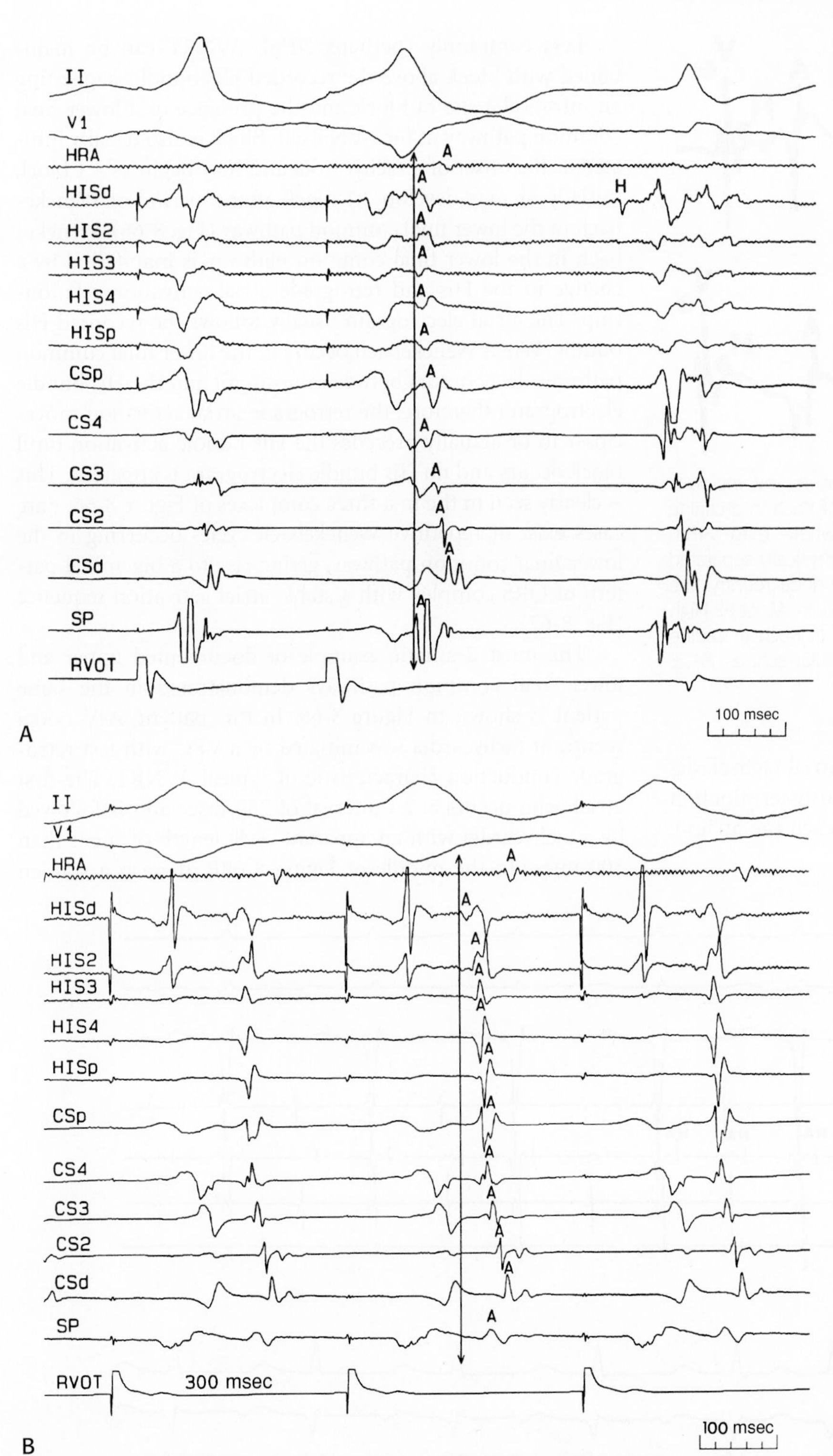


**FIGURE 8-61** *Discordant atrial activation during AVNRT and ventricular pacing.* The figure is organized identically to Figure 8-32. **A:** Two VPDs are delivered during AVNRT to expose atrial activation, which demonstrates a broad pattern of activation along the HBE and simultaneous activation at the SP (i.e., multiple breakthroughs). **B:** During ventricular pacing atrial activation shows a single sequential activation pattern. See text.

observed during typical AVNRT, we have reported atypical AVNRT associated with both A-V nodal and infra-His block (Fig. 8-64).[28] Initiation of the tachycardia associated with A-V block occurred whether stimulation was performed at the high-right atrium or coronary sinus. The finding of block in the node or below the His, in this case of a long R-P tachycardia, suggests atypical AVNRT as the diagnosis and excludes the slowly conducting bypass tract, which it can mimic.[63–65] However, one must prove that this rhythm is not atrial tachycardia by demonstrating its initiation with ventricular stimulation and the ability to reset or entrain the tachycardia with ventricular stimulation, while maintaining the exact same retrograde sequence as the tachycardia and demonstrating a V-A-V response (see discussion later in this chapter on responses to

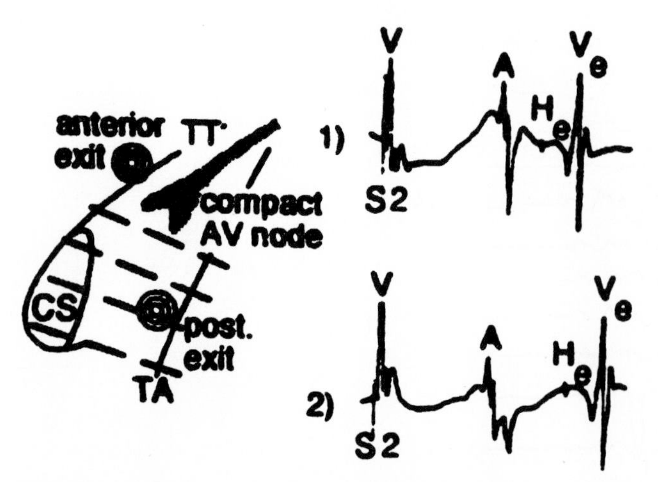


**FIGURE 8-62** *Failure to prevent A-V nodal reentry by incisions through the triangle of Koch.* Schema of triangle of Koch in a canine model of A-V nodal reentry. *Dashed lines* show where 1- to 3-mm deep incisions were made. These incisions which physically separated the "fast" and "slow" pathways failed to prevent A-V nodal reentry. See text for discussion. (From Loh P, de Bakker JMT, Hocini M, et al. High resolution mapping and dissection of the triangle of Koch in canine hearts: evidence for subatrial reentry during ventricular echoes. *PACE* 1997;20:1080 [abstract].)

overdrive ventricular pacing to distinguish atrial tachycardia from AVNRT or AVRT) (Fig. 8-65).[28] Obviously termination of the tachycardia by VPDs which do not reach the atrium, excludes atrial tachycardia.

Less commonly (perhaps 20%), AVNRT can be maintained with block above the recorded His bundle, suggesting an intranodal site of block and the presence of a lower final common pathway in the AVN itself. Block is also usually initiated at the onset of a tachycardia and may begin as 2:1 block initially or may develop 2:1 block after a period of Wenckebach in the lower final common pathway (Fig. 8-66). Wenckebach in the lower final common pathway is manifested by a change in the His and retrograde atrial activation relationship. The atrial electrogram usually follows the recorded His bundle. When Wenckebach occurs in the lower final common pathway, delay occurs between the circuit and the His bundle electrogram; therefore, the retrograde atrial activation moves closer to or actually precedes the His bundle activation until block occurs and no His bundle electrogram is apparent. This is clearly seen in the first three complexes of Figure 8-66. Rare cases exist of repetitive Wenckebach cycles occurring in the lower final common pathway, giving rise to a bigeminal pattern of QRS complex with a stable atrial activation sequence (Fig. 8-67).

The most dramatic example of documented upper and lower final common pathways demonstrated in the same patient is shown in Figure 8-68. In this patient, A-V nodal reentrant tachycardia was initiated by a VPC with fast retrograde conduction characteristic of typical AVNRT. The first atrial echo occurs at an interval of 280 msec and is followed by a tachycardia with an apparent cycle length of more than 500 msec. In the middle of Figure 8-68B, there is a sudden

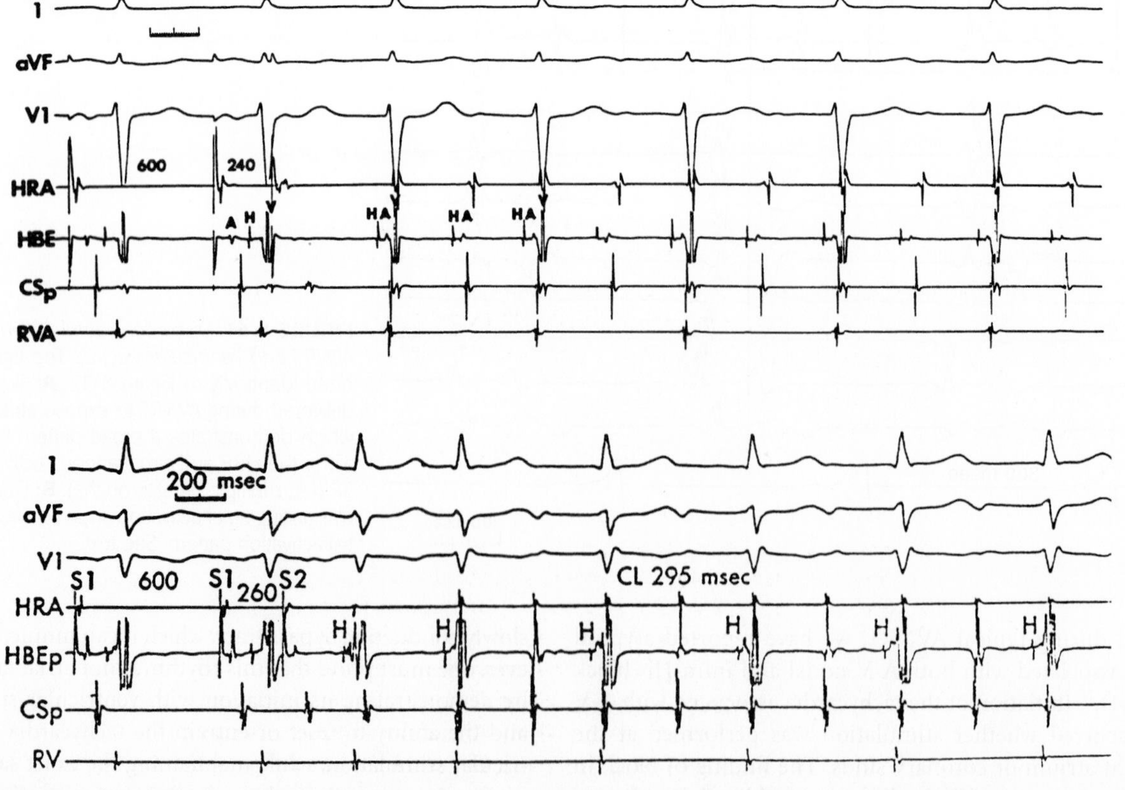


**FIGURE 8-63** *Typical AVNRT with infranodal and intranodal block.* In both panels typical AVNRT is induced by a single APD. In the **top panel** 2:1 A-V block occurs below the His. In the **bottom panel** 2:1 block appears in the A-V node after a period of 3:2 Wenckebach.

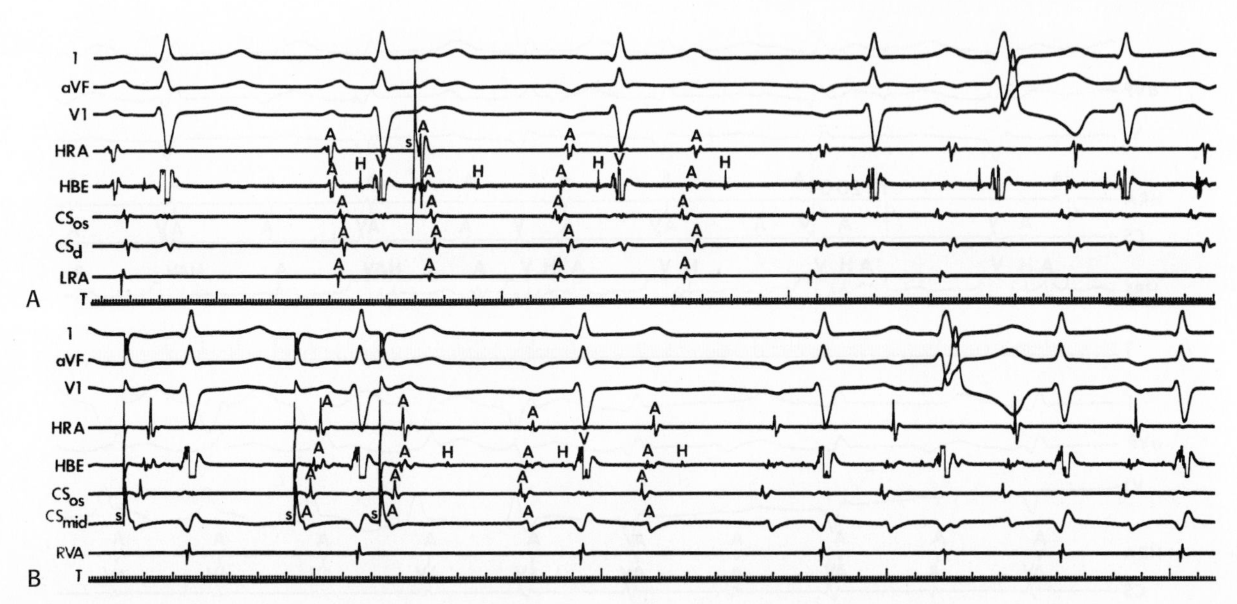


**FIGURE 8-64** *Infra-His block during atypical A-V nodal reentry.* Both panels are organized from top to bottom as leads 1, aVF, $V_1$, and electrograms from the HRA, HBE, os and distal CS, and low-right atrium (LRA). **A:** An APD delivered from the HRA during sinus rhythm initiates atypical A-V nodal reentry. Block below the His is observed on the initiating complex on the third and on the second complex of the tachycardia. **B:** An APD delivered from the mid-CS produces the exact same phenomenon. In contrast to typical A-V nodal reentry with infra-His block, with atypical A-V nodal reentry, the retrograde A precedes the blocked His potential. See text for discussion.

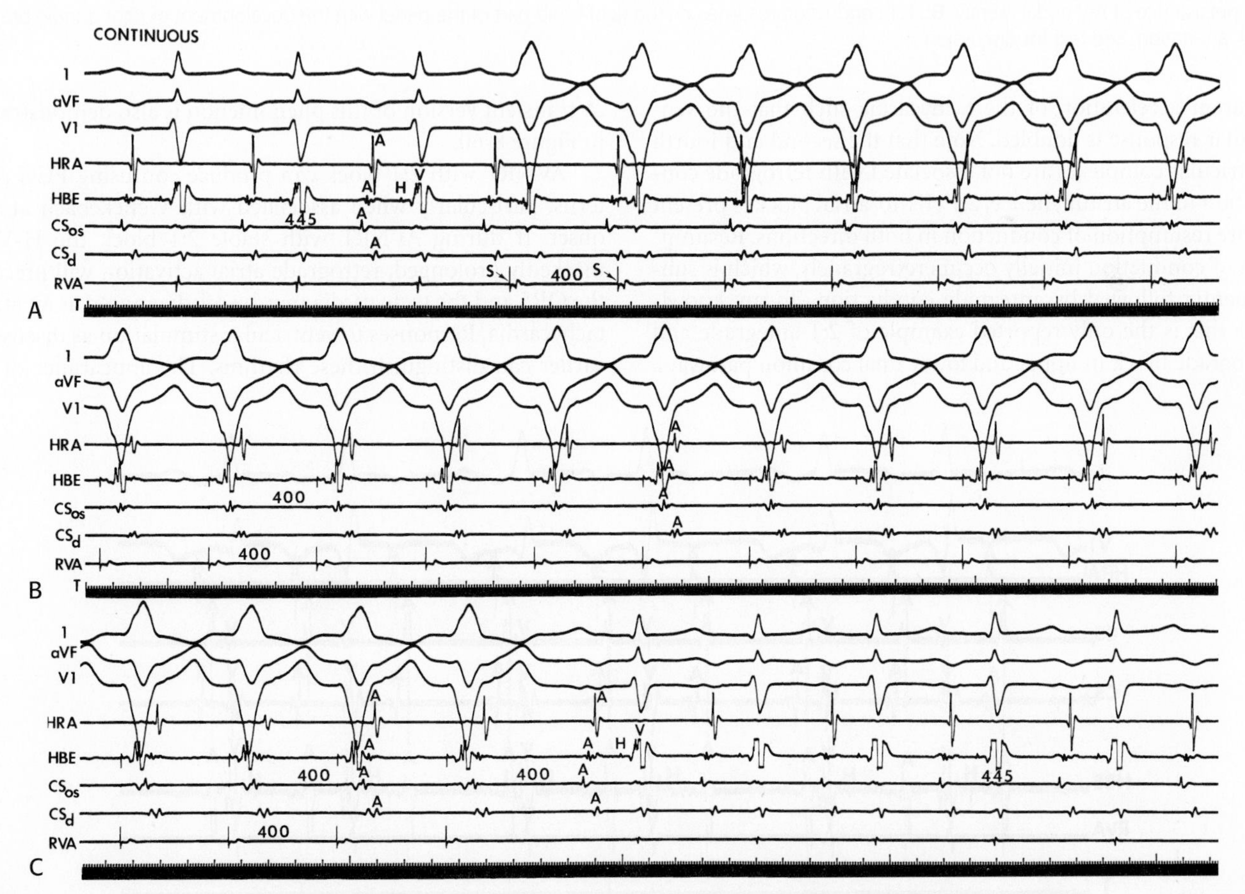


**FIGURE 8-65** *Entrainment of atypical A-V nodal reentry.* **A:** Atypical A-V nodal reentry is present in the first three complexes at a cycle length of 445 msec. Subsequently, ventricular pacing is begun at 400 msec with retrograde capture of the atrium from the third ventricular extrastimulus and through panel **B**. **C:** Pacing is discontinued and the first return cycle of atypical A-V nodal reentry is 400 msec, thereby demonstrating entrainment of that rhythm. See text for discussion.

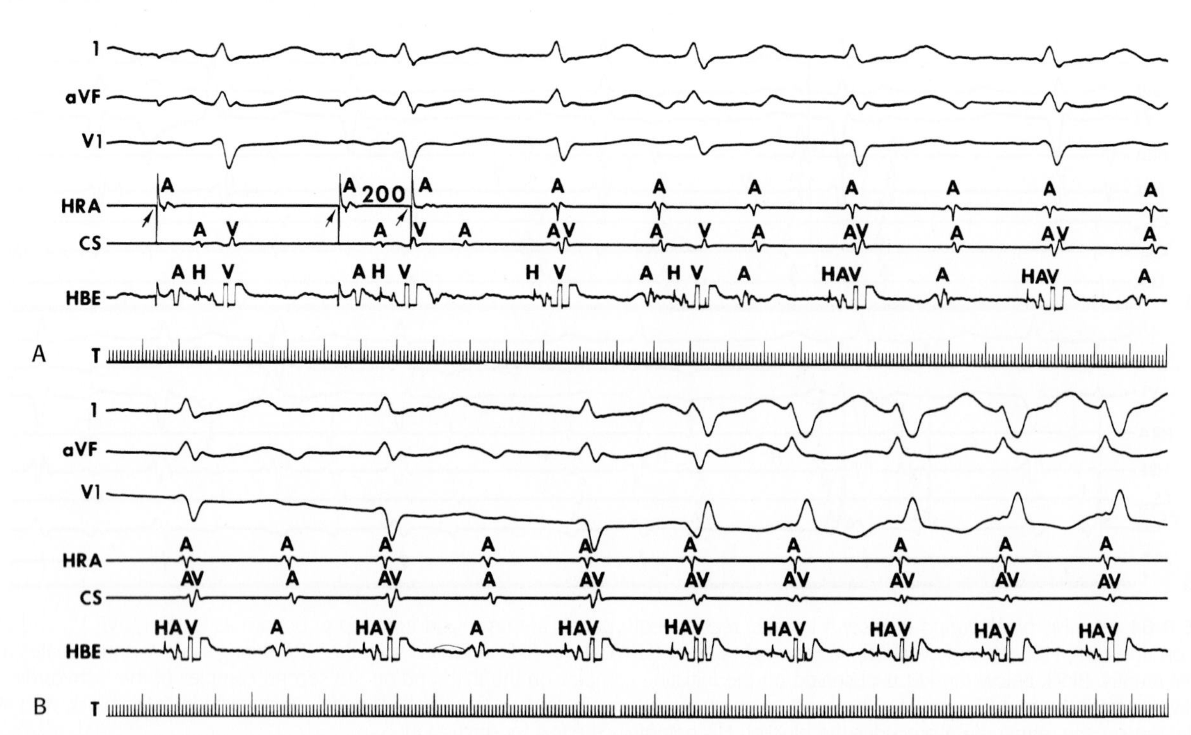


**FIGURE 8-66** *A-V nodal block during A-V nodal reentrant SVT.* From top to bottom, panels are arranged as leads 1, aVF, $V_1$, HRA, CS, and HBE. **A:** At a paced cycle length of 500 msec, a single atrial extrastimulus at 200 msec initiates A-V nodal reentrant SVT. The first three complexes demonstrate Wenckebach in a lower final common pathway culminating in the development of 2:1 A-V nodal block below the reentrant circuit with persistence of A-V nodal reentry. **B:** 1:1 conduction resumes on the right-hand part of the panel with the development of right bundle branch block aberration. See text for discussion.

apparent acceleration of the tachycardia such that the ventricular response is doubled. Note that the second and fourth ventricular complexes are not associated with retrograde conduction to the atrium; hence, 2:1 His-to-atrial block is present before resumption of conduction in both directions. Resumption of conduction initially occurs retrogradely, which is subsequently followed by antegrade conduction. To my knowledge this is the only reported example of 2:1 antegrade and retrograde block in upper and lower final common pathways. .A transient version of this phenomenon is also demonstrated in Figure 8-60.

AVNRT with 2:1 block can produce confusing ECG patterns, particularly when associated with Wenckebach at the onset. If during AVNRT with stable 2:1 block the H-V is markedly prolonged, retrograde atrial activation will precede the QRS and the tachycardia may be misdiagnosed as an atrial tachycardia. Responses to ventricular stimulation as discussed earlier can distinguish these rhythms. The appearance of an

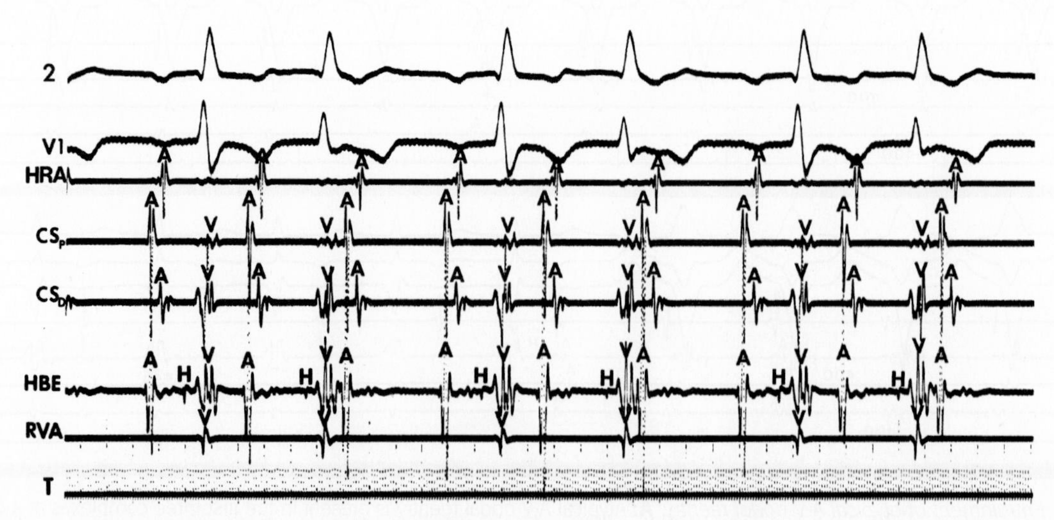


**FIGURE 8-67** *A-V nodal Wenckebach during A-V nodal reentry.* Leads 2 and $V_1$ are shown with electrograms from the HRA, proximal and distal CS, HBE, and RVA. A-V nodal reentry is present with a 3:2 Wenckebach pattern below the reentrant circuit in the A-V node. Persistence of the tachycardia with this repetitive Wenckebach cycle reveals the presence of a lower final common pathway.

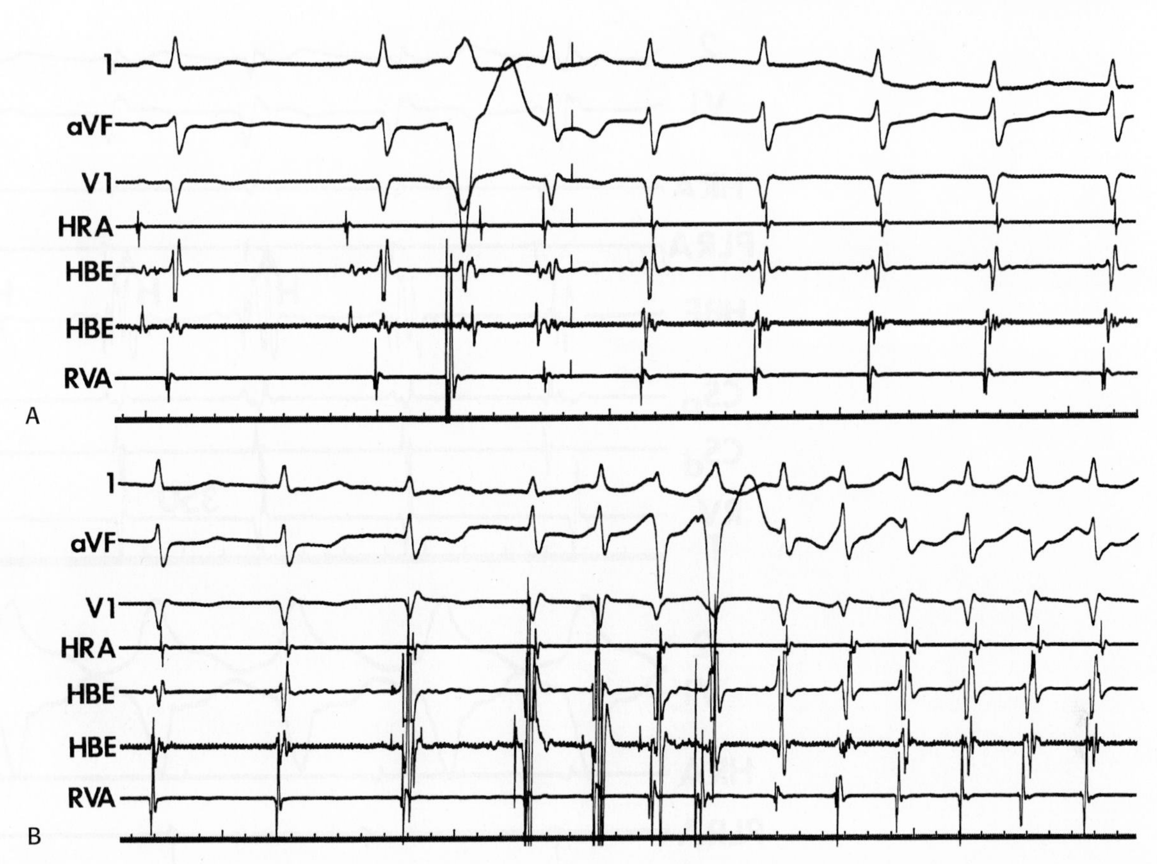


**FIGURE 8-68** *A-V nodal reentry with block in upper and lower final common pathways simultaneously.* **A:** Leads 1, aVF, and $V_1$ are shown with electrograms from the HRA, HBE, and RVA. Following two sinus complexes, a VPD conducting over the fast pathway initiates A-V nodal reentry. The first complex of the A-V nodal reentry has a cycle length of approximately 260 msec, and thereafter a tachycardia with an apparent cycle length of 250 msec. **B:** In the middle of the tracing, there is sudden resumption of 1:1 conduction to the ventricles at a cycle length of approximately 280 msec. Note that the first several complexes are associated with 2:1 block to the atrium despite 1:1 conduction to the ventricles. Ventricular premature stimulus produces a fusion of the fourth ventricular complex with persistence of the tachycardia. After the fifth complex of 1:1 ventricular conduction, 1:1 conduction resumes between the circuit and the atrium. Thus, this patient demonstrates A-V nodal reentrant SVT, initially with block in an upper and lower final common pathway, followed by conduction through the lower common pathway with persistence of block in the upper final common pathway, eventually followed by 1:1 conduction through both upper and lower final common pathways. See text for discussion.

apparent typical AVNRT (simultaneous atrial and ventricular activation) at the same cycle length upon normalization of the QRS also is consistent with the diagnosis of AVNRT but does not exclude atrial tachycardia with a long P-R producing simultaneous atrial and ventricular activation.

The occurrence of spontaneous block is not rare. In our laboratory, we have observed A-V block during EP study in 233 of 1,798 (13%) patients with AVNRT. If one analyzes the incidence of A-V block in reference to the total number of spontaneous or induced episodes of SVT, it decreases markedly. Most commonly, block is observed at the initiation of a tachycardia, but it has also been observed during acceleration of the tachycardia rate and following spontaneous or induced VPDs. Resumption of 1:1 conduction is always associated with at least transient aberration and slight lengthening of the AVNRT cycle length. Although A-V block was initially considered merely a laboratory phenomenon, we have observed a 12% incidence of A-V block (2:1 or Wenckebach type) at the onset of ***spontaneously occurring*** AVNRT. Thus, this is certainly not a rare event.

### *The Role of Atrial or Ventricular Pacing in Analyzing Upper and Lower Final Common Pathways*

Theoretically, if antegrade and/or retrograde Wenckebach periodicity or block could be demonstrated at a cycle length approximating the cycle length of the tachycardia, this would be evidence of upper and/or lower final common pathways (Fig. 8-69).[18,62,96] Conclusions based on these observations must be tempered by the absence of sympathetic tone during sinus rhythm, which is normally present during AVNRT. Another analysis that can be useful is to compare the A-H interval during SVT (as measured in the His bundle electrogram) to that produced by atrial pacing at the same cycle length as the SVT. If an upper final common pathway is absent, the A-H intervals will be equal. If an upper final common pathway is present, the A-H interval during the tachycardia will be less than that during atrial pacing and will reflect the difference produced by retrograde conduction through the upper common pathway and simultaneous antegrade conduction over the slow pathway. Quantitation of the extent of the upper

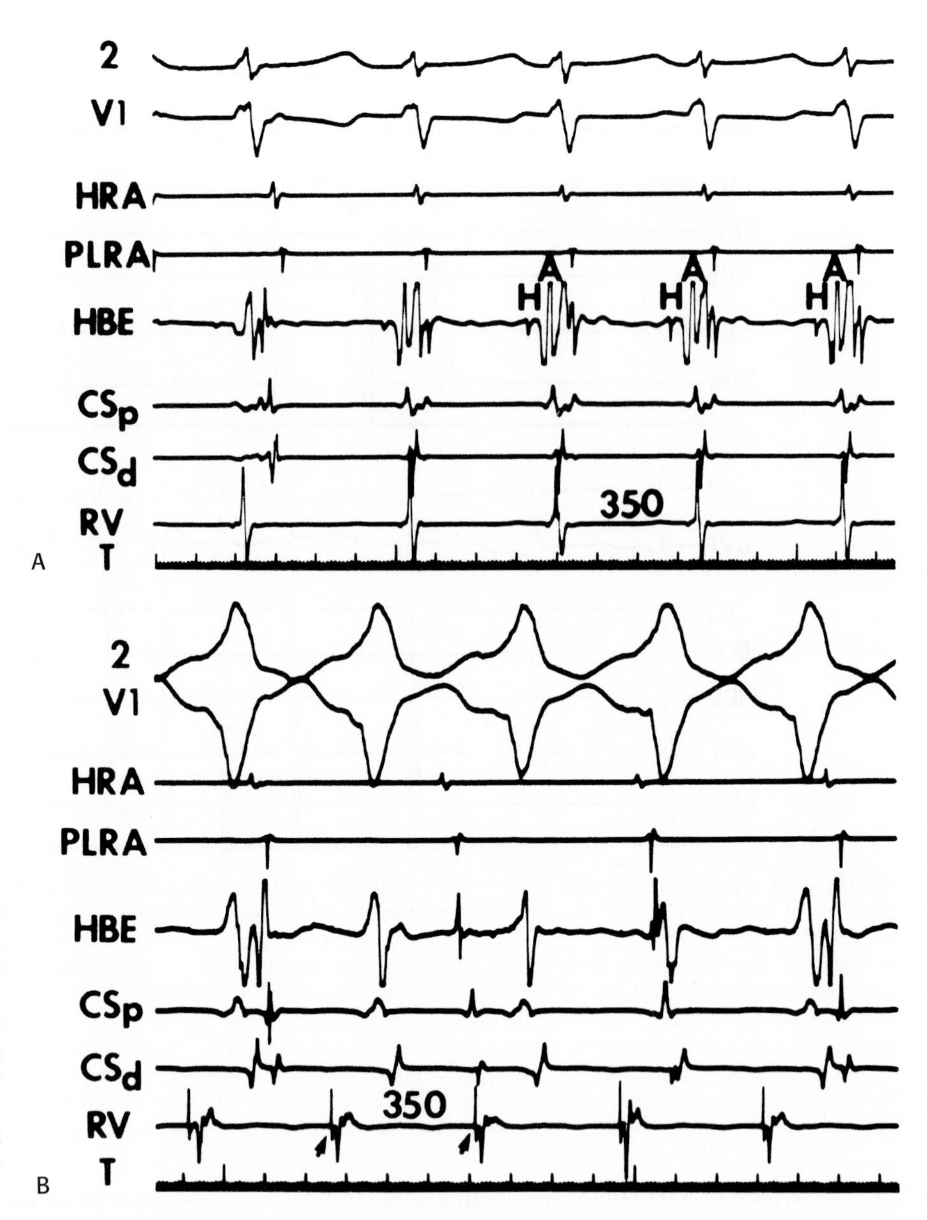


**FIGURE 8-69** *Demonstration of lower final common pathway by demonstration of no V-A conduction at the same cycle length as SVT.* (The figure is arranged the same as Figure 8-22.) **A:** SVT is present at a cycle length of 350 msec. **B:** Ventricular pacing at a comparable cycle length demonstrates A-V dissociation. The ability to manifest SVT at a similar cycle length associated with V-A block suggests that the block is in a lower final common pathway. See text for discussion.

common pathway can be made by recording the A-H interval during pacing from the end of the atrial electrogram to the onset of the His bundle deflection (this gives the shortest A-H possible), and the A-H during the tachycardia is measured from the onset of the atrial electrogram (because conduction must occur from the node to the atrium) to the onset of the His deflection. This is schematically shown in Figure 8-70.

Miller et al.[18,62,96] observed A-V Wenckebach at a rate at least 10 beats slower than that of the tachycardia in 6 of 28 consecutively studied patients, suggesting an upper final common pathway. Two additional patients had significantly longer A-H intervals measured during pacing than during the SVT. In 15 patients, pacing at the cycle length of SVT was associated with A-H intervals shorter than that during SVT and no Wenckebach because conduction was occurring over the fast pathway. This response precluded determination of the presence or absence of an upper common pathway. This problem can be overcome if the investigator paces more rapidly to induce block in the fast pathway and cause conduction to proceed over the slow pathway. At that point, the rate of pacing can be decreased below that of the tachycardia, while maintaining slow-pathway conduction. Using this method, we observed findings consistent with an upper final common pathway (i.e., A-H during pacing greater than A-H during SVT) in approximately 80% of patients. In many patients, Wenckebach cycles eventually lead to the induction of the tachycardia before the actual manifestation of A-V nodal block. If the cycle lengths producing a jump from the fast to the slow pathway with progressive slowing of conduction in the slow pathway before inducing SVT were longer than the cycle lengths of SVT, this also could be included as a manifestation of an upper final common pathway (Fig. 8-6). Using criteria of Wenckebach cycles inducing SVT exceeding the cycle length of SVT, and A-H intervals over the slow pathway during pacing at the cycle

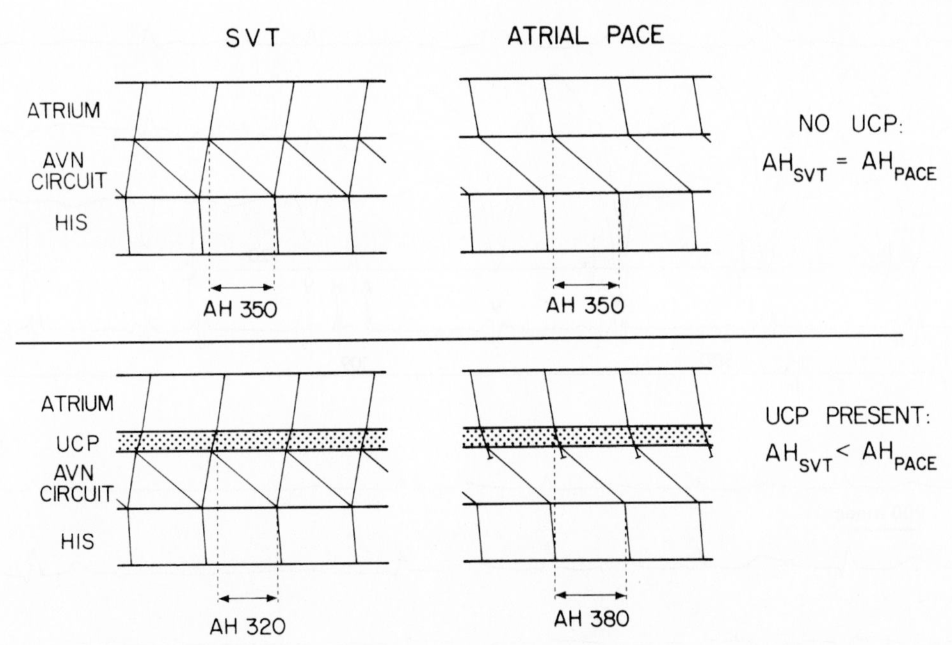


**FIGURE 8-70** *The effect of atrial pacing on A-H intervals in the presence and absence of an upper final common pathway.* Ladder diagrams portray the atrium, A-V nodal reentrant circuit, and His bundle with and without an upper final common pathway (UCP). In the absence of an upper final common pathway (**top panel**), the A-H interval during the tachycardia should equal the A-H interval during atrial pacing at the same cycle length as the tachycardia, assuming similar inputs and outputs of the atrium. In the **bottom panel**, the effect of atrial pacing in the presence of a UCP is shown. If a UCP is present, conduction antegradely and retrogradely occurs in the A-V node so that the "A-H" interval during SVT will be shorter than the A-H interval during pacing because during atrial pacing the UCP conduction time must be added to the antegrade conduction time over the slow pathway. See text for discussion. (From Miller JM, Rosenthal ME, Vassallo JA, et al. Atrioventricular nodal reentrant tachycardia: studies on upper and lower 'common pathways'. *Circulation* 1987;75:930–940.)

length of SVT exceeding the A-H during SVT, nearly 85% of patients will manifest one of these findings consistent with an upper final common pathway. This obviously requires that the investigator ensure that antegrade conduction proceeds over the slow pathway before any assessment of upper final common pathway in typical AVNRT. This is not necessary with atypical AVNRT, in which antegrade conduction proceeds over the fast pathway. Examples of A-H intervals that are greater during pacing than during tachycardia are shown in Figures 8-71 and 8-72. These conclusions are also limited by the absence of

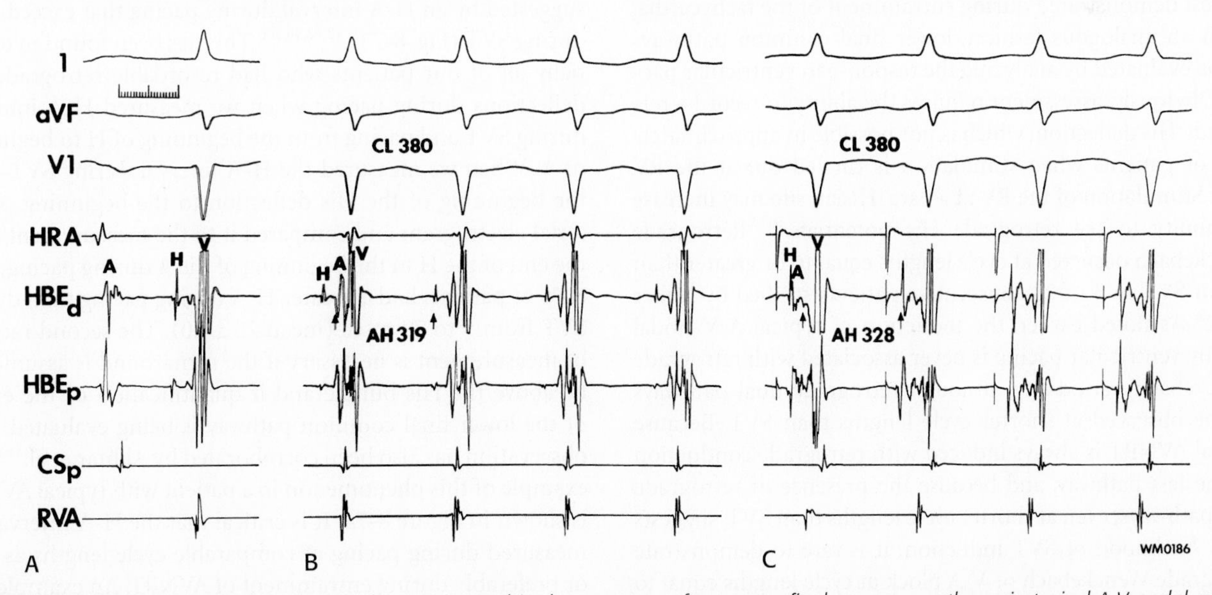


**FIGURE 8-71** *Influence of atrial pacing on the A-H interval in the presence of an upper final common pathway in typical A-V nodal reentry.* The tracing is arranged as in prior tracings **(A)** sinus rhythm, **(B)** A-V nodal reentry, **(C)** atrial pacing. During A-V nodal reentry at a cycle length of 380 msec, the A-H interval *(arrows)* measures 319 msec. During pacing at a comparable cycle length measuring from the era of the A to the beginning of the H, the A-H interval is longer at 328 msec. See text for discussion. (From Miller JM, Rosenthal ME, Vassallo JA, et al. Atrioventricular nodal reentrant tachycardia: studies on upper and lower 'common pathways'. *Circulation* 1987;75:930–940.)

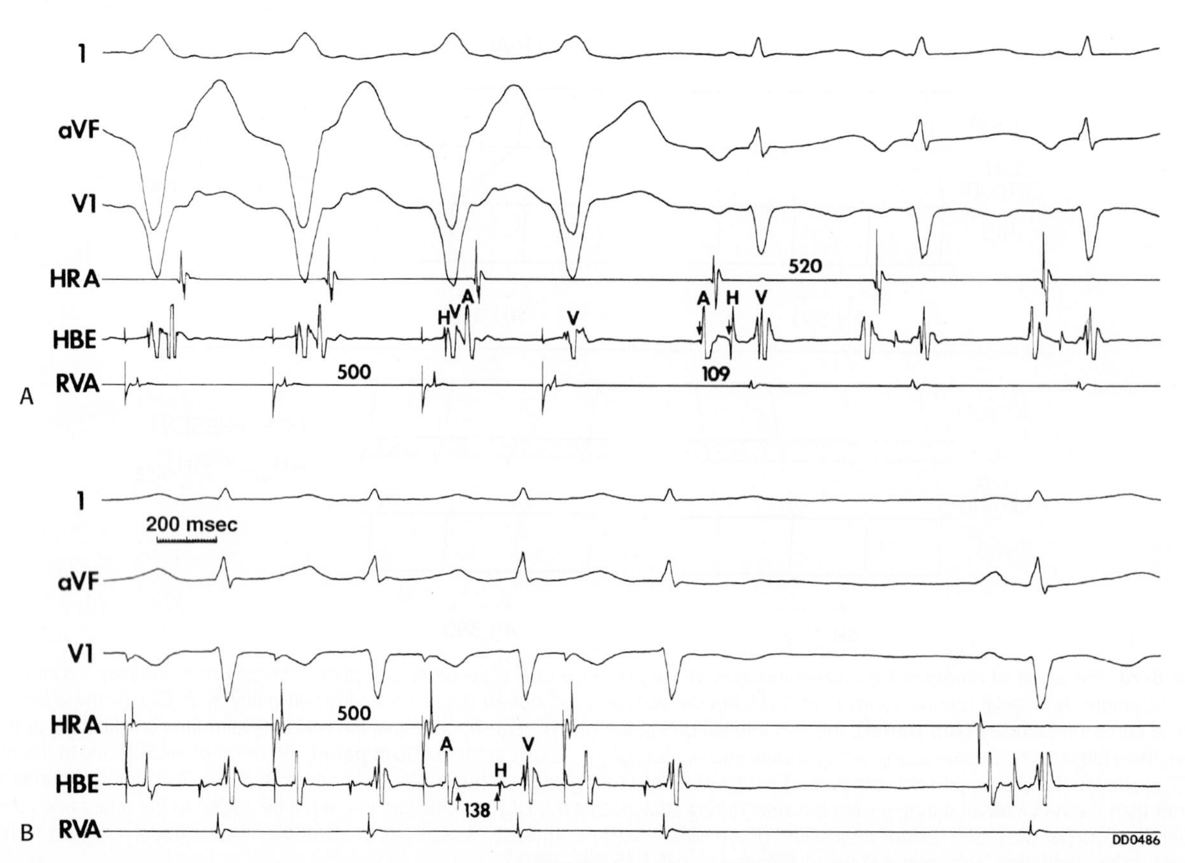


**FIGURE 8-72** *Comparison of A-H intervals during pacing and SVT in atypical A-V nodal reentry.* **A:** Atypical A-V nodal reentry is initiated by ventricular pacing. During atypical A-V nodal reentry, the A-H interval is 109 msec from the beginning of the A to the beginning of the H (i.e., assuming an upper final common pathway). **B:** During atrial pacing at a comparable cycle length, the A-H interval measured from the end of the A to the beginning of the H is almost 20 msec longer. See text for discussion. (From Miller JM, Rosenthal ME, Vassallo JA, et al. Atrioventricular nodal reentrant tachycardia: studies on upper and lower 'common pathways'. *Circulation* 1987;75:930–940.)

comparable autonomic tone during pacing and SVT, and thus are best demonstrated during entrainment of the tachycardia.

In an analogous fashion, lower final common pathways can be evaluated by analyzing the response to ventricular pacing. Obviously, assessment requires the ability to record a retrograde His deflection, which is not possible in approximately 15% of patients when stimulation is carried out at the RV apex. Stimulation of the RV at a para-Hisian site may increase the ability to see retrograde His potentials.[105] Retrograde Wenckebach occurred at cycle lengths equal to or greater than that of SVT in 3 of 28 consecutive patients studied by Miller et al.[96] As noted earlier, the induction of typical A-V nodal SVT by ventricular pacing is never associated with retrograde Wenckebach periodicity, although retrograde dual pathways can be observed at shorter cycle lengths than SVT. Because typical AVNRT is always induced with retrograde conduction up the fast pathway, and because the presence of retrograde dual pathways, even at shorter cycle lengths than SVT, suggests a low likelihood of SVT induction, it is rare to demonstrate retrograde Wenckebach or V-A block at cycle lengths equal to or greater than SVT (Fig. 8-69).

However, measurement of retrograde H-A intervals during SVT and ventricular pacing, particularly during entrainment of AVNRT, provides useful criteria for diagnosing a lower final common pathway. A lower common pathway is suggested by an H-A interval during pacing that exceeds that during SVT (Fig. 8-73).[18,62,96,106] This has been found in essentially all of our patients who had recordable retrograde His deflections during pacing when we measured H-A intervals during SVT and pacing from the beginning of H to beginning of A. When we measured the H-A interval during SVT from the beginning of the His deflection to the beginning of the atrial electrogram and compared it to the measurement from the end of the H to the beginning of the A during pacing, only 84% of patients had a greater H-A during pacing than during SVT from 5 to 79 msec (mean 25 ± 20). The second method of measurement is necessary if the turnaround is assumed to be above the His bundle and if quantification of the extent of the lower final common pathway is being evaluated. This observation has also been corroborated by Akhtar et al.[18,62] An example of this phenomenon in a patient with typical AVNRT is shown in Figure 8-74. It is critical that the H-A intervals be measured during pacing at comparable cycle lengths as SVT or preferably during entrainment of AVNRT. An example of a greater H-A during entrainment of AVNRT than AVNRT itself is shown in Figure 8-75. This supports the presence of a lower final common pathway in the AVN. Only one group has ever reported opposite observations during ventricular pacing.[105]

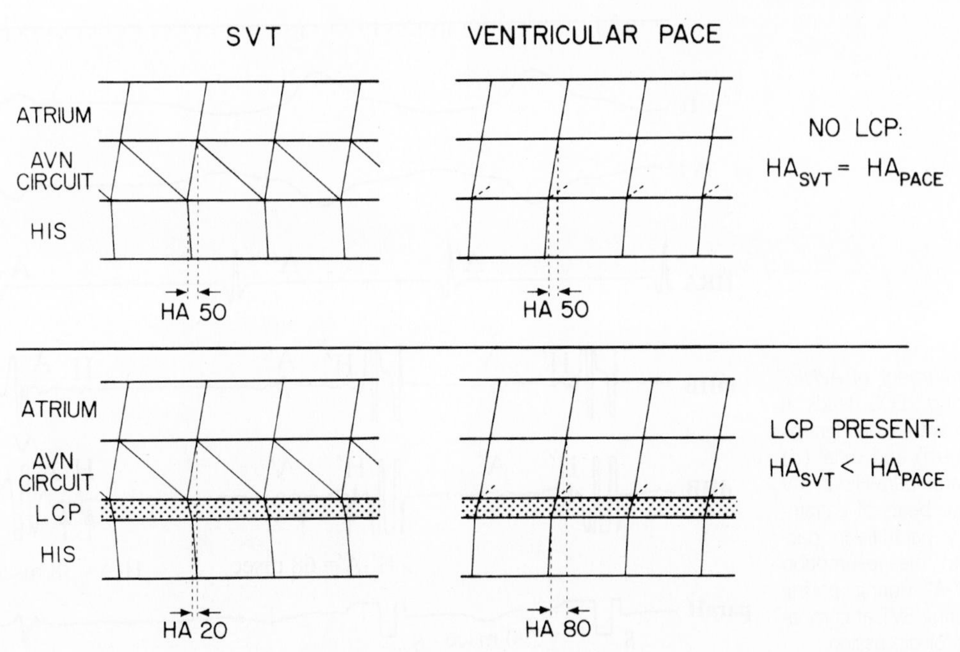


**FIGURE 8-73** *Schematic representation of effects of ventricular pacing on H-A intervals in the presence and absence of a lower final common pathway.* The atrium, A-V nodal circuit, and His bundle are shown in the presence and absence of a lower final common pathway (LCP). In the absence of a lower final common pathway, the H-A interval would be similar during SVT and ventricular pacing at a comparable cycle length. In the presence of an LCP, however, because the H-A interval is determined by retrograde conduction to the atria and simultaneous antegrade conduction to the His bundle, the H-A interval would be shorter than that during ventricular pacing, which requires retrograde conduction through the LCP as well as through the fast pathway. See text for discussion. (From Miller JM, Rosenthal ME, Vassallo JA, et al. Atrioventricular nodal reentrant tachycardia: studies on upper and lower 'common pathways'. *Circulation* 1987;75:930–940.)

The explanation for this difference remains elusive but may be related to the site at which the His bundle was recorded. Other investigators[80,83] have reported comparable H-A intervals during SVT and during ventricular stimulation and thus suggested the presence of a His-to-atrial connection. Those authors, however, used the response to ventricular extrastimuli for analysis. This method gives an inaccurate assessment of retrograde conduction through the AVN, because during ventricular stimulation the input into the AVN is limited by His–Purkinje refractoriness. This results in a flat $H_1$-$H_2$ interval and therefore a flat $H_2$-$A_2$ interval because the input to the AVN remains the same owing to slowing of His–Purkinje conduction in response to premature stimuli (see Chapter 3). This is the very reason VPDs rarely initiate typical AVNRT. Analysis

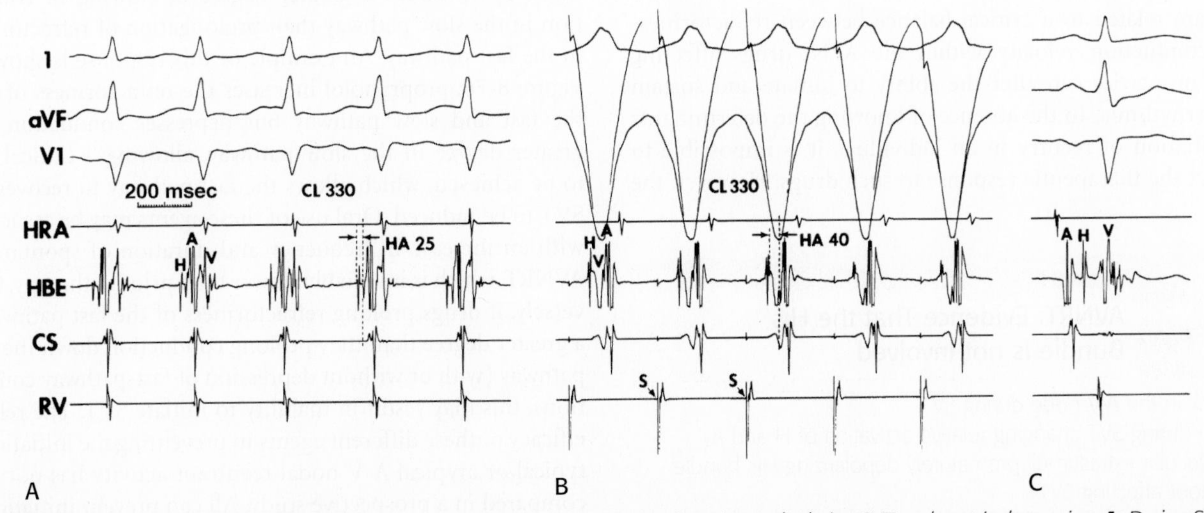


**FIGURE 8-74** *Demonstration of lower final common pathway by comparison of H-A intervals during SVT and ventricular pacing.* **A:** During SVT at a cycle length of 330 msec, the H-A interval is 25 msec (*dotted lines* and *arrows*). **B:** During ventricular pacing at the same cycle length, a retrograde His bundle is clearly seen. Measurements from the end of the H to the beginning of the A (*dotted lines* and *arrows*) is longer than the H-A intervals during SVT, diagnosing the presence of a lower final common pathway. **C:** Sinus rhythm. See text for discussion. (From Miller JM, Rosenthal ME, Vassallo JA, et al. Atrioventricular nodal reentrant tachycardia: studies on upper and lower 'common pathways'. *Circulation* 1987;75:930–940.)

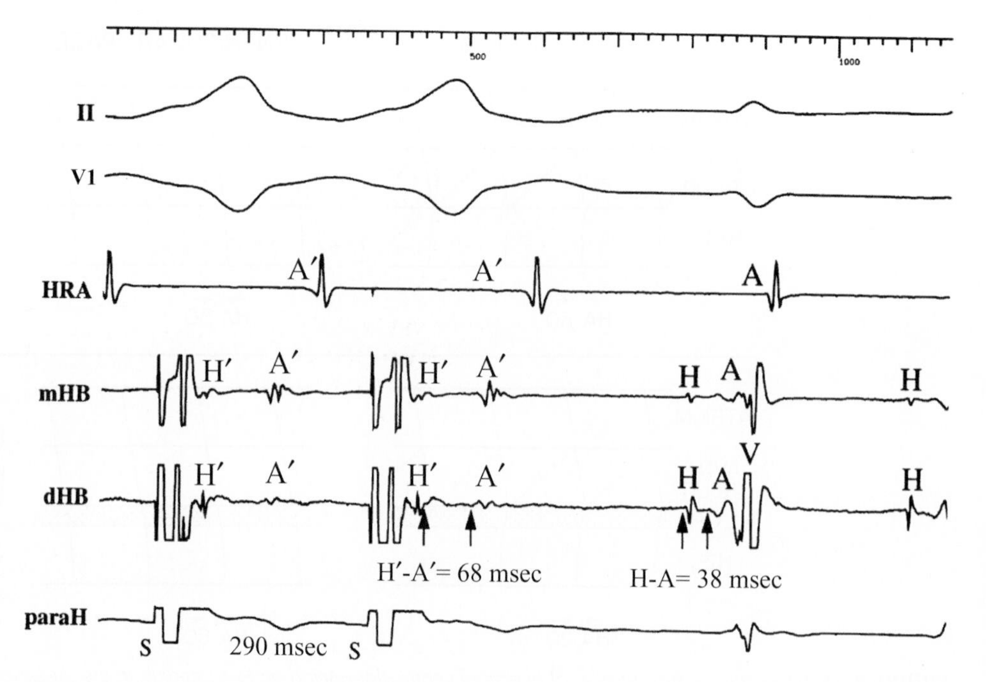


**FIGURE 8-75** *Entrainment of AVNRT by ventricular pacing.* ECG leads II and $V_1$ are shown with electrograms from the HRA, mid (m) and distal (d) His bundle (HB), and para-Hisian RV (paraH). The last two beats of entrainment of AVNRT by para-Hisian pacing are shown with the resumption of AVNRT. The H′-A′ during pacing exceeds the H-A during SVT at comparable rates. See text for discussion.

of H-A intervals should be measured only during pacing at a cycle length comparable to that of SVT, or preferably during entrainment of AVNRT. The data supporting a lower final common pathway are given in Table 8-4. Thus, based on spontaneously occurring phenomena, response to programmed stimulation, and recent experimental data, I believe AVNRT is a subatrial reentrant circuit confined to nodal (compact and transitional) tissue. Functional differences based on nonuniform anisotropy, and not specific anatomic structures, form the pathophysiologic basis for AVNRT.

### *Pharmacologic and Physiologic Maneuvers*

Because initiation and maintenance of A-V nodal reentrant SVT are related to a critical balance between refractoriness and conduction velocity within the AVN, drugs affecting these properties can alter the ability to initiate and sustain this arrhythmia. In the absence of knowing the determinants of initiation of reentry in an individual, it is impossible to predict the therapeutic response to such drugs. However, the

**TABLE 8-4 AVNRT: Evidence That the His Bundle is not Involved**

- Block in the A-V node during SVT
- APD during SVT changing relative activation of H and A
- Ventricular extrastimuli prematurely depolarizing His bundle without affecting SVT
- Ventricular pacing at SVT cycle length produces a greater "H-A" interval than "H-A" during SVT
- Ventricular pacing produces retrograde A-V nodal Wenckebach at a cycle length > SVT cycle length

physiologic effects of various agents have been studied. Digitalis, beta blockers, and calcium blockers prolong A-V nodal conduction and refractoriness in both the fast (beta) and slow (alpha) pathways.[18,58–61,107–112] Because the determinants for sustained AVNRT can be due to abnormalities of either retrograde or antegrade conduction, the therapeutic response in individual patients may vary. Occasionally, these drugs enable the investigator to demonstrate dual pathways that were not demonstrable before their administration. Moreover, these drugs may actually prolong the echo or tachycardia zone in response to APDs and may result in the ability to initiate echoes or sustained AVNRT that was not possible before their administration. These responses may occur if the drugs produce a greater degree of slowing of conduction in the slow pathway than prolongation of refractoriness in the fast pathway. An example of this response is shown in Figure 8-76: propranolol increases the refractoriness of both the fast and slow pathway but depresses conduction to a greater degree in the slow pathway, allowing a critical A-H to be achieved, which allows the fast pathway to recover and SVT to be induced. Oral use of these agents may be associated with an increase in frequency and duration of spontaneous AVNRT, which is invariably slower than prior to therapy. Conversely, if drugs prolong refractoriness of the fast pathway to a greater degree than they prolong conduction down the slow pathway (with or without depression of fast-pathway conduction), this may result in inability to initiate SVT. The relative efficacy of these different agents in preventing the initiation of typical or atypical A-V nodal reentrant activity has not been compared in a prospective study. All can prevent initiation of the arrhythmia, particularly when the major determinant is the slow pathway, that is, by preventing repetitive reentrance down the slow pathway because of prolonging its refractoriness. It is my impression, however, that calcium blockers have

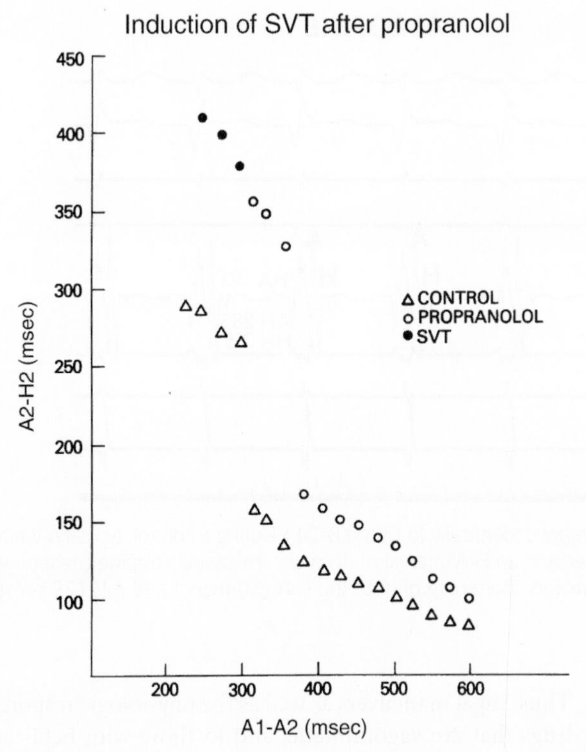


**FIGURE 8-76** *Influence of propranolol on induction of SVT.* Coupling intervals of atrial extrastimuli ($A_1$-$A_2$) are plotted on the *horizontal axis,* and resultant $A_2$-$H_2$ intervals, on the *vertical axis.* During the control state (*triangles*), fast- and slow-pathway conduction are seen, with the effective refractory period of the fast pathway at 310 msec. No A-V nodal reentry, however, is induced, even though $A_2$-$H_2$ intervals reached 290 msec. Following propranolol (*circles*), the dual-pathway curves are shifted upward and to the right, such that the A-H interval at all coupling intervals is longer than the control. The effective refractory period of the fast pathway is increased to 380 msec. Conduction over the slow pathway is markedly increased. When slow-pathway conduction reaches 375 msec and greater, SVT (*closed circles*) is induced.

the most potent effects on the AVN with verapamil being the most potent of this class of agents. In the past decade, adenosine has become the pharmacologic agent of choice for acute termination of AVNRT.[113–115] The mechanism by which this drug works is complex. It produces block in the slow pathway by indirectly inhibiting catecholamine-induced, adenylcyclase-mediated $Ca^{++}$ conductance. It also activates specific $K^+$ channels ($I_{K\text{-}Ado}$), which slow conduction and prolong refractoriness in the AVN.

The major effect of calcium and beta blockers as well as digitalis appears to be on the slow pathway. Some investigators have suggested that the retrograde fast pathway behaves like an A-V nodal bypass tract[80,83] because of its rapid and relatively fixed retrograde conduction, and the observation that it appears to be little affected by beta blockers and calcium blockers. These are weak arguments. Data relative to the presence of upper and final lower common pathways that are intranodal have been presented. The failure of these investigators to demonstrate a significant effect of these drugs on retrograde conduction has been primarily due to their techniques. Ventricular extrastimuli (as mentioned in Chapter 2 and earlier in this chapter) do not achieve as comparable an input into the AVN as the tachycardia or during rapid ventricular pacing. Assessment of retrograde conduction over the fast pathway by ventricular extrastimuli therefore yields misleading information. When studied by rapid pacing, the effects of verapamil, digitalis, and propranolol on retrograde fast-pathway conduction are similar to their effects on antegrade slow-pathway conduction; that is, they prolong it.[18,109–111] All of these drugs have been demonstrated to block retrograde fast-pathway conduction in individual patients and to terminate the arrhythmias in addition to their more frequent production of block in the slow pathway. Thus, these drugs unequivocally affect retrograde fast-pathway conduction in a manner qualitatively similar to their effect on the slow pathway, a behavior further suggesting that the retrograde fast pathway is composed of A-V nodal tissue. Responses to agents such as atropine and isoproterenol provide additional support for this conclusion.[8,68–70,116] As noted, these agents can facilitate induction of arrhythmias by improving retrograde fast-pathway conduction and/or antegrade slow-pathway conduction.[18,68–70] These agents are particularly useful in facilitating induction of typical AVNRT in patients exhibiting retrograde dual pathways, V-A Wenckebach, or complete V-A block during ventricular pacing in the baseline state. An example of the effect of atropine on A-V nodal reentrant SVT is shown in Figure 8-77. In this patient atropine increases the rate of SVT, which is associated with increase in both antegrade conduction over the slow pathway (shorter A-H) and retrograde conduction over the fast pathway (shorter H-A). As stated previously, atropine can manifest demonstrable effects on retrograde fast-pathway conduction when assessed by rapid pacing.

Class IA agents, such as procainamide, quinidine, and disopyramide can produce block in the fast pathway retrogradely to prevent and/or terminate SVT.[117–121] As such, these drugs may be effective in terminating as well as preventing the arrhythmia. Their effects on antegrade slow-pathway conduction are variable, particularly in the case of the Class IA agents, due in part to their vagolytic effects. Class IC agents, flecainide, and propafenone have more potent effects on both the fast and slow pathways. Amiodarone appears to affect both the fast and slow pathway, producing block retrogradely in the fast pathway and terminating and, of course, preventing tachycardias. Sotalol's effect on the AVN is similar to other beta blockers. Class I agents may also be of value in defining the mechanism of SVT. The production of infra-His block by these agents without termination of the arrhythmia excludes circus movement tachycardia using a concealed atrioventricular bypass tract (see following).

Termination of typical A-V nodal reentrant SVT by carotid sinus massage and other vagal maneuvers almost always occurs by gradual slowing and then antegrade block in the slow pathway.[16,122] Thus, in most instances, the tachycardia is terminated by a nonconducted atrial echo (Fig. 8-78A). Occasionally, in typical AVNRT, carotid sinus pressure (CSP) can produce slowing in the slow pathway and oscillations

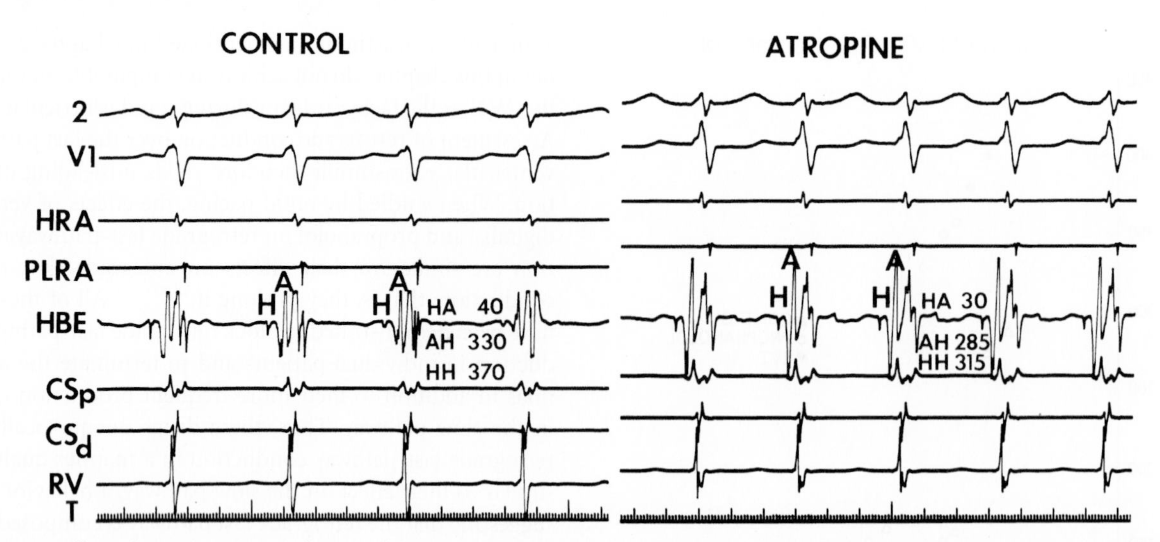


**FIGURE 8-77** *Effect of atropine on typical A-V nodal reentry.* (The figure is arranged identically to Figure 8-24.) During a control, typical A-V nodal reentry is present with a cycle length of 370 msec and A-H interval of 330 msec and an H-A interval of 40 msec. Following atropine (right panel), the tachycardia cycle length is shortened to 315 msec. This is as a consequence to shortening of both the H-A (30-msec) and A-H (285-msec) intervals.

with termination in the fast pathway, but this is uncommon. This has also been observed using neck collar suction with or without additional vagomimetic agents. In all instances, retrograde block appears at cycle lengths far in excess of atrial refractoriness supporting an A-V nodal site of block. In contrast, in atypical AVNRT, termination by vagal maneuvers, adenosine, beta- or calcium blockers is always in the retrograde slow pathway. In such instances termination occurs with gradual V-A prolongation, then block following a QRS without a retrograde P wave (Fig. 8-78B).

Thus, vagal maneuvers as well as the physiologic responses to drugs that are vagomimetic, and to those with beta- and calcium-blocking effects, all suggest that AVNRT is confined to the AVN. Manipulation of antegrade and retrograde conduction can facilitate induction of the arrhythmia and can enhance the rate of arrhythmia or can terminate the arrhythmia. The effects of these drugs depend on the critical balance of conduction and refractoriness in both the fast and slow pathways. Electrophysiologic characteristics of AVNRT are listed in Table 8-5.

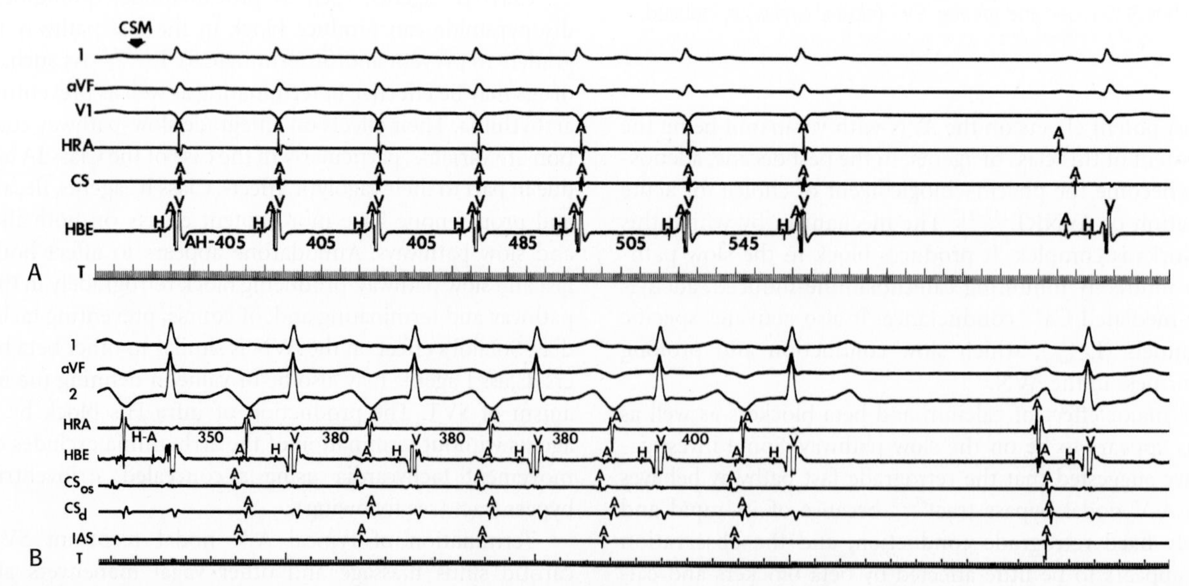


**FIGURE 8-78** *Termination of A-V nodal reentry by carotid sinus massage (CSM).* **A:** Termination of typical A-V nodal reentry by CSM. CSM (*arrow*) is applied during typical A-V nodal reentry. Progressive slowing that is due to A-H prolongation is seen before termination by block in the slow pathway. **B:** Termination of atypical A-V nodal reentry by CSM. The figure is organized as leads 1, aVF, and 2, and electrograms from the HRA, HBE, os of the CS, distal CS, and intra-atrial septum (IAS). Atypical A-V nodal reentry is present, and the carotid sinus pressure is applied. There is progressive slowing of the tachycardia associated with prolongation of retrograde conduction over the slow pathway (H-A intervals) until block occurs in the retrograde slow pathway, terminating the tachycardia.

TABLE 8-5 Criteria for A-V Nodal Reentrant SVT

**Typical A-V Nodal Reentry**

Initiation and termination by APDs, VPDs, or atrial pacing during A-V nodal Wenckebach cycles.
Dual A-V nodal refractory curves in response to APDs or atrial pacing.
Initiation dependent on *critical* A-H interval during slow-pathway conduction.
Retrograde atrial activation caudocephalad with variable activation of the triangle of Koch (V-A = −42 to +70 msec). Multiple atrial breakthroughs are possible.
Can be initiated, terminated, or reset without atrial activation.
Retrograde P wave within the QRS, distorting terminal portion of the QRS.
Atrium, His bundle, and ventricle not required, vagal maneuvers slow and then terminate SVT.

**Uncommon A-V Nodal Reentry**

Initiation and termination by APDs, VPDs, or ventricular pacing during retrograde A-V Wenckebach cycles.
Retrograde dual A-V nodal refractory curves.
Initiation dependent on critical H-A during retrograde slow-pathway conduction.
Retrograde atrial activation sequence caudocephalad with earliest activity usually at the posterior triangle of Koch or at the os of the coronary sinus. Multiple atrial breakthroughs are possible.
Retrograde P wave with long R-P interval.
Atrium, His bundle, and ventricle not required; vagal maneuvers slow and then abruptly terminate SVT, always in the retrograde slow pathway.

## SUPRAVENTRICULAR TACHYCARDIA RESULTING FROM CONCEALED ATRIOVENTRICULAR BYPASS TRACTS

The second most common mechanism of paroxysmal SVT is reentry using the normal A-V pathway as the antegrade limb and an A-V bypass tract for the retrograde limb. These bypass tracts cannot conduct antegradely, even when atrial pacing is performed at a site near the pathway. The presence of such concealed A-V bypass tracts, which are only capable of retrograde conduction, was not appreciated until the mid-1970s, despite almost a decade of experience with the Wolff–Parkinson–White syndrome. The evolution of intracardiac stimulation techniques, coupled with endocavitary mapping, led to the recognition of these bypass tracts, which are functionally silent during sinus rhythm and clinically unsuspected. The more carefully the mechanisms of SVT are analyzed, the greater the recognition of CBTs as the underlying mechanism. Atrioventricular reentry using a CBT was the mechanism of 1,349 of 3,550 (38%) consecutively studied patients with SVT in the absence of pre-excitation (Table 8-2). Other investigators also found this mechanism to be rather common, with an incidence ranging from 15% to 50%.[15–18,49,60,123–125] In the 1980s, it became apparent that concealed A-V bypass tracts may be of two varieties: one in which V-A conduction is rapid, analogous to the situation with overt pre-excitation, and one in which the bypass tract is slowly conducting and has decremental properties analogous to that of the AVN.[18,63–66,126–130] The former gives rise to a tachycardia with a short R-P interval and the latter with a long R-P interval. In addition, the fast-conducting bypass tracts usually participate in paroxysmal arrhythmias, whereas the slowly conducting bypass tracts are frequently associated with incessant tachycardias. Fast-conducting bypass tracts are 10 times more common than slowly conducting bypass tracts (Table 8-2).

SVT using a CBT has no sexual predilection. Although it occurs more frequently in younger patients than in those with AVNRT, overlap is great. We have observed cases in childhood throughout adult life. The oldest patient we have studied with SVT that was due to a CBT was 88 years old. It is however, very unusual to have the first episode occur after age 40. This is similar to patients with overt pre-excitation. Obviously, in youth, organic heart disease is absent; however, in older patients with tachycardias that are due to CBTs, the usual spectrum of cardiac disease is present. In patients with incessant SVT associated with slowly conducting bypass tracts, a cardiomyopathy may develop that is reversible upon cure of the tachycardia.[131,132] The mean cycle lengths of SVT using a CBT tend to be shorter than A-V nodal reentrant SVT (330 vs. 355 msec, respectively) but overlap is considerable. Although the majority of episodes of SVT with rates exceeding 225 bpm use a CBT, we have seen occasional examples of equally fast AVNRT.

### Mechanism of Initiation

Most cases of SVT using a fast-conducting CBT are initiated by APDs (Fig. 8-79). In contrast to the situation in typical AVNRT, the onset of the tachycardia is unrelated to A-V nodal delay specifically but is related to the total A-V time. The degree of A-V delay must be great enough to allow both the ventricular and atrial ends of the bypass tract to be capable of retrograde excitation. As expected, most commonly the delay is in the AVN; however, the delay may be anywhere in the His–Purkinje system or in the ventricular myocardium. An example of initiation of circus movement tachycardia using a left-sided bypass tract in which the delay providing recovery of excitability of the bypass tract is localized both in the His–Purkinje system (increase in H-V to 135 msec) and in the ventricular myocardium (presence of left bundle branch block) is shown in Figure 8-80. The importance of bundle branch block in initiation of the tachycardia is discussed further in subsequent paragraphs. Clearly, however, block in the bundle branch ipsilateral to a free-wall bypass tract will provide an additional amount of intramyocardial conduction delay, which will allow the bypass tract and/or its atrial insertion (i.e., atrial refractoriness) to recover excitability. Thus, the site

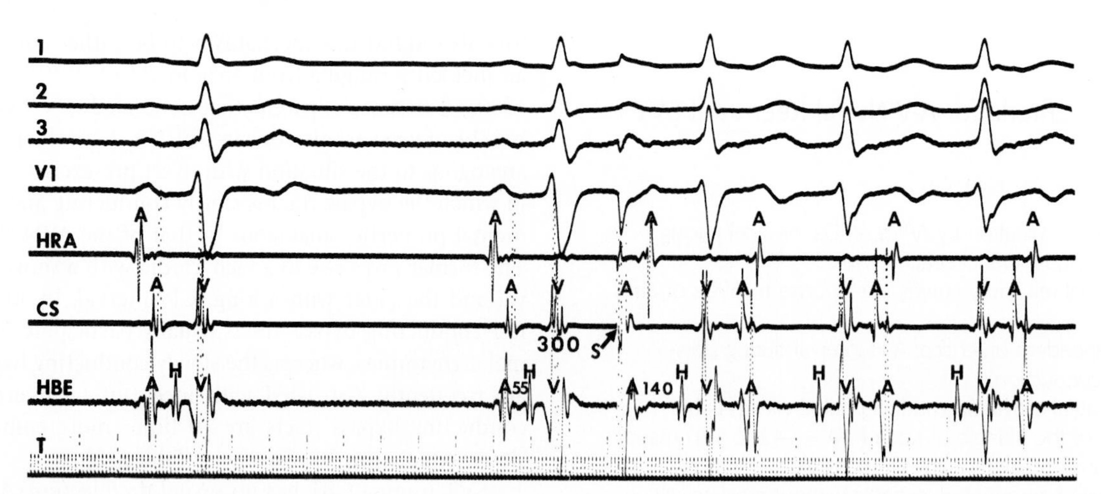


**FIGURE 8-79** *Initiation of SVT resulting from a CBT by an APD.* The second sinus beat is followed by an APD delivered from the CS (S, *arrow*) at a coupling interval of 300 msec. This produces enough A-V nodal delay (A-H is 140 msec) to allow the bypass tract to be successfully engaged retrogradely and initiate SVT. Note that the earliest onset of retrograde atrial activation is recorded in the CS. See text for discussion.

of A-V delay is unimportant; it may be localized primarily to the AVN, the His bundle, the more distal His–Purkinje system, the ventricles, or any combination of these sites. Therefore, curves relating the coupling intervals of the APD ($A_1$-$A_2$) to A-V nodal or total A-V delay and the development of SVT are typically smooth (Fig. 8-81). Dual A-V nodal pathways may occasionally be noted as a concomitant but unrelated finding. The incidence of dual pathways in patients with CBTs in our experience is nearly 40%.[123] In these cases, either the slow or fast intranodal pathway or both may be used as the antegrade limb of the tachycardia (Fig. 8-82). This may lead to an alternation of antegrade conduction over the slow and the fast pathway, resulting in a regularly irregular rate of SVT (alternating long and short cycles) or two separate stable SVT cycle lengths. We have also seen dual A-V nodal pathways with 1:2 conduction initiating A-V reentry that is due to a CBT (Fig. 8-83). In this case, conduction over the fast pathway did not produce enough delay to initiate the tachycardia; only after simultaneous conduction over the slow pathway was enough A-V delay encountered to allow for initiation of the tachycardia.

The site of atrial stimulation may also be important, particularly if the limiting factor is atrial refractoriness prohibiting the impulse to traverse the bypass tract and excite the atrium. To obviate this limitation, one must stimulate near the site of the bypass tract. That is, because the atrial insertion of the bypass tract would be activated earlier, it would

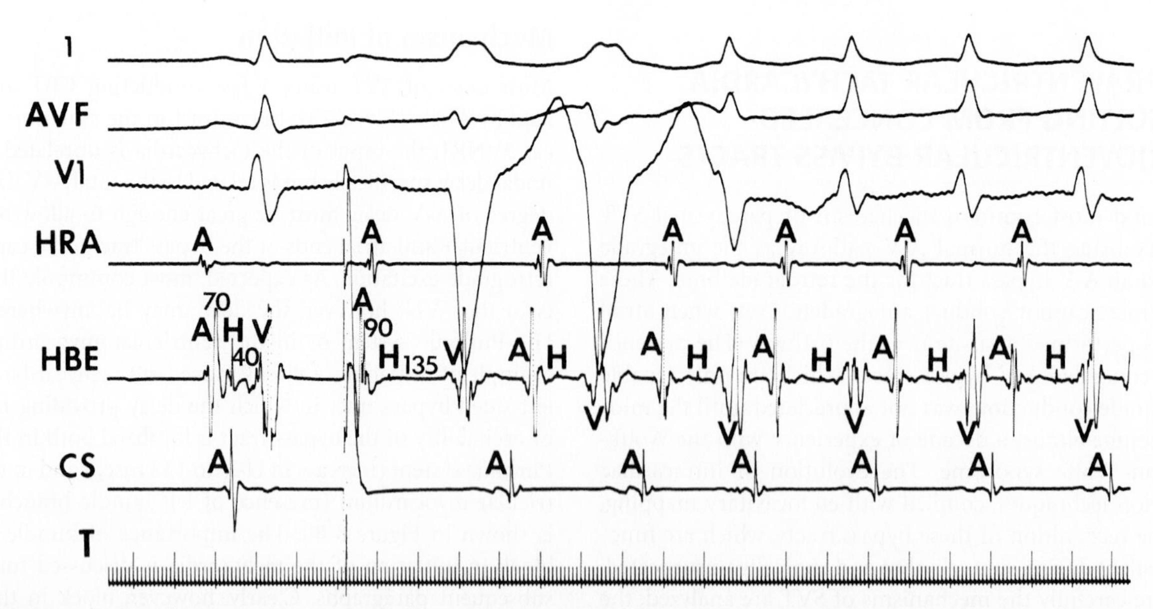


**FIGURE 8-80** *Induction of reentry using a concealed bypass tract owing to delay in the His–Purkinje system and ventricular myocardium.* Leads 1, AVF, and $V_1$ are shown along with HRA, HBE, and CS electrograms. Following one sinus complex, an APD is delivered, which initiates SVT using a CBT. No significant A-H delay is present; however, delay in the His–Purkinje system (H-V 135) and in the left ventricular myocardium left bundle branch block provides enough A-V delay to allow the retrograde refractory period of the bypass tract to recover. Stimulation from the CS also allows the atrial refractory period at the atrial insertion site of the bypass tract to recover. See text for discussion. T, time line.

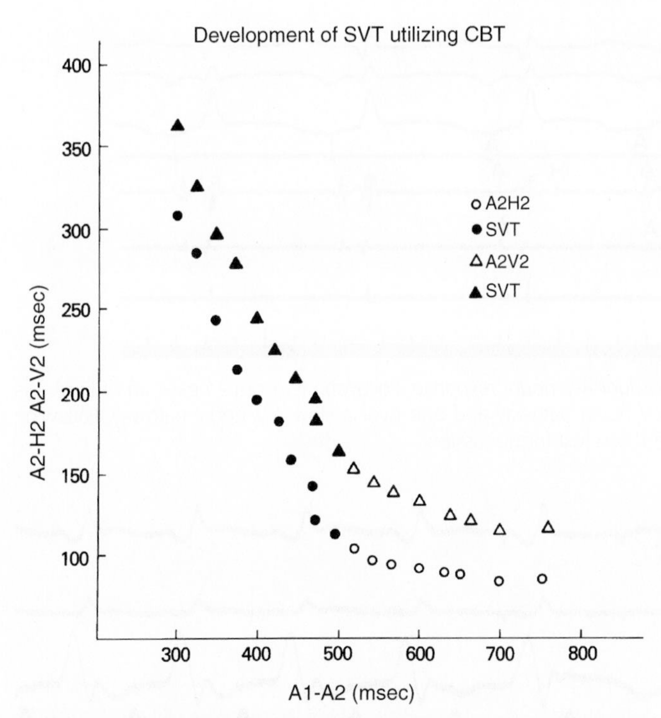


**FIGURE 8-81** *Relationship of APD coupling interval to A-V nodal and A-V conduction time and the development of SVT-CBT.* The APD coupling interval (A1-A2)is on the abscissa and A-V nodal (*circles*) and A-V (*triangles*) conduction times are on the ordinate. SVT (*solid circles* and *triangles*) appears after minimal A-V nodal or A-V conduction delay, and the curves are smooth.

recover earlier and thus make reexcitation easier. Therefore, atrial stimulation at the site of the bypass tract may initiate SVT, whereas stimulation at a distant site may fail to do so (Fig. 8-84). Because of earlier recovery of atrial refractoriness at the site of the bypass tract, it is even possible to initiate the tachycardia with little or no A-V nodal delay merely by providing more time for the atrium to recover (Fig. 8-85; also see Fig. 8-80). Another reason that the stimulation site may be important relates to the known differences in A-V nodal conduction and refractoriness based on stimulation site.[54,55] This is clearly demonstrated in Figure 8-86, in which stimulation from the high-right atrium results in block in the AVN, while stimulation from the coronary sinus at an identical coupling interval conducts through the AVN and the His–Purkinje system to excite the ventricles and (because of delay in interatrial conduction) allow reexcitation of the atrium over a left-sided bypass tract. Occasionally, a single APD, even when delivered from the atrial insertion of the bypass tract, does not result in SVT because enough delay has not resulted to allow the bypass tract or the atrium time to recover. This may be due to enhanced A-V nodal conduction, with which CBTs may be associated.[123,133,134] In such cases, rapid atrial pacing or the use of multiple atrial extrastimuli may produce enough A-V nodal delay and/or decrease of atrial refractoriness to allow for initiation of the tachycardia (Fig. 8-87).

The mode of initiation differs in tachycardias due to a slowly conducting CBT. Because conduction in the bypass tract is always slow, the tachycardia is often incessant and initiated by spontaneous shortening of the sinus cycle length (Fig. 8-88). This phenomenon has three potential mechanisms: (a) a rate-related decrease in the retrograde refractory period of the bypass tract; (b) a rate-related decrease in atrial refractoriness that allows the impulse to reactivate the atrium retrogradely over a functioning bypass tract; and (c) a concealed Wenckebach-type block with block at the atrial bypass tract junction terminating the Wenckebach cycle, relieving any antegrade concealed conduction that may have prevented retrograde conduction up the bypass tract. The latter mechanism is most likely operative in these patients. This conclusion is based on the fact that such slowly conducting bypass tracts actually demonstrate decremental conduction at rapid rates and that, in most instances, the atrial refractory period at the site of insertion of the bypass tract is less than the R-P interval. Thus, some sort of antegrade

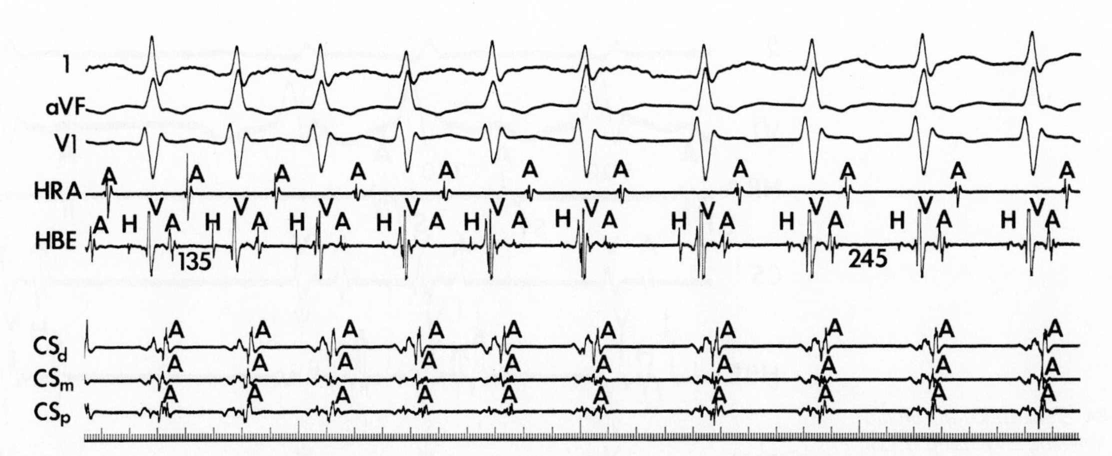


**FIGURE 8-82** *Alternations in cycle length of SVT using a CBT by the presence of dual A-V nodal pathways.* The panel is arranged from top to bottom as leads 1, aVF, and $V_1$ and electrograms from the HRA, HBE, and distal (d), mid (m), and proximal ($CS_p$) CS. In the left-hand panel, SVT that is due to a left-sided CBT (earliest site $CS_p$) is shown with a cycle length of 305 msec and an A-H interval of 235 msec. In the middle of the tracing, block of the fast pathway occurs and conducts and proceeds over the slow pathway with an A-H interval of 245 msec, thereby prolonging the cycle length of the tachycardia to nearly 400 msec.

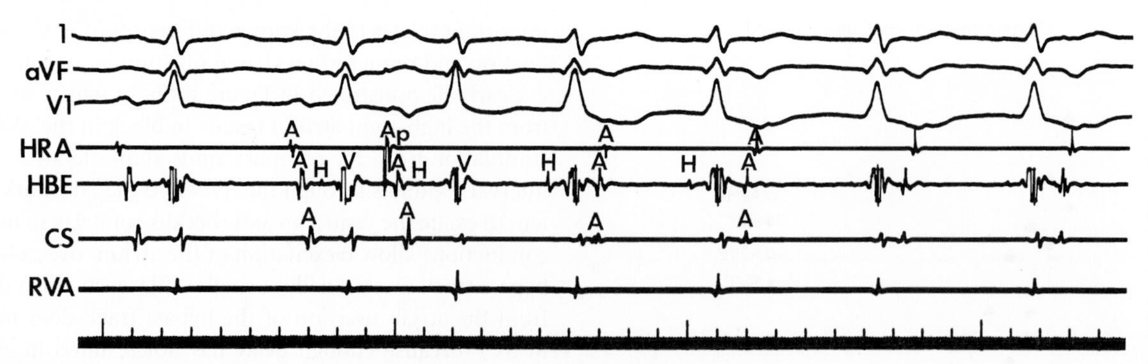


**FIGURE 8-83** *Induction of SVT using a CBT by an APD demonstrating a dual A-V nodal response.* Following two sinus beats, an APD ($A_p$) is introduced, which results in two ventricular responses, one over a fast A-V nodal pathway and one over a slow A-V nodal pathway. Following conduction of the impulse over the slow A-V nodal pathway, SVT is initiated. See text for discussion.

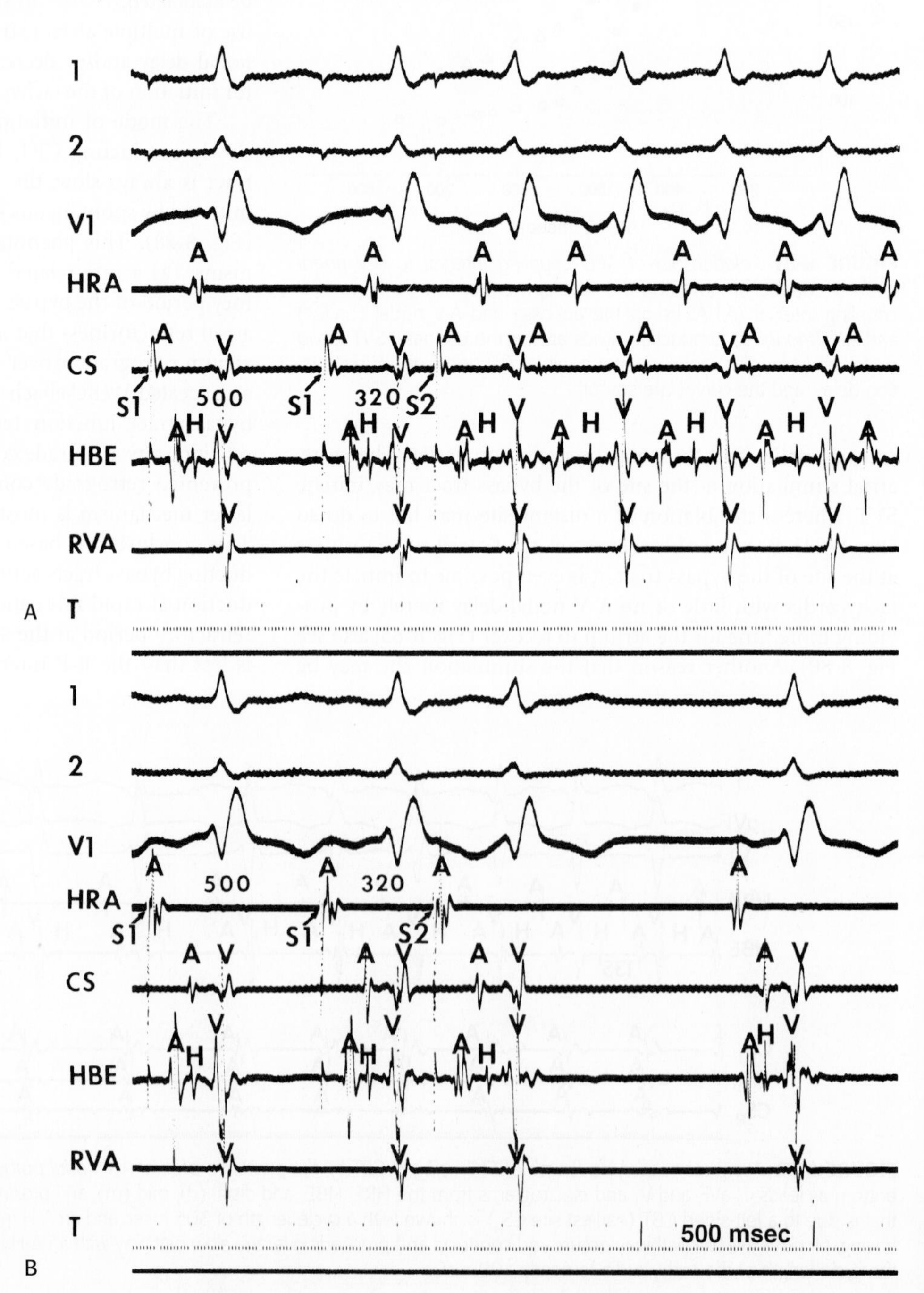


**FIGURE 8-84** *Significance of stimulation site in initiating SVT using a CBT.* **A:** SVT using a left-sided CBT is initiated by an APD delivered from the CS at a coupling interval of 320 msec. **B:** Identical stimulation from the HRA fails to induce SVT.

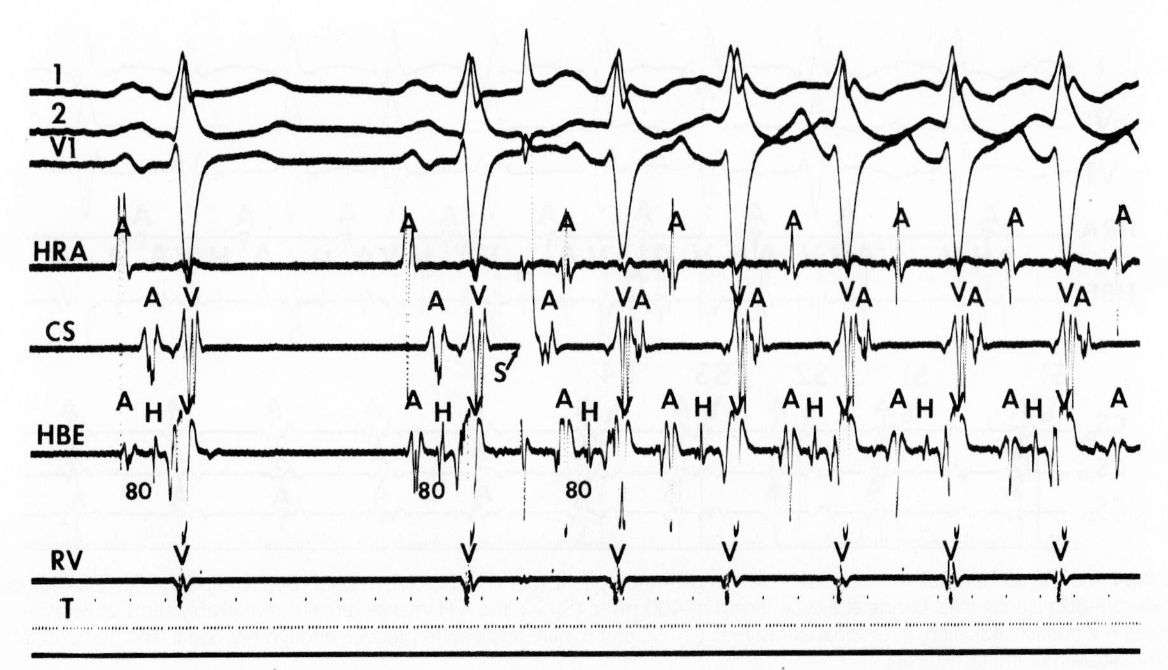


**FIGURE 8-85** *Initiation of SVT resulting from a CBT in the absence of A-V nodal delay.* After the second sinus complex, an (APD) (S, *arrow*) introduced from the CS resulting in SVT in the absence of A-V nodal delay (no A-H prolongation). The earliest onset of atrial activation seen in the CS is typical of a left-sided A-V bypass tract. See text for discussion.

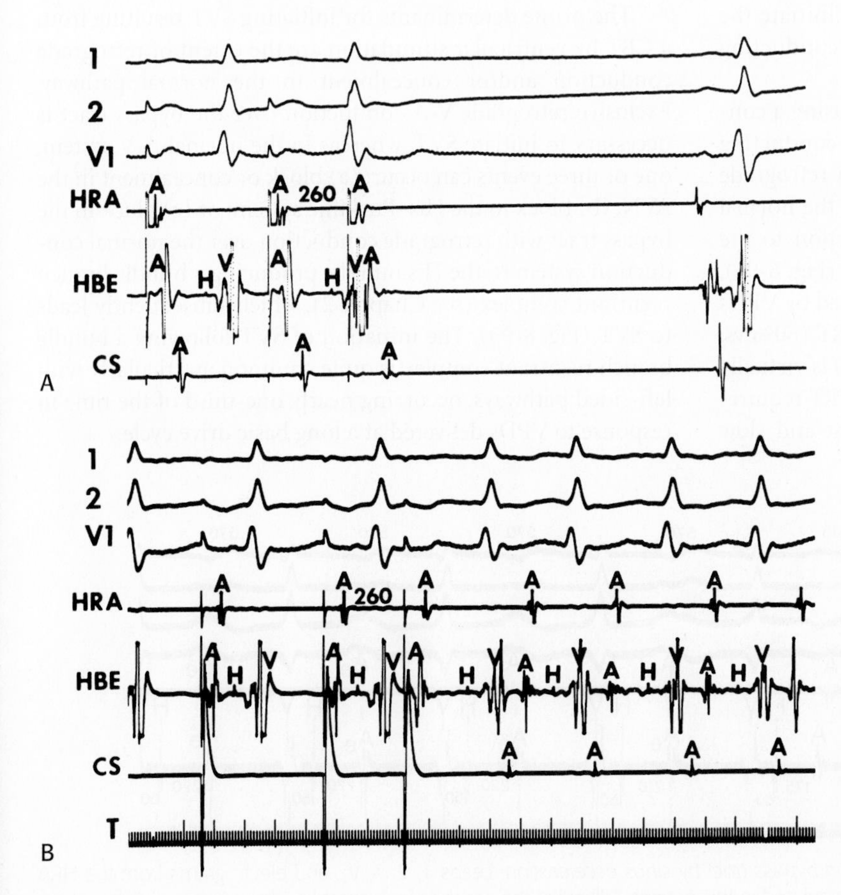


**FIGURE 8-86** *Effect of stimulation site on initiation of SVT that is due to CBT based on differences in A-V nodal conduction.* **A:** Atrial extrastimuli are delivered from the HRA. At a coupling interval of 260 msec, the atrial extrastimulus blocks in the A-V node and therefore no SVT using a CBT can be initiated. **B:** At an identical coupling interval from the CS, conduction through the A-V node can occur, and SVT ensues. Thus, differences in A-V nodal conduction dependent on atrial stimulation can influence the ability of induction of SVT using a CBT. See text for discussion.

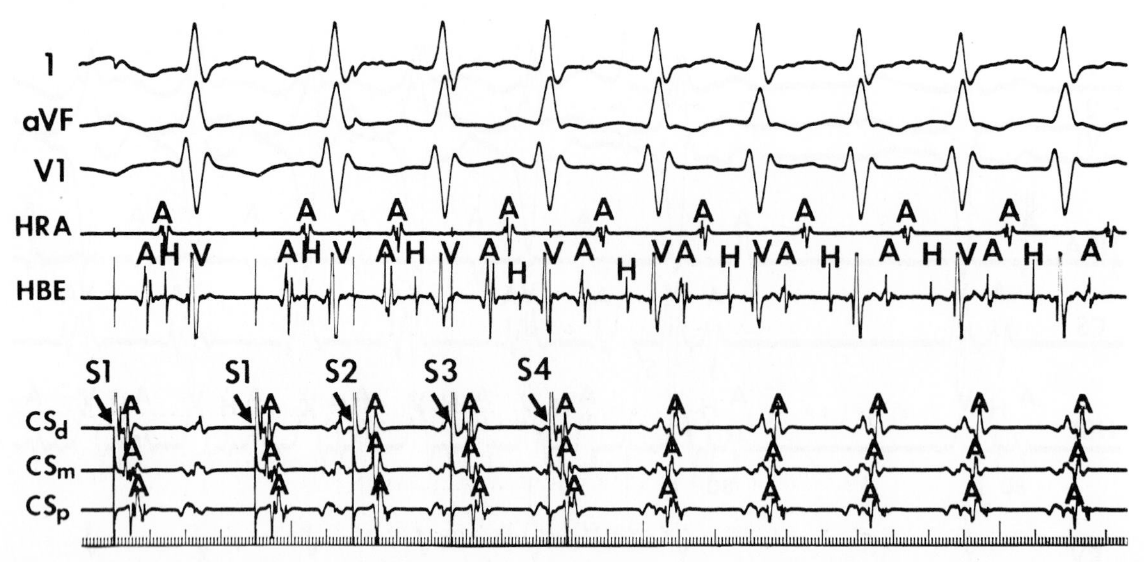


**FIGURE 8-87** *Multiple extrastimuli to induce SVT using a CBT in a patient with enhanced A-V nodal conduction.* (The figure is arranged identically to Figure 8-80.) During atrial pacing at a cycle length of 400 msec ($S_1$-$S_1$), the A-H interval remains remarkably short, at 65 msec. Because of enhanced A-V nodal conduction, three atrial extrastimuli ($S_2$, $S_3$, and $S_4$) are required to produce enough A-V nodal, and hence, total A-V delay to allow for initiation of the tachycardia.

concealment during sinus rhythm in the bypass tract must be operative, preventing tachycardia from always occurring. It is therefore not surprising that pacing-induced decreases in cycle length and even late-coupled APDs can initiate the tachycardia quite readily in patients with slowly conducting bypass tracts (Figs. 8-89 and 8-90).

Ventricular stimulation can also initiate SVT using a concealed A-V bypass tract. In patients with a rapidly conducting bypass tract this occurs with little or no delay in retrograde conduction because block and/or concealment in the normal A-V conduction system must occur and conduction to the atrium must proceed solely over the bypass tract (Fig. 8-91). In our experience, SVT using a CBT can be initiated by VPDs much more readily than SVT that is due to AVNRT (60% vs. 10%). The initiation of SVT by a late-coupled VPD is virtually pathognomic for a CBT because initiation of AVNRT requires a very closely coupled VPD to dissociate the fast and slow pathways. Ventricular pacing also more frequently initiates SVT that is due to a CBT than to AVNRT, with success rates of 75% to 80% versus 40%, respectively (Fig. 8-92).

The prime determinants for initiating SVT resulting from a CBT by ventricular stimulation are the extent of retrograde conduction and/or concealment in the normal pathway. Exclusive retrograde V-A conduction over the bypass tract is necessary to initiate SVT, whereas in the normal A-V system, one of three events can occur: (a) block or concealment in the AVN; (b) block in the His–Purkinje system; or (c) block in the bypass tract with retrograde conduction over the normal conduction system to the His bundle, producing a bundle branch reentrant complex (see Chapter 2), which subsequently leads to SVT (Fig. 8-93). The initiation of SVT following a bundle branch reentrant complex is quite common, particularly with left-sided pathways, occurring nearly one-third of the time in response to VPDs delivered at a long basic drive cycle.

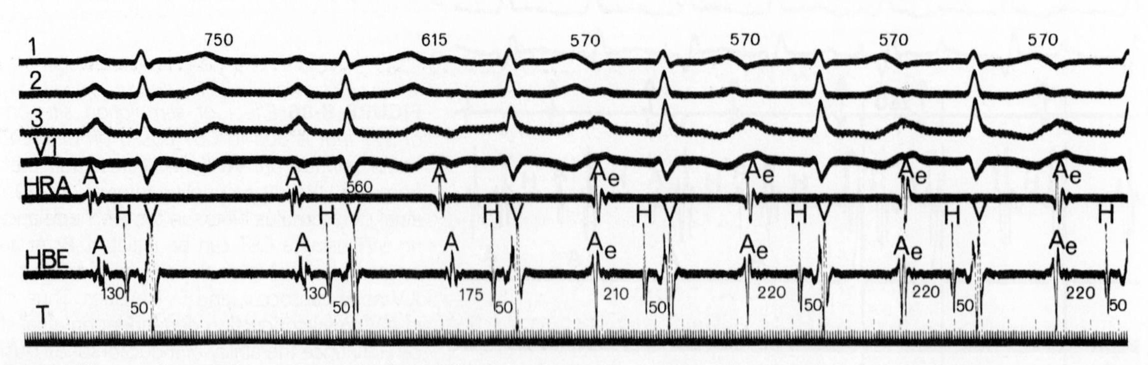


**FIGURE 8-88** *Initiation of SVT using a slowly conducting bypass tract by sinus acceleration.* Leads 1, 2, 3, $V_1$, and electrograms from the HRA and HBE are shown. The coronary sinus could not be cannulated in this patient. Following the second sinus complex, there was a slight acceleration of the sinus node to 560 msec, which was followed abruptly by the tachycardia using a slowly conducting left-sided bypass tract. The bypass tract is left sided because of the negative P wave in lead 1. See text for discussion.

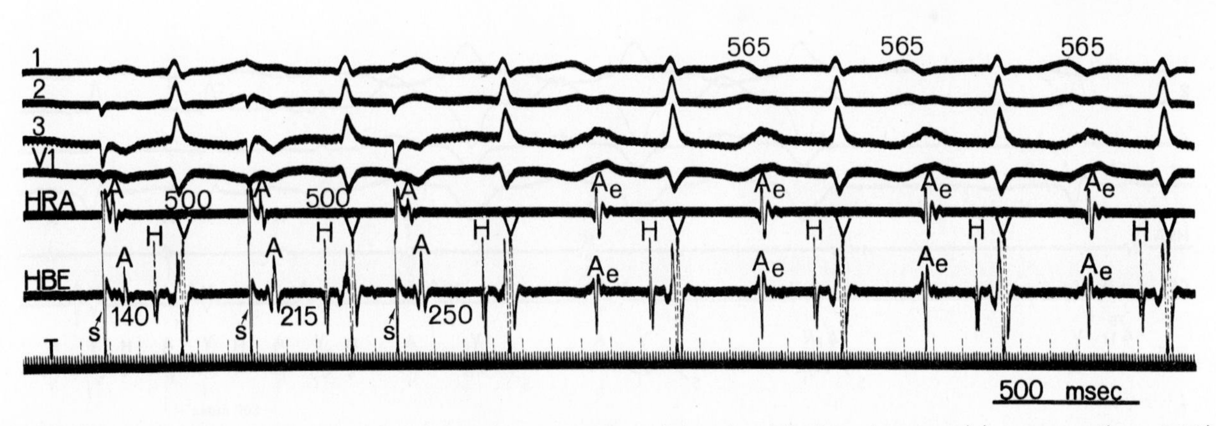


**FIGURE 8-89** *Initiation of SVT using a slowly conducting bypass tract by atrial pacing.* (The figure is arranged the same as Figure 8-84.) Atrial pacing at a cycle length of 500 msec producing modest A-H prolongation initiates SVT that is due to a left-sided slowly conducting bypass tract.

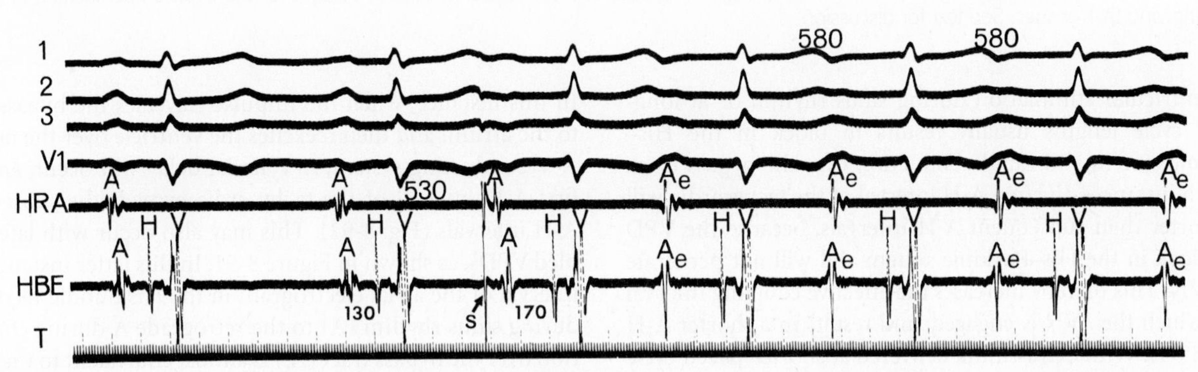


**FIGURE 8-90** *Initiation of SVT that is due to a slowly conducting bypass tract by a late-coupled APD.* (The figure is arranged identically to prior figures.) Following two sinus complexes, a late APD with a coupling interval of 530 msec initiates SVT to a slowly conducting bypass tract despite the fact that there is a minimal A-H delay.

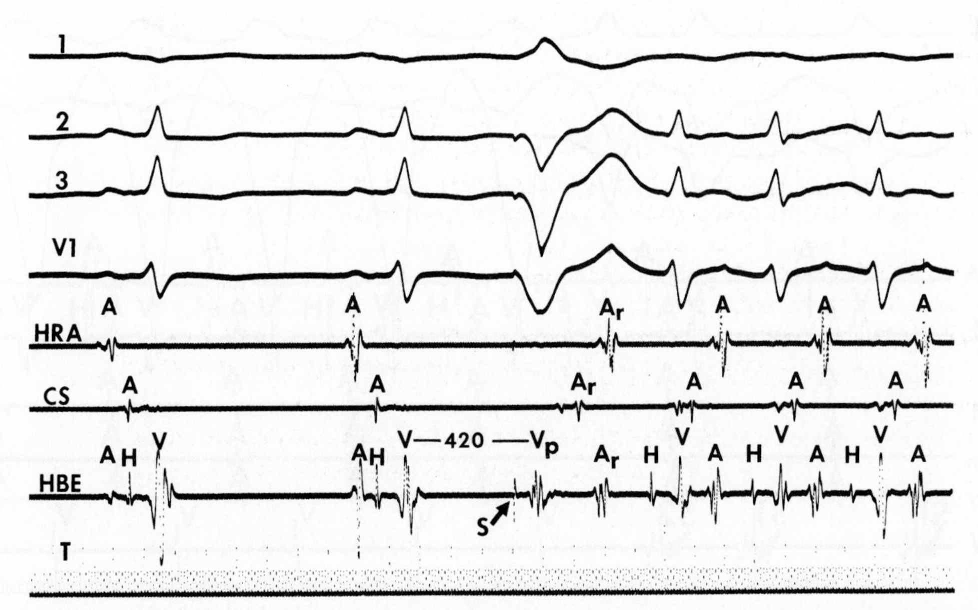


**FIGURE 8-91** *Initiation of SVT using a CBT by ventricular stimulation.* A VPD delivered at a coupling interval of 420 msec initiates SVT that is due to a left-sided CBT. See text for discussion.

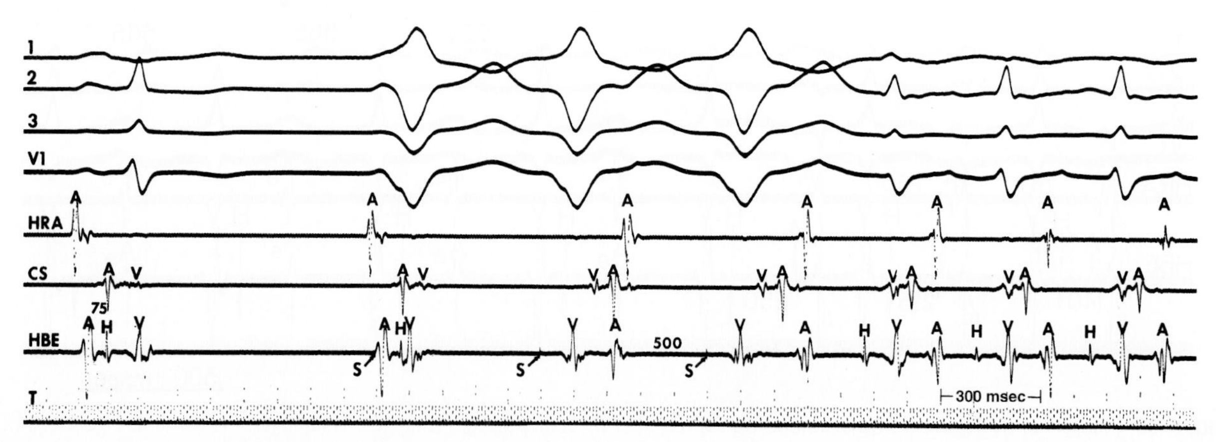


**FIGURE 8-92** *Initiation of SVT using a CBT by ventricular pacing.* Following a sinus complex, ventricular pacing is initiated at a cycle length of 500 msec. At the time of the first ventricular stimulus, atrial activation is purely sinus. On the second ventricular extrastimulus, atrial activation is a fusion of conduction over a left-sided bypass tract and over the A-V node. Following the third ventricular extrastimulus, block in the A-V node occurs as manifested by a prolongation of the V-A interval in the HBE, and conduction proceeds solely over the bypass tract located in the CS recording, and SVT ensues. See text for discussion.

Ventricular stimulation during sinus rhythm or at long-paced cycle lengths usually results in block in the His–Purkinje system and rapid conduction over the bypass tract. In such instances, the first A-H interval of the tachycardia will be shorter than subsequent A-H intervals, because the VPD will block in the His–Purkinje system and will not penetrate the AVN. This thereby increases the effective coupling interval with which the AVN is engaged, and results in a shorter A-H (Fig. 8-94). With extrastimuli delivered at shorter-paced cycle lengths, or during rapid ventricular pacing, both of which shorten HPS refractoriness, penetration to the AVN usually occurs, producing some retrograde concealment in the AVN. In this instance, when the impulse traverses the bypass tract to the atrium and then reexcites the ventricle over the normal A-V conducting system, A-V nodal delay will occur, and the first A-H interval of the tachycardia exceeds the subsequent A-H intervals (Fig. 8-92). This may also occur with late-coupled VPDs, as shown in Figure 8-91. In this latter instance, the interval of the atrial electrogram in the His bundle recording during sinus rhythm (A) to the retrograde A during conduction over the bypass tract ($A_r$) is almost equivalent to the sinus interval, yet the $A_r$-H interval (the first of the tachycardia) exceeds the sinus A-H interval by more than 100 msec. This demonstrates that the VPD penetrated the AVN and did not

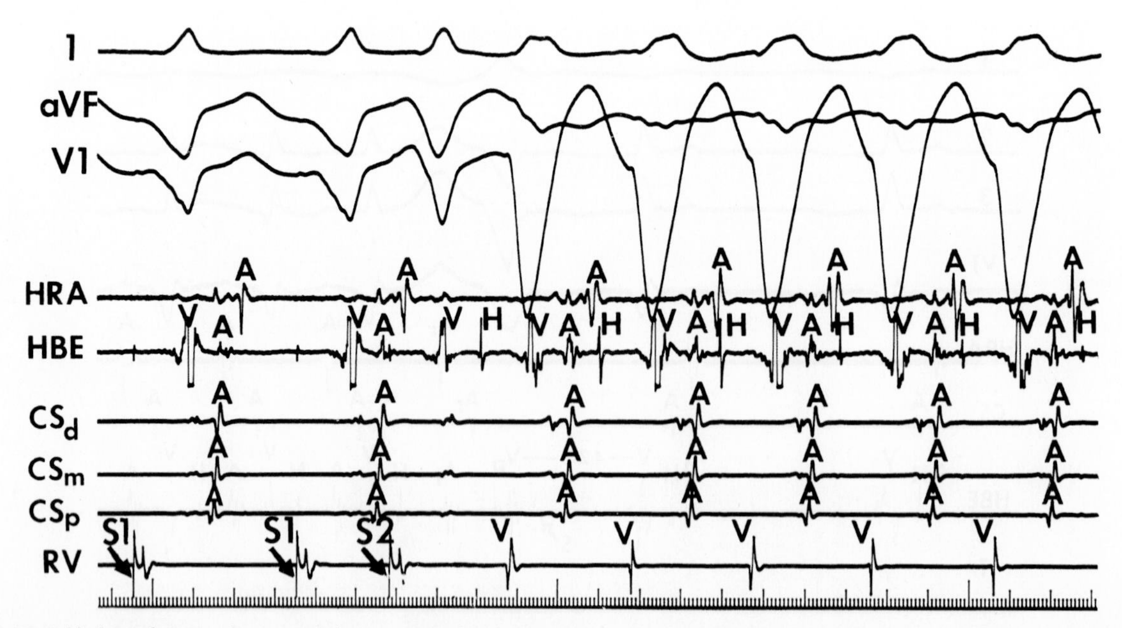


**FIGURE 8-93** *Initiation of SVT using a CBT by a ventricular extrastimulus producing bundle branch reentry.* (The figure is arranged as in Fig 8-60.) During ventricular pacing at 400 msec, a ventricular extrastimulus ($S_2$) is delivered at a coupling interval of 230 msec. This results in retrograde block in both the bypass tract and A-V node but is associated with a bundle branch reentrant complex. Following the bundle branch reentrant complex, which obviously has a left bundle branch block appearance, SVT over a left-sided bypass tract occurs. Note the presence of left bundle branch block aberration at the onset of the tachycardia. See text for discussion.

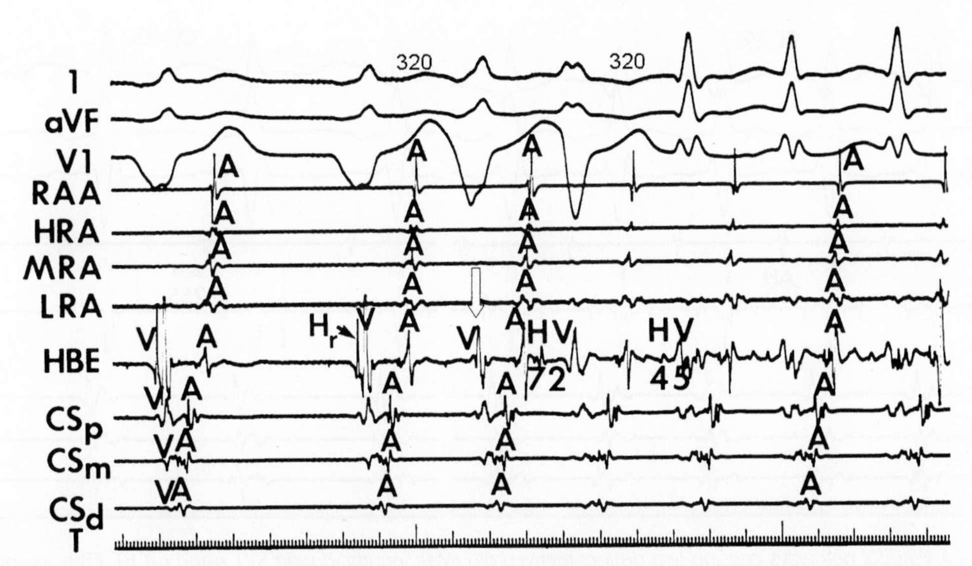


**FIGURE 8-94** *Initiation of SVT using a CBT by VPDs producing block in the His–Purkinje system.* (The figure is arranged similarly to others in this chapter.) During RV pacing at a cycle length of 600 msec simultaneous conduction to the His ($H_r$, *solid arrow*) and over a left lateral bypass tract is seen. The ventricular extrastimulus, delivered at 320 msec, is associated with block in the His–Purkinje system (*hollow arrow*) so that conduction proceeds solely over the bypass tract and then down the A-V node. Because the block occurred in the His–Purkinje system, the A-V node had time to recover. This results in a shorter A-H interval of the initiating complex than the A-H intervals during the tachycardia. Note that this occurs even though the initiating A-A interval, as measured in the CS, is similar to that during the tachycardia. See text for discussion.

block in the His–Purkinje system. In contrast, in Figure 8-94, a VPD initiates SVT and first beat of the tachycardia has an A-H of 72 msec, which is nearly 100 msec shorter than subsequent A-H intervals. One can see that the second VPD blocks in the His–Purkinje system (absence of $H_r$).

Although ventricular stimulation can readily initiate SVT using a typical, fast-conducting bypass tract, less commonly, the uncommon, long R-P tachycardia is initiated by ventricular stimulation. This most likely is a result of the already impaired conduction in that bypass tract such that ventricular extrastimuli produce block in the bypass tract if they are too premature. However, ventricular extrastimuli delivered virtually simultaneously with the spontaneously occurring sinus beat when the His bundle is refractory can initiate the long R-P tachycardia in certain circumstances. In fact, the ability to initiate the tachycardia by a VPD when the His bundle is refractory is diagnostic of a slowly conducting bypass tract and distinguishes it from the uncommon form of AVNRT.[126] With fast-conducting bypass tracts, once a VPD initiates the SVT, the tachycardia continues until either (a) the retrograde refractory period of the bypass tract is reached and V-A conduction fails or (b) the atrial input over the bypass tract reaches the AVN or His–Purkinje system when it is refractory and block occurs in the antegrade direction.

We have also seen adults with sick sinus syndrome who have marked bradycardia with junctional escape beats that initiate tachycardias. Tachycardias are initiated because the His bundle rhythm conducts normally in the antegrade direction and poorly if at all retrogradely. This allows this circulating wavefront to return to the atrium via the bypass tract and to reach an AVN capable of antegrade conduction. These patients frequently manifest the bradycardia–tachycardia syndrome. The initiation of SVT by junctional escapes in children may also represent a similar mechanism, although these patients have not been studied in great detail.[134]

### *Atrial Activation Sequence and P–QRS Relationship During Supraventricular Tachycardia*

During SVT using a CBT, the ventricle must be depolarized before retrograde conduction up the bypass tract. Atrial activation must therefore always follow ventricular activation at the insertion of the bypass tract and thus typically follows inscription of the QRS complex. With rapidly conducting bypass tracts, the conduction time over the bypass tract, as measured by the local V-A interval at the site of the earliest retrograde atrial activation, is usually 30 to 60 msec; thus, the R-P interval is short when measured on the surface ECG (90 to 160 msec). In SVTs using a rapidly conducting bypass tract, the R-P interval is typically shorter than the P-R interval, giving an R-P/P-R ratio of less than 1. This is obviously not the case in SVTs using slowly conducting bypass tracts in which the R-P interval is longer than the P-R interval (R-P/P-R, greater than 1). One of the hallmarks of a fast-conducting bypass tract is that the R-P interval remains fixed, regardless of the tachycardia cycle length, oscillations in cycle length from whatever cause, or changes in the P-R (or A-H) intervals. The tachycardia cycle length is most closely associated with the P-R interval (antegrade conduction). Because the R-P interval remains fixed, the R-P/P-R ratio can obviously change, depending on A-V conduction and tachycardia cycle length. For example, a patient with an SVT having a cycle length of 350 msec and an R-P interval of 150 msec will have an R-P ratio of 0.75 (150/200). If, however, the tachycardia cycle

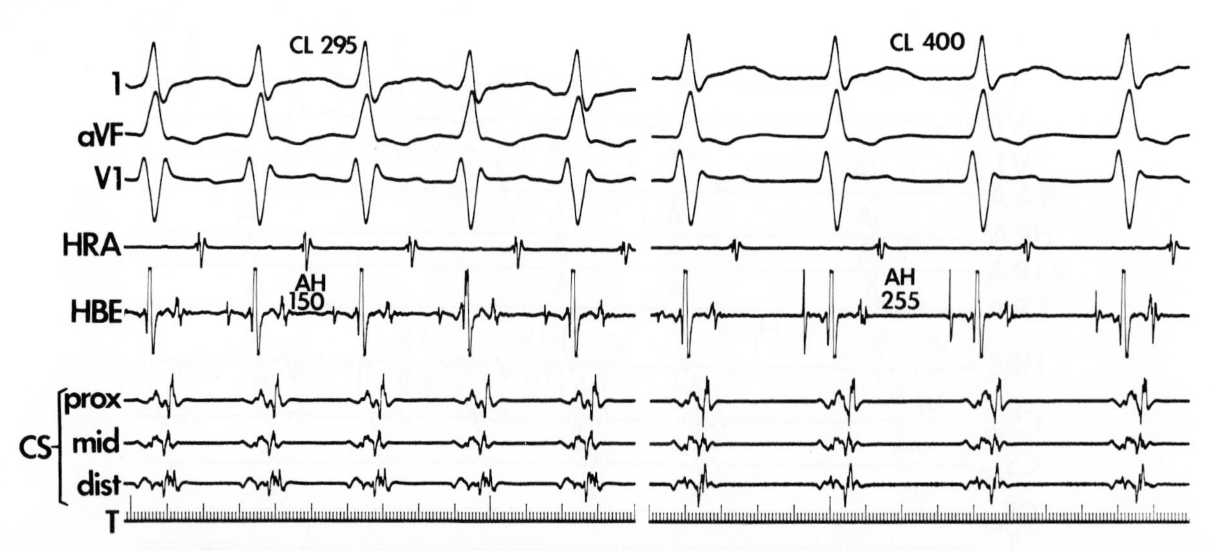


**FIGURE 8-95** *Dual A-V nodal pathways causing two distinct tachycardia cycle lengths during SVT using a CBT.* (The tracing is organized as in Figure 8-80.) On the left, a tachycardia is present with a cycle length of 295 msec as antegrade conduction proceeds over the fast A-V nodal pathway. In the right-hand panel, the second tachycardia with a cycle length of 400 msec is present with an identical retrograde activation sequence and identical R-P intervals. The tachycardia is slower because antegrade conduction proceeds over the slow A-V nodal pathway. The R-P interval remains fixed, regardless of changes in cycle length. See text for discussion.

length is reduced to 250 msec, then the R-P/P-R ratio will be 1.5 (150/100). Thus, the absolute value of R-P interval, and its fixed relationship to the preceding QRS, is more important diagnostically than R-P/P-R ratios, particularly when cycle lengths are less than 300 msec (i.e., heart rates greater than 200 bpm). An example of an SVT with two different cycle lengths that are due to two different P-R intervals secondary to dual A-V nodal pathways is shown in Figure 8-95. During the short cycle length of 295 msec, the R-P/P-R ratio is approximately 1, whereas during the slow tachycardia with a cycle length of 400 msec, the R-P/P-R ratio is much less than 1. In both cases, retrograde conduction (i.e., the V-A interval) is identical. Only the difference in antegrade conduction over either the fast- or slow-conducting A-V nodal dual pathways alters the tachycardia cycle length and the R-P/P-R ratio.

In the presence of a CBT, the relationship of atrial activation and/or the P wave to the QRS complex is generally constant over a wide range of ventricular-paced rates and coupling intervals of VPDs and during SVT cycle lengths in the absence of aberration. Small increases in the V-A interval may appear in response to early coupled VPDs or very rapid pacing because of several reasons. First, at short coupling intervals or paced cycle lengths, intramyocardial conduction delay can occur, producing a prolonged V-A interval. Second, short cycle lengths or coupling intervals may encroach on the refractoriness of the bypass tract, causing some decremental conduction. Third, rarely, one can observe longitudinal dissociation in the bypass tract such that it can exhibit a short and long conduction time. Finally, an increased V-A interval is the rule when one stimulates from the chamber contralateral to a free-wall bypass tract (e.g., right ventricular stimulation with a left-sided bypass tract). This phenomenon is identical to the spontaneous effect of bundle branch block ipsilateral to the bypass tract (see following). An increase in the V-A conduction time in response to ventricular pacing has been used as a diagnostic criterion for a free-wall bypass tract in the ventricle contralateral to the site of stimulation. Weiss et al.[135] demonstrated an increase in V-A intervals of 15 to 65 msec (46 ± 15 msec) during right ventricular stimulation in patients with a left-sided bypass tract but no change in those with septal bypass tracts. Paradoxically shorter V-A intervals may be observed during right ventricular stimulation in the presence of right free-wall bypass tracts. To distinguish intramyocardial delay from delay in the bypass tract, one must analyze the atrial and ventricular electrograms at the bypass tract site (e.g., the coronary sinus electrogram for left-sided bypass tracts). In the majority of patients in whom the V-A interval increases in response to rapid pacing or VPDs, the local V-A interval at the site of the bypass tract does not significantly change, although some change may be noted if the bypass tract has a slanted course from ventricle to atrium (see Chapter 10). In this latter instance, the change is related to a different activation wavefront approaching the ventricular insertion of the bypass tract. Once engaged from a different direction, there will be a change in local V-A interval, which thereafter remains fixed regardless of the paced rate. This suggests that in those instances in which a V-A delay occurs in response to ventricular stimulation, the delay results from a change in intramyocardial activation. The V-A remains constant if ventricular activation remains unchanged.

Although the presence of persistently short and fixed V-A intervals at rapid paced rates is the rule when fast-conducting bypass tracts are operative, similar rapid and apparently fixed V-A conduction can be observed in typical AVNRT. Thus, this finding alone should not be considered diagnostic of a bypass tract, as some investigators have suggested.[83] Analysis of the pattern and timing of atrial, His, and ventricular electrograms during SVT and pacing can clearly distinguish the

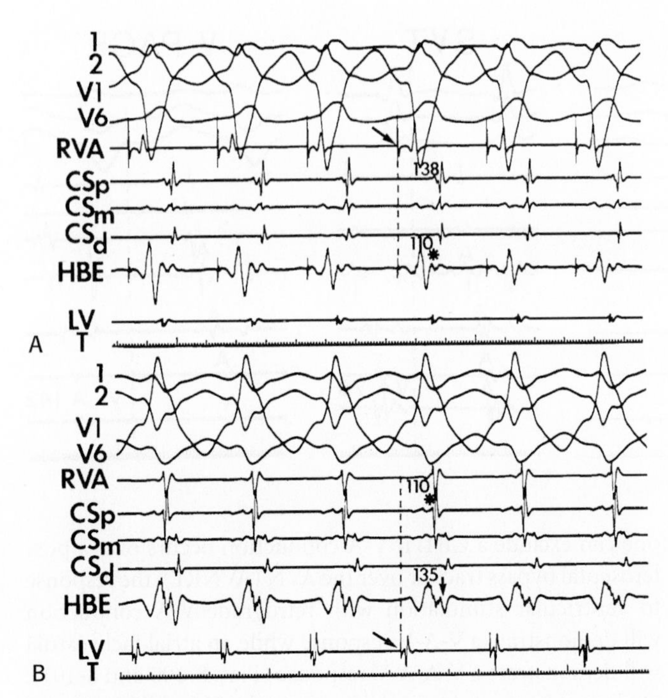


**FIGURE 8-96** *Use of left ventricular pacing to diagnose a left-sided bypass tract.* **A:** RV pacing demonstrates retrograde conduction with earliest activation in the HBE at 110 msec. **B:** Left ventricular pacing results in earlier activation in the CS than the HBE. See text for explanation.

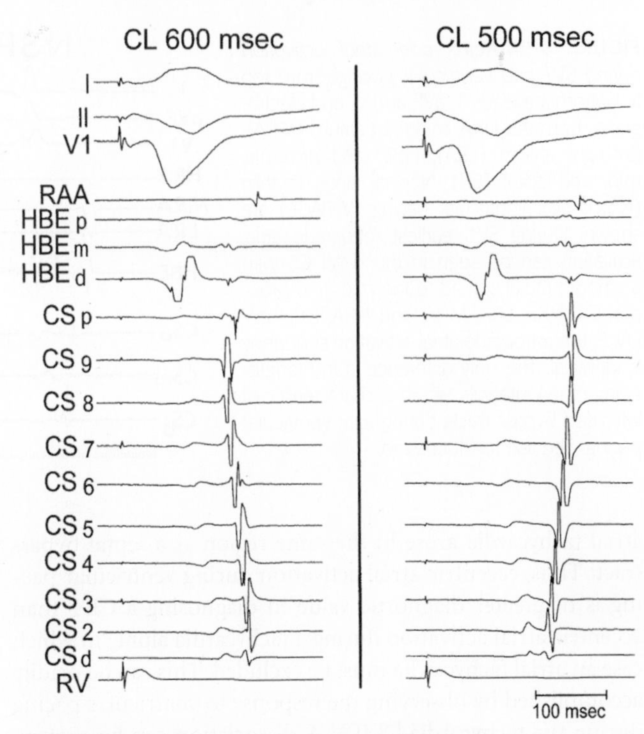


**FIGURE 8-97** *Use of rapid ventricular pacing to produce A-V nodal block in order to observe activation over a left-sided bypass tract.* On the left, during RV pacing at a cycle length of 600 msec retrograde conduction is over the A-V node with breakthroughs at the HBE and CS9. When the paced cycle length is reduced to 500 msec (**right panel**) A-V nodal block is produced allowing manifest retrograde conduction over a left lateral bypass tract. See text for discussion.

two. The retrograde atrial activation sequence will be eccentric if the bypass tract is located on the free wall of atria, that is, if it is nonseptal. Detailed atrial mapping is of paramount importance in evaluating SVT. The atrial activation sequence during SVT using a CBT and ventricular pacing at comparable cycle lengths to the SVT should be identical. Thus, if SVT cannot be induced, one may analyze the retrograde atrial activation sequence during ventricular pacing to localize the site of atrial insertion of the CBT. The investigator, however, should be aware that during ventricular pacing activation to the atria may proceed over both the normal atrioventricular conduction system and the bypass tract, leading to a fusion of atrial activation. If retrograde A-V nodal conduction is very rapid, stimulation in the contralateral ventricle (e.g., RV pacing in presence of a left-sided bypass tract) may produce retrograde activation only over the normal conduction system (Fig. 8-96). The investigator can pace at shorter cycle lengths in order to produce A-V nodal conduction delay or block in order to promote conduction over the bypass tract (Fig. 8-97). However retrograde conduction may persist over the normal AVCS even at paced cycle lengths comparable to the SVT cycle length. The activation sequence during ventricular pacing then would be misleading. Therefore, when using the atrial activation sequence during ventricular pacing to localize the bypass tract, it is necessary to demonstrate that retrograde conduction proceeds solely over the bypass tract during ventricular pacing. Occasionally, the use of verapamil or adenosine may be required to produce block in the AVN, thereby ensuring that retrograde conduction proceeds only over the bypass tract.

Analysis of retrograde activation during SVT is preferred because atrial fusion is not possible if a single bypass tract is present. An example of a comparison of retrograde activation during SVT in ventricular pacing is shown in Figure 8-98. It can be readily seen that retrograde atrial activation in both the right and left atrium is identical during SVT and ventricular pacing. Demonstration of fusion of atrial activation during SVT suggests the presence of multiple bypass tracts (see Chapter 10). Changes in atrial activation, either spontaneously or in response to ventricular stimulation, can demonstrate the presence of multiple bypass tracts (Fig. 8-99). Eccentric atrial activation during SVT and during ventricular pacing is diagnostic of CBT of the free wall of the right or left ventricle. If the bypass tract is opposite the site of ventricular stimulation, the V-A interval prolongs during pacing.

Although an atrial tachycardia usually has "eccentric" atrial activation, the earliest site of atrial activation during SVT using a CBT is always adjacent to the mitral or tricuspid annulus and is identical to that produced by ventricular stimulation. Atrial tachycardias are less commonly located near the annuli, and retrograde atrial activation over the AVN shows a "normal" midline pattern during ventricular stimulation, which differs from the pattern during an eccentric atrial tachycardia. Of course, a similar pattern of activation could be produced if

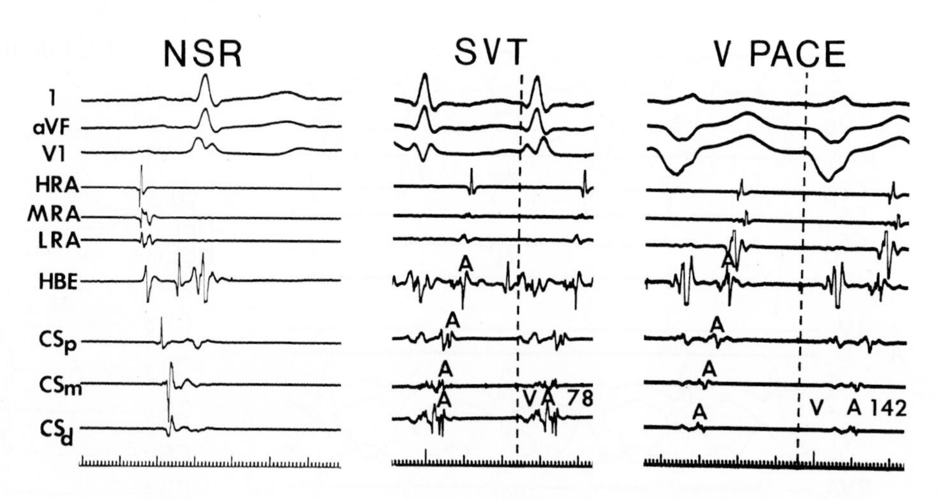


**FIGURE 8-98** *Retrograde atrial activation during SVT and ventricular pacing.* From top to bottom are leads 1, aVF, and $V_1$ and electrograms from the HRA, mid right atrium (MRA), low-right atrium (LRA), HBE, and proximal, mid, and distal (CS). Normal sinus rhythm (NSR), SVT, ventricular pacing (V PACE) are shown. During SVT, earliest retrograde atrial activation can be seen in the distal CS with a smooth radial spread to the mid- and proximal CS, HBE, LRA, MRA, and HRA. During V PACE, the retrograde atrial activation sequence is identical. The only difference is the lengthening of V-A intervals, which is characteristic of left-sided bypass tracts during right ventricular pacing. See text for discussion.

atrial tachycardia arose in the same region as a septal bypass tract. Thus, eccentric atrial activation during ventricular pacing is of greater diagnostic value in diagnosing a CBT than eccentric atrial activation during a tachycardia alone; in which case an atrial tachycardia must be excluded. This can be readily accomplished by observing the response to ventricular pacing during the tachycardia.[136] If V-A dissociation can be proven, one can exclude a CBT. If V-A conduction occurs over a posteroseptal bypass tract or over the AVN (AVNRT), the response to ventricular stimulation with retrograde V-A conduction will demonstrate a V-A-V response while an atrial tachycardia will demonstrate a V-A-A-V response (Figs. 8-100 and 8-101). One must be careful to exclude a "pseudo–V-A-A-V response" produced by a very long V-A, which exceeds the paced cycle

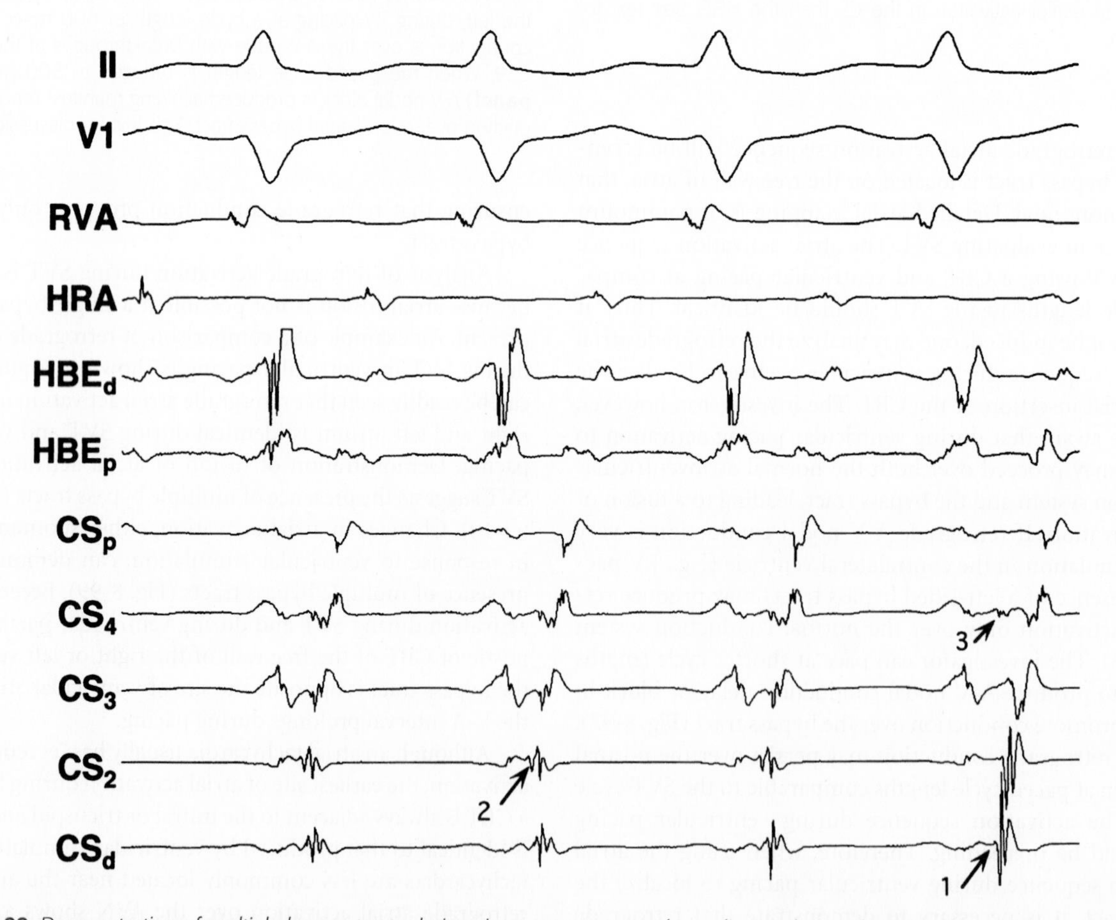


**FIGURE 8-99** *Demonstration of multiple bypass tracts during circus movement tachycardia.* Leads II and $V_1$ are shown with electrograms from the HRA, distal (d) and proximal (p) HBE and proximal to distal CS. For the first two complexes atrial activation in CS2 is earliest. On the fourth complex block occurs at CS2 and earliest activity occurs simultaneously at CSd and CS4. These findings suggest the presence of three bypass tracts.

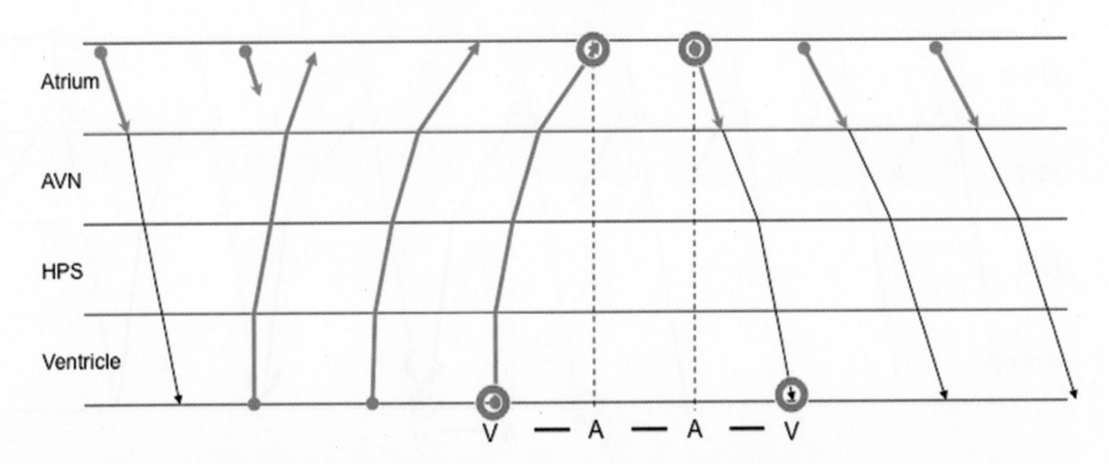
Ventricular pacing during atrial tachycardia
Atrium
AVN
HPS
Ventricle
V — A — A — V
VAAV response after cessation of ventricular pacing occurs because of the presence of a single retrograde and antegrade tachycardia limb. The same pattern would not be expected in AVNRT or in AVRT
Focal AT source
Block in AV conducting system
Ventricular Pacing
A

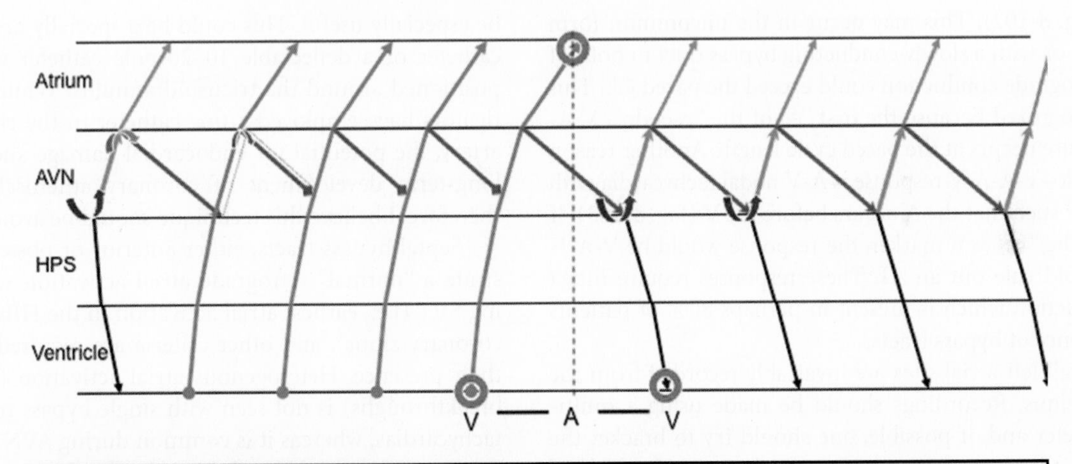
Ventricular pacing during AVNRT
Atrium
AVN
HPS
Ventricle
V — A — V
VAV response after cessation of ventricular pacing occurs because of the presence of separate retrograde and antegrade tachycardia limbs. The same pattern would be expected in AVRT but not in atrial tachycardia
Retrograde "fast" pathway
Antegrade "slow" pathway
Indicates reentrant mechanism
Ventricular pacing
B

**FIGURE 8-100** *Patterns of response to overdrive ventricular pacing in atrial tachycardia **(A)**, AVNRT **(B)**, and AVRT **(C)**.* In each panel ventricular overdrive pacing demonstrating retrograde conduction is shown in *blue.* In **A** (AT) following cessation of pacing, two P waves precede the next H and QRS. In **B** and **C** there is a V-A-V response. See text. *(continued)*

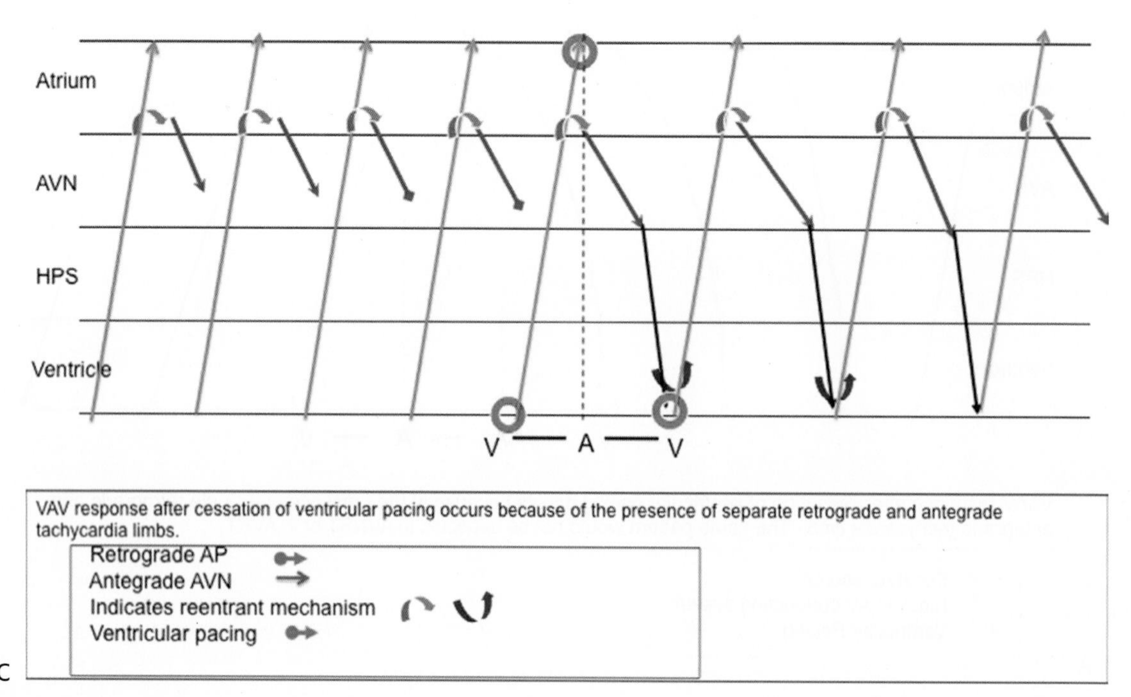
Ventricular pacing during AVRT
Atrium
AVN
HPS
Ventricle
V — A — V
VAV response after cessation of ventricular pacing occurs because of the presence of separate retrograde and antegrade tachycardia limbs.
Retrograde AP
Antegrade AVN
Indicates reentrant mechanism
Ventricular pacing
C

**FIGURE 8-100** *(Continued)*

length (Fig. 8-102). This may occur in the uncommon form of AVNRT or with a slowly conducting bypass tract in both of which retrograde conduction could exceed the paced CL. This can be recognized because the first "A" of the "pseudo"–V-A-A-V response occurs at the paced cycle length. Another reason for a pseudo–V-A-A-V response is A-V nodal tachycardia with a long H-V such that the A occurs before the V (Fig. 8-103). If one used the "H" as a marker, the response would be V-A-H which would rule out an AT. These responses require intact V-A conduction which is present in perhaps 80% of patients in the absence of bypass tracts.

Free-wall left atrial sites are invariably recorded from the coronary sinus. Recordings should be made using a multipolar catheter and, if possible, one should try to bracket the earliest; that is, demonstrate later activation on either side of the earliest site. This may not be possible if the most distal coronary sinus is not reached. In such cases more distal left atrial sites must be mapped through a patent foramen ovale or via a transseptal approach (Fig. 8-104). Mapping the right atrium along the tricuspid valve is more difficult. If careful mapping is not performed in patients with a right lateral CBT, the high-right atrium might be activated earlier than the atrium recorded in the His bundle electrogram, producing an "apparent" high–low activation sequence, and may result in a misdiagnosis of sinus node reentrant SVT or intra-atrial reentrant SVT. Thus, careful mapping of multiple sites around the tricuspid and mitral valves is required for proper diagnosis. This may require a superior vena cava approach and/or the use of catheters with deflectable tips. Specially designed multipolar catheters that can record around the tricuspid ring can be especially useful. This could be a specially designed "halo" catheter or a deflectable 10–20-pole catheter which can be positioned around the tricuspid annulus. While some investigators have employed a fine catheter in the right coronary artery, the potential for endocardial damage and subsequent long-term development of coronary atherosclerosis exists; therefore, I believe this technique should be avoided.

Septal bypass tracts, either anterior or posterior, demonstrate a "normal" retrograde atrial activation sequence during SVT (i.e., earliest atrial activation in the HBE or os of the coronary sinus), and other criteria are required to ascertain their presence. Heterogenous atrial activation (i.e., multiple breakthroughs) is not seen with single bypass tracts or atrial tachycardias, whereas it is common during AVNRT. Thus, the presence of multiple breakthroughs should suggest a diagnosis of AVNRT or multiple bypass tracts. Because SVT using a CBT must first go to the ventricle before returning to the atrium, the R-P and hence V-A interval is longer than that in typical AVNRT in which the atria and ventricle are activated nearly simultaneously. However, in atypical AVNRT, as well as intermediate forms of AVNRT, the R-P interval may overlap with that observed in SVT using a CBT. As expected, the V-A intervals measured from intracardiac electrograms are more accurate than R-P intervals. Using the earliest atrial activation measured in either the high-right atrium, coronary sinus, or A-V junction, the shortest V-A intervals during typical AVNRT ranged from –40 to +75 msec. In atypical AVNRT, the R-P and the V-A are long, with earliest activation usually exceeding 150 msec. In patients with a single, rapidly conducting CBT used as the retrograde limb of the tachycardia, the earliest

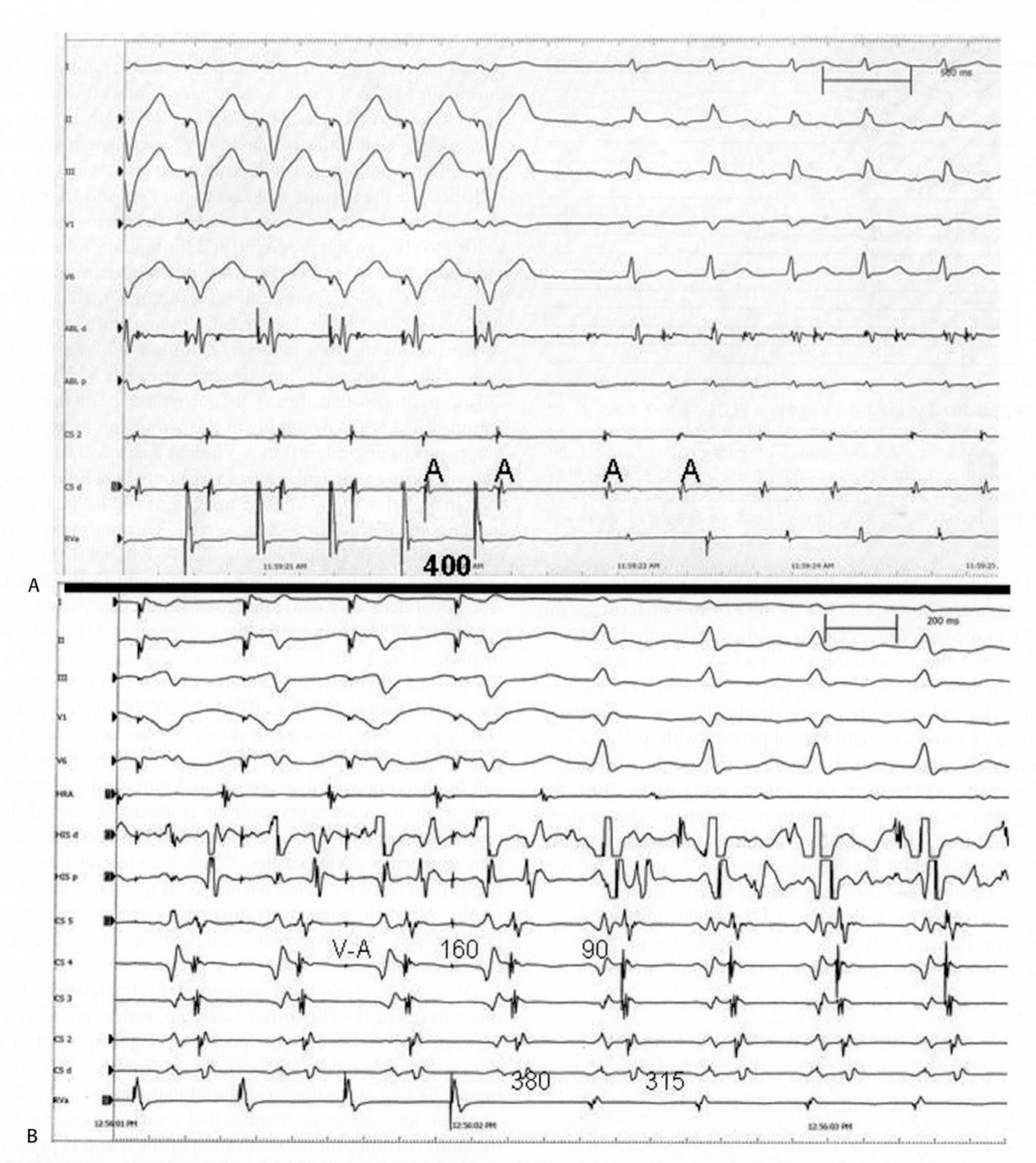


**FIGURE 8-101** *Use of ventricular pacing to distinguish atrial tachycardia from circus movement tachycardia.* **A:** Ventricular pacing at 400 msec demonstrates one-to-one retrograde conduction. Upon cessation of pacing there is a V-A-A-V response prior to resumption of the tachycardia. **B:** Ventricular pacing is associated with retrograde conduction, but upon cessation of pacing the tachycardia resumes following a V-A-V response. The former response is diagnostic of atrial tachycardia, and the latter excludes it. See text for discussion.

retrograde atrial activation we have recorded is 58 msec with a range of 58 to 172 msec during normal ventricular activation. It is of interest that in SVT caused by CBT, the shortest V-A intervals we have seen were in patients with left free-wall bypass tracts (Fig. 8-105). The shortest V-A interval we have observed in a septal bypass tract in an adult patient is 70 msec. Thus the earliest septal activation during any AVRT is 70 msec.

In our experience a cutoff of V-A for the shortest V-A measured anywhere of 65 msec provided the best discriminative value, with a positive predictive value of 95% for both typical AVNRT (<65 msec) and SVT using a CBT (>65 msec). However, these criteria misclassified 3% of SVTs in CBTs and 5% of patients with typical AVNRT. If we were to use a 70-msec cutoff, we could separate septal CBT from AVNRT, but we would

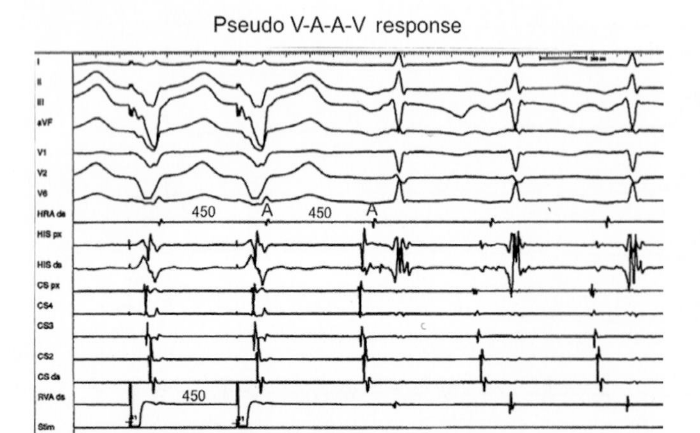


**FIGURE 8-102** *Pseudo–V-A-A-V response.* ECG leads 1, 2, 3, aVF, V1, V2, and V6 are shown with EGMs from the HRA, His (proximal-px, and distal-ds), CS px to ds, and RVA. Cessation of RVA pacing at 450 msec is associated with an apparent V-A-A-V response in the HRA. However the first A and next A occur at the PCL suggesting the second A was caused by the last paced complex. This is then a V-A-V response. See text for discussion.

misclassify 8% of nonseptal CBTs. Thus, 70 msec is a better discriminator for septal CBT at the expense of accuracy for CBT located elsewhere. This is nearly identical to the data of Ross and Uther,[124] who found that a V-A interval of 60 msec was the best value to discriminate between the two. Using a value above 60 msec, they correctly identified 98% of patients with SVT using CBTs and 89% of patients with AVNRT. Conversely, they misclassified 11% of patients with AVNRT and 2% of circus movement tachycardias using CBTs. Thus, the V-A interval is a useful diagnostic measurement. These values; however, can only be applied to adults or adult-sized patients. The normal values for children, who can have very narrow QRS, depending on their size, has not been established.

A variety of methods are available to distinguish A-V nodal tachycardia from AVRT using a septal bypass tract (Table 8-6). An easy way to do this is to note the response to ventricular

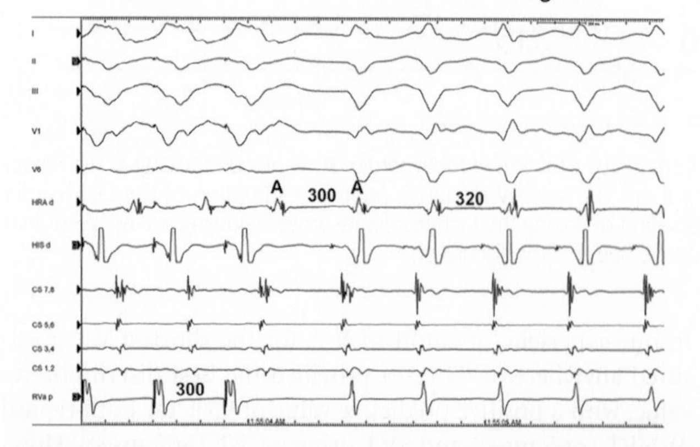


**FIGURE 8-103** *Pseudo–V-A-A-V in AVNRT with a long H-V.* Overdrive ventricular pacing at 300 msec is delivered during AVNRT. There is an apparent V-A-A-V response because the H-V is longer than the H-A (RBBB and LAH is present). The V-A-H response rules out AT. See text.

stimulation during the tachycardia.[137,138] Since the ventricle is part of the reentrant circuit in AVRT, right ventricular pacing during the SVT will result in a postpacing interval which will be within 60 to 80 msec of the SVT cycle length as long as pacing is just slightly faster than the SVT cycle length. AVNRT will demonstrate a return cycle >100 msec more than the SVT cycle because the impulse must get to the RBB and His before engaging the circuit and then return over the normal AVCS (V to RBB to His, around the circuit and through the lower common pathway, His, and HPS). These differences are shown in Figure 8-106. An exception to this can occur if there are dual A-V nodal pathways and ventricular pacing shifts antegrade conduction to the slow pathway, yielding a long postpacing cycle. This can be sorted out by comparing the V-A interval during pacing to that during the tachycardia. For the same reasons listed at the beginning of this paragraph to explain a longer postpacing interval in A-V nodal tachycardia, the V-A interval during ventricular pacing will only be a little longer than in SVT due to a CBT (<85 msec), but will be >100 msec longer compared to the V-A in AVNRT. This finding is obviously unaltered by the presence of dual A-V nodal pathways.

Another way to account for an increment in PPI due to A-V nodal delay as a consequence of ventricular pacing is to correct the PPI by subtracting the increment in AH produced by pacing (Fig. 8-107).[137] Comparing basal versus apical pacing in sinus rhythm (or preferably during SVT) is a useful method of distinguishing AVRT versus AVNRT. Finally, para-Hisian pacing can be used to document the presence of an accessory pathway; when a septal pathway is present the St-A will be the same with His capture and pure ventricular capture; while if an accessory pathway is absent, a marked difference between stimulus to A when His capture is lost and pure ventricular pacing ensues.[139] This is unnecessary and difficult to do since RV apical pacing yields qualitatively similar results. All of the maneuvers discussed above are not useful in the presence of very decremental pathways or left free-wall pathways.

We have also found that comparing the differences in H-A intervals (using the His-to-right atrial appendage electrogram between SVT and ventricular pacing during sinus rhythm at the same rate) provides excellent discrimination for identifying the SVTs that are due to CBT and that are due to AVNRT. The basis for this measurement is that ventricular pacing during sinus rhythm produces activation of the A and H in series in AVNRT but is parallel in patients with bypass tracts; the opposite is true during SVT (Fig. 8-108).[140] As a result, the delta H-A interval ($H\text{-}A_{svt} - H\text{-}A_{pace}$) can distinguish SVT that is due to AVNRT from septal bypass tract. In Figure 8-108 (top), one can see that if a delta H-A more negative than 0 msec is used as a cutoff, the mechanism of the tachycardia could be correctly identified as AVNRT in 100% of cases. In the presence of a septal accessory pathway the difference always is more positive than 30 msec. A limitation of this method is that the H-A interval cannot be measured during ventricular pacing in approximately 15% of cases. In that situation, one can compare the H-A interval in SVT and the V-A

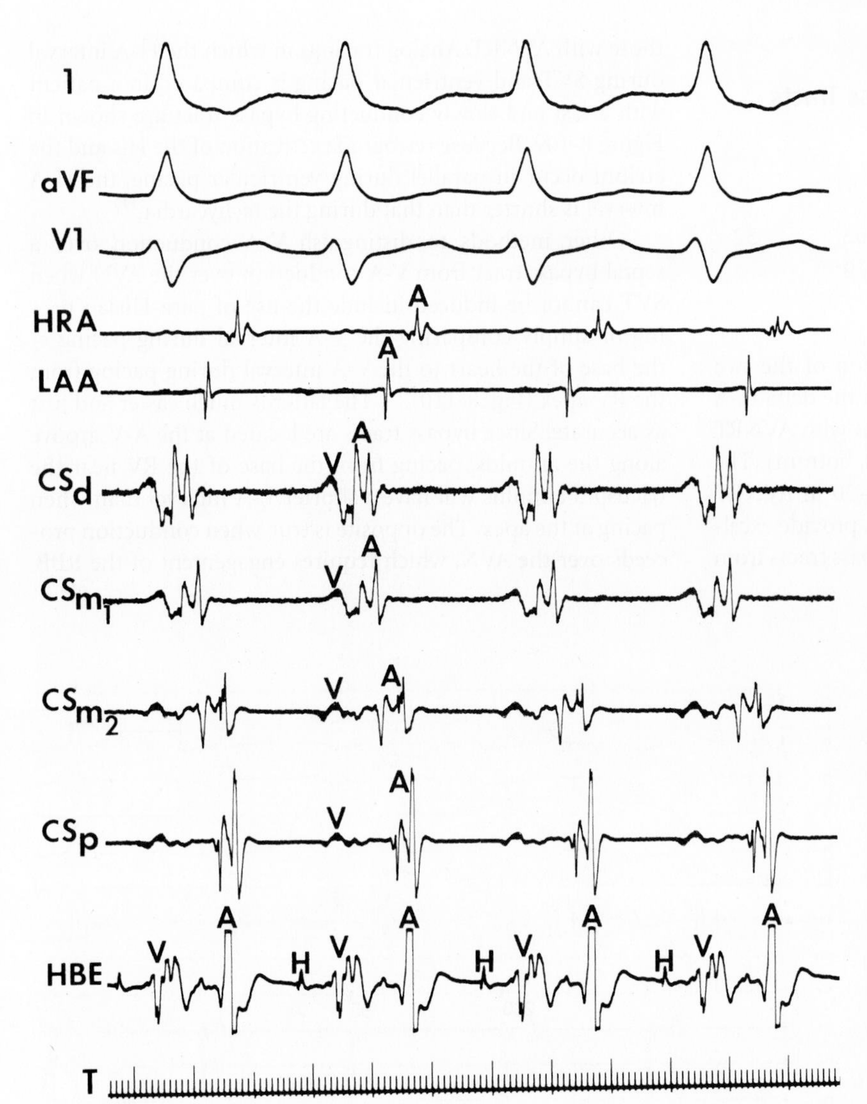


**FIGURE 8-104** *Use of multiple CS and left atrial recordings to localize a bypass tract.* From top to bottom are leads 1, aVF, and $V_1$ and electrograms from the four bipolar electrograms obtained from the CS from a catheter that could only pass through a lateral wall. Recordings from the superior left atrium cannot be obtained from the CS and must be acquired via a patent foramen ovate to record near the superior entrance of the left atrial appendage (LAA). Note earliest activation is in the lateral left atrium with spread to the superior and inferior left atrium thereafter. Note the extremely short V-A interval of 70 msec despite the lateral location of the bypass tract.

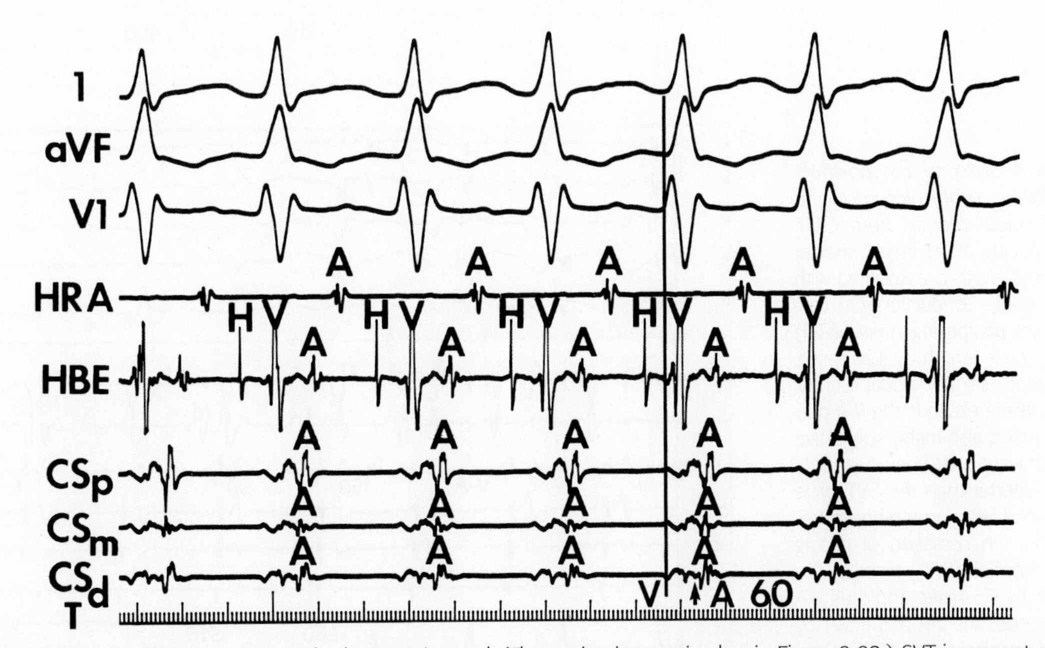


**FIGURE 8-105** *SVT using a CBT at an extremely short V-A interval.* (The tracing is organized as in Figure 8-82.) SVT is present at a cycle length of 310 msec, with earliest activation recorded in the distal CS. The V-A interval is 60 msec, showing within a range of 5% of patients with A-V nodal reentry. See text for discussion.

**TABLE 8-6 Location of Concealed Bypass Tracts (1,349 Patients)**

| | LFW | PS | RFW | AS |
|---|---|---|---|---|
| Fast CBT (1,200) | 625 | 450 | 93 | 32 |
| Slow CBT (149) | 51 | 82 | 9 | 7 |

interval during pacing. Although the separation of the two types of SVT is not quite as good as that when the delta H-A is used, no overlap occurs between the patients with AVNRT and those with septal bypass tracts (Fig. 8-108, bottom). The $HA_{SVT} - VA_{pace}$ is always more negative than –30 in AVNRT and less negative in AVRT. Thus, both methods provide excellent criteria for distinguishing patients with bypass tracts from those with AVNRT. Analog tracings in which the H-A interval during SVT and ventricular pacing is compared in a patient with a fast and slowly conducting bypass tract are shown in Figure 8-109. Because retrograde activation of the His and the atrium occur in parallel during ventricular pacing, the H-A interval is shorter than that during the tachycardia.[140]

Other methods to distinguish V-A conduction over a septal bypass tract from V-A conduction over the AVN when SVT cannot be induced include the use of para-Hisian pacing or simply comparing the V-A interval during pacing at the base of the heart to the V-A interval during pacing from the RV apex (Fig. 8-110).[141] The latter is much easier and just as accurate. Since bypass tracts are located at the A-V groove along the annulus, pacing from the base of the RV near the tricuspid annulus will have a shorter V-A interval than when pacing at the apex. The opposite is true when conduction proceeds over the AVN, which requires engagement of the RBB.

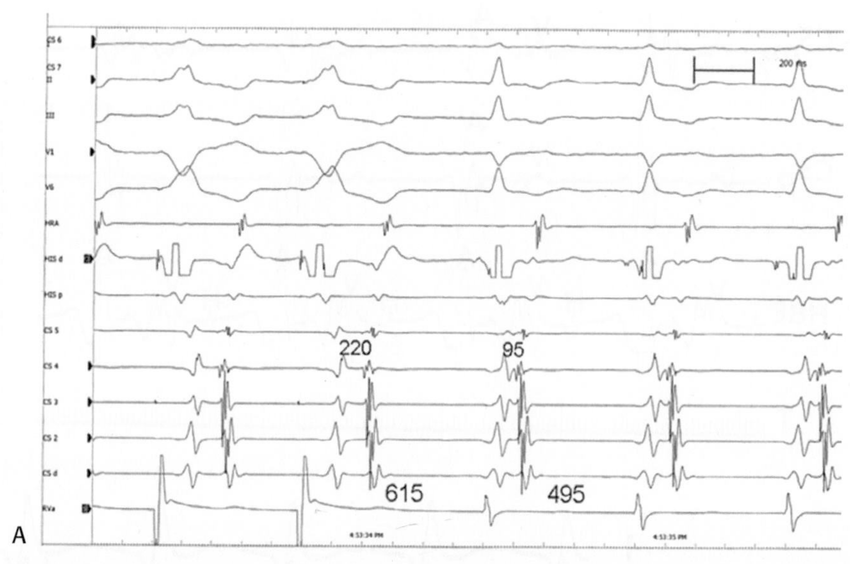


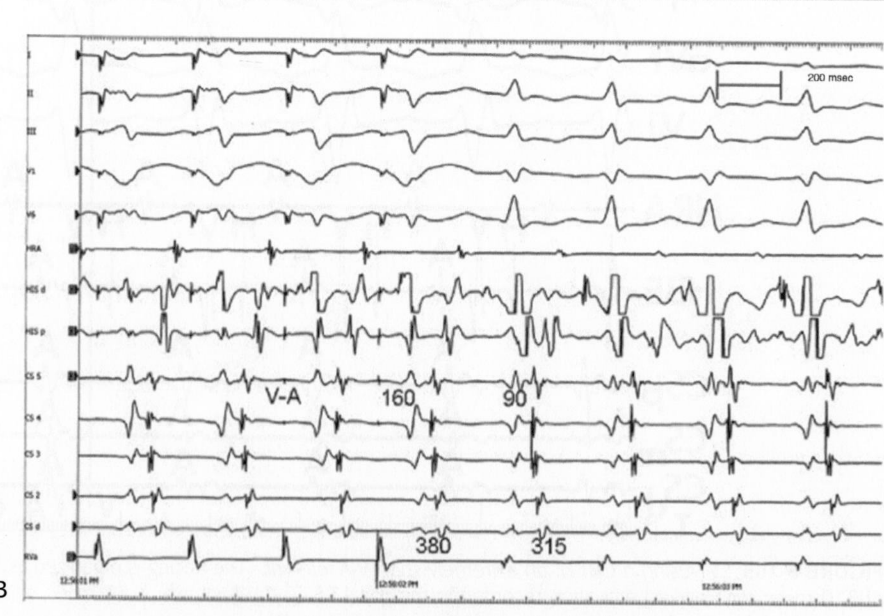


**FIGURE 8-106** *Analysis of the postpacing interval following ventricular pacing to distinguish A-V nodal reentry from CMT.* **A:** Ventricular pacing at 20 msec shorter than the SVT cycle length is associated with one-to-one retrograde conduction. On cessation of pacing the postpacing interval (PPI) exceeds the SVT cycle length by 120 msec, which is consistent with A-V nodal reentry. The V-A during pacing exceeds the V-A during SVT by 125 msec, also highly suggestive of A-V nodal tachycardia. **B:** Ventricular pacing at 15 msec shorter than the SVT cycle length is associated with one-to-one retrograde conduction. On cessation of pacing the postpacing interval (PPI) exceeds the SVT cycle length by 65 msec and thus V-A during pacing exceeds the V-A of the SVT by 70 msec. This is diagnostic of AVRT. See text for discussion.

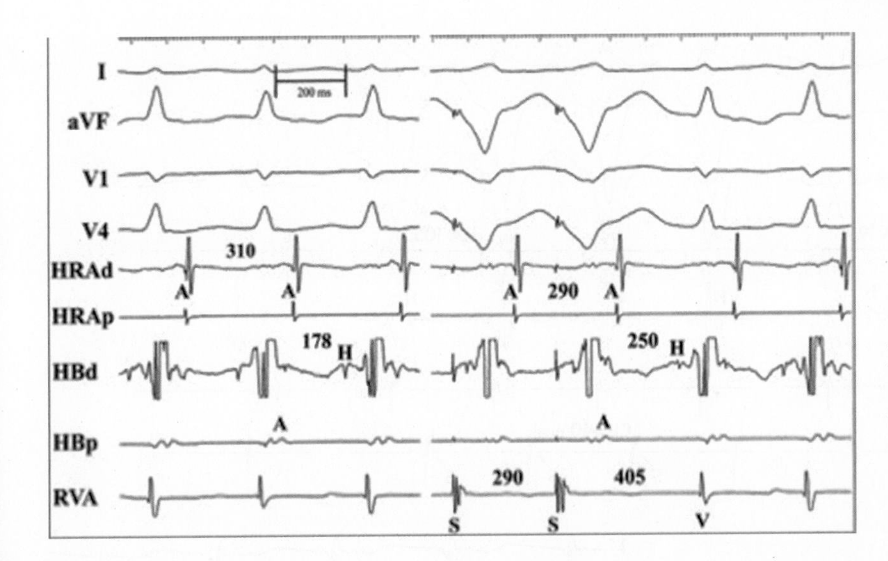


**FIGURE 8-107** *PPI correction factor for A-V nodal slowing.* SVT is shown on the left and response to ventricular pacing is shown on the right. The A-H during the SVT is178 msec but is 72 msec longer following ventricular pacing. The resultant PPI is 72 msec longer than it would have been without A-V nodal delay. Absence of this correction may result in a PPI that falls into the "AVNRT diagnostic zone." See text.

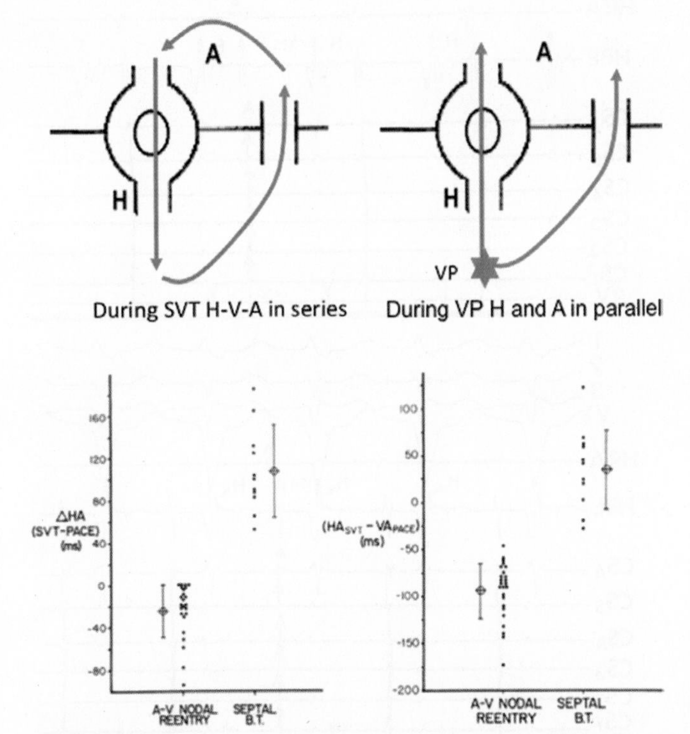


**FIGURE 8-108** *Use of the difference of H-A intervals during SVT in pacing to distinguish A-V nodal reentry and septal bypass tracts.* On **top** is a schema showing the differences in H-A interval during AVRT (**left**) and pacing (**right**). On the **bottom left** the difference in H-A intervals during SVT and ventricular pacing are shown in patients with A-V nodal reentry and those with septal bypass tracts. There is a large separation between the two groups. A delta H-A interval of +10 msec would accurately identify all patients with A-V nodal reentry and those with septal bypass tracts with no false-positives. When a retrograde His deflection cannot be seen during ventricular pacing, one can use the H-A interval minus V-A interval during ventricular pacing to distinguish A-V nodal reentry from septal bypass tracts. The difference between the H-A interval during SVT and the V-A interval during ventricular pacing accurately separates those patients with A-V nodal reentry and separate bypass tracts if one uses a value of –30 msec (**bottom right**). See text for discussion.

This comparison is even more accurate when pacing is carried out during the SVT when entrainment is present. Para-Hisian pacing is used to compare the retrograde activation sequence and timing during pacing at the RV base using low current and during capture of the His bundle at high current.[105] If the V-A remains fixed regardless of whether or not the His bundle is retrogradely activated, a bypass tract is present (Fig. 8-111, top). If the atrial activation sequence and timing move in tandom with the His bundle, conduction over the AVN is present (Fig. 8-111, bottom). If there is a change in activation depending upon whether or not the His bundle is captured, conduction over both the AVN and a bypass tract is present. I believe this technique has limitations because of the possibility of simultaneous atrial and His bundle capture during high current stimulation and the possibility that the atrial activation over the AVN may change if the His is captured early. Moreover it is not useful in the presence of decremental pathways and should not be used if a decremental bypass tract is a possibility. This is because retrograde conduction up the normal conducting system is faster than over the decremental bypass tract (Fig. 8-112). In the presence of a left-sided pathway, it is unnecessary and can be very misleading. Finally the mode of initiation with ventricular extrastimuli may be very helpful. Initiation with a V-H-A response from the RV apex is diagnostic of AVNRT if the retrograde H follows the QRS.[142] A theoretical situation in which a V-H-A response could be seen with a bypass tract is if the retrograde H was over the RBB (prior to the His V electrogram), blocks in the AVN, goes over the bypass tract to the atrium, and the AVN recovers for antegrade conduction. This is extremely rare. Once retrograde conduction over the HPS is over the LBB and the His follows the His bundle ventricular electrogram, block in the AVN is very unlikely to occur at slow basic paced cycle lengths.

One of the most important methods of diagnosing the presence and participation of retrogradely conducting bypass tracts during SVT is the ability of a VPD to depolarize the atrium, with the same atrial activation sequence as SVT when

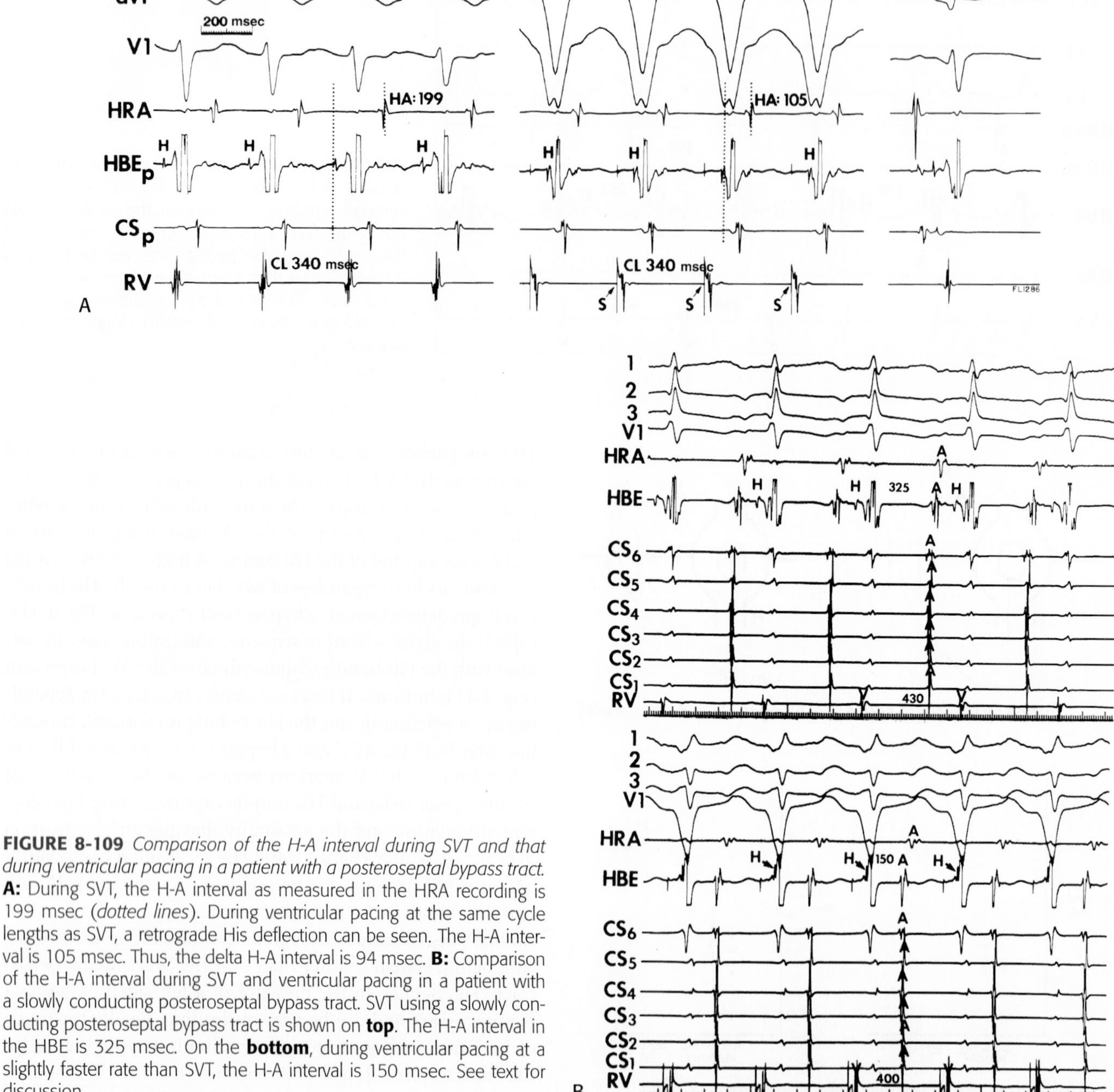


**FIGURE 8-109** *Comparison of the H-A interval during SVT and that during ventricular pacing in a patient with a posteroseptal bypass tract.* **A:** During SVT, the H-A interval as measured in the HRA recording is 199 msec (*dotted lines*). During ventricular pacing at the same cycle lengths as SVT, a retrograde His deflection can be seen. The H-A interval is 105 msec. Thus, the delta H-A interval is 94 msec. **B:** Comparison of the H-A interval during SVT and ventricular pacing in a patient with a slowly conducting posteroseptal bypass tract. SVT using a slowly conducting posteroseptal bypass tract is shown on **top**. The H-A interval in the HBE is 325 msec. On the **bottom**, during ventricular pacing at a slightly faster rate than SVT, the H-A interval is 150 msec. See text for discussion.

the His bundle is refractory.[18,64,65,123,124,126,143] This will be discussed in subsequent paragraphs.

The locations of CBT are similar to those in overt pre-excitation (Table 8-6). Of 1,349 patients with SVT due to a CBT, we found evidence of more than one bypass tract (five with three CBTs) in 109 patients. Of the 1,349 bypass tracts, 1,200 were rapidly conducting, and 149 CBT were slowly conducting. The locations of the fast-conducting CBT were left free wall, 625 (52%); posteroseptal, 450 (38%); anteroseptal, 32, (3%); and right free wall, 93 (8%). Of the 149 slowly conducting CBT, 51 were left free wall (left lateral or left posterior), 82 posteroseptal, 9 right free wall, and 7 anteroseptal. Thus, the most common site of slowly conducting CBTs is septal, but they can occur anywhere. Of note, we have almost as many left free wall slowly conducting bypass tracts as septal. Although the distribution of bypass tracts in patients with and without pre-excitation is similar, we have a much higher incidence of multiple bypass tracts in patients with overt pre-excitation (25% vs. 10%). This may merely be a selection bias of referred patients.

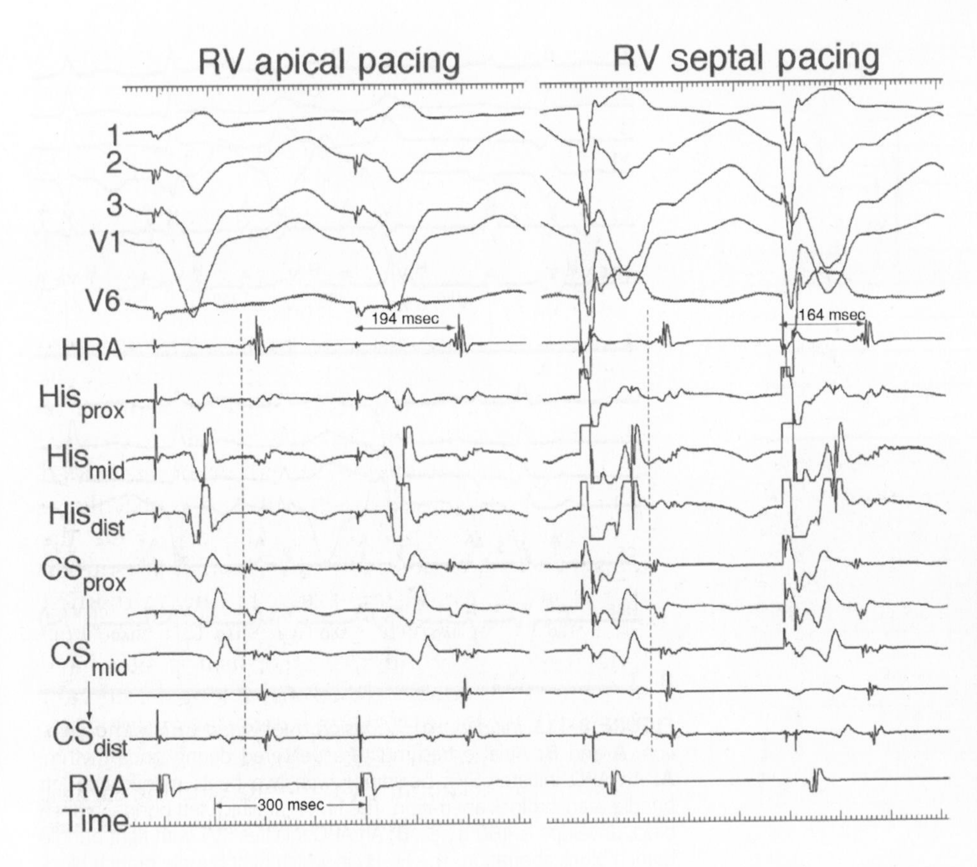


**FIGURE 8-110** *Affect of RV pacing site on ventriculoatrial conduction.* The ventriculoatrial (V-A) conduction time during RV septal apical pacing (**left**) is compared to inferobasal pacing (**right**) in a patient with a septal bypass tract. The V-A interval is longer during apical pacing than basal pacing because of proximity of the ventricular insertion of the bypass tract to the tricuspid annulus. (From John Miller, with permission.)

### Effect of Bundle Branch Block During Supraventricular Tachycardia Using Concealed Bypass Tracts

Patients with CBTs have a higher incidence of developing bundle branch block at the onset of tachycardia than do patients with AVNRT. These findings are consistent with data from other investigators[15,16,123,124,144] and are particularly true with left bundle branch block aberration. In our experience paroxysmal SVT with sustained left bundle branch block aberration results from a CBT 90% of the time. The high incidence of bundle branch block in SVT resulting from CBT induced by APDs is multifactorial. Some patients with CBTs may have relatively short A-H intervals with rapid A-V nodal conduction and/or longer His–Purkinje refractoriness. In these patients, an APD will be more likely to encroach on the refractory period of the His–Purkinje system, causing bundle branch block. In Figure 8-113, both left and right bundle branch block are induced in the same patient. Note the short A-H interval during sinus rhythm (60 to 70 msec). Left bundle branch block develops at a relatively long $H_1$-$H_2$ of 460 msec. In both instances, aberration rapidly diminishes, suggesting a normal response of His–Purkinje system refractoriness to shortened cycle length. The ability to achieve short $H_1$-$H_2$ intervals due to enhanced A-V nodal conduction may be responsible for the development of aberration when His–Purkinje refractoriness is normal.

In contrast, a relatively low incidence of bundle branch block at the onset of the AVNRT is most likely due to the fact that typical AVNRT develops only during slow-pathway conduction, which results in an input to the His–Purkinje system that exceeds its relative refractory period. As such, bundle branch block would be expected to be an uncommon finding. Another possible explanation, particularly in the case of left bundle branch block, is that the patient population is selected. Because most CBTs are left sided, the left bundle branch block may provide the necessary slowing of conduction required for SVT. Thus, these patients come to our attention only because of their SVT, which requires left bundle branch block for the critical delay necessary to sustain reentry.

The mode of initiation also plays an important role in determining the incidence and type of bundle branch block. Aberration is more likely when stimulation is performed during sinus rhythm or during long drive cycle lengths during which His–Purkinje refractoriness is longest and A-V nodal conduction and refractoriness are shortest. In addition, during atrial stimulation, right bundle branch block is twice as common as left bundle branch block, while during right ventricular stimulation, the type of aberration is almost always left bundle branch block. The response to atrial stimulation merely reflects the normal differences of refractoriness of the right and left bundle branch. During right ventricular stimulation, initiation of left bundle branch block aberration, either directly from $V_2$ or from a bundle branch reentrant complex, results from retrograde concealment in the left bundle branch (Fig. 8-93). In this situation, the left bundle branch will always recover after the right bundle branch; therefore, if aberration occurs it will always take the form of left bundle branch block

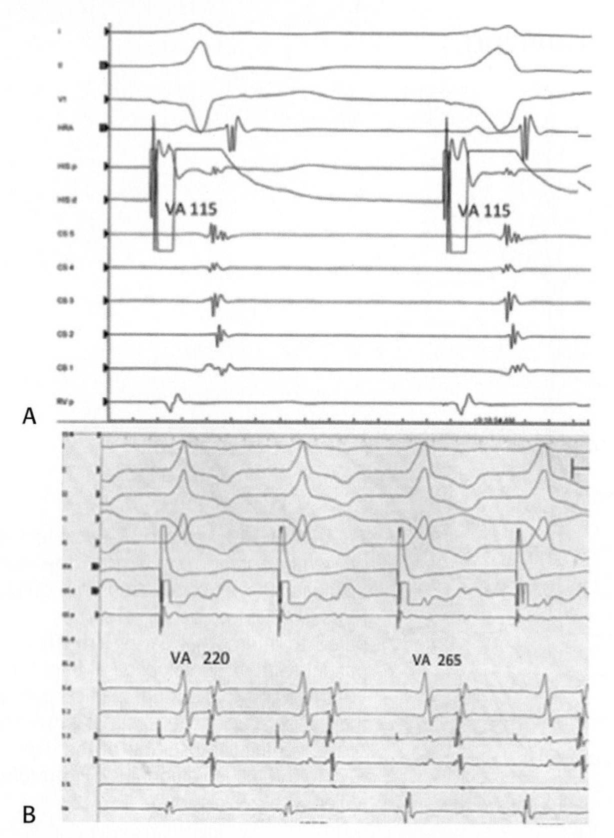


**FIGURE 8-111** *Use of Para-Hisian pacing.* **A:** During Para-Hisian pacing the V-A interval and activation pattern are the same when there is simultaneous His and RV capture (left complex) compared to that during pure RV capture (right complex). This demonstrates the presence of a bypass tract. **B:** Simultaneous His and ventricular pacing (first 2 complexes) produced a V-A time of 220 msec and with pure ventricular pacing (complexes 3 and 4) retrograde conduction is delayed to 265 msec. Atrial activation is the same. This is compatible with conduction over the A-V node. See text for discussion.

or conduction delay. The incidence of aberration is greater with ventricular stimulation (75%) than with atrial stimulation (50%). Lehmann et al.[144] found virtually identical results in patients with pre-excitation and orthodromic SVT. Our

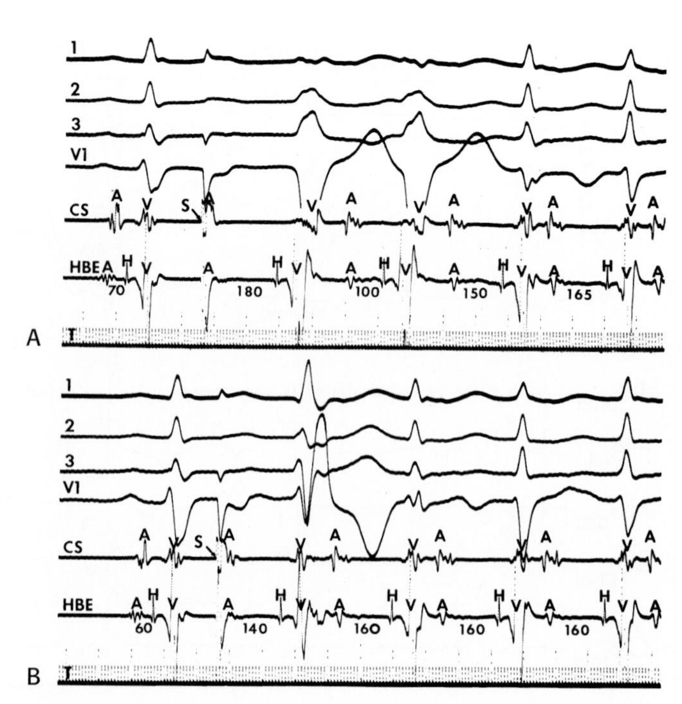


**FIGURE 8-113** *Initiation of SVT using a left-sided CBT with aberration.* **A** and **B:** Atrial extrastimuli are delivered during sinus rhythm. **A:** An APD initiates SVT, beginning with two beats manifesting left bundle branch block aberration. The $H_1$-$H_2$ at which left bundle branch block develops is 460 msec. **B:** An APD initiates SVT with right bundle branch block aberration. The $H_1$-$H_2$ in which right bundle branch block occurs is 370 msec. See text for discussion.

incidence of aberration with APDs is slightly higher because we delivered APDs during sinus rhythm as well as during atrial pacing.

Because part of the ventricles is a required component of the reentrant circuit, bundle branch block on the same side as the bypass tract usually produces a slowing of the tachycardia secondary to a lengthening of the size of the reentrant circuit resulting from lengthening of the V-A conduction time.[15,16,18,49,60,123,124,145–147] An example of this phenomenon is given in Figure 8-114, where the earliest site of atrial activation is in the left atrium. The local V-A time remains the

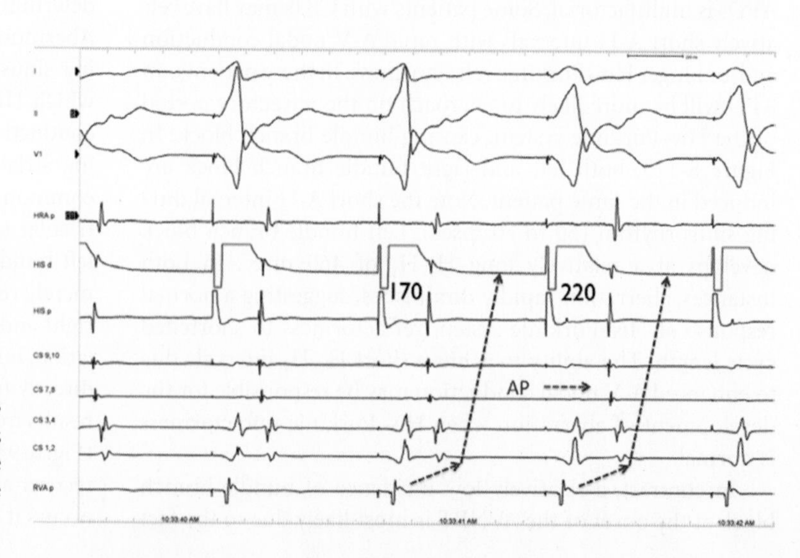


**FIGURE 8-112** *Limitation of Para-Hisian pacing in the presence of a slowly conducting CBT.* Para-Hisian pacing is performed as in Figure 8-111. Conduction proceeds over the A-V node because conduction over the RBB and A-V node is faster than over the bypass tract. See text for discussion.

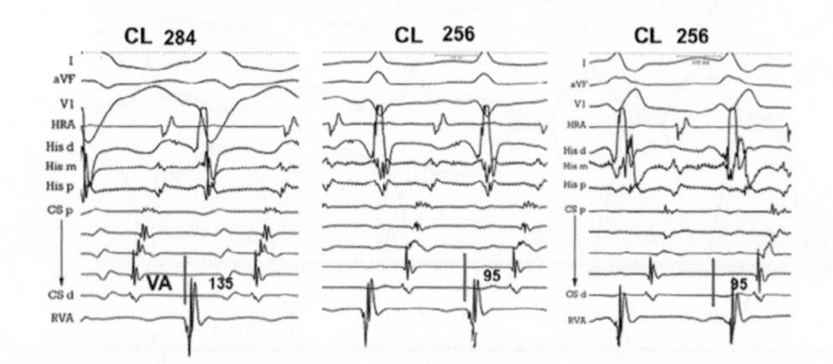


**FIGURE 8-114** *Effect of bundle branch block on V-A interval in SVT using a left-sided CBT.* **A:** SVT with LBBB (**left**), normal conduction (**middle**), and RBBB (**right**) are compared. SVT cycle length and V-A conduction are prolonged by 28 and 40 msec, respectively (284 vs. 256 msec and 135 vs. 95 msec) during LBBB, a phenomenon that is diagnostic of a left-sided bypass tract. Note that during RBBB there is no effect on tachycardia cycle length or V-A interval. **B:** Changes in antegrade conduction can effect the SVT cycle length. See text for discussion.

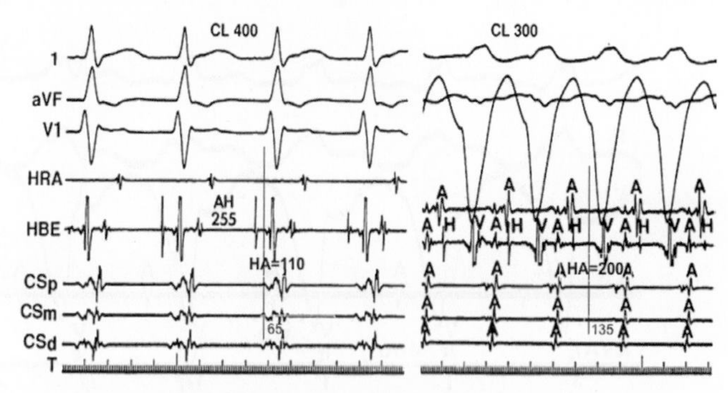


**FIGURE 8-115** *Shortening of SVT cycle length on developing ipsilateral bundle branch block despite lengthening of the V-A interval.* The figure is organized as is Figure 8-97. During narrow complex tachycardia (**left**) using a left-sided bypass tract the cycle length is 400 msec and the V-A interval is 65 msec. On the right, during LBBB, the V-A lengthens to 135 msec, but the cycle length is paradoxically shortened due to switch in conduction to the fast A-V nodal pathway. Notice there is also an increase in H-A with an increase in H-V. Both the effect of ipsilateral BBB on the V-A and H-V on H-A are diagnostic of a bypass tract that is participating in the tachycardia. See text for discussion.

same whether or not left bundle branch block is present. However, the V-A interval measured from the onset of the QRS is prolonged by 40 msec in the presence of a left bundle branch block (135 vs. 95 msec). Note that the tachycardia cycle length changes only by 28 msec (284 vs. 256 msec). This results because the longer V-A interval during left bundle branch block produces a shorter A-H interval than during conduction with a narrow QRS. When the initial input into the AVN is shorter, it results in an increase in the A-H interval. Thus, despite the 10 msec increase in the H-V interval during left bundle branch block, the decrement in the A-H interval overcompensates for this. In fact, a paradoxic shortening of tachycardia cycle length during bundle branch block can be seen if marked shortening in A-V nodal conduction occurs in response to the prolonged changing V-A intervals.[124] For example, the sudden earlier input to the AVN with normalization of the QRS could result in a dual-pathway response, resulting in a lengthening of the tachycardia cycle length during normal QRS. We have observed this phenomenon several times. A dramatic example of this phenomenon is shown in Figure 8-115 in which SVT with LBBB is associated with fast-pathway conduction and a short cycle length. However, the V-A interval is long because of the presence of a left free-wall bypass tract. Slow-pathway conduction is associated with SVT with a narrow QRS, resulting in a longer cycle length, but a shorter V-A interval. Most often, the tachycardia cycle length increases in concordance with the V-A interval; however, because of compensatory changes in A-V nodal and potentially also in His–Purkinje conduction, changes in tachycardia cycle length are diagnostically less useful. Thus a change in V-A is obligatory with the development of ipsilateral bundle branch block, and is necessary to prove it even if the tachycardia cycle length prolongs with the bundle branch block. In addition there is an increase in H-A dependent on the increase in H-V (20 msec), supporting the role of the HPS in the circuit.

Lengthening of the SVT cycle length, and more specifically the V-A interval, by ≥35 msec on development of bundle branch block is diagnostic of a free-wall bypass tract located on the same side as the blocked bundle.[16,17,124,145,146] If bundle branch block develops on the side of the heart contralateral to the bypass tract, the V-A interval will not change. This can be seen in Figure 8-114, in which SVT using a left-sided CBT is shown during right bundle branch block (left), normal conduction (middle), and left bundle branch block (right) aberration. Thus, patients with left-sided bypass tracts show prolongation of V-A interval with left bundle branch block, and those with right-sided bypass tracts show a V-A prolongation with right bundle branch block. Bundle branch block during SVT using septal CBTs produces either no increase in the V-A interval or an increase ≤25 msec.[145,146] Although a prolongation of tachycardia cycle length of ≥35 msec usually accompanies ipsilateral bundle branch block, the cycle length may be not as great as the change in V-A interval due to a shortening of the A-H interval because of the longer V-A interval and subsequent longer cycle length. In rare cases the tachycardia cycle length can be shorter during ipsilateral bundle branch block due to a shift from slow-pathway conduction to fast-pathway conduction (Fig. 8-115). Kerr et al.[146] demonstrated that, in the case of posteroseptal bypass tracts, left bundle branch block can produce a small increase in the V-A interval (13 ± 8 msec), whereas in those with anteroseptal bypass tracts, right bundle branch block is associated with a small increase in the V-A interval (16 ± 9 msec). In a few patients, they observed changes between 25 and 35 msec during SVT using bypass tracts that they determined were septal in origin. As stated, it is the change in V-A interval that is critical. Because bundle branch block contralateral to a free-wall CBT or associated with septal bypass tracts results in insignificant changes in the V-A interval, the P wave may fall inside the widened QRS. This can be mistaken for AVNRT by surface

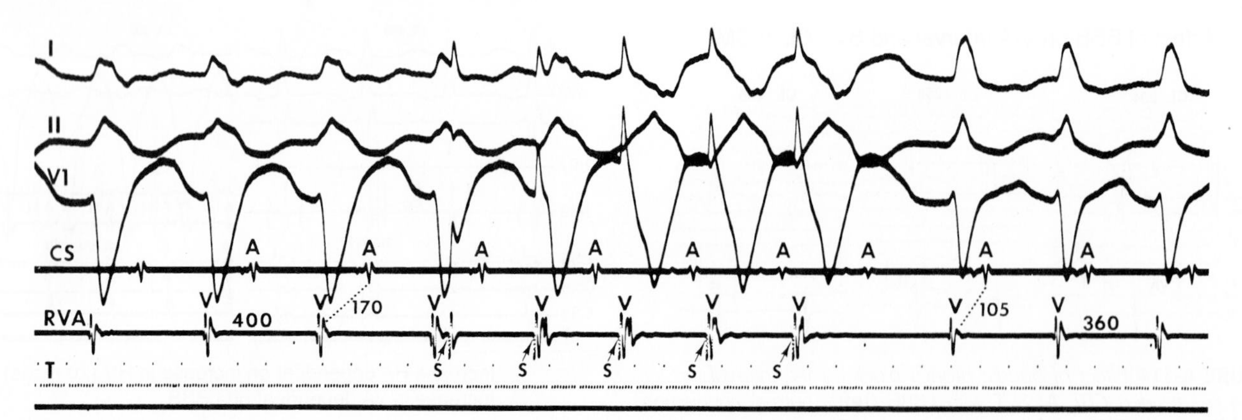


**FIGURE 8-116** *Use of ventricular stimulation to normalize aberrant conduction during SVT.* SVT with LBBB is present in the first four complexes. A short burst of ventricular pacing (S, *arrow*) at 300 msec results in a normalization of the QRS complex, which is associated with a decrease in SVT cycle length (from 400 msec to 360 msec) and abbreviation of V-A conduction. Those findings are consistent with a left-sided bypass tract. See text for discussion.

ECG criteria. Intracardiac studies are necessary to make the correct diagnosis.

Programmed ventricular stimulation can be used to demonstrate the effect of bundle branch block if it is not present during the tachycardia. An increase in the V-A interval of >45 msec during right ventricular stimulation is diagnostic of a left-sided free-wall bypass tract.[135] The increased time to reach the bypass tract is the reason for failure of a right ventricular extrastimulus to pre-excite the atrium during SVT using a left lateral bypass tract. In effect, right ventricular stimulation is an "artificial" left bundle branch block. Moreover, both the development and abolition of bundle branch block by single or multiple ventricular extrastimuli during SVT is another means of assessing the effects of functional bundle branch block on SVT.[147] This technique is of particular value if bundle branch block persists during the tachycardia and results from repetitive retrograde concealed conduction. The abolition of bundle branch block should result in a shortening of the V-A interval if the bundle branch block is ipsilateral to the bypass tract (Fig. 8-116). As stated, because a shorter V-A interval may lengthen subsequent A-H and/or H-V intervals, a balanced situation may be created, and no change in cycle length or, paradoxically, an increase in cycle length may be noted.

### *Requirement of Atrium and Ventricle During Supraventricular Tachycardia Using Concealed Bypass Tracts*

The reentrant circuit responsible for SVT using a CBT incorporates the atria and ventricles. Continuation of a tachycardia in the presence of A-V or V-A block, regardless of the site of block, rules out a CBT as a functioning part of the reentrant circuit. Conversely, in patients with clinical episodes of SVT, the failure to initiate a tachycardia by APDs that block in the AVN or His–Purkinje system may be the first clue that a CBT is operative. If APDs are delivered during a long basic drive cycle length, or during sinus rhythm, which increases His–Purkinje refractoriness and decreases A-V nodal refractoriness (see Chapter 2), infra-nodal block may result and prevent initiation of the tachycardia. This mechanism for failure to initiate the tachycardia can be overcome by repeating the stimulation protocol at a shorter drive cycle length, which will both shorten His–Purkinje refractoriness and increase A-V nodal refractoriness, thereby allowing conduction of the APD to ventricle and reentry over the CBT. Of note, in virtually all patients in whom tachycardias using CBTs cannot be initiated by APDs delivered at long drive cycle lengths because of His–Purkinje block, SVT can be initiated by ventricular stimulation, which requires retrograde His–Purkinje block to develop circus movement tachycardia. Thus, during sinus rhythm, initiation of tachycardia from the ventricle is often easier than from the atrium. On the other hand, if atrial stimulation is performed using too short a basic drive cycle length, the APDs may block in the AVN, and SVT then cannot be initiated. In this case, SVT may be induced by repeating the study at longer drive cycle lengths or after administration of drugs that will facilitate A-V nodal conduction by decreasing A-V nodal refractoriness (e.g., atropine).

After the tachycardia is initiated, the investigator can evaluate how much of the atria and ventricles are requisite components of the reentrant circuit in SVT using a CBT. This can be done by analyzing the extent of the atria that can be depolarized by APDs or atrial pacing without disturbing the tachycardia. Those areas, which can be captured without influencing the SVT, can be considered not necessary. We uniformly found that, in patients using left-sided bypass tracts, we can capture the right atrial electrograms without influencing the tachycardia (Fig. 8-117). This is confirmed by lack of influencing left atrial activation. Compensatory A-V nodal delay in response to a single APD may, however, not effect the V-V interval mimicking a response that suggests failure to influence the tachycardia. In this case the left atrial electrograms would be advanced. Thus, in the absence of left atrial electrograms, failure of a right APD to influence the SVT cycle length should be demonstrated over a range of coupling intervals, or for several consecutive paced beats at cycle lengths shorter

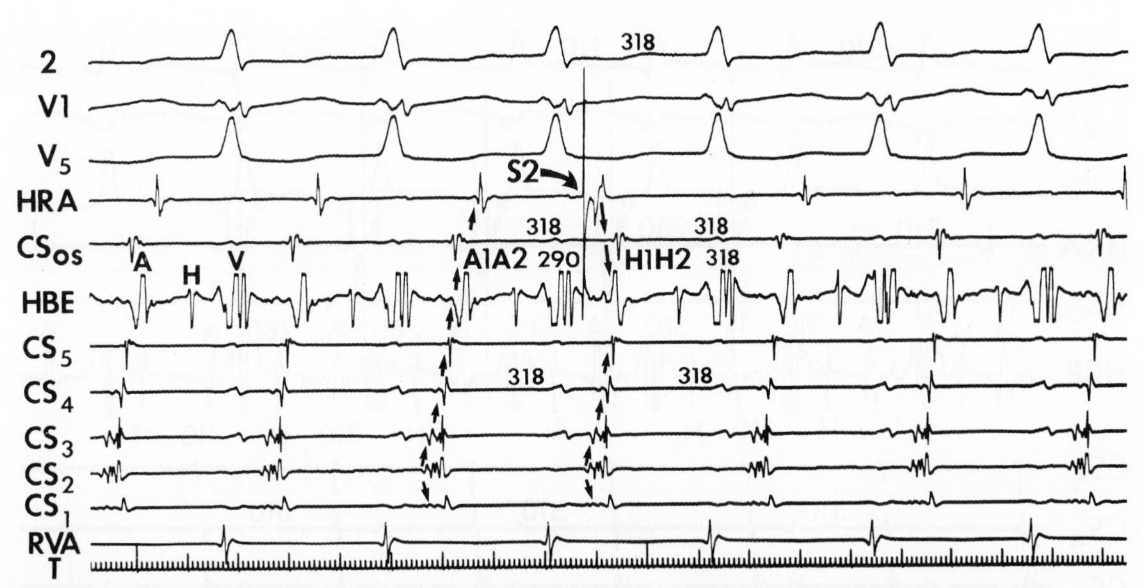


**FIGURE 8-117** *Use of an atrial stimulus to demonstrate right atrial activation is unnecessary to maintain tachycardias using a left-sided CBT.* Leads 2, $V_1$, and $V_5$ are shown with electrograms from the HRA, the os of the CS, the HBE, and five other bipolar electrograms from the CS, $CS_1$ being distal and $CS_5$ being proximal. SVT is present at a cycle length of 318 msec, with the site of earliest activation in bipolar pair 2 in the CS. Atrial activation spreads from there, as shown following the second QRS complex. An $S_2$ is delivered from the HRA, captured in the HRA and the atrium at the A-V junction in the HBE prematurely, as shown by the *down arrows.* The $A_1$-$A_2$ in the HBE is advanced to be 290 msec. Retrograde activation in the left atrium, as manifested by activation sequence in the CS electrograms is unchanged, as is the $H_1$-$H_2$ interval and the tachycardia cycle length. See text for discussion.

than the tachycardia, because in either of these cases, exact compensatory A-V nodal delay over the entire range of intervals or consecutive paced complexes would be highly unlikely (Fig. 8-118). In an analogous fashion we have been able to capture left atrial sites in patients with right free-wall and anteroseptal bypass tracts. We have not been able to dissociate all electrograms in the A-V junction (i.e., at the os of the coronary sinus or proximal His bundle recording site) during posteroseptal tachycardias. These findings suggest that differential input to the AVN occurs and that only parts of the atrium ipsilateral to the bypass tract are requisite components of the reentrant circuit. Morady et al.[148,149] also demonstrated lack of contralateral atrial tissue participating in the reentrant circuit. In contrast to our observations they reported that the low septal right atrial (in the His bundle electrogram) and coronary sinus os electrograms could be simultaneously dissociated from orthodromic tachycardia in two of six patients with right posteroseptal bypass tracts and suggested that little or no atrial myocardium is required for SVT in such patients.[148] However, on close measurement of the data purporting to demonstrate this finding (see Fig. 4 in Reference 141), when the coronary sinus electrogram was captured, both the His bundle and ventricular electrograms were slightly advanced. This therefore represents resetting of the SVT with atrial fusion; a finding diagnostic of a macroreentrant arrhythmia, in this case, AVRT. As such, there is no adequate documentation that the atrial tissues surrounding the AVN can be dissociated from SVT using a right posterior septal CBT.

Analysis of how much of the ventricles is involved is also possible. It is well known that right ventricular extrastimuli often fail to influence SVT using a left free-wall bypass tract. As noted, this occurs because the ventricular stimulus is delivered far from the tachycardia circuit. The local ventricular refractory period, intraventricular conduction time to the circuit, and tachycardia cycle length all influence the ability of the right ventricular stimulus to reach the reentrant circuit to influence it. Saoudi et al.[150] demonstrated dissociation of the right ventricle from the tachycardia circuit during attempts at entrainment of circus movement tachycardias using left-sided bypass tracts. Conversely, Ormaetxe et al.[151] demonstrated that RV pacing, which entrains SVT using a left-sided CBT, can never manifest fusion because the LV must be captured by the stimulated impulse in order to produce entrainment. This preempts LV activation over the left bundle branch, so that no fusion is possible. In contrast, fusion is possible if septal bypass tracts are operative.[151]

Both Benditt et al.[143] and Miles et al.[152] also noted the inability of single ventricular extrastimuli delivered over a wide range of coupling intervals to influence tachycardias with bypass tracts contralateral to the stimulation site. Thus, only parts of atria and ventricle ipsilateral to the CBT are requisite components of orthodromic tachycardias using CBT. The atrium and ventricle contralateral to the bypass tract seems unnecessary to maintain circus movement tachycardia. As noted, the development of bundle branch block ipsilateral to the bypass tract increases the extent of ventricular participation such that the contralateral ventricle becomes required to maintain the arrhythmia. In that situation contralateral ventricular stimuli can reset the tachycardia. Thus, the tachycardia circuit can change size based on physiologic changes in

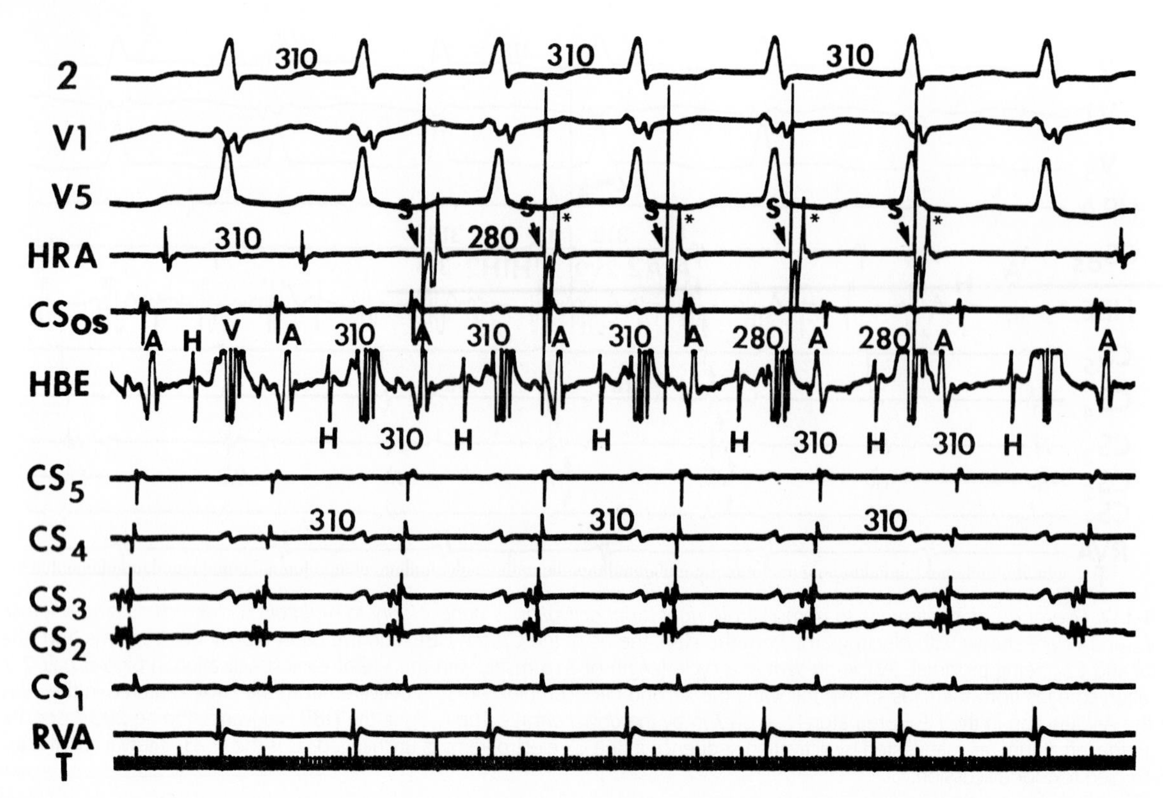


**FIGURE 8-118** *Use of rapid pacing to dissociate right and left atrial electrograms during SVT using a left-sided bypass tract.* (The figure is organized the same as Figure 8-117). The tachycardia cycle length at this time is 310 msec. Following the second QRS, high-right atrial pacing is begun at a cycle length of 280 msec for five complexes. Not only is the HRA captured but the fourth and fifth atrial extrastimuli also capture the low septal atrium and the His bundle recording. The His bundle activation remains unchanged, as does activation in all CS electrograms. The sequential capture of the right atrium, including that recorded in the HBE, fails to alter the tachycardia, suggesting lack of necessity of these right atrial sites.

ventricular, and theoretically, atrial activation patterns. Other specific responses to programmed stimulation during the tachycardia in the presence or absence of bundle branch block are discussed subsequently.

## Electrical Stimulation During Supraventricular Tachycardia Using a Concealed Bypass Tract

Because the reentrant circuit in orthodromic tachycardia using a CBT involves part of both the atria and ventricles, stimulation from either chamber can affect tachycardias, even rapid ones (e.g., rates greater than 200 bpm). The ability to alter the tachycardia is related to the proximity of the stimulation site to the reentrant circuit. In patients with SVT due to CBTs, it is difficult to depolarize both atria prematurely without affecting the tachycardia. Although we and others have demonstrated that all the atrium is not necessary for a given circus movement tachycardia,[148,149] in most patients, APDs delivered over a range of coupling intervals can reset the tachycardia by penetrating the normal A-V conducting system before it would have been depolarized by the atrial wavefront resulting from retrograde conduction via the bypass tract (Fig. 8-119). Atrial activation in this instance is usually a fusion of antegrade activation produced by the APD and retrograde activation produced via the bypass tract. Depending on the resultant A-H interval produced by the APD that resets the tachycardia, the next QRS may be early or late. An example of fusion of atrial activation during resetting is shown in Figure 8-120. In this instance, the first of two consecutively delivered APDs initiates circus movement tachycardia using a left-sided bypass tract, as demonstrated by early activation in the coronary sinus atrial electrogram. The second APD preempts retrograde activation of the right atrium by the bypass tract and conducts antegradely down the right atrium to the low atrial septum and the AVN to capture the His bundle prematurely, thus resetting the tachycardia and advancing it. Therefore, following the second stimulus, atrial activation is a fusion of antegrade depolarization by the stimulated APD and retrograde depolarization (CS electrogram) over the bypass tract. Occasionally, the APD can actually penetrate the CBT antegradely and still reset the SVT. In this case, the atria are activated only by the APD—no fusion is present.

Earlier APDs can terminate CMTs by multiple mechanisms: (a) production of block in the AVN or His–Purkinje system with atrial fusion; (b) depolarization of the atria so as to render it refractory to the impulse returning via the accessory pathway, thereby creating a form of V-A block; (c) penetration of the bypass tract antegradely, resulting in collision with the returning impulse; and (d) antegrade conduction capturing the ventricle prematurely such that the QRS is advanced and the impulse reaches ventricular insertion of the bypass tract when it is refractory; or, alternatively, if retrograde conduction

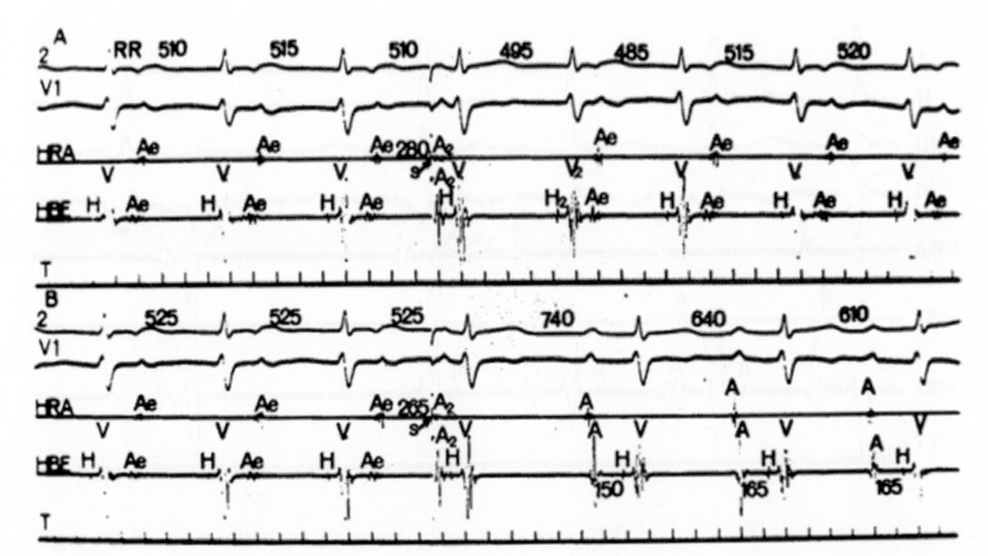

**FIGURE 8-119** *Resetting and termination of SVT using a CBT by an APD.* SVT is present as a cycle length between 510 and 515 msec. Following a third complex, an APD is introduced from the HRA at 280 msec, which penetrates the tachycardia and resets it without terminating it. In the **bottom panel**, an earlier APD terminates the tachycardia by blocking in the A-V node.

can occur, block subsequently appears antegradely as in the first three mechanisms. In each of the first three mechanisms there is antegrade block in the AVCS. Mechanism 3 is by far the most common mode of termination (Fig. 8-121). With each of mechanisms 2 to 4, termination is usually associated with failure of retrograde conduction over the bypass tract. Multiple mechanisms can be operative in an individual patient, depending on the coupling interval of the APD, the A-V conduction time, and the intra-atrial conduction delay. The fourth mechanism is not uncommon in the presence of enhanced A-V conduction and/or during tachycardias with short cycle lengths, both of which are closely related.

The use of ventricular stimulation during SVT allows one to demonstrate that the ventricles are components of the reentrant circuit as well as proving the functional role of the bypass tract. This is of particular value in three situations: (a) patients with septal bypass tracts who exhibit normal retrograde atrial activation and failure of V-A prolongation on the development of bundle branch block during SVT; (b) patients with slowly conducting bypass tracts to distinguish them from ectopic atrial rhythms and the atypical form of AVNRT (see prior discussion of stimulation during AVNRT); and (c) patients whose coronary sinus and left atrium cannot be catheterized for technical reasons, making detailed atrial mapping impossible. Responses to VPDs that demonstrate the presence of a bypass tract include (a) capture of the atrium at a coupling interval identical to that of the VPD (exact capture phenomenon); (b) paradoxically premature captures; (c) atrial capture when the His–Purkinje system is refractory, that is, retrograde atrial activation following antegrade His bundle depolarization of a prior tachycardia complex; and (d) an increase in the V-A interval during entrainment produced by stimulating the

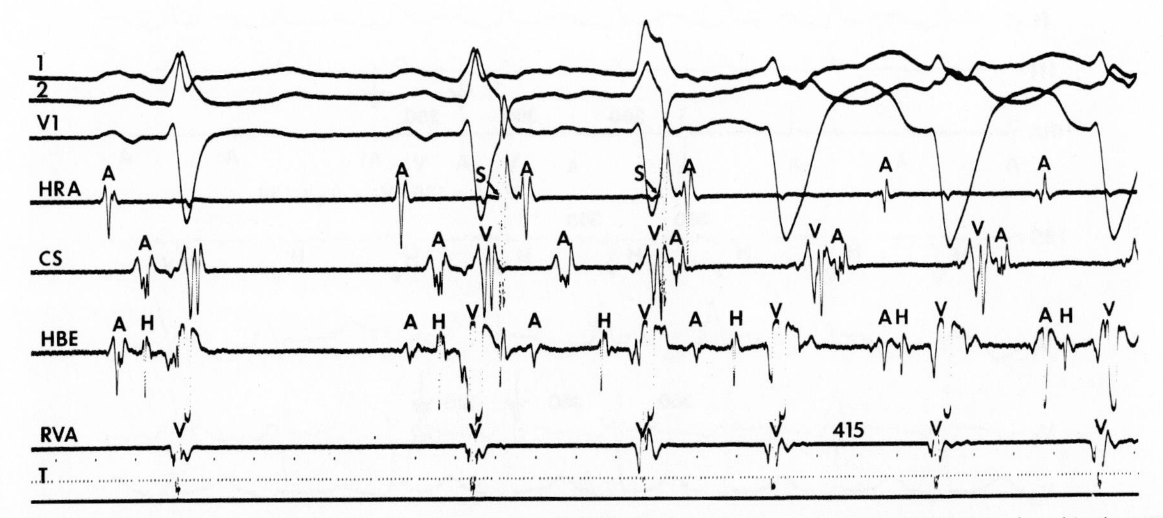

**FIGURE 8-120** *Initiation and resetting of SVT using two extrastimuli.* Following two sinus complexes, an APD is introduced in the HRA, which initiates SVT using a left-sided bypass tract. See the early activation of CS atrial electrogram following QRS. A second extrastimulus is introduced simultaneous with the QRS, which captures the HRA and conducts through the A-V node to reset the tachycardia, which continues with left bundle branch block aberration. During the second extrastimulus, two wavefronts are present in the atrium, one from the initiated SVT and one from the atrial extrastimulus. See text for discussion.

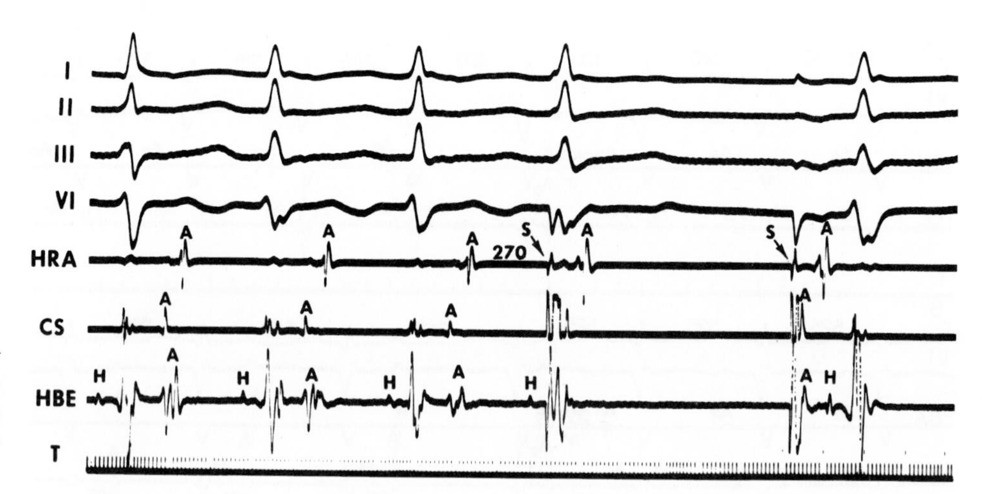


**FIGURE 8-121** *Termination of SVT-CBT by an APD. SVT-CBT is terminated by an APD (S, arrow) delivered at a coupling interval of 270 msec that blocks in the A-V node.*

ventricle contralateral to the bypass tract.[18,63,64,123,124,126,143,153] This latter phenomenon is analagous to the influence of ipsilateral bundle branch block on the V-A interval.

If the VPD can prematurely depolarize the atria at the exact coupling interval at which it was delivered, one must assume that the stimulation site is within the reentrant circuit, because if intervening tissue were involved, the V-A interval would increase, and subsequently the A-A interval would exceed the coupling interval of the VPD. The ability to capture the atrium producing an A-A interval less than the coupling interval of the VPD (paradoxical capture) suggests that the VPD was delivered not only within the reentrant circuit but closer to the bypass tract than the initial site of ventricular depolarization via the normal A-V pathway. This phenomenon confirms incorporation of a bypass tract in the SVT and demonstrates the presence of an excitable gap within the reentrant circuit. It is easiest to demonstrate with right-sided bypass tract with stimulation of the base of the right ventricle, because with a normal QRS, the earliest activation of the ventricles is on the left side of the septum (Fig. 8-122). Analogously, if left bundle branch block develops in a patient with a left-sided bypass tract, left ventricular stimulation is likely to produce a paradoxic capture, because during left bundle branch block, the earliest activation of the ventricle is in the right ventricle. The premature atrial activation in each instance results from a shortened V-A conduction time during the VPD, which is due to greater proximity of the stimulation site to the bypass tract than the site of initial ventricular activation during SVT. This situation is somewhat analogous to that in which V-A conduction changes from prolonged to short on normalization of bundle branch block ipsilateral to the site of the bypass tract.

The response most commonly seen and easiest to demonstrate is atrial capture by VPDs when the His–Purkinje system

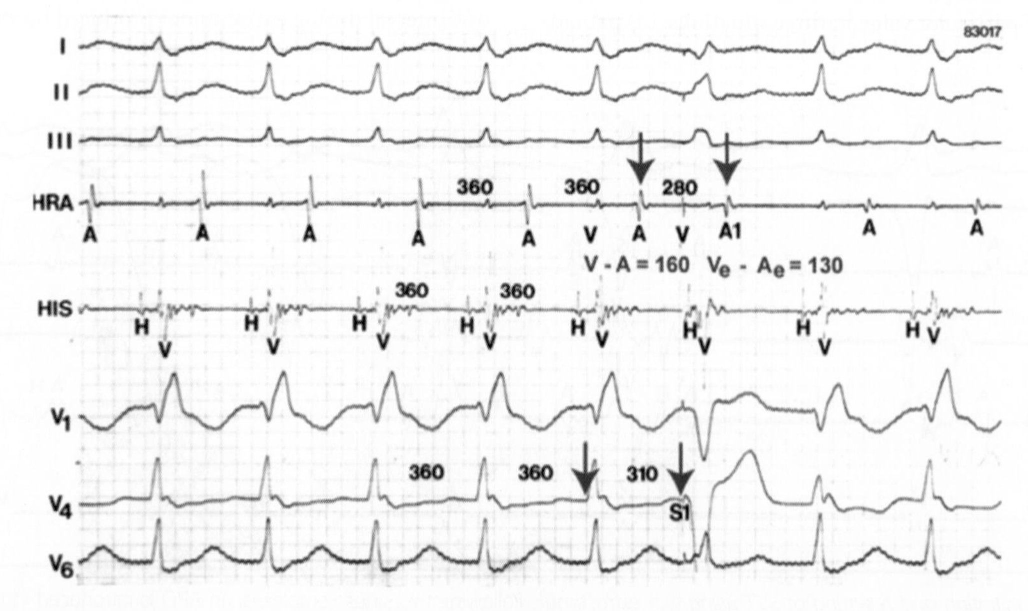


**FIGURE 8-122** *Paradoxical capture by a His-refractory VPC.* SVT with RBBB is shown at a cycle length of 360 msec. An RV extrastimulus ($S_1$) is delivered when the His is refractory at a coupling interval of 310 msec. This result in premature activation of the atrium ($A_1$) at an interval of 280 msec. This "paradoxical" capture occurs because the RV is closer to the bypass tract than the LV septum, the earliest site of activation during RBBB. See text for discussion.

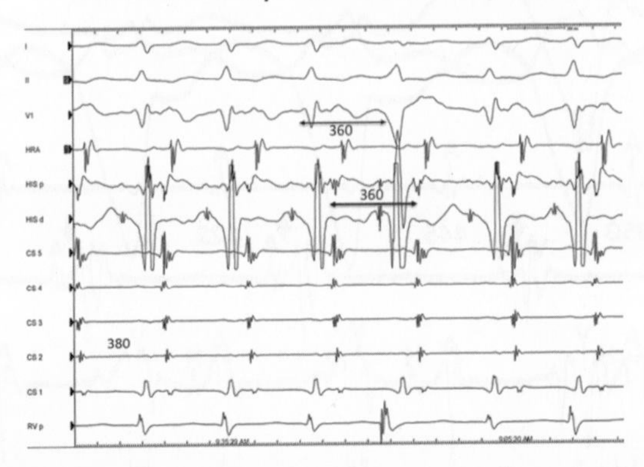


**FIGURE 8-123** *His Refractory VPC pre-exciting the atrium using a septal CBT.* SVT at a cycle length of 380 msec using a septal CBT is shown. A single, His Refractory VPC is delivered at a coupling interval of 360 produces an exact capture of the atrium.

is known to be refractory, that is, when antegrade His bundle depolarization is already manifested (Fig. 8-123). As long as the antegrade His bundle deflection is not influenced by ventricular stimulation, excitation of the atria by a ventricular premature beat must be over a bypass tract. It is possible to deliver the stimulus 35 to 55 msec before the inscription of the His deflection because retrograde conduction from ventricle-to-His invariably exceeds the H-V interval (see Chapter 2). Pre-excitation of the atrium when the His bundle is refractory may not always be possible by right ventricular stimulation if the bypass tract is left sided.[123,124,143,153] This is related to the fact that stimulation in the right ventricle is distant from the ventricular insertion of the bypass tract. The conduction time from the right ventricular stimulation site to the site of the bypass tract, the cycle length of the tachycardia, and local right ventricular refractory period determine the ability of right ventricular stimulation to reach the reentrant circuit before ventricular activation over the normal pathway. Closely coupled VPDs, usually ≤75% of the SVT cycle length, are required,[152] and in many cases, this requires stimulation before antegrade activation of the His bundle. We have seen patients in whom ventricular stimuli delivered more than 100 msec prematurely fail to pre-excite the atrium. One can use double extrastimuli to overcome the limitations of local ventricular refractoriness (Fig. 8-124). In this case, the first extrastimulus shortens right ventricular refractoriness and allows a second to be delivered much more prematurely. Despite the fact that the stimulus is delivered 100 msec before inscription of the His bundle, the His bundle is activated antegradely; thus, atrial pre-excitation must occur over a bypass tract. However, if LBBB aberration is present during AVRT using a left-sided bypass tract, a single His refractory RV VPC can pre-excite the atrium because under these conditions the RV is part of the reentrant circuit (Fig. 8-125). The site of stimulation relative to the site of bypass tract, as well as the rate of the tachycardia are the main determinants of the ability to pre-excite the atrium, as noted. Both Benditt et a1.[143] and Miles et al.[152] have demonstrated that stimulation close to the bypass tract allows one to pre-excite the atrium when the His bundle is refractory in virtually all instances. Miles et al.[152] have developed a pre-excitation index (analyzing the coupling interval of the premature ventricular stimulus as a percentage of the tachycardia cycle length) that may be useful in determining the location of the bypass tract. Atrial pre-excitation by right ventricular stimuli at coupling intervals >90% of the tachycardia cycle length invariably means the presence of a septal or right-sided bypass tract. If the

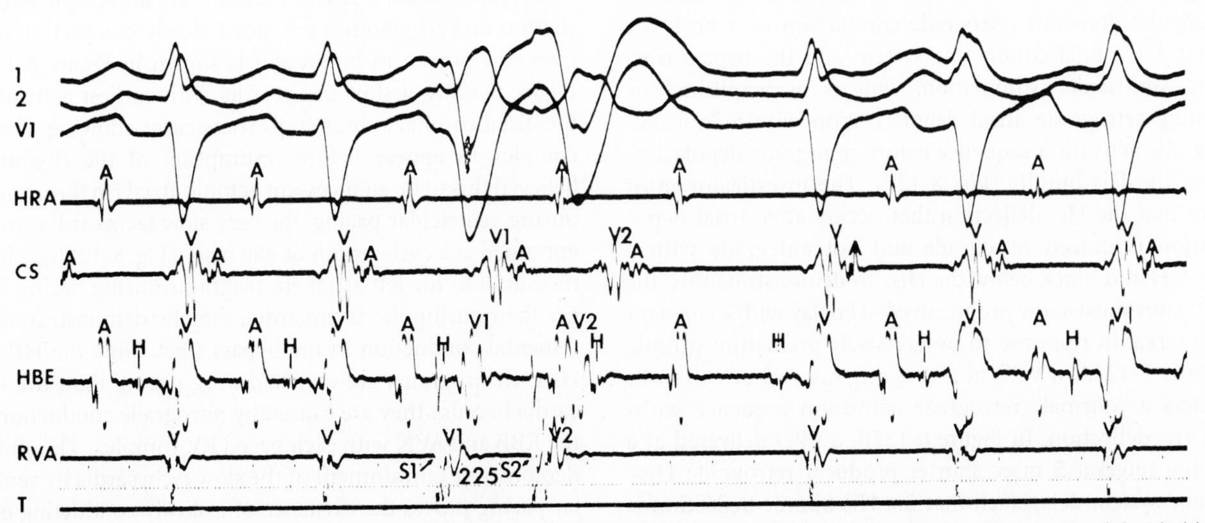


**FIGURE 8-124** *Requirement of two right ventricular stimuli to pre-excite the atrium while the His bundle is refractory in a left-sided bypass tract.* Following two complexes of a tachycardia using a left-sided bypass tract, a ventricular extrastimulus ($S_1$) is delivered without pre-exciting the atrium. The first extrastimulus altered refractoriness at the right ventricular pacing site so that, when a second extrastimulus ($S_2$) is delivered at 225 msec, it conducts back to the atrium. Because the His bundle deflection just behind $V_2$ is unaltered, such that the first four complexes have identical A-H intervals and H-H intervals, the atrium must have been activated over a bypass tract. See text for discussion. (From Farshidi A, Josephson ME, Horowitz LN. Electrophysiologic characteristics of concealed bypass tracts: clinical and electrocardiographic correlates. *Am J Cardiol* 1978;41:1052.)

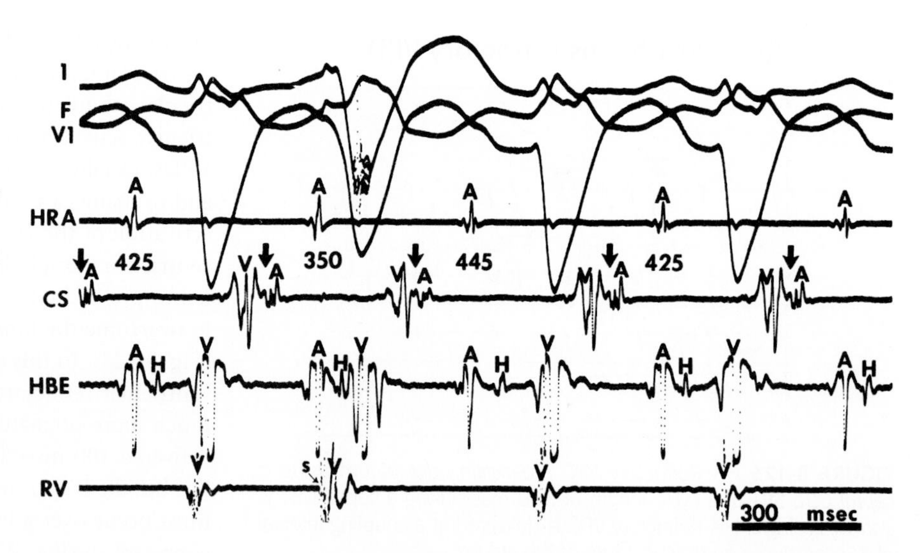


**FIGURE 8-125** *Atrial pre-excitation by a single VPD during SVT using a left side CBT during LBBB.* A VPD (S, *arrow*) is introduced at a coupling interval of 350 msec during SVT (cycle length of 425 msec) after the His bundle has been antegradely depolarized (i.e., the second His bundle deflection occurs on time), resulting in atrial capture. Because the His bundle must have been refractory, ventriculoatrial conduction must occur over an accessory atrioventricular pathway. In contrast to SVT with a normal QRS, the LBBB makes the RV part of the circuit, so atrial pre-excitation is possible. See text for discussion.

investigator performs stimulation from both ventricles and/or uses multiple ventricular extrastimuli, atrial pre-excitation when the His bundle is refractory should be demonstrated in almost all patients with SVT using a CBT.

In patients with slowly conducting bypass tracts, the response to ventricular stimulation during the tachycardia may be totally opposite. Because the slowly conducting bypass tracts have decremental properties,[63–65,126] the response to premature ventricular stimuli results in slowing of V-A conduction, which, if marked, can actually retard the return cycle (Fig. 8-126). This would be a form of postexcitation, or delay of excitation, in response to a VPD when the His bundle is refractory. Clearly, any disturbance of atrial activation by a VPD delivered during antegrade conduction over the His bundle is diagnostic of the presence of a bypass tract.

Septal bypass tracts may also be diagnosed by demonstrating simultaneous retrograde conduction over both the normal A-V nodal conducting system and the bypass tract during ventricular stimulation. This is accomplished by recording retrograde atrial depolarization with a "normal" retrograde activation sequence before retrograde depolarization of the His bundle (Fig. 8-127). The investigator must ensure that the His deflection that occurs after atrial depolarization is indeed retrograde and not antegrade with a short A-H and block below the His. To demonstrate this, the investigator must show progressive V-H delay with a constant V-A interval in response to progressively premature stimuli. In Figure 8-127A, a VPD at a coupling interval of 340 msec produces a "normal" retrograde activation sequence without a His deflection. In Figure 8-127B, a VPD delivered at a coupling interval 5 msec shorter produces retrograde His–Purkinje system delay such that the His bundle deflection is seen with a long V-H interval. The V-A interval is identical in both panels. The His bundle deflection is most likely retrograde because it was absent at the slightly longer coupling interval. It is less likely to be antegrade because the apparent "A-H" is too short to have been conducted. Para-Hisian pacing, described earlier in this chapter, and differences in the V-A interval depending on the site of RV stimulation (apex vs. base) are other methods to demonstrate the presence of a rapidly conducting septal bypass tract.

SVTs using posteroseptal slowly conducting bypass tracts must be differentiated from the atypical form of AVNRT and ectopic atrial rhythms. When the retrograde atrial activation sequence is eccentric, only ectopic atrial rhythms need to be excluded, because typical AVNRT has a specific retrograde activation sequence, which is usually earliest at the os of the coronary sinus. Ventricular stimulation is paramount to making a distinction between an ectopic atrial rhythm and a concealed, slowly conducting bypass tract. If ventricular pacing produces the same retrograde atrial activation sequence and/or the tachycardia can be entrained by ventricular pacing,[10,150] then a bypass tract can be diagnosed. An example of a patient who had a rhythm resembling an ectopic left atrial rhythm and in whom a left-sided slowly conducting bypass tract was proven to be present is shown in Figure 8-128. In Figure 8-128A, a slow tachycardia with earliest activation at the distal coronary sinus stops transiently, allowing one sinus complex to appear before resumption of the rhythm. We believed this to be an incessant ectopic atrial rhythm; however, during ventricular pacing, the very slow tachycardia could be entrained at a cycle length of 450 msec (Fig. 8-128B). The V-A measured to the left atrial electrograms during pacing is longer than during the tachycardia, thereby demonstrating decremental conduction in the bypass tract. Note the HRA and HBE electrograms are earlier during pacing than the tachycardia because they are caused by retrograde conduction over the RBB and AVN with each paced RV complex. The ability to demonstrate entrainment of the slow tachycardia by ventricular pacing proves the existence of a slowly conducting bypass tract and excludes an atrial tachycardia.

In order to distinguish the uncommon form of A-V nodal tachycardia from a slowly conducting posteroseptal bypass tract (both can have identical retrograde activation sequences) ventricular stimulation or para-Hisian pacing as described earlier in this section must be used (Table 8-7). Figure 8-100

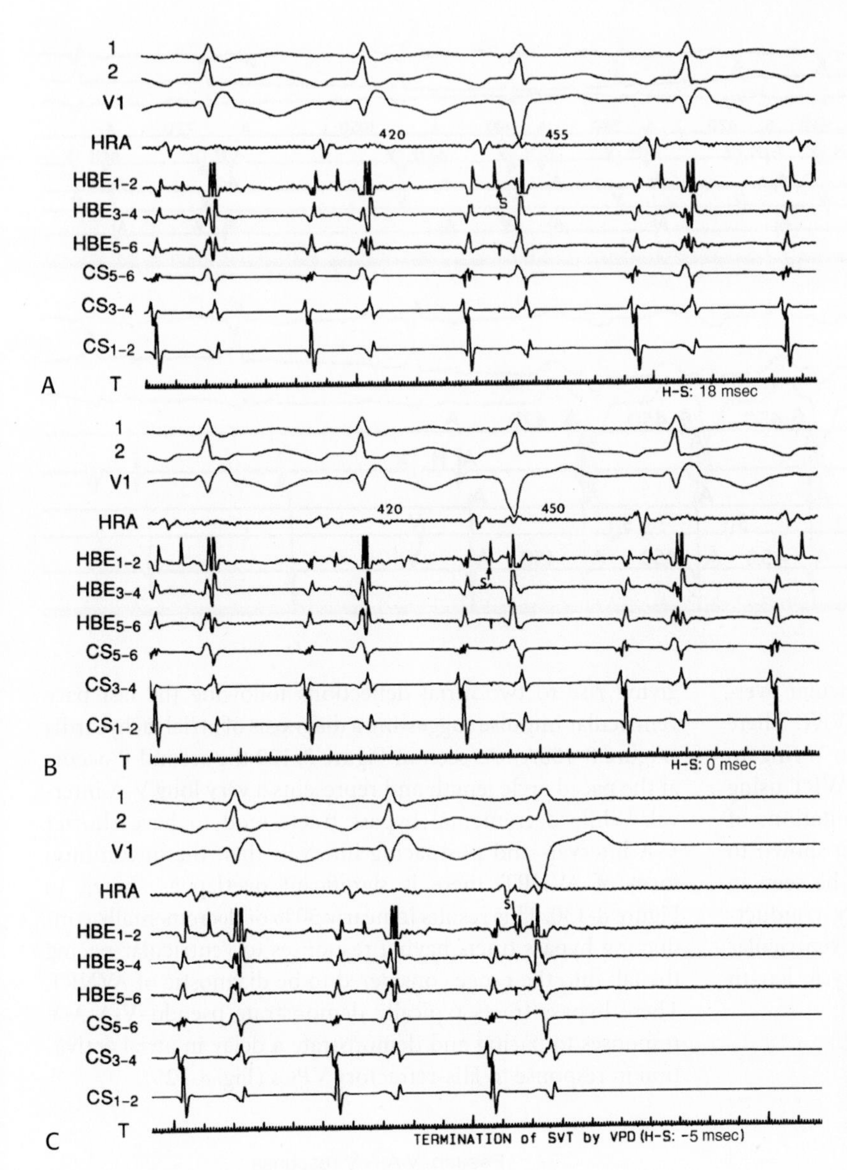


**FIGURE 8-126** *Delay and termination of SVT using a slowly conducting left posterior bypass tract by ventricular stimulation when the His bundle is refractory.* ECG leads 1, 2, and $V_1$ are displayed with distal (1–2) to proximal (5–6) HBE, and the distal three pair of electrodes from a decapolar catheter in the CS. **A** and **B:** Ventricular extrastimuli delivered when the His is refractory reset SVT using a left posterior bypass tract and delay subsequent to atrial activation. **C:** A ventricular extrastimulus delivered when the His is refractory terminates SVT. See text for explanation.

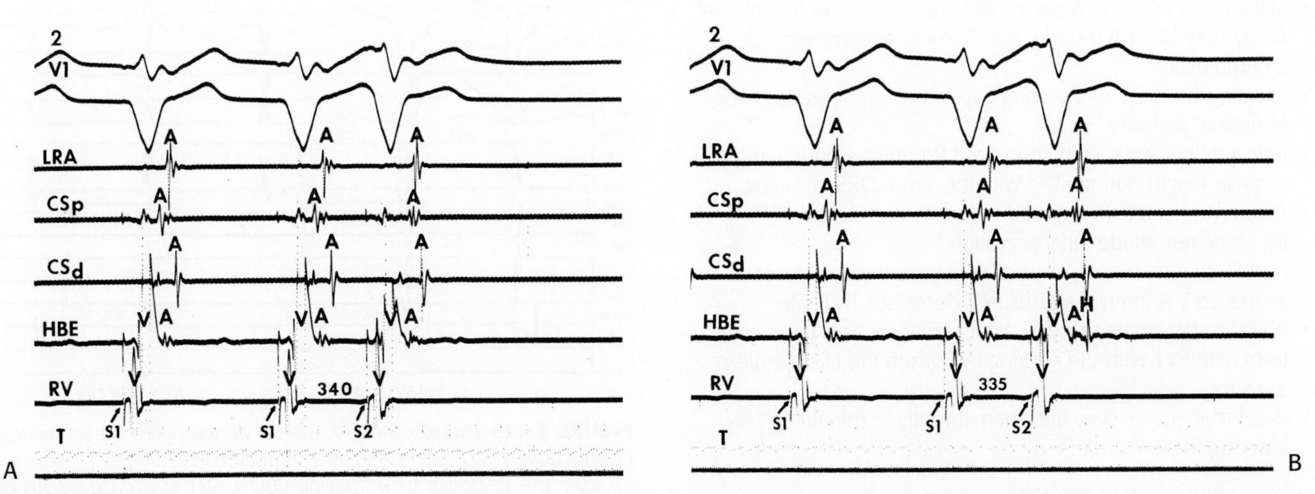


**FIGURE 8-127** *Demonstration of a septal bypass tract by simultaneous retrograde activation of the bypass tract and the normal A-V conduction system.* **A:** VPD ($S_2$, *arrow*) conducts retrogradely to the atrium with no V-A delay and a normal retrograde activation sequence. **B:** The presence of a septal bypass tract is confirmed when an earlier VPD retrogradely depolarizes the His bundle after retrograde atrial activation. See text for further discussion.

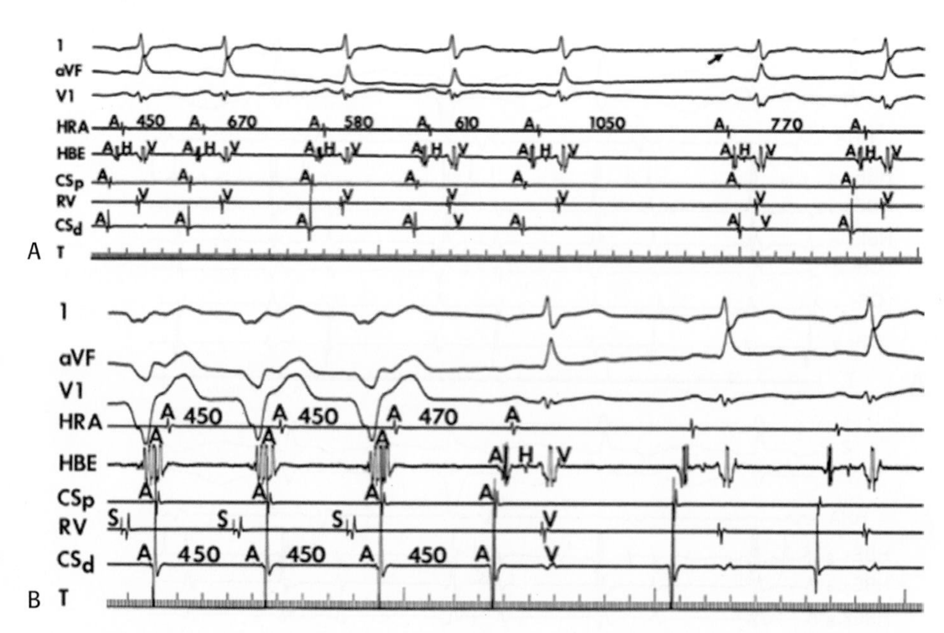


**FIGURE 8-128** *Slowly conducting left-sided bypass tract mimicking ectopic atrial rhythm.* **A:** The first five complexes appear to show an oscillatory left atrial rhythm with earliest activation in the distal coronary sinus ($CS_d$). One beat of sinus rhythm follows a pause, and the tachycardia again resumes. **B:** Ventricular pacing is used to distinguish automatic left atrial rhythm from circus movement tachycardia using a slowly conducting bypass tract. Ventricular pacing at 450 msec captures the atrium retrogradely with the same activation sequence as the tachycardia. On cessation of pacing, the first return cycle in the distal CS is 450 msec, thereby demonstrating entrainment of the tachycardia. This is diagnostic of a reentrant rhythm using a slowly conducting bypass tract. See text for discussion.

showed the mechanisms of the responses to ventricular overdrive pacing in atrial tachycardia, AVNRT, and AVRT. There are, however, limitations to these methods when trying to distinguish the uncommon form of AVNRT and AVRT using a decrementally conducting bypass tract. The limitations of para-Hisian pacing has been discussed above and shown in Figure 8-112. A pseudo–V-A-A-V response may be seen in either the atypical AVRNRT or a decrementally conducting bypass tract (Fig. 8-129). During overdrive ventricular pacing the V-A interval may exceed the paced cycle length giving rise to two atrial deflections following the last pace ventricular impulse suggesting a diagnosis of atrial tachycardia (Figure 8-100A). As seen in Figure 8-129 the second P occurs at the paced cycle length and represents a very long V-A interval. While decremental bypass tracts tend to have shorter V-A intervals and postpacing intervals than the uncommon form of AVNRT, there is significant overlap as shown in Figure 8-130. This results in nearly 50% of decrementally conducting bypass tracts having responses to ventricular pacing the fall into the range considered to be diagnostic of AVNRT. These bypass tracts typically demonstrate pseudo–V-A-A-V responses to pacing and demonstrate a delay in atrial activation in response to His-refractory VPCs (Fig. 8-125).

## TABLE 8-7 Criteria for A-V Reentrant SVT

- Initiation and termination by APDs, VPDs, or pacing.
- Initiation by APDs or A pacing depends on critical A-V interval. Delay may be in A-V node, His–Purkinje system, ventricle, or a combination.
- Initiation by VPDs or V pacing depends on retrograde block in normal pathway.
- Retrograde P wave with short-fixed R-P interval independent of cycle length during SVTs with the same QRS complex.
- Atrium and ventricle required to initiate and sustain SVT. Eccentric retrograde atrial activation.[a]
- Bundle branch block ipsilateral to bypass tract produces increased V-A interval and usually decreases SVT rate.[a]
- Ability to pre-excite or delay atrial activation, and/or to terminate SVT with VPD during SVT when the His bundle is refractory.
- Vagal maneuvers slow and then abruptly terminate SVT by blocking the A-V node.[b]

[a]Unless septal, retrograde atrial activation is "normal," and no change occurs with development of bundle branch block.

[b]When slowly conducting bypass tract is operative, vagal maneuvers can produce block in bypass tract in 30% of cases.

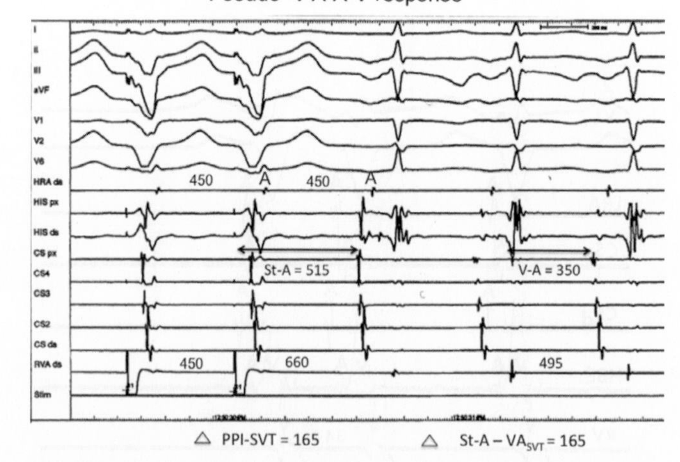


**FIGURE 8-129** *Pseudo–V-A-A-V interval during overdrive ventricular pacing during SVT using a decrementally conducting left paraseptal CBT.* The response to RV pacing during SVT at a cycle length of 495 msec using a decrementally conducting CBT is shown. The postpacing interval (PPI) is 165 msec longer than the SVT cycle length and the stimulus A is 165 msec longer than the $VA_{SVT}$ by 165 msec, both of which suggest AVNRT. See text for discussion.

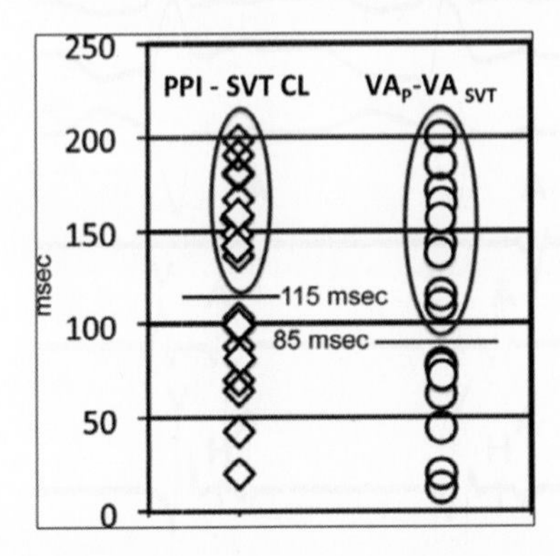


**FIGURE 8-130** *Postpacing responses of AVRT using a decremental septal accessory pathway.* Differences in PPI versus SVT-CL and $VA_P$ and $VA_{SVT}$ in 18 patients with septal decrementally conducting CBT. More than 50% of CBTs using decrementally conducting CBT meet PPI and V-A interval criteria that would suggest AVNRT. See text for discussion. (Data are a combination of those reported in Bennet M Te atl Circulation: Arrhythmia and Electrophysiology. 2011;4:506–509 and our laboratory.)

Termination of SVT using a CBT by ventricular extrastimuli results when the VPD blocks in the accessory pathway and collides with the antegradely conducting impulse somewhere in the normal conduction system or pre-excites the atrium with subsequent block of the atrial impulse in the AVN or His–Purkinje system either because of the prematurity of the atrial impulse (i.e., which encroaches on A-V nodal or His–Purkinje refractoriness) or due to retrograde concealment by the VPD, or both (Figs. 8-131 and 8-132). Block antegradely in the A-V conducting system is the most common finding because block in the accessory pathway retrogradely requires that the VPD encroach on the refractory period of the bypass tract. The ability of the VPD to block retrogradely in the CBT is determined by (a) the local refractory period at the site of stimulation, (b) the distance from the site of stimulation to the bypass tract, (c) the conduction time from the stimulus to the bypass tract, and (d) the retrograde refractory period of the bypass tract. Thus, termination of SVT by retrograde block in the bypass tract often requires early coupled VPDs, particularly when right ventricular stimulation is being used in a patient with a left-sided bypass tract (Fig. 8-132). In many patients, however, termination is possible by either modality (Fig. 8-133). VPD termination of an SVT is much more likely for a tachycardia using a CBT than for AVNRT. Termination by a single VPD is virtually pathognomonic of a bypass tract participating in the reentrant circuit in two circumstances: (a) termination of SVT by a late-coupled VPD (>80% of the SVT cycle length) and (b) termination of a single VPD of an SVT with a cycle length ≤300 msec. If SVT can be terminated by a VPD delivered when the His bundle is refractory, a CBT is necessarily operative.

In summary, termination of SVT using a CBT by atrial and/or ventricular stimulation may be quite complex because of the many potential sites of block. In a given tachycardia, block may occur at different sites, depending on the prematurity of the atrial or ventricular extrastimulus. In addition, block may occur following several complexes after the stimulated impulse. The changes in conduction and refractoriness produced by the premature impulse may set up oscillations that eventually find one component of the reentrant circuit refractory, and termination ensues. For example, a ventricular premature beat introduced during functional bundle branch block can normalize the tachycardia. Block will not occur in response to the premature beat, but the shortened cycle length that results from a decreased V-A interval during normalization of the QRS may result in block, either retrogradely or antegradely, one or more complexes after the VPD was delivered.

The mechanisms of termination that can be seen in response to ventricular and atrial extrastimuli may be seen spontaneously.[154–156] Obviously, the presence of multiple bypass tracts, dual A-V nodal pathways, and development or loss of functional bundle branch block play a major role in the variability of spontaneous termination. In general, however, spontaneous termination with retrograde block in the bypass tract without any perturbations usually results during very

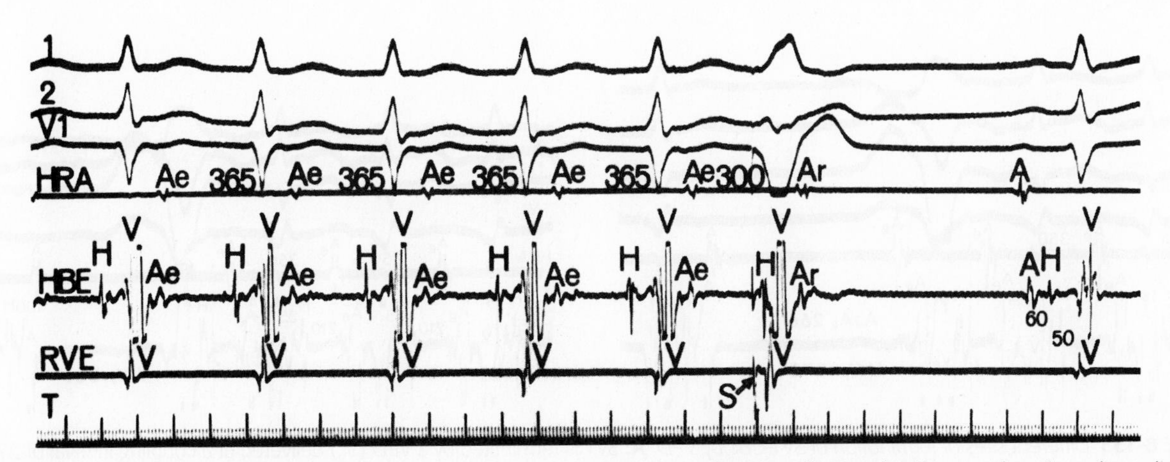


**FIGURE 8-131** *Termination of SVT using a CBT by a VPD when the His bundle is refractory.* Following the fifth complex of a tachycardia, a VPD is introduced when the His bundle is refractory. This pre-excites the atrium. Because of the prematurity of the atrial activation, block in the A-V node occurs, and the tachycardia terminates.

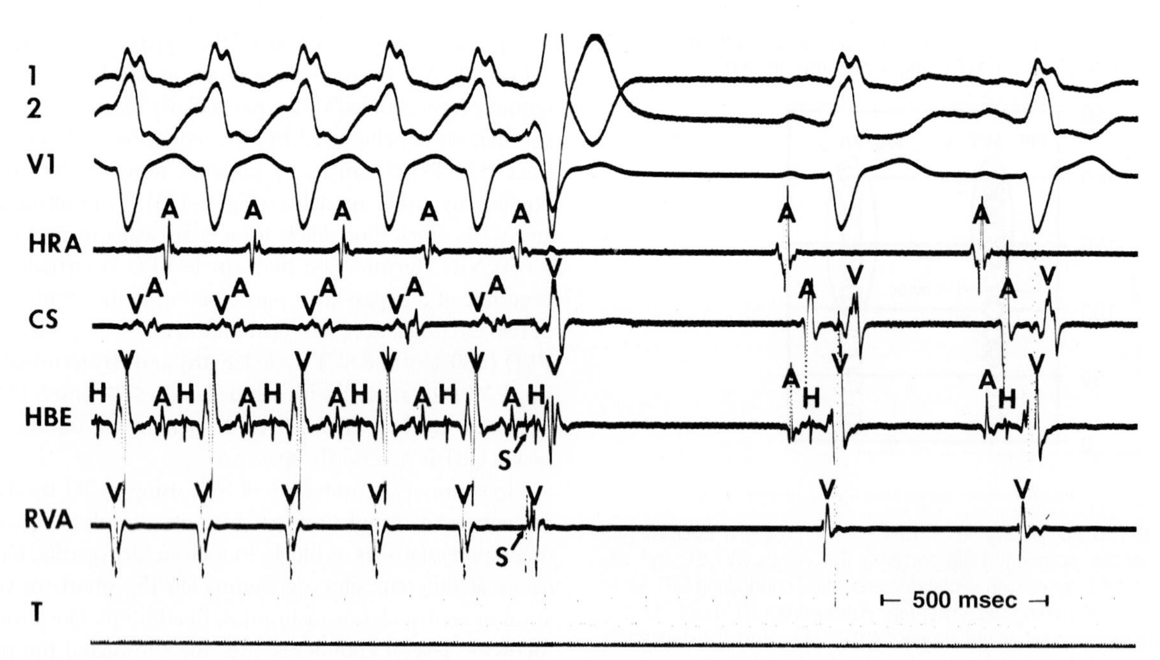


**FIGURE 8-132** *Termination of SVT by a VPD producing block in the bypass tract.* Following five complexes of a rapid SVT (270 msec), a VPD is introduced when the His bundle is refractory. Its ventricular extrastimulus blocks in the bypass tract retrogradely to terminate the tachycardia.

rapid tachycardias (Fig. 8-134) or with a sudden shortening cycle length as which might occur following loss of ipsilateral bundle branch block (Fig. 8-135). In our experience, antegrade block is more common as the cause of spontaneous termination. Usually, a gradual delay occurs before block, which may be associated with an oscillating cycle length with alternate complexes demonstrating a Wenckebach periodicity (Fig. 8-136). This type of termination is also common after administration of pharmacologic agents affecting A-V nodal conduction (see below).

## Effects of Pharmacologic and Physiologic Maneuvers During Supraventricular Tachycardia

The effects of pharmacologic agents in the treatment of SVT that results from CBT are unpredictable because many of the available drugs have differential actions on the bypass tract and on the AVN such that in some situations the agents may help perpetuate the arrhythmia. Diagnostically, however, if the administration of an agent produces infra-His block resulting in termination of the arrhythmia, one can infer that the ventricles were required to maintain the tachycardia and a CBT was operative. Perpetuation of the tachycardia in the presence of A-V nodal block does not exclude atrial tachycardias or AVNRT. The only relatively selective agents available are those primarily affecting the AVN. These drugs include calcium blockers (verapamil and diltiazem), a variety of beta blockers, digoxin, and adenosine. All of the agents prolong A-V nodal conduction and refractoriness and virtually always terminate SVT using a CBT by producing block in the AVN.[60,108,109,112–115,157–161] Verapamil rarely terminates SVT by blocking retrograde conduction over the bypass tract[162]; when it does, block is usually preceded by oscillation produced

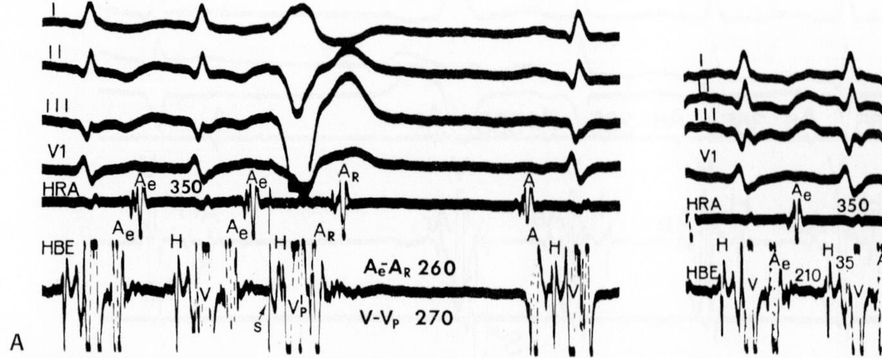


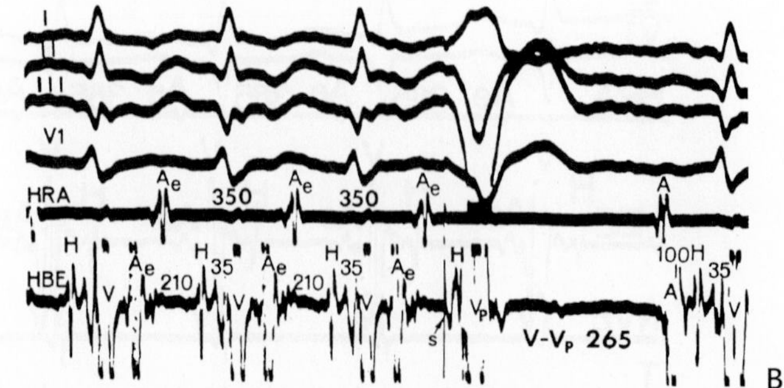


**FIGURE 8-133** *Different sites of termination of SVT-CBT by VPD.* **A:** SVT is terminated by a VPD ($V_p$) delivered at a coupling interval of 270 msec after antegrade depolarization of the His bundle (H appears on time). The atria are pre-excited ($A_e$-$A_r$ = 260 msec) and SVT terminates due to block of $A_r$ in the A-V node. **B:** When $V_p$ is introduced at a coupling interval of 265 msec, block occurs in the bypass tract (no retrograde conduction), terminating the tachycardia. See text for further discussion.

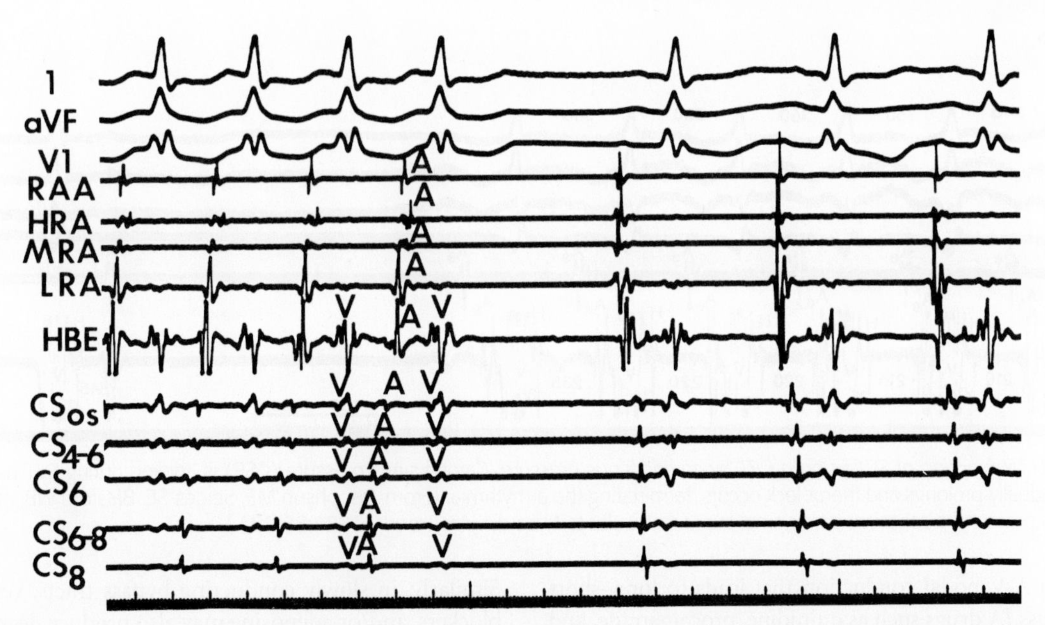


**FIGURE 8-134** *Spontaneous termination of SVT by retrograde block in the bypass tract.* The figure is arranged from top to bottom as leads 1, aVF, and electrograms from the right atrial appendage (RAA), HRA, mid-right atrium (MRA), low-right atrium (LRA), HBE, and five bipolar electrograms from the os of the $CS_{os}$, to the lateral margin of the CS. SVT utilizing a left lateral bypass tract is present at a short cycle length of 250 msec. The fourth QRS complex suddenly blocks in the bypass tract, terminating the tachycardia.

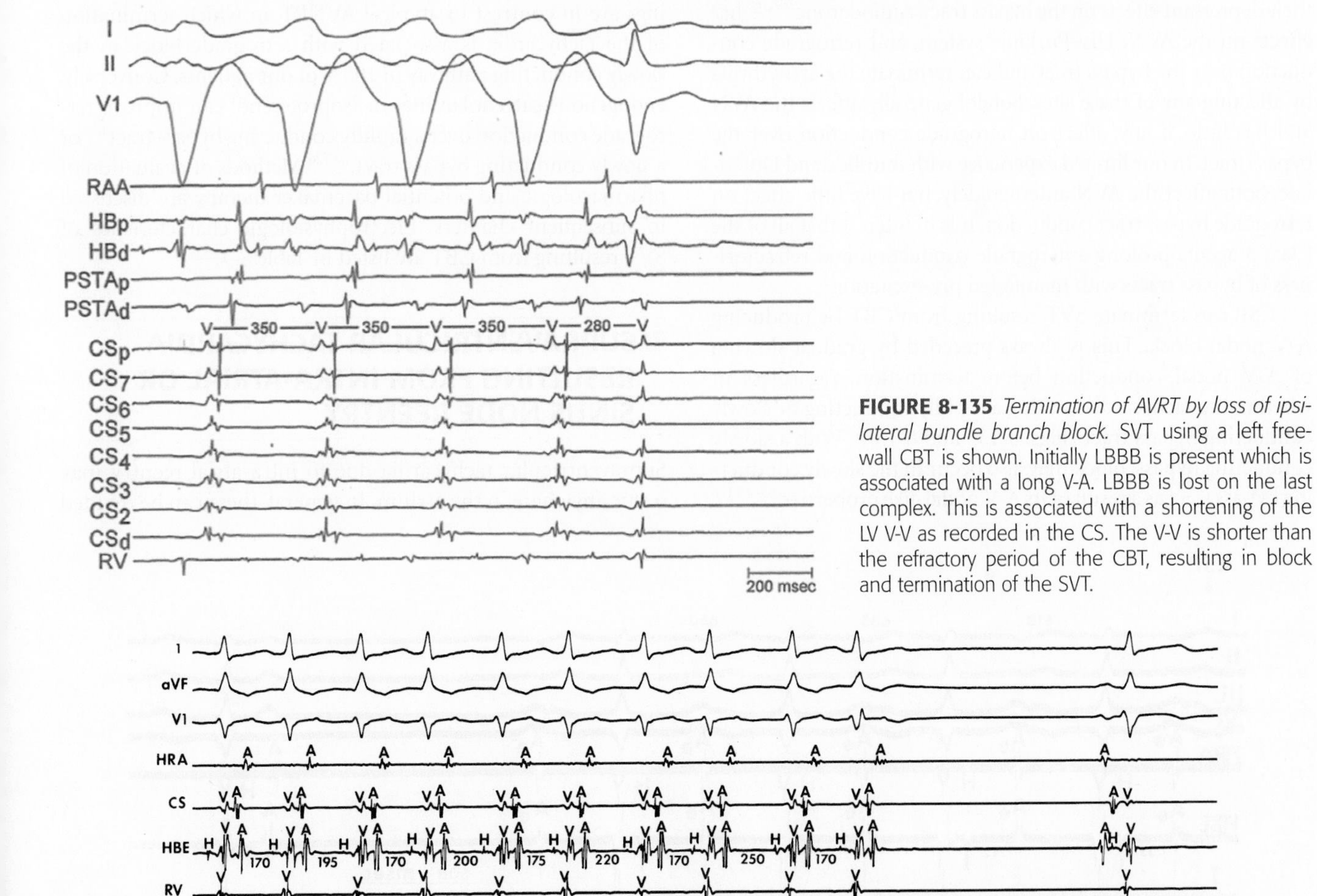


**FIGURE 8-135** *Termination of AVRT by loss of ipsilateral bundle branch block.* SVT using a left free-wall CBT is shown. Initially LBBB is present which is associated with a long V-A. LBBB is lost on the last complex. This is associated with a shortening of the LV V-V as recorded in the CS. The V-V is shorter than the refractory period of the CBT, resulting in block and termination of the SVT.

**FIGURE 8-136** *Termination of SVT using a CBT by A-V nodal block.* SVT using a left-sided CBT is shown with an oscillating cycle length demonstrating alternate beat Wenckebach phenomena. Every other A-H interval becomes progressively longer until it finally blocks in the A-V node, terminating the tachycardia.

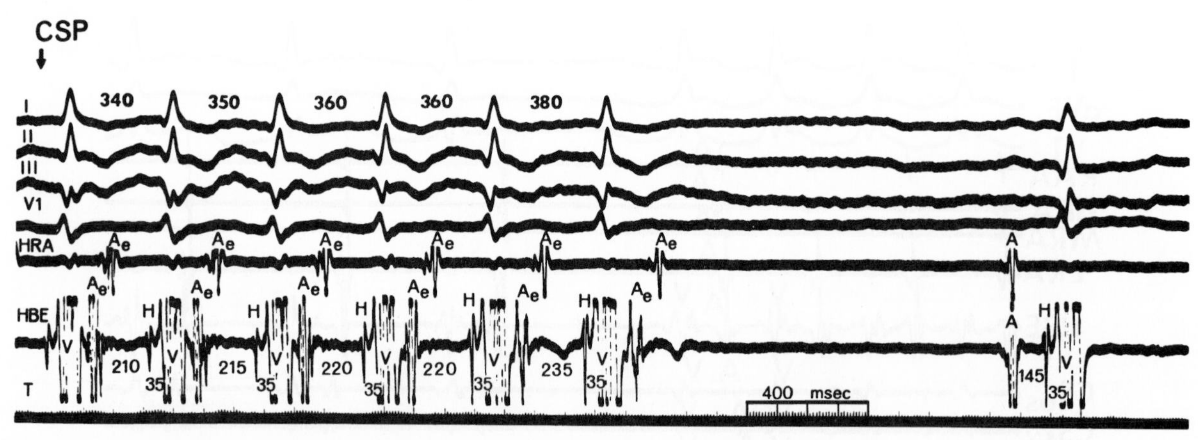


**FIGURE 8-137** *Termination of SVT using a CBT by carotid sinus pressure.* Carotid sinus pressure (CSP) is applied during SVT using a CBT. The A-H interval gradually prolongs and then block occurs, terminating the arrhythmia. (From Josephson ME, Seides SE, Batsford WB, et al. The effects of carotid sinus pressure in reentrant paroxysmal supraventricular tachycardia. *Am Heart J* 1974;88:694.)

by changes in A-V nodal conduction that leads to long–short sequences. Class IA drugs such as quinidine, procainamide, and disopyramide and Class IC drugs such as propafenone and flecainide are primarily effective by producing block in the bypass tract.[163–166] However, they have variable effects on A-V nodal and His–Purkinje conduction, both of which may counterbalance their depressant effects on the bypass tract. Amiodarone[167,168] has effects on the AVN, His–Purkinje system, and retrograde conduction over the bypass tract and can terminate the arrhythmia by affecting any of these sites. Sotalol generally affects the AVN and has little, if any, effect on retrograde conduction over the bypass tract. In our limited experience with Ibutilide and Dofetilide, both affect the AVN anterogradely, but have little effect on retrograde bypass tract conduction. It is of interest that all of the Class 3 agents prolong anterograde conduction and refractoriness of bypass tracts with manifested pre-excitation.

CSP can terminate SVT resulting from CBT by producing A-V nodal block. This is always preceded by gradual slowing of A-V nodal conduction before termination, regardless of whether the tachycardia is using a rapidly conducting or slowly conducting bypass tract (Figs. 8-137 and 8-138). With a slowly conducting bypass, block may also occur in the slowly conducting bypass tract as a result of its A-V nodal-like properties.[63–65,126] Similarly, in slowly conducting bypass tracts, verapamil, beta blockers, and/or adenosine may also produce decremental conduction and block. Overall, in our experience, CSP terminates SVT using slowly conducting bypass tracts by producing antegrade block in the AVN in almost two-thirds of the patients and in the bypass tract in the remaining one-third. These findings are in contrast to atypical AVNRT, in which termination of the tachycardia is associated with retrograde block in the slowly conducting pathway in 100% of our patients. Conversely, endogenous catecholamines or isoproterenol can improve retrograde conduction over a rapidly conducting bypass tract[156] or a slowly conducting bypass tract.[64,126] Methods of evaluation of pharmacologic and potential pacemaker therapy are discussed in subsequent chapters. Electrophysiologic characteristics of SVT resulting from CBT are listed in Table 8-7.

## SUPRAVENTRICULAR TACHYCARDIA RESULTING FROM INTRA-ATRIAL OR SINUS NODE REENTRY

Supraventricular tachycardia due to intra-atrial reentry may occur anywhere in the atrium. In general, these can be divided

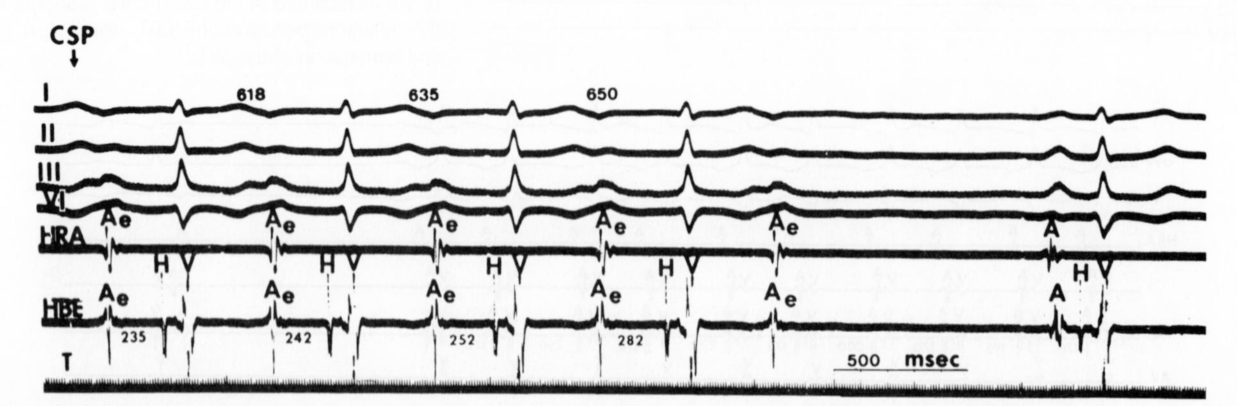


**FIGURE 8-138** *Termination of SVT using a slowly conducting bypass tract by carotid sinus pressure.* CSP is applied during a slow tachycardia using a slowly conducting left lateral bypass tract. Tachycardia termination occurs by progressive prolongation and then block in the A-V node. See text for discussion.

into those that have an activation sequence similar if not identical to that of the sinus node (termed sinus node reentry) and those that arise elsewhere in the atrium (intra-atrial reentry). Whether or not sinus node reentry should be distinguished from intra-atrial reentry is a matter of debate; however, because of its characteristic P-wave morphology and atrial activation sequence, sinus node reentry can be addressed as a selected subset of intra-atrial reentrant arrhythmias.

The possibility that reentry within the sinus node could be a mechanism for SVT was first suggested by Barker et al.[169] more than 55 years ago. Subsequently, experimental studies in animals, both in vitro and in vivo, and in humans have clearly shown that the sinus node can potentially function as a site of reentry in an analogous fashion to the AVN.[17,18,170–174] Most of these studies, however, have based diagnosis of sinus node reentry on indirect evidence dependent on atrial activation patterns comparable or similar to that of sinus rhythm. Only the in vitro study of Allessie and Bonke[170] actually mapped the reentrant pathway and localized it to the sinus node. More recent studies by the same group,[175] however, have cast doubt on the possibility of sustained reentry occurring solely within the sinus node based on the wave length (product of conduction velocity and refractory period), which would be necessary for a tachycardia using the sinus node. Thus, whether or not reentry localized solely within the sinus node can cause sustained, paroxysmal SVTs is not firmly established. From a practical standpoint, however, paroxysmal reentrant arrhythmias localized to the region of sinus node are considered "sinus node reentry" here. In all likelihood, the sinus node and/or perinodal tissue does *participate* in reentrant phenomena, probably by providing the slow conduction required for reentry. This is not surprising in light of the fact that the sinus node and perinodal tissue show certain electrophysiologic similarities to AVN. Although in most instances so-called sinus node reentry is limited to a single echo, sustained reentry resulting in clinical SVT has been demonstrated from the region of the sinus node.[17,18,174,176–178] In our experience, SVT secondary to so-called sinus node reentry accounts for only 1% of the arrhythmias in patients presenting with paroxysmal SVT, although 10% to 15% of patients undergoing electrophysiologic evaluation will exhibit isolated sinus node echoes. It is obviously difficult to distinguish "sinus node reentry" from arrhythmias arising in the region of the high crista. Intra-atrial reentry occurring at sites distant from the region of the sinus node is more common than sinus node reentry, occurring in approximately 5% of our patient population. In my experience the majority of intra-atrial reentrant SVTs arise in the right atrium or septum, in contrast to other types of atrial tachycardias which can arise in either atrium. Electrophysiologic features of sinus node and intra-atrial reentry are described in Tables 8-8 and 8-9.

Atrial reentrant arrhythmias tend to occur in patients with heart disease, particularly those with intra-atrial reentry distant from the sinus node. The rates of atrial reentrant arrhythmias vary, with sinus node reentry rates tending to be slower than other forms of atrial reentry, averaging approximately 130 bpm. Intra-atrial reentry outside the sinus node usually tends to be faster, with rates ranging from 120 to 240 bpm. The rates of these different tachycardias exhibit significant overlap, part of which is due to our inability to distinguish intra-atrial reentrant tachycardias from reentry localized to the sinus node. This is one reason why many investigators lump these arrhythmias under the term intra-atrial reentry.

**TABLE 8-8 Criteria for "Sinus Node" Reentrant SVT**

- Initiation and termination by APDs, VPDs, atrial pacing, and ventricular pacing independent of IACD or AVNCD.
- P waves identical to sinus in morphology and activation sequence.
- P-R related to SVT rate.
- A-V nodal block may exist without affecting SVT.
- Vagal maneuvers and adenosine slow and then abruptly terminate SVT.

AVNCD, A-V nodal conduction delay; IACD, intra-atrial conduction delay.

### *Mechanism of Initiation of Supraventricular Tachycardias Resulting from Intra-atrial Reentry*

As with the forms of reentrant SVT, both sinus node reentry and intra-atrial reentry are most frequently initiated by APDs or atrial pacing (Figs. 8-139 to 8-143).[17,18,174–178] However, unlike SVT resulting from AVNRT and SVT using a CBT, no A-V delay is required. Such delays may occur as a part of the normal response to APDs but are not necessary for initiation. Of diagnostic importance is the frequent initiation of intra-atrial reentry in the presence of A-V block (Fig. 8-143). This rules out the AVRT. Intra-atrial reentry can often be initiated over a wide range of coupling intervals ($A_1$-$A_2$) of APDs. This broad range depends on (a) the intrinsic degree of inhomogeneity in conduction and/or refractoriness in the atrium, sinus node, and perinodal tissue (factors not precisely quantifiable in humans) and (b) the distance of the stimulation site from the site of reentry. With regard to sinus node reentry, the slower the conduction in the sinus node and the closer the site of stimulation to the sinus node, the wider the tachycardia zone (i.e., the zone of coupling intervals of APDs that initiate SVT). Theoretically, a similar situation exists for other intra-atrial reentrant

**TABLE 8-9 Criteria for Intra-atrial Reentrant SVT (Distant from the Sinus Node)**

- Initiation by APDs only during atrial RRP resulting in IACD
- Atrial activation sequence different from sinus P-R related to SVT rate
- AVN block may exist without affecting SVT
- Vagal maneuvers or adenosine do not usually or reproducibly terminate SVT (may produce AVN block)

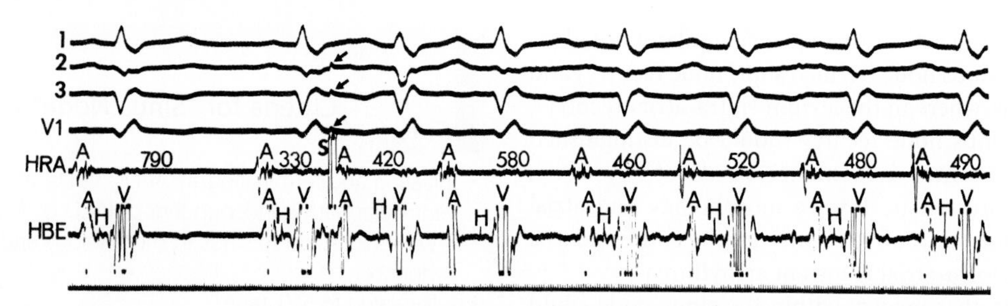


**FIGURE 8-139** *Initiation of sinus node reentrant SVT by an APD from the high-right atrium.* An APD (S, *arrow*) delivered at a coupling interval of 330 msec results in SVT in the absence of atrial latency. The P waves and atrial activation sequence during SVT are similar to sinus rhythm. Note the oscillation of cycle length at the onset of SVT.

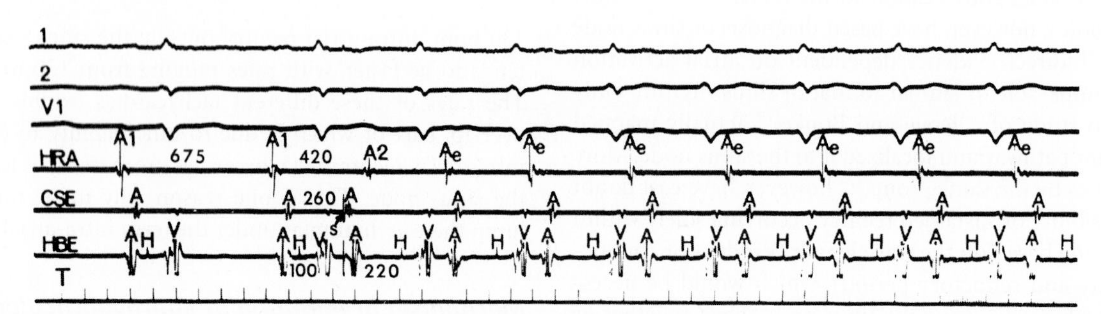


**FIGURE 8-140** *Initiation of sinus node reentrant SVT by an APD from the coronary sinus.* During sinus rhythm, an APD (S, *arrow*) is delivered from the coronary sinus (CSE) at a coupling interval of 260 msec. This impulse reaches the high-right atrium ($A_2$) at a coupling interval of 420 msec and results in SVT with a typical "sinus" atrial activation sequence.

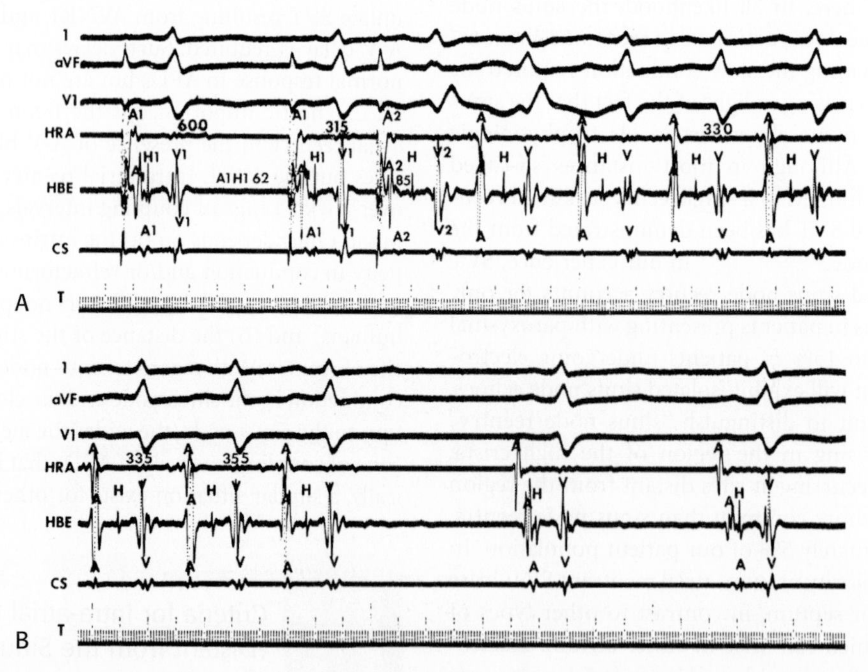


**FIGURE 8-141** *Initiation and termination of intra-atrial reentrant SVT.* **A:** An APD ($A_2$) is delivered from the high-right atrium (HRA) at a coupling interval of 315 msec during a basic paced cycle length ($A_1$-$A_1$) of 600 msec, initiating SVT. The atrial activation sequence during the SVT shows simultaneous atrial activation in the HRA, HBE, and CS, which is distinctly different from sinus rhythm as seen in **(B)** after spontaneous termination. Termination of SVT occurs abruptly after a slight prolongation of the tachycardia cycle length.

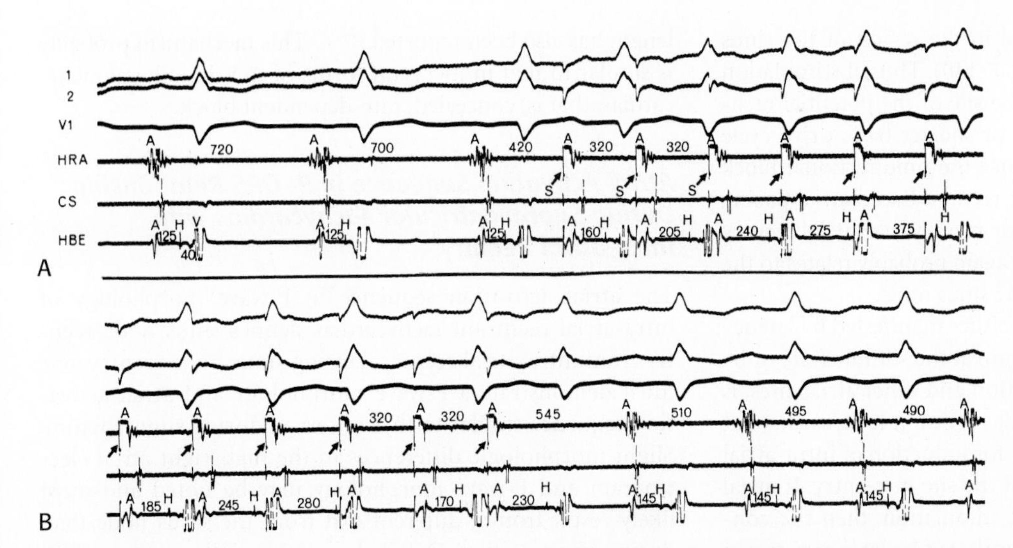


**FIGURE 8-142** *Initiation of sinus node reentrant SVT by atrial pacing.* The two panels are continuous. **A:** Atrial pacing at a cycle length of 320 msec is begun after two sinus beats. Pacing at this cycle length is associated with A-V nodal Wenckebach block (block in A-V node of the last P wave shown in **A** and the fourth P wave shown in **B**.) When pacing is discontinued, SVT is present with an atrial activation sequence similar to that of sinus rhythm.

sites. Although overlap in APD coupling intervals required for initiation of sinus node and intra-atrial tachycardias is considerable, atrial tachycardias outside the region of sinus node usually require APD coupling intervals shorter than those required for sinus node reentry. This may be related to the inherent slow conduction within the sinus node and perinodal tissues, which provides one of the important substrates required for reentry that may be absent in other parts of the atria. In other parts of the atria the mechanism of slow conduction differs (e.g., nonuniform anisotropy), and the size of the circuit may be in part determined by anatomic factors. In the absence of a critical role of nonuniform anisotropy in initiation of SVT, regardless of the site of stimulation, it is assumed that the coupling intervals required for initiation would be relatively constant if measured at the site of reentry. In most cases, this can be demonstrated only in sinus node reentry, where the measurements from the high-right atrial electrogram placed in the vicinity of the sinus node can be readily obtained. Although intra-atrial reentry of any type can be initiated from any region in the heart, the more distant the site of stimulation is from the site of reentry, the shorter the coupling intervals required for initiation. This finding explains why intra-atrial reentry (which can occur far from the sinus node in either atria) requires coupling intervals closer than that required for sinus node reentry during high-right atrial stimulation. When coronary sinus stimulation is used to initiate sinus node reentry, early coupled APDs are required

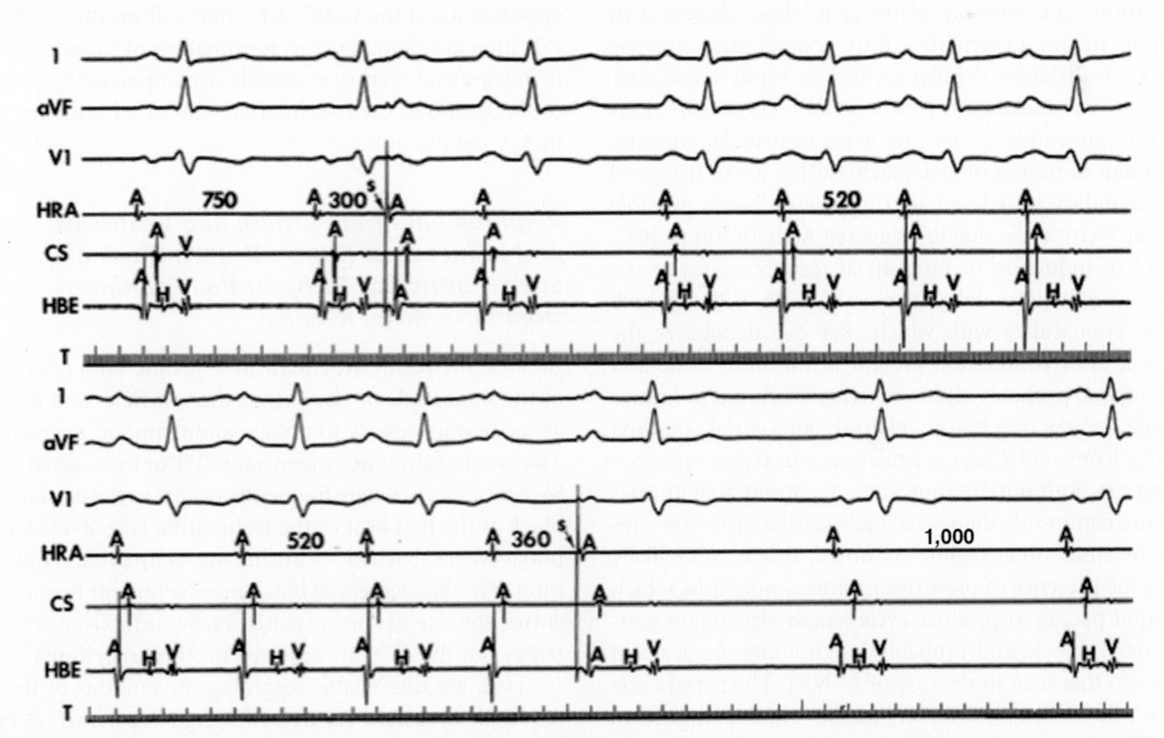


**FIGURE 8-143** *Initiation of AT in the presence of A-V block.* A single APD at a coupling interval of 300 msec blocks in the A-V node while initiating a tachycardia. The tachycardia continues with Wenckebach but is terminated with an APD.

to obtain the critical A-A interval in the region of the sinus node required to initiate SVT (Fig. 8-140). Thus, if stimulation is carried out very distant from the site of the potential reentrant circuit, two or more APDs or shorter basic drive cycle lengths may be required to produce the unidirectional block and slow conduction required for reentry. Rapid atrial pacing can more reliably induce sinus node reentry than atrial reentry from other sites (Fig. 8-142). This again probably relates to the pre-existent slow conduction in the sinus node.

Intra-atrial conduction delay, either manifested by latency from the stimulus to the electrogram at the stimulus site or by delay between the site of stimulation and other atrial sites, is not necessary to initiate sinus node reentrant tachycardia, but it is associated with and necessary for induction of intra-atrial reentry, particularly if recorded at the site of reentry. If atrial reentry is localized to the site of stimulation, then the conduction delay required will be manifested by latency between the stimulus spike in the local atrial electrogram noted before the onset of initiation of the tachycardia. In most instances, one does not initiate reentry at the site of stimulation. In such cases it is difficult to ascertain the site of conduction delay in the atrium. Multiple recording sites in both atria are required to record the site of critical conduction delay and/or block necessary for the development of atrial tachycardias distant from the site of stimulation. Thus, observation of block and/or slow conduction required for reentry distant to stimulation site has been rarely reported.[18]

Initiation of intra-atrial reentrant rhythms by ventricular stimulation is uncommon except in the presence of a retrogradely conducting bypass tract, in which case, retrograde atrial activation is very rapid, and coupling intervals of ventricular stimuli are virtually identical to those delivered in the atrium. In our experience, sinus node reentry may be induced by ventricular depolarizations or rapid ventricular pacing.[174,178] The initiation of intra-atrial reentry in regions outside the sinus node is very rare using ventricular stimulation although initiation of atrial tachycardia due to triggered activity secondary to delayed afterdepolarizations is possible (see "Atrial Tachycardia due to Triggered Activity" on p. 268). The rarity of induction of intra-atrial reentry relates to the retrograde conduction delay associated with VPDs, which limits the prematurity with which they can depolarize the atrium. The slow conduction present in the sinus node and perinodal tissue probably allows ventricular stimuli to induce sinus node reentry despite the relatively long atrial coupling that results from ventricular stimulation. Atrial and ventricular pacing can both initiate sinus node reentrant arrhythmias much more commonly than atrial tachycardias arising at sites outside the sinus node region. As noted, this is most likely related to the presence of pre-existent slow conduction, which allows rapid pacing to produce cycle length–dependent conduction delay, block, and probably longitudinal dissociation analogous to that seen in the case of AVNRT. The paced cycle lengths at which sinus node reentry can be induced range from 300 to 660 msec. Initiation of sinus node reentrant tachycardia associated with spontaneous shortening of the sinus cycle length has also been reported.[177,179] This mechanism probably is similar to that in incessant forms of A-V junctional tachycardias, that is, concealed, rate-dependent block.

### *Atrial Activation Sequence in P–QRS Relationship During Supraventricular Tachycardias with Intra-atrial Reentry*

The atrial activation sequence in P-wave morphology of intra-atrial reentrant tachycardias defines sinus node reentry from intra-atrial reentry. During sinus node reentry, one must demonstrate a P-wave morphology and atrial activation sequence similar to that observed during sinus rhythm. Slight morphologic differences in the high-right atrial electrogram and P-wave morphology may be noted and most likely result from a different exit from the sinus node than during sinus rhythm. Detailed mapping of the entire atrium still shows an activation sequence similar to the atrial activation sequence during sinus rhythm. In intra-atrial reentry localized to regions outside the sinus node, the atrial activation sequence will differ, as will the P-wave morphology (Fig. 8-144). The differences may be marked, such as reentry originating in the left atrium, or may merely show a right atrial or septal origin that has a distinctly different intra-atrial activation sequence.

The P-R and A-H intervals during the tachycardia are appropriate for the rate. In most cases, the P-R is shorter than the R-P interval; however, in the presence of pre-existent A-V nodal conduction delay, the P-R may be longer than the R-P and may even fall within the QRS and mimic AVNRT from the surface ECG (Fig. 8-145). Right atrial pacing at rates approximating the tachycardia rate will produce comparable P-R intervals. Spontaneous termination of sinus node reentry or intra-atrial reentry is usually accompanied by progressive prolongation of the A-A interval with or without any changes in A-V conduction.

### *Requirement of the Atrium and Ventricles and Influence of Bundle Branch Block on Supraventricular Tachycardia Resulting from Intra-atrial Reentry*

Because the reentrant circuit involves the atria (in the region of the sinus node or elsewhere), the ventricles and most of the atria are unnecessary to initiate and maintain the tachycardia. The onset of sinus node reentrant SVT or intra-atrial reentrant SVT located elsewhere frequently occurs in the presence of A-V block at the first beat of the tachycardia (Fig. 8-143), and A-V nodal Wenckebach block during the tachycardia is not uncommon. Variable degrees of block may be present throughout the entire episode of the sustained tachycardia. Neither the ventricles nor the AVN are required for this arrhythmia.

Data are unavailable regarding the amount of the atrium required to sustain reentry. Although experimental evidence initially suggested that reentry could occur in the sinus node alone,[170] doubt was cast on this finding in later experiments.[175]

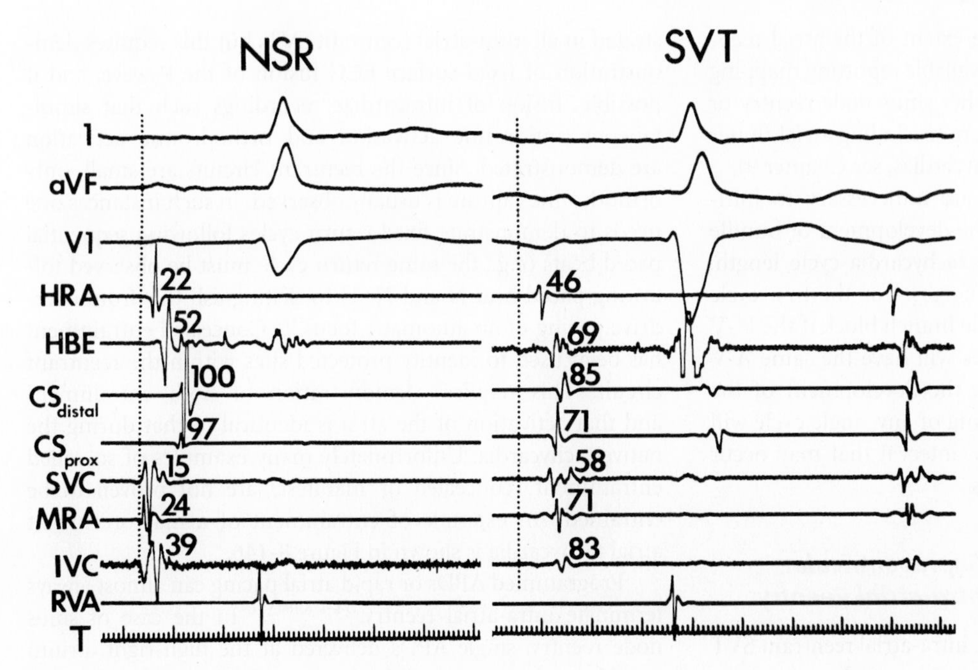


**FIGURE 8-144** *Comparison of atrial activation during normal sinus rhythm and during SVT that is due to intra-atrial reentry.* Leads 1, aVF, and $V_1$ are shown with electrograms from the HRA, HBE, distal and proximal CS, superior vena cava (SVC), mid-right atrium (MRA), inferior vena cava (IVC), and right ventricular apex (RVA). The P wave also differ. See text for discussion.

Probably no more than a few square centimeters are necessary to sustain reentry, and therefore the remaining atrial tissue is unnecessary. The extent of atrial participation can be evaluated by introducing APDs from different sites in the atrium and seeing how much of the atrium can be depolarized without influencing the tachycardias. In sinus node reentry, the mid- and low-right atrium and entire left atrium can be depolarized without affecting the tachycardia, confirming that the tachycardia is localized to an area high in the right atrium. Detailed stimulation from areas closer to the sinus node with high-density mapping in that region would be necessary to ascertain the actual extent of reentrant circuit. Similarly, the extent of atrial tissue required for intra-atrial reentry can be grossly defined. It is even more difficult, however, to map a region of reentry with atrial tachycardias localized outside the region of the sinus node in humans. High-density mapping during

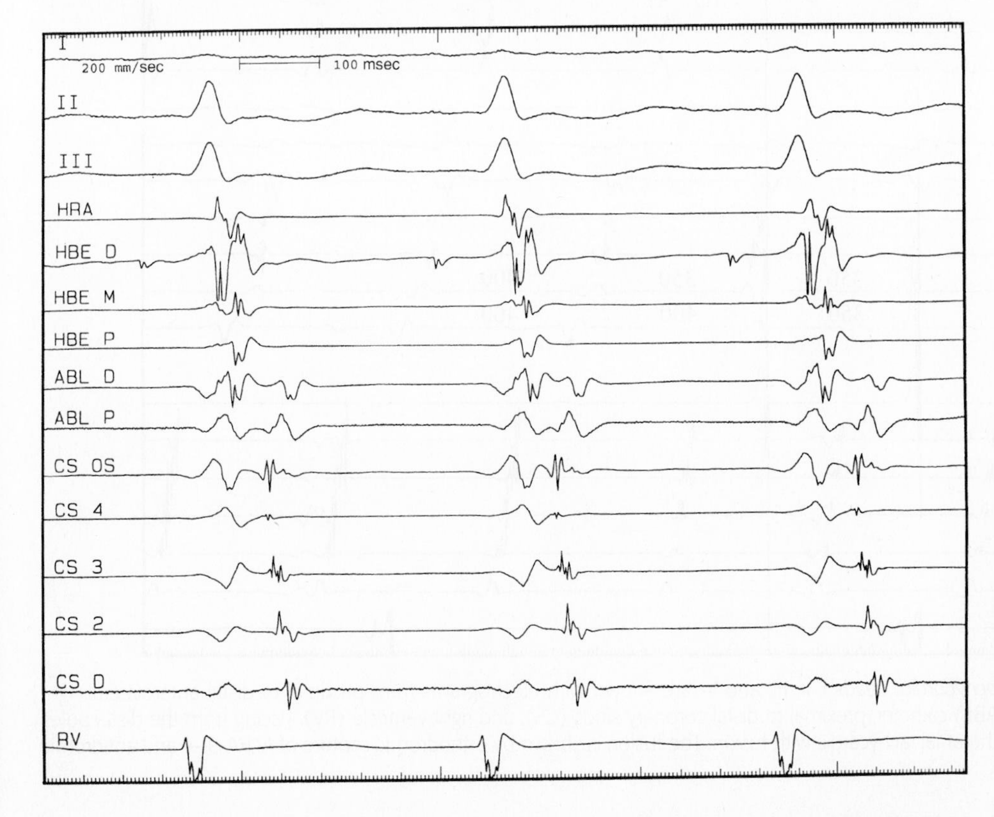


**FIGURE 8-145** *Intra-atrial reentrant SVT with simultaneous activation of the atrium and ventricle, mimicking AVNRT.* ECG leads I, II, III are shown with electrograms from the HRA, distal (D), mid (M), and proximal (P) HBE, distal and proximal ablation (ABL) CS OS to CS distal. SVT at a cycle length of 360 msec is present. Atrial tachycardia (high to low activation sequence) is associated with a long P-R due to conduction down a slow A-V nodal pathway resulting in simultaneous atrial and ventricular activation, mimicking AVNRT.

tachycardias is needed to define the extent of the atrial reentrant circuit. Currently, no data are available reporting mapping of the entire reentrant circuit of either sinus node reentry or intra-atrial reentry localized elsewhere (excluding atrial flutter and other macroreentrant atrial tachycardias, see Chapter 9).

Because infra-atrial structures are unnecessary to initiate and maintain the tachycardia, the development of bundle branch block has no effect on the tachycardia cycle length. The P-R interval may transiently increase for the first cycle following the development of bundle branch block if the H-V interval increases. Subsequent cycles will have the same A-V conduction as cycle lengths before the development of the bundle branch block. The lengthening of any single cycle will always equal the increment in H-V interval that may occur when bundle branch block develops.

### *Effects of Stimulation During Supraventricular Tachycardias Resulting from Intra-atrial Reentry*

As with other reentrant arrhythmias, intra-atrial reentrant SVT can be reset and entrained.[180,181] Resetting can demonstrate a fully excitable gap as manifested by a flat or mixed (flat and increasing) return cycle, or a partially excitable gap manifested by an increasing return cycle.[180] Entrainment can be demonstrated in all intra-atrial reentrant SVTs but this requires demonstration of fixed surface ECG fusion of the P wave, and if possible, fusion of intracardiac recordings such that simultaneous antidromic activation and orthodromic activation are demonstrated. Since the reentrant circuits are small, only orthodromic capture is usually observed. In such instances one needs to demonstrate fixed return cycles following sequential paced beats (e.g., the same return cycle must be observed following paced beat N and N+1) to distinguish this from overdrive pacing of an automatic focus.[182] Concealed entrainment has been used to identify protected sites within the reentrant circuit. This requires demonstration of both entrainment and that activation of the atria is identical to that during the native tachycardia. Unfortunately many examples of so-called entrainment (concealed or manifest) are not proven to be entrained. An example of entrainment of a macroreentrant atrial tachycardia is shown in Figure 8-146.

Programmed APDs or rapid atrial pacing can almost always terminate intra-atrial reentry.[174–178,180,181] In the case of sinus node reentry, single APDs delivered at the high-right atrium are almost always successful, whereas two APDs or rapid pacing may be needed if stimulation is performed from a site distant to the sinus node (e.g., left atrium). An analogous situation occurs when intra-atrial reentry occurs elsewhere in the atrium. In this

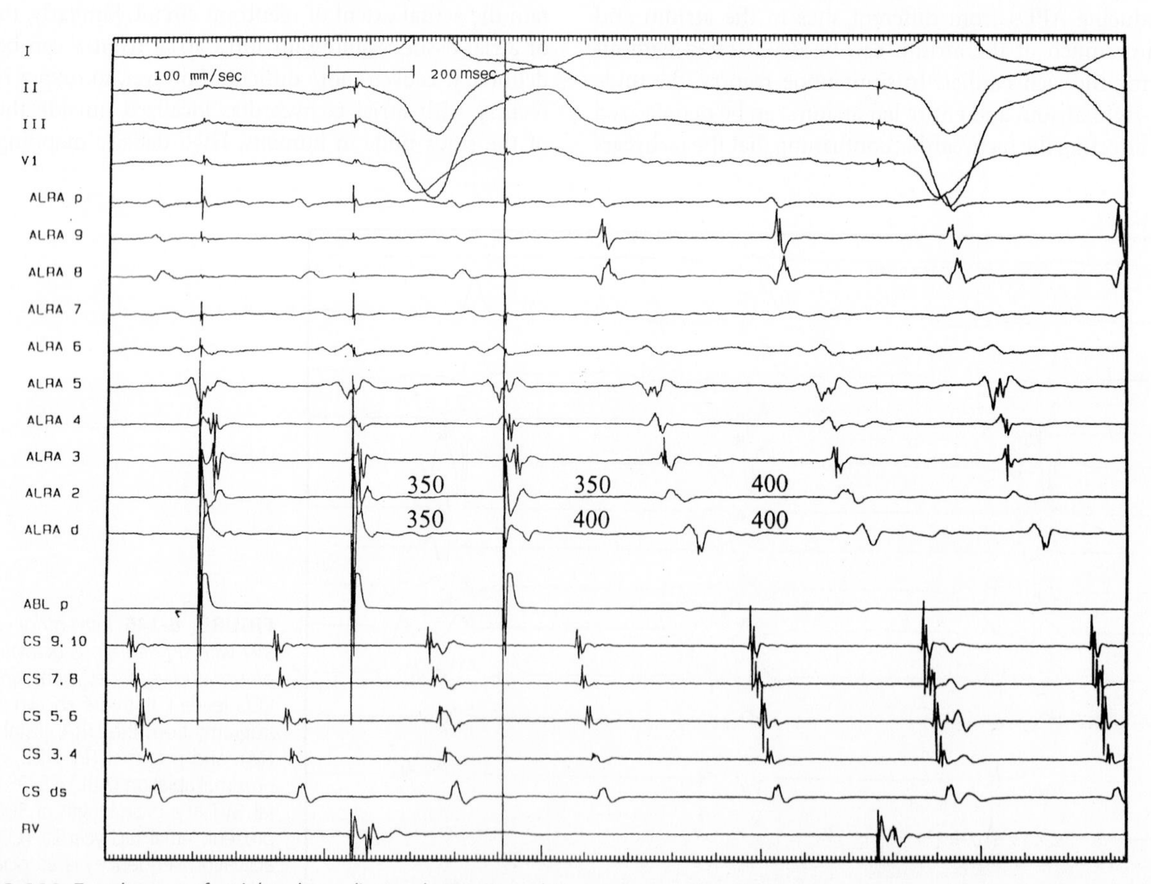


**FIGURE 8-146** *Entrainment of atrial tachycardia.* Leads I, II, III, and $V_1$ are shown with electrograms from proximal to distal anterolateral right atrium (ALRA p, ALRA d), the ablation (ABL) catheter, proximal to distal coronary sinus (CS), and right ventricle (RV). Pacing from the distal poles of the ABL catheter (not seen) entrains the atrial tachycardia with fusion. The fusion is shown by orthodromic capture of ALRA 9–4 and antidromic capture of ALRA d, 2, 3.

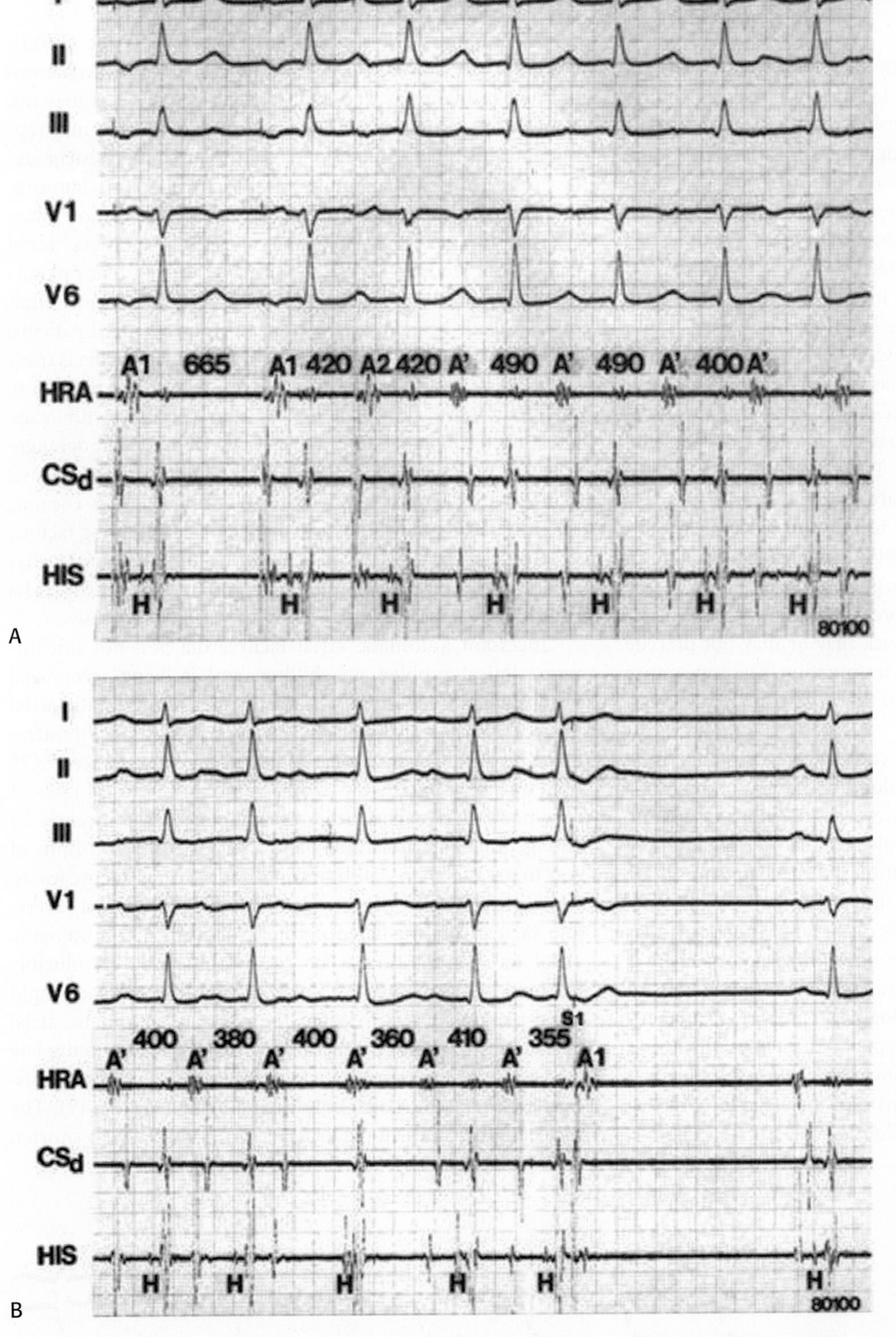


**FIGURE 8-147** *Initiation and termination of right atrial tachycardia from the coronary sinus.* Both panels are arranged from top to bottom as ECG leads I, II, III, $V_1$, and $V_6$ and electrograms from the HRA, CS distal, and HIS. **A:** During a paced cycle length of 665 msec a single premature CS complex initiates a right atrial tachycardia which is slightly irregular. **B:** During SVT a CS premature complex at an interval of 355 msec terminates the tachycardia.

instance, stimulation closest to the earliest site of atrial activation will be more likely to terminate the arrhythmia than if stimulation occurs distant from that site. Initiation and termination of intra-right atrial reentry can be accomplished by stimuli from the right (Fig. 8-143) and left atrium (Fig. 8-147). Ventricular pacing and VPDs theoretically can terminate these arrhythmias if 1:1 V-A conduction is present and continues at rapid pacing rates.[174] Sinus node reentry or those atrial tachycardias due to triggered activity (see subsequent discussion) are more likely to be terminated than intra-atrial reentry by ventricular stimulation. This finding probably is related to the tachycardia cycle length. VPDs rarely can terminate intra-atrial reentrant rhythms, because retrograde V-A delay and/or block limits the prematurity at which the retrograde atrial impulse can reach the area of reentry.

### *Physiologic and Pharmacologic Maneuvers During Supraventricular Tachycardias Resulting from Intra-atrial Reentry*

CSP reproducibly slows and terminates sinus node reentrant tachycardias (Fig. 8-148). These tachycardias also respond to other vagal maneuvers and adenosine. Intra-atrial reentry outside the region of the sinus node shows a variable response to CSP. We have found that 15% of atrial reentrant tachycardias arising outside the sinus node can also be terminated by CSP or adenosine. These tachycardias were distinguished from those that could not be interrupted by CSP or adenosine by the fact that they were all localized to the right atrium and tended to have longer cycle lengths (mean cycle length of intra-atrial SVT responding was 430 msec). The mechanisms by which these tachycardias are terminated is unclear, but the right atrial location suggests some role of the muscarinic or adenosine receptors either directly (on $K^+$ channels) or indirectly via adenyl cyclase. These arrhythmias must be distinguished from atrial tachycardias due to triggered activity which are typically able to be terminated by vagal maneuvers and adenosine. Whenever CSP or adenosine terminate an intra-atrial reentrant tachycardia, gradual slowing of the atrial cycle length typically occurs before termination. Atrioventricular conduction delay and/or block may or may not precede or be associated with tachycardia termination. The appearance of A-V block with maintenance of the SVT strongly suggests a supranodal origin.

No large studies have been conducted to systematically determine the effect of pharmacologic manipulation on intra-atrial reentrant arrhythmias. However, intravenous verapamil, digitalis, amiodarone, and beta blockers can terminate these arrhythmias.[177,178] While termination is the rule for sinus node reentry, reentry remote from the sinus node may also respond. In my experience approximately one-third of tachycardias distant from the sinus node respond to these agents. There is some disagreement in the literature about responsiveness of intra-atrial reentry to pharmacologic and physiologic maneuvers.[180,181] Reasons for this discrepancy include (a) inclusion of atrial flutter; (b) excluding sinus node reentry; (c) failing to adequately define the mechanism of the atrial tachycardia; and (d) different patient populations.

## AUTOMATIC ATRIAL TACHYCARDIA

Although the vast majority of paroxysmal SVT is due to reentry, enhanced automaticity is the most common mechanism of atrial tachycardias studied in our laboratory. This may not represent its frequency in the general population, but may represent the fact that automatic atrial tachycardia is persistent and less easily treated than other atrial tachycardia mechanisms. As a consequence, it is more symptomatic so it is more often referred for electrophysiologic evaluation. Automatic atrial tachycardia tends to be either chronic and persistent or transient and related to specific events.[17,18,180,183–185] In most adult cases, organic heart disease is present. In hospitalized patients, the most common form of automatic atrial tachycardia is transient. This is most often associated with myocardial infarction, exacerbation of chronic lung disease, especially with acute infection, alcohol ingestion, and a variety of metabolic derangements (e.g., hypokalemia). Specifically, catecholamine release, hypoxia, atrial stretch, and drugs (e.g., amphetamines, cocaine, caffeine, and theophylline) are important precipitating factors. Because most hospitalized patients with automatic atrial tachycardia are severely ill, the studies of automatic atrial tachycardia have only been performed in incessant and chronic cases.

Incessant automatic atrial tachycardia is a not uncommon clinical problem in children and is being recognized more frequently in adults.[184,185] The rates of automatic atrial tachycardia at rest are usually slower than those of intra-atrial reentrant tachycardia. Typically, they never exceed 175 bpm and may be as slow as 100 bpm. However, the rates of automatic atrial tachycardias are influenced significantly by endogenous catecholamines and can go from 100 bpm at rest to greater than 250 bpm on exercise. Such tachycardias, when present for long periods of time, can lead to a reversible tachycardia-mediated cardiomyopathy.[186–188] Automatic atrial tachycardia cannot be predictably and reproducibly initiated or terminated by single or multiple APDs or rapid atrial pacing.[16–18,183–185] When the onset of automatic atrial tachycardia is observed, the first complex usually occurs late in the cardiac cycle and is therefore unassociated with significant atrial or A-V nodal conduction delay (Fig. 8-149). The cycle length of the ectopic focus tends to progressively shorten

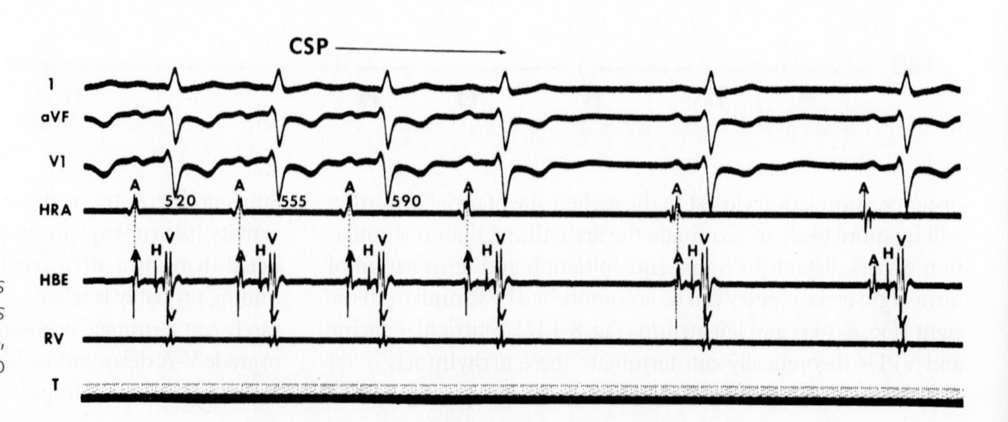


**FIGURE 8-148** *Termination of sinus node reentrant SVT by carotid sinus pressure (CSP).* CSP gradually slows, then abruptly terminates SVT due to sinus node reentry.

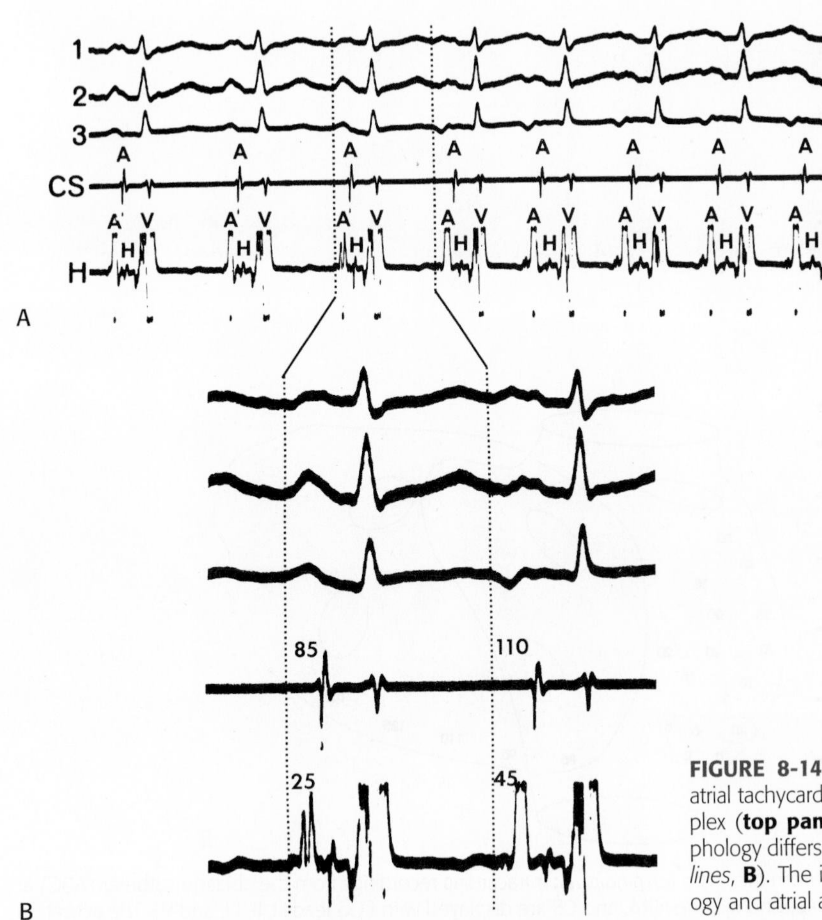


**FIGURE 8-149** *Initiation of automatic atrial tachycardia.* Automatic atrial tachycardia (AAT) begins spontaneously after the third sinus complex (**top panel**). No A-H prolongation is required. The P-wave morphology differs from sinus, as does the atrial activation sequence (*dotted lines*, **B**). The initial and subsequent P waves have the same morphology and atrial activation sequence. See text for further discussion.

for several cycles until its ultimate rate is achieved (warm-up). Because the rhythm is initiated by enhanced automaticity of a single focus, the first and subsequent P-wave and atrial activation sequences are identical. The same is true for triggered atrial tachycardias. This is in contrast to most forms of **reentrant** SVT, in which the initial and subsequent P waves differ. The initial and subsequent P waves of a reentrant SVT can be the same only if the reentrant circuit is very small and is localized near the site of stimulation or during incessant tachycardias induced by sinus node acceleration where concealed block is produced by sinus node acceleration and slow conduction is already present. The atrial activation sequence during automatic atrial tachycardia depends on the site of the automatic focus but always differs from normal sinus rhythm. The most common sites of origin of automatic tachycardias are along the crista terminalis, the atrial appendages, the triangle of Koch, the pulmonary veins, and the coronary sinus. Most early sites exhibit multicomponent electrograms suggesting poor coupling in the region of enhanced impulse formation. Whether or not the uncoupling is necessary to allow automaticity to occur is unknown. Examples of an atrial tachycardia arising from the crista terminalis and the os of the coronary sinus are shown in Figures 8-150 and 8-151.

The P-R and A-H intervals during automatic atrial tachycardia are directly related to the rate of the tachycardia; the faster the rate, the longer the intervals. As with other SVTs originating in the atria, automatic atrial tachycardia can exist in the presence of A-V block, and most of the chronic SVTs associated with A-V block are probably examples of automatic atrial tachycardia. The physiologic maneuvers such as CSP that selectively produce A-V block do not generally affect the automatic focus, and automatic atrial tachycardia continues (Fig. 8-152). However, in the majority of our patients (particularly with atrial tachycardias localized to the crista and the low atrial septum) adenosine produces transient slowing of the atrial tachycardia, but does not terminate it (Fig. 8-153). Of all the pharmacologic agents only beta blockers have been useful in transient cases. Incessant atrial tachycardia responds poorly to antiarrhythmic agents and therapy is either a curative ablation (see Chapter 15) or rate control. Because the focus is in the atrium, bundle branch block also does not influence the tachycardia, and unless the H-V interval prolongs on the development of bundle branch block, the QRS intervals will also be unchanged. Marked prolongation of the H-V interval, however, may alter the cycle at which bundle branch block first developed.

The effects of stimulation during automatic atrial tachycardia are similar to those reported for other automatic tissues (e.g., the sinus node).[180,183–185] APDs delivered at long coupling intervals, especially from sites distant to the automatic focus, do not affect the focus, and full compensatory pauses result. More premature APDs reset the automatic focus (Fig. 8-154). The pauses during resetting are less than compensatory. After

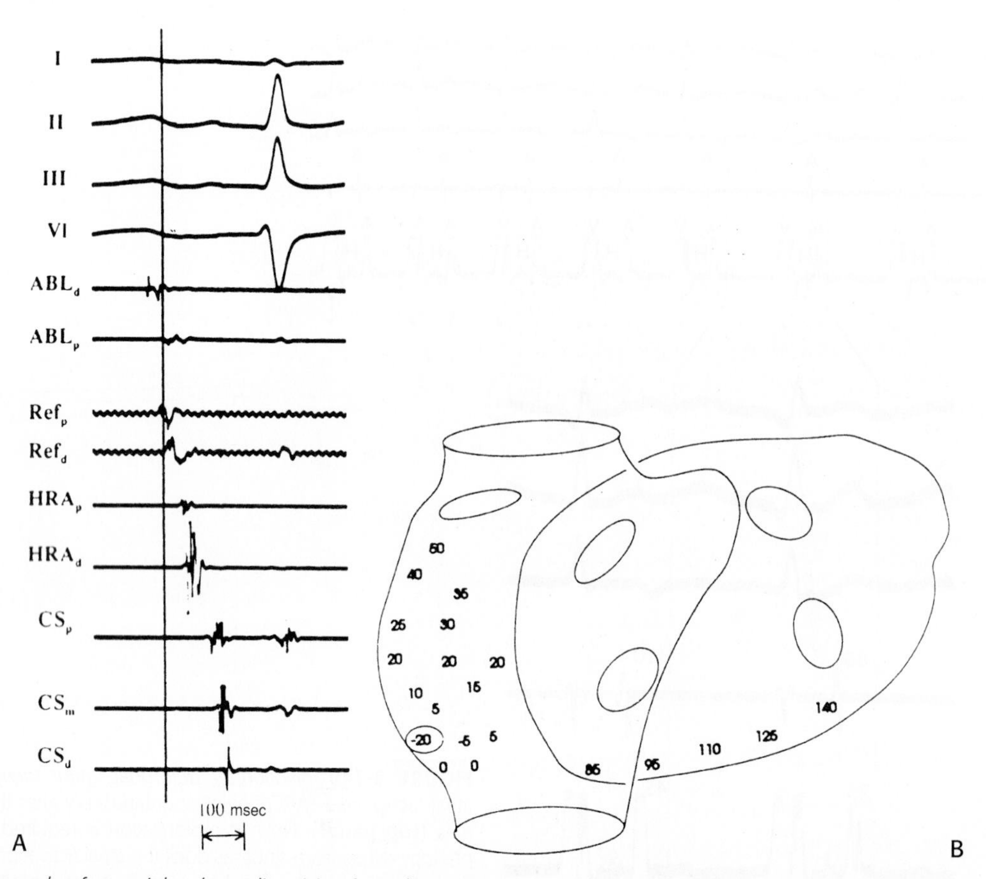


**FIGURE 8-150** *Example of an atrial tachycardia arising from the crista terminalis.* **A:** Intracardiac recordings from the ablation catheter (ABC) at the low crista terminals, a reference (Ref) catheter in the appendage, the HRA, and CS are displayed with ECG leads I, II, III, and $V_1$. The activation times are schematically depicted in **B**.

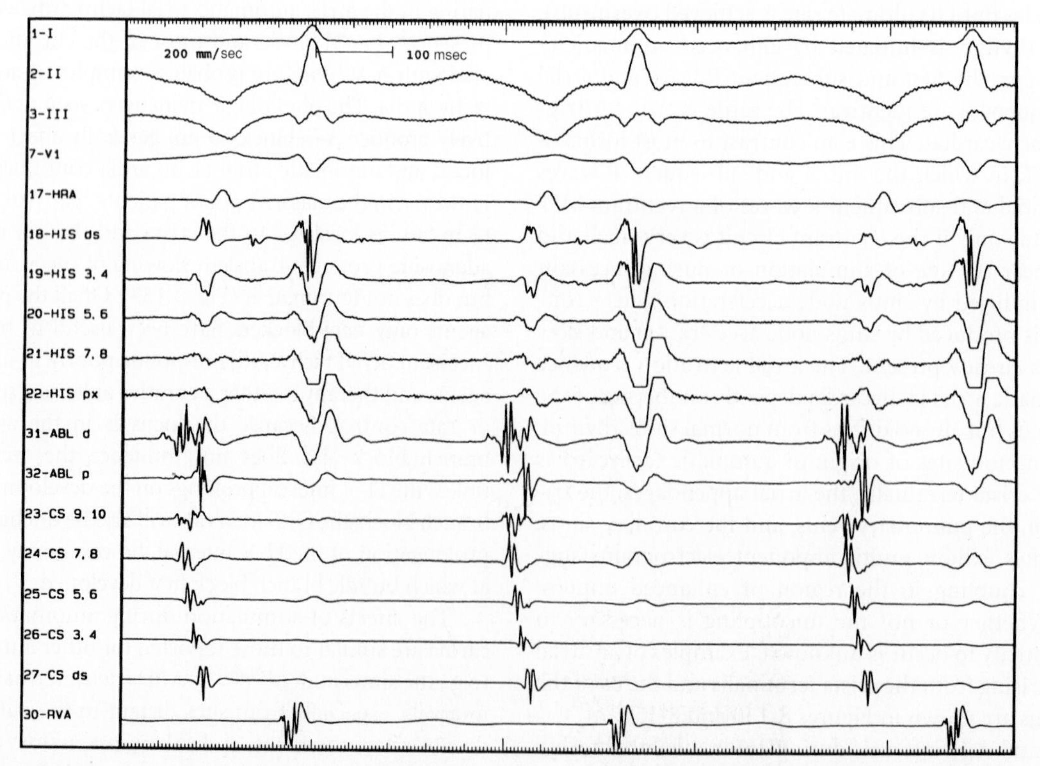


**FIGURE 8-151** *Example of an atrial tachycardia arising from the os of the coronary sinus.* ECG leads I, II, III, and $V_1$ are shown with intracardiac recordings from the His, the ablation catheter (ABL), CS, and RVA. Earliest activation is recorded in the distal ABL at the os of the CS, 45 msec prior to the P wave on the ECG.

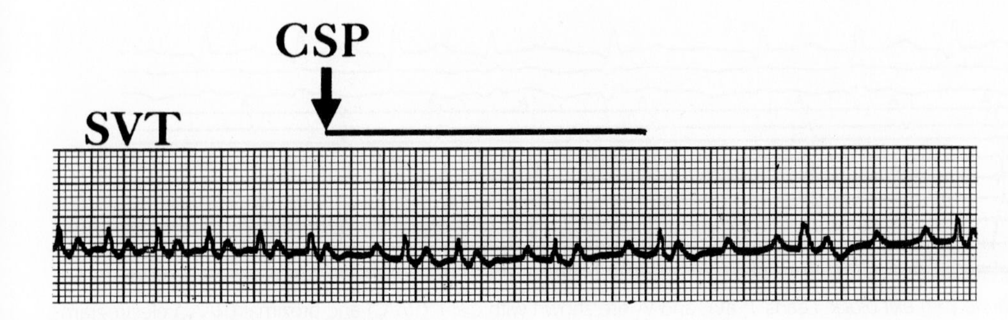


**FIGURE 8-152** *Effect of carotid sinus pressure on automatic atrial tachycardia (AAT).* CSP applied during AAT at a cycle length of 300 msec results in a 2:1 A-V block without affecting the AAT cycle length. See text for further discussion.

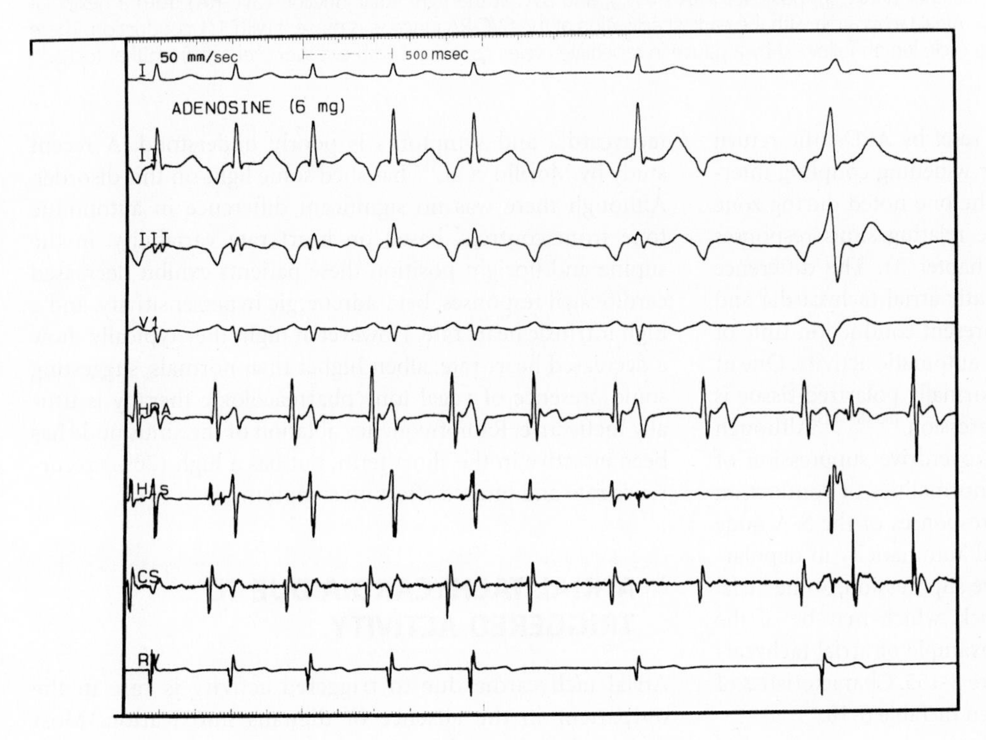


**FIGURE 8-153** *Adenosine produces transient slowing of the atrial tachycardia, but does not terminate it.* ECG leads I, II, II, and $V_1$ are shown with electrograms from the HRA, His, CS, and RV. Adenosine is administered during a long tachycardia. A-V block occurs with persistence of a slower atrial tachycardia. The N-V intervals depend on the A-A intervals. See text for discussion.

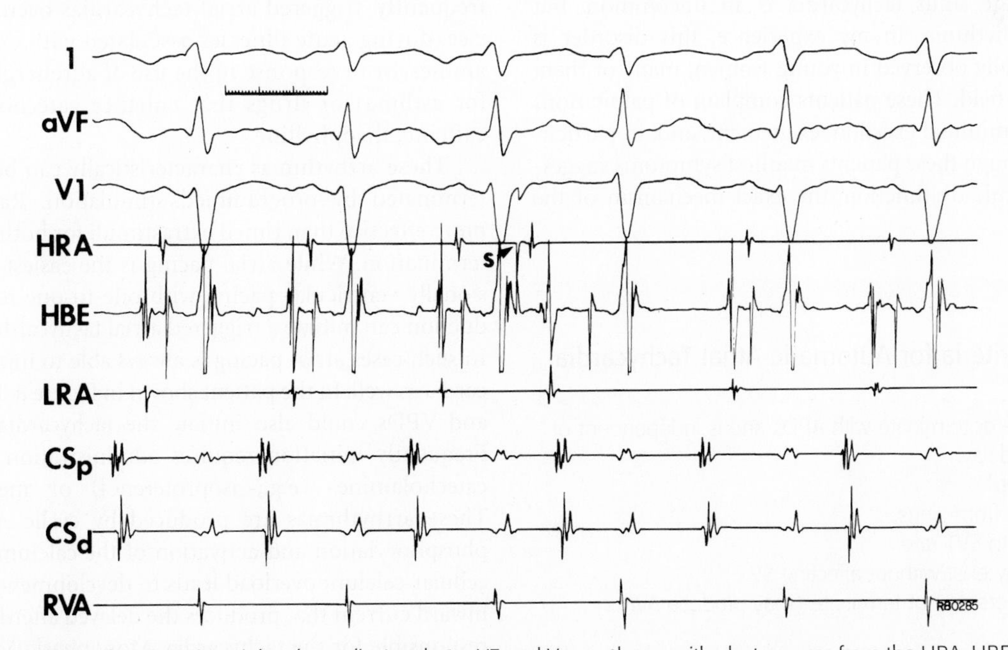


**FIGURE 8-154** *Resetting of automatic atrial tachycardia.* Leads 1, aVF, and $V_1$ are shown with electrograms from the HRA, HBE, low-right atrium (LRA), proximal, and distal CS, and RVA. Following three beats of a low-left atrial rhythm (earliest activation in $CS_p$), an APD is introduced from the HRA, which resets the tachycardia, advancing it by 20 msec. See text for discussion.

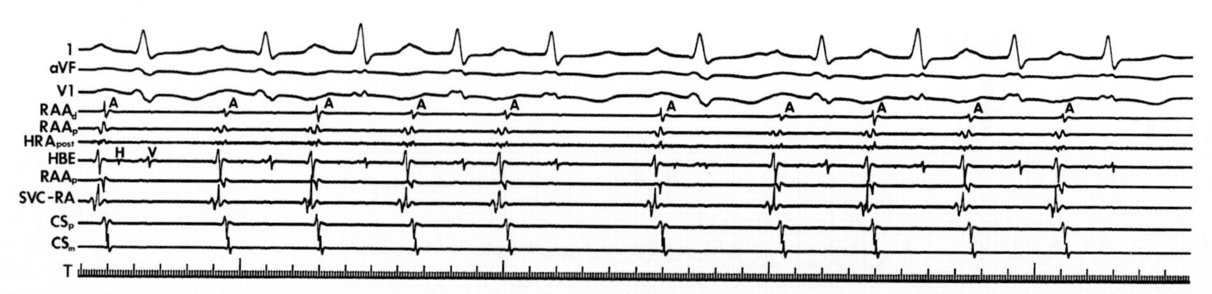

**FIGURE 8-155** *Automatic atrial tachycardia with exit block.* Leads 1, aVF, and $V_1$ are shown with distal ($RAA_d$) and proximal ($RAA_p$) electrograms from the right atrial appendage (RAA), posterior ($HRA_{post}$), posterior RAA ($RAA_p$), and SVC at the right atrial junction (SVC-RA) from a hexipolar catheter, HBE, and proximal and mid-$CS_m$. Atrial tachycardia with the earliest activation at the SVC-RA junction is present with 1:1 conduction. There is a gradual shortening of the tachycardia cycle length followed by a pause in repetitive cycles consistent with exit Wenckebach from that focus.

the automatic atrial tachycardia is reset by APDs, the return cycle usually remains constant over widening coupling intervals. This plateau is analogous to the one noted during zone 2 (the zone of reset) of the curve relating sinus responses to APD coupling intervals (see Chapter 3). The difference between cycle length of the automatic atrial tachycardia and the "fixed" pause is assumed to represent conduction time of the APD into and out of the area of automatic activity. One of the hallmarks of automaticity in normally polarized tissue is that pacing produces overdrive suppression.[180,183–185] Although this is primarily felt to be due to overdrive suppression of automaticity, it may also reflect abnormalities of conduction out of the focus analogous to the responses of the S-A node to overdrive suppression. Abnormal automaticity in depolarized tissue may not exhibit overdrive suppression. Some atrial tachycardias also manifest exit block, which may be of the Mobitz I or Mobitz II variety. An example of atrial tachycardia with exit block is shown in Figure 8-155. Characteristics of automatic atrial tachycardia are given in Table 8-10.

Inappropriate sinus tachycardia is an uncommon, but frustrating arrhythmia. In my experience, this disorder is almost universally observed in young women, many of them in the medical field. These patients complain of palpitations in response to minimal exertion, excitement, and, in particular, stress. Although these patients manifest symptoms suggestive of autonomic dysfunction, the exact mechanism of the tachycardia and symptoms is poorly understood. A recent study by Morillo et al.[189] has shed some light on this disorder. Although there was no significant difference in autonomic tone from controls, based on heart rate variability, in the supine and upright position these patients exhibit decreased cardiovagal responses, beta-adrenergic hypersensitivity, and a high intrinsic heart rate. However at night they typically show a decreased heart rate, albeit higher than normals, suggesting some presence of vagal tone pharmacologic therapy is usually ineffective. Radiofrequency ablation of the sinus node has been effective in the short term, but has a high (70%) recurrence rate and limited effect on symptoms.

**TABLE 8-10 Criteria for Automatic Atrial Tachycardia**

- Cannot initiate or terminate with APDs and is independent of IACD or AVN delay.
- SVT "warms up."
- P wave differs from sinus.
- P-R is related to SVT rate.
- AVN block may exist without affecting SVT.
- Vagal maneuvers do not terminate (may produce AVN block).
- Adenosine frequently transiently slows.
- Usually (but not always) exhibit overdrive suppression.

## ATRIAL TACHYCARDIA DUE TO TRIGGERED ACTIVITY

Atrial tachycardia due to triggered activity is rare in the outpatient in the absence of digitalis intoxication. Most frequently, triggered atrial tachycardias occur during exercise, during acute illnesses associated with excess catecholamines, or in response to the use of adrenergic agents (e.g., for asthma) or drugs that enhance catecholamines (e.g., caffeine, theophylline).

These arrhythmias characteristically can be initiated and terminated by programmed stimulation. Rapid pacing is more effective than timed extrastimuli for both initiation and termination. While atrial pacing is the easiest method occasionally ventricular pacing with one-to-one retrograde conduction can initiate a triggered atrial tachycardia (Fig. 8-156). In such cases atrial pacing is always able to initiate the tachycardia as well. In the patient shown in Figure 8-156 both APDs and VPDs could also initiate the tachycardia (Fig. 8-157). Frequently initiation requires administration of exogenous catecholamines (e.g., isoproterenol) or methylxanthines. These arrhythmias are produced by cyclic AMP-mediated phosphorylation and activation of the calcium channel. The cellular calcium overload leads to development of a transient inward current that produces the delayed afterdepolarizations responsible for the tachycardia. Monophasic action potential recordings can be used to detect afterdepolarizations, but care must be taken to exclude artifact.[180] These rhythms are

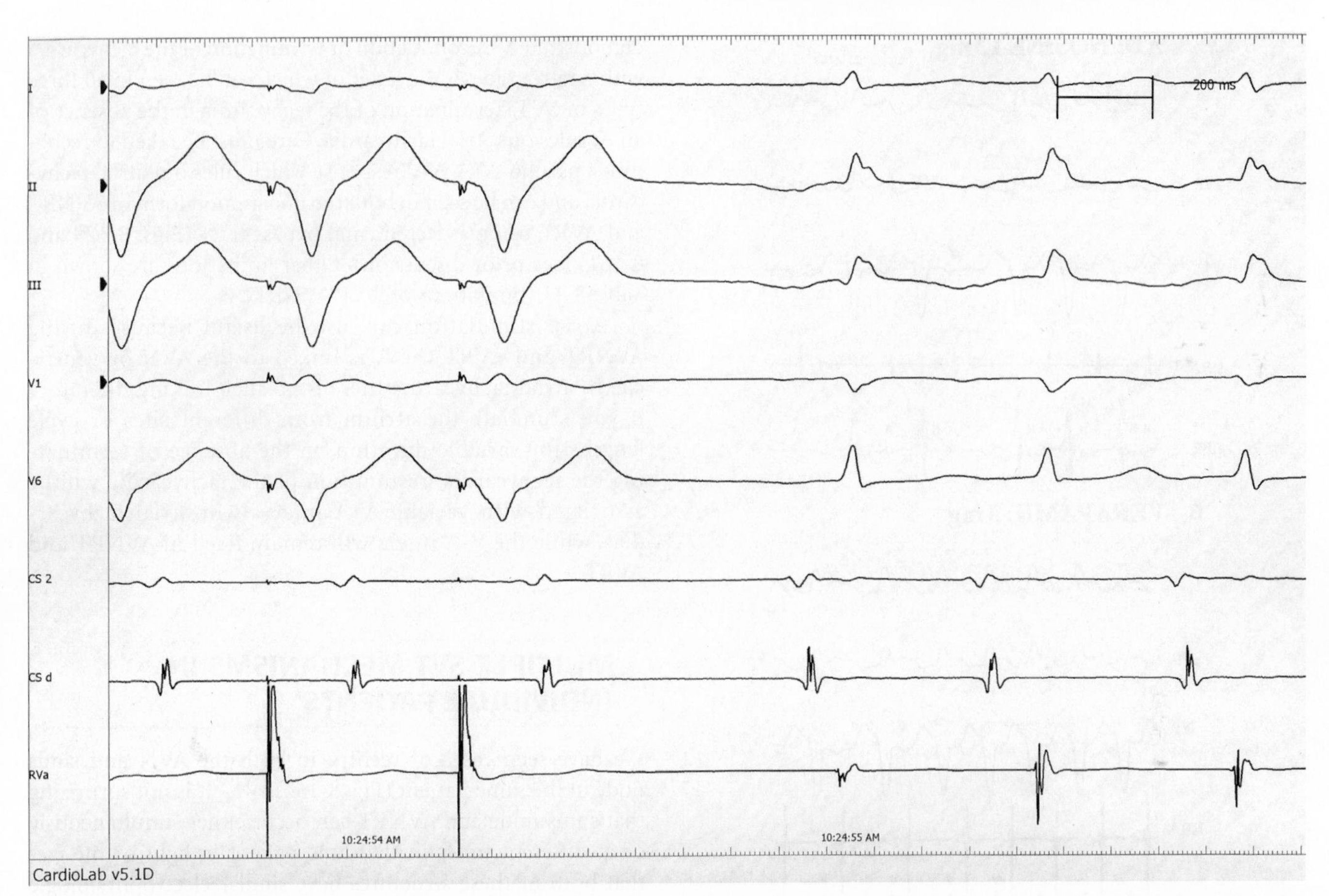


**FIGURE 8-156** *Initiation of a triggered atrial tachycardia by ventricular pacing with retrograde conduction.* The first three complexes show RV pacing with one-to-one retrograde conduction. Upon cessation of pacing a triggered atrial tachycardia begins. Note the V-A-A-V response. See text.

extremely sensitive to a variety of perturbations. CSP and other vagal maneuvers, adenosine, verapamil, and beta blockers can all terminate these arrhythmias (Fig. 8-158).[180,181] Sodium channel blocking agents can also suppress the arrhythmias.

The response of the arrhythmias to programmed stimulation is often characteristic. As shown in Figure 8-159 overdrive pacing produces acceleration of the tachycardia and a shortening of the interval to the first beat of the tachycardia and the paced cycle length is decreased.

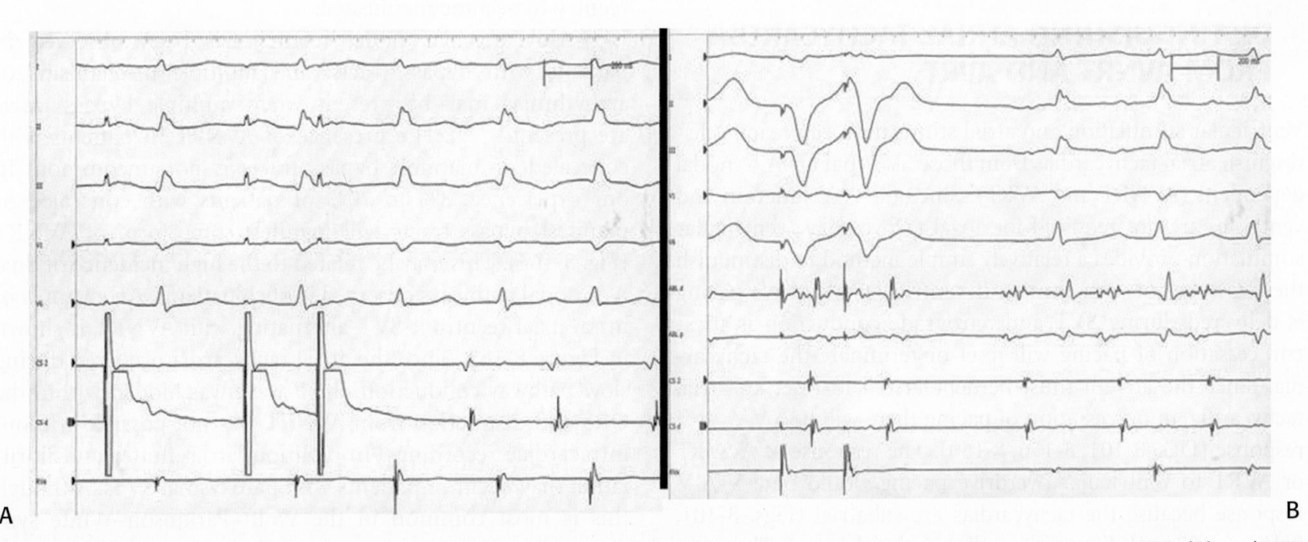


**FIGURE 8-157** *Triggered atrial tachycardia initiated by APDs and VPDs.* This is the same patient as in Figure 8-156. An APD **(A)** and VPD **(B)** initiate the same atrial tachycardia. See text for discussion.

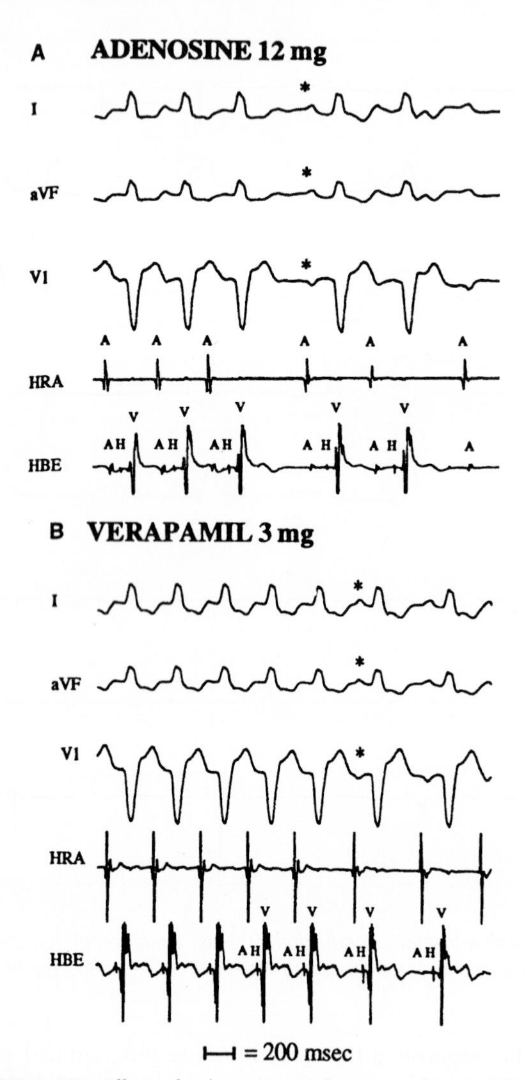


**FIGURE 8-158** *Effect of adenosine and verapamil on atrial tachycardia due to cyclase-mediated triggered activity.* Catecholamine-triggered atrial tachycardia is present in both panels. Adenosine **(A)** and verapamil **(B)** terminate SVT.

## DISTINGUISHING ATRIAL TACHYCARDIA FROM AVNRT AND AVRT

Ventricular stimulation and atrial stimulation can readily distinguish atrial tachycardias from those SVT that are A-V nodal dependent (AVNRT and AVRT). Since the A-V junction and ventricles are not required for atrial tachycardias, ventricular stimulation provides a relatively simple method to distinguish the two types of arrhythmias. If ventricular overdrive pacing is delivered during SVT and retrograde conduction is present, cessation of pacing will reset or terminate the tachycardia. Since the atrium must be depolarized to reset an atrial tachycardia, upon cessation of pacing there will be a V-A-A-V response (Figs. 8-101, 8-156, 8-160). The response of AVNRT or AVRT to ventricular overdrive pacing would be a V-A-V response because the tachycardias are subatrial (Figs. 8-101, 8-106, 8-107 and discussion earlier in the chapter). There are several limitations of this method, most obviously failure to demonstrate V-A conduction or termination of the tachycardia with a retrograde A, the latter of which can be seen in all three types of SVT. Termination of the tachycardia in the absence of an A, rules out atrial tachycardia. Care must be taken to recognize a pseudo–V-A-A-V response which rules out atrial tachycardia and can be seen in both the uncommon form of AVNRT and AVRT using a decremental bypass tract (Figs. 8-129 and 8-161) (see prior discussion). Other limitations are shown in Table 8-11 (limitations of OVP AVNRT).

Atrial stimulation can also be useful because during AVNRT and AVRT the A is linked to the AVN or ventricle. In atrial tachycardia there is no such linking; therefore if you stimulate the atrium from different sites or cycle lengths for variable duration, in the absence of terminating the tachycardia, resumption of the tachycardia will be associated with variable V-A intervals in atrial tachycardias, while the V-A inters will remain fixed in AVNRT and AVRT.

## MULTIPLE SVT MECHANISMS IN INDIVIDUAL PATIENTS

We have seen cases of reentry in both the AVN and sinus node in the same patient (Fig. 8-162).[174,179] It is not surprising that sinus node and AVNRT can occur either simultaneously or at different times in the same patient in light of the fact that both of these structures have similar electrophysiologic properties. In addition, single complexes of one form of reentry may initiate sustained arrhythmias of a different variety. In Figure 8-163, atypical AVNRT is initiated by a sinus node reentrant echo. In several patients we observed both sinus and A-V nodal SVT at different times. Paulay et al.[179] was the first to describe a simultaneous occurrence of sinus and A-V nodal reentrant SVT, with one form of SVT concealing the presence of the other. The development of A-V nodal block, which terminated the A-V nodal tachycardia, allowed the sinus node reentry to become manifested.

Atrioventricular nodal reentry has been observed in patients with bypass tracts, and multiple mechanisms of arrhythmias may be present when multiple bypass tracts are present.[190–192] The presence of AVNRT in patients with concealed or manifest bypass tracts is not uncommon. In our experience, 8% to 10% of patients with concealed or manifest bypass tracts will manifest some form of AVNRT (Fig. 8-164). This may be related to the high incidence of dual A-V nodal pathways observed in such patients. An example of intra-atrial reentrant SVT alternating with AVNRT is shown in Figure 8-165. Since the atrial tachycardia occurred during slow-pathway conduction, the P wave was hidden within the QRS and distinction from AVNRT was not possible without intracardiac recordings. In addition, atrial flutter and fibrillation may occur in patients with paroxysmal SVTs. Although this is most common in the Wolff–Parkinson–White syndrome during circus movement tachycardia (see Chapter 10), we have seen atrial flutter and/or fibrillation develop in the

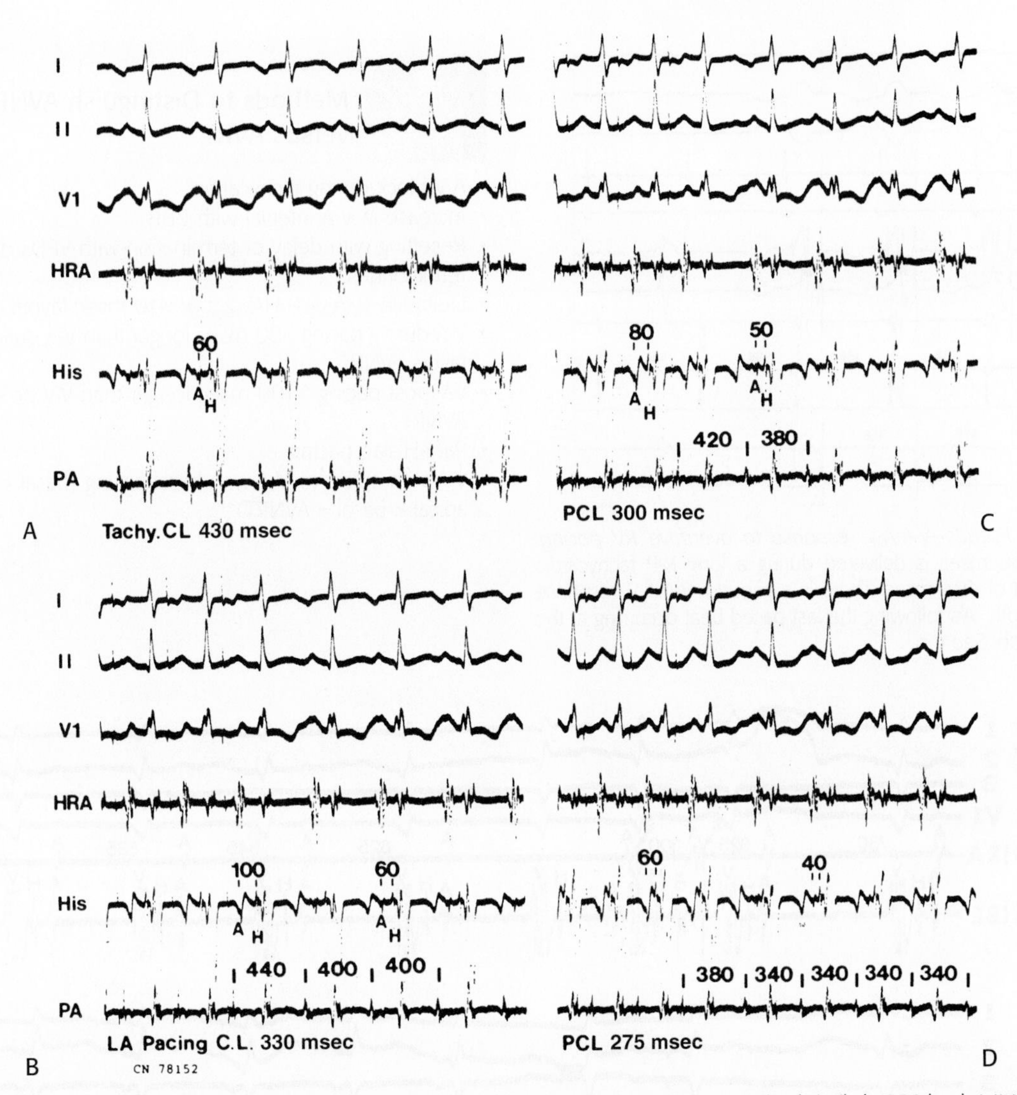


**FIGURE 8-159** *Effect of overdrive pacing on atrial tachycardia due to triggered activity.* **A–D** are organized similarly. ECG leads I, II, $V_1$ and recordings from the HRA, His, and pulmonary artery (PA). **A:** Atrial tachycardia is present with a cycle length of 430 msec. **B–D:** PA pacing at progressively shorter cycle lengths is associated with a shortening to the first unpaced cycle and initial tachycardia cycle length. Overdrive acceleration is characteristic of triggered rhythms.

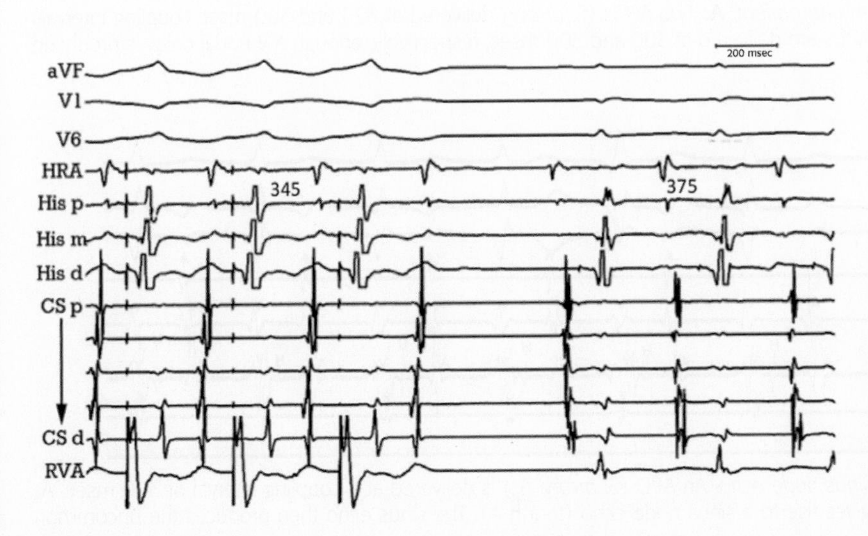


**FIGURE 8-160** *Response of atrial tachycardia to ventricular overdrive pacing.* Ventricular overdrive pacing at a cycle length of 345 msec is delivered during AT. Retrograde conduction is over a left-sided CBT (note early CS activation). Upon cessation of pacing there is a V-A-A-V response with the appearance of a right atrial tachycardia.

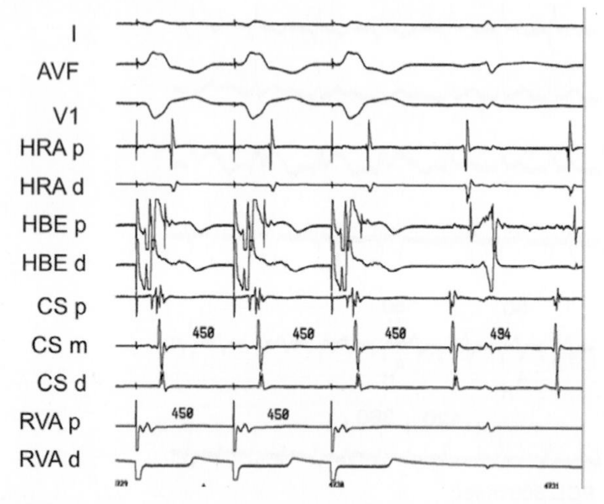


**FIGURE 8-161** *Pseudo–V-A-A-V response to overdrive RV pacing.* RV pacing at 450 msec is delivered during a long R-P tachycardia at a cycle length of 494 msec. There is a pseudo–V-A-A-V response diagnosed by "both" A's following the last paced beat occurring at the paced cycle length. See text.

**TABLE 8-11 Methods to Distinguish AVNRT versus AVRT**

- A-V block during tachycardia
- Increase in V-A interval with BBB
- Resetting with delay or termination with VPDs during His refractoriness
- Delta HA ($HA_{SVT} - HA_{pace/nsr}$): >10 msec favors AVRT
- V-A during pacing >90 msec longer than V-A during tachycardia favors AVNRT
- V-V post pacing >100 msec longer than V-V or SVT favors AVNRT
- Para-Hisian pacing
- V-A with apical vs. V-A with basal pacing (basal < apical = BPT; apical < basal = AVNRT)

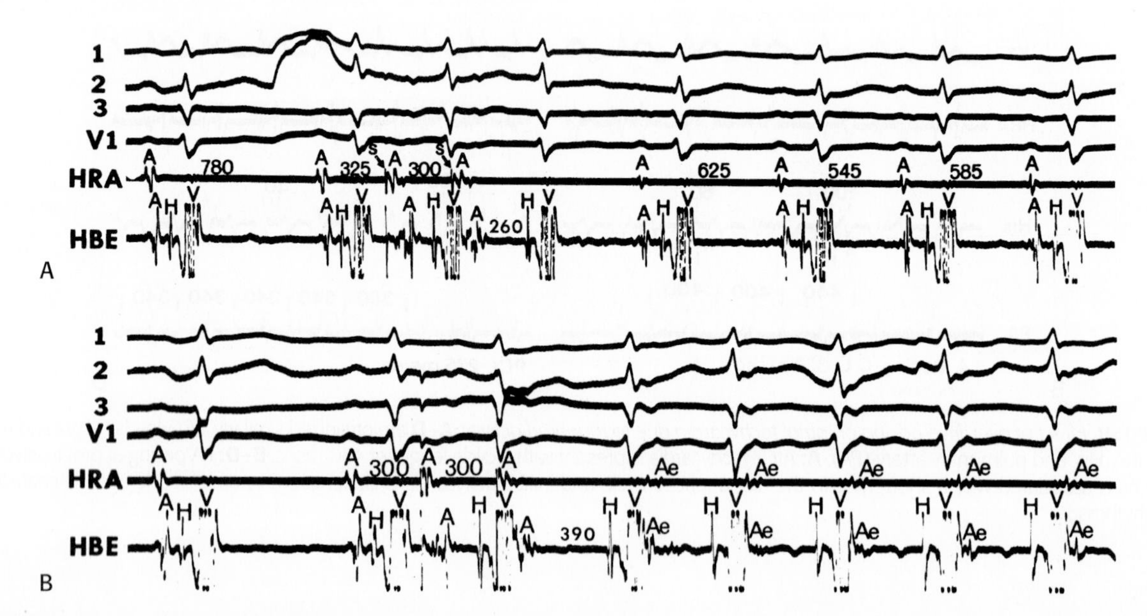


**FIGURE 8-162** *Sinus and A-V nodal reentrant SVT in one patient.* **A:** Two APDs (S, *arrow*) delivered at 325 and 300 msec coupling intervals result in sinus node reentrant SVT. **B:** When the two APDs are delivered at 300 and 300 msec, respectively, enough A-V nodal delay is produced (A-H = 390 msec) to initiate A-V nodal reentrant SVT.

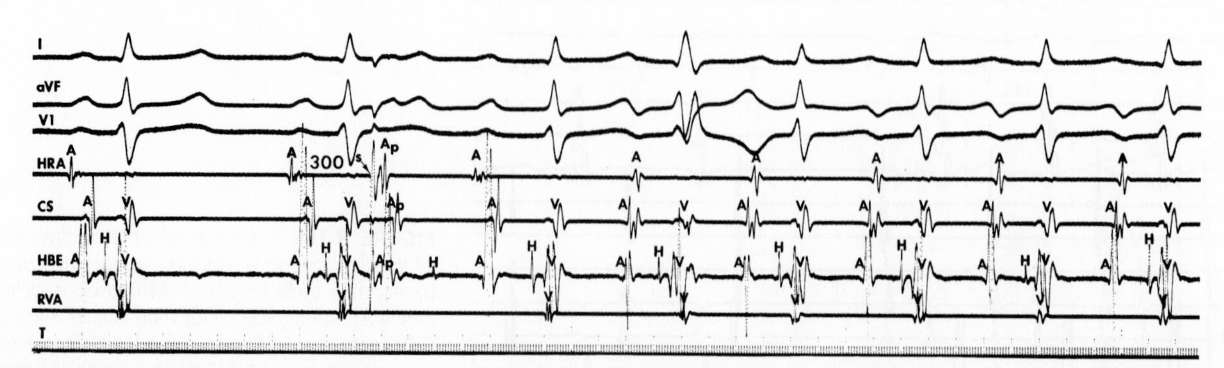


**FIGURE 8-163** *Initiation of A-V nodal reentry by a sinus node echo.* An APD (S, *arrow*, $A_p$) is delivered at a coupling interval of 300 msec. $A_p$ blocks below the His bundle, and it simultaneously gives rise to a sinus node echo (fourth A). The sinus echo then produces the uncommon form of A-V nodal reentrant SVT.

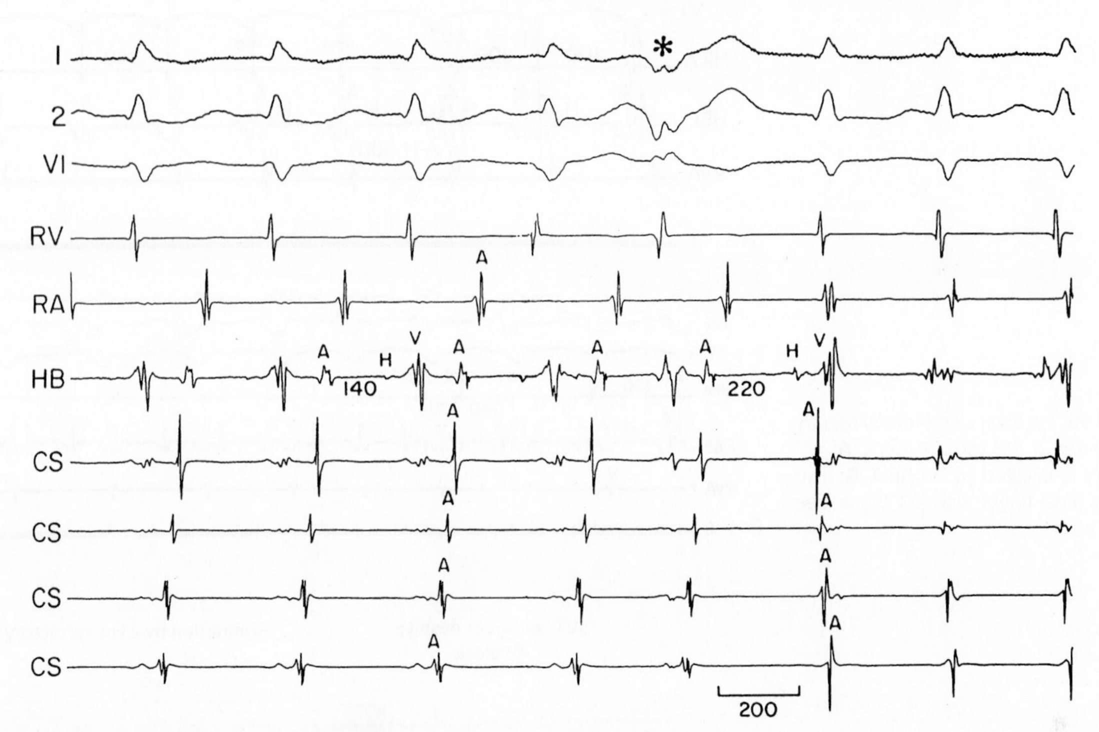


**FIGURE 8-164** *Coexistence of SVT using a concealed bypass tract and AVNRT.* ECG leads 1, 2, and $V_1$ are shown with electrograms from the RV, right atrium (RA), His bundle (HB), and CS proximal to distal (**top** to **bottom**). The first four complexes are SVT using a concealed left lateral bypass tract. A left ventricular VPD pre-excites the atrium over the bypass tract to produce block in the fast pathway and conduction down the slow pathway, which initiates AVNRT.

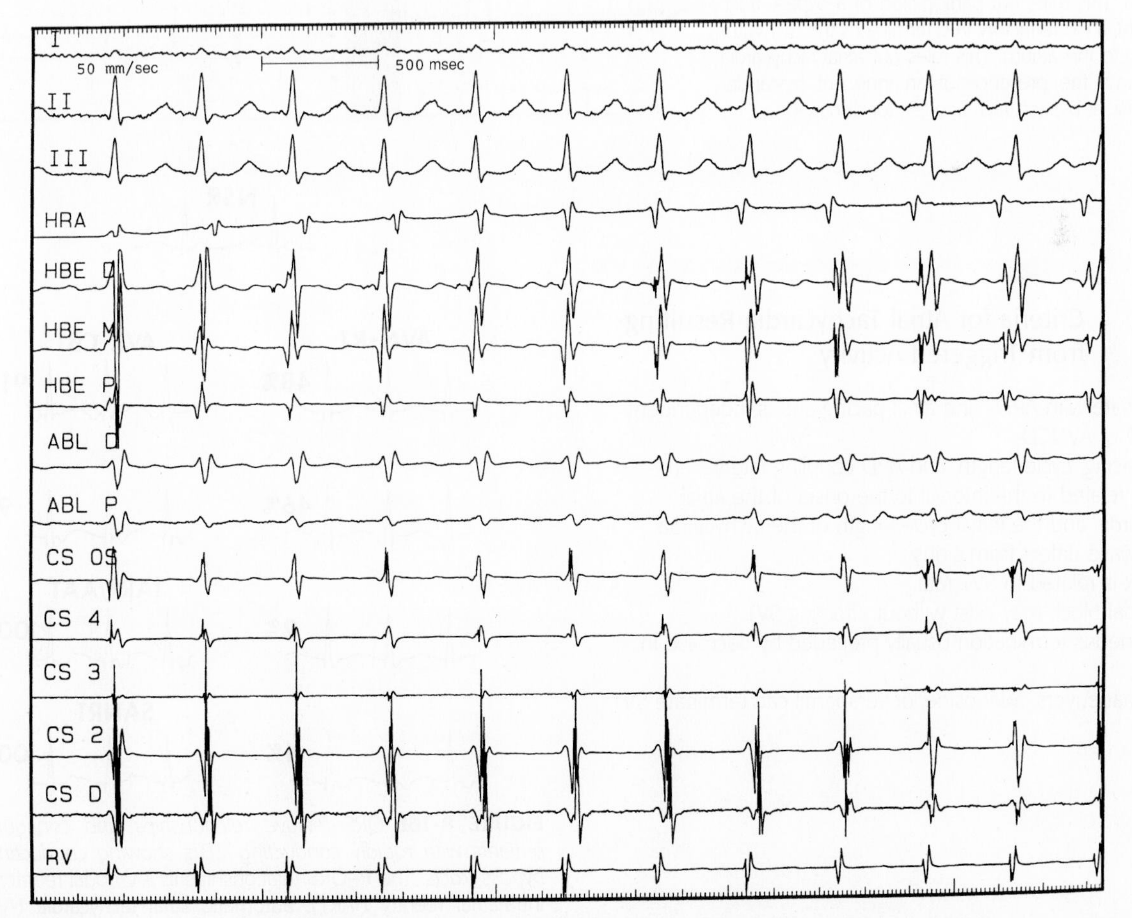


**FIGURE 8-165** *Simultaneous presence of atrial tachycardia and AVNRT.* The figure is from the same patient as in Figure 8-137. AVNRT is present during the first half of the tracing, following which atrial tachycardia takes over. Note change in atrial activation sequence.

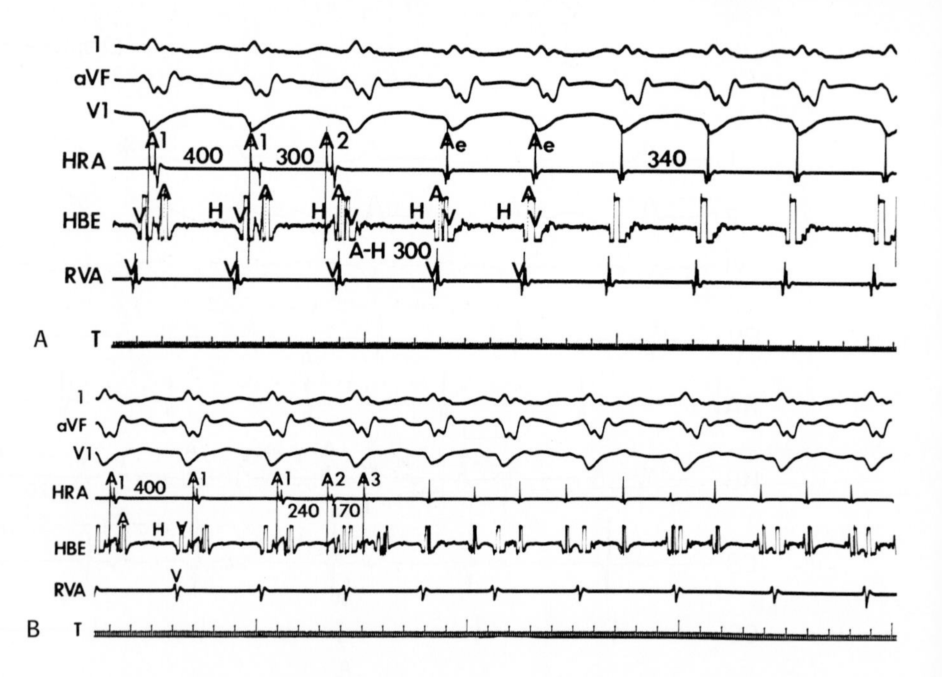


**FIGURE 8-166** *Initiation of A-V nodal reentry and atrial flutter in the same patient.* **A:** A-V nodal reentry is initiated by an APD. **B:** Two APDs initiate atrial flutter with 2:1 block. See text for discussion.

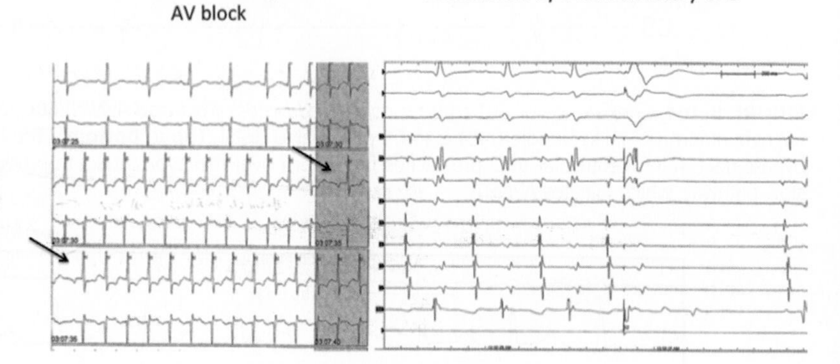


**FIGURE 8-167** *AVNRT with innocent bystander nodoventricular pathway.* The spontaneous SVT is shown on the left. *Arrows* point to periods of A-V block during the tachycardia. This rules out participation of a bypass tract. On the right, a His refractory VPC terminates the SVT without getting to the atrium. This rules out atrial tachycardia and confirms the presence of an innocent bystander nodoventricular bypass tract. See text for discussion.

## TABLE 8-12 Criteria for Atrial Tachycardia Resulting from Triggered Activity

- Can initiate with APDs and atrial pacing and is independent of IACD or AVNCD.
- Atrial pacing, cycle length, and APD coupling interval are directly related to the interval to the onset of the atrial tachycardia and the initial cycle length of the tachycardia.
- The P wave differs from sinus.
- The P-R is related to SVT rate.
- A-V nodal block may exist without affecting SVT.
- Spontaneous termination usually preceded by decrease in rate.
- Vagal maneuvers, adenosine, or verapamil can terminate SVT.

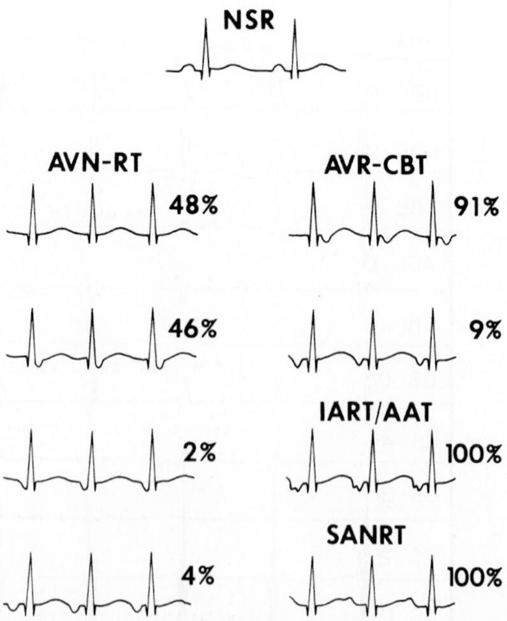

NSR

AVN-RT 48% 46% 2% 4%

AVR-CBT 91% 9%

IART/AAT 100%

SANRT 100%

**FIGURE 8-168** *QRS–P-wave relationships and configurations in patients with rapidly conducting CBTs showing conducting ("sick") bypass tracts.* The P–QRS relationships in A-V nodal reentry (AVNRT), intra-atrial reentry (IART), automatic atrial tachycardia (AAT), sinus node reentry tachycardia (SANRT), and atrioventricular reentry (AVR) using a CBT. See text for discussion.

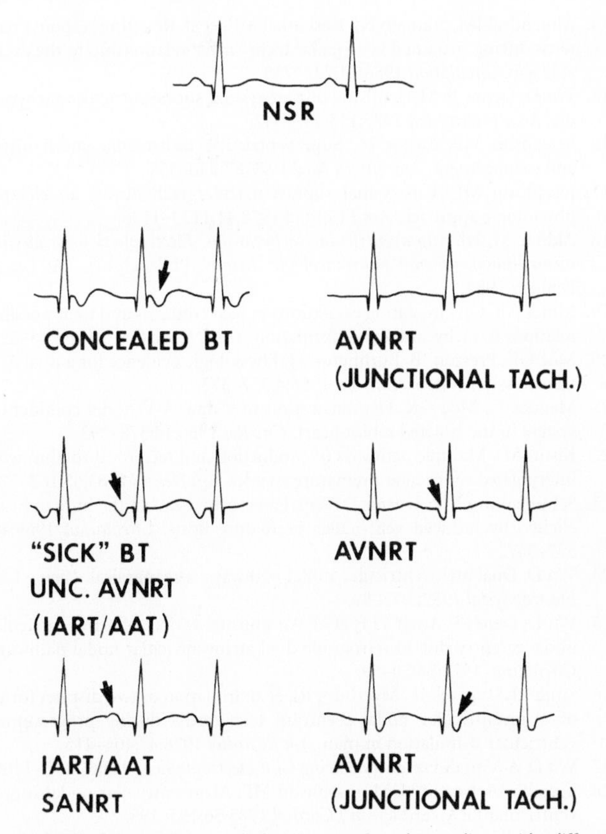


**FIGURE 8-169** *Differential diagnosis of tachycardias with different R-P/P-R relationships and P-wave configurations.*

course of SVTs that are due to many mechanisms and as an independent arrhythmia (Fig. 8-166). The incidence of atrial fibrillation may be as high as 10% in patients with SVT, but is obviously influenced by both age and the presence of organic heart disease. Occasionally AVNRT can exist with an innocent bystander nodoventricular pathway (Fig. 8-167). In the case shown in Figure 8-167 SVT is present and persists with A-V block (arrows, left panel); this rules out a bypass tract participating in the tachycardia. On the right, a His refractory VPC terminates the tachycardia without reaching the atrium. These findings suggest the SVT was due to AVNRT but the response to the VPC suggest the presence of a bypass tract not participating in the tachycardia.

## OVERVIEW

Programmed stimulation and intracardiac recording techniques have resulted in the reclassification of SVT. The incidence of the various types of SVT listed in Table 8-2 is representative of most laboratories. Although specific diagnostic criteria during electrophysiologic studies for most of the forms of SVT are listed in Tables 8-5 through 8-12, certain clues are available on the surface ECG (Figs. 8-168 and 8-169).[17,193–195] A systematic approach to the ECG will provide much of this information. The first step in analyzing the ECG is to localize atrial activity. The P-wave morphology and the relationship of the P wave to the QRS complex during SVT can be readily ascertained in most patients. If P waves during a paroxysmal SVT are identical to sinus P waves, the SVT most likely uses a sinus node reentry. P waves that are inverted in the inferior leads can represent reentry using the A-V junction (i.e., either AVNRT or A-V reentry using a posteroseptal CBT) or a low atrial tachycardia. Reentry using a CBT almost always has a shorter R-P interval than P-R, with the exception of slowly conducting bypass tracts. The short R-P interval helps distinguish it from intra-atrial reentrant tachycardias (R-P > P-R) and from AVNRT in which the P wave is usually buried within the QRS or results only in a slurring of the terminal QRS. A pseudo-Q wave may be seen in the inferior leads in AVNRT if there is delay below the circuit so that retrograde conduction over the fast pathway precedes ventricular activation (Fig. 8-170). Other locations of CBT can give rise to different P-wave morphologies, but a fixed and short R-P, regardless of changes in cycle length, always maintaining a 1:1 V-A relationship, is most compatible with SVT using a CBT. Paroxysmal SVT in which no P waves can be seen is almost always due to AVNRT, with the possible exception of atrial arrhythmias with P-R intervals that are so prolonged as a result of A-V nodal disease that the P wave is inscribed during the prior QRS. Junctional tachycardia can also mimic AVNRT,

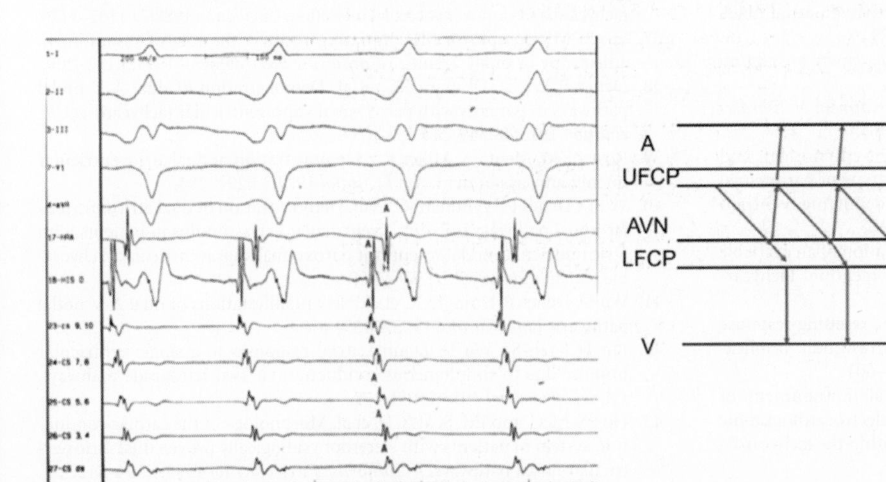


**FIGURE 8-170** *Mechanism of pseudo-Q wave in typical AVNRT.* On the left is AVNRT with "Q waves" in the inferior leads. As shown in the ladder diagram on the right, delay below the circuit (in this case the lower part of the A-V node) results in retrograde activation of the atrium prior to the ventricle. See text for discussion.

but it is nonparoxysmal and usually is related to drug toxicity (i.e., digitalis), metabolic derangements, or infarction, or is a consequence of valvular surgery.

Alternation of the QRS complexes also can provide some help in recognizing the mechanism of SVT.[193–195] During relatively slow tachycardias, alternation is almost always related to SVT using a CBT. During SVT with very rapid rates, alternation still is most common in SVT using CBT; however, it may be seen with other types of SVT as well. The R-P and P-R patterns and their relative incidence are summarized in Figures 8-158 and 8-159. The observation of A-V dissociation or A-V block during SVT rules out the existence of a functioning CBT and makes AVNRT unlikely (although this can occur). The use of drugs and/or CSP to produce A-V block can help the physician determine the mechanism of the SVT.

Successful therapy of SVT, whether medical, electrical, or ablation, depends on the knowledge of the underlying mechanisms and site of origin of the arrhythmia. Patients with recurrent SVT should undergo electrophysiologic evaluation and therapy chosen on the basis of a drug's ability to prevent the initiation or to aid in the termination of the arrhythmia. The manner in which such sequential studies are performed is described in Chapter 12. Obviously, studies are required to localize the origin of the tachycardia for catheter ablation as well as to determine the tachycardia-terminating stimulation mode for antitachycardia pacing.

## REFERENCES


1. Rosen MR, Hoffman BF, eds. *Electrophysiologic determinants of normal cardiac rhythms and arrhythmias.* Boston, MA: Martinus Nijhoff; 1983.
2. Frame LH, Hoffman BF, eds. *Mechanisms of tachycardia.* Boston, MA: Martinus Nijhoff; 1984.
3. Jalife J, Antzelevitch C. Pacemaker annihilation: diagnostic and therapeutic implications. *Am Heart J* 1980;100:128–130.
4. Malfatto G, Rosen TS, Rosen MR. The response to overdrive pacing of triggered atrial and ventricular arrhythmias in the canine heart. *Circulation* 1988;77:1139–1148.
5. Cranefield PF. Action potentials, afterpotentials, and arrhythmias. *Circ Res* 1977;41:415–423.
6. Wit AL, Cranefield PF. Triggered and automatic activity in the canine coronary sinus. *Circ Res* 1977;41:434–445.
7. Johnson N, Danilo P, Jr., Wit AL, et al. Characteristics of initiation and termination of catecholamine-induced triggered activity in atrial fibers of the coronary sinus. *Circulation* 1986;74:1168–1179.
8. Brugada P, Wellens HJ, eds. *The role of triggered activity in clinical arrhythmias.* Boston, MA: Martinus Nijhoff; 1983.
9. Waldo AL, ed. *Cardiac pacing: Role in diagnosis and treatment of disorders of cardiac rhythm.* Boston, MA: Martinus Nijhoff; 1963.
10. Waldo AL, Plumb VJ, Arciniegas JG, et al. Transient entrainment and interruption of the atrioventricular bypass pathway type of paroxysmal atrial tachycardia. A model for understanding and identifying reentrant arrhythmias. *Circulation* 1983;67:73–83.
11. Rosenthal ME, Miller JM, Josephson ME. Demonstration of an excitable gap in the common form of atrioventricular nodal reentrant tachycardia. *J Electrophysiol* 1987;1:334.
12. Stamato NJ, Rosenthal ME, Almendral JM, et al. The resetting response of ventricular tachycardia to single and double extrastimuli: implications for an excitable gap. *Am J Cardiol* 1987;60:596–601.
13. Almendral JM, Gottlieb CD, Rosenthal ME, et al. Entrainment of ventricular tachycardia: explanation for surface electrocardiographic phenomena by analysis of electrograms recorded within the tachycardia circuit. *Circulation* 1988;77:569–580.
14. Almendral JM, Stamato NJ, Rosenthal ME, et al. Resetting response patterns during sustained ventricular tachycardia: relationship to the excitable gap. *Circulation* 1986;74:722–730.
15. Wu D, Denes P. Mechanisms of paroxysmal supraventricular tachycardia. *Arch Intern Med* 1975;135:437–442.
16. Josephson ME, Kastor JA. Supraventricular tachycardia: mechanisms and management. *Ann Intern Med* 1977;87:346–358.
17. Josephson ME. Paroxysmal supraventricular tachycardia: an electrophysiologic approach. *Am J Cardiol* 1978;41:1123–1126.
18. Akhtar M, ed. *Supraventricular tachycardias. Electrophysiologic mechanisms, diagnosis, and pharmacologic therapy.* Philadelphia, PA: Lea & Febiger; 1984.
19. Mines GR. On circulating excitations in heart muscles and their possible relations to tachycardia and fibrillation. *Trans R Soc Can* 1914;4:43–52.
20. Moe GK, Preston JB, Burlington H. Physiologic evidence for a dual A-V transmission system. *Circ Res* 1956;4:357–375.
21. Mendez C, Moe GK. Demonstration of a dual A-V nodal conduction system in the isolated rabbit heart. *Circ Res* 1966;19:378–393.
22. Kistin AD. Multiple pathways of conduction and reciprocal rhythm with interpolated ventricular premature systoles. *Am Heart J* 1963;65:162–179.
23. Schuilenburg RM, Durrer D. Ventricular echo beats in the human heart elicited by induced ventricular premature beats. *Circulation* 1969;40: 337–347.
24. Wu D. Dual atrioventricular nodal pathways: a reappraisal. *Pacing Clin Electrophysiol* 1982;5:72–89.
25. Wu D, Denes P, Amat YLF, et al. An unusual variety of atrioventricular nodal re-entry due to retrograde dual atrioventricular nodal pathways. *Circulation* 1977;56:50–59.
26. Sung RJ, Styperek JL, Myerburg RJ, et al. Initiation of two distinct forms of atrioventricular nodal reentrant tachycardia during programmed ventricular stimulation in man. *Am J Cardiol* 1978;42:404–415.
27. Wu D. A-V nodal re-entry. *Pacing Clin Electrophysiol* 1983;6:1190–1200.
28. Vassallo JA, Cassidy DM, Josephson ME. Atrioventricular nodal supraventricular tachycardia. *Am J Cardiol* 1985;56:193–195.
29. Jalife J. The sucrose gap preparation as a model of AV nodal transmission: are dual pathways necessary for reciprocation and AV nodal "echoes"? *Pacing Clin Electrophysiol* 1983;6:1106–1122.
30. Antzelevitch C, Moe GK. Electrotonically mediated delayed conduction and reentry in relation to "slow responses" in mammalian ventricular conducting tissue. *Circ Res* 1981;49:1129–1139.
31. de CA, de AD. Spread of activity through the atrioventricular node. *Circ Res* 1960;8:801–809.
32. Merideth J, Mendez C, Mueller WJ, et al. Electrical excitability of atrioventricular nodal cells. *Circ Res* 1968;23:69–85.
33. Spach MS, Miller WT, 3rd, Miller-Jones E, et al. Extracellular potentials related to intracellular action potentials during impulse conduction in anisotropic canine cardiac muscle. *Circ Res* 1979;45:188–204.
34. Spach MS, Kootsey JM. The nature of electrical propagation in cardiac muscle. *Am J Physiol* 1983;244:H3–H22.
35. Dillon SM, Allessie MA, Ursell PC, et al. Influences of anisotropic tissue structure on reentrant circuits in the epicardial border zone of subacute canine infarcts. *Circ Res* 1988;63:182–206.
36. Cardinal R, Vermeulen M, Shenasa M, et al. Anisotropic conduction and functional dissociation of ischemic tissue during reentrant ventricular tachycardia in canine myocardial infarction. *Circulation* 1988;77:1162–1176.
37. Spach MS, Josephson ME. Initiating reentry: the role of nonuniform anisotropy in small circuits. *J Cardiovasc Electrophysiol* 1994;5:182–209.
38. Denes P, Wu D, Dhingra RC, et al. Demonstration of dual A-V nodal pathways in patients with paroxysmal supraventricular tachycardia. *Circulation* 1973;48:549–555.
39. Rosen KM, Mehta A, Miller RA. Demonstration of dual atrioventricular nodal pathways in man. *Am J Cardiol* 1974;33:291–294.
40. Wu D, Denes P, Wyndham C, et al. Demonstration of dual atrioventricular nodal pathways utilizing a ventricular extrastimulus in patients with atrioventricular nodal re-entrant paroxysmal supraventricular tachycardia. *Circulation* 1975;52:789–798.
41. Wu D, Denes P, Dhingra R, et al. New manifestations of dual A-V nodal pathways. *Eur J Cardiol* 1975;2:459–466.
42. Lin FC, Yeh SJ, Wu D. Double atrial responses to a single ventricular impulse due to simultaneous conduction via two retrograde pathways. *J Am Coll Cardiol* 1985;5:168–175.
43. Ho SY, McComb JM, Scott CD, et al. Morphology of the cardiac conduction system in patients with electrophysiologically proven dual atrioventricular nodal pathways. *J Cardiovasc Electrophysiol* 1993;4:504–512.

44. Janse MJ, Anderson RH, McGuire MA, et al. "AV nodal" reentry: Part I: "AV nodal" reentry revisited. *J Cardiovasc Electrophysiol* 1993;4:561–572.
45. McGuire MA, Janse MJ, Ross DL. "AV nodal" reentry: Part II: AV nodal, AV junctional, or atrionodal reentry? *J Cardiovasc Electrophysiol* 1993;4:573–586.
46. Jackman WM, Beckman KJ, McClelland JH, et al. Treatment of supraventricular tachycardia due to atrioventricular nodal reentry, by radiofrequency catheter ablation of slow-pathway conduction. *N Engl J Med* 1992;327:313–318.
47. Haissaguerre M, Gaita F, Fischer B, et al. Elimination of atrioventricular nodal reentrant tachycardia using discrete slow potentials to guide application of radiofrequency energy. *Circulation* 1992;85:2162–2175.
48. McGuire MA, de Bakker JM, Vermeulen JT, et al. Origin and significance of double potentials near the atrioventricular node. Correlation of extracellular potentials, intracellular potentials, and histology. *Circulation* 1994;89:2351–2360.
49. Wu D, Denes P, Amat-y-Leon F, et al. Clinical, electrocardiographic and electrophysiologic observations in patients with paroxysmal supraventricular tachycardia. *Am J Cardiol* 1978;41:1045–1051.
50. Goldreyer BN, Damato AN. The essential role of atrioventricular conduction delay in the initiation of paroxysmal supraventricular tachycardia. *Circulation* 1971;43:679–687.
51. Baker JH, 2nd, Plumb VJ, Epstein AE, et al. PR/RR interval ratio during rapid atrial pacing: a simple method for confirming the presence of slow AV nodal pathway conduction. *J Cardiovasc Electrophysiol* 1996;7:287–294.
52. Ross DL, Brugada P, Bar FW, et al. Comparison of right and left atrial stimulation in demonstration of dual atrioventricular nodal pathways and induction of intranodal reentry. *Circulation* 1981;64:1051–1058.
53. Josephson ME. Unpublished observations, 2015.
54. Batsford WP, Akhtar M, Caracta AR, et al. Effect of atrial stimulation site on the electrophysiological properties of the atrioventricular node in man. *Circulation* 1974;50:283–292.
55. Aranda J, Castellanos A, Moleiro F, et al. Effects of the pacing site on A-H conduction and refractoriness in patients with short P-R intervals. *Circulation* 1976;53:33–39.
56. Chen SA, Tai CT, Lee SH, et al. AV nodal reentrant tachycardia with unusual characteristics: lessons from radiofrequency catheter ablation. *J Cardiovasc Electrophysiol* 1998;9:321–333.
57. Tai CT, Chen SA, Chiang CE, et al. Multiple anterograde atrioventricular node pathways in patients with atrioventricular node reentrant tachycardia. *J Am Coll Cardiol* 1996;28:725–731.
58. Wu D, Denes P, Dhingra R, et al. The effects of propranolol on induction of A-V nodal reentrant paroxysmal tachycardia. *Circulation* 1974;50:665–677.
59. Hartel G, Hartikainen M. Comparison of verapamil and practolol in paroxysmal supraventricular tachycardia. *Eur J Cardiol* 1976;4:87–90.
60. Spurrell RA, Krikler DM, Sowton E. Concealed bypasses of the atrioventricular mode in patients with paroxysmal supraventricular tachycardia revealed by intracardiac electrical stimulation and verapamil. *Am J Cardiol* 1974;33:590–595.
61. Wellens HJ, Duren DR, Liem DL, et al. Effect of digitalis in patients with paroxysmal atrioventricular nodal tachycardia. *Circulation* 1975;52:779–788.
62. Akhtar M, Damato AN, Ruskin JN, et al. Antegrade and retrograde conduction characteristics in three patterns of paroxysmal atrioventricular junctional reentrant tachycardia. *Am Heart J* 1978;95:22–42.
63. Coumel P. Junctional reciprocating tachycardias. The permanent and paroxysmal forms of A-V nodal reciprocating tachycardias. *J Electrocardiol* 1975;8:79–90.
64. Farre J, Ross D, Wiener I, et al. Reciprocal tachycardias using accessory pathways with long conduction times. *Am J Cardiol* 1979;44:1099–1109.
65. Brugada P, Farre J, Green M, et al. Observations in patients with supraventricular tachycardia having a P-R interval shorter than the R-P interval: differentiation between atrial tachycardia and reciprocating atrioventricular tachycardia using an accessory pathway with long conduction times. *Am Heart J* 1984;107:556–570.
66. Wu D, Kou HC, Yeh SJ, et al. Determinants of tachycardia induction using ventricular stimulation in dual pathway atrioventricular nodal reentrant tachycardia. *Am Heart J* 1984;108:44–55.
67. Denes P, Wu D, Amat-y-Leon F, et al. The determinants of atrioventricular nodal re-entrance with premature atrial stimulation in patients with dual A-V nodal pathways. *Circulation* 1977;56:253–259.
68. Strasberg B, Swiryn S, Bauernfeind R, et al. Retrograde dual atrioventricular nodal pathways. *Am J Cardiol* 1981;48:639–646.
69. Wu D, Denes P, Bauernfeind R, et al. Effects of atropine on induction and maintenance of atrioventricular nodal reentrant tachycardia. *Circulation* 1979;59:779–788.
70. Brugada P, Heddle B, Green M, et al. Initiation of atrioventricular nodal reentrant tachycardia in patients with discontinuous anterograde atrioventricular nodal conduction curves with and without documented supraventricular tachycardia: observations on the role of a discontinuous retrograde conduction curve. *Am Heart J* 1984;107:685–697.
71. Bauernfeind RA, Swiryn S, Strasberg B, et al. Analysis of anterograde and retrograde fast pathway properties in patients with dual atrioventricular nodal pathways: observations regarding the pathophysiology of the Lown-Ganong-Levine syndrome. *Am J Cardiol* 1982;49:283–290.
72. Anselme F, Frederiks J, Papageorgiou P, et al. Nonuniform anisotropy is responsible for age-related slowing of atrioventricular nodal reentrant tachycardia. *J Cardiovasc Electrophysiol* 1996;7:1145–1153.
73. Josephson ME, Scharf DL, Kastor JA, et al. Atrial endocardial activation in man. Electrode catheter technique of endocardial mapping. *Am J Cardiol* 1977;39:972–981.
74. Amat-y-Leon F, Dhingra RC, Wu D, et al. Catheter mapping of retrograde atrial activation. Observations during ventricular pacing and AV nodal re-entrant paroxysmal tachycardia. *Br Heart J* 1976;38:355–362.
75. Sung RJ, Waxman HL, Saksena S, et al. Sequence of retrograde atrial activation in patients with dual atrioventricular nodal pathways. *Circulation* 1981;64:1059–1067.
76. Anselme F, Papageorgiou P, Monahan K, et al. Presence and significance of the left atrionodal connection during atrioventricular nodal reentrant tachycardia. *Am J Cardiol* 1999;83:1530–1536.
77. Anselme F, Hook B, Monahan K, et al. Heterogeneity of retrograde fast-pathway conduction pattern in patients with atrioventricular nodal reentry tachycardia: observations by simultaneous multisite catheter mapping of Koch's triangle. *Circulation* 1996;93:960–968.
78. Josephson ME. *Artioventricular nodal reentry; What have we learned from ablation techniques?.* Great Britain: Kluwer Academic Publishers, 1998.
79. McGuire MA, Bourke JP, Robotin MC, et al. High resolution mapping of Koch's triangle using sixty electrodes in humans with atrioventricular junctional (AV nodal) reentrant tachycardia. *Circulation* 1993;88:2315–2328.
80. Ross DL, Johnson DC, Denniss AR, et al. Curative surgery for atrioventricular junctional ("AV nodal") reentrant tachycardia. *J Am Coll Cardiol* 1985;6:1383–1392.
81. Katritsis DG, Camm AJ. Classification and differential diagnosis of atrioventricular nodal re-entrant tachycardia. *Europace* 2006;8:29–36.
82. Katritsis DG, Josephson ME. Classification of electrophysiological types of atrioventricular nodal re-entrant tachycardia: a reappraisal. *Europace* 2013;15:1231–1240.
83. Gomes JA, Dhatt MS, Damato AN, et al. Incidence, determinants and significance of fixed retrograde conduction in the region of the atrioventricular node. Evidence for retrograde atrioventricular nodal bypass tracts. *Am J Cardiol* 1979;44:1089–1098.
84. Josephson ME, Kastor JA. Paroxysmal supraventricular tachycardia: is the atrium a necessary link? *Circulation* 1976;54:430–435.
85. Wellens HJ, Wesdorp JC, Duren DR, et al. Second degree block during reciprocal atrioventricular nodal tachycardia. *Circulation* 1976;53:595–599.
86. Ko PT, Naccarelli GV, Gulamhusein S, et al. Atrioventricular dissociation during paroxysmal junctional tachycardia. *Pacing Clin Electrophysiol* 1981;4:670–678.
87. Portillo B, Mejias J, Leon-Portillo N, et al. Entrainment of atrioventricular nodal reentrant tachycardias during overdrive pacing from high right atrium and coronary sinus. With special reference to atrioventricular dissociation and 2:1 retrograde block during tachycardias. *Am J Cardiol* 1984;53:1570–1576.
88. Wellens HJ. Unusual examples of supraventricular re-entrant tachycardias. *Circulation* 1975;51:997–1002.
89. Hariman RJ, Chen CM, Caracta AR, et al. Evidence that AV nodal re-entrant tachycardia does not require participation of the entire AV node. *Pacing Clin Electrophysiol* 1983;6:1252–1257.
90. Bauernfeind RA, Wu D, Denes PO, et al. Retrograde block during dual pathway atrioventricular nodal reentrant paroxysmal tachycardia. *Am J Cardiol* 1978;42:499–505.
91. Shimizu A, Ohe T, Takaki H, et al. Narrow QRS complex tachycardia with atrioventricular dissociation. *Pacing Clin Electrophysiol* 1988;11:384–393.

92. Josephson ME, Miller JM. Atrioventricular nodal reentry: evidence supporting an intranodal location. *Pacing Clin Electrophysiol* 1993;16:599–614.
93. Miles WM, Hubbard JE, Zipes DP, et al. Elimination of AV nodal reentrant tachycardia with 2:1 VA block by posteroseptal ablation. *J Cardiovasc Electrophysiol* 1994;5:510–516.
94. Schuger CD, Steinman RT, Lehmann MH. Unmasking and modulation of the excitable gap in atrioventricular nodal reentrant tachycardia: new insight into the microreentry substrate. *J Am Coll Cardiol* 1988;11:115A.
95. Ross DL, Brugada P, Vanagt EJ, et al. Delayed termination of re-entrant atrioventricular nodal tachycardia. *Pacing Clin Electrophysiol* 1983; 6:104–112.
96. Miller JM, Rosenthal ME, Vassallo JA, et al. Atrioventricular nodal reentrant tachycardia: studies on upper and lower 'common pathways'. *Circulation* 1987;75:930–940.
97. Scherlag BJ, Patterson E, Nakagawa H, et al. Changing concepts of A-V nodal conduction: basic and clinical correlates. *Primary Cardiol* 1995; 21:13–21.
98. Loh P, de Bakker JMT, Hocini M, et al. High resolution mapping and dissection of the triangle of Koch in canine hearts: evidence for subatrial reentry during ventricular echoes. *Pacing Clin Electrophysiol* 1997;20:1080.
99. DiMarco JP, Sellers TD, Belardinelli L. Paroxysmal supraventricular tachycardia with Wenckebach block: evidence for reentry within the upper portion of the atrioventricular node. *J Am Coll Cardiol* 1984;3: 1551–1555.
100. Schmitt C, Miller JM, Josephson ME. Atrioventricular nodal supraventricular tachycardia with 2:1 block above the bundle of His. *Pacing Clin Electrophysiol* 1988;11:1018–1023.
101. Man KC, Brinkman K, Bogun F, et al. 2:1 atrioventricular block during atrioventricular node reentrant tachycardia. *J Am Coll Cardiol* 1996; 28:1770–1774.
102. Lee SH, Chen SA, Tai CT, et al. Electrophysiologic characteristics and radiofrequency catheter ablation in atrioventricular node reentrant tachycardia with second-degree atrioventricular block. *J Cardiovasc Electrophysiol* 1997;8:502–511.
103. Willems S, Shenasa M, Borggrefe M, et al. Atrioventricular nodal reentry tachycardia: electrophysiologic comparisons in patients with and without 2:1 infra-His block. *Clin Cardiol* 1993;16:883–888.
104. Yeh SJ, Yamamoto T, Lin FC, et al. Atrioventricular block in the atypical form of junctional reciprocating tachycardia: evidence supporting the atrioventricular node as the site of reentry. *J Am Coll Cardiol* 1990;15:385–392.
105. Hirao K, Otomo K, Wang X, et al. Para-Hisian pacing. A new method for differentiating retrograde conduction over an accessory AV pathway from conduction over the AV node. *Circulation* 1996;94:1027–1035.
106. Wah JYL, Friday K, Sakurai M, et al. Is the His bundle part of the AV nodal reentrant circuit? (Abstract). *Circulation* 1985;72:271.
107. Wu D, Wyndham C, Amat-y-Leon F, et al. The effects of ouabain on induction of atrioventricular nodal re-entrant paroxysmal supraventricular tachycardia. *Circulation* 1975;52:201–207.
108. Wu D, Kou HC, Yeh SJ, et al. Effects of oral verapamil in patients with atrioventricular reentrant tachycardia incorporating an accessory pathway. *Circulation* 1983;67:426–433.
109. Sakurai M, Yasuda H, Kato N, et al. Acute and chronic effects of verapamil in patients with paroxysmal supraventricular tachycardia. *Am Heart J* 1983;105:619–628.
110. Hamer AW, Zaher CA, Peter T, et al. Verapamil effects in AV node reentry tachycardia with intermittent supra-Hisian AV block. *Am Heart J* 1984; 107:431–439.
111. Reddy CP, McAllister RG Jr. Effect of verapamil on retrograde conduction in atrioventricular nodal reentrant tachycardia. *Am J Cardiol* 1984;54:535–543.
112. Yeh SJ, Lin FC, Chou YY, et al. Termination of paroxysmal supraventricular tachycardia with a single oral dose of diltiazem and propranolol. *Circulation* 1985;71:104–109.
113. DiMarco JP, Sellers TD, Berne RM, et al. Adenosine: electrophysiologic effects and therapeutic use for terminating paroxysmal supraventricular tachycardia. *Circulation* 1983;68:1254–1263.
114. Belhassen B, Pelleg A. Acute management of paroxysmal supraventricular tachycardia: verapamil, adenosine triphosphate or adenosine? *Am J Cardiol* 1984;54:225–227.
115. Belhassen B, Glick A, Laniado S. Comparative clinical and electrophysiologic effects of adenosine triphosphate and verapamil on paroxysmal reciprocating junctional tachycardia. *Circulation* 1988;77:795–805.
116. Akhtar M, Damato AN, Batsford WP, et al. Induction of atrioventricular nodal reentrant tachycardia after atropine. Report of five cases. *Am J Cardiol* 1975;36:286–291.
117. Wu D, Denes P, Bauernfeind R, et al. Effects of procainamide on atrioventricular nodal re-entrant paroxysmal tachycardia. *Circulation* 1978;57: 1171–1179.
118. Bauernfeind RA, Wyndham CR, Dhingra RC, et al. Serial electrophysiologic testing of multiple drugs in patients with atrioventricular nodal reentrant paroxysmal tachycardia. *Circulation* 1980;62:1341–1349.
119. Swiryn S, Bauernfeind RA, Wyndham CR, et al. Effects of oral disopyramide phosphate on induction of paroxysmal supraventricular tachycardia. *Circulation* 1981;64:169–175.
120. Brugada P, Wellens HJ. Effects of intravenous and oral disopyramide on paroxysmal atrioventricular nodal tachycardia. *Am J Cardiol* 1984; 53:88–92.
121. Garcia-Civera R, Sanjuan R, Morell S, et al. Effects of propafenone on induction and maintenance of atrioventricular nodal reentrant tachycardia. *Pacing Clin Electrophysiol* 1984;7:649–655.
122. Josephson ME, Seides SE, Batsford WB, et al. The effects of carotid sinus pressure in re-entrant paroxysmal supraventricular tachycardia. *Am Heart J* 1974;88:694–697.
123. Farshidi A, Josephson ME, Horowitz LN. Electrophysiologic characteristics of concealed bypass tracts: clinical and electrocardiographic correlates. *Am J Cardiol* 1978;41:1052–1060.
124. Ross DL, Uther JB. Diagnosis of concealed accessory pathways in supraventricular tachycardia. *Pacing Clin Electrophysiol* 1984;7:1069–1085.
125. Josephson ME, Wellens HJ, eds. *Electrophysiologic evaluation of supraventricular tachycardia*. Philadelphia, PA: WB Saunders; 1997.
126. Brugada P, Bar FW, Vanagt EJ, et al. Observations in patients showing A-V junctional echoes with a shorter P-R than R-P interval. *Am J Cardiol* 1981;48:611–622.
127. Sung RJ. Incessant supraventricular tachycardia. *Pacing Clin Electrophysiol* 1983;6:1306–1326.
128. Bardy GH, Packer DL, German LD, et al. Paradoxical delay in accessory pathway conduction during long R-P' tachycardia after interpolated ventricular premature complexes. *Am J Cardiol* 1985;55:1223–1225.
129. Critelli G, Gallagher JJ, Monda V, et al. Anatomic and electrophysiologic substrate of the permanent form of junctional reciprocating tachycardia. *J Am Coll Cardiol* 1984;4:601–610.
130. Okumura K, Henthorn RW, Epstein AE, et al. "Incessant" atrioventricular (AV) reciprocating tachycardia utilizing left lateral AV bypass pathway with a long retrograde conduction time. *Pacing Clin Electrophysiol* 1986;9:332–342.
131. Packer DL, Bardy GH, Worley SJ, et al. Tachycardia-induced cardiomyopathy: a reversible form of left ventricular dysfunction. *Am J Cardiol* 1986;57:563–570.
132. Cruz FE, Cheriex EC, Smeets JL, et al. Reversibility of tachycardia-induced cardiomyopathy after cure of incessant supraventricular tachycardia. *J Am Coll Cardiol* 1990;16:739–744.
133. Holmes DR, Jr., Hartzler GO, Maloney JD. Concealed retrograde bypass tracts and enhanced atrioventricular nodal conduction. An unusual subset of patients with refractory paroxysmal supraventricular tachycardia. *Am J Cardiol* 1980;45:1053–1060.
134. Levy AM, Bonazinga BJ. Sudden sinus slowing with junctional escape: a common mode of initiation of juvenile supraventricular tachycardia. *Circulation* 1983;67:84–87.
135. Weiss J, Brugada P, Roy D, et al. Localization of the accessory pathway in the Wolff-Parkinson-White syndrome from the ventriculo-atrial conduction time of right ventricular apical extrasystoles. *Pacing Clin Electrophysiol* 1983;6:260–267.
136. Knight BP, Zivin A, Souza J, et al. A technique for the rapid diagnosis of atrial tachycardia in the electrophysiology laboratory. *J Am Coll Cardiol* 1999;33:775–781.
137. Gonzalez-Torrecilla E, Arenal A, Atienza F, et al. First postpacing interval after tachycardia entrainment with correction for atrioventricular node delay: a simple maneuver for differential diagnosis of atrioventricular nodal reentrant tachycardias versus orthodromic reciprocating tachycardias. *Heart Rhythm* 2006;3:674–679.
138. Michaud GF, Tada H, Chough S, et al. Differentiation of atypical atrioventricular node re-entrant tachycardia from orthodromic reciprocating tachycardia using a septal accessory pathway by the response to ventricular pacing. *J Am Coll Cardiol* 2001;38:1163–1167.
139. Reddy VY, Jongnarangsin K, Albert CM, et al. Para-Hisian entrainment: a novel pacing maneuver to differentiate orthodromic atrioventricular

reentrant tachycardia from atrioventricular nodal reentrant tachycardia. *J Cardiovasc Electrophysiol* 2003;14:1321–1328.
140. Miller JM, Rosenthal ME, Gottlieb CD, et al. A new criterion reliably distinguishes atrioventricular nodal reentrant from septal bypass tract tachycardias. *J Am Coll Cardiol* 1987;9:12A.
141. Martinez-Alday JD, Almendral J, Arenal A, et al. Identification of concealed posteroseptal Kent pathways by comparison of ventriculoatrial intervals from apical and posterobasal right ventricular sites. *Circulation* 1994;89:1060–1067.
142. Owada S, Iwasa A, Sasaki S, et al. "V-H-A Pattern" as a criterion for the differential diagnosis of atypical AV nodal reentrant tachycardia from AV reciprocating tachycardia. *Pacing Clin Electrophysiol* 2005;28:667–674.
143. Benditt DG, Benson DW, Jr., Dunnigan A, et al. Role of extrastimulus site and tachycardia cycle length in inducibility of atrial preexcitation by premature ventricular stimulation during reciprocating tachycardia. *Am J Cardiol* 1987;60:811–819.
144. Lehmann MH, Denker S, Mahmud R, et al. Electrophysiologic mechanisms of functional bundle branch block at onset of induced orthodromic tachycardia in the Wolff-Parkinson-White syndrome. Role of stimulation method. *J Clin Invest* 1985;76:1566–1574.
145. Pritchett EL, Tonkin AM, Dugan FA, et al. Ventriculo-atrial conduction time during reciprocating tachycardia with intermittent bundle-branch block in Wolff-Parkinson-White syndrome. *Br Heart J* 1976;38:1058–1064.
146. Kerr CR, Gallagher JJ, German LD. Changes in ventriculoatrial intervals with bundle branch block aberration during reciprocating tachycardia in patients with accessory atrioventricular pathways. *Circulation* 1982;66:196–201.
147. Spurrell RA, Krikler DM, Sowton E. Retrograde invasion of the bundle branches producing aberration of the QRS complex during supraventricular tachycardia studied by programmed electrical stimulation. *Circulation* 1974;50:487–495.
148. Morady F, Wang YS, Scheinman MM, et al. Extent of atrial participation in atrioventricular-reciprocating tachycardia. *Circulation* 1983;67:646–650.
149. Morady F, Scheinman MM, Winston SA, et al. Dissociation of atrial electrograms by right and left atrial pacing in patients with atrioventricular reciprocating tachycardia. *J Am Coll Cardiol* 1984;4:1283–1289.
150. Saoudi NC, Castellanos A, Zaman L, et al. Attempted entrainment of circus movement tachycardias by ventricular stimulation. *Pacing Clin Electrophysiol* 1986;9:78–90.
151. Ormaetxe JM, Almendral J, Arenal A, et al. Ventricular fusion during resetting and entrainment of orthodromic supraventricular tachycardia involving septal accessory pathways. Implications for the differential diagnosis with atrioventricular nodal reentry. *Circulation* 1993;88:2623–2631.
152. Miles WM, Yee R, Klein GJ, et al. The preexcitation index: an aid in determining the mechanism of supraventricular tachycardia and localizing accessory pathways. *Circulation* 1986;74:493–500.
153. Sellers TD, Jr., Gallagher JJ, Cope GD, et al. Retrograde atrial preexcitation following premature ventricular beats during reciprocating tachycardia in the Wolff-Parkinson-White syndrome. *Eur J Cardiol* 1976;4:283–294.
154. Ross DL, Farre J, Bar FW, et al. Spontaneous termination of circus movement tachycardia using an atrioventricular accessory pathway: incidence, site of block and mechanisms. *Circulation* 1981;63:1129–1139.
155. Brugada P, Bar FW, Vanagt EJ, et al. Observations on mechanisms of circus movement tachycardia in the Wolff-Parkinson-White syndrome. Role of different tachycardia circuits and sites of block in maintenance of tachycardia. *Pacing Clin Electrophysiol* 1981;4:507–516.
156. Waxman MB, Cupps CL. Spontaneous termination of paroxysmal supraventricular tachycardia following disappearance of bundle branch block ipsilateral to a concealed atrioventricular accessory pathway: the role of autonomic tone in tachycardia diagnosis. *Pacing Clin Electrophysiol* 1986;9:26–35.
157. Wellens HJ, Tan SL, Bar FW, et al. Effect of verapamil studied by programmed electrical stimulation of the heart in patients with paroxysmal re-entrant supraventricular tachycardia. *Br Heart J* 1977;39:1058–1066.
158. Horio Y, Matsuyama K, Morikami Y, et al. Blocking effect of verapamil on conduction over a catecholamine-sensitive bypass tract in exercise-induced Wolff-Parkinson-White syndrome. *J Am Coll Cardiol* 1984;4:186–191.
159. Chang MS, Sung RJ, Tai TY, et al. Nadolol and supraventricular tachycardia: an electrophysiologic study. *J Am Coll Cardiol* 1983;2:894–903.
160. Betriu A, Chaitman BR, Bourassa MG, et al. Beneficial effect of intravenous diltiazem in the acute management of paroxysmal supraventricular tachyarrhythmias. *Circulation* 1983;67:88–94.
161. Klein GJ, Gulamhusein S, Prystowsky EN, et al. Comparison of the electrophysiologic effects of intravenous and oral verapamil in patients with paroxysmal supraventricular tachycardia. *Am J Cardiol* 1982;49:117–124.
162. Rosenthal M, Oseran DS, Gang E. Verapamil-induced retrograde conduction block in a concealed atrioventricular bypass tract. *Am J Cardiol* 1985;55:1222–1223.
163. Kou HC, Hung JS, Lee YS, et al. Effects of oral disopyramide phosphate on induction and sustenance of atrioventricular reentrant tachycardia incorporating retrograde accessory pathway conduction. *Circulation* 1982;66:454–462.
164. Abdollah H, Brugada P, Green M, et al. Clinical efficacy and electrophysiologic effects of intravenous and oral encainide in patients with accessory atrioventricular pathways and supraventricular arrhythmias. *Am J Cardiol* 1984;54:544–549.
165. Brugada P, Abdollah H, Wellens HJ. Suppression of incessant supraventricular tachycardia by intravenous and oral encainide. *J Am Coll Cardiol* 1984;4:1255–1260.
166. Kunze KP, Kuck KH, Schluter M, et al. Effect of encainide and flecainide on chronic ectopic atrial tachycardia. *J Am Coll Cardiol* 1986;7:1121–1126.
167. Alboni P, Shantha N, Pirani R, et al. Effects of amiodarone on supraventricular tachycardia involving bypass tracts. *Am J Cardiol* 1984;53:93–98.
168. Haines DE, Lerman BB, DiMarco JP. Repetitive supraventricular tachycardia: clinical manifestations and response to therapy with amiodarone. *Pacing Clin Electrophysiol* 1986;9:130–133.
169. Barker PS, Wilson FN, Johnston FD. The mechanism of auricular paroxysmal tachycardia. *Am Heart J* 1943;26:435–445.
170. Allessie MA, Bonke FI. Direct demonstration of sinus node reentry in the rabbit heart. *Circ Res* 1979;44:557–568.
171. Paulay KL, Varghese PJ, Damato AN. Sinus node reentry. An in vivo demonstration in the dog. *Circ Res* 1973;32:455–463.
172. Childers RW, Arnsdorf MF, De la Fuente DJ, et al. Sinus nodal echoes. Clinical case report and canine studies. *Am J Cardiol* 1973;31:220–231.
173. Paulay KL, Weisfogel GM, Damato AN. Sinus nodal reentry. Effect of quinidine. *Am J Cardiol* 1974;33:617–622.
174. Weisfogel GM, Batsford WP, Paulay KL, et al. Sinus node re-entrant tachycardia in man. *Am Heart J* 1975;90:295–304.
175. Kirchhof C, Bonke FIM, Allessie MA, eds. *Sinus node reentry—Fact or fiction?* Mt. Kisco, NY: Futura Publishing; 1987.
176. Wu D, Amat-y-leon F, Denes P, et al. Demonstration of sustained sinus and atrial re-entry as a mechanism of paroxysmal supraventricular tachycardia. *Circulation* 1975;51:234–243.
177. Curry PV, Evans TR, Krikler DM. Paroxysmal reciprocating sinus tachycardia. *Eur J Cardiol* 1977;6:199–228.
178. Gomes JA, Hariman RJ, Kang PS, et al. Sustained symptomatic sinus node reentrant tachycardia: incidence, clinical significance, electrophysiologic observations and the effects of antiarrhythmic agents. *J Am Coll Cardiol* 1985;5:45–57.
179. Paulay KL, Ruskin JN, Damato AN. Sinus and atrioventricular nodal reentrant tachycardia in the same patient. *Am J Cardiol* 1975;36:810–816.
180. Chen SA, Chiang CE, Yang CJ, et al. Sustained atrial tachycardia in adult patients. Electrophysiological characteristics, pharmacological response, possible mechanisms, and effects of radiofrequency ablation. *Circulation* 1994;90:1262–1278.
181. Engelstein ED, Lippman N, Stein KM, et al. Mechanism-specific effects of adenosine on atrial tachycardia. *Circulation* 1994;89:2645–2654.
182. Callans DJ, Hook BG, Josephson ME. Comparison of resetting and entrainment of uniform sustained ventricular tachycardia. Further insights into the characteristics of the excitable gap. *Circulation* 1993;87:1229–1238.
183. Scheinman MM, Basu D, Hollenberg M. Electrophysiologic studies in patients with persistent atrial tachycardia. *Circulation* 1974;50:266–273.
184. Gillette PC, Garson A, Jr. Electrophysiologic and pharmacologic characteristics of automatic ectopic atrial tachycardia. *Circulation* 1977;56:571–575.
185. Mehta AV, Sanchez GR, Sacks EJ, et al. Ectopic automatic atrial tachycardia in children: clinical characteristics, management and follow-up. *J Am Coll Cardiol* 1988;11:379–385.

186. Chen SA, Yang CJ, Chiang CE, et al. Reversibility of left ventricular dysfunction after successful catheter ablation of supraventricular reentrant tachycardia. *Am Heart J* 1992;124:1512–1516.
187. Rabbani LE, Wang PJ, Couper GL, et al. Time course of improvement in ventricular function after ablation of incessant automatic atrial tachycardia. *Am Heart J* 1991;121:816–819.
188. Corey WA, Markel ML, Hoit BD, et al. Regression of a dilated cardiomyopathy after radiofrequency ablation of incessant supraventricular tachycardia. *Am Heart J* 1993;126:1469–1473.
189. Morillo CA, Klein GJ, Thakur RK, et al. Mechanism of 'inappropriate' sinus tachycardia. Role of sympathovagal balance. *Circulation* 1994;90:873–877.
190. Denes P, Kehoe R, Rosen KM. Multiple reentrant tachycardias due to retrograde conduction of dual atrioventricular bundles with atrioventricular nodal-like properties. *Am J Cardiol* 1979;44:162–170.
191. Amat-y-Leon F, Wyndham C, Wu D, et al. Participation of fast and slow A-V nodal pathways in tachycardias complicating the Wolff-Parkinson-White syndrome. Report of a case. *Circulation* 1977;55:663–668.
192. Heddle WF, Brugada P, Wellens HJ. Multiple circus movement tachycardias with multiple accessory pathways. *J Am Coll Cardiol* 1984;4:168–175.
193. Bar FW, Brugada P, Dassen WR, et al. Differential diagnosis of tachycardia with narrow QRS complex (shorter than 0.12 second). *Am J Cardiol* 1984;54:555–560.
194. Chen SA, Tai CT, Chiang CE, et al., eds. *Role of the surface electrocardiogram in the diagnosis of patients with supraventricular tachycardia.* Philadelphia, PA: WB Saunders; 1997.
195. Josephson ME, Wellens HJ. Differential diagnosis of supraventricular tachycardia. *Cardiol Clin* 1990;8:411–442.

CHAPTER

9

# Atrial Flutter and Fibrillation

Atrial fibrillation and its cousin, atrial flutter (typical and atypical), are the most common arrhythmias with which we must deal clinically, yet they are the group of arrhythmias about which we know the least. For the past decade, experimental data as well as clinical electrophysiology studies have allowed a better, but still incomplete, understanding of these arrhythmias. It appears that they represent a heterogeneous group of disorders that are markedly influenced by the functional and anatomic structures of the right and left atrium as well as the autonomic nervous system. Atrial fibrillation and flutter frequently coexist and can appear spontaneously or can be induced in the same patient. As such, this chapter will deal with these arrhythmias.

The clinical and electrophysiologic definitions of atrial fibrillation and flutter are hard to decipher. More recently, atrial fibrillation has been divided into paroxysmal (self-terminating within 7 days), persistent (lasting greater than 1 week or requiring electrical or pharmacologic cardioversion), and permanent (failed cardioversion or not attempted).[1] Others have tried to categorize atrial fibrillation by assumed mechanisms, such as a focal atrial fibrillation, vagally mediated atrial fibrillation, sympathetically mediated atrial fibrillation, etc. Atrial fibrillation has also been classified based on whether or not it appears as an isolated electrical phenomenon (lone atrial fibrillation) or whether it is associated with some form of organic disease. All of these classifications have limitations. The fact that there are so many definitions attests to our lack of total understanding of this arrhythmia.

Atrial flutter, about which we know more, is also heterogeneously defined. Typical flutter is a term now used to describe both "classic" counterclockwise flutter in which the inferior leads demonstrate a sawtooth-like undulating baseline with positive flutter waves in lead $V_1$ and negative flutter waves in $V_6$, and clockwise flutter, which has positive, notched flutter waves in the inferior leads and in $V_6$ and negative flutter waves in $V_1$. Both of these patterns are currently believed to be due to reentry with opposite directions of activation (counterclockwise and clockwise) in the same anatomic circuit. The term "atypical" flutter is currently applied to any macrorentrant atrial tachycardia that is different from these two. This might involve an organized rhythm related to prior surgery in the right atrium, around the pulmonary veins (PVs), postablation, or potentially even around a repaired atrial septal defect. Moreover, it is now well recognized that automatic atrial tachycardia can produce an ECG quite similar to that of atrial flutter. Therefore, the differentiation between atrial flutter and atrial tachycardia on the surface ECG alone is often based primarily on rate. As such, the differentiation between "atrial flutter" and atrial tachycardia is really based on whether the tachycardia has a macroreentrant or focal mechanism, something undefinable by ECG alone. It is therefore necessary to distinguish a reentrant mechanism from an automatic mechanism to diagnose "atrial flutter" versus atrial tachycardia when tachycardia rates are 250 to 320 beats per minute (bpm) in the absence of drugs. I prefer to use the terms macrorentrant and focal atrial tachycardia; the term "flutter" is too often misused and incorrect. The term typical flutter should be used to describe macroreentrant, tricuspid-caval isthmus-dependent atrial tachycardia.

Given all these variables, this chapter will discuss the role of electrophysiology studies in evaluating these arrhythmias. Programmed atrial stimulation and endocardial activation mapping techniques have been used to (a) analyze the electrophysiologic substrates of atrial conduction, refractoriness, and ectopic atrial impulse formation that may be responsible for the initiation of either macroreentrant atrial tachycardia (i.e., typical and atypical atrial flutter) or atrial fibrillation; (b) establish the electrophysiologic mechanism and clinical significance of spontaneous and induced macrorentrant atrial tachycardia or fibrillation; (c) provide a method of evaluating the site of origin of ectopic impulse formation (if present) and/or the site and size of the reentrant circuit (if present) of macroreentrant atrial tachycardia by defining patterns of atrial activation during flutter; (d) characterize the presence and extent of an excitable gap in reentrant atrial tachycardia or during atrial fibrillation; (e) provide information concerning the ability to terminate macrorentrant atrial tachycardia by pacing; (f) define sites required for successful ablation of macroreentrant atrial tachycardias and develop electrophysiologic and/or anatomically based procedures to prevent atrial fibrillation; (g) evaluate the effect of pharmacologic agents on initiation and/or maintenance of fibrillation or macroreentrant atrial tachycardia; and (h) define a role of preventative pacing and atrial defibrillation as therapeutic options for atrial flutter and fibrillation. Additional benefits of an electrophysiologic study are the ability to determine the nature of wide complex rhythms during these tachycardias, which can have clear-cut diagnostic and therapeutic implications.

## ELECTROPHYSIOLOGIC AND ANATOMIC SUBSTRATES OF MACROREENTRANT ATRIAL TACHYCARDIA (TYPICAL AND ATYPICAL ATRIAL FLUTTER) AND FIBRILLATION

Atrial fibrillation occurs in many disease states, but can occur in the absence of disease, that is, lone atrial fibrillation. Microscopic abnormalities can be found in patients with and without atrial fibrillation which may be part of normal aging. Even in those cases of lone atrial fibrillation, pathologic studies have demonstrated a variety of abnormalities including myocardial hypertrophy, vacuolar degeneration, ultrastructural evidence of fibrillolysis, lymphocytic infiltrates, and patchy fibrosis, all of which suggest a myopathic process with various degrees of inflammation.[2] While none of these abnormalities are specific for patients developing spontaneous atrial fibrillation, similar findings were not observed in patients undergoing open heart surgery for Wolff–Parkinson–White syndrome with no history of atrial fibrillation. Moreover, the anatomy of the atria is very complex, as it is derived from regions with trabeculated myocardium (free wall of right and left atrium), multiple orifices (superior and inferior vena cava), coronary sinus (CS), ostia of the PVs, the mitral and tricuspid annulae, and the multilayered region of the fossa ovalis. The atria are a complex three-dimensional structure with many anatomic obstacles as well as variable oriented muscle fiber adjacent to and overlying one another on both the endocardial and epicardial surfaces, particularly in the left atrium (Fig. 9-1). This is most marked around the ostia of the PVs and the adjacent posterior wall (see section on Atrial Fibrillation). These multiple adjoining regions, in and of themselves, produce abnormalities of propagation in the absence of differing electrophysiologic properties. However, to complicate matters, the cellular electrophysiology of the various parts of the atrial tissue vary. For example, along the crista terminalis, cells possess phase 4 depolarization and a prolonged phase 2 following a transient outward current.[3] Septal myocardial cells do not show diastolic depolarization and have triangulated action potentials. Other areas in the atrium show postrepolarization refractoriness due to different recovery kinetics of potassium currents and/or impaired excitability. Thus, there is heterogeneity of recovery of excitability or functional refractoriness throughout the atria. Anisotropic propagation is nonuniform and gets progressively more nonuniform with age. Spach et al.[4,5] have shown that with aging there is loss of side-to-side connections along the thick muscle of the crista terminalis, which provides a substrate for reentrant excitation in very small areas. The atria are also markedly influenced by cholinergic as well as sympathetic innervation. This has also been shown to occur in a heterogeneous fashion.[6] There are several ganglionic plexuses around the atria (Fig. 9-2).[7] Thus, the atria have anatomic, electrophysiologic, and neurologic heterogeneity to such an extent that it is surprising why everybody does not have atrial arrhythmias.

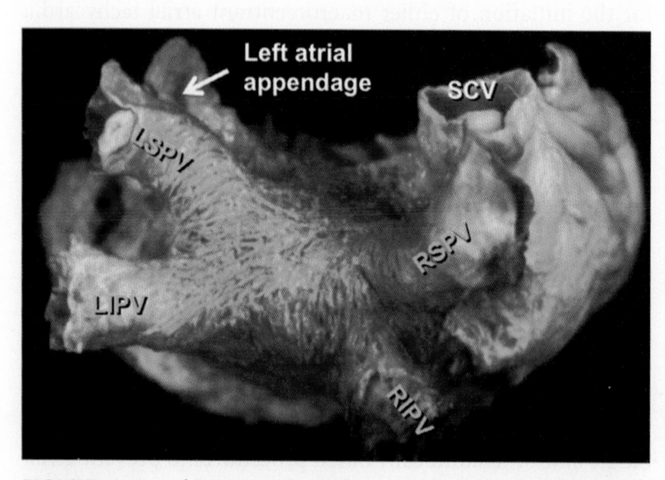


**FIGURE 9-1** *Architecture of atrial musculature in the left atrium.* The left atrium is viewed in the posterior view. The right and left superior and inferior veins (*LSPV, LIPV, RSPV, RIPV*) are shown. Note the relationship between the left atrial appendage and the LSPV and the superior vena cava (*SVC*) and the RSPV. Their proximity can lead to far-field signals from these structures recorded in the pulmonary veins. Note the complex arrangement of the left atrial musculature.

Clinical electrophysiologic observations in our laboratory[8–11] and those of others[12–15] have clearly pointed out certain common abnormalities of conduction and refractoriness present in patients who have macrorentrant atrial tachycardias and/or fibrillation. These are enumerated below.

### Conduction Defects in Patients with Atrial Fibrillation and Flutter

Many patients with atrial fibrillation and macroreentrant, tricuspid-caval isthmus-dependent atrial tachycardia (i.e., typical flutter) flutter have significant intra-atrial conduction defects manifested on the surface electrocardiogram by broad (110 msec or greater) and notched P waves in the inferior leads, a negative P terminal force of 1 mm in depth and duration in $V_1$, and/or a delayed terminal positive force in aVL. These are characteristic findings of so-called left atrial abnormality and are present in the vast majority of patients with atrial flutter or fibrillation, regardless of the underlying etiology. The broad notched P wave in the inferior leads is the most common abnormality, while the exaggerated negative terminal force in $V_1$ is the next most common. One or more of these abnormalities are seen in 80% to 85% of patients with these arrhythmias. A third electrocardiographic sign is terminal positivity of the P wave in aVL. In nearly two-thirds of patients, the P-wave duration exceeds 120 msec when all 12 leads are assessed simultaneously. We have now mapped more than 200 patients with left atrial abnormality using standard recordings from the high-right atrium (HRA), the low septal right atrium at the A-V junction, and at the proximal, lateral, and anterior

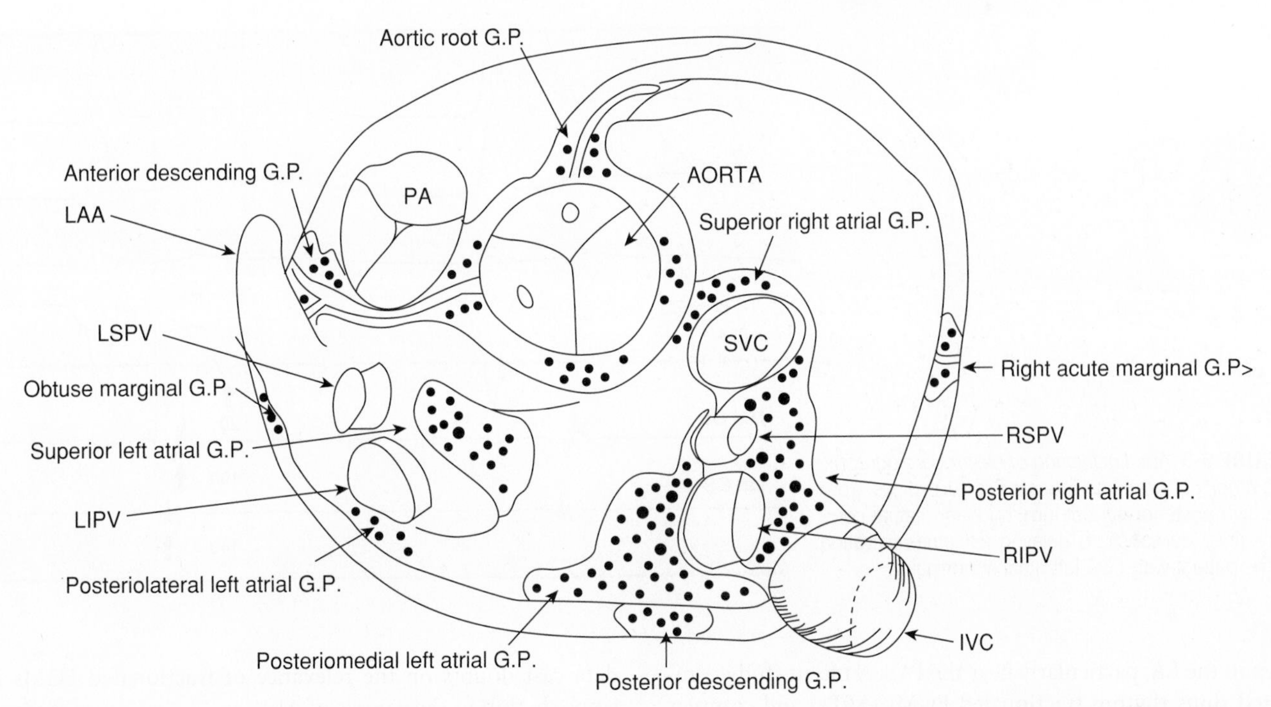


**FIGURE 9-2** *Ganglionated plexus around the atria in the superior view. PA, pulmonary artery; LAA, left atrial appendage; LSPV, left superior pulmonary vein; LIPV, left inferior pulmonary vein; RSPV, right superior pulmonary vein; RIPV, right inferior pulmonary vein; SVC, superior vena cava; IVC, inferior vena cava.* (Modified from Armour JA, Murphy DA, Yuan BX, et al. Gross and microscopic anatomy of the human intrinsic cardiac nervous system. *Anat Rec* 1997;247:289–298.)

sites in the CS, and relating the local activation time to the onset of the P wave. As noted in Chapter 2, normal right atrial activation is 35 to 55 msec and activation from the P wave to the CS ranges from 60 to 90 msec.[16] For patients with so-called left atrial abnormalities, right atrial conduction time is normal in 80% of patients with a mean right atrial conduction time of less than 50 msec. For the remaining patients, right atrial conduction time was only modestly prolonged except for six patients with dilated cardiomyopathy who had prolonged right atrial conduction times exceeding 62 msec. In contrast, intra-atrial conduction time, as measured from the P wave to the left lateral atrium recorded from the mid- or distal CS was prolonged in nearly 94% of our patients (Fig. 9-3). Where the site of delay is located is unclear, but there appears to be delay between the right and left atrium at the region of Bachmann bundle as well as at the lower septum. A more detailed analysis of intra-atrial conduction during sinus rhythm in patients with atrial fibrillation is important to assess the potential role, if any, of intra-atrial conduction disturbances in the pathogenesis of atrial fibrillation. Detailed mapping with the Carto system (Biosense, Cordis/Johnson and Johnson, see Chapter 3) has been of value in this regard. Correct interpretation of intra-atrial and interatrial conduction requires mapping along the posterior left atrium and left atrial septum in order to more specifically localize the sites of delay.

Other investigators[3,17,18] have described the electrophysiologic characteristics of atrial endocardial electrograms from the right atrium. They have quantified them in terms of duration and number of fragmented deflections as defined by the number of negative deflections in the electrogram. Normal electrograms were 74 ± 11 msec in duration with 3.9 ± 1.3 negative deflections. Abnormal electrograms were defined as those with a duration of ≥100 msec and/or eight or more fragmented deflections. Mapping was only performed in the right atrium in all of these studies. Twelve atrial sites, including anterior, lateral, posterior, and septal sites were measured at the high-, mid-, and low-right atrium. Only 23% of control patients had any fractionated electrograms while 68% of patients with paroxysmal, lone atrial fibrillation and 83% of patients with atrial fibrillation/flutter and sick sinus syndrome had abnormal electrograms. Those with the longest duration and the most fractionation were seen in patients with atrial fibrillation and flutter and sick sinus syndrome, and two-thirds of the abnormal electrograms were found in the HRA either posteriorly or laterally. The absence of any left atrial mapping data limited the ability to establish a causal relationship of these abnormal electrograms to the presence of atrial flutter or fibrillation. These electrograms, however, do represent marked nonuniform anisotropy and suggest an increased amount of fibrosis in those patients with these electrograms and atrial fibrillation. Whether these abnormalities are casually related to atrial fibrillation is unknown, but they may represent a potential substrate under specific circumstances.

More recently abnormal, multicomponent electrograms have been recorded in the LA near the antrum of the PVs. Pacing either the RA or LA increases the fragmentation, suggesting a prominent role of nonuniform anisotropy and the three-dimensional structure with variable fiber orientation

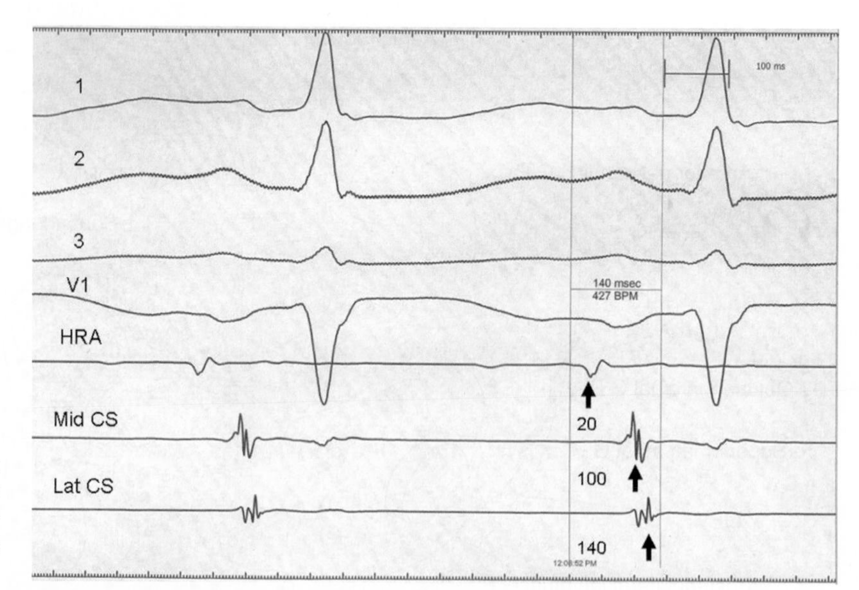


**FIGURE 9-3** *Atrial activation of electrocardiographic left atrial abnormality.* Intracardiac recordings from the high posterior right atrium, mid, and lateral coronary sinus demonstrate delayed left atrial activation in the patient with ECG left atrial abnormality.

seen in the LA, particularly near the PVs. A recent study compared sinus rhythm fractionated EGMs (SRFs) and complex fractionated EGMs (CAFÉs) during AF in the LA in patients with persistent AF and normals.[19] The investigators showed no difference in the distribution of fractionated EGMs in sinus rhythm between patients with AF and controls and no correlation between CAFEs and SRFs. Most SRFs were recorded in areas of collision of activation wavefronts. These data cast doubts on the relevance of fractionated EGMs in sinus rhythm to the genesis of AF.

We and others have been interested in evaluating the response of intra-atrial conduction to atrial extrastimuli during atrial pacing at cycle lengths of 600 and 450 msec.[9–12] In our initial studies[9] we analyzed standard recordings from the HRA, the His bundle recording site, and the midcoronary sinus to evaluate intra-atrial conduction times, maximum intra-atrial

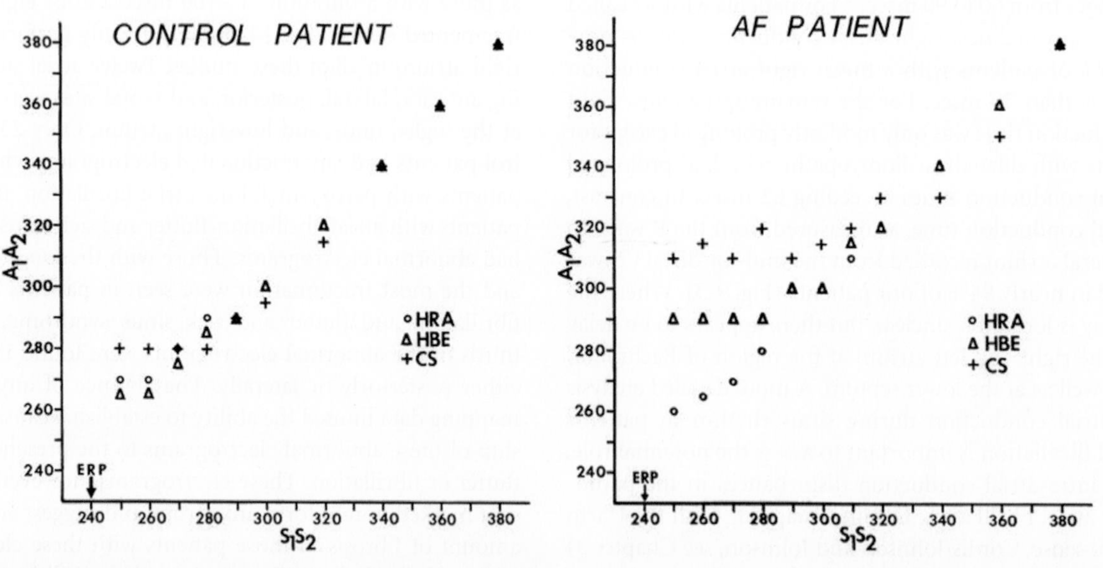


**FIGURE 9-4** *Response of intra-atrial conduction to premature stimuli in a control patient (left) and a patient with spontaneous atrial flutter (AF, right).* $S_1$-$S_2$ represents coupling intervals of extrastimuli to the last beat of an eight-beat drive at paced cycle lengths of 600 msec for each patient. $A_1$-$A_2$ represents conduction times to recording sites at the high-right atrium (HRA), His bundle electrogram (HBE), and coronary sinus (CS). Note the large zone of coupling intervals over which conduction delay is observed to recording sites at HBE and CS in the patient with a history of atrial flutter and/or fibrillation (**right panel**) and the greater degree of conduction delay at each recording site in the patient with atrial dysrhythmia. Stimulation in each patient was performed at the right atrial appendage at a drive cycle length of 600 msec. ERP, atrial effective refractory period. (From Buxton AE, Waxman HL, Marchlinski FE, et al. Atrial conduction: effects of extrastimuli with and without atrial dysrhythmias. *Am J Cardiol* 1984;54:755–761.)

conduction delay at both the A-V junction and midcoronary sinus, and the zone of coupling intervals over which delays were noted. No conduction delays were noted in response to late coupled extrastimuli in both control patients and those with atrial fibrillation or flutter. However, as extrastimuli were delivered with increasing prematurity, progressive intra-atrial conduction delay occurred. In patients without a prior history of arrhythmias (controls), intra-atrial conduction delays only occurred at coupling intervals just above refractoriness, whereas in those patients with a history of atrial flutter and or fibrillation, conduction delays occurred at much longer coupling intervals (Figs. 9-4 and 9-5). The differences in response to atrial extrastimuli between control patients and those with atrial flutter or fibrillation are shown in Figures 9-3 and 9-4. While in the control patients there was very little conduction delay up to atrial refractoriness, in patients with a prior history of typical tricuspid-caval isthmus-dependent atrial flutter of fibrillation these atrial conduction delays were seen beginning 50 msec above refractoriness. There are no data available in patients with other macroreentrant atrial tachycardias, although the association with atrial fibrillation suggests they would respond similarly. Thus, the relative refractory period (RRP) of the atrium is longer in patients with a history of typical atrial flutter or fibrillation. Although the degree of

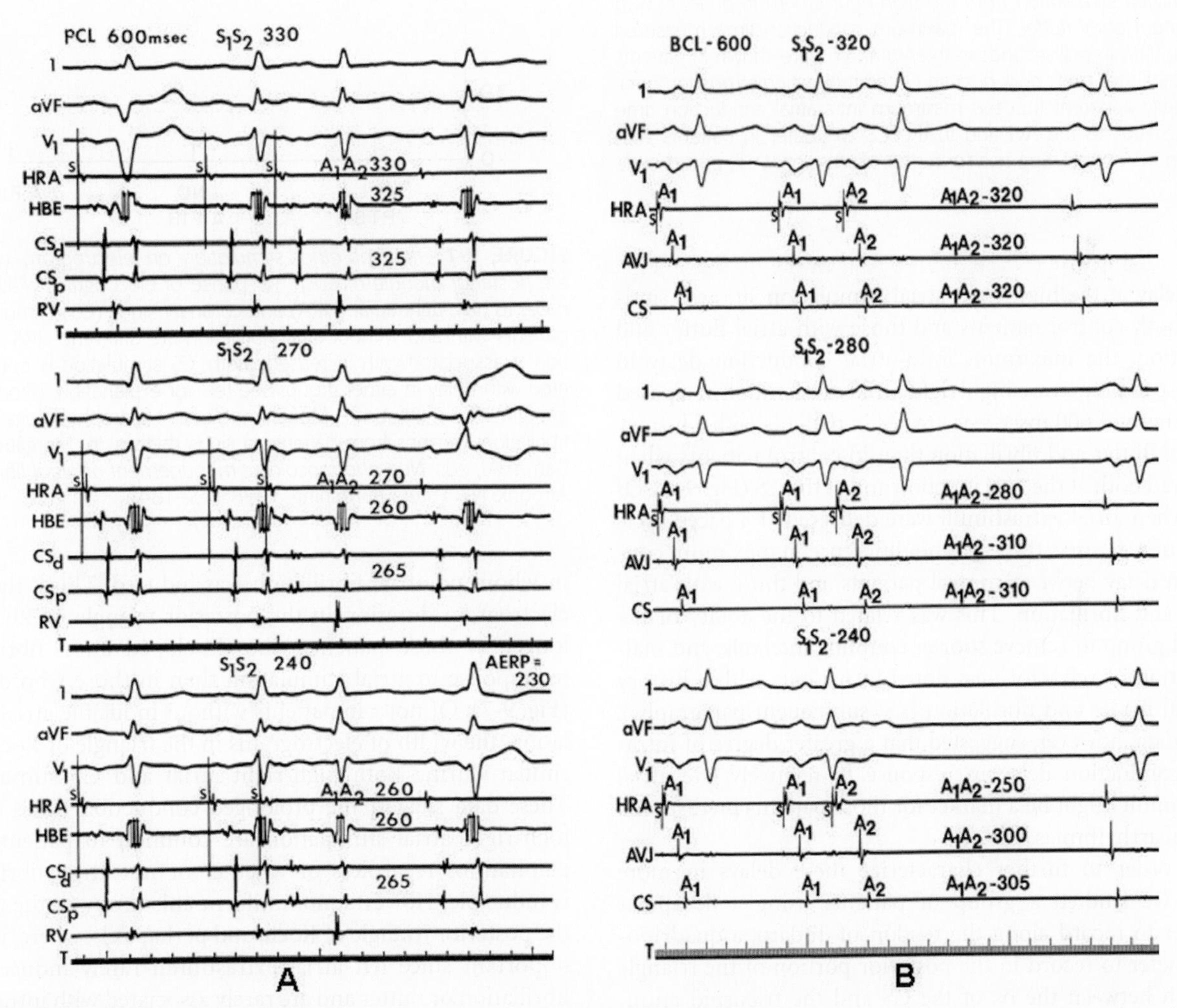


**FIGURE 9-5** *Response of intra-atrial conduction to premature stimulation at a paced cycle length (PCL) of 600 in a patient with and without a history of atrial flutter/fibrillation.* **A:** Response of intra-atrial conduction to premature stimulation at a paced cycle length (PCL) of 600 in a patient without a history of atrial flutter/fibrillation. From top to bottom, leads 1, aVF, $V_1$, electrograms from the HRA, HBE, distal ($CS_d$), proximal ($CS_p$), and RV. The atrial effective refractory period (AERP) in this patient was 230 msec. Premature atrial extrastimuli $S_1$-$S_2$ are delivered during a PCL of 600 msec. Progressively premature extrastimuli only produce slight intra-atrial conduction delays of 20 to 25 msec at coupling intervals just above atrial refractoriness. T, time line. **B:** Response of intra-atrial conduction to premature stimulation at a basic cycle length (BCL) of 600 msec in a patient with a history of atrial flutter and/or fibrillation. The atrial ERP in this patient was 230 msec. Progressive intra-atrial conduction delay occurs in response to increasing prematurity of extrastimuli. The maximal intra-atrial conduction delay observed to the atrioventricular junction (AVJ) recording site was 60 msec, and the maximal intra-atrial conduction delay observed to the CS recording site was 65 msec at an $S_1$-$S_2$ interval of 240 msec (C). HRA, high-right atrium; T, time line. (From Buxton AE, Waxman HL, Marchlinski FE, et al. Atrial conduction: effects of extrastimuli with and without atrial dysrhythmias. *Am J Cardiol* 1984;54:755–761, with permission.)

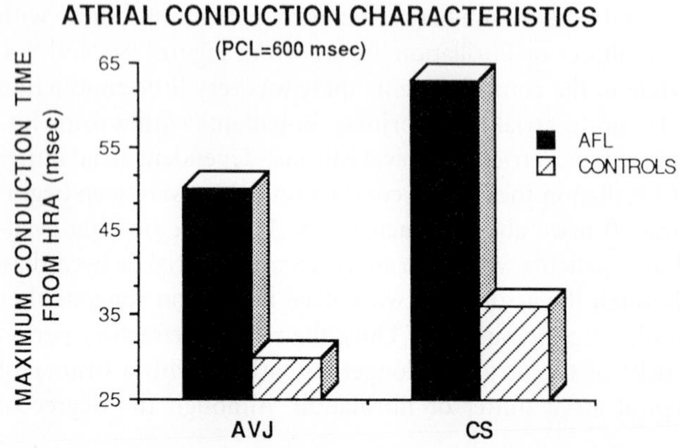

**FIGURE 9-6** *Comparison of atrial conduction time in response to programmed stimulation from the high-right atrium in patients with and without atrial flutter.* The maximum conduction time measured from the HRA in milliseconds to the AVJ and CS are shown in patients with atrial flutter (AFL, *dark bar*) and in control patients (*hashed bar*). It is readily apparent that the maximum intra-atrial conduction time from the HRA to the AVJ and to the CS is greater in patients with AFL than in controls. See text for further discussion. PCL, paced cycle length.

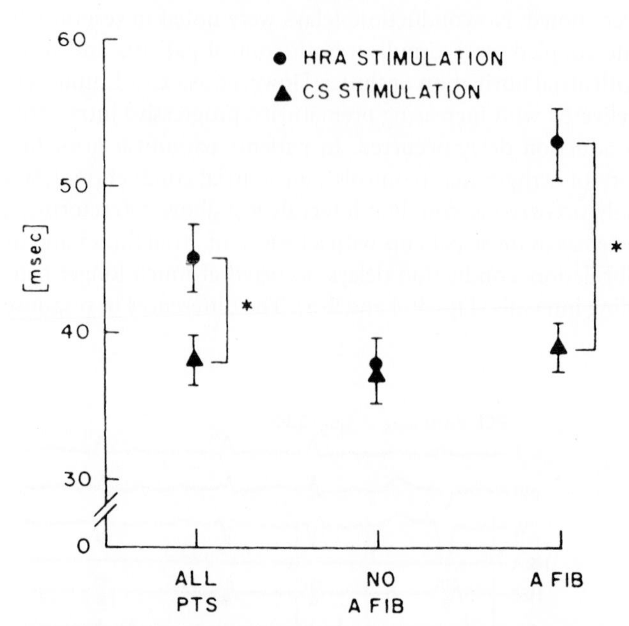


**FIGURE 9-7** *Effect of atrial stimulation on electrogram width in the posterior triangle of Koch.* Response of electrogram width (ordinate) to high-right atrial (HRA) and coronary sinus (CS) stimulation in patients with and without atrial fibrillation are different. HRA stimulation is associated with increased width. CS stimulation is not associated with delay in either group. See text for explanation. (From Papageorgiou P, Zimetbaum P, Monahan K, et al. Electrophysiology of atrial fibrillation. Lessons from patients in sinus rhythm. In: Murgatroyd FD, Camm AJ, eds. *Non-pharmacologic management of atrial fibrillation.* Armonk, NY: Futura Publishing, 1998:173–184.)

local delay at the high-right atrial stimulation site was similar in both control patients and those with atrial flutter and fibrillation, the maximum intra-atrial conduction delay in response to premature high-right atrial extrastimuli at a paced cycle length of 600 msec was greater in patients with a history of atrial flutter and fibrillation than in control patients when measured both at the A-V junction and at the CS (Fig. 9-6). Of note, when atrial extrastimuli were delivered at a paced cycle length of 450 msec, there was no difference in maximum conduction delay between control patients and those with atrial flutter and fibrillation. This was related to the ability of the control group to achieve shorter coupling intervals, and maladaptation of refractoriness noted in patients with a history of atrial flutter and fibrillation (see subsequent paragraphs). These data, however, suggested that a greater degree of intra-atrial conduction delay in response to relatively late atrial extrastimuli might be a marker for those patients predisposed to atrial arrhythmias.[9,12]

In order to further characterize these delays in more detail, we studied a group of patients using a decapolar catheter to record along the tendon of Todaro, a quadripolar catheter to record in the posterior portion of the triangle of Koch between the os of the CS and the tricuspid annulus, and a decapolar catheter in the CS to record the broader area in the left atrium.[10] These studies demonstrated several important findings. First, high-right atrial stimulation was associated with intra-atrial conduction delays at the triangle of Koch and the CS at coupling intervals as much as 60 msec above refractoriness while stimulation of the CS in the same patients produced no such delays. Second, in those patients in whom atrial fibrillation was induced, a greater degree of delay was noted in the triangle of Koch than in those patients in whom no atrial fibrillation was induced. Third, the local electrogram duration in the posterior triangle of Koch was longer in those patients who developed atrial fibrillation in response to atrial stimulation than in those who did not (Fig. 9-7). Of note, in patients without inducible atrial fibrillation, the width of electrograms in the triangle of Koch were similar during both high-right atrial and CS stimulation. These data suggest the prolonged conduction times during high-right atrial stimulation are common to patients with palpitations regardless of whether or not atrial fibrillation is inducible. However, nonuniform anisotropy in the area of the posterior triangle of Koch, and perhaps elsewhere, is quite important since left atrial extrastimuli rarely induce atrial fibrillation or flutter and are rarely associated with intra-atrial conduction delay, particularly in the posterior triangle of Koch (Fig. 9-8). Additional studies using high-density mapping in both atrial chambers would be critical to decide if any particular site of conduction delay is necessary for initiation of atrial fibrillation and/or flutter.

Another important area of conduction block, which seems requisite to the induction of atrial flutter, is that along the crista terminalis.[20–23] Studies of transverse cristal conduction are best performed using a 20-pole catheter placed along the

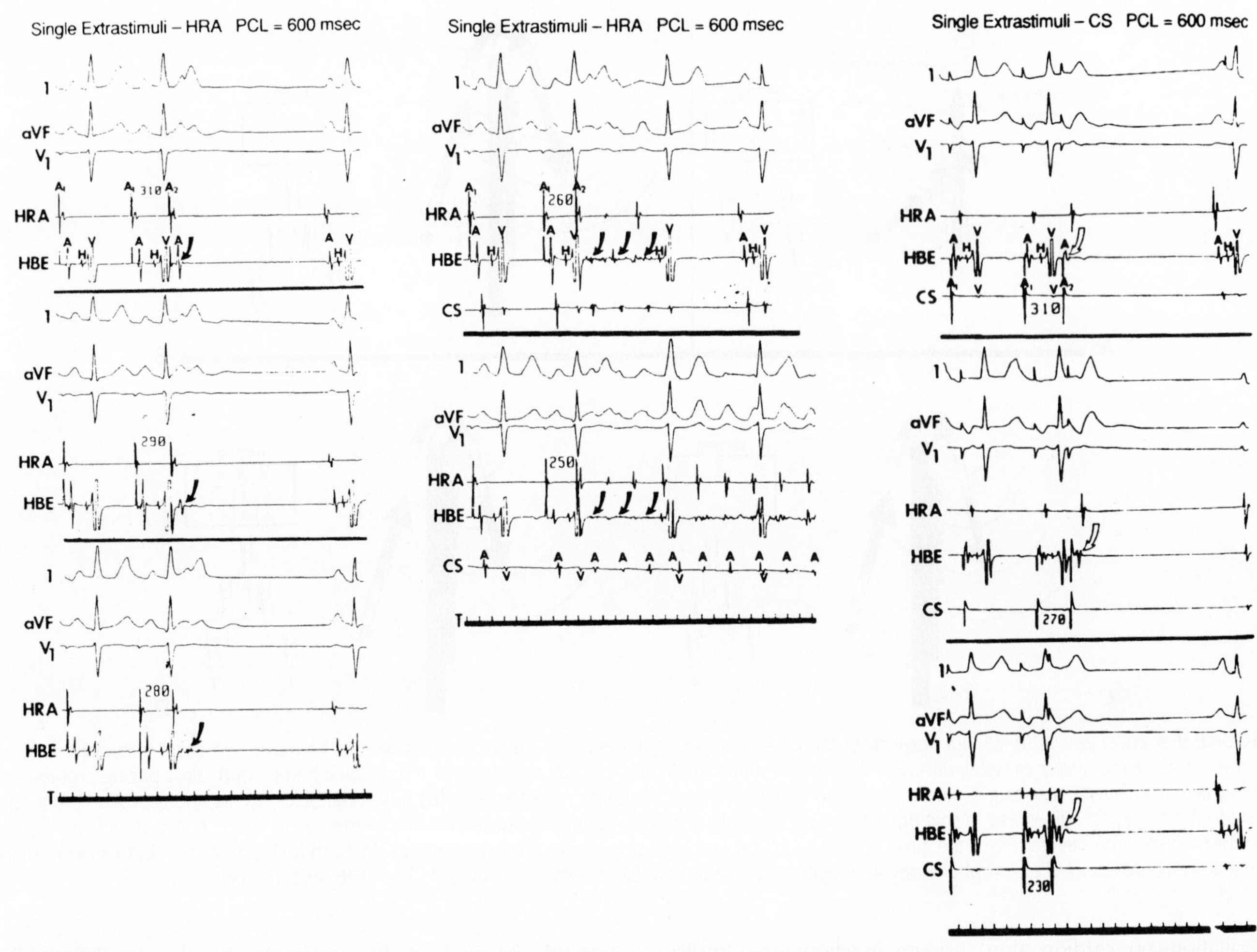


**FIGURE 9-8** *Influence of anisotropy on initiation of atrial flutter/fibrillation.* Three panels are shown with ECG leads 1, aVF, $V_1$ and intracardiac recordings from the high-right atrium (HRA) and His bundle (HBE). Atrial extrastimuli are delivered from the HRA (**two left panels**) and the coronary sinus (CS) at a paced cycle length of 600 msec. Extrastimuli from the HRA are associated with fragmentation in the HBE at a coupling interval of 280 msec and initiates nonsustained and sustained atrial flutter/fibrillation (AFL/AF) at coupling intervals of 260 and 250 msec, respectively. Stimulation from the CS at comparable coupling intervals neither produces fragmentation of the HBE or initiation of AFL/AF. See text for discussion.

crista terminalis with atrial activation rhythm evaluated during pacing at a variety of cycle lengths from the posterior right atrium medial to the crista and the trabeculated right atrium lateral to the crista. Such studies suggest that the crista forms a functional arc of block in most cases. The difference between fixed and functional block is shown in Figure 9-9. During slow pacing from these areas, no split potentials are usually seen; however, during rapid pacing from the low posterior right atrium split potentials with opposite activation sequences are seen.[20,21,23] In patients with a history of atrial flutter, transcristal block appears during pacing at longer cycle lengths (mean 638 ± 119 msec) than during pacing in a patient without a history of atrial flutter (214 ± 23 msec).[20] The opposite activation sequence reflects activation caudocranially from the posterior to the crista terminalis and craniocaudally lateral to the crista terminalis. The longest cycle length at which transverse cristal block appeared was increased slightly by propranolol and to a greater extent by procainamide.[20] A study from Almendral's group[23] demonstrated block in the crista at longer-paced cycle lengths from the posterior wall or CS os than from the lateral wall in patients with typical, counterclockwise, isthmus-dependent flutter. They suggested that this is the reason that counterclockwise flutter is more frequent than clockwise flutter. However, other factors must be involved since counterclockwise flutter is also induced in transplanted hearts in which the crista terminalis cannot play a role.[24]

We have recently evaluated the presence and degree of anisotropy on intra-atrial conduction velocity measured from a high-density (240 poles; 2.2-mm intraelectrode distance) plaque placed perpendicular to the tricuspid annulus. Intra-atrial conduction velocity was measured in 16 radii during pacing from the center of the plaque at 600 msec, the fastest rate of 1:1 conduction (F max), and at a rate just above local atrial refractoriness. We found no differences in the degree of anisotropy in patients with chronic atrial

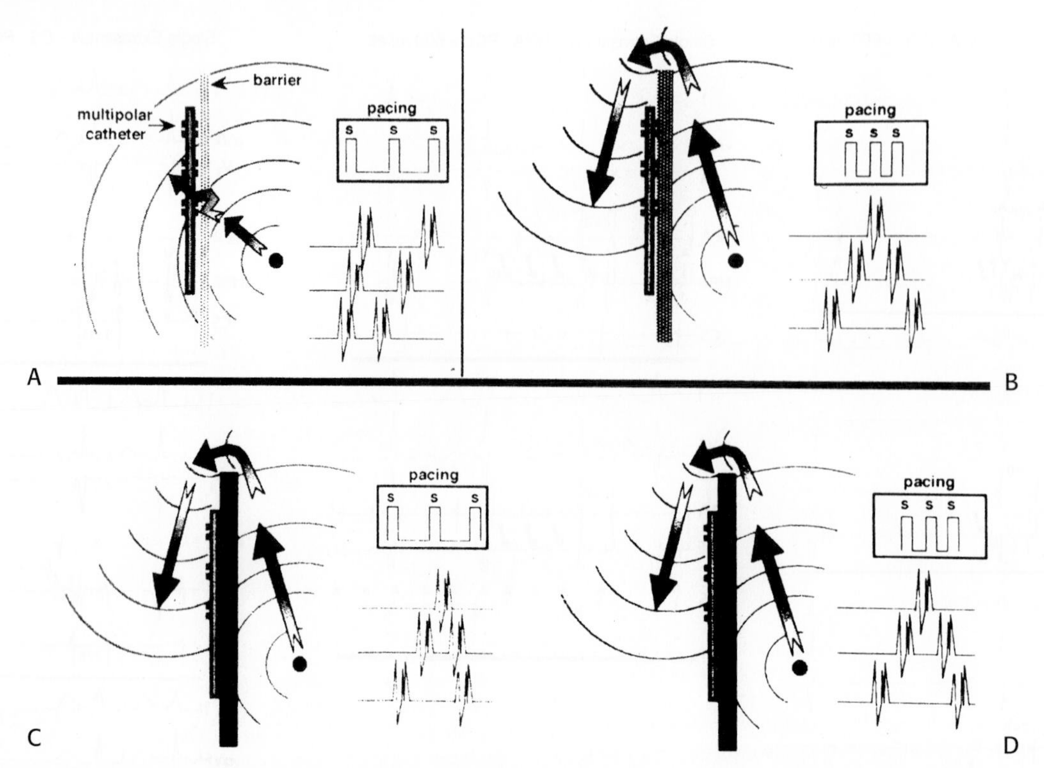


**FIGURE 9-9** *Fixed versus functional barriers.* In the diagrams, pacing is delivered medial to the potential barrier of the crista terminalis. Lateral to the crista is a multipolar catheter. Pacing is delivered at a rate depicted by "S." **A** and **B** depict a functional barrier. In **A**, slow pacing propagates slowly across the crista, resulting in parallel activation on both sides of the crista. At faster rates **(B)** functional block occurs and activation proceeds around the block. This gives rise to split potentials with opposite activation sequences on either side of the line of block. **C** depicts a fixed barrier in which conduction never crosses the crista regardless of the rate of pacing. (From Olgin JE, Kalman JM, Lesh MD. Conduction barriers in human atrial flutter: correlation of electrophysiology and anatomy. *J Cardiovasc Electrophysiol* 1996;7:1112–1126, with permission.)

fibrillation (postcardioversion), patients in whom atrial fibrillation could be induced, and those in whom no atrial fibrillation could be induced. The ratio of fast/slow conduction velocity was 2.1 to 2.3 in the patients during pacing at 600 msec and gradually decreased as the velocity was measured at more rapid-paced rates. This reduction was specifically related to a decrease in conduction velocity parallel to fiber orientation (in the so-called rapidly conducting direction) (Table 9-1). All patients showed significant direction-dependent conduction (anisotropy) with the fastest conduction perpendicular to the A-V groove (Fig. 9-10). The relationship to this pattern of conduction to the activation patterns during atrial fibrillation will be discussed subsequently.

**TABLE 9-1 Intra-atrial Conduction Velocity in Patients With and Without Atrial Fibrillation**

| | 600 msec | | | $F_{MAX}$ | | | ERP | | |
|---|---|---|---|---|---|---|---|---|---|
| Pacing (cm/sec) | $CV_F$ | $CV_S$ | R | $CV_F$ | $CV_S$ | R | $CV_F$ | $CV_S$ | R |
| **CAF** | 69 | 32 | 2.3 | 56 | 31 | 1.9 | 45 | 30 | 1.6 |
| **NSAF** | 76 | 36 | 2.2 | 67 | 36 | 2.0 | 44 | 28 | 1.6 |
| **SR** | 69 | 33 | 2.1 | 65 | 34 | 5.0 | 44 | 28 | 1.7 |
| **pD** | n.s. | n.s. | n.s. | n.s. | n.s. | n.s. | n.s. | n.s. | n.s. |

The conduction velocity (CV) in the fast (F) and slow (S) directions based on tissue anisotropy and their ratio (r) measured during a paced cycle length of 600 msec, the most rapid rate at which 1:1 intra-atrial propagation occurred (Fmax), and at the closest coupled APC just above refractoriness (ERP) are shown in patients with chronic atrial fibrillation (CAF), induced nonsustained AF (NSAF), and those in whom no AF was induced. Note there is no significant difference among patient groups. Conduction is only slowed at ERP with a greater degree of slowing in $CV_F$.

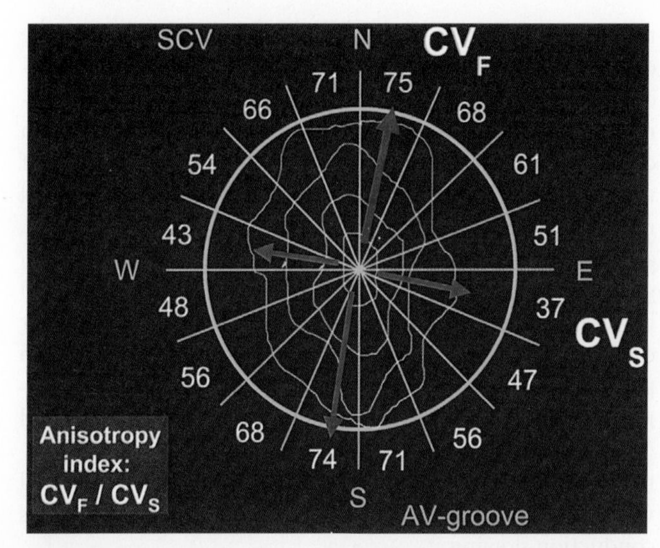


**FIGURE 9-10** *Anisotropic conduction over the epicardial free wall of the right atrium.* An isochronic map and conduction velocities in 16 radii in response to central stimulation from a 240-pole plaque are shown. The plaque is positioned perpendicular to the A-V groove with superior vena cava (*SVC*) on top. The isochronic map shows an elliptical pattern with rapid conduction perpendicular to the A-V groove and slow conduction parallel to it. The numbers represent conduction velocities ($CV_S$) along each radius. The ratio of fast ($CV_F$) to slow ($CV_S$) conduction, the anisotropy index, is ≈2. These findings suggest the presence of uniform anisotropy.

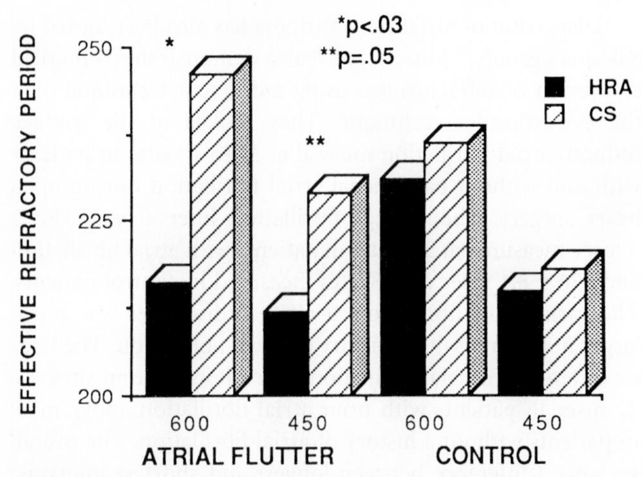


**FIGURE 9-11** *Comparison of the effective refractory period from the high-right atrium and coronary sinus in patients with and without atrial flutter.* The effective refractory period is plotted on the *vertical axis* in milliseconds. The refractory periods were performed from both the HRA (*dark bars*) and CS (*hashed bars*) at paced cycle lengths of 600 and 450 msec in patients with atrial flutter and in controls. The refractory period determined from the HRA was significantly shorter than that from the CS in patients with atrial flutter (216 vs. 246 msec) but not in control subjects. In addition, the effective refractory period at the HRA at a paced cycle length of 600 msec is shorter in patients with atrial flutter than in controls. At a cycle length of 450 msec, the effective refractory period of the HRA was shorter than from the CS in flutter patients (212 vs. 229 msec, $p = 0.05$). The control group had comparable effective refractory periods at the HRA and CS. See text for further discussion.

## Atrial Refractoriness

Changes in atrial refractoriness could and should have a marked influence on development of reentrant arrhythmias. Patients with a history of paroxysmal fibrillation or flutter appear to have different characteristics of refractoriness than in control subjects.[8,9,11,12] The right atrial refractory period is shorter in those patients in whom there is a history of paroxysmal atrial fibrillation or flutter than in controls (Fig. 9-11). Similar observations have been noted in patients in whom atrial fibrillation is inducible.[10,15] In addition, the high-right atrial refractory periods are shorter than those recorded in the CS at both cycle lengths of 450 and 600 msec (Fig. 9-11) in patients with atrial arrhythmias. Thus, patients with a history of atrial fibrillation or flutter, or those in whom it could be inducible, have not only shorter refractory periods than control subjects, but there is a difference in the refractory periods measured in the right and left atrium via the CS. Of particular note is the fact that while the effective refractory period at both high-right atrial and CS sites were shorter at a basic cycle length of 450 msec than at that determined at 600 msec, the degree to which the ERP shortened was different in those with a history of atrial fibrillation and flutter and those without (Fig. 9-12). In patients with a history of atrial arrhythmias, the effective refractory period of the HRA failed to shorten as much at shorter-paced cycle lengths as controls. In contrast, a decrease in refractoriness during CS stimulation was comparable in both the control and fibrillation/flutter groups. Thus, patients with a history of atrial fibrillation and flutter are characterized by a failure of adaptation of high-right atrial refractoriness when short and long cycle lengths are compared. These findings are similar to patients in whom atrial fibrillation was induced, as described by our group[8] and Attuel et al.[15] This failure of rate adaptation was noted even though many patients had been in sinus rhythm for days to weeks.

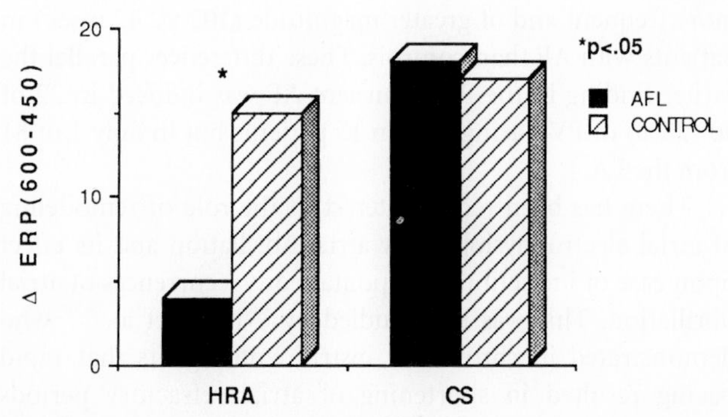


**FIGURE 9-12** *The effect of cycle length on atrial refractoriness.* The difference in effective refractory period ([trio] ERP) at cycle lengths of 600 and 450 msec is shown when stimulation is performed at the HRA and CS in patients with atrial flutter (AFL, *dark bar*) and in controls (*hashed bars*). It is apparent that the ERP measured at the HRA fails to shorten in response to a decreased cycle length. This blunting of cycle length responsiveness of HRA refractoriness is characteristic of patients with AFL. See text for further discussion.

Dispersion of atrial refractoriness has also been noted by Saksena's group.[25] Misier et al.[26] also demonstrated a marked dispersion of refractoriness using a different technique than the extrastimulus technique. They looked at the average induced atrial fibrillation interval at 35 to 40 sites in patients with and without paroxysmal atrial fibrillation during open heart surgery. The average fibrillation interval was 152 ± 3 msec measured at 247 sites in patients with atrial fibrillation and 176 ± 8.1 msec at 118 sites measured in control patients. The variance of fibrillation at all recording sites was much larger in patients with a history of atrial fibrillation. The largest difference in atrial fibrillation intervals in adjacent sites was 22 msec in patients with prior atrial fibrillation and 7 msec in patients without a history of atrial fibrillation. The overall variance (difference between longest and shortest intervals) in 4-second snapshots was 31.2 versus 11.5 msec. While this measurement of refractoriness and dispersion refractoriness is much different than that of standard measurements, these investigators showed a linear relationship between the atrial fibrillation intervals and the refractory period determined by the extrastimulus technique at four of the measured sites. However, not surprisingly, the fibrillatory intervals were much shorter than the measured refractory periods determined by the extrastimulus technique. Thus, while the fibrillation interval does not measure the local refractory period, it is an indirect measure of refractoriness. Both methods demonstrate greater heterogeneity in patients with a history of atrial fibrillation.

In the last 15 years there has been active investigation of left atrial and PV electrophysiology. Jais et al.[27] found shorter PV ERPs shorter in patients with AF (185 + 71) than control patients (283 + 45) while LA ERPs were similar (253 + 21 in AF vs. 253 + 41 controls). In AF patients the PV ERP was shorter than the LA ERP while in control patients the PV ERP exceeded the LA ERP. The PV ERPs varied from vein to vein and patient to patient although the superior PVs had shorter ERPs. Conduction delays during premature PV stimulation between the PV to the LA, measured on the Lasso, were more frequent and of greater magnitude (102 vs. 42 msec) in patients with AF than controls. These differences parallel the earlier finding in the RA. Transient AF was induced in 22 of 90 (25%) of PV pacing sites in 15 patients but in only 1 of 81 from the LA.

There has been recent interest in the role of remodeling of atrial electrophysiology by atrial fibrillation and its effect upon ease of induction and spontaneous recurrences of atrial fibrillation. This was first studied by Wijffels et al.[28,29] who demonstrated in chronically instrumented goats that rapid pacing resulted in shortening of atrial refractory periods which was progressive over time. This was correlated with an increased ease of inducibility and duration of atrial fibrillation. Following short periods of pacing for minutes only, brief episodes of atrial fibrillation could be induced as the refractory period shortened. By 24 hours of pacing, the refractory period had shortened maximally as measured by the standard atrial extrastimulus technique and by the fibrillation interval method described by Misier et al.[26] In Wijffels's study these changes were not affected by autonomic blockade, glibenclamide in doses to block the ATP sensitive potassium current, or atrial pressure. Goette et al.[30] found similar results in closed-chest dogs. They found that during short periods of up to 7 hours of atrial pacing at 800 bpm, the effective atrial refractory period shortened despite autonomic blockade, absence of changes in atrial pressure, and pretreatment with glibenclamide. They found that the remodeling was blocked by verapamil and accentuated by hypercalcemia. Intracellular calcium loading during rapid atrial activation is believed to play an important role in remodeling, with subsequent downregulation in L-type calcium channels as well as sodium and (transient outward current) potassium channels.[31] This channel remodeling may lead to shortening of the action potential with subsequent shortening of refractory periods as well as conduction slowing.

Others,[27,28,32,33] have demonstrated a reduction of tachycardia-induced electrical remodeling by verapamil. Daoud et al.[28] demonstrated that Class I antiarrhythmic agents failed to prevent remodeling. While not systematically evaluated, Daoud et al.[28] noted persistent inducibility of atrial fibrillation in patients who were treated with saline or procainamide in whom remodeling was still present and diminished inducibility in those patients pretreated with verapamil. Tieleman et al.[32,33] on the other hand, systematically studied the effects of verapamil on inducibility. While verapamil blocked the remodeling phenomenon, there was a minimal effect of inducibility of atrial fibrillation by verapamil. Thus, while it is tempting to speculate that rapid pacing as well as atrial fibrillation causes remodeling, which begets atrial fibrillation, remodeling may be merely a secondary phenomenon and not causally related to atrial fibrillation. However, it is certainly true that short refractoriness, particularly with dispersion of refractoriness, associated with the abnormalities of conduction present in patients with atrial fibrillation, can be proarrhythmic. Certainly verapamil is not an effective agent for preventing or terminating atrial fibrillation, while Class I agents, which do not affect remodeling, are most potent in terminating and preventing the atrial fibrillation. This suggests that there are other factors responsible for initiating atrial fibrillation that may include microscopic anatomic derangements, genetic predisposition to atrial fibrillation, variation in size, number, and thickness of pectinate bands in both atria, and the structure and function of the crista terminalis.

## Atrial Vulnerability

It has been demonstrated both experimentally and in humans that premature right atrial impulses falling in the RRP of the atria may produce one or more repetitive responses and may even induce atrial flutter or fibrillation.[28,29,34–45] Potential mechanisms for these observations include (a) the premature impulse triggers delayed afterdepolarizations, which result in one or more repetitive responses due to triggered activity in the RA, LA, or PVs;[46–48] (b) the premature impulses initiate one or more reentrant circuits, which lead to repetitive firing, or (c) combinations of the two; that is, repetitive responses lead to triggered beats and/or reentrant circuits which further induce additional areas of impulse formation, reentry, and fibrillatory conduction. Several investigators[28,29,36–45] have demonstrated a relationship between the ability of atrial premature depolarizations (APDs) to initiate atrial fibrillation and/or flutter in isolated tissue preparations or intact experimental animal models (dogs and goats) when dispersion of atrial refractoriness and/or conduction is present. Much of the recent work in remodeling has suggested that dispersion of atrial refractoriness may be more important, although this has not been demonstrated to be causally related to initiation of repetitive responses or sustained atrial fibrillation in humans. The bulk of evidence suggests that most instances of repetitive responses induced by atrial premature impulses are due to reentry. Extensive mapping of more sustained repetitive responses using data, simultaneously collected from several hundred sites, has confirmed that long-lasting repetitive responses are due to reentry.[39,40,49] Although the initial reentrant response may be due to an episode of circus movement, it may shift from a slow, single macroreentrant circuit (atrial flutter), or rapid, small circuit, into multiple "daughter" wavelets that characterize atrial activation seen in most cases of atrial fibrillation. The creation of such "daughter" wavelets depends on the initial or subsequent impulses encountering areas of insufficiently recovered tissue, creating secondary reentrant vortices distant from the initial site of reentry. Allessie et al.[40,41] using extensive simultaneous multisite mapping to analyze activation times and conduction velocities, have shown that atrial premature complexes that initiate atrial flutter and fibrillation have characteristic wavelengths, with the wavelength for flutter being longer than that for fibrillation.

It has also been demonstrated that atrial foci, which are rapidly firing, can lead to atrial fibrillation in patients with paroxysmal atrial fibrillation. In these patients, repetitive PACs or runs of atrial tachycardia from a single focus precede initiation of atrial fibrillation.[50–52] In such cases, the atrial ectopic activity may be targeted for curative ablation of atrial fibrillation (see Chapter 13). This recent observation has led some people to suggest that the demonstration of induced repetitive atrial responses, particularly when they produce short runs of atrial fibrillation, may be a useful marker of propensity to spontaneous atrial fibrillation. I disagree with this assumption, which is not based on any prospective studies. Haisseguerre[51] was the first to show that spontaneous firing of PV foci frequently initiate paroxysmal AF. This suggests that the initial RA repetitive response has little to do with AF itself but may trigger PV firing in patients predisposed to AF. Nevertheless, the ability to perform programmed atrial stimulation allows the investigator to evaluate the nature of repetitive responses to atrial extrastimuli in a controlled fashion and relate that to the presence or absence of spontaneous atrial arrhythmias. It has long been recognized that there is a zone of coupling intervals during which atrial extrastimuli are followed by repetitive responses and that the incidence of such responses increases as the coupling intervals are decreased (Fig. 9-13). Repetitive atrial responses are observed in 10% to 20% of patients undergoing atrial stimulation during sinus rhythm using stimuli that are twice diastolic threshold and 1 to 2 msec in duration. In our experience, repetitive responses will commonly occur when the extrastimuli are delivered in the HRA, particularly in the area at the superior crista terminalis near the sinus node or just inside the right atrial appendage. Occasionally, other atrial sites (e.g., the CS or the low-right atrium) may also result in repetitive firing, even when stimulation of the HRA fails to produce such responses. The data from Jais et al.[27] and Haissaguerre et al.[51] noted above suggest primary role of the PV in triggering paroxysmal AF. Increasing the amplitude or pulse duration of delivered extrastimuli increases the frequency of repetitive responses regardless of site of stimulation. This results because (a) increasing the current results in the ability to achieve shorter coupling intervals and encroachment on the local RRP that is due to well-known strength–interval relationships and (b) increase in the voltage and duration of the impulse depolarizes local tissue, causing slow conduction and localized reentry at the site of stimulation.

Repetitive atrial responses may have activation sequences that are similar to those produced by the paced stimulus or may have a totally different atrial activation sequence regardless of the site of stimulation. How similar they are may depend on how many simultaneous sites of atrial activation are being recorded and whether or not they trigger atrial extrasystoles from distant sites. Those repetitive responses that originate at or near the site of stimulation are usually associated with conduction delay between the site of stimulation and the local electrogram recorded from the proximal electrodes on a quadripolar catheter (i.e., so-called latency). This can be seen following the atrial extrastimulus in Figure 9-13. Those RA repetitive reponses have little to do with spontaneous AF initiation. Conduction delays at the initiation of repetitive responses occurring distant from the site of stimulation require recording from multiple intra-atrial sites. In such cases, intra-atrial delay (i.e., conduction delay to sites distant from the site of stimulation or at those sites), with or without local delay at the stimulation site, will be present. These local or intra-atrial conduction delays most likely result because the stimulus is delivered during the RRP of the atria. Nonuniform atrial anisotropy, demonstrated by Spach et al.[4,5] in experimental models and in patients may also be responsible for the production of such delays in response to premature stimuli. The role of anisotropy in human arrhythmias has also been demonstrated as previously discussed. This may say more about the ability to develop fibrillatory conduction in response to spontaneous PV firing.

In the electrophysiology laboratory, the RRP is usually defined by the longest $S_1$-$S_2$ interval at which latency is observed; that is, the coupling interval of $S_1$-$S_2$ at which the $A_1$-$A_2$ exceeds the $S_1$-$S_2$ interval. An earlier study in our

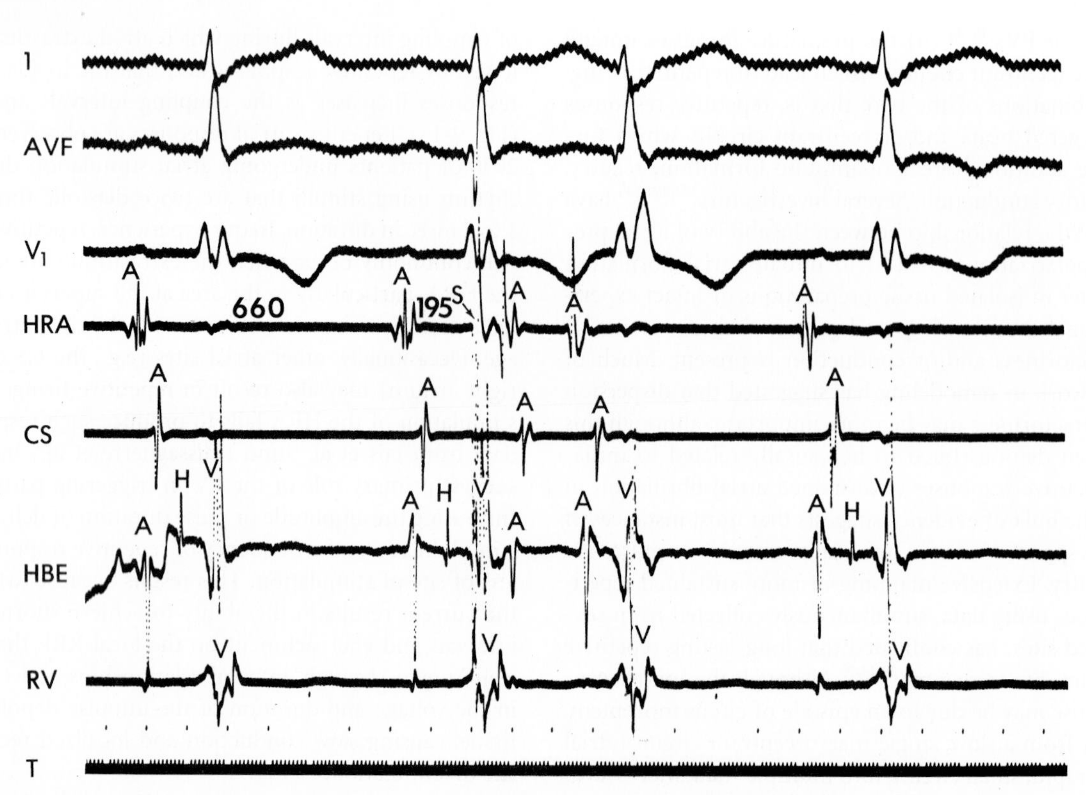


**FIGURE 9-13** *Repetitive atrial response initiated by a single atrial extrastimulus.* From **top** to **bottom:** ECG leads 1, aVF, and $V_1$ and electrograms from the high-right atrium (HRA), coronary sinus (CS), area of His bundle recording (HBE), and right ventricle (RV). An atrial extrastimulus (S, *arrow*) is delivered from the HRA at a coupling interval of 195 msec from the preceding sinus impulse. The stimulus is associated with latency (S-to-A delay) and is followed by an early atrial response. T, time line.

laboratory[30] evaluating atrial strength–interval relationships demonstrated that the RRP, defined by the onset of local intra-atrial conduction delay in response to atrial extrastimuli, was similar to that defined in a more traditional manner; that is, the requirement of increased current above threshold to produce a propagated response as a coupling interval is shortened. Our studies, therefore, suggest that latency, as measured clinically, is related to impingement on the atrial RRP. In patients without a history of atrial fibrillation or flutter, the RRP, as defined by either local latency or intra-atrial conduction delay in response to premature stimuli, occurs over a narrow range, usually within 20 to 30 msec above the atrial effective refractory.[53] In patients with atrial flutter and fibrillation the duration of this zone is increased. This may be the factor that makes AF coexist with flutter; flutter can become the initiator of fibrillatory conduction and atrial fibrillation.

Repetitive atrial responses to high RA stimuli must be distinguished from sinus node or A-V nodal echoes. By convention, the interval from the stimulated response to the first repetitive response must be less than 250 msec and must be unrelated to the presence of dual A-V nodal pathways or marked A-V nodal conduction delay. In most instances, this is not a difficult distinction to make, particularly if one records multiple atrial electrograms. Of note, when multiple atrial repetitive responses occur, the activation sequence and inter-atrial electrogram intervals may vary, particularly during initial responses.

In our experience, atrial vulnerability, as defined by the ability of single APDs to initiate repetitive atrial responses, is increased when atrial extrastimuli are delivered during pacing (as compared to during sinus rhythm), particularly at short drive cycle lengths (Fig. 9-14). Approximately 30% of patients manifest repetitive atrial responses when atrial extrastimuli are delivered from the HRA at paced cycle lengths of 600 to 450 msec. Similar data have been reported by others.[54–56] Cosio et al.[56] demonstrated that repetitive responses not only were facilitated by pacing, but, as we have shown, were particularly frequent as the basic drive cycle length was decreased (i.e., the paced rate was higher). The repetitive responses initiated during the decreased drive cycle length were associated with a decrease in the ERP. Thus, shorter $S_1$-$S_2$ and $A_1$-$A_2$ intervals were achieved, and intra-atrial conduction delays were observed at these shorter coupling intervals. In their series, repetitive responses occurred in 40% to 50% of patients without a prior history of atrial tachyarrhythmias (many of these patients, however, had structural heart disease).

The mechanism of enhanced vulnerability at short drive cycle lengths could theoretically have several explanations: (a) a cycle length–dependent decrease in the atrial ERP to a greater extent than in the RRP; (b) an actual increase in vulnerability (i.e., a shift in the onset of repetitive firing to longer coupling intervals or the appearance of repetitive responses at similar $A_1$-$A_2$ coupling intervals that previously failed to induce repetitive responses); or (c) the development of triggered activity.

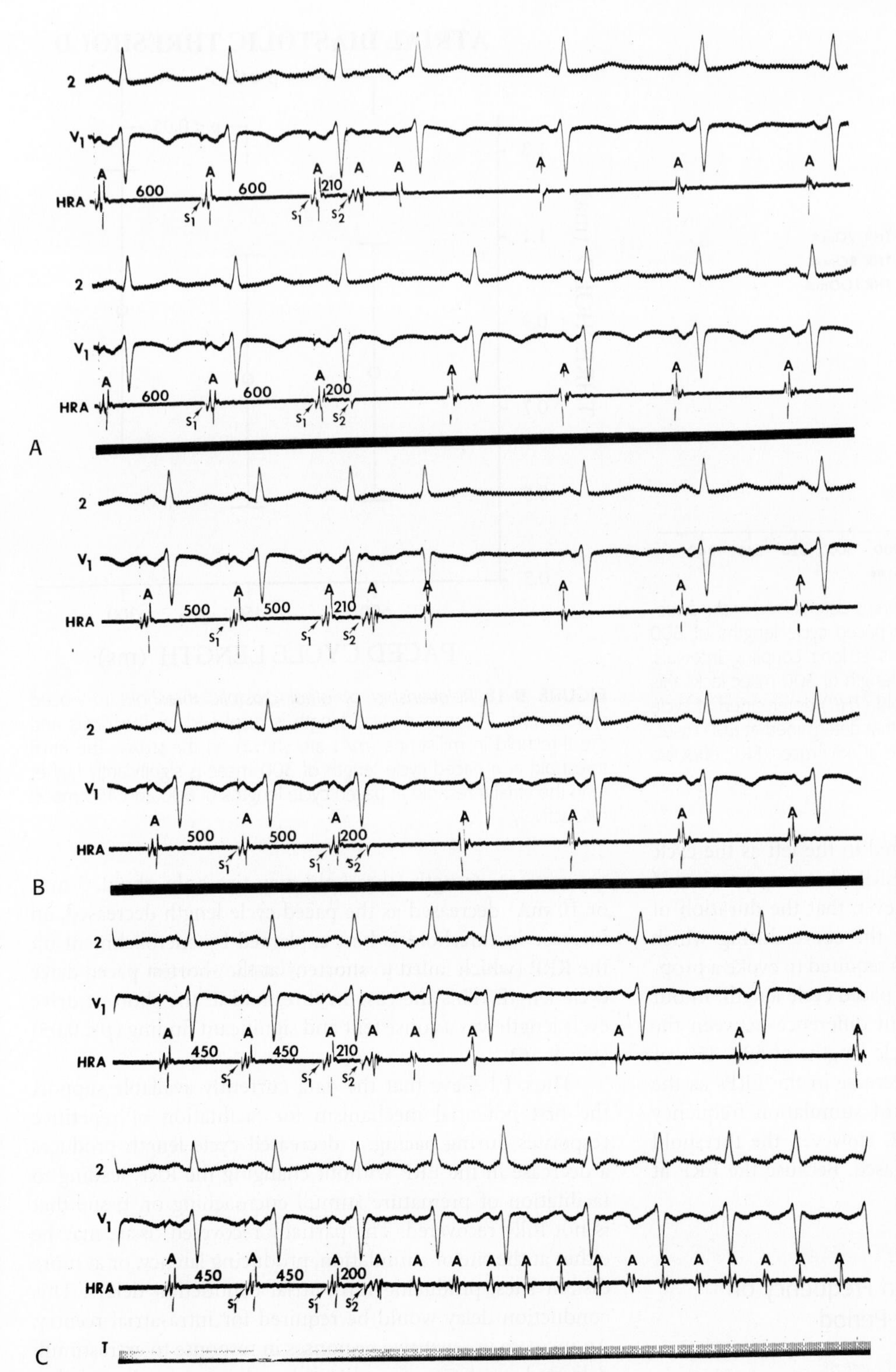


**FIGURE 9-14** *Effect of cycle length on atrial vulnerability.* **A:** A cycle length of 600 msec, an atrial extrastimulus ($S_2$, *arrow*) delivered at a coupling interval of 210 msec produces a single repetitive response. When $S_1$-$S_2$ is shortened to 200 msec, atrial refractoriness is reached. At a shorter drive cycle length of 500 msec **(B)**, atrial extrastimuli ($S_2$) delivered at identical coupling intervals ($S_1$-$S_2$ 210 and 200 msec) produce a response identical to that shown in **A. C:** However, when the cycle length is decreased to 450 msec, an $S_2$ delivered at 210 msec produces two repetitive responses. When $S_1$-$S_2$ is shortened to 200 msec, atrial flutter is initiated. See text for further discussion. (From Watson RM, Josephson ME. Atrial flutter. I. Electrophysiologic substrates and modes of initiation and termination. *Am J Cardiol* 1980;45:732, with permission.)

Most data point to reentry and not triggered activity as the mechanism of repetitive responses.[36–40]

Although an actual increase in vulnerability may occur in occasional instances, I believe the most important factor is that short drive cycle lengths decrease the ERP without a significant change in the RRP. Thus, the closer coupling intervals that were achievable would be more likely to encroach on the atrial RRP. This has been convincingly demonstrated in a study from our laboratory in which the strength–interval relationship was studied at multiple drive cycle lengths in 20 patients.[53] The drive cycle lengths we evaluated included 600, 450, and 300 msec, a much broader range than studied in any prior investigation. An example of strength–interval curves at these three cycle lengths is shown in Figure 9-15.

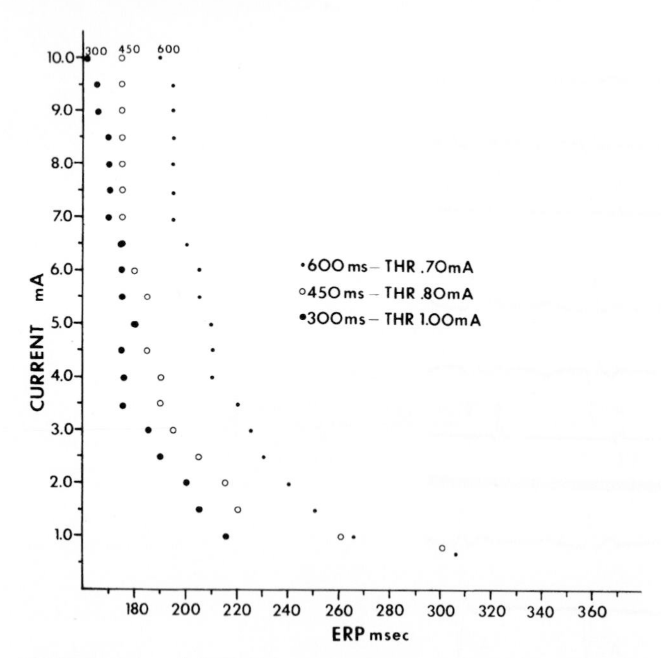


**FIGURE 9-15** *Atrial strength–interval curves determined in the baseline state.* In this patient, the curves at paced cycle lengths of 600 and 450 msec have horizontal portions at long coupling intervals. The curve determined at a paced cycle length of 300 msec lacks this horizontal portion. Note that the threshold (*THR*) determined at cycle length 300 msec is 0.3 mA higher than that determined at 600 msec, and 0.2 mA higher than that determined at 450 msec. ERP, effective refractory period.

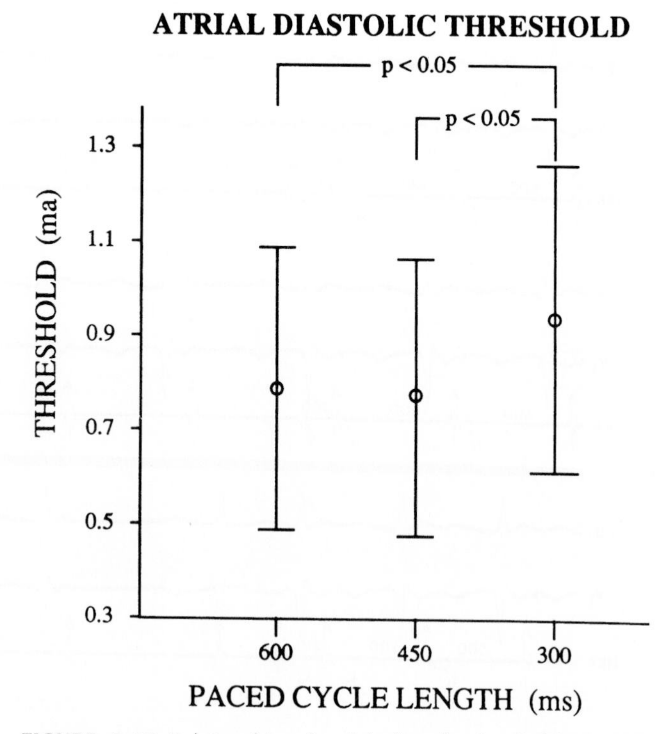


**FIGURE 9-16** *Relationship of atrial diastolic threshold to paced cycle length.* The paced cycle length is displayed on the *x-axis* and the threshold in milliamps (*mA*) are shown on the *y-axis.* The atrial threshold at a paced cycle length of 300 msec is significantly higher than the atrial threshold at paced cycle lengths of 600 and 450 msec, respectively.

As can be seen, the curves are shifted to the left as the cycle length is decreased, such that the ERP (the steep portion of the curve) is decreased. Note, however, that the duration of the RRP—that is, that portion of the curve during which increased current above threshold is required to evoke a propagated response—is similar at each paced cycle length. In our 20 patients, we found no significant difference between the durations of the RRPs at paced cycle lengths of 600, 450, or 300 msec. However, we noted a decrease in the ERPs as the current was increased. The effect of stimulation frequency on the ERP is shown in Table 9-2. However, the threshold increased as the cycle length decreased. Because the ERP at any current strength (threshold, two times threshold, 5 mA, or 10 mA) decreased as the paced cycle length decreased, an increase in threshold is best explained by encroachment on the RRP (which failed to shorten) at the shortest paced drive cycle length. This increase in threshold at the shortest drive cycle length was a consistent and significant finding ($p < 0.05$) (Fig. 9-16).

**TABLE 9-2 Effect of Stimulation Frequency on Effective Refractory Period**

| Cycle Length (msec) | Baseline Current | | | |
|---|---|---|---|---|
| | Thr | 2 × Thr | 5 mA | 10 mA |
| 600 | 287 ± 46 | 245 ± 24 | 212 ± 22 | 200 ± 22 |
| 450 | 279 ± 46 | 230 ± 24 | 197 ± 21 | 182 ± 21 |
| 300 | 241 ± 23 | 205 ± 17 | 175 ± 14 | 163 ± 13 |

Values are mean ± standard deviation for effective refractory periods (msec).
Thr, diastolic threshold.

Thus, I believe that the data currently available support the first potential mechanism for facilitation of repetitive responses during pacing: a decreased cycle length produces a decrease in the ERP without changing the RRP, leading to facilitation of premature stimuli encroaching on tissue that is not fully recovered. The partially recovered tissue may be either at the site of stimulation, producing latency, or at more distant sites, producing intra-atrial conduction delays. This conduction delay would be required for intra-atrial reentry. An increase in repetitive responses in response to extrastimuli delivered at a shorter-paced cycle length is not a universal phenomenon. Effects of autonomic tone, myocardial disease, and anisotropy are factors that can potentially influence the site- and rate-dependent effects on the production of repetitive response.

The relationship of local intra-atrial repetitive responses to spontaneous atrial fibrillation and flutter is uncertain. In my opinion, local repetitive responses may serve as additional "extrastimuli" to produce block and slow conduction at critical sites necessary to induce atrial fibrillation based on reentry or produce triggered activity in the PV which then initiates AF. Where such necessary conduction delays must occur to initiate atrial fibrillation or flutter has been under investigation (see discussion below). While some investigators[28,29] use repetitive responses as a surrogate marker for atrial fibrillation inducibility in goats, in humans the relationship of repetitive responses to spontaneous atrial fibrillation has not been shown. At this point in time, repetitive responses and even nonsustained atrial fibrillation induced by programmed stimulation in man should not be considered specific for predicting the clinical occurrence of atrial fibrillation or flutter.

## ATRIAL FLUTTER

Tricuspid-caval isthmus-dependent atrial flutter is one of the most unique arrhythmias because of its nearly constant rate of 250 to 300 bpm (in the absence of drugs) regardless of the clinical setting. Other forms of macroreentrant atrial tachycardias are not that well characterized, except for mitral annular flutter that will be discussed in Chapter 14. Most patients with atrial flutter have some form of heart disease, with hypertension, coronary artery disease, and cardiomyopathy most commonly found in the patient population in our laboratory. We have also frequently seen this rhythm in patients with chronic lung disease, atrial septal defects (pre- and postoperatively) and in nearly 5% of patients in whom sodium channel-blocking agents have been administered to treat atrial fibrillation. While the definition of atrial flutter as a supraventricular rhythm with a regular rate between 250 and 300 bpm is generally accepted, there are many classifications of the types of flutter that have evolved as our understanding of this rhythm has improved. In the past, flutter has been defined as either the "typical" or "common" type, which is characterized by a predominantly negative, sawtooth-like atrial activation pattern in the inferior leads with positive atrial deflections in lead $V_1$ and negative deflections in lead $V_6$, or the "uncommon" or "atypical" form characterized by predominantly positive, notched deflections in the inferior leads with negative deflections in $V_1$ and positive deflections in $V_6$ (Fig. 9-17). Atrial activation mapping of these two types of flutter have demonstrated that they represent opposite activation of the same reentrant circuit whose boundaries include the tricuspid annulus, the crista terminalis, the inferior vena cava, Eustachian ridge, CS, and probably the fossa ovalis.[10,22,57–60] Activation during counterclockwise or "typical" flutter proceeds up the septal side of the tricuspid annulus toward the crista terminalis, moves cephalocaudad along the anterolateral wall of the right atrium to reach the lateral annulus, then propagates through the isthmus defined by the inferior vena cava, the CS, and the tricuspid valve. The clockwise (atypical) flutter demonstrates activation in the opposite direction with clockwise activation from the isthmus caudocephalad along the anterior wall, around the crista terminalis and down the septum to reach the isthmus in the clockwise fashion. Documentation of such activation sequences requires use of a multipolar catheter that can be positioned to record nearly 60% of the tricuspid annulus involved in the flutter circuit, a CS catheter, and frequently a catheter using 10 to 20 poles along the crista terminalis (Fig. 9-18).

Although typical electrocardiographic patterns have been described for isthmus-dependent flutter, these ECG characteristics are not always present. We have recently reviewed

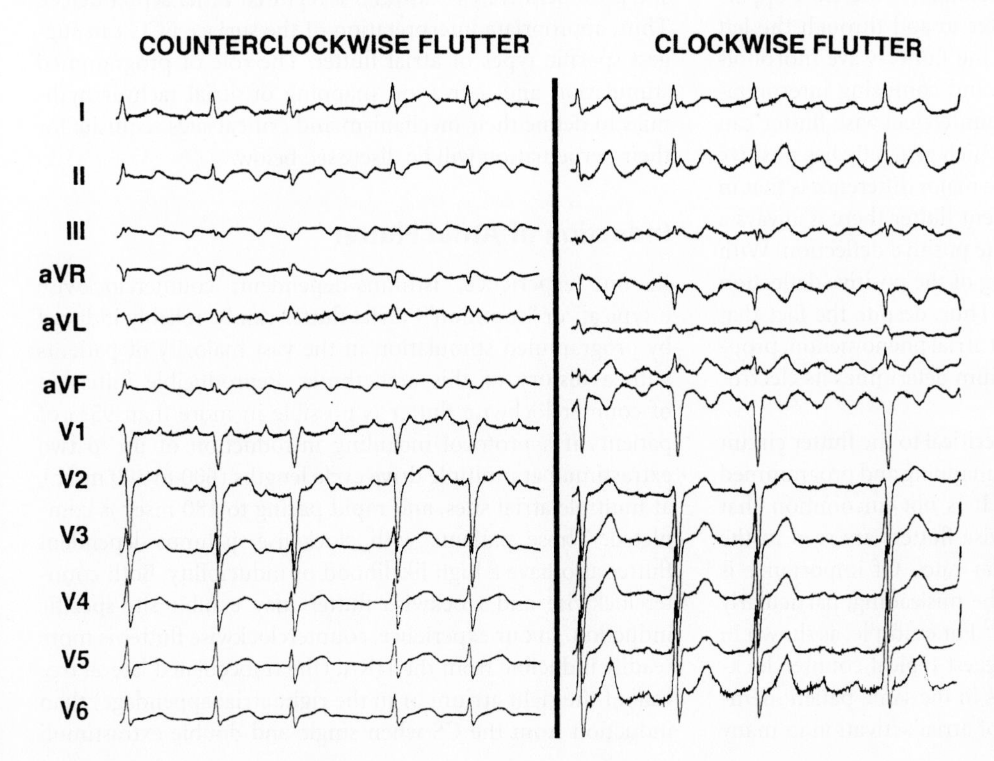


**FIGURE 9-17** *Electrocardiographic characteristics of counterclockwise and clockwise isthmus-dependent flutter.* Typical ECG patterns of isthmus-dependent flutters are shown. See text for description. (From Olgin JE, Miles W. Ablation of atrial tachycardias. In: Singer I, Barold SS, Camm AJ, eds. *Non-pharmacologic therapy of arrhythmias in the 21st century*. Armonk, NY: Futura Publishing, 1998:197–217, with permission.)

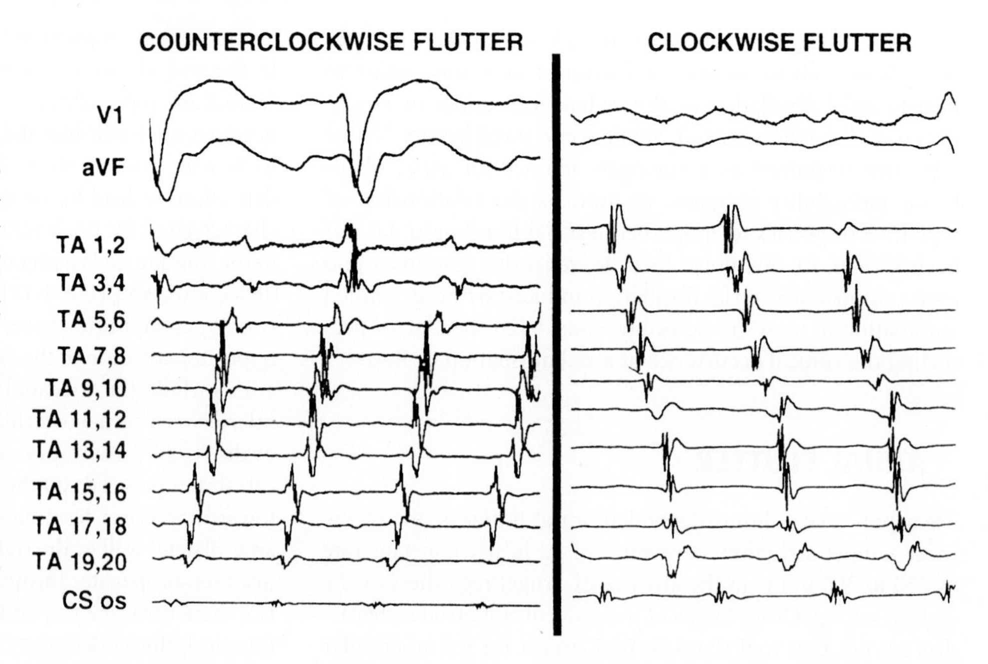


**FIGURE 9-18** *Endocardial activation during counterclockwise and clockwise flutter.* Activation during counterclockwise (**left**) and clockwise (**right**) flutter are shown with surface ECG leads $V_1$ and aVF. Electrograms are recorded around the tricuspid annulus (TA) using a 20-pole halo catheter with pole 1, 2 positioned at the isthmus and from the os of the coronary sinus (*CS*). Activation around the TA is counterclockwise on the **left** and clockwise on the **right**. See text for details. (From Olgin JE, Miles W. Ablation of atrial tachycardias. In: Singer I, Barold SS, Camm AJ, eds. *Non-pharmacologic therapy of arrhythmias in the 21st century*. Armonk, NY: Futura Publishing, 1998:197–217, with permission.)

156 consecutive cases of isthmus-dependent flutter in which the distal and/or proximal CS activation was recorded along with right atrial activation.[61] Counterclockwise flutter (the more common variety) may be characterized by pure negative deflections in the inferior leads, negative followed by positive deflections that are approximately of equal size, or a small negative deflection followed by a positive deflection of greater amplitude. These three varieties coexist with tall positive P waves, smaller positive P waves, or biphasic P waves in $V_1$, respectively. The degree to which positivity in the inferior leads is present appears to be related to the coexistence of heart disease and an enlarged left atrium. It is therefore apparent that propagation of atrial flutter to and through the left atrium is a major determinant of the flutter-wave morphology. This may lead to misleading and confusing interpretations of the electrocardiogram. Counterclockwise flutter can be mistaken for clockwise flutter, which generally has positive deflections in the inferior leads. The major difference is that in counterclockwise, isthmus-dependent flutter there is always a negative deflection that precedes the positive deflection. With clockwise flutter, there is a notching of the positive deflection in the middle of the flutter wave. Thus, despite the fact that isthmus-dependent flutter is a right atrial phenomenon, propagation to and through the left atrium determines its electrocardiographic appearance.

The exact sites involved in and critical to the flutter circuit can be determined using activation mapping and programmed stimulation (see page 300).[22,57–59] It is not uncommon that both clockwise and counterclockwise flutters are seen in the same patient and often have similar rates. Of importance is the fact that the surface ECG can be misleading, particularly if only the standard leads are used.[62] For example, as shown in Figure 9-19, the standard leads suggest typical counterclockwise flutter. Intracardiac recordings in the same patient demonstrate a change in the sequence of atrial activation in many areas, a finding more characteristic of atrial fibrillation or multiple reentrant atrial circuits. Atypical ECG patterns suggest atypical varieties of flutter or "organized" atrial fibrillation. Atrial tachycardias can arise from the left atrium, particularly from the PVs, and mimic atrial flutter. However, since their location is usually in the superior PVs, the P-wave morphology will be positive in the inferior leads, but would also be positive in $V_1$ and $V_2$ due to the posterior-anterior activation of the heart. Obviously, atrial mapping during the tachycardia is necessary to prove this. In a similar fashion, atypical morphologies may be seen when flutter arises at an atriotomy scar site postoperatively or around a repaired atrial septal defect. Thus, appropriate interpretation of the surface ECG can suggest specific types of atrial flutter. The role of programmed stimulation and activation mapping of atrial tachyarrhythmias to define their mechanism and critical sites requisite for their perpetuation will be discussed below.

## Induction of Atrial Flutter

In our experience, isthmus-dependent, counterclockwise ("typical" or "common") atrial flutter can be reliably induced by programmed stimulation in the vast majority of patients with a history of this arrhythmia. Reproducible initiation of counterclockwise flutter is possible in more than 95% of patients if a protocol including introduction of up to two extrastimuli at multiple drive cycle lengths (600 to 300 msec), at multiple atrial sites, and rapid pacing to 180 msec is completed. Those patients with clockwise, isthmus-dependent flutter also have a high likelihood of inducibility. Both counterclockwise and clockwise flutter may exhibit site-specific induction. In our experience, counterclockwise flutter is more readily inducible from the HRA, (the trabeculated lateral free wall of the right atrium or in the right atrial appendage) than induction from the CS when single and double extrastimuli

A

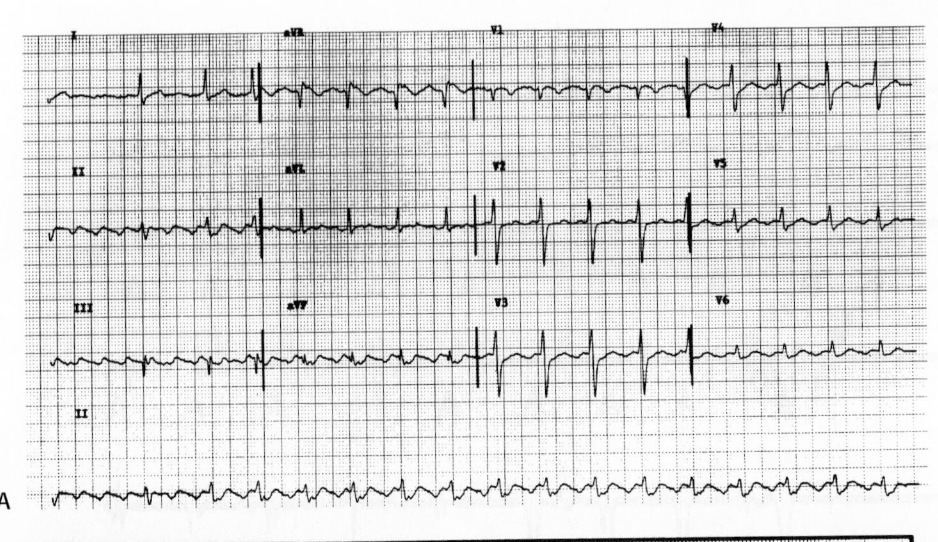

B

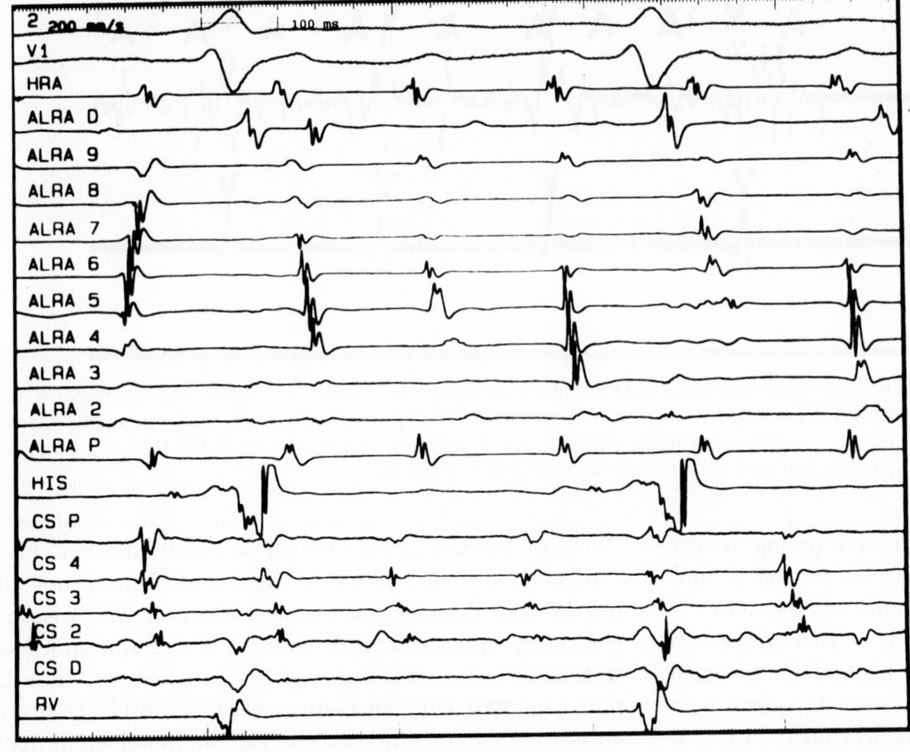


**FIGURE 9-19** *Inadequacy of ECG in predicting endocardial activation during apparent atrial flutter.* **A:** On **top** is a 12-lead ECG of what appears to be atrial flutter. **B:** In the **bottom panel** the atrial activation pattern is disorganized, consistent with atrial fibrillation. Recordings are from a 20-pole catheter placed along the anterolateral right atrium (ALRA) with the distal (D) pair at 8 o'clock in the LAO view and the proximal (P) pair at the anterior septum, the HBE, and the $CS_P$ to $CS_d$ with $CS_p$ located just inside the os. RV, right ventricle. See text for discussion. (From Huang DT, Monahan KM, Zimetbaum PJ, et al. Hybrid pharmacologic and ablative therapy: a novel and effective approach for the management of atrial fibrillation. *J Cardiovasc Electrophysiol* 1998;9:462–469, with permission.)

are used.[8] This is in contrast to Olgin et al.[63] who suggested that stimulation at the posterior septal smooth right atrium is more likely to initiate counterclockwise flutter, and that stimulation at the trabeculated free wall of the right atrium, lateral to the crista terminalis, is more likely to induce clockwise flutter. The reason for the discrepancy of these results is unclear, but in both cases the site of block appears to be in the isthmus between the CS, inferior vena cava, and the tricuspid valve.[63–65] One explanation for the discrepancies may be that Olgin et al.[63] did not evaluate the CS as a site of induction, and they excluded all patients in whom atrial flutter evolved after going through an early period of fractionation of electrograms in the triangle of Koch (A-V junction or os of the CS) or transient atrial fibrillation (Fig. 9-20). The reason for this early fractionation and period of what appears to be atrial fibrillation or impure atrial flutter may be the instability prior to formation of a line of block along the tendon of Todero and/or the Eustachian ridge. Such irregularity is extremely common in our experience[8,6] and that of Waldo and colleagues [66,67]

Rapid atrial pacing is more likely to initiate atrial flutter than the use of single HRA extrastimuli. Data from our laboratory[8,6] and from Olgin et al.[63] have demonstrated that double extrastimuli and rapid atrial pacing were also more effective than the use of a single extrastimulus in initiating flutter. While the overall frequency of any single extrastimulus or two extrastimuli initiating atrial flutter is low (less than 10%), the ability to initiate atrial flutter in any individual with a prior history of atrial flutter exceeds 90%. In our experience at the University of Pennsylvania atrial flutter was inducible in the laboratory by programmed stimulation using either one

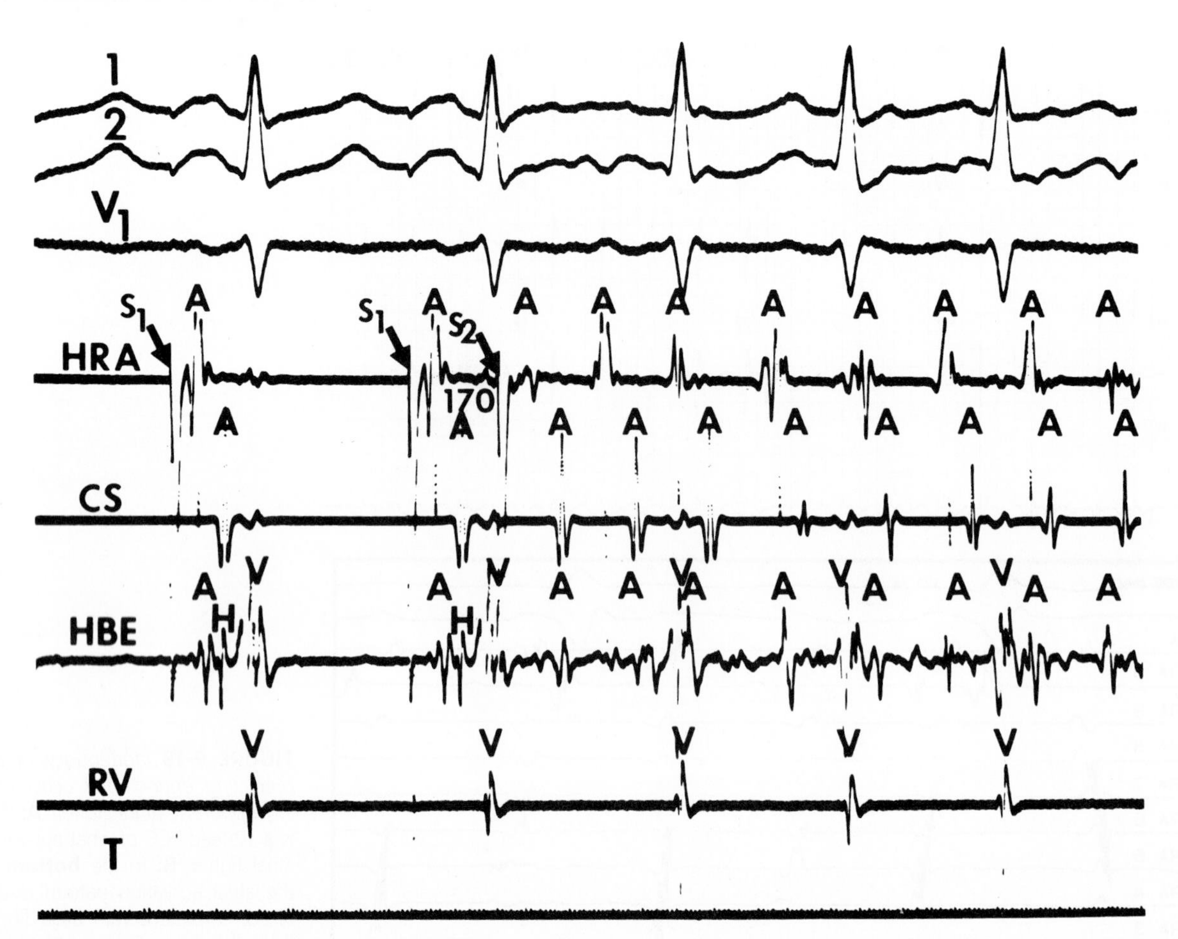


**FIGURE 9-20** *Induction of atrial flutter with a single atrial extrastimulus.* From top to bottom are ECG leads 1, 2, and $V_1$ and electrograms from the HRA, CS, His bundle (HBE), and right ventricle (RV). A single atrial premature depolarization ($S_2$) delivered at a coupling interval of 170 msec during a basic drive cycle length ($S_1$-$S_1$) of 600 msec induces atrial flutter. Note the initial irregularity of electrograms in the HRA and CS as well as fragmentation of the HBE. This rhythm eventually stabilized to counterclockwise flutter. T, time line.

or two atrial extrastimuli and/or rapid atrial pacing in 90% of 80 consecutive patients studied from 1980 to 1986. A similar incidence of inducibility of atrial flutter was found in 524 consecutive patients with a prior history of that arrhythmia studied at the Beth Israel Deaconess Medical Center from 1994 to 2011. The inducibility rate was 95% in patients who ultimately were proven to have isthmus-dependent flutter. Of note, the more rapid atrial pacing that is performed and the closer coupled atrial extrastimuli are delivered, the more likely atrial fibrillation (usually self-terminating) is induced, though the incidence of sustained atrial fibrillation is less than 10%. The significance of induction of atrial fibrillation in these patients is uncertain. Thus, failure to induce atrial flutter is rare in patients who have a history of atrial flutter as long as a complete stimulation protocol is employed. However, because of the induction of atrial fibrillation, in some patients atrial flutter may not be inducible.

The induction of atrial flutter appears to be a relatively specific response. Its induction in a patient without a prior history of atrial flutter or fibrillation is extremely rare. It is of interest that when counterclockwise and clockwise flutter are induced in the same patient, the cycle lengths are similar, although in our experience the cycle lengths of counterclockwise flutter may occasionally be slightly shorter. This is consistent with the findings of Olgin et al.,[63] and is not surprising since the anatomic circuit that counterclockwise and clockwise, isthmus-dependent flutter use is the same (see section on activation mapping and programmed stimulation, page 300). Differences in cycle length must be related to anisotropy and/or differences in electrophysiologic properties within the circuit, which are activated at different points in time during initiation and maintenance of flutter.

Although Olgin et al.[63] have described the site of block required for initiation of flutter being between the os of the CS, the inferior vena cava, and the tricuspid valve, they excluded those patients in whom fragmentation, fractionation, and oscillation of atrial electrograms in the His bundle electrogram and throughout the triangle of Koch were recorded prior to stabilization to atrial flutter (Fig. 9-20). It is of note that such oscillations and fragmentation are rarely seen during CS stimulation, but are very frequent during high-right atrial stimulation. Such delays in fragmentation are also seen in patients who develop atrial fibrillation (see section on activation mapping and programmed stimulation, page 300 and Fig. 9-8). The absence of such fragmentation during CS stimulation is associated with the lack of induction of atrial flutter or fibrillation and suggests a role

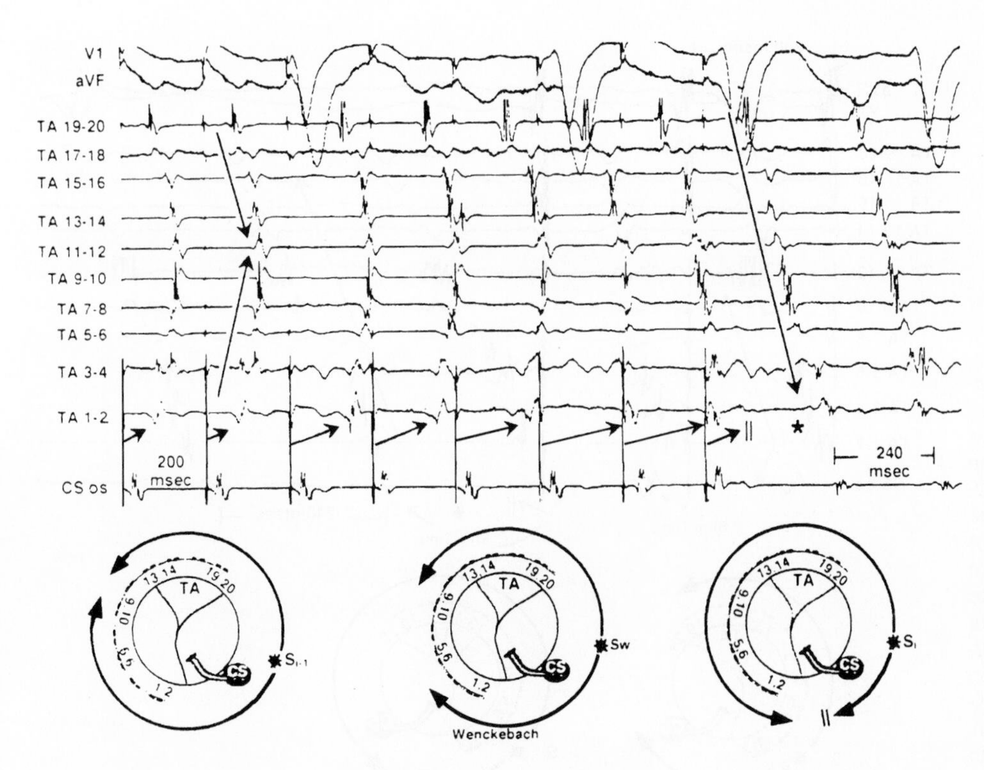


**FIGURE 9-21** *Initiation of counterclockwise flutter by rapid pacing from the smooth septal right atrium.* **A:** Surface ECG leads $V_1$ and aVF and intracardiac recordings are shown during initiation of counterclockwise flutter. The panel is arranged as in Figure 9-18. **B:** Diagram of activation of electrodes. Initial paced beats show simultaneous counterclockwise and clockwise activation of the right atrium (see *arrows* on second beat). Progressive delay to TA 1, 2 following activation of the CS occurs in a Wenckebach fashion. The eighth paced beat blocks between the CS and TA 1, 2, resulting in subsequent initiation of counterclockwise flutter. See text for discussion. (From Olgin JE, Kalman JM, Saxon LA, et al. Mechanism of initiation of atrial flutter in humans: site of unidirectional block and direction of rotation. *J Am Coll Cardiol* 1997;29:376–384, with permission.)

of nonuniform anisotropy in the development of unidirectional block and slow conduction associated with the development of these arrhythmias. It is of note that when rapid atrial pacing is used to initiate the arrhythmia, the efficacy of inducibility from both sites is comparable. The relative absence of fractionation in the triangle of Koch using rapid atrial pacing (particularly from the CS) suggests that there may be a different mechanism for the development of unidirectional block during rapid atrial pacing than during atrial extrastimuli. Decremental conduction, which has been demonstrated in the isthmus, may be critical when rapid atrial pacing is used to initiate atrial flutter, while nonuniform anisotropy may be more important during single and double extrastimuli. Further investigation of these concepts is necessary to clarify the role of nonuniform anisotropy, dispersion of refractoriness, and abnormalities of propagation in the isthmus in initiation of atrial flutter during different stimulation techniques. Regardless of mechanism, the site of block required for initiation of flutter appears to be in the isthmus (Figs. 9-21 and 9-22).

As stated earlier, the initiation of flutter, particularly that produced by the use of HRA extrastimuli, is often associated with fragmentation, fractionation, and oscillation of atrial electrograms in the His bundle electrogram and/or in the posterior triangle of Koch before ultimate stabilization of atrial activity is achieved. In many patients such fractionation appears required for initiation of flutter. As stated above this is primarily observed during high lateral right atrial stimulation and not during CS stimulation (Fig. 9-8). This transient appearance of what could be considered local atrial fibrillation may in fact reflect the setting up of lines of block that form the barriers necessary to define the flutter circuit. The size of these barriers will be discussed in subsequent paragraphs. Olgin et al.[63] excluded such patients from their study, although they also observed similar "fibrillatory" activity prior to organization to typical flutter.

While the isthmus is the site of block regardless of whether or not clockwise or counterclockwise flutter is induced, the direction of rotation may be dependent on the site of stimulation. In Olgin's study[63] counterclockwise flutter was always induced from the smooth right atrium and clockwise flutter was always induced from the anterolateral right atrium. This is not our experience. We have found a greater difficulty in initiation of flutter by extrastimuli delivered from the CS when compared to the anterolateral right atrium, but regardless of the successful site of stimulation, the most common form of flutter initiated had a counterclockwise rotation. Moreover, Olgin et al.[63] found an equal incidence of induction of clockwise and counterclockwise rotations, while in our experience counterclockwise flutter was initiated nearly three times as commonly as the clockwise flutter. We did note, however, that clockwise flutter was almost always induced from the anterolateral right atrium or right atrial appendage, which is in full accordance with Olgin et al.[63] The explanation for these differences is uncertain. One of the reasons for differences is their exclusion of patients with irregular atrial rhythms in transition to stable atrial flutter. An additional explanation is that Olgin et al.[63] stimulated from the posterior smooth atrium or os of the CS and we stimulated from deep in the CS, which in fact is the left atrium. Of interest is the fact that atrial flutter induced in transplanted hearts always has a counterclockwise rotation regardless of the site of stimulation and the absence of any role of the crista terminalis.[24] This suggests that additional factors help determine inducibility and rotation.

While Olgin et al.[63] suggested that induction of flutter was difficult, since only 5% to 10% of induction attempts

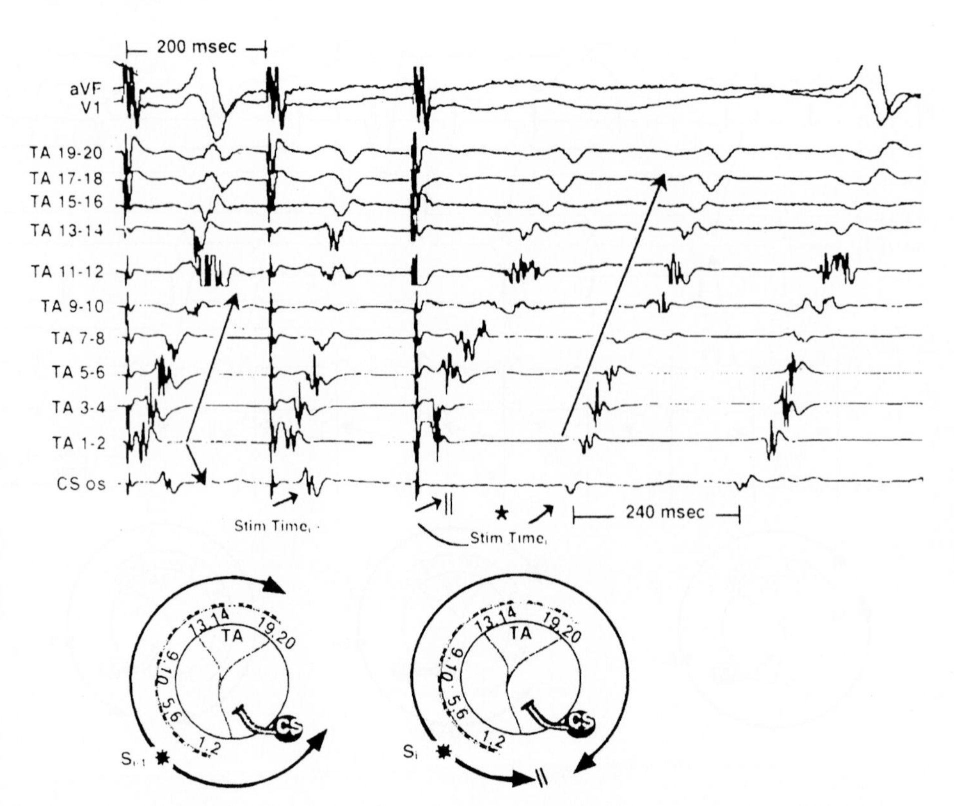


**FIGURE 9-22** *Initiation of clockwise flutter by rapid pacing from the trabeculated free wall of the right atrium.* The figure is organized as is Figure 9-21. During the first two paced beats the isthmus and CS os are activated counterclockwise and the right atrial free wall (TA 1,2–TA 19,20) is activated clockwise. On the third beat block in the isthmus occurs leading to initiation of clockwise flutter. See text for discussion. (From Olgin JE, Kalman JM, Saxon LA, et al. Mechanism of initiation of atrial flutter in humans: site of unidirectional block and direction of rotation. *J Am Coll Cardiol* 1997;29:376–384, with permission.)

were associated with induction of flutter, in fact atrial flutter was induced in 100% of patients who had flutter clinically. In addition, it can be induced reproducibly in such patients. Thus, it is misleading for electrophysiologists to think that flutter is difficult to induce. One needs to use relatively short coupled atrial extrastimuli at shorter-paced cycle lengths or rapid atrial pacing to induce the rhythm. If the late coupled atrial premature complexes and the "slow" rates of rapid atrial pacing are excluded, the chance of initiating flutter is high. Certainly it is reproducible and, in my opinion, is a reasonable, albeit not perfect, end point for judging the therapeutic efficacy of pharmacologic or ablative interventions. These will be discussed in subsequent chapters.

Induction of true atypical flutters (non–isthmus-dependent flutters) is more highly variable and may require sites of stimulation that are different from those used for the induction of isthmus-dependent flutter. This may be particularly true in flutters that arise in the left atrium or are associated with prior surgical interventions.

## Activation Mapping and Programmed Stimulation During Flutter

Characterization of the reentrant circuit in isthmus-dependent flutter has evolved over the past decade. This has been a result of more detailed mapping of the right atrium and sometimes the left atrium during flutter, in combination with programmed stimulation. Mapping techniques leading to these advances have incorporated multipolar catheters to record the anterolateral right atrium, the crista terminalis, the septum, the triangle of Koch, the CS, the Eustachian ridge, and roving catheters for stimulation and recording at specific sites. In addition, the recent use of the Carto system (Biosense, Cordis Webster; Johnson and Johnson; see Chapter 2) has allowed acquisition of several hundred sequentially mapped sites that are then plotted as both an isochronic activation map and a propagation map. Both mapping presentations clarify the reentrant circuit used for isthmus-dependent clockwise and counterclockwise flutters (Fig. 9-23). Use of this system has also been valuable in analyzing atypical flutters arising from the left atrium or prior surgical incisions (Fig. 9-24). Noncontact mapping (Navix, St Jude Medical) and the use of multipolar basket catheters also have great potential for furthering our knowledge of different atrial flutters. The most important catheters for characterizing isthmus-dependent flutters have been the use of multipolar standard or deflectable catheters with 10 to 20 poles. We actually prefer to use separate decapolar catheters for the anterolateral tricuspid annulus and the CS. The anterolateral tricuspid annulus catheter is placed near the tricuspid annulus with the distal tip placed at approximately 7 to 8 o'clock in the LAO view. Some investigators use a deflectable catheter that can be positioned in the anterolateral right atrium, cavotricuspid isthmus, and CS, but this usually requires a superior vena caval approach. Depending on the catheter used, the proximal poles may actually record from the septum and the middle poles the anterior right atrium. The CS catheter is useful to define left atrial activation during atrial flutter. Many laboratories no longer use a catheter along the crista terminalis or a separate catheter placed along the Eustachian ridge for clinical purposes, but they were critical in defining sites of block

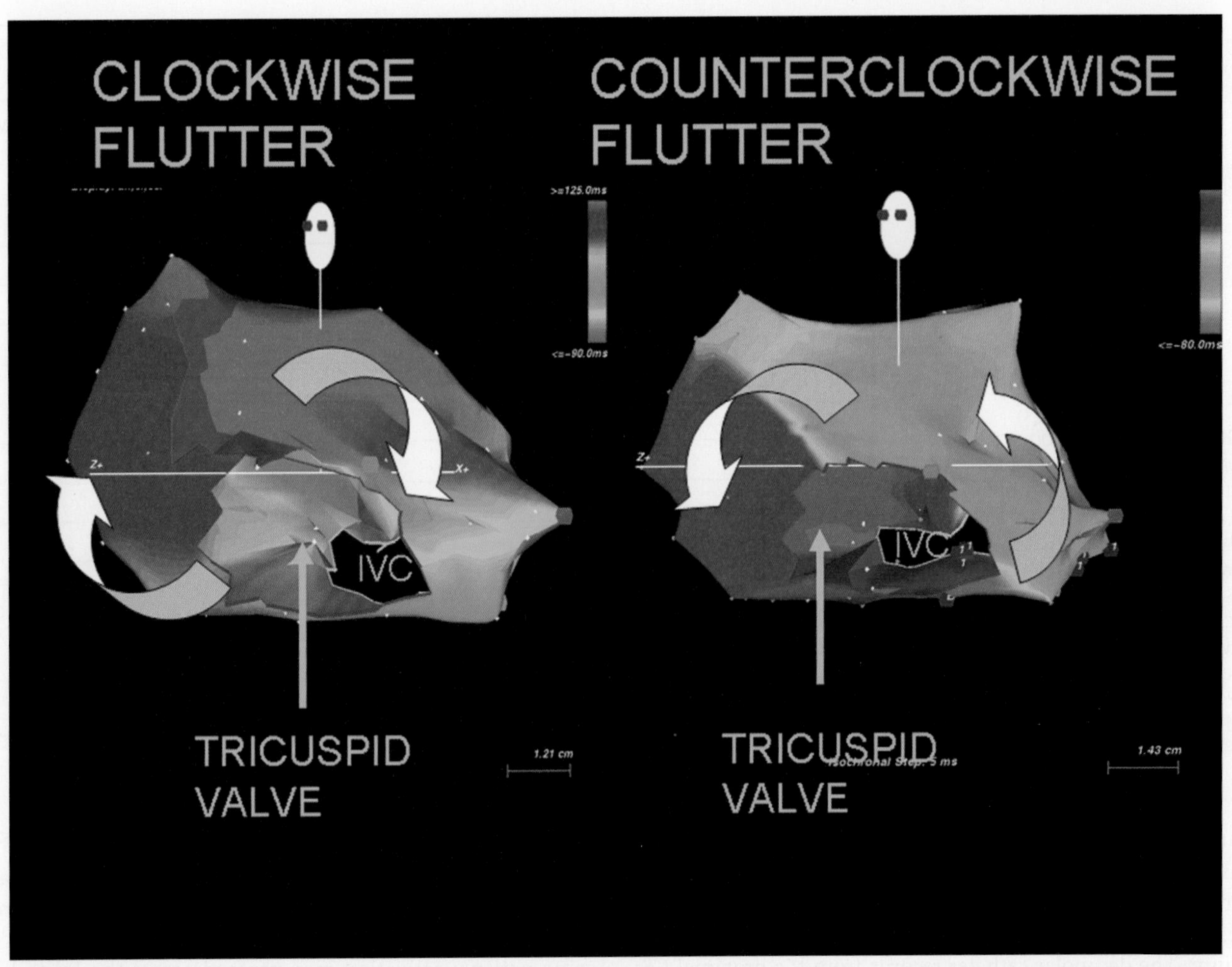


**FIGURE 9-23** *Activation of the atrium during counterclockwise and clockwise flutter using the Carto system.* Activation mapping of counterclockwise flutter is displayed on the right in colored isochrones with "earliest" activation in *red* and "latest" in *purple.* The *burgundy* demarcates adjacent earliest and latest sites. A full counterclockwise reentrant circuit is seen around the tricuspid annulus. Activation mapping of clockwise flutter is displayed on the left in colored isochrones with "earliest" activation in *red* and "latest" in *purple.* The *burgundy* demarcates adjacent earliest and latest sites. A full clockwise reentrant circuit is seen around the tricuspid annulus.

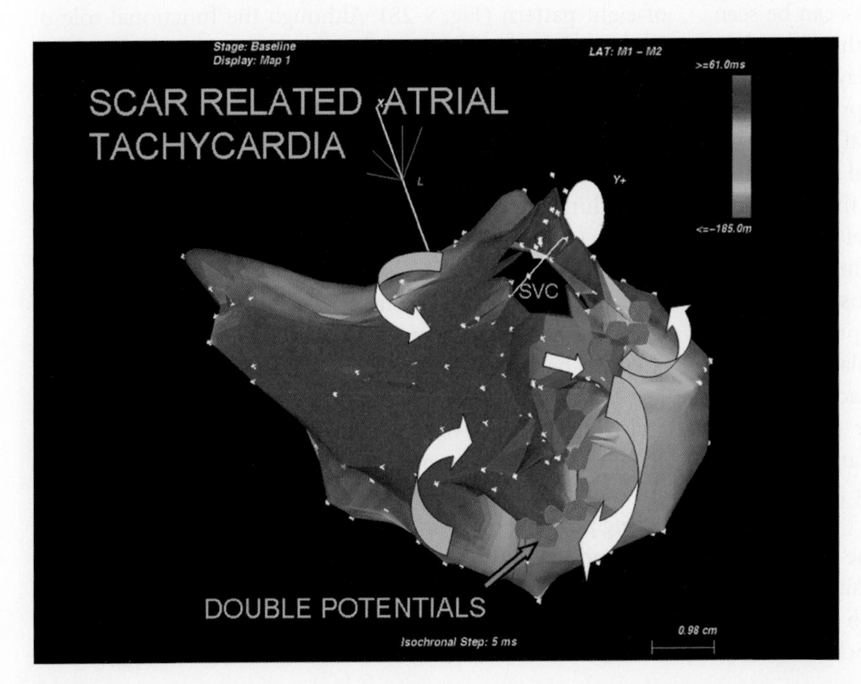


**FIGURE 9-24** *Activation of the atrium during atrial tachycardia around an atriotomy scar using the Carto system.* Activation mapping of tachycardia around a prior atriotomy scar is displayed in colored isochrones with "earliest" activation in *red* and "latest" in *purple.* A full reentrant circuit is seen around the scar with an isthmus between the edges of the scar. The *gray dots* are double potentials.

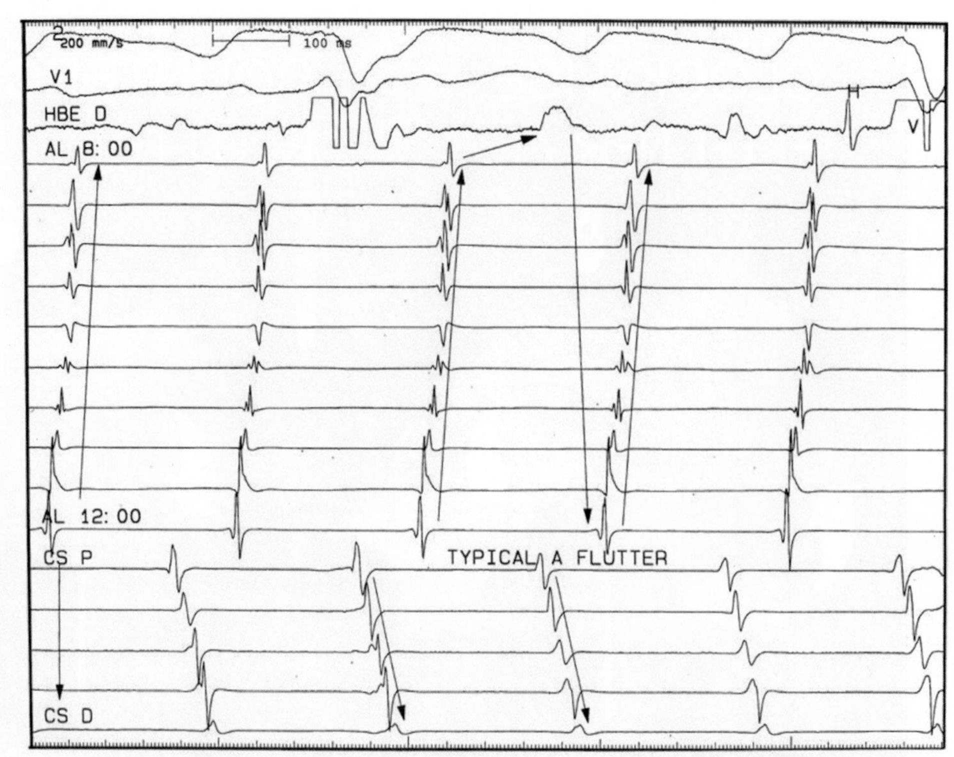


**FIGURE 9-25** *Activation mapping of counterclockwise flutter.* ECG leads 2 and $V_1$ are shown with recordings from the HBE, anterolateral right atrium (AL) with the distal tip at 8 o'clock in the LAO view and proximal pair at 12 o'clock and $CS_P$ to $CS_d$. Activation proceeds counterclockwise (cephalocaudad) along the AL wall with a delay between the distal AL and the HBE and CS P. *Arrows* show direction of activation in the right atrium and in the CS.

that created barriers that determined the flutter circuit. Typical counterclockwise flutter is shown in Figure 9-25. The distal tip in this patient is placed at 7 to 8 o'clock in the LAO view and the proximal electrode is recorded at noon in the anterior right atrium. The decapolar catheter records from the proximal CS (i.e., the os) to the distal CS, which is lateral. A single electrogram from the His bundle catheter is shown as well. Counterclockwise flutter characteristically shows sequential activation of the septum, the anterior wall and the anterolateral wall, the latter being activated craniocaudally. A delay can be seen between the lateral border of the isthmus and the atrial electrogram in the HIS bundle recording. This delay is localized to the isthmus. Note that left atrial activation proceeds from proximal to distal CS. In clockwise (old "atypical") flutter the activation sequence is reversed with caudocranial spread along the anterolateral wall going down the septum to the atrial electrogram in the His bundle recording, with a delay appearing between the His bundle atrial activity and the isthmus between the CS and the distal anterolateral electrograms (Fig. 9-26). Note in this figure that left atrial activation also proceeds from proximal to distal CS. More commonly, particularly if the CS catheter is positioned deep in the great cardiac vein, distal to proximal activation is observed. The similar proximal CS activation sequence in both counterclockwise and clockwise flutter suggests the left atrium is unnecessary for the reentrant circuit used for these arrhythmias.

Double potentials are seen not only along the crista terminalis where their activation sequence is in opposite directions, but are also seen along the Eustachian ridge. Both of these sites are anatomic structures along which lines of block are formed that may be fixed or functional. While some authors[10,22,57–59] believe these lines of block are fixed, pacing at variable rates has demonstrated change in conduction properties across the crista at different rates (see preceding paragraphs).[20,23] In some patients activation may proceed across the Eustachian ridge to form a lower circuit,[68] yielding an atypical accelerated flutter (Fig. 9-27). More often, a potential lower loop is seen, in which activation around the posterior IVC merges with activation around the tricuspid annulus to form a figure-of-eight pattern (Fig. 9-28). Although the functional role of lower-loop activation in maintaining the reentrant circuit is not always clear, both loops can be simultaneously entrained from the isthmus (Fig. 9-29). Thus, while in general these barriers are constant and help force the flutter circuit to the region of the tricuspid valve, they are not fixed. Figure-of-eight flutter may be seen any time two fixed boundaries are present (e.g., scar and tricuspid valve or IVC) (Fig. 9-30).

Occasionally the ECG looks like typical isthmus-dependent flutter, but intracardiac activation maps show parts of the atria have disorganized atrial activity (Fig. 9-18). Such rhythms behave more like atrial fibrillation than flutter, but can occasionally be converted to true flutter by Class I antiarrhythmic agents or amiodarone. Less commonly a focal atrial tachycardia can mimic atrial flutter. Figure 9-31 shows an example of an atrial tachycardia from a PV in a patient taking propafenone. Craniocaudal activation of both the septum and lateral wall is present. This finding should suggest a focal tachycardia from the left atrium (if precordial P waves are positive), or less commonly, the HRA (P wave biphasic in V1).

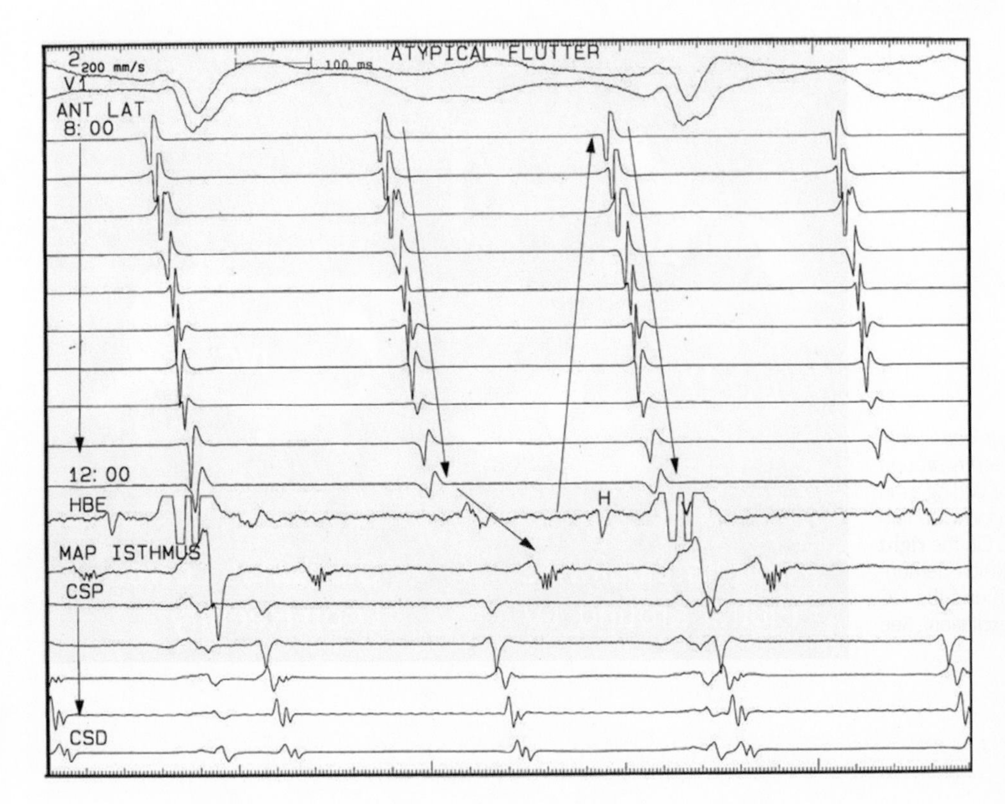


**FIGURE 9-26** *Activation mapping of clockwise flutter.* ECG leads 2 and $V_1$ are shown with recordings from the HBE, anterolateral right atrium (AL) with the distal tip at 8 o'clock in the LAO view and proximal pair at 12 o'clock. $CS_p$ to $CS_d$, and a mapping catheter in the isthmus. Activation proceeds clockwise (caudocephalad) along the AL wall with a delay between the distal HBE and recording site in the isthmus. *Arrows* show direction of activation in the right atrium.

## Characterization of the Reentrant Circuit in Atrial Flutter

Programmed stimulation has been critical in allowing us to determine those sites in the atrium that are part of the reentrant circuit and those that are not.[21,22,57–59,69–72] In addition, use of resetting or entrainment mapping has allowed us to localize the critical isthmus that is now the target of ablative therapy for this arrhythmia. Toward this end we have used resetting phenomena and entrainment in order to determine which parts of the atria are definitely parts of the reentrant circuit as well as to quantify the extent of the excitable gap in the circuit. The protocol for resetting involves the use of single extrastimuli at various sites in the atrium and analyzing the return cycles. The sites that are within the circuit demonstrate resetting at very long coupling intervals with the return cycle equal to the tachycardia cycle length (Fig. 9-32). When stimulation is carried out at sites distant from the circuit, the return cycle exceeds the tachycardia cycle length; moreover, the distance from the

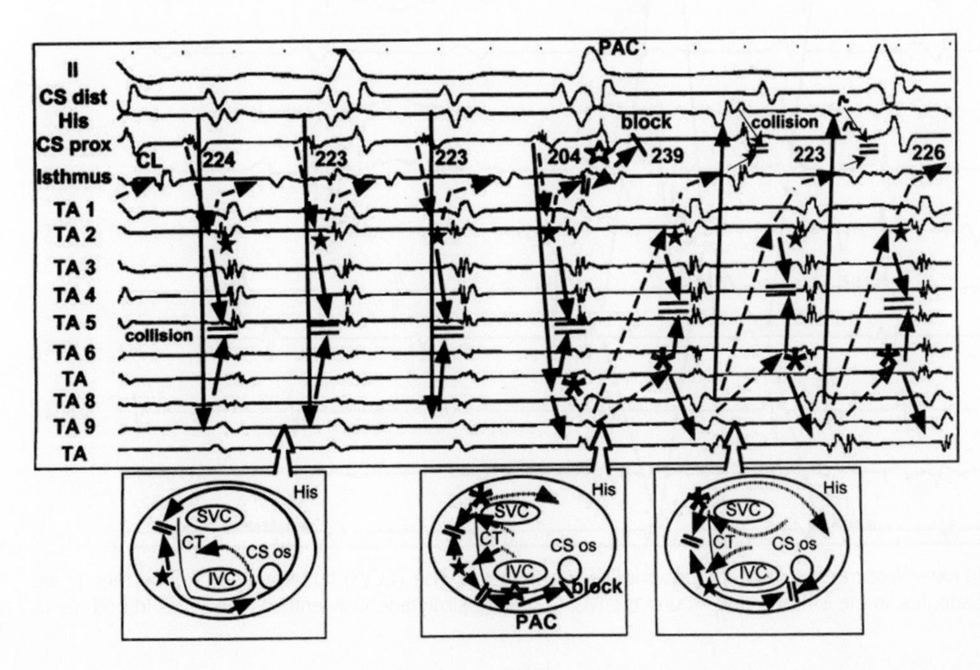


**FIGURE 9-27** *Transient lower-loop reentry.* (From Cheng J, Scheinman MM. Characteristics of double wave reentry induced by programmed stimulation in patients with typical atrial flutter. *Circulation* 1998;97:1589–1596, with permission.)

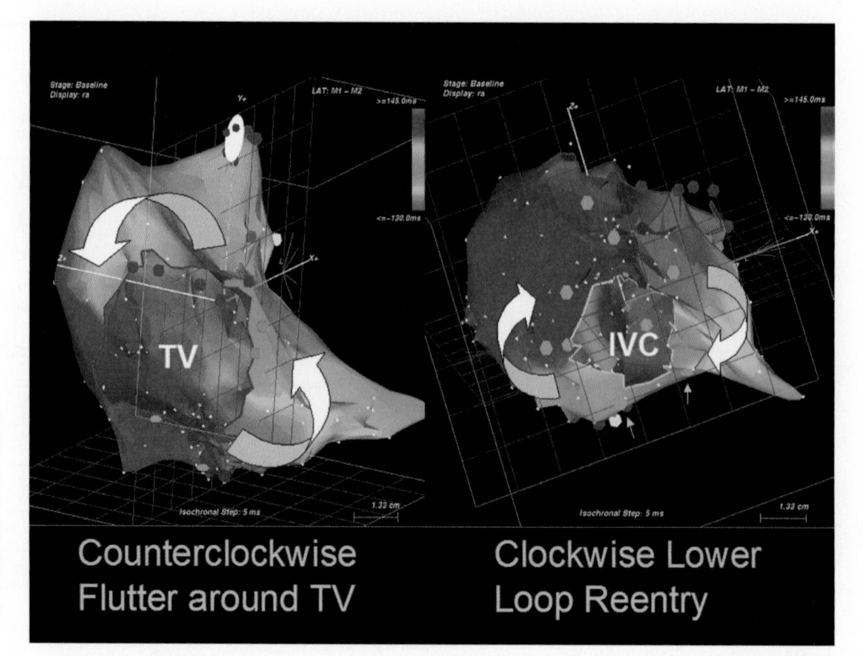


**FIGURE 9-28** *Counterclockwise isthmus-dependent flutter with a figure-of-eight lower-loop reentry around the IVC.* The maps are organized in color coding as in Figure 9-23. On the **left** typical counterclockwise flutter is shown as described in Figure 9-23. On the **right** is an inferior view of the right atrium which demonstrate simultaneous clockwise reentry around the IVC producing a figure-of-eight reentrant excitation. See text for discussion.

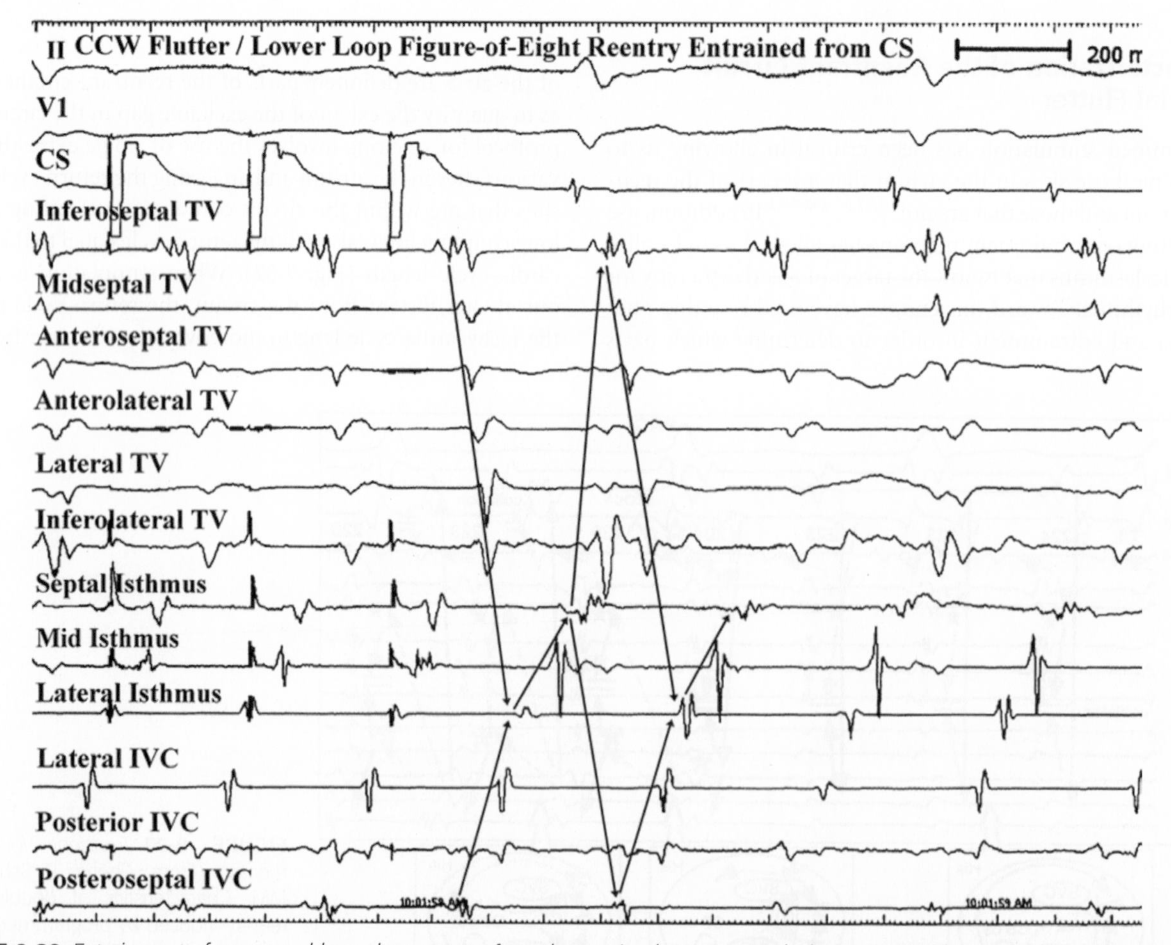


**FIGURE 9-29** *Entrainment of upper and lower-loop reentry from the proximal CS.* Counterclockwise (CCW) flutter and lower-loop reentry are present. EGMs from around the tricuspid annulus, in the isthmus, and around the IVC. CS pacing simultaneously entrains the EGMs in both reentrant circuits (*arrows*). See text.

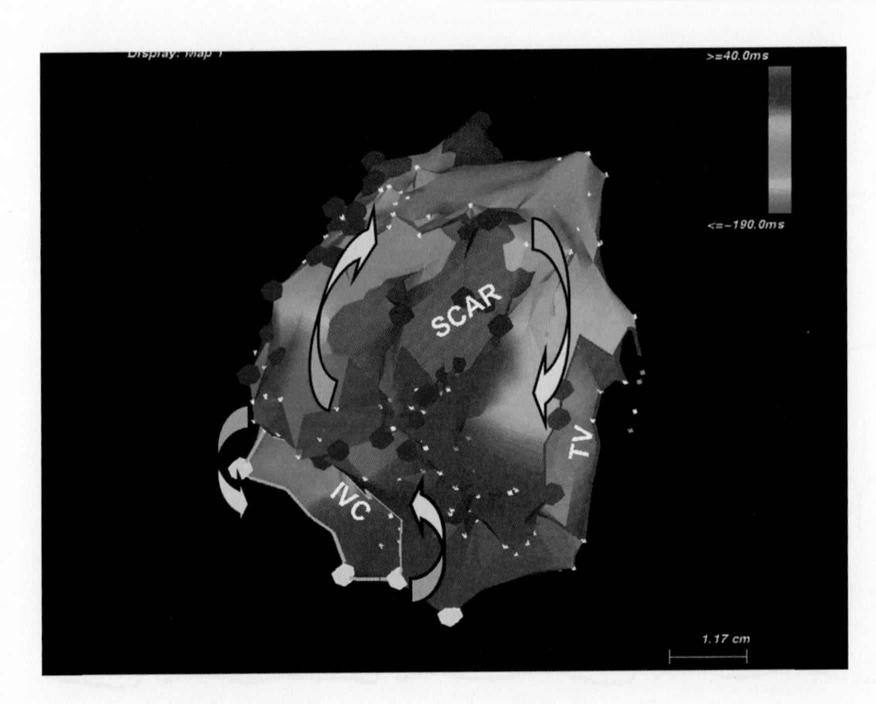


**FIGURE 9-30** *Figure-of-eight reentry around a scar and the IVC.* A scar from a prior atriotomy is shown in gray. Clockwise reentrant excitation is shown around the scar *(arrows)* and counterclockwise reentry is shown around the IVC *(arrows).* Note that no reentrant excitation is seen around the tricuspid valve.

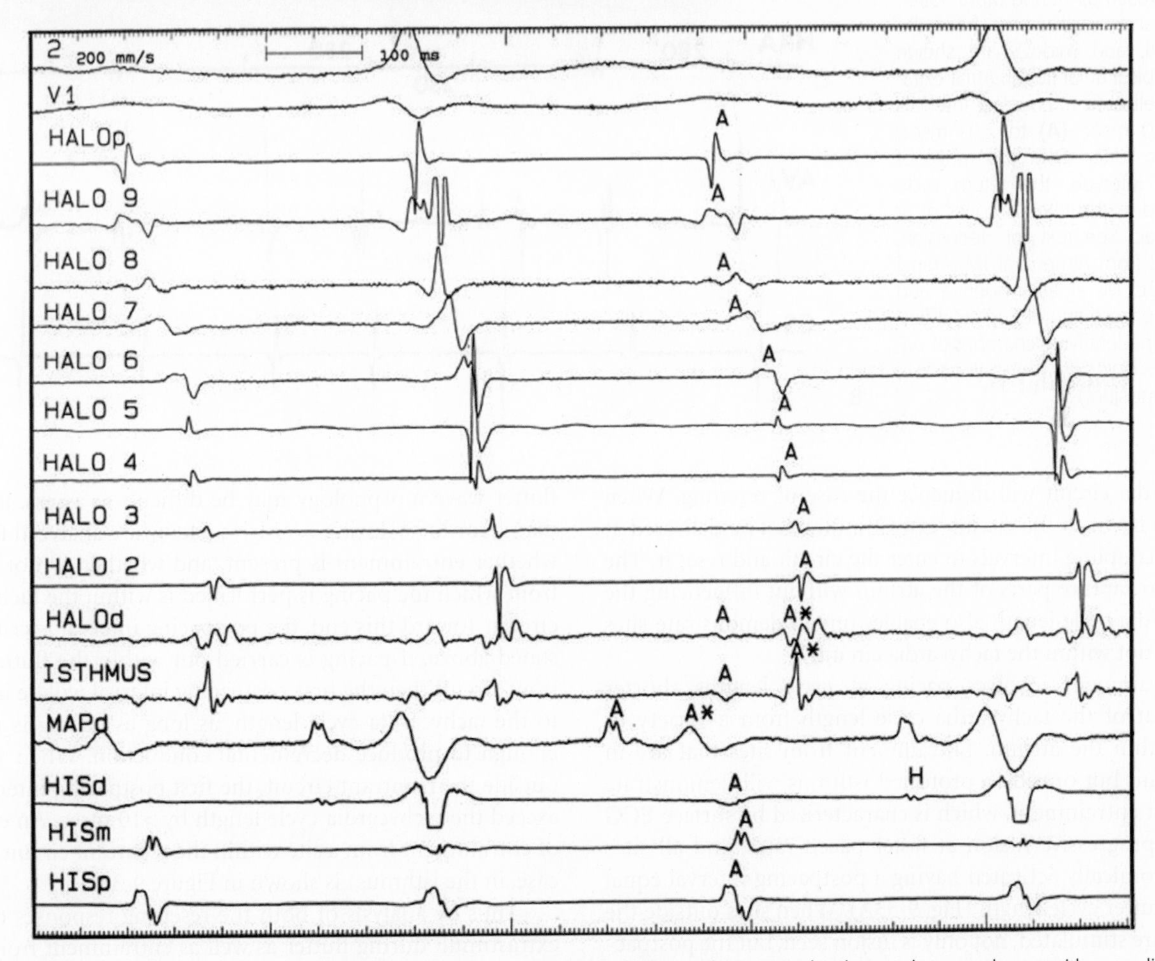


**FIGURE 9-31** *Atrial tachycardia from superior pulmonary vein mimicking clockwise flutter.* ECG leads 2 and $V_1$ are shown with recordings from the anterolateral right atrium using, a HALO catheter with the distal pair of electrodes (HALOd) in the isthmus, the septum from the distal (d), mid (m), and proximal (p) HIS, and a mapping catheter (MAPd) in the left superior pulmonary vein during a drug-slowed atrial tachycardia. The surface ECG mimicked clockwise, but the intracardiac electrograms showed nearly simultaneous activation of the septum (HISd,m,p) and anterolateral right atrium (HALO 7,8,9,p), which excludes a clockwise reentrant circuit. Earliest activity was found in the left superior pulmonary vein where a split potential was seen, with the first potential recorded 75 msec prior to the P wave. See text for discussion.

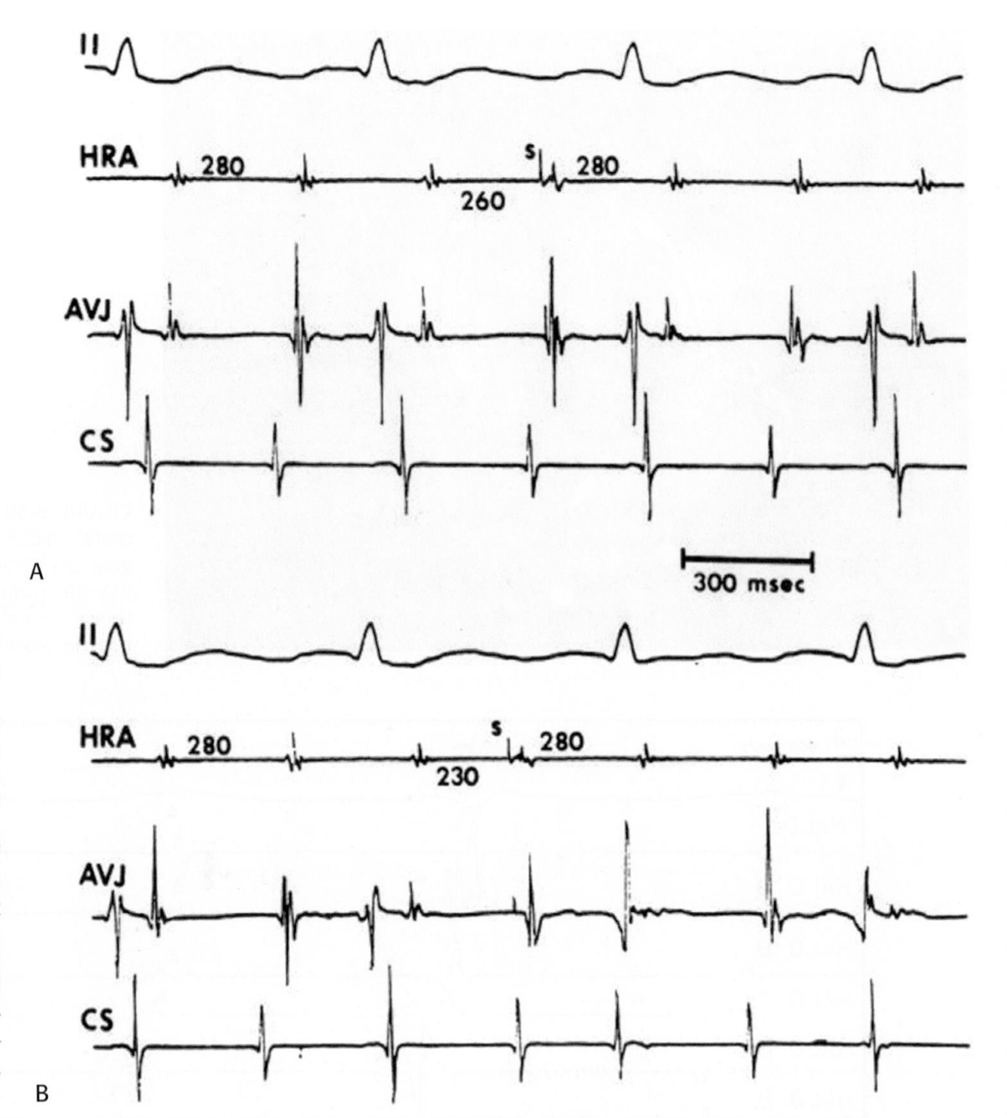


**FIGURE 9-32** *Demonstration of a flat resetting curve in response to atrial extrastimuli during atrial flutter.* Lead II and electrograms from the HRA, AVJ, and mid-CS are shown during typical atrial flutter. Atrial extrastimuli delivered at coupling intervals from 260 msec **(A)** to 230 msec, **(B)** reset flutter. Over this range of coupling intervals, the return cycle measured in the HRA is constant at 280 msec. See text for discussion. (Adapted from Almendral JM, Arenal A, Abeytus M, et al. Incidence and patterns of resetting during atrial flutter: role in identifying chamber of origin. *J Am Coll Cardiol* 1987;9:153A, with permission.)

tachycardia circuit will influence the ease of resetting. When sites are far from the circuit, extrastimuli must be delivered at shorter coupling intervals to enter the circuit and reset it. The ability to capture parts of the atrium without influencing the tachycardia cycle length also enables one to demonstrate sites that are not within the tachycardia circuit.

Entrainment involves pacing at cycle lengths shorter than that of the tachycardia cycle length from a variety of sites within the atrium. Entrainment from sites that are in the circuit but outside a protected isthmus will demonstrate manifest entrainment, which is characterized by surface ECG fusion, progressive fusion at faster paced rates, and all sites orthodromically activated having a postpacing interval equal to the flutter cycle length (Fig. 9-33A). When sites outside the circuit are stimulated, not only is fusion seen, but the postpacing interval will exceed the flutter cycle length by >10 msec (Fig. 9-33B). Concealed entrainment is said to occur when the paced atrial waveform on the surface QRS looks identical to the spontaneous flutter morphology. An example of concealed entrainment is shown in Figure 9-34. Since the flutter-wave morphology may be difficult to assess, intracardiac recordings during overdrive pacing are analyzed to assess whether entrainment is present, and whether or not the site from which the pacing is performed is within the tachycardia circuit. Toward this end, the postpacing interval is critical. As stated above, if pacing is carried out within the flutter reentrant circuit then the first postpacing interval will be identical to the tachycardia cycle length, as long as pacing is not fast enough to produce decremental conduction. When sites are outside the reentrant circuit, the first postpacing interval will exceed the tachycardia cycle length by >10 msec. An example of entrainment from a site within the reentrant circuit (in this case, in the isthmus) is shown in Figure 9-35.

Thus by analysis of both the resetting responses of atrial extrastimuli during flutter as well as entrainment from those sites, one can confirm the diagnosis of a reentrant mechanism and determine those sites that are within the reentrant circuit. This requires (a) comparing the relative ease of resetting of flutter from different sites, (b) comparing return cycles during either resetting or entrainment, and (c) analyzing the resetting

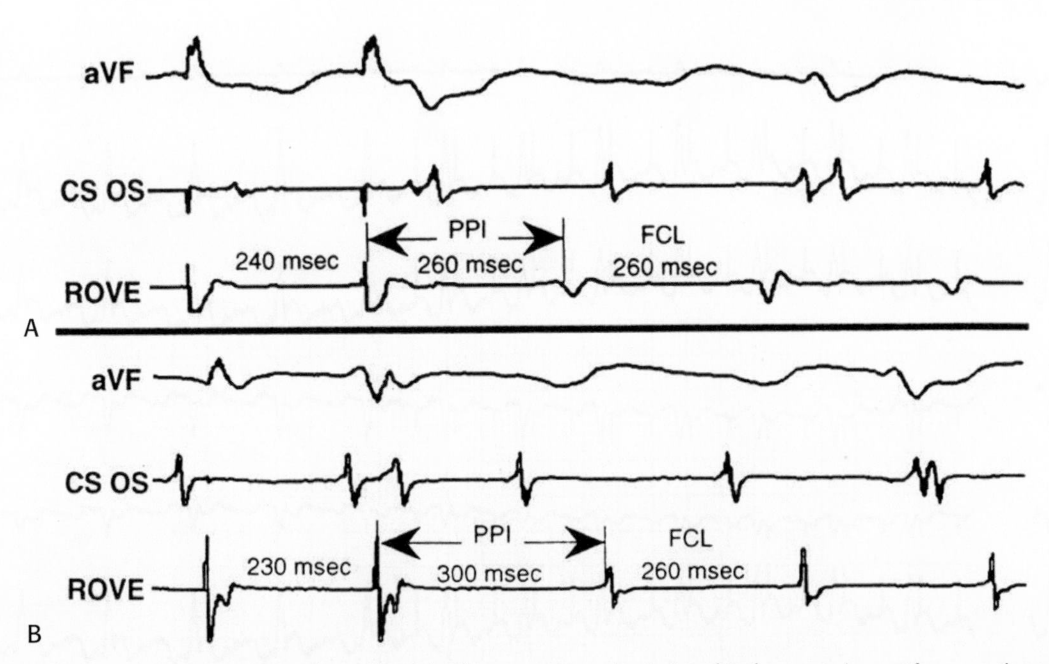


**FIGURE 9-33** *Entrainment from sites within and outside of the flutter reentrant circuit.* **A** and **B** show entrainment from a roving catheter (ROVE) at a site within **(A)** and outside **(B)** of the flutter circuit. Surface ECG lead aVF and an electrogram from the CS os and the ROVE are displayed. Entrainment from sites within the circuit will have a postpacing interval (PPI) equal to the flutter cycle length, while entrainment from sites outside the circuit will have a PPI greater than the flutter cycle length. See text for discussion. (From Olgin JE, Miles W. Ablation of atrial tachycardias. In: Singer I, Barold SS, Camm AJ, eds. *Nonpharmacologic therapy of arrhythmias in the 21st century*. Armonk, NY: Futura Publishing, 1998:197–217, with permission.)

patterns to determine the characteristics of the excitable gap of atrial flutter.[69–72]

Atrial stimuli delivered at the right atrial appendage, the smooth posterior septal atrium, including the fossa ovalis, and the left atrium via the CS have all been able to manifest local capture without influencing atrial flutter, suggesting that all these sites are outside the flutter reentrant circuit (Fig. 9-36). Since the left atrium appears unnecessary for typical atrial flutter, it is sometimes possible to capture left atrial sites with double extrastimuli without influencing the tachycardia circuit (Fig. 9-37). The closeness of the site of stimulation to the atrial flutter reentrant circuit will determine whether or not resetting can occur at all, and if so, with what coupling intervals. Sites farther from the circuit require extrastimuli delivered at shorter coupling intervals to perturb the circuit than those nearer the circuit. Regardless of whether flutter is clockwise or counterclockwise, stimulation from right atrial sites can reset the flutter at longer coupling intervals than sites in the left atrium, further supporting evidence that isthmus-dependent flutter is localized in the right atrium. In Figure 9-38 a comparison of stimulation from the high lateral right atrium and the CS during atrial flutter is shown. During late coupled extrastimuli from the HRA, the flutter is reset with the return cycle equal to the flutter cycle length, suggesting that this site is in the tachycardia circuit. Even when the coupling interval is reduced to 220 msec, the return cycle remains fixed. As discussed below, this suggests an excitable gap of at least 45 msec. In contrast, when the CS is stimulated distally, a single extrastimulus at a coupling interval of 220 msec does not reset the tachycardia. It is only when double extrastimuli are introduced that the tachycardia is reset. Note that the return cycle exceeds that of the tachycardia cycle length by more than 100 msec, suggesting that this site is very distant from the tachycardia circuit. Using this resetting model, the entire left atrium, the atrial septum from the fossa ovalis posteriorly to the superior vena cava and medial to the crista terminalis, and the right atrial appendage do not appear to be part of the reentrant circuit. Nevertheless, stimulation at these right atrial sites is able to reset the tachycardia at shorter coupling intervals than left atrial sites (none of which are in the reentrant circuit of typical flutter), further supporting the concept that this rhythm is localized to the right atrium. The high lateral anterior sites, low lateral anterior sites, and regions around the os of the CS and triangle of Koch are all within the reentrant circuit.

More recently, entrainment mapping has been used by several groups in order to precisely define the borders of the circuit and the site of the reentrant circuit.[21,22,57–59] These investigators have elegantly demonstrated that during entrainment the return cycles were identical to the tachycardia cycles (within 10 msec) all along the tricuspid annulus and down the free wall of the anterolateral right atrium (trabeculated right atrium), but that the septum and right atrial appendage as well as left atrium were not involved. Moreover, these entrainment studies demonstrated that the Eustachian ridge and the crista terminalis form posterior barriers to the circuit, which is forced through a narrow isthmus bordered by the inferior vena cava, Eustachian ridge, CS, and tricuspid valve. This has

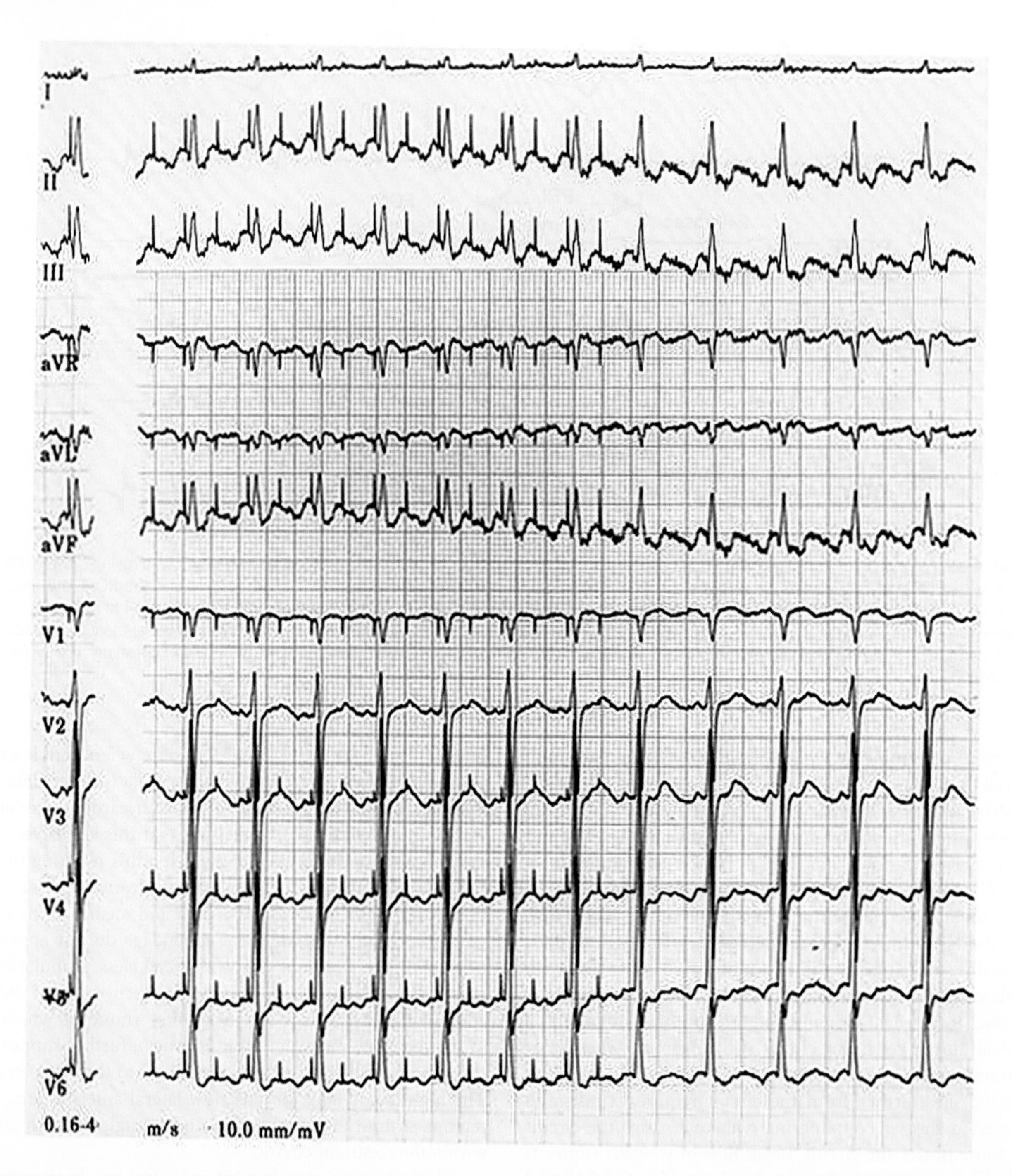


**FIGURE 9-34** *Surface ECG of atrial flutter during concealed entrainment.* A 12-lead ECG is shown during concealed entrainment of atrial flutter resulting from pacing in the isthmus. Note that the paced "flutter" waves are identical to the spontaneous flutter waves and the postpacing interval equals the flutter cycle length.

become the target site for ablative procedures (see Chapter 14). Of note, the double potentials that are noted on either side of the Eustachian ridge reflect activation in opposite directions. The smooth septum above the Eustachian ridge is not part of the reentrant circuit in the vast majority of cases. Occasionally, breakthroughs have been noted across the Eustachian ridge and lower crista terminalis by some investigators[68] suggesting that it is not always fixed. These breakthroughs may be associated with atypical forms of flutter; however, in most patients these areas of block seem to be functionally fixed. The tendon of Todaro forms another functionally determined line of block in typical isthmus-dependent flutter. We have noted double potentials along the tendon of Todaro, which is an extension of the Eustachian ridge, but neither systematic resetting nor entrainment mapping studies at this level of the triangle of Koch have been performed. Thus it appears that

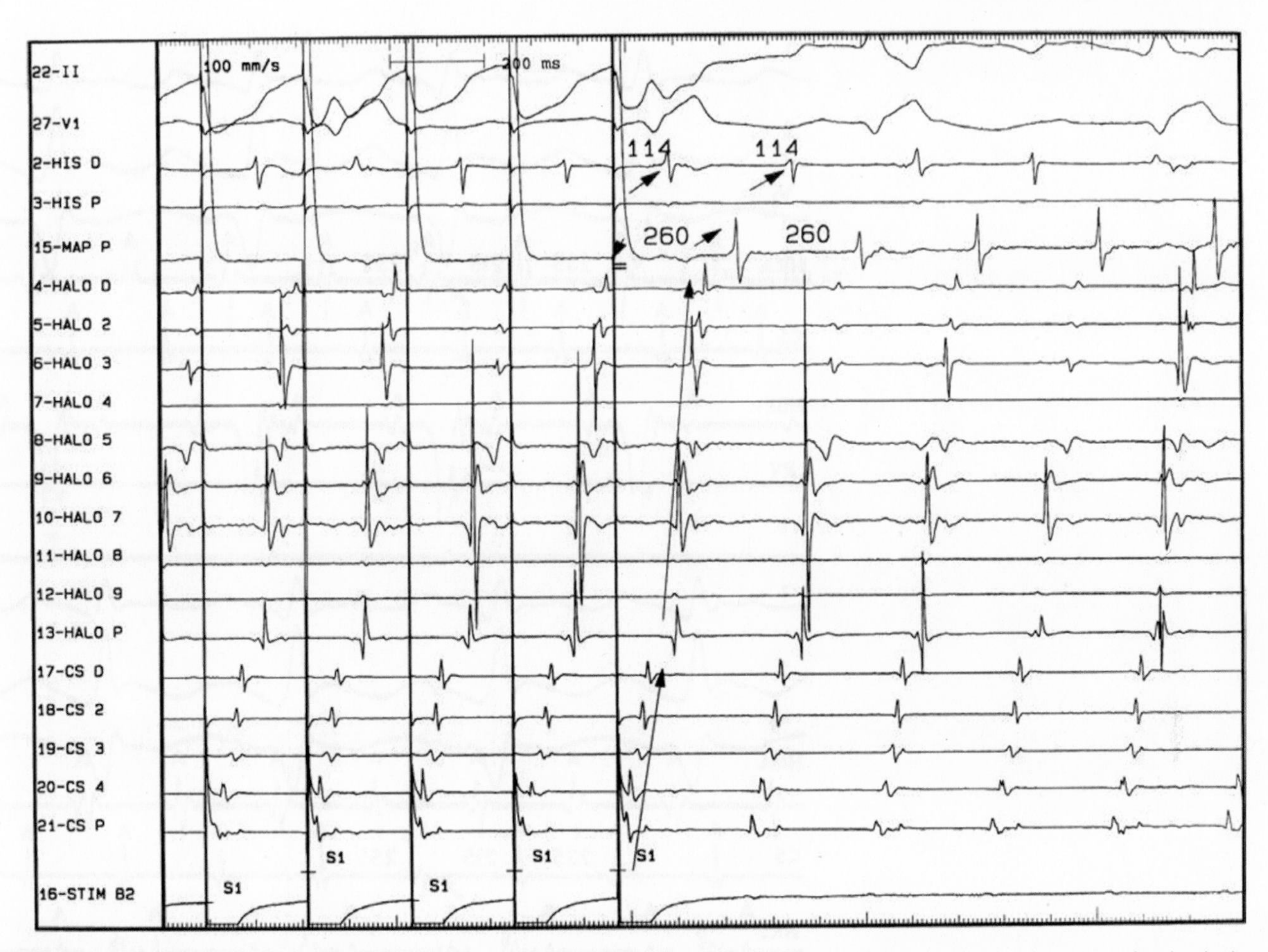


**FIGURE 9-35** *Intracardiac recordings during concealed entrainment.* ECG leads 2 and $V_1$ are displayed with recordings from the distal (d) and proximal (p) His bundle catheter, a 20-pole Halo catheter along the anterolateral right atrium with Halo D positioned at 8 o'clock and Halo P at 12 o'clock, a CS catheter ($CS_p$ positioned just inside the os), and a mapping catheter (MAPp) in the isthmus. Counterclockwise flutter is present at a cycle length of 260 msec. Pacing is performed from the isthmus (MAP) at 240 msec, resulting in entrainment with orthodromic capture of the HALO electrodes and antidromic activation of the HIS electrodes. The orthodromic activation is identical to spontaneous flutter, and the stimulus to HIS interval is identical to that seen in spontaneous flutter (114 msec). The return cycle at the pacing site equals the flutter cycle length. See text for discussion.

the tricuspid annulus forms the anterior border of isthmus-dependent flutters (either counterclockwise or clockwise), while the posterior border occurs at a variable distance from this anterior border. It is narrowest in the region of the Eustachian ridge and widest in the anterior part of the right atrium.

While conduction appears to be slowest through the isthmus defined by the inferior vena cava, Eustachian ridge, and CS as impulses travel around the tricuspid annulus in either a clockwise or counterclockwise direction, we have observed a fully excitable gap during resetting studies in both of these types of flutter. During resetting, a fully excitable gap is believed to be present if the return cycle is flat (i.e., there is no change in return cycle) as the coupling intervals are decremented. As the impulse encroaches on the refractory period of tissue within the circuit or on areas of poor excitability, the conduction time will increase. Thus the response to atrial extrastimuli may appear flat (no change for at least 20 msec range of coupling intervals), increasing, or mixed (initially flat followed by an increase in return cycles as the coupling intervals of extrastimuli are decreased). In almost all cases, a fully excitable gap, manifested by a flat curve of ≥20 msec can be demonstrated (Fig. 9-31). The range of the fully excitable gap appears to be between 30 and 65 msec in the absence of drugs, and in my experience, may exceed 100 msec if flutter is slowed by Class I agents. However, since the properties of atrial tissue may vary in different locations, these results may vary somewhat depending on where the stimulation is carried out. It would be of interest to repeat both resetting and entrainment studies from multiple sites around the tricuspid annulus to see how different the resetting curves would be. Preliminary data from our laboratory have shown similar curves and excitable gaps when stimulation is performed from the isthmus, os of the CS, fossa ovalis, and anterior and lateral tricuspid annulus. Thus, a relatively large fully excitable gap is present in typical isthmus-dependent flutter.

While entrainment from sites outside the isthmus are almost always associated with changes in the flutter-wave morphology (i.e., fusion) based on the spread of activity

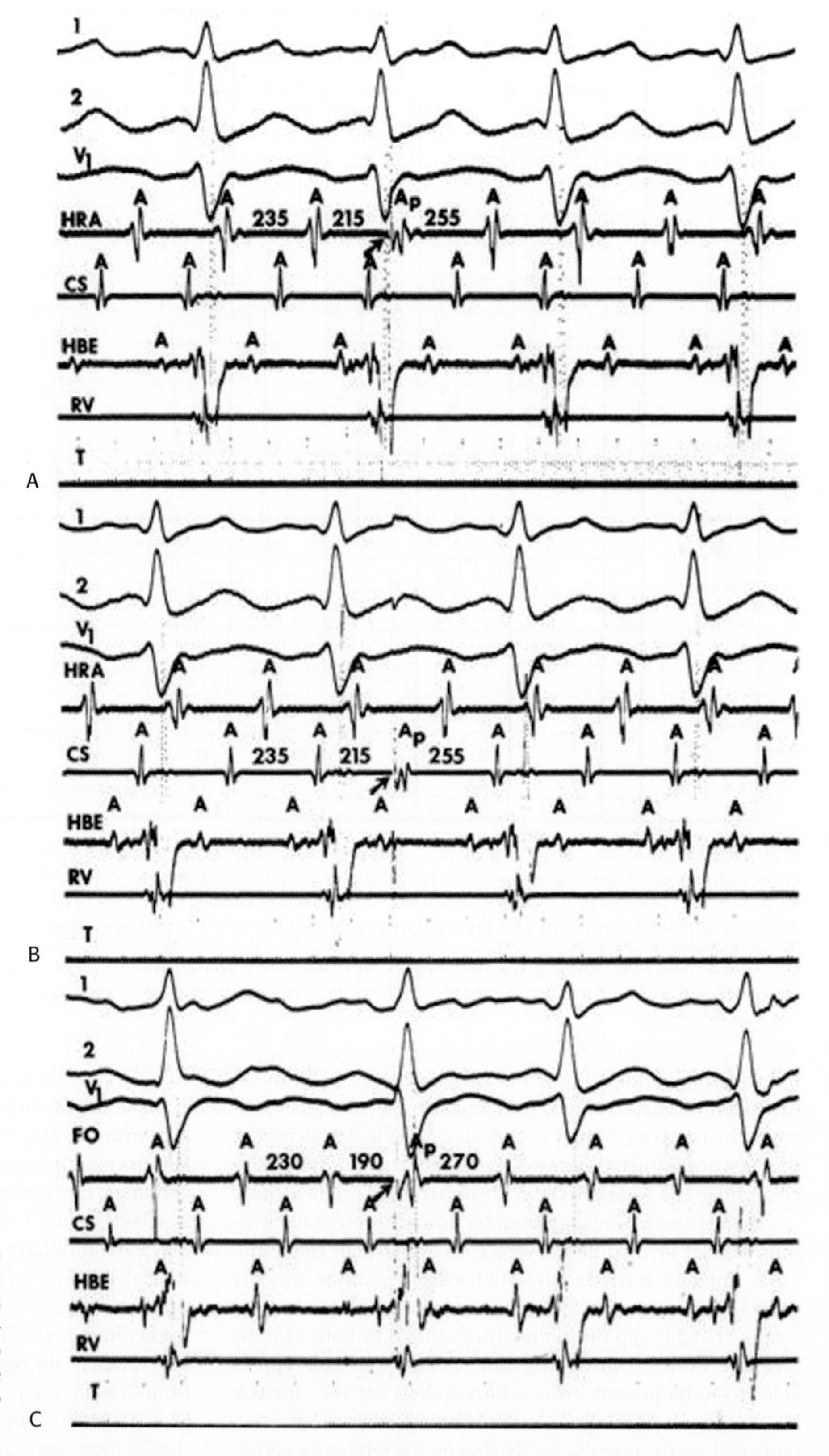


**FIGURE 9-36** *Failure to influence flutter during atrial stimulation.* Atrial premature (Ap) stimuli are delivered from the HRA **(A)**, CS **(B)**, and fossa ovalis (FO) **(C)** without influencing the flutter cycle length. The ability to depolarize large areas without affecting the flutter suggests these sites are not critical to the flutter circuit.

antidromically and orthodromically inside and outside of the circuit, stimulation from the isthmus produces concealed entrainment in which the flutter wave is unchanged. Examples of concealed entrainment are shown in Figures 9-34 and 9-35. Entrainment allows one to define the relative activation sequence and significance of split potentials.[57,59,65,73] Using this technique one can show that the Eustachian ridge forms a barrier in most cases with propagation of the impulse recorded in the isthmus followed by another that is recorded on the opposite side of the Eustachian ridge propagating in the opposite

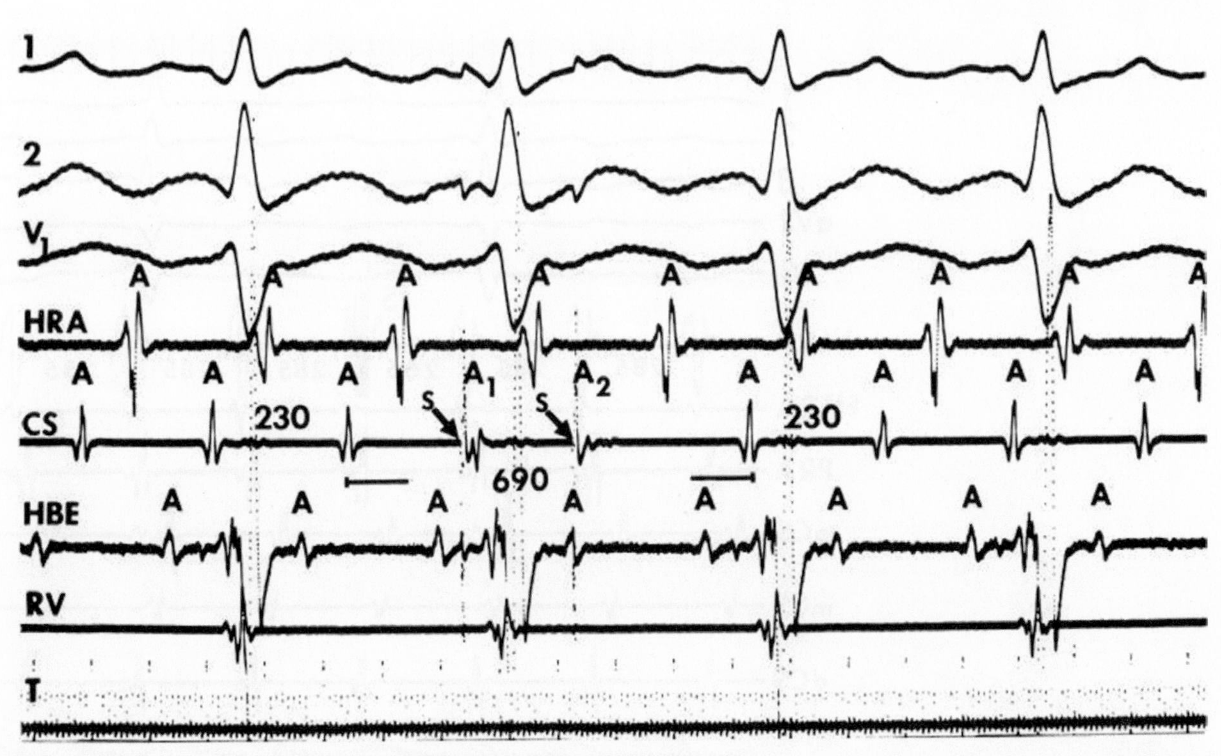


**FIGURE 9-37** *Failure of two extrastimuli from the left atrium to influence classic flutter.* Leads 1, 2, and $V_1$ are shown with electrograms from the HRA, mid-CS, HBE, and RV. Atrial flutter is present at a cycle length of 230 msec. Two atrial extrastimuli (shown by S, *arrows*) are delivered in the mid-CS, capturing the atrium locally but failing to influence the flutter cycle length. The atrial electrograms observed in the HBE and HRA remain unaffected and with the same activation sequence to each other as during spontaneous flutter. This suggests that the left atrium is passively activated and is not required to maintain flutter. See text for discussion. T, time line.

direction.[57–59] With pacing in the isthmus and recording from the proximal pair across the Eustachian ridge one can see antidromic and orthodromic capture of the two components of the electrogram in the Eustachian ridge. Therefore, the proposed circuit of isthmus-dependent flutter is shown in Figure 9-39 from Olgin et al.

Intra-isthmus reentry, a variant form of "typical atrial flutter" involving the septal isthmus and CS, can be seen as a de novo arrhythmia or may occasionally be seen after ablation of isthmus-dependent flutter.[74] The surface ECG pattern of this flutter resembles typical counterclockwise atrial flutter. Detailed entrainment mapping reveals concealed entrainment only from the portion of the isthmus adjacent to the septum and from the CS (Fig. 9-40). Pacing from the anterolateral portion of the isthmus produces manifest fusion with a prolonged postpacing interval. The postulated circuit travels around the CS os, bordered by the tricuspid annulus and Eustachian ridge, with an area of slow conduction adjacent to the CS os, possibly including the Eustachian ridge itself. The septum and anterolateral walls are passively activated in a caudocranial fashion. We have recently seen several cases of this in our laboratory which appeared to be typical atrial flutter on the surface ECG but proved to be reentry around the CS based on detailed entrainment mapping. All such tachycardias had negative "flutter waves" in leads 2, 3, and aVF with a short (<100 msec) intraisthmus conduction time. All were successfully treated with ablation (see chapter 14).

Lower-loop reentry is another variant form of typical flutter which may be transient or persistent during typical isthmus-dependent flutter (Figs. 9-27 to 9-30). Whether they truly form a figure-of-eight reentry or nearly complete second circuit, requires high-density mapping of the lateral isthmus. As stated earlier, the lower loop is entrainable during typical flutter (Fig. 9-30). Both share the tricuspid-caval isthmus which when ablated, abolishes both circuits (see Chapter 14).

When "atypical flutters" (macroreentrant atrial tachycardias) arises elsewhere in the atria, similar techniques can help define the borders of that flutter circuit.[21] The turning points around barriers are defined by approximation of split potentials, which get farther apart as the middle of a line of block is defined. The distance between that turning point and another fixed barrier defines an isthmus through which the impulse travels. An example of a right atrial scar-related flutter is shown in Figure 9-25. Left atrial macroreentrant flutter may occur on the septum, around the PV, the atrial appendage, or the mitral annulus. These tachycardias are often a consequence of ablation for atrial fibrillation (see Chapter 14). The frequent use of linear lesions leaves gaps in "lines" which serve as an area of slow conduction and/or block leading to reentry. The ECG of mitral annular flutter can look similar to tricuspid-caval isthmus-dependent typical flutter but activation mapping and the response to pacing is diagnostic. As shown in Figure 9-41, mitral annular flutter pacing from the distal CS and proximal CS have identical return cycles to the

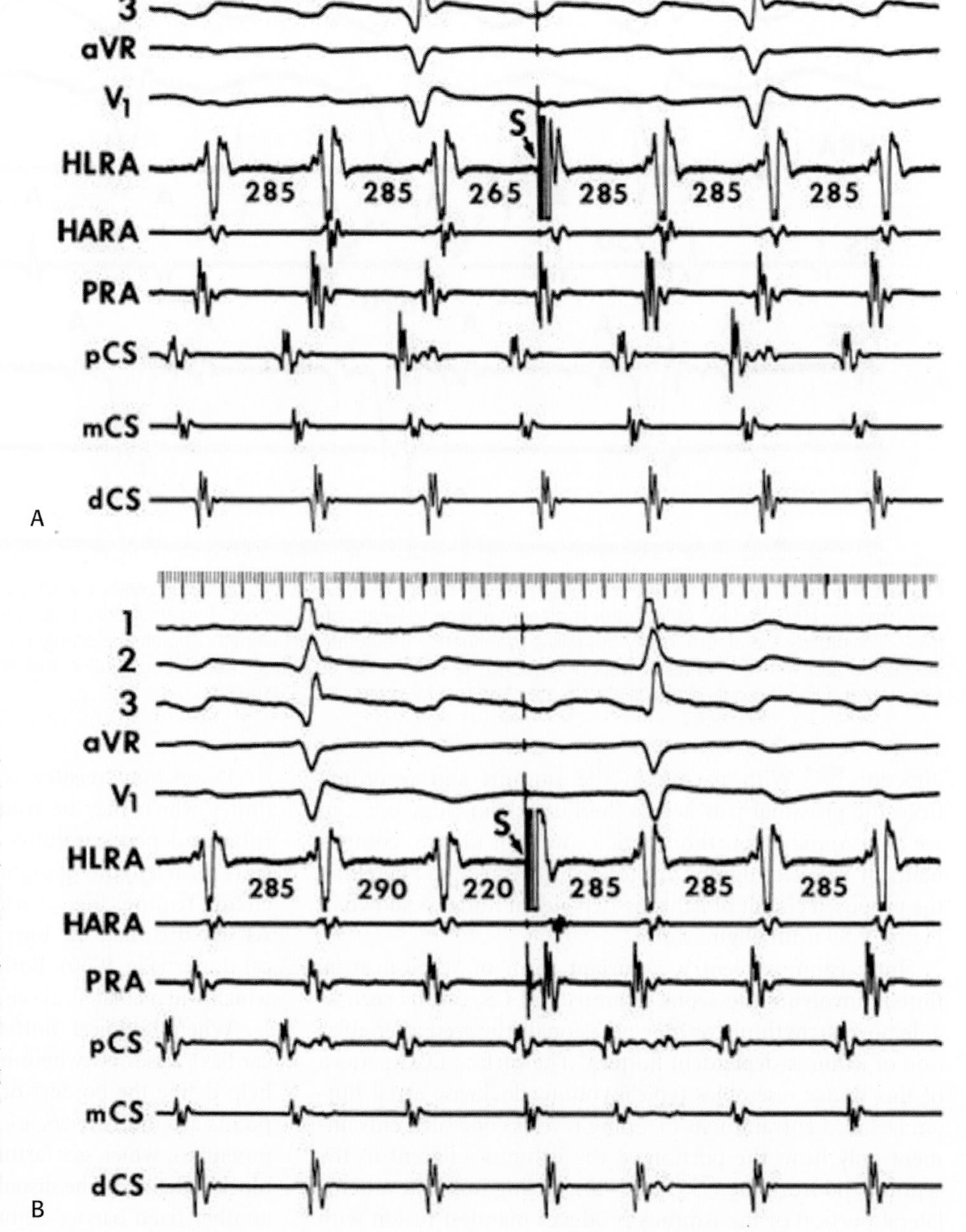


**FIGURE 9-38** *Relative ease of resetting from the right atrium and coronary sinus (CS).* All panels are arranged from top to bottom as ECG leads 1, 2, 3, aVR, and $V_1$ and intracardiac recordings from the high lateral right atrium (HLRA), high anterior right atrium (HARA), posterior right atrium (PRA), and proximal, mid, and distal coronary sinus (pCS, mCS, dCS). In all tracings, basic atrial flutter cycle length is 260 to 290 msec. **A** and **B:** Single atrial extrastimuli delivered from a long coupling interval of 265 msec, **A** (S, *arrow*), to shorter coupling intervals of 220 msec, **B** (S, *arrow*), reset atrial flutter with a flat resetting response curve having a return cycle of 285 msec.

tachycardia, suggesting they are both in the circuit, which must involve the mitral annulus.

## Termination of Atrial Flutter

Since both isthmus-dependent and scar-related types of atrial flutter are associated with fully excitable gaps, it is not surprising that termination of these arrhythmias by rapid atrial pacing is possible. The size of the excitable gap (which is 15% to 30% of the tachycardia cycle length) makes it possible for single atrial extrastimuli to enter the circuit and reset it. However, intra-atrial conduction delays and atrial refractoriness make it very difficult for a single atrial extrastimuli to terminate the flutter when delivered from unselected atrial sites. As noted above, systematic studies of the effects of stimulation in the isthmus during isthmus-dependent atrial flutter have not been performed. Such stimulation should have the highest likelihood of terminating flutter, since stimulation and capture could be achieved down to the refractory period of the tissue at the critical site. In fact, spontaneous termination

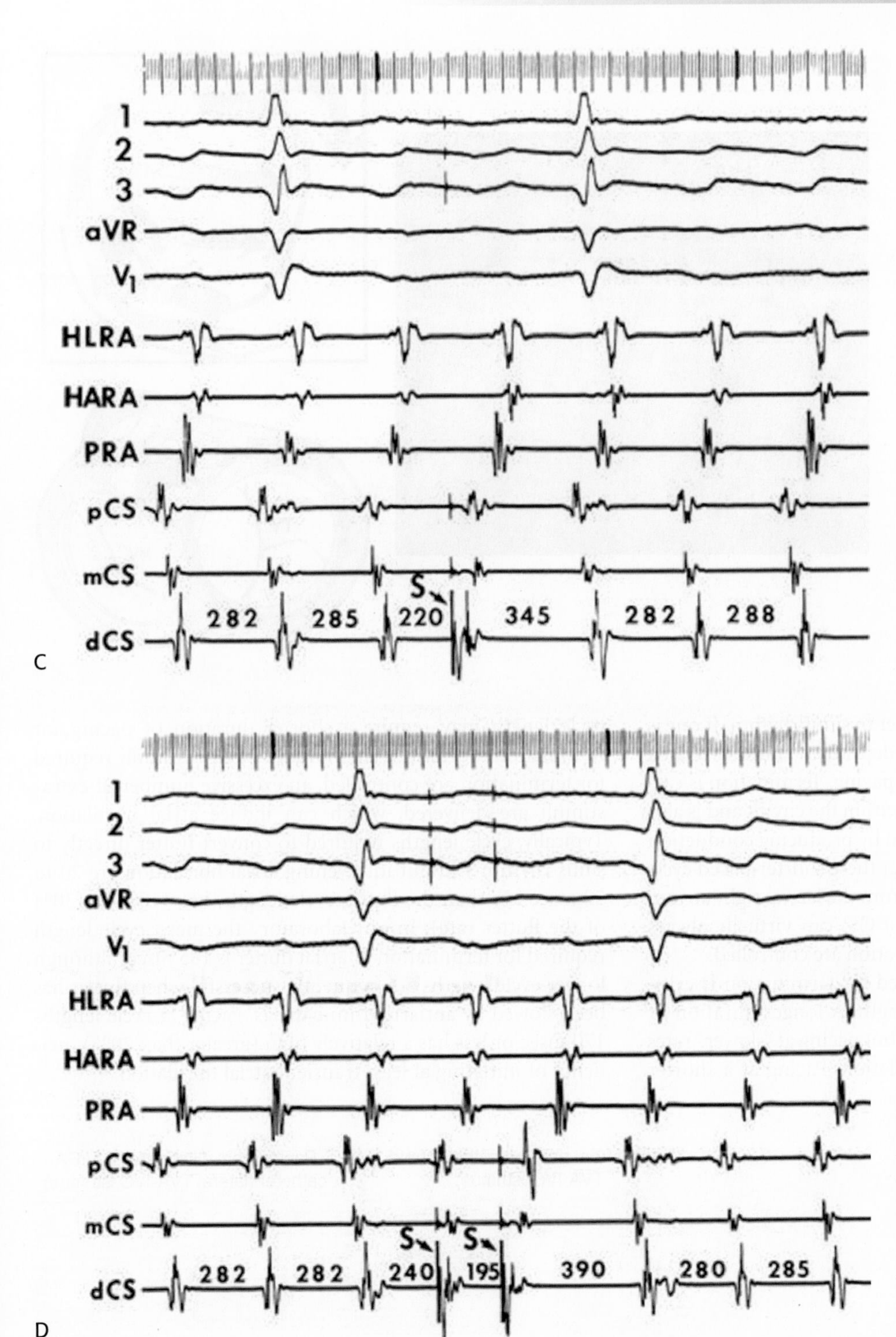


**FIGURE 9-38** (*Continued*) **C:** When stimulation is carried out from the most distal CS, the shortest atrial extrastimulus that produces capture (220 msec) fails to reset atrial flutter because the full compensatory pause is observed. **D:** It is only when double atrial extrastimuli are delivered with the second being short, at 195 msec, that atrial flutter is reset. The return cycle in this panel measured in the dCS is less than compensatory. See text for discussion.

of isthmus-dependent flutter always occurs in the isthmus in either counterclockwise or clockwise flutter.

Rapid pacing from either the right atrium or CS has been used clinically to terminate flutter, although the reported success of this intervention is variable.[8,75–78] Much of the variability of these reports, I believe, is related to the fact that arrhythmias other than isthmus-dependent flutter were included. When flutter is solely defined by the surface ECG, a variety of different arrhythmias with different mechanisms, all not reentrant, are possible. It is therefore not surprising to have a lack of uniformity of results. However, if one is dealing with isthmus-dependent or scar-related flutter, termination by rapid pacing is almost always successful if stimulation is appropriately performed. Waldo et al.[75] were the first to systematically demonstrate the reproducibility of termination of flutter by rapid atrial pacing. Successful termination of flutter is critically dependent on the rate and duration of pacing. Bursts of very rapid pacing frequently induces atrial fibrillation and,

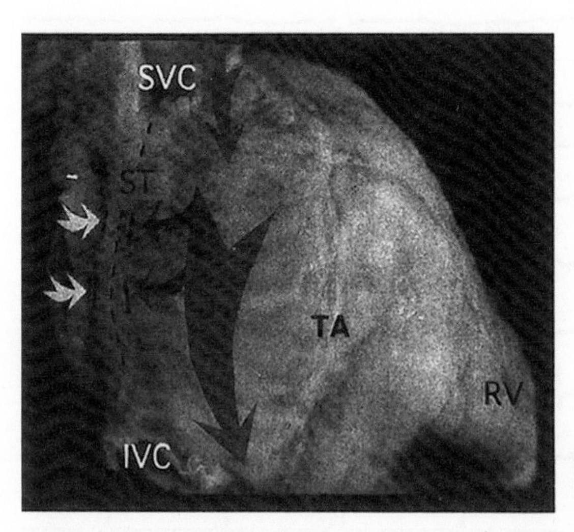


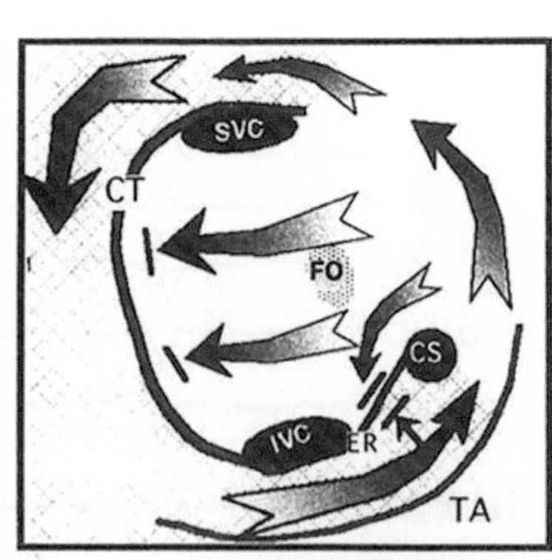


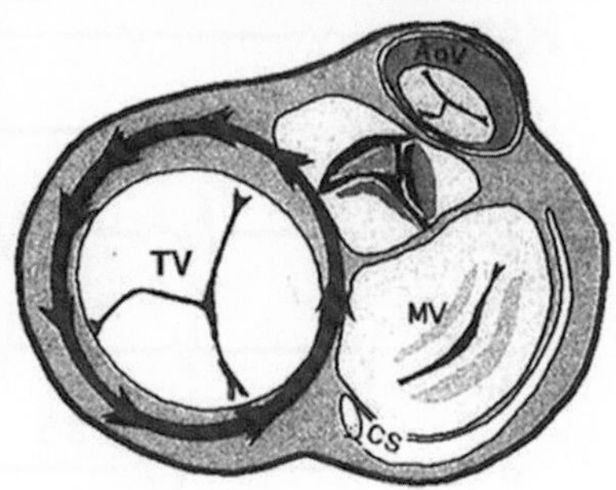


**FIGURE 9-39** *Schema of proposed reentrant circuit in counterclockwise flutter.* Activation proceeds around the tricuspid annulus with the crista terminalis (*CT*) and Eustachian ridge (*ER*) acting as posterior boundaries. The smooth septum posterior to the fossa ovalis and above the ER are not part of the circuit. See text for discussion. (From Olgin JE, Miles W. Ablation of atrial tachycardias. In: Singer I, Barold SS, Camm AJ, eds. *Nonpharmacologic therapy of arrhythmias in the 21st century.* Armonk, NY: Futura Publishing, 1998:197–217, with permission.)

therefore, fails to convert atrial flutter to sinus rhythm. If one is careful, more than 95% of isthmus-dependent and scar-related flutters can be terminated by rapid pacing. Termination is easier when stimulation is performed within the circuit and is also less likely to induce atrial fibrillation by producing conduction delay and block outside the circuit at these shorter-paced cycle lengths. In our experience, pacing from the lateral right atrium or CS (particularly in the proximal CS) can virtually always terminate flutter if the rate and duration are controlled.

The duration of pacing required for termination is critically dependent upon the cycle length. A longer duration of pacing is necessary at a slower rate, but pacing at "slower" rates is less likely to initiate atrial fibrillation. Pacing at a shorter cycle length may require a shorter duration of pacing for termination, but unless the number of extrastimuli required for termination are controlled, an excessive number of extrastimuli are delivered, which can induce atrial fibrillation. Typically, cycle lengths required to convert flutter directly to sinus rhythm without intervening atrial fibrillation are 20 to 50 msec less than the flutter cycle length (i.e., 110% to 130% of the flutter rate). In our laboratory the mean cycle length required for termination of atrial flutter is 185 msec, although longer cycle lengths are frequently successful when flutter has been slowed by antiarrhythmic drugs. Pacing at cycle lengths 170 msec or less has a relatively high (greater than 20%) incidence of initiating at least transient atrial fibrillation.

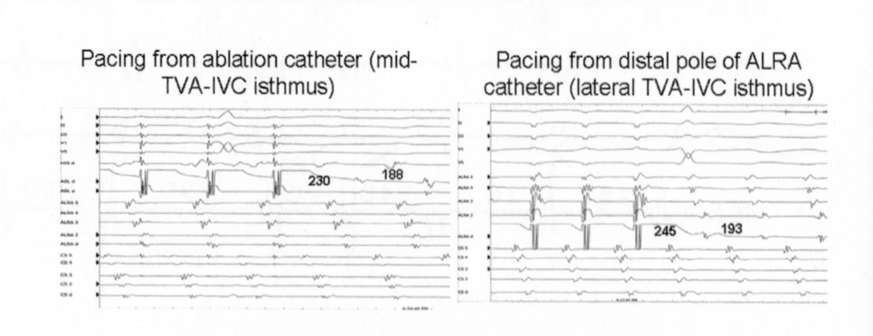


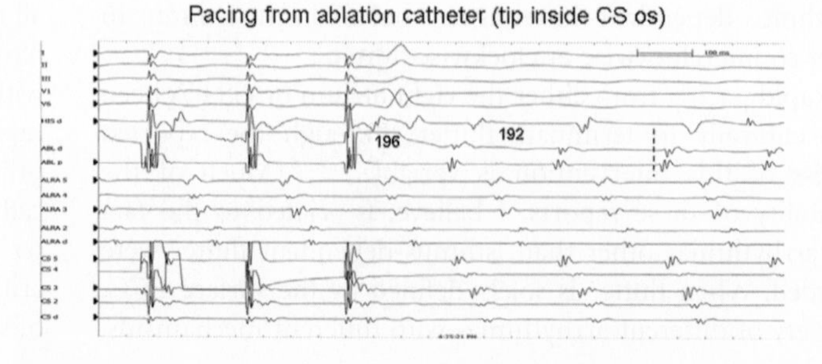


**FIGURE 9-40** *Intraisthmus reentry.* The ECG appears to show counterclockwise flutter. The cycle lengthy is short at ~190 msec and the intraisthmus conduction also appears to short at 80 msec.(ALRAd to CS os). Pacing from the midisthmus and lateral isthmus results in long postpacing intervals. Pacing from the os of the CS shows a postpacing interval comparable to the tachycardia cycle length suggesting it is in the circuit. See text for explanation.

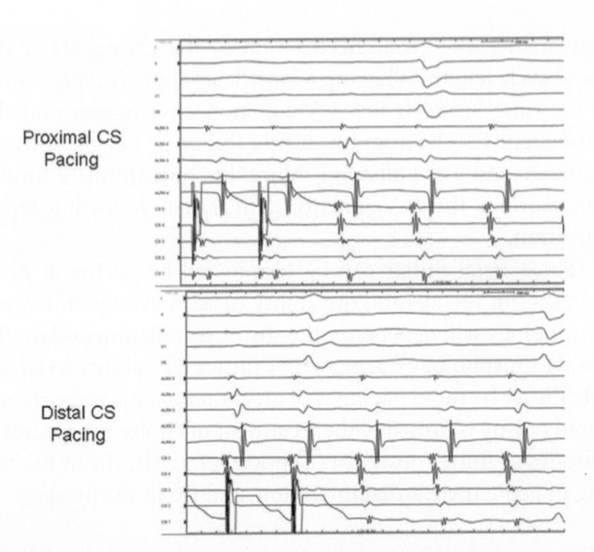


**FIGURE 9-41** *Pacing during mitral annular flutter.* Leads I, II, III, and V1 are shown with electrograms from the anterolateral RA (ALRA) and CS. Pacing from the proximal CS has an identical activation sequence as the flutter with a return cycle equal to the flutter cycle. The last paced complex occurs at the same time as the ALRA is activated by the next to last paced complex. In the **bottom panel** pacing from the distal CS is associated with collision with the proximal CS electrograms (activated from proximal to more distal) and has a return cycle identical to the flutter cycle length. This is diagnostic of mitral annular flutter. See text.

Direct termination to sinus rhythm is observed at cycle lengths shorter than those producing entrainment (i.e., continuous resetting) of atrial flutter.[66,79] The criteria for recognizing entrainment originally proposed by Waldo et al.[75] suggested that during entrainment the reentrant circuit responsible for flutter is repetitively engaged by the paced impulses. Thus all electrograms orthodromically activated by the last paced stimulus occur at the paced cycle length; and the first unpaced cycle at the pacing site occurs at the flutter cycle length, depending on whether or not it is in the circuit (see discussion on localizing atrial flutter earlier in this section). During pacing the flutter-wave morphology is a fusion between the amount of atrial tissue depolarized in the orthodromic and antidromic directions within and outside the circuit. Fusion may not be easily seen on the surface ECG in flutter that has a 2:1 conduction ratio, but antidromically and orthodromically captured wavefronts are easily seen during intracardiac mapping studies (Fig. 9-35). However, during high-right atrial pacing during counterclockwise flutter, the sudden change to an upright P wave in the inferior leads, as suggested by Waldo et al.[66,75,79] and Josephson et al.[72] often predict when termination will occur (Fig. 9-42). This sudden change reflects block in the flutter circuit (almost always in the isthmus) followed by activation of the atrium and subsequent activation of the atrium from the HRA alone. This results in simultaneous

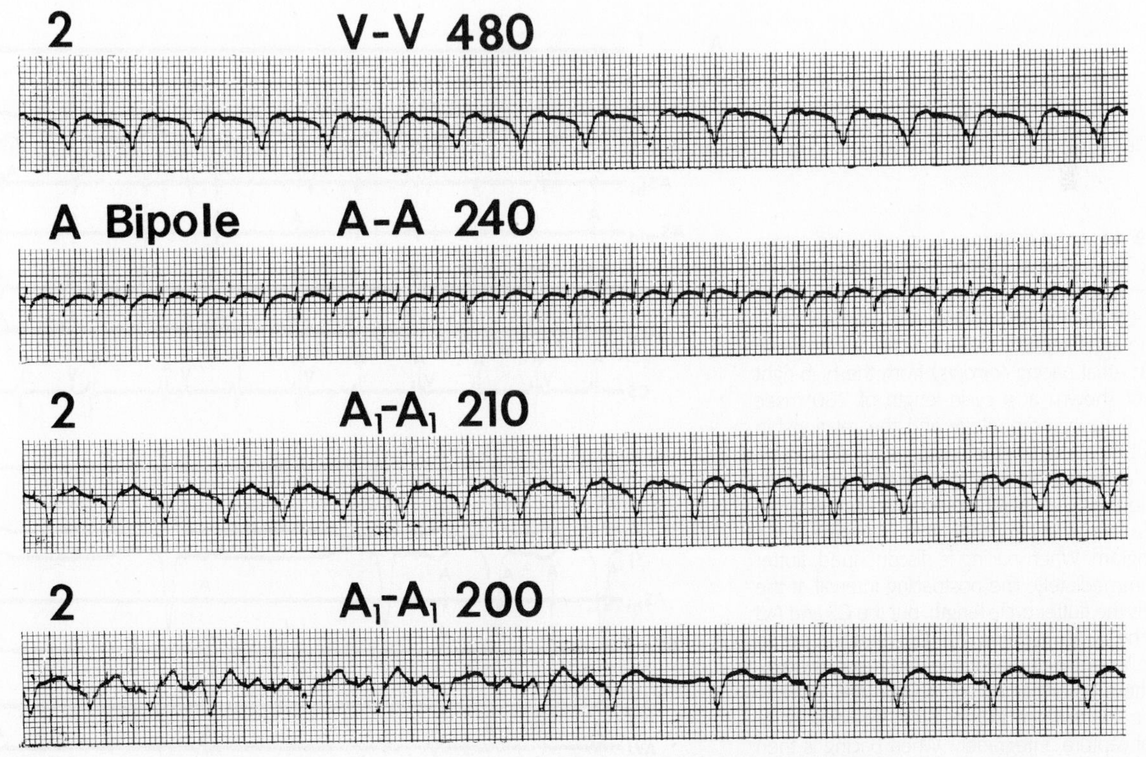


**FIGURE 9-42** *Entrainment and termination of atrial flutter.* Surface ECG 2 is shown during atrial flutter and during pacing at cycle lengths of 210 and 200 msec. A bipolar atrial A electrogram is also shown with a flutter cycle length (A-A) of 240 msec. The ventricular response (V-V) is 480 msec, as shown on the **top**. Atrial pacing ($A_1$-$A_1$) of 210 msec produces fusion of the flutter P wave, which is fixed as flutter is entrained. In the **bottom panel**, when the paced cycle length ($A_1$-$A_1$) is reduced to 200 msec, there is an abrupt change in the flutter morphology to an upright P wave. When pacing is discontinued, the flutter is terminated directly to sinus rhythm. See text for discussion.

activation of the septum and lateral wall in a craniocaudal direction. In some instances, particularly if flutter has a large fully excitable gap, a large mass of right atrial tissue can be captured by the stimulated impulse, producing a marked change in P-wave morphology, such that the P waves appear similar to the sinus P waves, without terminating flutter. Only when block in the isthmus occurs, and the sequence of activation between the os of the CS and the A-V junction at the His bundle recording site is changed, will flutter be terminated. This is shown in Figure 9-43 in which termination only occurs in the orthodromic directions when the os of the CS and A-V junction are captured antegradely. During counterclockwise flutter the A-V junction is activated after the CS by almost an entire revolution of the flutter cycle length. This can be seen in panel B in Figure 9-43 in which, following the last pacing stimulus (last arrow), the atrial electrogram in the CS occurs at the paced cycle length following a long delay approximately equal to the time between the A-V junction electrogram and the subsequent CS electrogram during flutter or during entrainment (A and B). Following block in the isthmus stimulation captures the A-V junction antegradely following septal activation.

Since atrial flutter can be terminated by pacing at multiple sites in the atrium, the ability to see a change in P-wave morphology will depend on the site of stimulation and on the P-wave morphology during native flutter. The ability to terminate flutter by rapid pacing is of great therapeutic importance. Rapid pacing is probably the treatment of choice for recurrent episodes of flutter observed (a) postoperatively, (b) in the setting of acute myocardial infarction, and (c) in the presence of

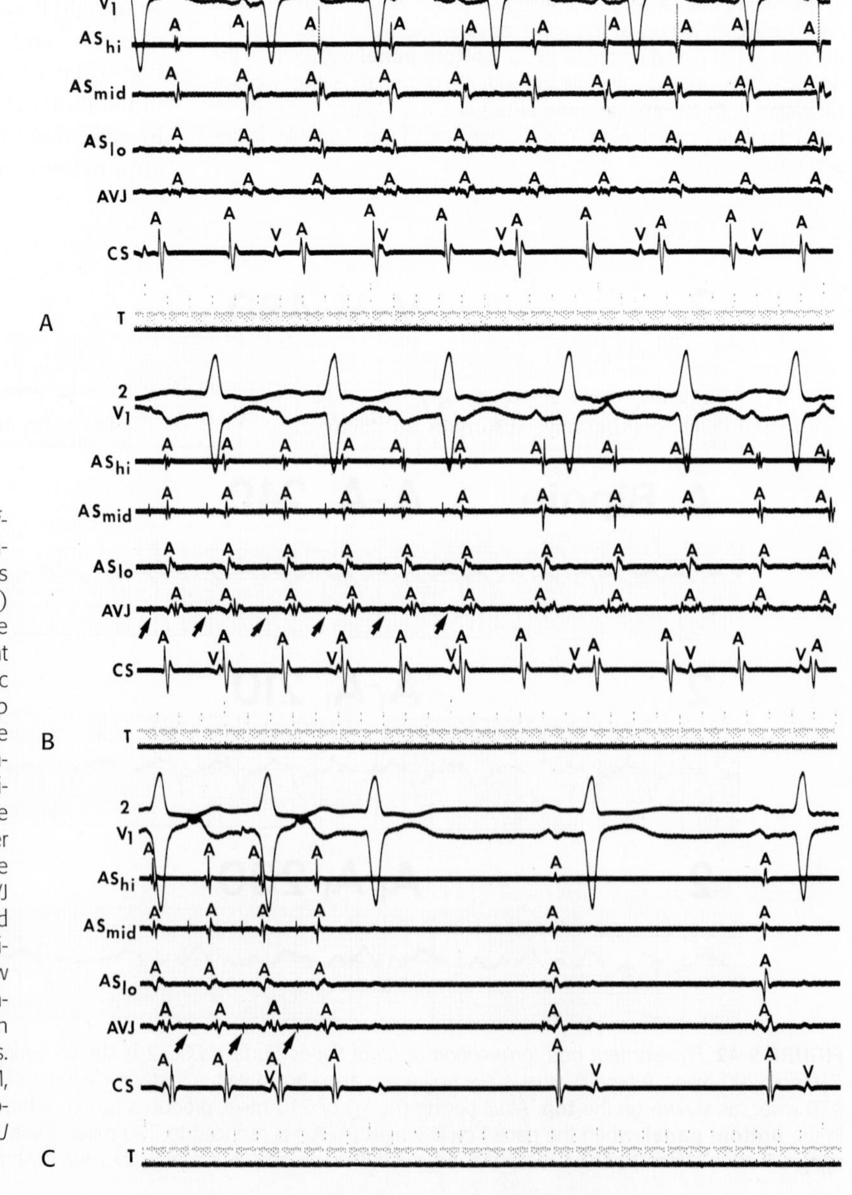


**FIGURE 9-43** *Atrial flutter: entrainment and termination.* **A:** Typical flutter (slowed by the prior administration of quinidine) is shown. Activation proceeds from the CS (at the os) to the A-V junction (AVJ) and up the atrial septum (AS) in a counterclockwise fashion. **B:** Atrial pacing *(arrows)* from the high-right atrium (not shown) at a cycle length of 260 msec alters the P-wave morphology and the relationship of the right atrial electrograms with each other. Note the AS is activated high to low (antidromic activation), while the CS and AVJ are activated orthodromically with a long delay from the stimulus spike to the CS electrogram. When pacing is discontinued, flutter resumes immediately. The postpacing interval at the AS exceeds the flutter cycle length, but the CS and AVJ return at the flutter cycle length. **C:** When the paced atrial cycle length is decreased to 240 msec, the activation pattern is further altered so that the CS now follows the electrogram in the AVJ, suggesting complete atrial capture antegradely. When pacing is then discontinued, sinus rhythm immediately resumes. See text for further discussion. (From Watson RM, Josephson ME. Atrial flutter. I. Electrophysiologic substrates and modes of initiation and termination. *Am J Cardiol* 1980;45:732, with permission.)

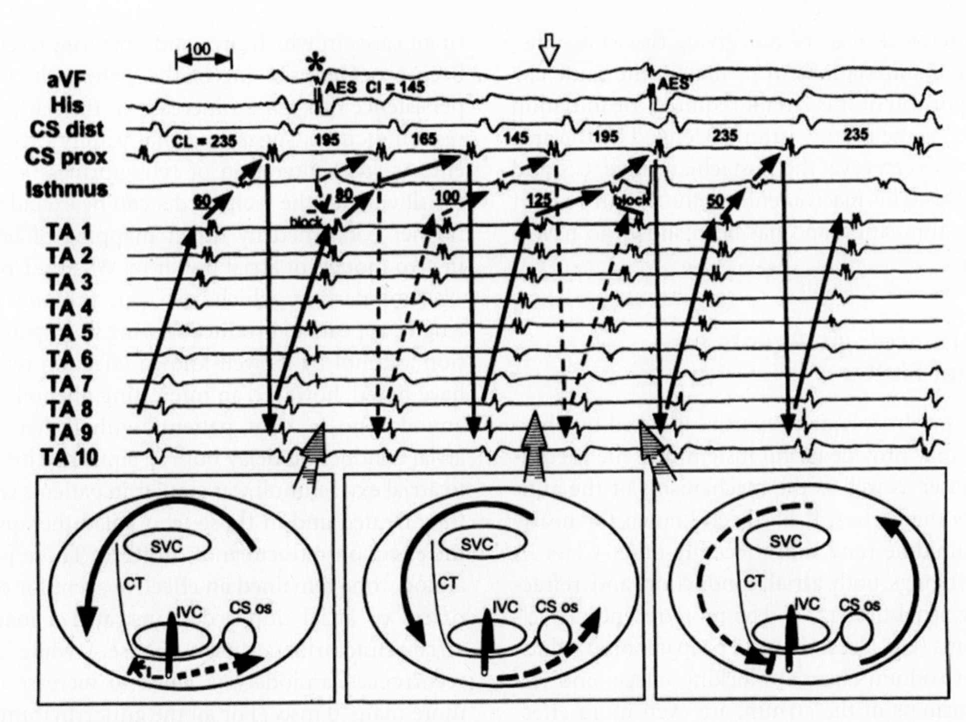


**FIGURE 9-44** *Initiation of transient double wave reentry.* Surface lead aVF and intracardiac recordings from the His bundle, distal and proximal coronary sinus ($CS_d$, $CS_p$), the isthmus, and from a halo catheter around the tricuspid annulus (TA) with T1 at the inferolateral right atrium and T10 at the high septum. Counterclockwise flutter is present at a cycle length (CL) of 235 msec. A critical atrial extrastimulus (AES) from the isthmus at a coupling interval of 145 msec produces acceleration of flutter due to initiation of double wave reentry. The *solid lines* indicate the original flutter wavefront and the *dashed line* the second wavefront. Note that the superior right atrium (TA 5–7) is activated simultaneously with the isthmus. Wenckebach block occurs in the isthmus resulting in restoration of a single wave counterclockwise flutter. SVC, superior vena cava; IVC, inferior vena cava; CT, crista terminalis. (From Cheng J, Scheinman MM. Characteristics of double wave reentry induced by programmed stimulation in patients with typical atrial flutter. *Circulation* 1998;97:1589–1596, with permission.)

digitalis intoxication manifesting A-V block and/or enhanced junctional or fascicular rhythms. With the development of implantable devices that have automatic antitachycardia atrial pacing, the ability to terminate atrial flutter provides the opportunity to use such a device in lieu of long-term antiarrhythmic therapy, which is expensive, variably effective, and associated with side effects.[77–80]

As stated above, the reasons for failure to terminate "atrial flutter" by rapid atrial pacing are (a) nonpenetration of the flutter focus; (b) apparent flutter on the surface ECG was actually flutter/fibrillation (impure flutter), a state in which parts of the atria have regular activity and others have chaotic fibrillatory activity; and (c) the mechanism of flutter was abnormal automaticity, which cannot be terminated by pacing. In our experience, the most common cause of failure to terminate apparent flutter is that the underlying rhythm was not pure reentrant flutter but flutter/fibrillation. This rhythm should actually be considered fibrillation during which parts of the atrium exhibit regular activity (see discussion below on atrial fibrillation). We have never been able to convert this rhythm by pacing.

Occasionally, stimulation during atrial flutter will produce two different types of transient accelerated rhythms. One of these is the so-called double wave reentry in which atrial flutter with an extremely large excitable gap can have a second wave introduced into the flutter circuit.[81] This rarely lasts more than a few beats but can be recognized by having simultaneous activation of the superior and inferior regions of the tricuspid annulus with all the activation being sequential (Fig. 9-44).[81] Another transient arrhythmia discussed earlier in this chapter occurs due to a breakdown of the inferior-posterior boundaries produced by the Eustachian ridge and lower crista terminalis. In this instance the rhythm may then revolve around the inferior vena cava, across the Eustachian ridge, and through the crista terminalis conducting slowly because of transverse activation through that structure. Alternatively, this rhythm may actually not break through the Eustachian ridge but exit at the apex of the triangle of Koch and come behind the Eustachian ridge to break through across the crista terminalis behind the inferior vena cava and then return to the isthmus. This accelerated rhythm is usually transient and stops by itself or can either terminate atrial flutter or initiate atrial fibrillation.[68] Both of these latter transient rhythms are uncommon and appear much less frequently than pacing-initiated atrial fibrillation.

In summary, stimulation during flutter, in combination with activation mapping of flutter, has demonstrated that typical isthmus-dependent flutter is produced by a macroreentrant circuit that goes around the tricuspid annulus, which forms the anterior border, with the posterior boundaries defined by the Eustachian ridge, the crista terminalis, and the fossa ovalis. This reentrant circuit can be activated in a clockwise or counterclockwise fashion, giving rise to two distinct morphologic manifestations of reentry in the same circuit. The critical portion of this circuit required for initiation and/or termination is the narrow isthmus defined by the area between the inferior vena cava, the Eustachian ridge, CS, and the tricuspid annulus. This macroreentrant flutter can be reset and entrained by stimulation and has been shown to have a large excitable gap.

## Effects of Pharmacologic Agents on Reentrant Atrial Flutter

Alterations in electrophysiologic properties induced by pharmacologic agents may provide useful insight into the mechanisms of atrial flutter as well as the mechanisms of the antiarrhythmic agents themselves. It has been known for nearly a century that quinidine (and more recently other Class IA agents), which prolongs both atrial conduction and refractoriness, can slow atrial flutter.[82–86] The more recently developed Class IC agents (e.g., flecainide and propafenone), which have more potent sodium channel-blocking effects and less effects on refractoriness in the atrium, are even more effective at slowing atrial flutter.[86] Of these IC agents, flecainide was the first to be approved for use in atrial arrhythmias in the United States, but propafenone is now also approved and widely used. Slowing of atrial flutter by the sodium channel-blocking agents is accompanied by a marked increase in the flutter-wave duration due to intra-atrial conduction delay. As noted earlier in this chapter, sodium channel-blocking drugs can decrease the paced cycle length required to produce block transversely across the crista terminalis, thereby facilitating induction of atrial flutter.[20] An example of atrial flutter slowed by quinidine is shown in Figure 9-45. One of the dangers of these agents is the possibility of 1:1 atrioventricular conduction and, therefore, when administered, A-V nodal-blocking agents should be given. The prolongation of the flutter cycle length by these agents does not correlate at all with any effect on refractoriness. The proof that these drugs act by slowing conduction comes from noting their effect on resetting curves. In all cases in which pre- and postdrug resetting curves have been observed, slowing of the tachycardia is associated with persistence or even an increase of the flat component of the resetting curve, suggesting that a fully excitable gap is present. As such, alteration of refractoriness as the determinant for slowing of the tachycardia can be excluded. This has been further confirmed by direct mapping of both in vitro and in vivo models of atrial flutter by Wu and Hoffman.[87]

Amiodarone, which also can prolong the flutter cycle length, appears to produce slowing by impairment of conduction and not by its well-known effect on refractoriness.[88] We have noted, however, an interesting phenomenon when using amiodarone to treat patients with flutter. Although intra-atrial conduction delay both in sinus rhythm and in response to atrial extrastimuli was similar in patients who were successfully treated and in those who failed therapy with this drug, the effect on refractoriness differed. Those patients in whom amiodarone remained an effective agent for preventing recurrences of atrial flutter demonstrated a marked increase in atrial refractoriness (mean 40 msec), while in those who had recurrences, amiodarone failed to increase refractoriness by more than 10 msec. For all the antiarrhythmic agents we have studied, prolongation of refractoriness was a property necessary to prevent induction of atrial flutter, while impairment of conduction was the most important factor in determining the flutter cycle length. In addition, termination of flutter by antiarrhythmic agents usually results in block in the isthmus. Since termination is most frequently achieved by drugs that slow conduction and maintain a persistent fully excitable gap, the effect on termination must be due to altered excitability and/or coupling.

The relative roles of conduction and refractoriness on initiation and or maintenance of the arrhythmia may be related to the concept that a critical wavelength is necessary for initiation of the tachycardia.[40] In any model of reentry, the wavelength of the circulating impulse, which is defined by the product of conduction velocity and refractoriness, is critical for initiation and perhaps maintenance of reentrant excitation. In a canine model of atrial arrhythmias, induction of atrial flutter required

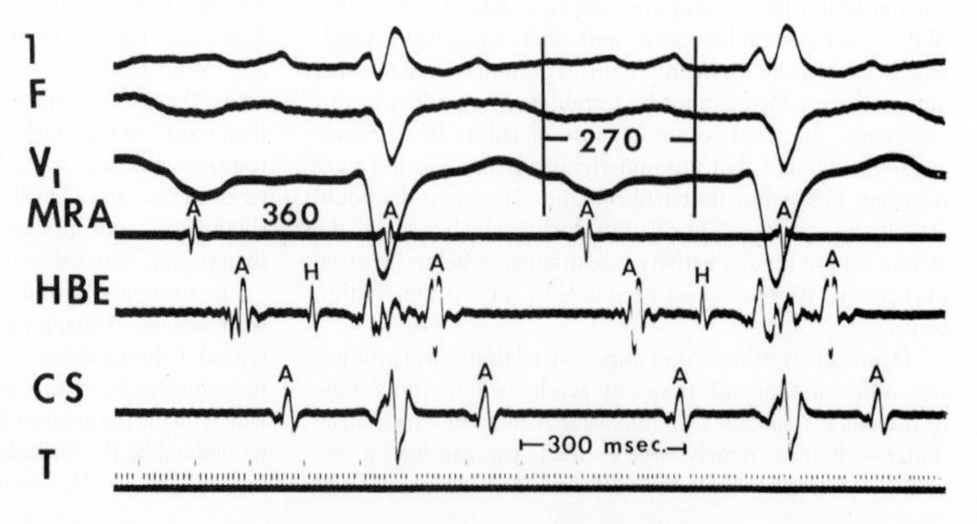


**FIGURE 9-45** *Atrial flutter: effect of quinidine.* Quinidine has slowed the flutter cycle length from 220 to 360 msec. That occurred coincident with a change in the flutter-wave duration from 150 to 270 msec (*vertical solid lines*). The atrial effective refractory period determined at a cycle length of 400 msec was 325 after the administration of quinidine (plasma level was 4.6 g/mL). See text for further discussion.

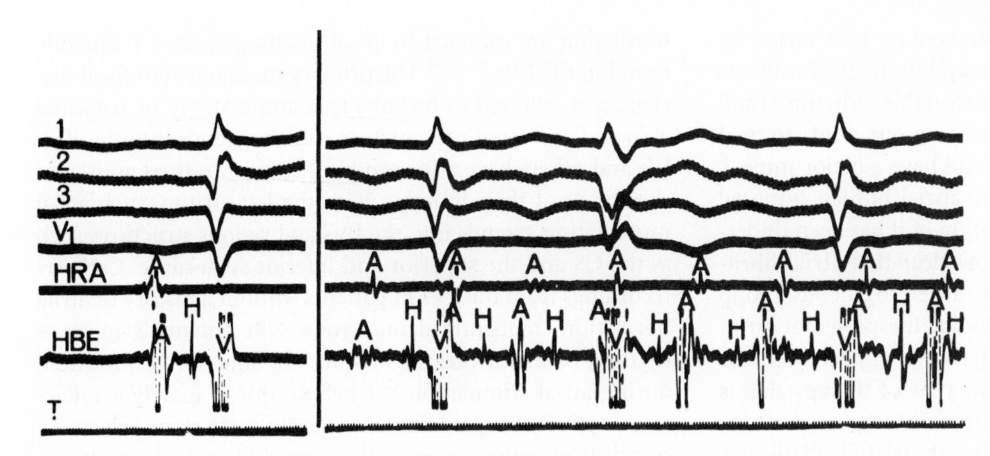


**FIGURE 9-46** *Infra-His block during atrial flutter.* Despite a normal H-V interval (45 msec) during sinus rhythm (the complex on the left), infra-His block is present during atrial flutter. This does not indicate impaired His–Purkinje function. See text.

a wavelength of 8 to 12 cm.[41] An increase in the wavelength would necessarily require a larger area of block around which the impulse must circulate to initiate reentry. Antiarrhythmic agents that alter the wavelength can prevent initiation. Thus, drugs that primarily prolong refractoriness without significantly affecting conduction (e.g., sotalol), and therefore increase wavelength, may be theoretically useful in preventing atrial flutter. Antiarrhythmic agents rarely increase conduction velocity so that prolongation of refractoriness may be the mechanism by which wavelength is increased by these agents. As in the case of amiodarone, if refractoriness was not increased (particularly if conduction is slowed), recurrences of flutter are seen with the cycle length prolonged by the effect of the drug on conduction velocity. Although the concept of a critical wavelength seems attractive as far as initiation is concerned, because of the need for a greater zone of unidirectional block, the application of this concept to termination of a sustained episode is not tenable. Drugs that have a pure effect on refractoriness based on blocking potassium channels (Class III agents) are relatively ineffective at terminating atrial flutter, even though they would be expected to prolong the wavelength. This is not surprising since, as discussed above, atrial flutter is associated with a fairly large excitable gap that would not be expected to be closed by the amount of prolongation of the wavelength. In addition, agents that shorten atrial refractoriness such as vagal stimulation or adenosine[86,88–91] have no effect on the cycle length of isthmus-dependent atrial flutter, although they can change it to atrial fibrillation. Ibutilide, a Class III agent which has a more complex mechanism of prolonging refractoriness (increasing inward sodium current) is very effective in terminating atrial flutter. Perhaps this works by decreasing excitability in the isthmus. In my experience, carotid sinus pressure, another vagal maneuver, has no effect on the flutter cycle length. Thus, the response to antiarrhythmic agents is consistent with the concept that the reentrant pathway in isthmus-dependent flutter is primarily anatomically determined, although the initiation of that rhythm can be altered by changes in conduction and/or refractoriness in critical parts of the circuit. Adenosine has no effect on macroreentrant atrial tachycardias based on anatomic structures, but may accelerate functional circuits by shortening atrial refractoriness.

## Atrioventricular Conduction During Flutter

Most commonly, 2:1 A-V conduction is present during atrial flutter. Variable A-V conduction (particularly alternate beat Wenckebach) and/or longer multiples (e.g., 4:1 or 6:1) are not uncommon, particularly in patients treated with digitalis, beta-blockers and/or calcium channel blockers. In the vast majority of such patients the nonconducted flutter-wave blocks in the A-V node. Occasionally multilevel block is present either spontaneously or after antiarrhythmic drugs, and block below the His can be observed (Fig. 9-46). This is more likely to occur in the presence of type 1 agents, which prolong His–Purkinje refractoriness, or during Wenckebach cycles in the A-V node, which lead to long-short activation of the His–Purkinje system. This phenomenon is not uncommon during alternate beat Wenckebach cycles in which the proximal site of block may be in the A-V node. In such instances, intra- or infra-His block does not have the same implications as the development of such block during sinus rhythm. Intra- or infra-His block during atrial flutter is usually physiologic because refractoriness in the His–Purkinje system exceeds the flutter cycle length. Intra- or infra-His block is less commonly seen during atrial flutter than atrial tachycardia because the short cycle length of atrial flutter produces consistent block in the A-V node such that impulses never reach the His–Purkinje system while it is refractory. Intra- or infra-His block during flutter would be more likely to occur if enhanced A-V nodal conduction were present, allowing each flutter impulse to encroach on the refractory period of the His–Purkinje system. Occasionally, with the presence of Class I agents that slow atrial flutter to rates of 300 msec or more, block in the His–Purkinje system (the refractoriness of which is also increased by these agents) can be seen.

# ATRIAL FIBRILLATION

Atrial fibrillation is the most frequent arrhythmia for which patients are hospitalized. It is associated with an increase in overall mortality, sudden cardiac death, congestive heart failure, an increase in stroke risk (up to 30% of strokes over age 70), and impaired quality of life because of a variety of symptoms associated with it. Currently, hundreds of millions of dollars are being spent annually to treat this arrhythmia and its complications. Thus, even small steps in our ability to treat this disorder and its complications will have a major impact. Because of the great medical and financial burden imposed by this arrhythmia, intense investigation of it has been undertaken over the past decade. It is now clear that atrial fibrillation is not just one disorder but a heterogeneous group of disorders. From a clinical standpoint the presentation of atrial fibrillation—paroxysmal self-terminating, persistent, or chronic—dictates to some degree the type of therapy that is employed. Theoretically, it would be more important to be able to target the specific mechanism of atrial fibrillation. A better understanding of the mechanism of atrial fibrillation in any individual could direct specific therapy for that specific mechanism. There are several potential mechanisms for initiating and maintaining atrial fibrillation. Sources of impulse initiation and factors enhancing them are accepted triggers of AF, the mechanism of maintenance of AF remains highly controversial; single source versus multiple sources. Some of the proposed mechanisms are shown in Figure 9-47.

One of the most important discoveries in the last decade has been the observation that many cases of paroxysmal atrial fibrillation are initiated by focal discharges, most frequently found in the PVs.[50–52,92] The primary mechanism of focal discharges is believed to be enhanced automaticity or triggered activity from atrial musculature, which extends into the PVs. We and others have also seen local reentry in these muscular sheaths or at their junction with the left atrium, such atrial musculature extends into the PVs and venous structures such as the CS and the superior and inferior vena cavae. Catheter recordings from the PVs in patients without a history of atrial fibrillation frequently demonstrate split potentials in sinus rhythm, or if not present in sinus rhythm can be produced during atrial stimulation.[92] I believe this is merely a reflection of poorly coupled fiber and the ability to record electrical signals from one or more of these atrial fibers and simultaneously record from the atrial musculature of the left atrium. However, a study of the PVs of subjects with atrial fibrillation has shown that these structures possess altered electrophysiologic properties compared with controls.[27] The refractory periods of the PVs (as assessed with single extrastimuli) were are shorter in the PVs than in the left atrium in patients with AF, while the refractory periods were longer in the PVs than in the atrium in control subjects. The action potential duration of the PVs is extremely short, and recent work has suggested that an increased calcium transient combined with rapidly

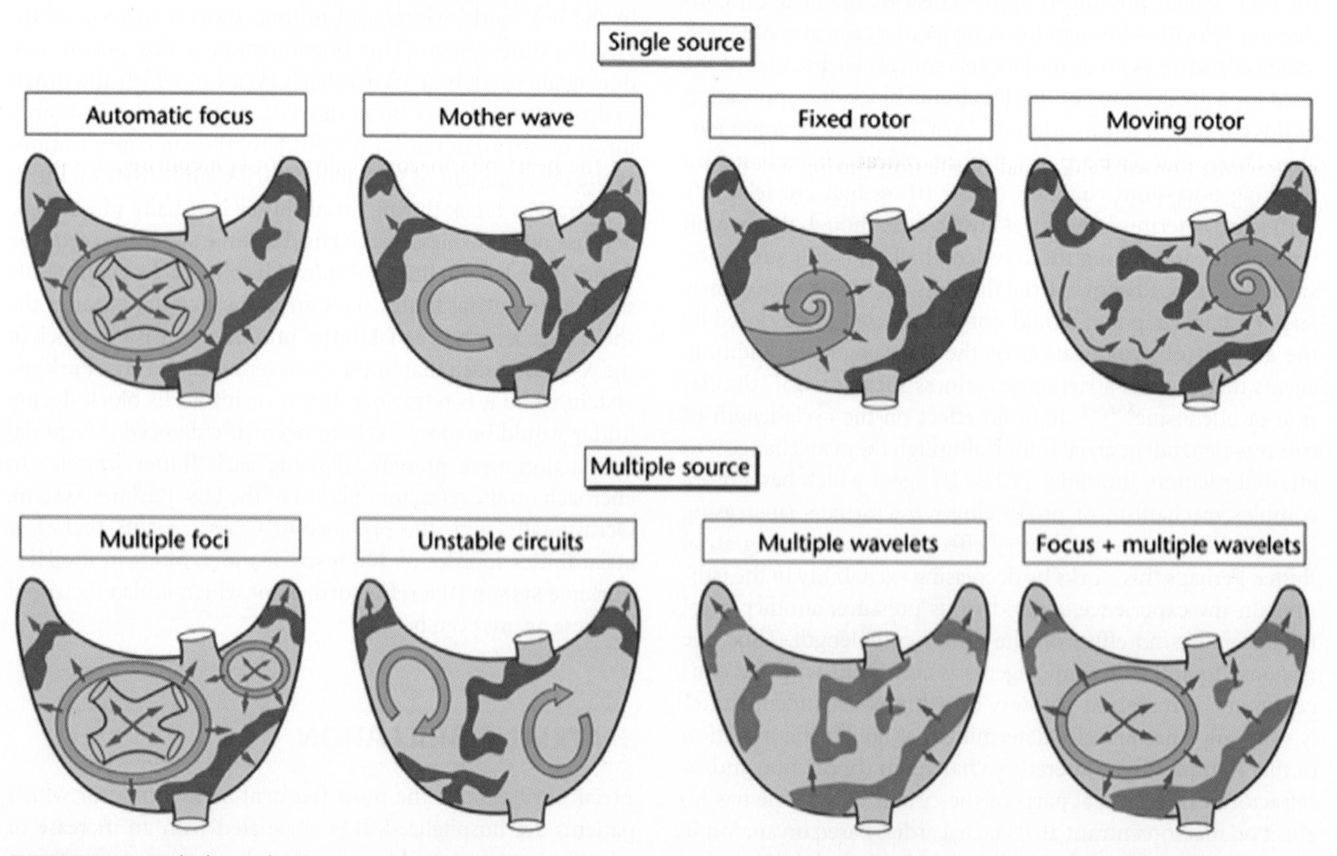


**FIGURE 9-47** *Multiple mechanisms of atrial fibrillation.* Potential mechanisms of fibrillation arising from a single source or multiple sources are diagrammatically depicted. (Courtesy of M. Shenasa.)

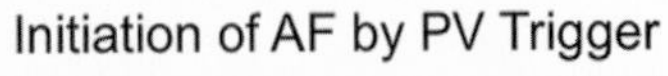


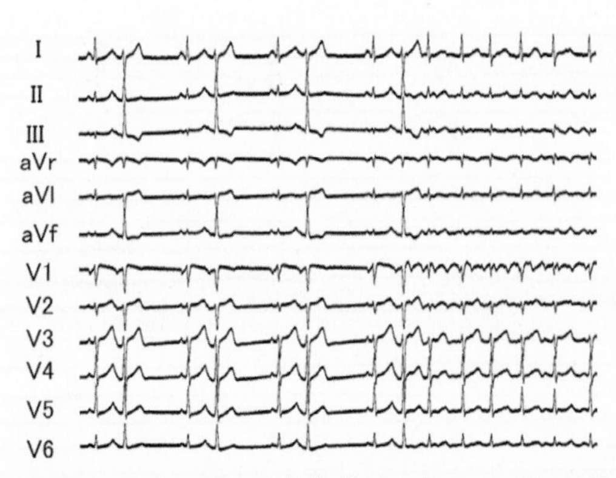


**FIGURE 9-48** *Initiation of atrial fibrillation by repetitive APDs from the right superior pulmonary vein.* Atrial bigeminy from the right superior pulmonary vein (P in II peaked and taller than III) eventually initiate atrial fibrillation.

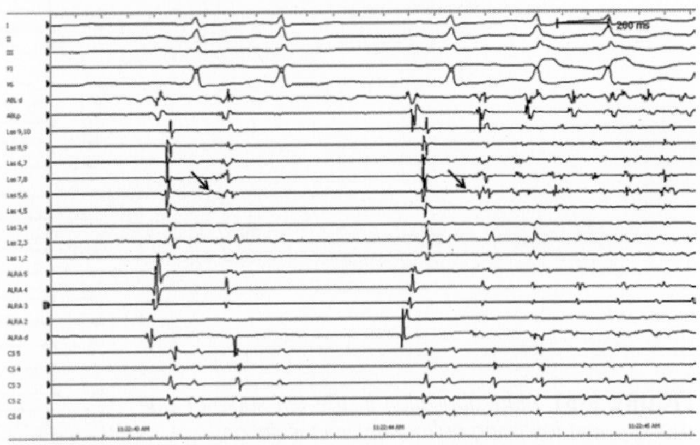


**FIGURE 9-49** *Spontaneous initiation of atrial fibrillation by ectopic beats originating in the pulmonary vein.* This patient has atrial fibrillation (AF) initiated from atrial ectopic beats originating in the left superior pulmonary vein. Note that the ectopic beats initating AF (*arrows*) arise from the area recorded by Lasso pole 5–6.

repolarized tissue may lead to early afterdepolarizations and triggered activity in the PVs.[93]

Not all people, however, develop spontaneous atrial arrhythmias from these sites. Even when they do, this is usually only a trigger for atrial fibrillation, although repeated discharges can be responsible for maintenance of the arrhythmia. A substrate has to be present that facilitates the development of atrial fibrillation in response to these triggers. These atrial foci demonstrate split potentials in sinus rhythm, and during the ectopic impulse formation, the second component, which arises distal in the PV, becomes the first component. Repetitive atrial foci can lead to an atrial tachycardia with subsequent degeneration to atrial fibrillation. An example of such a focus is shown in Figures 9-48 and 9-49. Atrial foci may also lead to rhythms mimicking atrial flutter. Atrial fibrillation or rapid atrial firing can also be seen during sinus rhythm within a PV (posttermination of ECG atrial fibrillation during ablation). This is the ultimate proof of concept that the PVs can be the actual source of triggering and maintaining atrial fibrillation (Figs. 9-50 and 9-51).

How one identifies patients with so-called "focal" atrial fibrillation is uncertain. One must certainly have a suspicion of a potential focal trigger of atrial fibrillation if one sees repetitive APCs or atrial tachycardia having the same P-wave morphology repeatedly initiating atrial fibrillation. The problem with identifying such atrial activity is that it is unpredictable and is therefore rarely recorded. The patient usually already is in atrial fibrillation when he or she presents. If demonstration of frequent ectopy or atrial tachycardia is necessary to recognize atrial fibrillation with a focal trigger, then perhaps only 2% to 3% of patients with paroxysmal atrial fibrillation fulfill criteria for this mechanism. In earlier investigations of focal triggers, Haissaguerre et al. were aggressive in[19] such patients. Using multiple catheters placed in the PVs, if ectopic activity was not present at baseline, they would stimulate the heart pharmacologically with epinephrine, atropine, isoproterenol, and/or adenosine (Haissaguerre, personal communication). If atrial fibrillation is present, cardioversion was performed and subsequent to cardioversion ectopic impulses from the PV could be detected. Whether this was a sensitive method of detecting such foci or an artifact of cardioversion

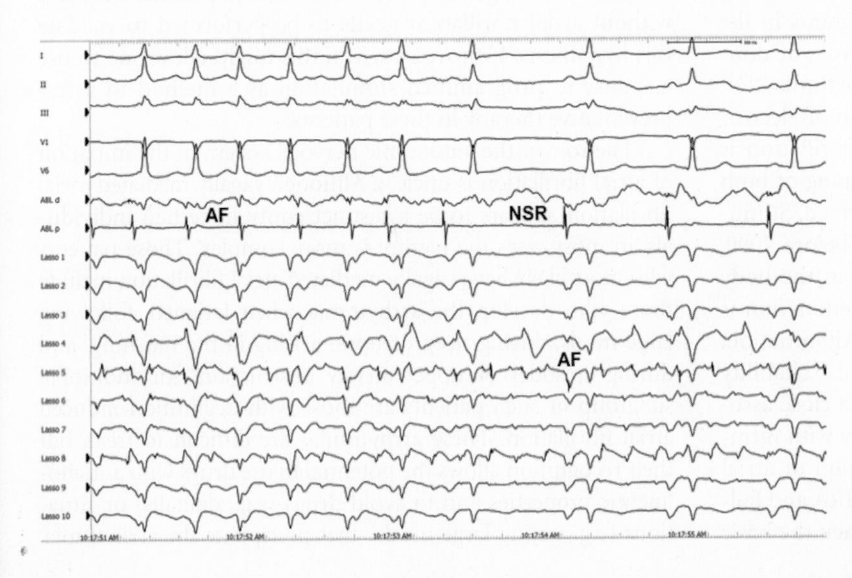


**FIGURE 9-50** *Atrial fibrillation recorded in the right superior pulmonary vein following pulmonary vein isolation.*

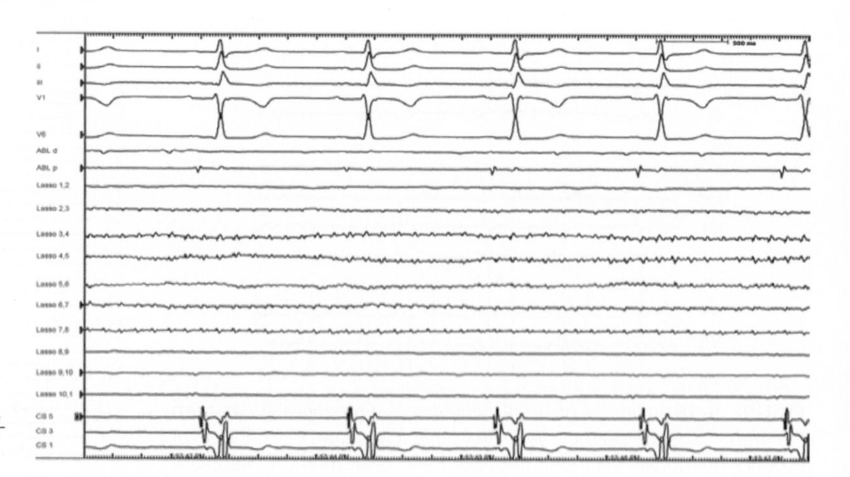

**FIGURE 9-51** *Atrial fibrillation in the left superior pulmonary vein following pulmonary vein isolation.*

with catheters irritating foci because of their prior placement in the PVs requires prospective study. Nevertheless, the concept of a trigger for atrial fibrillation, which could be treated specifically, has been demonstrated. Other arrhythmias such as circus movement tachycardia using a bypass tract or even A-V nodal tachycardia can also initiate fibrillation, and their successful treatment often results in freedom from atrial fibrillation. However, there needs to be a substrate upon which this trigger can act for fibrillation to ensue.

Since the initial observation by Haft et al.[34] in 1968 that atrial fibrillation could be induced by closely coupled atrial extrastimuli, programmed stimulation has been used to assess the propensity for atrial fibrillation. While repetitive responses and nonsustained atrial fibrillation are frequent, the induction of sustained atrial fibrillation with a single extrastimulus usually occurs in patients with a prior history of documented atrial fibrillation, atrial flutter, or palpitations consistent with these arrhythmias. As with atrial flutter, there is a high incidence of intra-atrial conduction defects during sinus rhythm, prolonged intra-atrial conduction in response to atrial extrastimuli, and a failure of adaptation of refractory periods to varying drive cycle lengths.[9,12,15,53] The greater the ease of induction from the HRA than from the CS and the association of induction with fractionation of atrial electrograms in the posterior triangle of Koch suggest a prominent role of nonuniform anisotropy in the initiation of this arrhythmia.[8,10,11] Whether or not other sites manifest fractionation of electrograms coincident with the initiation of atrial fibrillation is unknown since complete biatrial activation mapping of both atria at the time of initiation has not been performed. Stimulation from the PVs, which was not performed before 2000, can more easily initiate AF than stimulation from the body of the LA.[27] Studies by Saghy et al.[19] suggest fractionation is functional and not specific for a critical site of AF initiation. Simpson et al.[13] also showed abnormalities of atrial excitability in patients prone to atrial fibrillation and noted a close association of these abnormalities of atrial excitability with intra-atrial conduction defects. An example of induction of atrial fibrillation with a single extrastimulus from the HRA and failure to induce it at identical coupling intervals when the basic drive is carried out from the CS is shown in Figure 9-52. The difference in the ability to initiate AF from the CS versus the RA or PV may relate to the fact that the ERP of the CS is longer than the atrium so block and slow conduction are less likely to occur.

While abnormalities of conduction and refractoriness are common in patients with either atrial flutter or fibrillation, Allessie et al.[40] believe that the wavelength of the stimulated impulse determines the arrhythmia that is induced.[92] Atrial fibrillation requires a much shorter wavelength (<8 cm) than atrial flutter (8 to 12 cm). The shorter refractory period observed in the HRA as compared to the CS[8,10,11,72] associated with similar intra-atrial conduction compared to the CS facilitates induction of atrial fibrillation from the right atrium compared to the CS. This is a relatively consistent observation during electrophysiology studies in patients with atrial fibrillation. When right atrial stimulation is associated with greater conduction delay than during stimulation from the CS, the relative ease of initiating atrial fibrillation from the right atrium is more understandable. While I believe that the reproducible initiation of sustained atrial fibrillation by single right atrial extrastimuli, particularly at coupling intervals >200 msec, is clinically meaningful, a prospective study in patients with and without atrial fibrillation needs to be performed to validate this hypothesis. If proven correct, this might allow one to use response to programmed stimulation as a method to assess preventative therapy in these patients.

The role of the autonomic nervous system in the initiation of atrial fibrillation is unclear. Although vagally mediated atrial fibrillation appears to be a distinct entity in certain individuals, in most cases the picture is more complex. Those patients who most likely have vagally mediated atrial fibrillation include those who develop the arrhythmia when fatigued, following large meals, during sleep or upon arising in the morning, and during episodes of upper airway obstruction. An additional subgroup of such patients are those with deglutition-induced atrial fibrillation. These arrhythmias are difficult to treat, but their recognition allows the potential to use drugs with anticholinergic properties and to avoid drugs (e.g., digitalis) or situations (e.g., eating large meals) that precipitate the arrhythmia.

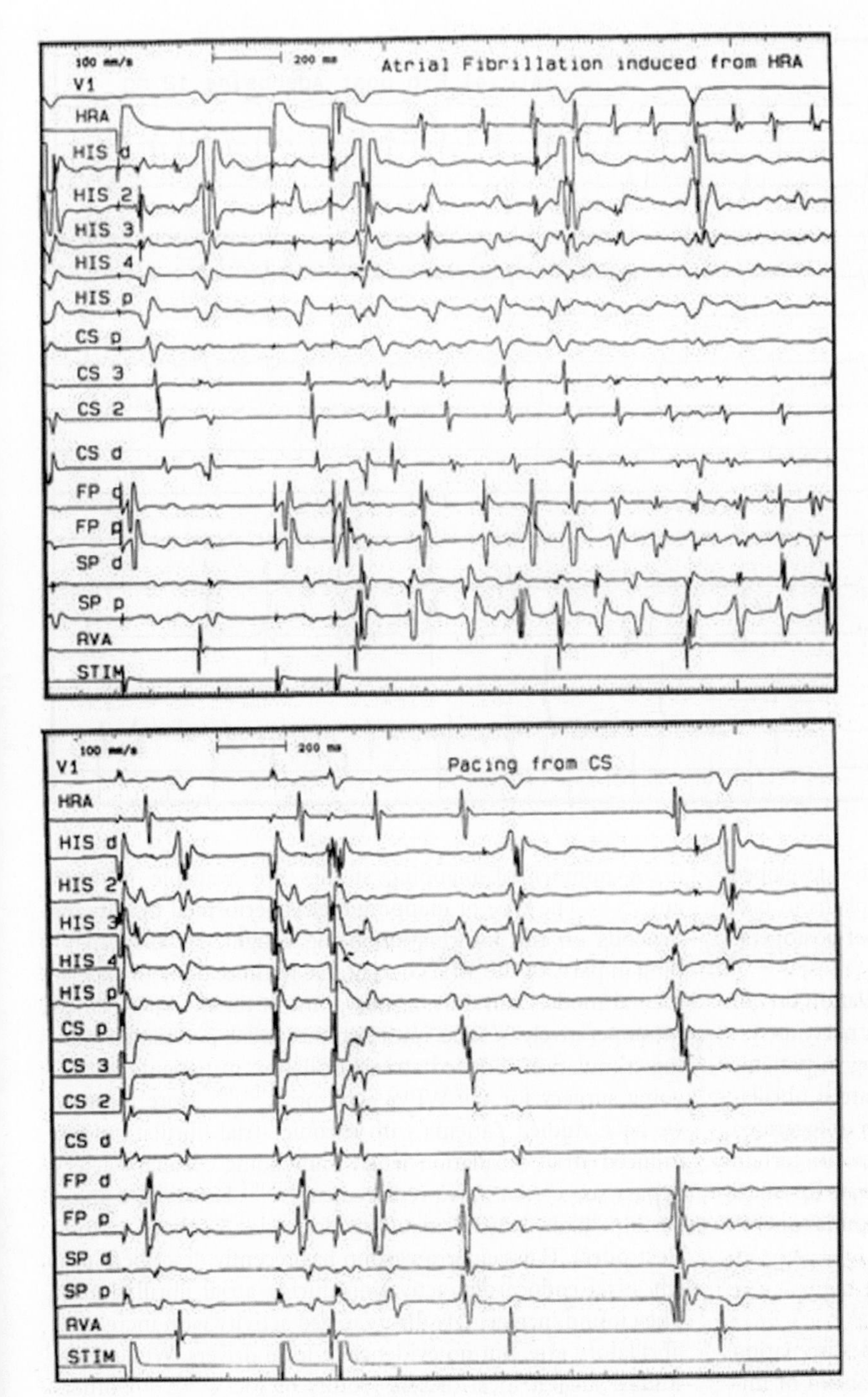


**FIGURE 9-52** *Prevention of induction of atrial fibrillation by high-right atrial stimuli by pacing the coronary sinus.* (From Papageorgiou P, Anselme F, Kirchhof CJ, et al. Coronary sinus pacing prevents induction of atrial fibrillation. *Circulation* 1997;96:1893–1898.)

We have used adenosine as a stress test for patients we believe have vagally mediated atrial fibrillation. While adenosine (12 mg IV) induces atrial fibrillation in a high percentage of such patients (Fig. 9-53), it can occasionally induce atrial fibrillation in patients who have never had the arrhythmia. This usually occurs in young people in whom enhanced sympathetic tone allows adenosine to demonstrate accentuated antagonism. It is of interest that there appears to be an increase in heart rate variability prior to the onset of idiopathic (lone) atrial fibrillation in 50% of patients and a decrease in heart rate variability in two-thirds of patients with organic heart disease prior to atrial fibrillation. In young, healthy athletes, the combination of enhanced sympathetic activity followed by reflex vagal activity is often responsible for atrial fibrillation, particularly at the end of or just following peak activity.[94] Thus, the influence of the autonomic nervous system on atrial fibrillation is unpredictable. Olgin et al.[6] demonstrated that heterogeneous sympathetic denervation produced by phenol in canines is associated with ease of induction of atrial fibrillation. The sympathetic nervous system seems to play an important role in postoperative atrial fibrillation, particularly in those in whom beta-blockers were stopped at the time of surgery. We have previously documented

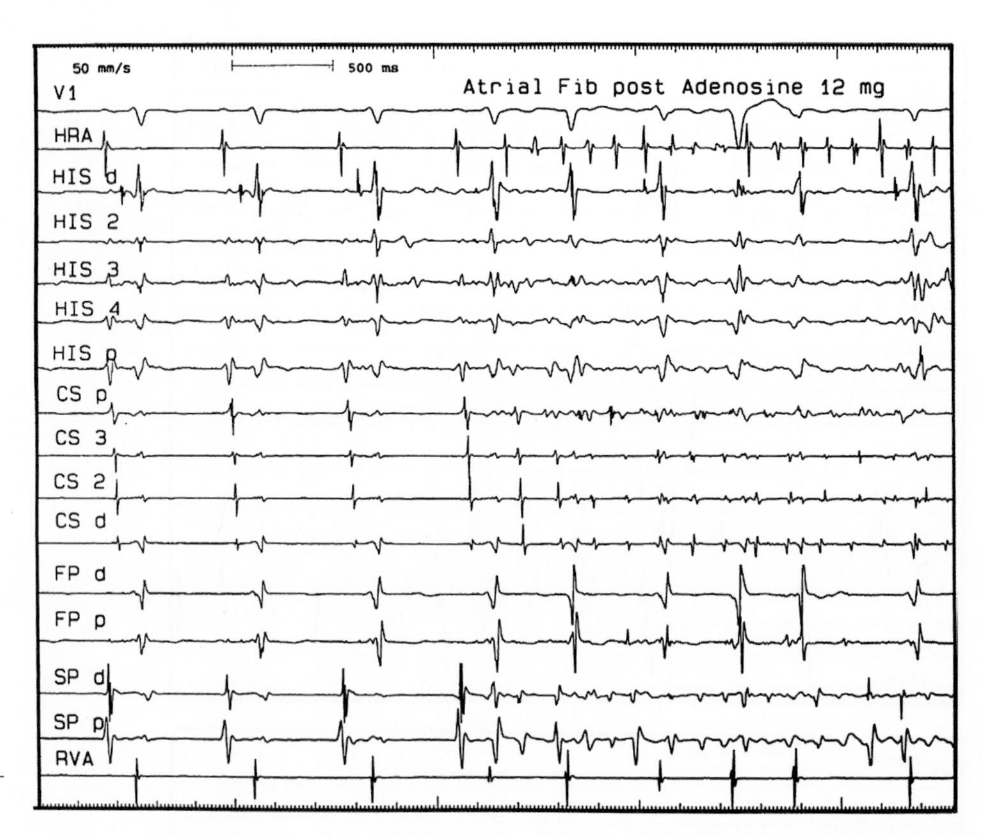


**FIGURE 9-53** *Initiation of atrial fibrillation by adenosine.*

an upregulation of beta-receptors in patients who developed postoperative atrial fibrillation.[95] This finding explains in part the efficacy of beta-blockers in the management of postoperative atrial fibrillation.

In general, however, patients with atrial fibrillation do not seem to have any abnormality of their autonomic nervous system. There is no difference in autonomic testing in patients with vagally mediated or nonvagally mediated atrial fibrillation and controls. This suggests that there is an exaggerated response to a normal autonomic nervous system in certain patients who are likely to have a persistent substrate for atrial fibrillation that is triggered by a change in autonomic tone.

## Mapping During Atrial Fibrillation

While analysis of the response to programmed stimulation may provide some information about the mechanism of initiation of atrial fibrillation, mapping during atrial fibrillation can provide insight into the mechanism of maintenance or perpetuation of the arrhythmia. Experimental mapping studies have demonstrated both random reentrant wavelets, which occasionally anchor at pectinate muscle bundles, and very rapid single and small reentrant circuits (rotors), which initiate the multiple wavelets by activating the atria at rates in excess of local refractory periods or conduction capabilities.[49,92,96–101] There seems in many cases to be a dominant frequency gradient between the left and right atrium, particularly in paroxysmal AF. Other studies also show that persistent atrial fibrillation is more complex and should be considered random reentry in a three-dimensional arrhythmia.[97,102,103]

A number of mapping studies are available in hum ans.[102–115] The type of mapping that is performed in humans depends on the information being sought. Detailed mapping in parts of the atria comparable to those done in experimental models can only, at this point in time, be performed intraoperatively.[109] The initial studies were performed during stimulation-induced atrial fibrillation in patients undergoing surgery for the WPW syndrome.[104–106] More recently, we have studied patients with chronic atrial fibrillation and induced atrial fibrillation when undergoing coronary artery bypass surgery or valve replacement.[102,107] However, using a custom "high-density" mapping electrode (5-splines with 20 electrodes), Haissaguerre's group has recently described local left atrial endocardial activation during atrial fibrillation.[108] They found increasingly disorganized activity with increasing fibrillatory rate, but no evidence of focal drivers. While some studies suggest focal drivers (rotors or foci),[114,116–119] others have shown no rotors but a markedly complex situation with three-dimensional activation.[102–104,111–113] In addition the left to right atrial dominant frequency gradient seen in paroxysmal AF is not seen in persistent AF, suggesting different mechanism for persistence of AF in the two forms.[89,119,120]

Catheter studies have been useful for a few reasons. First, using monophasic action potentials to map atrial fibrillation, one can observe a great variation in the amplitude and duration of the signals. More importantly, a separation of "action potentials" with clear diastolic intervals has been observed in all of our patients (Fig. 9-54).[121] This suggests the presence of fully excitable gaps during atrial fibrillation. Secondly, the organization of atrial activity during atrial fibrillation is

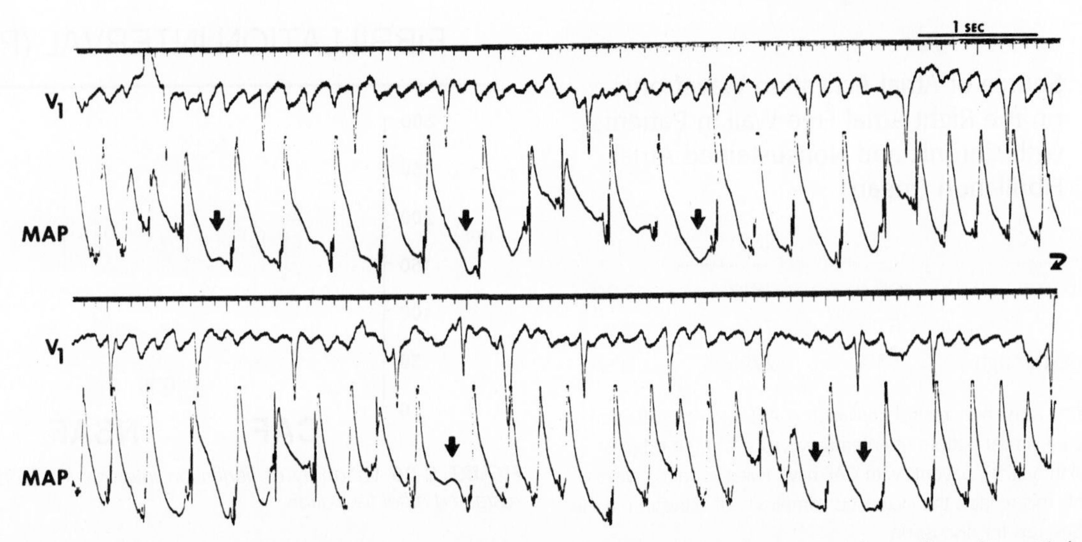


**FIGURE 9-54** *Demonstration of a fully excitable gap in atrial fibrillation using monophasic action potential recordings.* (From Kirchoff C, Josephson ME. Role of anisotropy in human arrhythmias. In: Spooner PM, Joyner RW, Jalife J, eds. *Discontinuous conduction in the heart.* Armonk, NY: Futura Publishing, 1997:135–157, with permission.)

highly variable. While broad, smooth wavefronts can be seen in the trabeculated right atrium and trabeculated left atrium, as well as in the CS, the region of the crista terminalis, the intra-atrial septum, and the region between the PVs demonstrate fragmented and chaotic activity. The more organized the atrial activity, the larger the fibrillatory waves seen on the surface ECG.[122] These patterns of atrial activation, particularly on the trabeculated free wall of the right atrium, have counterparts observed during detailed intraoperative mapping (see below).[102,104] The temporal and spatial organization can be evaluated by analyzing the space constants of electrical activation along decapolar catheters. Using a signal processing technique to quantify the correlation between adjacent atrial activation sequences along decapolar catheters at multiple sites in the right atrium, Botteron and Cain[106] demonstrated a shortening of the space constant in chronic atrial fibrillation and larger space constants in acute atrial fibrillation. While the range of values for space constants overlap, the shorter space constants in chronic atrial fibrillation correlate with more complex atrial activation patterns observed during intraoperative mapping (see below).

Intraoperative mapping has been performed using two different mapping techniques. One method provides a broad but less detailed overview of activation of both atria. This technique used by Schuessler et al.[97] incorporates 156 bipolar electrodes over both atria with the highest density in the region of the terminal crest of the right atrium. The left atrium is less well covered by the mapping electrodes. Schuessler et al.[97] studied 13 patients with stimulation-induced atrial fibrillation who were undergoing WPW surgery using this technique. They demonstrated reentrant circuits with large wavefronts in the right atrium with revolution times of approximately 200 msec. Reentrant excitation was rarely seen in the left atrium, possibly due to incomplete mapping of that chamber. Left atrial mapping appeared to show fibrillatory conduction from reentrant wavefronts in the right atrium.

The second method employs a plaque of 128 to 256 electrodes. Allessie's group and our laboratory used a spoon-shaped mapping electrode with 240 unipolar electrodes (2.2-mm interelectrode distance) placed manually on the free wall of the right atrium. This technique provides more detailed information, but it is limited to one atrial free wall. Konings et al.[104] used this technique to study stimulation-induced atrial fibrillation in 25 patients undergoing surgical division of atrioventricular bypass tracts. These investigators characterize three patterns of atrial activation during the atrial fibrillation based on the spatial complexity of activation wavefronts recorded by the spoon electrode. A type I pattern (10 patients) was one in which the atrium underneath the mapping plaque was activated by a single uniform wavefront without conduction delay. A type II pattern (8 patients) was characterized by either a single wavefront with markedly prolonged conduction or two separate wavefronts separated by a line of block. A type III pattern (7 patients) was characterized by three or more simultaneous wavefronts and multiple lines of block, as well as regions of markedly slow conduction. This classification, which was based on the dominant pattern underneath the plaque, is limited by the fact that there was frequently a change from one pattern to another during the short period of atrial fibrillation in which mapping was performed. These investigators also noted that the fibrillation interval (the mean FF interval) in all leads was shorter during type III ($136 \pm 16$ msec) than type II ($150 \pm 14$ msec), than type I ($174 \pm 18$ msec), respectively. In addition, the more complex the activation patterns, the greater the variability of fibrillation intervals and the slower the conduction velocity.

Using the identical mapping technique as Konings et al.[104] we performed high-density mapping in patients with organic heart disease undergoing open heart surgery in whom chronic atrial fibrillation was present (8 patients) and in pacing-induced atrial fibrillation (10 patients).[102,107] Our mapping was carried out on the right atrium. We performed a spatial

**TABLE 9-3 Source of Atrial Activation Wavefronts on the Right Atrial Free Wall in Patients with Chronic and Nonsustained Atrial Fibrillation (mean)**

| | CAF | NSAF | p |
|---|---|---|---|
| waves/sec | 29.9 | 14.6 | <0.001 |
| Edge | 67% | 73% | n.s. |
| Epicardial breakthrough | 33% | 27% | n.s. |

Although patients with chronic atrial fibrillation (CAF) and nonsustained AF (NSAF) have a similar pattern of entering waves (from the edge or epicardial breakthroughs), patients with CAF have twice as many waves at any moment. This reflects the increased complexity of activation in the CAF patients. See text for discussion.

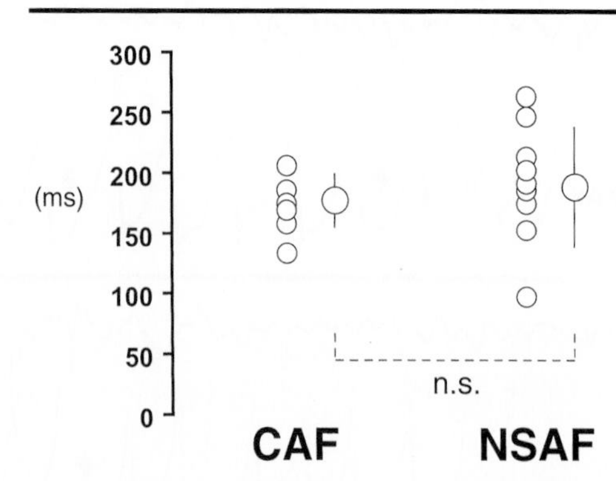


**FIGURE 9-56** *Variability of fibrillation intervals in chronic and nonsustained atrial fibrillation.*

and temporal quantification of arcs of conduction block, fibrillation waves, and evidence of random and complete reentry as well as characterization of AF complexity in a similar fashion as Konings et al.[104] In both chronic atrial fibrillation and pacing-induced atrial fibrillation (which was always nonsustained) approximately 70% of the wavefronts entered the atrium under the plaque from the edges while approximately 30% of the wavefronts were generated by epicardial breakthroughs (Table 9-3). The number of waves per second, however, was nearly twice as great in the chronic atrial fibrillation patients (29.9 waves per second) than in the nonsustained atrial fibrillation group (14.6 waves per second) (Table 9-3). The complexity of atrial fibrillation was highly variable in the nonsustained atrial fibrillation group with two patients each demonstrating type I and type III patterns and six patients demonstrating type II patterns (Fig. 9-55). All patients with a chronic AF, however, manifested a type III pattern. The mean fibrillation intervals, however, in both groups were approximately the same: 176 (21 msec in the chronic atrial fibrillation group) versus 188 (47 msec in the nonsustained atrial fibrillation group). The variability in intervals, however, was significantly greater in the chronic AF group with type III complexities than in the nonsustained group (Fig. 9-56 and Table 9-4).

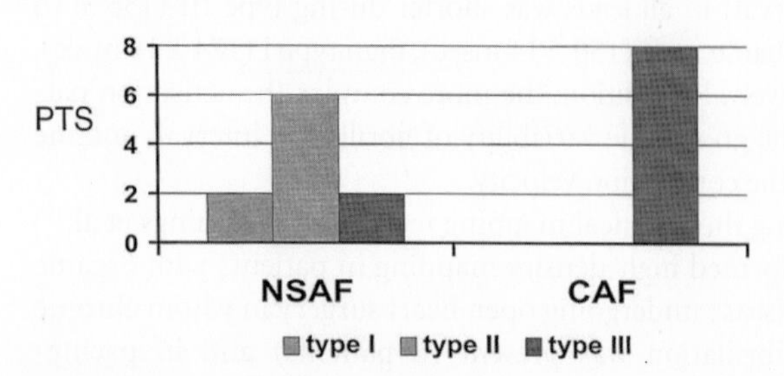


**FIGURE 9-55** *Complexity of atrial fibrillation in patients with nonsustained and sustained atrial fibrillation.*

The number of arcs of blocks per second was nearly twice as great in patients with chronic AF than in those with nonsustained AF: 44.5 ± 10.8 versus 24.4 ± 10.3; $p < 0.001$ (Table 9-5). This is not surprising since all chronic AF patients manifested type III complexity. However, the length of the arcs of block were not significantly different, both averaging about 11 mm. Of interest was that the orientation of lines of block was similar in both groups and was in general perpendicular to the tricuspid annulus suggesting a significant role of anisotropy in the formation of these lines of block. Of extreme interest was the fact that following conversion of chronic atrial fibrillation by cardioversion and cessation of nonsustained atrial fibrillation, the refractory periods, measured by programmed stimulation, at five sites were not different in both groups.[107] The effective refractory periods determined at a paced cycle length of 600 msec and at the fastest rate at which one-to-one conduction could be maintained were not different in both groups of patients. This lack of difference in refractoriness suggested that there was no evidence of electrophysiologic remodeling in these patients with chronic atrial fibrillation. This is markedly different than the studies by Wijffels et al.[28,29] in their goat model or in studies in the electrophysiology laboratory in humans.[30,32,33] The reason for these discrepant observations is unclear and requires further study.

**TABLE 9-4 Fibrillation Intervals in Patients with Chronic and Nonsustained Atrial Fibrillation (ms; mean + SD)**

| | CAF | NSAF | p |
|---|---|---|---|
| Median | 176 ± 21 | 188 ± 47 | |
| $P_{95\text{-}5}$ | 148 ± 25 | 96 ± 43 | 0.008 |
| *N* | 8 | 10 | |

While the median fibrillation intervals in patients with CAF and NSAF are similar, the range of intervals is greater in patients with CAF.
*N*, number of patients. See text for discussion.

TABLE 9-5 Incidence and Length of Conduction Block in Patients with Chronic and Nonsustained Atrial Fibrillation (mean ± SD)

| | CAF | NSAF | p |
|---|---|---|---|
| Blocks/sec | 44.5 ± 10.8 | 24.4 ± 10.3 | < 0.001 |
| Length (mm) | 10.8 ± 1.3 | 11.2 ± 2.8 | n.s. |

Although the lengths of lines of block are similar in CAF and NSAF, there were nearly twice as many lines of block per second in patients with CAF. See text for discussion.

More recent studies by Allessie's group[103,112,113] and Kalman's laboratory[111] mapping both right and left atria have shown virtually identical data as our study. Multiple random wavefronts with a varying degree of epicardial breakthroughs were the dominant finding. Only Lee et al.[111] demonstrated any rotor activity, which was transient and very rare (~8%). Even though wavefronts appeared random, there were repetitive activation wavefronts entering and within the mapping field. This suggests the presence of functional barriers driving the path of wavefronts. It is interesting how similar these data are regardless of where the recordings were taken (RA or LA) or the type of underlying heart disease. A limitation of all these high-density mapping studies is that the mapping plaque covered only 10% to 20% of the atrial surface during any data acquisition.

In summary, in humans with organic heart disease undergoing open heart surgery, right atrial activation during chronic atrial fibrillation shows a significantly higher degree of complexity than during electrically induced atrial fibrillation. During chronic atrial fibrillation the number of independent fibrillation waves and arcs of functional conduction block are twice as high as during electrically induced atrial fibrillation. However, both during chronic and electrically induced atrial fibrillation the lines of functional conduction block are similar in length and show preferential orientation perpendicular to the A-V groove. The preferential orientation of conduction block suggests tissue anisotropy plays an important role in the maintenance of chronic atrial fibrillation. Frequent epicardial breakthroughs in both chronic atrial fibrillation and paced-induced atrial fibrillation suggest that this rhythm should be considered a three-dimensional arrhythmia and suggest a role of the pectinate muscles as a source of epicardial breakthrough and a mechanism for perpetuation of atrial fibrillation. The lack of evidence of electrical remodeling of refractoriness in chronic atrial fibrillation needs further investigation but may be related to the anatomic remodeling and remodeling of gap junctions as associated with chronic atrial fibrillation. Alternatively, this may be a reflection of the small number of patients studied and the influence of the operative environment (e.g., anesthesia, temperature, etc.).

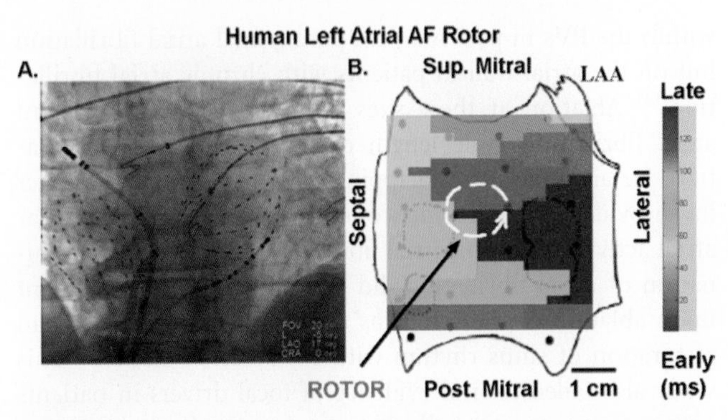


**FIGURE 9-57** *Demonstration of a left atrial rotor using Topera mapping system.* Mapping both atria with 64-pole basket catheters, specialized software has been able to detect apparently stable rotors during persistent atrial fibrillation. Such maps have been used to guide ablation (see Chapter 14). (Courtesy of Sanjay Narayan.)

Recently Narayan et al.[114,115,123] simultaneously mapped the RA and LA during long persistent atrial fibrillation using two 64-pole basket catheters. This method provides a much lower density of mapping and is also limited by contact issues. Nevertheless, these investigators reported apparently stable macroreentrant rotors in the left and/or right atrium in >95% of patients with persistent AF (Fig. 9-57). Targeting these rotors in addition to standard PV isolation had impressive short-term results in keeping patients free of atrial fibrillation (see Chapter 14). They also demonstrated the lack of relationship of CAFEs to the rotor core, further confirming the passive nature of these signals. More data are necessary to confirm these data, which have not been reproduced. It may mean that less dense mapping can separate the "forest from the trees" and that the larger view gives a more accurate global view of what is happening.

Relative "high density" catheter mapping of the atrium during atrial fibrillation has also revealed focal sites of rapid activation with centrifugal activation of the atrium, most commonly in the posterior left atrium, at the PV atrial junctions. The presence of "drivers" of atrial fibrillation, defined as focal sites of regular rapid atrial activity that may play a role in the maintenance of atrial fibrillation, has recently been studied intensively.[108–110,124] Sahadevan et al.,[109] performed epicardial mapping from large arrays containing over 400 electrodes placed on the surface of the right and left atria in nine patients with chronic AF undergoing cardiac surgery. Seven of the nine patients demonstrated a type I pattern in specific areas of the LA, with monomorphic atrial electrograms with a constant short cycle length (ranging from 137 to 288 msec). These areas, generally localized to the base of the LA appendage and lateral to the left PVs, had the shortest cycle lengths recorded in either atria, and were hypothesized to represent "drivers" of atrial fibrillation. In the two other patients studied, there was no regular activation in either atrium found. The mechanism of this focal activity could not be determined.

Haissaguerre's group performed mapping of these sites and created "three-dimensional" dominant frequency maps which demonstrated that the focal sites tend to be located within the PVs in patients with paroxysmal atrial fibrillation but on the atrial wall in patients with chronic atrial fibrillation.[124] Ablation at these sites often slowed the dominant atrial fibrillation cycle length or terminated atrial fibrillation. Detailed left atrial mapping with a multipolar catheter has provided further evidence of focal sites of rapid, regular atrial activation during atrial fibrillation. Interestingly, termination of atrial fibrillation did not appear to be dependent upon ablation of these foci, as the majority of patients had restoration of sinus rhythm with PV ablation alone.[110] This study also failed to find evidence of focal drivers in patients with permanent atrial fibrillation, though they were commonly found in patients with paroxysmal and persistent atrial fibrillation. Another recent study has identified a subset of patients with a higher dominant atrial fibrillation cycle length in the right atrium, originating near the SVC, with fibrillatory conduction to the rest of the right and left atria.[125] While the majority of patients have atrial fibrillation initiated by focal triggers in the left atrium, it is important to consider right atrial sources for initiation and maintenance of atrial fibrillation. Lazar et al.[119,120] also found dominant frequency analysis was only meaningful in paroxysmal atrial fibrillation which is generally accepted to be driven by PV firing. There is no dominant frequency in persistent fibrillation.

Mapping of fractionated electrograms during atrial fibrillation reveals multiple areas of complex fractionated electrograms (CAFEs) in the left atrium. In fact these electrograms are frequently used to identify "dominant frequency." However, the appearance of fractionated electrograms is consistently preceded by local acceleration of the fibrillation cycle length, and therefore appears to be a secondary effect due to local anisotropy or multiple colliding wavefronts.[108] The areas of fractionation tend to be dynamic with return to baseline after acceleration; therefore they cannot ipso facto be considered as critical to the genesis of atrial fibrillation. Such changes were commonly seen in paroxysmal atrial fibrillation which were mapped intraoperatively with high-density mapping (greater than 200 electrodes) described in preceding paragraphs. The passive nature of the electrograms was further demonstrated by Saghy et al.[19] and Narayan et al.[115] As a consequence, I believe CAFEs in the left atrium (or anywhere) during atrial fibrillation represent functional characteristics of the atrial tissue leading to abnormal electrograms at rapid rates, but are not necessarily in critical to the maintenance of atrial fibrillation.

## Stimulation During Atrial Fibrillation

The presence of excitable gaps in atrial fibrillation allows for the possibility of capture of the atrium during atrial fibrillation. Kirchhof et al.[126] demonstrated capture of the atrium by rapid pacing in the canine model of atrial fibrillation. These investigators were able to show capture of a relatively large area of up to 4 cm by the stimulated wavefront. The area of capture was limited by intra-atrial conduction block and collision with incoming fibrillatory waves. Pacing too slowly would fail to capture and pacing too rapidly would produce fibrillatory activity. Thus there was a critical time interval in which the atrium could be captured. In none of their dogs was atrial fibrillation terminated. These findings were not surprising to clinicians who have not infrequently observed that regularized rhythms could appear in one atrium and fibrillation could appear in the other atrium. Thus, it is not surprising that parts of the atrium can be captured by atrial stimulation while other areas remain in fibrillation (Fig. 9-58). We

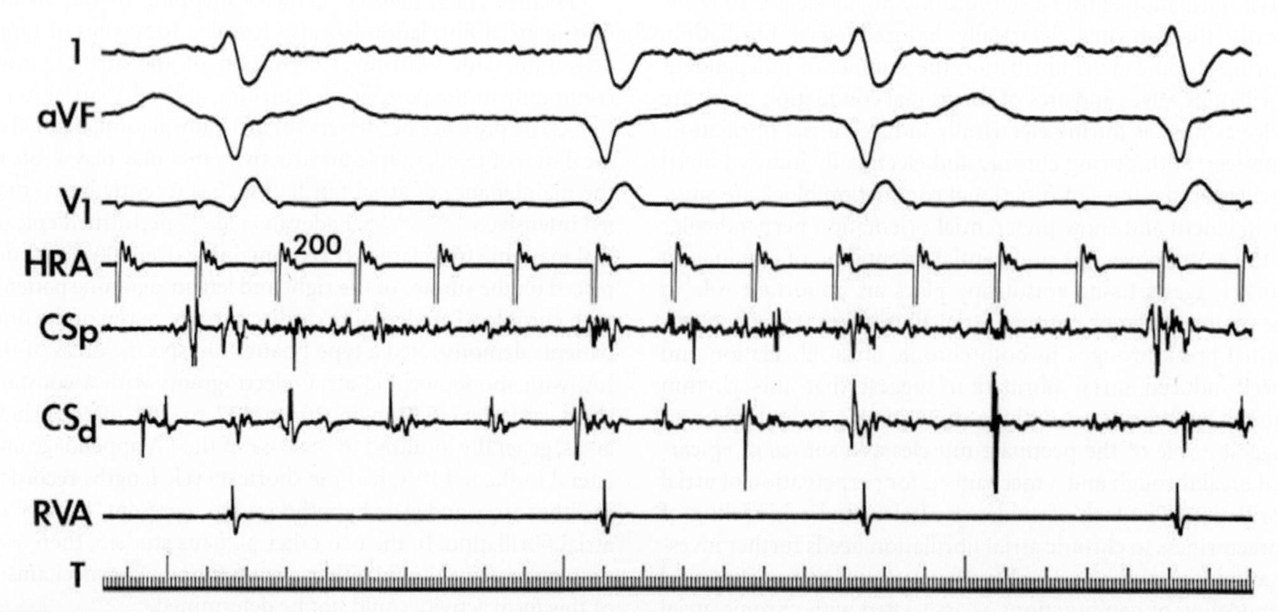


**FIGURE 9-58** *Failure of atrial pacing to terminate atrial flutter/fibrillation.* Leads 1, aVF, and $V_1$ are shown with electrograms from the HRA, proximal and distal CS ($CS_p$, $CS_d$), and the RVA. Although pacing at a cycle length of 200 msec captures the HRA electrogram, it does not influence the fibrillatory activity noted in the CS. The presence of flutter/fibrillation is associated with failure of pacing to terminate the arrhythmia. See text for discussion.

have never been able to terminate atrial fibrillation by pacing, even using multiple simultaneous sites in both atria. While it is conceivable that bursts of atrial pacing delivered immediately at the onset of atrial fibrillation could cause so much disorganization that it would be too unstable to perpetuate itself and thus terminate, once atrial fibrillation is sustained we have never seen it terminated by pacing.[127] It is uncertain whether stimulation at five or six sites simultaneously would be able to terminate fibrillation, but this may not be practical or feasible in a clinical situation. One potential advantage of atrial stimulation is that by capturing significant areas of the atrium one could decrease the number of wavefronts active in the heart at any given time and decrease atrial defibrillation thresholds. This may be important if atrial defibrillation is considered a potential therapeutic option since the fewer number of wavefronts one has, the lower the defibrillation threshold.

## Relationship Between Atrial Flutter and Fibrillation

Atrial flutter and fibrillation frequently coexist in the same patient. They may exist as separate individual arrhythmias at different times or can exist as one arrhythmia, which then undergoes a transition to the other arrhythmia. As stated previously in this chapter, during atrial fibrillation organized wavefronts of activation can be noted. This most commonly is seen in the trabeculated free wall of the right atrium.[122] Organization of electrical signals in the right atrial free wall produces large wavefronts that usually move in a craniocaudal direction during atrial fibrillation.[102,104] These wavefronts are similar to those seen in counterclockwise flutter. When this occurs, fibrillatory waves demonstrate greater amplitude than when intracardiac recordings demonstrate less organized activity. This is best seen in ECG lead $V_1$ which, when craniocaudal-organized activity is seen in the right atrium, demonstrates a positive F (fibrillation) wave that correlates with reasonable accuracy to the cycle length of the intracardiac electrograms observed in the right atrial free wall.[122] Thus, the organization of atrial fibrillation explains to some degree "coarse" and "fine" fibrillation on the surface ECG. This organized activity, which resembles that seen in counterclockwise flutter, may be produced by activation of the right atrium from the septum, which produces transverse block in the crista and forces the wavefront of excitation to move along a trabeculated right atrium in the manner in which it does in flutter. Such a hypothesis favors the septum and/or the left atrium as perpetuators of atrial fibrillation. The critical role of the septum in the conversion of atrial flutter to fibrillation is shown in Figure 9-59.[67] During flutter on the left, atrial activity is organized along the halo recordings in the anterolateral right atrial wall and along the posterior septum at the os of the CS, the midseptum and the septum at the site of the His bundle electrogram. Atrial fibrillation begins when the septal electrograms become disorganized. Disorganization of electrograms in the septum and left atrium, while the right atrium remains organized, is also not uncommon during fibrillation (Fig. 9-60). The conversion from fibrillation to flutter is associated with reorganization of septal activation so that it once again moves in a counterclockwise direction (caudocranial) (Fig. 9-61). In experimental models with detailed mapping, fibrillation turns to flutter when large arcs of block are formed to create a single broad wavefront.[98] While this block always appears to involve the crista terminalis in man, whether or

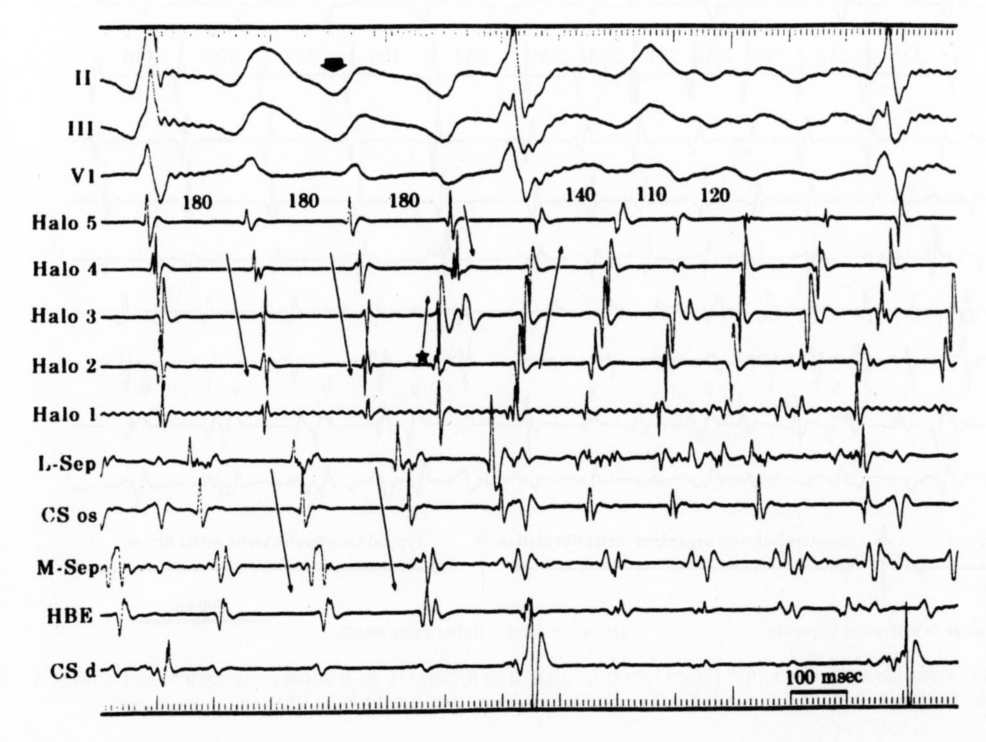


**FIGURE 9-59** *Transition of atrial flutter to atrial fibrillation.* (From Emori T, Fukushima K, Saito H, et al. Atrial electrograms and activation sequences in the transition between atrial fibrillation and atrial flutter. *J Cardiovasc Electrophysiol* 1998;9:1173–1179.)

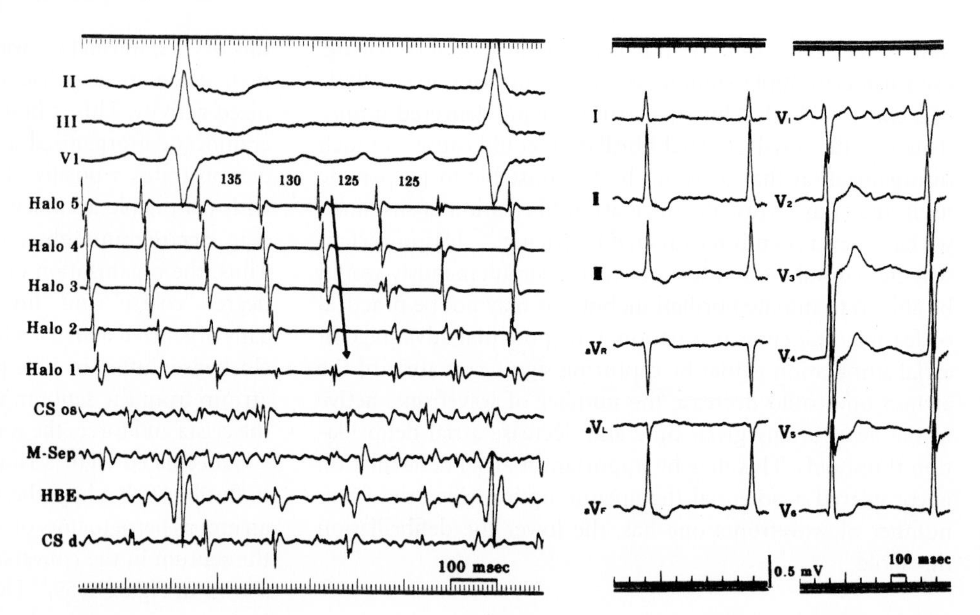


**FIGURE 9-60** *Dissociation of organized activity in the right atrium and disorganized activity in the septum and left atrium during atrial fibrillation.* (From Emori T, Fukushima K, Saito H, et al. Atrial electrograms and activation sequences in the transition between atrial fibrillation and atrial flutter. *J Cardiovasc Electrophysiol* 1998;9:1173–1179, with permission.)

not it requires block in the septum and left atrial sites as well as depends on how many wavelets are present during atrial fibrillation at any given moment in time. The transition from atrial fibrillation to flutter in response to a type I antiarrhythmic agent in man is not uncommon and is associated with the formation of a fixed line of block along the crista terminalis.[20] No catheter or intraoperative mapping involving the septum and left atrium during this phenomenon has been performed, thus the exact sites and extent of lines of block produced by these drugs is not clearly understood. The length of the line of block also appears critical.[98] In the canine pericarditis model, the length of the line of block required to change atrial fibrillation to atrial flutter was 24 ± 4 mm and occurred over several beats. This phenomenon, however, is of great clinical importance because atrial flutter can be simply and successfully ablated, thus forming the basis for a hybrid therapy

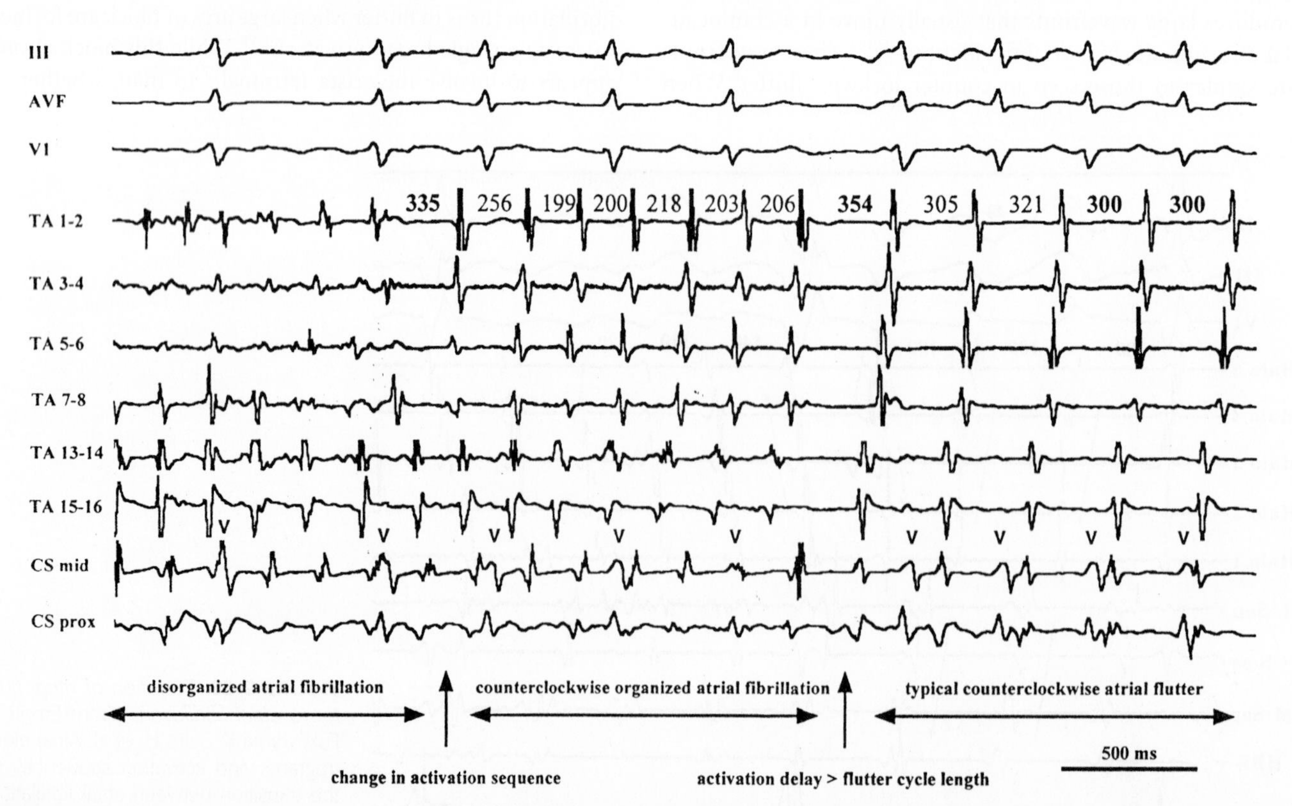


**FIGURE 9-61** *Spontaneous conversion of atrial fibrillation to flutter.* (From Emori T, Fukushima K, Saito H, et al. Atrial electrograms and activation sequences in the transition between atrial fibrillation and atrial flutter. *J Cardiovasc Electrophysiol* 1998;9:1173–1179, with permission.)

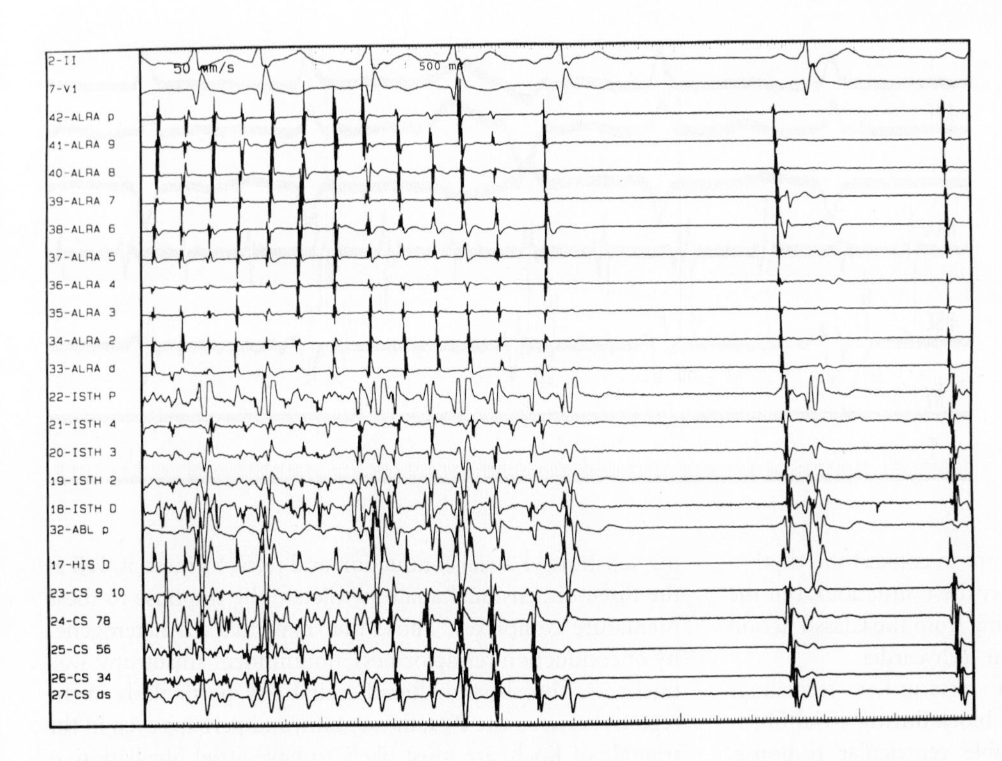


**FIGURE 9-62** *Spontaneous conversion of atrial fibrillation to sinus rhythm.*

(drugs and ablation) for some cases of atrial fibrillation (see Chapter 14).[62] Of note, termination of atrial fibrillation is frequently preceded by organization of atrial activity (Fig. 9-62).

## Miscellaneous Uses of Electrophysiology Studies

Wide QRS complexes are common during atrial fibrillation. Although several surface ECG criteria have been established to distinguish aberrant supraventricular impulses from those of ventricular origin, none is uniformly accurate. As such, intracardiac recordings may provide the only method of diagnosing the site of origin of these abnormal wide QRS complexes. Recording His bundle electrograms during these complexes is the single most accurate way of determining their origin. An abnormal QRS associated with an H-V interval greater than or equal to that with a normal QRS morphology is diagnostic of a supraventricular impulse with aberration (Fig. 9-63). In this particular instance, there was no long-short coupling to initiate the wide complex tachycardia, yet intracardiac recordings confirm supraventricular origin on this wide complex rhythm associated with infra-His conduction delay and the appearance of a left bundle branch block. Wide complex rhythms associated with no His bundle potentials or with retrograde His bundle potentials (H-V intervals less than that of those associated with normal A-V conduction, or His potentials following the QRS) (see Chapter 7) are considered to be ventricular in origin (Fig. 9-64). In occasional patients therapeutic interventions may be inappropriately withheld or inappropriately administered because of the incorrect diagnosis of the wide QRS complex. This is not uncommon during digitalization for control of the ventricular response during atrial fibrillation, in which case fascicular (ventricular) rhythms, which are relatively narrow, could be mistaken for aberration and further digitalis may be given. Another situation in which wide complexes are common is when Class I agents are given

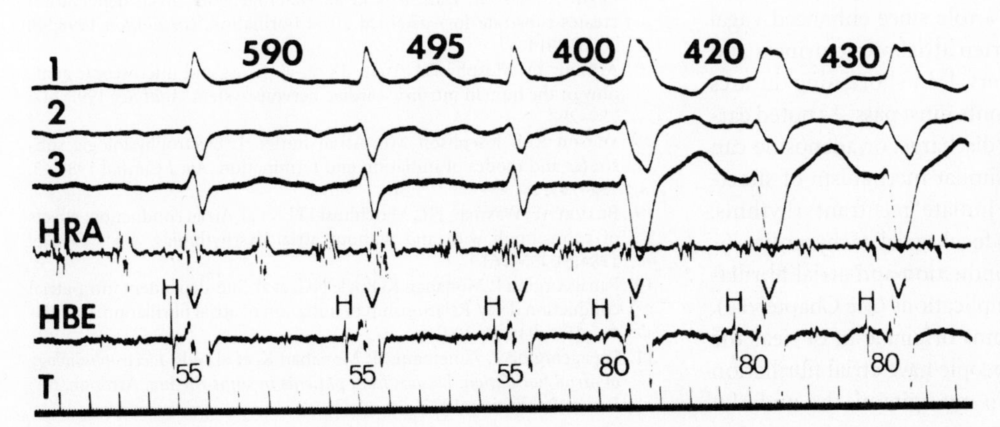


**FIGURE 9-63** *Left bundle branch block during atrial fibrillation.* During atrial fibrillation, the QRS complexes on the right have become broad, with the appearance of a left bundle branch block pattern. Analysis of the His bundle electrogram reveals those complexes to be supraventricular aberrations because they are associated with an increase in the H-V interval from 55 (the normal complex is on the left) to 80 msec.

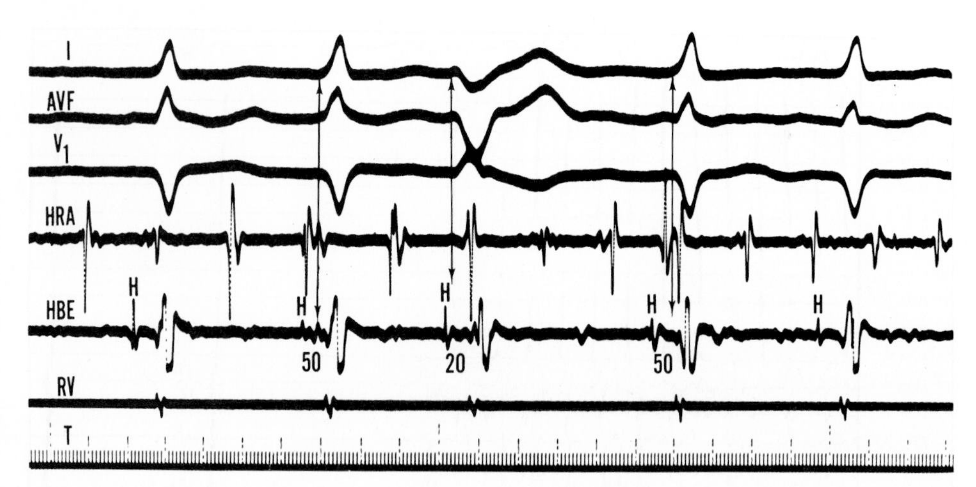


**FIGURE 9-64** *Fascicular premature depolarization during atrial flutter fibrillation.* The third complex shown in the panel demonstrates a right bundle branch block pattern with left-axis deviation. Analysis of the His bundle electrogram reveals this to be a fascicular premature depolarization as documented by the shortened H-V interval of 20 msec. In this instance, the His bundle deflection represents retrograde activation from the site of origin in the posterior fascicle of the left bundle branch.

during atrial fibrillation in an attempt to convert the rhythm to sinus. Aberration can occur under these situations, but the wide bizarre QRS complexes resulting from the Class I action may be misinterpreted as ventricular tachycardia.

Another situation for which intracardiac recordings are useful is to document a site of block during atrial fibrillation or atrial flutter with variable ventricular response. While in most cases the block is in A-V node, an occasional patient's block may be infra-His. This finding does not indicate impaired His–Purkinje function since the input to the His–Purkinje system may be quite rapid in the presence of enhanced A-V nodal conduction. The fact that Class IA agents also have vagolytic properties makes aberration likely since they also impair conduction and prolong refractoriness in the His–Purkinje system.

## SUMMARY

It is apparent that atrial flutter and fibrillation are certainly related arrhythmias. Both coexist and frequently transit from one to the other. These observations attest to the functional nature of lines of block in the atrial myocardium that determine whether or not atrial fibrillation or atrial flutter is present and whether or not they are perpetuated or terminated. Drugs can alter these electrophysiologic properties and convert atrial fibrillation to atrial flutter. In addition, the autonomic nervous system may play a role since enhanced vagal tone or sympathetic tone can shorten atrial refractoriness and increase the rate of fibrillatory intervals by shortening the arcs of block around which the wavefronts must pass. As noted earlier, vagal discharge, sympathetic discharge, or adenosine can all induce atrial fibrillation by a similar mechanism of shortening refractoriness enough to initiate reentrant rhythms. The important observation that focal atrial tachycardias or rotors can result in fibrillatory conduction and atrial fibrillation has important therapeutic implications (see Chapter 14). That many of these ectopic rhythms originate in or near the PVs is of interest, but why some people have atrial fibrillation and others do not is uncertain. In my opinion, the underlying substrate of atrial conduction and refractoriness as well as the three-dimensional anatomy dictate the response to these premature complexes. Those that have marked heterogeneity of conduction refractoriness, nonuniform anisotropy, wall thickness, fibrosis, and altered excitability, particularly in the regions between the PVs, the septum, and perhaps even in the triangle of Koch, are most likely to have atrial fibrillation. A greater understanding of this substrate using newer mapping techniques may lead to different therapeutic options that target the substrate and not the triggers of these arrhythmias.

## REFERENCES

1. January CT, Wann LS, Alpert JS, et al. 2014 AHA/ACC/HRS Guideline for the Management of Patients with Atrial Fibrillation: Executive Summary. *J Am Coll Cardiol.* 2014:64;2246–2280.
2. Frustaci A, Chimenti C, Bellocci F, et al. Histological substrate of atrial biopsies in patients with lone atrial fibrillation. *Circulation* 1997;96:1180–1184.
3. Hashiba K, Centurion OA, Shimizu A. Electrophysiologic characteristics of human atrial muscle in paroxysmal atrial fibrillation. *Am Heart J* 1996;131:778–789.
4. Spach MS, Miller WT, 3rd, Dolber PC, et al. The functional role of structural complexities in the propagation of depolarization in the atrium of the dog. Cardiac conduction disturbances due to discontinuities of effective axial resistivity. *Circ Res* 1982;50:175–191.
5. Spach MS, Dolber PC. Relating extracellular potentials and their derivatives to anisotropic propagation at a microscopic level in human cardiac muscle. Evidence for electrical uncoupling of side-to-side fiber connections with increasing age. *Circ Res* 1986;58:356–371.
6. Olgin JE, Sih HJ, Hanish S, et al. Heterogeneous atrial denervation creates substrate for sustained atrial fibrillation. *Circulation* 1998;98:2608–2614.
7. Armour JA, Murphy DA, Yuan BX, et al. Gross and microscopic anatomy of the human intrinsic cardiac nervous system. *Anat Rec* 1997;247:289–298.
8. Watson RM, Josephson ME. Atrial flutter. I. Electrophysiologic substrates and modes of initiation and termination. *Am J Cardiol* 1980;45:732–741.
9. Buxton AE, Waxman HL, Marchlinski FE, et al. Atrial conduction: effects of extrastimuli with and without atrial dysrhythmias. *Am J Cardiol* 1984;54:755–761.
10. Papageorgiou P, Monahan K, Boyle NG, et al. Site-dependent intra-atrial conduction delay. Relationship to initiation of atrial fibrillation. *Circulation* 1996;94:384–389.
11. Papageorgiou P, Zimetbaum P, Monahan K, et al., eds. *Electrophysiology of atrial fibrillation. Lessons from patients in sinus rhythm.* Armonk, NY: Futura Publishing, 1997.

12. Cosio FG, Palacios J, Vidal JM, et al. Electrophysiologic studies in atrial fibrillation. Slow conduction of premature impulses: a possible manifestation of the background for reentry. *Am J Cardiol* 1983;51:122–130.
13. Simpson RJ, Jr., Foster JR, Mulrow JP, et al. The electrophysiological substrate of atrial fibrillation. *Pacing Clin Electrophysiol* 1983;6:1166–1170.
14. Cosio FG, Arribas F, Palacios J, et al. Fragmented electrograms and continuous electrical activity in atrial flutter. *Am J Cardiol* 1986;57:1309–1314.
15. Attuel P, Childers R, Cauchemez B, et al. Failure in the rate adaptation of the atrial refractory period: its relationship to vulnerability. *Int J Cardiol* 1982;2:179–197.
16. Josephson ME, Scharf DL, Kastor JA, et al. Atrial endocardial activation in man. Electrode catheter technique of endocardial mapping. *Am J Cardiol* 1977;39:972–981.
17. Tanigawa M, Fukatani M, Konoe A, et al. Prolonged and fractionated right atrial electrograms during sinus rhythm in patients with paroxysmal atrial fibrillation and sick sinus node syndrome. *J Am Coll Cardiol* 1991;17:403–408.
18. Centurion OA, Fukatani M, Konoe A, et al. Different distribution of abnormal endocardial electrograms within the right atrium in patients with sick sinus syndrome. *Br Heart J* 1992;68:596–600.
19. Saghy L, Callans DJ, Garcia F, et al. Is there a relationship between complex fractionated atrial electrograms recorded during atrial fibrillation and sinus rhythm fractionation? *Heart Rhythm* 2012;9:181–188.
20. Tai CT, Chen SA, Chen YJ, et al. Conduction properties of the crista terminalis in patients with typical atrial flutter: basis for a line of block in the reentrant circuit. *J Cardiovasc Electrophysiol* 1998;9:811–819.
21. Olgin JE, Kalman JM, Lesh MD. Conduction barriers in human atrial flutter: correlation of electrophysiology and anatomy. *J Cardiovasc Electrophysiol* 1996;7:1112–1126.
22. Olgin JE, Miles W, eds. *Ablation of atrial tachycardias.* Armonk, NY: Futura Publishing, 1998.
23. Arenal A, Almendral J, Alday JM, et al. Rate-dependent conduction block of the crista terminalis in patients with typical atrial flutter: influence on evaluation of cavotricuspid isthmus conduction block. *Circulation* 1999;99:2771–2778.
24. Arenal A, Almendral J, Munoz R, et al. Mechanism and location of atrial flutter in transplanted hearts: observations during transient entrainment from distant sites. *J Am Coll Cardiol* 1997;30:539–546.
25. Pfeiffer D, Prakash A, Giorgberidze I, et al., eds. *Electrophysiology of Atrial Flutter/Fibrillation.* 2nd ed. Armonk, NY: Futura Publishing, 1996.
26. Misier AR, Opthof T, van Hemel NM, et al. Increased dispersion of "refractoriness" in patients with idiopathic paroxysmal atrial fibrillation. *J Am Coll Cardiol* 1992;19:1531–1535.
27. Jais P, Hocini M, Macle L, et al. Distinctive electrophysiological properties of pulmonary veins in patients with atrial fibrillation. *Circulation* 2002;106:2479–2485.
28. Wijffels MC, Kirchhof CJ, Dorland R, et al. Atrial fibrillation begets atrial fibrillation. A study in awake chronically instrumented goats. *Circulation* 1995;92:1954–1968.
29. Wijffels MC, Kirchhof CJ, Dorland R, et al. Electrical remodeling due to atrial fibrillation in chronically instrumented conscious goats: roles of neurohumoral changes, ischemia, atrial stretch, and high rate of electrical activation. *Circulation* 1997;96:3710–3720.
30. Goette A, Honeycutt C, Langberg JJ. Electrical remodeling in atrial fibrillation. Time course and mechanisms. *Circulation* 1996;94:2968–2974.
31. Yue L, Melnyk P, Gaspo R, et al. Molecular mechanisms underlying ionic remodeling in a dog model of atrial fibrillation. *Circ Res* 1999;84:776–784.
32. Tieleman RG, De Langen C, Van Gelder IC, et al. Verapamil reduces tachycardia-induced electrical remodeling of the atria. *Circulation* 1997;95:1945–1953.
33. Daoud EG, Knight BP, Weiss R, et al. Effect of verapamil and procainamide on atrial fibrillation-induced electrical remodeling in humans. *Circulation* 1997;96:1542–1550.
34. Haft JI, Lau SH, Stein E, et al. Atrial fibrillation produced by atrial stimulation. *Circulation* 1968;37:70–74.
35. Abildskov JA, Millar K, Burgess MJ. Atrial fibrillation. *Am J Cardiol* 1971;28:263–267.
36. Allessie MA, Bonke FI, Schopman FJ. Circus movement in rabbit atrial muscle as a mechanism of trachycardia. *Circ Res* 1973;33:54–62.
37. Allessie MA, Bonke FI, Schopman FJ. Circus movement in rabbit atrial muscle as a mechanism of tachycardia. II. The role of nonuniform recovery of excitability in the occurrence of unidirectional block, as studied with multiple microelectrodes. *Circ Res* 1976;39:168–177.
38. Allessie MA, Bonke FI, Schopman FJ. Circus movement in rabbit atrial muscle as a mechanism of tachycardia. III. The "leading circle" concept: a new model of circus movement in cardiac tissue without the involvement of an anatomical obstacle. *Circ Res* 1977;41:9–18.
39. Boineau JP, Mooney CR, Hudson RD, et al., eds. *Observations on reentrant excitation pathways and refractory period distributions in spontaneous and experimental atrial flutter in the dog.* Baltimore, MD: University Park Press, 1976.
40. Allessie MA, Lammers WJ, Bonke IM, et al. Intra-atrial reentry as a mechanism for atrial flutter induced by acetylcholine and rapid pacing in the dog. *Circulation* 1984;70:123–135.
41. Smeets JL, Allessie MA, Lammers WJ, et al. The wavelength of the cardiac impulse and reentrant arrhythmias in isolated rabbit atrium. The role of heart rate, autonomic transmitters, temperature, and potassium. *Circ Res* 1986;58:96–108.
42. Boineau JP, Schuessler RB, Mooney CR, et al. Natural and evoked atrial flutter due to circus movement in dogs. Role of abnormal atrial pathways, slow conduction, nonuniform refractory period distribution and premature beats. *Am J Cardiol* 1980;45:1167–1181.
43. Frame LH, Page RL, Hoffman BF. Atrial reentry around an anatomic barrier with a partially refractory excitable gap. A canine model of atrial flutter. *Circ Res* 1986;58:495–511.
44. Boyden PA, Hoffman BF. The effects on atrial electrophysiology and structure of surgically induced right atrial enlargement in dogs. *Circ Res* 1981;49:1319–1331.
45. Frame LH, Page RL, Boyden PA, et al. Circus movement in the canine atrium around the tricuspid ring during experimental atrial flutter and during reentry in vitro. *Circulation* 1987;76:1155–1175.
46. Wit AL, Cranefield PF. Triggered activity in cardiac muscle fibers of the simian mitral valve. *Circ Res* 1976;38:85–98.
47. Wit AL, Cranefield PF. Triggered and automatic activity in the canine coronary sinus. *Circ Res* 1977;41:434–445.
48. Johnson N, Danilo P, Jr., Wit AL, et al. Characteristics of initiation and termination of catecholamine-induced triggered activity in atrial fibers of the coronary sinus. *Circulation* 1986;74:1168–1179.
49. Schuessler RB, Grayson TM, Bromberg BI, et al. Cholinergically mediated tachyarrhythmias induced by a single extrastimulus in the isolated canine right atrium. *Circ Res* 1992;71:1254–1267.
50. Jais P, Haissaguerre M, Shah DC, et al. A focal source of atrial fibrillation treated by discrete radiofrequency ablation. *Circulation* 1997;95:572–576.
51. Haissaguerre M, Jais P, Shah DC, et al. Spontaneous initiation of atrial fibrillation by ectopic beats originating in the pulmonary veins. *N Engl J Med* 1998;339:659–666.
52. Hwang C, Karagueuzian HS, Chen PS. Idiopathic paroxysmal atrial fibrillation induced by a focal discharge mechanism in the left superior pulmonary vein: possible roles of the ligament of Marshall. *J Cardiovasc Electrophysiol* 1999;10:636–648.
53. Buxton AE, Marchlinski FE, Miller JM, et al. The human atrial strength-interval relation. Influence of cycle length and procainamide. *Circulation* 1989;79:271–280.
54. Engel TR, Gonzalez AD. Effects of digitalis on atrial vulnerability. *Am J Cardiol* 1978;42:570–576.
55. Wyndham CR, Amat-y-Leon F, Wu D, et al. Effects of cycle length on atrial vulnerability. *Circulation* 1977;55:260–267.
56. Cosio FG, Llovet A, Vidal JM. Mechanism and clinical significance of atrial repetitive responses in man. *Pacing Clin Electrophysiol* 1983;6:53–59.
57. Olgin JE, Kalman JM, Fitzpatrick AP, et al. Role of right atrial endocardial structures as barriers to conduction during human type I atrial flutter. Activation and entrainment mapping guided by intracardiac echocardiography. *Circulation* 1995;92:1839–1848.
58. Kalman JM, Olgin JE, Saxon LA, et al. Activation and entrainment mapping defines the tricuspid annulus as the anterior barrier in typical atrial flutter. *Circulation* 1996;94:398–406.
59. Nakagawa H, Lazzara R, Khastgir T, et al. Role of the tricuspid annulus and the eustachian valve/ridge on atrial flutter. Relevance to catheter ablation of the septal isthmus and a new technique for rapid identification of ablation success. *Circulation* 1996;94:407–424.
60. Cosio FG, Arribas F, Lopez-Gil M, et al. Atrial flutter mapping and ablation. I. Studying atrial flutter mechanisms by mapping and entrainment. *Pacing Clin Electrophysiol* 1996;19:841–53.
61. Milliez P, Richardson AW, Obioha-Ngwu O, et al. Variable electrocardiographic characteristics of isthmus-dependent atrial flutter. *J Am Coll Cardiol* 2002;40:1125–32.

62. Huang DT, Monahan KM, Zimetbaum P, et al. Hybrid pharmacologic and ablative therapy: a novel and effective approach for the management of atrial fibrillation. *J Cardiovasc Electrophysiol* 1998;9:462–469.
63. Olgin JE, Kalman JM, Saxon LA, et al. Mechanism of initiation of atrial flutter in humans: site of unidirectional block and direction of rotation. *J Am Coll Cardiol* 1997;29:376–384.
64. Feld GK, Fleck RP, Chen PS, et al. Radiofrequency catheter ablation for the treatment of human type 1 atrial flutter. Identification of a critical zone in the reentrant circuit by endocardial mapping techniques. *Circulation* 1992;86:1233–1240.
65. Olshansky B, Okumura K, Hess PG, et al. Demonstration of an area of slow conduction in human atrial flutter. *J Am Coll Cardiol* 1990;16:1639–1648.
66. Waldo AL. Some observations concerning atrial flutter in man. *Pacing Clin Electrophysiol* 1983;6:1181–1189.
67. Emori T, Fukushima K, Saito H, et al. Atrial electrograms and activation sequences in the transition between atrial fibrillation and atrial flutter. *J Cardiovasc Electrophysiol* 1998;9:1173–1179.
68. Cheng J, Cabeen WR, Jr., Scheinman MM. Right atrial flutter due to lower loop reentry: mechanism and anatomic substrates. *Circulation* 1999;99:1700–1705.
69. Almendral JM, Arenal A, Abeytus M, et al. Incidence and patterns of resetting during atrial flutter: role in identifying chamber of origin. *J Am Coll Cardiol* 1987;9:153A.
70. Disertori M, Molinis G, Inama G, et al. Overdrive and programmed atrial electrostimulation in the study of the electrogenetic mechanism of atrial flutter in man. *Pacing Clin Electrophysiol* 1981;4:133–147.
71. Disertori M, Inama G, Vergara G, et al. Evidence of a reentry circuit in the common type of atrial flutter in man. *Circulation* 1983;67:434–440.
72. Josephson ME, Buxton AE, Almendral JM, et al., eds. *Electrophysiologic characteristics of atrial flutter and their therapeutic implications.* Mt. Kisco, NY: Futura Publishing, 1989.
73. Olshansky B, Okumura K, Henthorn RW, et al. Characterization of double potentials in human atrial flutter: studies during transient entrainment. *J Am Coll Cardiol* 1990;15:833–841.
74. Yang Y, Varma N, Keung EC, et al. Reentry within the cavotricuspid isthmus: an isthmus dependent circuit. *Pacing Clin Electrophysiol* 2005; 28:808–818.
75. Waldo AL, MacLean WA, Karp RB, et al. Entrainment and interruption of atrial flutter with atrial pacing: studies in man following open heart surgery. *Circulation* 1977;56:737–745.
76. Greenberg ML, Kelly TA, Lerman BB, et al. Atrial pacing for conversion of atrial flutter. *Am J Cardiol* 1986;58:95–99.
77. Luderitz B, d'Alnoncourt CN, Steinbeck G, et al. Therapeutic pacing in tachyarrhythmias by implanted pacemakers. *Pacing Clin Electrophysiol* 1982;5:366–371.
78. Wyndham CR, Wu D, Denes P, et al. Self-initiated conversion of paroxysmal atrial flutter utilizing a radio-frequency pacemaker. *Am J Cardiol* 1978;41:1119–1122.
79. Waldo AL, Henthorn RW, Plumb VJ, eds. *Atrial flutter—recent observations in man.* Philadelphia, PA: Lea & Febiger, 1984.
80. Schoels W, Swerdlow CD, Jung W, et al. Worldwide clinical experience with a new dual-chamber implantable cardioverter defibrillator system. *J Cardiovasc Electrophysiol* 2001;12:521–528.
81. Cheng J, Scheinman MM. Acceleration of typical atrial flutter due to double-wave reentry induced by programmed electrical stimulation. *Circulation* 1998;97:1589–1596.
82. Hordof AJ, Edie R, Malm JR, et al. Electrophysiologic properties and response to pharmacologic agents of fibers from diseased human atria. *Circulation* 1976;54:774–779.
83. Josephson ME, Caracta AR, Ricciutti MA, et al. Electrophysiologic properties of procainamide in man. *Am J Cardiol* 1974;33:596–603.
84. Josephson ME, Seides SF, Batsford WP, et al. The electrophysiological effects of intramuscular guinidine on the atrioventricular conducting system in man. *Am Heart J* 1974;87:55–64.
85. Josephson ME, Caracta AR, Lau SH, et al. Electrophysiological evaluation of disopyramide in man. *Am Heart J* 1973;86:771–780.
86. Zipes DP, ed. *Management of cardiac arrhythmias: pharmacologic, electrical and surgical techniques.* Philadelphia, PA: WB Saunders, 1997.
87. Wu KM, Hoffman BF. Effect of procainamide and N-acetylprocainamide on atrial flutter: studies in vivo and in vitro. *Circulation* 1987;76:1397–1408.
88. Buxton AE, Doherty JU. Amiodarone: correlation of electrophysiologic effects with control of atrial arrhythmias. *Circulation* 1985;72:III-32.
89. Zipes DP, Mihalick MJ, Robbins GT. Effects of selective vagal and stellate ganglion stimulation of atrial refractoriness. *Cardiovasc Res* 1974;8:647–655.
90. Hordof AJ, Spotnitz A, Mary-Rabine L, et al. The cellular electrophysiologic effects of digitalis on human atrial fibers. *Circulation* 1978;57:223–229.
91. Prystowsky EN, Naccarelli GV, Jackman WM, et al. Enhanced parasympathetic tone shortens atrial refractoriness in man. *Am J Cardiol* 1983;51:96–100.
92. Allessie MAA, Lammers W, Rensma PL, et al., eds. *Flutter and fibrillation in experimental models: what has been learned that can be applied to humans?* New York, NY: Futura Publishing, 1987.
93. Patterson E, Lazzara R, Szabo B, et al. Sodium-calcium exchange initiated by the Ca2+ transient: an arrhythmia trigger within pulmonary veins. *J Am Coll Cardiol* 2006;47:1196–1206.
94. Lok NS, Lau CP. Abnormal vasovagal reaction, autonomic function, and heart rate variability in patients with paroxysmal atrial fibrillation. *Pacing Clin Electrophysiol* 1998;21:386–395.
95. Hedberg A, Kempf F, Jr., Josephson ME, et al. Coexistence of beta-1 and beta-2 adrenergic receptors in the human heart: effects of treatment with receptor antagonists or calcium entry blockers. *J Pharmacol Exp Ther* 1985; 234:561–568.
96. Wu TJ, Yashima M, Xie F, et al. Role of pectinate muscle bundles in the generation and maintenance of intra-atrial reentry: potential implications for the mechanism of conversion between atrial fibrillation and atrial flutter. *Circ Res* 1998;83:448–462.
97. Schuessler RB, Kawamoto T, Hand DE, et al. Simultaneous epicardial and endocardial activation sequence mapping in the isolated canine right atrium. *Circulation* 1993;88:250–263.
98. Ortiz J, Niwano S, Abe H, et al. Mapping the conversion of atrial flutter to atrial fibrillation and atrial fibrillation to atrial flutter. Insights into mechanisms. *Circ Res* 1994;74:882–894.
99. Mansour M, Mandapati R, Berenfeld O, et al. Left-to-right gradient of atrial frequencies during acute atrial fibrillation in the isolated sheep heart. *Circulation* 2001;103:2631–2636.
100. Mandapati R, Skanes A, Chen J, et al. Stable microreentrant sources as a mechanism of atrial fibrillation in the isolated sheep heart. *Circulation* 2000;101:194–199.
101. Jalife J, Berenfeld O, Mansour M. Mother rotors and fibrillatory conduction: a mechanism of atrial fibrillation. *Cardiovasc Res* 2002;54:204–216.
102. Kirchhof CJH, Saltman AE, Krukenkamp IB, et al. High-density mapping of chronic atrial fibrillation in man. *Circ* 1996;94:555.
103. Allessie MA, de Groot NM, Houben RP, et al. Electropathological substrate of long-standing persistent atrial fibrillation in patients with structural heart disease: longitudinal dissociation. *Circ Arrhythm Electrophysiol* 2010;3:606–615.
104. Konings KT, Kirchhof CJ, Smeets JR, et al. High-density mapping of electrically induced atrial fibrillation in humans. *Circulation* 1994;89:1665–1680.
105. Cox JL, Canavan TE, Schuessler RB, et al. The surgical treatment of atrial fibrillation. II. Intraoperative electrophysiologic mapping and description of the electrophysiologic basis of atrial flutter and atrial fibrillation. *J Thorac Cardiovasc Surg* 1991;101:406–426.
106. Botteron GW, Cain ME, eds. *Lessons from mapping atrial fibrillation in humans: implications for ablation.* Armonk, NY: Futura Publishing, 1997.
107. Kirchhof CJH, Saltman AE, Krukenkamp IB, et al. Lack of evidence of electrical remodeling in patients with chronic atrial fibrillation. *Circ* 1996;94:554.
108. Rostock T, Rotter M, Sanders P, et al. High-density activation mapping of fractionated electrograms in the atria of patients with paroxysmal atrial fibrillation. *Heart Rhythm* 2006;3:27–34.
109. Sahadevan J, Ryu K, Peltz L, et al. Epicardial mapping of chronic atrial fibrillation in patients: preliminary observations. *Circulation* 2004;110:3293–3299.
110. Takahashi Y, Hocini M, O'Neill MD, et al. Sites of focal atrial activity characterized by endocardial mapping during atrial fibrillation. *J Am Coll Cardiol* 2006;47:2005–2012.
111. Lee G, Kumar S, Teh A, et al. Epicardial wave mapping in human long-lasting persistent atrial fibrillation: transient rotational circuits, complex wavefronts, and disorganized activity. *Eur Heart J* 2014;35:86–97.
112. de Groot NM, Houben RP, Smeets JL, et al. Electropathological substrate of longstanding persistent atrial fibrillation in patients with structural heart disease: epicardial breakthrough. *Circulation* 2010;122:1674–1682.
113. Eckstein J, Maesen B, Linz D, et al. Time course and mechanisms of endo-epicardial electrical dissociation during atrial fibrillation in the goat. *Cardiovasc Res* 2011;89:816–824.

114. Narayan SM, Krummen DE, Shivkumar K, et al. Treatment of atrial fibrillation by the ablation of localized sources: CONFIRM (Conventional Ablation for Atrial Fibrillation With or Without Focal Impulse and Rotor Modulation) trial. *J Am Coll Cardiol* 2012;60:628–636.
115. Narayan SM, Wright M, Derval N, et al. Classifying fractionated electrograms in human atrial fibrillation using monophasic action potentials and activation mapping: evidence for localized drivers, rate acceleration, and nonlocal signal etiologies. *Heart Rhythm* 2011;8:244–253.
116. Pandit SV, Jalife J. Rotors and the dynamics of cardiac fibrillation. *Circ Res* 2013;112:849–862.
117. Vaquero M, Calvo D, Jalife J. Cardiac fibrillation: from ion channels to rotors in the human heart. *Heart Rhythm* 2008;5:872–879.
118. Atienza F, Almendral J, Moreno J, et al. Activation of inward rectifier potassium channels accelerates atrial fibrillation in humans: evidence for a reentrant mechanism. *Circulation* 2006;114:2434–2442.
119. Lazar S, Dixit S, Marchlinski FE, et al. Presence of left-to-right atrial frequency gradient in paroxysmal but not persistent atrial fibrillation in humans. *Circulation* 2004;110:3181–3186.
120. Lazar S, Dixit S, Callans DJ, et al. Effect of pulmonary vein isolation on the left-to-right atrial dominant frequency gradient in human atrial fibrillation. *Heart Rhythm* 2006;3:889–895.
121. Kirchoff C, Josephson ME, eds. *Role of anisotropy in human arrhythmias.* Armonk, NY: Futura Publishing, 1997.
122. Roithinger FX, SippensGroenewegen A, Karch MR, et al. Organized activation during atrial fibrillation in man: endocardial and electrocardiographic manifestations. *J Cardiovasc Electrophysiol* 1998;9:451–461.
123. Narayan SM, Krummen DE, Clopton P, et al. Direct or coincidental elimination of stable rotors or focal sources may explain successful atrial fibrillation ablation: on-treatment analysis of the CONFIRM trial (Conventional ablation for AF with or without focal impulse and rotor modulation). *J Am Coll Cardiol* 2013;62:138–147.
124. Sanders P, Berenfeld O, Hocini M, et al. Spectral analysis identifies sites of high-frequency activity maintaining atrial fibrillation in humans. *Circulation* 2005;112:789–797.
125. Lin YJ, Tai CT, Kao T, et al. Frequency analysis in different types of paroxysmal atrial fibrillation. *J Am Coll Cardiol* 2006;47:1401–1407.
126. Kirchhof C, Chorro F, Scheffer GJ, et al. Regional entrainment of atrial fibrillation studied by high-resolution mapping in open-chest dogs. *Circulation* 1993;88:736–749.
127. Giorgberidze I, Saksena S, Mongeon L, et al. Effects of high-frequency atrial pacing in atypical atrial flutter and atrial fibrillation. *J Interv Card Electrophysiol* 1997;1:111–123.

CHAPTER

# 10 Preexcitation Syndromes

Preexcitation exists when, in relation to atrial events, all or some part of the ventricular muscle is activated by the atrial impulse sooner than would be expected if the impulse reached the ventricles only by way of the normal atrioventricular (A-V) conduction system.[1] The clinical significance of the preexcitation syndromes relates primarily to the high frequency of associated arrhythmias and to the various bizarre and often misleading associated electrocardiographic patterns. Understanding the pathophysiologic basis for arrhythmias in these disorders provides much of our knowledge concerning the mechanism of reentrant arrhythmias.

The preexcitation syndromes previously were classified on the basis of proposed anatomic connections described by the eponyms Kent fibers, James fibers, and Mahaim fibers. The major objection to this classification was that it was imprecise and did not allow sufficient flexibility in explaining accumulated electrophysiologic and pathologic observations. As a consequence, many of these eponyms were inappropriately applied to various forms of preexcitation. Consequently, the European Study Group for Preexcitation devised a new classification of the preexcitation syndromes, based on their proposed anatomic connections.[2] These connections are (a) A-V bypass tracts forming direct connections between the atria and ventricles,[3–7] (b) nodoventricular fibers connecting the A-V node to the ventricular myocardium,[4,8–10] (c) fasciculoventricular connections from the His–Purkinje system to the ventricular myocardium,[11] and (d) A-V nodal bypass tracts, direct communications from the atrium to the His bundle,[3,12] or from the atrium to the lower A-V node via a specialized internodal tract,[9] or via specialized intranodal tracts with rapid conduction.[13,14] Subsequently, connections defined pathophysiologically as atriofascicular and nodofascicular (i.e., from the atrium or A-V node to the right bundle branch or adjacent myocardium) have been described and distinguished from nodoventricular fibers.[15–20] Pathologic examination of a surgically excised specimen revealed what appeared to be an accessory A-V nodal–His-like conducting system structure.[21,22] A schema of these pathways is shown in Figure 10-1.

Physiologic (to be distinguished from anatomic) A-V connections produce the classic Wolff–Parkinson–White (WPW) syndrome; nodoventricular, atriofascicular, nodofascicular, and fascicular ventricular connections (which were frequently referred to as "Mahaim fibers") produce WPW variants, and A-V nodal bypass tracts may produce the so-called Lown–Ganong–Levine syndrome. Of note is that many of the fibers actually described by Mahaim have been demonstrated to exist anatomically in the absence of electrophysiologic function.[2,4,10] Hence, anatomic descriptors will be retained but applied only when the accessory pathways demonstrate electrophysiologic function. Because these pathways appear to represent developmental abnormalities, it is not surprising that multiple types of accessory pathways may exist in any individual patient.

## ATRIOVENTRICULAR BYPASS TRACTS

The A-V bypass tract is the most frequently encountered type of preexcitation, and it is the only type for which a reproducible correlation has been demonstrated between electrophysiologic function and anatomic structure. Functioning A-V bypass tracts produce the typical WPW ECG pattern of a short P-R interval (≤0.12 seconds), a slurred upstroke of the QRS complex (delta wave), and a wide QRS complex (≥0.12 seconds). The first accurate description of the mechanism of the WPW Syndrome was by Wolferth and Wood in 1933.[23] They beautifully described the mechanism of the QRS complex and the SVT in the disorder. The typical QRS pattern results because the atrial impulse bypasses the normal delaying site (A-V node) and initiates ventricular depolarization earlier than expected. The length of the P-R interval and the degree of preexcitation (which may be variable) depend on several factors: (a) A-V nodal and His–Purkinje conduction time; (b) conduction time of the sinus impulse to the atrial insertion of the bypass tract, which in turn depends on the distance between the bypass tract and the sinus node as well as on intra-atrial conduction and refractoriness; and (c) conduction time through the bypass tract, which is a function of its structure (length and thickness), the quality of input to the bypass tract, and the spatial–geometric arrangement between the atrium and ventricles, which determines the quality of the electrical input and output of the bypass tract.[21,24] Hence, the P-R interval occasionally exceeds 0.12 sec if intra-atrial conduction delay or prolonged conduction over the bypass tract is present. Moreover, if these delays are marked, preexcitation of the ventricles can occur after the onset of the QRS complex

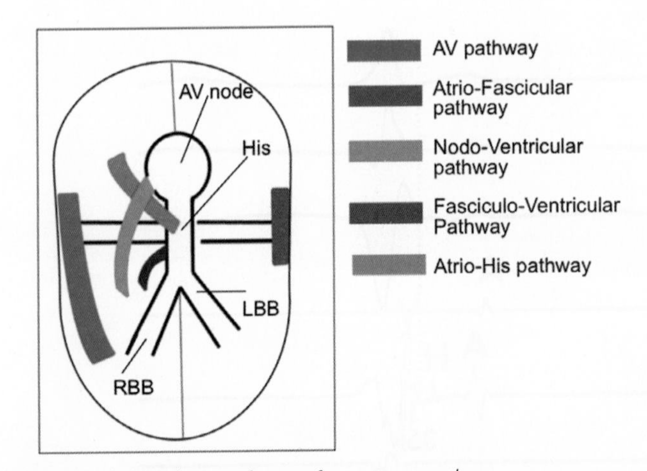


**FIGURE 10-1** *Schema of type of accessory pathways.*

and fail to produce the classic delta wave or wide QRS complex, yet still activate that part of the ventricles in which the bypass tract inserts earlier than it would have been activated over the normal pathway. Delayed input into the bypass tract resulting in this apparent paradox is most likely to occur in left lateral A-V bypass tracts. Enhanced A-V nodal conduction and/or slow conduction over the bypass tract are additional mechanisms for inapparent preexcitation. An example of this phenomenon is shown in Figure 10-2. During sinus rhythm (Fig. 10-1A), the P-R interval and QRS complex are normal; no evidence of preexcitation is apparent. However, during two beats of a junctional rhythm at a cycle length of 600 msec, with the same H-V interval, the QRS complex differs significantly, with diminution of the Q wave in lead 1, the appearance of a Q wave and loss of the slurred upstroke in lead aVF, and a decrease in the amplitude of the R wave in V1. Earliest retrograde activation is seen in the coronary sinus, which is concordant with a left-sided anterograde conduction over a left-sided bypass tract (exaggerated q in lead I and r in V1). The shorter V-A than A-V suggests that antegrade conduction over the bypass tract is rather slow. These findings suggest that during sinus rhythm part of the ventricle is activated earlier than expected but occurs simultaneously with or just after the initial activation of the ventricles over the normal pathway. The presence of preexcitation is recognized only when the QRS in sinus rhythm is compared to the QRS during SVT, which is produced by ventricular activation solely over the normal A-V conducting system. Therefore, any combination of delayed input to the bypass tract, slow conduction over the bypass tract, or fast conduction over the A-V conducting system may result in inapparent preexcitation.

The incidence of A-V bypass tracts detected electrocardiographically has been variously reported as 0.1 to 3.1/1,000, and it has been noted in people of all ages, although its incidence decreases with increasing age.[25–27] However, there appears to be an increased familial incidence of the disorder. Recent study by Vidaillet et al.[28] demonstrated a 3.4% incidence of accessory pathways in first-degree relatives of patients with preexcitation, an incidence significantly higher than that of the general population ($p < 0.0001$). The incidence may even be higher if one could obtain evidence of concealed accessory pathways (see Chapter 8). In fact, we have seen several families in whom various members have evidence of overt preexcitation while other relatives have concealed bypass tracts. This is not surprising, considering that bypass tracts are thought to result from developmental abnormalities of the A-V ring. It is important to recognize that evidence of preexcitation may disappear. In a longitudinal study of patients with symptomatic WPW, Chen et al.[29] noted a loss of antegrade preexcitation of 22.5% over a 10-year follow-up. Whether or not the likelihood of loss of preexcitation is higher in asymptomatic patients is unknown.

Functioning A-V bypass tracts are associated with certain congenital abnormalities, particularly Ebstein's anomaly of the tricuspid valve. Patients with Ebstein's anomaly have a 10% incidence of preexcitation, which invariably have at least one anatomic right-sided (to the anatomic right ventricle) insertion.[5,30,31] This remains the case with corrected transposition, in which Ebstein's anomaly of the left (tricuspid) valve is asssociated with bypass tracts to the functioning systemic ventricle (anatomic right ventricle). Furthermore, multiple bypass tracts are frequently observed in Ebstein's anomaly. Conversely, of patients with WPW syndrome presenting with SVT early in childhood, only 5% have Ebstein's anomaly, despite the fact that it is the most common form of congenital heart disease associated with WPW. Interestingly, Deal et al.[30] found that children with left-sided bypass tracts infrequently have structural heart disease (5%), while in contrast, 45% of patients with right-sided bypass tracts have associated heart disease. In their study, structural heart disease was present in only 20% of the patients presenting with the WPW syndrome in the first 4 months of life.

In adults, an association with the left-sided bypass tracts and mitral valve prolapse has been noted.[32,33] Left-sided bypass tracts appear to be the most common, however, and because mitral valve prolapse is also common in the patient population, their association may in fact represent the coexistence of two relatively common conditions. Although several other disorders have been said to be associated with the WPW syndrome, the true incidences are unknown because of the lack of electrophysiologic studies in all these patient populations. For example, of 30 patients with hypertrophic obstructive cardiomyopathy (HOCM) specifically referred for electrophysiology study because of surface ECGs suggestive of WPW, none had electrophysiologic evidence of A-V bypass tracts. In fact, I have seen only two patients with HOCM who had the WPW syndrome, and both patients presented with SVT. Recently other forms of cardiomyopathy have been described with "WPW" syndrome, but these are not associated with previously mapped and reported defects associated with classic HOCM. The most well studied are mutations in PRKAG2, an enzyme modulating glucose uptake and glycolysis. Blair et al.,[34] Golub et al.,[35] and Arad et al.[36] have described a glycogen storage hypertrophic cardiomyopathy associated with WPW in patients with PRKAG2 mutations. The ECGs presented in some of these patients do not appear to be

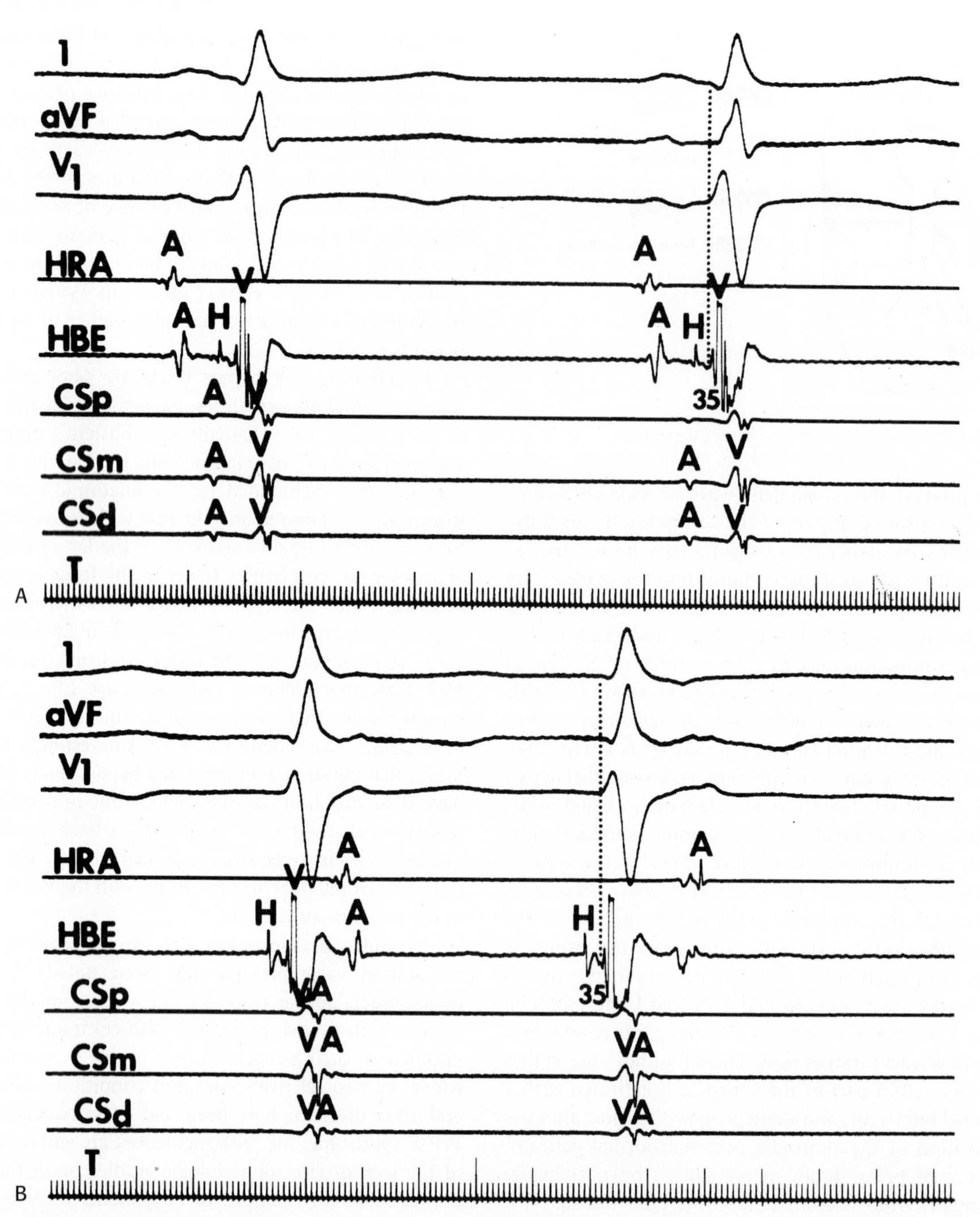


**FIGURE 10-2** *Inapparent preexcitation.* Both panels are organized from **top** to **bottom** as leads 1, aVF, and $V_1$ and electrograms from the HRA, HBE, proximal (CSp), mid- (CSm), and distal (CSd) coronary (CS) electrodes (all in first 4 cm of the CS), and time lines (T). **A:** Sinus rhythm with a normal A-H and H-V interval. The PR-R interval and QRS duration are normal, and there is no obvious preexcitation. **B:** During a junctional rhythm, antegrade activation proceeds solely over the normal A-V conducting system. Retrograde atrial activation is a fusion of sinus and retrograde conduction over a left lateral bypass tract; the second complex shows retrograde activation solely over the left-sided bypass tract. During conduction over the normal A-V system, one sees loss of the slurring of the upstroke lead 2, the development of a small q wave in lead 2 and the diminution of a broad Q wave in lead 1. These findings suggest that during sinus rhythm **(A)** preexcitation of the ventricle occurred at or just after the onset of ventricular activation over the normal conducting system, because the H-V intervals are the same but the QRS differs. See text for further discussion.

classic AV bypass tracts. More recently Yang et al.[37] described a skeletal myopathy and LVH associated with WPW due to mutations in the gene encoding the lysosome-associated protein-2 (LAMP-2). Nevertheless, in the vast majority of young patients with A-V bypass tracts, no heart disease is present.

As noted, the clinical significance of WPW syndromes is the high frequency of arrhythmias and the sometimes-confusing electrocardiographic patterns that can mimic bundle branch block and infarction. Forty to eighty percent of patients with A-V bypass tracts manifest tachyarrhythmias, the most common of which is a circus movement tachycardia (orthodromic SVT) using the normal A-V conducting system as the antegrade limb and the bypass tract as the retrograde limb of the reentrant circuit.[32,38] A reversed pattern of circus movement tachycardia (antidromic SVT) occurs when antegrade conduction proceeds over the bypass tract and retrograde conduction occurs over the normal A-V pathway or, in many instances, an additional bypass tract.[38–42] Clinically, antidromic tachycardias are much less frequent than orthodromic tachycardias (see following discussion). Atrial flutter and fibrillation are less common presenting arrhythmias but are potentially more life threatening, because they can result in extremely rapid ventricular rates that precipitate ventricular tachycardia and/or fibrillation.[32,43,44] Atrial flutter-fibrillation may be the presenting arrhythmia in 5% to 10% of patients with A-V bypass tracts and occurs even more commonly when orthodromic or antidromic tachycardia also is present. As many as 50% of patients with symptomatic arrhythmias have been reported to develop atrial fibrillation of variable duration at some time.[45,46] It is much lower in my experience. The incidence of atrial flutter and/or fibrillation does appear to be higher in patients with A-V bypass tracts than in the normal population, the explanation of which is not understood. We have not found hemodynamic differences during tachycardias, atrial activation sequences that are related to bypass tract location, or tachycardia rate to be critically important in developing atrial fibrillation. Another interesting observation is that atrial fibrillation appears to be five times more common when overt preexcitation (i.e., WPW) is present than in patients with concealed bypass tracts at similar locations and similar rates of tachycardias. Patients with atrial fibrillation have a higher incidence of inducible atrial fibrillation than those without the arrhythmia. Others have made similar observations.[45,46] The mechanisms of atrial fibrillation and tachycardias are discussed later in the chapter. In patients who are asymptomatic the incidence of sudden cardiac death (assumed secondary to atrial fibrillation) is virtually nil.[29,47] While patients over 40 years who have never had symptomatic arrhythmias related to their accessory pathway remain asymptomatic, for those younger than 40 there is a 30% chance of developing symptoms, that is, SVT.[47]

## ELECTROPHYSIOLOGIC PROPERTIES OF A-V BYPASS TRACTS

Unlike the A-V node, conduction over an A-V bypass tract usually behaves in an all-or-none fashion. Rapid pacing or atrial premature depolarizations (APDs) either conduct without delay (no change in P-to-delta wave) or block suddenly (Fig. 10-3). Progressive slowing of conduction over an A-V bypass tract in response to APDs or atrial pacing has been documented in patients with assumed rapidly conducting bypass tracts (P-to-delta ≤0.12 seconds) or in whom a diagnosis of atriofascicular, nodofascicular, or nodoventricular bypass tracts was suspected.[18,21,22,24,48,49] Slowly conducting

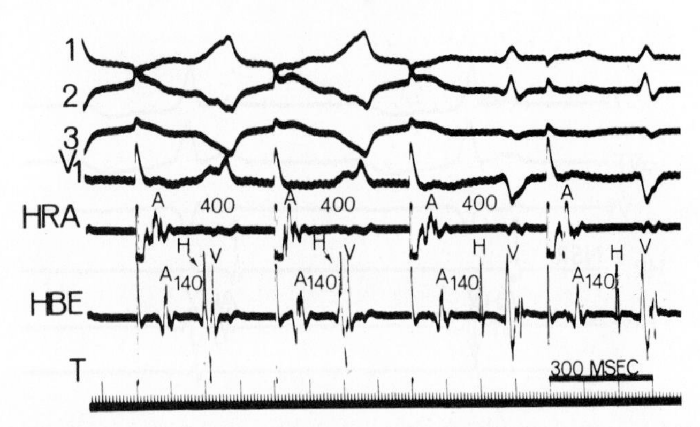


**FIGURE 10-3** *Effect of atrial pacing on conduction over an A-V bypass tract.* From **top** to **bottom** are ECG leads 1, 2, 3, and V1, a high-right atrial electrogram (HRA), a His bundle electrogram (HBE), and time lines (T). The atria are paced at a cycle length of 400 msec. The first two complexes show marked preexcitation with the antegrade His bundle potential (H) buried in the QRS complex. Sudden block in the bypass tract results in normalized QRS morphologies and constant A-H intervals.

atrioventricular bypass tracts are rare (<1%) in patients with preexcitation over an apparent atrioventricular bypass tract. These are most commonly found at the right anterior free wall. Decremental conduction (i.e., prolonged P–delta wave) in response to APDs or atrial pacing with persistence of preexcitation can also be due to intra-atrial conduction delay between the site of stimulation and the bypass tract. Wenckebach-type second-degree block in a bypass tract in response to pacing is rarely observed. When it does occur, it is most commonly in the presence of an atriofascicular bypass tract (see subsequent discussion of bypass tracts with decremental conduction).

Not uncommonly, intermittent conduction over a bypass tract is observed. This is to be distinguished from inapparent preexcitation that is due to prolonged intra-atrial conduction, accelerated A-V conduction, prolonged conduction over a bypass tract, or any combination of these. Four specific conditions can produce intermittent preexcitation (i.e., presence and absence of preexcitation on the same tracing during sinus rhythm or pacing at 60 to 100 beats per minute [bpm]): (a) acceleration-dependent and deceleration-dependent (phase 4) block in the accessory pathway (Fig. 10-4);[50–52] (b) A-V bypass tracts with long refractory periods and supernormal conduction;[53,54] (c) antegrade or retrograde concealed conduction produced by APDs, ventricular premature depolarizations (VPDs), or atrial tachyarrhythmias[55–57] and a long bypass tract refractory period with a gap phenomenon in response to APDs.

To recognize the phase 4 block and phase 3 block, one must demonstrate absence of preexcitation at long cycle lengths followed by evidence of preexcitation at shorter paced cycle lengths and sudden block again at even shorter paced cycle lengths (Fig. 10-4). One must exclude rapid A-V conduction over the normal A-V conduction system during slow rhythms that would reach the ventricles before the bypass tract, thereby preventing manifest preexcitation. Subsequently, pacing at

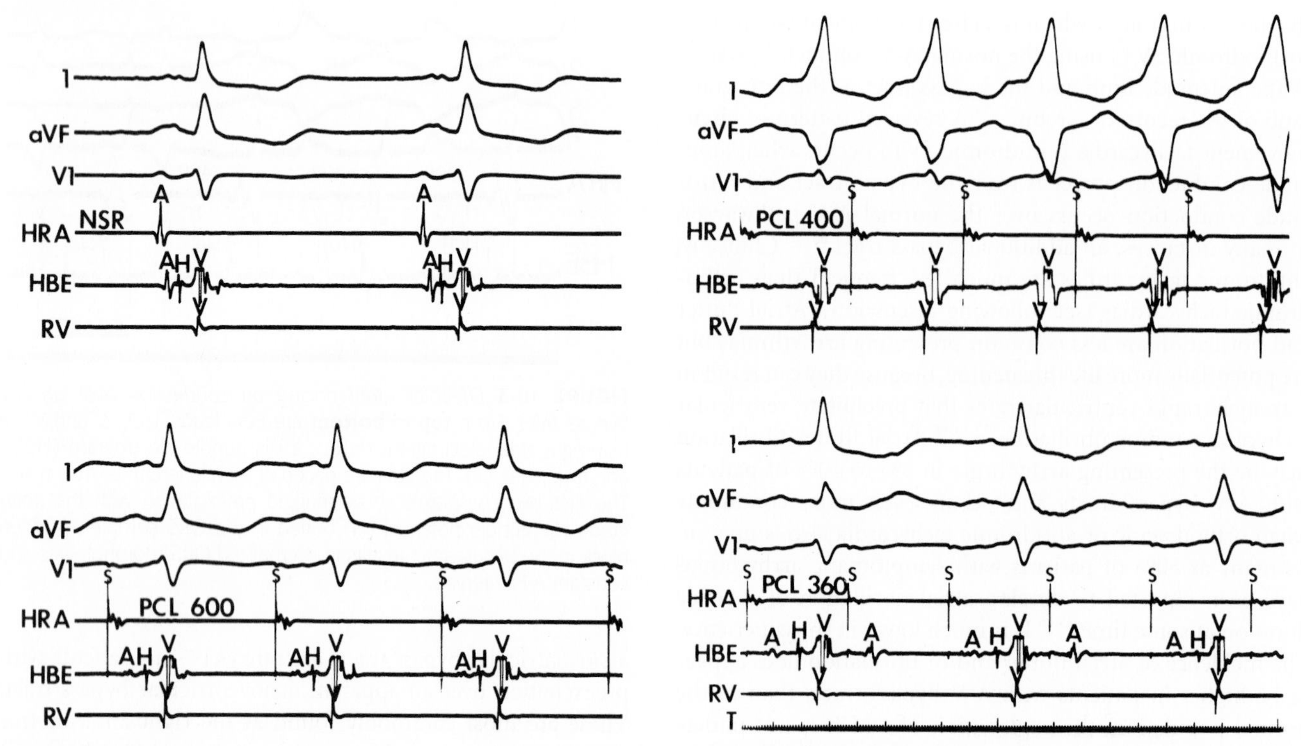


**FIGURE 10-4** *Phase 4 block in the accessory pathway.* Leads 1, aVF, and V1 and electrograms from the HRA, HBE, and RV are shown during normal sinus rhythm (NSR, **top**) and during incremental paced cycle lengths (PCL) from the HRA. During sinus rhythm and a PCL of 600, no preexcitation is present. When the cycle length is decreased to 400 msec, preexcitation occurs, which disappears once again as the PCL is further reduced to 360 msec and 2:1 A-V block with a normal QRS is evident. The absence of preexcitation at long cycle lengths, presence at middle cycle lengths, and absence again at short cycle lengths suggest that phase 4 block is responsible for the absence of preexcitation during sinus rhythm. See text for discussion. (From Lerman BB, Josephson ME. Automaticity of the Kent bundle: confirmation by phase 3 and phase 4 block. *J Am Coll Cardiol* 1985;5:996.)

increasing rates produces prolonged A-V conduction time over the normal pathway, which allows preexcitation to become manifest. A second piece of evidence that supports the presence of phase 4 block is observation of premature complexes with a similar configuration of the preexcited complex (Fig. 10-5).[50] These premature complexes are a direct manifestation of automaticity in the bypass tract.

For diagnosis of supernormal conduction, one should demonstrate preexcitation at long cycle lengths followed by block at shorter (but still relatively long) cycle lengths, and long bypass tract refractory periods. At even shorter coupling intervals or shorter paced cycle lengths, preexcitation once again appears. No change should occur in the P-to-delta intervals during both periods of preexcitation (i.e., at long and short cycle lengths). This criterion is needed to exclude "pseudo"-supernormal phenomena that are due to a gap phenomenon, as discussed in Chapter 6. If gap phenomenon was responsible for "pseudo-supernormal" conduction, the conducted beat at a shorter cycle length should have a longer P to delta due to proximal to ventricle delay in the bypass tract. Although most cases of intermittent preexcitation have not been well studied, the clinical implications are that they generally have long refractory periods and are incapable of rapid repetitive conduction down the bypass tract, hence slower ventricular response, during atrial flutter-fibrillation.[38,58] Of note, some patients with intermittent preexcitation can have improved antegrade conduction over the bypass tract, causing persistent preexcitation, following administration of isoproterenol, which shortens the refractory period of the bypass tract.[38,59] Shortening of the refractory period of the bypass tract may allow conduction to resume at cycle lengths 200 msec shorter, but these cycle lengths are still in the range of 300 to 400 msec, and thus, not potentially lethal. Demonstration of concealed conduction causing absence of preexcitation requires demonstration of APD that is nonconducted over the bypass tract or a VPD influencing antegrade conduction over the bypass tract on subsequent beats. This is quite common as a mechanism for runs of overt preexcitation followed by runs of absent preexcitation during atrial fibrillation.

The vast majority of A-V bypass tracts conduct both anterogradely and retrogradely. Less than 5% of patients with preexcitation have bypass tracts that conduct only antegradely.[60] This is much less common than the converse situation of retrogradely conducting bypass tracts in the absence of antegrade preexcitation (i.e., so-called concealed bypass tracts). In patients who manifest only antegrade conduction over their bypass tract, spontaneous circus movement

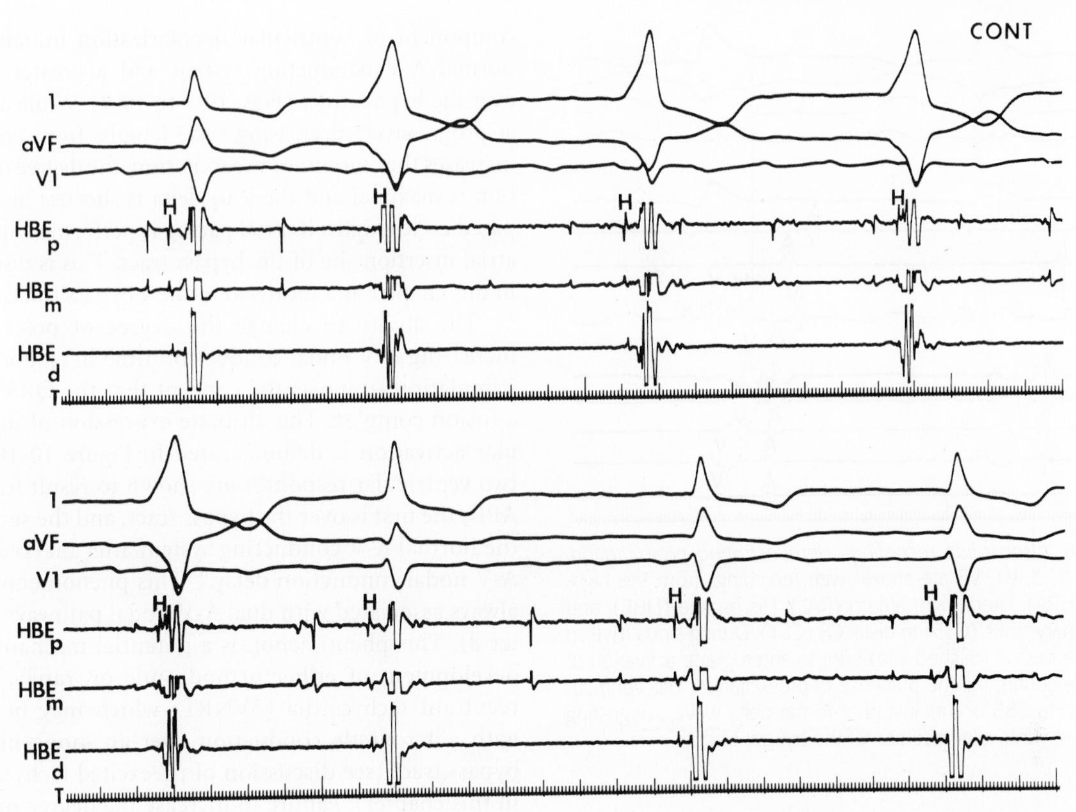


**FIGURE 10-5** *Enhanced automaticity of bypass tract.* Surface leads 1, aVF, and $V_1$ are shown with proximal ($HBE_p$), mid- ($HBE_m$) and distal ($HBE_d$) HBEs. An accelerated regular wide-complex rhythm is seen during atrial fibrillation. The morphology of this wide complex is similar to that of preexcited complexes shown in Figure 10-3. This most likely represents enhanced automaticity in the bypass tract. See text for discussion.

tachycardia, either antidromic or orthodromic, is not usually observed, but when it is, it is antidromic. The primary rhythm disturbance they manifest is atrial fibrillation, in which case, the bypass tract is not related to the mechanism of the fibrillation but serves as a conduit of rapid conduction to the ventricles.[60] A caveat to this estimate of bypass tracts that conduct only antegradely is that patients studied in electrophysiology laboratories are a selected group of patients. It is estimated by some that if a populational study of all asymptomatic patients with a WPW ECG were studied, the percent of patients with antegrade only conduction might be as high as 40% to 50%.[61]

As noted earlier, over time antegrade conduction over an atrioventricular bypass tract may disappear. Chen et al.[29] noted a loss of preexcitation in one-fifth of symptomatic patients with WPW. Only 7.8% lost retrograde conduction. Spontaneous loss of preexcitation has been observed in one-fifth to one-half of children with WPW.[30,62] In my experience, spontaneous loss of preexcitation occurs in less than 10% of adults (i.e., >18 years old), and loss of retrograde conduction is noted in <2% of patients. Data from our laboratory is limited by selection bias, which is a result of our university status and our early use of surgery and catheter ablation. The long-term natural history of patients with the WPW syndrome is currently virtually impossible to define in the Western world because of early intervention.

## ELECTROPHYSIOLOGIC EVALUATION IN PATIENTS WITH WOLFF–PARKINSON–WHITE SYNDROME

Electrophysiologic studies in patients with WPW are useful for (a) confirming the diagnosis; (b) studying the mode of initiation of tachycardias; (c) localizing the bypass tract; (d) demonstrating that the bypass tract participates in the tachycardias; (e) evaluating the refractoriness of the bypass tract and its implication for risk of life-threatening arrhythmias; (f) terminating tachycardias; and (g) aiding the development of pharmacologic, pacing, or ablative therapy for arrhythmias associated with WPW syndrome.

### Diagnosis of an A-V Bypass Tract

By definition, if an A-V bypass tract is present, activation of some part of the ventricles begins earlier than expected, so that the H-V interval (in this case, the His-to-delta-wave interval) is less than normal at rest and/or can be made less than normal by various maneuvers (Fig. 10-6). Because the QRS complex is a fusion complex of conduction (usually all-or-none) down a rapidly conducting bypass tract and conduction down the A-V node–His–Purkinje system, slowing of

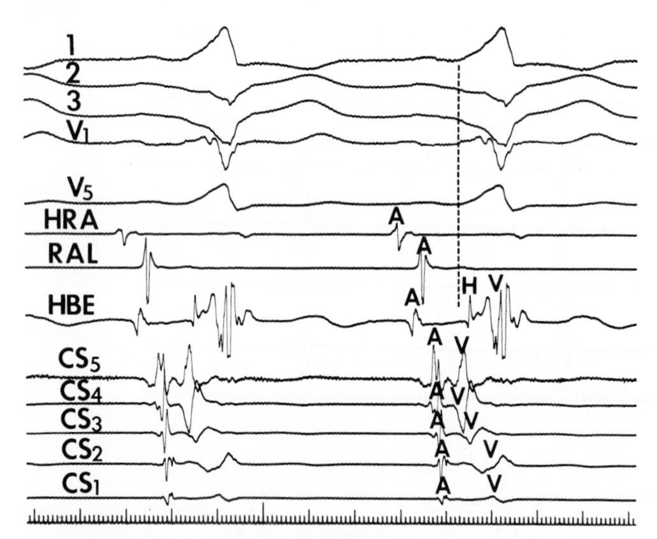


**FIGURE 10-6** *Intracardiac recordings demonstrating preexcitation.* ECG leads 1, 2, 3, V1, V5 are shown with recordings from the high-right atrium (HRA), lateral right atrium (RAL), His bundle (HBE), and proximal coronary sinus (CS5) to distal CS (CS1). During sinus rhythm the delta wave begins (dashed line) prior to anterograde activation of the His bundle confirming the presence of preexcitation. The ventricular electrogram in CS5 occurs just prior to the delta wave, suggesting proximity to the ventricular insertion of the bypass tract.

conduction down the normal pathway results in an increasing degree of preexcitation. Such slowing can make preexcitation manifest when it was inapparent during sinus rhythm. This can be achieved pharmacologically, by carotid sinus massage, or by atrial stimulation. Typically, atrial pacing or APDs, which prolong A-V nodal conduction, cause a greater degree of preexcitation because while the P-to-delta-wave interval remains constant, the P-to-His increases, resulting in a smaller component of ventricular depolarization initiated over the normal A-V conducting system and a greater component over the bypass tract (Figs. 10-7 to 10-9). While atrial pacing at progressively decreasing cycle lengths from any atrial site increases the amount of preexcitation, the degree of preexcitation is maximal and the P-to-delta is shortest at comparable paced cycle lengths if atrial pacing is performed at or near the atrial insertion site of the bypass tract. This is discussed later in this chapter as a means to locate a bypass tract.

The ability to change the degree of preexcitation by increasing A-V nodal conduction time in response to atrial stimulation supports the concept that the QRS complex is a fusion complex. The ultimate expression of dual ventricular activation is demonstrated in Figure 10-10, in which two ventricular responses are shown to result from a single APD: the first is over the bypass tract, and the second is over the normal A-V conducting system after marked antegrade A-V nodal conduction delay.[63] This phenomenon is almost always associated with dual A-V nodal pathways (see Chapter 8). This phenomenon is a potential mechanism for the development of either orthodromic or, rarely, A-V nodal reentrant tachycardia (AVNRT) which may be associated with anterograde conduction over an innocent bystander bypass tract (see discussion of preexcited tachycardias later in this chapter). Failure to increase the degree of preexcitation by atrial pacing or atrial extrastimuli may be due to (a) an additional A-V nodal bypass tract or markedly enhanced A-V nodal conduction, which prevents A-V nodal delay; (b) pacing-induced block in the A-V bypass tract that is due to a long refractory period exceeding that of the A-V node; or (c) total preexcitation that is present in the basal state as a result of prolonged or absent A-V conduction over the normal pathway.

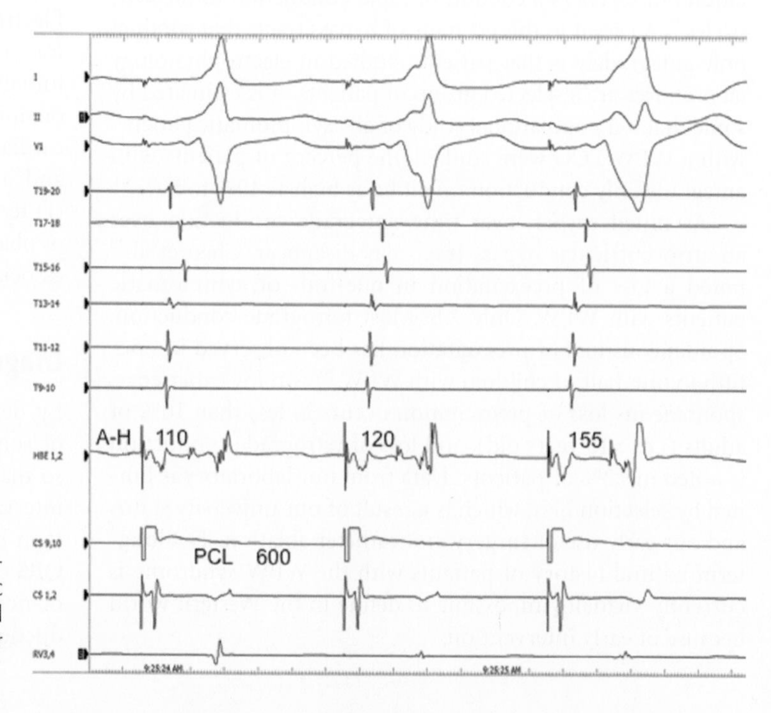


**FIGURE 10-7** *Effect of pacing on degree of Preexcitation.* Initiation of atrial pacing from the coronary sinus at 600 msec produces prolongation of the A-H interval which is associated with increasing preexcitation over a right anterior atrioventricular bypass tract. Note the constant p-delta.

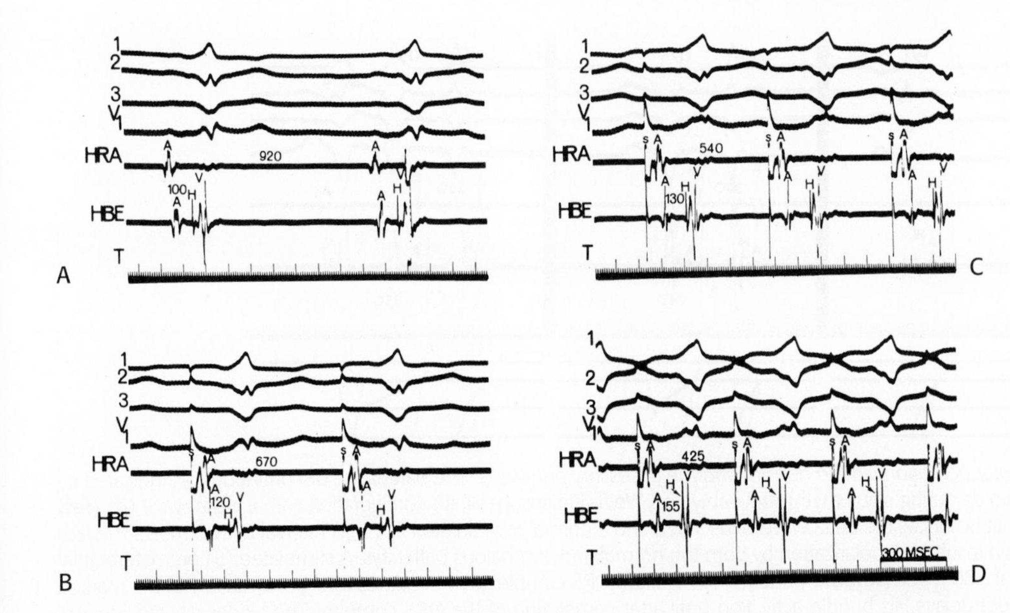


**FIGURE 10-8** *Effect of atrial pacing on the degree of preexcitation.* **A:** During sinus rhythm, a slight degree of preexcitation is present. **B–D:** With atrial pacing at decreasing cycle lengths, the degree of preexcitation increases due to progressive A-V nodal delay. See text for further details.

Pharmacologic and/or physiologic maneuvers that can alter A-V nodal conduction may also be used to alter the degree of preexcitation, therefore confirming the presence of a bypass tract and the concept of a fusion complex. Isoproterenol and atropine can decrease the degree of preexcitation by shortening A-V nodal conduction. This allows more of the ventricles to be activated over the normal pathway owing to enhanced A-V conduction and consequently reducing the component of ventricular activation over the bypass tract. Carotid sinus pressure, digoxin, beta blockers, calcium blockers, or adenosine can increase the degree of preexcitation by prolonging A-V nodal conduction so that most of the ventricles are activated over the bypass tract. Carotid sinus pressure may also result in transient A-V nodal block with a His bundle escape rhythm. This escape rhythm should manifest a normal (narrow) QRS complex if preexcitation were caused by an A-V connection (Fig. 10-11), but would not alter preexcitation if a bypass tract originated below the A-V node, as it would in a fasciculoventricular bypass tract (see discussion of Fasciculoventricular Bypass Tracts). Similar findings (i.e., normal QRS) would also be observed during His bundle pacing or during spontaneous His bundle extrasystoles (Fig. 10-12). Normalization of the QRS during a His bundle rhythm, particularly in the presence of drug or in response to a physiologic maneuver (e.g., carotid sinus pressure induced A-V block), confirm the origin of the bypass tract above the site of impulse formation of the escape rhythm, that is, in the high A-V node or in the atrium, with direct connection to the ventricle. While adenosine is widely used to produce transient A-V slowing or block in order to maximize preexcitation, it may induce atrial fibrillation, which may be associated with a rapid ventricular response.

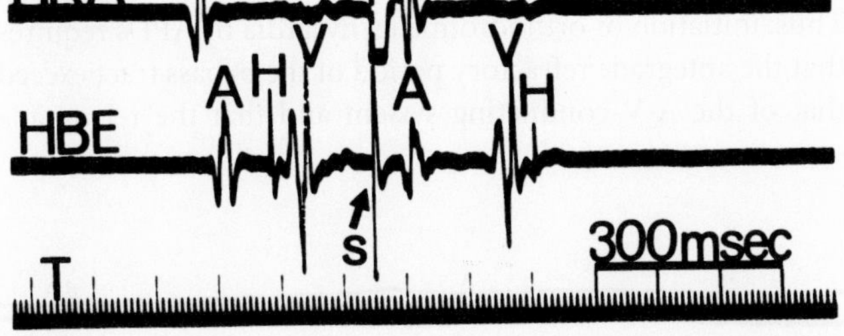

**FIGURE 10-9** *Effect of an (APD) on preexcitation.* Following the first complex during sinus rhythm, an APD is delivered, which produces marked A-V nodal conduction delay such that the antegrade H is inscribed within the terminal part of the QRS. Total ventricular preexcitation results over the bypass tract because completion of ventricular activation occurs before arrival of the impulse propagating over the normal conducting system.

## MODE OF INITIATION OF TACHYCARDIAS

As noted, the most common tachycardias associated with the WPW syndrome are the circus movement tachycardias, 95% of which are orthodromic; that is, they conduct antegradely down the normal A-V conducting system and retrogradely up the bypass tract. The relationship of conduction and refractoriness of the normal A-V conducting system and the bypass tract, as well as the site of stimulation, determine both the ability to initiate circus movement tachycardia and, theoretically, the type of circus movement tachycardia.[38,64,65] Conduction and refractoriness of the bypass tracts in most cases behave like working muscle; therefore, bypass tracts demonstrate rapid conduction, and have refractory periods that tend to shorten at decreasing paced cycle lengths. The WPW syndrome allows one to actually see all the requirements for

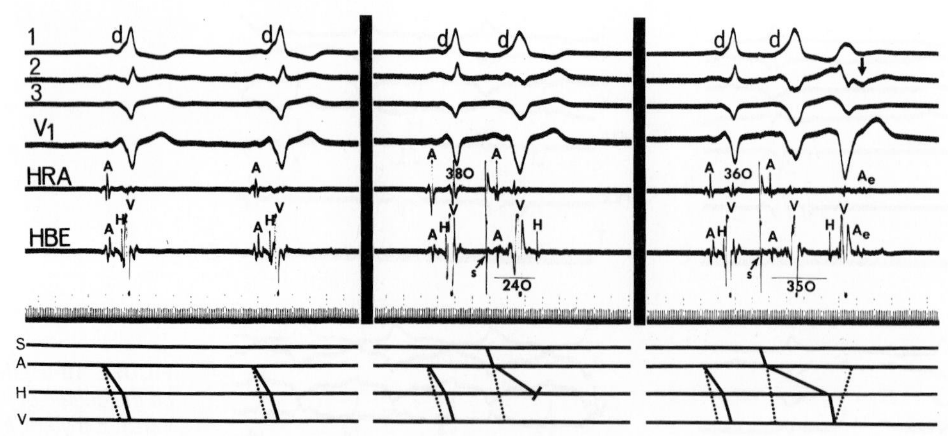


**FIGURE 10-10** *APD resulting in ventricular activation via the normal and the accessory pathways.* The panels are discontinuous, as indicated by the heavy black vertical lines. Control records during sinus rhythm reveal typical Wolff–Parkinson–White configuration with a delta wave (d) (**left** panel). Note the His bundle deflection that occurs as the delta wave is inscribed and a normal stimulus-to-His (S-H) interval of 100 msec. The ladder diagram depicts the QRS complex as a result of depolarization by both the normal and anomalous pathways. A stimulated (S) premature atrial beat is introduced at a coupling interval of 380 msec (**middle** panel). The resultant QRS complex demonstrates total preexcitation as the marked A-V nodal delay (S-H interval = 240 msec) delays His bundle activation until after completion of the QRS complex. The ladder diagram depicts the dissociation of conduction between both pathways in response to the atrial premature beat. The stimulated (S) atrial beat is delivered at 360 msec (**right** panel). The first QRS complex results from excitation solely over the anomalous pathway. A-V nodal conduction is greatly prolonged (S-H interval = 350 msec) so that the ventricle can be reexcited over the normal pathway. The second ventricular response demonstrates aberrant conduction with an H-V interval of 50 msec. An atrial echo (Ae), manifested as an inverted P wave in lead 2 (*arrow*), results from retrograde conduction over the anomalous pathway, as shown in the ladder diagram. In the ladder diagrams, S, stimulus; A, atrium; H, His bundle; and V, ventricle. Anomalous pathway conduction is depicted by dotted lines, and normal A-V conduction is depicted by solid lines. (From Josephson ME, Seides SF, Damato AN. Wolff-Parkinson-White syndrome with 1:2 atrioventricular conduction. *Am J Cardiol* 1976;37:1094.)

a reentrant rhythm: (a) two anatomic or functionally determined pathways of conduction; (b) unidirectional block in one of the pathways (in this instance, either in the accessory pathway or in the A-V nodal His pathway); (c) sufficient slowing in part of the circuit to overcome refractoriness ahead of the circulating impulse; and (d) conduction time of the impulse must exceed the longest effective refractory period of any component in the circuit. Both antegrade and retrograde refractory periods of the accessory pathway are major determinants of (a) the ability to initiate and sustain circus movement SVT, and (b) the ventricular responses to atrial tachyarrhythmias (e.g., atrial fibrillation, atrial flutter, and atrial tachycardia).

## ORTHODROMIC TACHYCARDIA

The most common tachyarrhythmia in patients with WPW is orthodromic circus movement SVT in which antegrade conduction proceeds down the normal A-V conducting system and retrograde conduction occurs over the bypass tract, with intervening atrial and ventricular tissue completing the reentrant circuit. This is the identical circuit observed in reentrant SVT using a concealed bypass tract (described in detail in Chapter 8). As with patients with concealed bypass tracts, patients with WPW have orthodromic tachycardia initiated most commonly in response to spontaneous or stimulated APDs. The only difference between orthodromic tachycardias in patients with concealed bypass tracts and those with overt preexcitation is that antegrade block is already present in patients with concealed bypass tracts. In patients with WPW, the APD serves a dual purpose: (a) It produces block in the accessory pathway, and (b) it conducts slowly enough down the normal A-V conducting system and ventricles to allow that bypass tract and the atrium to recover excitability. Thus, initiation of orthodromic tachycardia by APDs requires that the antegrade refractory period of the bypass tract exceed that of the A-V conducting system and that the retrograde

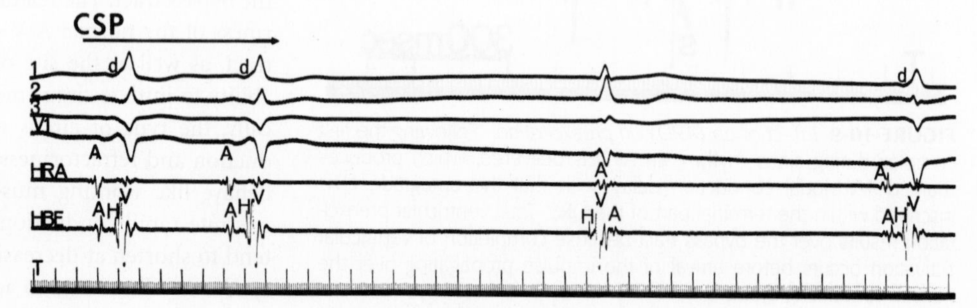


**FIGURE 10-11** *Use of carotid sinus pressure to diagnose an A-V bypass tract.* Carotid sinus pressure (CSP) produces sinus slowing with a His bundle escape complex with a normal QRS complex. Normalization of the QRS complex during a His bundle rhythm rules out a fasciculoventricular bypass tract. See text for discussion.

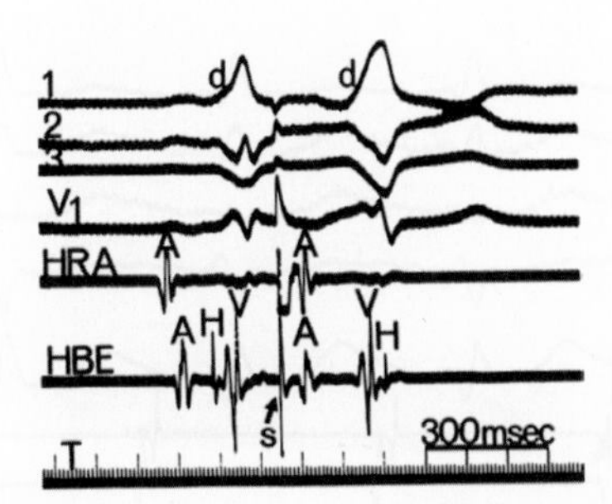
1
2
3
V1
HRA
HBE
T
d
d
A
A
H
V
A
V
H
S
300msec

**FIGURE 10-12** *Effect of a His extrasystole on preexcitation.* A sinus complex with preexcitation is shown on the **left**. Note that the onset of the delta wave (d) begins simultaneously with activation over the His bundle. This is followed by a His extrasystole, which has a normal QRS and a normal H-V. Retrograde atrial activation occurs simultaneously with a QRS. The loss of preexcitation with a His extrasystole suggests the origin of the bypass tract above the site of impulse formation.

refractory period of the bypass tract and the refractory period of the atrium recover by the time the ventricle is activated antegradely over the A-V conducting system. This sequence is schematically shown in Figure 10-13.

The coupling interval of APDs required to initiate SVT in the WPW syndrome is somewhat shorter than that required for induction of circus movement tachycardia in patients with concealed bypass tract. This is a consequence of the fact that block in the bypass tract is required for initiation of the tachycardia. Because block is already present in patients with concealed bypass tracts, APDs delivered at longer coupling intervals may be sufficient to produce the requisite delay for reentry to occur. In our experience, the antegrade effective refractory period of the bypass tract (determined at a mean paced cycle length of 600 msec) in the majority of patients presenting with orthodromic tachycardia lies between 250 and 350 msec with a mean of just over 300 msec and a range of 180 to 600 msec. These data are comparable to those of Wellens and Brugada.[38] In patients with bypass tracts demonstrating long antegrade effective refractory periods, particularly those with intermittent preexcitation, tachycardias can be more readily induced by late coupled APDs. Once block in the bypass tract is accomplished and antegrade conduction proceeds to the ventricle over the normal A-V conducting system, it is primarily the retrograde refractory period of the bypass tract and recovery of atrial refractoriness at the atrial insertion site of the bypass tract that determines whether or not a circus movement tachycardia will be initiated. For orthodromic tachycardia to occur, the retrograde refractory period of the bypass tract must be less than the conduction time over the A-V conducting system and through the ventricles. In addition, the refractory period of the atrium at the atrial site of insertion of the bypass tract must be shorter than that of the conduction time through the normal A-V conduction system, ventricle, and bypass tract to complete the circuit. Perpetuation of the tachycardia requires that the refractory period of any part of the tachycardia circuit be shorter than that of the tachycardia cycle length.

With this in mind, initiation of orthodromic SVT by APDs obviously requires some degree of A-V delay to allow recovery of the bypass tract, the atrium into which it is inserted, and the A-V node. As expected, the site of critical delay required

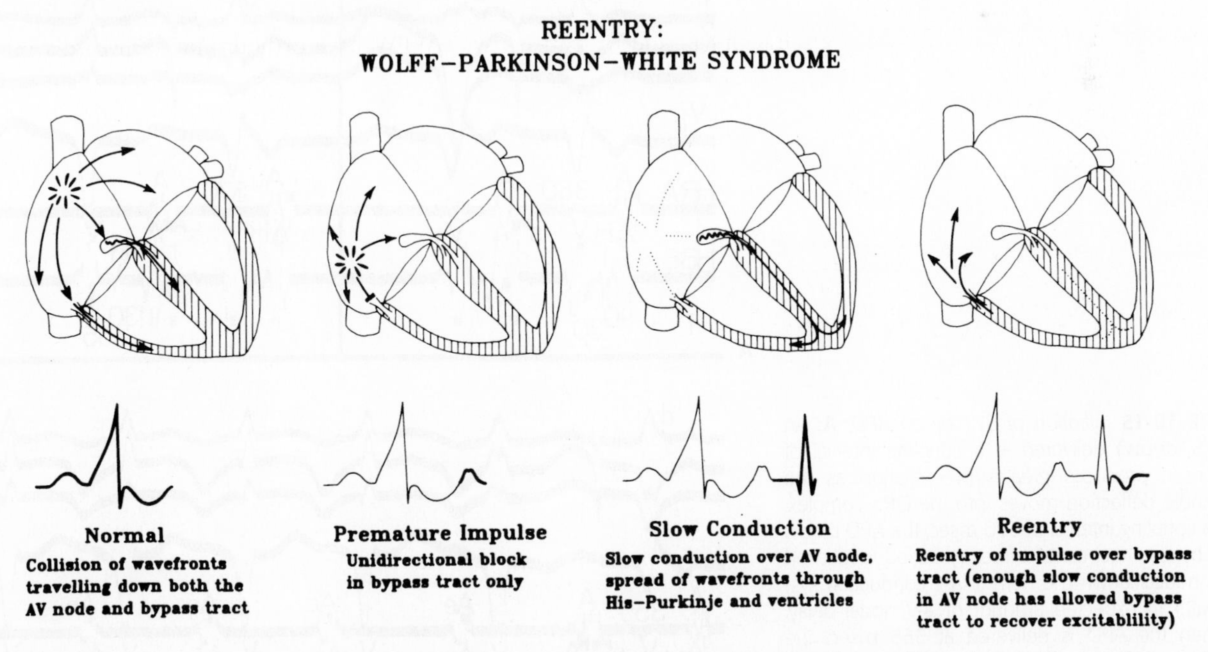
REENTRY:
WOLFF–PARKINSON–WHITE SYNDROME
Normal
Collision of wavefronts travelling down both the AV node and bypass tract
Premature Impulse
Unidirectional block in bypass tract only
Slow Conduction
Slow conduction over AV node, spread of wavefronts through His–Purkinje and ventricles
Reentry
Reentry of impulse over bypass tract (enough slow conduction in AV node has allowed bypass tract to recover excitablility)

**FIGURE 10-13** *Mechanism of initiation of SVT by an APD in WPW syndrome.* An ECG lead 2 is shown with a schema of intracardiac events. The first complex is sinus and represents a fusion with ventricular depolarization produced by activation over the normal and the accessory pathways. In the second complex, an APD blocks in the accessory pathway, and in the third complex the atrial impulse conducts slowly to the ventricles over the normal conducting system, giving rise to a normal QRS complex. In the fourth complex the reentrant circuit is completed by retrograde conduction over the bypass tract. See text for discussion.

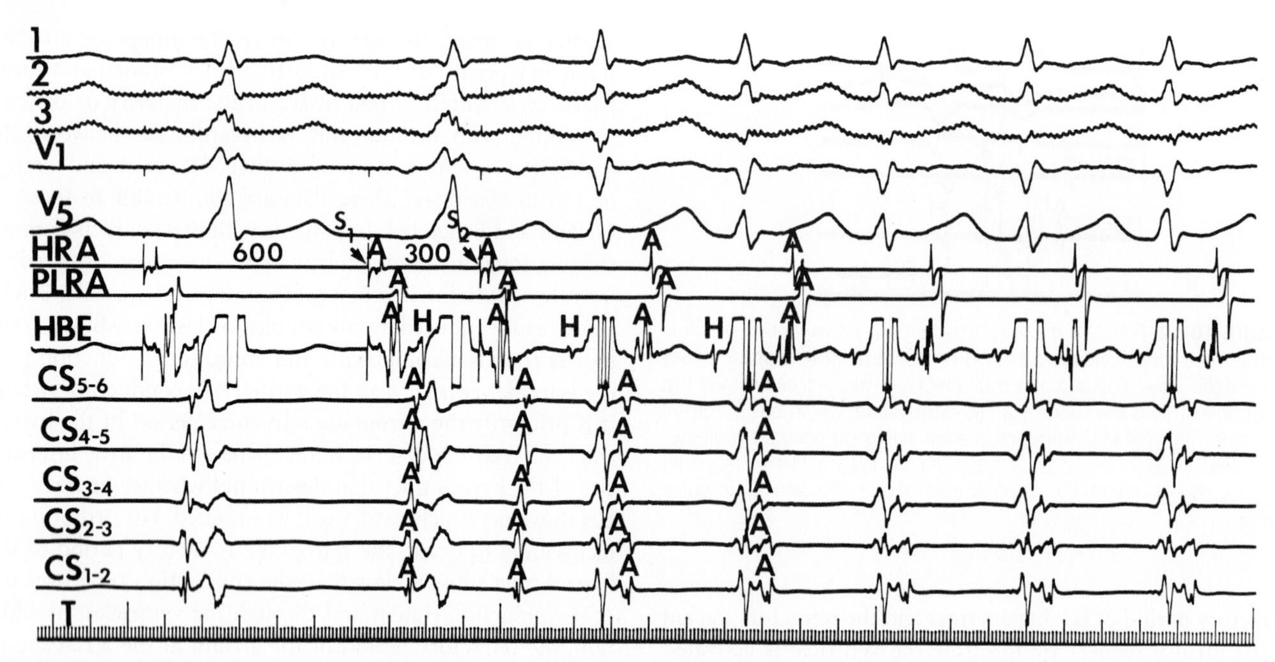


**FIGURE 10-14** *Initiation of orthodromic SVT immediately on developing antegrade block on the bypass tract.* Leads 1, 2, 3, V1, and V5 are shown with electrograms from the HRA, posterolateral RA (PLRA), HBE, and five bipolar CS electrograms. The electrode pairs from which the recordings are made are shown with each CS recording: 1, the distal electrode; 6, the most proximal electrode. During pacing at a cycle length of 600 msec, block in the bypass tract occurred at a coupling interval (S1-S2) of 300 msec. The modest increase in the A-H interval observed at this time is enough to provide time for the bypass tract to recover excitability and conduct retrogradely to initiate the tachycardia.

for initiation is most commonly in the A-V node; however, the delay may also occur anywhere in the His–Purkinje system, bundle branches, or ventricular myocardium. Most often, enough delay is already present at the coupling interval at which the bypass tract blocks for initiation of the tachycardia (Fig. 10-14). If A-V delay is not sufficient to allow the bypass tract to recover, further shortening of atrial coupling intervals is required to initiate the tachycardia (Fig. 10-15). However,

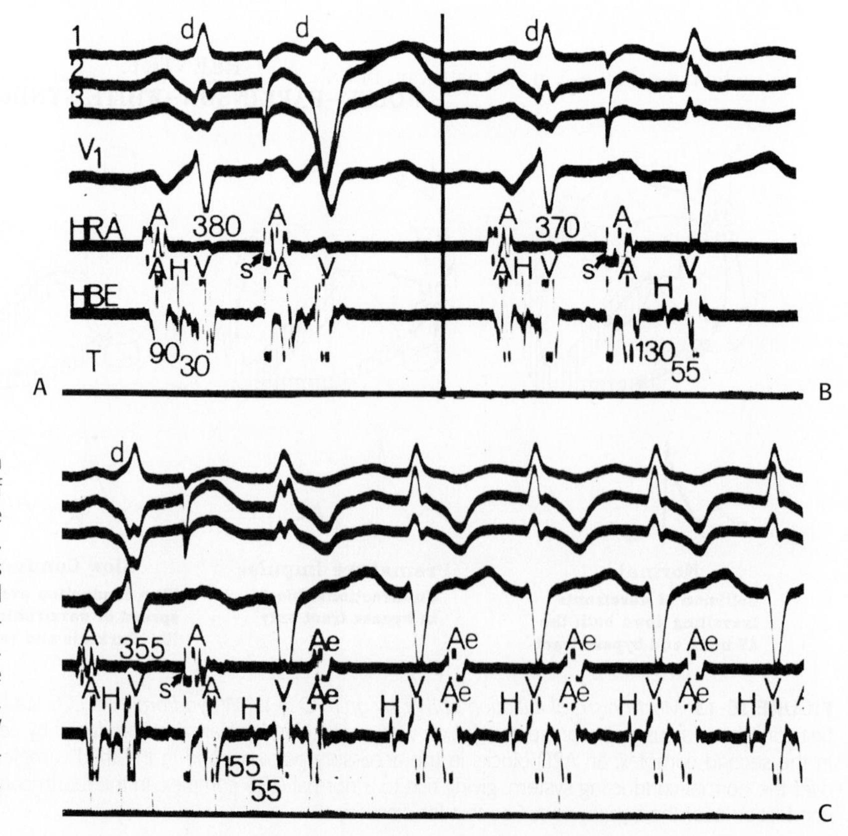


**FIGURE 10-15** *Initiation of SVT by an APD.* **A:** An APD (S, *arrow*) delivered at a coupling interval of 380 msec produces greater preexcitation as the His bundle deflection moves into the QRS complex. **B:** At a coupling interval of 370 msec, the APD blocks in the bypass tract as its refractory period is reached and conducts down the normal A-V conduction system with an expected amount of A-V nodal delay. **C:** When the APD is delivered at 355 msec, the impulse again blocks in the bypass tract; however, since it conducts antegradely with slightly more A-V nodal delay, the recovered bypass tract can be depolarized retrogradely, completing the reentrant circuit, thereby resulting in SVT. See text for discussion.

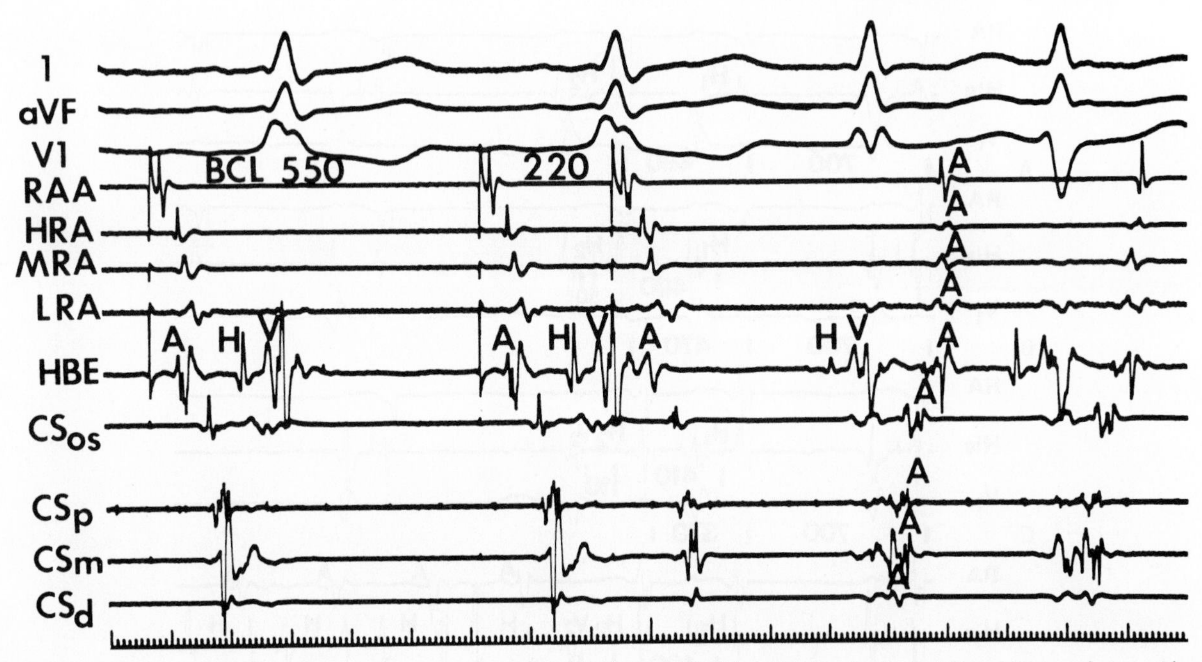


**FIGURE 10-16** *Initiation of orthodromic tachycardia in a patient with dual A-V nodal pathways.* Leads 1, aVF, and V1 are shown with electrograms from the right atrial appendage (RAA), HRA, mid- and low-right atrium (MRA, LRA), HBE, and four recordings from the CS beginning most proximally at the os ($CS_{os}$). During pacing at a basic cycle length (ECL) of 550 msec, conduction to the A-V node is over the fast pathway with an A-H of approximately 100 msec. Minimal preexcitation over a left lateral bypass tract is seen. Block in the bypass tract occurred at 270 msec, but not enough anterograde delay occurred to allow the bypass tract to recover. This was due to the intra-arterial conduction delay in addition to conduction over the fast pathway. When the coupling interval reached 220 msec, a jump to the slow pathway was observed, with marked prolongation of the A-H interval to 300 msec. This was more than enough time to allow the left-sided bypass tract time to recover and initiate SVT.

as noted, because the coupling intervals of APDs required to produce block in the bypass tract are usually short, enough A-V nodal delay is usually present so that the tachycardia is initiated at the onset of block. This is particularly true in patients who have dual A-V nodal pathways but no A-V nodal reentry. Early coupled APDs conduct over the "slow" pathway, providing more than enough A-V delay to initiate the tachycardia (Fig. 10-16). The critical requirement of His–Purkinje delay to initiate the tachycardia is shown in Figure 10-17. The importance of bundle branch block in initiation of tachycardias has been discussed in detail in Chapter 8 and is discussed again subsequently in this chapter. Basically, block in the bundle branch ipsilateral to a free wall bypass tract provides an additional amount of intramyocardial conduction delay, which allows the bypass tract or its atrial insertion time to recovery excitability. Thus, the site of delay is unimportant; all that matters is that all tissues in advance of the circulating impulse have recovered excitability.

The site of stimulation may also be important, particularly if the limiting factor for initiation of the tachycardia is atrial refractoriness (i.e., atrial refractoriness prohibits the impulse from traversing the fully excitable bypass tract and activating the atrium). To obviate this limitation, one must stimulate near the atrial insertion of the bypass tract. This facilitates initiation for two reasons: (a) the closer the stimulation to the bypass tract, the easier it is to encroach on the refractory period of the bypass tract and achieve block; and (b) the earlier the atrium (or the bypass tract) is activated, the earlier it will recover, thereby facilitating reentry. Thus, one may actually require less antegrade delay if recovery of excitability is shifted earlier in time. This is shown in Figure 10-18, in which stimulation from the high-right atrium had failed to initiate a tachycardia, but stimulation from the coronary sinus initiated the tachycardia with minimal prolongation of A-V nodal conduction (A-H = 130 msec).

Occasionally, single atrial extrastimuli cannot induce block and/or enough delay to initiate tachycardia, and other modes of initiation are required. These include the induction of sinoatrial, intra-atrial, or A-V nodal echoes, which then either block in the bypass tract and/or produce enough conduction delay down the normal pathway to reenter the atria via the bypass tract. Similarly, rapid atrial pacing or the use of multiple extrastimuli can produce sudden block in the bypass tract and initiate SVT where single extrastimuli cannot. In some patients, drug-induced block in the bypass tract or drug-induced prolongation of the bypass tract refractory periods enables an increase in sinus rate to induce block in the bypass tract. This latter mechanism may lead to incessant SVT. Finally, atrial extrastimuli also can initiate tachycardias by a variety of 1:2 conduction phenomena (see Fig. 10-10); an atrial impulse conducts both over the bypass tract and over the normal A-V system. In Figure 10-19, stimulation at the distal coronary sinus (not shown) conducts over the bypass tract and through the A-V node, but conduction down the A-V conducting system initially cannot occur because either the His–Purkinje system or ventricles are encountered during

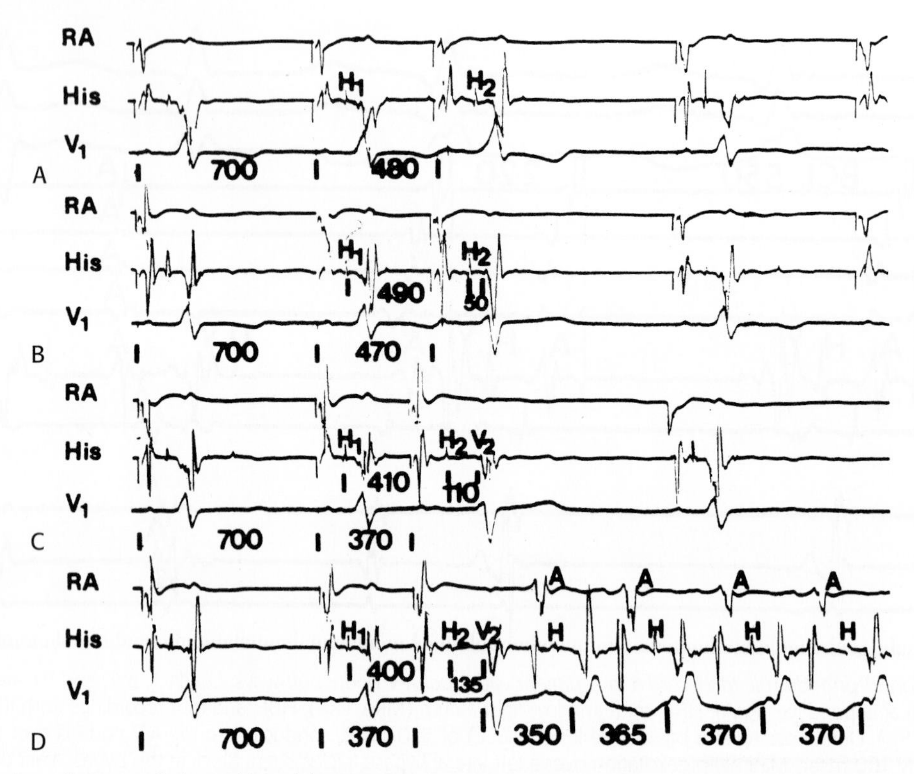


**FIGURE 10-17** *Critical requirement of His–Purkinje delay to initiate circus movement tachycardia.* **A–D:** Right atrial (RA) pacing is carried out at a cycle length of 700 msec, and progressively premature atrial extrastimuli are delivered. **A:** Antegrade conduction proceeds over the bypass tract (note broad delta wave in V1). **B:** When the atrial coupling interval is reduced to 470 msec, block in the bypass tract occurs with a normal A-H and H-V interval. No retrograde conduction over the bypass tract is noted. **C:** A coupling interval of 370 msec results in minimal prolongation of the A-H interval but an increase in the infra-His conduction time to 110 msec. Despite this delay, retrograde conduction over the bypass tract is still not possible. **D:** Despite similar coupling intervals, a slightly shorter H1-$H_2$ interval results, which leads to an increase in the H2-V2 interval. Only after the H2-V2 interval reaches a critical value of 135 msec is retrograde conduction over the bypass tract is possible and tachycardia is initiated. (From Wellens HJJ, Brugada P. Value of programmed stimulation of the heart in patients with the Wolff-Parkinson-White syndrome. In: Josephson ME, Wellens HJJ, eds. *Tachycardias: mechanisms and management.* Philadelphia: Lea & Febiger, 1962:199.)

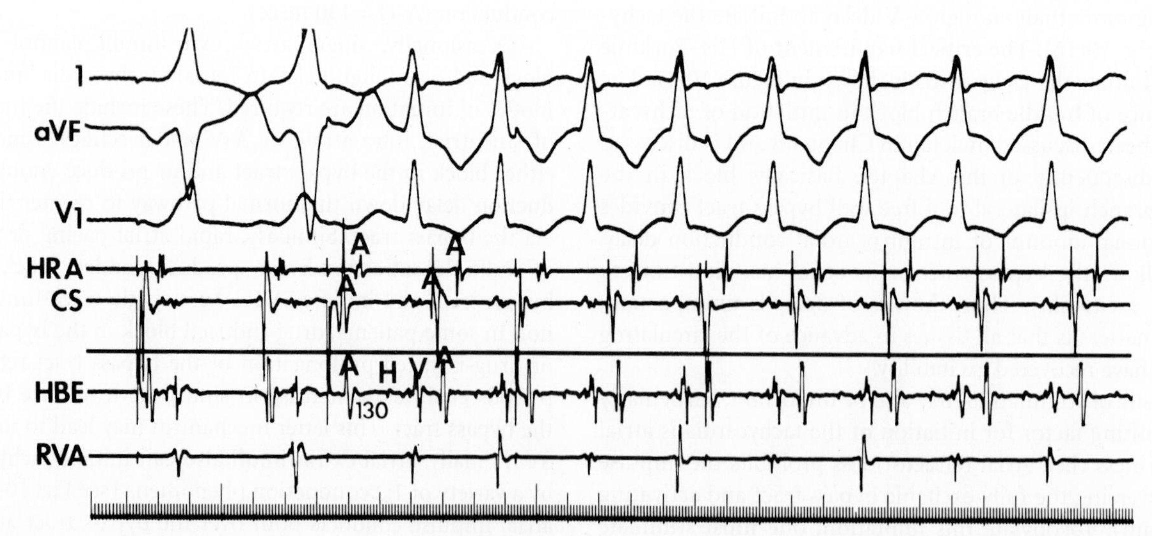


**FIGURE 10-18** *Effect of site of stimulation on initiation of a tachycardia.* In this patient with a left posterior bypass tract, stimulation from the HRA failed to initiate a tachycardia despite being able to block in the bypass tract. Stimulation from the CS, at the site of the bypass tract, initiated SVT despite only a modest increase in A-H interval to only 130 msec. The ability of CS stimulation to initiate the tachycardia is based on the fact that the earlier the site of the bypass tract is activated, the earlier it will recover. Therefore, at comparable coupling intervals of atrial extrastimuli, the bypass tract will always be able to recover more easily when stimulation is initiated from the site of the bypass tract (see text for discussion). RVA, right ventricular apex.

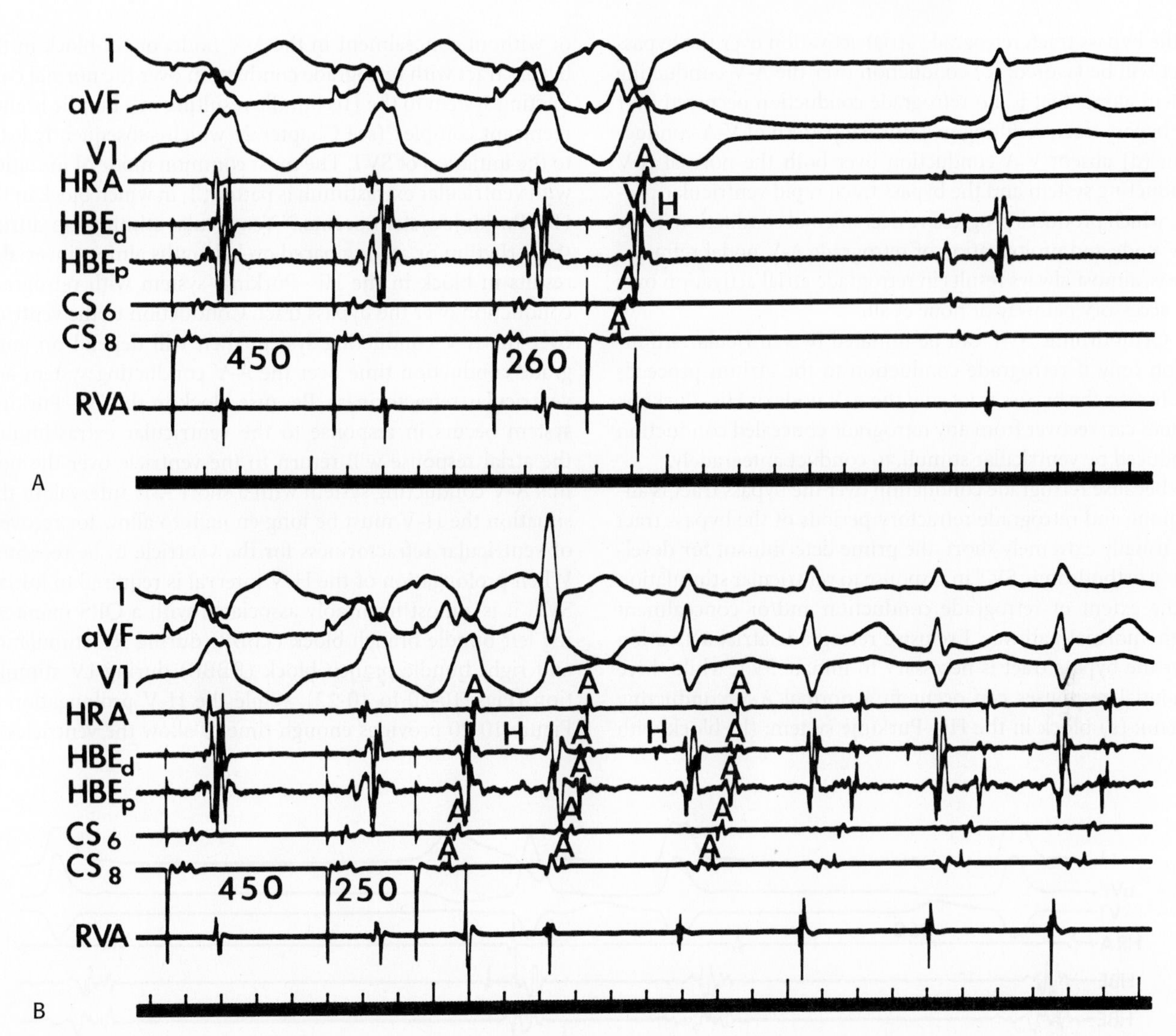


**FIGURE 10-19** *Initiation of orthodromic tachycardia by 1:2 conduction phenomenon to the A-V node.* Leads 1, aVF, and V1 and electrograms from the HRA, $HBE_d$, and $HBE_p$, the mid-posterior (CS6) and left lateral (CS8) coronary sinus, and RVA. **A:** During a paced cycle length of 450 msec, an atrial extrastimulus delivered from the distal CS (not shown) produces delay in the A-H so that the antegrade His deflection occurs after completion of the totally preexcited QRS complex. Antegrade conduction cannot proceed to the ventricles, because they have just been depolarized and are refractory. **B:** At a coupling interval 10 msec earlier, the A-H is sufficiently prolonged that the ventricles are no longer refractory and the antegrade impulse can result in a second ventricular activation over the normal A-V conducting system and can initiate SVT. See text for discussion.

a refractory state. When the coupling interval is reduced to 250 msec, both A-H and H-V prolongation allow conduction to proceed to the ventricles, with the subsequent development of reentry over the left-sided bypass tract. Stimulation from the coronary sinus also allowed the left atrial insertion site of the bypass tract to recover excitability earlier than if right atrial stimulation had been employed. This was an additional factor in facilitating initiation of circus movement tachycardia.

Initiation of orthodromic circus movement tachycardia by ventricular stimulation is possible in 80% of patients. Modes of initiation and incidence of initiation are identical to tachycardia induction by ventricular stimulation in patients with concealed bypass tracts (see Chapter 8). Several patterns of V-A conduction can be observed during ventricular pacing and ventricular extrastimuli:[38,66,67] (a) Conduction over the accessory pathway alone (the most common pattern at short paced cycle lengths and short coupling intervals); the V-A conduction time is the same over a wide range of VPD coupling intervals and paced cycle lengths in the absence of intraventricular conduction delay or the presence of additional bypass tracts; (b) conduction over both the accessory pathway and the A-V conducting system; this is particularly common when right ventricular pacing is performed at long drive cycle lengths or right ventricular extrastimuli are delivered at long coupling intervals in patients with left-sided bypass tracts. This occurs because it is easier to engage the right bundle branch and conduct retrogradely through the A-V node than it is to reach a distant left-sided bypass tract. The atrial activation pattern depends on the relative refractoriness and conduction times over both pathways and usually exhibits a variable degree of atrial fusion. If the retrograde refractory period and/or conduction time of any of the components of the A-V conducting system exceeds that of the bypass tract, retrograde atrial activation over the bypass tract will be favored; (c) conduction over the A-V conducting system alone; that is, no retrograde conduction occurred over the bypass tract, resulting in a normal pattern of V-A conduction; (d) absent V-A conduction over both the normal A-V conducting system and the bypass tract; rapid ventricular pacing, which produces progressive decremental conduction in the A-V node and prolongation of retrograde A-V nodal refractoriness, almost always results in retrograde atrial activation over the accessory pathway or none at all.

Orthodromic SVT can be initiated by ventricular stimulation only if retrograde conduction to the atrium proceeds solely over the bypass tract, and the A-V node or His–Purkinje system can recover from any retrograde concealed conduction produced by ventricular stimuli, to conduct antegradely.

Because retrograde conduction over the bypass tract is all-or-none and retrograde refractory periods of the bypass tract are usually extremely short, the prime determinant for developing orthodromic SVT in response to ventricular stimulation is the extent of retrograde conduction and/or concealment in the normal pathway. Exclusive retrograde atrial activation over the bypass tract is necessary to initiate SVT, while three potential responses can occur in a normal A-V conducting system: (a) block in the His–Purkinje system; (b) block with or without concealment in the A-V node; or (c) block in the bypass tract with retrograde conduction over the normal conducting system to the His bundle resulting in a bundle branch reentrant complex (see Chapter 2) which subsequently leads to the initiation of SVT. The most common mode of initiation with ventricular extrastimuli is pattern 1, in which block in the His–Purkinje system occurs.[66] Ventricular stimulation during sinus rhythm or at long paced cycle lengths almost invariably results in block in the His–Purkinje system with retrograde conduction over the bypass tract. Conduction to the ventricle over the A-V conducting system then will depend on antegrade conduction time over the A-V conducting system and ventricular refractoriness. Because block in the His–Purkinje system occurs in response to the ventricular extrastimulus, the atrial response will return to the ventricle over the normal A-V conducting system with a short A-H interval. In this situation the H-V must be long enough to allow for recovery of ventricular refractoriness for the ventricle to be reexcited. When prolongation of the H-V interval is required to initiate SVT, it is almost invariably associated with a QRS manifesting left bundle branch block (LBBB) during RV stimulation and right bundle branch block (RBBB) during LV stimulation (Figs. 10-20 to 10-22). While the H-V prolongation in Figure 10-20 provides enough time to allow the ventricles to

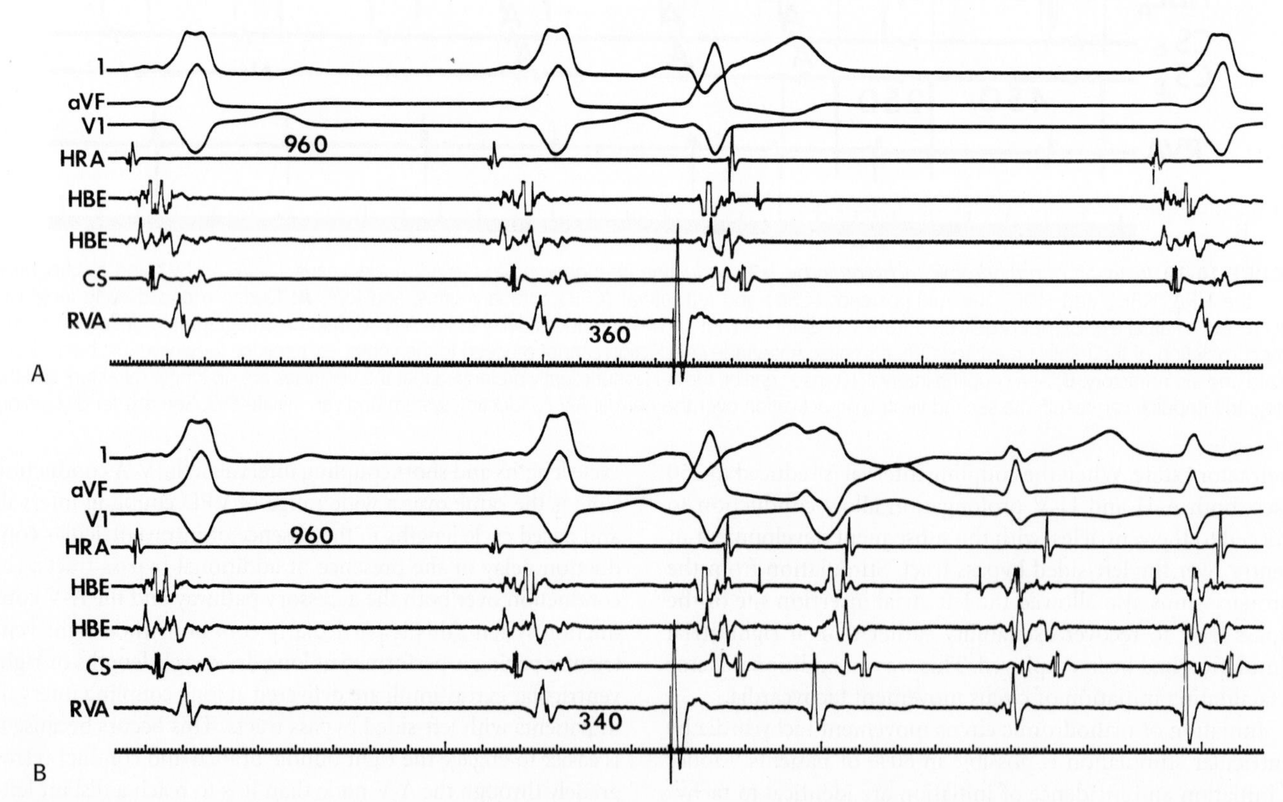


**FIGURE 10-20** *Initiation of orthodromic SVT by a VPD during sinus rhythm.* **A:** Following the first two sinus complexes, which conduct over an anteroseptal bypass tract, a VPD is delivered at a coupling interval of 360 msec. This blocks in the His–Purkinje system and conducts retrogradely solely over the anteroseptal bypass tract. Antegrade conduction, however, fails because of block below the His. **B:** When the coupling interval is reduced to 340 msec, antegrade conduction is associated with a marked H-V prolongation, which allows the ventricle to be reexcited and to initiate SVT. The left bundle branch block pattern of the first complex does not provide additional delay for this anteroseptal bypass tract to recover. See text for discussion.

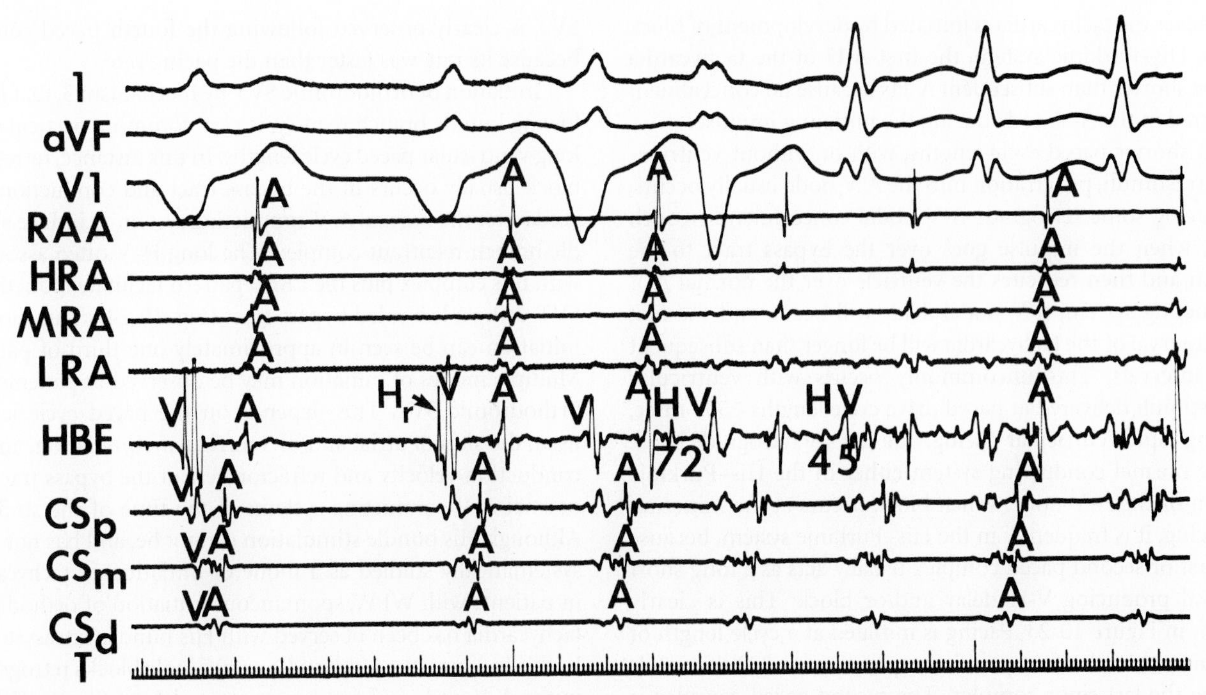


**FIGURE 10-21** *Initiation of orthodromic SVT by a VPD during ventricular pacing.* During ventricular pacing from the (RV) (not shown), at a paced cycle length of 600 msec, a ventricular extrastimulus delivered at 320 msec initiates SVT. The initiating VPD produces block in the His–Purkinje system (note loss of retrograde His deflection) and conduction retrogradely over a left lateral bypass tract. The impulse then returns antegradely over the normal A-V conducting system to initiate the tachycardia. The initiation depends on H-V prolongation, which is modest, and left bundle branch block (LBBB), both of which allow enough time for the left lateral bypass tract to recover excitability and to initiate the tachycardia. Neither H-V prolongation nor LBBB is necessary to maintain the tachycardia. See text for discussion.

recover, the shorter amount of H-V prolongation shown in Figures 10-21 and 10-22 suggests that the intraventricular conduction delay produced by LBBB aberration associated with the first echo provides the critical amount of delay, which allows for atrial reexcitation over the bypass tract to initiate the tachycardia. In Figure 10-20 perpetuation of the SVT is ensured by marked A-V nodal conduction delay associated with dual A-V nodal pathways. In Figure 10-22 perpetuation of the tachycardia probably also requires the LBBB pattern, because both the A-H and H-V intervals remain fairly short.

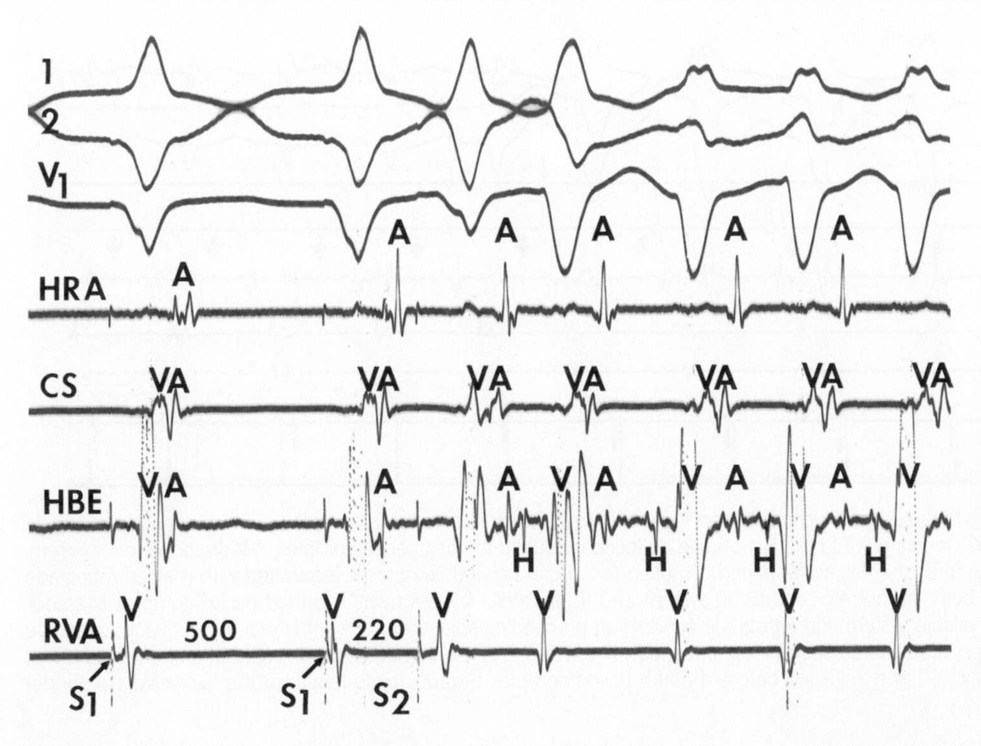


**FIGURE 10-22** *Initiation of orthodromic SVT by ventricular stimulation.* During ventricular pacing (V1-V1), a VPD (V2) is introduced at a coupling interval of 220 msec. Retrograde conduction of V2 proceeds over a left-sided bypass tract and initiates SVT. The A-H and H-V intervals of the initiating beat are short, suggesting that the LBBB provides the critical delay, allowing the left-sided bypass tract to recover excitability. Moreover, the maintenance of this tachycardia, which is associated with rather short A-H and H-V intervals, is also facilitated by the LBBB. See text for discussion.

Whenever the tachycardia is initiated by development of block in the His–Purkinje system, the first A-H of the tachycardia will be shorter than subsequent A-Hs because no concealment occurred in the A-V node during the initiating impulse.

At shorter paced cycle lengths, with or without ventricular extrastimuli, penetration into the A-V node usually occurs, producing some retrograde A-V nodal concealment. In such cases, when the impulse goes over the bypass tract to the atrium and then reexcites the ventricle over the normal A-V conducting system, A-V nodal delay will occur, and the first A-H interval of the tachycardia will be longer than subsequent A-H intervals. This uncommonly occurs with ventricular extrastimuli delivered at paced drive cycle lengths ≥500 msec. During rapid ventricular pacing, one can see retrograde block in the normal conducting system either in the His–Purkinje system or the A-V node. When block occurs at the initiation of pacing, it is frequently in the His–Purkinje system, because the first or second paced complex usually acts as a long short interval producing V-H delay and/or block. This is clearly shown in Figure 10-23. Pacing is initiated at a cycle length of 400 msec, but the first paced complex occurs 800 msec following the last sinus complex. The second paced complex is associated with a long V-H interval owing to block in the right bundle branch retrogradely with conduction over the left bundle branch system (see Chapter 2). Simultaneously, the ventricular stimulus conducts solely over a left-sided bypass tract to the atrium. SVT does not develop because of retrograde concealment in the A-V node. Following the third paced complex, complete block in the His–Purkinje system occurs, and an antegrade His bundle deflection follows atrial activation, which resulted from conduction over the bypass tract. The fourth paced complex preempted the ability to see SVT, which would have been initiated at that time, but orthodromic SVT is clearly observed following the fourth paced complex because its rate was faster than the pacing rate.

Initiation of orthodromic SVT by mechanism 3, that is, following bundle branch reentry, is very common, particularly at long ventricular paced cycle lengths. In this instance, retrograde block usually occurs in the bypass tract and conduction proceeds over the normal A-V conducting system to induce a bundle branch reentrant complex. The long H-V often associated with this complex plus the LBBB pattern facilitate induction of SVT using a left-sided bypass tract (Fig. 10-24). This mode of initiation can be seen in approximately one-third of patients. Multiple modes of initiation may be observed in patients with orthodromic SVT. This depends on the paced cycle lengths used, the sites of atrial and/or ventricular stimulation, and the conduction velocity and refractoriness of the bypass tract and normal A-V conducting systems at the time of the study.[38,68] Although His bundle stimulation cannot be, and has not been, systematically studied as a mode of initiation of tachycardias in patients with WPW, spontaneous initiation of orthodromic tachycardia has been observed with His bundle extrasystoles.[39] In this instance, the His bundle extrasystole blocks retrogradely in the A-V node and conducts antegradely to the ventricles to retrogradely conduct over the bypass tract, reexcite the atrium, and return to the ventricles over the normal A-V conducting system. In this case, owing to retrograde concealment, the first A-H interval of the tachycardia will usually be slightly longer than that of subsequent complexes (Fig. 10-25).

## PREEXCITED TACHYCARDIAS

Preexcited circus movement tachycardias are much less frequent, perhaps occurring spontaneously in 5% to 10% of

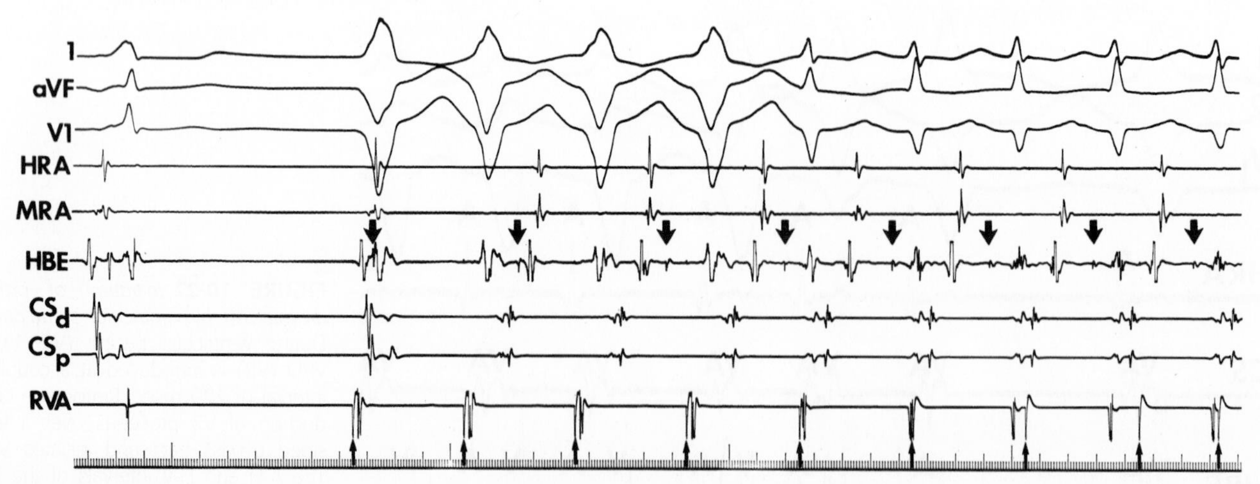


**FIGURE 10-23** *Initiation of orthodromic tachycardia by ventricular pacing.* Following the first spontaneous complex, ventricular pacing at a cycle length of 400 msec is initiated. The *dark arrows* point to the His bundle deflections. During the first paced complex, A-V dissociation is present, but the His bundle is retrogradely captured by the ventricular paced complex. The second paced complex is associated with marked retrograde His–Purkinje delay and conduction up both the normal conducting system and a left lateral bypass tract. The third paced complex is associated with retrograde block in the His–Purkinje system and retrograde conduction proceeding solely over the left lateral bypass tract. Antegrade conduction over the normal conducting system can be seen by the antegrade H (*arrow*). SVT would have been initiated at that time but it was preempted by the fourth paced complex. SVT is manifested before the fifth paced complex because cycle length of the tachycardia is shorter than the paced cycle length.

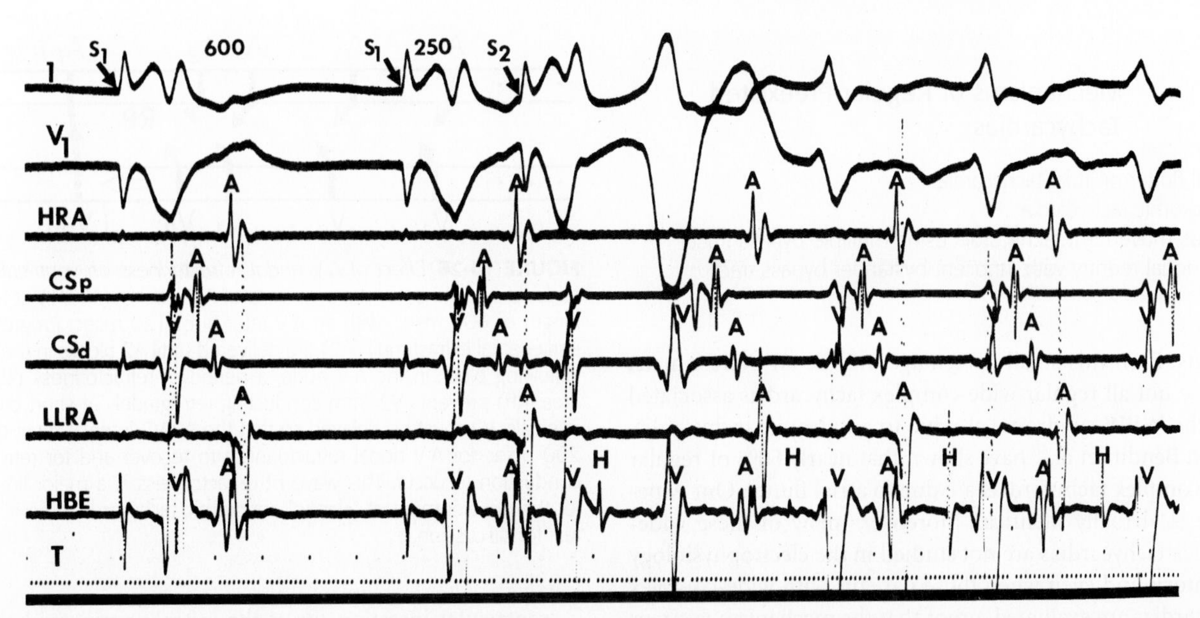


**FIGURE 10-24** *Initiation of orthodromic tachycardia by bundle branch reentry.* At a paced cycle length of 600 msec, a ventricular extrastimulus delivered at an S1-S2 of 250 msec results in retrograde block in a left lateral bypass tract and initiation of a bundle branch reentrant complex (see Chapter 2). The long H-V and LBBB morphology associated with the bundle branch reentrant complex allow the left-sided bypass tract time to recover, allowing retrograde excitation and initiation of SVT. LLRA, low lateral right atrium.

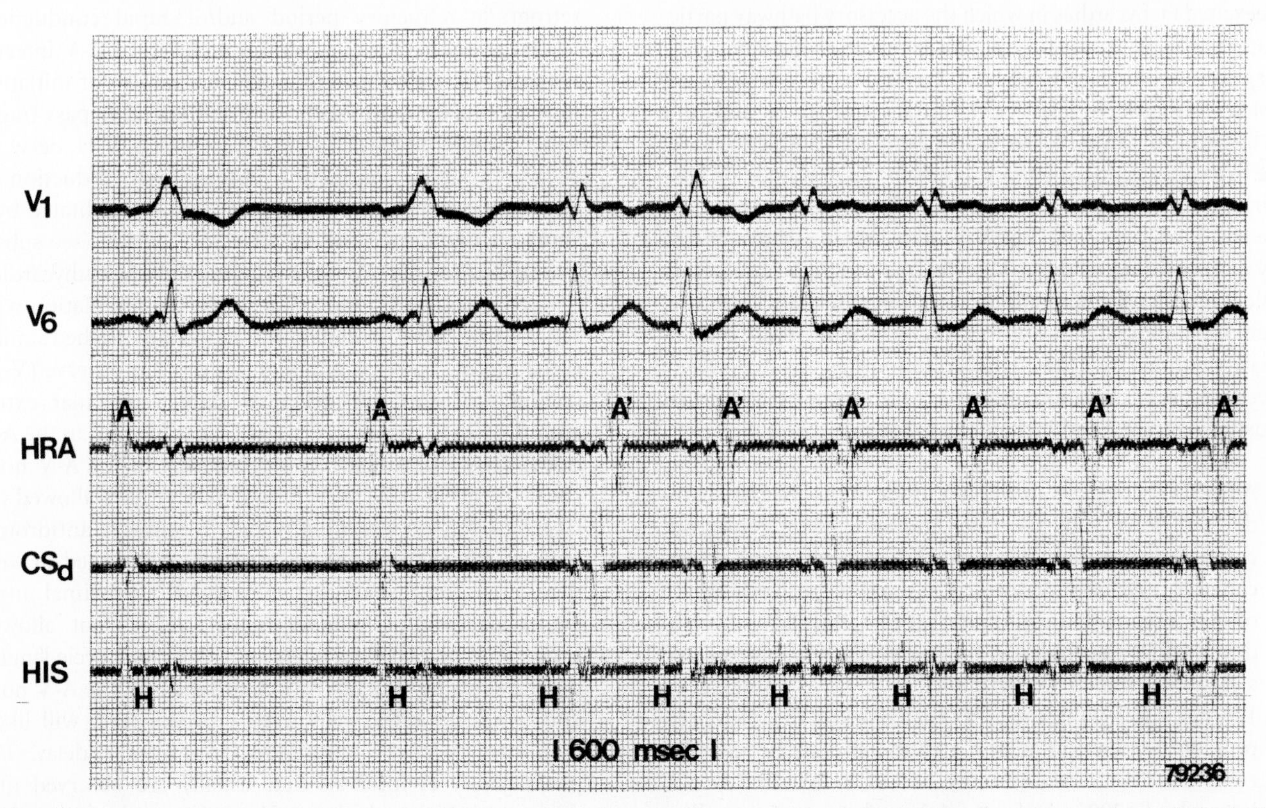


**FIGURE 10-25** *Initiation of orthodromic tachycardia by a spontaneous His extrasystole.* Following the first two sinus impulses, which conduct over a left lateral bypass tract, a spontaneous His extrasystole initiates SVT. The His extrasystole is associated with retrograde block in the A-V node, but the normal QRS, which ensues, conducts retrogradely over the left lateral bypass tract to initiate SVT. (From Wellens HJJ, Brugada P. Value of programmed stimulation of the heart in patients with the Wolff-Parkinson-White syndrome. In: Josephson ME, Wellens HJJ, eds. *Tachycardias: mechanisms and management.* Philadelphia, PA: Lea & Febiger, 1962:199.)

TABLE 10-1 Mechanisms of Regular Preexcited Tachycardias

- Atrial flutter or atrial tachycardia
- Antidromic tachycardia
- Circus movement tachycardia using multiple bypass tracts
- A-V nodal reentry with innocent bystander bypass tract

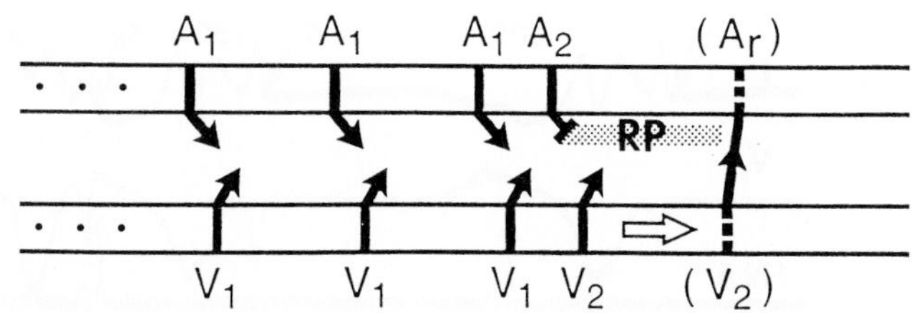


**FIGURE 10-26** *Effect of A-V nodal refractoriness on ventriculoatrial conduction.* The basic drive consists of A-V pacing (A1-V1) at a cycle length of 600 msec, with an A-V interval of 120 msec. Progressively earlier atrial extrastimuli (A2) are delivered until A2 blocks in the node. Following block in the A-V node, a period of refractoriness (stippled area, RP) prevents V2 from conducting retrogradely at short coupling intervals. V2 must be delayed so that the A2-V2 interval must exceed 200 msec for A-V nodal refractoriness to recover and for retrograde conduction to occur. This wave of refractoriness is a major limitation for the development of "classic" antidromic tachycardia by APDs. See text for discussion.

patients. Even this small percentage may be an overestimate, because not all regular wide-complex tachycardias associated with the WPW syndrome are due to antidromic tachycardia. In fact, Benditt et al.[40] have shown that nearly 60% of regular wide-complex tachycardias are due to atrial flutter. Our experience is virtually identical. Moreover, many of these wide-complex tachycardias are not studied in the electrophysiology laboratory, and even when those patients with wide-complex tachycardias are evaluated, proof that the mechanism is circus movement antidromic tachycardia is not always available. Initiation of preexcited tachycardias in the laboratory is at least twice as frequent as their spontaneous occurrence. The causes of regular preexcited tachycardias are given in Table 10-1. Antidromic tachycardia is the most common mechanism of preexcited tachycardias in which the accessory pathway participates in the reentrant circuit. This tachycardia uses the accessory pathway anterogradely and the normal A-V conducting system retrogradely. Classically, initiation of true antidromic tachycardia by an APD requires (a) intact conduction over the bypass tract, (b) antegrade block in the A-V node or His–Purkinje system, and (c) intact retrograde conduction over the His–Purkinje system and A-V node, which assumes recovery of excitability of the A-V node for retrograde conduction following partial antegrade penetration. This latter requirement is a limiting factor for this "classic" mode of initiation of this arrhythmia by APDs. This limitation suggests that several mechanisms of initiation and types of preexcited tachycardias must be operative and include the following:

1. An APD that blocks in the A-V node with antegrade conduction down a bypass tract and subsequent retrograde conduction through the normal A-V conducting system can occur. We have performed A-V pacing at a cycle length of 600 msec with an A-V interval of 120 msec and introduced APDs that block in the node. When we introduced a right ventricular extrastimulus with an A-V interval of 120 msec following the APD that blocked the node, retrograde conduction to the atrium never occurred. The right ventricular extrastimulus had to be delivered at A-V intervals of ≥200 msec for the A-V node to recover to allow retrograde conduction to the atrium (Fig. 10-26). Perhaps ventricular stimulation at a site farther from the His–Purkinje system would have been associated with a longer V-H interval, and retrograde conduction would have occurred. This may in fact be the case during antegrade preexcitation because ventricular excitation begins at the ventricular insertion site at the mitral or tricuspid annuli, which are farther from the conduction system than when stimulation is performed at the right ventricular apex. This may provide an additional 50 msec delay to allow the A-V node to recover for retrograde conduction, but this may not be enough time unless the A-V node has a short retrograde refractory period and/or rapid conduction. Nevertheless, because in antidromic SVT, the A-V interval remains relatively short, this first mechanism of initiation must be uncommon except with left lateral bypass tracts, which would potentially provide enough V-H delay to allow retrograde conduction. Alternatively, induction of antidromic tachycardia by APDs would be facilitated by a short retrograde A-V nodal refractory period (see subsequent discussion), a common finding in these tachycardias.

Lehmann et al.[69] looked at a selected population with rapid retrograde A-V nodal conduction and reached similar conclusions. However, although we did not observe (V-A) conduction when we delivered right ventricular extrastimuli at ≥120 msec after the APD that blocked in the A-V node, early APDs that block proximally in the A-V node (near the atrial-A–V node junction) may have allowed the tissue to recover excitability and to support antidromic reentry. Alternatively, the same study performed at long drive cycle lengths could have resulted in proximal intraventricular and/or interventricular delays that allowed earlier A-V nodal recovery. As a result of long cycle lengths during sinus rhythm, an APD that blocks in the A-V node and conducts antegradely over a bypass tract will likely manifest "effective" retrograde His–Purkinje delay. The prolonged V-H intervals that usually are observed may represent intraventricular and/or interventricular conduction delay as well as delay in the ipsilateral or contralateral bundle branch used for retrograde conduction. This delay provides the A-V node time to recover. In our experience as well as that of Lehmann et al.[69] and Packer et al.,[70] the delay from the atrial insertion of the bypass tract to the retrograde His deflection must be at least 150 msec for initiation of antidromic tachycardia. This is most likely to occur with left lateral bypass tracts, which are the sites of bypass tracts most frequently involved in true antidromic tachycardias (Fig. 10-27). Another potential mechanism of induction of a preexcited tachycardia with a His deflection inscribed shortly after the QRS is that the APD blocks below the His and conducts anterogradely down a contralateral accessory pathway. Retrograde conduction over an ipsilateral pathway would complete the circuit. His–Purkinje refractoriness would limit the ability to return over the normal conducting system. It is always important to prove that the recorded His potential is retrogradely activated; this is confirmed by

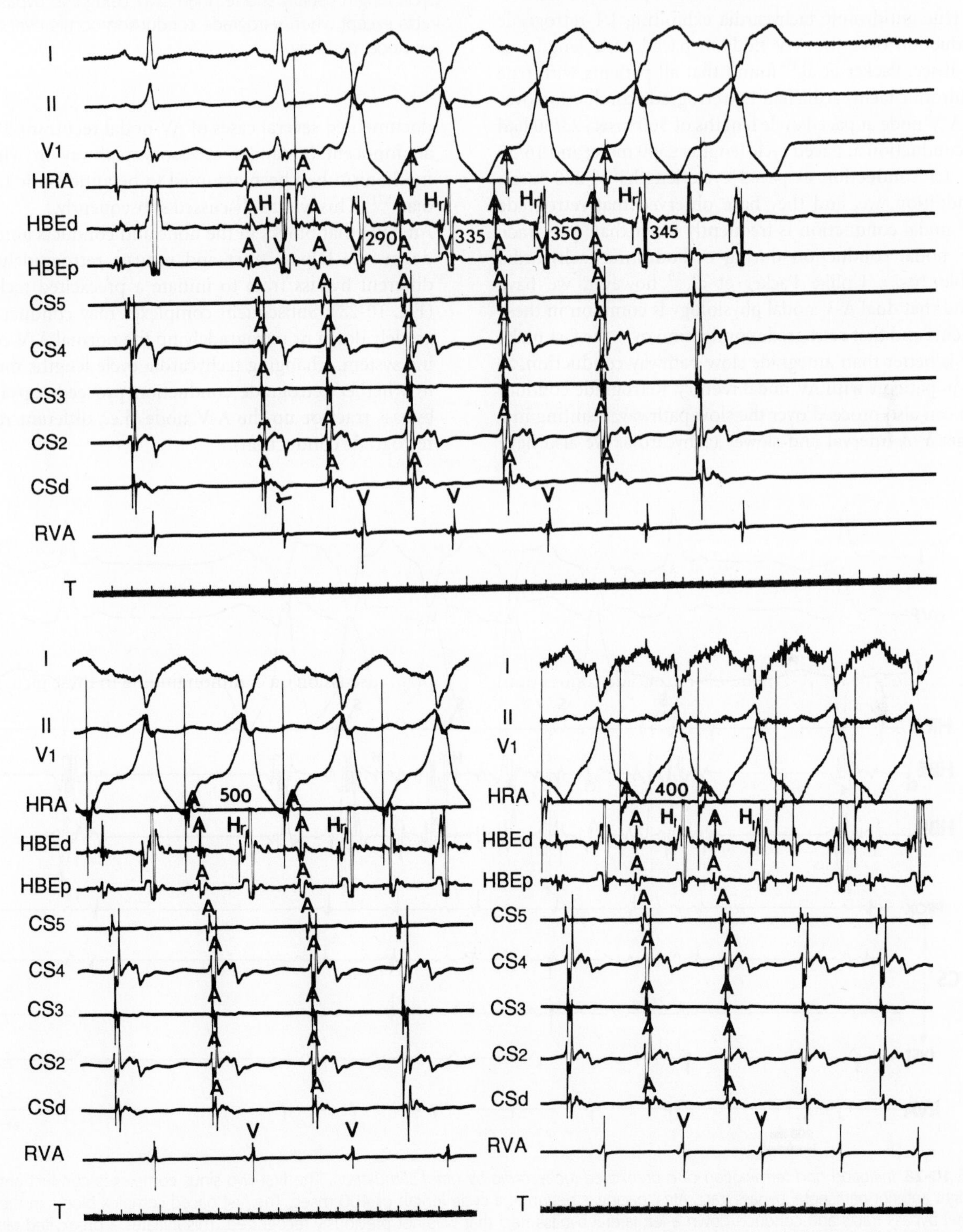


**FIGURE 10-27** *Initiation of antidromic tachycardia.* An APD blocks in the A-V node and conduction occurs over the left lateral accessory pathway (AP), initiating antidromic tachycardia The delta-to-His interval is 80 msec during antidromic tachycardia. $H_r$ is a retrograde His potential. This is supported by the fixed relation of the His to the V (and A) despite atrial pacing at shorter cycle lengths. See text for explanation.

a fixed V-H interval during incremental atrial pacing and/or a similar V-H interval when pacing from the ventricular insertion site of the bypass tract (Fig. 10-27B and C).

Retrograde A-V nodal conduction in these patients therefore must be excellent. In fact, in patients with true antidromic tachycardia, retrograde A-V nodal conduction is remarkably good, with the majority of patients manifesting true antidromic tachycardia exhibiting 1:1 retrograde conduction over the A-V node at paced cycle lengths of 300 msec. Packer et al.[70] found that all patients with true antidromic tachycardia had 1:1 retrograde conduction over the A-V node at paced cycle lengths of 360 msec; 23/30 had 1:1 conduction at paced cycle lengths ≤300 msec; and 16/30 had 1:1 conduction at paced cycle lengths of 260 msec. In addition, we, and they have observed that retrograde A-V nodal conduction is frequently faster than antegrade A-V nodal conduction during orthodromic tachycardia (Table 10-2). Unlike Packer et al.,[70] however, we have found that dual A-V nodal physiology is common in these patients and that retrograde conduction over the fast pathway is better than antegrade slow pathway conduction, as it is in patients with AV nodal reentry. Retrograde conduction can also proceed over the slow pathway, resulting in a longer V-A interval and slower tachycardia. We also have documented several cases of AV nodal reentrant SVT with an innocent bystander accessory pathway in whom the mechanism had been assumed to be antidromic tachycardia.[42,71] (This will be discussed subsequently.)

2. An APD that blocks in the node and conducts antegradely down one bypass tract and returns retrogradely over a different bypass tract to initiate a preexcited tachycardia (Fig. 10-28): Subsequent complexes may conduct anterogradely down or retrogradely up the normal A-V conducting system. Changing tachycardia cycle lengths may relate to whether retrograde conduction proceeds up a second bypass tract or up the A-V node (i.e., different routes of retrograde conduction).

**TABLE 10-2 Electrophysiologic Substrate of Antidromic Tachycardia**

- Good retrograde A-V nodal conduction
- Bypass tract is usually free wall
- Cycle length usually shorter than CMT using two bypass tracts except when retrograde conduction occurs over a slow A-V nodal pathway

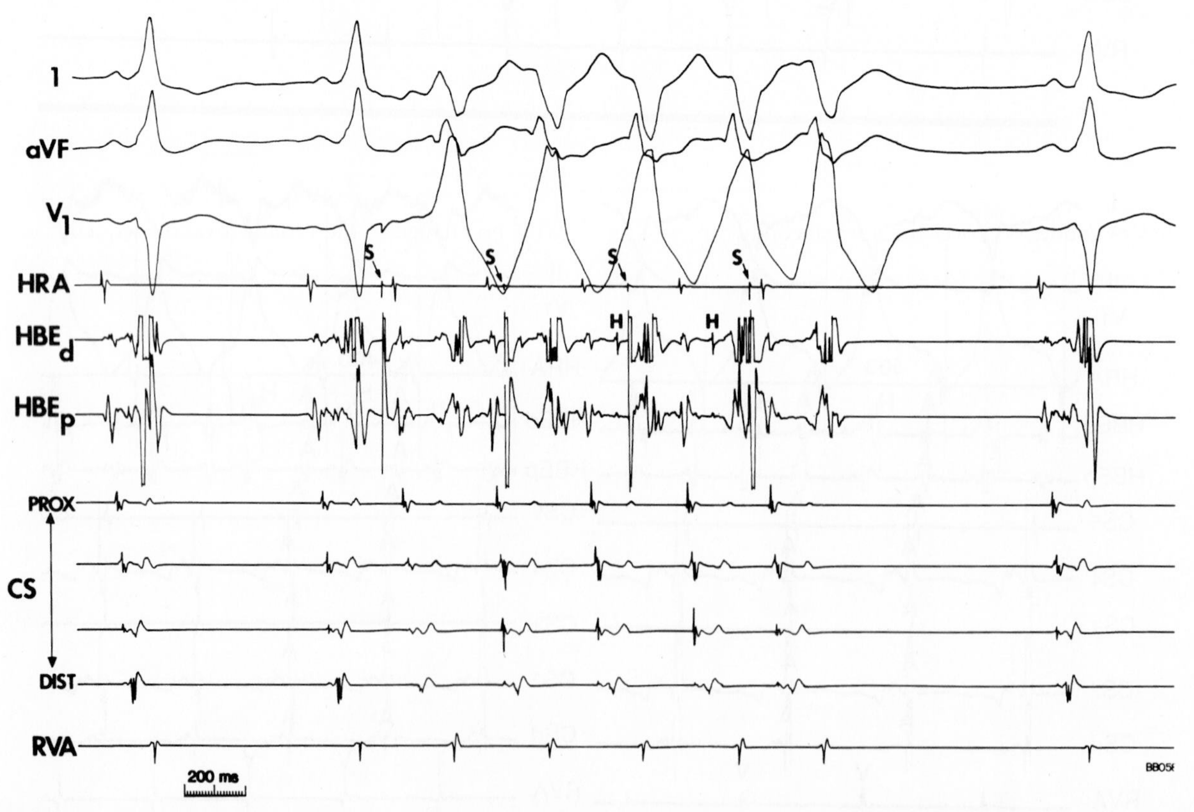


**FIGURE 10-28** *Initiation and termination of a preexcited tachycardia by atrial stimulation.* The first two sinus complexes conduct antegradely over a right anterior paraseptal bypass tract. Atrial pacing is begun at a cycle length of 400 msec. The first paced complex blocks in the anterior paraseptal bypass tracts and conducts down a left lateral bypass tract that was not previously recognized. This initiates a preexcited tachycardia using the right anterior paraseptal bypass tract retrogradely and a left lateral bypass tract antegradely. This lasts for three complexes (note atrial activation in HRA precedes stimulus artifact) until the fourth atrial stimulus captures the right atrium early and terminates the arrhythmia. See text for discussion. DIST, distal; PROX, proximal.

3. An APD that conducts over the bypass tract and simultaneously over the slow pathway of a dual A-V nodal pathway situation: Conduction beyond the His bundle to the ventricles is not possible owing to ventricular inexcitability, yet an A-V nodal echo to the atrium can occur. This atrial echo can then go down the bypass tract antegradely, when the ventricles will have recovered excitability, and initiate a preexcited tachycardia. An example of an APD with such 1:2 conduction owing to dual pathways initiating A-V nodal reentry with an innocent bystander bypass tract is shown in Figure 10-29. A-V nodal reentry may or may not persist or be preempted by retrograde conduction up the fast A-V nodal pathway caused by premature ventricular excitation over the bypass tract. In that situation the location of His potentials would depend on whether or not they were antegrade or retrograde. While this situation is theoretically possible, I have never seen it. One could distinguish A-V nodal reentry from classic antidromic reentry, which uses the His–Purkinje system retrogradely, by analyzing the H-A intervals during documented V-A conduction over the normal pathway during ventricular pacing and that during initiation and maintenance of the tachycardia. One must recognize, however, that if ventricular pacing is initiated during sinus rhythm, the H-A interval may not be due to retrograde conduction over the node but may be due to retrograde conduction exclusively over the bypass tract or fusion over the normal system and the bypass tract. Therefore, I prefer to analyze the H-A interval during entrainment of the tachycardia to eliminate the possibility of a fusion of atrial activation. As noted in Chapter 8, the H-A interval during A-V nodal echoes or A-V nodal reentry would be shorter than that resulting from retrograde V-A conduction over the normal conduction system in response to ventricular pacing (Fig. 10-30). In our experience, H-A intervals of ≤60 msec were never seen in true antidromic tachycardias. A more sensitive and specific criterion is the difference in the H-A interval observed during ventricular pacing (in sinus rhythm or during entrainment of the preexcited tachycardia) and the H-A interval during the preexcited tachycardia.[71] In A-V nodal reentry, the difference is always >0 msec, while in other preexcited tachycardias, it is always ≤0 msec (Fig. 10-31). Another finding consistent with AVNRT is the failure of an APD delivered during a preexcited tachycardia at the time the atrium at the A-V junction (AVJ) is refractory to affect the H-H and A-A even though it advances the preexcited V (Fig. 10-32). This response is also seen in atrial tachycardia. When true antidromic tachycardia or a preexcited tachycardia using two accessory pathways is present, a similarly timed APD will advance the V and subsequently A, demonstrating the A is caused by the V (Fig. 10-33). Electrophysiologic features of preexcited tachycardias due to A-V nodal reentry are shown in Table 10-3.

Furthermore, in my experience, when atrial stimulation induces preexcited tachycardias, multiple bypass tracts are often operative. Whether or not they are operative throughout the tachycardia (i.e., integral components of the reentrant circuit) depends on (a) the relative retrograde activation times over additional bypass tracts and the normal A-V conducting system and (b) the varying degrees of antegrade and/or retrograde concealment into the additional bypass tracts and/or the normal A-V conduction system during the tachycardia.

APDs with 1:2 conduction with A-V nodal echoes provide an initiating mechanism of preexcited tachycardias that has heretofore been unrecognized. Initiation of A-V nodal reentry with innocent bystander preexcited tachycardias by ventricular premature complexes (VPCs) is also possible (Fig. 10-34). The ability to induce A-V nodal reentry by VPDs in these patients is higher than in the general population of patients with A-V nodal reentry (see Chapter 8). This, however may represent a patient selection bias of patients with preexcited tachycardia, since the only reason the tachycardia was seen was because it was inducible. In addition, in the presence of a bypass tract, if A-V nodal reentry is induced with block below the His, a preexcited tachycardia can ensue (Fig. 10-34). The actual frequency of apparent antidromic tachycardia that is due to A-V nodal reentry with passive conduction over a bypass tract is unknown. Proof of A-V nodal reentry as the mechanism of preexcited tachycardias may be difficult. The most clear-cut proof would be demonstration of A-V nodal reentry following spontaneous or drug-induced block in the bypass tract at the same cycle length, with the same H-A interval, and the same retrograde activation sequence as during the preexcited tachycardia (Fig. 10-35). Other criteria supporting A-V nodal reentry are the induction of A-V nodal reentry by atrial or ventricular extrastimuli with subsequent conduction over the bypass tract owing to His–Purkinje delay or block, with no change in the atrial activation sequence or H-A. A more detailed description of A-V nodal reentry with innocent bystander bypass tract is given later in this section.

Although APDs producing antegrade block in the node, antegrade conduction over the bypass tract, and retrograde conduction over the normal His–Purkinje system with long V-H intervals can initiate antidromic tachycardia,[41] this has been surprisingly uncommon as the mechanism of preexcited circus movement tachycardias. Approximately 50% of our patients in whom atrial stimulation has induced a preexcited tachycardia have had true antidromic tachycardias. The remainder have had either preexcited tachycardias using multiple bypass tracts or A-V nodal reentry with an innocent bystander bypass tract. An example of an APD initiating a preexcited tachycardia using multiple bypass tracts is shown in Figure 10-28. In this patient, an anterior paraseptal bypass tract is present during sinus rhythm. Atrial stimulation from the high-right atrium is initiated at a paced cycle length of 400 msec. The first atrial extrastimulus blocks in the right anterior paraseptal bypass tract and conducts over a left lateral bypass tract. Before the next stimulus, retrograde conduction is manifest over the previously blocked right anterior bypass tract. The presence of His potentials during this tachycardia probably represents simultaneous antegrade conduction over

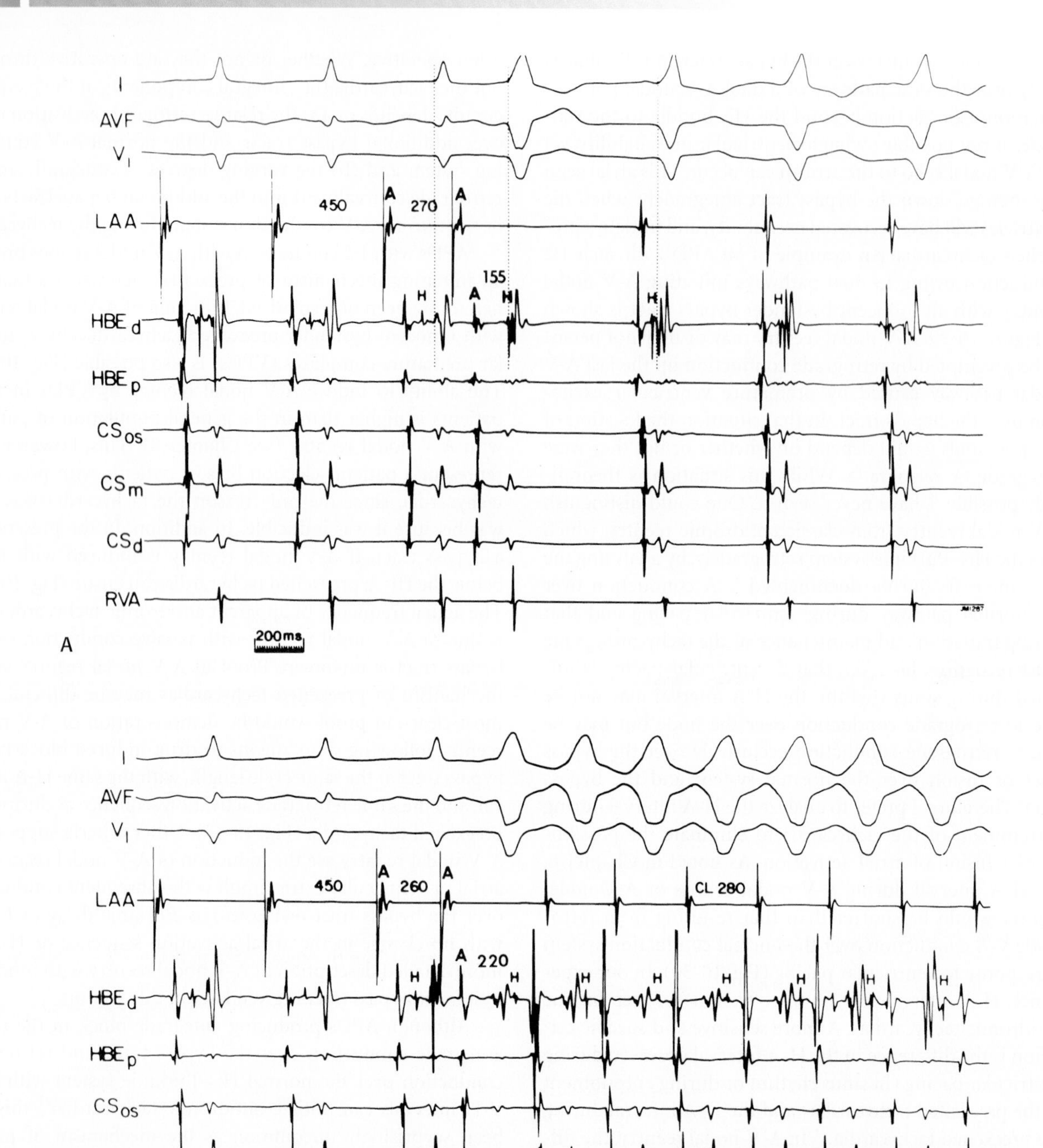


**FIGURE 10-29** *A-V nodal tachycardia with an innocent bystander bypass tract initiated with 1:2 atrial to ventricular conduction.* **A:** An APD delivered at a coupling interval of 270 msec conducts along both the A-V node and a right paraseptal bypass tract. The His is seen just within the preexcited QRS (H-H = 155 msec). **B:** A more premature atrial depolarization at 260 msec produces block in the fast A-V nodal pathway with anterograde conduction over the slow A-V nodal pathway (with an A-H of 220 msec), initiating A-V nodal reentrant tachycardia (AVNRT). This APD also conducts anterogradely along the bypass tract (i.e., 1:2 conduction). Following initiating of AVNRT, there is subsequent bystander activation of the accessory pathway during the tachycardia. CL, cycle length. LAA, left atrial appendage.

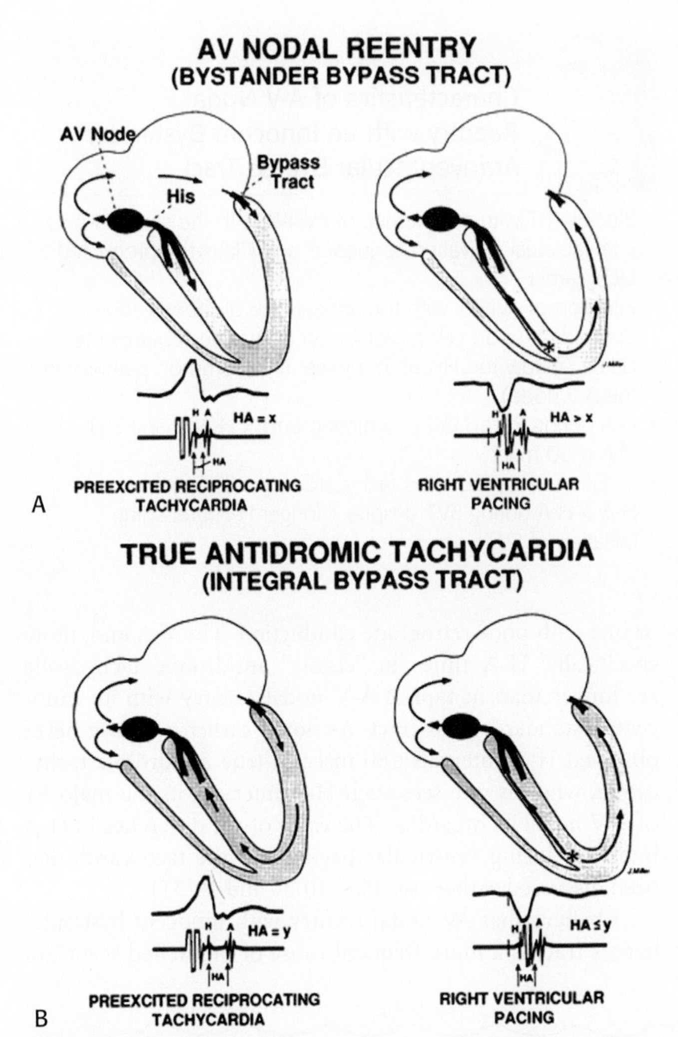


**FIGURE 10-30** *H-A intervals during right ventricular pacing and during preexcited tachycardia.* **A:** During AVNRT with bystander bypass tract, the His and the atria will be activated simultaneously (HA = x), while during right ventricular pacing, the His and the atria will be activated in sequence (HA > x). **B:** During antidromic reciprocating tachycardia (ART), the His and the atria are activated in sequence (HA = y), the same as, or in some instances less than, during right ventricular pacing (HA = y). See text for full discussion. *, stimulation.

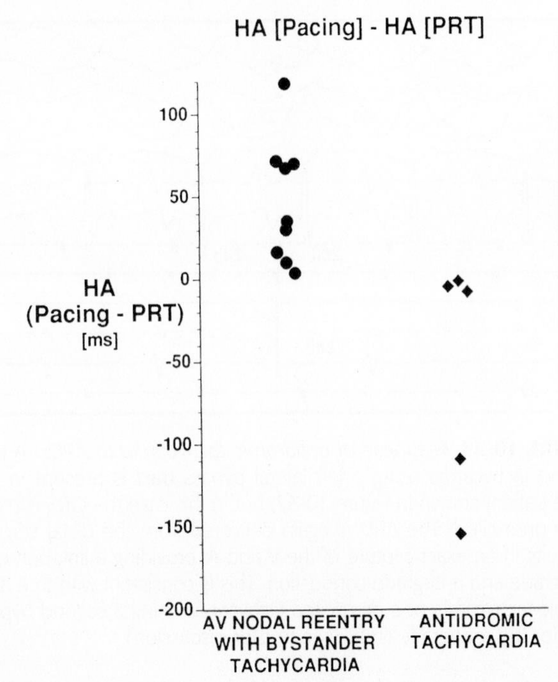


**FIGURE 10-31** *The difference between H-A intervals during right ventricular pacing and preexcited tachycardias.* Circles, A-V nodal reentry with innocent bystander bypass tract. Diamonds, antidromic tachycardia (n = 4) or preexcited tachycardia using multiple bypass tracts. See text for discussion. PRT, preexcited reciprocating tachycardia.

the normal A-V conducting system as conduction proceeds over the left lateral bypass tract. This is supported by the fact that the fourth atrial extrastimulus terminates the tachycardia by retrograde block in the right anterior bypass tract owing to the premature capture of the ventricles over the left-sided pathway (in the absence of a His deflection) and anterograde concealment into the right-sided pathway. The failure to see a His deflection implies that the extrastimulus either blocked in the AV node or was associated with AV nodal delay resulting in obscuration of the His by the preexcited QRS.

In our experience, "classic" antidromic tachycardias using a single A-V bypass tract can also be initiated by ventricular

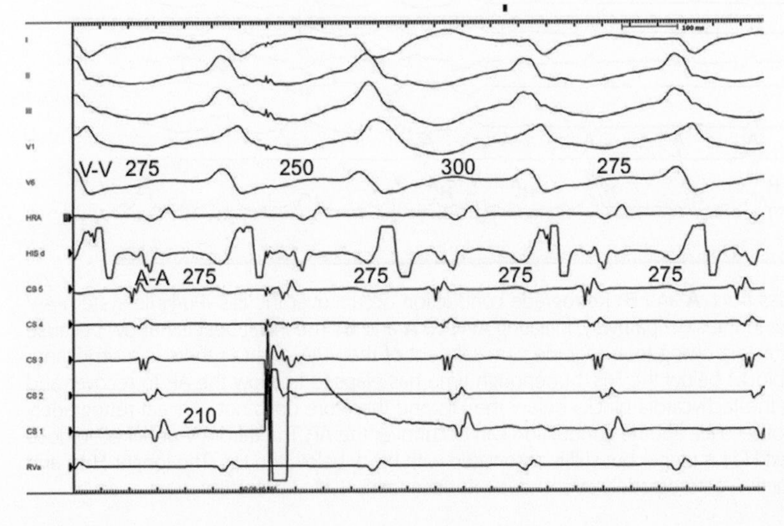


**FIGURE 10-32** *A-V nodal reentry with an innocent bystander left lateral bypass tract.* A preexcited tachycardia over a left lateral bypass tract is present. The QRS is not totally preexcited. An atrial premature beat is delivered from the distal coronary sinus (CS1) which advances the QRS with an increased amount of preexcitation, demonstrating antegrade conduction over an accessory pathway. The atrial activity remains unaffected, excluding antidromic tachycardia. The failure to advance the "A" is consistent with A-V nodal reentry with an innocent bystander accessory pathway. See text for discussion.

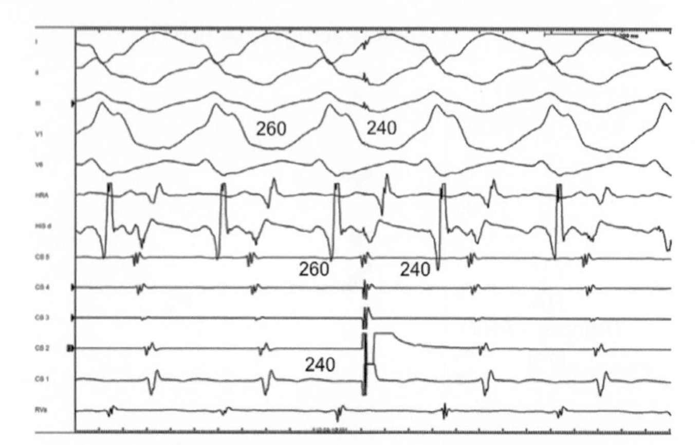


**FIGURE 10-33** *Response of antidromic tachycardia to APDs.* A preexcited tachycardia using a left lateral bypass tract is present in the same patient shown in Figure 10-32, but in this case the QRS is maximally preexcited. The APD is again delivered from the distal CS, but it results in an exact capture of the V and A, providing a link between retrograde and antegrade conduction. This is consistent with true antidromic tachycardia or a preexcited tachycardia using a second bypass tract for the retrograde limb. (see text for discussion)

stimulation. In this instance, retrograde block in the bypass tract must occur and retrograde conduction proceeds only over the normal A-V conduction system. This is manifested by a prolonged V-H-A activation sequence, which subsequently initiates the tachycardia with antegrade conduction down the bypass tract and repetitive retrograde conduction up the normal pathway (Fig. 10-36). This mechanism is most likely to occur in patients with an antegrade conducting only pathway

**TABLE 10-3 Characteristics of A-V Nodal Reentry with an Innocent Bystander Atrioventricular Bypass Tract**

- Block in BT with persistence of AVNRT with the same H-A interval, atrial activation sequence, and CL as the preexcited tachycardia
- Initiation of AVNRT with the appearance of preexcitation dependent upon H-V prolongation or 2:1 block below the circuit (below the His or in a lower final common pathway in the A-V node)
- H-A during RVP (NSR on entrainment) > H-A during SVT
- H-A ≤ 60 msec
- Initiation of a preexcited tachycardia by a VPC with an H-A > H-A during SVT despite a longer H-H preceding initiation of SVT

or one with poor retrograde conduction. The V-A and, more specifically, H-A times in "classic" antidromic tachycardia are longer than in typical A-V nodal reentry with an innocent bystander bypass tract. As noted earlier, we have never observed H-A intervals ≤60 msec in true antidromic tachycardia, whereas one sees such H-A intervals in the majority of A-V nodal tachycardias. The value of the difference in H-A intervals during ventricular pacing and the tachycardia has been discussed earlier (see Figs. 10-30 and 10-31).

I believe that AV nodal reentry with innocent bystander bypass tract is a more frequent cause of preexcited reentrant

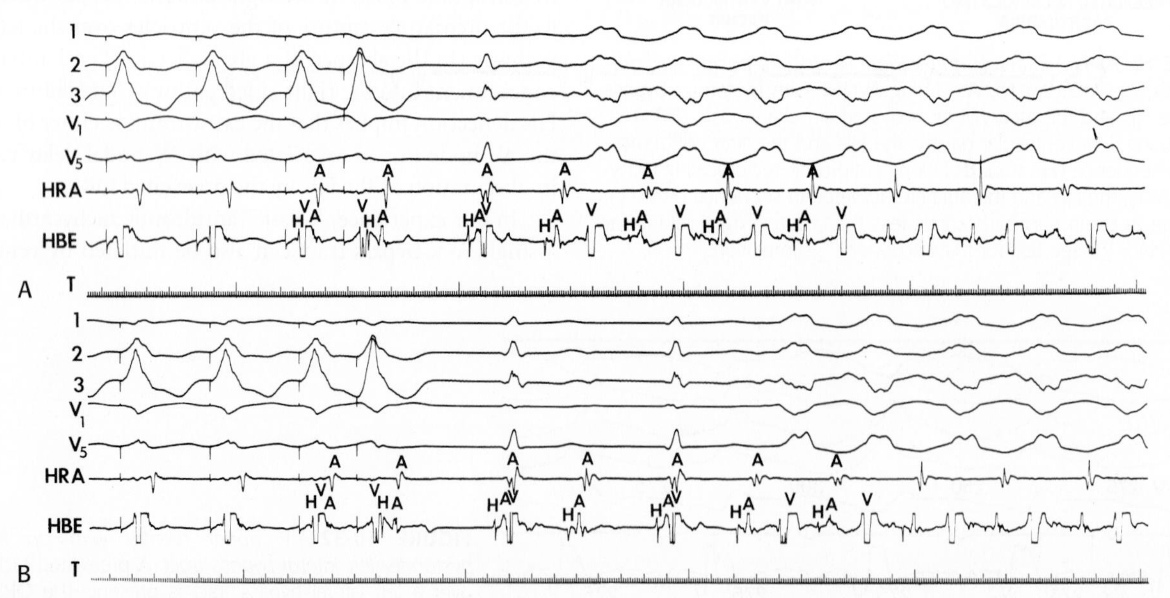


**FIGURE 10-34** *A-V nodal tachycardia with a bystander bypass tract.* **A** and **B:** Retrograde conduction occurs over the His–Purkinje system A-V node during right ventricular pacing at 400 msec. A VPD blocks in the slow pathway, initiating AVNRT. **A** and **B:** The initial beat is narrow because (l) the retrograde A over the fast pathway finds the AP still refractory owing to retrograde concealment of the VPD, and (2) there is a simultaneous A and V in the first echo. **A:** The second A-V nodal echo blocks below the His, but enough time has elapsed to allow the AP to recover and conduct anterogradely as a bystander. **B:** The second beat of the tachycardia blocks below the His and therefore does not conceal retrogradely into the AP. However, because the H-H is short, the AP does not recover, and no conduction can occur over the AP. The third A-V nodal echo does not conduct, owing to simultaneous A and V activation. The next H-H is longer but still is associated with block below the His. The longer H-H, and hence longer A-A, allows the next beat of the AVNRT to conduction anterogradely over the AP. Surface leads 1, 2, 3, V1, V5.

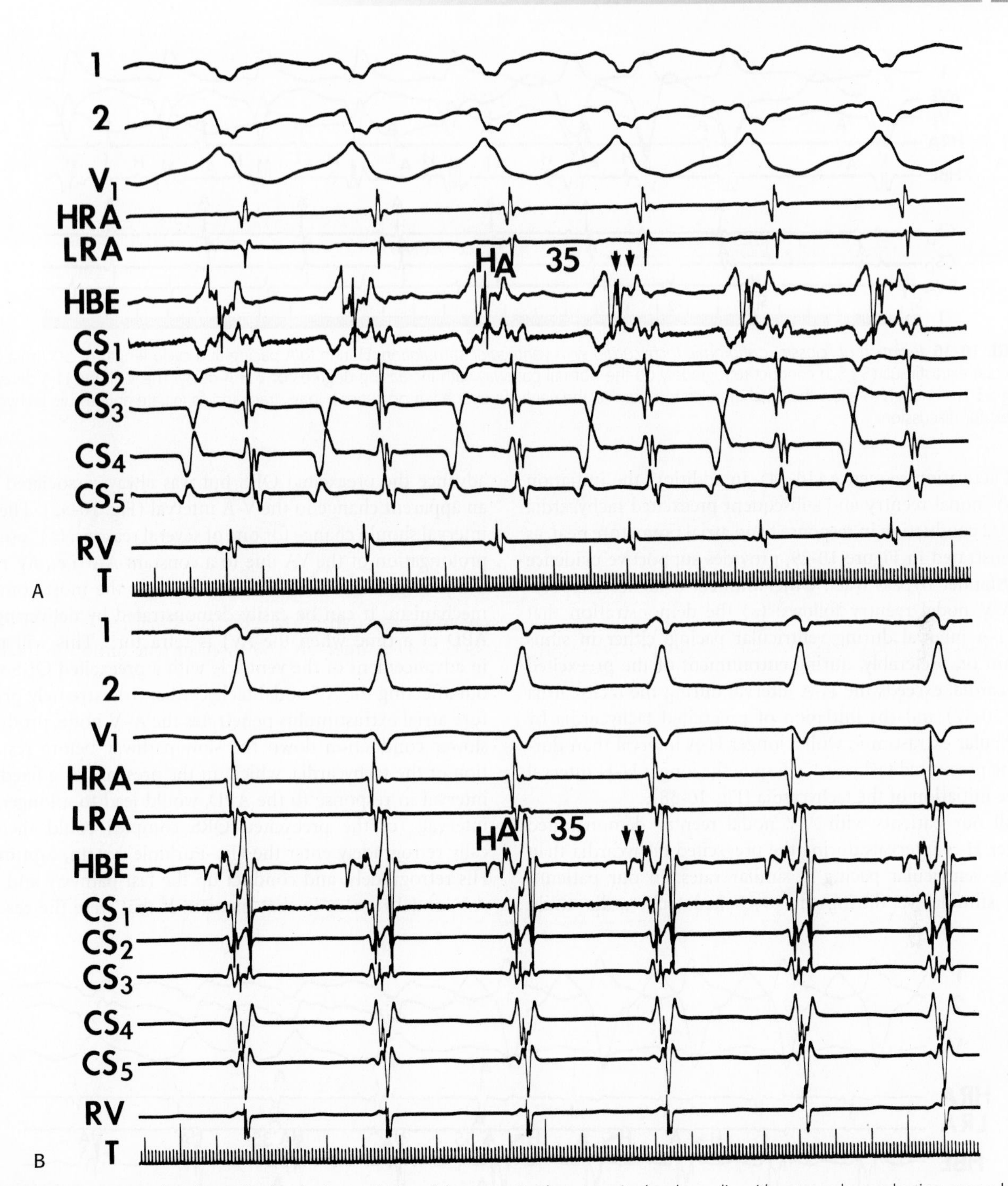


**FIGURE 10-35** *Preexcited tachycardia that is due to A-V nodal reentry.* **A:** The preexcited tachycardia with antegrade conduction over a left lateral bypass tract. **B:** Following block in the bypass tract produced by procainamide, A-V nodal reentry continues with a narrow QRS complex. Note the identical H-A interval and retrograde activation sequence in the narrow and preexcited tachycardia. See text for discussion.

tachycardia than previously recognized. Features are listed in Table 10-3. We have documented A-V nodal reentry as the mechanism of 13 of 56 cases of preexcited tachycardias, unrelated to atrial tachyarrhythmias which I have studied over the last 40 years. The diagnosis of A-V nodal reentry as the mechanism of the tachycardia primarily depended on the persistence of typical A-V nodal reentry with and without activation over a bypass tract. In six cases, this was due to block in the bypass tract by antiarrhythmic agents with persistence of a tachycardia with an identical H-A interval and atrial activation sequence, all of which were compatible with A-V nodal reentry (Fig. 10-35). In other instances, typical A-V nodal reentry, induced by APDs or VPDs, subsequently developed into a preexcited tachycardia with the appearance of delay and/or block below the His bundle with persistence of the preexcited tachycardia having an identical H-A interval and

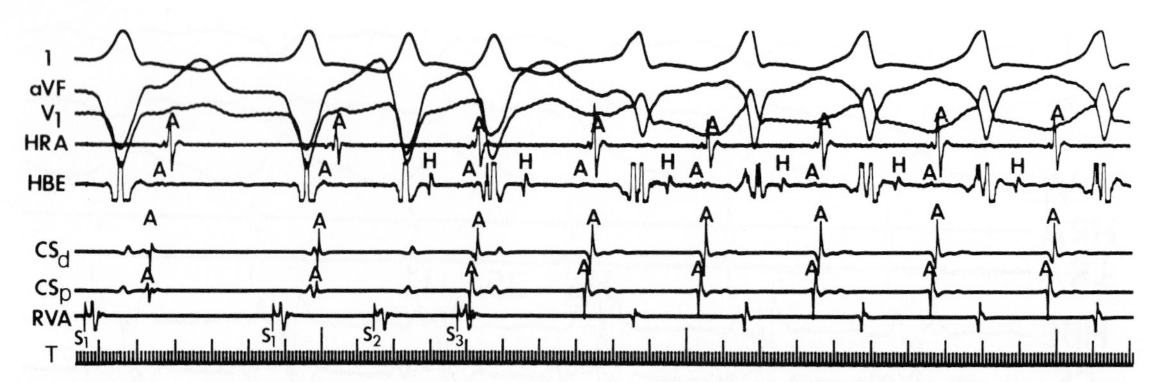


**FIGURE 10-36** *Initiation of "classic" antidromic tachycardia with ventricular stimulation.* During RVA pacing at a cycle length of 500 msec, two ventricular extrastimuli (S2,S3) conduct retrogradely up the normal pathway with increasing degrees of V-H-A delay. The V-H and H-A delays following S3 are enough to allow the atrial impulse to return to the ventricle over a left posterior bypass tract and to initiate antidromic tachycardia. See text for discussion.

atrial activation sequence (10-34). In addition, the initiation of A-V nodal reentry and subsequent preexcited tachycardia with 1:2 conduction in response to an atrial premature beat, as demonstrated in Figure 10-29, provides supportive evidence of bystander bypass tract. Other indirect evidence supporting A-V nodal reentry follows: (a) the demonstration that the H-A interval during ventricular pacing, either in sinus rhythm or, preferably, during entrainment of the preexcited tachycardia, exceeds the H-A interval during the tachycardia (Fig. 10-37) and (b) initiation of preexcited tachycardia by ventricular extrastimuli with a longer H-A interval than during the preexcited tachycardia despite the longer H-H interval before initiation of the tachycardia (Fig. 10-38).

All our patients with A-V nodal reentry demonstrated shorter H-A intervals during the preexcited tachycardia than during ventricular pacing at similar rates. In our patients, atrial stimulation during the preexcited tachycardia could advance the preexcited QRS but was always associated with an apparent change in the V-A interval (Fig. 10-32). The V-A interval should change for one of several reasons: (a) "pseudo" prolongation of the VA due to a constant AA (i.e., AV nodal tachycardia remained unaffected); this is the most common mechanism. It can be easily demonstrated by delivering the APD at a time when the AVJ is refractory. This will result in advancement of the ventricle with a preexcited QRS without affecting the AV nodal tachycardia; (b) extremely premature atrial extrastimulus penetrates the A–V node, producing slower conduction down the slow pathway before resumption of the tachycardia, which, in the presence of a fixed A-V interval in response to the APD, would lead to a longer V-A interval; (c) the preexcited QRS complex could theoretically retrogradely enter the His–Purkinje system, capture the His retrogradely, and conduct up the fast pathway and reset A-V nodal reentry in that manner. If that were the case, for

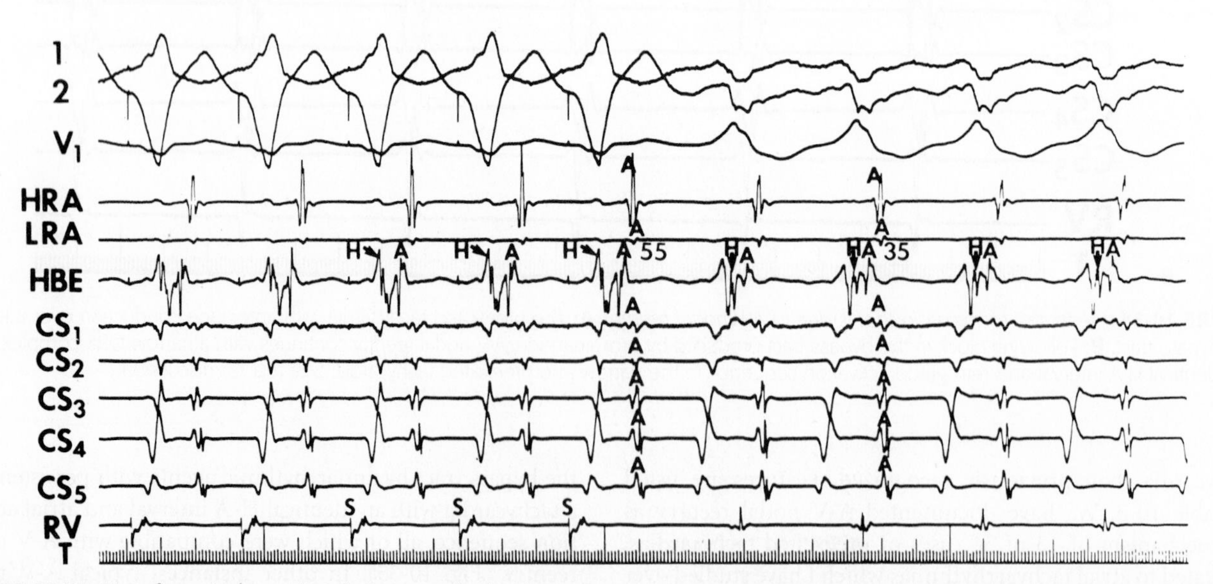


**FIGURE 10-37** *Use of ventricular pacing during preexcited tachycardia to recognize A-V nodal reentry.* Surface leads 1, 2, and V1 are displayed with multiple intracardiac recordings. (See Fig. 10-32.) During ventricular pacing (first five complexes) the H-A interval is 55 msec. While on resumption of the preexcited tachycardia the H-A is 35 msec with an identical actual activation sequence. A longer H-A during RV pacing than during the tachycardia supports A-V nodal reentry with innocent bystander bypass tract as the mechanism of the preexcited tachycardia. See text for discussion.

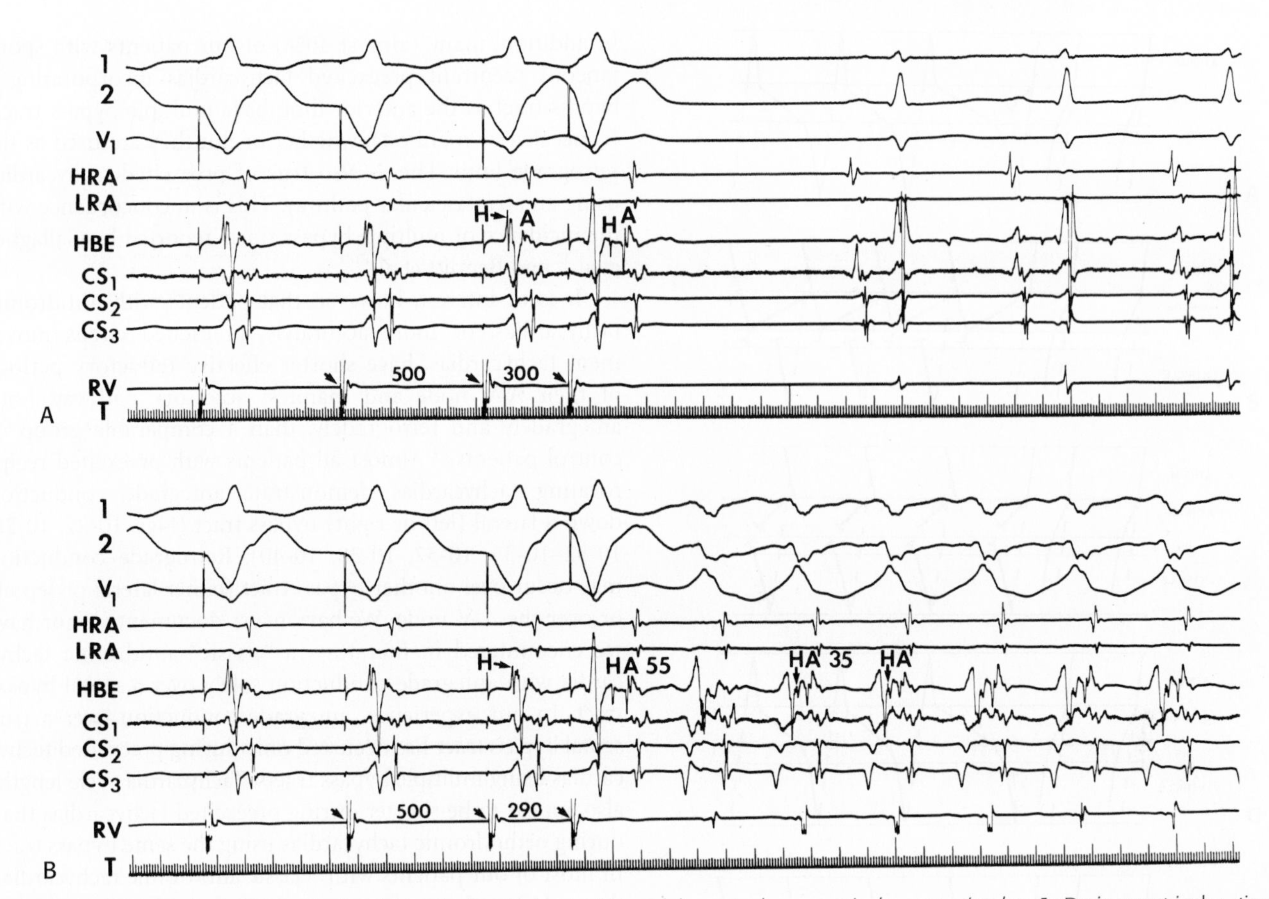


**FIGURE 10-38** *Initiation of preexcited tachycardia that is due to A-V nodal reentry by a ventricular extrastimulus.* **A:** During ventricular stimulation, a VPD at a coupling interval of 300 msec produces V-H prolongation with a very short H-A interval without any tachycardia. **B:** When the coupling interval is reduced to 290 msec, the increased V-H is associated with retrograde conduction up a fast A-V nodal pathway, which turns around to conduct down the slow pathway and simultaneously activate the atria. Atrial activation reaches a left lateral bypass tract, through which it conducts antegradely to the ventricle before the impulse reaches the His bundle over the slow pathway. A-V nodal reentry continues, but the QRS is always preexcited because of antegrade conduction over the bypass tract, preempting conduction over the slow pathway and normal His–Purkinje system. Note the H-A interval on the initiating complex is longer than the H-A interval during the tachycardia despite the fact that the H1-H2 interval exceeds the cycle length of the tachycardia. See text for discussion.

the same V-A interval to be present, the retrograde conduction time (the V-H interval) of the preexcited QRS complex plus the H-A interval in response to this complex should add up to the same V-A interval of an undisturbed A-V nodal reentry. I personally have never seen the last mechanism, which is analogous to failure of a single, late VPD to affect a rapid AV nodal tachycardia (see Chapter 8). Even if this unlikely event occurred, the H-A interval of that preexcited complex would necessarily exceed that during the rest of the tachycardia. Observations that could exclude A-V nodal reentry are shown in Table 10-4.

Cycle length alterations dependent on changing V-H intervals – thereby demonstrating requisite participation of the His-Purkinje system in the tachycardia circuit – are not uncommon in true antidromic tachycardias.[41] This is one of the diagnostic features of true antidromic tachycardias and rules out AVNRT with an innocent bystander accessory pathway. We never saw this phenomenon in any of our patients with A-V nodal reentry and innocent bystander bypass tracts. Documentation of A-V nodal reentry as the underlying mechanism of a preexcited tachycardia is of critical importance in planning ablative therapy to cure the arrhythmia. As noted above the mere presence of an H-A interval of <70 msec should suggest A-V nodal tachycardia.

Thus, preexcited tachycardias have multiple mechanisms. The term **antidromic tachycardia** should be reserved for tachycardias that use an A-V bypass tract antegradely and the normal A-V conducting system retrogradely. A schema of some of the potential mechanisms of preexcited tachycardias

**TABLE 10-4 Methods to Exclude A-V Nodal Reentry as a Cause of a Preexcited Tachycardia**

- Exact A and V capture by APC delivered when AVJ is depolarized
- Failure of entrainment by AP or VP to influence V-A during tachycardia
- H-A tachycardia > H-A RVP

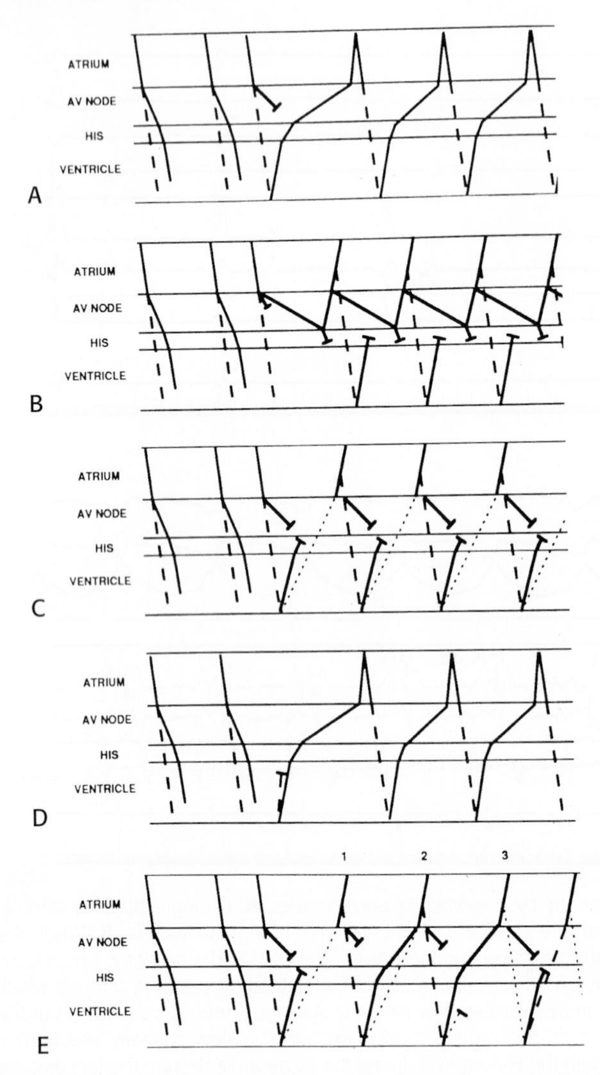


**FIGURE 10-39** *Schema of multiple mechanisms of preexcited tachycardias.* **A:** The top ladder diagram shows "classic" antidromic tachycardia initiated by an APD, blocks in the node and conducts over the same bypass tract observed during atrial pacing. Retrograde conduction proceeds with marked V-H-A delay to initiate a preexcited tachycardia. **B:** A-V nodal reentry (block in the fast and conduction down the slow pathway is shown) with 1:2 conduction. The slow pathway fails to excite the ventricles, because they remain refractory owing to excitation over the bypass tract in response to A2. When the atrial echo reaches the bypass tract, however, antegrade conduction is possible. A-V nodal reentry perpetuates itself, but the QRS is always caused by excitation over the bypass tract, which prevents antegrade activation over the normal A-V conducting system. **C:** An atrial premature complex initiating preexcited tachycardia using a second bypass tract for retrograde conduction. **D:** Classic antidromic tachycardia being initiated by ventricular premature stimulus. **E:** Multiple complicated routes of activation when two bypass tracts are operative. See text for discussion.

is given in Figure 10-39. The difficulty in recording clear retrograde or antegrade His potentials during atrial or ventricular stimulation in the presence of preexcitation makes establishment of the exact initiating and sustaining mechanisms of preexcited tachycardias difficult to ascertain. Nevertheless, in our experience, ~23% of preexcited tachycardias are due to A-V nodal reentry with an innocent bystander bypass tract. In addition, many (almost 40%) of our patients with spontaneous reentrant preexcited tachycardias incorporating a bypass tract as the anterior limb have multiple bypass tracts (concealed or manifest), whether or not they are used as the retrograde limb. This is also true of preexcited tachycardias using an atriofascicular pathway. This is in concordance with the incidence of multiple bypass tracts reported by Gallagher et al.[32] and Benditt et al.[40]

It is of interest, however, that patients with antidromic tachycardias, or more accurately, preexcited circus movement tachycardias, have shorter effective refractory periods of their A-V node and manifest accessory pathway, both antegradely and retrogradely, than a comparable group of control patients.[70] Almost all patients with preexcited reciprocating tachycardias demonstrate antegrade conduction down a lateral (left or right) bypass tract (Figs. 10-27, 10-28, 10-32–10-35, 10-37, 10-38, 10-40). Retrograde conduction may occur over another bypass tract (either lateral or septal) or over the A-V node. We have never documented, nor have we encountered in literature, a "classic" antidromic tachycardia with antegrade conduction solely over a septal bypass tract. In our experience, antegrade conduction over a true septal bypass tract has occurred only during preexcited tachycardias using multiple bypass tracts. Tachycardia cycle lengths also appear to be shorter during preexcited tachycardias than during orthodromic tachycardias using the same bypass tract. In most of our patients with "classic antidromic tachycardia," the cycle length was longer than the orthodromic tachycardia in the same patient. This may not be the case if dual A-V nodal physiology is present and if the orthodromic tachycardia uses the slow pathway antegradely while the antidromic

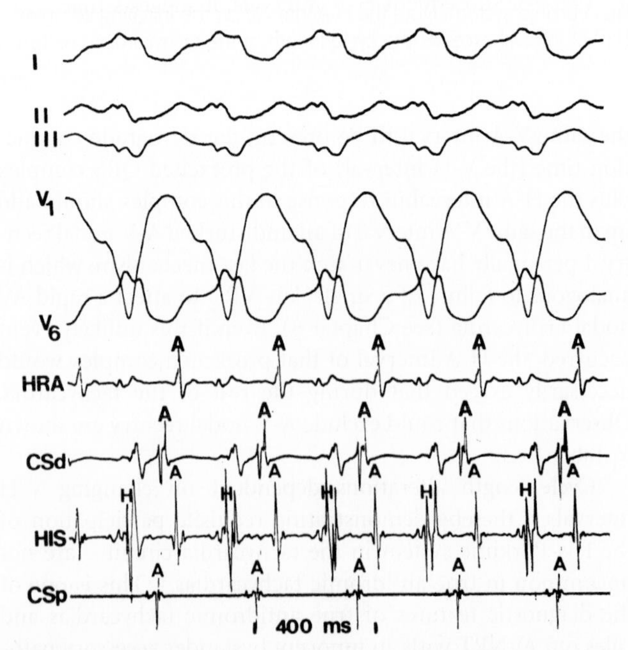


**FIGURE 10-40** *Preexcited tachycardia using two bypass tracts.* A preexcited tachycardia is present using a right lateral bypass tract antegradely and a left posterior free wall bypass tract retrogradely (earliest retrograde activation, CSp).

**TABLE 10-5 Rate Changes During Preexcited Tachycardias Due to Changes in Retrograde Conduction**

**RATE CHANGE ASSOCIATED WITH**

- Change in V-H interval: antidromic tachycardia
- Change in H-A interval: antidromic tachycardia
- Change in V-A: antidromic tachycardia or CMT using two bypass tracts

tachycardia uses the fast pathway retrogradely. This situation may explain why Packer et al.[70] found the cycle length of antidromic tachycardia to be shorter than orthodromic tachycardia in the same patient. In our experience, preexcited tachycardias using two or more bypass tracts tend to have longer cycle lengths than orthodromic tachycardias or the "classic" antidromic tachycardia. This is due to the fact two bypass tracts are typically in opposite chambers and are incorporated in a larger reentrant circuit than one involving a midline, rapidly conducting A-V node.

Finally, it is important to recognize that preexcited tachycardias may be irregular, particularly classic antidromic tachycardia. Rate changes are most commonly due to changes in retrograde conduction (Table 10-5). This is often due to changing retrograde conduction over different fascicles, with different V-H intervals, in patients with classic antidromic tachycardia (Fig. 10-41).[41] Obviously, one also may see such irregularities whenever different routes of retrograde and/or antegrade conduction use different bypass tracts. However, if the change in cycle length can be ascribed to a change in V-H and/or subsequent H-A intervals, it suggests that retrograde conduction occurs over the normal A-V conducting system (Fig. 10-42). This is evidence diagnostic of classic antidromic tachycardia. More rarely, rate changes can occur due to a change in A-V intervals; this may relate to decremental

**TABLE 10-6 Rate Changes During Regular Preexcited Tachycardias Due to Changes in Anterograde Conduction**

- Rate change associated with a change in A-V interval with the same QRS
- Two closely located bypass tracts with different conduction properties
- One bypass tract with longitudinal dissociation
- Atrial flutter with changing A-V conduction over a single bypass tract

antegrade conduction of the bypass tract (Table 10-6). Carotid sinus stimulation may be of help in distinguishing the mechanism of preexcited tachycardias if the rhythm terminates (Table 10-7).

The site of stimulation not only plays an important role in inducibility of circus movement tachycardia (see preceding discussion) but also may determine the type of circus movement tachycardia. Wellens and Brugada[38] (demonstrated that APDs at the same coupling intervals could induce antidromic or orthodromic tachycardia, depending on the stimulation site (Fig. 10-43). The closer the stimulation site is to the bypass tract, the more likely block in the bypass tract will occur and orthodromic tachycardia result. Conversely, antidromic tachycardia is more likely to occur with APDs delivered close to the A-V node.

## ATRIAL FIBRILLATION

Atrial fibrillation occurs in approximately 50% of patients with WPW syndrome, and in approximately 10% is the presenting arrhythmia (although perhaps not the initial arrhythmia). Its clinical importance is the fact that extremely rapid

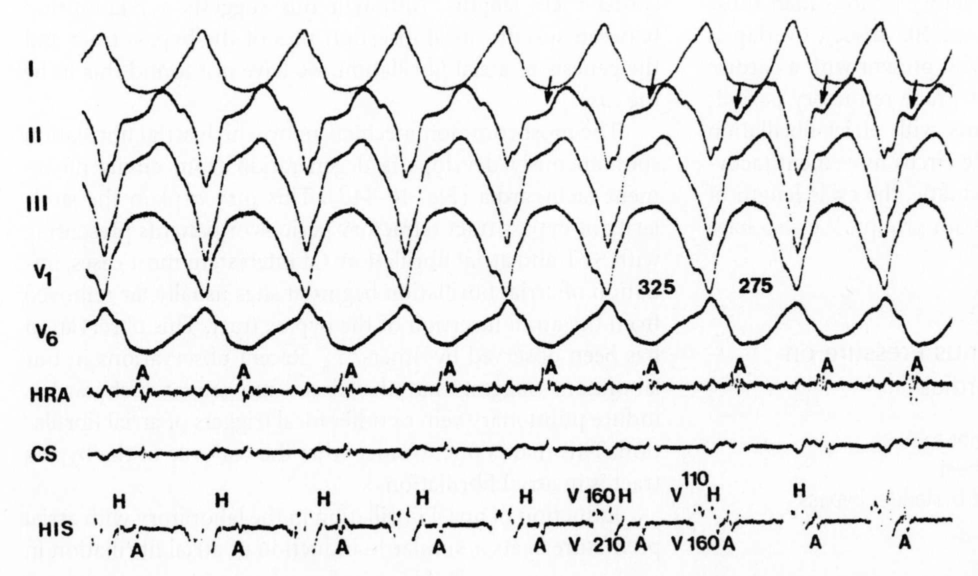


**FIGURE 10-41** *Antidromic tachycardia with an irregular ventricular response.* ECG leads I, II, II, V1, and V6 are shown with recordings from the HRA, CS, and His bundle. Antidromic tachycardia is present with anterograde conduction over a right paraseptal bypass tract. The change in cycle length is related to a change in V-H and consequently V-A intervals (*arrows*). See text for discussion. (From Kuck KH, Brugada P, Wellens HJJ. Observations on the antidromic type of circus movement tachycardia in the Wolff-Parkinson-White syndrome. *J Am Coll Cardiol* 1983;2:1003.)

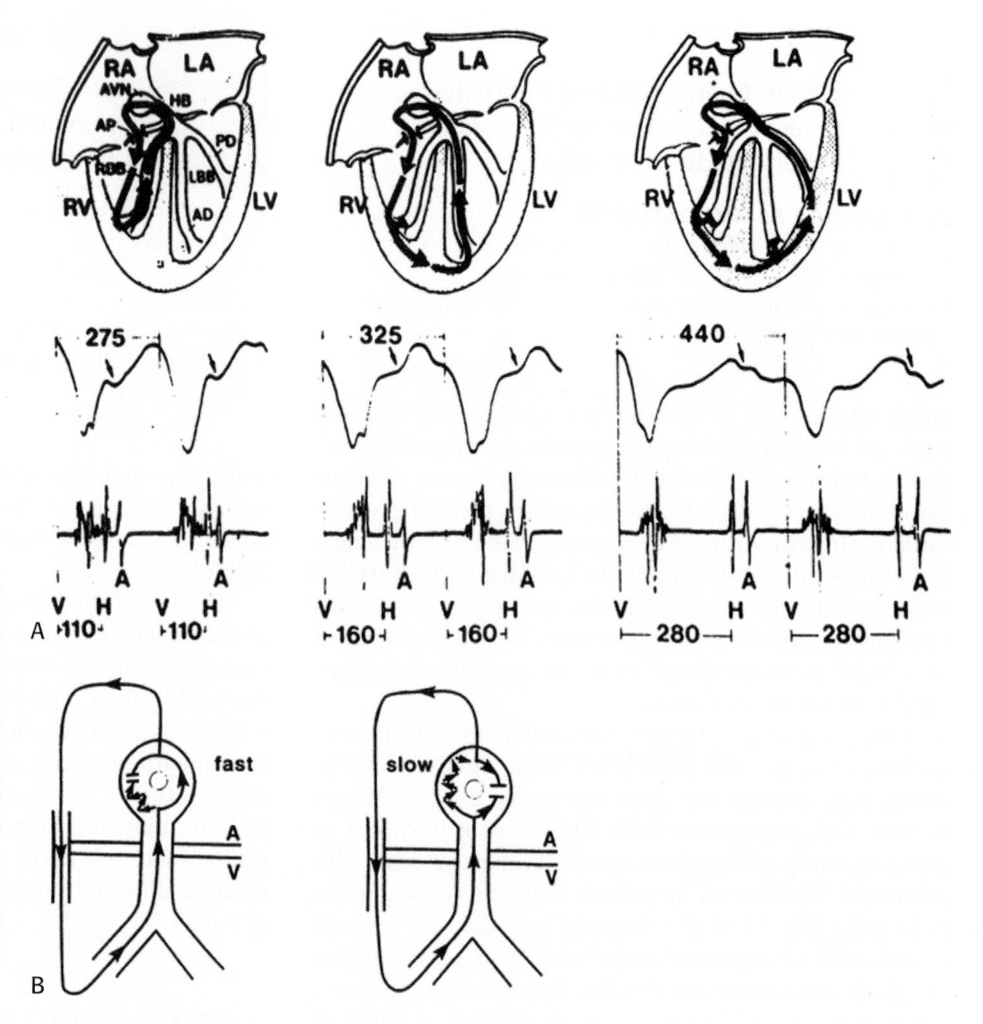


**FIGURE 10-42** *Mechanisms of change in cycle length during antidromic tachycardia due to altered ventriculoatrial conduction.* During antidromic tachycardia the cycle length can prolong if the route of retrograde conduction changes as manifested by a change in V-H interval (**A, top**) or there is a change in retrograde conduction through the A-V node (**B, bottom**). See text for discussion. (Adapted from Wellens HJJ, Josephson, ME. Preexcited tachycardias. In: Josephson ME, Wellens HJJ, eds. *Tachycardias: mechanisms and management.* Mount Kisco, NY: Futura Publishing, 1993:313–333.)

rates can occur over the bypass tract leading to ventricular fibrillation (Fig. 10-44A). In our experience, no clinical features or bypass tract locations distinguish patients with preexcitation and atrial fibrillation from those without atrial fibrillation. Although patients with atrial fibrillation have somewhat shorter bypass tract refractory periods than those with orthodromic SVT only (260 vs. 305 msec), overlap is considerable. Only those patients who present with a cardiac arrest have significantly shorter antegrade refractory periods (mean, 225 msec). Whereas patients with atrial fibrillation have a higher incidence of inducible circus movement tachycardia than those who are asymptomatic, the cycle length of induced tachycardias is similar in both groups. We also have

### TABLE 10-7 Effect of Carotid Sinus Pressure on Preexcited Tachycardias

- Antidromic tachycardia-terminate prior to A
- CMT using two bypass tracts—no effect
- A-V nodal tachycardia with innocent bystander bypass tract—terminate after A

not found atrial pressure during circus movement tachycardia to differ in the two groups. As stated earlier, for unclear reasons, patients with overt preexcitation do have a higher incidence of atrial fibrillation than those with concealed bypass tracts despite comparable bypass tract locations and tachycardia cycle lengths. Although this suggests a relationship between specific atrial insertion sites of the bypass tract and the genesis of atrial fibrillation, we have not found this to be the case.

The most common mechanism by which atrial fibrillation spontaneously develops is degeneration from circus movement tachycardia (Fig. 10-44B). This may explain the similarity of bypass tract refractory periods of patients presenting with SVT and atrial fibrillation. Of interest, in most cases, initiation of atrial fibrillation begins at sites usually far removed from the atrial insertion of the bypass tract. This observation has been observed by others.[72–75] Recent observations in our laboratory suggest that the circus movement tachycardias induce pulmonary vein or other focal triggers of atrial fibrillation. This makes one wonder what the real role of the bypass tract is in atrial fibrillation.

Induction of atrial fibrillation in the laboratory with atrial premature beats is similar to induction of atrial fibrillation in

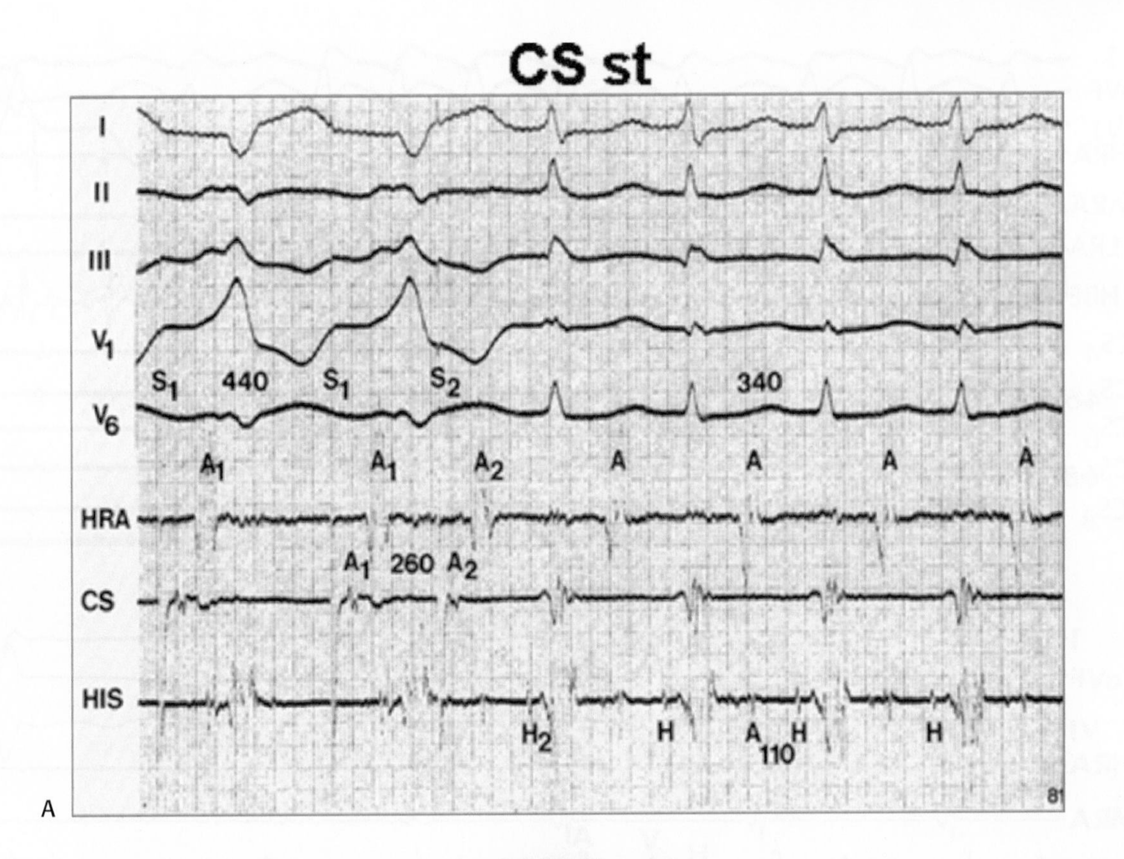


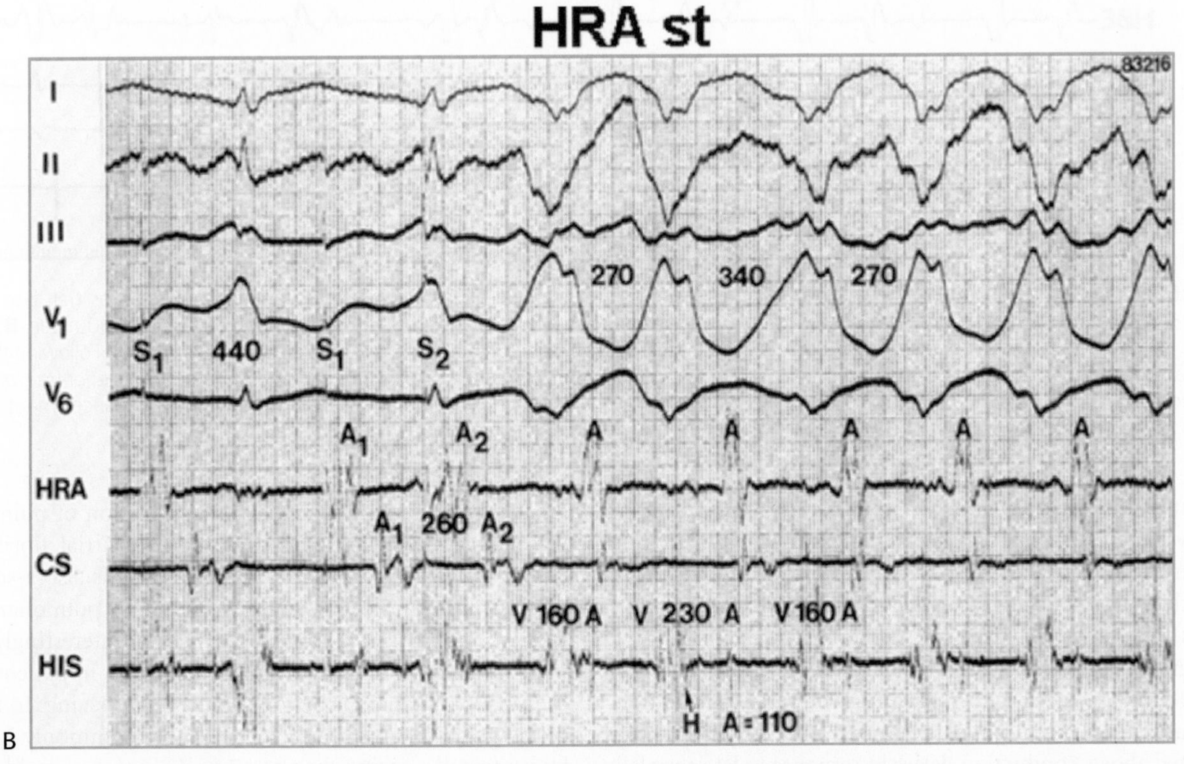


**FIGURE 10-43** *Effect of site of stimulation on the mechanism of induced arrhythmias.* **A:** During HRA stimulation, an APD delivered at an A1-A2 of 260 msec blocks in the A-V node and conducts totally over a left lateral bypass tract. Retrograde conduction goes over the normal His–Purkinje system to initiate a classic antidromic tachycardia. Note that the V-H and H-A intervals are directly related to the cycle length of the tachycardia complexes supporting use of the His–Purkinje system for retrograde conduction. **B:** When stimulation is performed near the site of the bypass tract in the CS, block of the bypass tract occurs at the identical A1-A2 interval that produced A-V nodal block when HRA stimulation was used. With block in the bypass tract, conduction proceeds over the normal conducting system to initiate classic orthodromic tachycardia. See text for discussion.

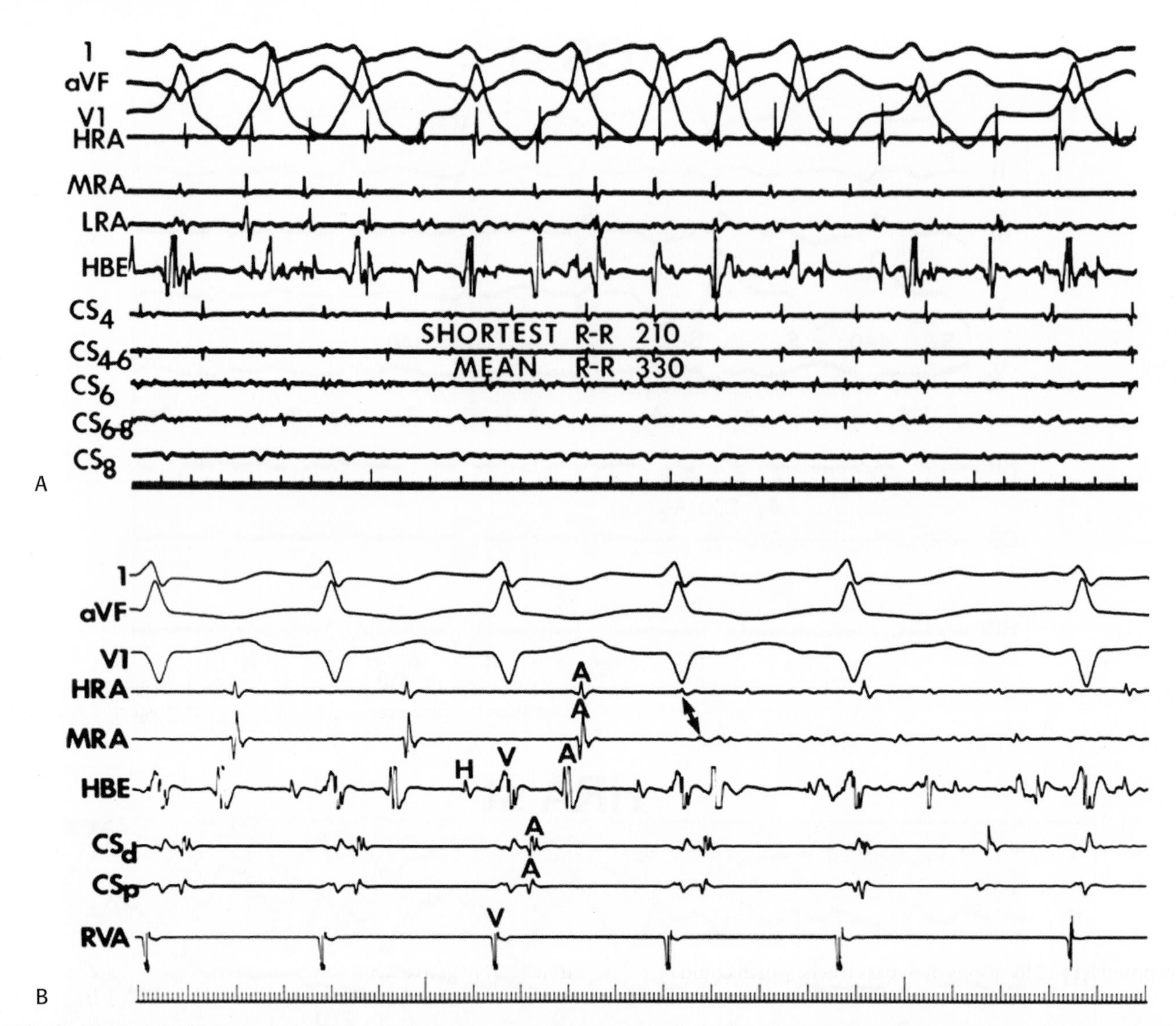


**FIGURE 10-44** *Atrial fibrillation in WPW.* **A:** Ventricular response during atrial fibrillation with preexcited ventricular complexes (left free wall) is usually faster than when complexes are not preexcited. Here, the shortest R-R interval is 210 msec, and the mean R-R is 330 msec. **B:** Orthodromic tachycardia using a left free wall bypass tract (earliest atrial activation in CSp) is present for the first three complexes. Following the third complex, degeneration to atrial fibrillation is observed. Note that despite the fact that the bypass tract is located in the left posterior free wall, atrial fibrillation begins in the right atrium. At initiation of the tachycardia, the QRS complexes are normal, because of retrograde concealment into the bypass tract. See text for discussion.

patients with atrial fibrillation without preexcitation. The electrophysiologic substrate (prolonged intra-atrial conduction in response to APDs, failure of refractoriness to adapt to changes in cycle length, and higher percent of fractionated electrograms) is discussed in Chapter 9. Vulnerability to induction of >1 minute of atrial fibrillation by one or two APDs is observed in 50% to 85% of patients presenting with atrial fibrillation compared to <10% in patients without atrial fibrillation.[45,46] As noted above, conduction delays in response to late coupled APDs are similar to those observed in patients with lone atrial fibrillation in the absence of preexcitation. The significance of a shorter anterograde refractory period of the bypass tract in patients with atrial fibrillation may have to do with the necessity of earlier APDs required to produce block in the bypass tract to initiate SVT. The earlier APD would be associated with greater atrial conduction delays and initiation of pulmonary vein triggers, which would predispose to atrial fibrillation. Circus movement orthodromic tachycardia is also associated with cannon A waves which may result in pulmonary vein triggers and enhanced vagal discharge. An interestingly common mode of induction of atrial fibrillation in patients with the WPW syndrome is by rapid ventricular pacing. In fact, in our experience, atrial fibrillation is more commonly induced by ventricular pacing than atrial pacing at comparable rates. For this particular mode of induction, intra-atrial pressure may play a role in induction of the arrhythmia. Because spontaneous induction of the arrhythmia from circus movement SVT is the most common mechanism, surgical and catheter ablation of the bypass tract apparently cures atrial fibrillation (at least over a 5-year period) in the vast majority (>90%) of patients. Of some concern is the persistent vulnerability to atrial fibrillation that has been noted by Haissaguerre et al.[46] of 56%. This may be due to easier formation of pulmonary vein triggers in these patients. Others have also noted persistent vulnerability.[45] We have also observed that the response to APDs described above is also unaltered by surgical or catheter ablation. This is also consistent with the hypothesis that pulmonary vein triggers require an appropriate substrate in order to initiate atrial fibrillation; cure of SVT which appears to be a trigger of pulmonary vein firing may be what prevents atrial fibrillation in the short term. However removal of the initiating trigger does not affect the underlying substrate. Perhaps these people will develop lone atrial fibrillation at a later age. The answer to this problem will require a 20- to 40-year follow-up. In the patients who are not cured by ablative procedures, primary atrial abnormalities may be responsible for atrial fibrillation in a similar fashion as they are in patients without preexcitation. A study is required to evaluate whether the ability to initiate atrial fibrillation predicts a substrate that will not be changed by cure of WPW ablative therapy and hence, likely recurrence of fibrillation during long-term follow-up.

## LOCALIZATION OF THE BYPASS TRACT

Although the initial suggestion of Rosenbaum et al.[76] that bypass tracts could be divided into Type A and Type B (based on the major QRS forces in V1 and V2), the results of catheter endocardial and intraoperative epicardial mapping suggested a variety of locations of bypass tracts exists. Based on the results of epicardial mapping, Gallagher et al.[32] and Tonkin et al.[77] proposed 8 to 12 locations of bypass tracts, which could be recognized by the initial 40-msec vector of the delta wave during maximal preexcitation. Similar complex algorithms have been proposed in the "ablation" era to attempt to precisely localize the accessory pathway to 12 sites around the A-V valves as well as epicardial sites within the coronary sinus.[78–82] They have actually attempted to distinguish mid-septal (right and left), para-Hisian, and anteroseptal bypass tracts, which arise within 1.5 cm of each other using ECG criteria.[81,83] Although these electrocardiographic and vector-cardiographic criteria may be useful during maximal preexcitation, for the most part, during sinus rhythm, the QRS complex is a fusion and total preexcitation is not present. One cannot arbitrarily use the initial 20 or 40 msec of the QRS or the ratio of R/S in any lead in the absence of total preexcitation to pinpoint the location of a bypass tract. The site of transition of the precordial leads is also flawed by variable lead placement, variations of body shape and/or size, and variations in heart size, location in the chest, and extent of fibrosis or other disease process. As such, I believe a simple approach to regionalize accessory pathways is most reasonable. Lindsay et al.[84] and Milstein et al.[85] have developed more practical ECG criteria to localize the general region of bypass tracts. Milstein et al.[85] divided bypass tracts into four general locations, which represent the

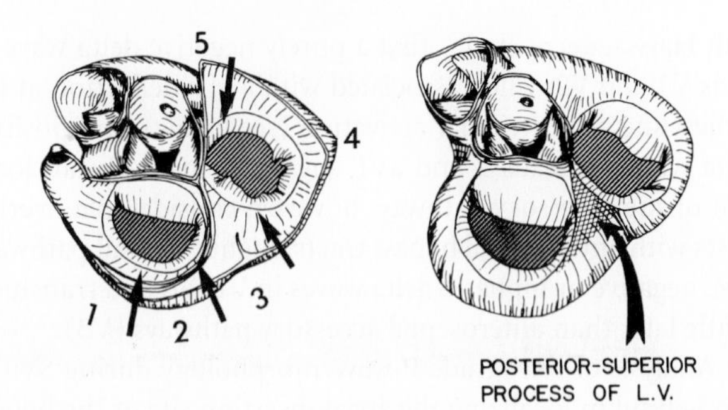


**FIGURE 10-45** *Schema of bypass tract locations used for ECG analysis.* On the left the heart is opened at the midatrial level, and on the right the atria have been removed. The regions we find useful for ECG classification of bypass tracts are shown on the left. Region 1 is left lateral, region 2 is left posterior free wall, region 3 is posterior septal, region 4 is right free wall, and region 5 is anterior septal. The area between 3 and 5 along the tricuspid valve incorporates what are now referred to as mid-septal pathways. See text for discussion.

four surgical approaches (anteroseptal, right free wall, posteroseptal, and left free wall) used to cure WPW. I prefer to divide the location of bypass tracts into five regions: an anteroseptal region, right free wall region, posteroseptal region, a posterior free wall region, and left lateral region. I do this because of significant differences in the ECG of left posterior free wall and true left lateral bypass tract. One could potentially divide the right free wall into two areas – anterior and lateral – but these bypass tracts are insufficiently common to justify this. The schema of locations that we use is shown in Figure 10-45. Basically, left lateral bypass tracts are characterized by negative delta waves in leads 1 and L and by positive delta waves in inferior leads and all the precordial leads. Left posterior (inferior) free wall bypass tracts usually have isoelectric delta waves in lead 1, negative delta waves in inferior leads, isoelectric or slightly positive (closer to posteroseptal location) delta in aVL, and strongly positive delta waves in the right precordial leads. This group may be difficult to distinguish from left posteroseptal bypass tracts, which have positive delta waves in 1 and L. Right posteroseptal bypass tracts are characterized by negative delta waves in the inferior leads (although lead 2 may be isoelectric or biphasic), a left superior axis, and an R/S ratio less than 1 in V1. In general the more negative the delta in lead 2 the more leftward the location. While Arruda et al.[78] state that a negative delta in lead 2 suggests an epicardial CS location, this is not true in the majority of cases. I have seen many right inferior free wall accessory pathways with negative delta waves in leads 2, 3, and aVF. It is, however, true that the larger the negative delta wave in lead 3 relative to lead 2, the more likely this will be a posteroseptal bypass tract that is approachable from the right side. Right free wall bypass tracts generally have biphasic or negative delta waves in both V1 and V2, and positive delta waves in leads 1 and 2, with usually a variably negative delta wave in lead 3 depending on superior versus inferior location. Anteroseptal bypass tracts have positive delta waves in lead 1, inferiorly directed delta waves that are positive in lead 2 and aVF greater than lead 3, and precordial leads with primarily negative or biphasic (40 msec) delta waves. I agree with Haissaguerre et al.[83] that a purely negative delta wave in leads V1 and V2, when associated with a His deflection at the earliest site of ventricular activation (see below), and positive delta waves in leads 2 and aVF suggests a para-Hisian location of the accessory pathway; however, considerable overlap exists with anteroseptal bypass tracts. Right free wall pathways have negative or biphasic delta waves in V1–V3 and transition a little later than anteroseptal accessory pathways (V3).

Analysis of retrograde P-wave morphology during SVT is also helpful in localizing the atrial insertion site of the bypass tracts used for retrograde conduction during SVT. Posteroseptal bypass tracts have inverted P waves in the inferior leads and positive P waves in aVR and aVL. Posterior left free wall bypass tracts have a simliar P-wave morphology in the inferior leads, but the P wave in aVR is more positive than in aVL (which is often isoelectric) and the P wave in lead 2 is more negative than the P wave in lead 3. Left lateral bypass tracts have negative P waves in leads 1 and aVL with a tendency for positive P waves in lead 3 to be greater than those in lead aVF, which are greater than those in lead 2 as the location of the bypass tracts moves more superiorly. In left superior atrial insertion sites the P wave will be more positive in lead 3 than in lead 2, while the opposite is true for right anterior free wall bypass tracts.

Despite claims as to the accuracy of a variety of schemas to precisely localize the ventricular, they all have many limitations and pitfalls. These include the influence of prior infarction, conduction defects, hypertrophy, drug and/or electrolyte imbalance, congenital heart disease, and postoperative changes, which can all influence the electrocardiogram. Moreover, the potential for multiple bypass tracts, the absence of maximal preexcitation, variable lead positions across the precordium, and variations in the position of the heart relative to the recording electrodes, make precise localization merely a guess. Nevertheless, the ECG can help regionalize the site of the bypass tract. Other techniques are required to more accurately and precisely identify the location of the bypass tract.

Several intracardiac mapping and stimulation techniques have been used: (a) determination of the relationship of the delta wave to local ventricular electrograms, (b) pacing from multiple atrial sites, (c) analysis of the retrograde atrial activation pattern during orthodromic tachycardia and/or ventricular stimulation, (d) evaluation of the effect of bundle branch block on V-A conduction during SVT, and (e) direct recording of electrical potentials from the bypass tract.

## RELATION OF LOCAL VENTRICULAR ELECTROGRAMS TO DELTA WAVE

Theoretically, if one could map the ventricles along the mitral and tricuspid rings, the earliest site of ventricular activation and, therefore, the ventricular insertion of the bypass tract could be localized. Aside from technical considerations that may limit this approach, particularly in the left ventricle, whether the bypass tract is epicardial (they usually are) or truly endocardial may influence the relative timing of the local ventricular electrogram, because conduction across the muscle wall will be markedly influenced by anisotropic properties of the ventricle. Because the right ventricle bypass tracts are in some instances endocardial,[86] analysis of multiple-site right ventricular electrograms extending from just cephalad to the tricuspid valve at the His bundle recording site and moving anterolaterally, laterally, and inferoposteriorly can provide considerable information. Use of a Halo catheter or other multipolar catheter to record circumferentially around the tricuspid annulus is extremely useful in regionalizing the bypass tract. Analysis of left ventricular electrograms in the coronary sinus recording provides similar information. We used quadripolar, hexapolar, octapolar, decapolar, and occasionally, dodecapolar catheters for coronary sinus recordings. When the entire coronary sinus cannot be recorded by the electrodes on a single catheter, we move the catheter within the coronary sinus to record a total of 8 to 12 sites. We record bipolar electrograms using either 2-mm or 5-mm interelectrode distances. We usually use all poles for adjacent recordings (i.e., we obtain recordings from poles 1 and 2, 2 and 3, 3 and 4, 4 and 5, and 5 and 6 in a hexapolar catheter) when electrodes have a 5-mm interelectrode distance. Unipolar recordings (unfiltered and filtered) are used to assess which pole is closest to the bypass tract. This is of particular value in guiding the ablation catheter. An example of this technique is shown in Figure 10-46, in which we used a decapolar catheter

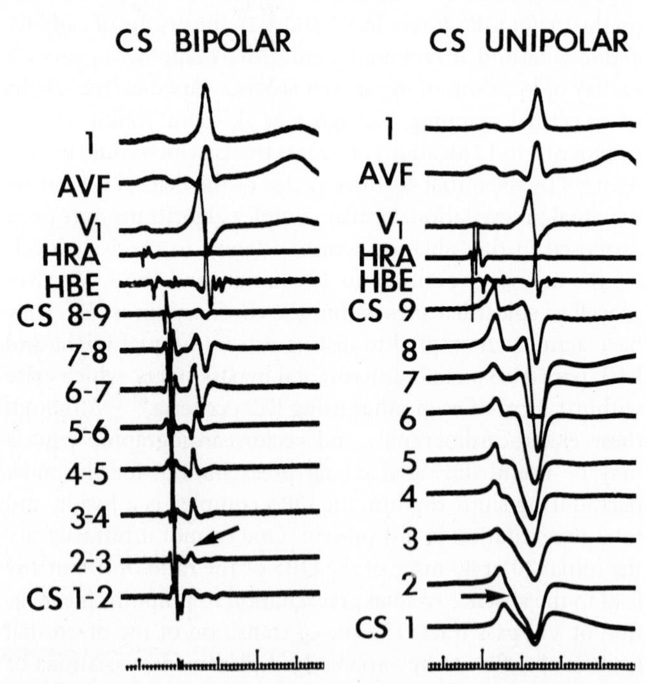


**FIGURE 10-46** *Use of unipolar and bipolar recordings to localize ventricular insertion of the bypass tract in the left ventricle.* Bipolar and unipolar recordings from a decapolar catheter in the CS are shown. The tenth pole is not recorded. Note the earliest bipolar recording is recorded from between poles 2 and 3 of the CS catheter. Using unipolar recordings, the earliest intrinsicoid deflection is in pole 2, defining that pole as closest to the site of ventricular insertion of the bypass tract. See text for discussion.

(tenth pole not shown) in the coronary sinus. One can clearly see that the second bipolar pair provides the earliest electrogram in the filtered signal, and the unipolar recordings reveal that the second pole is the closest to the ventricular insertion site. Although the theoretical advantage of unipolar electrograms is the ability to distinguish contributions of individual poles, frequently the electrograms are so large, and the intrinsicoid deflections not easily determinable, that the ability to distinguish the fastest of a slow-moving waveform is problematic. This is particularly relevant when the coronary sinus is away from the annulus, a frequent problem in the posteroseptal and posterior region (on the atrial side of the annulus) and the distal coronary sinus (ventricular side of the annulus). The variability of the anatomic relationship of the coronary sinus and mitral annulus is an important limitation to the use of electrograms recorded in the coronary sinus to identify the atrial insertion site of the accessory pathway.[87] The relationship of the earliest atrial activation and earliest ventricular activation also must be determined to determine the presence or absence of a slanted bypass tract (see subsequent discussion). As such, ultimately the recordings from the ablation catheter determine the site of ablation. As stated above, the use of both unipolar and bipolar recordings is important to precisely localize the ventricular insertion of the bypass tract for catheter ablation. It is critical to demonstrate that the tip electrode of the ablation/mapping catheter is recording the earliest activity since it will be the electrode through which radiofrequency energy is delivered. Recordings from the LV mapping electrode are compared to those in the coronary sinus to ensure recording of the earliest atrial activity and earliest ventricular activity. The ability to use the coronary sinus catheter to assess left ventricular preexcitation should not be neglected. The limitations imposed by anatomic variations apply for the ventricular insertion site as well, but are less significant. Normally, the basal aspects of the left ventricle recorded from the coronary sinus are activated late in the normal QRS complex. In the presence of a left-sided bypass tract, the base of the heart is activated early, simultaneously with the delta wave (Fig. 10-46). Early activation usually can be distinguished in one bipolar electrogram with an accuracy of 1 cm if 5-mm interelectrode distances are used. The accuracy improves to <5 mm when unipolar recordings are used. Obviously, the most precise method of determining the site of ventricular preexcitation is via a left ventricular mapping catheter. The ventricular insertion site usually has a close relationship with the atrial insertion site, as shown by comparing the site of antegrade preexcitation with retrograde atrial activation mapping (Fig. 10-47), although they may be disparate by up to 2 cm if the bypass tract crosses the A-V sulcus at an angle (see Chapter 14). Changes in local V-A interval due to changes in the wavefront of activation suggest a slanted bypass tract. In my experience, when a slanted bypass tract is present, the ventricular insertion is inferior to the atrial insertion when the bypass tracts are located at the lower half of the mitral and tricuspid annuli and superior to the atrial insertion when located superiorly (viewed in the LAO position). In both cases, the ventricular insertion is usually more medial than the atrial insertion. This has also been observed by Jackman (personal communication; Fig. 10-48). This is most often seen with left-sided bypass tracts when local activation in the CS is compared during LBBB, normal QRS, and RBBB. With LBBB the A and V merge, and with normal or RBBB QRSs' they separate (Fig. 10-49 and see Chapter 14).

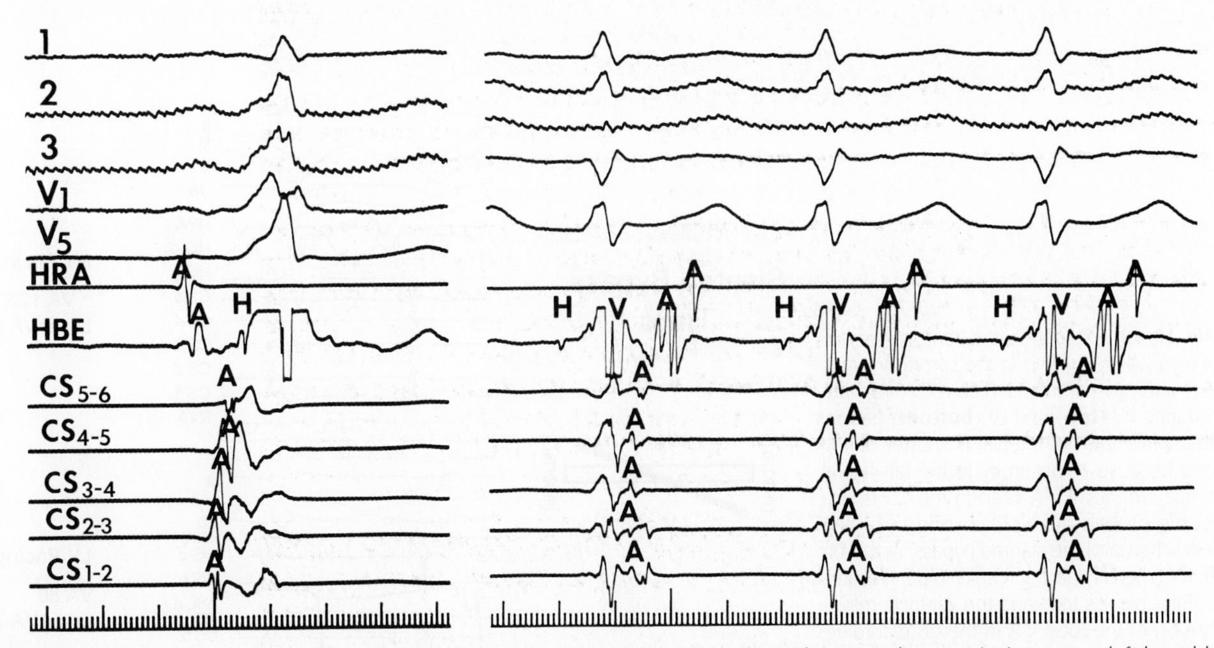


**FIGURE 10-47** *Orthodromic tachycardia with left lateral bypass tract.* A sinus complex with antegrade preexcitation over a left lateral bypass tract is documented by ventricular activation before the delta wave in the next to last bipolar electrode from a hexapolar coronary sinus catheter (CS2-3). Orthodromic tachycardia is shown on the right. Earliest retrograde atrial activation is also recorded in electrode CS2-3. The CS electrodes bracketing the earliest activity (i.e., CS1-2 and CS3-4) confirm CS2-3 as earliest. Thus the site of the ventricular insertion of the bypass tract matches the atrial insertion site.

Slanted AP

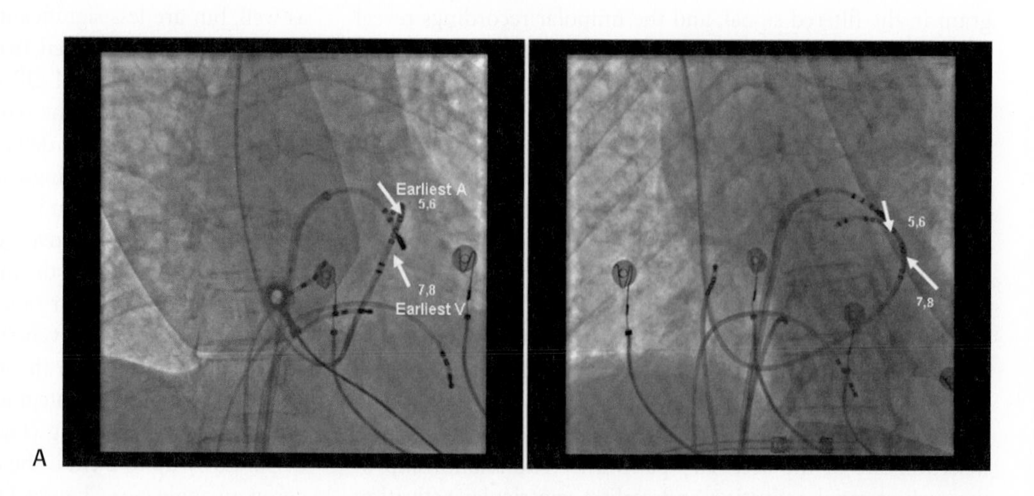


A

Right Anterior
2/4 pts
(50%)
Anteroseptal and
Right Anterior Paraseptal
5/6 pts (83%)
Left
Anterolateral
11/15 pts
(73%)
HB
Right
Lateral
8/14 pts
(57%)
TA
MA
Left
Lateral
27/35 pts
(77%)
Right Posterior
4/4 pts
(100%)
Posteroseptal
19/21 pts
(90%)
Left Posterior
12/15 pts
(80%)

B

**FIGURE 10-48** *Direction of slant of bypass tracts.* An x-ray of slanted left lateral bypass tract. **A:** On the RAO (**left panel**) and LAO (**right panel**) projections are displayed. *Arrows* point to the site of earliest atrial and ventricular activity. **B:** The direction of slant between atrial and ventricular bypass tracts. See text for discussion. (From NASPE/ACC electrophysiology board review course, with permission.)

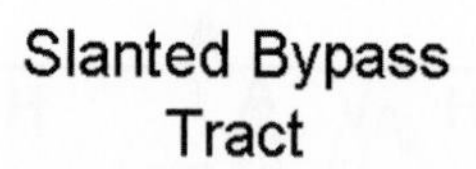


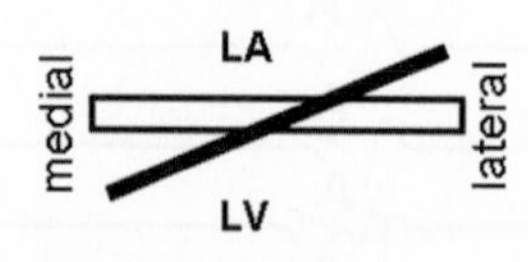


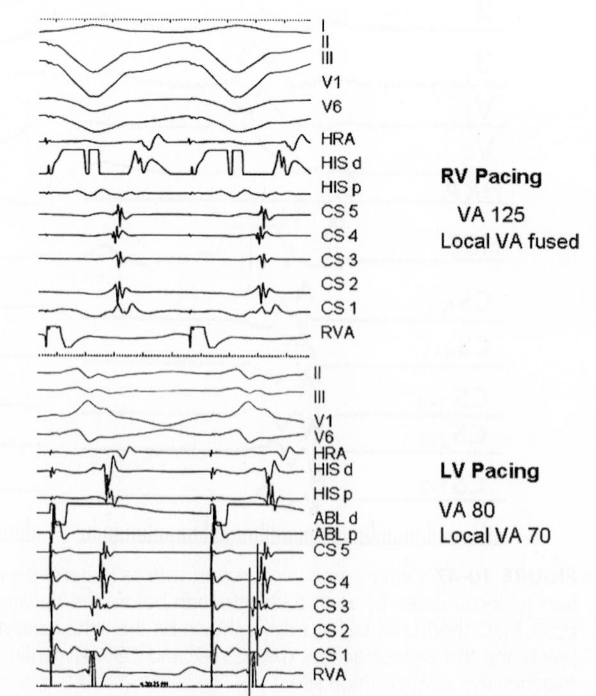


**FIGURE 10-49** *Effect of wavefront of activation on local V-A recording in the coronary sinus.* The ECG and several intracardiac recordings are shown during RV (**top**) and LV (**bottom**) pacing. Note that while the V-A interval is shorter during LV pacing because of proximity to the left lateral bypass tract, the local V-A seen in the CS is longer (70 msec) than during RV pacing (local V-A fused). A schema of the slanted bypass tract is on the left. RV (medial) pacing results in parallel activation of the bypass tract and the ventricle resulting in fusion of the local V-A in the CS recording. Lateral LV pacing results in sequential activation of the LV and the bypass tract producing a V-A equal to the time it takes to get to the LV insertion of the bypass tract and the conduction time over the bypass tract to the atrium.

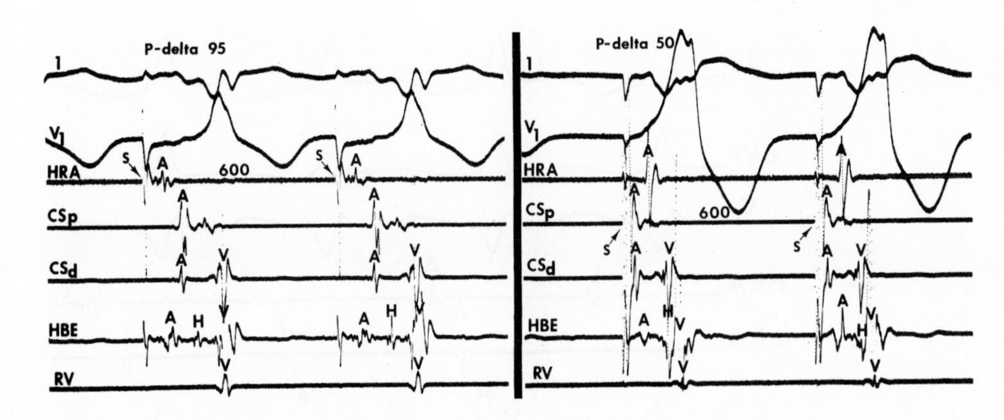


**FIGURE 10-50** *Effect of atrial pacing site on the degree of preexcitation.* In the **left** panel, HRA pacing at a cycle length of 600 msec is associated with a P-delta interval of 95 msec and with significant preexcitation. However, when atrial pacing is carried out from the CS at the identical cycle length, more marked preexcitation and a shorter P-delta (50 msec) interval result, giving evidence of a left-sided bypass tract. See text for further discussion.

## PACING FROM MULTIPLE ATRIAL SITES

As discussed earlier, the closer the stimulation site is to the atrial insertion of the bypass tract, the more rapidly the impulse will reach the bypass tract relative to the A-V node. Thus, the greater the proximity to the atrial insertion site of the bypass tract during atrial pacing, the greater the degree of preexcitation and the shorter the P-to-delta-wave interval will be.[32,88] This response occurs because the effects of intra-atrial and interatrial conduction delays are minimized, particularly when dealing with left-sided bypass tracts. For example, if activation of the atrial insertion of the bypass tract begins 80 msec after the high-right atrial depolarization, pacing the atrium at or near the site of the bypass tract will shorten that interval by approximately 80 msec. This will decrease the P-to-delta-wave time by approximately 80 msec and will produce a greater degree of ventricular preexcitation because the ventricles will begin depolarization earlier via the bypass tract. An example of how this technique can be used to localize the bypass tract is shown in Figure 10-50 in which high-right atrial pacing results in preexcitation with a P-to-delta-wave interval of 95 msec, while coronary sinus pacing produces a shortening of the P-to-delta-wave interval to 50 msec and a greater degree of preexcitation. This effect is particularly valuable in localizing the bypass tract if it is incapable of retrograde conduction, thereby prohibiting localization by atrial mapping during SVT or ventricular pacing (see following discussion).

## RETROGRADE ATRIAL ACTIVATION

The demonstration of eccentric retrograde atrial activation during ventricular stimulation and/or orthodromic circus movement SVT is evidence of a retrogradely conducting A-V bypass tract.[32,89,90] Because retrograde atrial activation during orthodromic circus movement tachycardia proceeds from the atrial insertion of the bypass tract, localization of the earliest site of the retrograde atrial activation identifies the atrial insertion site of the bypass tract. Therefore, it is imperative that electrograms from around both the tricuspid and mitral valves be evaluated. A Halo catheter or other type of multipolar (10 to 20 poles) placed around the tricuspid annulus may be useful to guide precise mapping of right-sided pathways. A multipolar catheter recording from the os to the distal coronary sinus (near the aortic valve) can be used to guide left atrial mapping with the limitations of coronary sinus anatomy taken into consideration. In addition, one must determine whether the bypass tract insert directly into the CS musculature or into the left atrium. CS muscle sleeves are usually detected as high frequency recordings which can precede or follow a lower-frequency left atrial electrogram, depending on the insertion site (Figs. 10-14, 10-16, 10-47, and 10-51). Although Antz et al.[91] state that the LA-CS connection is 2.5 cm from the CS os, we have found the connections of the CS and left atrium are also variable. This is not surprising because of the variable relationship of the CS to the A-V ring. Furthermore, the multiple component electrograms may also reflect nonuniform anisotropic conduction from the insertion site and not separate CS and left atrial recordings. Thus, a detailed assessment of CS electrograms is required to localize the atrial insertion site. Precise mapping should be performed with a deflectable tip catheter in both the right and left atrium or via the retrograde aortic approach to the LV. Occasionally mapping of the veins off the coronary sinus is necessary to precisely localize epicardial pathways. These are not infrequently associated with structural abnormalities in the coronary sinus, for example, coronary sinus diverticulum. Mapping can be performed during ventricular pacing but, preferably, should be done during orthodromic SVT to eliminate the confusion resulting from simultaneous retrograde activation over the normal conduction system. Both right and left atrial catheters can be moved to record along the entire circumference of the tricuspid and mitral valves to precisely ascertain the site of earliest atrial activation. This is critically important, particularly when multiple bypass tracts are suspected (see following discussion).

In normal patients and in those with A-V nodal reentrant SVT, the earliest site of retrograde atrial activation during ventricular pacing is usually at the apex or base of the triangle of Koch. In many patients multiple breakthrough sites are seen with simultaneous activation of the apex and base of the triangle of Koch or even the coronary sinus[92,93] (see Chapter 8). The remainder of the right atrium and the more distal sites of

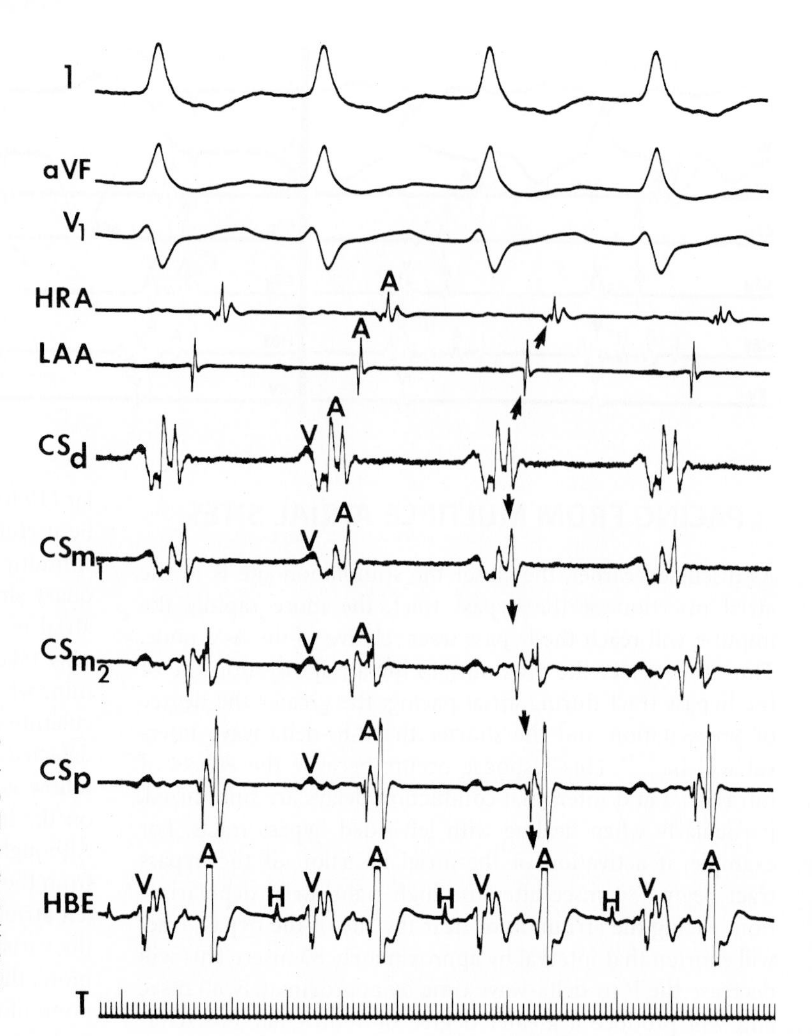


**FIGURE 10-51** *Use of direct left atrial recording to localize a left lateral bypass tract.* Orthodromic tachycardia is present. The coronary sinus catheter can be advanced only to the inferolateral portion of the CS. Although this site showed the shortest ventriculoatrial activation and earliest atrial activation, the catheter could not be advanced to evaluate more distal left atrial sites. Direct left atrial catheterization through a patent foramen ovate enabled recording atrial activity at the level of the LAA and showed that it was later than the atrial electrogram from the CSd. This, therefore, bracketed the earliest site, proving it came from the midlateral wall.

the coronary sinus are activated later.[89,90,92–94] In patients with retrogradely functioning free wall A-V bypass tracts, the atria are activated eccentrically during SVT and during ventricular pacing, if retrograde conduction in the latter instance proceeds over the bypass tract preferentially. Consequently, the left atrium will be depolarized first in the presence of a left free wall bypass tract, and the free wall of the right atrium will be depolarized first in the presence of a right free wall bypass tract (Figs. 10-47, 10-51 to 10-55). Thus, the retrograde atrial activation sequence during ventricular pacing is usually similar to that during SVT, particularly during fast-paced rates which favor conduction over the accessory pathway. Atrial fusion due to simultaneous activation over the A-V node and bypass tract must be excluded. Failure to do so can be misleading. This can be done by pharmacologic block of the A-V node or the use of VPDs. Furthermore, as stated earlier, the retrograde atrial activation sequence during ventricular stimulation and the comparative antegrade activation sequence during sinus rhythm occur near each other, with some differences based on whether the bypass tract is slanted.

In patients with retrogradely functioning septal bypass tracts, atrial excitation may appear similar to "normal" atrial activation located in the anterior, mid, or posterior triangle of Koch, as shown in Figures 10-56 and 10-57. With posteroseptal bypass tracts, the electrogram at the os of the coronary sinus or base of the triangle of Koch will usually be slightly earlier than that recorded at the apex of the triangle of Koch. With anteroseptal, para-Hisian, or mid-septal bypass tracts, the electrogram at or near the apex or midportion of the triangle of Koch will be earlier than the base of the triangle of Koch or coronary sinus. Because both these patterns of atrial activation can be seen in an A-V nodal reentry, other methods must be used to show whether retrograde conduction is occurring over a bypass tract. Ventricular extrastimuli or pacing can help resolve the issue of what is conducting retrogradely with a "normal" retrograde atrial activation sequence. The most obvious situation is when ventricular extrastimuli clearly can dissociate retrograde conduction over a septal bypass tract from that over the normal A-V conducting system. This requires observation of conduction over both pathways simultaneously during ventricular stimulation (Fig. 10-58). This figure additionally demonstrates phase 4 (cycle lengths >1,000 msec) and acceleration dependent (cycle lengths <900 msec) block in an anteroseptal bypass tract (see preceding discussion of electrophysiologic properties of A-V bypass tracts). As noted above, ventricular pacing or ventricular extrastimuli from the right

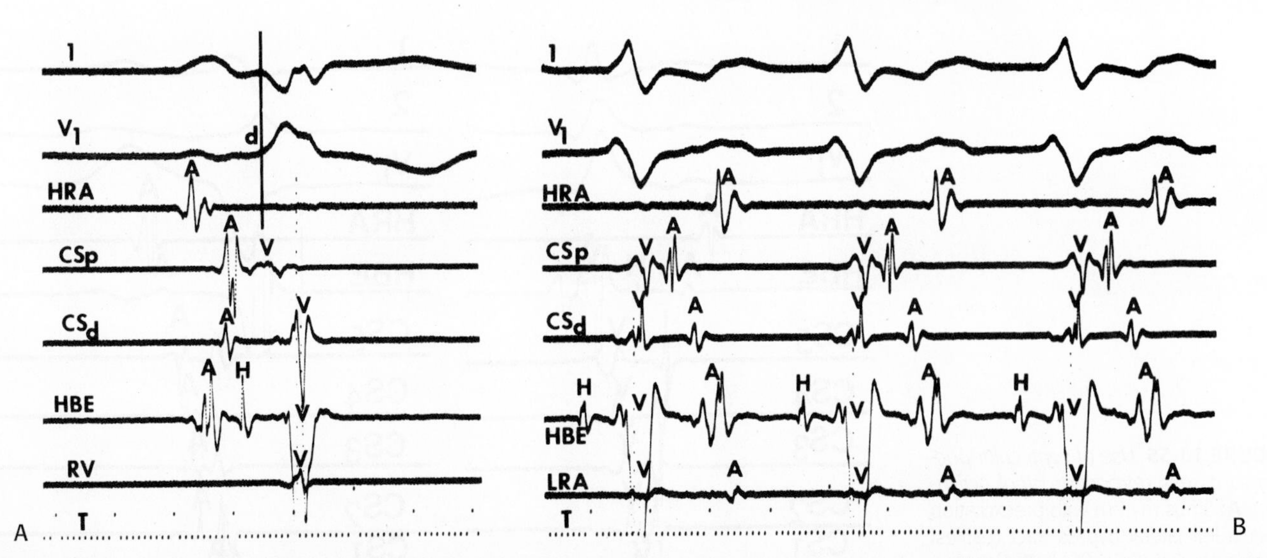


**FIGURE 10-52** *Retrograde atrial activation during orthodromic tachycardia using a left posterior free wall bypass tract.* **A:** A sinus complex. **B:** Orthodromic tachycardia. Earliest ventricular activity during NSR is shown in the CSp, which is in the midposterior free wall of the left atrium. This corresponds to the earliest site of atrial activation during orthodromic tachycardia. Later activation in both the CSd and HBE confirms the posterior free wall at the site of the bypass tract.

ventricle can result in fusion of retrograde atrial activation over both the normal A-V conducting system and a left-sided bypass tract, giving the impression of "normal" retrograde conduction. In such instances, stimulation from the left ventricle can demonstrate the presence of a left-sided bypass tract where right ventricular stimulation yields confusing results. This is demonstrated in Figure 10-59, in which left ventricular pacing demonstrated a left free wall bypass tract, which is distinguished from a left lateral bypass tract by the earliest retrograde atrial activation being recorded in the midposterior coronary sinus and not the distal coronary sinus. This demonstrates the limitations of analyzing retrograde conduction during RV pacing during sinus rhythm to document the presence and location of a bypass tract. Use of adenosine or other drugs that impair A-V nodal conduction is another means of ensuring retrograde conduction up the bypass tract, thereby allowing one to localize the bypass tract.

Three other methods of ventricular stimulation during sinus rhythm are useful for distinguishing septal bypass tracts from "normal" retrograde conduction as seen in A-V nodal reentry. The easiest is to compare the V-A interval during

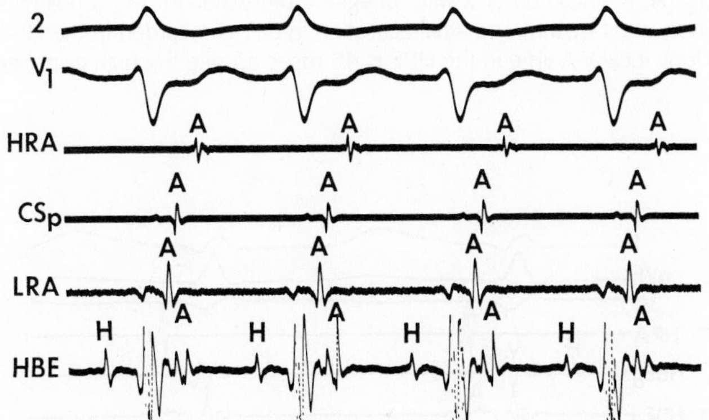

**FIGURE 10-53** *Atrial activation during orthodromic tachycardia using a right posterior lateral bypass tract.* During orthodromic tachycardia, the atrial electrogram at the LRA precedes atrial activation at the CSp and the HBE.

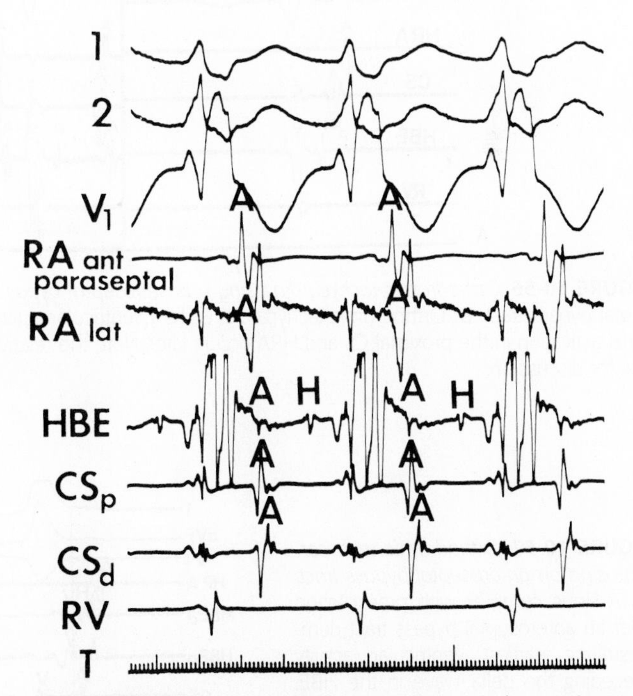


**FIGURE 10-54** *Orthodromic tachycardia using a right anterior paraseptal bypass tract.* Orthodromic tachycardia with a right bundle branch block morphology is present. Earliest atrial activation appears in the anterior right atrium and is followed by atrial activation in the anterolateral right atrium and HBE. Left atrial activation as measured in the CS occurs later. RAant, anterolateral right atrium; RAlat, lateral right atrium.

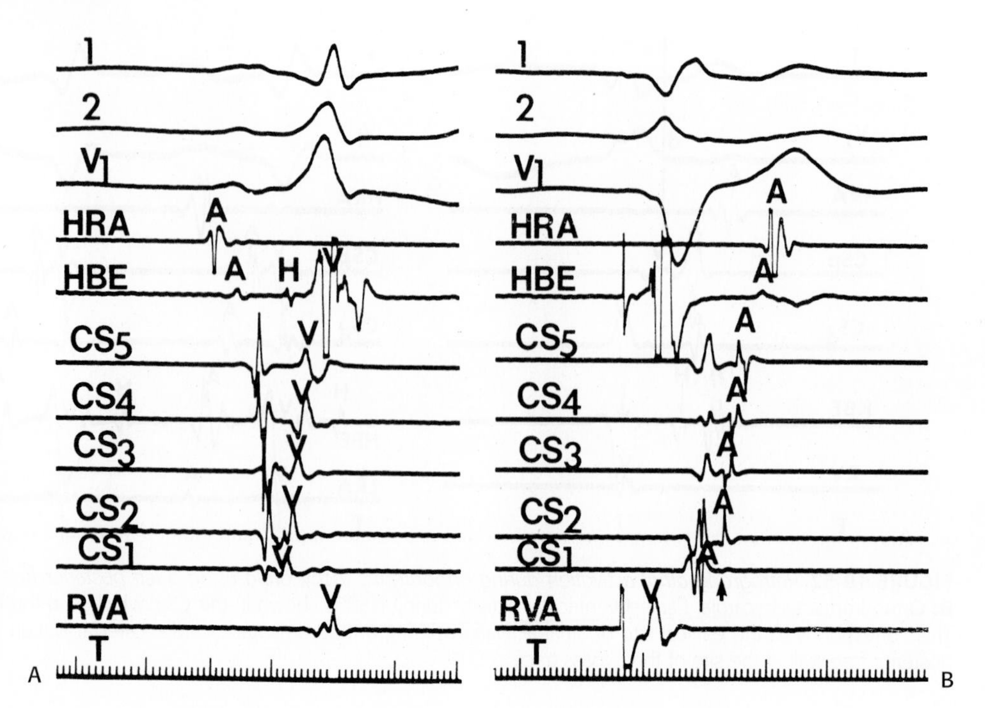


**FIGURE 10-55** *Use of ventricular pacing to assess retrograde atrial activation.* **A:** Sinus rhythm with preexcitation over a left lateral bypass tract (earliest ventricular activity in CS1). **B:** Ventricular pacing produces a retrograde atrial activation sequence that matches the site of antegrade preexcitation with the earliest atrial activation in the CS1.

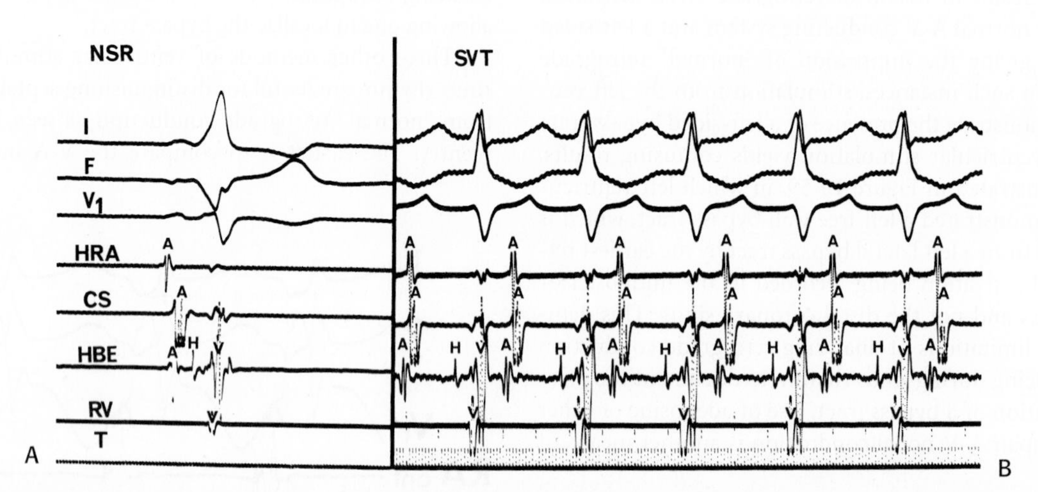


**FIGURE 10-56** *Orthodromic tachycardia using a posteroseptal bypass tract.* **A:** A sinus complex with antegrade preexcitation over a posterior septal bypass tract. **B:** Orthodromic tachycardia. Earliest ventricular activation in sinus rhythm and atrial activation in SVT is recorded in the HBE. Atrial activation in the proximal CS and HRA occurs later. Note the relatively long local V-A time in the HBE is 45 msec despite the high gain. See text for discussion.

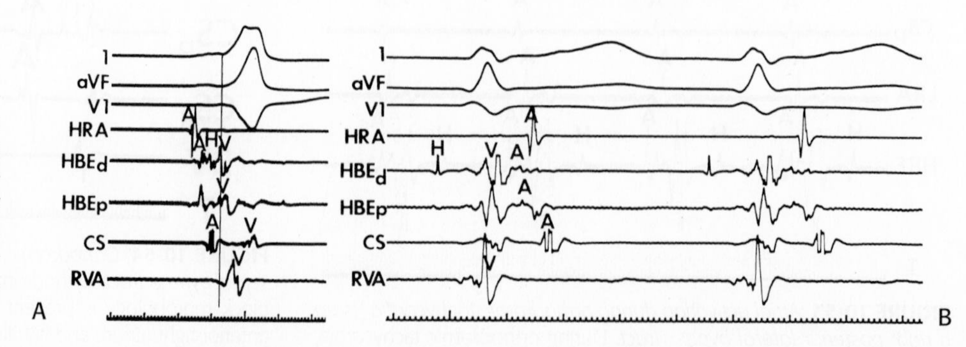


**FIGURE 10-57** *Orthodromic tachycardia using an anteroseptal bypass tract.* **A:** A sinus complex with preexcitation over an anteroseptal bypass tract demonstrating earliest ventricular activity preceding the delta wave in the HBE. **B:** During orthodromic tachycardia, earliest retrograde activation also occurs in the HBE.

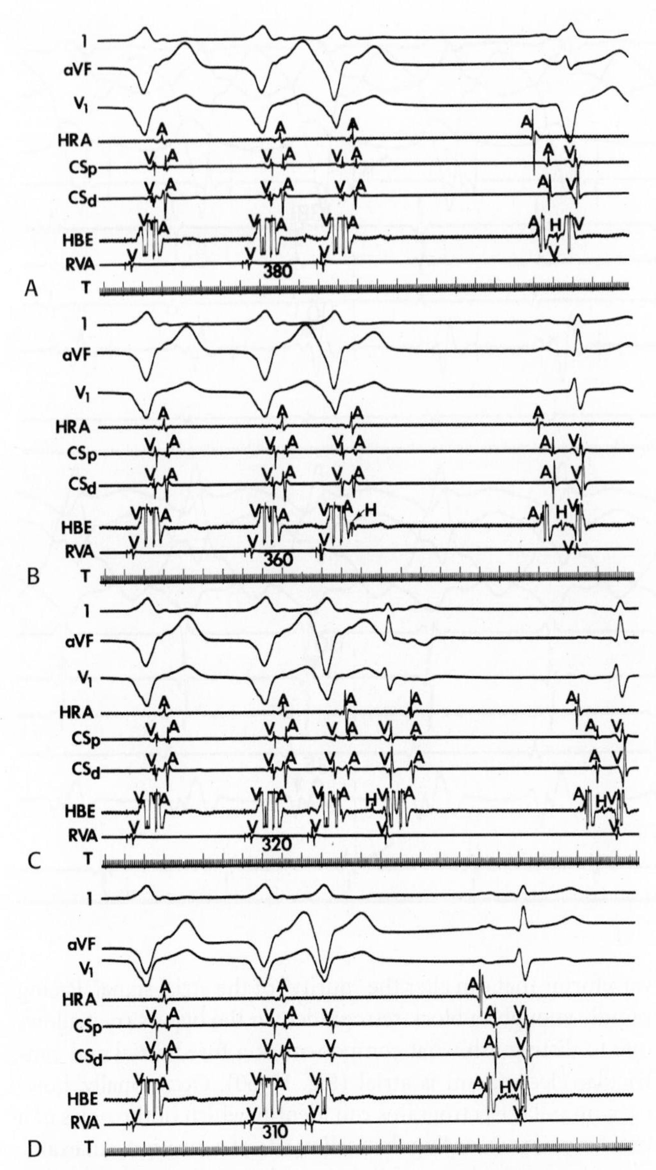


**FIGURE 10-58** *Use of ventricular extrastimuli to distinguish retrograde conduction over an anteroseptal bypass tract from retrograde conduction over the normal A-V conducting system.* **A–D:** Ventricular pacing at a basic cycle length of 600 msec is shown with progressively premature ventricular extrastimuli delivered. **A:** A ventricular extrastimulus is delivered at 380 msec and conducts retrogradely to the atrium with no V-A delay and a "normal" retrograde atrial activation sequence with earliest activity recorded in the HBE. **B:** When the coupling interval is reduced to 360 msec, a septal bypass tract is confirmed by a retrograde His bundle depolarization, which occurs after retrograde atrial activation with the same retrograde atrial activation sequence and timing. **C:** When a ventricular extrastimulus is delivered at 320 msec, block in the His–Purkinje system occurs and V-A conduction proceeds solely over the septal bypass tract. The retrograde atrial activation can now conduct antegradely down the normal conducting system to produce an echo complex. **D:** Block in the bypass tract and in the His–Purkinje system is observed. See text for discussion.

ventricular pacing from the RV apex and the RV inflow tract adjacent to the triangle of Koch. Since accessory pathways traverse the tricuspid annulus, pacing adjacent to the annulus will be associated with shorter V-A intervals than pacing from the RV apex. The opposite is true for A-V nodal tachycardia in which retrograde conduction must proceed over the right bundle branch, which is engaged earliest at the RV apex. A second method mentioned in Chapter 8 is to compare the H-A interval during SVT and the H-A interval during ventricular pacing initiated during sinus rhythm. This analysis can virtually always separate septal bypass tracts from the A-V nodal reentry, as can the absolute value of the V-A interval as well as the difference in V-A intervals during SVT and RV pacing. As mentioned in Chapter 8, the H-A interval during ventricular pacing will always be less than that during SVT when a septal bypass tract is operative (sequential activation during SVT and parallel activation during pacing) and will always be longer than that recorded during A-V nodal reentry in which the presence of a lower final common pathway in the A-V node is documented.[95] Since a retrograde His deflection is not universally recorded during RV pacing, comparing the VA during SVT with that during RV pacing may be useful in separating a septal pathway from AVNRT. If the VA is more than 90 msec longer during pacing than SVT, AV nodal tachycardia is almost always present. Since the ventricle is part of the tachycardia circuit, RV pacing will show much less of a difference (usually 50 to 75 msec). As discussed in Chapter 8, the difference between the post-pacing interval (PPI) and SVT cycle length >100 to 115 msec favors A-V nodal reentry, but this may be confounded by marked slowing of antegrade A-V nodal conduction (with or without dual pathways) produced by pacing too fast. Moreover, as stated in Chapter 8, these differences in PPI and V-A intervals are not valid in tachycardias with long V-A intervals. Moreover, as mentioned earlier in Chapter 8, an absolute value of the V-A interval measured in the septum of <70 msec will separate septal bypass tracts from A-V nodal reentry. Benditt et al. have demonstrated that if one uses the electrogram at the high-right atrium, the V-A interval recorded to the high-right atrium always exceeds 95 msec during circus movement tachycardia.[96] We have observed that the shortest V-A intervals are found in left lateral bypass tracts, with the shortest V-A interval we have observed being 58 msec (range 58 to 172). The shortest V-A interval reported by Benditt et al.[97] was 61 msec. The third method is by para-Hisian pacing. Changes in the atrial activation sequence and timing dependent on capturing the His bundle can distinguish normal retrograde conduction and that over a bypass tract (Table 10-8).[98]

It is imperative that one recognizes that, as with antegrade conduction, bypass tracts almost always behave in an all-or-none fashion during retrograde conduction. Thus, the V-A interval should remain constant despite oscillations of cycle length if a bypass tract is used. Alterations of the V-A interval can occur rarely, owing to concealed antegrade conduction in response to APDs or occasionally in response to a very early VPD at initiation of the tachycardia or during orthodromic tachycardia. Rarely, a bypass tract appears to exhibit longitudinal dissociation, resulting in two distinct V-A intervals with identical, eccentric, retrograde activation sequences. In general, however, the observation of changing V-A intervals

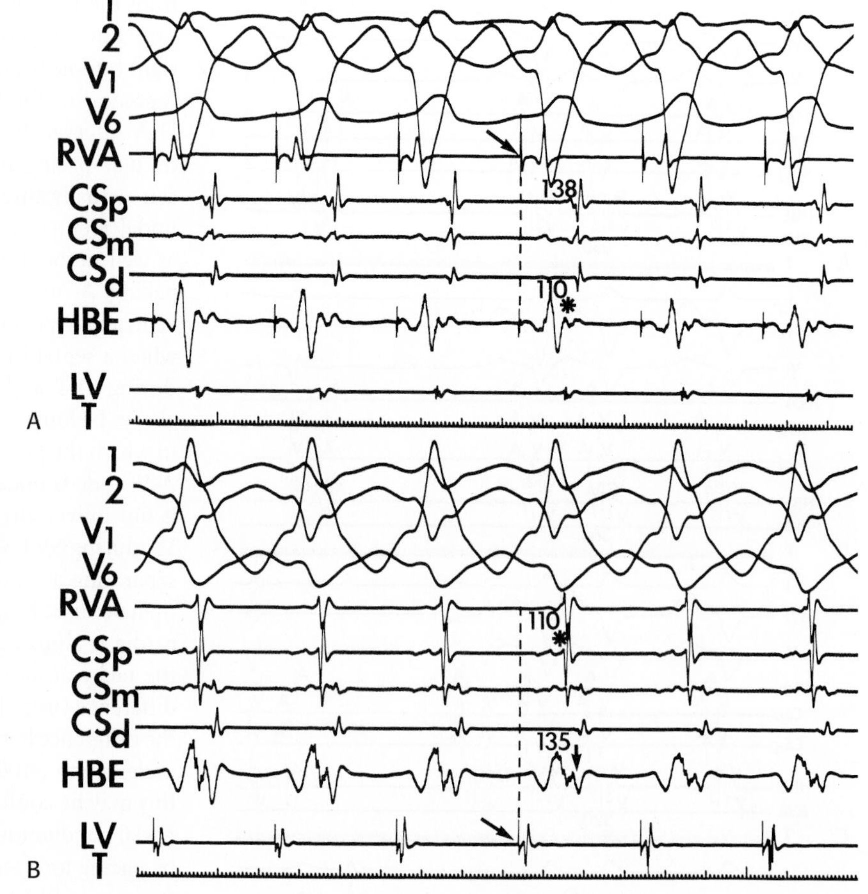


**FIGURE 10-59** *Use of left ventricular pacing to diagnose left-sided bypass tract.* **A:** During right ventricular pacing, retrograde atrial activation appears "normal" with earliest atrial activity recorded in the HBE, 110 msec following the QRS (*). **B:** When pacing is carried out from the left ventricle, earliest retrograde atrial activation is observed in the CSp with a V-A time of 110 msec (*). Note that, with left ventricular pacing, atrial activation in the HBE occurs significantly later, at 135 msec. Thus, in the presence of rapid V-A conduction over the normal A-V conducting system, stimulation from the left ventricle may be necessary to demonstrate the presence of a left-sided bypass tract.

usually means that multiple bypass tracts are operative (see following discussion) or that a different mechanism of the tachycardia exists. Differences in retrograde atrial activation sequence should be sought during these changes.

Gallagher et al.[32] and Farre et al.[99] suggested that unipolar recordings may be extremely useful in determining the location of the bypass tract. Although unipolar recordings, if clear and discrete from ventricular recordings, can have localizing value, more often than not the atrial electrogram, particularly if the signal is unfiltered, is obfuscated by the local ventricular electrogram, which produces depolarization and repolarization waveforms that can alter the "purity" of the atrial signal. Pacing rapidly enough to block retrogradely in the bypass tract allows one to distinguish what component of a fused atrial and ventricular electrogram is atrial (Fig. 10-60). Occasionally, however, unipolar electrograms can identify which of the poles of a bipolar pair is recording the earliest site of activation. An example of how unipolar recordings can identify the earliest bipolar signal at which the distal (tip) electrode records earlier activity than the proximal pole is shown in Figure 10-61 (Courtesy of Warren Jackman). This becomes critical when performing transcatheter ablation of bypass tracts (see Chapter 14).

**TABLE 10-8 Methods of Distinguishing a Bypass Tract from Normal Retrograde Conduction Due to A-V Nodal Reentry**

**During Tachycardia**

- Preexcite or postexcite the atrium, or terminate SVT by VPC when His is refractory

**During NSR**

- V-A shorter during VP near annulus than from apex
- H-A during SVT is less than H-A (or V-A) during VP
- Para-Hisian pacing with a change in H-A with or without a change in V-A with capture and no capture

## EFFECT OF BUNDLE BRANCH BLOCK DURING ORTHODROMIC TACHYCARDIA

Prolongation of both the tachycardia cycle length, and more importantly, the V-A interval, by more than 35 msec following the development of bundle branch block is diagnostic of a free wall bypass tract ipsilateral to the conduction defect.[24,32,90,100–104] The mechanism for this phenomenon (discussed in detail in Chapter 8) lies in the fact that at least some part of the ventricles is a required component of the reentrant circuit. The V-A interval thus includes the time the circulating impulse exits from the His–Purkinje system to the ventricular myocardium to the time it reaches the bypass

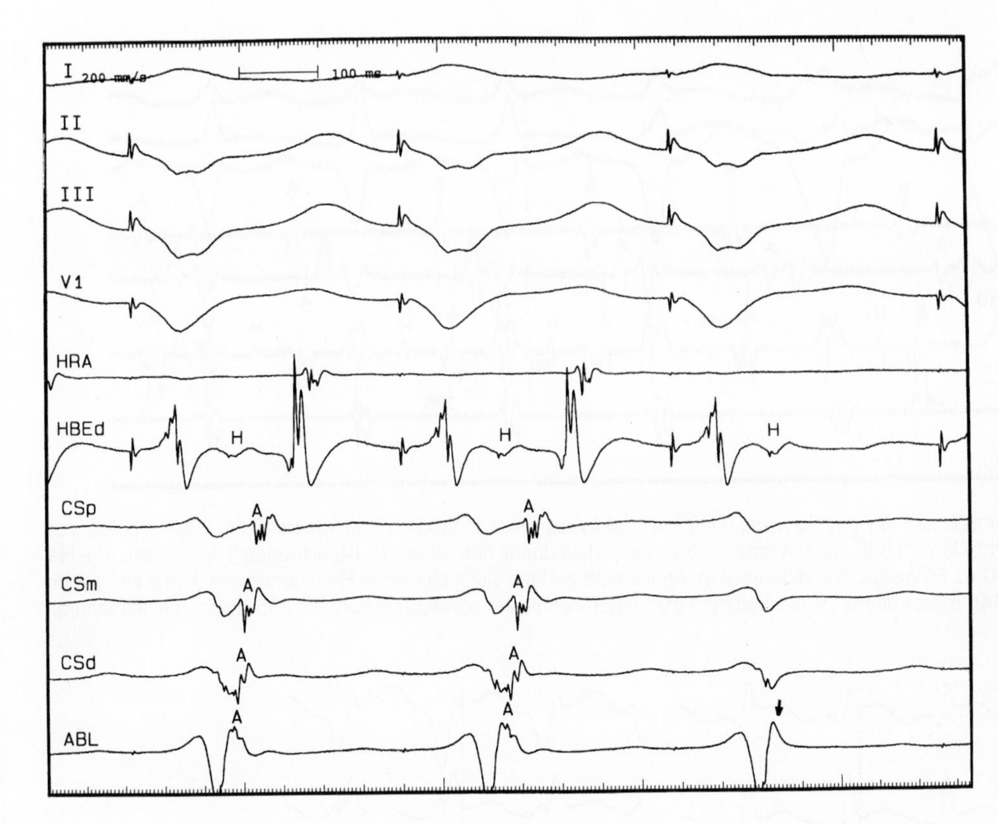


**FIGURE 10-60** *Use of rapid ventricular pacing to distinguish atrial activity which is fused in the ventricular electrogram.* Surface leads I, II, III, V1 are shown with electrograms from the HRA, $HBE_d$ (distal HBE), proximal (p), mid (m), and distal (d) CS and the ablation catheter. During ventricular pacing the atrial electrogram is fused with the ventricular electrogram in the first two beats. The third paced complex blocks retrogradely in the bypass tract allowing precise definition of the atrial electrogram. See text for discussion.

tract. Therefore, patients with left free wall bypass tracts will show prolongation of the V-A interval with the development of LBBB, and those with right-sided bypass tracts show a V-A prolongation with RBBB. In both instances, ipsilateral bundle branch block increases the size of the reentrant circuit by extending the amount of intraventricular conduction required to reach bypass tract. Bundle branch block developing on the contralateral side to the bypass tract has no influence on the V–A interval or cycle length of the tachycardia (Figs. 10-62 to 10-64). In patients with anteroseptal or posteroseptal bypass tracts,

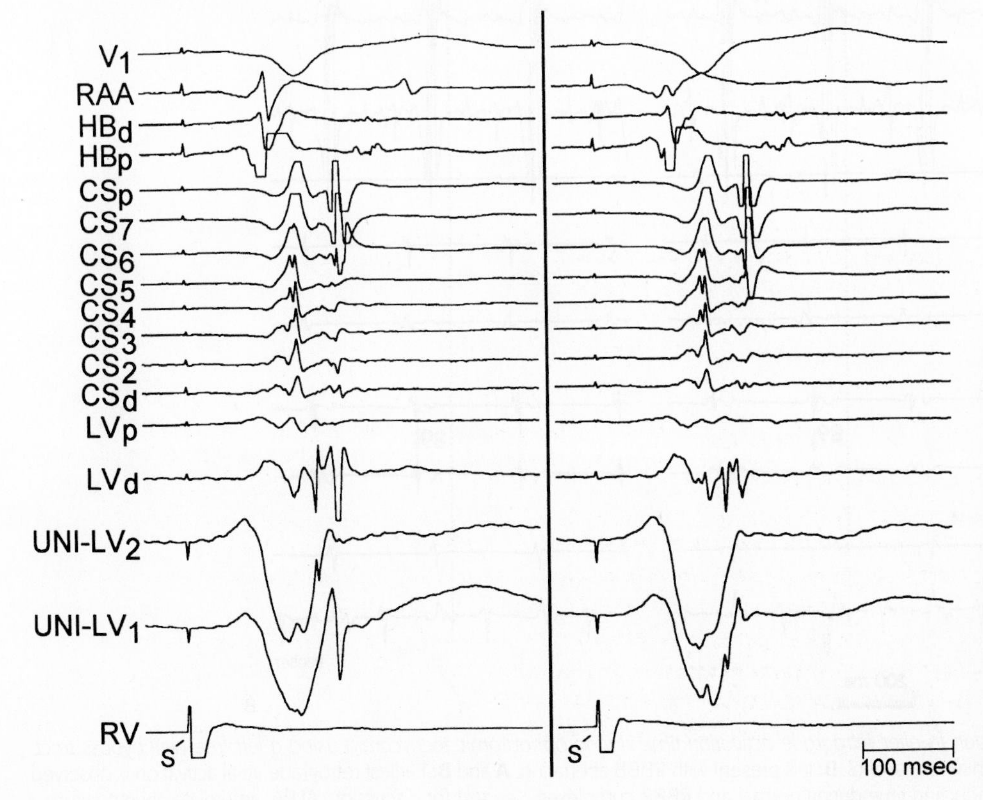


**FIGURE 10-61** *Importance of unipolar recordings.* Atrial activation is recorded during right ventricular pacing from the right atrial appendage (RAA), proximal and distal His bundle ($HB_{d,p}$), 10 bipolar signals from the CS, a bipolar signal and unipolar signals from the distal (UNI-LV1) and second pole (UNI-LV2) of the LV mapping catheter. In the left panel the earliest component of the bipolar signal is recorded at UNI-LV1, which is not appropriate if ablation is to be performed. The ideal site is shown on the right at which the UNI-LV1 signal is responsible for the earliest component of the bipolar signal. See text for discussion. (Courtesy of Warren Jackman.)

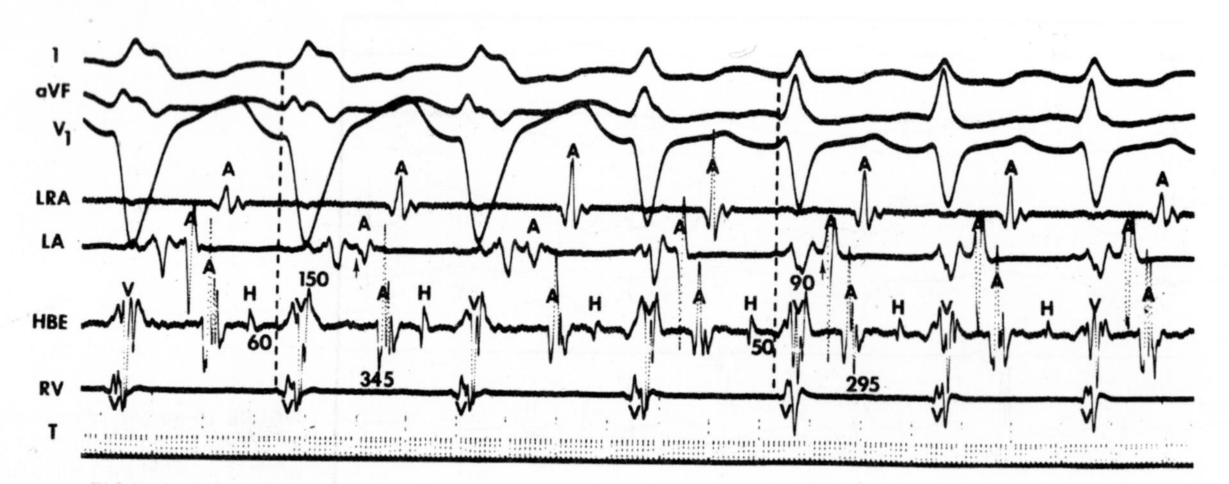


**FIGURE 10-62** *Effect of LBBB during orthodromic tachycardia using a left free wall bypass tract.* Orthodromic tachycardia with LBBB is present on the left and with a normal QRS on the right. During LBBB, the V-A time is 150 msec, while during normal ventricular activation it is 90 msec. The H-V is also slightly prolonged during LBBB (60 vs. 50 msec). The difference in V-A intervals and the slight change in H-V intervals result in a tachycardia cycle length that is significantly slower (345 msec) during LBBB aberration than when ventricular activation is normal (295 msec). LA, left atrium.

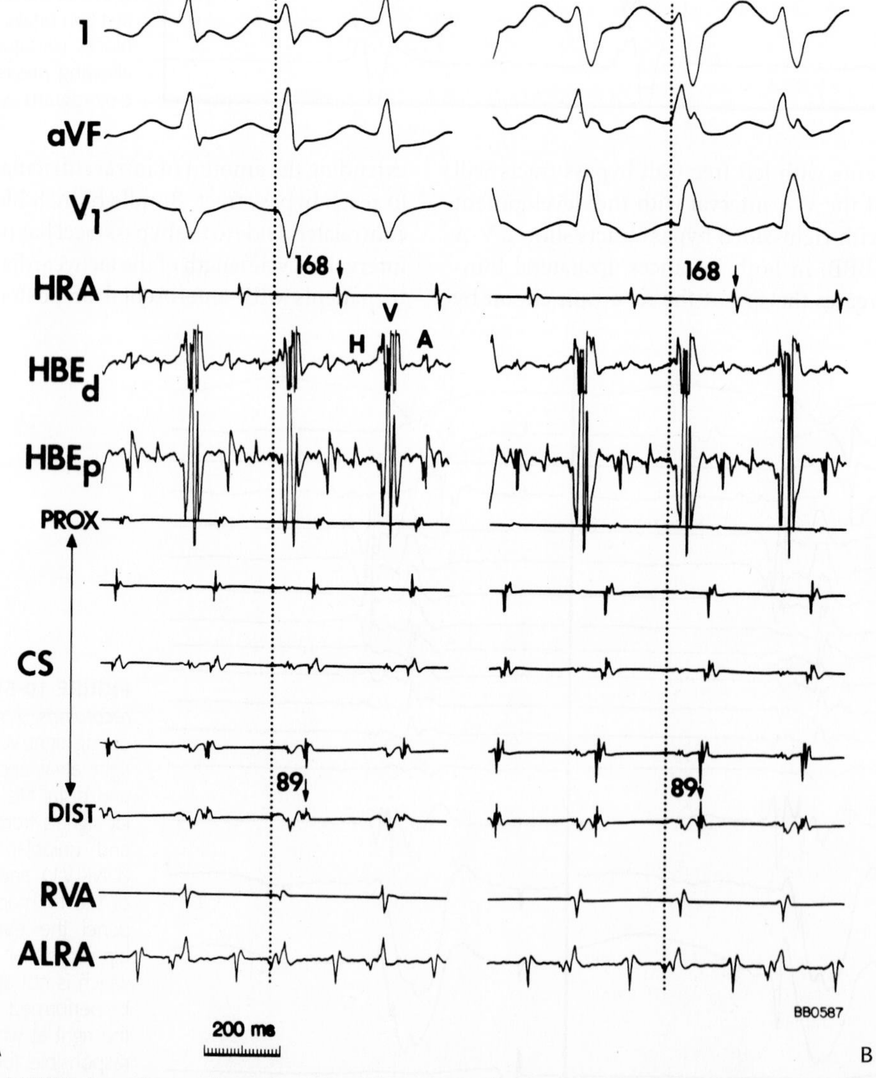


**FIGURE 10-63** *Failure of RBBB aberration to alter retrograde activation time during orthodromic tachycardia using a left free wall bypass tract.* **A:** Orthodromic tachycardia is present with a normal QRS. **B:** It is present with RBBB aberration. **A** and **B:** Earliest retrograde atrial activation is observed in the distal CS. Note an identical V-A conduction time during normal and RBBB complexes. See text for discussion. ALRA, anterolateral right atrium.

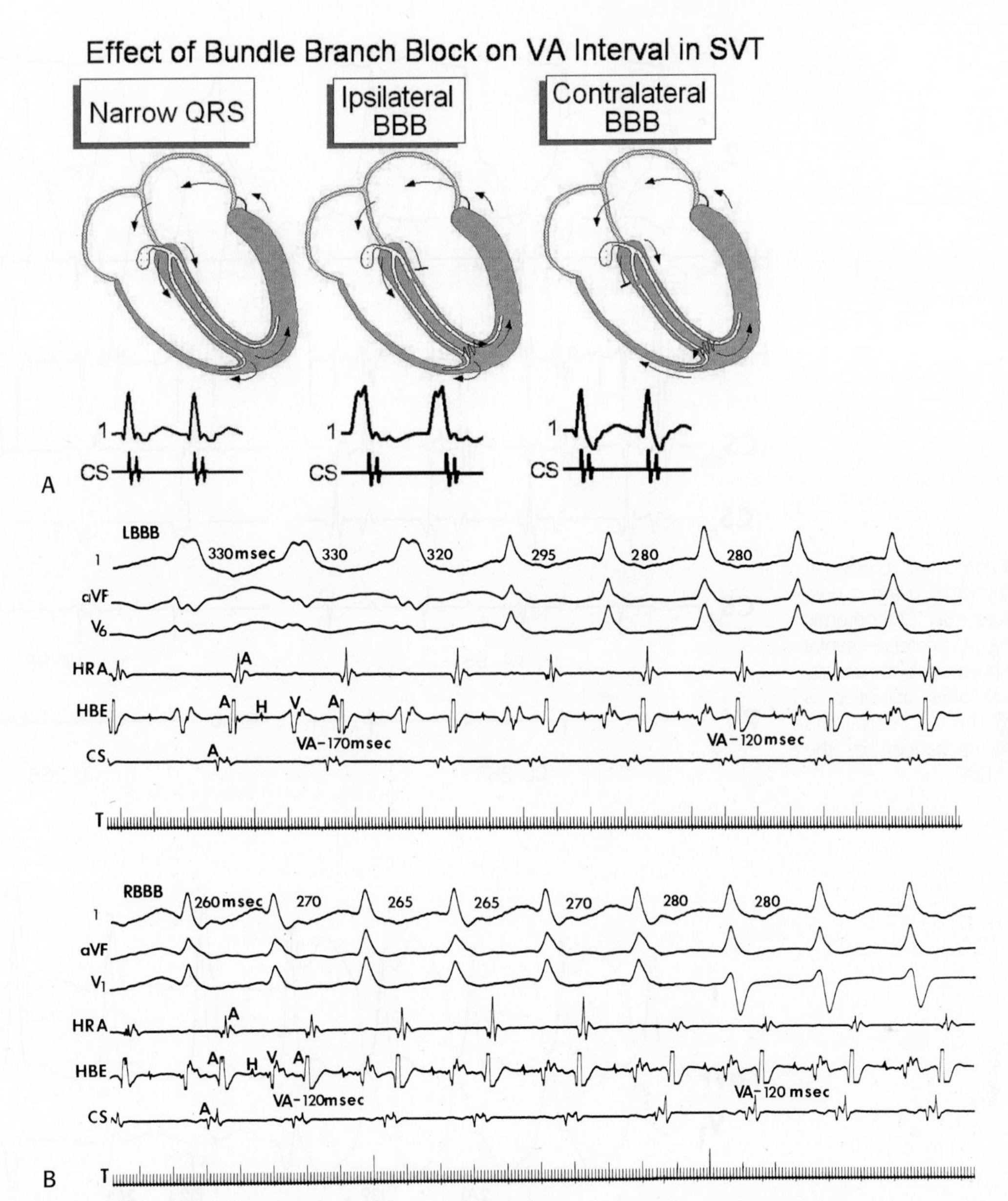


**FIGURE 10-64** *Effect of bundle branch block on V-A interval during SVT.* **A:** Circus movement tachycardia over a left-sided bypass tract is schematically show during a normal QRS, ipsilateral BBB, and contralateral BBB. Note that the V-A interval during a normal QRS and contralateral BBB (RBBB) have the same V-A. Ipsilateral BBB (LBBB) produces a longer VA interval because of the increase in time to reach the ventricular end of the bypass tract from the RV. **B:** Alternating bundle branch block during orthodromic tachycardia using a left-sided bypass tract. Leads 1, aVF, and V6 **(A)** and leads 1, aVF, and V1 **(B)** are shown with intracardiac recordings. Orthodromic tachycardia is present in both panels. **A:** The first three complexes manifest LBBB aberration and have a V-A interval of 170 msec and a cycle length of 330 msec. This converts to a normal QRS with a V-A interval of 120 msec and a cycle length of 280 msec. **B:** Recorded shortly thereafter, RBBB is present (qR in V1), which has the same V-A interval of 120 msec as when the tachycardia manifested normal QRS. The slight change in cycle length in this instance is due to changing A-H intervals. See text for discussion.

the development of bundle branch block produces either no increase in the V-A interval or an increase ≤25 msec.[101,103] In patients with orthodromic tachycardia using a posteroseptal bypass tract, LBBB may produce a small increase in the V-A interval (13 ± 8 msec), while in those using anteroseptal bypass tracts, RBBB may be associated with a small increase in V-A interval (16 ± 9 msec).[101] Examples of the effect of LBBB and RBBB on the V-A intervals and cycle lengths in patients with orthodromic tachycardias and posteroseptal bypass tracts and anteroseptal bypass tracts, respectively, are shown in Figures 10-65 and 10-66. We have also observed that the development of anterior fascicular block can alter V-A intervals during free wall left-sided bypass tracts with or without the presence of bundle branch block. Jazayeri et al.[105] studied this phenomenon in a large group of patients. These investigators demonstrated a 15- to 35-msec increase in the V-A interval with the development of left anterior hemiblock, regardless of whether it occurred with a normal QRS or with either

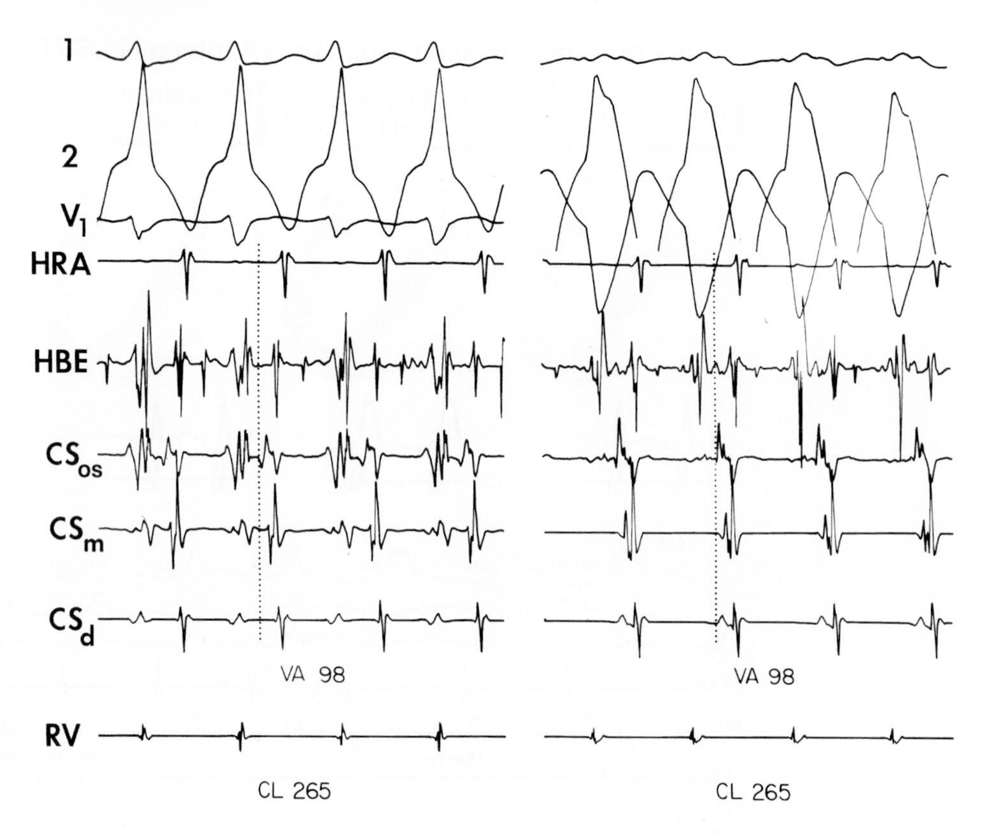


**FIGURE 10-65** *Effect of LBBB on orthodromic tachycardia using a posterior septal bypass tract.* Orthodromic tachycardia using a posterior septal bypass tract is shown in both panels. Earliest retrograde atrial activation is seen at the $CS_{OS}$. The V-A interval and cycle length are unchanged by the development of LBBB.

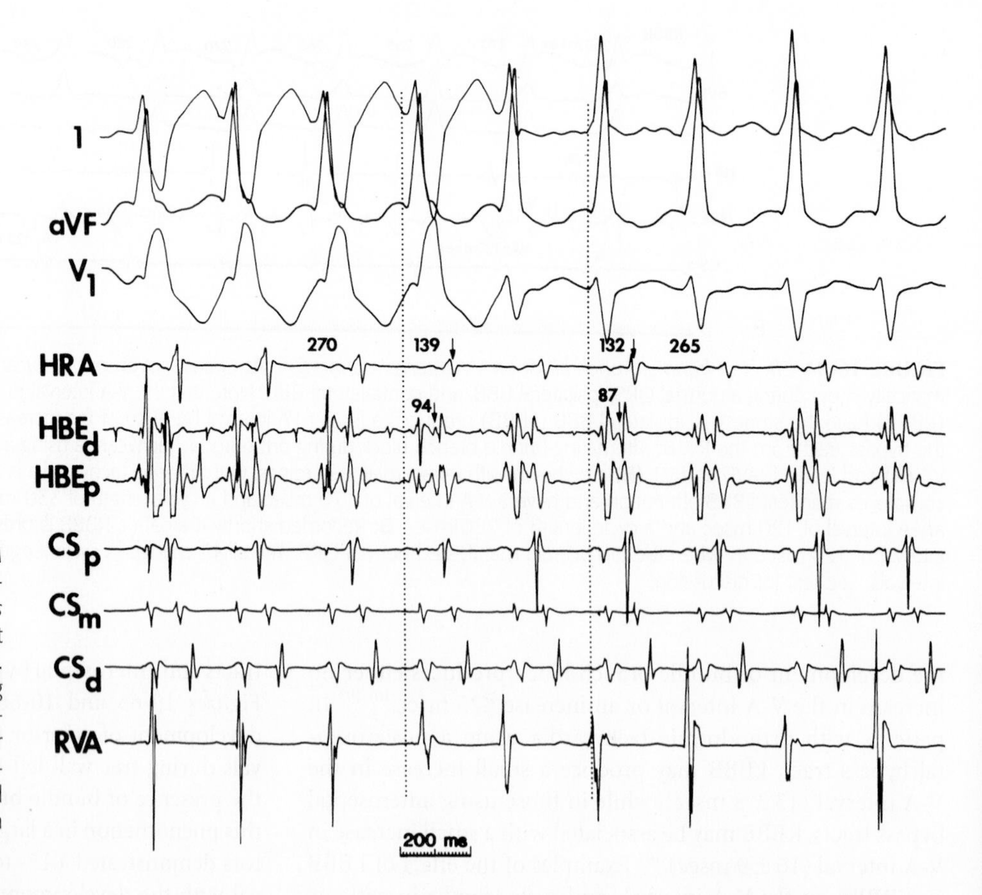


**FIGURE 10-66** *Effect of RBBB on V-A conduction during orthodromic tachycardia using an anteroseptal bypass tract.* Orthodromic tachycardia is present with RBBB aberration and a normal ORS. Earliest retrograde atrial activation during both is in the $HBE_d$. During RBBB aberration, the V-A interval is slightly greater than that during normal ventricular activation (94 vs. 87 msec). This is associated with a minimal difference in tachycardia cycle length. See text for discussion.

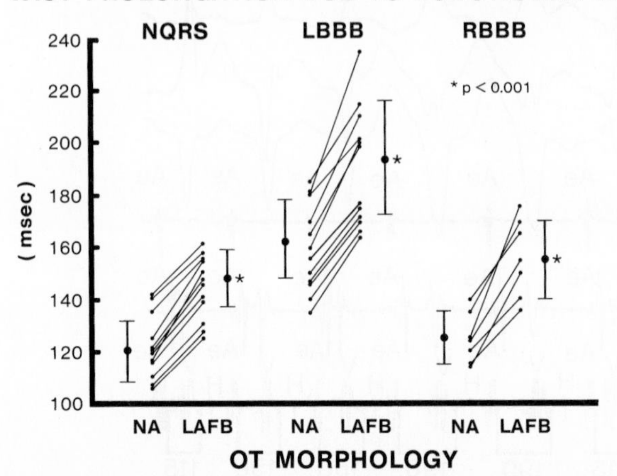


**FIGURE 10-67** *Effect of left anterior fascicular block (LAFB) on V-A intervals during orthodromic tachycardia.* Three patient groups were studied during orthodromic SV using a left lateral bypass tract: those with normal QRS (NQRS), those with LBBB, and those with RBBB. In all three groups, the V-A interval is compared during normal axis (NA) and during LAFB. Note an increase in the V-A interval in each patient group with the development of LAFB. See text for discussion. OT, orthodromic tachycardia; VACT, V-A conduction time. (From Jazayeri MR, Caceres J, Tchou P, et al. Electrophysiologic characteristics of sudden QRS axis deviation during orthodromic tachycardia: role of functional fascicular block in localization of accessory pathway. *J Clin Invest* 1989;83:952.)

right or LBBB (Fig. 10-67). Examples of the effect of anterior hemiblock on V-A intervals during aberration produced by either ventricular stimulation or atrial stimulation are shown in Figures 10-68 and 10-69. Varying degrees of anterior hemiblock may produce different V-A intervals. The effect of the development of anterior hemiblock on V-A intervals is most marked in the presence of superolateral free wall left-sided bypass tracts. As noted in Chapter 8, these phenomena result because conduction disturbances in one or both fascicles of the conducting system ipsilateral to the bypass tract enlarge the reentrant circuit by forcing the initial site of ventricular activation farther away from the bypass tract (Figs. 10-64 and 10-70). These observations are useful in localizing bypass tracts to the free wall or septal regions of the heart when detailed atrial mapping cannot be performed.

## DIRECT RECORDING OF BYPASS TRACT POTENTIALS

Recent observations suggest that one might be able to record electrical signals directly from the bypass tract using catheters.[106–109] Although bypass tract potentials have been recorded using standard catheters more often from the right side of the heart (Fig. 10-71), we have also recorded such potentials from left-sided bypass tracts using standard catheters positioned in the coronary sinus (Figs. 10-72 and 10-73). Jackman et al.[107]

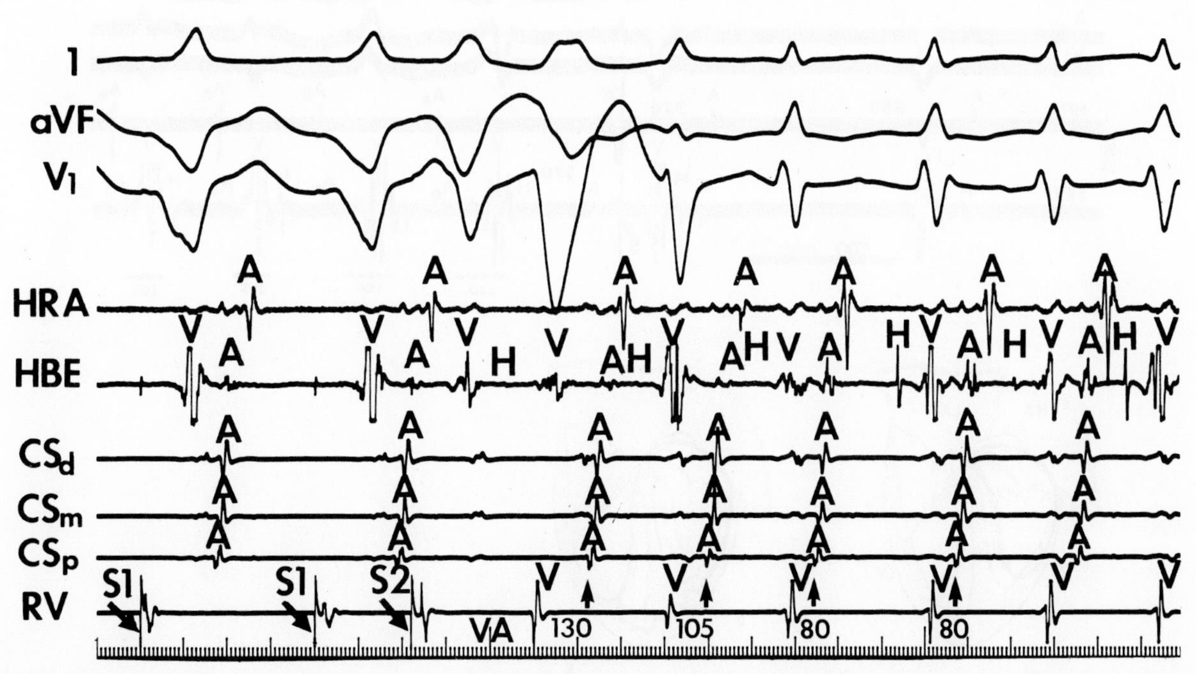


**FIGURE 10-68** *Effect of left anterior hemiblock and LBBB on orthodromic tachycardia using a left lateral bypass tract.* Orthodromic tachycardia is initiated by a ventricular extrastimulus (S2) delivered at coupling interval of 220 msec during a basic drive cycle length of 400 msec. The tachycardia is initiated via bundle branch reentry. The bundle branch reentrant complex functions as a left bundle left axis deviation complex and has a V-A interval of 130 msec. This is followed by a complex that has a narrower QRS but left axis deviation. The V-A interval during left axis deviation with a normal QRS is 105 msec. When the QRS normalizes both in axis and duration, the V-A interval is 80. The last three complexes demonstrate normal axis with incomplete RBBB, and the V-A interval remains fixed at 80 msec. See text for discussion.

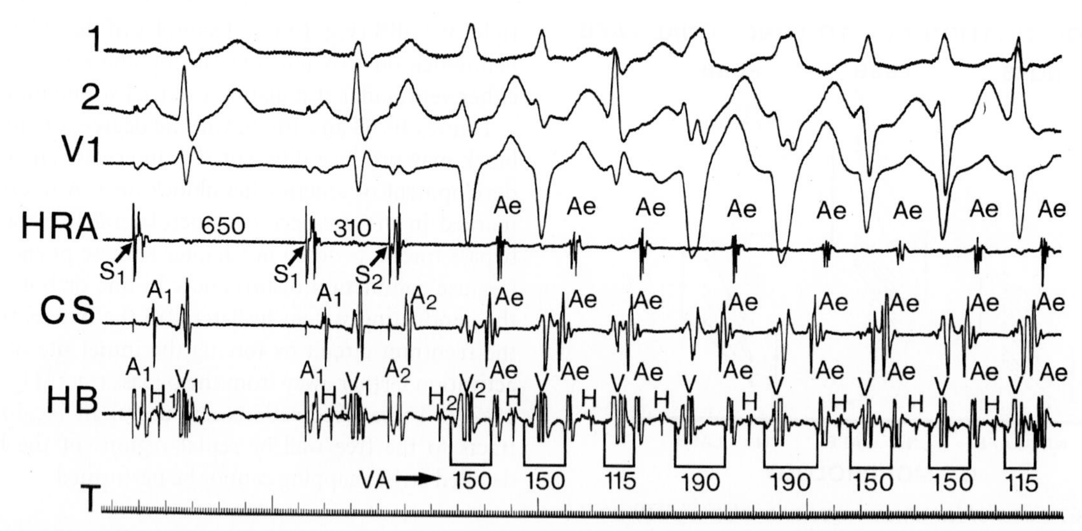


**FIGURE 10-69** *Effect of left anterior hemiblock and on V-A intervals in orthodromic tachycardias induced by atrial stimulation.* Orthodromic tachycardia is induced by an atrial extrastimulus delivered from the HRA at a coupling interval of 310 msec. The first two complexes manifest left anterior hemiblock and have V-A intervals of 150 msec. The third complex results in a normal axis but RBBB and has a V-A interval of 115 msec. The fourth and fifth complexes manifest complete LBBB with left axis deviation and have a V-A interval of 190 msec. The next two complexes have left anterior hemiblock, and the V-A interval returns to 150 msec. Finally, the last complex has a normal QRS and a normal axis and has a V-A interval of 115 msec, identical to that of the third QRS complex, which manifests RBBB and a normal axis. See text for discussion. (From Jazayeri MR, Caceres J, Tchou P, et al. Electrophysiologic characteristics of sudden QRS axis deviation during orthodromic tachycardia: role of functional fascicular block in localization of accessory pathway. *J Clin Invest* 1989;83:952.)

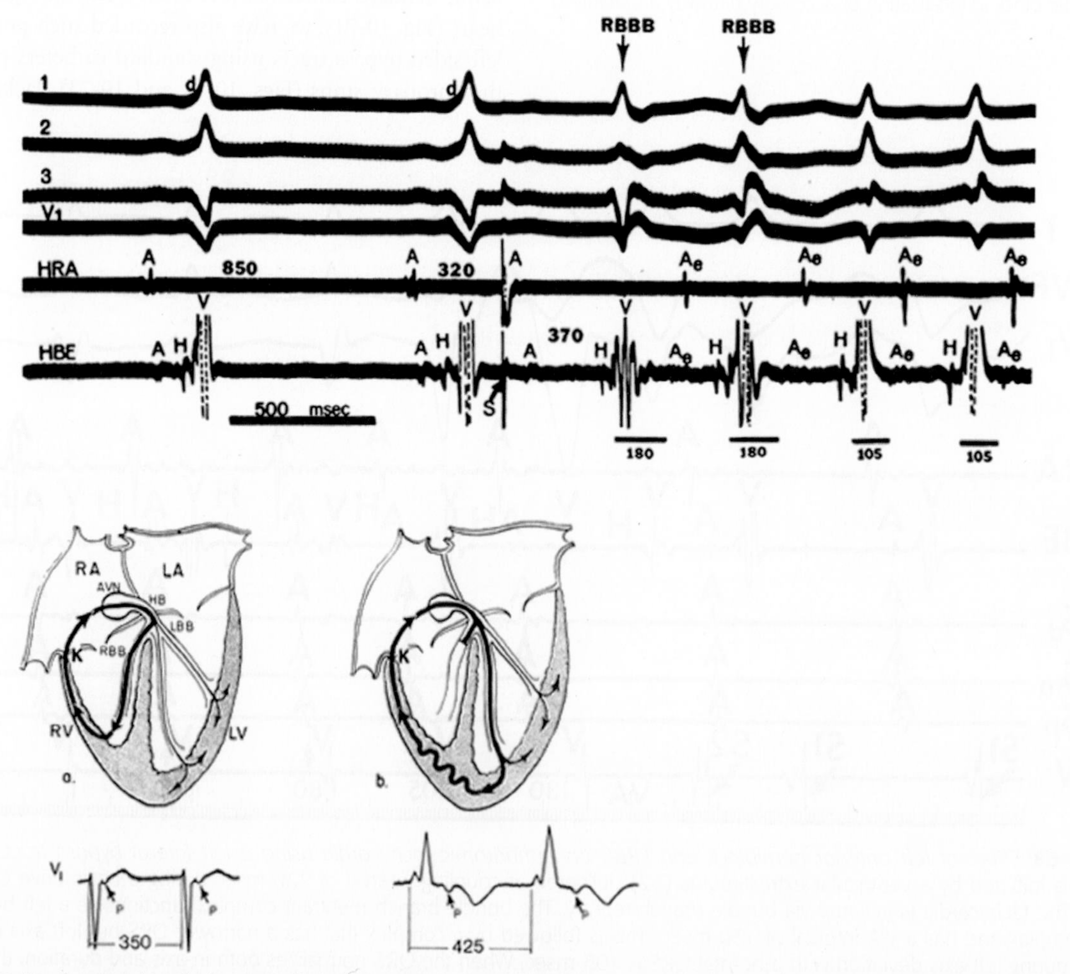


**FIGURE 10-70** *Mechanism by which RBBB during SVT using a right-sided bypass tract influences the V-A interval cycle length.* **A:** SVT with RBBB has a longer cycle length and V-A conduction time than SVT with a normal QRS complex (425 and 180 msec vs. 350 and 105 msec, respectively). This phenomenon is diagnostic of a right-sided bypass tract. **B:** Schematic explanation. See text for discussion.

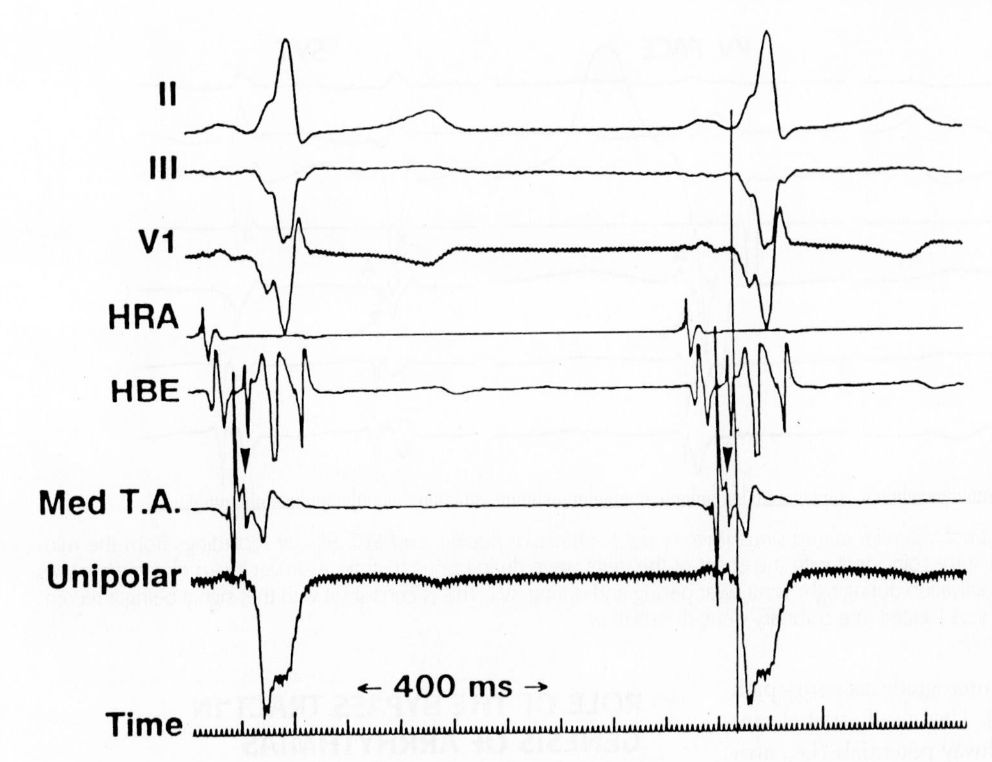


**FIGURE 10-71** *Recording a right-sided bypass tract potential.* Leads II, III, and V1 are shown with electrograms from the HRA, HBE, and bipolar and unipolar (tip) recordings from the medial tricuspid annulus (Med T.A.) between the os of the coronary sinus and the HBE. Note the sharp spike of the bypass tract potential is observed on the unipolar and bipolar signals and precedes the local ventricular electrogram and the delta wave.

suggested that an orthogonal catheter electrode array might facilitate recording bypass tract potentials from the left side of the heart and believes that, by using this technique, one can routinely record bypass tract potentials. The technique has several limitations, however. Validation that the "spike" that is recorded between atrium and ventricle is indeed due to activation over a bypass tract is required. Bypass tract potentials should be manifested as a sharp spike 10 to 30 msec before the onset of the delta wave during antegrade recordings. Validation that the spike is indeed recording bypass tract potentials and not a component of atrial and/or ventricular electrograms is critical and, in our opinion, has been lacking in many of the examples that have been reported. Thus, initially one must record a sharp rapid deflection between the atrial and ventricular electrograms at the earliest site of retrograde atrial activation during reciprocating tachycardia, right ventricular pacing, as well as during sinus rhythm. In order to exclude that this sharp deflection is really a component of the ventricular electrogram requires that it disappear with premature ventricular stimulation without affecting the remaining ventricular electrogram or the QRS complex, with simultaneous disappearance of the atrial activation. Proof that the electrogram is not part of the atrial electrogram requires its persistence with elimination of the atrial electrogram during retrograde block. Both criteria should be met; however, in most reported cases, validation has not been attempted or satisfactorily accomplished. Niebauer et al.[110] evaluated the pacing

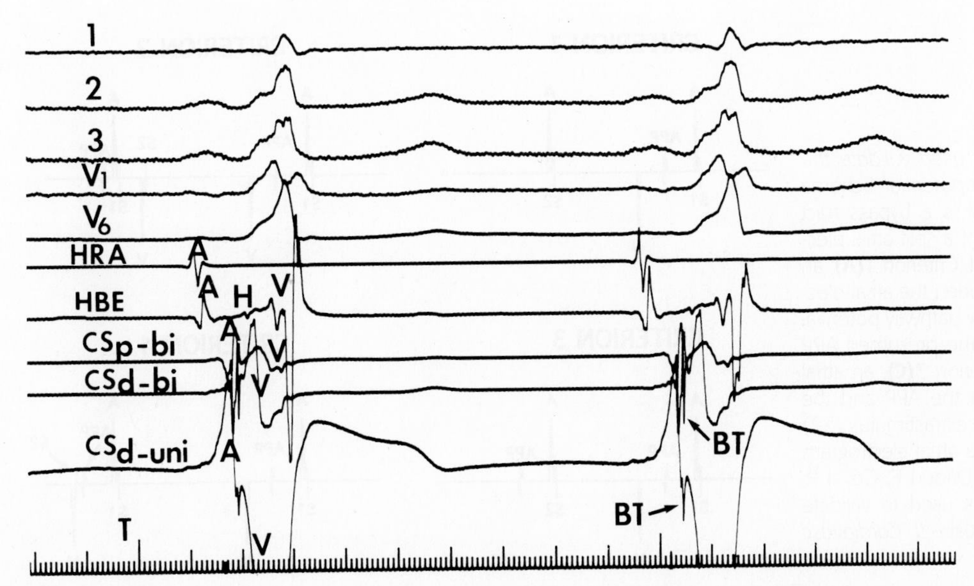


**FIGURE 10-72** *Recording of a left-sided bypass tract potential during sinus rhythm.* CS bipolar and unipolar recordings demonstrate a sharp spike, which represents a bypass tract (BT) potential, which appears 20 msec before the delta wave. This was recorded with a standard quadripolar catheter with electrodes spaced at 5 mm. $CS_{d\text{-}bi}$, distal bipolar CS; $CS_{p\text{-}bi}$, proximal bipolar CS; $CS_{d\text{-}uni}$, distal unipolar CS.

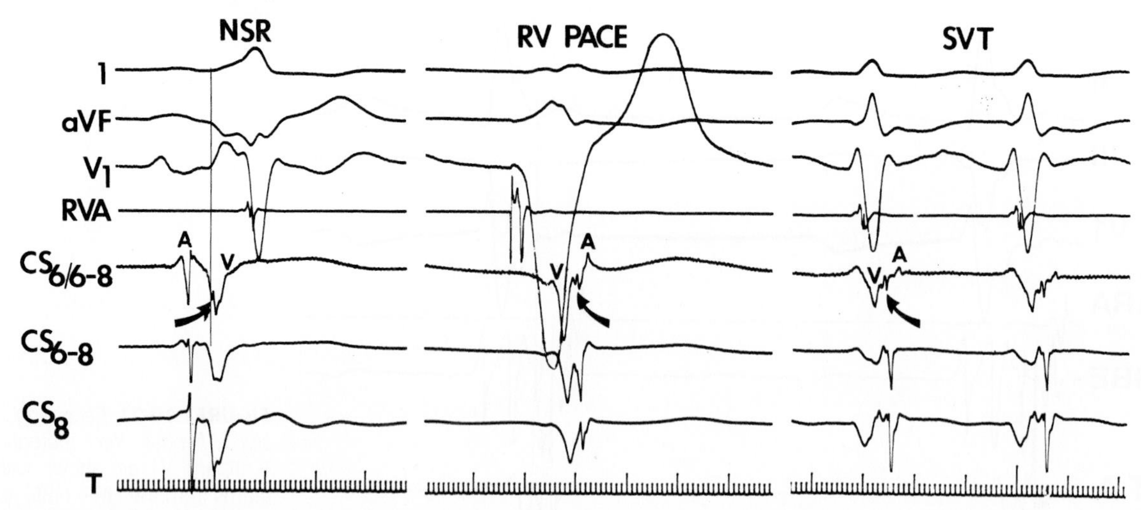


**FIGURE 10-73** *Recording of a bypass tract potential during sinus rhythm, right ventricular pacing, and SVT.* Bipolar recordings from the mid-posterior CS (CS6/6-8) demonstrated a spike coincident with the onset of the delta wave during sinus rhythm. A similar sharp electrogram was observed between ventricular and atrial activation during right ventricular pacing and during SVT. This is consistent with that signal being a recording of a left posterior bypass tract which was located in a coronary sinus diverticulum.

maneuvers proposed to validate an anterograde accessory pathway potential (Figs. 10-74 to 10-78). They used atrial electrograms that simulated accessory pathway potentials (i.e., atrial electrograms manifesting split potentials separated by at least 30 msec) and assessed their response to atrial and ventricular extrastimuli. All but one of the proposed criteria was seen in response to atrial and ventricular stimulation. The only observation they never made was block between the first and second components of the atrial electrogram simulating block between the atrium and the bypass tract. This latter observation has never been convincingly demonstrated in our laboratory. Although bypass tract recordings can be obtained and may serve as a marker for a catheter ablation of the bypass tracts, proof that the electrical signal interpreted as a bypass tract potential is a bypass tract potential, in my opinion, is rarely achieved. Most often it is not possible to distinguish a component of the atrial or ventricular electrogram from a bypass tract potential.

## ROLE OF THE BYPASS TRACT IN GENESIS OF ARRHYTHMIAS

The most common arrhythmia in patients with A-V bypass tracts is circus movement tachycardia using a bypass tract, most commonly in the retrograde direction (i.e., orthodromic tachycardia). However, there is no a priori reason that a patient with an antegradely functioning bypass tract must use that pathway during SVT. Because the presence of an A-V bypass tract does not confer on that patient immunity from other arrhythmias, patients with WPW are no less susceptible to other forms of arrhythmias. Therefore, demonstration that the bypass tract plays a critical role in the genesis of the arrhythmia is imperative and is essential for appropriate therapy, especially catheter ablation or surgery. As noted earlier, atrial fibrillation is a common rhythm in patients with

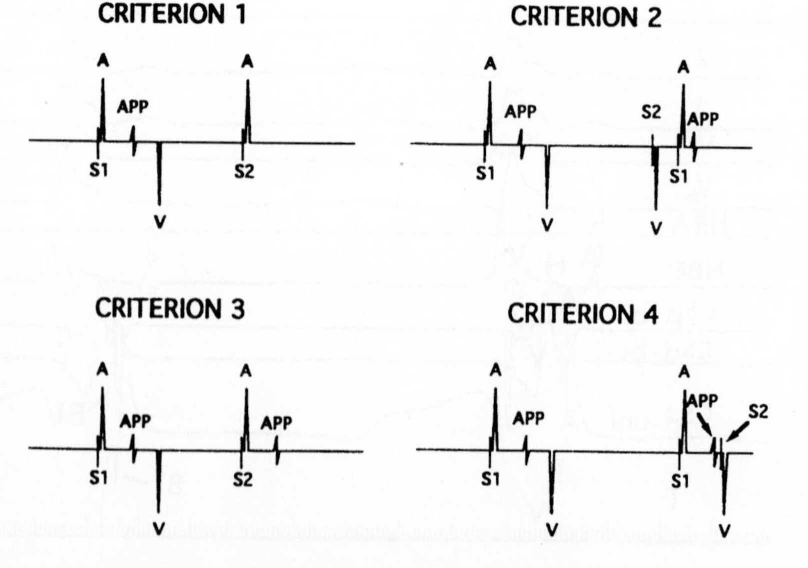


**FIGURE 10-74** *Evaluation of methods used validate the presence of an anterograde bypass tract potential.* Schema of pacing maneuvers to prove a signal is a bypass tract potential using the second component of a split atrial electrogram to mimic a bypass tract potential. Criterion 1**(A)**, an atrial extrastimulus (S2) that blocks between the atrial electrogram **(A)** and the presumed accessory pathway potential (APP). Criterion 2**(B)**, advancement of the presumed APP by a ventricular extrastimulus (S2). Criterion 3**(C)**, an atrial extrastimulus (S2) that blocks between the APP and the ventricle (V). Criterion 4**(D)**, a ventricular extrastimulus (S2) that advances the V without affecting the atrial electrogram or presumed APP. (From Niebauer MJ, Daoud E, Goyal R, et al. Assessment of pacing maneuvers used to validate anterograde accessory pathway potentials. *J Cardiovasc Electrophysiol* 1995;6:350–356.)

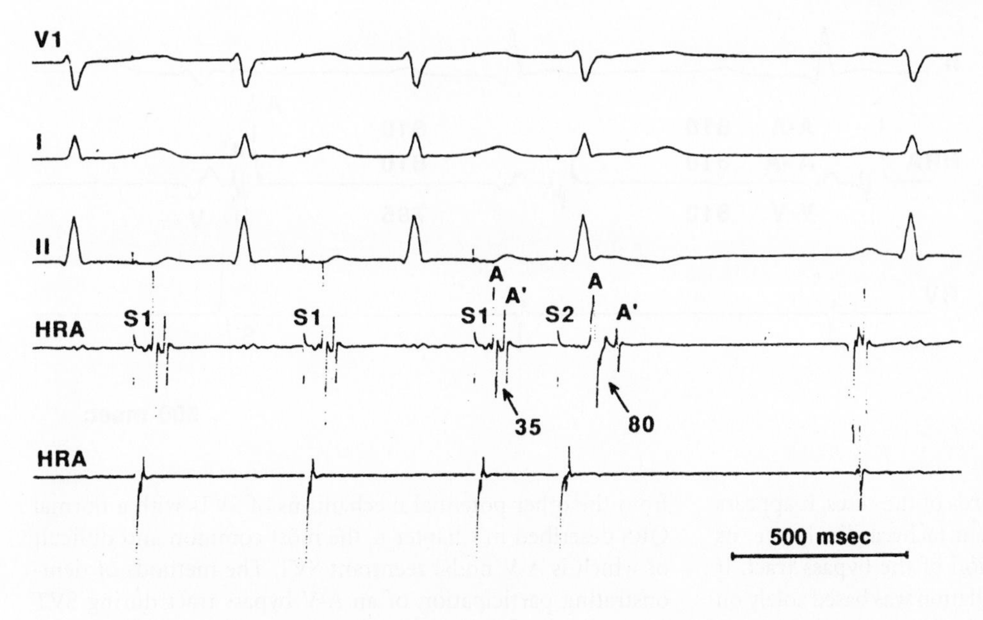


**FIGURE 10-75** *Evaluation of Criterion 1.* ECG leads V1, I, and II are shown with two electrograms from the HRA, the top showing a split atrial electrogram and the bottom from the pacing site. During atrial pacing the atrial electrogram is (A and A′) with an isoelectric interval of 35 msec. The shortest coupled atrial extrastimulus that captured produced an increase in A-A′ to 80 msec. Complete block between A and A′ was never observed in this or any other patient. (From Niebauer MJ, Daoud E, Goyal R, et al. Assessment of pacing maneuvers used to validate anterograde accessory pathway potentials. *J Cardiovasc Electrophysiol* 1995;6:350–356.)

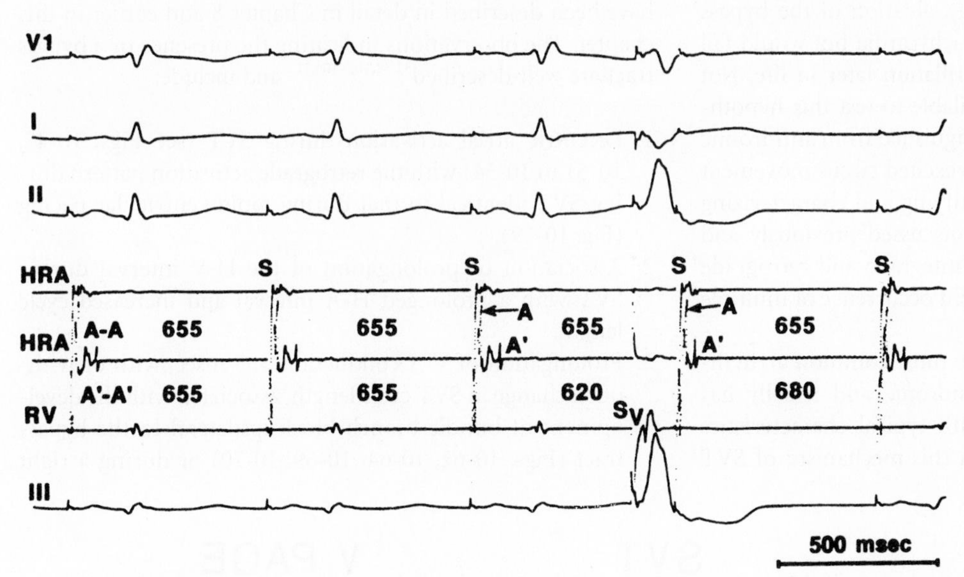


**FIGURE 10-76** *Evaluation of Criterion 2.* Surface leads V1, I, II, and III are shown with two electrograms from the HRA; the top from the atrial pacing site and the bottom from a nearby site with a split atrial electrogram (A and A′). An RV electrogram is also shown. During atrial pacing at 655 msec a ventricular extrastimulus is delivered (SV), which advances A′ (the presumed accessory pathway potential) by 35 msec without affecting A. See text for discussion. (From Niebauer MJ, Daoud E, Goyal R, et al. Assessment of pacing maneuvers used to validate anterograde accessory pathway potentials. *J Cardiovasc Electrophysiol* 1995;6:350–356.)

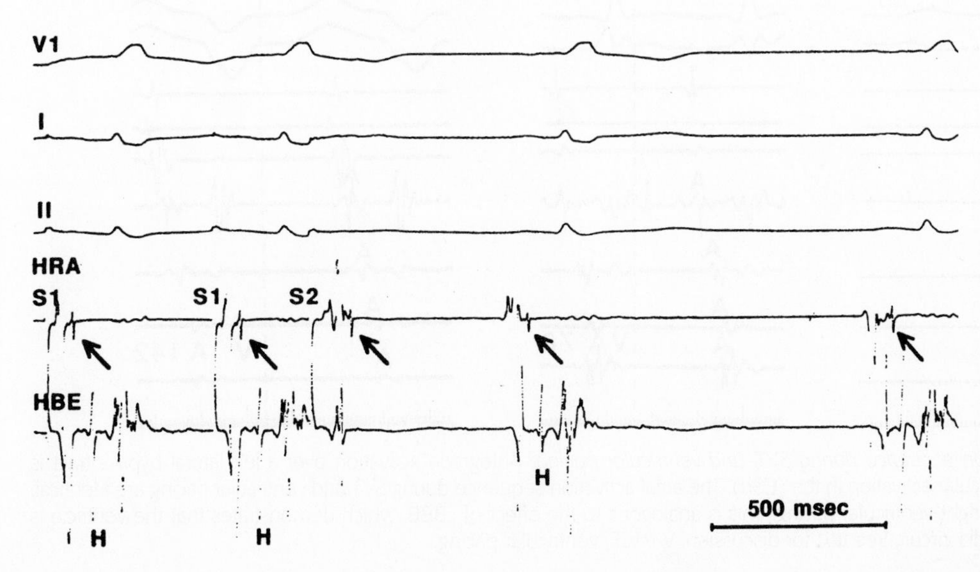


**FIGURE 10-77** *Evaluation of Criterion 3.* ECG leads V1, I, and II are shown with a split atrial electrogram from the HRA and an HBE. During atrial pacing (S1-S1) at a cycle length of 500 msec an atrial extrastimulus (S2) was delivered, which depolarizes both components of the split electrogram mimicking block between the accessory pathway and the ventricle. (From Niebauer MJ, Daoud E, Goyal R, et al. Assessment of pacing maneuvers used to validate anterograde accessory pathway potentials. *J Cardiovasc Electrophysiol* 1995;6:350–356.)

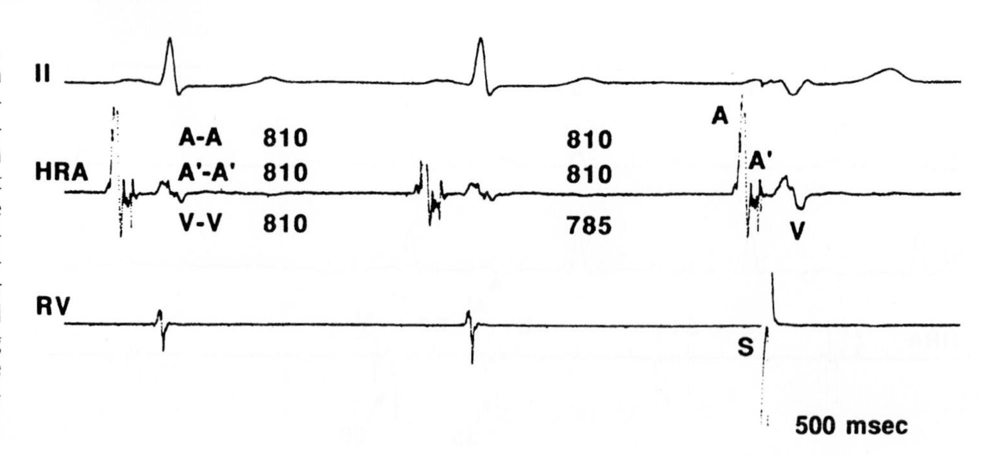


**FIGURE 10-78** *Evaluation of criterion 4.* Lead II and a split atrial electrogram from the HRA are shown with an RV electrogram. During sinus rhythm an extrastimulus from the RV is delivered, which advances the RV by 25 msec without affecting the second component of the atrial electrogram, thus mimicking dissociation of the ventricle from the simulated accessory pathway. See text for discussion. (From Niebauer MJ, Daoud E, Goyal R, et al. Assessment of pacing maneuvers used to validate anterograde accessory pathway potentials. *J Cardiovasc Electrophysiol* 1995;6:350–356.)

the WPW syndrome, and in two-thirds of the cases, it appears to be related to the circus movement tachycardia; hence, its cure is possible with surgical ablation of the bypass tract. If the propensity to develop atrial fibrillation was based solely on primary intra-atrial pathophysiology, ablation of the bypass tract could cure circus movement tachycardia but would fail to prevent recurrences of atrial fibrillation later in life. Not enough long-term follow-up is available to test this hypothesis. Atrial tachycardia must be distinguished from antidromic tachycardia, or more accurately, "preexcited circus movement tachycardia." The problems in identifying and characterizing preexcited tachycardias have been discussed previously and include the difficulty in recording antegrade and retrograde His bundle potentials and the frequent occurrence of multiple bypass tracts.

Because orthodromic SVT is the most common arrhythmia associated with the WPW syndrome and usually has a normal QRS complex or one with typical characteristics of aberration, one must distinguish this mechanism of SVT from the other potential mechanisms of SVTs with a normal QRS described in Chapter 8, the most common and difficult of which is A-V nodal reentrant SVT. The methods of demonstrating participation of an A-V bypass tract during SVT have been described in detail in Chapter 8 and earlier in this chapter. The observations indicating the presence of a bypass tract are well-described[32,38,102–104,111] and include:

1. Eccentric atrial activation during SVT (see Figs. 10-47, 10-51 to 10-54) with the retrograde activation pattern during SVT identical to that during rapid ventricular pacing (Fig. 10-79).
2. Association of prolongation of the H-V interval during SVT with a prolonged H-A interval and increased cycle length.
3. Prolongation of V-A conduction >35 msec, with or without a change in SVT cycle length, associated with the development of bundle branch block ipsilateral to the bypass tract (Figs. 10-62, 10-64, 10-69, 10-70) or during a right

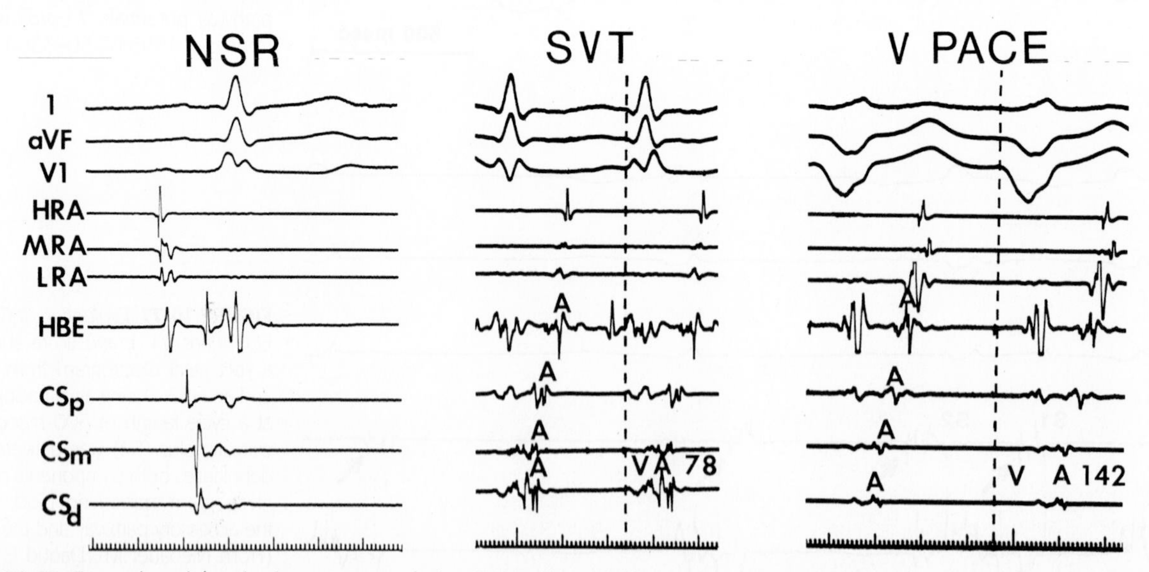


**FIGURE 10-79** *Eccentric atrial activation sequence during SVT, and ventricular pacing.* Antegrade activation over a left lateral bypass tract is shown on the left, with the earliest ventricular activation in the (CSd). The atrial activation sequence during SVT and ventricular pacing are identical, but the V-A interval is prolonged during right ventricular pacing. This is analogous to the effect of LBBB, which demonstrates that the ventricle is an essential component of the tachycardia circuit. See text for discussion. V PACE, ventricular pacing.

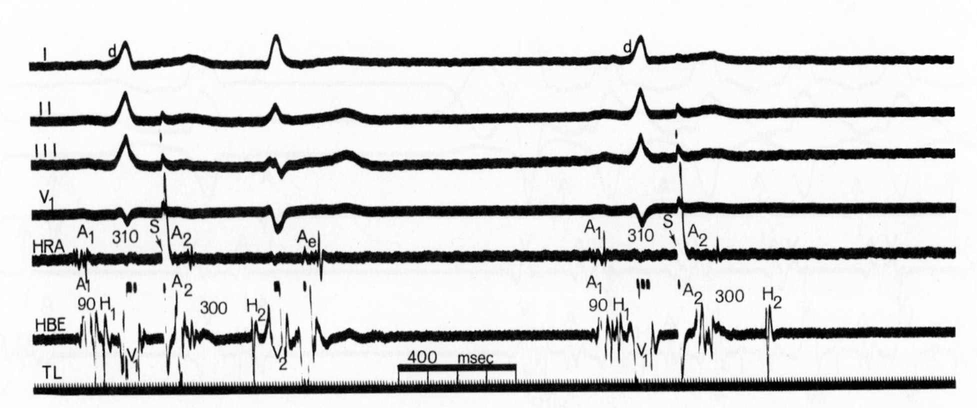


**FIGURE 10-80** *Effect of A-V block on the ability to initiate reentry.* On the left, an APD (S, *arrow,* A2) delivered at a coupling interval of 310 msec blocks in the bypass tract and conducts down the normal A-V conduction system, with an A-H of 300 msec to produce a normal QRS complex. The amount of A-V delay allows the bypass tract to recover and an atrial echo (Ae) results from retrograde conduction over the bypass tract. The next sinus complex is followed by an APD delivered at an identical coupling interval. That impulse conducts slowly through the A-V node (A-H 300 msec) but blocks below the recorded His bundle deflection. No echo results despite an identical A-H interval as the first APD. Thus, the ventricle is a requisite component of the reentrant circuit. See text for discussion.

ventricular stimulation in the presence of a left free wall bypass tract (Fig. 10-79).[103]

4. The inability to initiate and/or sustain SVT in the presence of A-V block (Fig. 10-80).
5. The ability to preexcite the atrium during SVT when the His bundle has been depolarized and is therefore refractory to the retrograde impulse (Fig. 10-81), or the depolarization of the atria by a VPD delivered during ventricular pacing before retrograde activation of the His bundle (Fig. 10-58) with a V-A-V return cycle and an identical V-A interval on the return beat as during SVT.
6. Termination or delay of orthodromic tachycardia in the absence of atrial activation by a VPD delivered when the His bundle is refractory to retrograde activation (Fig. 10-82).
7. Entrainment of SVT by ventricular pacing with each paced V occurring just after an antegrade His with or without ventricular fusion (Fig. 10-83).

Obviously the ability to preexcite the atrium when the His bundle is refractory requires that the VPD reach the bypass tract prior to the time it would be activated over the normal

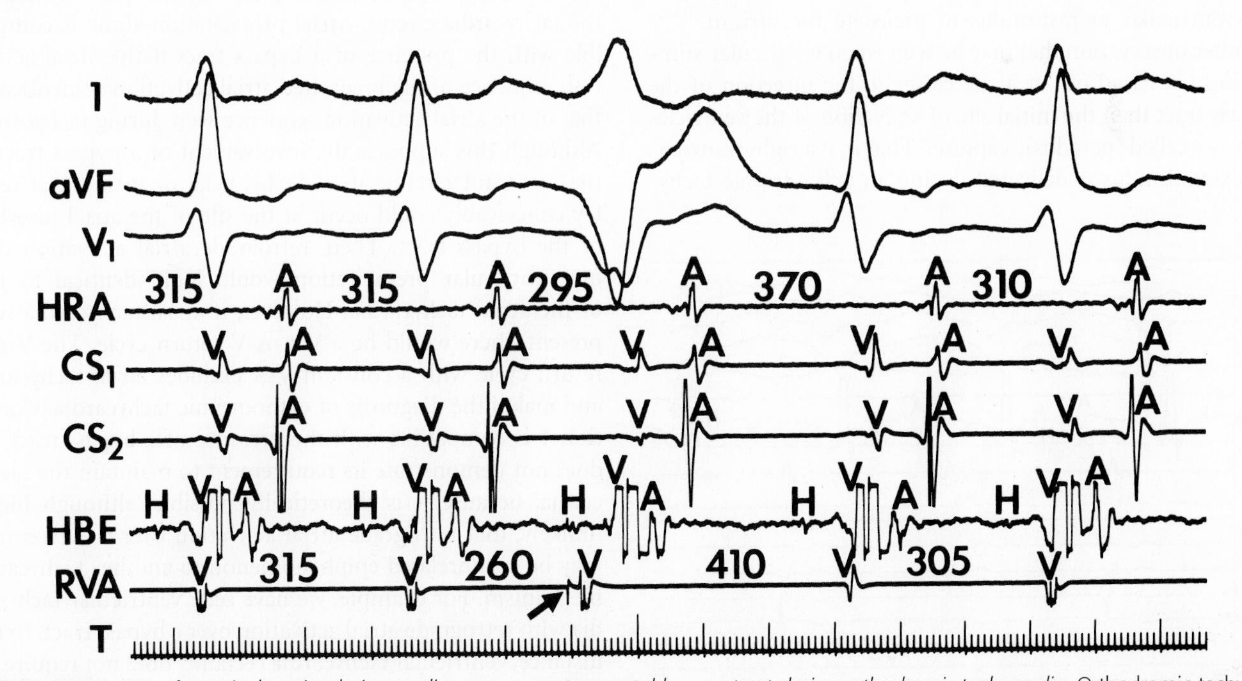


**FIGURE 10-81** *Use of ventricular stimulation to diagnose a posteroseptal bypass tract during orthodromic tachycardia.* Orthodromic tachycardia is present with a "normal" atrial activation sequence. A ventricular extrastimulus introduced from the RVA at a coupling interval of 260 msec preexcites the atrium when the His bundle is refractory with the same atrial activation sequence as that noted during orthodromic tachycardia. This early activation of the atrium then resets the tachycardia with a longer A-H and a delay in the return cycle. The ability to preexcite the atria when the His bundle is refractory with the same atrial activation sequence as seen during the orthodromic tachycardia confirms the presence of functioning posteroseptal bypass tract.

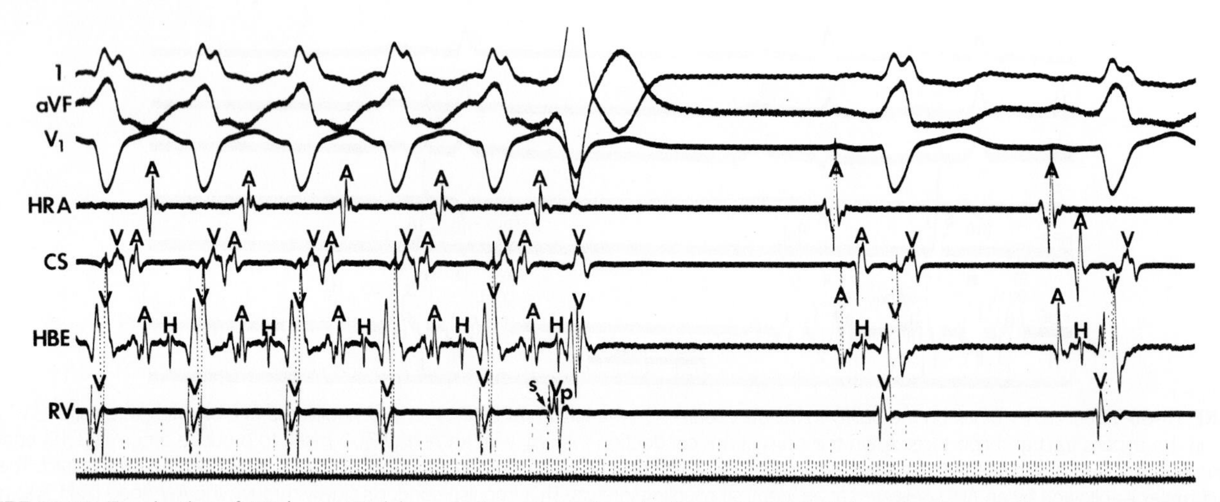


**FIGURE 10-82** *Termination of SVT by a VPD delivered after antegrade activation to the His bundle.* Orthodromic tachycardia with LBBB aberration using a left-sided bypass tract is terminated by a ventricular extrastimulus delivered simultaneously with antegrade His bundle activation. The tachycardia terminates by retrograde block in the bypass tract when the His is refractory. This confirms the necessary participation of the bypass tract in the tachycardia circuit. See text for discussion.

conducting system. Thus, during rapid tachycardias, a single right ventricular stimulus might not reach a left lateral bypass tract in time to preexcite the atrium. In such instances two extrastimuli are required to demonstrate this phenomenon. This is shown in Figure 10-84, in which the first of two ventricular extrastimuli fails to affect retrograde atrial activation while the second can terminate the tachycardia. (This phenomenon was also discussed in Chapter 8.) The tachycardia cycle length and the site of the ventricular extrastimulus with respect to the bypass tract markedly influence the ability of the ventricular extrastimulus to preexcite the atrium.[100,112] Another observation that may be seen when ventricular stimulation is carried out at a site closer to the insertion of the bypass tract than the initial site of activation of the ventricles is the so-called "paradoxic capture." That is, if a right ventricular extrastimulus is delivered during an orthodromic tachycardia using a right free wall bypass tract, the V-A interval associated with atrial preexcitation will be shorter than that during the tachycardia. This occurs because the earliest site of ventricular activation during a normal QRS complex is the left side of the septum, which is farther from the bypass tract than the right ventricular stimulus. This is even more evident if RBBB is present (Fig. 10-85).

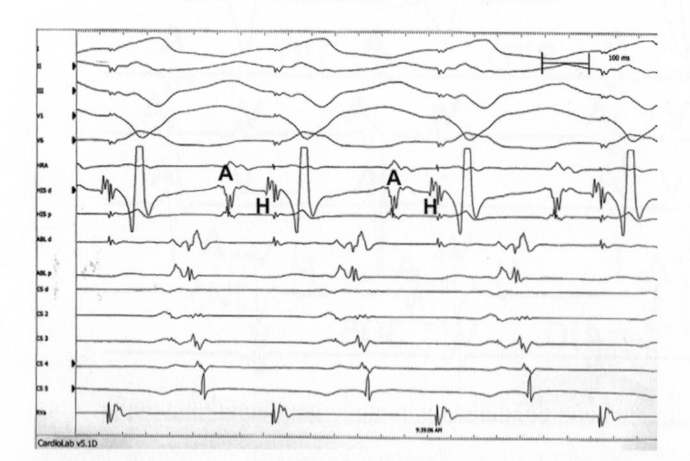


**FIGURE 10-83** *Entrainment of SVT by RV pacing with manifest fusion in the His–Purkinje system.* During SVT RV pacing produces retrograde conduction over a left-sided pathway with simultaneous antegrade conduction over the A-V node and His bundle. This proves the presence of CMT. See text.

Only conditions 2, 3, 5, 6, and 7 absolutely demonstrate participation of the bypass tract in the reentrant circuit, because they demonstrate requirement of the ventricle in the tachycardia circuit. Atrial preexcitation alone is compatible with the presence of a bypass tract if the atrial activation sequence of the preexcited atrial activation is identical to that of the atrial activation sequence seen during tachycardia. Although this supports the involvement of a bypass tract in the reentrant circuit, atrial tachycardia or intra-atrial reentry conceivably could occur at the site of the atrial insertion of the bypass tract. Then, retrograde atrial activation during ventricular preexcitation would look identical to that of the atrial tachycardia. However, if atrial tachycardia were present, there would be a V-A-A-V return cycle. The V-A-V return cycle with a constant V-A excludes atrial tachycardia and makes the diagnosis of orthodromic tachycardia. Condition 1 is compatible with the presence of a bypass tract but does not demonstrate its requirement to maintain the tachycardia, because it is theoretically possible, although highly unlikely, that retrograde atrial activation over a bypass tract may be an unrelated epiphenomenon to another tachycardia mechanism. For example, we have seen ventricular tachycardia with retrograde atrial activation over a bypass tract. In this instance, ventricular tachycardia certainly does not require the bypass tract for its persistence. The inability to initiate SVT in the presence of A-V block may be fortuitous and can also be seen in A-V nodal reentry. These are theoretical possibilities; however, in the vast majority of cases, all the conditions mentioned are useful in diagnosing the presence of a bypass tract.

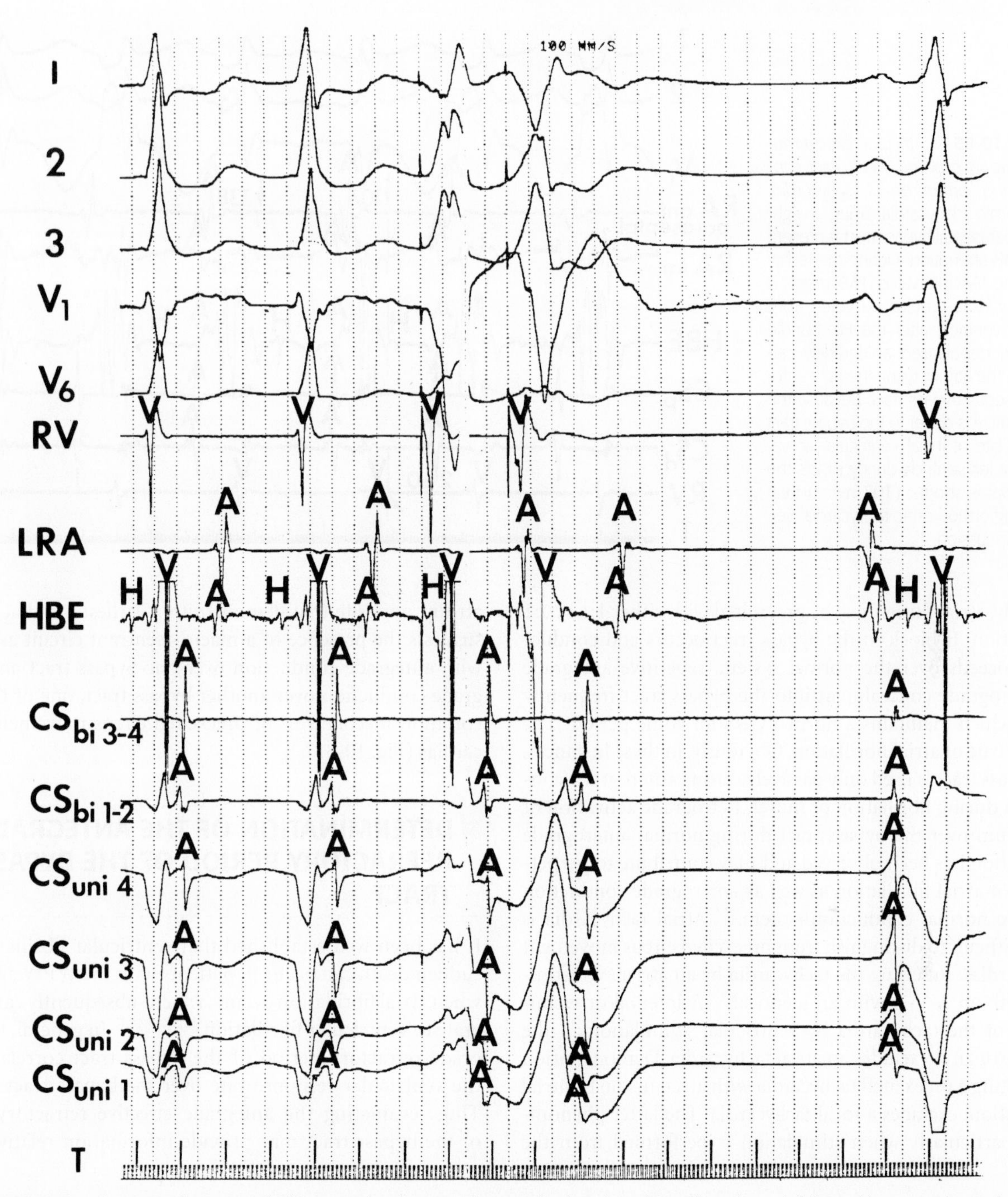


**FIGURE 10-84** *Requirement of two ventricular extrastimuli to terminate orthodromic tachycardia using a left lateral bypass tract.* Orthodromic tachycardia using a left lateral bypass tract, with earliest activity in the bipolar coronary sinus ($CS_{bi\ 1\text{-}2}$) and unipolar coronary sinus ($CS_{uni\ 1}$) is present in the first two complexes. The first ventricular extrastimulus fails to affect the tachycardia with the antegrade His and retrograde atrial activation over the bypass tract being unaltered. The second extrastimulus, which is introduced earlier in the cardiac cycle, conducts over the bypass tract retrogradely. The premature atrial excitation results in antegrade block in the node. The inability of a right ventricular extrastimulus to affect circus movement tachycardia demonstrates the lack of requirement of the right ventricle in tachycardias using a left-sided bypass tract. See text for discussion.

Comparison of H-A intervals during ventricular pacing and SVT as well as V-A intervals during pacing from the RV apex and inflow tract have been discussed in Chapter 8 and earlier in this chapter as a means to further distinguish septal bypass tracts from A-V nodal reentry when none of the preceding criteria are fulfilled.

As noted earlier, the most common rhythm associated with a regular preexcited tachycardia is atrial flutter or atrial tachycardia.[40] Whether or not conduction proceeds over the bypass tract is obvious by the appearance of a typical preexcited complex. Usually, there are runs of total preexcitation and/or runs of normal ventricular activation (Fig. 10-86).

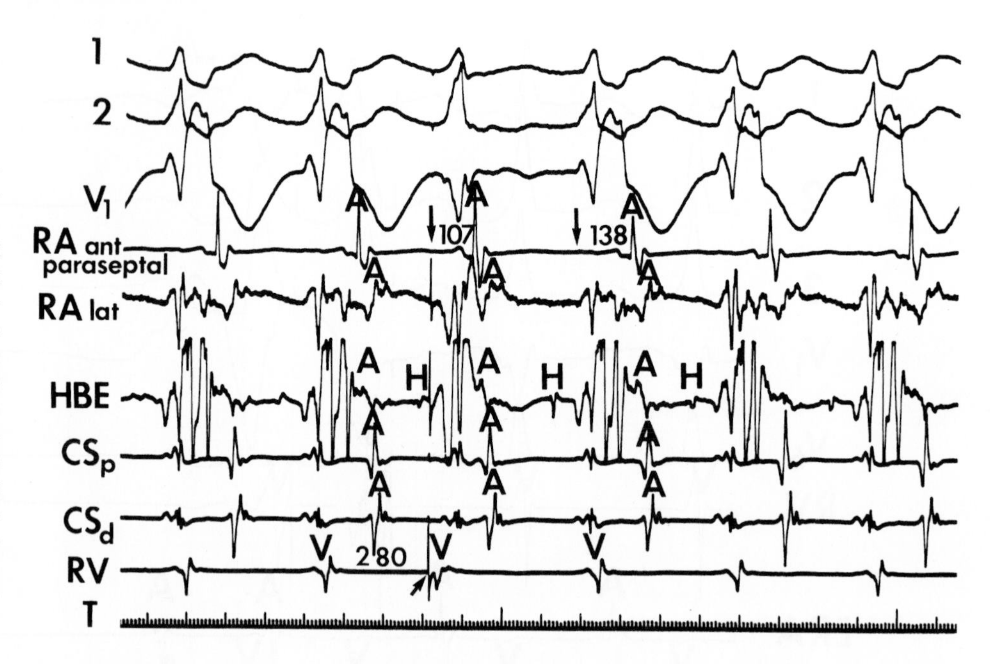


**FIGURE 10-85** *Ventricular extrastimulus producing a paradoxical atrial capture during orthodromic tachycardia.* Orthodromic tachycardia using a right anterior paraseptal bypass tract is present with RBBB aberration. During the tachycardia, the V-A interval is 138 msec. A ventricular extrastimulus delivered from the right ventricle after the His bundle has been depolarized antegradely can preexcite the atrium using the right anterior paraseptal bypass tract. Because the right ventricle is closer to the bypass tract than the site of initial ventricular activation in the left ventricle during RBBB, the V-A interval is shorter (107 msec) than it is during orthodromic tachycardia. See text for discussion.

Typically, atrial flutter may be preexcited with either 1:1 or 2:1 conduction. If block in the bypass tract occurs and conduction proceeds over the normal system, repetitive antegrade and retrograde concealment into the bypass tract frequently occur, which maintains a normal QRS for some period. The same is true of atrial fibrillation. Obviously, in these instances, the bypass tract is used only passively during anterograde conduction during fibrillation or flutter. Retrograde activation of the atrium over the bypass tract during normal anterograde conduction has been observed and may contribute to perpetuation of atrial fibrillation as well as anterograde conduction over the normal conduction system.[113] Atrial tachycardia is more difficult to distinguish from preexcited circus movement tachycardias. Resetting the tachycardia by an atrial extrastimulus with an A-V-A with an identical V-A interval or termination of the tachycardia by ventricular stimulation in the absence of an A excludes an atrial tachycardia. Demonstration of resetting a preexcited tachycardia with atrial fusion by atrial stimulation, excludes a focal tachycardia. The latter phenomenon, particularly when stimulation is performed from the atrium opposite that demonstrating earliest atrial activation, suggests the presence of a macro-reentrant circuit associated with antegrade conduction over one bypass tract and retrograde conduction over another bypass tract, one of the more common mechanisms of preexcited circus movement tachycardias (Fig. 10-87).

## DETERMINATION OF THE ANTEGRADE REFRACTORY PERIOD OF THE BYPASS TRACT

It has been well established that ventricular fibrillation and sudden death can occur in patients with the WPW syndrome when atrial fibrillation occurs, which subsequently can degenerate to ventricular fibrillation.[32,38,43,44,73] In general, the antegrade refractory period of the bypass tract correlates with the ventricular response rate over the bypass tract.[44,65,73,114] Thus, evaluating the antegrade effective refractory period of the bypass tract may provide information relative to the

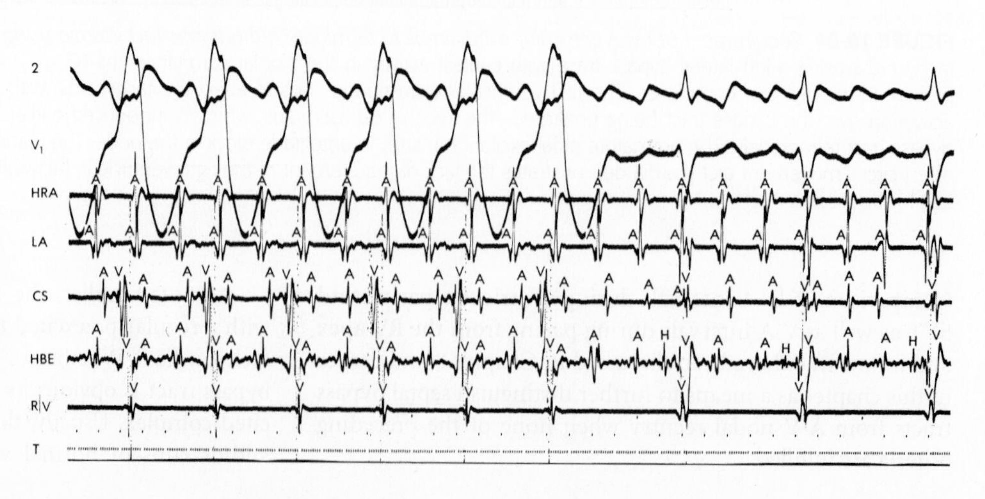


**FIGURE 10-86** *Atrial flutter demonstrating antegrade conduction over the bypass tract.* During atrial flutter, antegrade conduction usually occurs over the bypass tract, resulting in marked preexcitation (first six complexes). When conduction proceeds over the normal pathway (last three complexes), the ventricular response is usually slower because of a higher degree of concealment without block in the A-V node than in the bypass tract, which tends to function in an all-or-nothing fashion.

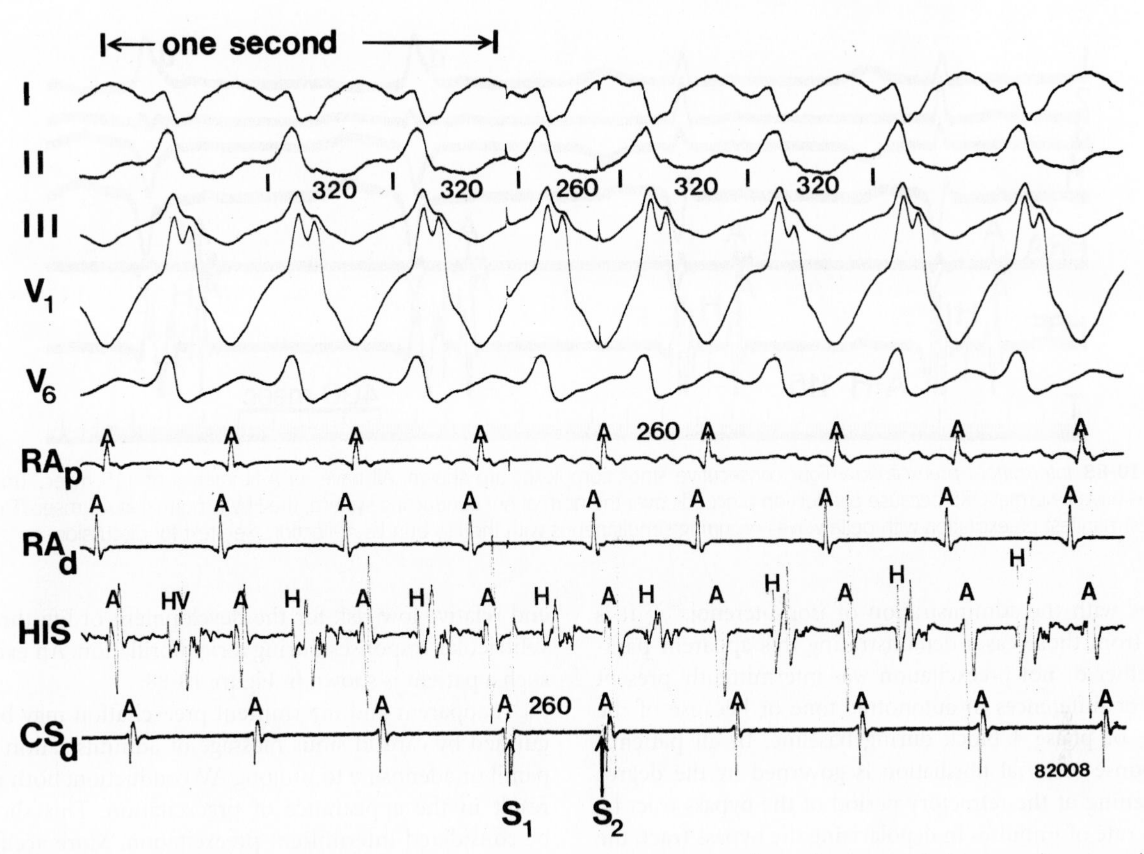


**FIGURE 10-87** *Resetting of a preexcited tachycardia to prove it is a circus movement tachycardia.* A preexcited tachycardia using a left lateral bypass tract antegradely and a right free wall bypass tract retrogradely is shown. Atrial extrastimuli from the CS are delivered, the second of which resets the tachycardia without influencing atrial activation in the RA or His bundle (i.e., atrial fusion is present). This S2 produces an exact capture of the ventricles with antegrade conduction over the bypass tract and retrograde atrial activation equal to the exact capture of the ventricle. This proves that the ventricle is responsible for atrial activation. This excludes an atrial tachycardia and confirms the diagnosis of preexcited circus movement tachycardia using two bypass tracts. See text for discussion. $RA_d$, distal; $RA_p$ = proximal RA.

life-threatening potential for atrial arrhythmias. Factors associated with atrial–fibrillation-induced ventricular fibrillation include male gender, septal location of the bypass tract, short refractory period of the bypass tract (shortest R-R <220 msec), and heightened adrenergic state. More controversial factors are multiple bypass tracts and use of digitalis. Conversely, we are probably better able to predict those patients who are at low risk for lethal ventricular responses during atrial flutter and fibrillation by demonstrating a long effective refractory period of the bypass tract. As mentioned earlier in this chapter, asymptomatic patients with WPW have a negligible incidence of sudden cardiac death (approximating that in the general population) although an episode of sudden death is the first symptom of WPW in half of the patients. Patients who have reached the age of 40 without symptoms are unlikely to ever experience symptoms due to WPW.

Methods by which one can evaluate the refractory period of the bypass tracts include (a) demonstration of intermittent preexcitation,[38,58,59] (b) assessing the ability of antiarrhythmic agents to produce antegrade block in the bypass tracts,[115–117] (c) the response of the delta wave to exercise,[38,118–120] and (d) programmed electrical stimulation.

## INTERMITTENT PREEXCITATION

Intermittent preexcitation is a term used differently by different investigators. Although some have included patients who manifest preexcitation on one day and none on another day,[58,59] we and others[38] require that intermittent preexcitation be observed on the same rhythm strip and always be associated with a prolongation of the P-R interval. Changes in autonomic tone on different days can influence conduction over the A-V node and can decrease the manifestations of preexcitation daily. The P-R interval, however, will remain short. Loss of preexcitation should reflect properties of the bypass tract, and therefore, factors producing enhancement of conduction over the normal pathway must be excluded. Despite the differences of definition, intermittency of preexcitation, however defined, is correlated with a long effective refractory period, long cycle lengths maintaining 1:1 conduction over the pathway antegradely, and prolonged preexcited R-R intervals during atrial fibrillation. This would therefore suggest a low risk for the spontaneous occurrence of rapid rates during atrial fibrillation. However, occasional patients with intermittent preexcitation have been noted to have atrial fibrillation, with the shortest preexcited R-R interval being less than

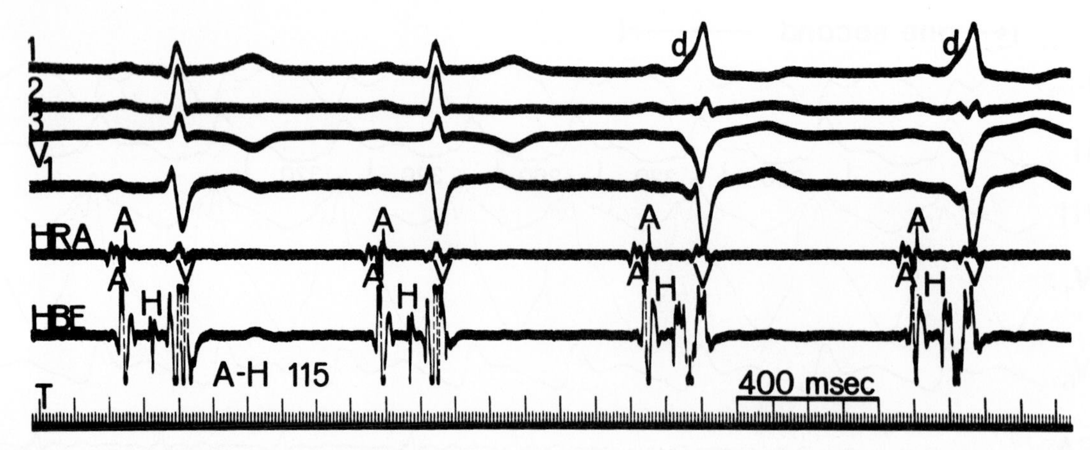


**FIGURE 10-88** *Intermittent preexcitation.* Four consecutive sinus complexes are shown. All have an A-H interval of 115 msec. The first two complexes have a normal QRS because conduction proceeds over the normal A-V conducting system; the H-V is normal at 45 msec. The last two complexes manifest preexcitation with delta waves occurring simultaneous with the His bundle deflection. See text for discussion.

250 msec with the administration of isoproterenol.[58,59] It is unclear from those cases demonstrating this apparent paradox whether or not preexcitation was intermittently present because of differences in autonomic tone or because of the presence of phase 4 block during baseline. In all patients, the response to atrial fibrillation is governed by the degree of shortening of the refractory period of the bypass tract by the high rate of impulses in depolarizing the bypass tract, the degree of antegrade decremental conduction and concealed conduction in the bypass tract, and the effects of accompanying sympathetic tone on shortening the refractory period of both the bypass tract and the A-V node. In our experience, patients who truly have intermittent preexcitation (i.e., on the same tracing) rarely develop life-threatening responses during atrial fibrillation, particularly when the arrhythmia is not associated with enhanced sympathetic tone. Even in the presence of exercise, life-threatening responses in these patients remain a rare event. These patients also commonly exhibit block in the bypass tract during exercise (see following discussion). The patients with alleged intermittent preexcitation who have been reported to develop a rapid ventricular response during atrial fibrillation usually showed marked catecholamine enhancement of conduction over both the bypass tract and the A-V node, but they rarely demonstrated intermittent preexcitation on the same electrocardiogram.[58,59,120] The degree to which catecholamines can influence bypass tract refractoriness is remarkable[121] they can even produce life-threatening ventricular responses in patients with relatively prolonged refractory periods in the baseline state. However, if one compares a group of patients with intermittent preexcitation on the same tracing with those showing persistent preexcitation or inapparent preexcitation, the ventricular response during induced atrial fibrillation, even during isoproterenol administration, is slower in patients with intermittent preexcitation. Thus, our experience parallels that of Wellens and Brugada[38] intermittent preexcitation (sudden loss of delta wave with prolongation of the P-R interval) is an indication of prolonged refractoriness over the bypass tract and relative low risk for the development of life-threatening ventricular responses during atrial fibrillation. An example of such a patient is shown in Figure 10-88.

Inapparent and intermittent preexcitation may be distinguished by carotid sinus massage or administration of verapamil or adenosine to prolong AV conduction; both methods result in the appearance of preexcitation. This should not be considered intermittent preexcitation. More accurately, it should be described as inapparent or a latent preexcitation. These patients may, in fact, develop life-threatening responses, and the inappropriate inclusion of these patients in a series of patients with alleged intermittent preexcitation has probably been responsible for the imperfect correlation between "intermittent preexcitation" and slow ventricular responses during atrial fibrillation. Caution should be used if adenosine is administered since it can cause atrial fibrillation.

## EFFECT OF ANTIARRHYTHMIC AGENTS ON PREEXCITATION

Wellens et al.[116,117] and Brugada et al.[115] demonstrated that ajmaline, procainamide, and amiodarone may produce block in the bypass tract in patients who have relatively long refractory periods of the bypass tract (i.e., >270 msec). These investigators also demonstrated the importance of the initial refractory period of the bypass tract as a determinant for drug responsiveness: The shorter the refractory period of the bypass tract, the less likely that block in the bypass tract can be achieved by antiarrhythmic agents.[122] However, although antegrade block may be produced in patients with relatively long antegrade refractory periods, this in no way reflects a similar effect on retrograde refractory periods. Thus, patients with production of antegrade block in their bypass tract by any of these antiarrhythmic agents may still have readily inducible circus movement tachycardia (Fig. 10-89). Others, however, contend that block in the bypass tract by antiarrhythmic agents does not accurately identify patients who

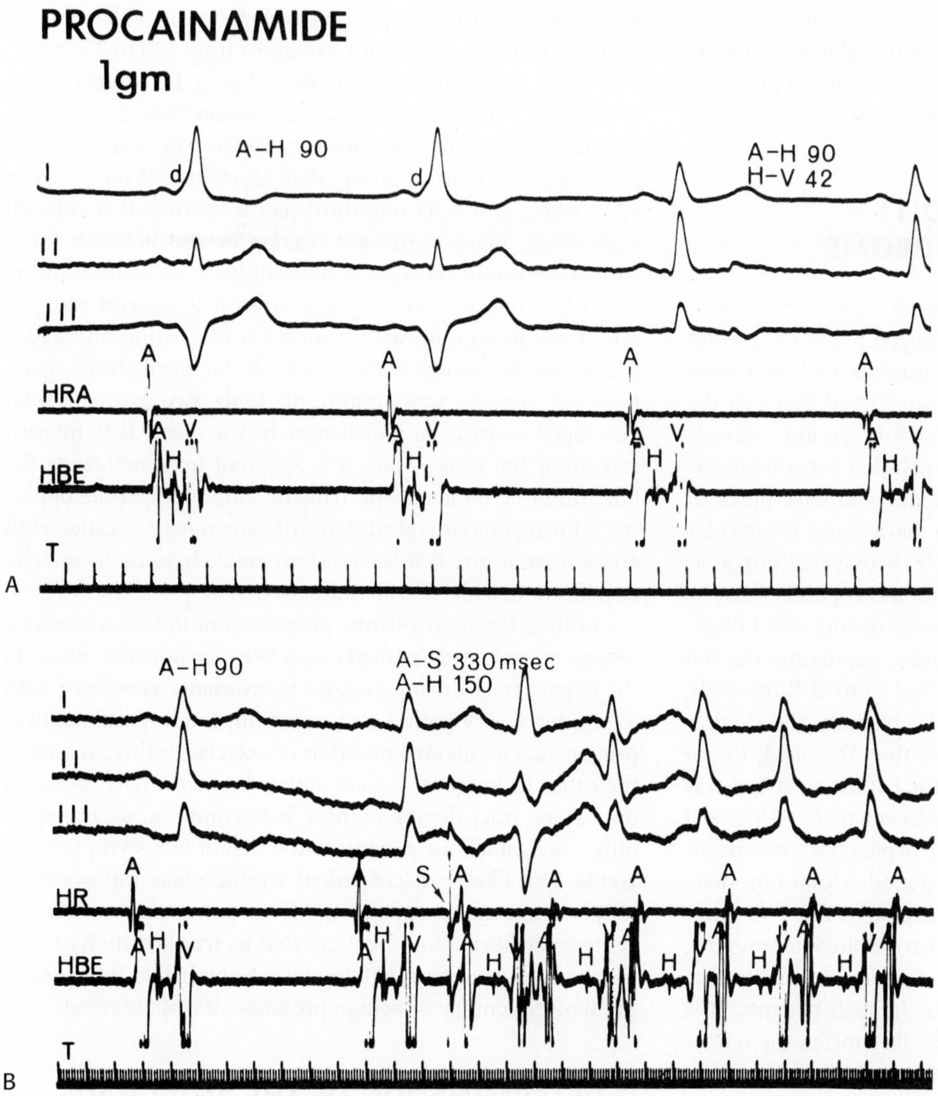

**FIGURE 10-89** *Induction of antegrade block in the bypass tract with procainamide.* **A:** Four sinus complexes following the administration of 1 g of procainamide intravenously. The first two complexes demonstrate obvious preexcitation. Following the procainamide, sudden loss of delta wave and preexcitation occur, and the last two complexes show normal activation over the His–Purkinje system. Although antegrade block in the bypass tract suggests a long antegrade refractory period of the bypass tract and a slower ventricular response during atrial fibrillation, it does not predict the ability to induce SVT. **B:** This is demonstrated in B where, following antegrade block in the bypass tract, orthodromic tachycardia is induced by a single atrial premature impulse. See text for discussion. HR, High right atrium.

are incapable of manifesting life-threatening ventricular responses during atrial fibrillation.[121,123] Some of this discrepancy is related to patient selection, while an additional explanation may be related to mode of administration of procainamide. Wellens et al.[116,117] delivered the agent directly into a central vein more rapidly than other investigators. Of interest, despite the fact that Fananapazir et al.[123] regard the procainamide test as inadequate, the *p*-value for the effect of procainamide on the antegrade effective refractory period and its relationship to the shortest R-R interval during atrial fibrillation was significant at $p < 0.01$. The investigator's concern was the scatter that was observed. Thus, even the major detractors of this test have demonstrated a statistically significant correlation between antegrade block in the bypass tract and the effective refractory period with the shortest R-R interval during atrial fibrillation.

In our laboratory, we have found that block in the bypass tract by drugs has almost always been observed in patients with baseline antegrade effective refractory periods that exceeded 300 msec. These findings were true regardless of the class of antiarrhythmic agent used (i.e., Class 1A [e.g., procainamide, quinidine], Class 1B [i.e., lidocaine], Class 1C [flecainide, propafenone], Class 3 [e.g., ibutilide, dofetilide], or amiodarone). In our experience, the major limitation of this test is the relatively small number of patients in whom block does occur; thus, the test appears to have a good predictive value for prolonged effective refractory periods, but its sensitivity and specificity are not great. Differences in patient population are most likely responsible for the low sensitivity in our patients. Nevertheless, it is my impression that antegrade block in the bypass tract produced by an antiarrhythmic agent correlates with a relatively prolonged antegrade refractory period and relatively long minimal preexcited R-R interval during atrial fibrillation. It therefore remains a reasonably good indicator of a relatively low-risk patient. Conversely, in our experience, failure to produce block in the bypass tract has not been a good predictor for those at risk of developing rapid ventricular responses during atrial fibrillation. The implications of our inability to predict a short antegrade effective refractory period and rapid ventricular response during induced atrial fibrillation are discussed later. In general, identifying a patient who is unlikely to develop a rapid ventricular response is valuable and is the object of this test. The ability to predict a patient at high risk is moot (see following discussion).

## EXERCISE TESTING IN WOLFF–PARKINSON–WHITE SYNDROME

Block in the accessory pathway during exercise has been reported to be associated with a prolonged refractory period of the bypass tract.[118–120] This is consistent with our own experience. All our patients who demonstrated block in the bypass tract during exercise had refractory periods exceeding 300 msec. Other investigators suggest that occasional discrepancies occur, and that some patients who have block in the bypass tract during exercise may have rapid ventricular responses during atrial fibrillation.[58,121] If one carefully analyzes the reported discrepancies, however, two points must be made: (a) The mean ventricular response during atrial fibrillation in these patients was relatively long, approximating 300 msec, and only occasional complexes had short R-R intervals, which suggests that, in these particular patients, the rhythm may not have in fact been life threatening; (b) block in the bypass tract was not truly block in the bypass tract but was "pseudo"-normalization that was due to enhanced A-V nodal conduction. To document block in the bypass tract, one needs to record all 12 leads and demonstrate a sudden loss of the delta wave, which is associated with an increase in the P-R interval. In many cases reported to demonstrate block on exercise, these criteria have not been met. It is conceivable, that in rare cases, life-threatening responses occur in such patients. It is known that catecholamines can markedly shorten the refractory period of the bypass tract[124] so that marked enhancement of catecholamine output during severe stress may override the "apparent" refractory period manifested by block in the bypass tract at lesser exercise stresses. Nevertheless, it is my opinion that this is the best test because it yields a determinant of maximum 1:1 conduction over the bypass tract in the presence of catecholamines. Although there may be patients who manifest block in the bypass tract during exercise but who demonstrate an occasional short R-R interval (<220 msec) during atrial fibrillation, the mean ventricular response is almost always >300 msec, persistently short R-R intervals are uncommon, and occasional normalization of the QRS is often observed. Despite the fact that outliers may occasionally demonstrate very short R-R intervals during induced atrial fibrillation, it is highly unlikely that this signifies a life-threatening response, because the mean ventricular response usually is in the order of 300 msec, a value not too different from patients with atrial fibrillation who do not develop ventricular fibrillation. Klein et al.[44] demonstrated many years ago that the shortest R-R interval and mean R-R intervals in patients with ventricular fibrillation evolving from atrial fibrillation were significantly shorter than in those patients who did not develop ventricular fibrillation. These investigators found that the mean shortest R-R interval in the group who developed ventricular fibrillation was 180 ± 29 msec, with a range of from 140 to 250 msec, which was significantly shorter than that in the control group of patients without ventricular fibrillation (240 ± 63 msec). Overlap was considerable, however, because in nearly half the patients in the control group, their shortest R-R interval was <250 msec, and fully one-third had a shortest R-R interval <200 msec. Thus, significant overlap existed between those with and without ventricular fibrillation. In an analysis of the mean R-R intervals, the average mean R-R interval was 269 ± 62 msec in a group with ventricular fibrillation and 340 ± 8 msec in the group without ventricular fibrillation; again, however, overlap was significant. Only two patients who developed ventricular fibrillation had a mean R-R interval exceeding 300 msec. Thus, it is apparent from reviewing the literature that patients who truly develop block in the bypass tract during exercise (abrupt loss of delta wave associated with an increase in the P-R interval) are unlikely to be those who develop ventricular fibrillation.

In sum, I remain a strong proponent of the use of exercise testing in evaluating patients with WPW syndrome. Block in the bypass tract during exercise is invariably associated with a long refractory period and, more importantly, an excellent prognosis. The major limitation of exercise testing, as well as the other techniques, is their rather low sensitivity. Block in the bypass tract during exercise is uncommon, occurring in only <10% of all our patients and <25% of our asymptomatic adults. This likely reflects patient selection bias, but nonetheless, because the vast majority of our patients never develop ventricular fibrillation, I believe that its true sensitivity is low for predicting patients with low risk. Nonetheless, it has a high predictive accuracy of benign prognosis if it is observed.

## DETERMINATION OF THE ANTEGRADE REFRACTORY PERIOD OF THE BYPASS TRACT BY PROGRAMMED STIMULATION

One of the major determinants of the rate of conduction over the bypass tract during atrial fibrillation or flutter is the antegrade refractory period of that bypass tract. Wellens and Durrer[114] showed many years ago that the refractory period of the bypass tract exhibited a strong relationship with the shortest R-R or mean R-R interval during atrial fibrillation. Other investigators have shown a less exact but statistically significant correlation. As noted earlier, patients who develop ventricular fibrillation have shorter effective refractory periods than those who do not develop ventricular fibrillation.[44] Although values such as 250 to 270 msec have been used to separate short from long refractory periods, this is artificial, owing to the extreme overlap. Clearly, however, patients whose refractory periods exceed 300 msec, and whose cycle length at which maximum 1:1 conduction over the bypass tract occurs exceeds 300 msec, have an extremely low likelihood of developing ventricular fibrillation. As noted earlier, patients with SVT but no atrial fibrillation have a mean effective refractory period of just

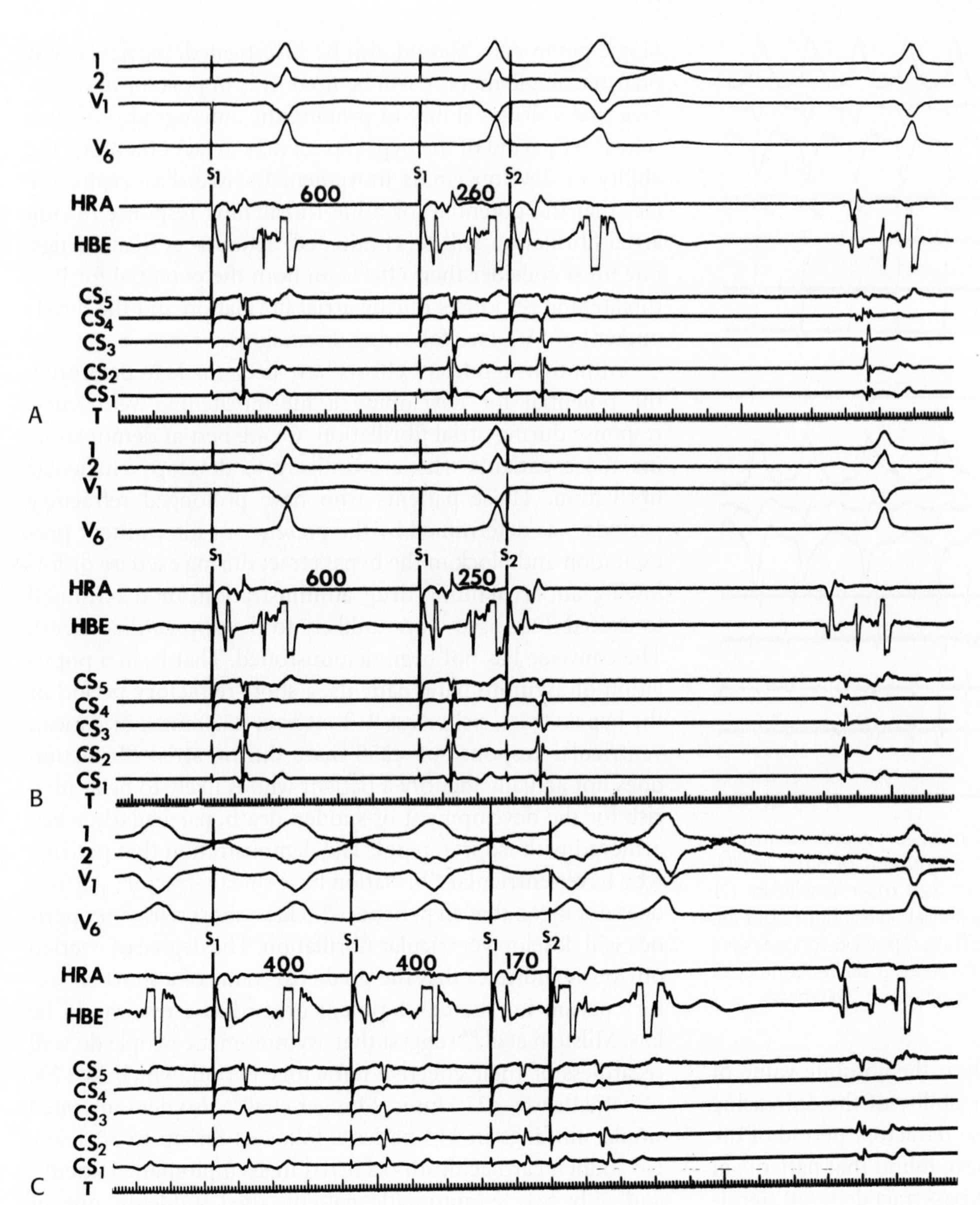


**FIGURE 10-90** Effect of cycle length on antegrade refractory period of the bypass tract. **A**, **B**, and **C** are arranged simultaneously. **A** and **B:** Refractory period determinations are made at a drive cycle length (S1-S1) of 600 msec. **B:** The effective refractory period (ERP) of the bypass tract is 250 msec. **C:** When the drive cycle length is shortened to 400 msec, antegrade conduction persists at shorter coupling intervals than ERP at the longer drive cycle lengths. See text for discussion.

over 300 msec, those with circus movement tachycardia and atrial fibrillation have a mean effective refractory period of 290 msec, those who present with atrial fibrillation but no cardiac arrest have a mean effective refractory period of 260 msec, and those who present with a cardiac arrest have a mean effective refractory period of 225 msec. However, in our experience as well as others, overlap is significant. Nonetheless, no single patient in our series who had an antegrade refractory period >300 msec and who failed to conduct 1:1 at cycle lengths <300 msec developed ventricular fibrillation. In our experience, the mean ventricular response during atrial fibrillation correlates best with the maximum rate of 1:1 conduction over the bypass tract, while the shortest R-R interval correlates somewhat better with the effective refractory period of the bypass tract. One must, however, perform refractory period studies at multiple cycle lengths, because the effective refractory period of the bypass tract shortens with decreasing cycle lengths.[32,125] Thus, the refractory period should be determined at a rapid cycle length, preferably 400 msec or less. An example of how the refractory period of the bypass tract was shortened when determined at 600 and 400 msec is shown in Figure 10-90. The effective refractory period in this figure shortened from 250 msec at a basic paced cycle length of 600 msec to 220 msec at a paced cycle length of 400 msec.

The maximum rate at which 1:1 ventricular conduction proceeds over the bypass tract should be determined as well as the induction of atrial fibrillation for completeness (Fig. 10-91). The refractory period should be determined at the atrial site approximate to the insertion of the bypass tract to obviate the effect of intra-atrial conduction delay and to allow appropriate determination of the bypass tract. As noted, cycle length can influence the refractory period, and the refractory period determinations should therefore be performed at multiple cycle lengths, including at least one cycle

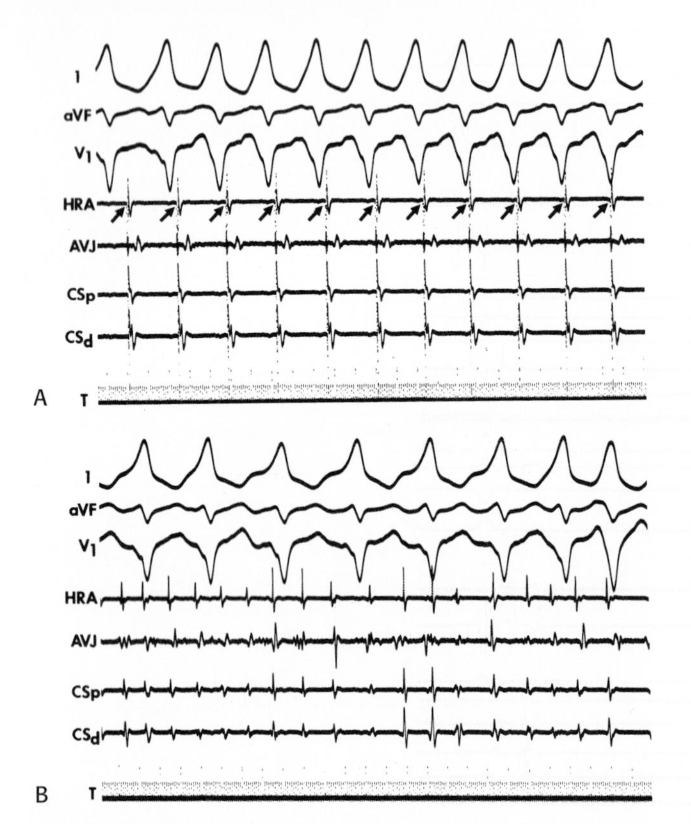


**FIGURE 10-91** *Determining the potential for rapid ventricular responses by atrial pacing and elective conduction of atrial fibrillation.* **A:** Atrial pacing at a cycle length of 220 msec results in 1:1 conduction over the bypass tract. **B:** Atrial fibrillation is induced but the fastest ventricular response is 230 msec. Thus, repetitive concealment in the bypass tract during atrial fibrillation causes a slower ventricular response than would atrial flutter at a cycle length of 220 msec.

length of 400 msec or less. Not only is the absolute value of the refractory period useful, but the ability of the decreasing cycle length to cause a decrease in the refractory period of the bypass tract is also important. We have found that patients in whom the refractory period of the bypass tract does not significantly decrease when determined at decreasing cycle lengths have slower ventricular responses during atrial fibrillation than those patients in whom the effective refractory period of the bypass tract shortens with shortening of the paced cycle length. Because catecholamines can markedly influence the effective refractory period of the bypass tract, and thus the ventricular response during atrial fibrillation, some investigators suggest performing programmed stimulation (i.e., determining the effective refractory period of the bypass tract, the maximum rate of 1:1 conduction over the bypass tract, and the shortest R-R interval and mean R-R interval during induced atrial fibrillation) following isoproterenol. In our experience, the use of isoproterenol to achieve sinus acceleration of 25% can produce marked shortening of the refractory period, and can increase in the ventricular response during atrial fibrillation so much, that most patients in whom atrial fibrillation is induced can manifest potentially life-threatening responses. Thus, the ability to interpret the results is limited. The effect of antiarrhythmic agents on these electrophysiologic parameters should also be investigated, particularly if pharmacologic therapy will be used. It is important to recognize that a drug's ability to prolong the anterograde effective refractory period of the bypass tract may in fact potentiate the ability to develop circus movement tachycardia despite the fact that the potential for a life-threatening response during atrial fibrillation will be eliminated. Thus, to evaluate drugs, one must consider their effects on both the potential for life-threatening responses during atrial fibrillation and the development of SVT (see following discussion).

Although significant efforts have been made to determine the potential for developing a life-threatening ventricular response during atrial fibrillation, we are best at demonstrating those patients who are unlikely to develop ventricular fibrillation. Those patients who have prolonged refractory periods – as determined by the presence of intermittent preexcitation and block in the bypass tract during exercise or following antiarrhythmic drug administration, or determined to exceed 300 msec – are unlikely to develop cardiac arrest. The converse has not been demonstrated. That is, in a population of asymptomatic patients, a short refractory period of the bypass tract, a shortest R-R interval <220 msec or a mean ventricular response of <250 msec during atrial fibrillation **does not** actually identify a patient who is likely to be at high risk for the development of sudden death, particularly when achieved with isoproterenol. The demonstration that patients who have ventricular fibrillation have short refractory periods does not mean that all patients who have short refractory periods will develop ventricular fibrillation. The degree of overlap obviously indicates that the predictive value of a short refractory period for the development of cardiac arrest would be low. Milstein et al.[64] suggest that asymptomatic people do well regardless of their effective refractory period, which in 17% of patients was <270 msec. Munger et al.[47] also demonstrated similar findings in 113 patients followed for up to 35 years. No sudden cardiac death occurred in asymptomatic patients, and only two symptomatic patients died suddenly, one of whom was an athlete with a grossly enlarged and hypertrophied heart (520 g) at autopsy. Wellens has undertaken a prospective study in a group of 142 asymptomatic patients with WPW (Wellen HJJ, personal communication). He divided the patients into 52 with effective refractory periods ≤240 msec and 90 patients with effective refractory periods >240 msec and followed them for more than 20 years. The incidence of sudden death in these groups did not differ. Only two patients in both groups died suddenly, and in only one patient in each group did atrial fibrillation seem a likely cause. Thus, the overwhelming evidence suggests that one cannot use the antegrade effective refractory period measurements to predict patients at risk for development of sudden death. It also does not appear that the use of the ventricular response during induced atrial fibrillation, particularly in asymptomatic patients, is useful. It is my personal bias that regardless of the presence or absence of symptoms, these measurements are poor predictors of patients at risk. Patients with syncope do not have distinct clinical or electrophysiologic features that differ from patients who never develop life-threatening arrhythmias.[126] Thus, I believe that we cannot predict patients at high risk for sudden death but we are able to select patients at low risk for sudden death. This is useful because it has implications for lifestyle recommendation for these patients. The widespread use of electrophysiologic studies to predict patients who are likely to die, and therefore have limitations placed on their lifestyle, seems totally unjustified at this point. The only things we can do are (a) assure people who are totally asymptomatic that they are unlikely to experience sudden cardiac death and, if less than 30 years old, are likely to remain asymptomatic regardless of their effective refractory periods and (b) reassure those patients who have prolonged refractory periods as assessed by any method that they are extremely unlikely to develop ventricular fibrillation regardless of whether symptoms are present or not. Finally, one must remember that freedom from developing life-threatening ventricular response during atrial fibrillation or the demonstration of a long antegrade refractory period of the bypass tract is of no value in predicting the likelihood of developing orthodromic tachycardia.

## TERMINATION OF ORTHODROMIC TACHYCARDIA

Because the reentrant circuit in orthodromic tachycardia is large and incorporates both the atrium and ventricles, premature stimuli from either chamber can almost always penetrate the circuit, even during tachycardias with rapid rates. More rapid rates may necessitate the introduction of multiple electrical stimuli to reach either the normal A-V conducting system or the bypass tract during its refractory state. Thus, in most tachycardias with cycle lengths exceeding 300 msec, single atrial and/or ventricular extrastimuli can terminate the arrhythmia (Fig. 10-92). Termination of a supraventricular

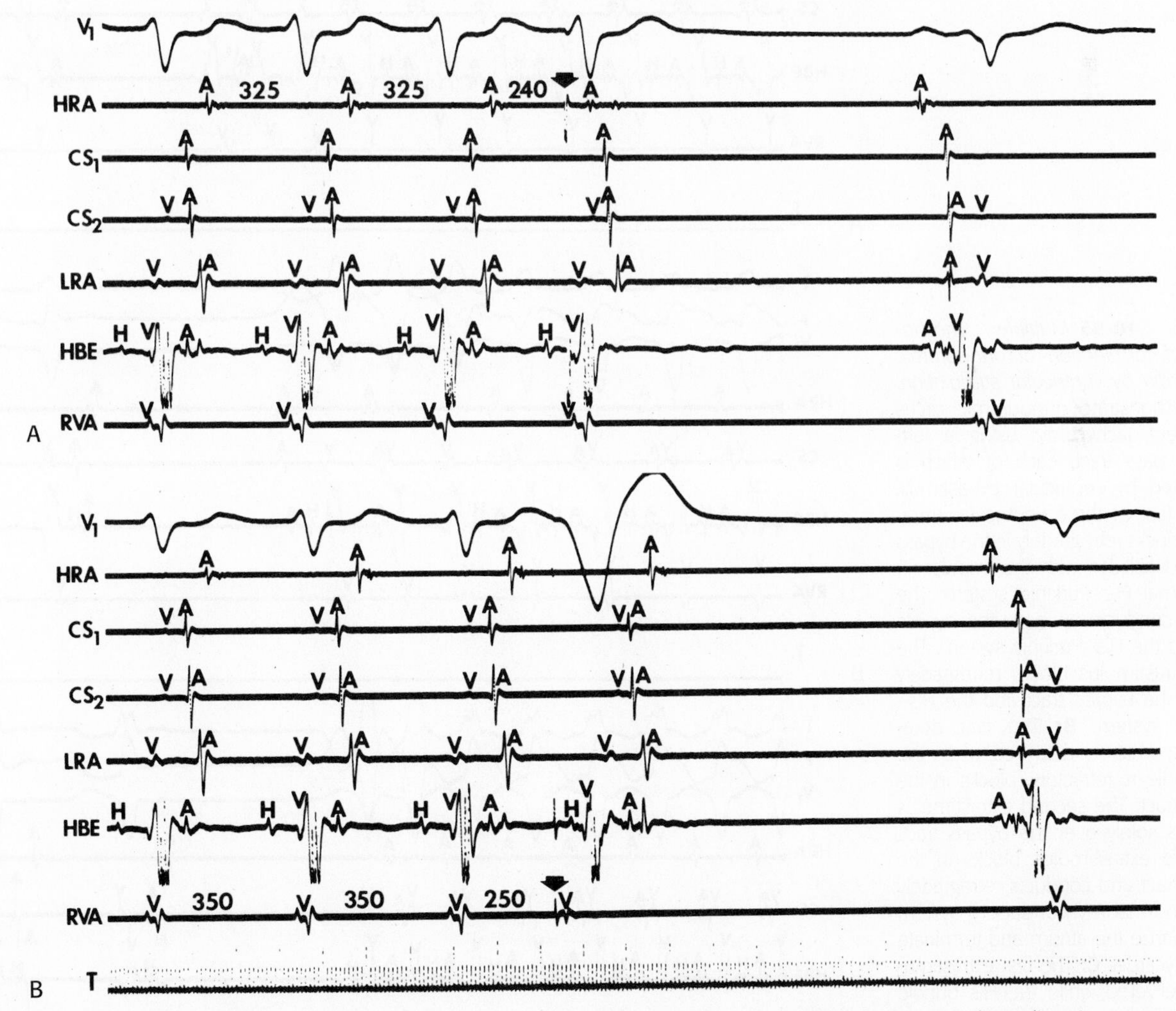


**FIGURE 10-92** *Termination of orthodromic tachycardia by atrial and ventricular stimuli.* **A** and **B:** Orthodromic tachycardia using a posteroseptal bypass tract is shown. **A:** A single atrial stimulus terminates the tachycardia by blocking in the A-V node. **B:** A ventricular extrastimulus preexcites the atrium with an activation sequence identical to that during SVT without disturbing the antegrade His bundle. This confirms the presence of a functioning bypass tract. The tachycardia is terminated when the early atrial impulse attempts to return to the ventricle but blocks antegradely in the A-V node.

arrhythmia by a ventricular premature beat in and of itself should suggest the presence of a bypass tract. The faster the rate, and the farther the extrastimulus is from the site of the bypass tract, the more premature or the greater the number of stimuli required to terminate the arrhythmia. Thus, in patients with right-sided or septal bypass tracts, single premature stimuli from the right atrium or the right ventricle will almost always terminate tachycardias with cycle lengths >300 msec. Ventricular extrastimuli then can result in termination of the tachycardia even when delivered when the His bundle is refractory (Fig. 10-92, also see Fig. 10-82). The most common mechanism of termination is by antegrade block in the A-V node. The response to ventricular extrastimuli, however, can vary greatly, depending on the coupling interval and number of ventricular extrastimuli needed. Thus, ventricular extrastimuli can terminate the tachycardia by (a) blocking retrogradely in the bypass tract; (b) conducting retrogradely up the normal A-V conducting system, with or without retrograde conduction up the bypass tract; or (c) retrograde conduction over the bypass tract with subsequent antegrade block in the A-V node, or occasionally below the His bundle (Fig. 10-93). Whereas orthodromic tachycardias can be reset

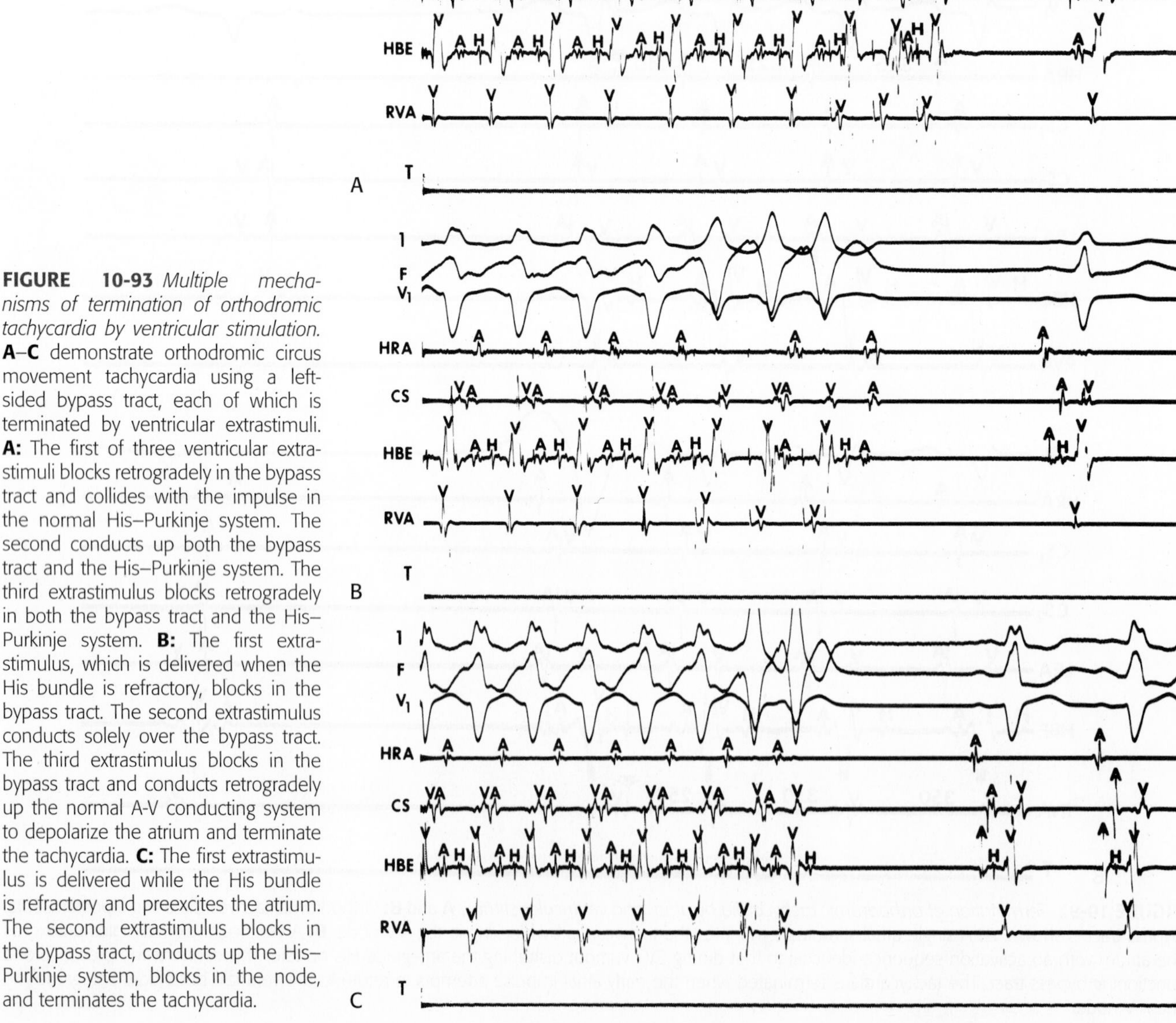


**FIGURE 10-93** *Multiple mechanisms of termination of orthodromic tachycardia by ventricular stimulation.* **A–C** demonstrate orthodromic circus movement tachycardia using a left-sided bypass tract, each of which is terminated by ventricular extrastimuli. **A:** The first of three ventricular extrastimuli blocks retrogradely in the bypass tract and collides with the impulse in the normal His–Purkinje system. The second conducts up both the bypass tract and the His–Purkinje system. The third extrastimulus blocks retrogradely in both the bypass tract and the His–Purkinje system. **B:** The first extrastimulus, which is delivered when the His bundle is refractory, blocks in the bypass tract. The second extrastimulus conducts solely over the bypass tract. The third extrastimulus blocks in the bypass tract and conducts retrogradely up the normal A-V conducting system to depolarize the atrium and terminate the tachycardia. **C:** The first extrastimulus is delivered while the His bundle is refractory and preexcites the atrium. The second extrastimulus blocks in the bypass tract, conducts up the His–Purkinje system, blocks in the node, and terminates the tachycardia.

and/or entrained by atrial or ventricular pacing, termination requires block in either the bypass tract or the A-V conducting system.[32,38,127,128]

## Multiple Bypass Tracts

Because A-V bypass tracts appear to be a congenital abnormality that is due to developmental defects in the A-V rings, it is not surprising that multiple A-V bypass tracts can be present in the same patient. These multiple bypass tracts may or may not be apparent, and their detection often requires (a) the use of detailed atrial mapping during programmed stimulation, during SVT in the catheterization laboratory, or during surgery; (b) the elimination of an apparent bypass tract by surgery, catheter ablation, or by pharmacologic agents; and/or (c) mapping of ventricular activation during pacing from both the right and left atrium.[39,63,129–133] During use of these techniques, the incidence of multiple bypass tracts ranges from 10% to 30%.[32,41,134] The highest incidence of multiple bypass tracts is from our laboratory. In the preablation era we recognized nearly one-third of the bypass tracts, unsuspected during the preoperative electrophysiology study, at the time of surgery. The wide range of incidence in multiple bypass tracts probably stems from differences in patient populations and methodologic differences in determining the presence of such bypass tracts. The incidence of multiple bypass tracts is higher in patients with antidromic tachycardia,[32,38,39,41,134] in patients in whom atrial fibrillation results in ventricular fibrillation,[44] and in patients with Ebstein's anomaly.[32,39] Electrocardiographic observations and findings during electrophysiologic studies that demonstrate or suggest the presence of multiple bypass tracts include (a) changing antegrade delta waves; (b) evidence of multiple routes of retrograde atrial activation; (c) orthodromic SVT with intermittent antegrade fusion (i.e., preexcited) complexes; (d) preexcited circus movement tachycardias, particularly if antegrade activation proceeds over a posteroseptal bypass tract and/or the tachycardia is slower than that of orthodromic tachycardia in the same patient; (e) atypical patterns of preexcitation; and (f) evidence of mismatch of antegrade preexcitation and the site of retrograde atrial activation observed during orthodromic SVT (Table 10-9).

The observation of changing antegrade delta waves – that is, changing patterns of preexcitation – is uncommon during sinus rhythm. Therefore, it was fortuitous that the first person I studied with WPW syndrome manifested two forms of preexcitation during sinus rhythm (Fig. 10-94).[132] Occasionally, following the use of Type I agents or amiodarone, block in one accessory pathway can lead to manifestation of antegrade conduction over a second accessory pathway.[38] Atrial fibrillation (either spontaneous or induced) may provide the opportunity to see different patterns of preexcitation, thereby allowing one to document the presence of multiple bypass tracts. This has been suggested as an indication for the deliberate induction of atrial fibrillation during an electrophysiologic study. Because aberration of the normal conducting system can occur during atrial fibrillation, it is imperative to carefully differentiate changing QRSs that are due to multiple bypass tracts from conduction over one bypass tract and over the normal conducting system with aberration. Because multiple bypass tracts are often located in the free walls of the right and left A-V grooves, the use of both right and left atrial pacing occasionally can document the presence of additional bypass tracts that are not manifested if only pacing from the one atrium is performed. This can be seen in Figure 10-95, where right atrial pacing produces ventricular activation over a right-sided bypass tract, and coronary sinus pacing produces ventricular activation over a left-sided bypass tract. In addition, the tachycardias initiated by stimulation at different sites can vary, resulting in two retrograde activation sequences, which document the presence of multiple bypass tracts (see following discussion).

The observation of multiple routes of retrograde atrial activation during SVT or ventricular pacing is an important clue to the presence of multiple bypass tracts. If a single bypass tract was present, the V-A interval should be fixed and the retrograde P-wave morphology constant during orthodromic tachycardia. If the V-A interval or P-wave morphology changes during orthodromic tachycardia, the presence of an additional bypass tract should be suspected. During the electrophysiology study, the presence of two distinct retrograde atrial activation patterns documents the presence of multiple bypass tracts and explains changing P-wave morphology and V-A intervals (see Fig. 10-95). In other cases, during orthodromic tachycardia, a single, fixed retrograde atrial activation pattern is observed in the presence of two or more bypass

**TABLE 10-9 Evidence of Multiple Bypass Tracts**

1. Changing antegrade delta waves
   a. NSR
   b. Following antiarrhythmic agents
   c. Atrial fibrillation
   d. Right and left atrial pacing
2. Evidence of multiple routes of retrograde atrial activation
   a. Changing retrograde P wave and/or V-A interval
   b. Multiple retrograde atrial activation during ventricular stimulation
   c. Failure to prolong contralateral atrial activation with the appearance of ipsilateral BBB
3. Orthodromic CMT with antegrade fusion
4. Preexcited tachycardias
   a. Antegrade conduction over a septal BT
   b. Preexcited tachycardia CL > orthodromic SVT CL
5. Atypical patterns of preexcitation
6. Mismatch of site of antegrade preexcitation and retrograde Atrial activation during orthodromic CMT.

BBB, bundle branch block; BT, bypass tract; CL, cycle length; CMT, circus movement tachycardia; NSR, normal sinus rhythm; SVT, supraventricular tachycardia; V-A, ventriculoatrial.

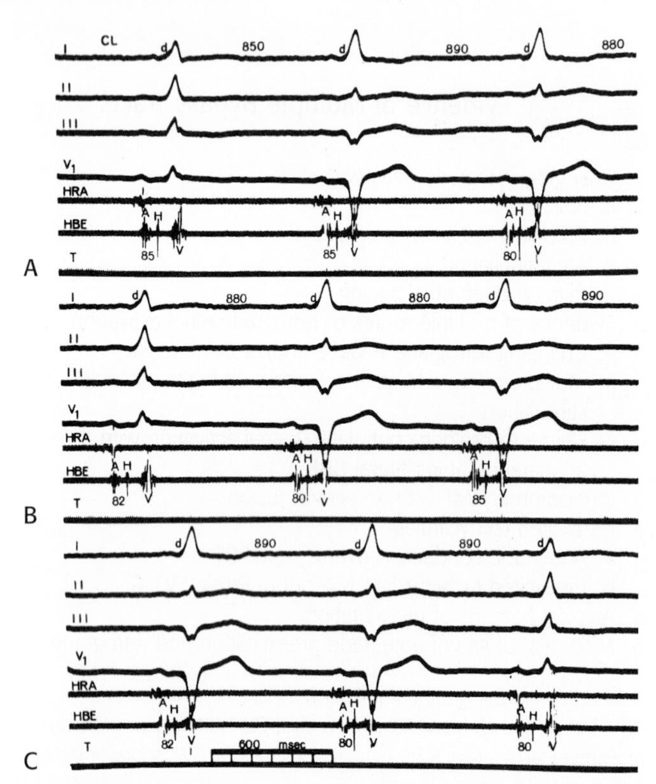


**FIGURE 10-94** *Alternating conduction over right- and left-sided bypass tracts.* **A–C:** Continuous ECGs demonstrate a change from antegrade activation over a left lateral bypass tract (first complex) to antegrade activation over a right lateral bypass tract (second complex). See text for discussion. (From Josephson ME, Caracta AR, Lau SH. Alternating type A and type B Wolff-Parkinson-White syndrome. *Am Heart J* 1974;87:363.)

tracts. In this instance, additional bypass tracts can be recognized by the appearance of more than one atrial breakthrough site. This is demonstrated in Figure 10-96, where the earliest retrograde atrial activation occurs in the distal coronary sinus, compatible with a left lateral bypass tract. If only a single bypass tract was present, activation of the atrium in the AVJ should follow atrial activation recorded at the os of the coronary sinus. In this instance, atrial activation in the His bundle recording precedes atrial activation of the os by 30 msec, suggesting a second pathway in the anterior septum.

Occasionally, multiple routes of retrograde atrial activation can be observed during the induction of a tachycardia by ventricular pacing. Analyzing the atrial activation sequence during ventricular pacing, during the ventricular extrastimulus that initiates SVT and during SVT, one often can observe that retrograde atrial activation during ventricular pacing is a fusion of activation over one or more bypass tracts and over the A-V node. With the introduction of a ventricular extrastimulus, retrograde activation may proceed over one bypass tract to initiate orthodromic tachycardia with retrograde conduction over an additional bypass tract (Fig. 10-97). The site of ventricular pacing is critical because retrograde atrial activation will preferentially proceed over a bypass tract adjacent to the site of stimulation as long as that bypass tract is capable of retrograde conduction. On the other hand, a very early atrial extrastimulus may block in the bypass tract closest to the stimulus site and conduct over a bypass tract at a more distant site (see Fig. 10-95). In either case, the induction sequence provides another opportunity to compare retrograde atrial activation sequences.

Another finding related to retrograde atrial activation that suggests a second bypass tract is the failure to prolong atrial activation at all sites with the development of bundle branch block ipsilateral to the bypass tract. For example, if during orthodromic tachycardia using an apparent left-sided bypass tract, LBBB develops, activation of both atria should be prolonged, with right atrial activation following left atrial activation. If following LBBB right atrial activation remains constant while left atrial activation prolongs, an additional right-sided bypass tract must be present.

In a similar vein, if one has orthodromic tachycardia and then develops fusion complexes consistent with preexcitation, an additional bypass tract must be operative. The V-A interval may simultaneously change and increase to the degree to which the QRS becomes preexcited and the ventricle activated earlier than it was when conduction proceeded solely over the normal A-V conducting system. Changes in the V-A interval occur with the appearance of antegrade fusion if impairment of A-V nodal or His–Purkinje conduction by drugs, cycle length oscillation, or retrograde concealment was responsible for the sudden appearance of fusion. Occasionally, a narrow QRS tachycardia can gradually develop into a preexcited tachycardia after going through various states of fusion. Examples of these phenomena are shown in Figure 10-98. Analogously, if a preexcited tachycardia demonstrates antegrade fusion, a second bypass tract must be used as the retrograde limb (Fig. 10-99). In this instance one must document that fusion is not caused by A-V nodal reentry with an innocent bystander accessory pathway (see Fig. 10-32). As stated earlier in the chapter (see discussion of antidromic tachycardia), the mere presence of a preexcited tachycardia should suggest the likely presence of multiple bypass tracts. Almost 40% of patients with preexcited circus movement tachycardias, incorporating a bypass tract as the antegrade limb, have multiple bypass tracts. Multiple bypass tracts are almost invariably present if the preexcited tachycardia demonstrates antegrade conduction over a posteroseptal bypass tract, because antegrade conduction over such a bypass tract has not been described with "classic antidromic tachycardia."[39] In addition, in our experience, in the absence of dual pathways with orthodromic tachycardia using the slow pathway, if the preexcited tachycardia is slower than orthodromic tachycardia in the same patient, multiple bypass tracts are likely to be present. Antidromic tachycardia is only slower than orthodromic tachycardia if retrograde conduction during antidromic tachycardia is slower than antegrade conduction during orthodromic tachycardia.

If the electrocardiographic pattern of preexcitation during a preexcited tachycardia or during sinus rhythm does not conform to an expected QRS morphology for a given location, one should evaluate the possibility that ventricular activation

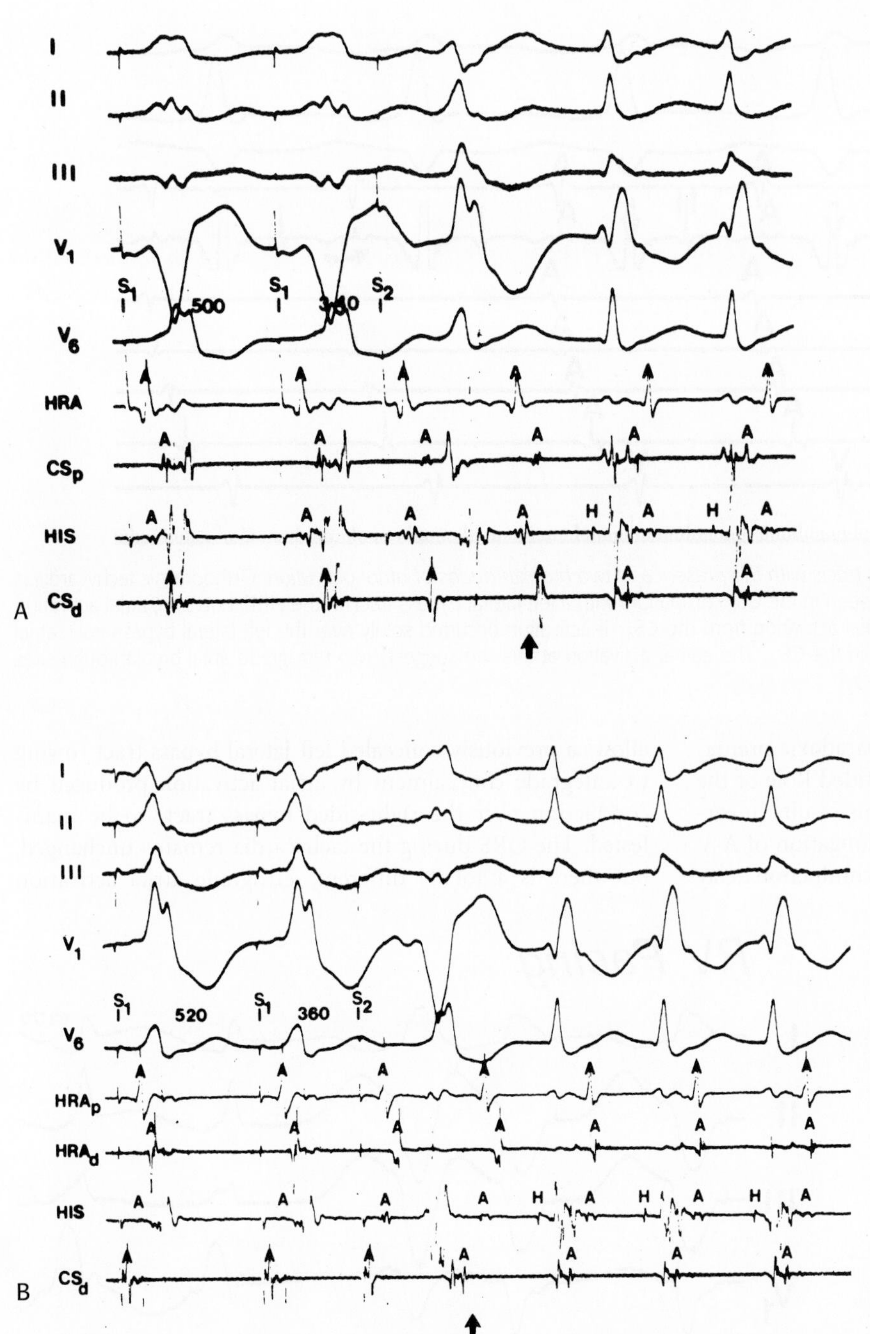


**FIGURE 10-95** *Effect of site of pacing on antegrade conduction over different bypass tracts.* **A:** During right atrial pacing, antegrade activation occurs over a right lateral bypass tract. When an extrastimulus (S2) is delivered from the HRA it blocks in the right-sided bypass tract and conducts over a left-sided bypass tract, which initiates an echo beat over the right-sided bypass tract. This atrial echo initiates orthodromic tachycardia with simultaneous retrograde atrial activation over both the left- and right-sided bypass tracts. **B:** Coronary sinus pacing produces antegrade activation over a left lateral bypass tract. A premature stimulus (S2) blocks in the left-sided bypass tract and conducts over a right lateral bypass tract, initiating an atrial echo over the left lateral bypass tract. This echo initiates orthodromic tachycardia with conduction antegradely over the normal conducting system and retrograde conduction over both the left lateral and right-sided bypass tracts. The fact that the right-sided bypass tract is used is suggested by the difference in retrograde atrial activation when conduction proceeds solely over the left-sided bypass tract following antegrade conduction over the right-sided bypass tract (*arrow*) in the last three complexes. $HRA_d$, distal HRA; $HRA_p$, proximal HRA. (Adapted from: Heddle WF, Brugada P, Wellens HJJ. Multiple circus movement tachycardias with multiple accessory pathways. *J Am Coll Cardiol* 1984;4:166.)

is actually a fusion of antegrade conduction over more than one bypass tract. Finally, if there is a mismatch between the site of antegrade preexcitation, as determined from either the ECG or electrophysiologic studies, and the site of earliest retrograde atrial activation during orthodromic tachycardia (again as determined either by retrograde P-wave morphology on the ECG or during electrophysiologic studies), a second bypass tract is most certainly operative.

Sometimes there will be no evidence of multiple bypass tracts during spontaneous sinus rhythm, induced atrial fibrillation, right or left atrial pacing, orthodromic tachycardia, or preexcited tachycardias. This most commonly occurs when additional bypass tracts are "concealed" both during sinus rhythm or circus movement tachycardia because of preferential activation over one bypass tract. These bypass tracts can often be recognized by performing atrial or ventricular stimulation during orthodromic tachycardia or, as stated previously, by assessing the effect of bundle branch block on retrograde atrial activation. Thus, it is important to introduce both atrial and ventricular extrastimuli during circus movement tachycardia to see if changing A-V times or retrograde routes of activation allows manifestation of an additional bypass tract. An example of how this stimulation can reveal the presence of additional bypass tracts is shown in Figure 10-100. Circus movement tachycardia using a right anterior bypass tract is present on the left. The introduction of a right VPC (RV

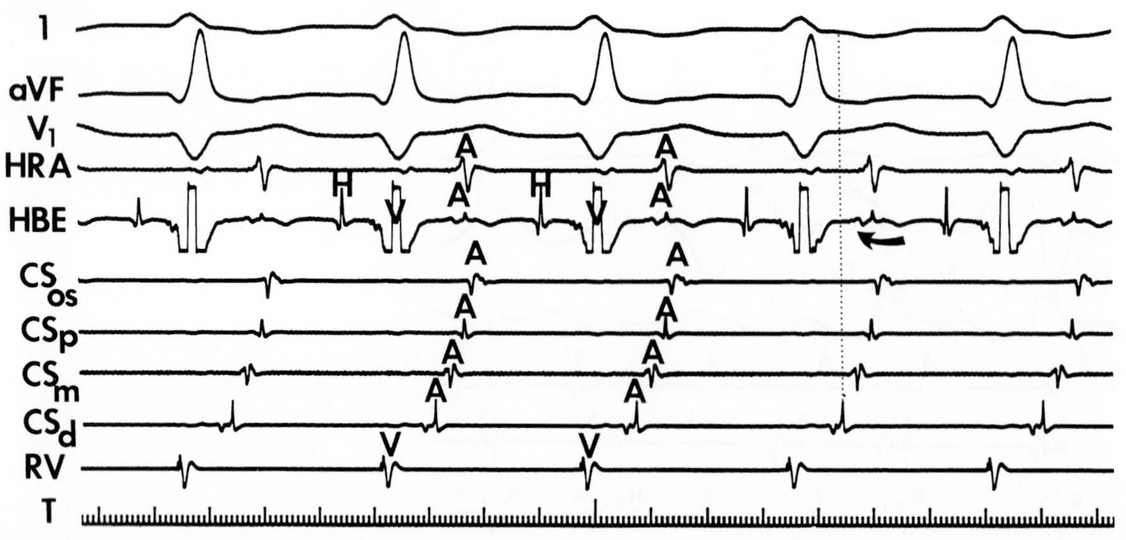


**FIGURE 10-96** *Demonstration of multiple bypass tracts with the presence of two breakthroughs of atrial activation.* Orthodromic tachycardia is present with the earliest retrograde atrial activation seen in the $CS_d$ compatible with a left lateral bypass tract. In the HBE, however, atrial activation occurs earlier than expected (*arrow*), preceding atrial activation from the $CS_{os}$. If activation occurred solely over the left lateral bypass tract, atrial activation in the HBE would follow atrial activation in the $CS_{os}$. The earlier activation at this site suggests two retrograde atrial breakthrough sites and two bypass tracts. See text for discussion.

electrogram not shown) produces a classic paradoxic premature atrial capture (see preceding section entitled Role of the Bypass Tract in Genesis of Arrhythmias). This results in earlier input to the A-V node, producing a prolongation of A-V nodal conduction. The additional A-V nodal conduction delay allows a previously concealed left lateral bypass tract (owing to antegrade concealment by atrial activation produced by conduction over the right-sided bypass tract) to be manifested. The QRS during the tachycardia remains unchanged, but there is a totally different retrograde atrial activation

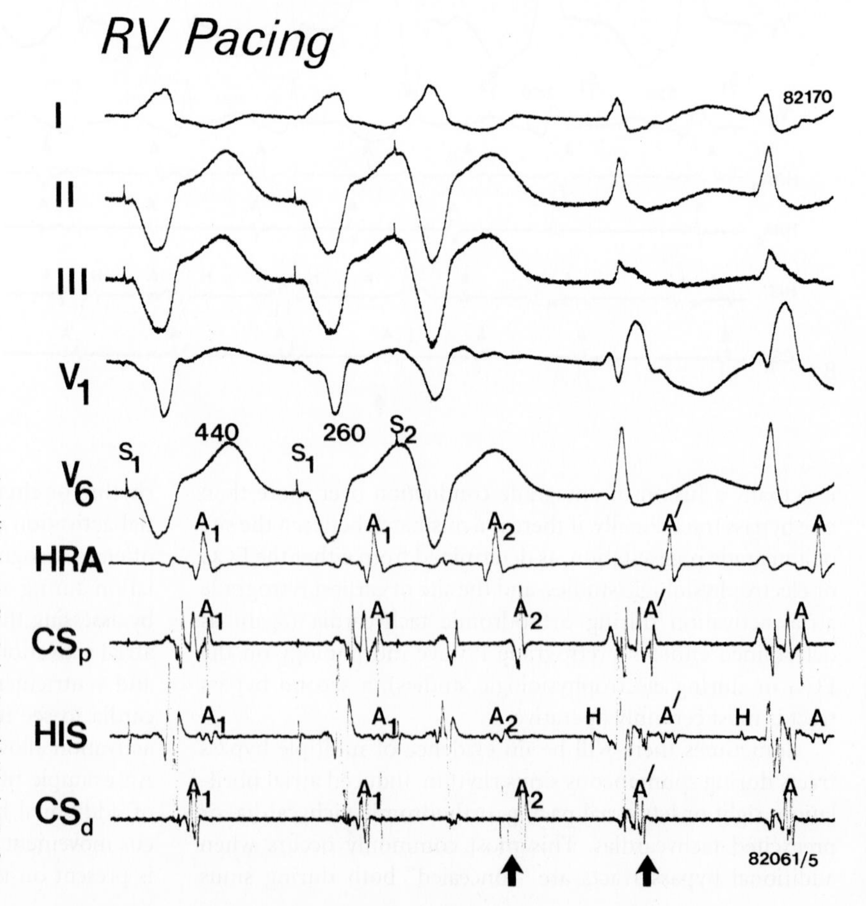


**FIGURE 10-97** *Demonstration of multiple retrograde activation sequences during ventricular stimulation.* During ventricular pacing at a cycle length of 440 msec, a ventricular extrastimulus (S2) is delivered, which initiates SVT. During ventricular pacing, atrial activation in the HRA, $CS_p$, HIS, and $CS_d$ are relatively simultaneous, suggesting a fusion complex. With S2, block occurs in a left-sided bypass tract, manifested by delayed activation of the CS electrogram. Retrograde conduction at this point proceeds over a right-sided bypass tract manifested A2 being earliest in the HRA followed by atrial activation in the HBE and CS. With the induction of orthodromic tachycardia, however, earliest retrograde activation appeared in the $CS_d$ (*second arrow*). The activation sequences suggest two bypass tracts. See text for discussion.

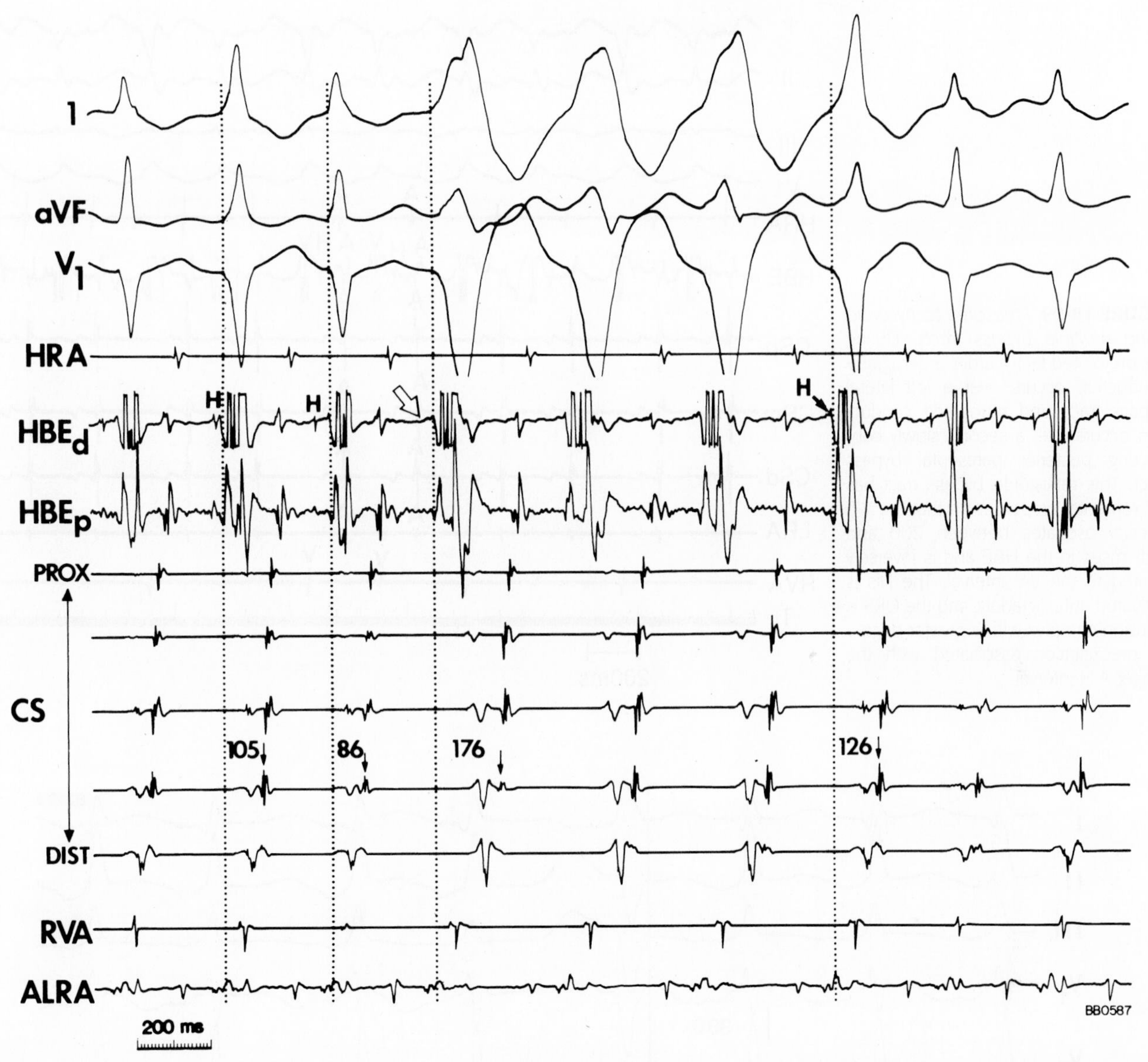


**FIGURE 10-98** *Antegrade fusion during orthodromic tachycardia.* During orthodromic tachycardia using a left lateral bypass tract – earliest activation in more distal pairs of CS electrograms – antegrade activation over a right anterior paraseptal bypass tract is seen. Fusion is seen in the second and seventh complexes, and total preexcitation over the anterior paraseptal bypass tract is seen in the fourth through sixth complexes. Note the difference in V-A intervals associated with different H-V intervals with various degrees of fusion. The change in V-A intervals is due to the relative activation of the ventricles over the bypass tract and the time that the normal conducting system activates the ventricles. See text for discussion.

sequence, with the earliest site of retrograde atrial activation being the left atrium. The V-A interval in the high-right atrial recording, however, remains the same as it did before the VPC on the first and third complexes. The second and fourth complexes show a change in morphology in both the HRA and HIS suggesting atrial fusion. Thus, following the VPC, antegrade conduction proceeds over the normal A-V conducting system, but retrograde atrial activation occurs over both a left- and a right-sided bypass tract. The high incidence of multiple bypass tracts noted in our laboratory (~25%) probably reflects both the care and detail with which we attempt to document the presence of additional bypass tracts as well as a selected patient population.

The presence of multiple bypass tracts has important clinical implications. Patients with multiple bypass tracts have been associated with a higher incidence of ventricular fibrillation according to some investigators, a higher incidence of preexcited tachycardias, and clearly, more complicated anatomy for catheter-based or surgical ablation. Thus, it is imperative that one make every effort to detect their presence during electrophysiologic studies. In the presence of multiple bypass tracts the complexity and number of the potential tachycardia circuits is large (Fig. 10-101). If one considers the fact that a given patient may have more than two A-V bypass tracts (20% of our patients with multiple bypass have three or more tracts), enhanced A-V nodal conduction,

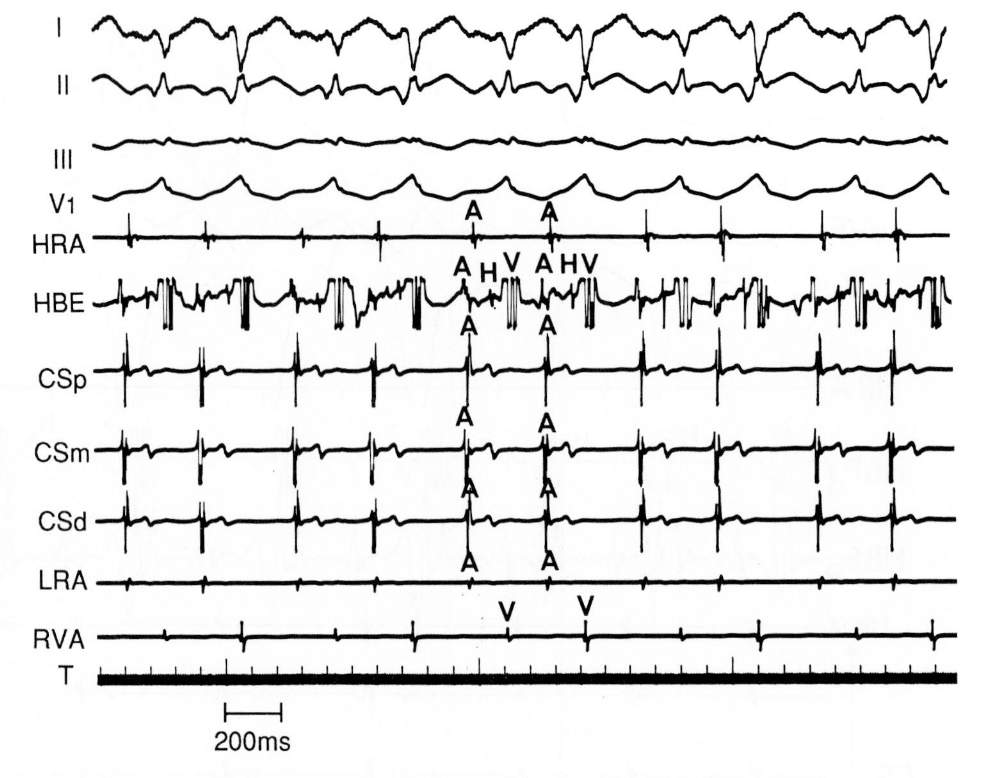


**FIGURE 10-99** *Preexcited tachycardia using multiple bypass tracts.* During the preexcited tachycardia, anterograde conduction occurs over a left lateral bypass tract, and retrograde conduction occurs over a second slowly conducting posterior paraseptal bypass tract. This retrograde bypass tract has decremental properties so that the V-A interval oscillates between 200 and 125 msec in the HBE and is inversely related to the V-V interval. The His is activated anterogradely, and the QRS is a fusion complex with a greater degree of preexcitation associated with the longer A-H interval.

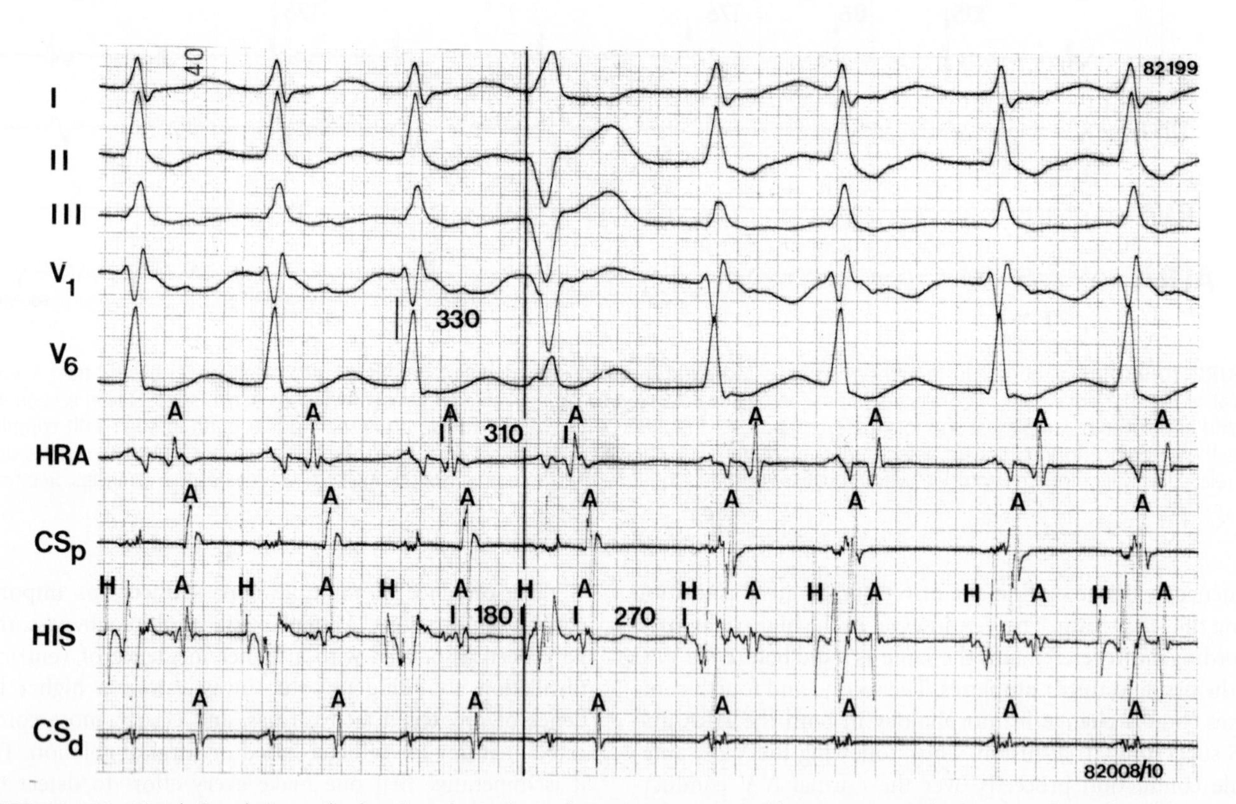


**FIGURE 10-100** *Stimulation during orthodromic tachycardia to demonstrate a second bypass tract.* Orthodromic tachycardia is present with conduction over an anterolateral bypass tract (earliest retrograde atrial activation in the HRA). A ventricular stimulus delivered when the His is refractory preexcites the atrium with a shorter V-A interval than during the first three complexes; thus, producing a paradoxical premature capture. This earlier retrograde atrial activation sequence results in subsequent delay of antegrade conduction through the A-V node. This delay allows for retrograde activation over a left lateral bypass tract to be manifested. This left lateral bypass tract was previously concealed by antegrade penetration into it by atrial activation that initiated over the right anterior bypass tract. Subsequently, orthodromic tachycardia appears to have a retrograde activation sequence over both a left lateral (early activation in $CS_d$) and right anterolateral bypass tract. See text for discussion.

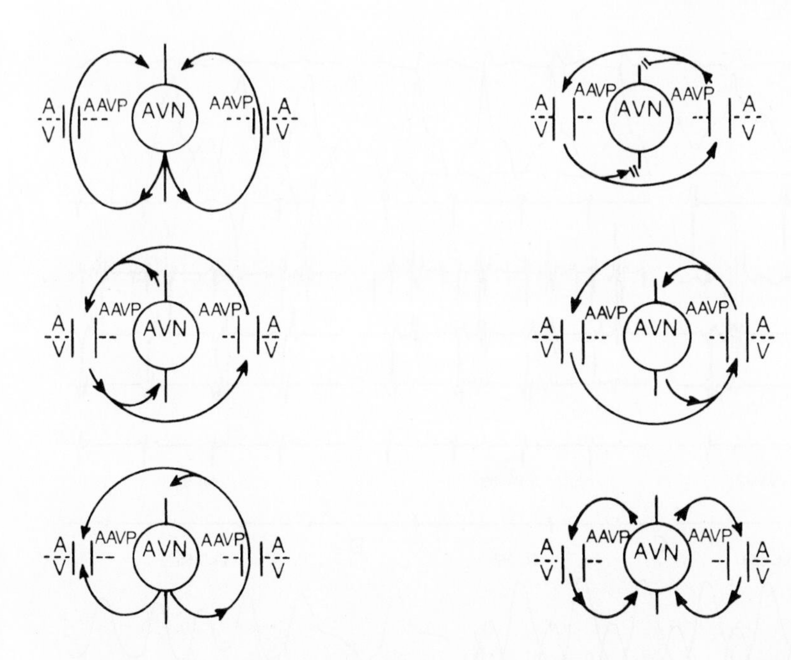


**FIGURE 10-101** *Multiple potential mechanisms of arrhythmias when two bypass tracts are present.* Schematically shown are six potential mechanisms of arrhythmias with two functioning atrioventricular bypass tracts. See text for discussion. AA-VP, accessory A-V pathway.

A-V nodal reentry, and/or other forms of preexcitation, the possibilities of tachyarrhythmias are mind-boggling. In nearly 10% of patients with preexcitation, A-V nodal reentry is present, and in some it is the only arrhythmia (Fig. 10-102). In Figure 10-103 a patient with multiple bypass tracts manifested several different tachyarrhythmias: circus movement tachycardia with a narrow QRS using a posteroseptal bypass tract (noted in normal sinus rhythm); the same orthodromic tachycardia but with antegrade fusion over an anteroseptal bypass tract; circus movement tachycardia with LBBB using

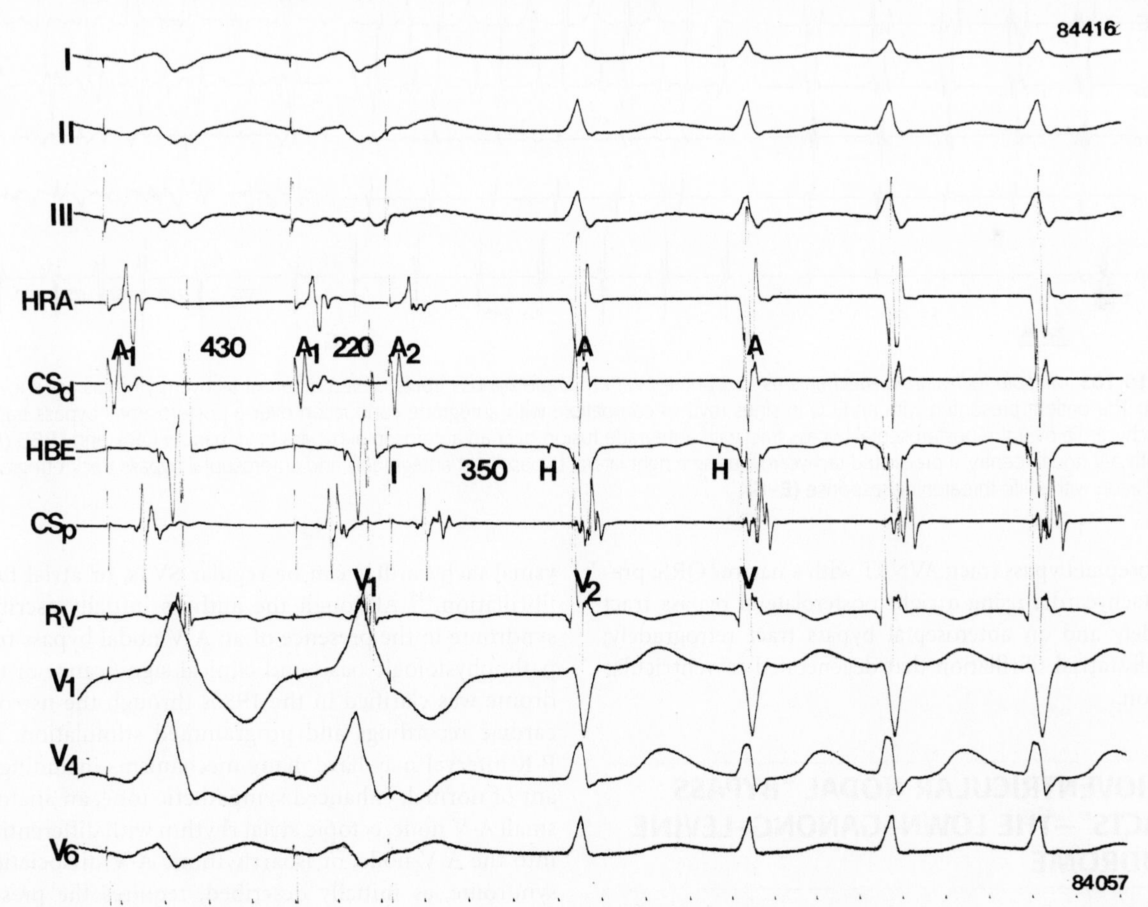


**FIGURE 10-102** *A-V nodal reentry as the mechanism of SVT in a patient with WPW.* ECG leads I, II, III, V1, V4, and V6 are shown with intracardiac recordings from the HRA, coronary sinus distal ($CS_d$) and proximal ($CS_p$), HBE, and RV. During atrial pacing from $CS_d$ preexcitation over a left lateral bypass tract is observed. Atrial extrastimuli only induced typical A-V nodal tachycardia; orthodromic tachycardia was never observed.

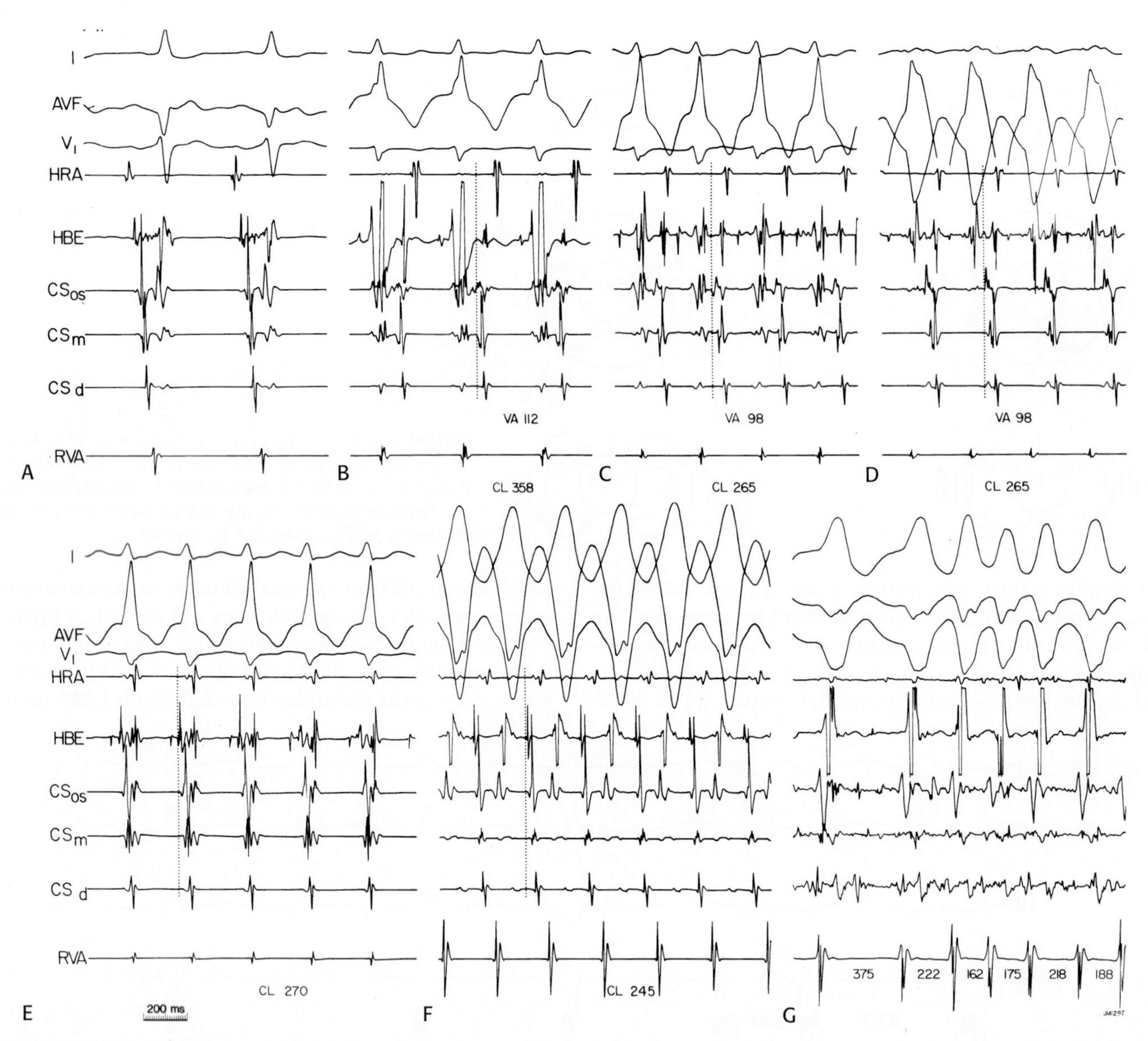


**FIGURE 10-103** *Multiple tachycardia mechanisms in a patient with multiple bypass tracts.* Seven different tachyarrhythmias are shown in this patient. **A:** The patient presented with an ECG in sinus rhythm compatible with antegrade conduction over a posteroseptal bypass tract. Orthodromic tachycardia over the posteroseptal bypass tract with antegrade fusion over an anteroseptal bypass tract, narrow QRS, and LBBB **(B–D)** are shown with A-V nodal reentry, a preexcited tachycardia using a right lateral bypass tract antegradely and anteroseptal bypass tract retrogradely, and atrial fibrillation with a life-threatening response **(E–G)**.

a posteroseptal bypass tract; AVNRT with a narrow QRS; preexcited tachycardia using a right posterolateral bypass tract antegradely and an anteroseptal bypass tract retrogradely; and finally, atrial fibrillation that degenerated to ventricular fibrillation.

## ATRIOVENTRICULAR NODAL "BYPASS TRACTS"—THE LOWN–GANONG–LEVINE SYNDROME

The Lown–Ganong–Levine syndrome is characterized by a short P-R interval, a narrow QRS complex, and a clinical syndrome of recurrent paroxysmal SVTs. These paroxysmal tachycardias can be regular SVTs, or atrial flutter or fibrillation.[135] Although the authors initially ascribed this syndrome to the presence of an A-V nodal bypass tract, the pathophysiologic basis and clinical significance of the syndrome was clarified in the 1980s through the use of intracardiac recordings and programmed stimulation. A short P-R interval may have many mechanisms including a variant of normal, enhanced sympathetic tone, an anatomically small A-V node, ectopic atrial rhythm with differential input into the A-V node, or isoarrhythmic A-V dissociation. The syndrome, as initially described, requires the presence of paroxysmal arrhythmias in addition to the short P-R interval. These arrhythmias give clinical significance to the syndrome. Three anatomic possibilities have been entertained as operative mechanistically. Most investigators believe that enhanced A-V nodal conduction (perhaps using specialized intranodal fibers) is responsible for the majority of cases[13,14,135–140] while a minority are associated with atrio-His connections.[3,5,139–141] In the former case, tachycardias using the A-V node alone or in conjunction with a concealed bypass tract are the most common mechanisms of arrhythmias. In the latter instance, atrial flutter and fibrillation with rapid ventricular responses are the clinical problem. Controversy still exists concerning the functional significance and the anatomic existence of the posterior intranodal tracts described by James,[9] which are the third possibility. Although there is no anatomic correlate of a specialized intranodal pathway, the complex structure of the A-V node, with areas of tightly packed, longitudinally arranged transitional fibers on the periphery of the node, and a lattice network of more loosely connected fibers around densely packed nodal tissue can provide an anatomic substrate for relatively fast and relatively slow conduction.

## Electrophysiologic Properties

The hallmark of patients with the so-called Lown–Ganong–Levine syndrome is enhanced or accelerated A-V conduction, which more than 90% of the time is due to accelerated conduction through the A-V node.[135–141] Thus, most patients with the clinical syndrome usually manifest a short A-H interval (≤60 msec) and normal intra-atrial and His–Purkinje conduction (Fig. 10-104). In the rare case where the A-V node is completely bypassed by an atrio-His connection, insertion of this bypass tract into the distal His bundle results in a short H-V or the absence of a His deflection with a normal QRS (Fig. 10-105).

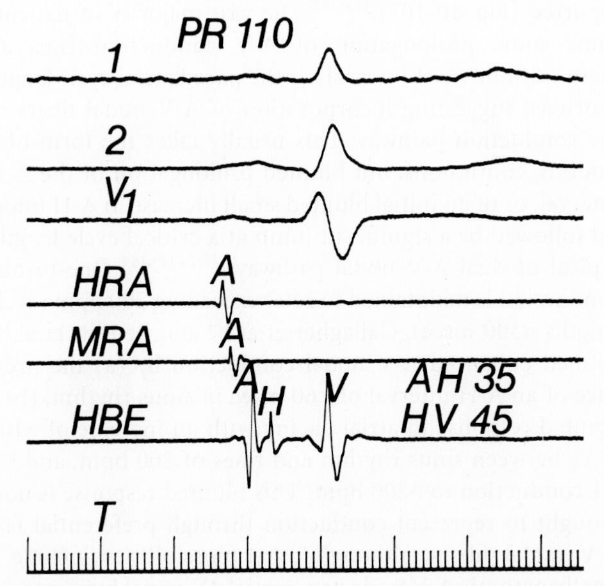


**FIGURE 10-104** *Intracardiac recording in a patient with a short P-R interval.* Typical of patients with short P-R intervals (110 msec), A-V nodal conduction time is short (A-H interval, 35 msec), and the H-V interval is normal (H-V = 45 msec). See text for discussion.

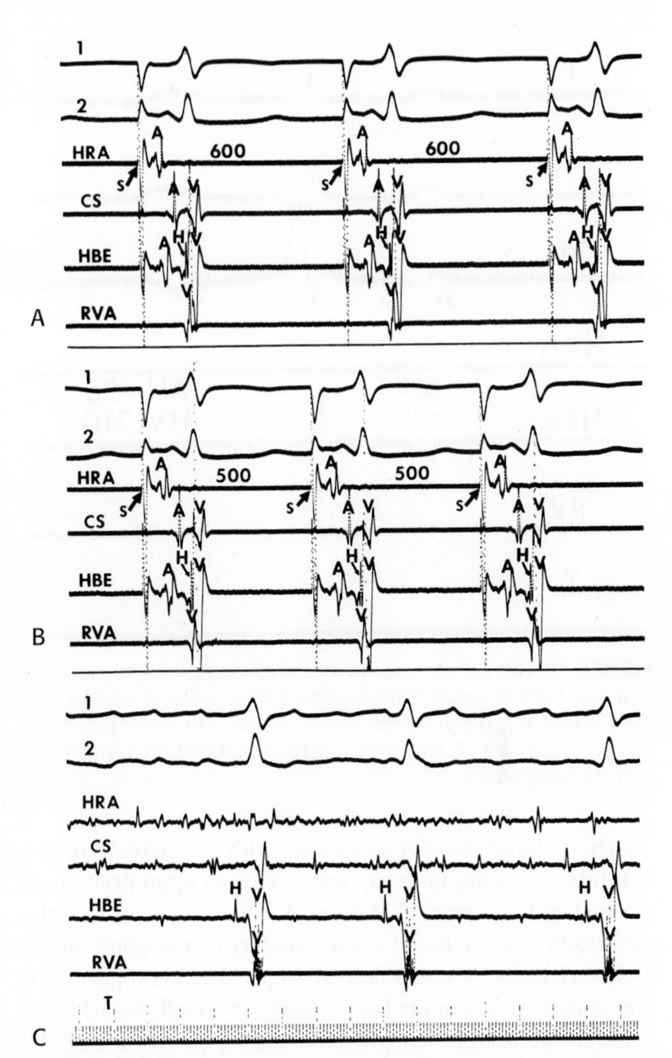


**FIGURE 10-105** *Atrio-His bypass tract inserting below the recording site of the His bundle deflection.* **A** and **B:** Atrial pacing does not affect the P-R interval, which remains fixed at 100 msec. Antegrade His bundle deflection (H) occurs at the beginning of the ventricular electrogram in the HBE because the bypass tract inserts distal to the His bundle recording site. **C:** Proof of that appears during atrial fibrillation in which block in the atrio-His bypass tract occurs and conduction proceeds over the normal pathways. Note that the His bundle deflection during atrial fibrillation is identical to the His bundle potentials shown in A and B and is associated with a normal H-V interval and an identical QRS complex to that observed in A and B.

The His bundle in this instance is retrogradely activated from the site of distal His insertion. The short H-V is due to the difference in conduction time from the site of insertion in the distal His bundle to the ventricle and to the conduction time from the site of insertion in the distal His bundle to the proximal His bundle. One must distinguish this "short H-V" from the recording of a distal right bundle branch potential, an anatomically shortened posterior division, or premature insertion of normal-sized bundle branch to the ventricular muscle. The latter would be a fascicular–ventricular bypass tract and have a slightly preexcited QRS (see subsequent discussion). To do this, one requires the observation of block in the bypass tract,

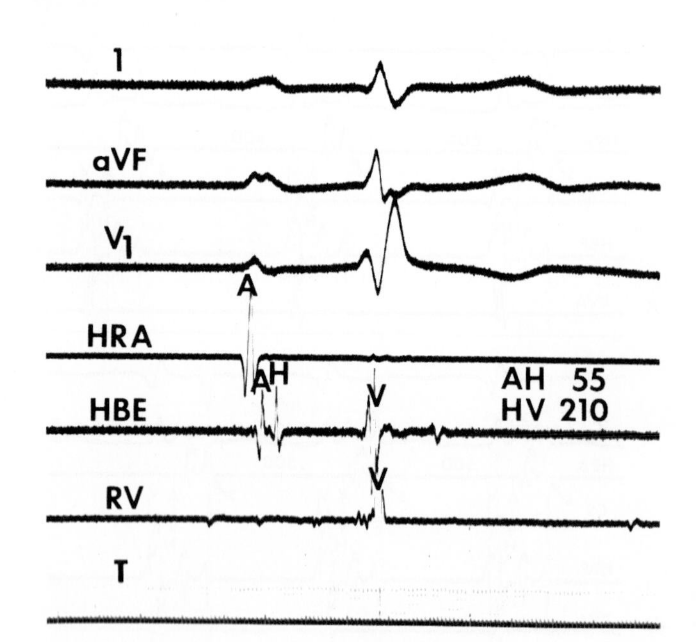


**FIGURE 10-106** *Accelerated A-V nodal conduction in the presence of a long P-R interval and an abnormal QRS complex.* A-V nodal conduction time is short (A-H = 55 msec), despite a markedly prolonged infranodal conduction time (H-V = 210 msec) and a QRS complex demonstrating RBBB.

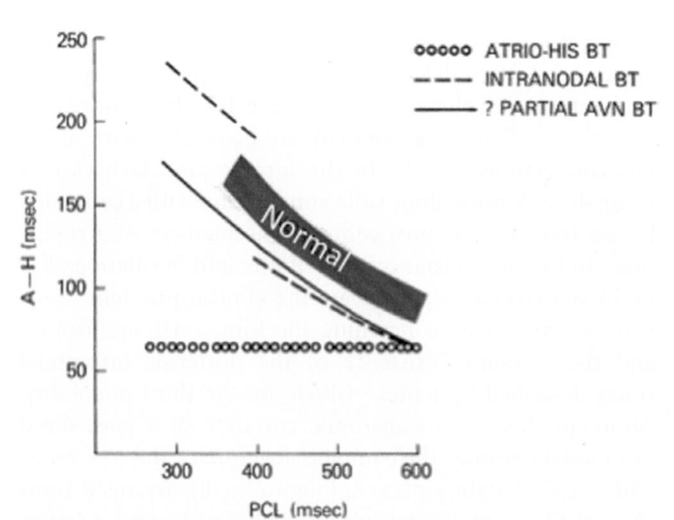


**FIGURE 10-107** *Patterns of A-V nodal conduction in response to atrial pacing in patients with short P-R intervals.* The atrial paced cycle length is shown on the abscissa, and the resultant A-H interval is on the ordinate. The response of patients with normal P-R intervals to atrial pacing is shown by the stippled area. Three patterns of response to atrial pacing are observed in patients with short P-R intervals: (1) no A-V nodal delay, characteristic of an atrio-His bypass tract (*circles*); (2) a dual-pathway response, characteristic of a preferential intranodal pathway (*dashed line*); and (3) a response qualitatively similar to normal but with a lesser degree of A-H prolongation, compatible with a partial A-V nodal bypass tract, a small A-V node, or an extremely rapid intranodal pathway (*solid line*).

which is simultaneously associated with an increase in the P-R interval owing to the appearance of an appropriate A-H interval and a normal H-V interval with maintenance of the same QRS (Fig. 10-105C), and/or absence of a response of the P-R, A-H, and H-V intervals to atrial pacing and programmed stimulation. Block in the bypass tract can usually be achieved through the use of antiarrhythmic agents or occasionally by the induction of atrial fibrillation. Because the essence of this syndrome is enhanced A-V conduction, most commonly A-V nodal conduction, two of the originally proposed criteria, a short P-R interval and a narrow QRS, need not be present. Intra-atrial conduction delays and/or H-V prolongation can produce a normal P-R interval without influencing A-V nodal conduction. In the same vein, the presence of bundle branch block in no way signifies an alteration in A-V nodal conduction. Thus, the P-R interval can be normal or even prolonged with a wide QRS in the presence of enhanced A-V nodal conduction (Fig. 10-106).

It is imperative to identify the mechanism and characteristics of the type of accelerated A-V conduction since the mechanism of enhanced A-V conduction determines the type of the spontaneous arrhythmias. This can be done by analyzing the response of the A-V conducting system to programmed stimulation and/or drug interventions. If accelerated conduction is due to enhanced A-V nodal conduction, patients should respond to such perturbations qualitatively similar to, but perhaps quantitatively less than, the normal A-V node. In contrast, if accelerated A-V conduction is due to an atrio-His bypass tract, responses characteristic of nodal tissue should not be present. The electrophysiologic characteristics of patients with enhanced A-V conduction are discussed in subsequent paragraphs.

## Atrial Pacing

Several types of responses to atrial pacing have been reported (Fig. 10-107).[135–142] The vast majority of patients show some prolongation of A-V conduction (i.e., an increase in the A-H interval) as the paced atrial cycle length shortens, suggesting incorporation of A-V nodal fibers in the conduction pathway. This usually takes the form of a smooth, continuous, but blunted prolongation of the A-H interval, or of an initial blunted small increase in A-H interval followed by a significant jump at a critical cycle length, typical of dual A-V nodal pathways.[13,14,143,144] One-to-one conduction is maintained to rates exceeding 200 bpm (cycle lengths <300 msec). Gallagher et al.[134] and Benditt et al.[136] defined enhanced A-V nodal conduction by (a) the presence of an A-H interval of <60 msec in sinus rhythm, (b) a blunted response to atrial pacing with an increase of <100 msec between sinus rhythm and rates of 200 bpm, and (c) 1:1 conduction to >200 bpm. This blunted response is now thought to represent conduction through preferential fast A-V nodal fibers, although other possibilities include a small anatomic A-V node or a partial AV nodal bypass tract. In patients with such blunted responses, the A-H interval is rarely >200 msec, and in the study by Benditt et al.,[136] the mean A-H during the fastest paced rate of 1:1 conduction was only 153 msec. The shortest cycle length maintaining 1:1 conduction is distinctly shorter in patients with short P-R intervals and SVT than in those with normal P-R intervals and SVT. In our experience, the mean cycle length of 1:1 conduction is approximately 270 msec in patients with short A-H intervals, whereas that in patients with SVT with normal P-R intervals is 325 msec. This is similar to the findings of Benditt et al.,[136] who found a mean cycle length in patients with enhanced A-V conduction to be 268 msec, whereas that in the next group of patients (some with and some without SVT) was 392 msec. These numbers may vary somewhat, depending on patient selection and adrenergic tone in the laboratory. It is of interest, however, that in both groups the maximum A-H before Wenckebach was similar.

In a second type of response, a small increase is followed by a jump in the A-H at a critical paced cycle length with a subsequent gradual increase while maintaining 1:1 conduction at cycle lengths of <300 msec. This is a characteristic of dual A-V nodal pathways. In such patients, the maximum A-H interval can exceed 200 msec, and the maximum increment in A-H interval will exceed 100 msec because conduction at shortest paced cycle lengths during 1:1 conduction is through the slow A-V nodal pathway. We have not found a statistically significant difference in the paced cycle length at which block in the fast pathway occurs in patients with short and normal P-R intervals and A-V nodal reentrant tachycardia, although there is a trend for the fast pathway to block at shorter cycle lengths in patients with short A-H intervals.

In the least common pattern, either minimal or no increase occurs in the A-H interval, even at short paced cycle lengths. Occasionally, 1:1 A-V conduction can be maintained to paced cycle lengths of 200 msec with only a minimally prolonged A-H interval.[141,142] In those patients in whom the A-H and H-V interval both remain fixed and short, an atrio-His bypass tract can be implicated. An atrio-His bypass tract also may be present, even if atrial pacing produces a slight prolongation of the "A-H" interval. In this case, "A-H" prolongation is an artifact of measurement and is due to delay in retrograde conduction from the site of distal insertion in the His to the proximal His bundle recording site and has nothing to do with A-V nodal conduction. In these cases, the His potential may be recorded within the QRS.

The site of atrial pacing can influence the response curves. It is well recognized that pacing from the coronary sinus is associated with shorter A-H intervals and, in 50% of cases, shorter paced cycle lengths to A-V nodal Wenckebach and shorter A-V nodal refractory periods. This suggests a preferential input into the A-V node in this latter group of patients, probably from the left atrial extension of A-V node. One must also exclude the possibility of heightened sympathetic tone as a cause of short A-H intervals and A-V nodal refractoriness. In the presence of high sympathetic tone, extremely rapid rates of 1:1 conduction are possible. As such, patients with enhanced A-V nodal conduction who are in a "high sympathetic state" – such as patients with chronic lung disease on theophylline, patients in whom isoproterenol or atropine are administered, and infants – should not be included in the group of patients who at baseline exhibit these abnormalities of enhanced conduction.

## Response to Atrial Premature Depolarizations

The introduction of progressively premature APDs produces patterns of A-V conduction analogous to those in response to atrial pacing. Most commonly, a smooth increase in the A-H interval or dual A-V nodal pathways is demonstrated. The finding of a dual A-V nodal pathway curve is more common in response to atrial extrastimuli than to pacing, particularly when the drive cycle length is shortened and multiple extrastimuli are used. We have found dual-pathway responses and A-V nodal reentry in all patients with narrow-complex reentrant SVT and short P-R intervals in whom a concealed bypass tract has been excluded (see Chapter 8).[14] Failure of the A-H to prolong in response to atrial extrastimuli corresponds to a flat curve during atrial pacing and most commonly is due to an atrio-His bypass tract (Fig. 10-108). In some instances, little or no change occurs in the A-H interval, but the H-V prolongs and block below the His may be observed. This can occur because His–Purkinje or His bundle refractoriness is encroached on, regardless of whether the mechanism of absence of an A-H response is an atrioproximal His bypass tract or extremely enhanced A-V nodal conduction. If both the A-H and H-V are borderline short, the response to atrial extrastimuli at multiple drive cycle lengths (particularly short drive cycle lengths) can also provide insight into the mechanism of enhanced A-V conduction. Some degree of A-H prolongation in response to APDs introduced during short drive cycle length, without a change in H-V, suggests that the bypass tract either inserts into the A-V node or is composed of A-V nodal tissues (i.e., preferentially rapidly conducting A-V nodal fibers).

The presence of a short A-H and H-V interval that fail to change in response to premature extrastimuli suggests an atrio-His bypass tract. In this instance, at short paced cycle lengths, a bypass tract composed of tissue comparable to atrial or ventricular muscle which has a short baseline refractory period that should further shorten, and therefore should show no prolongation of conduction until very short cycle lengths are used. Thus, at short basic paced cycle lengths (approximately 300 to 400 msec), the H-V interval should remain fixed and short because it is a retrograde His deflection (see preceding discussion), and the A-H interval should remain the same because it is not a linear measurement of A-V nodal conduction.

When one measures the effective refractory period of the A-V node, considerable overlap is seen between patients with normal and short P-R intervals, particularly those with SVT. The effective refractory period of the A-V node is somewhat shorter than that of the population at large, but there is great overlap. There is no significant difference of effective refractory periods

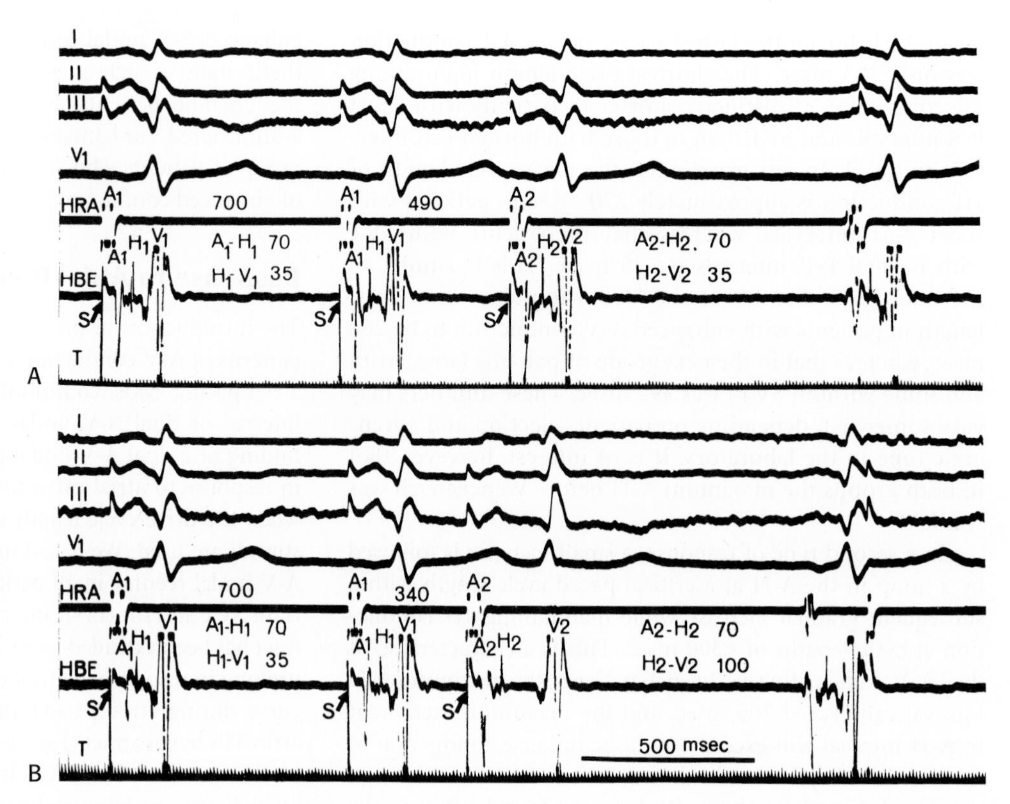


**FIGURE 10-108** *Response to APDs in a patient with an atrio-His bypass tract.* **A:** An APD (A2) at a coupling interval (A1-A2) of 490 msec produces no change in A2-H2 or H2-V2 intervals. **B:** An A1-A2 of 340 msec produces no change in A2-H2 but it markedly prolongs infranodal conduction time (H2-V2 100 msec). The lack of A-V nodal conduction delay is diagnostic p2399 of an atrio-His bypass tract. The A-H intervals of 70 msec are normal, suggesting that the bypass tract inserted in the distal His. See text for discussion.

in patients with SVT regardless of the P-R interval, although those patients having a short P-R interval have a tendency toward slightly shorter effective refractory periods. The functional refractory period, however, is definitely shorter in patients with enhanced A-V nodal conduction than in those with SVT with normal P-R intervals.

## Ventriculoatrial Conduction

Electrophysiologic evaluation of V-A conduction has not been studied in as much detail as antegrade conduction. However, patients with the Lown–Ganong–Levine syndrome can be divided into two groups. Those patients who have had accelerated A-V nodal conduction, with or without dual pathways, have extremely rapid V-A conduction. Two reasons explain this. First, in general the shorter the A-H, the better the retrograde conduction; because these patients by definition have enhanced A-V nodal conduction, rapid V-A conduction is not surprising. Furthermore, this is not surprising in the group of patients who have dual A-V nodal pathways who present with A-V nodal reentrant SVT. As described in Chapter 8, patients with A-V nodal reentry have rapid V-A conduction. It is the ability to conduct rapidly up the fast pathway retrogradely that allows these tachycardias to be initiated and maintained. In such instances the H-A interval remains relatively short with little increase as the ventricular pacing rate is increased. Another group of patients with enhanced A-V conduction who have rapid V-A conduction are those with antegradely concealed but retrogradely conducting bypass tracts. In this case, short and fixed V-A intervals are the rule, as they are with other bypass tracts, and retrograde conduction is often maintained at extremely short ventricular paced cycle lengths (<250 msec). The retrograde His and the A are activated in parallel, and the short H-A intervals seen are related to this phenomenon. The H-A intervals, however, tend to be slightly longer than the H-A intervals with retrograde conduction over a fast A-V nodal pathway, particularly at rather long paced cycle lengths. When ventricular cycle lengths are reduced, however, the H-A interval increases somewhat when retrograde conduction proceeds over an A-V nodal pathway. Then, the H-A interval can exceed the H-A interval in patients with retrograde conduction over concealed bypass tracts, because in the latter group the H-A does not reflect linear conduction but rather fixed conduction through both the His–Purkinje system and the bypass tract. Thus, at paced cycle lengths <300 msec, the H-A intervals in patients with concealed retrograde bypass tracts may be (but by no means universally so) shorter than the H-A intervals in those patients with conduction retrogradely through a fast A-V nodal pathway. The V-A intervals parallel these changes. In fact, the H-A interval in patients using fast A-V nodal pathways is typically shorter than the A-H interval at comparable paced cycle lengths. This is another characteristic typical of patients with dual A-V nodal pathways and A-V nodal reentry (see Chapter 8). In contrast, patients who manifest true atrio-His bypass tracts, as defined previously, have unpredictable V-A conduction. In many cases, we have observed that V-A conduction is absent. Even when present, V-A conduction in these patients is not as good as A-V conduction. Why this should be the case is unclear but certainly is consistent with the fact that these patients do not seem to have reentrant arrhythmias (see following section entitled Role of the Bypass Tract in Arrhythmias).

## Response to Pharmacologic and Physiologic Maneuvers

Patients with enhanced A-V nodal conduction behave differently than those with atrio-His bypass tracts that appear to be physiologically similar to A-V bypass tracts in their response to pharmacologic and physiologic maneuvers. As such, drugs and physiologic maneuvers that profoundly affect A-V nodal conduction without any significant effects on atrial tissue can be used to distinguish the mechanism of enhanced A-V conduction. An increase in the A-V interval in response to drugs such as digoxin, beta-blockers, calcium-blockers, or adenosine suggests that abbreviated A-V conduction is due to enhanced A-V nodal conduction, or if a bypass tract exists, it inserts into the A-V node (Figs. 10-109 and 10-110). An increase in P-R and A-H intervals in response to atrial extrastimuli suggests the same thing. Carotid sinus pressure and other vagal maneuvers may be used in an analogous fashion to demonstrate that conduction through the A-V node is responsible for the genesis of a short P-R. Castellanos et al.[142] demonstrated that carotid sinus pressure can produce A-V Wenckebach block in some patients with short P-R intervals, thereby proving that the accelerated A-V nodal conduction is responsible for the short P-R in those cases.

In patients with atrio-His bypass tracts, block of the bypass tract by pharmacologic agents usually requires the use of Type IA or Type IC agents, or amiodarone. In such cases, block in the bypass tract is associated with immediate prolongation of the A-H and H-V intervals to normal values without a change in QRS. The change differs markedly from that of the prolongation of A-H and H-V intervals that occurs with these agents in patients with enhanced A-V nodal conduction. With atrio-His bypass tracts, both the A-H and H-V intervals prolong suddenly and markedly, because the measured A-H interval during sinus rhythm actually reflects retrograde conduction to the recorded His bundle from the site of insertion of the bypass tract and does not reflect a linear measurement of either A-V nodal or His–Purkinje conduction.

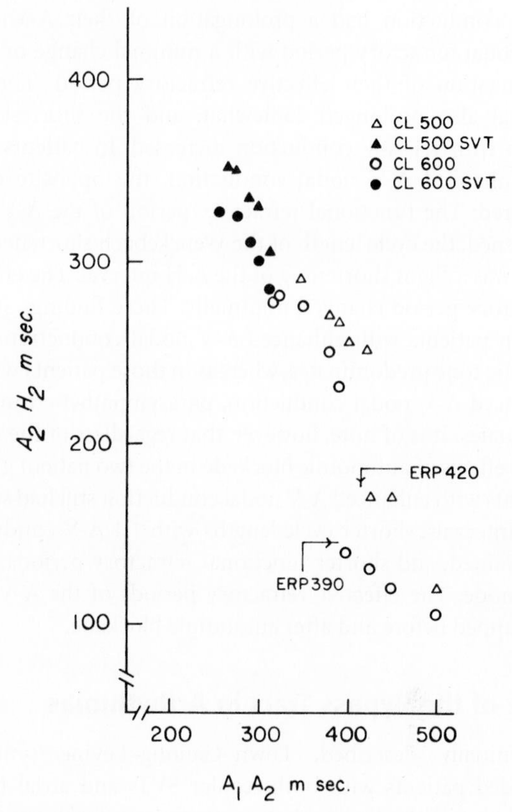


**FIGURE 10-109** *Effect of cycle length on A-V nodal conduction and refractoriness in a patient with an accelerated A-V nodal conduction and SVT.* The coupling interval of APDs (A1-A2) is shown on the abscissa, and the resulting A-H interval (A2-H2) is shown on the ordinate. Data from studies performed at a basic cycle length of 600 msec are shown in *circles,* and those from studies performed at 500 msec are shown in *triangles.* At every A1-A2 interval, the A2-H2 interval is longer at the shorter drive cycle length. The ERP of the "fast" pathway is prolonged by 30 msec (*arrow*) at a drive cycle length of 500 msec. (From Josephson ME, Kastor JA. Supraventricular tachycardia in Lown-Ganong-Levine syndrome: intranodal versus antinodal reentry. *Am J Cardiol* 1977;40:521.)

Benditt et al.[145] evaluated the effects of autonomic blockade in patients with enhanced A-V nodal conduction. They compared these results to a group of patients, with and without SVT, who did not have enhanced A-V nodal conduction. Following autonomic blockade, patients with enhanced A-V

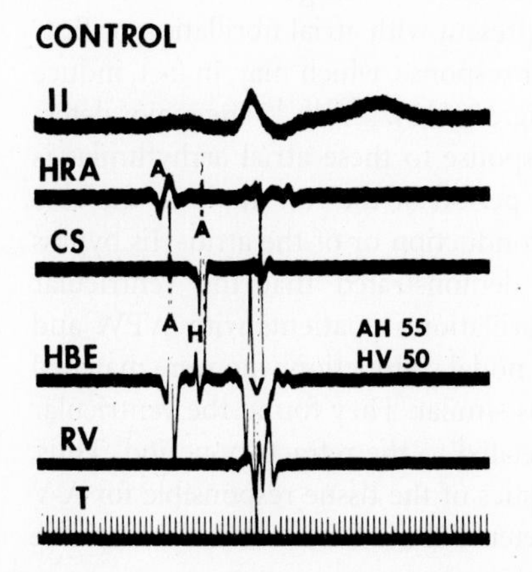


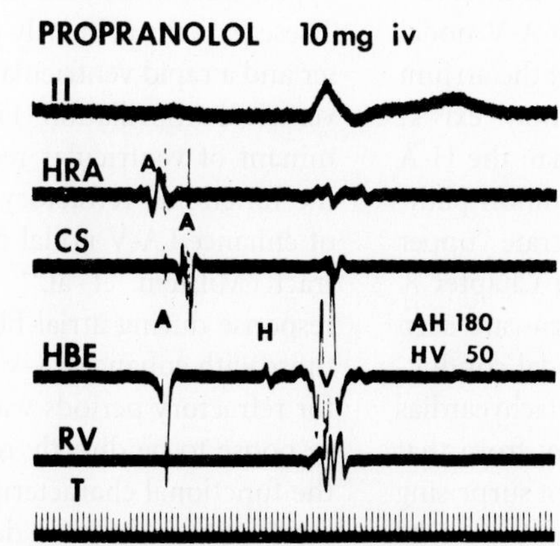


**FIGURE 10-110** *Effect of propranolol in a patient with accelerated A-V nodal conduction.* On the left is a control sinus beat demonstrating an A-H interval of 55 msec. After the administration of propranolol, 10 mg intravenously (IV), the basal A-H interval increased to 180 msec. (From Josephson ME, Kastor JA. Supraventricular tachycardia in Lown-Ganong-Levine syndrome: intranodal versus antinodal reentry. *Am J Cardiol* 1977;40:521.)

nodal conduction had a prolongation of their A-V nodal functional refractory period with a minimal change or slight prolongation of their effective refractory period. The A-H interval also prolonged somewhat, and the shortest cycle length with 1:1 A-V conduction increased. In patients without enhanced A-V nodal conduction, the opposite effects occurred: The functional refractory period of the A-V node shortened, the cycle length of the Wenckebach shortened, and there was a slight shortening of the A-H interval. The effective refractory period changed minimally. These findings suggest that in patients with enhanced A-V nodal conduction, sympathetic tone predominates, whereas in those patients without enhanced A-V nodal conduction, parasympathetic tone predominates. It is of note, however, that regardless of the differential effects of autonomic blockade in the two patient groups, patients with enhanced A-V nodal conduction still had shorter A-H intervals, shorter cycle lengths with 1:1 A-V conduction maintained, and shorter functional refractory periods of the A-V node. The effective refractory periods of the A-V node overlapped before and after autonomic blockade.

## Role of the Bypass Tract in Arrhythmias

As initially described, Lown–Ganong–Levine syndrome included patients with both regular SVTs and atrial flutter-fibrillation.[135] As discussed, there are two predominant groups of patients, based on mechanism of the short P-R interval. In patients in whom the short P-R interval is due to enhanced A-V nodal conduction, with or without dual pathways, the tachycardias that occur spontaneously are usually reentrant SVTs. In our experience, the mechanism of SVT in these patients does not appear to differ significantly from that of patients with normal P-R intervals. This has also been noted by several other investigators.[139,142,143] Thus, patients with dual A-V nodal pathways observed in response to single or multiple atrial extrastimuli, rapid atrial pacing, or ventricular extrastimuli have A-V nodal reentrant SVT. Another large group of patients has concealed A-V bypass tracts. Although the incidence of these two mechanisms may vary depending on patient population, one of these two mechanisms is the most common cause of regular narrow-complex SVTs. These findings are no different from the mechanisms of SVT in patients with normal P-R intervals (see Chapter 8). In patients with short P-R intervals and A-V nodal reentrant SVT, no evidence for an A-V nodal bypass tract exists. Thus, one can demonstrate that the atrium is not necessary (i.e., an "upper final common pathway" exists) and that the H-A during tachycardia is shorter than the H-A during ventricular pacing (i.e., a "lower final common pathway" exists). Details of studies that can demonstrate "upper and lower final common pathways" are given in Chapter 8. Heterogeneous retrograde atrial activation patterns are seen in these patients as in those with normal A-V nodal conduction.[92,93] The cycle length of A-V nodal reentrant tachycardias in patients with short P-R intervals is no different from that in patients with normal P-R intervals.[146] This is not surprising because the major determinant of cycle length of A-V nodal reentry is conduction down the slow pathway. In our experience, the slow-pathway conduction times and refractoriness in patients with normal and short P-R intervals are indistinguishable. On the other hand, the fast pathway in such patients is faster than in patients with normal P-R intervals; the A-Hs are shorter in sinus rhythm, and capability for retrograde conduction over the fast pathway is greater. This had led us and others[143] to suggest that patients with the Lown–Ganong–Levine syndrome and A-V nodal reentry are merely one end of the bell-shaped curve of patients with A-V nodal reentrant SVT. It is perhaps because the fast pathway is capable of such excellent retrograde conduction that such patients more commonly have SVT, which brings them to our attention. This makes sense since retrograde fast pathway conduction is the prime determinant for developing AV nodal reentry. Thus, the Lown–Ganong–Levine syndrome may merely reflect a bias caused by the characteristics of the fast pathway.

The bulk of evidence suggests that the fast pathway is composed of A-V nodal tissue but has more rapid conduction and shorter refractory periods.[14,136] The fast A-V nodal pathway in these patients demonstrates an inverse relationship of conduction and refractoriness to cycle length and response to drugs such as propranolol, verapamil, adenosine, and digoxin in a manner qualitatively similar to normal A-V nodal tissue. Thus, these patients appear to represent just one part of the spectrum of patients with A-V nodal reentry and normal P-R intervals. In contrast, the cycle length of tachycardias using concealed bypass tracts tends to be much shorter in patients with short P-R intervals than in patients with normal P-R intervals. This is not surprising because in patients with concealed bypass tracts antegrade conduction proceeds over the rapidly conducting A-V node, thereby abbreviating that limb of the reentrant circuit. In fact, enhanced A-V nodal conduction and reciprocating tachycardia using concealed bypass tracts should be considered in any individual with paroxysmal reciprocating tachycardias having cycle lengths ≤250 msec. In such patients, enhanced A-V nodal conduction makes aberration common, resulting in a high incidence of SVT with wide QRS complexes.

Patients with short P-R intervals that are due to either enhanced A-V nodal conduction or atrio-His bypass tracts may exhibit atrial flutter or fibrillation with a rapid ventricular response. We have never seen any patient with an atrio-His bypass tract who had a reentrant SVT using the AVJ as one limb. These patients primarily present with atrial fibrillation or flutter and a rapid ventricular response, which may, in fact, induce ventricular fibrillation (Fig. 10-111).[3,139,141,142] The major determinant of ventricular response to these atrial arrhythmias is the functional refractory period of the A-V node in the case of enhanced A-V nodal conduction or of the atrio-His bypass tract. Milstein et al.[147] demonstrated that the ventricular response during atrial fibrillation in patients with WPW and those with enhanced A-V nodal conduction who were matched for refractory periods was similar. They found the ventricular response to be directly related to the refractory period. Thus, the functional characteristics of the tissue responsible for A-V conduction is the main determinant of the ventricular response

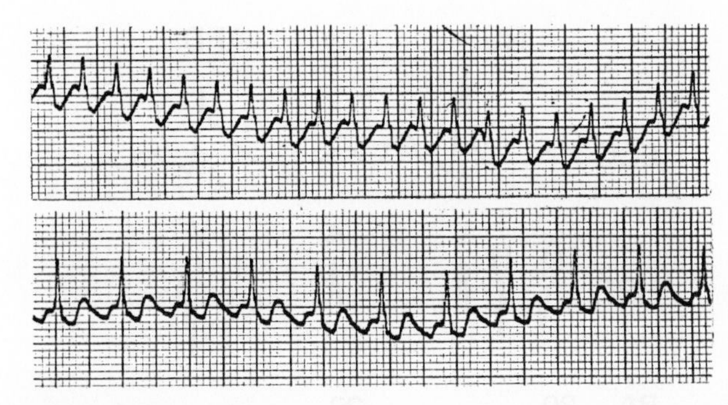

**FIGURE 10-111** *Atrial flutter with 1:1 conduction in a patient with atrio-His bypass tract.* **A:** Atrial flutter with 1:1 A-V conduction is present in a patient with an atrio-His bypass tract. **B:** 200 mg of lidocaine produced block in the bypass tract, resulting in 2:1 conduction down the normal pathway.

during atrial flutter or fibrillation, not the site of insertion of that tissue. Of note, in the group of patients with enhanced A-V nodal conduction who demonstrate dual A-V nodal pathways, the ventricular response is slower. This is a result of the fact that block in the fast pathway frequently occurs with conduction over the slow pathway and repetitive concealment into the fast pathway once conduction proceeds over the slow pathway.

### Therapeutic Implications

As with other types of recurrent SVT, therapy should be individualized. Because most of the reciprocating tachycardias are due to A-V nodal reentry or reentry using a concealed A-V bypass tract, treatment should be the same as that for patients with normal P-R intervals with these arrhythmias. Thus, in patients with SVT due to A-V nodal reentry or concealed A-V bypass tracts, although drugs may be useful, the potential cure by catheter ablation may be a reasonable choice of therapy for patients with recurrent symptoms. With the development of deflectable catheters and increased experience, radiofrequency ablation is the therapy of choice for most patients (see Chapter 14). Patients with atrio-His bypass tracts and atrial flutter and fibrillation with rapid ventricular responses require treatment with drugs that can suppress these bypass tracts and/or prevent the arrhythmia. These include Class I and 3 antiarrhythmic agents or amiodarone. In the case of atrial flutter (either as a primary arrhythmia or one created from atrial fibrillation by drugs) catheter ablation of flutter is possible and is highly successful (see Chapters 9 and 14). If these efforts are not successful, ablation of the AVJ may be considered. Catheter-delivered radiofrequency energy is the current method of choice to create A-V block (see Chapter 14).

## ACCESSORY PATHWAYS WITH ANTEROGRADE DECREMENTAL CONDUCTION AND FASCICULOVENTRICULAR PATHWAYS

At the beginning of this chapter, we assigned all the variants of preexcitation syndromes pathophysiologic names as opposed to the eponyms formerly applied. Thus, fibers initially considered under the rubric "Mahaim" fibers are now recognized as atriofascicular, nodofascicular, nodoventricular, and fasciculoventricular bypass tracts. Nodoventricular bypass tracts were initially described by Mahaim and Benatt in 1937 as conducting tissue extending from the A-V node to the ventricular myocardium.[148] Pathologically, fibers have been described from the node to the ventricle and from the fascicle to the ventricle, usually in or adjacent to the septum. Subsequently it was recognized that bypass tracts can arise in the A-V node and insert in the right bundle branch.[15,17–19] Such antegradely conducting nodofascicular fibers are clinically believed to be more common clinically than fibers from the A-V node inserting directly into the ventricle, but both are **extremely** rare. Concealed nodoventricular bypass tracts (i.e., retrograde conduction only) are more common than concealed nodofascicular pathways in my experience (see Chapter 8). Eventually it became clear that the majority of what were assumed to be antegradely conducting nodoventricular and nodofascicular bypass tracts were actually slowly conducting atrioventricular or atriofascicular bypass tracts.[18,20–22,48,49,148–150] All atriofascicular bypass tracts and all but three slowly conducting atrioventricular bypass tracts I have studied have inserted either into the right ventricle or right bundle branch. These may be difficult to distinguish from bypass tracts arising in the node from the surface ECG, but are readily distinguishable during electrophysiology study. In general if the ventricular insertion of these bypass tracts is in the ventricular myocardium, particularly, near the tricuspid annulus, they will tend to have relatively broader r waves in leads V2-V4 with slurring of the downstroke of the S wave. If they insert in or adjacent to the RBB, the QRS looks like typical LBBB, with small or no r wave in V1-V4 and a rapid downstroke. Although several types of arrhythmias have been described in patients with slowly conducting atrioventricular, nodoventricular, nodofascicular bypass tracts, and atriofascicular bypass tracts, fasciculoventricular bypass tracts have not been implicated in any reentrant arrhythmia.[15–19] The arrhythmias with which these fibers are associated are listed in Table 10-10. Importantly, any of these bypass tracts can act as either participants (with the exception of fasciculoventricular) or bystanders in reentrant arrhythmias. These arrhythmias, which appear electrocardiographically as wide-complex tachycardias with an LBBB morphology, may have A-V dissociation and therefore may be difficult to distinguish from some ventricular tachycardias. The electrophysiologic studies are critical to establishing the pathophysiologic substrate of these individual fibers and the mechanisms of the arrhythmias with which they are associated.

### Slowly Conducting Accessory Pathways

Anterograde decrementally conducting accessory pathways are not as uncommon as previously thought. In our experience, <3% of patients referred to us for ventricular preexcitation have such a pathway. A slightly higher percentage (6%) of

**TABLE 10-10 Tachycardias Using Decremental ("Mahaim") Fibers**

1. Nodofascicular or atriofascicular bypass tract
   a. A-V nodal reentry with innocent bystander bypass tract
   b. atriofascicular or nodofascicular nodal reentry
   c. atriofascicular or nodofascicular ventricular nodal reentry
   d. atriofascicular or nodofascicular—concealed AP reentry
2. Slowly conducting or nodoventricular A-V bypass tract
   a. A-V nodal reentry with innocent bystander bypass tract
   b. Antidromic tachycardia over a slowly conducting A-V bypass tract or nodoventricular-nodal reentry
   c. Preexcited tachycardia over a slowly conducting A-V bypass tract and retrograde conduction over a concealed BT
3. Fasciculoventricular bypass tract (no reentrant tachycardias)

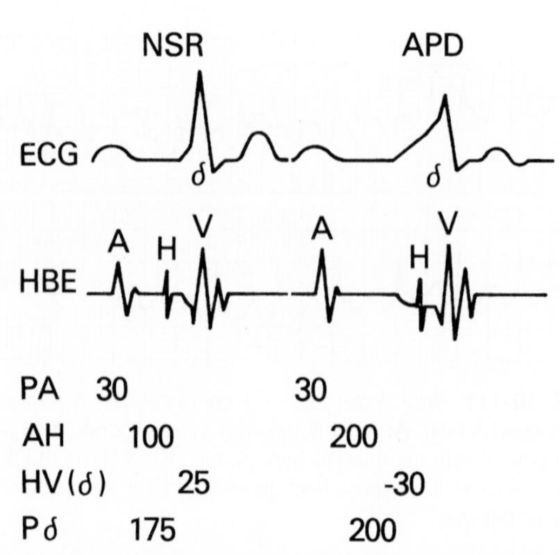


**FIGURE 10-112** *Electrophysiologic behavior of a decrementally conducting bypass tract.* During sinus rhythm (**left**), the degree of preexcitation depends on the relative conduction time down the decrementally conducting bypass tract and conduction time down the normal conducting system below the "takeoff" of the bypass tract. An APD (**right**) results in a greater degree of preexcitation owing to the production of an A-V nodal conduction delay below the site of the bypass tract. The increase in P-delta interval is due to conduction delay above the site of the takeoff.

patients presenting with SVT with an LBBB morphology have an atriofascicular, atrioventricular, or, very rarely, a nodofascicular bypass tract. It is not uncommon for these decrementally conducting accessory pathways to be associated with typical, rapidly conducting A-V accessory connections.[17–19,151] This is not surprising because both appear to represent congenital cardiac abnormalities. Ebstein's anomaly is the most common associated congenital heart lesion, as it is with typical A-V bypass tracts.[19]

## Electrophysiologic Manifestations

Electrocardiographic and electrophysiologic characteristics of decrementally conducting bypass tracts depend on the sites of insertion: either the atrium or the A-V node and the site of insertion in the ventricle. Those pathways that arise in the atrium more closely resemble a typical A-V bypass tract. Thus SVT with A-V dissociation excludes either an atriofascicular or slowly conducting atrioventricular bypass tract and suggests that the bypass tract arises from the A-V node. Both atriofascicular and slowly conducting atrioventricular pathways demonstrate greater preexcitation when atrial stimulation is performed closer to the bypass tract, whereas the degree of preexcitation observed over bypass tracts that arise from the A-V node is not influenced by the site of atrial stimulation. The conduction velocity down the bypass tract is an additional critical determinant of the degree of preexcitation. If the conduction time over the bypass tract to the ventricle (by whatever route) approximates that of the normal conduction system, little or no preexcitation may be present in the basal state (Fig. 10-112). Any perturbation – such as changing autonomic tone, or electrical or pharmacologic maneuvers that prolong conduction to the ventricles over the normal A-V normal conducting system (primarily the A-V node) to a greater degree than in the slowly conducting accessory pathway – will increase the degree of preexcitation. Since all of these accessory pathways exhibit decremental conduction, the P-delta (or P-R) will increase in response to atrial pacing.

Electrophysiologic studies are critical to document the presence and type of these slowly conducting accessory pathways and their participation in clinical arrhythmias. During sinus rhythm, the intra-atrial and A-H interval are usually normal. The H-V interval may be normal or decreased, depending on whether any evidence of preexcitation exists. Normalization of the H-V by His bundle pacing proves that the takeoff is from the node or the atrium and excludes a fasciculoventricular pathway (see below). Electrophysiologic studies have demonstrated that the vast majority (probably greater than 90%) of these decrementally conducting accessory pathways are atriofascicular or long atrioventricular pathways. Slowly conducting short atrioventricular pathways are a distant second with pathways arising in the A-V node being least common. Sites of 34 atriofascicular or long atrioventricular and 9 short atrioventricular pathways that I have studied are shown in Figure 10-110.

## Atriofascicular and Long Atrioventricular Bypass Tracts

As shown in Figure 10-113, atriofascicular and/or long atrioventricular pathways have their atrial insertion at the free wall of the right atrium. This location has been consistent in all studies.[22,48,49,149,150] Pathologic studies have demonstrated that the tissue is structurally similar to the normal AVJ with a node-like structure leading to a His-like structure.[21,22] This structure physiologically can be traced along the free wall of the right ventricle to the region where the moderator band and RBB usually inserts (see below). Insertion in more proximal

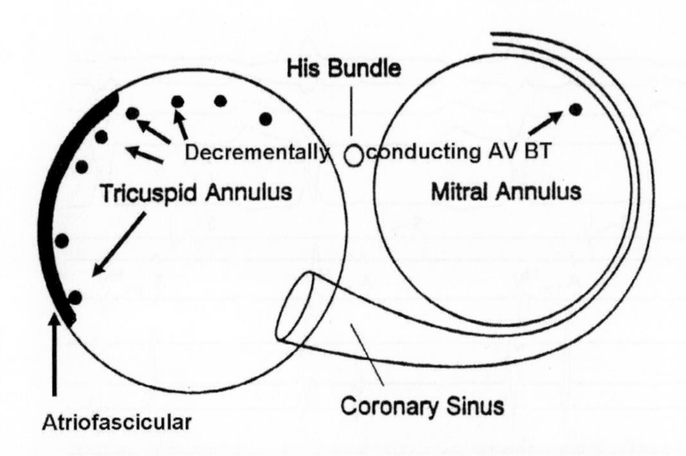


**FIGURE 10-113** *Sites of decrementally conducting atriofascicular and long and short atrioventricular accessory pathways.* Decrementally conducting atriofascicular and long atrioventricular pathways are located along the anterior and lateral free wall of the right ventricle (*solid line,* 35 patients). Short atrioventricular pathways are more variably located (*dots,* 12 at the right free wall and 3 at a left lateral site).

portions of the RBB (e.g., septal base of the moderator band) is likely in cases with a very short or slightly negative V-H during maximal preexcitation (e.g., V-H ≤10 msec). Changes in autonomic tone (Fig. 10-114) and atrial stimulation can increase the degree of preexcitation by slowing conduction in the A-V node. In the baseline state minimal or no preexcitation may be present; thus, the H-V interval may be normal (~60%) or short. Atrial pacing typically produces an expected prolongation of the A-H interval. Even a "normal" H-V may be shorter in the apparent absence of preexcitation. Subtle preexcitation may be suspected by absence of normal septal forces in leads 1, aVL, and V5-V6, which is a clue that minimal preexcitation is present. Recently Sternick et al.[152] have noted that an rS in lead 3, particularly when associated with absence of a septal Q in lead 1 predicted the presence of an atriofascicular pathway. During atrial pacing or atrial extrastimuli as the A-H interval prolongs, the QRS morphology gradually shifts progressively to a more preexcited LBBB morphology. The A-H interval will show a greater degree of prolongation than the A-V interval regardless of the morphology. The H-V interval decreases as the His deflection becomes progressively displaced into the QRS (Figs. 10-115 to 10-117). In the majority of cases the His will be inscribed 5 to 25 msec after the QRS (Figs. 10-115 and 10-116), and in a minority it is buried in the QRS (Fig. 10-117). When the His deflection is lost within the QRS, it is unclear whether or not conduction continues to proceed over the His bundle or whether block has occurred. In our experience, this occurs in <15% of patients. At the point of maximal preexcitation, the His–QRS relationship remains unaltered (resulting in a constant A-H and a short V-H interval) until block in the accessory pathway occurs (Fig. 10-118). The fixed V-H interval, despite shorter atrial paced cycle lengths and/or coupling intervals (Fig. 10-119), suggests the bypass tract inserts into or near the distal right bundle branch at the anterior free wall of the right ventricle with retrograde conduction to the His bundle. In my opinion, whenever the V-H is <20 msec insertion into the right bundle branch is likely. If the insertion were in the ventricle, the V-H would approximate the H-V minus the duration of the His (since it is activated retrogradely), plus the difference in the LBB-V and RBB-V, since conduction time over the LBB is normally shorter than over the RBB. Long atrioventricular bypass tracts inserting near the right bundle branch have been described by Haissaguerre et al.[20] During atrial pacing these fibers are associated with longer V-H intervals (mean 38 msec) and have a longer conduction time to the distal right bundle branch (V-RBB) than true atriofascicular tracts (25 vs. 3 msec). In my experience and that of others, most of these long fibers are consistent with slowly conducting atriofascicular tracts.[18,20–22,48,49,149,150,153]

Careful mapping of the tricuspid annulus and the anterior free wall of the right ventricle has demonstrated discrete potentials with complexes comparable to those recorded

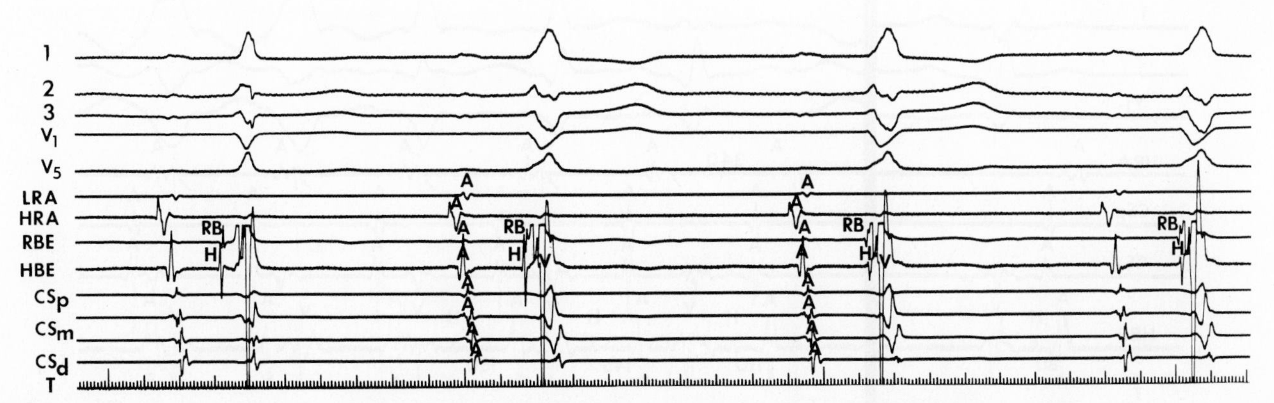


**FIGURE 10-114** *Spontaneous shifts in conduction over an atriofascicular bypass tract.* Four sinus complexes are shown. The first is a normal sinus complex with no evidence of conduction over the atriofascicular tract. Note the His bundle potential precedes right bundle potential. The second complex shows a slight change in the QRS, but the right bundle and the His bundle are activated nearly simultaneously with a shortened H-V interval. In the third and fourth complexes, conduction over the atriofascicular tract is present, and there is a reversal of activation sequences, with the right bundle potential occurring before the His bundle potential. This suggests that the atriofascicular bypass tract inserts into the right bundle branch and conducts retrogradely to the His bundle. See text for discussion. RBE, right bundle electrogram.

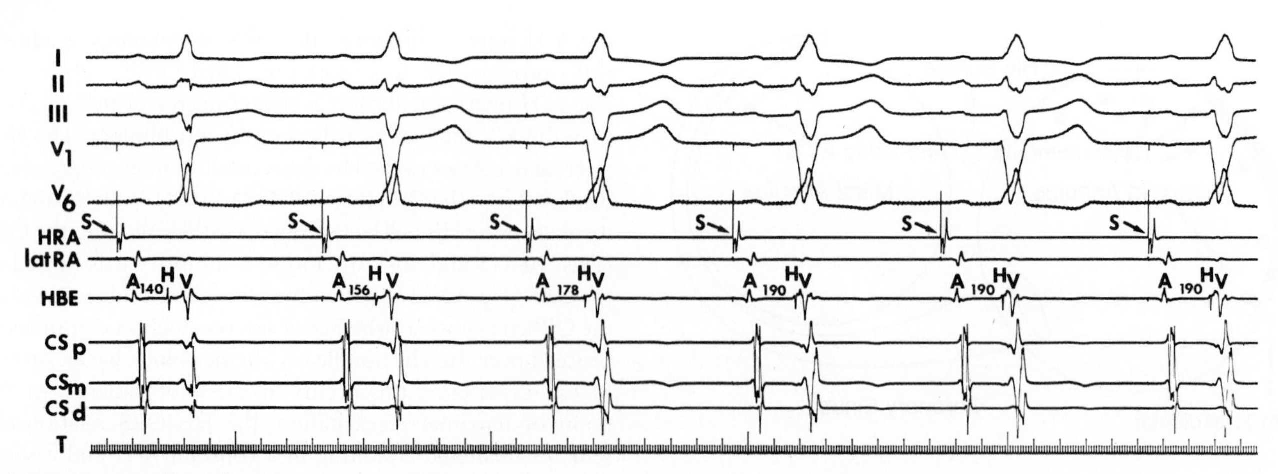


**FIGURE 10-115** *Effect of atrial pacing on atriofascicular bypass tract.* Atrial pacing at a cycle length of 800 msec produces the progressive development of preexcitation over an atriofascicular bypass tract. As preexcitation occurs, the A-H lengthens and the H-V shortens. Beginning with the fourth paced impulse, the A-H remains fixed with the His deflection shortly following the onset of the QRS. A fixed A-H with a short, retrograde V-H during atrial pacing is characteristic of an atriofascicular bypass tract.

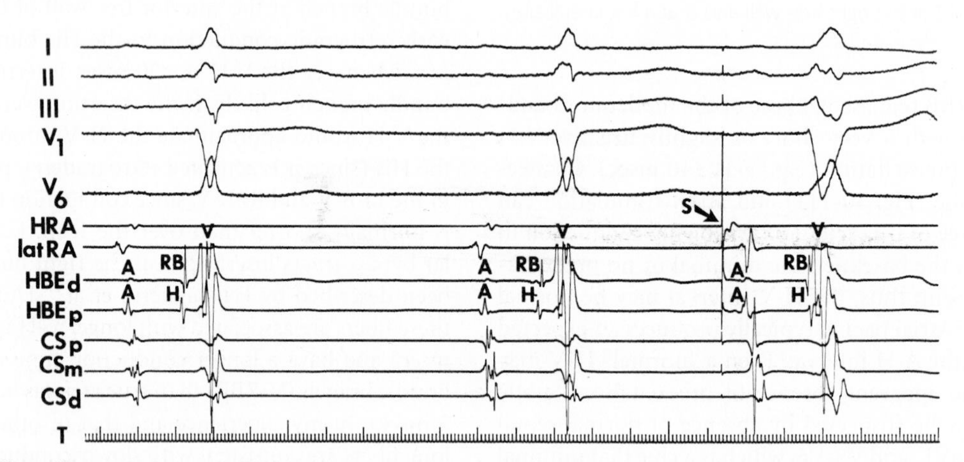


**FIGURE 10-116** *Effect of an APD on preexcitation over an atriofascicular bypass tract.* The first two complexes are sinus with the normal A-H and H-V intervals. Note that the His deflection precedes the right bundle deflection. Following the second sinus complex, an APD is delivered from the HRA. This results in manifest preexcitation with reversal of the RB and His potentials so that the RB is activated 20 msec before the His bundle. This suggests that the bypass tract inserts in the RB and conducts retrogradely to the His bundle.

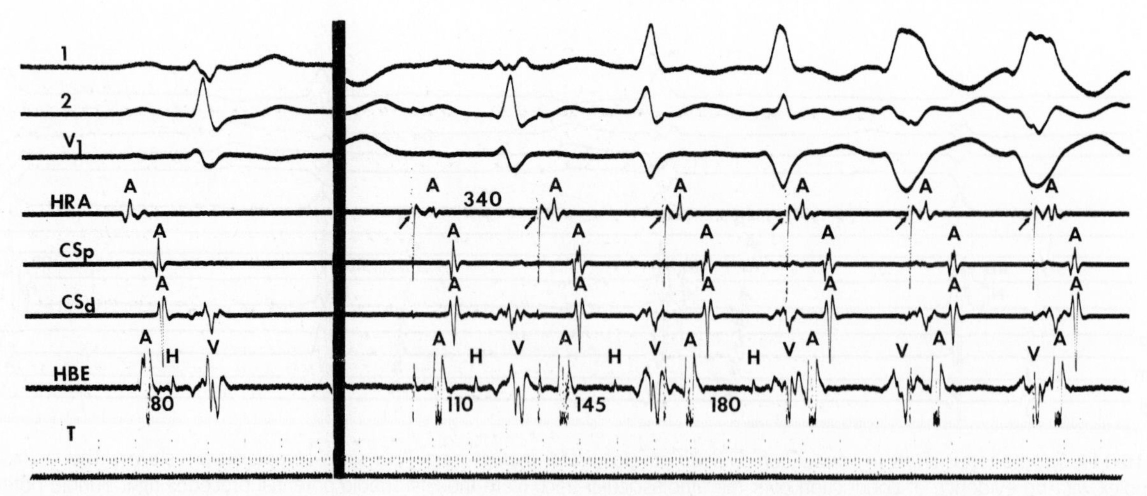


**FIGURE 10-117** *Effect of atrial pacing in a patient with a decrementally conducting atrioventricular ventricular bypass tract.* The sinus complex shown on the left gives no evidence of preexcitation. In the sinus complex shown on the right, during atrial pacing at a cycle length of 340 msec, as the A-H interval increases, there is a gradual change to an LBBB configuration, the degree of which depends on the amount of A-V nodal delay. The maximum change in QRS morphology appears as the antegrade His bundle deflection becomes cast within the QRS. See text for details.

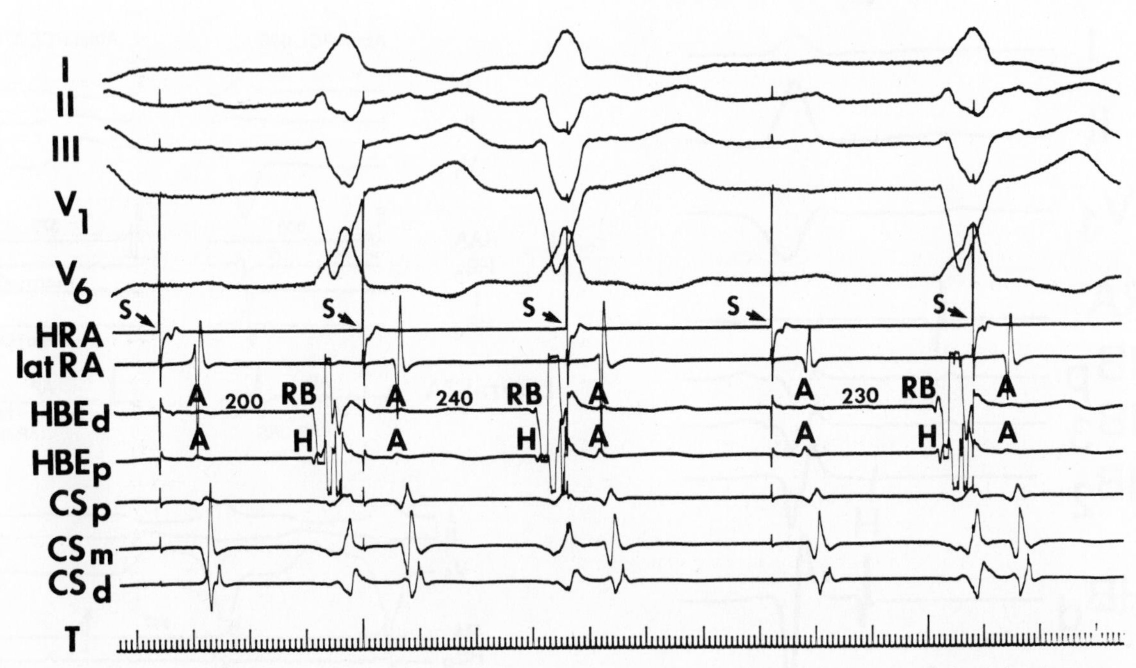


**FIGURE 10-118** *Atrial pacing producing A-V Wenckebach in a patient with an atriofascicular bypass tract.* Pacing from the HRA at a cycle length of 360 msec is associated with progressive prolongation of the P-R and A-H intervals and block in the A-V node. Note that the RB precedes the His during all conducted complexes. And the V-H remains fixed. This suggests that during conducted beats, antegrade conduction goes through an atriofascicular bypass tract, which enters the RB and captures the His retrogradely. A-V Wenckebach occurs in the atriofascicular bypass tract. See text for discussion.

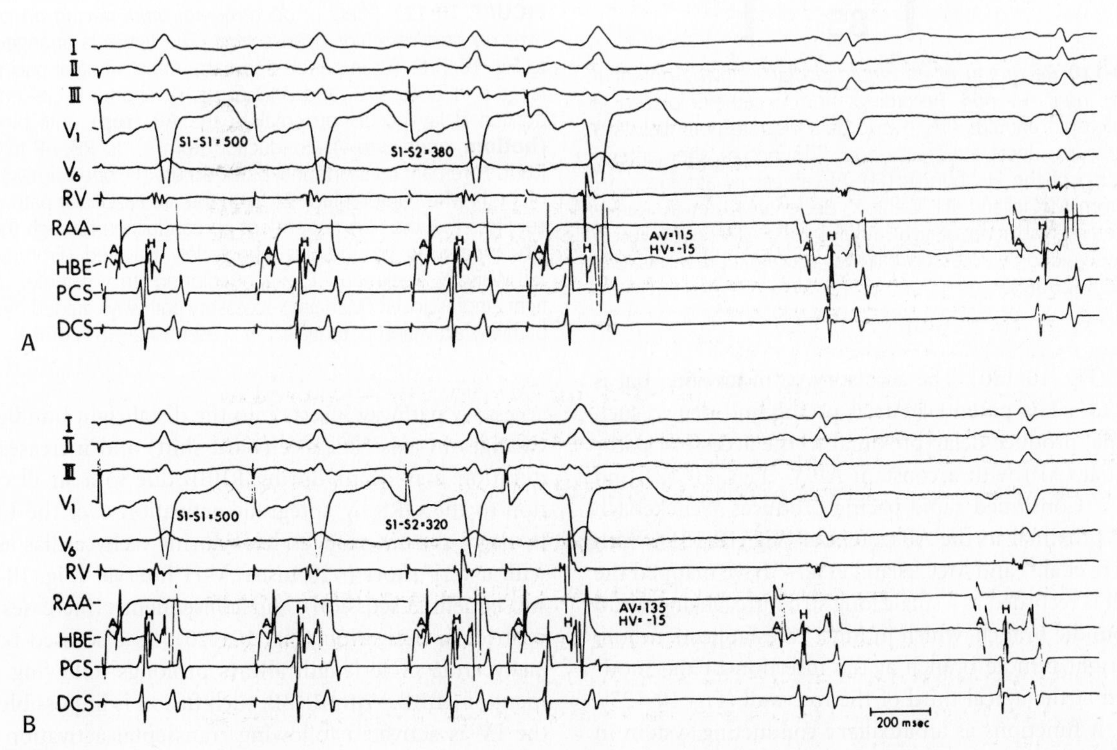


**FIGURE 10-119** *Effect of progressively premature atrial extrastimuli on A-V conduction in a patient with an atriofascicular bypass tract.* **A** and **B:** Atrial pacing at a drive cycle length of 500 msec is shown with progressively premature atrial extrastimuli. **A:** An APD delivered from the RAA at a coupling interval of 380 msec results in an A-V of 115 msec and an H-V of −15 msec. **B:** At an S1-S2 60 msec earlier (i.e., 320 msec), the A-V increases to 135 msec, but the H-V stays fixed at −15 msec. The increasing P-R interval with a fixed V-H and a constant degree of preexcitation provides supporting evidence of a decrementally conducting bypass tract that inserts in the right bundle branch. See text for discussion. DCS, distal coronary sinus; PCS, proximal coronary sinus. (From Ellenbogen KA, Ramirez NM, Packer DL, et al. Accessory nodoventricular (Mahaim) fibers: a clinical review. *Pacing Clin Electrophysiol* 1986;9:868–884.)

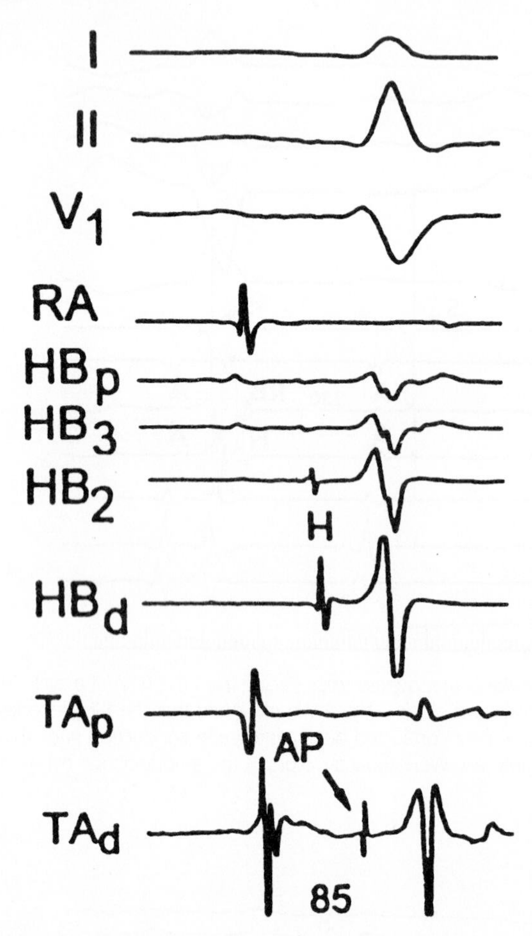


**FIGURE 10-120** *Recording of an atriofascicular pathway potential at the lateral right A-V ring.* Recordings from a catheter placed at the lateral tricuspid annulus ($TA_{p,d}$) records a discrete potential (AP) 85 msec following local atrial activation. This occurs after anterograde activation of the His bundle (H). AP, accessory atriofascicular pathway. (From McClelland JH, Wang X, Beckman KJ, et al. Radiofrequency catheter ablation of right atriofascicular (Mahaim) accessory pathways guided by accessory pathway activation potentials. *Circ* 1994;89:2655–2666.)

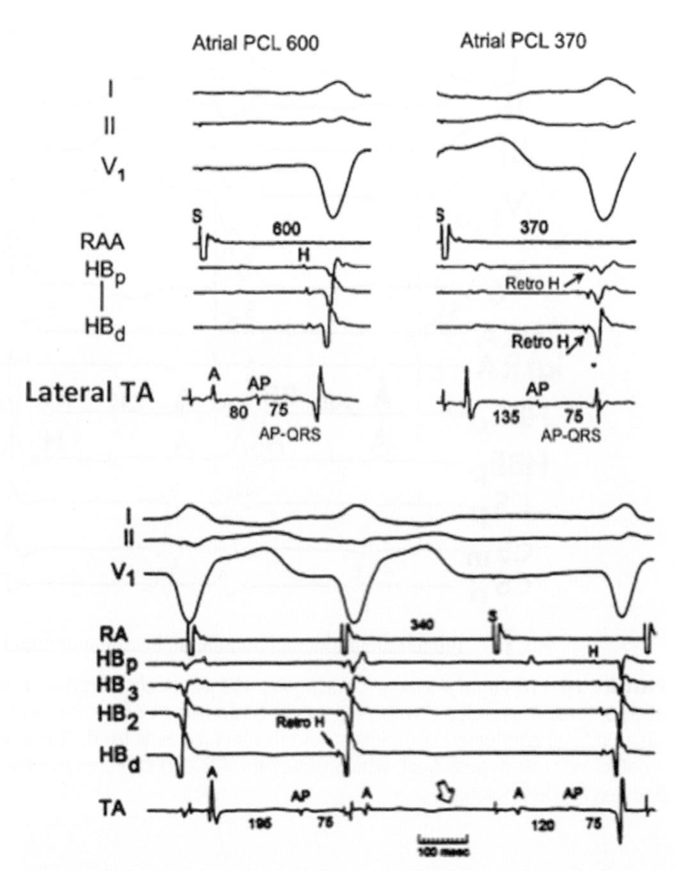


**FIGURE 10-121** *Effect of decremental atrial pacing on conduction over an atriofascicular bypass tract.* The figure is arranged similarly to Fig. 10-116. Three panels show the effect of atrial pacing at cycle lengths of 600, 370, and 340 msec. At shorter cycle lengths conduction delay occurs proximal to the AP (**top**) until block occurs (**bottom**, *open arrow*). Conduction from AP to RB, AP to QRS, and RB to H remain constant until block occurs (D, *open arrow*). Absence of the H when anterograde block in the atriofascicular pathway occurs confirms that the H is dependent on conduction through the atriofascicular pathway; i.e., the H is retrogradely activated. (From McClelland JH, Wang X, Beckman KJ, et al. Radiofrequency catheter ablation of right atriofascicular (Mahaim) accessory pathways guided by accessory pathway activation potentials. *Circ* 1994;89:2655–2666.)

at the AVJ (Fig. 10-120). The accessory pathway potential is analogous to a His potential. Atrial pacing and drugs, such as adenosine, produce delay proximal to the accessory pathway potential (AP) with a constant AP-V (Figs. 10-121 and 10-122).[20,150] Continued rapid pacing produces Wenckebach with block proximal to the AP potential (Fig. 10-121). Both Haissaguerre et al.[20] and McClelland et al.[150] have mapped the distal AP. It is recorded as a single long structure, analogous to the right bundle branch, which in most cases appears to join the distal right bundle branch at the insertion of the moderator band at the apical third of the free wall (Fig. 10-123). In essence, it functions as an auxiliary conducting system in parallel to the normal conduction system. During preexcitation propagation is traced anterogradely over the accessory pathway and retrogradely up the right bundle branch to the His bundle to give rise to the short V-H interval (Fig. 10-123). Transient or permanent proximal RBBB does not change the degree of preexcitation markedly and confirms that the accessory pathway inserts into the distal right bundle branch. Changes in axis (i.e., a leftward shift) and increases in QRS duration may occur during RBBB due to a small contribution to the QRS by antegrade activation over the LBB (particularly, the anterior fascicle) during tachycardias associated with a very short (<20 msec) V-H interval (Fig. 10-124 and subsequent discussion) and consequently increases in total ventricular activation (Fig. 10-125). As discussed below, the tachycardia cycle length always prolongs following development of RBBB. With RBBB, such fusion is impossible because the LV is activated following transseptal activation and the axis will shift to the left. In the presence of RBBB retrograde conduction to the His bundle occurs following transseptal engagement of the left bundle branch. In this instance, the His bundle is activated prior to the proximal right bundle branch, with anterograde conduction down the right bundle branch to the site of block. This is the mechanism of long and short

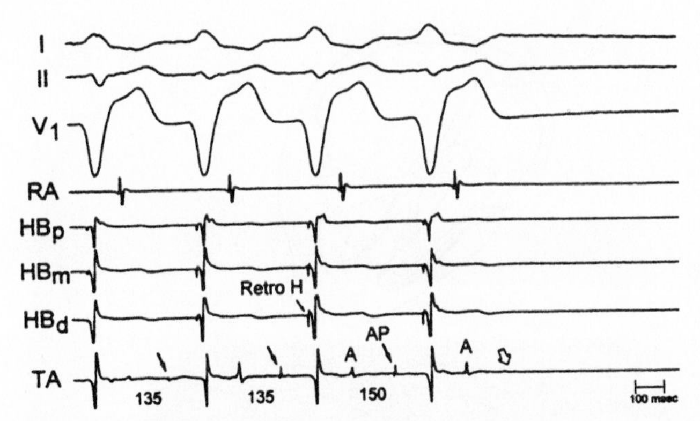


**FIGURE 10-122** *Effect of adenosine on conduction over an atriofascicular pathway.* The figure is arranged similarly to Figure 10-117. Supraventricular tachycardia with anterograde conduction over an atriofascicular pathway and retrograde conduction over the A-V node is present for the first four complexes. Adenosine was administered just prior to the recording. The adenosine produces progressive delay in the atriofascicular pathway (increasing A to AP) until block occurs proximal to the AP, terminating the tachycardia. Retrograde conduction through the A-V node is unaffected. See text for discussion. (From McClelland JH, Wang X, Beckman KJ, et al. Radiofrequency catheter ablation of right atriofascicular (Mahaim) accessory pathways guided by accessory pathway activation potentials. *Circ* 1994;89:2655–2666.)

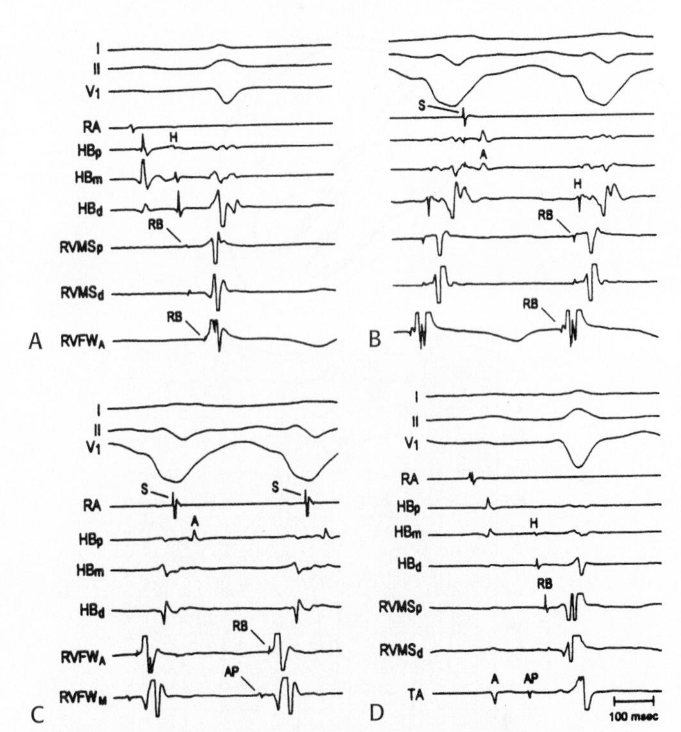


**FIGURE 10-123** *Recordings along an atriofascicular bypass tract and the normal conduction system during sinus rhythm and atrial pacing.* All panels show leads I, II, and V1 and recordings from the right atrium (RA), His bundle ($HB_{p,m,d}$), proximal and distal right ventricular mid septum ($RVMS_p$ and $RVMS_d$) and RV free wall near the apex ($RVFW_A$) at the site of earliest RV activation. **A:** During sinus rhythm there is minimal preexcitation. The RB at the RVMS is activated anterogradely following HB depolarization. The RVFWA is activated over the atriofascicular pathway (note relationship of RV electrogram at RVMS and RVFW). **B:** During atrial pacing producing full preexcitation, the RB and H are activated retrogradely. Note the change in activation sequence of the RVFW and RVMS compared to **(A)**. **C:** During atrial pacing as in **(B)** activation along the mid RVFW ($RVFW_M$) and $RVFW_A$ are shown. An atriofascicular pathway potential (AP) is seen at the $RVFW_M$ prior to the RB at the $RVFW_A$. The RV electrogram at this site is later than that at the apex suggesting that the AP is insulated until its insertion at the $RVFW_A$. **D:** During sinus rhythm as in panel **(A)**, RB activation occurs anterogradely along the RVMS. A recording along the lateral tricuspid annulus (TA) records the most proximal AP potential. (From McClelland JH, Wang X, Beckman KJ, et al. Radiofrequency catheter ablation of right atriofascicular (Mahaim) accessory pathways guided by accessory pathway activation potentials. *Circ* 1994;89:2655–2666.)

V-H tachycardias (see subsequent discussion). The onset of ventricular activation always occurs at the apical third of the right ventricular free wall regardless of the route of retrograde activation.

Rarely, one can see an obvious jump in A-H intervals before the His is inscribed within the QRS. Dual A-V nodal pathways are more readily appreciated using ventricular stimulation. During rapid ventricular pacing and ventricular extrastimuli, the retrograde conduction time is usually fast, compatible with conduction over a fast A-V nodal pathway. Initiation of tachyarrhythmias by ventricular stimulation (which we have observed in 85% of our patients) is virtually always associated with conduction up a relatively fast retrograde pathway followed by conduction down an antegrade slow pathway that is associated with preexcitation. The anterograde slow pathway can either be the accessory pathway or the slow A-V nodal pathway, in which case the accessory pathway acts as an innocent bystander during typical A-V nodal reentry. We have documented dual A-V nodal pathways (described in more detail later) in the majority of patients with atriofascicular pathways. In my opinion, the sudden appearance of preexcitation associated with a "jump" from fast to slow A-V nodal pathways with a His inscribed before ventricular activation or with a V-H ≤−10 msec (i.e., H-V ≥10 msec) strongly favors A-V nodal reentry. While one cannot exclude a slowly conducting atriofascicular tract that becomes manifest with a jump to the slow A-V nodal pathway, a consistent pattern of dual-pathway dependence and an "H-V" relationship too short to be retrograde from the distal right bundle branch would be fortuitous. Dual A-V nodal physiology has rarely been noted in atriofascicular pathways. Recently Sternick et al.[154] described an atriofascicular pathway which manifested a double response to APDs and a nonreentrant 1 to 2 tachycardia (Fig. 10-126).

During ventricular stimulation, if rapid and fixed V-A conduction is present, one must always exclude the presence of a separate A-V bypass tract. In my experience the incidence of additional bypass tracts is approximately 15% even in the absence of Ebstein's malformation, with which atriofascicular and/or long atrioventricular pathways are associated. Analysis of the retrograde atrial activation sequence and response to programmed stimulation during the tachycardia usually are sufficient to document the presence of an additional A-V bypass tract, as described earlier (see Chapter 8).

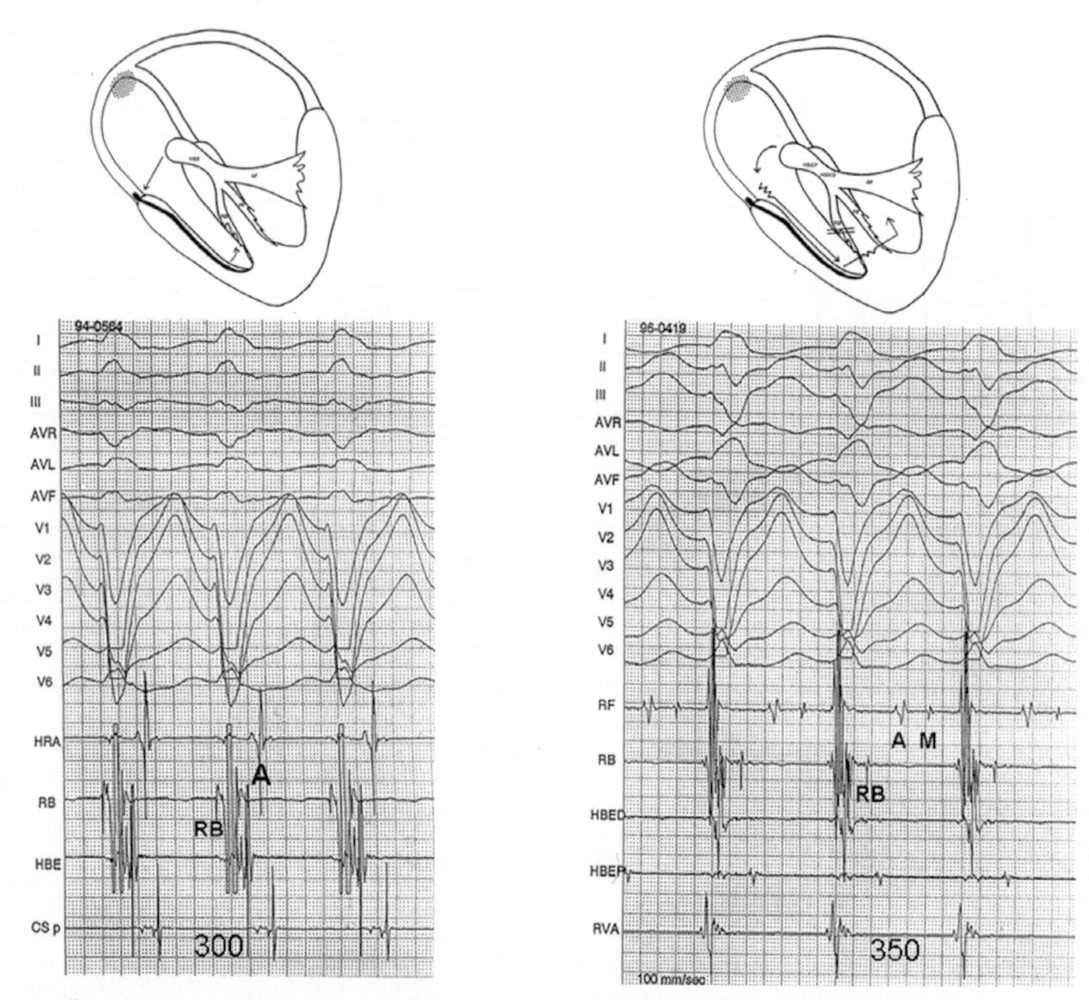


**FIGURE 10-124** *Effect of RBBB on V-H, QRS axis and width, and tachycardia cycle length during antidromic conduction over an atriofascicular bypass tract.* On the **left** is typical antidromic tachycardia over an atriofascicular pathway. The proximal RBB is activated at to onset of the QRS and the QRS is 110 msec with an axis of +30. The tachycardia cycle length is 300 msec. On the right is the tachycardia during RBBB. Retrograde activation is over the LBB and the RBB is activated after the QRS. Note that the QRS axis has shifted to the left (–45) and the QRS duration is 125 msec. This suggests the short V-RBB tachycardia results in a QRS that is a fusion of activation over the anterior division of the LBB and activation beginning at the RV free wall. See text for discussion.

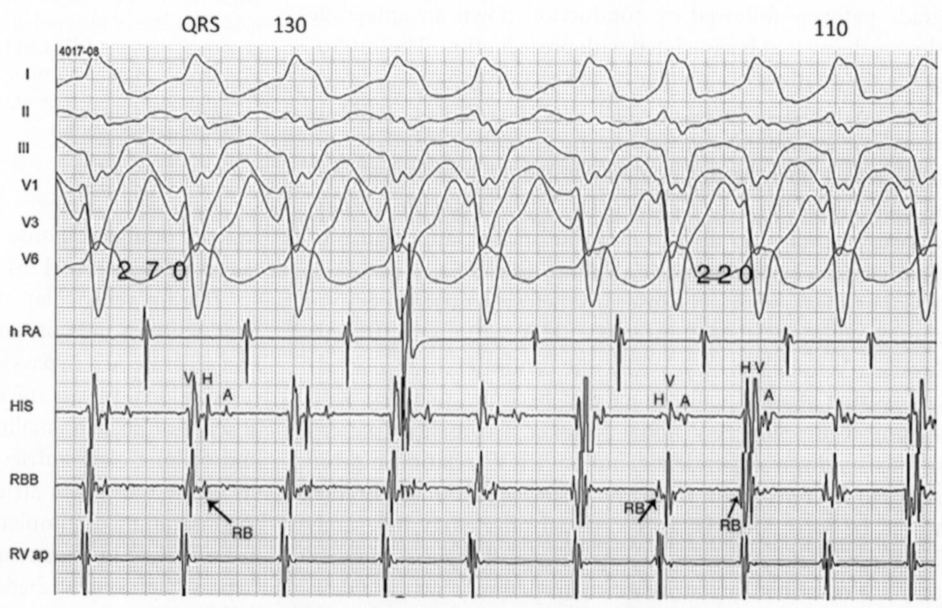


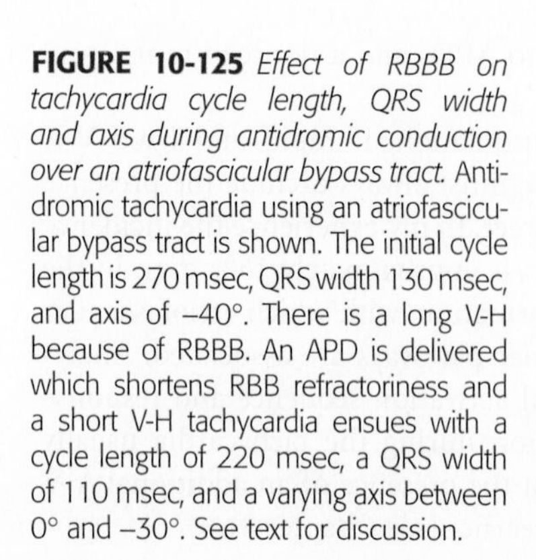
**FIGURE 10-125** *Effect of RBBB on tachycardia cycle length, QRS width and axis during antidromic conduction over an atriofascicular bypass tract.* Antidromic tachycardia using an atriofascicular bypass tract is shown. The initial cycle length is 270 msec, QRS width 130 msec, and axis of –40°. There is a long V-H because of RBBB. An APD is delivered which shortens RBB refractoriness and a short V-H tachycardia ensues with a cycle length of 220 msec, a QRS width of 110 msec, and a varying axis between 0° and –30°. See text for discussion.

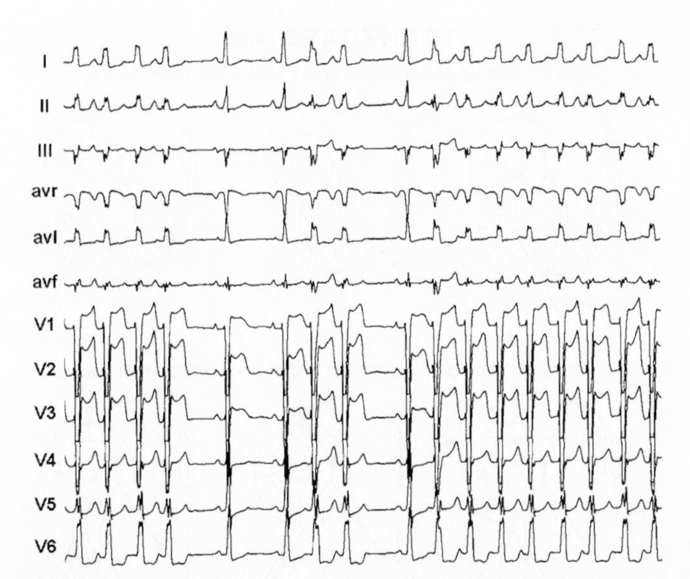


**FIGURE 10-126** *Atriofascicular pathway with dual pathway physiology and 1 to 2 conduction.* Each sinus beat on the right hand part of the tracing conducts over a fast and slow atriofascicular pathway to give rise to a 1 to 2 tachycardia. On the left conduction over the "slow" atriofascicular pathway is intermittent.

## Short Slowly Conducting Atrioventricular Bypass Tracts

These bypass tracts are less common than the atriofascicular or long atrioventricular pathways. They are analogous to decrementally conducting concealed bypass tracts (see Chapter 8) anatomically in that they bridge the A-V rings. As such the earliest ventricular activation occurs adjacent to the annulus. Gillette et al.[48] was the first to describe these pathways which, in contrast to concealed slowly conducting pathways, primarily arise at the right free wall. Twelve of fifteen such pathways I have seen were on the right free wall (see Fig. 10-113). As with other anterogradely decremental pathways, retrograde conduction is not seen. The amount of preexcitation is related to the relative conduction times over the A-V node and bypass tract. Retrograde conduction to the His bundle is only seen during antidromic tachycardias or following A-V block. In such instances conduction proceeds up either the right or left bundle branch, which is determined by whether or not RBBB is present. The V-H interval is longer than that observed with atriofascicular or long atrioventricular pathways due to the distance from the ventricular insertion site to the right bundle branch,[20] and the His is usually inscribed within the QRS (intermediate V-H). Additionally, the QRS widths are greater and have slower initial forces (i.e., delta waves) than those observed in atriofascicular pathways. Although these pathways demonstrate decremental conduction and Wenckebach-type block in response to rapid atrial pacing (Fig. 10-127), they appear less responsive to adenosine and vagal maneuvers than atriofascicular pathways, which suggests that this structure is not composed of A-V nodal like tissue.[20] This contention is supported by their sensitivity to lidocaine (Fig. 10-128).

## Nodofascicular and Nodoventricular Bypass Tracts

Bypass tracts that originate in the A-V node are rare. They should be considered anytime SVT, narrow complex or preexcited, with A-V dissociation is observed. Their presence as the retrograde limb of a narrow complex SVT with A-V dissociation is confirmed by ventricular stimulation during SVT which resets the tachycardia by stimuli delivered when the His bundle is refractory[18,87,153,155–158] (see subsequent discussion). Those fibers that are anterogradely conducting do not conduct retrogradely. Their presence is suggested if antidromic tachycardia is present with A-V dissociation. During the tachycardia the V-H may be short (nodofascicular) or intermediate

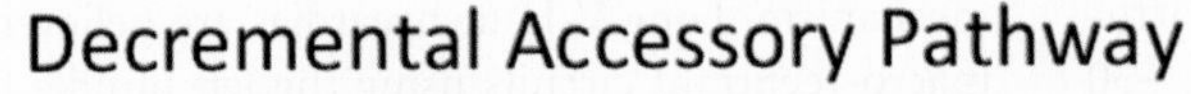


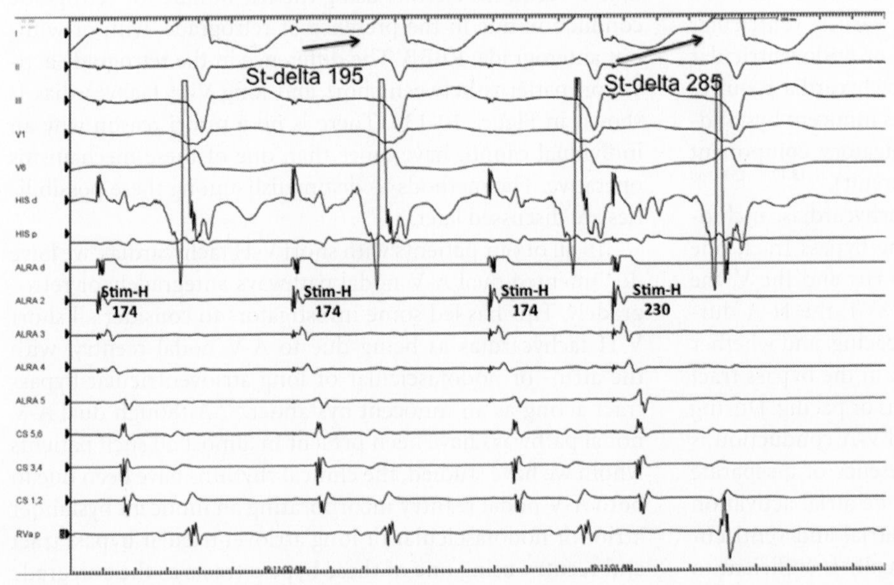


**FIGURE 10-127** *Response of a decremental atrioventricular pathway to APDs.* During atrial pacing at 600 msec the stimulus to delta is 195 msec, demonstrating slow conduction over this right free wall accessory pathway. An APD is introduced at 375 msec producing a minimal change in QRS but significant prolongation of the stimulus to delta wave to 285 msec in the absence of intra-atrial conduction delay. This confirms the decremental nature of the accessory pathway. The absence of changes in preexcitation suggests marked A-V nodal conduction delay or block at baseline.

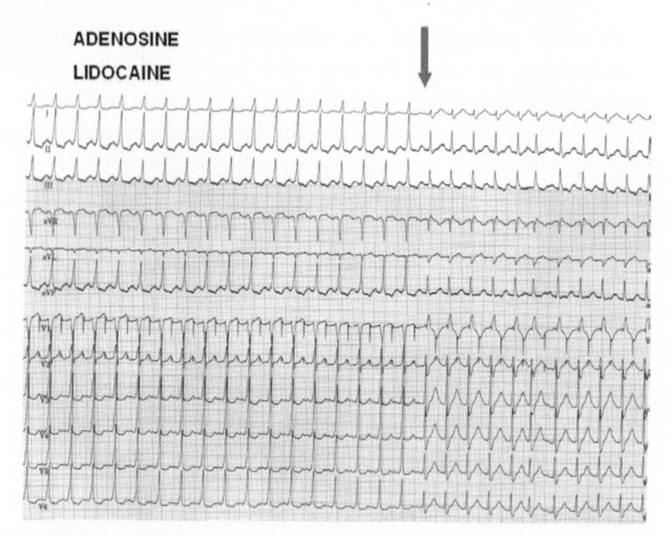


**FIGURE 10-128** *Response of decrementally conducting short A-V pathway to lidocaine.* Atrial pacing with a decrementally conducting anteroseptal pathway. Both lidocaine and adenosine produce antegrade block in the pathway.

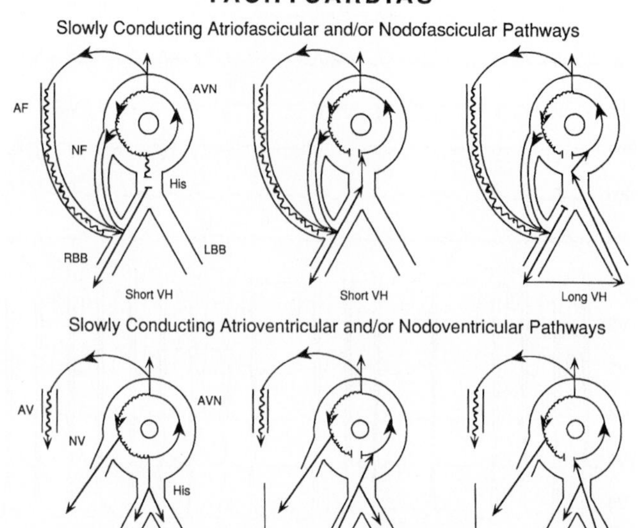


**FIGURE 10-129** Types of arrhythmias possible using atrio- or nodofascicular and nodoventricular or decrementally conducting A-V or slowly conducting A-V bypass tracts.

(50 to 80 msec, nodoventricular) during the tachycardias in the absence of RBBB (see earlier discussion). The distal insertion of nodofascicular pathways is in the proximal RBB so that earliest ventricular activation is at the apical third of the right ventricular free wall. The relatively normal axis reflects a contribution of conduction over the LBB to ventricular depolarization. Nodoventricular pathways insert directly into the ventricular myocardium in the region of the AVJ.

## Tachycardias Associated with Atriofascicular, Slowly Conducting A-V, Nodofascicular, and Nodoventricular Bypass Tracts

Virtually all patients with nodofascicular, decrementally conducting atriofascicular or A-V tracts, or true nodoventricular bypass tracts present with arrhythmias. Tachycardias virtually always have a LBBB pattern with an axis between, −30 and +60 degrees depending on the site of earliest ventricular activation. The role of the nodofascicular or nodoventricular fiber in initiating and maintaining the tachycardia requires detailed study, because the fibers can act as innocent bystanders during A-V nodal reentry or an obligatory component (antegrade limb of a macro-reentrant circuit).[15,18,19,87,155–158] To distinguish the mechanism of the tachycardias, including the site of ventricular insertion of the bypass tract, one needs to evaluate the relationship of the His and the V, the V-H during pacing and the V-H during SVT, the H-A during SVT, and the H-A during ventricular pacing, and whether or not the tachycardia persists after block in the bypass tract has been achieved by pharmacologic means or pacing. During ventricular stimulation, if rapid and fixed V-A conduction is present, one must always exclude the presence of a separate A-V bypass tract. Analysis of the retrograde atrial activation sequence and response to programmed atrial and ventricular stimulation during the tachycardia usually is sufficient to document the presence of an additional A-V bypass tract, as described earlier.

Tachycardias associated with atriofascicular and nodofascicular or nodoventricular or slowly conducting A-V bypass tracts can be divided into those with short and long V-H intervals. The types of arrhythmias theoretically possible with nodofascicular and nodoventricular pathways are schematically shown in Figure 10-129. Short V-H tachycardias may be due to A-V nodal reentry or use of an atriofascicular or nodofascicular bypass tract inserting into the right bundle branch. Positive H-V intervals or those ≤10 msec suggest A-V nodal reentry. An associated H-A ≤50 msec further supports this mechanism. Long V-H tachycardias are believed to represent macro-reentrant circuits using the left bundle for retrograde conduction due to the presence of retrograde, with or without anterograde, RBBB. The difference in the retrograde activation patterns between short and long V-H tachycardias is shown in Figure 10-130. There is no a priori reason why an individual cannot have more than one of these mechanisms operative. The methods to distinguish among these possibilities are discussed later.

In all of our patients with short V-H tachycardias, we have documented dual A-V nodal pathways antegradely or retrogradely. This has led some investigators to consider all short V-H tachycardias as being due to A-V nodal reentry, with the atrio- or nodofascicular or long atrioventricular bypass tract acting as an innocent bystander.[150] Although dual A-V nodal pathways have been present in almost all such patients whom we have studied, the clinical rhythms have been due to both A-V nodal reentry incorporating an innocent bystander atrio- or nodofascicular or long atrioventricular bypass tract and reentry using one of these bypass tracts as the antegrade

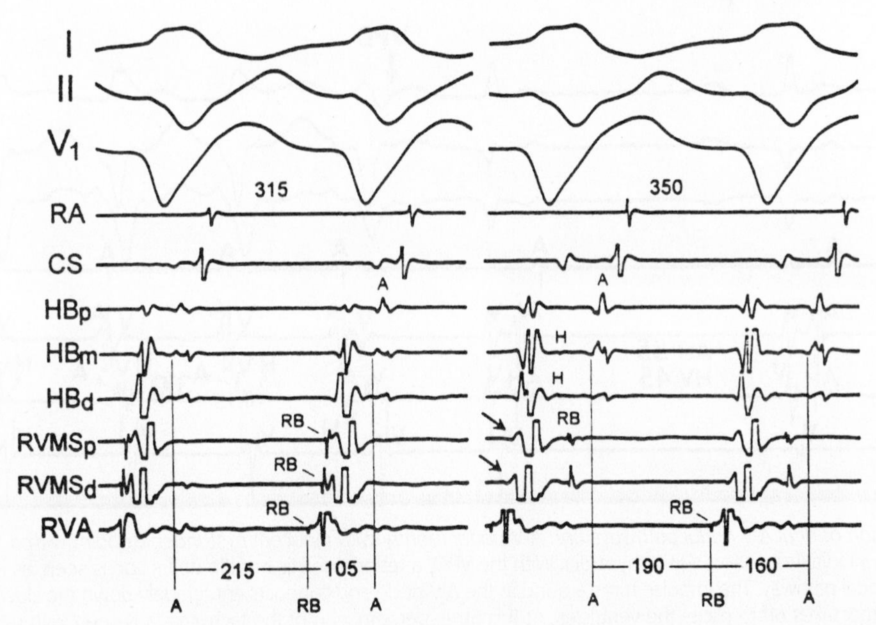


**FIGURE 10-130** *Effect of right bundle branch block on SVT using an atriofascicular pathway.* Leads I, II, and V1 are shown with recordings from the right atrium (RA), mid coronary sinus (CS), proximal (p), mid (m), and distal (d) His bundle (HB), and recordings of the right bundle (RB) at the proximal and distal mid RV septum ($RVMS_p$ and $RVMS_d$), and at the free wall of the RV near the apex (RVA). During the SVT on the **left (A)** conduction goes over the atriofascicular pathway to the RB at the RVA and retrogradely conducts to the HB giving rise to a short V-H SVT with a cycle length of 315 msec. Anterograde conduction down the pathway to the RB is 215 msec and from RVA to A in the HB is 105 msec. When right bundle branch block occurs **(B)** proximal to the RB at the RVA, transseptal activation occurs prior to retrograde activation over the left bundle branch with subsequent retrograde activation of the HB and anterograde activation of the proximal RB along the RVMS to the site of block. This results in a longer cycle length because of a longer route of retrograde conduction (RB – A = 160 msec). Anterograde conduction down the atriofascicular pathway is shorter due to the longer cycle length of the tachycardia. See text for discussion. (From McClelland JH, Wang X, Beckman KJ, et al. Radiofrequency catheter ablation of right atriofascicular (Mahaim) accessory pathways guided by accessory pathway activation potentials. *Circ* 1994;89:2655–2666.)

limb of the reentrant circuit. These mechanisms can be very difficult to distinguish, and both may be present in individual patients. Atrial or ventricular extrastimuli can initiate both tachycardia mechanisms. In patients with A-V nodal reentry, induction by atrial extrastimuli is always associated with a dual-pathway response, which may not be seen if the impulse traverses the atrio- or nodofascicular or long atrioventricular bypass tract antegradely and captures the His bundle retrogradely before it is antegradely activated by the impulse traversing the slow pathway. In most instances, a jump may be seen such that the antegrade His follows the QRS with a typical A-V nodal echo to initiate SVT. This is analogous to 1:2 conduction initiating preexcited tachycardias over an A-V bypass tract (see Fig. 10-29). In this instance, the first complex and all subsequent complexes are due to conduction over an atriofascicular or long atrioventricular bypass tract such that the impulse reaches the ventricle before the same impulse reaches the His bundle over the slow pathway. This results in ventricular activation over the bypass tract and atrial activation as a result of an A-V nodal echo. The process repeats, and sustained A-V nodal reentry is associated with a maximally preexcited tachycardia with a left bundle configuration. This mechanism is similar to that described previously in this chapter, with 1:2 conduction initiating orthodromic tachycardia or, more analogously, antidromic tachycardia.

This pattern is less likely to occur with a nodofascicular bypass tract because of early retrograde activation of the His bundle and A-V node that can preempt A-V nodal reentry. As demonstrated by the case shown in Figure 10-29, A-V nodal reentry can be associated with a "long V-H" or a "short V-H" tachycardia. No fusion is seen during the long V-H tachycardia, because the ventricles will be refractory to any activation over the normal pathway. Fusion is, however, possible during a short V-H tachycardia.

Initiation by ventricular extrastimuli more readily affords one the opportunity to assess whether or not the decrementally conducting bypass tract is an innocent bystander. In Figure 10-131, a VPD initiates SVT. The rapid V-A conduction over the His–Purkinje with turnaround down the slow pathway documents the presence of dual pathways. The question arises whether the nodofascicular bypass tract is an innocent bystander or is participating in the tachycardia. One of the important methods used to distinguish the two is by comparing the H-A interval during initiation of the tachycardia by ventricular extrastimuli or during ventricular pacing with the H-A interval during the tachycardia. In Figure 10-131, the H-A interval is longer with the initiating VPD than during the tachycardia. This occurs despite the fact that the interval from the last depolarization of the His bundle of the second sinus beat to the retrograde His bundle in response to VPD actually exceeds the H-H intervals during the tachycardia. Because the A-V node usually exhibits greater decremental conduction with

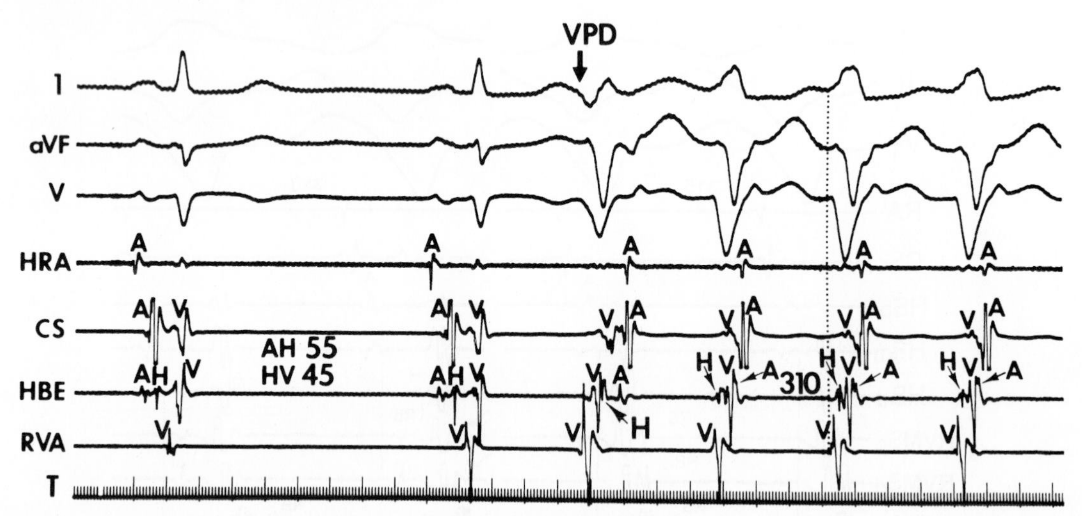


**FIGURE 10-131** *Initiation of dual A-V nodal pathways and A-V nodal reentry with innocent bystander Mahaim with a VPD.* Following two sinus complexes, a VPD (*arrow*) initiates a short V-H tachycardia. With the VPD, a retrograde His bundle deflection is seen, as is rapid conduction to the atrium over a fast A-V nodal pathway. The impulse turns around in the A-V node and conducts antegradely down the slow pathway from which the nodofascicular bypass tract takes off to excite the ventricles. At this time, perpetuation of the tachycardia is seen with retrograde conduction over the fast pathway and antegrade conduction over the slow pathway. Note that the H-A interval response to the VPD is longer than the H-A interval during the tachycardia, despite the fact that the tachycardia cycle length, and hence, input to the fast pathway, is shorter than the H-H interval at the time of the VPD. See text for discussion.

repetitive engagement of impulses than to a single impulse at similar coupling intervals, the more prolonged H-A with the initiating VPD suggests that the sustained arrhythmia is A-V nodal reentry. If an atriofascicular, nodofascicular, or decremental atrioventricular bypass tract were used as the anterograde limb of the circuit, the H-A interval during ventricular pacing or the ventricular extrastimulus initiating it (particularly at comparable coupling intervals as the cycle length of the tachycardia) should have the same H-A interval as that observed during the tachycardia. Another important distinguishing feature is the V-H interval. If the V-H interval during the tachycardia is significantly less than the H-V interval (i.e., <20 msec) and the V-H interval during pacing at the right ventricular apex, a nodoventricular or slowly conducting atrioventricular bypass tract (that inserts far from the right bundle branch) is excluded, because conduction from the ventricle back to the His always exceeds the H-V by the time it takes the impulse to reach the right bundle branch from the site of ventricular stimulation. Thus, in my opinion, a true nodoventricular or slowly conducting short atrioventricular fiber can never be obligatorily involved in a short V-H tachycardia. Atrial or ventricular extrastimuli can sometimes reveal that a short V-H tachycardia is due to A-V nodal reentry. This is shown in Figure 10-132, where A-V nodal reentry with an RBBB pattern

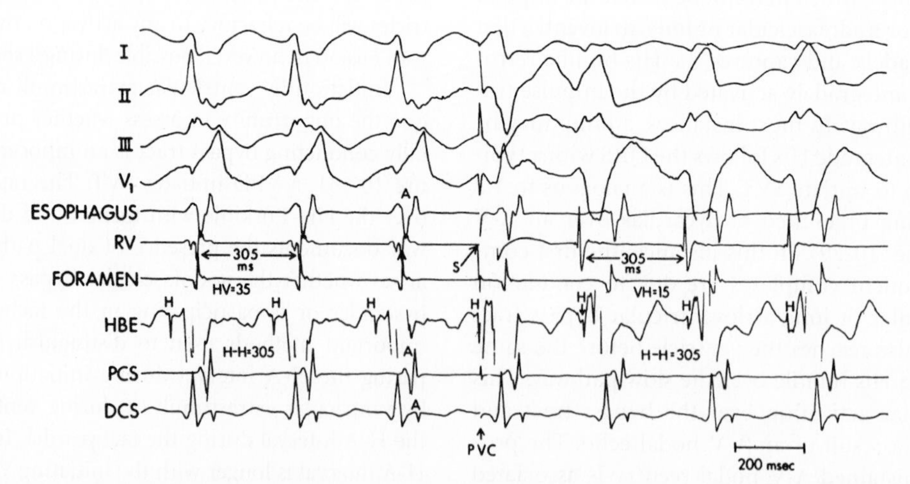


**FIGURE 10-132** *Demonstration of A-V nodal reentry with innocent bystander slowly conducting A-V bypass tract.* On the left, typical A-V nodal reentry is present with retrograde atrial activation occurring with the QRS, which manifests RBBB. The H-V is normal at 35 msec. Following a timed (PVC), conduction now proceeds antegradely over an atrioventricular bypass tract with a fixed V-H interval of 15 msec. The broader initial force during preexcitation than during RBBB aberration is evidence of a delta wave and presence of a decrementally conducting short A-V bypass tract. The H-H, H-A, and A-A intervals remain constant before and after the PVC. See text for discussion. (From Gallagher JJ, Selle JG, Sealy WC, et al. Variants of preexcitation. Update 1989. In: Zipes DP, Jaliffe J, eds. *Cardiac electrophysiology from cell to bedside.* Philadelphia: WB Saunders, 1990:460.)

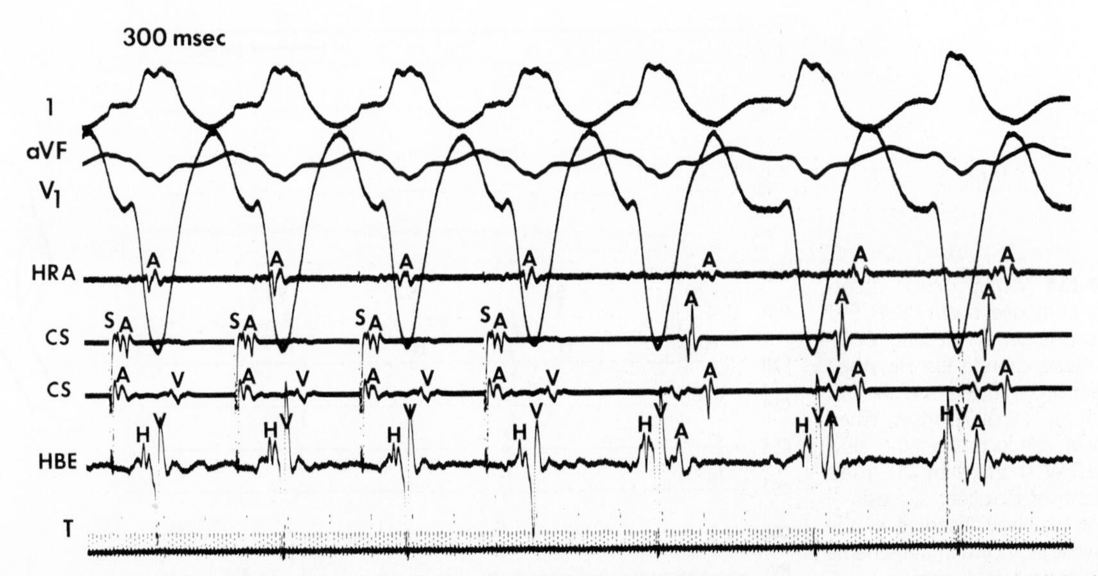


**FIGURE 10-133** *Entrainment of atriofascicular-nodal reentry.* Atrial pacing from the CS at a PCL of 300 msec is shown on the left. The V-H interval remains fixed. On cessation of pacing, in the middle of the panel, the return cycle is also 300 msec, with the V-H remaining fixed and short. The ability to entrain the tachycardia with a fixed V-H interval during pacing that is identical to that during the first unpaced tachycardia supports the diagnosis of an atriofascicular bypass tract participating in the circuit. See text for discussion.

is present on the left and is converted to an LBBB-type tachycardia (antegrade conduction over a decremental right-sided atrioventricular bypass tract) by a single ventricular complex without any change in the A-A interval. If an atriofascicular, decrementally conducting atrioventricular, or nodofascicular bypass tract were **incorporated** in the circuit in a patient with RBBB, a long V-H tachycardia should be present because the impulse cannot reach the His bundle over the right bundle branch. The presence of a short V-H tachycardia in such instances should suggest A-V nodal reentry with an innocent bystander bypass tract. A fixed short V-H during atrial pacing-induced entrainment of SVT (Fig. 10-133) suggests that a nodofascicular, atriofascicular bypass tract is present but does not exclude A-V nodal reentry with an innocent bystander bypass tract.

Of note, in patients with both long and short V-H antidromic atriofascicular tachycardias the QRS width and axis frequently are different, with wider QRSs and more leftward axis when a long V-H tachycardia is compared to the short V-H tachycardia (see Figs. 10-124 and 10-125). The QRS width is virtually always longer. Axis shifts may be subtle or marked. A significant axis shift suggests that fusion is taking place during the short V-H tachycardia due to some activation of the LV over the anterior fascicle of the LBB (Fig. 10-124). Loss of this left Purkinje contribution results in a wider QRS and an axis shift.

Tachycardias due to atriofascicular bypass tracts may be very difficult to distinguish from those due to nodofascicular bypass tracts. While V-A block or V-A dissociation excludes the participation of a slowly conducting atriofascicular bypass tract, this is a rare finding.[18,155–158] These patients can be recognized by AV dissociation with a typical LBBB pattern, short V-H, and could be terminated or reset by a His-refractory VPC. These are much rarer than atriofascicular pathways. I have personally studied three patients with nodofascicular reentrant tachycardia, in one of whom there was RBBB and the pathway came off the slow A-V nodal pathway and inserted in the distal His bundle (Fig. 10-134).

As previously noted, the relationship of preexcitation to dual pathways favors, but does not specifically diagnose, a nodofascicular tract. The presence of a slowly conducting atriofascicular bypass tract can be demonstrated if (a) the site of atrial pacing influenced the P-R interval without affecting the degree of preexcitation and/or (b) atrial stimulation from the free wall delivered after the A-V junctional atrium was depolarized could advance the tachycardia.[18,49] This latter finding, particularly when associated with maintenance of the V-H-A sequence of the reset complex, excludes A-V nodal reentry (Fig. 10-135). Of the mechanisms of reentry, "classic" fascicular-nodal (i.e., nodofascicular-nodal reentry or atriofascicular-nodal atrial reentry), and A-V nodal reentry with an innocent bystander nodofascicular tract are the most common.

Long V-H tachycardias are generally believed to represent a macro-reentrant circuit incorporating the left bundle branch retrogradely and either an atriofascicular, nodofascicular, slowly conducting A-V, or nodoventricular bypass tract anterogradely. Retrograde block in the proximal right bundle branch is associated with antegrade conduction over the distal right bundle branch or right ventricle with subsequent retrograde activation over the left bundle branch (see Figs. 10-124, 10-125, 10-129, and 10-130). However, A-V nodal reentry can theoretically also produce a long V-H tachycardia if a rapidly conducting nodoventricular bypass tract takes off from the proximal part of the slow pathway to activate the ventricles prior to the time the His is activated anterogradely.

Some patients may have several of these proposed mechanisms.[15,17–19] An example of a patient who had A-V nodal

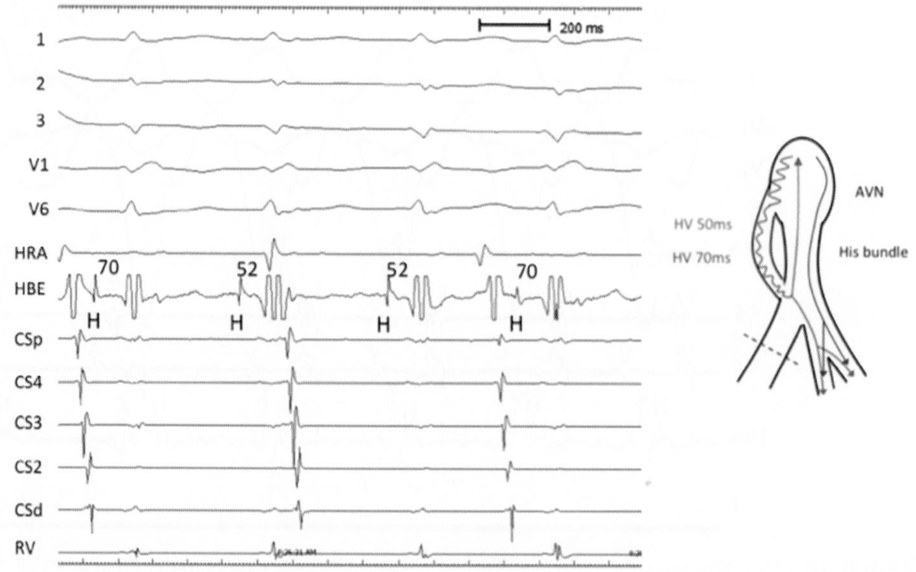

**FIGURE 10-134** *Nodofascicular accessory pathway in a patient with RBBB.* SVT with A-V dissociation is present. Occasional sinus beats capture the His when the sinus beat is conducted over the fast pathway, with an H-V of 70 msec. When the sinus beat conducts over the slow pathway, the H-V shortens by 20 msec. The consistent observation suggests a nodofascicular pathway inserting in the distal His bundle as shown in the schema on the right. See text for discussion

reentry with narrow QRS complexes, A-V nodal reentry with antegrade conduction over a bystander nodofascicular bypass tract, and typical short V-H nodofascicular reentry is shown in Figure 10-136. In this figure, although the V-A interval is longer, the H-A interval is the same when antegrade activation occurs over a bystander atriofascicular bypass tract compared to A-V nodal reentry with a normal QRS. When atriofascicular or nodofascicular nodal reentry occurs, both the V-H and the V-A (in the HBE) are longer than in A-V nodal reentry with a narrow complex. Nodoventricular fibers can theoretically have an intermediate V-H interval if conduction antegradely proceeds over the nodoventricular bypass tract and goes retrogradely to the atrium over the right bundle branch system. In this case, the V-H will be slightly longer than V-H during ventricular pacing from the midseptum. The identical pattern can be observed with a circuit using a decrementally conducting A-V bypass tract. Tables 10-11 and 10-12 review V-H criteria as a means of distinguishing tachycardia types, and Table 10-11 lists the specific criteria for the different tachycardia types discussed previously.

Fusion of the QRS can be seen during sinus rhythm and atrial pacing up to a point, but fusion is almost never apparent during SVT. Theoretically, fusion could result during A-V nodal reentry with an innocent bystander nodofascicular bypass tract if antegrade conduction through the A-V node and left bundle occurred with simultaneous antegrade ventricular activation

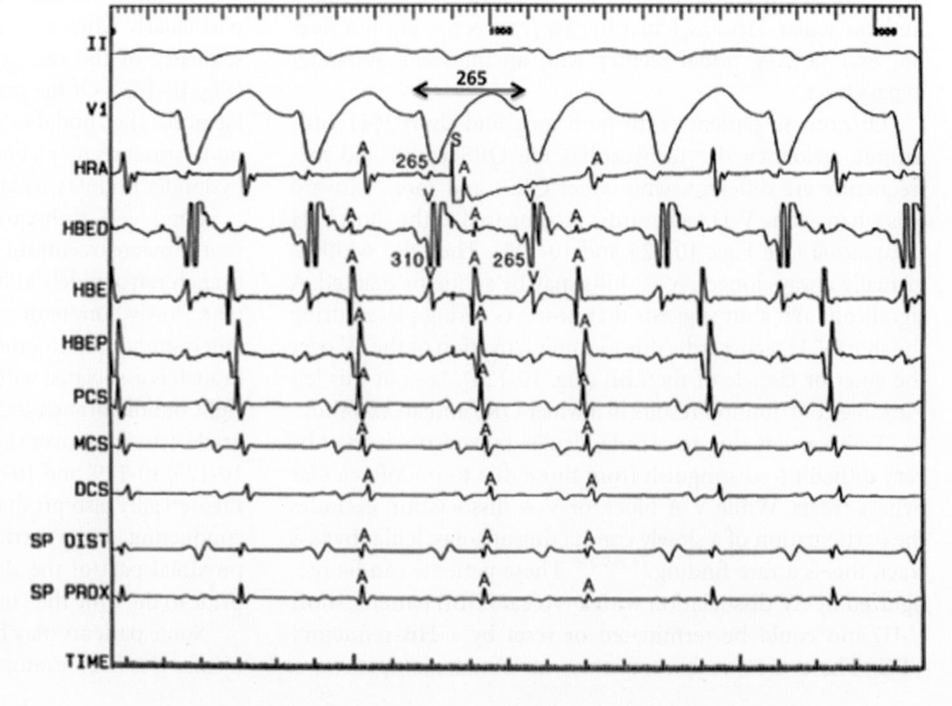


**FIGURE 10-135** *Proof of atriofascicular pathway participation in the reentrant circuit.* SVT with a left bundle branch block appearance is present with a short V-H interval. An APC is delivered from the HRA at 265 msec which advances the ventricular complex without altering atrial activation in the region of the A-V node (A in HBE, all CS recordings, and those from the "slow pathway"(SP) occur on time). Subsequent atrial activation follows the reset ventricular complex with the same activation sequence and timing.

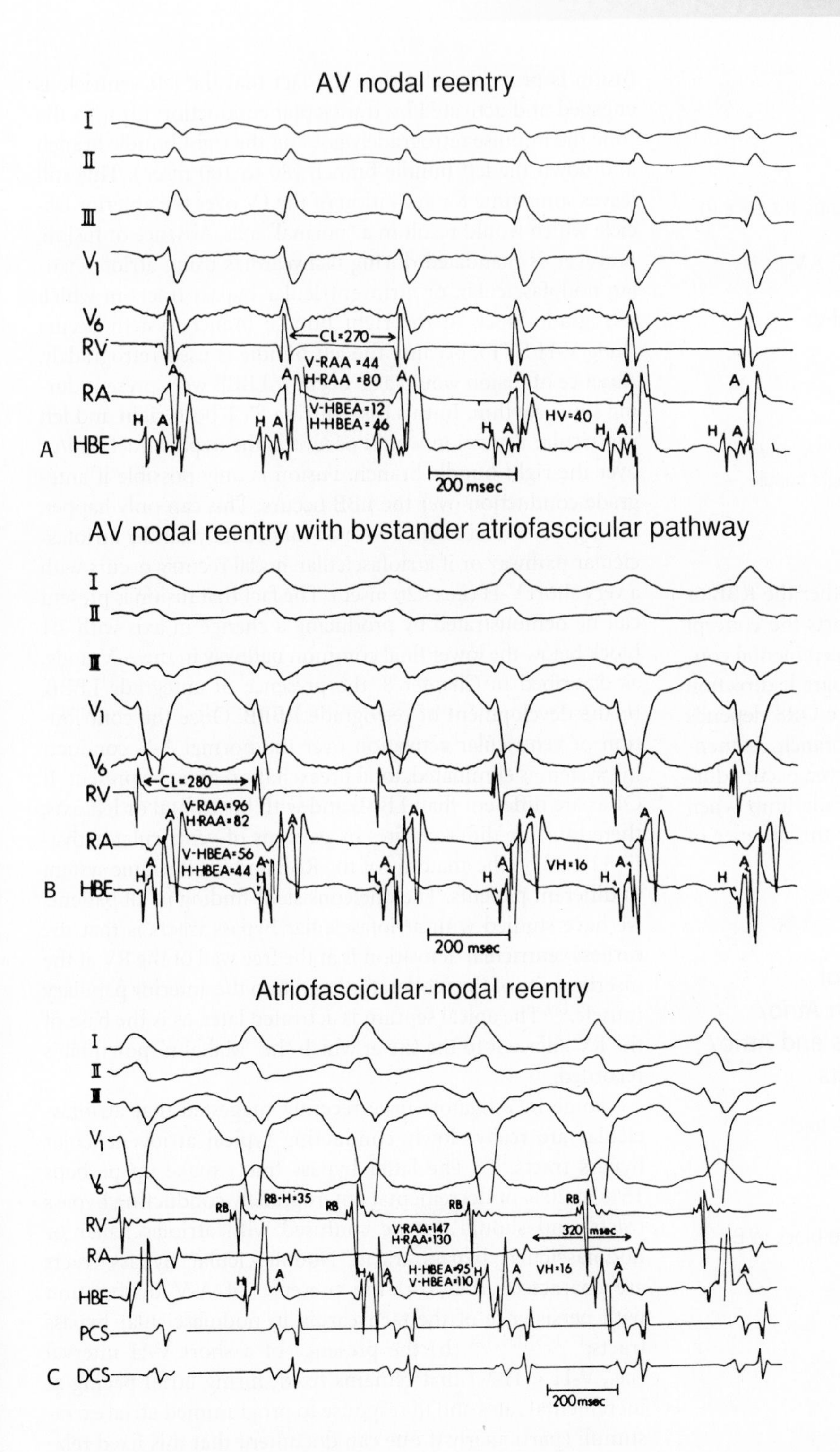


**FIGURE 10-136** *Innocent bystander atriofascicular bypass tract and participating atriofascicular bypass tract in reentrant SVT.* **A:** A-V nodal reentry is present with classic H-A and A-V relationships. **B:** The same tachycardia is present but with innocent bystander participation of an atriofascicular bypass tract. Note the H-A interval is identical with that during typical A-V nodal reentry in **(A)**. With bystander atriofascicular bypass tract, the V-H is 16 msec. **C:** Atriofascicular-nodal reentry using the atriofascicular bypass tract is shown in the same patient. Here, activation of the right bundle precedes His bundle activation. The H-A during this tachycardia is prolonged to 95 msec in the HBE, and the tachycardia cycle length is increased to 320 msec. See text for discussion.

over the right bundle branch via an atriofascicular or nodofascicular bypass tract. In that case, varying degrees of delay in the A-V node could result in varying degrees of activation of the left ventricle over the left bundle branch system. Fusion could be present, but inapparent if the His bundle was activated retrogradely during the tachycardia, such as in typical short V-H nodofascicular-nodal reentry (similar to reentry using an atriofascicular tract as stated above), if retrograde conduction from the site of insertion in the right bundle branch system reached the His bundle and conducted antegradely down the left bundle branch. This could be suggested by a more left and inferior axis. The fact that fusion is present is confirmed with a change in axis and/or QRS width with the development of RBBB (see prior discussion of atriofascicular bypass tracts and Figures 10-124 and 10-125. Total ventricular depolarization over an atriofascicular pathway inserting in the distal RBB should have a horizontal or left axis. Although one could postulate these ECG patterns represent different insertion sites of the RBB into

**TABLE 10-11 Tachycardia Types**

Short V-H tachycardia (V–H < H–V and < V–H during RV pacing)
 AF or NF → nodal reentry
A-V nodal reentry with innocent bystander AF, NF, A-V, or NV bypass tract
Intermediate V-H tachycardia (H in QRS, V-H ≥ H-V)
 A-V or NV → RBB → nodal reentry
Long V-H tachycardia (H after QRS, V-H > H-V)
 AF, NF, A-V or NV → LBB → nodal reentry

AF, slowly conducting atriofascicular; NF, nodofascicular; A-V, slowly conducting atrioventricular; NV, nodoventricular; RBB, right bundle branch; LBB, left bundle branch.

the RV, a change in axis dependent upon whether the RBB or LBB is used for retrograde conduction supports the concept of fusion during atriofascicular reentry. Any decremental conduction in the right bundle branch in the retrograde direction could influence the degree to which the entire QRS depends on antegrade activation over the right bundle branch. As mentioned earlier, however, overt fusion rarely, if ever, occurs during SVT using a bypass tract as the anterograde limb when the V-H exceeds 50 msec. The explanation for this absence of fusion is probably related to the fact that the left ventricle is engaged and activated by transseptal conduction prior to the time the impulse retrogradely goes up the right bundle branch and down the left bundle branch (80 to 100 msec). This still leaves some time for activation of the LV over the anterior fascicle which would result in a "normal" axis. Absence of fusion, however, is mandated during tachycardias using atriofascicular, nodofascicular, or atrioventricular bypass tracts in which retrograde block in the right bundle branch system occurs (long V-H SVT), because the left bundle is used retrogradely. Absence of fusion would also occur if LBBB were present during sinus rhythm. In this case, during SVT both right and left ventricular activation would occur via the bypass tract and/or over the right bundle branch. Fusion is only possible if antegrade conduction over the LBB occurs. This can only happen during A-V nodal reentry with an innocent bystander atriofascicular pathway or if atriofascicular-nodal reentry occurs with a very short V-H (i.e., <20 msec). The fact that fusion is present can be demonstrated by producing a change in axis with 2:1 block below the lower final common pathway in the A-V node, as described in Chapter 8, the presence of antegrade LBBB, or the development of retrograde RBBB. Once the contribution of ventricular activation over the normal A-V conducting system is eliminated, total preexcitation must be present. If QRSs are different than LBBB and with horizontal or left axis, there must be different sites or patterns of ventricular activation based on the anatomy of the RBB and RV Purkinje system in different patients. The one consistent finding in all patients we have studied with atriofascicular bypass tracts is that the earliest ventricular activation is at the free wall of the RV at the insertion site of the moderator band into the anterior papillary muscle.[159] The apical septum is activated later, as is the base of the RV adjacent to the site at which the "Mahaim" potential is recorded.

Some investigators have recently suggested that atriofascicular are really slowly conducting typical atrioventricular bypass tracts.[21,48] The latter bypass tracts make up perhaps 15% to 20% of decremental anterogradely conducting bypass tracts, and should not be confused with atriofascicular or nodofascicular bypass tracts. Nodofascicular bypass tracts are characterized by (a) the presence of A-V dissociation with persistence of the tachycardia in nodofascicular bypass tracts;[17–19,87,156–158] (b) the presence of a short V-H interval (i.e., V-H < H-V) that remains fixed during atrial pacing at incremental rates and in response to programmed atrial extrastimuli (particularly if one can document that this fixed relationship is associated with a reversal of the activation of the His and right bundle branch); (c) an increasing P-R interval with a fixed V-H and no change in the degree of preexcitation; and (d) most mapping studies demonstrate earliest excitation at the apical anterior right ventricular wall, where the right bundle branch usually initiates ventricular activation, and not at the A-V groove.[18,20,160] In contrast to short decrementally conducting atrioventricular bypass tracts, long, insulated bypass tract extending from the A-V ring to the midanterior wall (approximately 6 cm) have been documented by

**TABLE 10-12 Electrophysiologic Features of Tachycardias Associated with Atrio/Nodofascicular Bypass Tracts and Atrio/Nodoventricular Bypass Tracts**

A-V nodal reentry with innocent bystander bypass tract
- H-A SVT < H-A RVP
- H before or simultaneous with RB
- Fusion of QRS possible
- Continuation at same SVT-CL despite antegrade block in BT
- V-H SVT < V-H RVP and < H-V

Atriofascicular or nodofascicular reentry
- Common (Short V-H SVT)
 V-H SVT < V-H RVP
 RB before H
 H-A SVT = H-A RVP
- Uncommon (Long V-H SVT)
 V-H SVT > V-H RVP
 H before RB
 H-A SVT = H-A RVP

Nodoventricular or atrioventricular reentry
 V-H SVT slightly > V-H RVP (intermediate V-H SVT) or much > V-H RVP (long V-H SVT)
 RB before H during intermediate V-H SVT, H before RB during long V-H SVT
 H-A SVT = H-A RVP

BT, bypass tract; RB, right bundle branch; RVP, RV pacing.

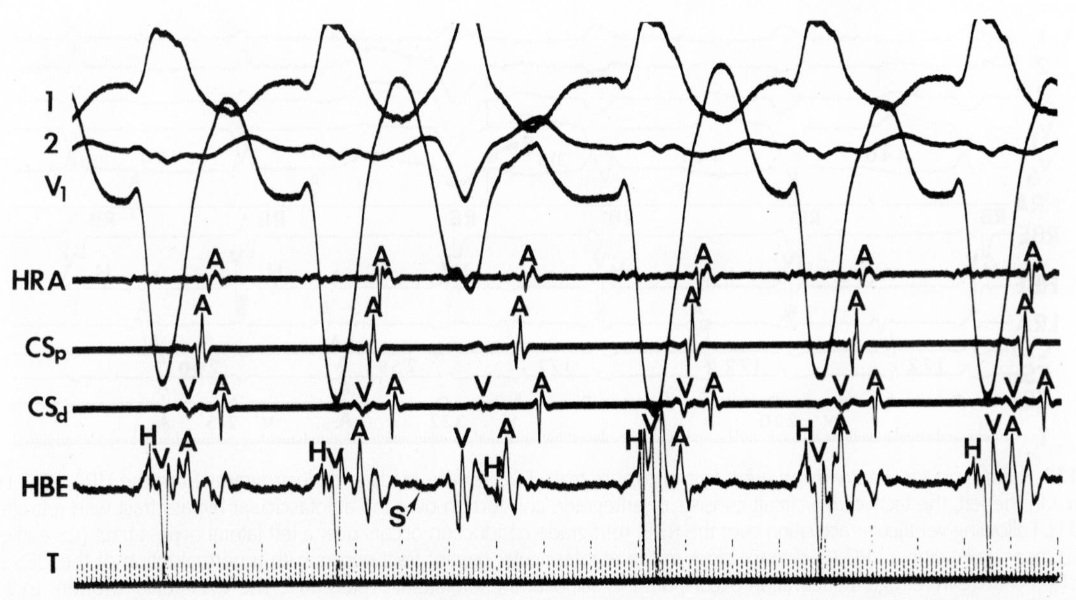


**FIGURE 10-137** *Circus movement tachycardia using a nodofascicular bypass tract antegradely and a posteroseptal bypass tract retrogradely.* A short V-H tachycardia is present during the first two complexes. Following the second complex, a ventricular extrastimulus (not shown) is delivered, which preexcites the atrium without influencing the antegrade His deflection. The tachycardia is reset, and the reset complex has the same V-H and H-A intervals as the rest of the SVT. The activation sequence suggests that a posteroseptal bypass tract is present and participates in the tachycardia circuit. (From Lerman BB, Waxman HL, Proclemer A, Josephson ME. Supraventricular tachycardia associated with nodoventricular and concealed atrioventricular bypass tracts. *Am Heart J* 1962;104:1097.)

Haissaguerre et al.,[20] but these are likely to be atriofascicular bypass tracts. Nodofascicular bypass tracts with antidromic reentry are associated with HV intervals 10-20 msec shorter than the HV because they insert in the distal His bundle or proximal RBB (see Fig. 10-134). HV intervals associated with atriofascicular reentry are much shorter and are negative (−10 to −25 msec during short V-H antidromic tachycardias). I personally have only studied three nodofascicular antidromic tachycardias in 42 years of performing EP studies. One had preexistent RBBB distal to the insertion of the pathway and appeared to exit the node from the slow pathway. When antegrade conduction proceeded over the slow pathway, the H-V interval was 18 msec shorter than when it proceeded over the fast pathway.(see Fig. 10-134). Ablation of the slow pathway prevented SVT and led to an H-V of 70, consistent with fast pathway conduction during the tachycardia (Fig. 10-142).

Slowly conducting short A-V bypass tracts demonstrate, by definition, earliest ventricular excitation should be located along the A-V ring.[18,160] Certainly, all slowly conducting concealed atrioventricular bypass tracts are located around the A-V rings. The vast majority of pathways that demonstrate earliest activation at the apical free wall of the right ventricle are slowly conducting atriofascicular bypass tracts. Rarely, nodofascicular tracts can be responsible for this type of ventricular activation.

Because rapidly and/or slowly conducting A-V bypass tracts (concealed or manifest) may also be present in individual patients with anterogradely decrementally conducting bypass tracts, complex reentrant circuits may be seen. We have observed additional A-V bypass tracts in 14/59 patients with decrementally conducting A-V (or fascicular) or nodoventricular (or fascicular) bypass tracts (Figs. 10-137 and 10-138).

The diagnosis of a retrogradely functioning nodoventricular or nodofascicular bypass tract is extremely difficult if one-to-one V-A association is present. It requires the demonstration of retrograde atrial preexcitation or postexcitation (delay of subsequent atrial activation) by ventricular extrastimuli introduced during SVT without disturbing the timing of the His bundle. This is analogous to stimulation during orthodromic tachycardia using A-V bypass tracts (see Chapter 8 and the preceding discussion of the role of the bypass tract in the genesis of arrhythmias). The V-H is longer in nodoventricular bypass tracts than nodofascicular pathways, but overlap may exist. Depending on the prematurity of the ventricular extrastimulus, V-A delay can occur because the impulse must traverse some portion of the A-V node. Therefore, instead of "preexcitation" of the atria, which is possible at long coupling intervals, V-H or V-A (if V-A conduction is present) prolongation would be likely to occur in response to an earlier ventricular extrastimulus. This in and of itself, however, is not diagnostic of a nodoventricular or a nodofascicular bypass tract, because slowly conducting concealed A-V bypass tracts behave in a similar fashion (see Chapter 8). If A-V dissociation is present advancement or delay of the next His and QRS with a VPC delivered when the His is refractory is diagnostic of a concealed nodoventricular or nodofascicular pathway. A clue to a nodofascicular pass tract is the slowing of the tachycardia with the development of spontaneous, catheter, or stimulation-induced right bundle branch block. Only the ability to demonstrate A-V dissociation with persistence

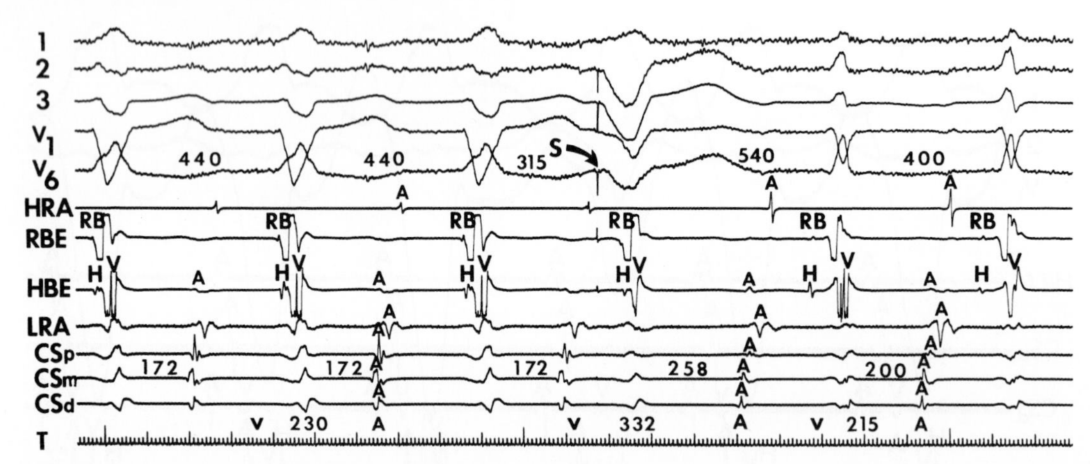


**FIGURE 10-138** *Atriofascicular reentry using a left lateral bypass tract.* Five surface leads and electrograms from the HRA, RBE, HBE, LRA, and CS are shown. On the left, the tachycardia circuit consists of antegrade conduction over the atriofascicular bypass tract with retrograde activation of the RB and H. Following ventricular activation over the RBB, retrograde conduction occurs over a left lateral bypass tract (CS earliest) with a V-A interval of 230 msec. Following a VPC (S, *arrow*), block in the atriofascicular bypass tract occurs with a normalization of the QRS and the H-RB sequence. A slight change in retrograde activation occurs, but it is still over the left lateral bypass tract. The V-A interval shortens to 215 msec with normalization of the QRS. See text for discussion.

of the tachycardia could distinguish a retrogradely conducting nodofascicular or nodoventricular bypass tract from a slowly conducting atrioventricular bypass tract as the retrograde limb of the circuit. If A-V block is spontaneously present during the tachycardia, advancement, delay, or termination of the tachycardia by a "His Refractory" VPC, suggests an innocent bystander concealed nodoventricular or nodofascicular pathway (see Chapter 8).

In sum, the bulk of evidence suggests that the vast majority of antegrade, decrementally conducting bypass tracts insert into or adjacent to the distal right bundle branch and arise from the atrium. They should therefore be more appropriately called slowly conducting atriofascicular or, theoretically, long atrioventricular bypass tracts. These can produce short V-H and long V-H tachycardias, and they can function as innocent bystanders during A-V nodal reentry. True nodoventricular or nodofascicular bypass tracts with insertion into the right ventricular myocardium or right bundle branch are less common. Slowly conducting short atrioventricular bypass tracts are of intermediate frequency. Although much attention has been focused on reentrant arrhythmias using a bypass tract – either passively as a bystander or incorporating it into the circuit – other arrhythmias can occur. Atrial flutter-fibrillation may occur in such patients, and varying degrees of preexcitation will be observed, depending on the site of takeoff from the A-V node of the bypass tract and the relative delays in the A-V node above and below the takeoff site.

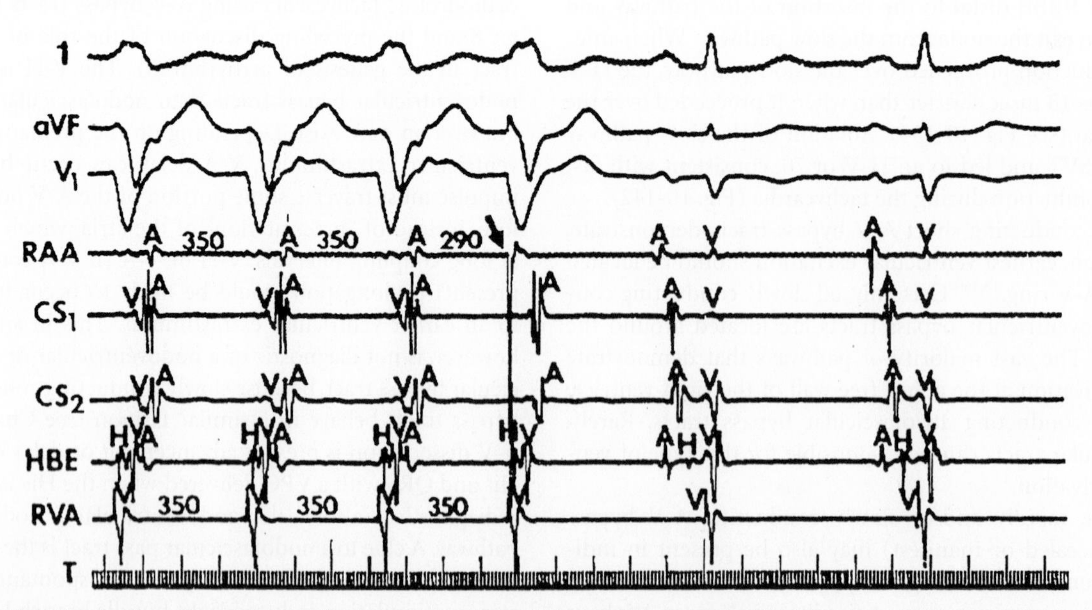


**FIGURE 10-139** *Termination of an atriofascicular reentrant tachycardia by an APD.* During the tachycardia using an atriofascicular bypass tract, an APD (*arrow*) delivered from the RAA terminates the tachycardia by block in the bypass tract.

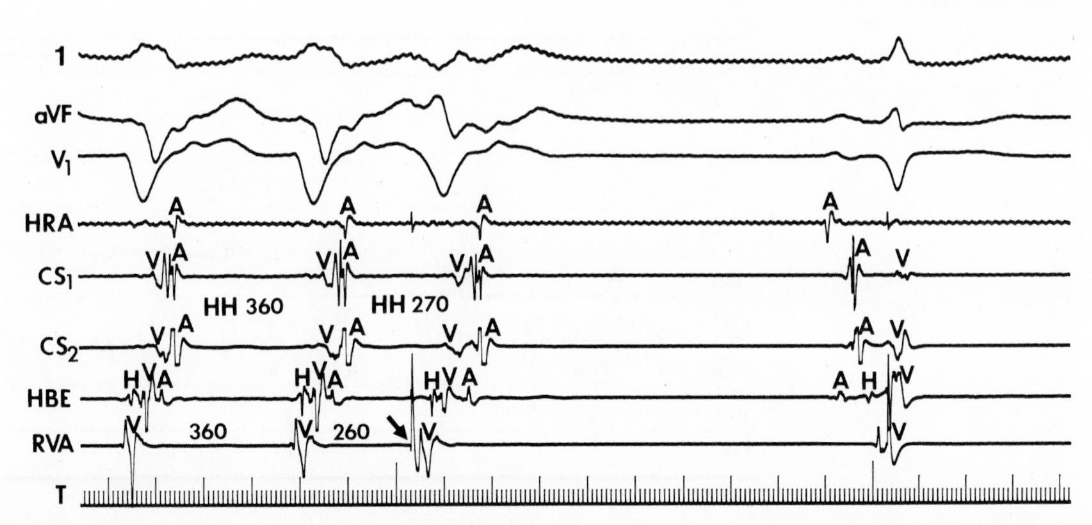


**FIGURE 10-140** *Termination of SVT using an atriofascicular bypass tract by a VPD.* Following two complexes of SVT, a ventricular extrastimulus delivered from the RVA retrogradely captures the His deflection and conducts to the atrium. The impulse then blocks antegradely in the atriofascicular pathway. See text for discussion.

## Therapeutic Implications

In the vast majority of patients with tachycardias using these "decrementally conducting" bypass tracts, the rhythm can be terminated by either atrial or ventricular pacing (Figs. 10-139 and 10-140). Antegrade block is always produced in the bypass tract with or without block in the A-V node. Although some authors[17,19] suggest that termination by ventricular extrastimuli only occurs when a retrograde His bundle is not seen, we have not found this to be the case. In Figure 10-140, retrograde capture of the His bundle and conduction over the fast A-V nodal pathway results in block in the atriofascicular pathway and perhaps in a slow pathway, if present, in response to early retrograde atrial activation, and termination of SVT. Ventricular stimulation produces antegrade block in the atriofascicular pathway due to retrograde invasion of the atriofascicular bypass tract and premature atrial activation over the A-V node. The ease of termination of programmed stimulation suggests that an antitachycardia pacemaker may be useful in management of this arrhythmia, but in our experience it is unnecessary. Ablation is the therapeutic intervention of choice (see Chapter 14). Ablation is usually guided by accessory pathway potentials.[17,20,149,150,155] Distal ablation of the ventricular insertion is less successful.[153] Ablation at the A-V ring for slowly conducting short A-V pathways and of

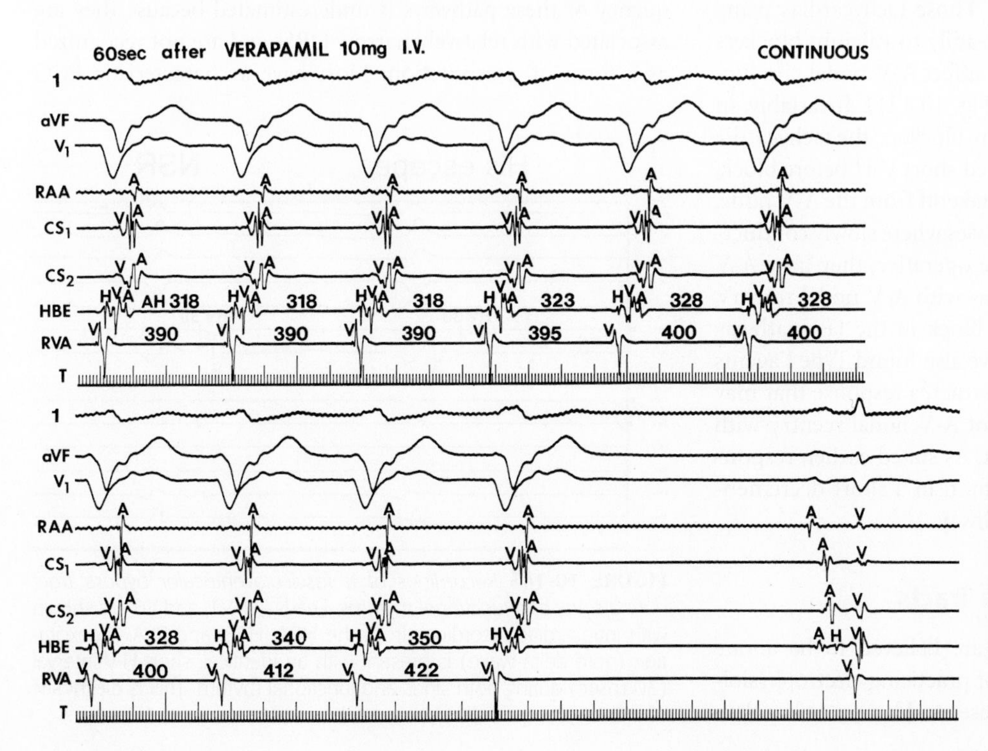


**FIGURE 10-141** *Termination of SVT using an atriofascicular bypass tract with verapamil.* The tracing is continuous. Following 10 mg of verapamil IV, the tachycardia slows gradually and terminates. Note that the tachycardia slowing is related to an increase in the P-R and A-H interval. The V-H and degree of preexcitation remain fixed. This suggests that the site of action of verapamil is in the atriofascicular bypass tract. See text for discussion.

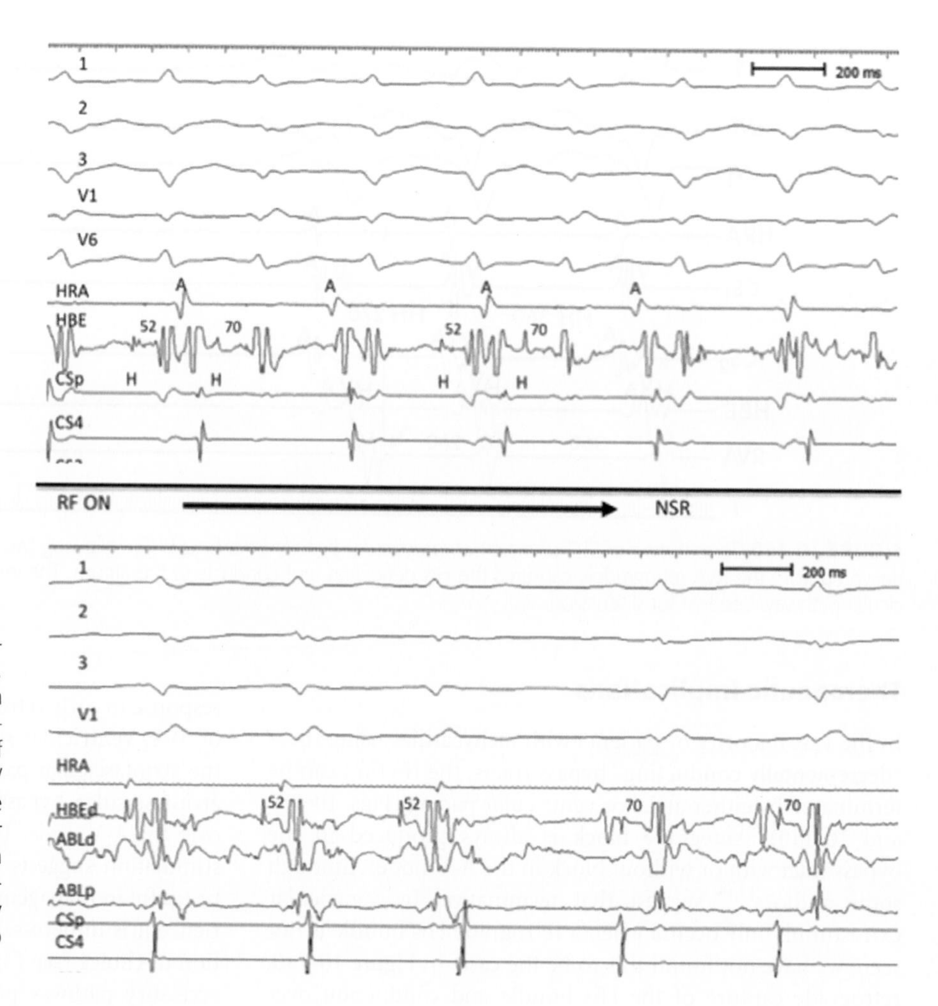


**FIGURE 10-142** *Ablation of the slow pathway to treat a nodofascicular tachycardia.* The tracings are from the same patient shown in Fig. 10-134. On **top** the SVT with A-V dissociation is seen. Intermittent conduction of sinus beats over the fast pathway has an H-V of and 0 msec while conduction over the slow pathway proceeds over a nodofascicular bypass tract to the distal His, giving rise to a shorter H-V. Ablation of the slow pathway produces conduction only over the fast pathway with an H-V of 70 msec. The patient has no recurrent SVT.

the ventricular septum adjacent to the AVJ for nodoventricular pathways have been described. Those tachycardias using atriofascicular pathways respond readily to calcium blockers (Fig. 10-141) and other drugs that affect A-V nodal conduction, for example, adenosine (see Fig. 10-121). Invariably, in response to beta-blockers or calcium-blockers, the tachycardia slows without any change in the fixed short V-H before block, which must occur above the site of takeoff from the A-V node. These findings also suggest that in cases where slowly conducting atriofascicular bypass tracts are operative, they have A-V nodal-like properties. Sometimes, as with A-V nodal reentry, Type I agents produce retrograde block in the fast pathway and prevent the arrhythmia. We have also found Type I agents to be useful in blocking the bypass tract, a response that may enable one to make the diagnosis of A-V nodal reentry with an innocent bystander bypass tract. As stated earlier, responsiveness to lidocaine is more common in a short decrementally conducting A-V accessory pathway.

## Fasciculoventricular Bypass Tracts

Fasciculoventricular bypass tracts are believed to be a rare form of preexcitation. In 41 years of practicing electrophysiology I have personally observed 15 cases and have seen less than two dozen others studied by colleagues. I believe that the frequency of these pathways is underestimated because they are associated with relatively narrow QRSs and are not recognized as a form of preexcitation. Most have a characteristic ECG

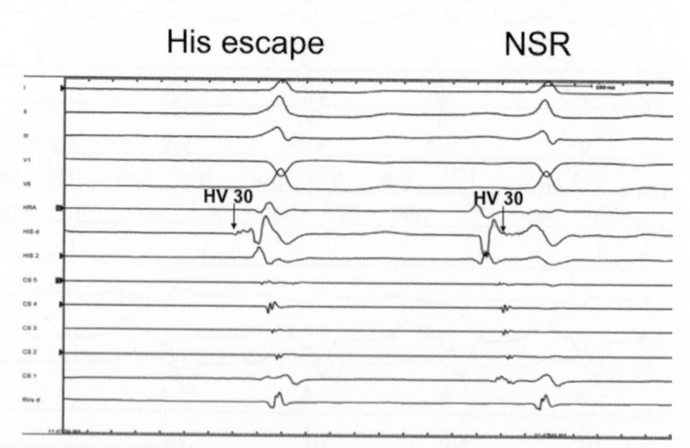


**FIGURE 10-143** *Recordings of a fasciculoventricular bypass tract during sinus and junctional rhythms.* Leads I, II, V1, and V6 are shown with intracardiac recordings from the HRA, HBE, and RVA. Preexcitation (note delta wave) is present with an identical, short H-V interval (30 msec) during both sinus and junctional rhythm. This is diagnostic of a fasciculoventricular bypass tract.

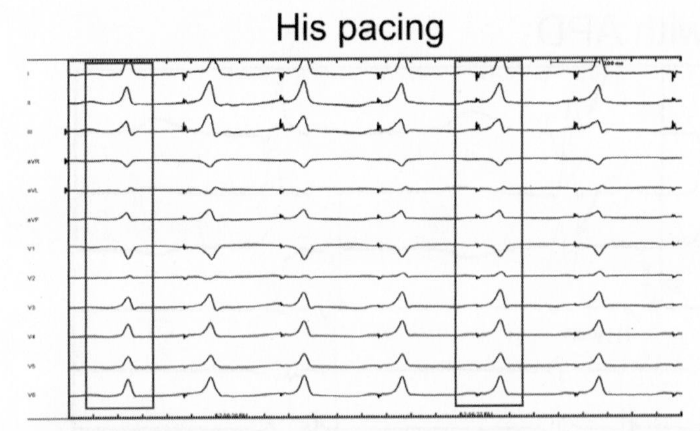


**FIGURE 10-144** *His bundle pacing in a patient with a fasciculoventricular pathway A 12 lead ECG is shown.* The first complex is sinus. His bundle pacing is initiated with a stimulus to V and QRS identical to the H-V and QRS in sinus. This is diagnostic of a fasciculoventricular pathway.

with a slight "delta wave", a left inferior axis, a QRS of 90 to 120 msec, and precordial R/S transition by V3 (Fig. 10-142). Gallagher et al.,[19] Sternick et al.,[154] and Ganz et al.[161] have electrophysiologically characterized such fibers, which should be easy to diagnose. Preexcitation should be present with normal P-R and A-H intervals and a short H-V (His-to-delta wave) interval. Atrial pacing prolongs the P-R interval owing to A-V nodal delay but will not change the degree of preexcitation because the fiber takes off from the His–Purkinje system. Junctional rhythms or His extrasystoles should be associated with a similar degree of preexcitation and short H-V interval (Fig. 10-143). In contrast to atrioventricular, atriofascicular, and nodofascicular bypass tracts, His bundle stimulation results in a preexcited QRS with a short H-V interval (Fig. 10-144). In a patient with preexcitation, if atrial pacing produces an increase in the A-H interval without a change in the short H-V interval (H before RB), and no change in the

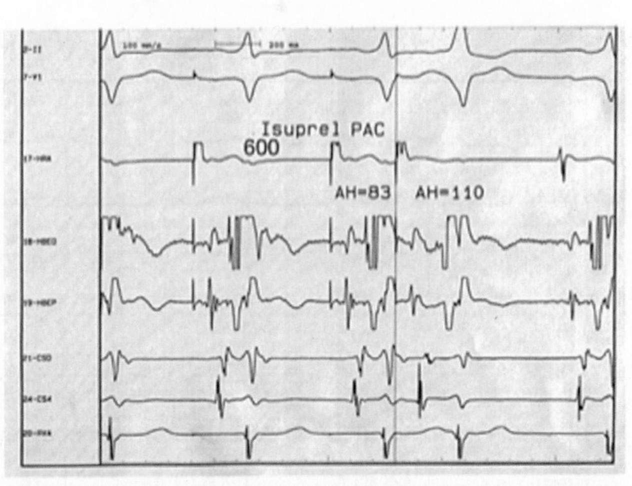


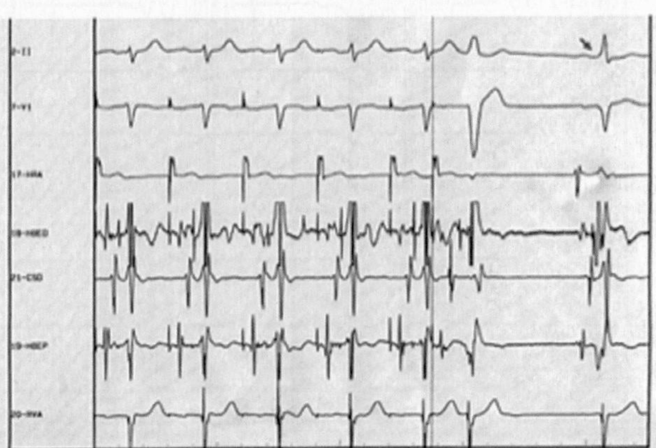

**FIGURE 10-146** *Change in preexcitation over a fasciculoventricular pathway with an APD producing LBB conduction delay or block.* Leads II and V1 are shown with recordings from the HRA, HBE, CS, and RVA. Atrial stimulation is present during an Isuprel infusion. An APC is delivered which demonstrates marked preexcitation ova fasciculoventricular pathway. The H-V is unchanged. This likely resulted from LBBB which was induced with a similar coupled APC delivered at a shorter drive cycle length (450 msec) which blocked in the bypass tract.

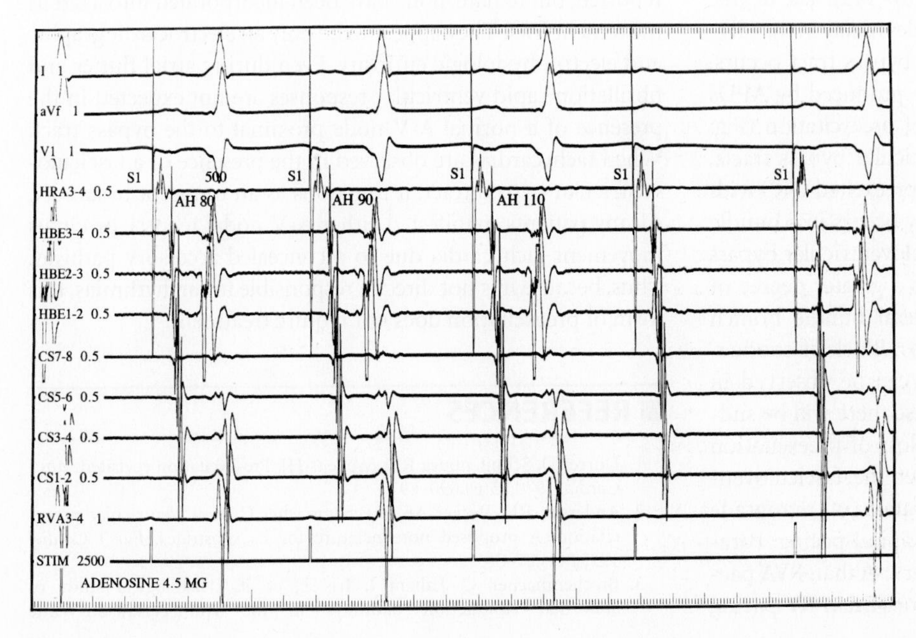


**FIGURE 10-145** *Loss of preexcitation over a fasciculoventricular bypass tract during pacing-induced A-V nodal Wenckebach.* The tracing is organized with leads 1, aVF, and V1 with multiple His bundle leads (HBE), HRA, 4 CS leads, and an EGM from the RVA. During atrial pacing at a cycle length of 500 msec results in A-V nodal Wenckebach. Preexcitation is lost with A-V nodal block. This is characteristic of a fasciculoventricular bypass tract. See text for discussion. (From Ganz LI, Elson JJ, Chenarides JG. Preexcitation in a child with syncope: where is the connection? *J Cardiovasc Electrophysiol* 1998;9:892–895.)

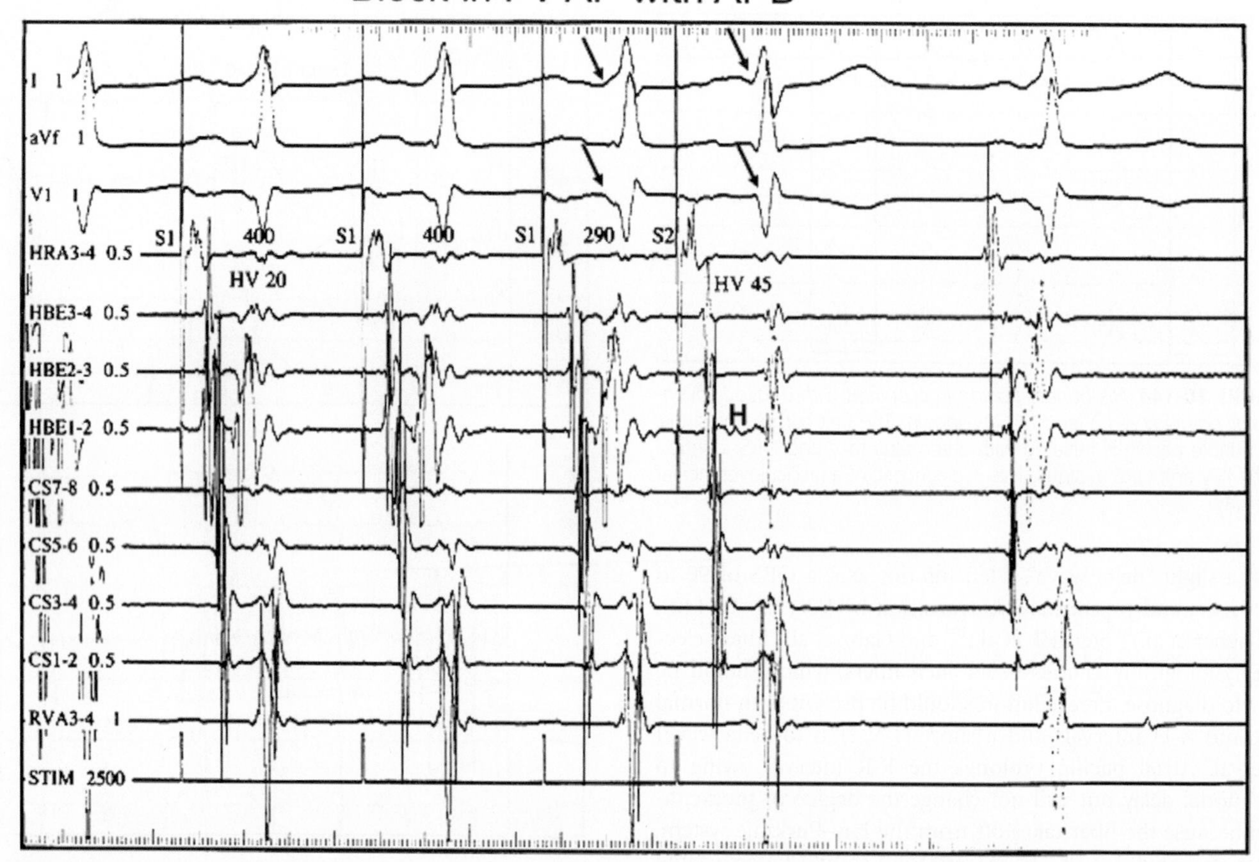


**FIGURE 10-147** *Effect of atrial stimulation on a fasciculoventricular bypass tract.* The figure is organized in Fig. 10-145. During atrial pacing (S1-S1) at a cycle length of 400 msec an atrial extrastimulus (S2) is delivered at a coupling interval of 290 msec. During the pacing drive (S1) preexcitation is present with an H-V interval of 20 msec. Following S2, block in the fasciculoventricular bypass tract occurs, which is associated with a prolongation of the H-V interval to 45 msec. See text for discussion. (From Ganz LI, Elson JJ, Chenarides JG. Preexcitation in a child with syncope: where is the connection? *J Cardiovasc Electrophysiol* 1998;9:892–895.)

degree of preexcitation, a fasciculoventricular bypass tract is present. A-V nodal Wenckebach should be associated with loss of preexcitation and A-V conduction (Fig. 10-145). The degree of preexcitation generally remains fixed, unless delay in the His–Purkinje system below the takeoff of the bypass tract occurs. Theoretically, such a delay, which may be produced by APDs or drugs, may result in a greater degree of preexcitation (Fig. 10-146). In contrast to A-V and nodofascicular bypass tracts, His bundle stimulation should result in a preexcited QRS with a short H-V interval. Theoretically, if delay occurs in a bundle branch proximal to the takeoff of a fasciculoventricular bypass tract, preexcitation will decrease owing to a greater degree of ventricular activation over the contralateral bundle branch (a situation which I have not encountered). Block of conduction in fasciculoventricular bypass tracts can be observed in response to atrial extrastimuli in which case there will be sudden H-V prolongation (to normal) with loss of preexcitation (Fig. 10-147). Retrograde conduction over the fasciculoventricular bypass tract is usual. Demonstration of retrograde conduction requires para-Hisian and RV apical pacing. Para-Hisian ventricular pacing will have a shorter V-A than RVA pacing with similar H-A. The V-H during para-Hisian RV pacing will have a shorter V-H (10 to 20 msec) than RVA pacing (45 to 70 msec). Few fasciculoventricular bypass tracts have been reported, but to date, none have been incorporated into a circus movement SVT. They appear to be only an electrocardiographic and electrophysiologic curiosity. Even during atrial flutter and fibrillation rapid ventricular responses are not expected in the presence of a normal A-V node proximal to the bypass tract. When tachycardias are observed in the presence of a fasciculoventricular bypass tract, it functions as an innocent bystander. All my patients manifested either A-V nodal reentry or circus movement tachycardia due to a concealed accessory pathway. Thus, because it is not directly responsible for arrhythmias, this form of preexcitation does not require treatment.

## REFERENCES


1. Durrer D, Schuilenburg RM, Wellens HJ. Pre-excitation revisited. *Am J Cardiol* 1970;25(6):690–697.
2. Anderson RH, Becker AE, Brechenmacher C, et al. Ventricular preexcitation. A proposed nomenclature for its substrates. *Eur J Cardiol* 1975;3(1):27–36.
3. Brechenmacher C, Laham J, Iris L, et al. [Histological study of abnormal conduction pathways in the Wolff-Parkinson-White

syndrome and Lown-Ganong-Levine syndrome]. *Arch Mal Coeur Vaiss* 1974;67(5):507–519.
4. Davies MJ. *Pathology of conducting tissue of the heart.* London: Butterworths, 1971.
5. Lev M, Gibson S, Miller RA. Ebstein's disease with Wolff-Parkinson-White syndrome; report of a case with a histopathologic study of possible conduction pathways. *Am Heart J* 1955;49(5):724–741.
6. Truex RC, Bishof JK, Downing DF. Accessory atrioventricular muscle bundles. 2. cardiac conduction system in a human specimen with Wolff-Parkinson-White syndrome. *Anat Rec* 1960;137:417–435.
7. Wood FC, Tasissa G, Butler J, et al. Histologic demonstration of accessory muscular connections between auricle and ventricle in a case of short P-R interval and prolonged QRS complex. *Am Heart J* 1943;25:454.
8. Anderson RH, Bouton J, Burrow CT, et al. Sudden death in infancy: a study of cardiac specialized tissue. *Br Med J* 1974;2(911):135–139.
9. James TN. Morphology of the human atrioventricular node, with remarks pertinent to its electrophysiology. *Am Heart J* 1961;62:756–771.
10. Truex RC, Bishof JK, Hoffman EL. Accessory atrioventricular muscle bundles of the developing human heart. *Anat Rec* 1958;131(1):45–59.
11. Mahaim I. Kent's fibers and the A-V para-specific conduction through the upper connections of the bundle of His-Tawara. *Am Heart J* 1947; 33:651.
12. Lev M, Leffler WB, Langendorf R, et al. Anatomic findings in a case of ventricular pre-excitation (WPW) terminating in complete atrioventricular block. *Circulation* 1966;34(5):718–733.
13. Denes P, Wu D, Dhingra RC, et al. Demonstration of dual A-V nodal pathways in patients with paroxysmal supraventricular tachycardia. *Circulation* 1973;48(3):549–555.
14. Josephson ME, Kastor JA. Supraventricular tachycardia in Lown-Ganong-Levine syndrome: atrionodal versus intranodal reentry. *Am J Cardiol* 1977;40(4):521–527.
15. Bardy GH, German LD, Packer DL, et al. Mechanism of tachycardia using a nodofascicular Mahaim fiber. *Am J Cardiol* 1984;54(8): 1140–1141.
16. Benditt DG, Epstein ML, Benson DW Jr. et al. Dual accessory nodoventricular pathways: role in paroxysmal wide QRS reciprocating tachycardia. *Pacing Clin Electrophysiol* 1983;6(3 Pt 1):577–586.
17. Ellenbogen KA, Ramirez NM, Packer DL, et al. Accessory nodoventricular (Mahaim) fibers: a clinical review. *Pacing Clin Electrophysiol* 1986; 9(6 Pt 1):868–884.
18. Gallagher JJ., Selle JG, Sealy WC, et al. Variants of preexcitation. Update 1989. In: Zipes DP, Jaliffe J, eds. *Cardiac electrophysiology from cell to bedside.* Philadelphia, PA: WB Saunders, 1990.
19. Gallagher JJ, Smith WM, Kasell JH, et al. Role of Mahaim fibers in cardiac arrhythmias in man. *Circulation* 1981;64(1):176–189.
20. Haissaguerre M, Cauchemez B, Marcus F, et al. Characteristics of the ventricular insertion sites of accessory pathways with anterograde decremental conduction properties. *Circulation* 1995;91(4):1077–1085.
21. De la Fuente D, Sasyniuk B, Moe GK. Conduction through a narrow isthmus in isolated canine atrial tissue. A model of the W-P-W syndrome. *Circulation* 1971;44(5):803–809.
22. Klein GJ, Guiraudon GM, Kerr CR, et al. "Nodoventricular" accessory pathway: evidence for a distinct accessory atrioventricular pathway with atrioventricular node-like properties. *J Am Coll Cardiol* 1988; 11(5):1035–1040.
23. Wolferth, CC, Wood F. The mechanism of production of short P-R intervals and prolonged QRS complexes in patients with presumably undamaged hearts: hypothesis of an accessory pathway of auriculo-ventricular conduction (Bundle of Kent). *Am Heart J* 1933;6(3):297–311.
24. Slama R, Coumel P, Bouvrain Y. Type A Wolff-Parkinson-White syndromes, inapparent or latent in sinus rhythm. *Arch Mal Coeur Vaiss* 1973; 66(5):639–653.
25. Chung KY, Walsh TJ, Massie E. Wolff-Parkinson-White syndrome. *Am Heart J* 1965;69:116–133.
26. Garson A Jr., Gillette PC, McNamara DG. Supraventricular tachycardia in children: clinical features, response to treatment, and long-term follow-up in 217 patients. *J Pediatr* 1981;98(6):875–882.
27. Mandel WJ, Laks MM, Fink B, et al. Comparative electrophysiologic features of the WPW syndrome in the pediatric and adult patient. *Am J Cardiol* 1974;33(1):155.
28. Vidaillet HJ Jr., Pressley JC, Henke E, et al. Familial occurrence of accessory atrioventricular pathways (preexcitation syndrome). *N Engl J Med* 1987;317(2):65–69.
29. Chen SA, Chiang CE, Tai CT, et al. Longitudinal clinical and electrophysiological assessment of patients with symptomatic Wolff-Parkinson-White syndrome and atrioventricular node reentrant tachycardia. *Circulation* 1996;93(11):2023–2032.
30. Deal BJ, Keane JF, Gillette PC, et al. Wolff-Parkinson-White syndrome and supraventricular tachycardia during infancy: management and follow-up. *J Am Coll Cardiol* 1985;5(1):130–135.
31. Giardina AC, Ehlers KH, Engle MA. Wolff-Parkinson-White syndrome in infants and children. A long-term follow-up study. *Br Heart J* 1972;34(8):839–846.
32. Gallagher JJ, Pritchett EL, Sealy WC, et al. The preexcitation syndromes. *Prog Cardiovasc Dis* 1978;20(4): 285–327.
33. Josephson ME, Horowitz LN, Kastor JA, et al. Paroxysmal supraventricular tachycardia in patients with mitral valve prolapse. *Circulation* 1978;57(1):111–115.
34. Blair E, Redwood C, Ashrafian H, et al. Mutations in the gamma(2) subunit of AMP-activated protein kinase cause familial hypertrophic cardiomyopathy: evidence for the central role of energy compromise in disease pathogenesis. *Hum Mol Genet* 2001;10(11):1215–1220.
35. Gollob MH, Green MS, Tang AS, et al. Identification of a gene responsible for familial Wolff-Parkinson-White syndrome. *N Engl J Med* 2001; 344(24):1823–1831.
36. Arad M, Moskowitz IP, Patel VV, et al. Transgenic mice overexpressing mutant PRKAG2 define the cause of Wolff-Parkinson-White syndrome in glycogen storage cardiomyopathy. *Circulation* 2003;107(22):2850–2856.
37. Yang Z, McMahon CJ, Smith LR, et al. Danon disease as an underrecognized cause of hypertrophic cardiomyopathy in children. *Circulation* 2005;112(11):1612–1617.
38. Wellens HJ, Brugada P, eds. *Value of programmed stimulation of the heart in patients with the Wolff-Parkinson-White syndrome. Tachycardias: mechanisms and management.* Philadelphia, PA: Lea & Febiger, 1962.
39. Bardy GH, Packer DL, German LD, et al. Preexcited reciprocating tachycardia in patients with Wolff-Parkinson-White syndrome: incidence and mechanisms. *Circulation* 1984;70(3):377–391.
40. Benditt DG, Pritchett EL, Gallagher JJ. Spectrum of regular tachycardias with wide QRS complexes in patients with accessory atrioventricular pathways. *Am J Cardiol* 1978;42(5):828–838.
41. Kuck KH, Brugada P, Wellens HJ., et al. Observations on the antidromic type of circus movement tachycardia in the Wolff-Parkinson-White syndrome. *J Am Coll Cardiol* 1983;2(5):1003–1010.
42. Wellens HJ, Josephson ME, eds. *Preexcited tachycardias. Tachycardias: mechanisms and management.* Mount Kisco, NY: Futura Publishing, 1993.
43. Cosio FG, Benson DW Jr, Anderson RW, et al. Onset of atrial fibrillation during antidromic tachycardia: association with sudden cardiac arrest and ventricular fibrillation in a patient with Wolff-Parkinson-White syndrome. *Am J Cardiol* 1982;50(2):353–359.
44. Klein GJ, Bashore TM, Sellers TD, et al. Ventricular fibrillation in the Wolff-Parkinson-White syndrome. *N Engl J Med* 1979;301(20):1080–1085.
45. Della Bella P, Brugada P, Talajic M, et al. Atrial fibrillation in patients with an accessory pathway: importance of the conduction properties of the accessory pathway. *J Am Coll Cardiol* 1991;17(6):1352–1356.
46. Haissaguerre M, Fischer B, Labbé T,, et al. Frequency of recurrent atrial fibrillation after catheter ablation of overt accessory pathways. *Am J Cardiol* 1992;69(5):493–497.
47. Munger TM, Packer DL, Hammill SC, et al. A population study of the natural history of Wolff-Parkinson-White syndrome in Olmsted County, Minnesota, 1953–1989. *Circulation* 1993;87(3):866–873.
48. Gillette PC, Garson A Jr, Cooley DA, et al. Prolonged and decremental antegrade conduction properties in right anterior accessory connections: Wide QRS antidromic tachycardia of left bundle branch block pattern without Wolff-Parkinson-White configuration in sinus rhythm. *Am Heart J* 1982;103(1):66–74.
49. Tchou P, Lehmann MH, Jazayeri M, et al. Atriofascicular connection or a nodoventricular Mahaim fiber? Electrophysiologic elucidation of the pathway and associated reentrant circuit. *Circulation* 1988;77(4):837–848.
50. Lerman BB, Josephson ME. Automaticity of the Kent bundle: confirmation by phase 3 and phase 4 block. *J Am Coll Cardiol* 1985;5(4):996–998.
51. Pick A, Katz LN. Disturbances of impulse formation and conduction in the preexcitation (WPW) syndrome; their bearing on its mechanism. *Am J Med* 1955;19(5):759–772.

52. Przybylski J, Chiale PA, Halpern MS, et al. Existence of automaticity in anomalous bundle of Wolff-Parkinson-White syndrome. *Br Heart J* 1978;40(6):672–680.
53. Chang MS, Miles WM, Prystowsky EN., et al. Supernormal conduction in accessory atrioventricular connections. *Am J Cardiol* 1987;59(8):852–856.
54. Przybylski J, Chiale PA, Sánchez RA, et al. Supernormal conduction in the accessory pathway of patients with overt or concealed ventricular pre-excitation. *J Am Coll Cardiol* 1987;9(6):1269–1278.
55. Klein GJ, Yee R, Sharma AD. Concealed conduction in accessory atrioventricular pathways: an important determinant of the expression of arrhythmias in patients with Wolff-Parkinson-White syndrome. *Circulation* 1984;70(3):402–411.
56. Prystowsky EN, Pritchett EL, Gallagher JJ. Concealed conduction preventing anterograde preexcitation in Wolff-Parkinson-White syndrome. *Am J Cardiol* 1984;53(7):960–961.
57. Svinarich JT, Tai DY, Mickelson J, et al. Electrophysiologic demonstration of concealed conduction in anomalous atrioventricular bypass tracts. *J Am Coll Cardiol* 1985;5(4):898–903.
58. Klein GJ, Gulamhusein SS. Intermittent preexcitation in the Wolff-Parkinson-White syndrome. *Am J Cardiol* 1983;52(3):292–296.
59. Easley AR Jr., Sensecqua JE, Mann DE, et al. Intermittent preexcitation: marked enhancement of anterograde conduction in the atrioventricular accessory pathway with isoproterenol. *Pacing Clin Electrophysiol* 1988; 11(3):349–354.
60. Hammill SC, Pritchett EL, Klein GJ, et al. Accessory atrioventricular pathways that conduct only in the antegrade direction. *Circulation* 1980;62(6):1335–1340.
61. Klein GJ, Gula LJ, Krahn AD, et al. WPW pattern in the asymptomatic individual: has anything changed? *Circ Arrhythm Electrophysiol* 2009;2(2):97–99.
62. Perry JC, Garson A Jr. Supraventricular tachycardia due to Wolff-Parkinson-White syndrome in children: early disappearance and late recurrence. *J Am Coll Cardiol* 1990;16(5):1215–1220.
63. Josephson ME, Seides SF, Damato AN. Wolff-Parkinson-White syndrome with 1:2 atrioventricular conduction. *Am J Cardiol* 1976;37(7):1094–1096.
64. Milstein S, Sharma AD, Klein GJ. Electrophysiologic profile of asymptomatic Wolff-Parkinson-White pattern. *Am J Cardiol* 1986;57(13): 1097–1100.
65. Rinne C, Klein GJ, Sharma AD, et al. Relation between clinical presentation and induced arrhythmias in the Wolff-Parkinson-White syndrome. *Am J Cardiol* 1987;60(7):576–579.
66. Akhtar M, Shenasa M, Schmidt DH. Role of retrograde His Purkinje block in the initiation of supraventricular tachycardia by ventricular premature stimulation in the Wolff-Parkinson-White syndrome. *J Clin Invest* 1981;67(4):1047–1055.
67. Wellens HJ, Durrer D. Patterns of ventriculo-atrial conduction in the Wolff-Parkinson-White syndrome. *Circulation* 1974;49(1):22–31.
68. Brugada P, Bar FW, Vanagt EJ, et al. Observations on mechanisms of circus movement tachycardia in the Wolff-Parkinson-White syndrome. Role of different tachycardia circuits and sites of block in maintenance of tachycardia. *Pacing Clin Electrophysiol* 1981;4(5):507–516.
69. Lehmann MH, Tchou P, Mahmud R, et al. Electrophysiological determinants of antidromic reentry induced during atrial extrastimulation. Insights from a pacing model of Wolff-Parkinson-White syndrome. *Circ Res* 1989;65(2):295–306.
70. Packer DL, Gallagher JJ, Prystowsky EN. Physiological substrate for antidromic reciprocating tachycardia. Prerequisite characteristics of the accessory pathway and atrioventricular conduction system. *Circulation* 1992;85(2):574–588.
71. Hurwitz JL, Miller JM, Josephson ME. The value of the HA interval in diagnosing preexcited tachycardias due to AV nodal reentry. *J Am Coll Cardiol* 1991;17:323A.
72. Bauernfeind RA, Wyndham CR, Swiryn SP, et al. Paroxysmal atrial fibrillation in the Wolff-Parkinson-White syndrome. *Am J Cardiol* 1981; 47(3):562–569.
73. Campbell RW, Smith RA, Gallagher JJ, et al. Atrial fibrillation in the preexcitation syndrome. *Am J Cardiol* 1977;40(4):514–520.
74. Sung RJ, Castellanos A, Mallon SM, et al. Mechanisms of spontaneous alternation between reciprocating tachycardia and atrial flutter-fibrillation in the Wolff-Parkinson-White syndrome. *Circulation* 1977;56(3):409–416.
75. Wathen M, Natale A, Wolfe K, et al. Initiation of atrial fibrillation in the Wolff-Parkinson-White syndrome: the importance of the accessory pathway. *Am Heart J* 1993;125(3):753–759.
76. Rosenbaum F, Lee CW, Hong MK, et al. The potential variations of the thorax and the esophagus in anomalous atrioventricular excitation (Wolff-Parkinson-White syndrome). *Am Heart J* 1945;29:281.
77. Tonkin AM, Wagner GS, Gallagher JJ, et al. Initial forces of ventricular depolarization in the Wolff-Parkinson-White Syndrome. Analysis based upon localization of the accessory pathway by epicardial mapping. *Circulation* 1975;52(6):1030–1036.
78. Arruda MS, Smith WM, Ideker RE, et al. Development and validation of an ECG algorithm for identifying accessory pathway ablation site in Wolff-Parkinson-White syndrome. *J Cardiovasc Electrophysiol* 1998;9(1):2–12.
79. Chiang CE, Chen SA, Teo WS, et al. An accurate stepwise electrocardiographic algorithm for localization of accessory pathways in patients with Wolff-Parkinson-White syndrome from a comprehensive analysis of delta waves and R/S ratio during sinus rhythm. *Am J Cardiol* 1995;76(1):40–46.
80. Fitzpatrick AP, Gonzales RP, Lesh MD, et al. New algorithm for the localization of accessory atrioventricular connections using a baseline electrocardiogram. *J Am Coll Cardiol* 1994;23(1):107–116.
81. Tai CT, Chen SA, Chiang CE, et al. Electrocardiographic and electrophysiologic characteristics of anteroseptal, midseptal, and para-Hisian accessory pathways. Implication for radiofrequency catheter ablation. *Chest* 1996;109(3):730–740.
82. Takahashi A, Shah DC, Jaïs P, et al. Specific electrocardiographic features of manifest coronary vein posteroseptal accessory pathways. *J Cardiovasc Electrophysiol* 1998;9(10):1015–1025.
83. Haissaguerre M, Marcus F, Poquet F, et al. Electrocardiographic characteristics and catheter ablation of parahissian accessory pathways. *Circulation* 1994;90(3):1124–1128.
84. Lindsay BD, Crossen KJ, Cain ME. Concordance of distinguishing electrocardiographic features during sinus rhythm with the location of accessory pathways in the Wolff-Parkinson-White syndrome. *Am J Cardiol* 1987;59(12):1093–1102.
85. Milstein S, Sharma AD, Guiraudon GM, et al. An algorithm for the electrocardiographic localization of accessory pathways in the Wolff-Parkinson-White syndrome. *Pacing Clin Electrophysiol* 1987;10(3 Pt 1): 555–563.
86. Guiraudon GM, Klein GJ, Sharma AD, et al. Surgery for Wolff-Parkinson-White syndrome: further experience with an epicardial approach. *Circulation* 1986;74(3):525–529.
87. Wu DL, Yeh SJ, Yamamoto T, et al. Participation of a concealed nodoventricular fiber in the genesis of paroxysmal tachycardias. *Am Heart J* 1990;119(3 Pt 1):583–591.
88. Denes P, Wyndham CR, Amat-y-Leon F, et al. Atrial pacing at multiple sites in the Wolff-Parkinson-White syndrome. *Br Heart J* 1977; 39(5):506–514.
89. Josephson ME, Scharf DL, Kastor JA, et al. Atrial endocardial activation in man. Electrode catheter technique of endocardial mapping. *Am J Cardiol* 1977;39(7):972–981.
90. Wellens HJ, Durrer D. The role of an accessory atrioventricular pathway in reciprocal tachycardia. Observations in patients with and without the Wolff-Parkinson-White syndrome. *Circulation* 1975;52(1):58–72.
91. Antz M, Otomo K, Arruda M, et al. Electrical conduction between the right atrium and the left atrium via the musculature of the coronary sinus. *Circulation* 1998;98(17):1790–1795.
92. Anselme F, Hook B, Monahan K, et al. Heterogeneity of retrograde fast-pathway conduction pattern in patients with atrioventricular nodal reentry tachycardia: observations by simultaneous multisite catheter mapping of Koch's triangle. *Circulation* 1996;93(5):960–968.
93. Anselme F, Papageorgiou P, Monahan K, et al. Presence and significance of the left atrionodal connection during atrioventricular nodal reentrant tachycardia. *Am J Cardiol* 1999;83(11):1530–1536.
94. Amat-y-Leon F, Dhingra RC, Wu D, et al. Catheter mapping of retrograde atrial activation. Observations during ventricular pacing and AV nodal re-entrant paroxysmal tachycardia. *Br Heart J* 1976;38(4):355–362.
95. Miller JM, Rosenthal ME, Gottlieb CD, et al. A new criterion reliably distinguishes atrioventricular nodal reentrant from septal bypass tract tachycardias. *J Am Coll Cardiol* 1987;9:12A.
96. Yamanouchi Y, Igawa O, Hisatome I., et al. Activation mapping from the coronary sinus may be limited by anatomic variations. *Pacing Clin Electrophysiol* 1998;21(11 Pt 2):2522–2526.
97. Benditt DG, Pritchett EL, Smith WM, et al. Ventriculoatrial intervals: diagnostic use in paroxysmal supraventricular tachycardia. *Ann Intern Med* 1979;91(2):161–166.

98. Hirao K, Otomo K, Wang X, et al. Para-Hisian pacing. A new method for differentiating retrograde conduction over an accessory AV pathway from conduction over the AV node. *Circulation* 1996;94(5):1027–1035.
99. Farre J., et al. *Atrial unipolar waveform analysis during retrograde conduction over left-sided accessory atrioventricular pathways. Cardiac arrhythmias: where to go from here?* Mount Kisco, NY, Futura Publishing 1987.
100. Coumel P, Attuel P. Reciprocating tachycardia in overt and latent preexcitation. Influence of functional bundle branch block on the rate of the tachycardia. *Eur J Cardiol* 1974;1:423.
101. Kerr CR, Gallagher JJ, German LD. Changes in ventriculoatrial intervals with bundle branch block aberration during reciprocating tachycardia in patients with accessory atrioventricular pathways. *Circulation* 1982;66(1):196–201.
102. Neuss H, Schlepper M, Thormann J. Analysis of re-entry mechanisms in the three patients with concealed Wolff-Parkinson-White syndrome. *Circulation* 1975;51(1):75–81.
103. Pritchett EL, Tonkin AM, Dugan FA, et al. Ventriculo-atrial conduction time during reciprocating tachycardia with intermittent bundle-branch block in Wolff-Parkinson-White syndrome. *Br Heart J* 1976; 38(10):1058–1064.
104. Zipes DP, DeJoseph RL, Rothbaum DA. Unusual properties of accessory pathways. *Circulation* 1974;49(6):1200–1211.
105. Jazayeri MR, Caceres J, Tchou P, et al. Electrophysiologic characteristics of sudden QRS axis deviation during orthodromic tachycardia. Role of functional fascicular block in localization of accessory pathway. *J Clin Invest* 1989;83(3):952–959.
106. Jackman WM, Friday KJ, Scherlag BJ, et al. Direct endocardial recording from an accessory atrioventricular pathway: localization of the site of block, effect of antiarrhythmic drugs, and attempt at nonsurgical ablation. *Circulation* 1983;68(5):906–916.
107. Jackman WM, Friday KJ, Yeung-Lai-Wah JA, et al. New catheter technique for recording left free-wall accessory atrioventricular pathway activation. Identification of pathway fiber orientation. *Circulation* 1988; 78(3):598–611.
108. Kuck KH, Geiger M. Accessory pathway conduction block: concordance of spontaneous, stimulation-induced and drug-induced site of block. *Circulation* 1987;76(Suppl 4):136.
109. O'Callaghan WG, Colavita PG, Kay GN, et al. Characterization of retrograde conduction by direct endocardial recording from an accessory atrioventricular pathway. *J Am Coll Cardiol* 1986;7(1): 167–171.
110. Niebauer MJ, Daoud E, Goyal R, et al. Assessment of pacing maneuvers used to validate anterograde accessory pathway potentials. *J Cardiovasc Electrophysiol* 1995;6(5):350–356.
111. Sellers TD Jr., Gallagher JJ, Cope GD, et al. Retrograde atrial preexcitation following premature ventricular beats during reciprocating tachycardia in the Wolff-Parkinson-White syndrome. *Eur J Cardiol* 1976; 4(3):283–294.
112. Benditt DG, Benson DW Jr, Dunnigan A, et al. Role of extrastimulus site and tachycardia cycle length in inducibility of atrial preexcitation by premature ventricular stimulation during reciprocating tachycardia. *Am J Cardiol* 1987;60(10):811–819.
113. Ong JJ, Kriett JM, Feld GK, et al. Prevalence of retrograde accessory pathway conduction during atrial fibrillation. *J Cardiovasc Electrophysiol* 1997;8(4):377–387.
114. Wellens HJ, Durrer D. Wolff-Parkinson-White syndrome and atrial fibrillation. Relation between refractory period of accessory pathway and ventricular rate during atrial fibrillation. *Am J Cardiol* 1974;34(7):777–782.
115. Brugada P, Dassen WR, Braat S, et al. Value of the ajmaline-procainamide test to predict the effect of long-term oral amiodarone on the anterograde effective refractory period of the accessory pathway in the Wolff-Parkinson-White syndrome. *Am J Cardiol* 1983;52(1):70–72.
116. Wellens HJ, Bär FW, Gorgels AP, et al. Use of ajmaline in patients with the Wolff-Parkinson-White syndrome to disclose short refractory period of the accessory pathway. *Am J Cardiol* 1980;45(1):130–133.
117. Wellens HJ, Braat S, Brugada P, et al. Use of procainamide in patients with the Wolff-Parkinson-White syndrome to disclose a short refractory period of the accessory pathway. *Am J Cardiol* 1982;50(5):1087–1089.
118. Levy S, Broustet JP. Exercise testing in the Wolff-Parkinson-White syndrome. *Am J Cardiol* 1981;48(5):976–977.
119. Levy S, et al. *Value of noninvasive techniques in the Wolff-Parkinson-White syndrome with particular reference to exercise testing. Cardiac arrhythmias: from diagnosis to therapy.* Mount Kisco, NY, Futura Publishing, 1984.
120. Strasberg B, Ashley WW, Wyndham CR, et al. Treadmill exercise testing in the Wolff-Parkinson-White syndrome. *Am J Cardiol* 1980;45(4):742–748.
121. Critelli G, Gallagher JJ, Perticone F, et al. Evaluation of noninvasive tests for identifying patients with preexcitation syndrome at risk of rapid ventricular response. *Am Heart J* 1984;108(4 Pt 1):905–909.
122. Wellens HJ, Bär FW, Dassen WR, et al. Effect of drugs in the Wolff-Parkinson-White syndrome. Importance of initial length of effective refractory period of the accessory pathway. *Am J Cardiol* 1980;46(4):665–669.
123. Fananapazir L, Packer DL, German LD, et al. Procainamide infusion test: inability to identify patients with Wolff-Parkinson-White syndrome who are potentially at risk of sudden death. *Circulation* 1988; 77(6):1291–1296.
124. Wellens HJ, Brugada P, Roy D, et al. Effect of isoproterenol on the anterograde refractory period of the accessory pathway in patients with the Wolff-Parkinson-White syndrome. *Am J Cardiol* 1982;50(1):180–184.
125. Tonkin AM, Miller HC, Svenson RH, et al. Refractory periods of the accessory pathway in the Wolff-Parkinson-White syndrome. *Circulation* 1975;52(4):563–569.
126. Yee R, Klein GJ. Syncope in the Wolff-Parkinson-White syndrome: incidence and electrophysiologic correlates. *Pacing Clin Electrophysiol* 1984;7(3 Pt 1):381–388.
127. Saoudi NC, Castellanos A, Zaman L, et al. Attempted entrainment of circus movement tachycardias by ventricular stimulation. *Pacing Clin Electrophysiol* 1986;9(1 Pt 1):78–90.
128. Waldo AL, Plumb VJ, Arciniegas JG, et al. Transient entrainment and interruption of the atrioventricular bypass pathway type of paroxysmal atrial tachycardia. A model for understanding and identifying reentrant arrhythmias. *Circulation* 1983;67(1):73–83.
129. Castellanos A, Agha AS, Befeler B, et al. Double accessory pathways in Wolff-Parkinson-White syndrome. *Circulation* 1975;51(6):1020–1025.
130. Denes P, Amat-Y-Leon F, Wyndham C, et al. Electrophysiologic demonstration of bilateral anomalous pathways in a patient with Wolff-Parkinson-White syndrome (type B preexcitation). *Am J Cardiol* 1976; 37(1):93–101.
131. Heddle WF, Brugada P, Wellens HJ. Multiple circus movement tachycardias with multiple accessory pathways. *J Am Coll Cardiol* 1984;4(1):168–175.
132. Josephson ME, Caracta AR, Lau SH. Alternating type A and type B Wolff-Parkinson-White syndrome. *Am Heart J* 1974;87(3):363–366.
133. Portillo B, Portillo-Leon N, Zaman L, et al. Quintuple pathways participating in three distinct types of atrioventricular reciprocating tachycardia in a patient with Wolff-Parkinson-White syndrome. *Am J Cardiol* 1982; 50(2):347–352.
134. Gallagher JJ, Sealy WC, Kasell J, et al. Multiple accessory pathways in patients with the pre-excitation syndrome. *Circulation* 1976;54(4): 571–591.
135. Lown B, Ganong WF, Levine SA. The syndrome of short P-R interval, normal QRS complex and paroxysmal rapid heart action. *Circulation* 1952;5(5):693–706.
136. Benditt DG, Pritchett LC, Smith WM, et al. Characteristics of atrioventricular conduction and the spectrum of arrhythmias in Lown-Ganong-Levine syndrome. *Circulation* 1978;57(3):454–465.
137. Caracta AR, Damato AN, Gallagher JJ, et al. Electrophysiologic studies in the syndrome of short P-R interval, normal QRS complex. *Am J Cardiol* 1973;31(2):245–253.
138. Castellanos A Jr., Castillo CA, Agha AS, et al. His bundle electrograms in patients with short P-R intervals, narrow QRS complexes, and paroxysmal tachycardias. *Circulation* 1971;43(5):667–678.
139. Castellanos A, Zaman L, Moleiro F, et al. The Lown-Ganong-Levine syndrome. *Pacing Clin Electrophysiol* 1982;5(5):715–740.
140. Coumel P, Waynberger M, Slama R, et al. The short P-R syndrome with normal QRS complex. Electrocardiographic peculiarities. *Arch Mal Coeur Vaiss* 1972;65(2):161–181.
141. Moleiro F, Mendoza IJ, Medina-Ravell V, et al. One to one atrioventricular conduction during atrial pacing at rates of 300/minute in absence of Wolff-Parkinson-White Syndrome. *Am J Cardiol* 1981;48(4):789–796.
142. Castellanos A, Zaman L, Luceri R, et al. Arrhythmias in patients with short PR intervals and narrow QRS complexes. In: Josephson ME, Wellen HJJ, eds.*Tachycardias: mechanisms and management.* Philadelphia, Lea & Febiger, 1984:171.
143. Bauernfeind RA, Swiryn S, Strasberg B, et al. Analysis of anterograde and retrograde fast pathway properties in patients with dual atrioventricular

nodal pathways: observations regarding the pathophysiology of the Lown-Ganong-Levine syndrome. *Am J Cardiol* 1982;49(2):283–290.
144. Iannone LA. Electrophysiology of atrial pacing in patients with short PR interval, normal QRS complex. *Am Heart J* 1975;89(1):74–78.
145. Benditt DG, Klein GJ, Kriett JM, et al. Enhanced atrioventricular nodal conduction in man: electrophysiologic effects of pharmacologic autonomic blockade. *Circulation* 1984;69(6):1088–1095.
146. Bauernfeind RA, Ayres BF, Wyndham CC, et al. Cycle length in atrioventricular nodal reentrant paroxysmal tachycardia with observations on the Lown-Ganong-Levine syndrome. *Am J Cardiol* 1980;45(6):1148–1153.
147. Milstein S, Klein GJ, Rattes MF, et al. Comparison of the ventricular response during atrial fibrillation in patients with enhanced atrioventricular node conduction and Wolff-Parkinson-White syndrome. *J Am Coll Cardiol* 1987;10(6):1244–1248.
148. Mahaim I, Benatt A. Nouvelles recherches sur les connections supericures de la branche du faisceau de His-Tawara avec cloison interventriculaire. *Cardiologia* 1937;1:61–102.
149. Klein LS, Hackett FK, Zipes DP, et al. Radiofrequency catheter ablation of Mahaim fibers at the tricuspid annulus. *Circulation* 1993;87(3):738–747.
150. McClelland JH, Wang X, Beckman KJ, et al. Radiofrequency catheter ablation of right atriofascicular (Mahaim) accessory pathways guided by accessory pathway activation potentials. *Circulation* 1994;89(6):2655–2666.
151. Lerman BB, Waxman HL, Proclemer A, et al. Supraventricular tachycardia associated with nodoventricular and concealed atrioventricular bypass tracts. *Am Heart J* 1982;104(5 Pt 1):1097–1102.
152. Sternick EB, Timmermans C, Sosa E, et al. The electrocardiogram during sinus rhythm and tachycardia in patients with Mahaim fibers: the importance of an "rS" pattern in lead III. *J Am Coll Cardiol* 2004;44(8):1626–1635.
153. Haissaguerre M, Warin JF, Le Metayer P, et al. Catheter ablation of Mahaim fibers with preservation of atrioventricular nodal conduction. *Circulation* 1990;82(2):418–427.
154. Sternick EB, Rodriguez LM, Gerken LM, et al. Electrocardiogram in patients with fasciculoventricular pathways: a comparative study with anteroseptal and midseptal accessory pathways. *Heart Rhythm* 2005;2(1):1–6.
155. Grogin HR, Lee RJ, Kwasman M, et al. Radiofrequency catheter ablation of atriofascicular and nodoventricular Mahaim tracts. *Circulation* 1994;90(1):272–281.
156. Haissaguerre M, Campos J, Marcus FI, et al. Involvement of a nodofascicular connection in supraventricular tachycardia with VA dissociation. *J Cardiovasc Electrophysiol* 1994;5(10):854–862.
157. Mark AL, Basta LL. Paroxysmal tachycardia with atrioventricular dissociation in a patient with a variant of pre-excitation syndrome. *J Electrocardiol* 1974;7(4):355–364.
158. Morady F, Scheinman MM, Gonzalez R, et al. His-ventricular dissociation in a patient with reciprocating tachycardia and a nodoventricular bypass tract. *Circulation* 1981;64(4):839–844.
159. Gandhavadi M, Sternick EB, Jackman WM, et al. Characterization of the distal insertion of atriofascicular accessory pathways and mechanisms of QRS patterns in atriofascicular antidromic tachycardia. *Heart Rhythm* 2013;10(9):1385–1392.
160. Murdock CJ, Leitch JW, Klein GJ, et al. Epicardial mapping in patients with "nodoventricular" accessory pathways. *Am J Cardiol* 1991;68(2):208–214.
161. Ganz LI, Elson JJ, Chenarides JG. Preexcitation in a child with syncope: where is the connection? *J Cardiovasc Electrophysiol* 1998;9(8):892–895.

CHAPTER

11

# Recurrent Ventricular Tachycardia

This chapter will be divided into discrete sections: (a) definitions; (b) pathophysiologic substrates and mechanisms of tachycardias; and (c) electrophysiologic studies (EPS)—modes of initiation, response to stimulation, effects of drugs, and localizing the origin of ventricular tachycardia (VT). VTs encompass a spectrum of arrhythmias that range from nonsustained, asymptomatic VT to sustained arrhythmias, which can produce hemodynamic compromise and cardiac arrest. These tachycardias may be uniform in morphology (i.e., monomorphic) or polymorphic. VT most often occurs in the setting of some form of cardiac disease. Although chronic ischemic heart disease, especially that associated with prior infarction and aneurysm formation, is the most common cardiac disorder associated with VT (particularly sustained, monomorphic VT), these arrhythmias can occur in patients with a variety of disorders, such as cardiomyopathy, congenital and valvular heart disease, drug toxicity, metabolic disorders, long QT interval syndromes, or even in structurally normal hearts. In contrast to patients with monomorphic sustained VT, which is primarily associated with coronary artery disease (≈90%), patients presenting with nonsustained arrhythmias (monomorphic or polymorphic) and cardiac arrest are more heterogeneous groups. Occasionally, any of these forms of VT can occur in patients with normal hearts.

Sustained monomorphic VT can be characterized by electrophysiologic techniques. The results of electrophysiologic testing in patients with nonsustained VT, polymorphic VT, and status post cardiac arrest are more difficult to interpret. In patients with coronary artery disease, particularly when associated with prior infarction, most VTs, regardless of the duration or morphology, appear to have a similar pathophysiologic substrate, and probably a similar mechanism. The evidence supporting this includes the ability to change either nonsustained monomorphic VT or polymorphic VT into sustained uniform VT by different modes of programmed stimulation and/or by the addition of drugs that slow conduction. These and other observations concerning mechanism are discussed in detail later in this chapter.

Over the past four decades, electrophysiologic studies have been responsible for a greater understanding of ventricular arrhythmias. This has led to major advances in their pharmacologic and nonpharmacologic therapy. The present chapter discusses the methods of studying ventricular arrhythmias.

Much of this chapter concentrates on electrophysiologic studies of sustained monomorphic VT. In addition, the application of electrophysiologic studies to patients who present with nonsustained VT or cardiac arrest is addressed. It is imperative that clinicians and clinical investigators recognize that the study of ventricular arrhythmias is still evolving. The clinical application of electrophysiologic studies has been established only for ventricular arrhythmias in patients with chronic ischemic heart disease and for those patients with nonsustained and sustained monomorphic VTs in the absence of coronary artery disease. The role of electrophysiologic studies in evaluating nonsustained and/or polymorphic arrhythmias associated with metabolic disorders, drug toxicity, cardiomyopathy, and so on is not yet established. A discussion of our current level of understanding of this issue is included and detailed later.

The expanded use of implantable cardioverter-defibrillators (ICDs) based on ejection fraction alone and the invasive nature of EPS is responsible for the apparent diminished interest in trying to understand the underlying mechanisms of ventricular arrhythmias.

The principal goals of the electrophysiologic study in the evaluation of VT are (a) confirming the diagnosis of VT, (b) defining the mechanism of arrhythmia, (c) localizing the site of origin, and (d) evaluating the efficacy of pharmacologic or nonpharmacologic (pacemaker, defibrillator, or ablation by either catheter or surgery) therapeutic methods. In this chapter we deal with the first three goals. The last goal is discussed in subsequent chapters.

## DEFINITIONS OF VENTRICULAR TACHYCARDIAS

The definitions employed by electrophysiology laboratories are arbitrary but provide a useful framework for both the clinician and the electrophysiologist to distinguish "pathologic" responses from "normal" expected responses.[1–3]

### Morphology

Monomorphic VT has a single, stable QRS morphology. Polymorphic or multiform VT has a changing QRS morphology. How often the complexes must change to qualify as polymorphic is unsettled. For practical purposes, we consider a tachycardia polymorphic if it has no constant morphology for more than five complexes, has no clear isoelectric baseline, or has QRS complexes that are asynchronous in multiple simultaneously recorded leads. Polymorphic VT may be seen with long or normal QT intervals. The term torsade de pointes was originally meant to be employed for a clinical syndrome that includes polymorphic tachycardia and long QT intervals, due to reversible causes such as hypokalemia, bradycardia, or drug toxicity.[4,5] These arrhythmias must be distinguished from polymorphic tachycardias with normal QT intervals and those associated with hereditary long QT intervals. Regardless of the cause, polymorphic VT frequently degenerates into ventricular fibrillation (VF). Rapid sustained monomorphic VT can also degenerate into VF, frequently following a stage of polymorphic tachycardia. This is a fairly common mechanism of sudden cardiac death recorded by Holter monitor.[6–8] This observation suggests a link between monomorphic sustained VT and VF and provides a rationale for using suppression of induced VT as a goal for therapy in patients with cardiac arrest (see Chapter 12).

### Duration

Most laboratories consider a tachycardia sustained if it lasts ≥30 seconds. Because many tachycardias require therapy before 30 seconds, some investigators have used 15 seconds as the duration required for a "sustained" VT. In point of fact, most tachycardias that last 15 seconds continue for 30 seconds. The requirement of a specified duration has practical significance with the development of ICDs, which can be programmed to deliver antitachycardia pacing (ATP), cardioversion, or defibrillation based on the duration of VT.

The number of complexes required to define a clinically relevant induced nonsustained VT is not established. Three consecutive complexes at a rate greater than 100 is sufficient for the diagnosis of a nonsustained VT noted on Holter monitor or on standard ECG. In the electrophysiology laboratory, we require five or six consecutive, nonbundle branch reentrant complexes, regardless of morphology, to qualify as a nonsustained VT. The frequency (≈50%) of bundle branch reentry in normal subjects in response to a single programmed ventricular extrastimulus (VES) (see Chapter 2) mandates our discounting such complexes. These bundle branch reentrant complexes have no relevance to clinical nonsustained VT. Repetitive polymorphic responses are also very common (up to 50%), particularly when multiple (≥3) extrastimuli are used with extremely short coupling intervals (<180 msec). The clinical significance of induced nonsustained polymorphic tachycardia is questionable and requires further evaluation to determine its relevance (to be discussed in subsequent paragraphs).

### Classification of Ventricular Tachycardia QRS Complexes

Monomorphic VT is usually classified as having either an LBBB or RBBB pattern based on a QRS morphology in lead $V_1$.[9,10] Left bundle branch block (LBBB) morphologies include a QS, rS, or a qrS in $V_1$. RBBB patterns are defined by rsR′, qR, RR′, RS, or monophasic R waves in $V_1$.[9,10] The clinical significance and results of electrophysiologic evaluations for these tachycardias are discussed in subsequent paragraphs. Patients may have more than one monomorphic VT, which can evolve one from the other or can occur individually at separate times.

## DIAGNOSIS OF VENTRICULAR TACHYCARDIA

Several electrocardiographic observations have been proposed as diagnostic of VT. These have been recently reviewed by Miller et al.[11] These include (1) QRS complexes exceeding 0.14 seconds in duration for RBBB VTs and 0.16 seconds for LBBB VTs in the absence of drugs, (2) a superior frontal plane QRS axis in RBBB VTs and a right inferior axis in LBBB VTs, (3) evidence of atrioventricular (A-V) dissociation, and (4) specific morphologic features of the QRS (Table 11-1).[12–14] Recently Vereckei et al.[15] have evaluated the use of aVR as a single lead for VT diagnosis. They reported good sensitivity and specificity, but I have not found it significantly better than $V_{1-2}$ criteria. Although all of these criteria have limitations, the presence of any of these criteria can correctly identify VT in more than 90% of the patients. Morphologic criteria are particularly important in the diagnosis of rapid VT (>180 bpm), as A-V dissociation, fusion complexes, or sinus captures are often absent.

With the use of intracardiac recording techniques, it has become clear that most of the preceding electrocardiographic features are not pathognomonic of VT. VT can be relatively narrow (even narrower than the sinus complex), and in ≈5% of VT the QRS may be <120 msec. Furthermore, A-V dissociation can be seen with supraventricular rhythms, fusion complexes can result from two ventricular ectopic foci, and morphologic and/or axis characteristics established for patients with normal

**TABLE 11-1 Characteristics of Wide Complex Tachycardia Favoring Diagnosis of VT**

- QRS complexes >0.14 s for RBBB and >0.16 s for LBBB tachycardias (in the absence of antiarrhythmic drugs)
- A superior frontal plane axis for RBBB, and a right inferior axis in LBBB tachycardias
- Evidence of A-V dissociation (fusion complexes, capture beats)
- Morphologic criteria, focusing on ECG leads $V_{1-2}$ and $V_6$
  - RBBB: monophasic R, qR, Rr′, and RS in V1 and RS ratio <1 in $V_6$
  - LBBB: initial r wave ≥0.04 s or an interval of ≥0.07 s from the QRS onset to the nadir of the S wave in $V_{1-2}$, notching of the down stroke of the S wave in $V_{1-2}$, or an initial q wave in $V_6$

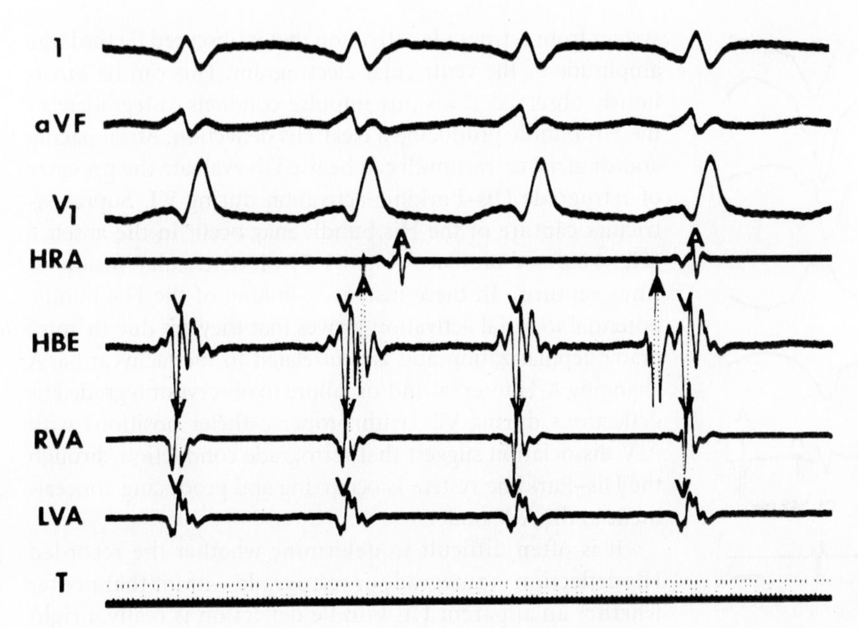


**FIGURE 11-1** Intracardiac recording during ventricular tachycardia. From **top** to **bottom:** ECG leads 1, aVF, and $V_1$, and electrograms from the high-right atrium (HRA), His bundle region (HBE), right ventricular apex (RVA), and left ventricular apex (LVA). T, time line. Note the absence of His bundle deflections and variable retrograde conduction. (From Josephson ME, Horowitz LN, Farshidi A, et al. Recurrent sustained ventricular tachycardia. 2. Endocardial mapping. *Circulation* 1978;57:440.)

QRS complexes in sinus rhythm are less specific in the presence of underlying conduction disturbances (≥30% of patients with VT and coronary artery disease). In such instances, intracardiac recording and stimulation techniques may be the only method by which the diagnosis of VT can be established definitively. Although some investigators have advocated the use of adenosine to facilitate the diagnosis of VT versus SVT, I strongly disagree. Because of the possibility of adenosine producing a coronary steal syndrome, which can cause VT to degenerate to VF, I do not believe adenosine should be given in the absence of the knowledge of the coronary anatomy.

## Use of His Bundle Recordings in Diagnosing Ventricular Tachycardia

The ability to directly record His bundle activity has permitted more precise differentiation of those events occurring proximal rather than distal to the His bundle. In the absence of pre-excitation a supraventricular impulse must pass through the His bundle and the specialized ventricular conducting system before initiating depolarization of the ventricles. This produces the normal H-V interval of 35 to 55 msec. It seems reasonable, therefore, to use the relationship of the His bundle deflection to the QRS as an immediate clue to the diagnosis of VT.

During VT, in many patients, no consistent His bundle deflections are noted (Fig. 11-1). This may result because no engagement of the His–Purkinje system by the ventricular impulse occurs (probably uncommon), or because retrograde His bundle activation occurs during ventricular activation and is obscured by the large ventricular deflection in the His bundle recording. His deflections can usually be observed if attention is given to catheter position. One may identify His bundle activity before ventricular activation (in this instance, the H-V interval is shorter than normal; e.g., 20 msec), or just after the onset of ventricular depolarization to produce a short V-H interval (Fig. 11-2). His potentials may also be seen in the terminal part of the QRS or following the QRS complex (Fig. 11-3). Intermittent conduction to the His bundle usually has a 2:1 pattern (Fig. 11-4), but Wenckebach patterns may also be observed (Fig. 11-5).

If His bundle deflections are not seen, one must differentiate the absence of retrograde activation of the His–Purkinje

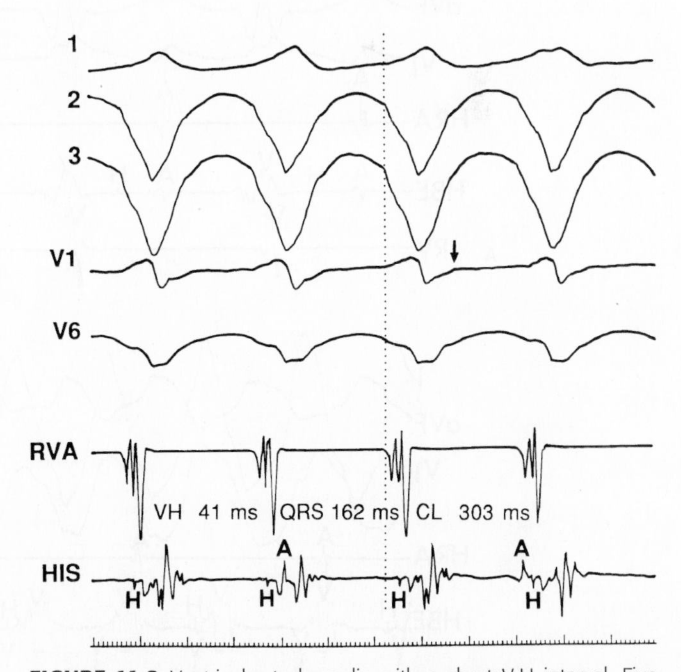


**FIGURE 11-2** Ventricular tachycardia with a short V-H interval. Five surface ECGs are shown with electrograms from the RVA and His bundle region (HIS). Note that the His bundle activation occurred 41 msec after the onset of QRS. Retrograde block in the A-V node is present because atrial activation is dissociated from the tachycardia. See text for discussion.

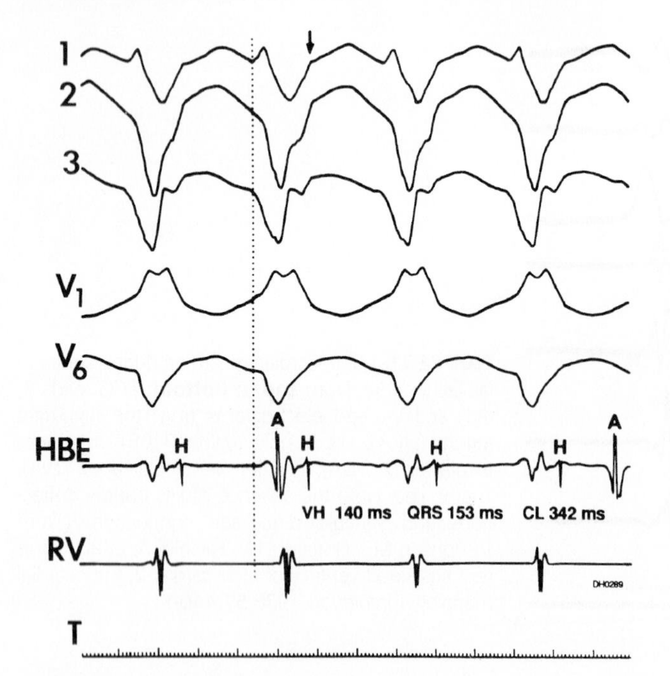


FIGURE 11-3 Ventricular tachycardia (VT) with a long V-H interval. VT with a right bundle branch block superior axis is shown with five ECG leads and intracardiac recordings from the HBE and right ventricle (RV). T is shown on the bottom. The dotted vertical line marks the onset of the QRS and the vertical *arrow* marks the offset. Note that the V-H interval during the tachycardia is seen 140 msec following the ORS. The QRS is 153 msec in duration, and the cycle length of the tachycardia is 342 msec. See text for discussion.

system from retrograde activation that is obscured by the large amplitude of the ventricular electrogram. This can be fortuitously observed if a sinus impulse conducts antegradely to the His bundle producing a clear His deflection. Atrial pacing and/or atrial extrastimuli can be used to evaluate the presence of retrograde His–Purkinje activation during VT. Supraventricular capture of the His bundle may occur in the absence (Fig. 11-6) or presence (Fig. 11-7) of ventricular fusion or sinus captures. In these instances, linking of the His bundle potential to atrial activation proves that they are due to antegrade depolarization and are unrelated to the tachycardia. A changing A-H interval and/or failure to observe antegrade His deflections during VT (with proper catheter position) with A-V dissociation suggest that retrograde conduction through the His–Purkinje system is occurring and producing concealment in the A-V node.

It is often difficult to determine whether the recorded His deflection is antegrade or retrograde—or for that matter whether an apparent His bundle deflection is really a right bundle branch potential. Two techniques that may be used to clarify the situation are (a) recording right and left bundle branch potentials to demonstrate that their activation begins before His bundle activation and (b) His bundle pacing producing a longer H-V interval than the one noted during the tachycardia. Both of these are extremely difficult to do but can help define the mechanism of His bundle activation and the tachycardia origin. The role of the

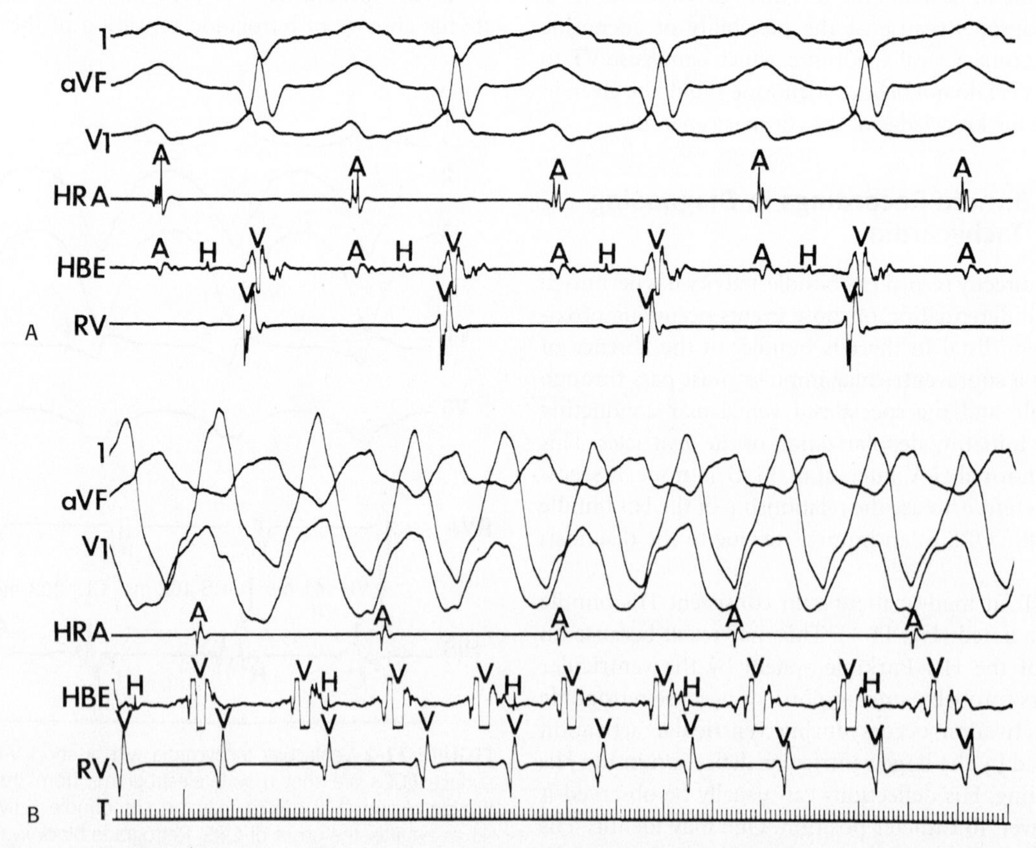


FIGURE 11-4 Two to one retrograde activation of the His bundle. Three surface leads and electrograms from the HRA, HBE, and RV are shown. **A:** Sinus rhythm is present. **B:** VT is present. Note that during VT 2:1 retrograde conduction to the His bundle is observed without conduction through the A-V node to the atrium.

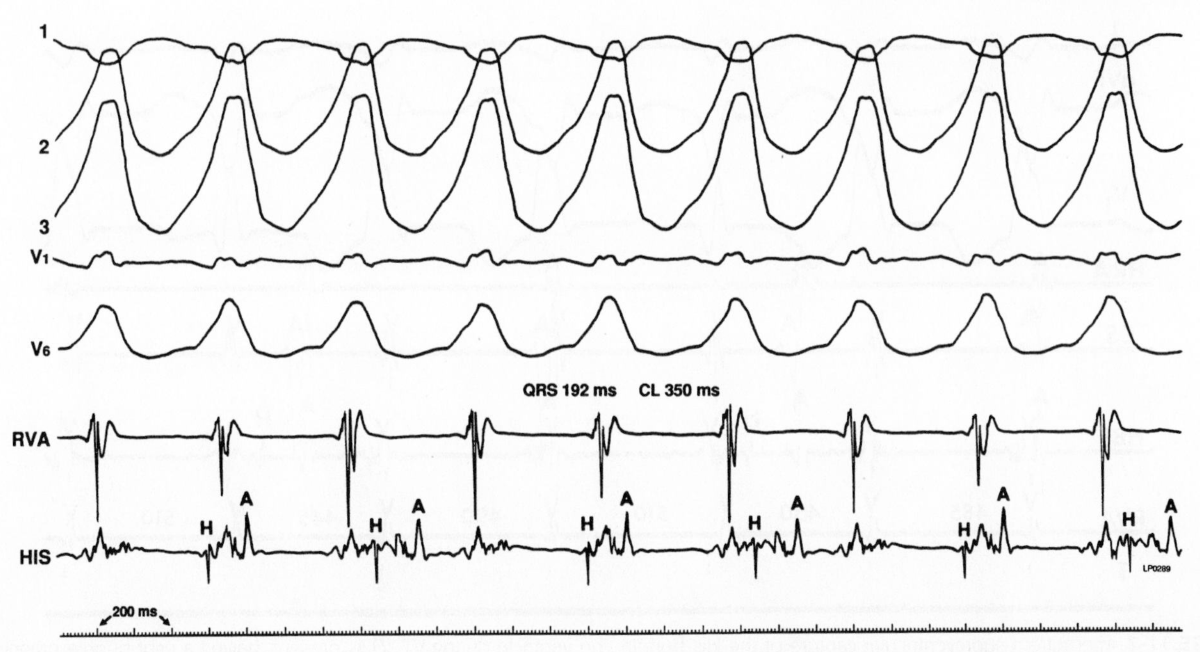


**FIGURE 11-5** Retrograde Wenckebach in the His–Purkinje system. VT is present. Five surface ECG leads are shown with electrograms from the RVA and His bundle region. The second, third, and fourth QRS complexes are associated with short V-H interval, a longer V-H interval, and no V-H interval as block occurs between the ventricle and the His bundle recording. The pattern is repeated in the next three complexes. Thus, 3:2 retrograde conduction to the His bundle is present. Note that this occurs without a change in the QRS morphology and duration or the VT cycle length.

His–Purkinje system in the genesis of VT is discussed in subsequent paragraphs.

### *Limitations of His Bundle Recordings for the Diagnosis of Ventricular Tachycardia*

Certain pitfalls are inherent in the use of His bundle recordings for the diagnosis of VT, as described in the following paragraphs.

(1) The inability to record His bundle potentials during the tachycardia most commonly reflects improper catheter position; therefore, verification of proper catheter position is mandatory. The simplest methods for verifying proper catheter position include the following: (a) the immediate appearance of His bundle deflections on termination of the tachycardia, or conversely, disappearance of the His bundle deflection on initiation of the tachycardia, without catheter manipulation; (b) spontaneously occurring or induced supraventricular capture of the His–Purkinje system (with or without ventricular capture) during the tachycardia with the sudden appearance of His bundle deflections; and (c) in the presence of supraventricular capture, H-V intervals comparable to those during sinus rhythm (Figs. 11-6 and 11-7). We have found that the use of more closely spaced bipolar electrodes (1 to 5 mm apart) facilitate identification of His bundle activity when it occurs within the ventricular electrogram. Using bipolar recordings

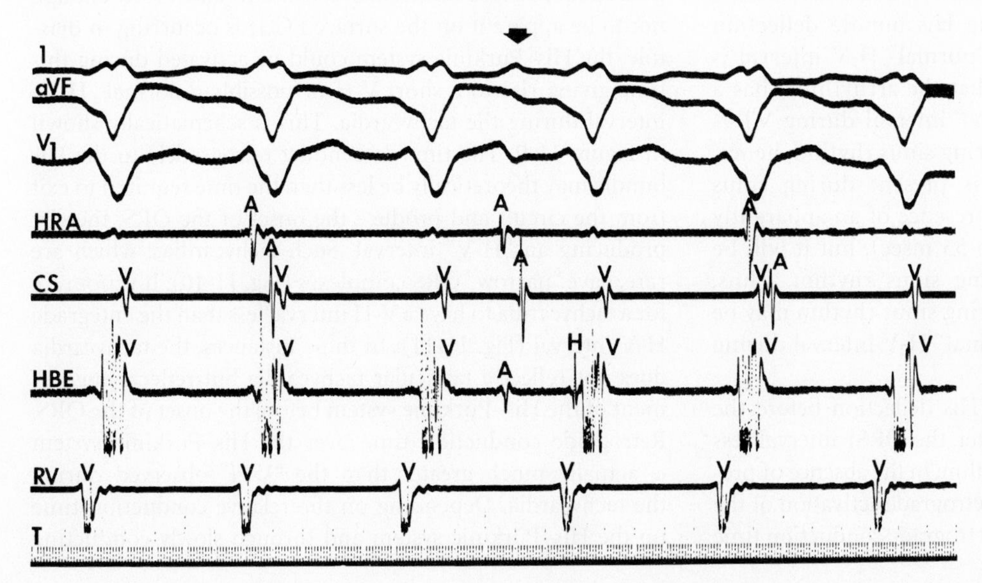


**FIGURE 11-6** Antegrade depolarization of the His bundle during VT. From **top** to **bottom**. ECG leads 1, aVF, and $V_1$, and electrograms from the HRA, coronary sinus (CS), HBE, and RVA. VT with A-V dissociation is present. The second atrial impulse (A) conducts through the His bundle but fails to alter the tachycardia. The first and third sinus complexes block in the A-V node due to retrograde concealment. T, time line.

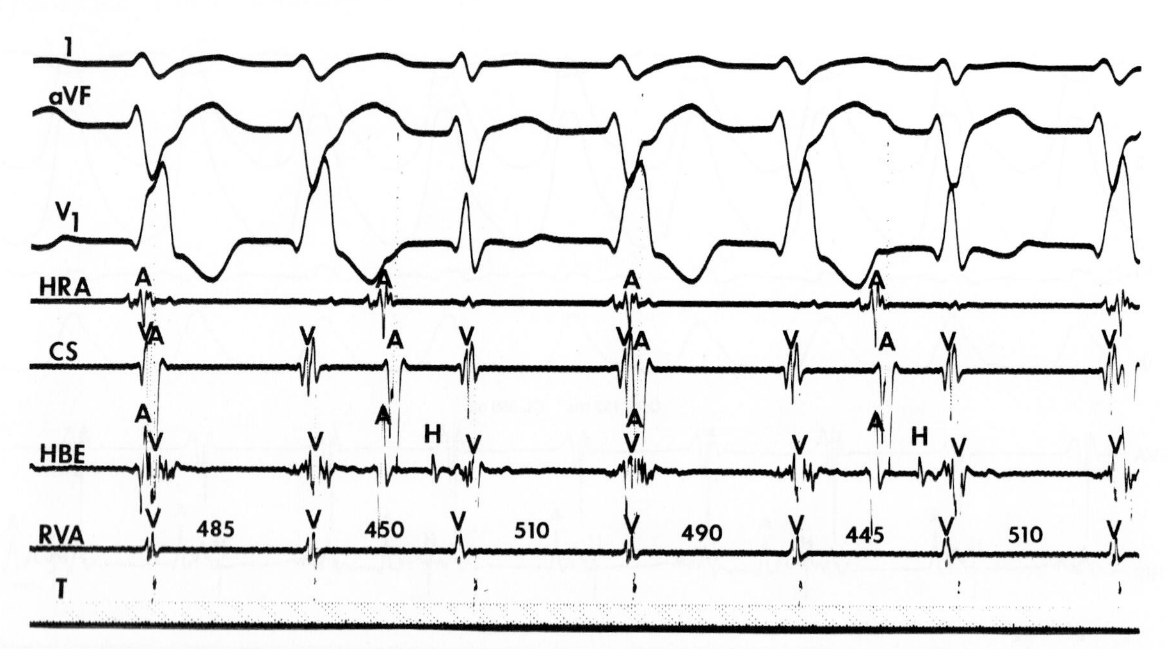


**FIGURE 11-7** Intermittent supraventricular capture of the His bundle and ventricle during VT. VT is present, having a right bundle branch block morphology with left axis deviation. Intracardiac recordings from the HRA, CS, HBE, and RVA are shown along with T. Following the second VT complex, the sinus impulse captures the His bundle and part of the ventricle to produce a supraventricular fusion. The next VT cycle returns on time. Two complexes later, another supraventricular fusion is observed, again without influencing the tachycardia. This demonstrates lack of requirement of the His bundle for perpetuation of the tachycardia. See text for discussion.

with an interelectrode distance of 5 mm, we have recorded His–Purkinje activity during the tachycardia in approximately 80% of patients.[16]

If His deflections are not spontaneously observed during the tachycardia, because of either poor position or obscuration of the His deflection by the ventricular electrogram, rapid atrial pacing can be used to clarify the issue in some cases. If rapid atrial pacing can produce supraventricular capture during the tachycardia—that is, changing the QRS to a sinus QRS—this is diagnostic of VT, regardless of whether the His deflection is seen (proper catheter position) or is not seen (inappropriate catheter position) (Fig. 11-8). Atrial pacing is an active maneuver that may be useful in diagnosing VT even in the absence of recording His bundle electrograms.

(2) The mere presence of the His bundle deflection before the QRS complex with a "normal" H-V interval is not absolutely reliable evidence that the arrhythmia has a supraventricular origin. The "H-V" interval during VT is usually less than that observed during sinus rhythm; hence, if infranodal conduction delay is present during sinus rhythm, the VT may exist in the presence of an apparently "normal" H-V interval (i.e., 35 to 55 msec), but it will be less than the H-V interval during sinus rhythm. Thus, knowledge of A-V conduction during sinus rhythm may be necessary to define what is a "normal" H-V interval during the tachycardia.

The occurrence of an "H-V" (His deflection before the QRS) or a V-H (His deflection after the QRS) interval less than that recorded during sinus rhythm, in the absence of pre-excitation, implies the presence of retrograde activation of the His bundle. It further implies that retrograde conduction time from the "origin" or exit of the tachycardia (as defined by the onset of the QRS) to the His bundle is less than "antegrade" conduction time to depolarize the ventricular myocardium. Some investigators[16,17] suggest that the site of origin of such a tachycardia is within the His–Purkinje system. These rhythms have generally been referred to as fascicular rhythms,[16,17] although proof that they originate in the fascicles of the conducting system and differ from other forms of VT is often lacking. As stated earlier, pre-excited tachycardia using either an A-V or nodoventricular bypass tract must be excluded (see Chapter 10).

Two specific circumstances may produce confusing data. The first is a reentrant VT occurring in the setting of a prior infarction. Because ventricular activation (albeit slow enough not to be apparent on the surface ECG) is occurring in diastole, the His–Purkinje system could be activated during this time giving rise to a short V-H or possibly a normal "H-V" interval during the tachycardia. This is schematically shown in Figure 11-9. The time to conduct retrogradely to the His bundle may theoretically be less than the time required to exit from the circuit and produce the onset of the QRS, thereby producing an "H-V" interval. Such tachycardias, which are rare, have "narrow" QRS complexes (Fig. 11-10). It is not rare for a tachycardia to have a V-H interval less than the antegrade H-V interval (Fig. 11-11). In these instances, the tachycardia does not reflect a fascicular tachycardia but reflects engagement of the His–Purkinje system before the onset of the QRS. Retrograde conduction time over the His–Purkinje system is actually much greater than the "V-H" observed during the tachycardia. Depending on the relative conduction time up the His–Purkinje system and through slowly conducting

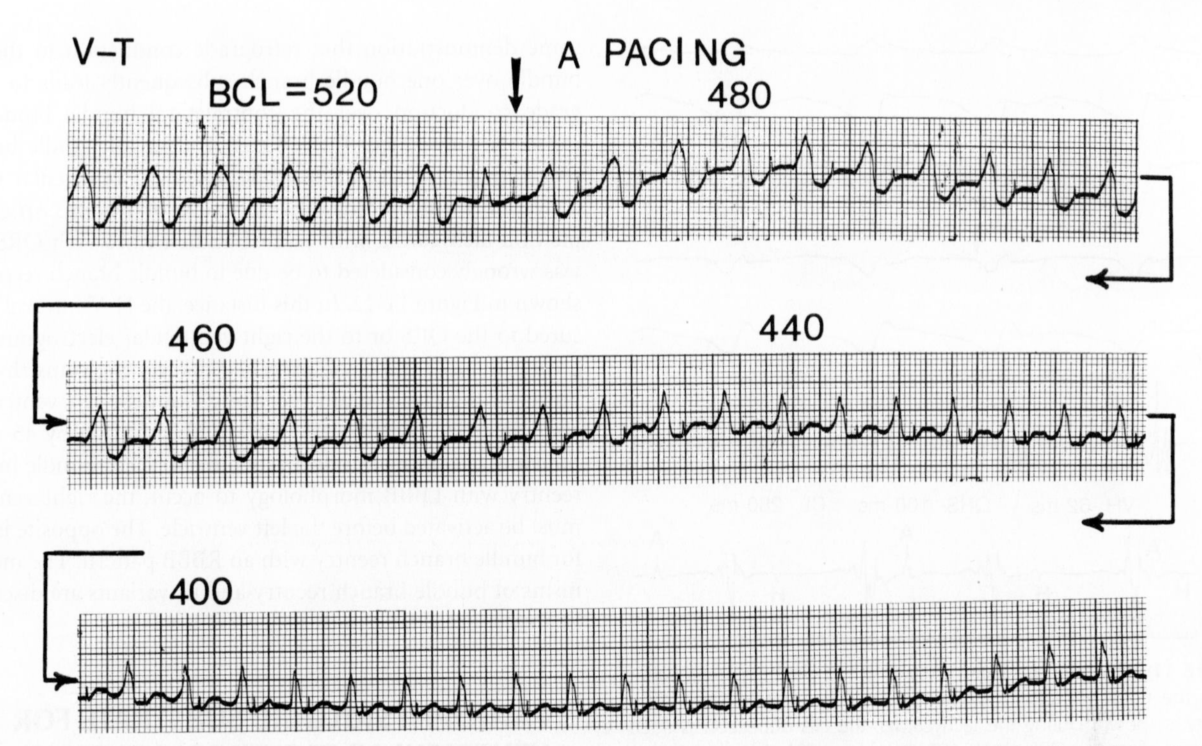


**FIGURE 11-8** Use of atrial pacing during a wide complex tachycardia to diagnose VT. VT is present on the upper left with a left bundle branch block pattern at a cycle length of 520 msec. Atrial pacing is begun *(arrow)* at a cycle length of 480 msec, which is gradually reduced to 400 msec. As the atrial-paced cycle length decreases, a greater degree of ventricular activation is produced via the normal conducting system. Finally, at 400 msec, the QRS is totally normalized. The ability to normalize the QRS with atrial pacing during a wide complex rhythm is diagnostic of VT. See text for discussion. BCL, basic cycle length.

muscle to give rise to the QRS, the His deflection can occur before, during, or after the QRS.

The second circumstance that can give rise to VT having an H-V interval greater than or equal to the H-V during sinus rhythm is bundle branch reentrant VT.[18,19] The mechanism, which is the same as isolated bundle branch reentry discussed in Chapter 2, is discussed in more detail in subsequent paragraphs. When bundle branch reentrant VT has an LBBB morphology, retrograde conduction occurs over the left bundle system with antegrade conduction over the right bundle branch. The His deflection typically occurs before the right bundle deflection with an H-V interval approximating the H-V interval during sinus rhythm. The "H-V" interval may be longer than sinus if there is antegrade conduction delay down the RBB. Theoretically, if there is prolonged retrograde conduction over the His–Purkinje system, producing a markedly delayed His deflection (very long V-H), the "in parallel" activation of the His bundle would appear as a "normal" H-V interval. In this case, one must demonstrate that the His deflection is not a requisite for subsequent ventricular activation and thus is not a reflection of bundle branch reentry. Certain criteria are necessary for the diagnosis of bundle branch reentry, all of which provide

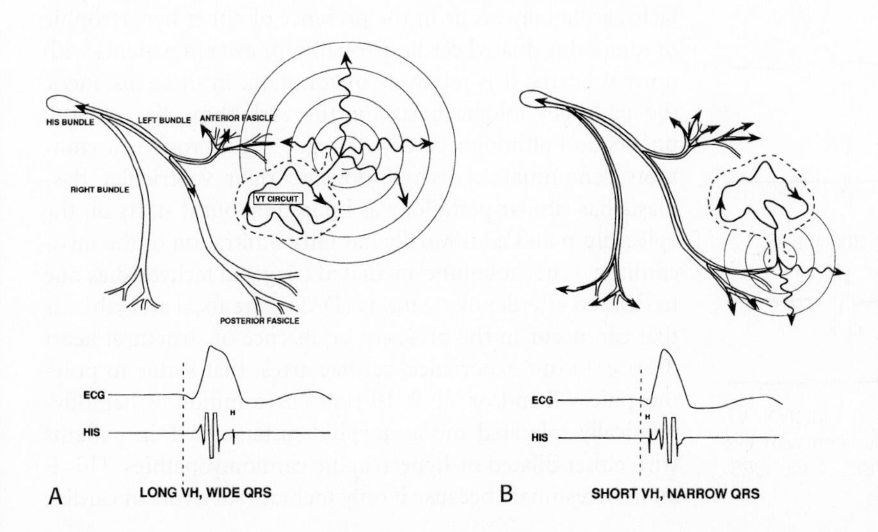


**FIGURE 11-9** Relationship of V-H interval to differences in conduction time to the His–Purkinje system and to the rest of the ventricular myocardium. **A:** A VT circuit is schematically shown surrounded by diseased tissue through which the impulse must propagate slowly before reaching the His–Purkinje system. This results in a long V-H interval. **B:** The schema shows that propagation of the impulse from the reentrant circuit to the His–Purkinje system is more rapid than that to the remainder of the myocardium, resulting in a short V-H interval. See text for discussion.

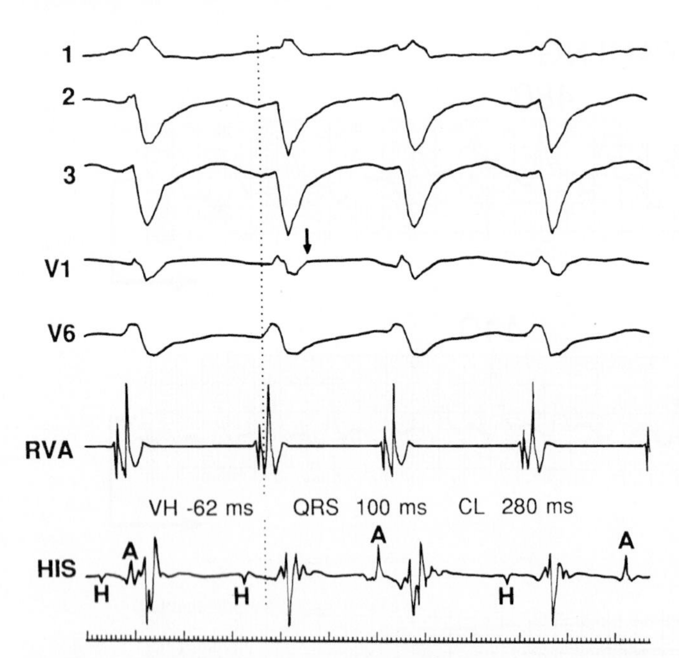


**FIGURE 11-10** Ventricular tachycardia with the His bundle activated before the QRS. VT with a left bundle branch block left axis morphology is shown. During the tachycardia, the His deflection is seen 62 msec before the QRS (H-V = 62 or V-H = −62). A-V dissociation is also present. In this instance, conduction to the His–Purkinje was far more rapid than that to the ventricular myocardium, resulting in early His–Purkinje activation. The His–Purkinje system then is used to activate distal ventricular myocardium, producing a narrow QRS. See text for discussion.

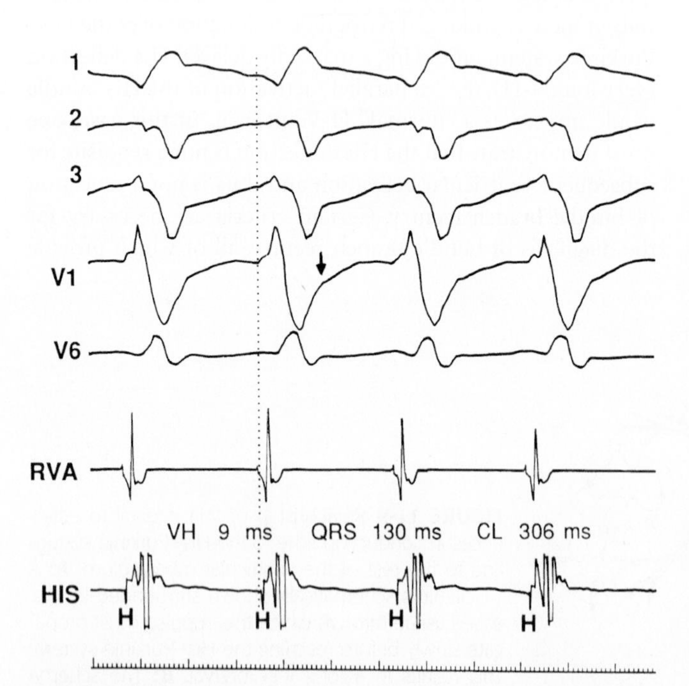


**FIGURE 11-11** Ventricular tachycardia with a short V-H interval. VT with a left bundle branch block left axis deviation is seen with His bundle activation occurring 9 msec following the onset of the QRS. See text for discussion.

some demonstration that retrograde conduction to the His bundle over one bundle branch subsequently leads to antegrade conduction over the contralateral bundle branch to cause the subsequent QRS. Thus, in cases of bundle branch reentry having an LBBB morphology, right ventricular septal activation must precede left ventricular activation. An example of a tachycardia with a His bundle before each QRS that was wrongly considered to be due to bundle branch reentry is shown in Figure 11-12. In this instance, the H-V interval measured to the QRS or to the right ventricular electrogram was greater than 75 msec and exceeded that during sinus rhythm; however, the electrogram recording from the left ventricular apex preceded right ventricular septal activation by 45 msec, therefore excluding bundle branch reentry. For bundle branch reentry with LBBB morphology to occur, the right ventricle must be activated before the left ventricle. The opposite is true for bundle branch reentry with an RBBB pattern. The mechanisms of bundle branch reentry and its variants are discussed in greater detail later in this chapter.

## PATHOPHYSIOLOGIC SUBSTRATE FOR VENTRICULAR TACHYARRHYTHMIAS

Nonsustained VT, hemodynamically tolerated sustained monomorphic VT, and arrhythmias producing cardiac arrest can have different anatomic and electrophysiologic substrates. These differences make it mandatory that these arrhythmias not be lumped together in terms of response to stimulation, effects of pharmacologic therapy, effectiveness of ablation, and clinical outcome.

### Anatomic Substrate

The most common anatomic substrate for all these arrhythmias is chronic coronary artery disease, usually associated with prior infarction. Arrhythmias that are due to coronary artery disease are the only ones for which we have a reasonable understanding of the pathophysiologic substrate required for their genesis. Although sustained uniform monomorphic tachycardia may occur in the presence of either hypertrophic or idiopathic dilated cardiomyopathy, or even in patients with normal hearts, it is relatively uncommon. In these instances, the pathophysiologic basis for the arrhythmia is not well understood although patchy or segmental fibrosis is a common denominator. Arrhythmogenic right ventricular dysplasia has similar pathology as infarction, but it starts on the epicardium and additionally has fatty infiltration of the myocardium. Catecholamine-mediated triggered tachycardias due to delayed afterdepolarizations (DADs) are focal arrhythmias that can occur in the presence or absence of structural heart disease. In our experience, cardiac arrest that is due to polymorphic VT and/or VF is 10 times as common as hemodynamically tolerated monomorphic sustained VT in patients with either dilated or hypertrophic cardiomyopathies. This is an underestimate because it only includes survivors of cardiac

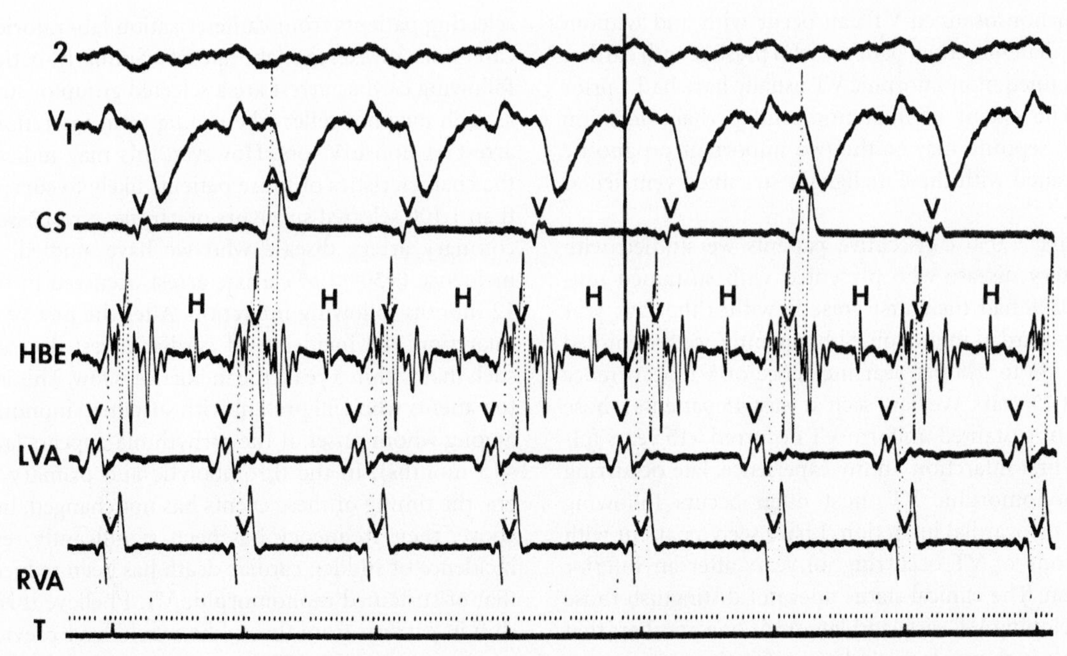


**FIGURE 11-12** Ventricular tachycardia with an apparent normal H-V interval mimicking bundle branch reentry. During VT with a left bundle branch block and left axis morphology, the His bundle is activated 75 msec before the QRS, which was similar to the HV in sinus rhythm. However, analysis of activation at the left ventricular apical septum (LVA), demonstrates that ventricular activation begins in the left ventricle. Thus, bundle branch reentry is impossible as the mechanism for this arrhythmia. See text for discussion.

arrest. This may occur because in most cases there is patchy fibrosis instead of the large areas of contiguous scar seen in infarction.

Regardless of the underlying cardiac pathophysiology, sustained monomorphic tachycardia can be studied electrophysiologically such that interpretation of the mechanism and development of therapy is possible. Nonsustained VT is found in patients with a variety of disorders; thus, the pathophysiologic substrate for this arrhythmia is variable, and the utility of programmed stimulation for spontaneous VT in these different disorders depends on the underlying substrate. Because the pathophysiologic substrate for arrhythmias associated with cardiomyopathies (with the exception of arrhythmogenic right ventricular dysplasia) or those in normal hearts is poorly understood, the role of programmed stimulation to study patients with cardiac arrest or nonsustained VT in such patients is not established. However, I believe that the induction of sustained monomorphic VT is probably clinically significant regardless of the underlying pathology.

Electrophysiologic studies are most useful in patients with coronary artery disease and prior infarction. The pathologic substrate for patients with ventricular tachyarrhythmias associated with coronary artery disease is usually a prior myocardial infarction resulting in wall motion abnormalities.[20–23] The greater the wall motion abnormalities, the higher the incidence of aneurysm formation, and the lower the ejection fraction, the more likely is the development of a sustained uniform VT. Patients who present with cardiac arrest appear to fall into two groups. Most commonly, these patients have prior infarction, although usually with less wall motion abnormalities and depression of myocardial function than patients with sustained uniform VT. Occasionally, patients have multiple prior myocardial infarctions. Although some investigators[22] suggest more severe ventricular dysfunction in patients with cardiac arrest than in those with sustained uniform VT, this is neither our experience nor that of others.[23] The second group of patients who present with a cardiac arrest are those who have severe coronary artery disease and relatively normal ventricular function; in this group the arrest is most likely due to acute ischemia. Electrophysiologic studies appear less useful in this latter group. Nonsustained VT, particularly when uniform, may occur in patients with normal ventricular function, with or without severe coronary disease, or in patients with severely abnormal ventricular function associated with multiple prior infarctions and/or ventricular aneurysms. In my experience, patients with prior infarction and uniform VT have the lowest ejection fractions (27%), while those with cardiac arrest and nonsustained VT have higher ejection fractions (35% and 39%, respectively). For nonsustained VT, this reflects a selection bias for patients with prior infarction and lower ejection fractions, because we tend not to treat, or study, patients with nonsustained VT and higher ejection fractions because they have a good progress. Thus, patients with cardiac arrest and nonsustained VT who are studied in our laboratory are anatomically similar. In the general population of patients with asymptomatic nonsustained VT, the majority will have normal left ventricular function. Our patient population is clearly selected so that we study patients with lower ejection fractions, recognizing that lower ejection fraction per se places a person at high risk for sudden death.

Although nonsustained VT can occur with and without prior myocardial infarction, patients who present with cardiac arrest or sustained monomorphic VT usually have had a prior infarction. The extent of infarction, and perhaps location involving the septum, may be the two important prognostic factors associated with these malignant sustained ventricular arrhythmias.[21,24]

Of the first 1,050 consecutive patients we studied with coronary artery disease who presented with sustained uniform VT, ≈25% had their first episode within the first year following myocardial infarction. Subsequently, we have noted a consistent 3% to 5% per year incidence of VT occurrence over the next 15 years. We have seen at least 45 patients whose first episode of sustained uniform VT occurred >15 years following their first infarction. In my experience, late occurring sustained monomorphic VT most often occurs following inferior wall myocardial infarction. I have seen a patient with his first episode of VT occurring 40 years after an inferior wall infarction. The clinical status does not distinguish those patients developing VT early and late from one another; that is, both have a high incidence of large infarction, severe ventricular dysfunction, the presence of an aneurysm, and significant coronary artery disease.[25] Clinical status does appear to an important factor in recurrent episodes of VT. Recurrences seem to be more frequent in the setting of overt heart failure, possibly because of electrolyte imbalance, high catecholamine state (increased calcium-mediated triggered activity acting as VT triggers), and drug toxicity.

The cycle lengths of the tachycardias occurring early after infarction, however, tend to be faster, and the tachycardia is more poorly tolerated. This may reflect evolving scar formation, which when ultimately completed, may be related to longer tachycardia cycle lengths, owing to abnormalities of conduction with which it is associated (see following discussion). Nonetheless, Roy et al.[26] demonstrated that tachycardias initiated 2 weeks after infarction (even if they had not been present clinically) can be replicated by programmed stimulation a year later. Thus, some components of the anatomic substrate must be relatively fixed once infarction has occurred. This is supported by inducibility at 10 and 100 days in an Ovine infarction model.[27] Moreover the ability of programmed stimulation to predict risk of sudden cardiac arrest and survival postinfarction lead credence to this hypothesis.[28] Since the introduction of thrombolysis and primary angioplasty for acute infarction, the incidence of sustained monomorphic VT has decreased remarkably. Only 1% of patients will experience an episode of sustained, tolerated VT in the year following infarction.

It is more difficult to assess the time from myocardial infarction when cardiac arrest or nonsustained VT occurs. As noted previously, nonsustained VT occurs with or without infarction, and one cannot truly estimate the incidence or timing of this arrhythmia with the degree of coronary stenosis and the presence of infarction or ischemia-induced myocardial dysfunction. Attempts to make these correlations are fraught with selection and/or entry bias, which is inherent in selecting patients from catheterization laboratories, coronary care units, or exercise laboratories. Similarly, patients studied following cardiac arrest are a selected group of survivors, and as such may not reflect the timing from infarction to cardiac arrest of nonsurvivors. However, this may indicate some of the characteristics of those patients likely to survive. Of more than 1,100 selected survivors of cardiac arrest associated with coronary artery disease who we have studied, the highest incidence (≈50%) of cardiac arrest occurred in the first 6 to 12 months following infarction. After the first year following infarction, the incidence of cardiac arrest decreases rapidly, such that within 3 years the incidence is low. This is in contrast to patients who will present with sustained monomorphic VT, among whom onset of the arrhythmia appears later (median ≈15 months). In the thrombolytic and primary angioplasty era, the timing of these events has not changed, but, as stated above, their frequency has been significantly reduced. The incidence of sudden cardiac death has been reduced less than that of sustained monomorphic VT. I believe this is due to a shift in patients from those who would have previously developed monomorphic VT to more presenting with cardiac arrest due to preservation of myocardium by early reperfusion.

The pathophysiologic substrate in disease states other than coronary artery disease is less clear. Hypertrophy and fibrosis characterize myopathic ventricles. Hypertrophy is associated with calcium overload, increased action potential duration (APD), a decrease in gap junctions, and alterations in their location, etc., all of which are potentially arrhythmogenic. These have been recently reviewed.[29]

## Electrophysiologic Substrate

The clinically measurable electrophysiologic consequences of infarction that are potentially arrhythmogenic include abnormalities of conduction and refractoriness, heterogeneity of conduction and refractoriness, enhanced automaticity, and areas of inexcitability. We found that abnormalities of conduction are most prominent. We described abnormalities of conduction in terms of patterns of endocardial activation and electrogram characteristics using filtered bipolar electrograms recorded by catheter and intraoperative mapping techniques during sinus rhythm in patients with nonsustained and sustained VTs to distinguish them from patients with normal ventricles and those with prior infarction but no ventricular arrhythmias.[30–36] We used filtered bipolar recordings to magnify near field signals and diminish far field signals (Fig. 11-13). We elected to look at the electrogram characteristics because of the observation that the VT often occurred at sites that demonstrated markedly abnormal electrograms manifesting multiple components, low-amplitude, prolonged duration, frequently occurring after the end of the QRS, and isolated late potentials (Fig 11-14). The areas of latest activation in sinus rhythm often become mid-diastolic activity during the VT (Fig 11-15). This observation led us to study ventricular activation and characterize electrograms in patients having sustained and nonsustained VTs.

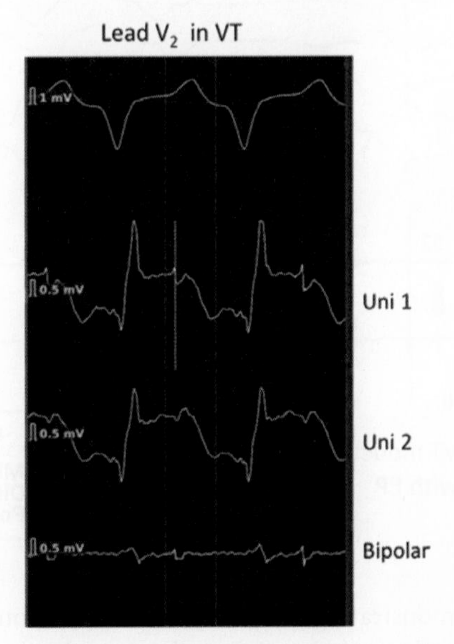


**FIGURE 11-13** Use of bipolar recordings to reduce the far field signals recorded with unipolar recordings. Unipolar (**top**) and bipolar (**bottom**) signals recorded with the Rhythmia mapping system. The bipolar signal removes the large farfield signal recorded in the two unipolar electrograms from which the bipolar signal is derived. The amplitude of the sharp, nearfield signal is minimally altered.

We developed criteria for normal, abnormal, and fractionated electrograms using bipolar signals recorded with a Bard Josephson catheter (see Fig. 1-1 bottom catheter) with a 2-mm tip and 1-mm ring electrode and both a 5- or 10-mm interelectrode distance according to our left ventricular mapping schema (Fig. 11-16).[30,31] Filtering was 30 to 500 Hz. Normal electrograms had sharp, biphasic, or triphasic spikes with amplitudes of ≥3 mV, durations of ≤70 msec, and/or an amplitude/duration ratio of ≥0.046. We considered all other electrograms abnormal. We considered an electrogram fractionated if it had an amplitude of ≤0.5 mV, a duration of ≥133 msec, and/or an amplitude/duration ratio of ≤0.005. We defined fractionated electrograms as abnormal electrograms that fell outside the 95% confidence limits of amplitude and duration of all abnormal electrograms. We defined an electrogram as late if any component extended beyond the end of the QRS. Examples of these electrograms are shown in Figure 11-17. The most common abnormalities were low voltage and increase in electrogram duration, both of which appear to be nonspecific markers of infarction or even poor contact. Multicomponent and fractionated electrograms, isolated late potentials and late electrograms were more closely related to arrhythmogenic sites; but the positive predictive value was only ~30%.[31] Only 14% of "sites of origin" came from sites that demonstrated normal electrograms. It should be obvious that since mapping catheters have different size electrode (tip and ring), normal and abnormal electrogram characteristics need to be defined for each catheter. Subsequent intraoperative studies using a 20 pole plaque electrode showed that successful surgery was associated with elimination of isolated late potentials and split potentials suggesting mechanistic significance (Fig. 11-18; see Chapter 13).[37] Note the different normal values for electrodes that were 0.5 mm in width and 2-mm interelectrode distance.

We defined local activation time (LAT) at any site as time from the onset of the surface QRS to the time that the largest, rapid deflection of a local electrogram crossed the baseline. We defined total endocardial activation as the time from the earliest local activation to the time of the latest local activation. We used the total endocardial activation time, the duration of the longest electrogram recorded, the presence of late electrograms (including late potentials), and the extent of abnormal

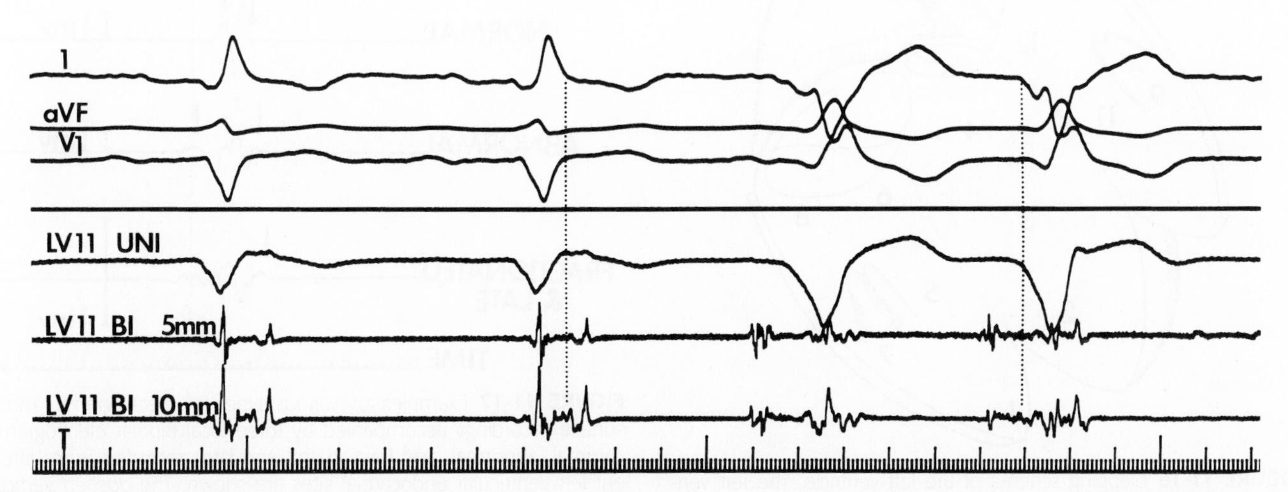


**FIGURE 11-14** Relationship of VT to fractionated late potentials. Three surface leads are shown with unipolar and 5- and 10-mm bipolar recordings from the anterior wall of the left ventricle (LV11, see Fig. 11-16 ). The first two complexes are sinus in origin and the left ventricular recordings show markedly abnormal electrograms. Multiple components are present, and the electrogram exceeds 160 msec in duration. Moreover, the electrogram extends beyond the end of the QRS, producing significantly delayed endocardial ventricular activation. VT spontaneously begins, and this left ventricular site, which was recording late activity during sinus rhythm, records electrical activity 90 msec before the onset of the QRS during VT. This suggests a relationship between abnormal, low-amplitude, multicomponent, and late potentials with the areas from which VT originate. See text for discussion. CS, coronary sinus; HBE, His bundle electrogram; LVA, left ventricular apex; RVA, right ventricular apex; T, time line.

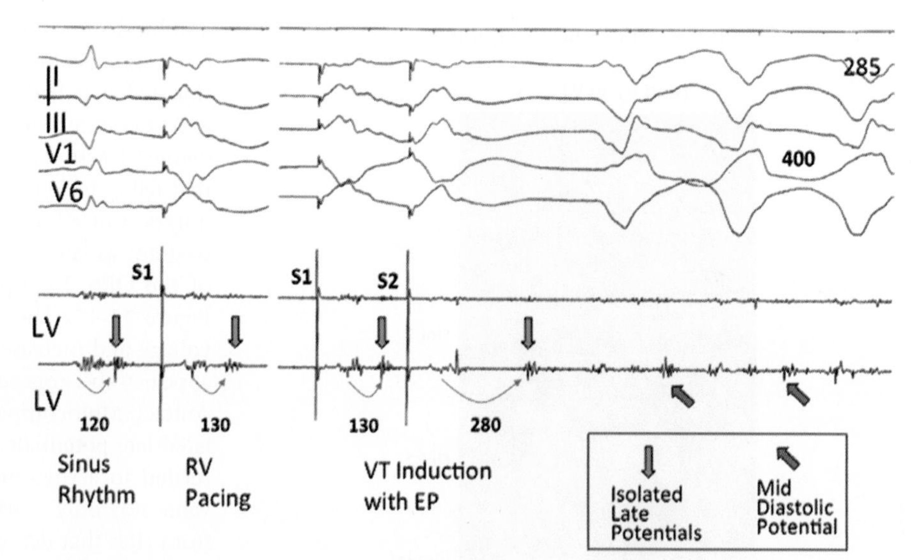


**FIGURE 11-15** Relationship of isolated late potentials to induction of ventricular tachycardia. Late potentials noted during sinus rhythm and RV pacing (*blue arrows*) become further delayed following an extrastimulus (S2) and initiate VT during which they become mid-diastolic potentials (*red arrows*). See text for discussion.

electrograms as indicators of abnormalities of conduction. As can be seen in Table 11-2, patients with nonsustained VT and those without tachycardia but prior infarction have similar conduction abnormalities. Patients with sustained uniform VT have the most abnormal electrograms, while endocardial activation in those patients with cardiac arrest falls between nonsustained VT and sustained VT. Analog records of a patient demonstrating normal activation without coronary disease, a patient with coronary disease and prior infarction without inducible arrhythmias, and a patient with sustained uniform VT are shown in Figure 11-19. In general, patients with infarction have abnormalities of local and total endocardial activation; however, those with sustained VT have a greater number of sites demonstrating abnormal electrograms

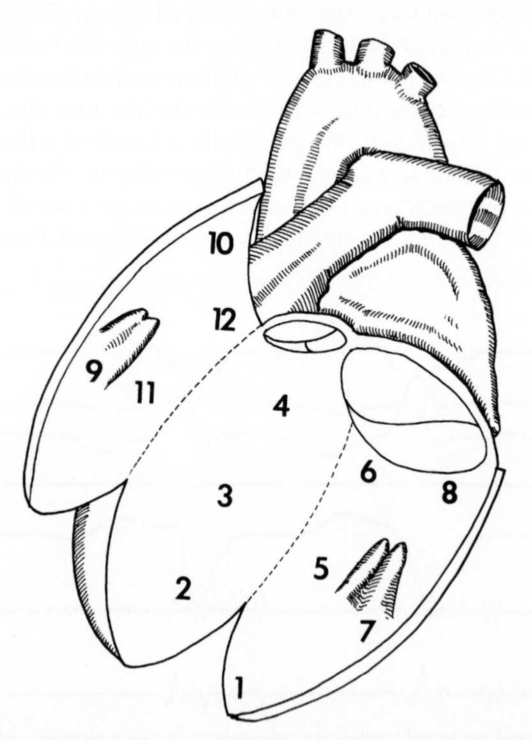


**FIGURE 11-16** Mapping schema of the left ventricle. The left ventricle is opened anterolaterally. Sites 2, 3, and 4 are the septum, 1 is the apex, 5 and 6 are the mid- and basal inferior wall, 8 is the inferoposterior wall, 9 is the apical anterolateral wall, 10 is the basal lateral wall, 11 is the midanterior wall, and 12 is the basal anterior wall. (From Cassidy DM, Vassallo JA, Miller JM, et al. Endocardial catheter mapping in patients in sinus rhythm: relationship to underlying heart disease and ventricular arrhythmias. *Circulation* 1986;73:645.)

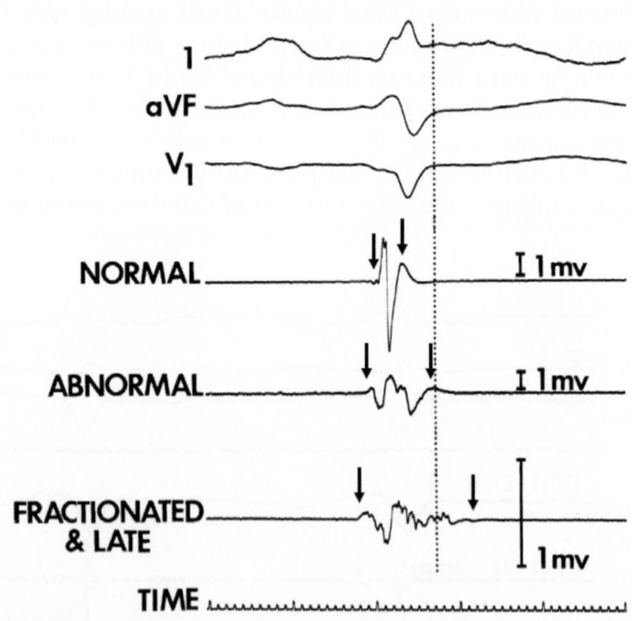


**FIGURE 11-17** Examples of various types of electrograms. Three surface recordings accompanied by three local bipolar electrograms (normal, abnormal, and fractionated and late) recorded from different left ventricular endocardial sites are shown. The *dashed vertical line* denotes the end of the surface QRS activity. The *arrows* show the onset and offset (characterized by the amplification signal decay artifact) of local electrical activity. One-millivolt calibrations are seen. See text for discussion. (From Cassidy DM, Vassallo JA, Miller JM, et al. Endocardial catheter mapping in patients in sinus rhythm: relationship to underlying heart disease and ventricular arrhythmias. *Circulation* 1986;73:645.)

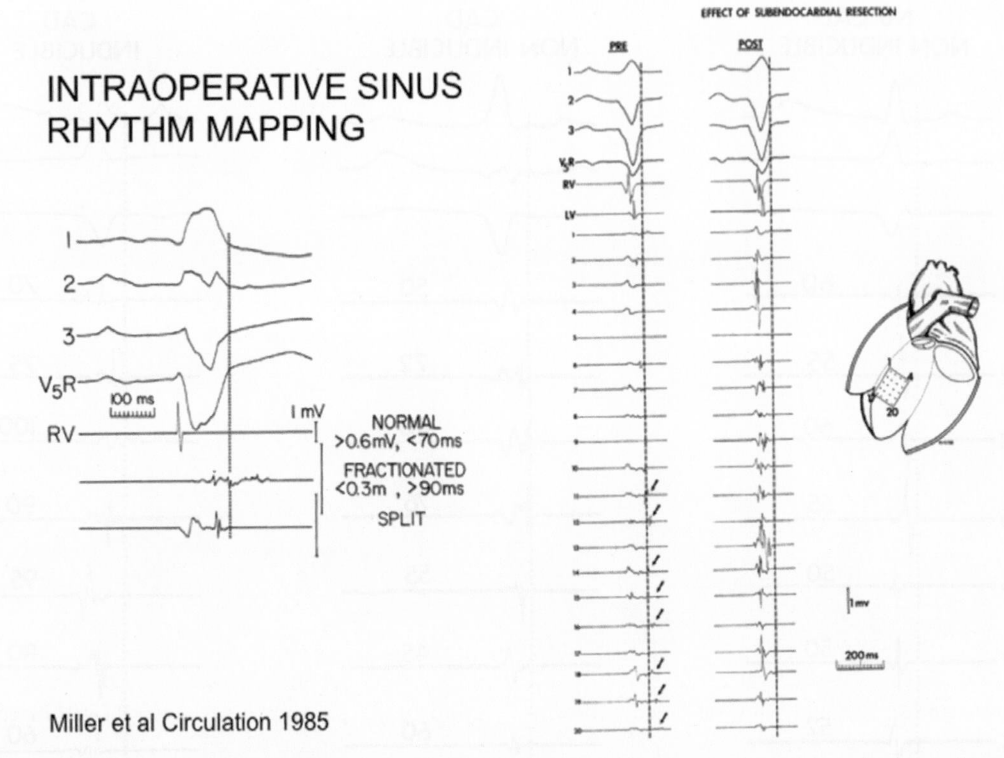


**FIGURE 11-18** Intraoperative sinus rhythm mapping using a plaque electrode with 0.5-mm electrodes and a 2-mm interelectrode distance. Normal values and abnormal electrograms recorded with this plaque are shown on the left. Pre- and postoperative signals from the septum are shown on the right. Note all late potentials are removed by surgery.

of lower amplitude and longer duration, fractionated and late electrograms than those with coronary artery disease and no VT or nonsustained VT.[32,35] Not surprisingly patients with inferior infarction have the latest onset and offset activation abnormalities normally: thus; with further delayed activation produced by inferior infarction, prolonged fractionated electrograms will be seen as late signals more easily than similar electrograms associated with anteroseptal infarction because activation begins earlier in the QRS.[36] This is reflected in the analysis of signal-averaged ECG (SAECG) in patients with VT

**TABLE 11-2 Influence of Coronary Artery Disease and Clinical Arrhythmia**

| | No VT | NSVT | CA | VT |
|---|---|---|---|---|
| Patient (*n*) | 9 | 15 | 38 | 70 |
| Normal sites (%) | 54 ± 25 | 63 ± 26 | 57 ± 27 | 42 ± 19[a] |
| Abnormal sites (%) | 45 ± 24 | 35 ± 23 | 37 ± 23 | 48 ± 17[b] |
| Fractionated sites (%) | 1 ± 3 | 2 ± 4 | 6 ± 12 | 10 ± 10[c] |
| Endocardial activation time (msec) | 52 ± 11 | 54 ± 23 | 54 ± 23 | 73 ± 32 |
| Duration of longest electrogram (msec) | 86 ± 12[d] | 102 ± 12 | 112 ± 34 | 129 ± 43[e] |
| Late sites (%) | 15 ± 15 | 11 ± 11 | 8 ± 12 | 15 ± 16 |

No VT, no ventricular tachycardia; NSVT, nonsustained ventricular tachycardia; CA, cardiac arrest; VT, ventricular tachycardia.

[a] $p < 0.005$, VT vs. NSVT.
[b] $p < 0.05$ VT vs. NSVT, CA.
[c] $p < 0.05$ VT vs. No VT, NSVT.
[d] $p < 0.05$ No VT vs. NSVT, CA.
[e] $p < 0.05$ VT vs. NSVT, CA.

From Cassidy DM, Vassallo JA, Buxton AE, et al. The value of catheter mapping during sinus rhythm to localize site of origin of ventricular tachycardia. *Circulation* 1984;69:1103.

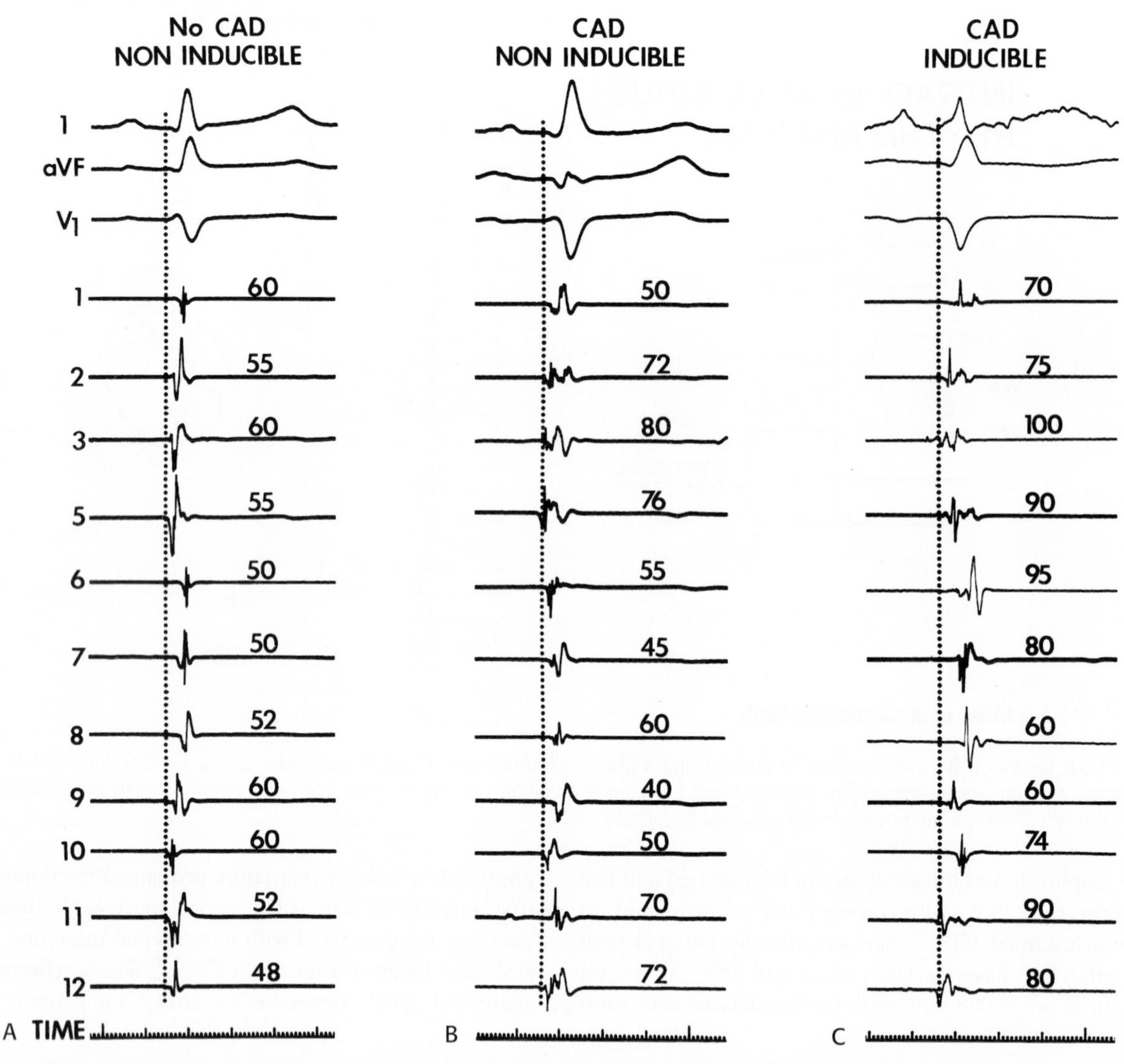


**FIGURE 11-19** Sinus rhythm maps in patients with and without coronary disease who have no inducible arrhythmias and with coronary artery disease and inducible VT. All three tracings are arranged in the same manner with three ECG leads (I, aVF, and $V_1$) and 11 of the 12 left ventricular mapping sites along with time lines. **A:** The patient with no coronary artery disease (CAD) and no inducible arrhythmias has relatively rapid endocardial activation, the electrograms have normal amplitude and duration. **B:** A sinus rhythm map is shown from a patient with CAD and prior infarction but no inducible arrhythmias. In this instance, the pattern of activation is normal but the electrograms are of broader duration and several have multiple components. None, however, are late. **C:** In a patient with prior infarction and inducible VT, many of the electrograms are abnormal and the sequence of activation is markedly distorted by areas of prior infarction. Many electrograms have multiple components, and several are recorded near the end of the QRS. See text for discussion.

and IMI versus AMI (see subsequent discussion of SAECG). These abnormalities of activation, whether recorded endocardially in the catheterization laboratory or intraoperatively, occur only in areas of prior infarction and significant wall motion abnormalities.[35,36,38,39] It is of note that patients with spontaneous nonsustained VT who have sustained monomorphic VT induced by programmed stimulation have a greater number of abnormal electrograms, which correlate with a greater extent of infarction, than those patients who do not have sustained monomorphic VT inducible. The characteristics of the spontaneous nonsustained VT have no predictive value in determining which patient will have sustained monomorphic VT induced.[40,41]

Although the anatomic substrate of patients presenting with cardiac arrest and sustained uniform VT is similar, tachycardias producing arrest have faster rates than tolerated VTs.[42] Rate of tachycardia, and not the location of prior infarction, ejection fraction, or extent of coronary disease is the only factor that determines clinical outcome. This has been corroborated by other studies.[22,23] Although the longer cycle length of hemodynamically tolerated monomorphic VT is associated with a greater extent of electrogram abnormalities on the endocardium, we have not demonstrated a correlation of VT cycle length to electrogram duration at the site of origin or any other specific electrogram characteristics observed during sinus rhythm mapping.[31,33] This may reflect either a limitation of extent of mapping (i.e., number of sites) in local regions, or that the cycle length of VT is more related to abnormalities of conduction that are anisotropic and not reflected by mapping during sinus rhythm.

We[43–45] and others[29,46–49] have analyzed the cause of these electrogram abnormalities associated with VT in humans. Clearly, these fragmented or fractionated electrograms are not an artifact of filtering or motion, because such electrograms can neither be created nor abolished by changing the filtering and can be recorded with uni- or bipolar recordings in fixed pieces of tissue or in nonmoving and infarcted regions during intraoperative mapping.[39,40,43] Anatomic studies of tissue removed from the site of origin of VT and sites distant from VT have demonstrated that abnormal electrograms are associated with a specific pathologic condition of viable muscle fibers imbedded in and separated by connective tissue.[43,44,48,50] These muscle fibers may be abnormal or normal, but they are alive and associated with normal or near-normal action potentials.[46–48] Recent studies using confocal microscopy and immunofluorescent staining of gap junctions showed an alteration in number, position, and, possibly, function of gap junctions.[29,51,52] The amplitude of the electrograms seems to be most closely related to the duration and complexity of activation underneath the electrode which is influenced by the number and orientation of viable muscle fibers under the recording electrode and degree of fibrosis (Fig. 11-20). The extent and location of fibrosis is a critical determinant of the electrogram amplitude, duration, complexity, and timing because of its effect on fiber orientation, curvature, connectivity, and anisotropy, all of which influence conduction.

Detailed mapping studies with microelectrodes in human tissue and in tissue from experimental canine tachycardia models[29,43,44,46–48,50,51–53] demonstrate that slow propagation of an impulse through areas from which fractionated electrograms are recorded is associated with relatively normal action potentials of the muscle fibers. Response of these local electrograms to antiarrhythmic agents is also compatible with relatively normal action potential characteristics.[54,55] Other studies have demonstrated that a reduced space constant and poor intercellular coupling caused by infarction lead to slow propagation of the cardiac impulse.[56] Computer models by Lesh et al.[57–59] and studies using dose-dependent changes in cellular resistance caused by heptanol[57,60] confirm that changes in intercellular resistivity can alter conduction and produce fractionated electrograms. Thus, anatomic abnormalities can produce functional abnormalities (poor cellular coupling, impedance mismatch, altered curvature, etc.), which produce slow conduction, one of the necessary factors required for

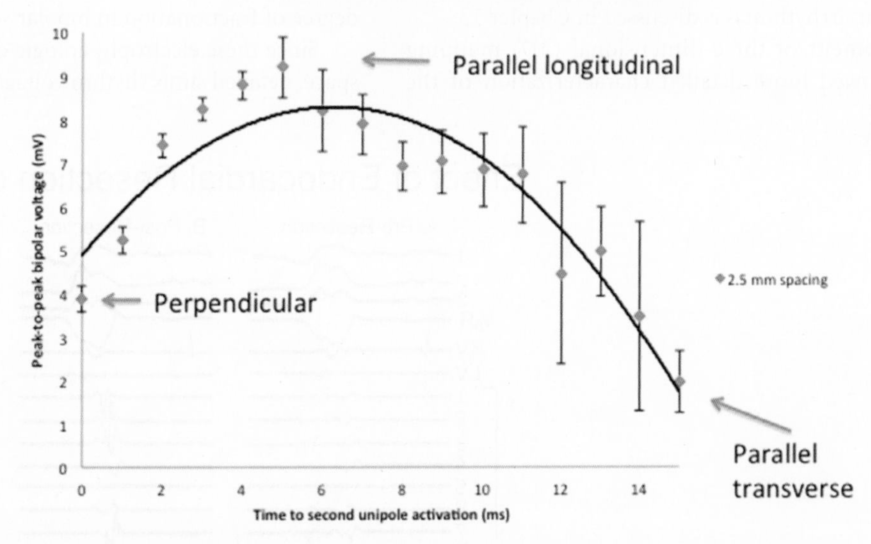


**FIGURE 11-20** Dependence of bipolar voltage on angle of contact and conduction time between the two unipolar electrograms from which the bipolar electrogram is derived. The peak-to-peak bipolar amplitude in mV is plotted against the interelectrode activation time. The electrodes are 0.4 $mm^2$ with a 2.5-mm interelectrode distance. When the bipolar pair of electrodes are more perpendicular to the tissue, the voltage is lower than when the electrodes are parallel to the surface with rapid activation between electrodes. When the wavefront is transverse to the bipoles, activation is slower and the amplitude of the bipolar electrogram is markedly reduced.

reentrant VT to occur spontaneously or to be initiated. Slow conduction produced by ischemia (low pH), hyperkalemia, or uniform depression of Na channels reduces the peak-to-peak unipolar voltage and duration. It has a similar effect on bipolar signals but duration is less affected because far field activity, a contributor of unipolar duration, is markedly reduced in bipolar, especially filtered bipolar, recordings. Thus the peak-to-peak voltage is a direct reflection of conduction velocity and not of tissue mass. Scar effects voltage by impacting the conduction velocity and activation time. Only a small amount of scar can produce markedly abnormal electrograms. We have shown that most of the cause of low-amplitude and fractionated electrograms and late potentials secondary to infarction is produced by ≈2 mm of endocardial scar.[37] Removal of that 2 mm scar by subendocardial resection (SER) eliminates late potentials and normalizes half of the subjacent electrograms.[37] The remaining electrograms still show low voltage and fractionation, but to a much lesser degree than prior to SER (Fig. 11-21). Thus, the scar also acts as an insulator of underlying electrograms. In summary, scar (even a small amount) slows conduction and some loss of tissue. Loss of tissue alone, without fibrosis induced changes in activation due to separation of myocytes would not produce fractionated, low-voltage electrograms or late potentials. The unipolar and bipolar signals would show low-voltage, broad electrograms without fractionation. These abnormalities of the electrograms are most closely related to fibrosis-dependent effects on conduction, **not** loss of tissue. The use of sinus rhythm mapping in localizing the arrhythmogenic substrate for ablation of untolerated ventricular arrhythmias is discussed in Chapter 13.

The development of three-dimensional (3D) mapping systems has allowed more detailed characterization of the electrophysiologic substrate of healed infarction, as a greater number of sites can be collected and the spatial relationships of these sites can be understood. Importantly, the use of different recording systems and catheter types requires standardization, particularly the establishment of a new set of normal values. For example, using the Carto XP system (Biosense, Johnson & Johnson) Marchlinski et al.[61] found normal bipolar voltage (4-mm tip electrode to the second pole, 2-mm proximal, filtered at 10 to 400 Hz) is ≈1.6 mV in the LV and 1.3 mV in the RV. This unusual filter setting is preset in the Carto XP system and is different from the 30 to 500 Hz settings used in our initial studies with a different catheter.[30] Normal values in our patients using the Carto system are similar (1.4 to 1.7 mV, apex and base of LV, respectively; and 1.3 mV in the RV). Unfortunately, no duration standards are available because of the lack of "fixed" gain recordings. The newer Carto 3 system has bipolar filters preset at 16 to 240 Hz; this filtering gives slightly different normal. In order to make meaningful comparisons among published data filter settings and catheter tip and ring electrode size and interelectrode distance must be comparable. We use standard filter settings (30 to 500 Hz for bipolar and 0.05 to 500 Hz for unipolar recordings) and identical catheters (3.5- to 4-mm tip, 2-mm ring and 1-mm interelectrode distance). Unfortunately while most laboratories use preset filter settings regardless of the system they use, other laboratories try to be systematic like us. Thus it is hard to interpret differences in data, particularly when those recordings are used to guide ablation (see Chapter 13). The high-pass filter markedly influence unipolar signals while the low pass setting influences the degree of fractionation in bipolar signals.

Since these electrophysiologic data can be displayed in 3D space, detailed sinus rhythm voltage mapping has been used to

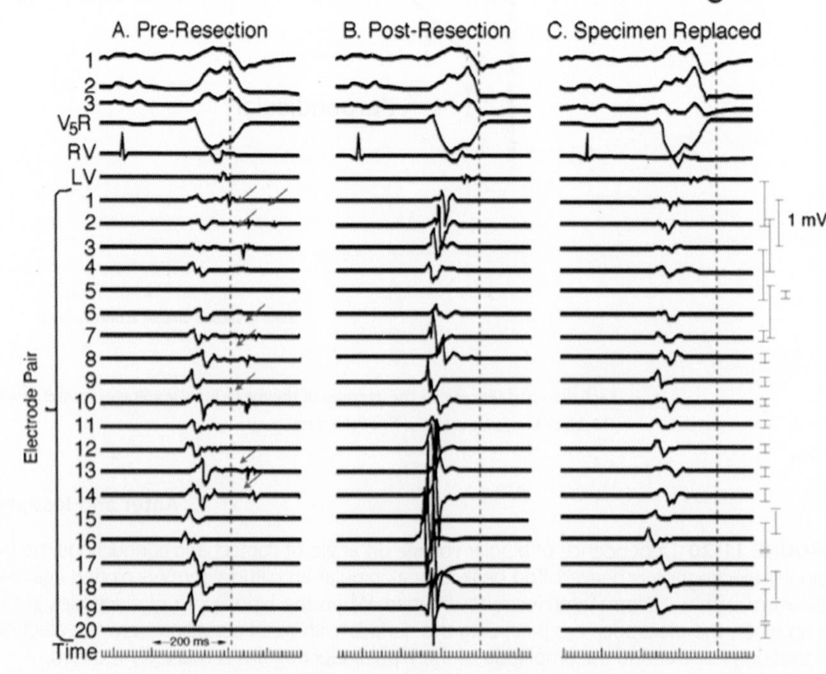


**FIGURE 11-21** Effect of subendocardial resection on bipolar electrograms. The electrograms are recorded with the same plaque used in Figure 11-18. Following removal of 2 to 3 mm of tissue the late potentials in sinus rhythm are removed and the amplitude of 50% of the underlying tissue normalizes. When the resected tissue is replace the voltage is reduced to preresection levels, without late potentials. See text for discussion.

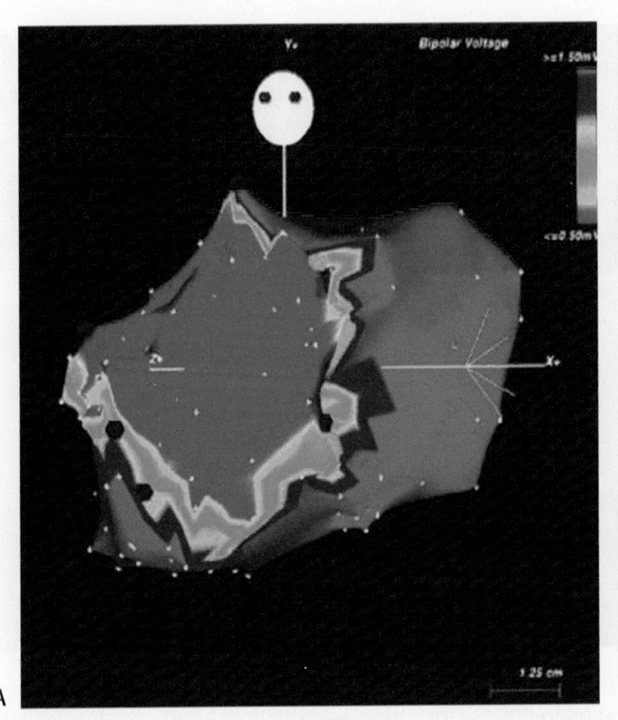


A

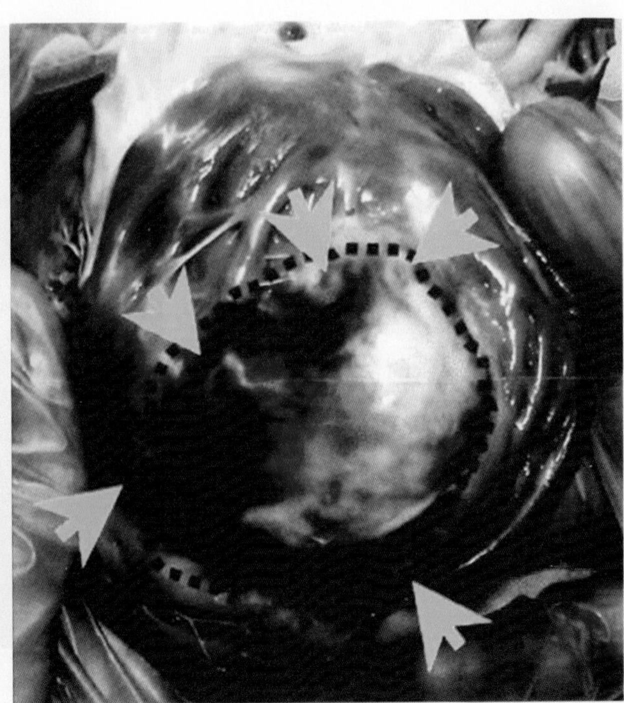

B

**FIGURE 11-22** Electroanatomic mapping in a porcine model of myocardial infarction. **A:** Sinus rhythm voltage map of the LV is shown in the AP projection, with *red color* denoting bipolar electrograms ≤0.5 mV denoting dense scar. *Red dots* denote sites of RV ablation lesions intentionally delivered at the infarct border. **B:** Gross pathology of the infarct and ablation lesions is shown. *Yellow arrows* denote the site of ablation lesions, which were consistently identified at the border of the dense scar. These data support the accuracy of sinus rhythm voltage mapping for representing the infarct anatomy. (From Wrobleski D, Houghtaling C, Josephson ME, et al. Use of electrogram characteristics during sinus rhythm to delineate the endocardial scar in a porcine model of healed myocardial infarction. *J Cardiovasc Electrophysiol* 2003;14:524.)

characterize infarct anatomy despite the fact that voltage reflects conduction/activation time, not tissue mass. Several studies in animal models[62,63] and in man[61,64,65] have demonstrated that bipolar endocardial voltage mapping in sinus rhythm provides a reasonable approximation of the infarct architecture (Fig 11-22). Contiguous areas of low voltage defines the endocardial extent of the infarct scar. In patients with VT in the setting of healed infarction, this area can be considerable. For example, in one study of such patients the mean infarct area in patients referred for VT ablation was 65 ± 24 $cm^2$ (range 51 to 110 $cm^2$).[61] It is critical the one realize that electrograms only reveal the properties of the first few millimeters of scar. In addition to allowing insight into the electrophysiologic substrate of VT in various forms of structural heart disease, substrate mapping has led to the development of substrate-based ablation for unmappable VTs (see Chapter 13).

Studies that have performed activation and entrainment mapping during VT in the context of sinus rhythm voltage mapping provides a further understanding of the relationship of the infarct border zone (1.0 to 1.5 mV as arbitrarily defined by Marchlinski et al.[61] using standard ablation catheter and the VT circuit). Dense scar was defined as voltage ≤ 0.5 mV. Virtually all of the VTs we have mapped have their critical isthmus within areas with voltage <0.5 mV, which is a reflection of the first 2 to 3 mm of endocardial tissue. Exits from the isthmus are rarely in the "border zone." Using higher resolution mapping with the Rhythmia system we have found many viable areas in what was presumed to be dense scar or even dead using standard ablation (3.5-mm tip). Many of isthmuses are found in regions of 0.1 to 0.5 mV using this higher resolution mapping system (Fig. 11-23). This observation is supported by intraoperative mapping and the effects of SER on diastolic pathways and late potentials as noted earlier.[36] Several investigators[66,67] have used combinations of sinus rhythm voltage mapping using different thresholds for dense scar (0.1 to 0.5 mV) and entrainment mapping during VT to determine that the VT circuit path follows relatively high-voltage "channels" within the infarct scar (Fig. 11-24) (see section on mapping below and in Chapter 13). While this sounds good and has resulted in successful ablation, the pathology of VT shows muscle bundles of 50 to 200 micron associated with late potentials in sinus rhythm and diastolic pathways during VT in tissue removed at successful surgery.[45] This is much smaller than the 1-cm pathways demonstrated by changing voltage criteria or using electrical inexcitability to define scar.[64] Catheter mapping using 3.5- to 4-mm tip electrodes does not have the resolution to detect such small viable fibers and usually record "normal or near-normal" voltage if adjacent large muscle bundles are present and dense scar in areas shown to be viable using much smaller electrodes.

Presently most endocardial voltage maps during sinus rhythm and activation maps during VT typically are acquired by point-by-point mapping using the Carto system. Recently

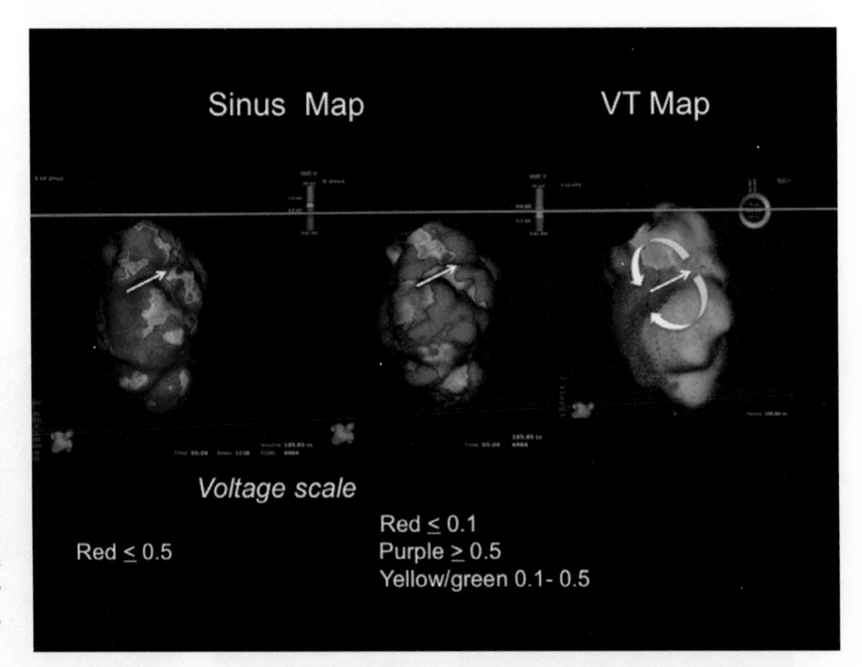


**FIGURE 11-23** Relationship of isthmus during VT to voltage recorded in sinus rhythm. Voltage maps are shown in the two maps on the left. The voltage scale is shown below each map. On the left *red* identifies sites less than 0.5 mV. In the middle *red* signifies tissue with less than 0.1 mV. On the right is an activation map during VT showing figure-of-eight reentry (*red* early, *purple* late). The *white arrow* identifies the site of the isthmus. See text for discussion.

St Jude's Navix system has been shown to be comparable to Carto for voltage and its underlying anatomic scar.[68] Detailed electroanatomic mapping can also be performed with noncontact techniques, which theoretically allow acquisition within a single beat.[69] Low-voltage areas corresponding to the infarct can be determined in sinus rhythm by "deflection" of the wavefront demonstrated on isopotential mapping (Fig. 11-25). In a porcine model of infarction, channels of preferential conduction out of the infarct can be identified when pacing inside the infarct.[70] These channels appear to identify sites that are essential to the VT circuit. Where these are in relation to the electroanatomically defined border has not been assessed. If confirmed in human VT, this observation could allow VT mapping without induction of specific VT morphologies. A major limitation is the imprecision with which these pathways are defined by noncontact methods. In addition sites behind the papillary muscles are hidden from the view of the recording catheter. The more recent use of multipolar contact mapping with small electrodes using the PentaRay Biosense catheter and the new Rhythmia mapping system (see Chapter 1) can detect small fiber bundles that are not detected by the standard 3.5- to 4-mm mapping/ablation catheters. These are invariably recorded in areas of scar with voltages between 0.1 and 0.5 mV.

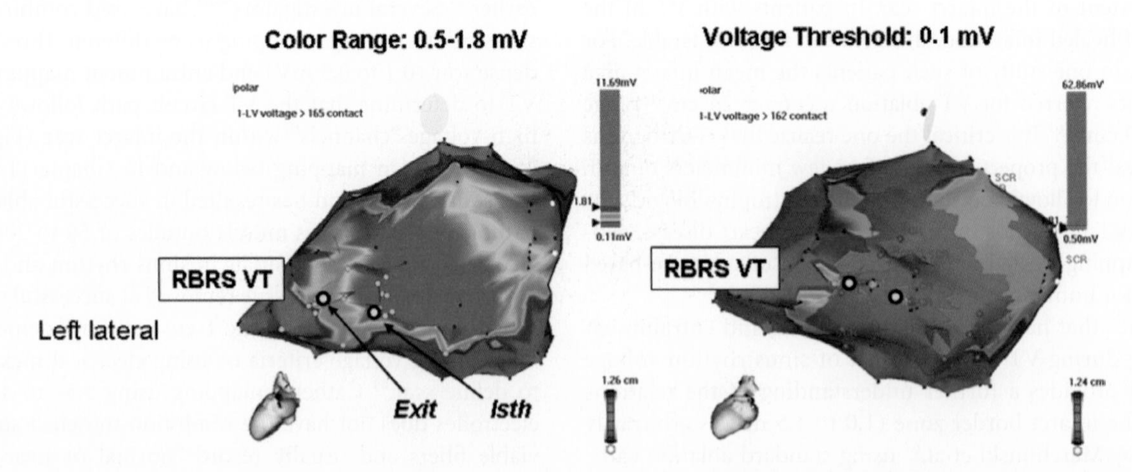


**FIGURE 11-24** Relatively high-voltage "channels" within the infarct may be important to conduction within the VT circuit. A left lateral view of a voltage map performed in sinus rhythm in a patient with a large posterolateral infarction is shown. In the left panel, a typical color pattern for voltage mapping is displayed. In addition, the results of entrainment mapping, showing sites demonstrating relationship to the VT circuit in light *blue dots* (exit; isth, isthmus site). By varying the color display on the voltage map as in the right panel (where sites ≤0.5 mV are shown in *gray* and sites >1.0 mV are shown in purple, it can be seen that the sites within the circuit (*blue dots*) are within a "channel" of relatively preserved voltage, compared to the rest of the infarct. (From Hsia H, Lin D, Sauer W. Anatomic characterization of endocardial substrate for hemodynamically stable reentrant ventricular tachycardia: Identification of endocardial conducting channels. *Heart Rhythm* 2005;3;503–512.)

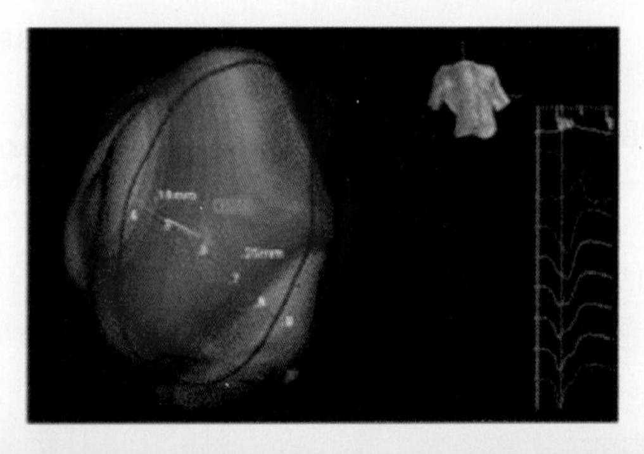

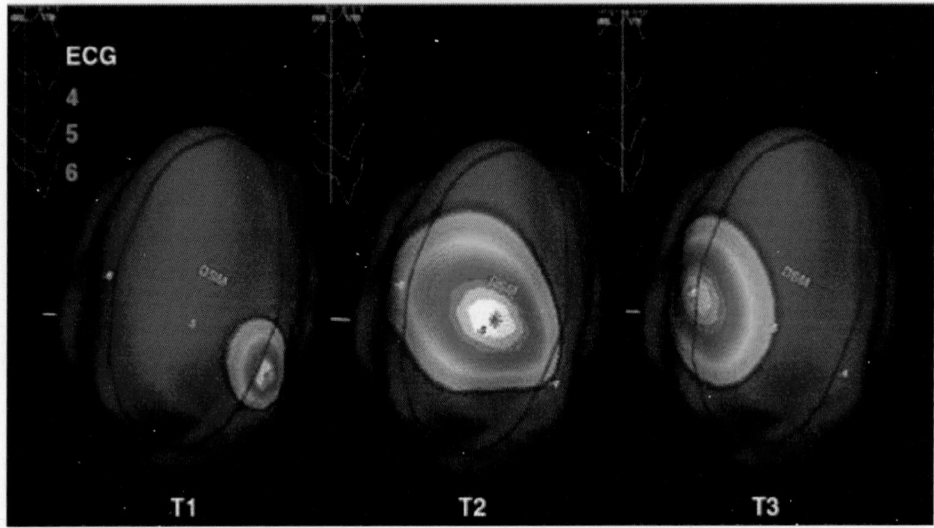


**FIGURE 11-25** Noncontact substrate mapping in a porcine model of anterior infarction. In this type of mapping, the infarct is identified (outlined by *black ellipse*) by low voltage and slow conduction during sinus rhythm and pacing around the borders of the infarct. Isopotential mapping, which tracts unipolar activation wavefronts, is denoted by the color display: sites depicted in *white* represent the activation wavefront, sites in *purple* are resting and colors in between represent sites with lower voltage unipolar electrograms, representing sites that are about to be activated or recovering from just being activated. Areas that appear to be important for conduction out of the infarct to normal tissue are identified by pacing within the substrate (**top panel**). In this example, there are two relatively discrete sites of exit from the substrate, occurring at 5:00 and 9:30 if the substrate is viewed as a clock face. As shown in the **bottom panel**, these same sites appear to be important for conduction during VT. T1, T2, T3 are frames taken in advancing time. T1 shows the activation wavefront during VT entering the substrate that 5:00 (one of the pacing exit sites) and sweeping across the substrate to exit at 9:30 (the other pacing exit site). See text for discussion. (From Jacobson J, Afonso VX, Eisenman G, et al. Characterization of the infarct substrate and ventricular tachycardia circuits with noncontact unipolar mapping in a porcine model of myocardial infarction. *Heart Rhythm* 2006;3:189–197.)

In patients with VT in the setting of LV cardiomyopathy, endocardial sinus rhythm mapping has not identified abnormalities as dramatic as those seen in patients with coronary artery disease.[32] For example, when patients with cardiomyopathy (either hypertrophic or dilated) and ventricular arrhythmias are compared to those with coronary artery disease, significant differences are noted (Table 11-3). Patients with cardiomyopathy in general have more normal endocardial activation and normal electrograms. Even when abnormal, the electrograms are rarely fractionated; in general, fractionated electrograms are observed only in patients with sustained VT, which is a relatively rare presenting arrhythmia in patients with LV cardiomyopathy (Table 11-4). Endocardial activation in patients with cardiomyopathy presenting with cardiac arrest and nonsustained VT does not differ significantly from that in normal individuals. Only ≈10% of sites will be abnormal, primarily because of the duration of the electrogram. When patients with cardiomyopathy are divided into those with and without arrhythmias, the only group of patients in whom significant abnormalities of activation and of conduction are noted are those with sustained uniform VT (Table 11-3). These patients have more abnormal sites and are the only patients with fractionated sites. In addition, the duration of the longest electrogram in patients with cardiomyopathy and sustained uniform VT is markedly prolonged when compared to patients with cardiomyopathy and other arrhythmias. Analysis of electrogram distribution in patients with nonsustained and sustained VT with coronary artery disease and cardiomyopathy is shown in Figure 11-26. Compared to patients with coronary artery disease and VT, patients with cardiomyopathy have fewer abnormal sites, fewer fractionated sites, and relatively normal overall endocardial activation with virtually no late sites. The data from these studies and those of Vassallo et al.[71,72] analyzing ventricular electrograms

**TABLE 11-3 Influence of Underlying Heart Disease**

| | CAD | CM |
|---|---|---|
| Patients (*n*) | 132 | 26 |
| Normal sites (%) | 50 ± 24 | 84 ± 18[a] |
| Abnormal sites (%) | 43 ± 21 | 15 ± 18[a] |
| Fractionated sites (%) | 7 ± 11 | 1 ± 3[b] |
| Endocardial activation time (msec) | 66 ± 30 | 49 ± 14[b] |
| Duration of longest electrogram (msec) | 118 ± 39 | 93 ± 25[b] |
| Late sites (%) | 12 ± 14 | 2 ± 6[a] |

CAD, coronary artery disease; CM, cardiomyopathy.
[a] $p < 0.001$.
[b] $p < 0.005$.
From Cassidy DM, Vassallo JA, Buxton AE, et al. The value of catheter mapping during sinus rhythm to localize site of origin of ventricular tachycardia. *Circulation* 1984;69:1103.

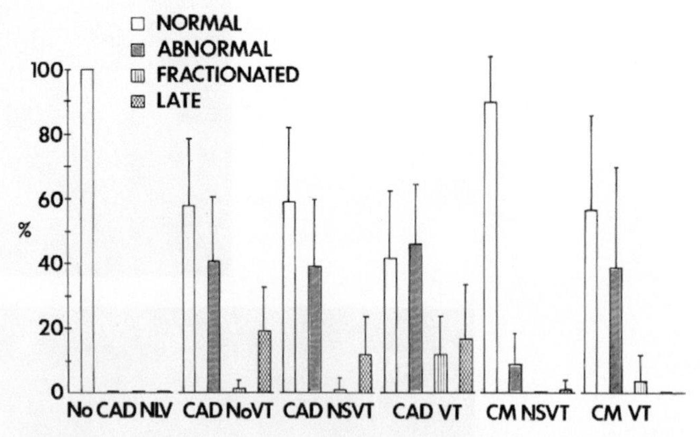


**FIGURE 11-26** Electrogram distribution in different patient populations. The incidence of normal, abnormal, fractionated, and late electrograms in patients with no heart disease and normal left ventricles (NLV), coronary artery disease (CAD) and no VT, CAD and nonsustained VT (NSVT), CAD and sustained VT, cardiomyopathy (CM) and NSVT, and CM with sustained VT. Patients with sustained VT have the highest incidence of abnormal electrograms as well as fractionated and late electrograms. Patients with prior infarction actually have more abnormal and late electrograms than patients with CM. See text for discussion.

and activation sequences in patients with LBBB in patients with coronary artery disease and cardiomyopathy suggest that endocardial activation is nearly normal in patients with cardiomyopathy.

In the subset of patients with dilated cardiomyopathy who have frequent episodes of uniform sustained VT, sinus rhythm voltage mapping abnormalities can be identified. Studies using electroanatomic mapping have demonstrated qualitatively similar, but quantitatively different endocardial areas of low-voltage and less fractionated electrograms and late potentials compared to patients with sustained VT due to healed infarction.[73] In 19 patients with VT in the setting of DCM, low-voltage areas were smaller in area than in patients with healed infarction and VT (20% vs. 42% of endocardial surface) and were typically confined to areas around the mitral and aortic annulae (Fig. 11-27). In patients with dilated cardiomyopathy caused by more focal insults (e.g., myocarditis, sarcoidosis), this predilection to the perivalvular area is not always observed (Fig. 11-28). Importantly, endocardial VT mapping demonstrated that areas of low voltage, fractionation, and late potentials provided the substrate that supported the VT circuit in this clinical setting as well. In patients with dilated cardiomyopathy sinus rhythm voltage

**TABLE 11-4 Influence of Cardiomyopathy and Clinical Arrhythmia**

| | No VT | NSVT | CA | VT |
|---|---|---|---|---|
| Patient (*n*) | | | | |
| Normal sites (%) | 87 ± 7 | 90 ± 10 | 91 ± 11 | 60 ± 25[a] |
| Abnormal sites (%) | 13 ± 7 | 10 ± 10 | 9 ± 11 | 37 ± 27[b] |
| Fractionated sites (%) | 0 ± 0 | 0 ± 0 | 0 ± 0 | 3 ± 7 |
| Endocardial activation sites (msec) | 43 ± 11 | 50 ± 16 | 43 ± 14 | 49 ± 14 |
| Duration of longest electrogram (msec) | 92 ± 5 | 95 ± 23 | 83 ± 14 | 109 ± 43 |
| Late sites (%) | 4 ± 6 | 5 ± 8 | 0 ± 0 | 0 ± 0 |

Abbreviations are as in Table 11-2.
[a] $p < 0.01$ VT vs. No VT, NSVT, CA.
[b] $p < 0.05$ No VT, NSVT, CA.
From Cassidy DM, Vassallo JA, Buxton AE, et al. The value of catheter mapping during sinus rhythm to localize site of origin of ventricular tachycardia. *Circulation* 1984;69:1103.

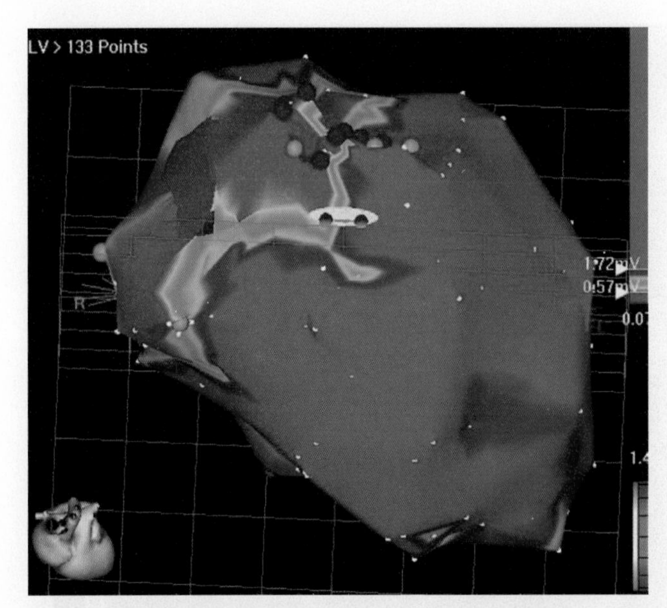


**FIGURE 11-27** Sinus rhythm voltage mapping in nonischemic cardiomyopathy. Voltage maps are shown in a coronal view. *Purple-colored areas* represent normal endocardium (voltage ≥1.8 mV), *red areas* represent dense scar (voltage ≤0.5 mV) with the border zone indicated by the intervening colors. Typically the endocardial voltage abnormalities observed in such patients are limited to the perimitral valve area.

and electrogram abnormalities may be more evident on the epicardium and VT circuits can be mapped to the epicardium preferentially (Fig. 11-29).[74] This observation is consistent with findings from intraoperative mapping of patients with cardiomyopathy undergoing defibrillator implantation or surgery which demonstrated transmural and/or epicardial conduction abnormalities. Recent studies by Sosa et al.[75,76] suggest epicardial abnormalities are present in patients with Chagas disease.

This has led to interest in detecting abnormalities deeper than the subendocardium. Unipolar mapping has gained popularity in defining intramural and/or subepicardial scar. As noted above electrogram abnormalities, either unipolar or bipolar, reflect propagation and not necessarily tissue mass. As such I consider electrogram abnormalities to reflect conduction abnormalities, which may be caused by functional or anatomic abnormalities. Hutchinson et al.,[77] using the Carto XP system with filtering set at 1 to 400 HZ defined "normal" unipolar voltage recorded from the LV endocardium was 8.3 mV. Other filter settings and systems (Carto 3) have been used by different investigators in populations with sustained VT associated with prior myocardial infarction and cardiomyopathy.[78,79] While the values for "normal" differ a little, these studies show a correlation between the low-voltage endocardial unipolar mapping and low-voltage epicardial bipolar mapping and gadolinium enhancement by MRI. Similar studies have not been performed in normal populations or in those with cardiomyopathy and no VT. We have used filtering at 0.05 to 500 in all Carto systems in patients with and without VT and have normal values of ~7.5 mV in the absence of hypertrophy. I have found a high incidence of false negatives in patients with hypertrophic cardiomyopathy (Fig. 11-30) and other hypertrophic states using delayed gadolinium enhancement as the marker of scar. Moreover, while the "intramural/subepicardial scar depicted by unipolar mapping in these highly selected patients appear to correlate with bipolar epicardial mapping, the interpretation that this represents "microfibrosis" is not proven. The presence of delayed enhancement defines **macro fibrosis**. Patients with dilated cardiomyopathy typically have patchy fibrosis, and large unipolar voltage in the precordial

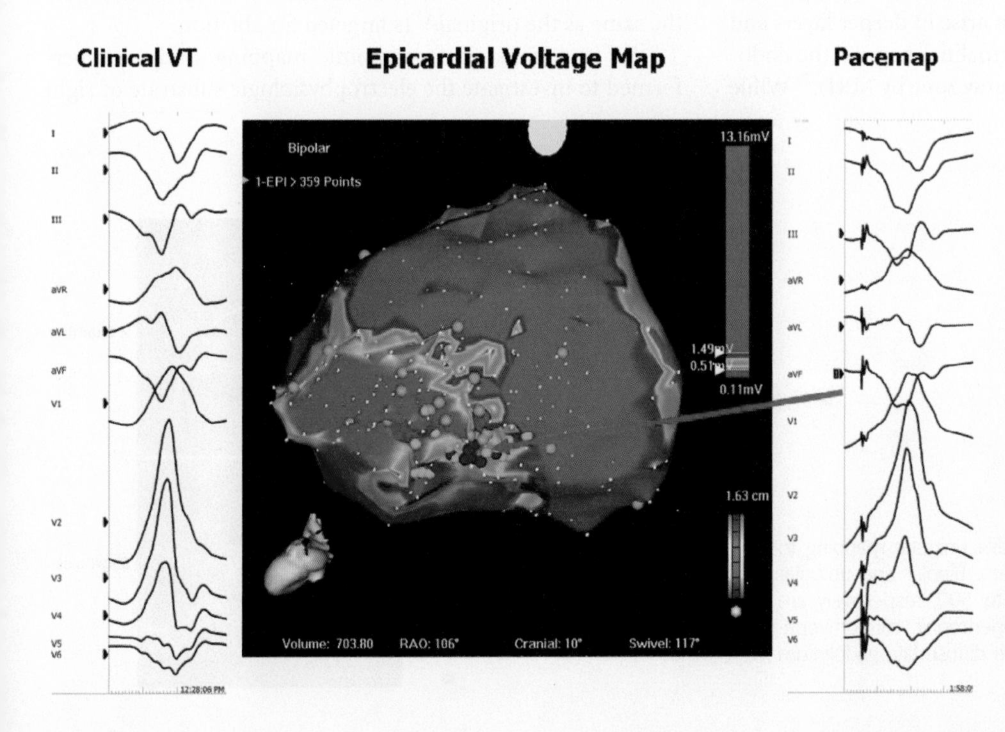


**FIGURE 11-28** Epicardial voltage mapping in a patient with cardiac sarcoid and sustained VT. The electroanatomic map is shown in posterior–anterior projection; the voltage scale is color coded so that normal tissue is displayed in *purple* (bipolar electrograms ≥1.5 mV) and dense scar in *red* (<0.5 mV). Unlike most patients with dilated cardiomyopathy and VT, where mapping demonstrates a perivalvular substrate, this patient had apical voltage map abnormalities. Pace mapping, performed to approximate the exit site of the VT circuit, also localizes the site of the circuit to the apical voltage abnormality. Ablation at this site resulted in prevention of clinical VT episodes.

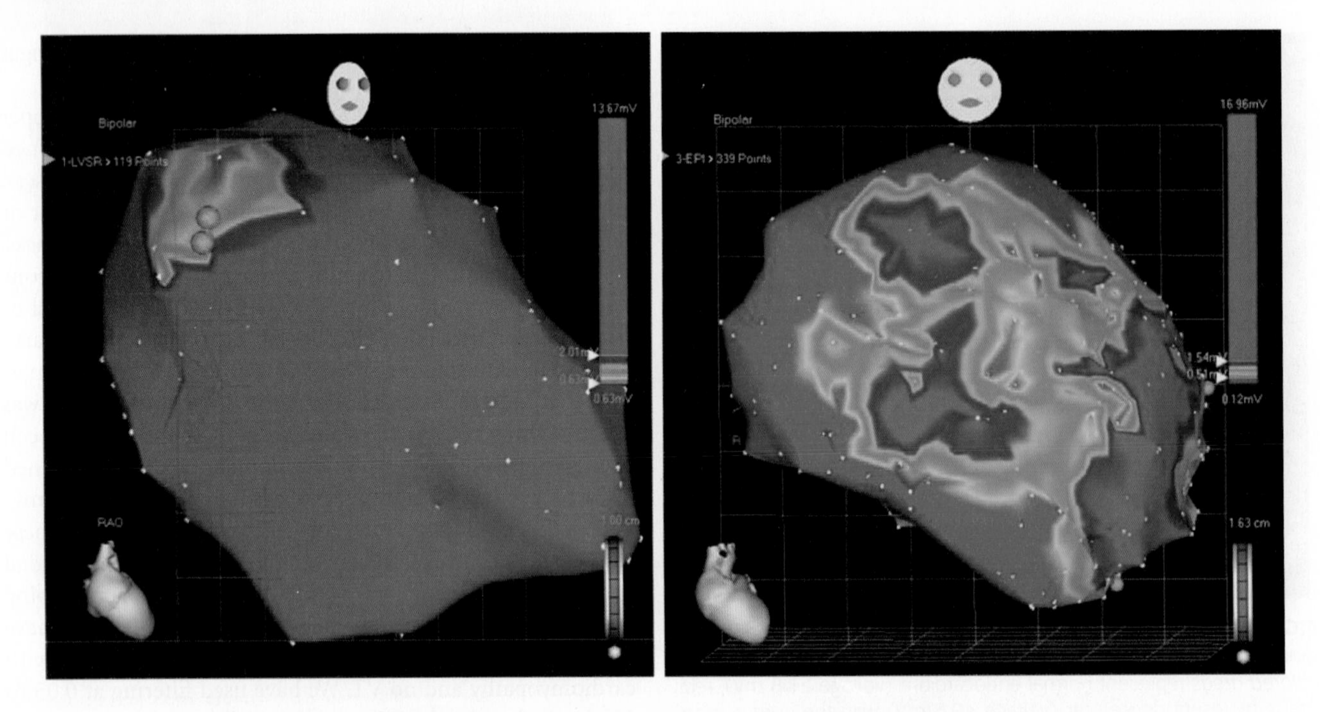


**FIGURE 11-29** Sinus rhythm voltage mapping in nonischemic cardiomyopathy. Endocardial mapping in this patient with recurrent uniform VT did not demonstrate electrogram abnormalities. Epicardial mapping demonstrated contiguous areas of low-voltage, abnormal electrograms that served as the substrate for reentrant VT.

leads and normal unipolar endocardial maps. This could in fact be recorded in the presence of microfibrosis. The signature of micro- or macrofibrosis is nonuniform anisotropic conduction, not decreased voltage. We still require methods to detect inapparent conduction abnormalities cause by microfibrosis. While sustained VT in cardiomyopathy appears to frequently have an intramural or subepicardial origin, patients with infarction-related VT may also arise in deeper layers and may be detected by unipolar abnormalities beyond the endocardial substrate (analogous to the gray zone by MRI).[79] While Hutchinson et al.[77] suggest this may explain the reason for failed endocardial ablation for infarct-related VT, these conclusions are fraught with many limitations. These include short follow-up (3 months), inadequate definition of the correlation between critical sites defined by pace-mapping versus entrainment mapping, proof of adequacy of determining critical sites, and the absence of ECGs of recurrent VTs to see if they were the same as the original VTs targeted for ablation.

An analogous electroanatomic mapping study was performed to investigate the electrophysiologic substrate of right

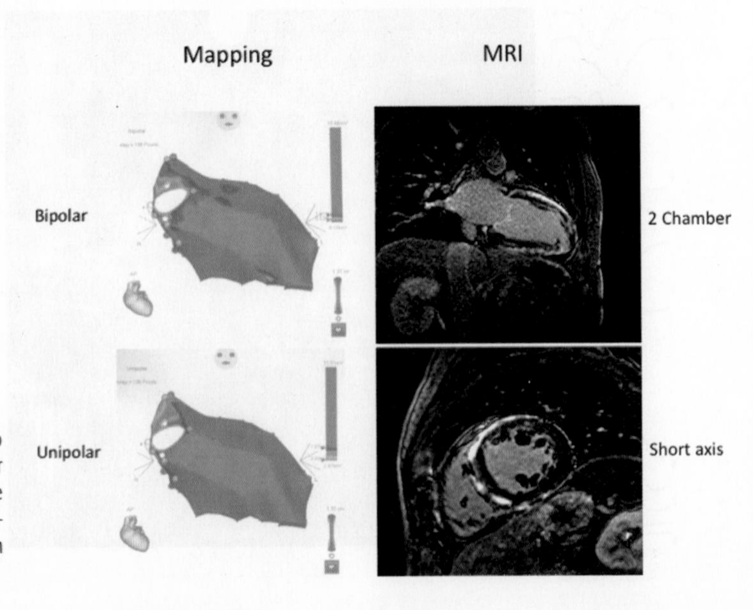


**FIGURE 11-30** Limitation of endocardial unipolar mapping to identify epicardial/subepicardial substrate. Bipolar and unipolar maps filtered at0.03 to 500 and 30 to 500, respectively are shown with MRI in a patient with hypertrophic cardiomyopathy. The unipolar map is normal despite diffuse late gadolinium enhancement. See text for discussion.

ventricular cardiomyopathy (RV dysplasia).[80] In 21 patients with recurrent VT, contiguous areas of low-voltage abnormal electrograms measured $55 \pm 37$ cm$^2$, representing 34% of the RV surface area. Areas of abnormal electrograms always involved the RV-free wall, spared the RV apex, and were said to include the intraventricular septum (15/21 patients). This observation differs from the accepted description of the "triad" of arrhythmogenic RV dysplasia (ARVD).[81] In addition, the majority of abnormal electrograms as well as VT sites of origin, were located in perivalvular areas—the tricuspid valve (5 patients), the pulmonic valve (6 patients), or both (10 patients) (Fig. 11-31). However, the "septal" areas were in the RVOT which has no abutting septum; the true septum appears normal. My experience in 24 cases studied prior to and during the electroanatomic mapping era is that abnormalities are in the RVOT, the RV-free wall, and the region of the tricuspid annulus. In some patients these areas were confluent. The true septum was, spared (Figs. 11-31 and 11-32). Of interest is that the region at the tricuspid annulus was the most frequently associated with VTs that I have mapped. Unipolar mapping has identified large epicardial abnormalities in this population,[82] the pathology of which has been known to have early epicardial involvement.[81] Such mapping has led to early epicardial approaches to ablate VTs in ARVD.

Hypertrophic cardiomyopathy, both with and without obstruction, is associated with a high incidence of sudden cardiac death. Although electrograms observed during sinus rhythm mapping appear similar to those in dilated cardiomyopathy, the response of these electrograms to ventricular extrastimuli (VES) may distinguish patients at risk. We initially observed fractionation of electrograms at the RV apex and RV outflow in response to VES in members of high-risk families with hypertrophic obstructive cardiomyopathy.[83] Saumarez et al.[84,85] have confirmed our findings and demonstrated that patients with lethal arrhythmias show a greater degree of fragmentation (i.e., longer duration) at longer coupling intervals (i.e., longer relative refractory periods) than in patients without such a history. As noted above, I have not found endocardial unipolar mapping to be of value in this population. Further work is necessary to characterize the sites and mechanism of conduction abnormalities in patients with all forms of cardiomyopathy.

If an epicardial substrate is suggested by endocardial unipolar mapping in a patient with cardiomyopathy and VT with ECG features suggesting epicardial origin, direct epicardial mapping of the substrate and VT is required (see Chapter 13). Epicardial fat hinders interpretation of epicardial substrate mapping using low voltage as a marker of abnormality because the fat decreases the EGM amplitude due to insulation of the tissue from the recording electrode. It does not; however, result in multicomponent or fractionated EGMs or late potentials, which are markers of fibrosis and abnormal myocardial activation.

Signal averaging techniques have been developed to record this substrate of prolonged, asynchronous conduction from the surface of the heart.[84–91] Basically orthogonal XYZ leads are used, and after signal averaging and high-pass (above 40 Hz) filtering, the leads are combined into a vector magnitude ($X^2 + Y^2 + Z^2$, RMS amplitude), a measurement that sums up the high-frequency information contained in all of these leads. This vector magnitude is often called the filtered QRS complex. The duration of the QRS and the amplitude of the high-frequency signals in the last 40 msec (so-called late potentials) have been used with the duration of terminal activity beneath 40 mV, as a measure of abnormalities of conduction associated with arrhythmias. Normal values are a

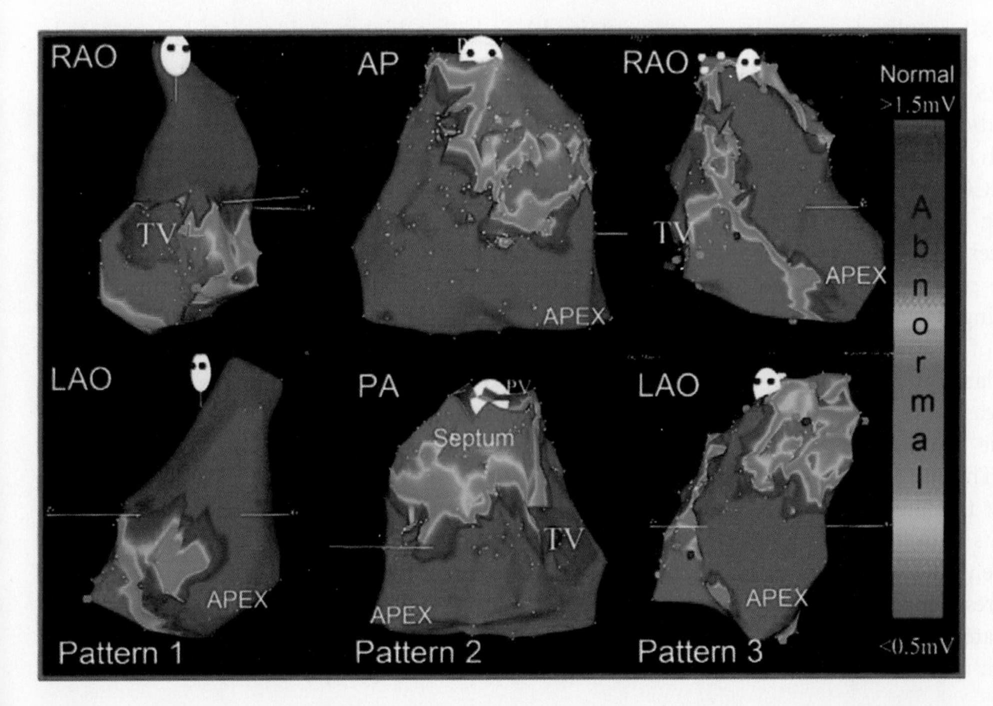


**FIGURE 11-31** Sinus rhythm voltage mapping in right ventricular cardiomyopathy and ventricular tachycardia. Patterns of voltage mapping abnormalities were typically related to perivalular areas: near the tricuspid valve (pattern 1), the pulmonic valve (pattern 2) or both (pattern 3). *Purple-colored areas* represent normal endocardium (voltage ≥1.8 mV), *red areas* represent dense scar (voltage ≤0.5 mV) with the border zone indicated by the intervening colors. (From Marchlinski FE, Zado EZ, Dixit S, et al. Electroanatomic substrate and outcome of catheter ablative therapy for ventricular tachycardia in the setting of right ventricular cardiomyopathy. *Circulation* 2004;110:2293–2298.)

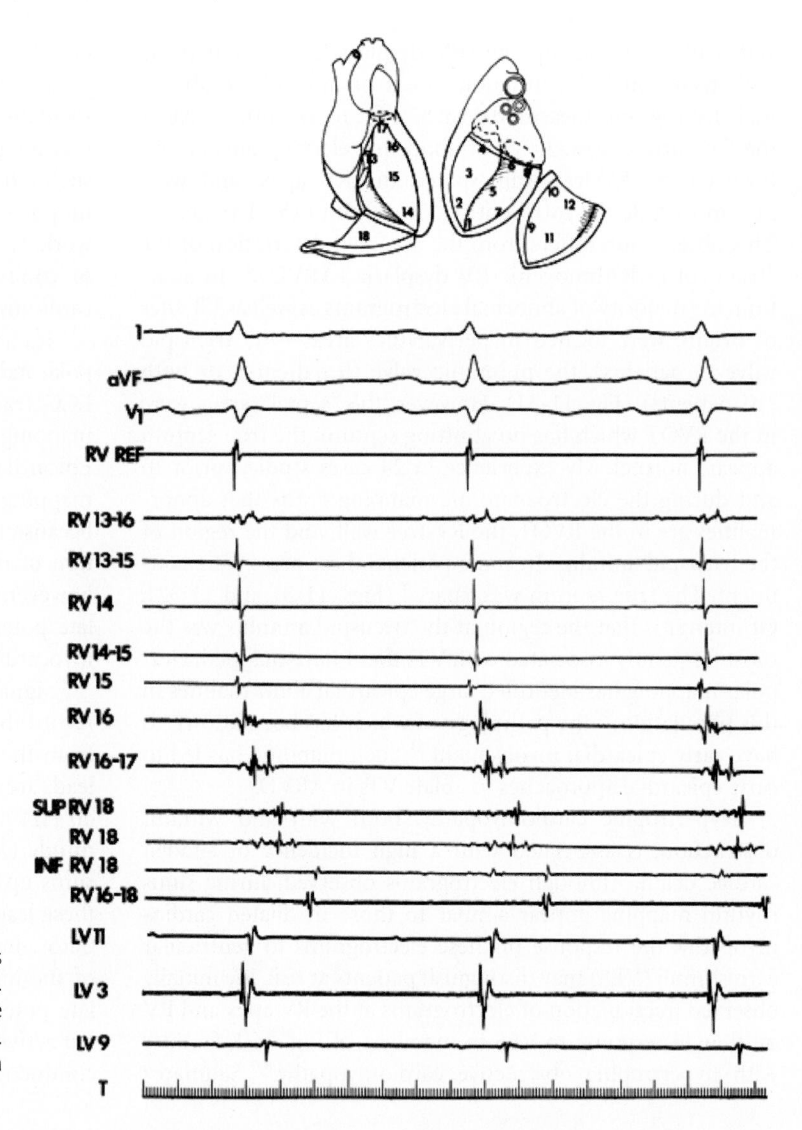


**FIGURE 11-32** Sinus rhythm mapping in ARVD. A sinus map in a patient with ARVD and sustained VT is shown. Markedly fragmented and delayed EGMs are seen in the RVOT and the free wall of the RV. The true septum is spared. The delayed activation correlates with the epsilon wave on the surface ECG.

QRS duration of ≤114 msec, an RMS amplitude in the last 40 msec of >20 μV, and a duration of the signal <40 μV of ≤38 msec. Of note, the filtered QRS duration is shorter for women than for men.[91] No systematic studies have validated the use of the SAECG in patients with IVCDs or bundle branch block. An example of a normal SAECG and an abnormal one from a patient with VT are shown in Figure 11-33. Studies in patients with VT and coronary artery disease have demonstrated that the low-amplitude late potentials are related to fragmented electrical signals extending beyond the QRS. Both the number of sites and duration of this fragmented activity influence the ability to record a late potential using signal averaging.[92] In coronary artery disease and prior infarction, 88% of signals recorded during the late potential are from the endocardium (Fig. 11-34).[93,94] The incidence of positive SAECGs (i.e., increased duration of the filtered QRS and/or late potentials) is highest in patients with infarction-related sustained uniform VT (approximately 85%) and is lower for patients presenting with cardiac arrest (approximately 55%) and nonsustained VT (approximately 50%).[84–86,88,90,91,95,96] Patients with inferior wall infarction (particularly those with nonsustained VT) have a higher incidence of late potentials than those with anterior infarction.[96] This is most likely related to the ease with which late potentials can be recorded from inferobasal sites of infarction, which are normally activated late in the QRS. These findings are directly related to the abnormal electrograms noted on the endocardium during sinus rhythm mapping.[92,93] These abnormalities of conduction recorded on the body surface have been evaluated and approved for predicting lethal arrhythmias postmyocardial infarction[97] as well as determining which patients with syncope might have ventricular arrhythmias as the cause.[97–100] In all studies the QRS duration appears to be the most sensitive measurement, the others being not independently predictive.

The primary use of signal-averaged electrocardiography has been in postinfarction patients.[90,91] Unfortunately it has a positive predictive value of ≈20%, although its negative predictive value approaches 95%. Similar good negative predictive values have been reported for patients with syncope,[98] but the gold standard for this clinical syndrome upon which sensitivity was based was inducibility of sustained VT. It is unclear whether inducible VT is an appropriate endpoint. The role of

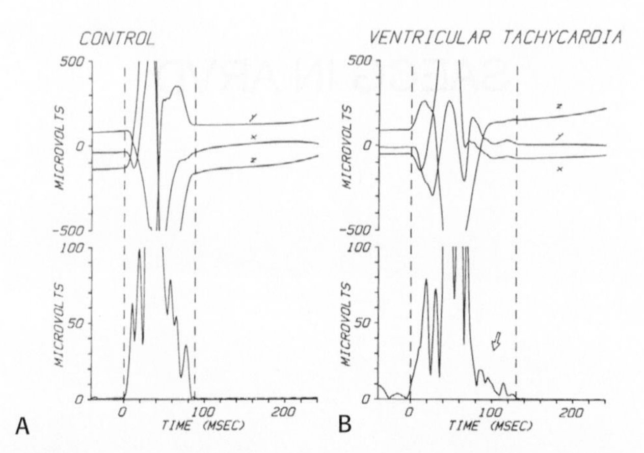


**FIGURE 11-33** Signal-averaged ECGs in patients with inferior infarction with and without VT. **A:** Control, a signal-averaged ECG is shown. The highly gained XYZ recordings are filtered above 40 Hz. Note the symmetric configuration of the filtered complex, which is 100 msec in duration. The mean voltage of the last 40 msec of the filtered QRS was 45 μV (normal >20 μV). **B:** A signal-averaged ECG from a patient with inferior infarction and VT. Note that the QRS duration is markedly prolonged to 117 msec and the terminal part of the filtered QRS shows a low-amplitude late potential (*arrow*). The mean amplitude of the last 40 msec was 10 μV. (From Simson MB. Use of signals in the terminal QRS complex to identify patients with ventricular tachycardia after myocardial infarction. *Circulation* 1981;64:235.)

the SAECG in predicting inducible sustained VT in patients with prior infarction and nonsustained VT and ejection fractions less than 40% has recently been evaluated in the Multicenter Unstained Tachycardia Trial (MUSTT). Despite earlier, nonrandomized studies that suggested utility of the SAECG, more recent studies[97] demonstrate that the SAECG could not predict inducibility of sustained VT in this population. Interestingly, the SAECG was an independent predictor of mortality and sudden cardiac death in subpopulations of MUSTT patients (unpublished observations). Obviously, the exact role of the SAECG, as well as other noninvasive risk stratifiers, needs to be determined. Current guidelines for use of the SAECG have been published in a consensus document of the American College of Cardiology.[101]

The natural history of development of these conduction abnormalities in coronary artery disease is uncertain, although they appear to develop gradually, 3 days to 2 weeks following infarction.[87,90,91,102] Once present, these late potentials do not disappear. This seems to support the observations of Roy et al.[26] that uniform VT induced 2 weeks after infarction can be reliably reproduced a year later. This was recently reproduced in an ovine model of infarction in which inducible VT in the first 2 weeks was reproduced at 100 days.[27] These findings form the basis for the use of programmed stimulation to determine the risk of sudden cardiac arrest postmyocardial infarction.

In patients with nonischemic dilated cardiomyopathy and VT, in whom endocardial activation is generally normal, the SAECG is often abnormal.[102] In patients who present with sustained VT or VF, the SAECG is both longer in duration and has a lower amplitude in the terminal (40 msec) than in

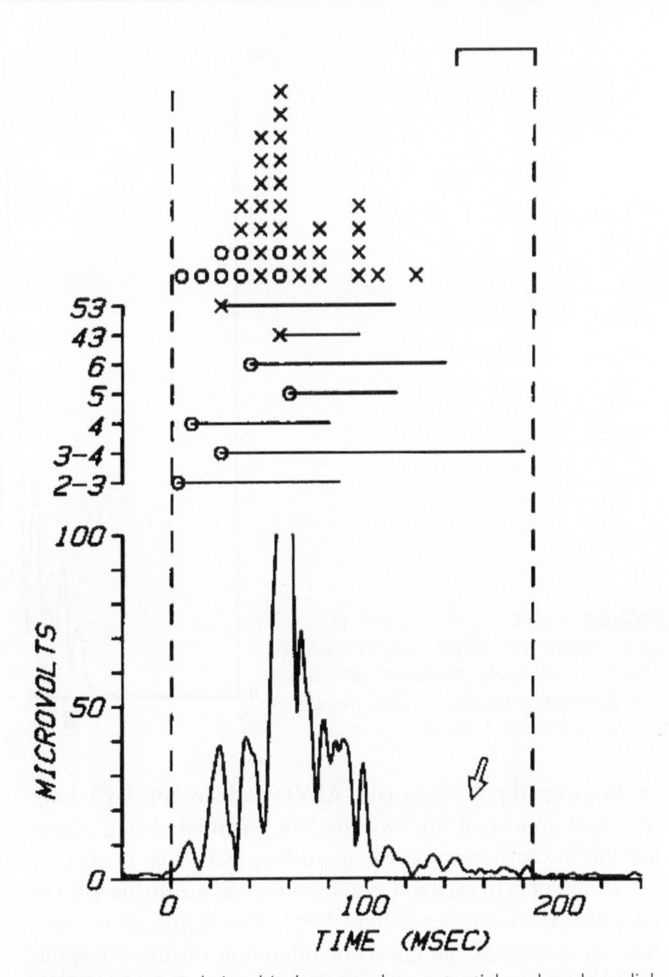


**FIGURE 11-34** Relationship between late potential and endocardial and epicardial recordings in a patient with VT. The filtered signal-averaged QRS is shown on the **bottom** and mapping sites on **top**. Sites 2–3, 3–4, 4, 5, and 6 are endocardial sites. Sites 43 and 53 are epicardial sites The bar represents duration of the electrogram. Other epicardial sites are shown as Xs, and endocardial sites are shown as Os. Note that the low-amplitude late potential (*arrow*) is associated with late endocardial activity from four sites and late epicardial activity from one site. See text for discussion. (From Simson MB, Untereker WJ, Spielman SR, et al. Relation between late potentials on the body surface and directly recorded fragmented electrograms in patients with ventricular tachycardia. *Am J Cardiol* 1983;51:105.)

comparable patients with cardiomyopathy and no malignant arrhythmia.[103] Although prolongation of duration seen in these patients may be a reflection of the abnormal QRS on the surface ECG, in the group of patients with sustained VT or fibrillation, 83% had a late potential, regardless of QRS duration. These data suggest that the substrate of slow conduction in patients with cardiomyopathy resides in the midmyocardium or epicardium. Data using epicardial mapping in Chagas disease support this hypothesis.[75] Although an early study by Middlekauff et al.[104] failed to demonstrate any utility of the SAECG in these patients, Mancini et al.[105] found a high correlation of positive SAECG with mortality and fibrosis. Further evaluation of signal averaging is necessary to establish whether it can provide a noninvasive method to recognize an arrhythmogenic substrate in patients with nonischemic dilated LV

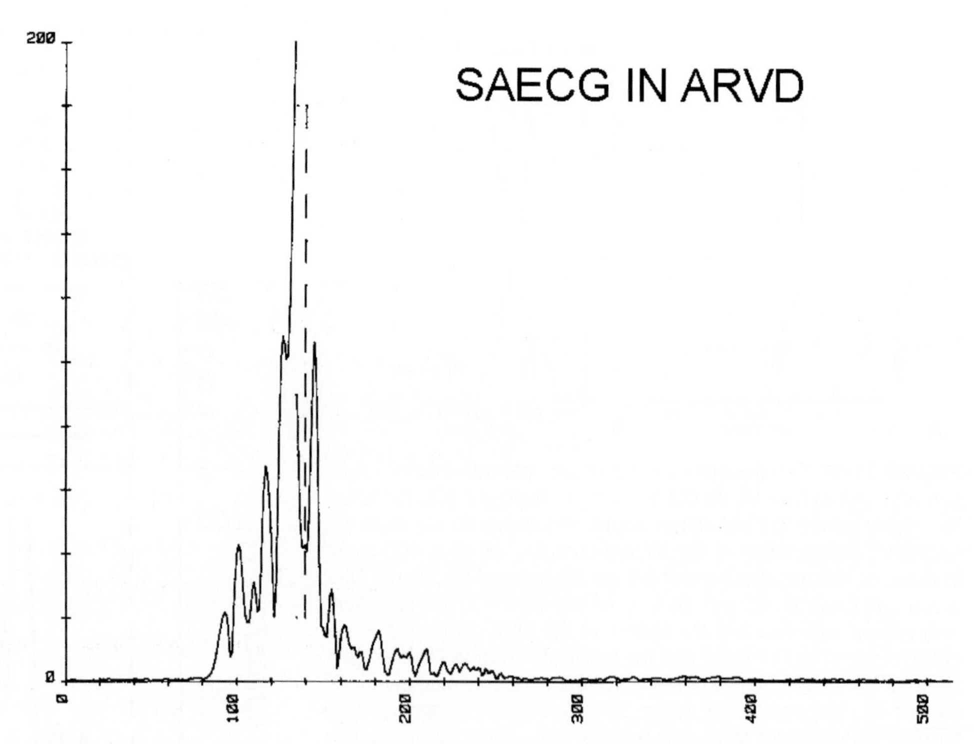


**FIGURE 11-35** Signal-averaged ECG in a patient with ARVD and VT. The SAECG is markedly abnormal with a late potential extended to 260 msec, with a duration of 110 msec.

cardiomyopathy. Patients with ARVD and sustained VT have the most abnormal SAECG; the late potentials being correlated to the epsilon waves on the surface ECG (Fig. 11-35).

Differences in excitability, refractoriness, and dispersion of refractoriness are other potential arrhythmogenic abnormalities. We evaluated the effects of infarction on the threshold of excitability, refractoriness, and strength-interval curves.[106] These studies demonstrated that sites of infarction characterized by abnormal electrograms have higher thresholds than normal sites in patients with infarction ($1.9 \pm 1$ vs. $0.7 \pm 0.4$ mA, $p < 0.05$) (Fig. 11-36). This higher threshold corresponds to a strength-interval curve that has shifted upward, particularly during late coupling intervals (Fig 11-37). Refractory periods determined at threshold were longer at sites of infarction, but the steep part of the strength-interval curves were not significantly different (Fig 11-38). Furthermore, the effect of change in cycle length of the refractory period measured as the steep part of the strength-interval curve was similar in normal sites and sites of infarction ($39 \pm 9$ vs. $32 \pm 8$ msec, $p$ = NS). The current at which the steep part of the strength-interval curve was achieved was also comparable.

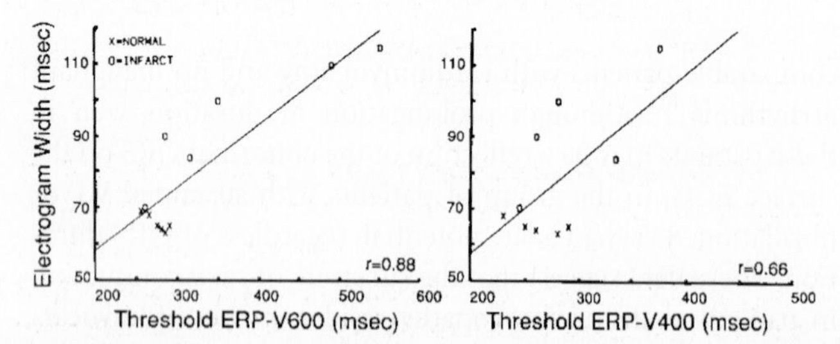


**FIGURE 11-36** Relation between local electrogram width and measured threshold effective refractory period (ERP). The local electrogram width during sinus rhythm is plotted against the ERP measured at threshold stimulus strength during ventricular pacing cycle length of 600 and 400 msec. The X denotes measurements from a normal site and O from an infarcted site from the infarct patient group. (From Kienzle MG, Doherty JU, Cassidy D, et al. Electrophysiologic sequelae of chronic myocardial infarction: local refractoriness and electrographic characteristics of the left ventricle. *Am J Cardiol* 1986;58:63.)

Because abnormalities of excitability and refractoriness are encountered in infarcted sites having abnormal electrograms, we evaluated whether dispersion of refractoriness, dispersion of activation, dispersion of total recovery (LAT plus local refractory periods) for the entire ventricle or for adjacent sites were arrhythmogenic.[107] Definitions are given in Table 11-5. We compared these parameters in patients with no arrhythmias and normal hearts, patients with long QT interval syndromes and recurrent VF, and patients with coronary artery disease status postmyocardial infarction who presented with sustained ventricular tachyarrhythmias. Examples of patients from each group are shown in Figures 11-39 to 11-41. These data, which are summarized in Tables 11-6 and 11-7, demonstrated that patients with long QT interval syndromes have a normal dispersion of activation and a significant dispersion of refractoriness and total recovery time, whereas patients with coronary artery disease and ventricular arrhythmias have normal dispersion of refractoriness but marked abnormalities of ventricular activation, which produce the consequent dispersion of total recovery. This was true whether or not the parameters were evaluated for the entire left ventricle or at adjacent sites. In view of the fact that in patients with sustained VT due to coronary artery disease arrhythmias can be reproducibly initiated by programmed stimulation and that in those with long QT syndromes arrhythmias are not inducible (see subsequent paragraphs on initiation of ventricular tachyarrhythmias), one must conclude that abnormalities of conduction

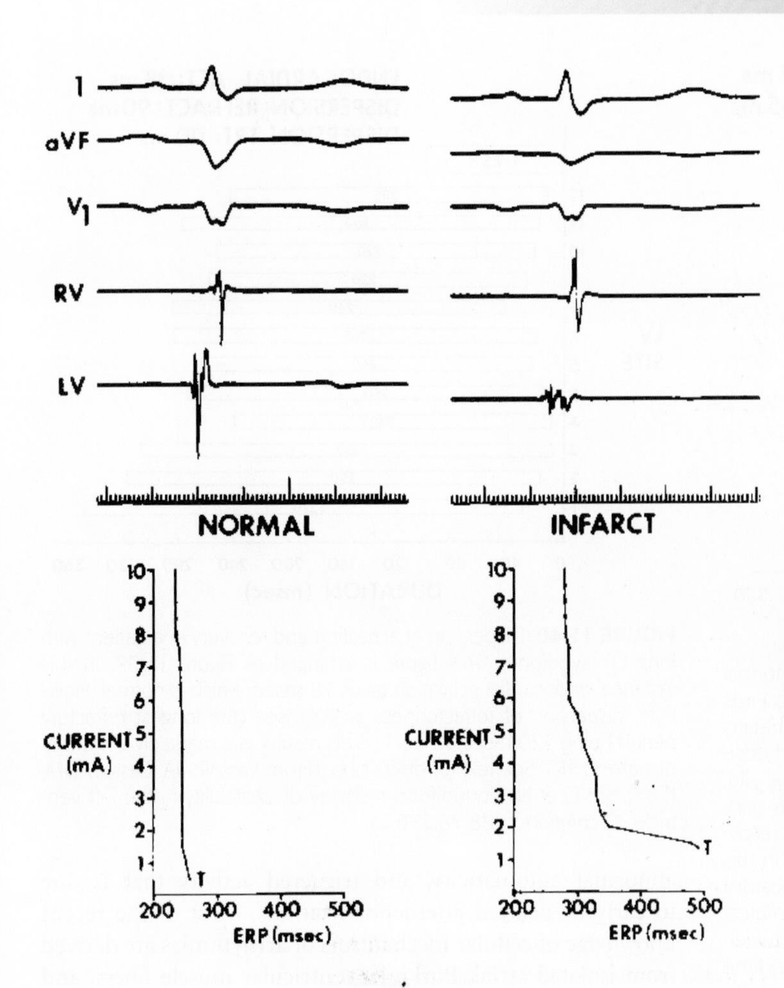


**FIGURE 11-37** Locally recorded electrograms and strength-interval curves from an infarct and noninfarct site in the same patient. Electrophysiologic leads 1, aVF, and $V_1$ are displayed with a right ventricular reference and left ventricular electrograms (RV and LV). Ten-msec time lines are shown below. The strength-interval curves measured at each site are also shown with the measured refractory period plotted from threshold to 10 mA. Alterations characteristic of chronic infarction are seen in both the local electrogram and strength-interval curve. (From Kienzle MG, Doherty JU, Cassidy D, et al. Electrophysiologic sequelae of chronic myocardial infarction: local refractoriness and electrographic characteristics of the left ventricle. *Am J Cardiol* 1986;58:63.)

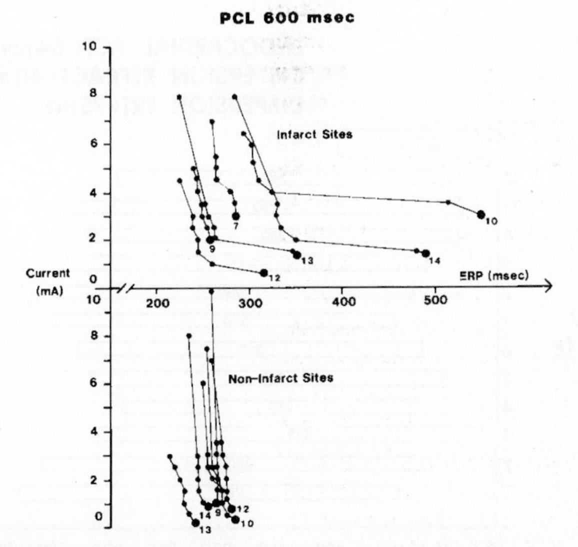


**FIGURE 11-38** Individual strength-interval curves from infarct and noninfarct sites from patients with previous myocardial infarction. Each curve consists of the ERP at threshold (*large filled circles*) and at each of the next five increments of current strength (*small filled circles*). The last point of each curve corresponds to the stimulus strength at which no further shortening of ERP occurred (first point of the steep portion of the strength-interval curve). The curved numbers refer to individual patients. PCL, pacing cycle length. (From Kienzle MG, Doherty JU, Cassidy D, et al. Electrophysiologic sequelae of chronic myocardial infarction: local refractoriness and electrographic characteristics of the left ventricle. *Am J Cardiol* 1986;58:63.)

**TABLE 11-5 Definitions**

**Local refractory period:** Longest $S_1$-$S_2$ coupling interval that failed to elicit a response after an eight-beat drive from each left ventricular site

**Local activation time:** Interval (msec) from the onset of the surface QRS complex to the point where the rapid deflection of the largest deflection of the local electrogram crossed the baseline

**Total endocardial activation time:** Duration (msec) from the earliest to the latest site of left ventricular activation

**Total recovery time:** Local activation time (relative to the surface QRS complex) and the local refractory period (msec) at each left ventricular site

**Dispersion of refractoriness:** The widest range of refractory periods within the left ventricle for each patient

**Dispersion of total recovery time:** The difference between the earliest and latest recovery times in the left ventricle for each patient

From Vassallo JA, Cassidy DM, Kindwall KE, et al. Nonuniform recovery of excitability in the left ventricle. *Circulation* 1988;78:1365.

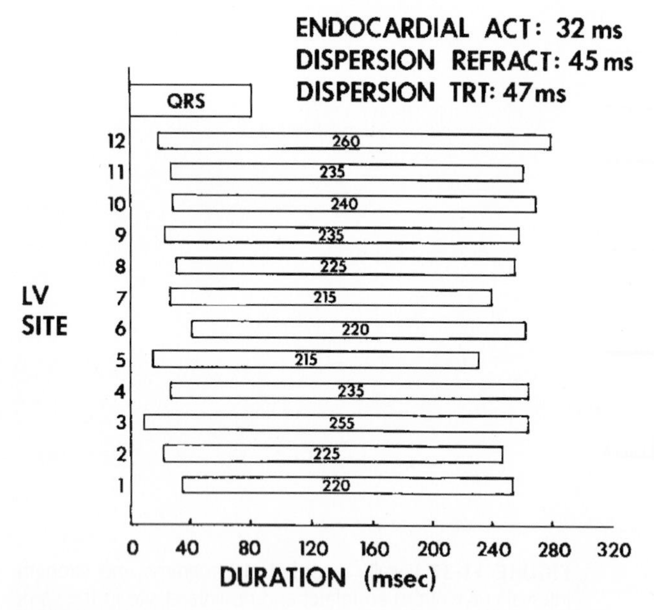


**FIGURE 11-39** Dispersion of activation and recovery in a normal patient. On the horizontal axis is time duration and on the vertical axis are the mapped left ventricular sites. The QRS displayed on top begins at 0 time and extends to approximately 80 msec. The left-hand edge of each bar represents the local activation time at the individual site, and the duration of the bar represents the local ERP (value in bar). The right-hand edge of each bar represents the end of total recovery time (the sum of activation time and local refractoriness). In this patient, one sees early breakthrough sites at 3, 5, and 12. Endocardial activation (ACT) time from the earliest onset (site 3) to the latest (site 6) is 32 msec. The dispersion refractoriness (difference between shortest and longest) is 45 msec, and dispersion of total recovery time (TRT) (the maximum difference between the right-hand edge of the rectangles) is 41 msec. These are all normal values. See text for discussion. (From Vassallo JA, Cassidy DM, Kindwall KE, et al. Nonuniform recovery of excitability in the left ventricle. *Circulation* 1988;78:1365.)

provide a more important reflection of inducible arrhythmias (which we assume to be a marker for reentry) than dispersion of refractoriness alone. Thus, one must consider abnormalities of conduction to be of primary importance in the genesis of sustained uniform ventricular arrhythmias. The greater these abnormalities, the more likely uniform tachycardias occur spontaneously or can be induced. Invasive or noninvasive methods to demonstrate abnormalities of conduction are, therefore, useful markers of an arrhythmogenic substrate. Patients with VF or nonsustained VT appear to have fewer conduction abnormalities (i.e., less slow conduction), and hence, their tachycardias remain either nonsustained or degenerate to VF. The relationship of these arrhythmias to sustained VT is discussed subsequently.

## MECHANISMS OF VENTRICULAR TACHYCARDIA

The mechanisms of VT have been under active investigation both experimentally and clinically in the past three decades. Potential mechanisms of VTs include reentry, normal and

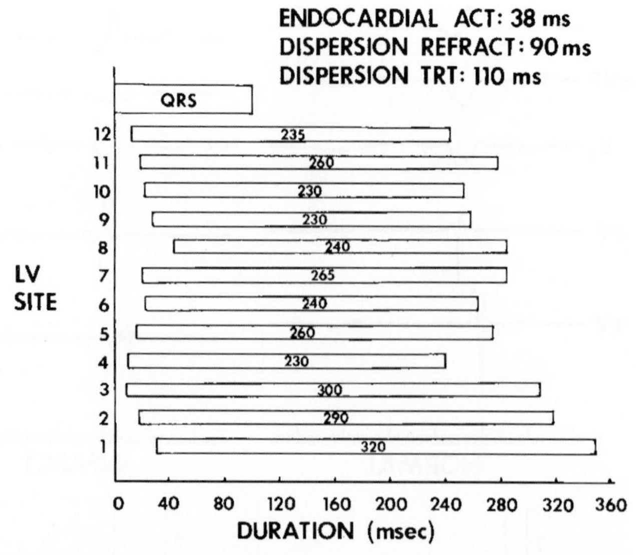


**FIGURE 11-40** Dispersion of activation and recovery in a patient with long QT syndrome. This figure is arranged as Figure 11-39. In this instance, endocardial activation takes 38 msec, which is normal. However, dispersion of refractoriness is 90 msec (the longest refractory period being 320 msec at site 1). This results in a markedly abnormal dispersion TRT. See text for discussion. (From Vassallo JA, Cassidy DM, Kindwall KE, et al. Nonuniform recovery of excitability in the left ventricle. *Circulation* 1988;78:1365.)

abnormal automaticity, and triggered activity that is due to early or delayed afterdepolarizations. Most of the recent knowledge of cellular mechanisms of arrhythmias are derived from isolated atrial, Purkinje, ventricular muscle fibers, and

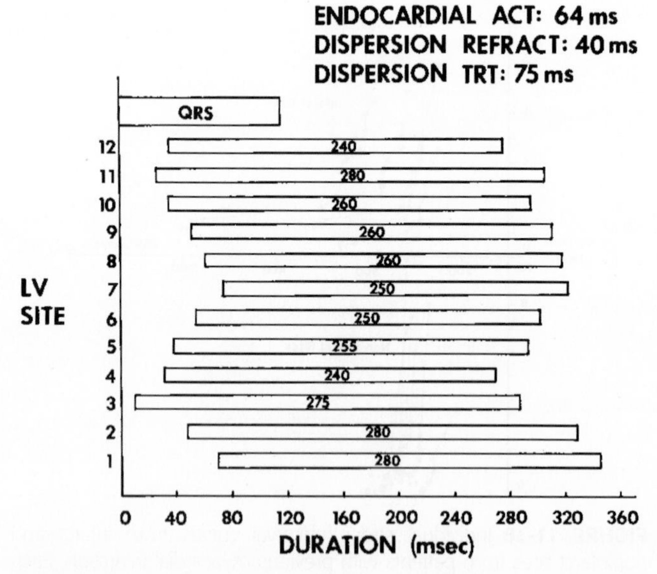


**FIGURE 11-41** Dispersion of activation and recovery in a patient with prior CAD and VT. This tracing is arranged as Figures 11-39 and 11-40. In this patient with VT and CAD, there is marked dispersion of endocardial activation, which requires 64 msec to complete. Dispersion of refractoriness is normal at 40 msec. Because of the irregular and prolonged activation times, there is prolongation of total dispersion of recovery of 15 msec. See text for discussion. (From Vassallo JA, Cassidy DM, Kindwall KE, et al. Nonuniform recovery of excitability in the left ventricle. *Circulation* 1988;78:1365.)

**TABLE 11-6 Data Based on Whole Left Ventricle Analysis**

| | Endocardial Activation Time (msec) | Dispersion of Refractoriness (msec) | Dispersion of Total Recovery Time (msec) |
|---|---|---|---|
| Normal left ventricle (no ventricular tachycardia) | 34 ± 9<br>75 ± 23 | 40 ± 14<br>53 ± 14 | 52 ± 14<br>90 ± 30 |
| Coronary artery disease (with ventricular tachycardia) | *p* <0.01 | NS | *p* <0.05 |
| Long QT interval | 42 ± 5<br>NS | 87 ± 27<br>*p* <0.01 | 114 ± 43<br>*p* <0.01 |

Data are mean ± standard deviation.
From Vassallo JA, Cassidy DM, Kindwall KE, et al. Nonuniform recovery of excitability in the left ventricle. *Circulation* 1988;78:1365.

segments of myocardium exposed to a variety of conditions. More recently molecular genetics has provided information relevant to the mechanisms of certain arrhythmias. Heterogeneity of local APD based on ion channel derangements are probably responsible for arrhythmias associated with the long QT syndromes and Brugada syndrome (idiopathic VF associated with ST elevation in $V_{1-3}$ and pseudo-RBBB), short QT syndrome, and catecholaminergic PMVT.[108–119] Such heterogeneity can lead to triggered or reentrant arrhythmias. Connexin dysfunction can also produce heterogeneity of APD but can lead to reentry due to their effect on conduction. The exact mechanism by which these ion channelopathies cause arrhythmias is unresolved and is under active investigation. Debate therefore continues as to the role of early afterdepolarizations, abnormal automaticity, and reentry in these polymorphic tachycardias that are the hallmark of these syndromes. This is particularly true in the Brugada syndrome in which controversy remains as to whether it is a problem of conduction or repolarization.[120,121]

Despite the differences in experimental design, in my opinion, generalizations regarding arrhythmia mechanisms can be made by comparing the mode of initiation of tachycardias and influence of stimulation during tachycardias in in vitro and in vivo experimental preparations to comparable situations in humans. In addition, activation mapping in humans and the effects of drugs on initiation and VT cycle length may provide important clues to the underlying mechanism. These phenomena can only be evaluated in induced, sustained uniform VT. The bulk of evidence derived from these studies, albeit indirect, suggests that reentry is the mechanism of sustained uniform tachycardias associated with coronary artery disease.[1,122,123] In addition, nonsustained VT and VT (particularly, uniform) producing cardiac arrest may have a similar mechanism because they have a qualitatively similar, although quantitatively less, substrate of abnormal conduction. Moreover, their response to programmed stimulation and pharmacologic agents suggests a common mechanism. As discussed later, the evidence supporting reentry is based on

**TABLE 11-7 Data Based on Adjacent Left Ventricle Sites**

| | Endocardial Activation Time (msec) | Dispersion of Refractoriness (msec) | Dispersion of Total Recovery Time (msec) |
|---|---|---|---|
| Normal left ventricle (no ventricular tachycardia) | 25 ± 7 | 32 ± 11 | 41 ± 14 |
| Coronary artery disease (with ventricular tachycardia) | 42 ± 11 | 75 ± 41 | 42 ± 20 |
| | *p* <0.01 | NS | NS |
| Long QT interval | 31 ± 9 | 77 ± 31 | 85 ± 33 |

Data are mean ± standard deviation.
From Vassallo JA, Cassidy DM, Kindwall KE, et al. Nonuniform recovery of excitability in the left ventricle. *Circulation* 1988;78:1365.

the ability to reproducibly initiate and terminate the tachycardia by programmed stimulation, the response of the tachycardia to stimulation, the effect of drugs on the tachycardia, and activation mapping demonstrating reentrant excitation. How these responses differ from those expected for other mechanisms is discussed in more detail subsequently.

The underlying mechanism for VF and for the entire spectrum of nonsustained and polymorphic ventricular arrhythmias in patients with cardiomyopathy, electrolyte imbalance, valvular disorders, and so on remains incompletely understood. However, in the vast majority of cases the mechanism of sustained uniform VT, regardless of underlying cardiac disorder, appears most consistent with reentry (including patients with congenital heart disease, cardiomyopathy, and those with no organic heart disease), based on similar observations as those noted for uniform VT observed in the setting of coronary artery disease. While infarction provides gross fibrosis and macro nonuniform anisotropy, abnormal propagation in cardiomyopathies with less fibrosis may be related to the abnormalities of gap junction number, structure, function, and location.

## Initiation of Ventricular Tachycardias

The ability to reproducibly initiate an arrhythmia by programmed electrical stimulation (PES) has been considered a hallmark of reentrant arrhythmia.[1,124] Arrhythmias that are due to automaticity, either normal or abnormal, are due to spontaneous depolarization and cannot usually be initiated by programmed stimulation.[125–127] Triggered activity that is due to DADs, under a number of different circumstances, can be initiated by programmed stimulation.[51,125–128] The modes of stimulation required to initiate triggered activity caused by DADs and the characteristics of the resultant rhythm as well as the influence of pharmacologic agents (e.g., isoproterenol, atropine, aminophylline, and procainamide) on initiation can be used to differentiate triggered activity from reentrant excitation. Tachyarrhythmias that are believed to be due to early afterdepolarization are bradycardia dependent, and although they can be initiated in the experimental laboratory, they are not well suited for study by programmed stimulation, which automatically necessitates a relative "tachycardic" state.[125,126,129,130] The so-called short-long-short sequence of early afterdepolarization initiation of triggered activity recently summarized by Cranefield and Aronson[130] suggests that unusual modes of stimulation, which have not heretofore been employed, may be useful in initiating such rhythms. However, this protocol of stimulation can easily facilitate reentrant excitation. As such I do not believe this mode of stimulation can distinguish triggered activity from reentrant rhythms.

### *Protocol of Programmed Stimulation*

One of the major limitations in evaluating reported results of programmed stimulation to initiate VT is that different protocols have been used in different laboratories. Another limitation is that the reported results of stimulation have included patients with sustained uniform VT, nonsustained VT, and those presenting with cardiac arrest, treated as a single group. Some even report the results in patients who have never had a sustained arrhythmia, but who might be at risk for its occurrence. As mentioned earlier in this chapter, the anatomic and electrophysiologic substrates of these arrhythmias differ.[22,23,32,89,95] It is not surprising that the response to programmed stimulation also differs. Therefore, sensitivity and specificity should only be applied to the use of programmed stimulation for a single arrhythmia type. The only arrhythmia for which such data exist is sustained monomorphic VT.

In addition to the type of arrhythmia and the underlying anatomic substrate, specific features of the methodology of programmed stimulation can influence the ability to initiate the tachycardia. These include the number of extrastimuli, paced cycle length (PCL), site of stimulation, and the current (or voltage and pulse width), and the reproducibility of the response. These parameters are methods used to overcome some general factors that may influence the ability to initiate VT. They include distance from the origin of the arrhythmia, refractoriness at the site of stimulation, and conduction to the potential site of the tachycardia circuit or focus. The lack of control of those variables related to the protocol of programmed stimulation as well as the inclusion of different arrhythmia subtypes and different disease states have led to a marked variability in reported sensitivity, specificity, and reproducibility of programmed stimulation in the study of VT.[131–136] This has led to confusion in interpreting results of programmed stimulation and misuse of this technique in the management of arrhythmias. Thus, although some generalities exist regarding the effects of increasing number of extrastimuli, altering drive cycle lengths, and increasing current, the investigator must interpret the response to programmed stimulation in light of the specific arrhythmia being evaluated or whether stimulation is being used for risk stratification postmyocardial infarction.

### *Number of Extrastimuli*

The appropriate number of extrastimuli used to evaluate programmed stimulation for sustained VT is not universally agreed upon. In general, the greater the number of extrastimuli employed, the increased sensitivity of induction of any arrhythmia; however, this is associated with a decreasing specificity of the technique (Fig. 11-42). The sensitivity of PES to initiate sustained uniform VT increases significantly with the addition of three VES, with little incremental benefit from the addition of a fourth extrastimulus or rapid pacing (Fig. 11-43). Hummel et al.[137] suggest that if one begins PES with four VES at a short drive– PCL, one can reach an endpoint of inducible monomorphic VT sooner than if one starts with single VES. However, whether or not the VT induced by Hummel's method is the same as the spontaneous VT was never clarified in their manuscript. The more aggressively one stimulates, the more likely a nonspecific response, usually a polymorphic VT

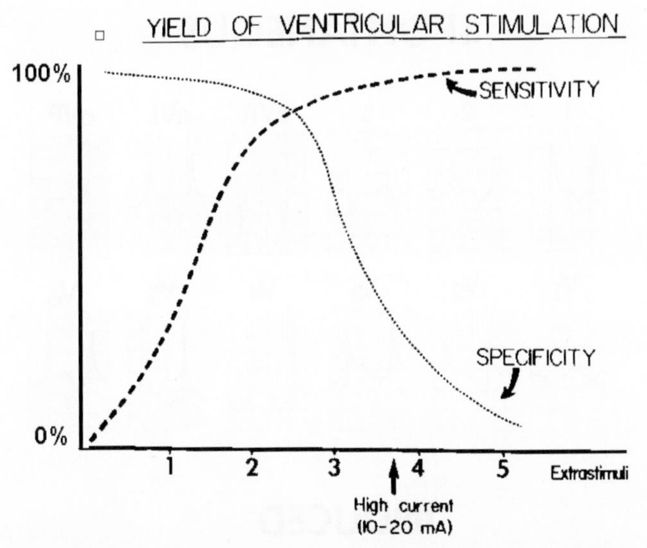


**FIGURE 11-42** Effect of aggressiveness of stimulation with sensitivity and specificity of responses. The various modes of initiation are shown on the horizontal axis from least to most aggressive, and the percentage of inducibility rate is shown on the vertical axis. It can be seen that the more aggressive the stimulation, the higher the sensitivity but the lower the specificity. A protocol involving three extrastimuli at twice diastolic threshold gives the best balance of sensitivity and specificity.

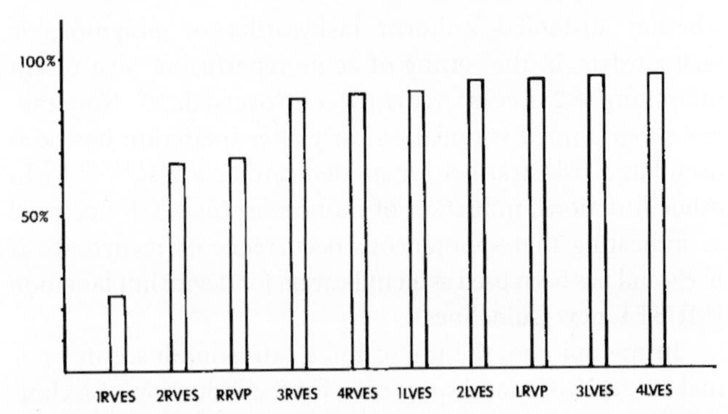


**FIGURE 11-43** Effect of number of extrastimuli and site of stimulation on inducibility. Increasing aggressiveness of right (RVES) then left ventricular stimulation (LVES) is shown on the horizontal axis, and the percentage of inducibility is shown on the left. It is clear that using three right ventricular extrastimuli there is approximately a 90% sensitivity. More aggressive modes of stimulation from the right or left ventricle add little to improve the sensitivity.

or VF, can result.[1,38,133,138–142] In general, the induction of VF or very rapid VT requires more VES, delivered at shorter coupling intervals than induction of sustained monomorphic VT. Moreover, the more abnormal the SAECG, the longer the coupling intervals of VES necessary to initiate either VT or VF.[142]

When sustained monomorphic VT is studied, the induction of polymorphic tachycardia must be considered a nonspecific response. Both nonsustained and sustained polymorphic arrhythmias, including VF, can be induced even in normal subjects without a history of VT or cardiac arrest. In our experience, the induction of polymorphic VT and/or VF in normal individuals usually requires multiple extrastimuli delivered at short coupling intervals, usually ≤180 msec (Fig. 11-44). Importantly, the initiating stimulus is associated with marked latency, compatible with local conduction delay at the stimulus site. In these people, these responses have no clinical significance. Thus, in patients without a prior history of sustained ventricular arrhythmias, we try to avoid using coupling intervals <180 msec.

The induction of polymorphic VT and/or VF in a patient who presents with cardiac arrest may have a different implication. By Baysean analysis, this response is more likely to have clinical significance in a patient population in whom similar arrhythmias are present. In other words, because a cardiac arrest may be initiated by a polymorphic tachycardia, the induction of a polymorphic VT in this patient population may be significant (although this is unproven). Despite this, one should always be circumspect when interpreting a polymorphic tachycardia as a clinically significant arrhythmia because, as noted previously, comparable arrhythmias can be induced in patients without any history of arrhythmia.

In contrast, the induction of a hemodynamically tolerated sustained monomorphic tachycardia (particularly with a cycle length ≥240 msec) only occurs in patients with spontaneous VT, cardiac arrest, or in the presence of a substrate known to be arrhythmogenic, such as a left ventricular aneurysm or recent myocardial infarction. It should be noted that the clinical significance of the induction of any arrhythmia,

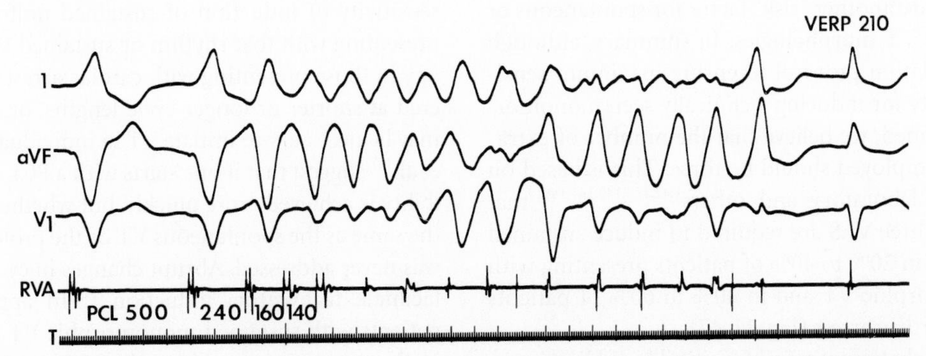


**FIGURE 11-44** Induction of nonsustained polymorphic VT. Nonsustained polymorphic VT is induced by triple extrastimuli delivered at extremely short coupling intervals. The last two coupling intervals are 160 and 140 msec, respectively, and are associated with local conduction delay (i.e., latency). Such responses have no clinical significance. See text for discussion. VERP, ventricular effective refractory period.

whether sustained uniform tachycardia or polymorphic tachycardias, in the setting of acute reperfusion or a recent infarction (<2 weeks) remains controversial.[25,26] Nonetheless programmed stimulation early after infarction has been useful as a risk stratifier for sudden cardiac arrest.[28,143–147] In other situations, induction of monomorphic VT is accepted as indicating that spontaneous occurrence or recurrence is likely and has been used as an indication for device implantation (MUSTT, new Guidelines).

In my opinion, the use of three extrastimuli seems optimal for sensitivity and specificity, for the induction of a clinically seen monomorphic VT due to prior infarction, with the recognition that in occasional patients a sustained monomorphic tachycardia requires four or more extrastimuli for its induction. In such a patient, the risk of additional extrastimuli producing nonspecific arrhythmias versus the benefit of being able to induce and, hence, develop therapy for a clinically relevant monomorphic VT should be considered. This is a reason for using multiple stimulation sites and drive cycle lengths (see below). When cardiac arrest is the presenting syndrome, we would not deliver more than three extrastimuli, because the additional extrastimuli would be more likely to induce polymorphic tachycardias than a uniform one (10:1), which if acted on would lead to the treatment of "nonspecific responses" in some individuals.

It is important that the induced arrhythmia be comparable to the spontaneous arrhythmia to ensure specificity of programmed stimulation. Although this is easily accomplished in the case of sustained monomorphic VT in which documentation of the spontaneous VT by a 12-lead ECG is possible (Fig. 11-45), it is nearly impossible in patients presenting with nonsustained VT or cardiac arrest in whom electrocardiographic documentation of the spontaneous arrhythmia is not available. Moreover, multiple morphologically distinct uniform sustained VT can be induced from the same or different sites (Fig. 11-46). These VT can often be changed back and forth by stimulation during VT (Fig.11-46), which is particularly common in patients treated with antiarrhythmic agents or early after myocardial infarction. In patients who present with recurrent sustained VT, these tachycardias are relevant. We found that these "additional" uniform VT are commonly responsible for recurrences.[148] In addition to antiarrhythmic drugs, aneurysms are another "risk" factor for spontaneous or inducible multiple VT morphologies. In summary, although the optimal stimulation protocol to ensure maximum sensitivity and specificity for inducing a clinically seen monomorphic VT is not defined, we believe that the number of extrastimuli generally employed should be three. This is based on studies from our laboratory and others[1,42,122,140,141,149] that demonstrate that three VES are required to induce sustained monomorphic VT in 20% to 40% of patients presenting with sustained monomorphic VT and in 40% to 60% of patients presenting with cardiac arrest (Fig. 11-47).

It is important that repetition of "critical" coupling intervals or the entire protocol is employed in order to define a true negative study.

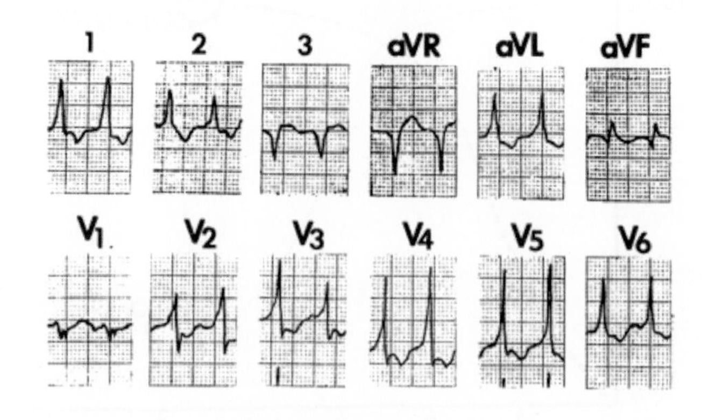


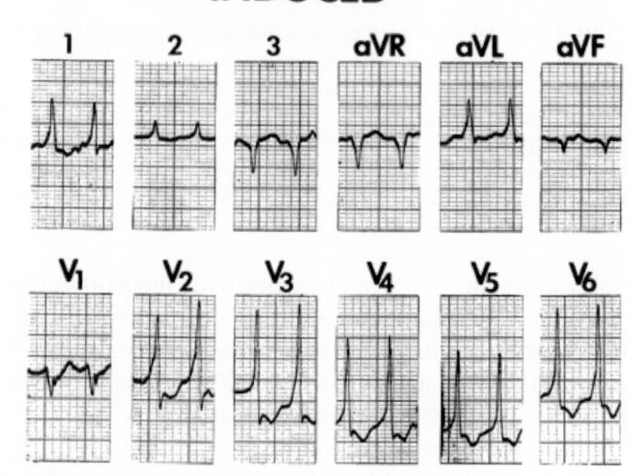


**FIGURE 11-45** Comparison of induced and spontaneous sustained VT. **Top:** Spontaneous left bundle branch block tachycardia with left inferior axis is shown. **Bottom:** The induced VT has a nearly identical morphology and cycle length to the spontaneous VT.

### *Influence of Drive Cycle Length*

Multiple investigators have evaluated whether changing the drive cycle length influences inducibility of VT.[1,42,122,137,149–155] Most studies demonstrate that the use of at least two cycle lengths (typically 600 and 400 msec) is required to enhance the sensitivity of induction of sustained uniform VT in patients presenting with that rhythm or sustained VT of any morphology in those presenting with cardiac arrest. Extrastimuli delivered at shorter or longer cycle lengths, or even sinus rhythm, may be necessary to initiate VT in individual patients. Hummel et al.[137] suggest that if one starts with a PCL of 350 msec, inducibility is achieved more quickly, but whether the induced VT is the same as the spontaneous VT or the protocol was completed was never addressed. Abrupt changes in cycle lengths also may facilitate tachycardia induction.[151] In approximately 5% of patients with sustained monomorphic VT (or, less commonly in those presenting with cardiac arrest), VT can be initiated only during sinus rhythm. In 10% to 15%, induction can be accomplished either during sinus rhythm or ventricular pacing.

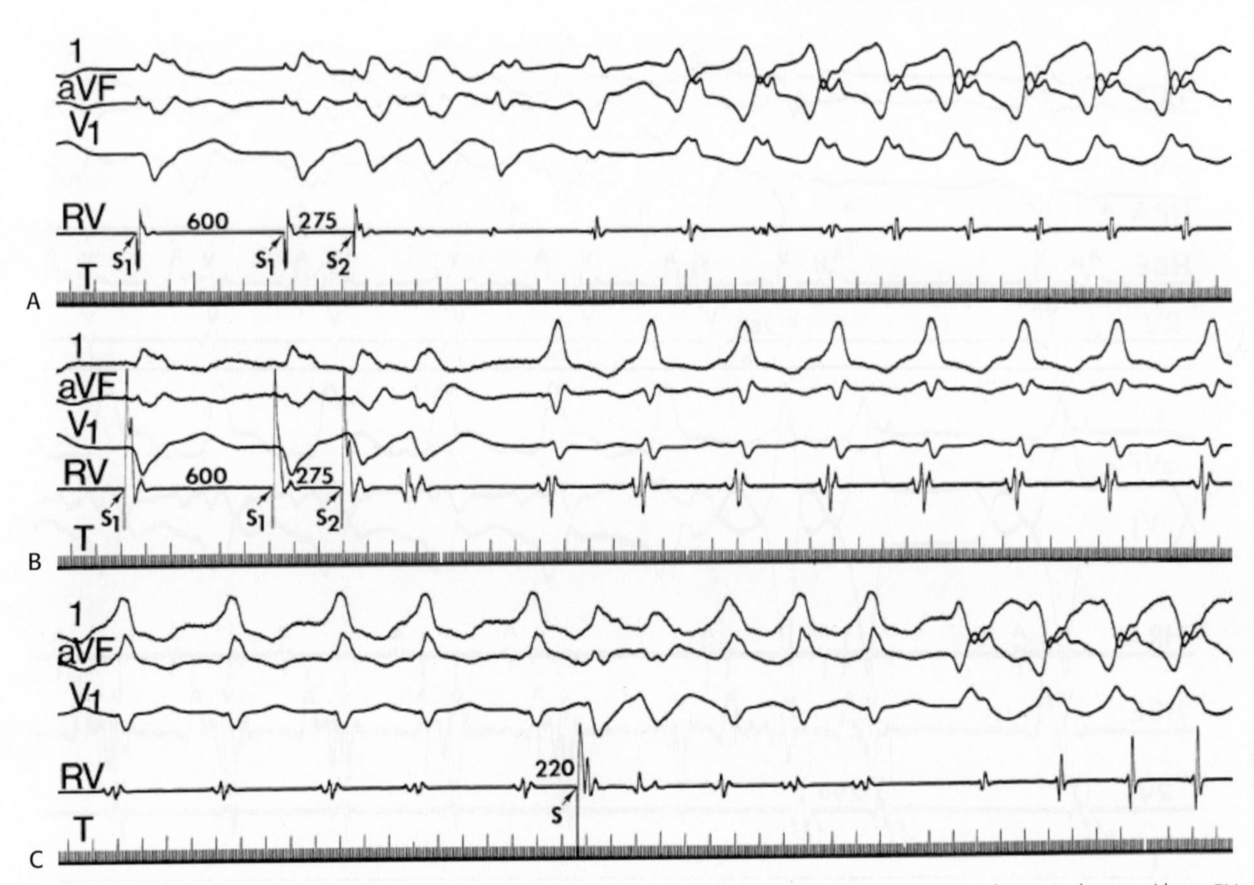


**FIGURE 11-46** Induction of multiple morphologically distinct tachycardias. **A–C:** The surface leads 1, aVF, and $V_1$ are shown with an RV electrogram. **A:** During a basic drive cycle length of 600 msec, a single RV extrastimulus induces a VT with right bundle branch block configuration. **B:** A single extrastimulus at the same coupling interval induces a left bundle branch block tachycardia. **C:** The left bundle branch block tachycardia is changed to the right bundle branch block tachycardia following the introduction of a single RV extrastimulus. See text for discussion.

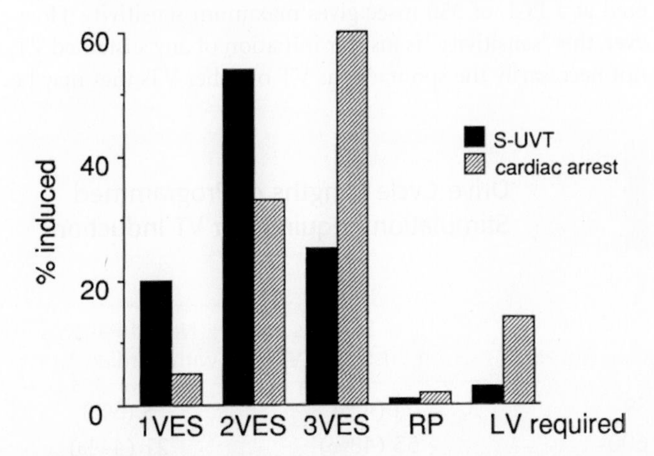


**FIGURE 11-47** Relationship of mode of induction of sustained VT to clinical presentation. The mode of induction of VT (*horizontal axis*) is compared to the percentage induced (*vertical axis*) in patients with sustained uniform VT (S-UVT) and those presenting with cardiac arrest. Patients with cardiac arrest more frequently require triple extrastimuli and left ventricular stimulation than those presenting with sustained uniform VT. See text for discussion. RP, refractory period; VES, ventricular extrastimuli.

Thus, most VT that can be induced during sinus rhythm can also be induced during ventricular pacing (Fig. 11-48). In such instances the coupling intervals required to initiate VT tend to be longer during ventricular pacing, but this is unpredictable in individual patients. In the remaining 80% to 85%, extrastimuli delivered during ventricular pacing successfully initiate VT. It is difficult to evaluate whether multiple drive cycle lengths or additional extrastimuli are more important to increasing the sensitivity of induction of VT.[152,153] Both tend to shorten the prematurity with which VES can be delivered.[151,152] The baseline right ventricular effective refractory period does not distinguish between VT requiring single, double, or triple extrastimuli for induction in patients presenting with sustained uniform VT or those with cardiac arrest (Table 11-8).[42]

The cycle length used can influence the number of extrastimuli required for induction. Theoretically, if one knew the drive cycle length that allows for induction of sustained VT with the least number of extrastimuli, one would use that cycle length, because the incidence of induction of nonspecific arrhythmias would be lower. Unfortunately, one cannot predict which cycle length will facilitate induction of the clinically relevant tachycardia. A standard protocol should include the use of at least two cycle lengths. In our laboratory, we routinely use drive cycle lengths of 600 and 400 msec in all patients as well

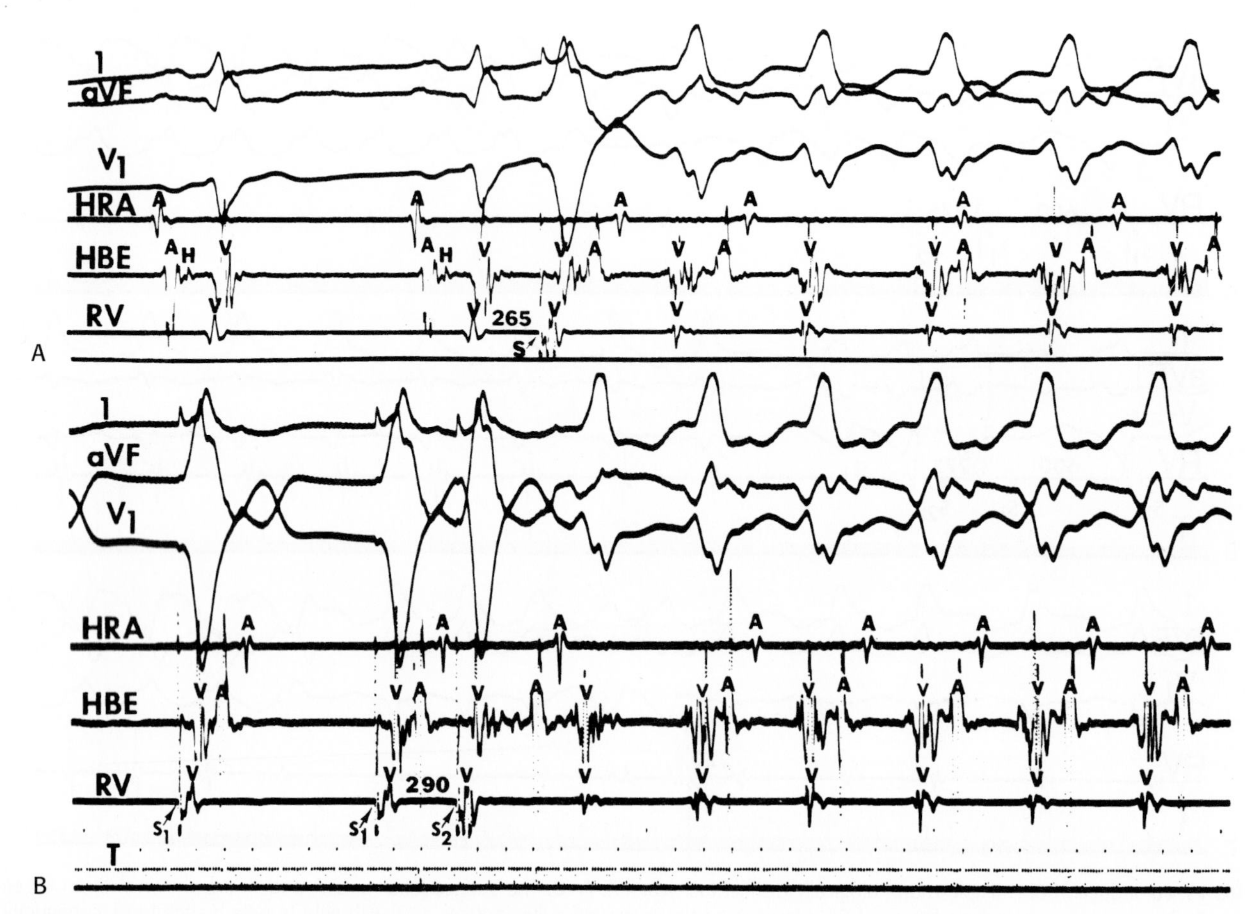


**FIGURE 11-48** Induction of VT by extrastimuli delivered during sinus rhythm and ventricular pacing. **A** and **B:** Three surface ECG leads and electrograms from the HRA, HBE, and RV are shown. **A:** During sinus rhythm, a single VES initiates a left bundle branch block–type tachycardia. **B:** During ventricular pacing, a single extrastimulus delivered at a longer coupling interval induces the same tachycardia. See text for discussion.

as stimulation during sinus rhythm. Additional cycle lengths may be employed if stimulation at these drive cycle lengths fails to initiate tachycardia. The relative success of different cycle lengths on the induction of sustained VT in patients presenting with uniform sustained VT or cardiac arrest is shown in Table 11-9. As noted above, Hummel et al.[137] suggest that initiating programmed stimulation using four VES delivered at a PCL of 350 msec gives maximum sensitivity. However, this "sensitivity" is just for initiation of any sustained VT, not necessarily the spontaneous VT or other VTs that may be

**TABLE 11-8 Relationship of Induction Mode to RVERP[a]**

| Group | S | D | T |
|---|---|---|---|
| Sustained ventricular tachycardia | 253 ± 21 | 242 ± 23 | 260 ± 26 |
| Cardiac arrest | 240 ± 107 | 250 ± 22 | 254 ± 25 |

RVERP, right ventricular effective refractory period.
[a]Values are expressed as msec (mean ± standard deviation). Refractory periods were measured at a drive cycle length of 600 msec in 107 patients in the ventricular tachycardia group and in 57 patients in the cardiac arrest group. Refractory periods were measured at a drive cycle length of 500 msec in six patients in the ventricular tachycardia group and in two patients in the cardiac arrest group.
From Buxton AE, Waxman HL, Marchlinski FE, et al. Role of triple extrastimuli during electrophysiologic study of patients with documented sustained ventricular tachyarrhythmias. *Circulation* 1984;69:532.

**TABLE 11-9 Drive Cycle Lengths of Programmed Stimulation Required for VT Induction**

| Patient Group | | |
|---|---|---|
| DCL (msec) | No. of Patients with Sustained VT | No. Of Patients with Cardiac Arrest |
| SR | 4 (4%) | 3 (6%) |
| 600 | 53 (48%) | 21 (44%) |
| 500 | 28 (25%) | 10 (21%) |
| Total | 109 | 47 |

DCL, drive cycle length; SR, sinus rhythm; VT, ventricular tachycardia.
From Buxton AE, Waxman HL, Marchlinski FE, et al. Role of triple extrastimuli during electrophysiologic study of patients with documented sustained ventricular tachyarrhythmias. *Circulation* 1984;69:532.

observed if a complete protocol were performed. Knowledge of all such monomorphic VTs is critical in developing pharmacologic, pacing, implantable defibrillator, or ablative therapy.

### Multiple Sites of Stimulation

Studies have demonstrated that using at least two sites of stimulation enhances the ability to initiate tachycardias.[1,42,140,156] In our experience, stimulation from a second site (i.e., other than the right ventricular apex) is needed to initiate sustained VT in patients presenting with sustained uniform VT and, even more importantly, in those with cardiac arrest. If three extrastimuli are delivered only from the right ventricular apex, 10% to 20% of patients will require the use of a second right ventricular or left ventricular site for initiation of sustained (Fig. 11-49). In a study by Doherty et al.,[156] in 58% of patients in whom triple extrastimuli at two cycle lengths failed to initiate a tachycardia from the right ventricular apex, a uniform sustained VT was induced from the right ventricular outflow tract. This accounted for 22% of the total inducible sustained VT. In approximately 60% of patients, the same sustained uniform VT was induced from both the right ventricular apex and right ventricular outflow tract (Fig. 11-50). We previously noted that neither drive cycle length nor ventricular refractory periods at either site was the determinant of mode of induction for patients presenting with sustained VT or cardiac arrest (Tables 11-8 and 11-9).[42] Thus, the inducibility appears related to the relationship of the wavefront of activation from the site of stimulation and the mechanism at the tachycardia origin. Site specificity for induction would suggest reentry as the underlying mechanism.

Because the number of extrastimuli required to initiate VT may differ depending on site of stimulation, the site that allows use of the lowest number of stimuli is preferred. While nonspecific responses (i.e., polymorphic VT or VF) are often induced with three VES, particularly when delivered at short coupling intervals, only specific responses (e.g., sustained monomorphic VTs) are likely to be induced using fewer stimuli. To determine the influence of stimulation site on the mode of induction and to allow for the safest stimulating protocol to induce the tachycardia (least number of extrastimuli), I recommend alternating stimulation from the right ventricular apex and outflow tract at each specified cycle length and number of extrastimuli. In approximately 20% of patients presenting with sustained uniform VT, a sustained uniform VT will be induced from one site with less stimuli than at another site, thereby preventing the use of a more aggressive stimulation protocol at the other site.[140,156] If stimulation from the right ventricular apex and outflow tract fails, despite use of multiple drive cycle lengths and up to three extrastimuli, left ventricular stimulation may be employed. The yield is small (2% to 5%) for patients with sustained VT, but because the response of induced sustained VT is relatively specific, it seems worthwhile to use left ventricular stimulation if right ventricular stimulation fails. If only two right VES are used from multiple sites and multiple cycle lengths, left ventricular stimulation may be required in approximately 10%.[157] Induction of sustained uniform VT in patients presenting with cardiac arrest is more likely to require left ventricular stimulation than those presenting with sustained uniform VT (Table 11-10).[42] The reason for this latter observation is unclear.

### Role of Increasing Current

Several investigators have evaluated the use of increasing current (5 to 20 mA) in the induction of sustained ventricular

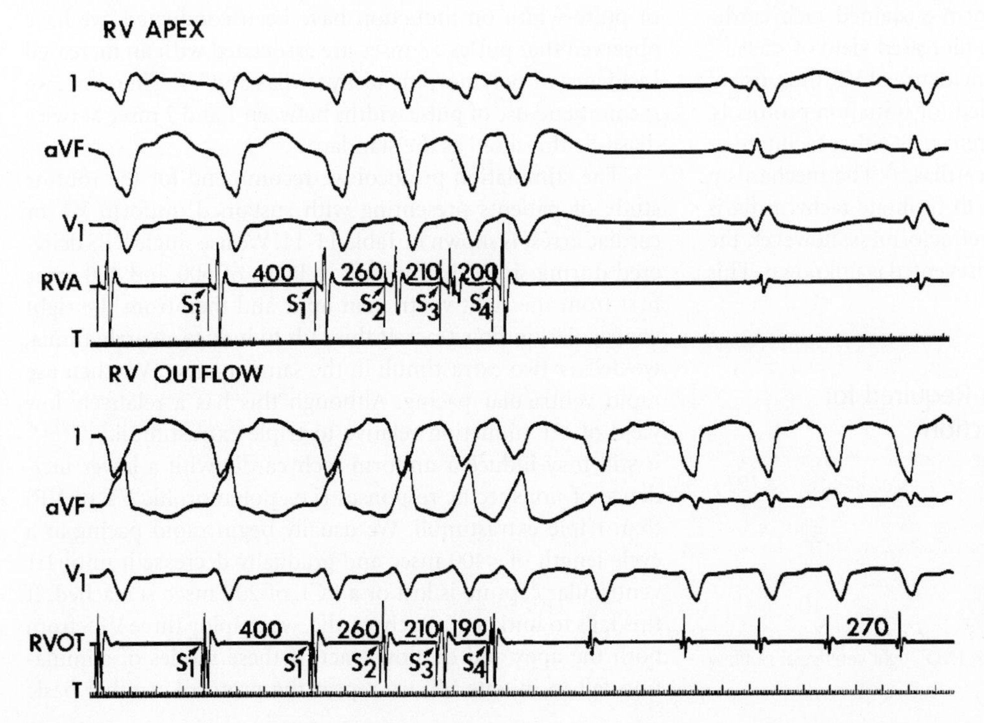


**FIGURE 11-49** Requirement of right ventricular outflow tract (RVOT) stimulation to initiate VT. **Top:** Triple extrastimuli delivered from the RVA at a drive cycle length of 400 msec failed to initiate VT. **Bottom:** Three extrastimuli from the RVOT at comparable coupling intervals initiate a sustained uniform VT. See text for discussion.

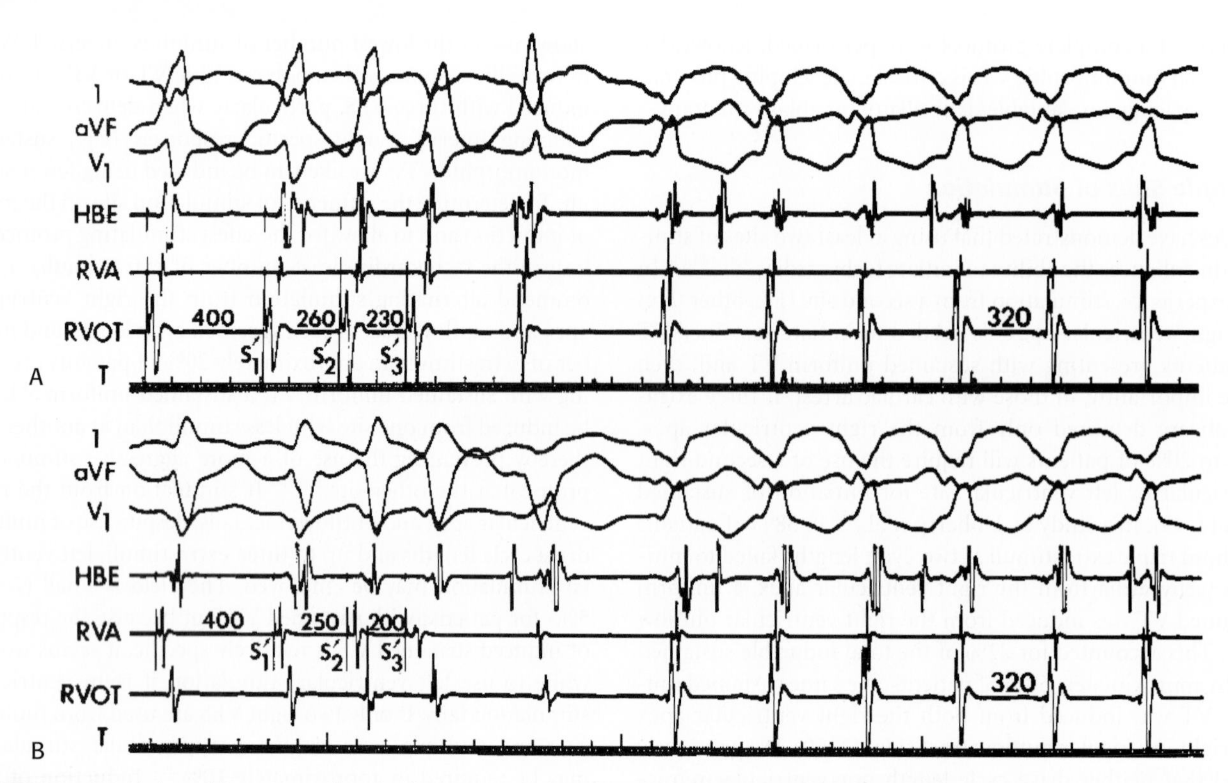


**FIGURE 11-50** Initiation of the same VT by stimulation at two right ventricular sites. **A:** VT with a right bundle right superior axis is initiated by two ventricular extrastimuli delivered from the RVOT. **B:** The same tachycardia is initiated by stimulation from the RVA.

arrhythmias.[133,140,141,158] All have found an increased incidence of VF when three or more extrastimuli at increased current are used compared to when twice diastolic threshold current is used. In one study, in 60% of patients who were given four extrastimuli at 10 mA, a nonclinical tachycardia (VF, polymorphic VT, nonsustained VT, or uniform VT of different morphology) was induced. Moreover, only a small increment in sensitivity of initiating a uniform sustained tachycardia occurs with increased current. The increased yield of <5%.[158] is far outweighed by the increased incidence of VF; thus, use of currents >5 mA is not recommended for initiation protocols. Even when used, the increased current may either facilitate or inhibit induction of certain tachycardias.[158] The mechanism by which increased current seems to facilitate tachycardia is by shortening the measured local refractoriness; however, the mechanism by which induction is prevented is unknown. This may reflect the lower reproducibility of induction of sustained VT when three extrastimuli are used to initiate a tachycardia. On the other hand, increased current could partially depolarize local tissue, causing slow conduction from the stimulation site such that a critical coupling interval at the VT site is not achieved or that local reentry leading to nonclinical VF is induced (Spear). Although no systematic studies of the effect of pulse width on induction have been conducted, we have observed that pulses >2 msec are associated with an increased incidence of polymorphic tachycardias and VF. Therefore, we recommend use of pulse widths between 1 and 2 msec at twice diastolic threshold as the standard.

TABLE 11-10 Site of Stimulation Required for Arrhythmia Conduction

| Site of Stimulation | S-VT (147) | Cardiac Arrest (83) |
|---|---|---|
| RVA | 125 | 52 |
| RVOT | 14 | 1 |
| LV | 3 | 10 |

LV, left ventricle; RVA, right ventricular apex; RVOT, right ventricular outflow tract, S-VT, sustained VT.

The stimulation protocol we recommend for the routine study of patients presenting with sustained uniform VT or cardiac arrest is shown in Table 11-11. We use single VES delivered during sinus rhythm and at PCLs of 600 and 400 msec first from the right ventricular apex and then from the right ventricular outflow tract. If this fails to induce an arrhythmia, we deliver two extrastimuli in the same manner. We then use rapid ventricular pacing. Although this has a relatively low yield of VT induction relative to triple extrastimuli,[1,42,122,159] it still may induce a uniform tachycardia with a lower incidence of nonspecific responses (i.e., polymorphic VT or VF) than triple extrastimuli. We usually begin rapid pacing at a cycle length of <400 msec and gradually decrease it until 1:1 ventricular capture is lost or a PCL of 200 msec is reached. If this fails to initiate the tachycardia, we employ three VES from both the apex and outflow tract. If these modes of stimulation fail to initiate VT, we repeat the protocol at other basic

**TABLE 11-11 Protocol of Programmed Stimulation for VT**

| |
|---|
| 1 VES—RVA, RVOT<br>NSR; PCL, 600 and 400 msec |
| 2 VES—RVA, RVOT<br>NSR; PCL, 600 and 400 msec<br>RVP—RVA 400 msec to loss of 1:1 capture |
| 3 VES—RVA, RVOT<br>NSR; PCL, 600 and 400 msec |
| Repeat protocol using: Other PCLs<br>Other RV sites<br>1–2 LV sites<br>Isoproterenol<br>Procainamide |

VT, ventricular tachycardia; VES, ventricular extrastimulation; RVA, right ventricular apex; RVOT, right ventricular outflow tract; NSR, normal sinus rhythm; PCL, paced cycle length; RVP, rapid ventricular pacing; RV, right ventricular; LV, left ventricular.

cycle lengths. If this fails, we repeat the protocol using other right ventricular or left ventricular sites. In addition, we may use isoproterenol or a Type I agent, such as procainamide, to facilitate induction of the tachycardia. We also perform atrial programmed stimulation and pacing, because occasionally, VT may be induced by these methods or SVT with aberration or pre-excited tachycardias may have been the spontaneous arrhythmia which was misdiagnosed as VT.

Although the use of isoproterenol to facilitate induction of VT has been reported by several investigators,[160–162] in our experience, it has a low yield in patients with postinfarction sustained uniform VT (<5%). In contrast to our experience, Freedman et al.[161] suggest that facilitation of VT induction by isoproterenol may be as high as 20%. Isoproterenol is useful in initiation of exercise-induced tachycardias or repetitive monomorphic tachycardia, which are usually nonsustained, that most often originate from the right ventricular outflow tract and are typically based on triggered activity due to DADs. Occasionally epinephrine, atropine, or aminophylline may work alone or in combination to facilitate induction of these rhythms when isoproterenol fails to spontaneously initiate or facilitate initiation by PES. The most common VT due to triggered activity that is clinically encountered arises at the RV outflow tract, but may occasionally arise in the LV outflow tract as well.[163] Tachycardias due to abnormal automaticity may also be initiated by catecholamines alone. Programmed stimulation cannot reproducibly initiate them, even in the presence of catecholamines.

The use of procainamide or other Type I agents to facilitate induction of a tachycardia is not as well recognized. Facilitation of induction of sustained VT is not uncommon in patients with coronary artery disease and prior infarction (with or without angina) in whom no arrhythmia or, more often, a nonsustained tachycardia (uniform or polymorphic) is induced in the baseline state, particularly if the clinical tachycardia, either sustained monomorphic VT or a cardiac arrest, occurred following drug administration (Fig. 11-51). Once monomorphic tachycardia is induced in such patients,

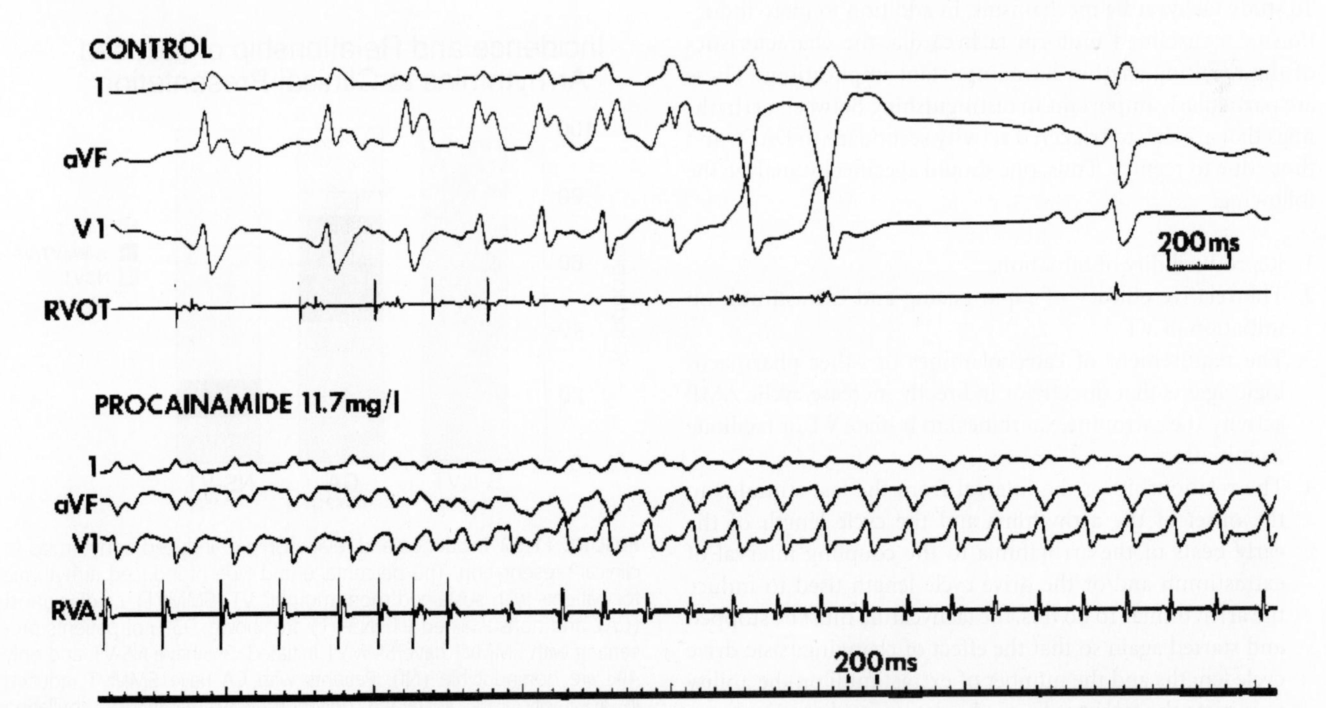


**FIGURE 11-51** Facilitation of induction of sustained VT by procainamide. In the control panel, three ventricular extrastimuli fail to initiate a sustained VT. Following the administration of 15 mg/kg of procainamide producing a plasma level of 11.7 mg/L, a sustained uniform VT is induced with three extrastimuli. Note that the morphology of the sustained arrhythmia is identical to the last beats of the nonsustained VT induced in the control. See text for discussion.

it behaves just as the other reentrant monomorphic tachycardias described later in this chapter. This is one of the observations that link the underlying mechanism of the previously mentioned arrhythmias to that of sustained uniform VT.

The response to programmed stimulation that is obviously most difficult to interpret is the induction of polymorphic VT in a patient who has experienced a cardiac arrest. As stated earlier, aggressive stimulation (e.g., triple extrastimuli) can induce similar arrhythmias in patients who have never had a cardiac arrest, or even in people with normal hearts. In such instances, the induction of polymorphic VT is a nonspecific response and lacks relevance. Therefore, we believe that the end point of programmed stimulation should be induction of the clinical arrhythmia or, in this instance, the assumed ventricular arrhythmia. In the case of patients presenting with a cardiac arrest, although doubt will always exist, I believe one must treat the reproducible induction of a polymorphic arrhythmia as a possible indicator of the clinical arrhythmia. It cannot, however, in and of itself help one to understand the mechanism of cardiac arrest, although some investigators have used the induction of polymorphic VT to guide therapy (see Chapter 12). Features that suggest a polymorphic VT may be mechanistically meaningful are (a) reproducible initiation of the same polymorphic template, particularly from different sites, and (b) the transformation of the polymorphic VT to a monomorphic VT by procainamide.[164,165]

## Initiation of Sustained Uniform Ventricular Tachycardia

To study tachycardia mechanisms, in addition to mere induction of a sustained uniform tachycardia, the characteristics of the resulting rhythm have important implications. These are particularly important in distinguishing between arrhythmias that are due to triggered activity secondary to DADs and those due to reentry. Thus, one should specifically analyze the following:

1. Reproducibility of initiation.
2. The relative efficacy of rapid pacing and extrastimuli on initiation of VT.
3. The requirement of catecholamines or other pharmacologic agents that directly or indirectly increase cyclic AMP activity (i.e., atropine, xanthines) to initiate VT or facilitate its initiation.
4. The relationship of the interval from the last stimulus to the onset of the arrhythmia and the cycle length of the early beats of the arrhythmia to the coupling interval of extrastimuli and/or the drive cycle length used to induce the arrhythmia: To do this, the tachycardia must be stopped and started again so that the effect of changing basic drive cycle lengths and the number of extrastimuli on the ability to initiate the tachycardia can be determined.
5. Site specificity of induction of VT.
6. The relationship of initiation of VT to conduction delay block and/or continuous electrical activity.

Variable inducibility rates have been reported for induction of sustained VT in patients with coronary artery disease, cardiomyopathy, valvular heart disease, and primary electrical disease.[162] This is primarily related to the inclusion of nonsustained VT, patients presenting with cardiac arrest (regardless of the specific tachycardia producing arrest), or documented polymorphic VT and VF under the rubric of sustained VT. In our laboratory, in ≈95% of patients presenting with sustained monomorphic VT, their tachycardia can be replicated, regardless of the underlying pathology with the exception of exercise-induced sustained VT. Patients presenting with cardiac arrest and nonsustained VT have a lower incidence of inducibility; therefore, their inclusion under the rubric of "VT" is responsible for the variable induction rates reported. This is depicted in Figure 11-52, which shows the incidence of inducible arrhythmia in patients presenting with sustained uniform VT, cardiac arrest, and nonsustained VT. If only patients with coronary artery disease are evaluated, little difference occurs in the percentage of inducible arrhythmias in patients presenting with sustained uniform VT (Fig. 11-53). However, the incidence of inducibility in patients presenting with cardiac arrest or nonsustained VT increases with coronary artery disease. Only in the latter two groups of patients does the disease process influence the ability to initiate the rhythm. Other researchers have also noted a high inducibility rate for patients presenting with sustained monomorphic VT with cardiomyopathy (idiopathic, hypertrophic, or arrhythmogenic right ventricular dysplasia), congenital heart disease, or no apparent heart disease.[81,163,166–175]

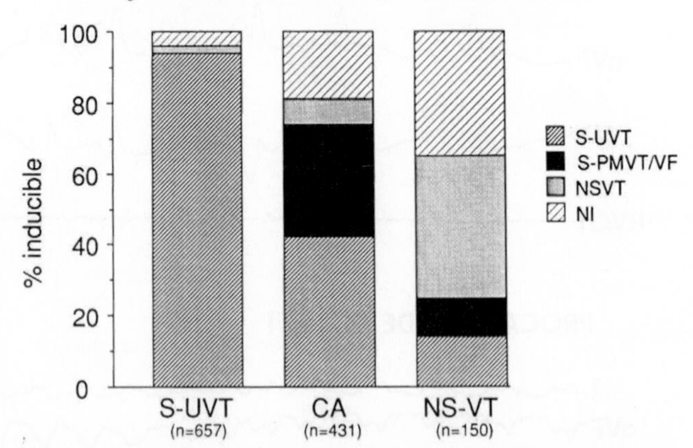


**FIGURE 11-52** Incidence and relationship of induced arrhythmias to clinical presentation. The percentage and type of induced arrhythmia for patients with sustained monomorphic VT (SMMVT), cardiac arrest (CA), and nonsustained VT (NS-VT) are shown: 93% of patients presenting with SMMVT have SMMVT initiated; 2% have NS-VT, and only 4% are noninducible (NI). Patients with CA have SMMVT induced in 40% of cases, sustained polymorphic VT/ventricular fibrillation (SPMVT/VF) in approximately 35%, NS-VT in 8%, and no inducible arrhythmias in 17%. In patients with NS-VT, 12% have SMMVT, approximately 10% have SPMVT/VF, 40% have NS-VT, and the remainder have no inducible arrhythmias. (Data as of June 1995.)

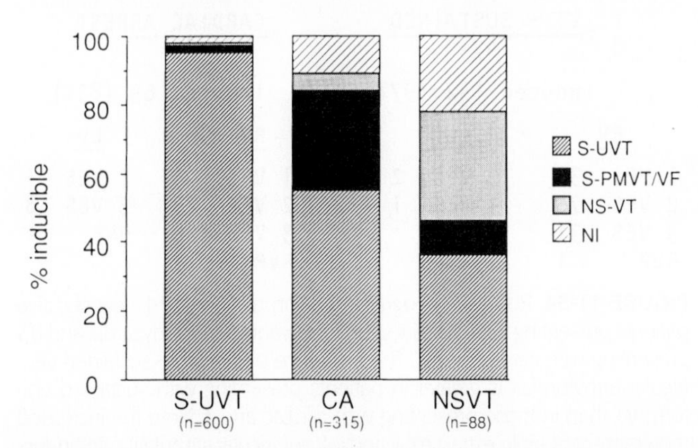


**FIGURE 11-53** Inducibility of VT associated with CAD. In patients with CAD, the most marked differences are in inducibility in patients presenting with CA and NS-VT. In patients presenting with SMMVT, 95% have an inducible sustained MMVT. In patients with CA, 57% have SMMVT, and 31% have SPMVT/VF induced. Only 12% are noninducible. In patients presenting with NS-VT, 37% have an SMMVT induced, 14% have SPMVT/VF, 26% have NS-VT induced, and only 23% are noninducible. (Data as of June 1995.)

Sustained monomorphic VT can be reproducibly initiated from day-to-day and year-to-year, particularly those with coronary artery disease and prior infarction.[1,26,131] Although some investigators question the reproducibility of induction of sustained VT,[132,176] particularly for arrhythmias requiring triple extrastimuli for induction, these investigators have lumped multiple tachycardia subtypes under the single heading of VT. If one deals only with sustained monomorphic VT, reproducibility of initiation is consistent: If the tachycardia can be induced on day 1, it will be induced on day 2, 10, or a year from the initial study. This is not to say that the exact mode of initiation is reproducible. For example, patients in whom double and triple extrastimuli are required for initiation during day 1 may have a different mode of initiation on day 2. Therefore, although the exact number of extrastimuli or site of stimulation may vary daily, the ability to initiate the arrhythmia does not. The mere repetition of stimulation, either longitudinally (by repeating the entire protocol) or horizontally (by repeating each coupling interval), enhances the sensitivity, and reproducibility of initiation.[134] We have studied patients over a 3-year period without any change in our ability to initiate the tachycardia. In patients with multiple morphologically distinct sustained monomorphic VTs, all VTs may not be reproducibly initiated on a given day, but one or more will.

In those tachycardias that can be initiated by single VES or atrial stimulation, the mode of initiation is also usually reproducible. Induction of VT by single VES may be seen in VT due to CAD and in patients with idiopathic LV, verapamil sensitive VT. This phenomenon perhaps reflects a substrate that is always "primed" for initiation. Although no specific anatomic characteristics influence the mode of stimulation, two electrophysiologic parameters, which are related, appear to influence the mode of initiation. These include slow tachycardias,[177] VT in patients with the most marked abnormalities of conduction noted by endocardial mapping or signal averaging (unpublished observations), and verapamil sensitive VT.[13,113,169–173] This suggests an important role for conduction abnormalities in initiation of the tachycardia, a finding that supports a reentrant mechanism (see following discussion). Distance of stimulation site from the site of origin or from a site of previous infarction does not appear to influence the number of extrastimuli required to initiate VT.[177]

The fact that sustained uniform VT can be reproducibly initiated excludes both normal and abnormal automaticity as the underlying mechanism. One must therefore differentiate triggered activity from reentry as the underlying mechanism because both can be initiated by programmed stimulation. Although there are numerous studies of the results of programmed stimulation on induction of sustained uniform VT, fewer data are available documenting the ability of stimulation to induce triggered activity associated with delayed or early afterdepolarizations.[125–130] VTs due to DADs often are related to a high catecholamine state. The most common clinical situation in which this occurs is RVOT and LVOT tachycardias. Induction of such ventricular arrhythmias is related to PCL, number of paced complexes, and prematurity of extrastimuli delivered and is facilitated by isoproterenol infusion, atropine, Calcium, and phosphodiesterase inhibitors.[163,178] These differ somewhat from triggered activity in atrial tissue superfused with nonphysiologic amounts of catecholamines.[125,126,128] Most of the experimental data related to triggered activity in ventricular tissue are from studies in digitalis-induced triggered rhythms in Purkinje fibers.[125,126] Although preliminary data on triggered activity in infarcted myocardial cells are available,[126,127,179] only one study demonstrated the ability to induce DADs in human Purkinje fibers obtained from explanted hearts superfused with ouabain or epinephrine.[179] In neither case was sustained rhythmic activity induced, only DADs. Human VTs due to digitalis intoxication have not been systematically studied.

The stimulation protocols used in experimental studies are similar to those used in humans, although rapid pacing and programmed extrastimuli are used in both. Regardless of preparation, rapid pacing is the most successful method of initiating sustained triggered activity that is due to DADs. The frequency of triggering increases as the basic PCL decreases. Most episodes of triggered activity induced by rapid pacing lasted less than 25 beats. Single, double, triple, or quadruple extrastimuli in the absence of prior pacing usually fails to initiate triggered activity in digitalis-intoxicated Purkinje fibers.[180] It is rare to induce triggered activity in this preparation in the absence of a train of impulses of less than 10 complexes. On the other hand, although extrastimuli rarely initiate triggered activity during sinus rhythm, they can if delivered during a basic drive cycle that exceeds 10 paced impulses. In this latter instance, at any given PCL, the frequency of triggering increases as the coupling interval of the premature stimulus decreases. In ouabain-perfused preparation, the cycle length of triggered activity induced by rapid pacing or extrastimuli is related to the PCL and coupling interval of the extrastimuli, such that the faster the paced rate, the faster the tachycardia.

The maximum reproducibility of initiation using all methods is <50% and most episodes are nonsustained.

Once a triggered rhythm is initiated, a period of quiescence is necessary to reinitiate the triggered rhythm. This is believed to be due to activation of the Na/K pump which hyperpolarizes the cells so that the DADs can no longer reach threshold. Thus, the ability to initiate, terminate, and reinitiate in sequence is uncommon. Sustained triggered activity also warms up, that is, it accelerates following initiation before reaching a stable cycle length and decelerates prior to termination. The rates of experimental triggered rhythms generally are much slower than the rates of spontaneous sustained, monomorphic VT in humans, even in the presence of catecholamines. In summary, triggered activity due to DADs is moderately difficult to reproducibly initiate, is most reliably initiated by rapid pacing, and the frequency of initiation is related to the rate of pacing and prematurity of extrastimuli. In addition, catecholamines (isoproterenol and epinephrine) or drugs that increase cyclic AMP directly or indirectly (atropine, xanthines, or other phosphodiesterase inhibitors) are frequently required to initiate sustained rhythmic activity that is due to DADs. Even when initiated by pacing alone, catecholamines facilitate initiation, increase the rate, and shorten the interval to the onset of the triggered rhythm.

Triggered activity that is due to early afterdepolarizations appears to be bradycardia dependent, regardless of the method by which they are induced. Only early afterdepolarizations that interrupt Phase 3 of repolarization appear to be able to initiate sustained arrhythmic activity.[129] Some investigators suggest that the sustained rhythmic activity following early afterdepolarizations in vitro is in fact abnormal automaticity based on its response to overdrive pacing (see following discussion). More recently Antzelevitch and colleagues[112] and El Sherif et al.[108] have suggested that reentrant excitation is the mechanism of polymorphic VTs associated with long QT intervals (i.e., torsade de pointes). Cranefield and Aronson have stressed that the short-long-short sequence initiating triggered activity that is due to early afterdepolarizations is the hallmark of that arrhythmia[126,130] and related it to clinical arrhythmias: torsade de pointes and repetitive monomorphic tachycardias in the right ventricular outflow tract. They predicted that routine stimulation, therefore, would not induce sustained arrhythmias, which can be sustained and uniform. Data in the subsequent paragraphs will make it obvious that the behavior of the vast majority of sustained monomorphic VTs, particularly in the setting of structural heart disease, is not compatible with triggered activity that is due to either delayed or early afterdepolarizations.

In patients presenting with sustained, hemodynamically stable, monomorphic VT, reproducible initiation by VES is the rule. In more than 90% of patients presenting with paroxysmal, sustained, monomorphic VT, the VT can be reproducibly initiated at the same study and at different times. In our experience, in the total population of patients presenting with sustained, tolerated monomorphic VT, or in only those with coronary artery disease and prior infarction, the inducibility rate of any sustained monomorphic VT is 95% (Figs. 11-52 and 11-53). Single and double VES initiate sustained VT in 60% to 85% of patients.[1,42,122,123,149] Moreover, once sustained uniform VT is initiated, it is often easier to reinitiate. As noted earlier, sustained monomorphic VT is induced in >50% of patients presenting with cardiac arrest in the setting of coronary artery disease (Fig. 11-53). In such patients, induction of sustained VT more often requires triple extrastimuli than in patients presenting with hemodynamically tolerated VT (Figs. 11-54 and 11-55). The major difference is the **cycle**

PROGRAMMED STIMULATION

VT - SUSTAINED 147 — Induced 142 (97%)

| RV | | LV | |
|---|---|---|---|
| 1 VES | 37 | 2 VES | 2 |
| 2 VES | 70 | 3 VES | 1 |
| 3 VES | 31 | | |
| RVP | 1 | | |

CARDIAC ARREST 83 — Induced 69 (83%)

| RV | | LV | |
|---|---|---|---|
| 1 VES | 5 | 2 VES | 1 |
| 2 VES | 23 | 3 VES | 8 |
| 3 VES | 28 | RVP | 1 |
| RVP | 3 | | |

**FIGURE 11-54** Results of programmed stimulation in 147 consecutive patients presenting with sustained uniform ventricular tachycardia and 83 presenting with cardiac arrest. The incidence of inducible sustained ventricular arrhythmias is greater in patients presenting with sustained uniform VT than in those presenting with cardiac arrest. Note the increased requirement of triple extrastimuli and left ventricular stimulation for induction of sustained arrhythmias in patients presenting with cardiac arrest. See text for further discussion. RVP, rapid ventricular pacing.

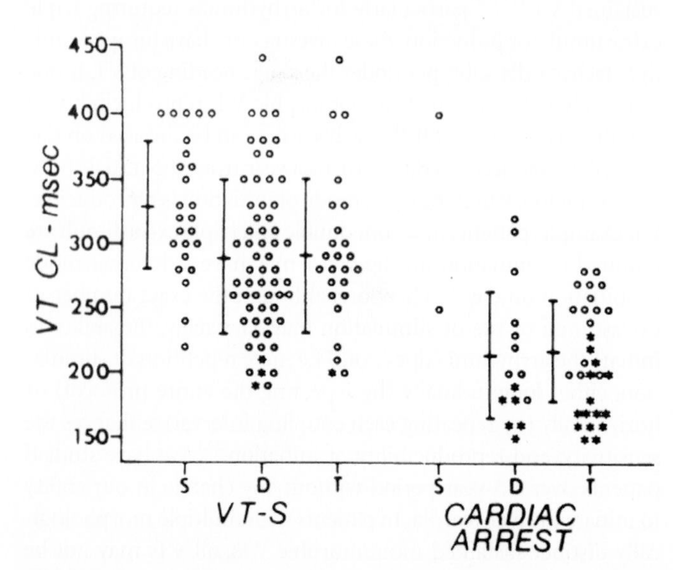


**FIGURE 11-55** Relationship of cycle length of induced tachycardias (VT CL) to mode of induction in the group of patients presenting with recurrent sustained VT (VT-S) and cardiac arrest. Horizontal and vertical bars denote mean values of induced tachycardia cycle length and standard deviations. *Open circles* represent induced tachycardias of uniform pattern, and *asterisks* represent polymorphic tachycardias. Regardless of mode of initiation, patients presenting with cardiac arrest have faster tachycardias induced than those presenting with VT-S. S, tachycardias induced by single ventricular extrastimuli; D, induction by double extrastimuli; T, induction by triple extrastimuli. (From Buxton AE, Waxman HL, Marchlinski FE, et al. Role of triple extrastimuli during electrophysiologic study of patients with documented sustained ventricular tachyarrhythmias. *Circulation* 1984;69:532.)

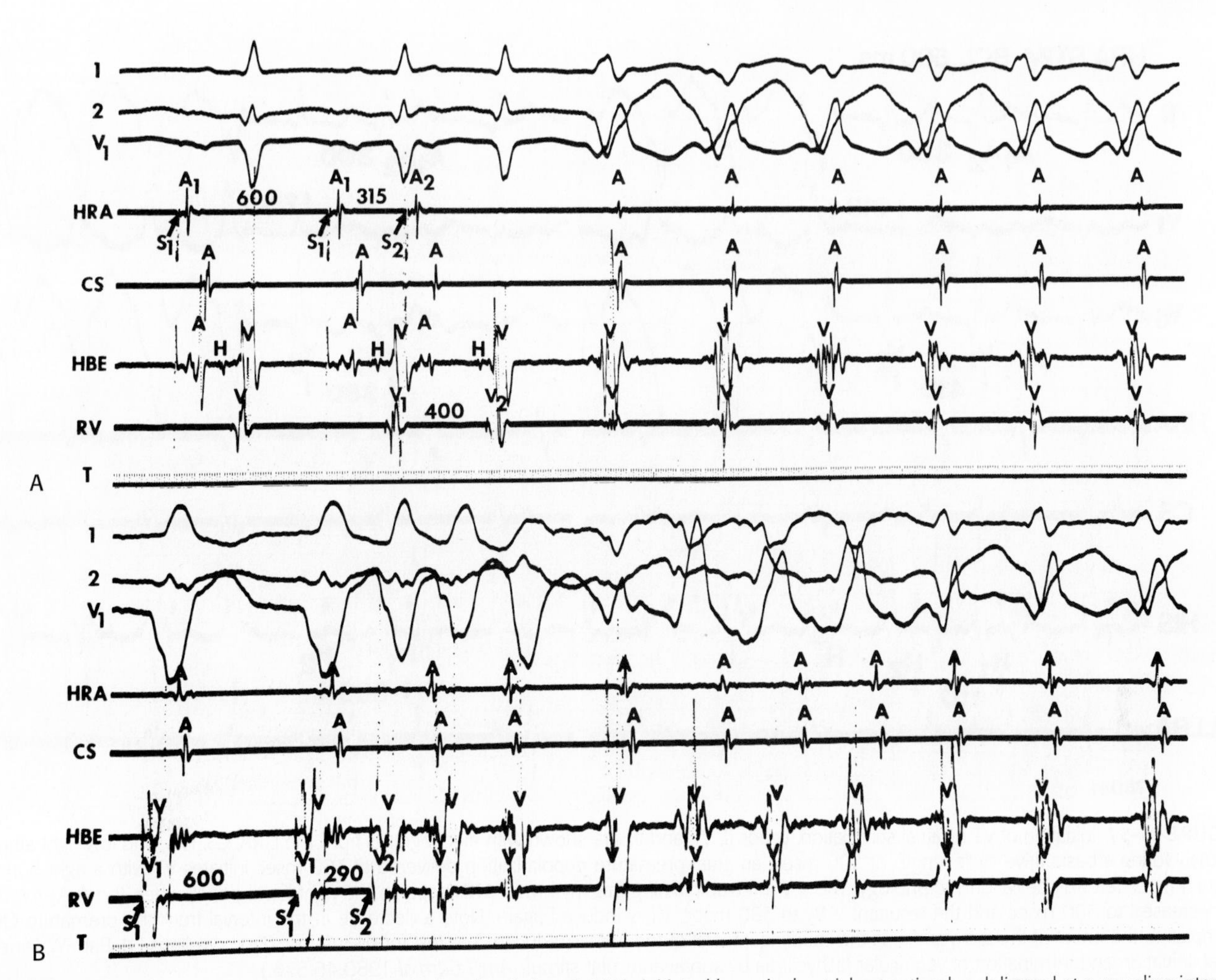


**FIGURE 11-56** Initiation of VT by atrial and ventricular stimulation. **A:** VT is initiated by a single atrial extrastimulus delivered at a coupling interval of 315 msec, producing a $V_1V_2$ interval of 400 msec. **B:** A ventricular extrastimulus at a shorter $V_1V_2$ interval (290 msec) is required to initiate the VT. See text for discussion.

**length of the VT**, which is shorter for patients presenting with cardiac arrest at comparable modes of initiation ($p < 0.05$, see Fig. 11-55). In patients presenting with cardiac arrest, initiation of VT by a single VES is rare.

Atrial extrastimuli can initiate VT in approximately 5% of patients with sustained uniform VT. Usually, but not always, these tachycardias can also be initiated by VES (Fig. 11-56). These VTs are usually slower and very reproducibly initiated over a broad zone of coupling intervals.[181] Initiation of sustained uniform VT by atrial stimulation is more common in patients without coronary disease.[169–173,181,182] One must assess the relationship of the coupling interval of the premature beat to the coupling interval of the first beat of the tachycardia. A direct relationship is characteristic of a triggered rhythm due to delayed afterdepolarizations (Fig. 11-57).

In experimental VT due to digitalis intoxication, sustained VT due to triggered activity could be reproducibly induced with single and double atrial or VES in only 25%.[180] Moreover, triggered rhythms were unable to be induced by stimulation during sinus rhythm or by extrastimuli delivered during a drive train of less than 8 to 10 paced complexes. All experimental studies on triggered activity demonstrate that the reproducibility is markedly affected by quiescence; that is, it is harder to induce triggered activity after a triggered rhythm has been just initiated. Human tachycardias believed to be due to DADs are inducible by PES in <65%, most commonly by rapid atrial or ventricular pacing, usually facilitated by catecholamines.[163] Induction of sustained monomorphic VT due to triggered activity by atrial pacing is more common in patients with noncoronary disease or without any heart disease.[169–173,181,182] These findings are in contrast to the clinical studies of sustained monomorphic VT that show a higher reproducibility rate of initiation, particularly with extrastimuli using paced cycles of eight complexes. Although triggered activity is most effectively initiated by rapid pacing, less than 5% of patients with recurrent sustained monomorphic VT due to reentry in the setting of old myocardial infarction require rapid ventricular pacing for initiation (Fig. 11-58). In a small percentage of patients, atrial pacing, atrial tachycardia, or atrial fibrillation can

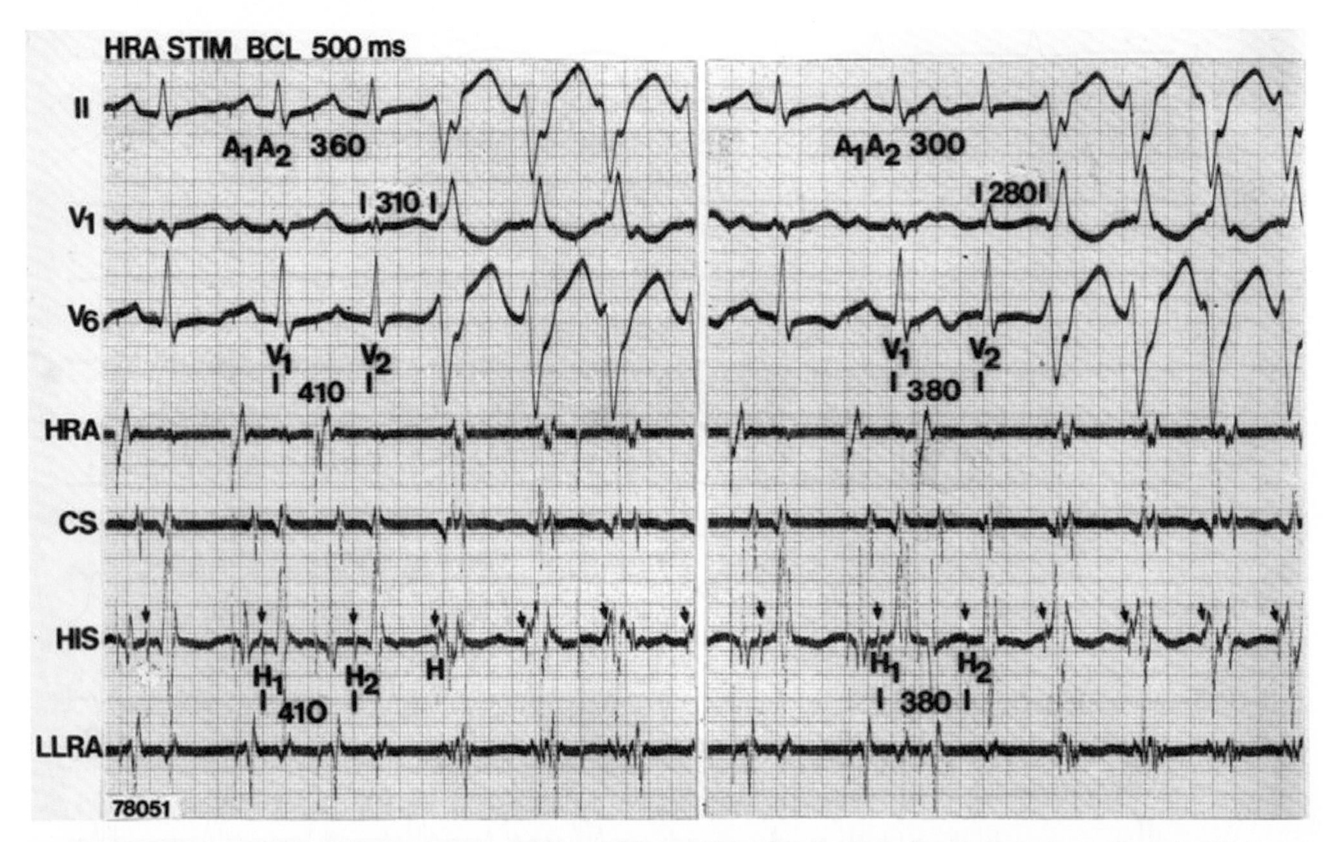


**FIGURE 11-57** Initiation of VT by atrial stimulation. Leads II, $V_1$, and $V_6$ are shown with electrograms from the HRA, CS, HIS, and low-right atrium (LRA). During a basic drive cycle length of 500 msec, an atrial premature depolarization delivered at 360 msec initiates VT with a right bundle branch block left axis deviation morphology. The V-V interval initiating this rhythm is 410 msec. In the right-hand panel, when the $A_1A_2$ interval is decreased to 300 msec and the resultant $V_1V_2$ to 380 msec, VT is induced again. Note a decrease in the interval from the premature QRS complex to the onset of the tachycardia as the coupling interval of the APD is reduced. See text for discussion. (From Wellens HJ, Bar FW, Farre J, et al. Initiation and termination of ventricular tachycardia by supraventricular stimuli. *Am J Cardiol* 1980;46:576.)

induce reentrant sustained monomorphic VT[181] in patients with prior infarction (Fig. 11-59). In such cases, single or double extrastimuli can also initiate VT. Use of triple extrastimuli is far more productive in initiating tachycardias than using rapid pacing; the former initiates tachycardias in >90% of patients. This has been tested in our laboratory using our protocol, which uses rapid pacing before the introduction of triple extrastimuli. In the 25% or so of patients with sustained VT who require triple extrastimuli for initiation, the use of rapid pacing has failed to initiate their tachycardia. Thus, rapid pacing only adds a few percent points to the overall inducibility rate.

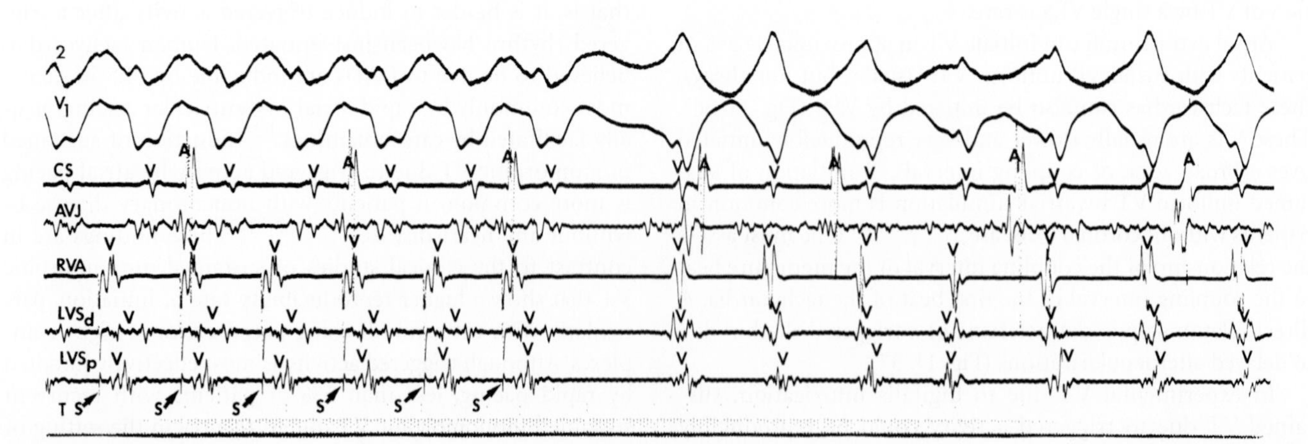


**FIGURE 11-58** Initiation of VT by rapid ventricular pacing. Leads 2 and $V_1$ are shown with electrograms from the CS, A-V junction (AVJ), RVA, and distal and proximal pairs of electrodes at the left ventricular septum ($LVS_d$, $LVS_p$). Burst pacing from the RVA initiates VT with a left bundle branch block configuration. S, *arrow* denotes stimulus artifact.

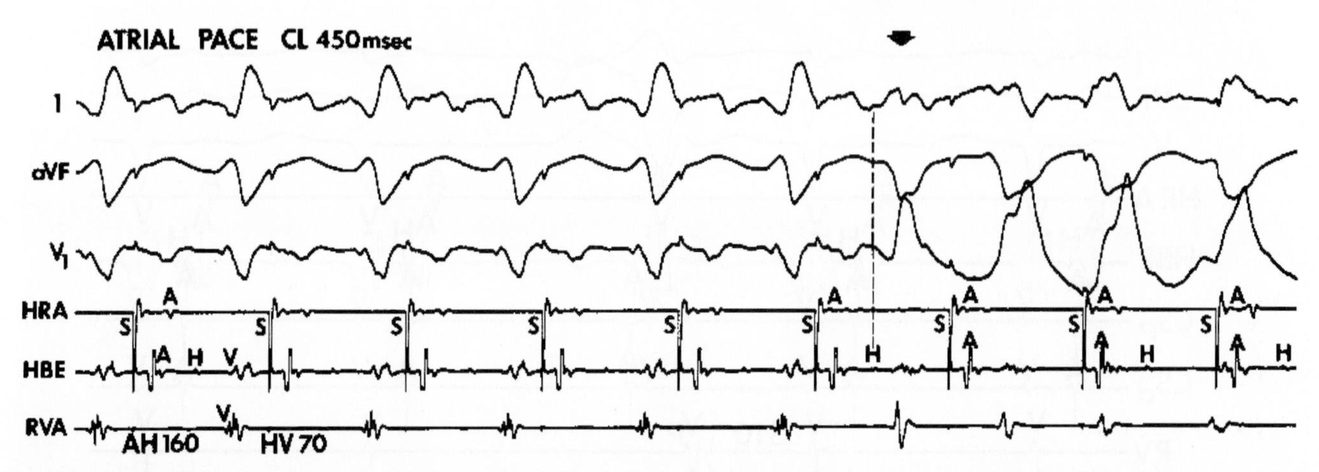


**FIGURE 11-59** Initiation of VT by atrial pacing in a patient with coronary artery disease. Atrial pacing at a cycle length (CL) of 450 msec initiates VT. Note the Q waves in leads 1 and $V_1$ from a prior anteroseptal infarction. The H-V interval is also prolonged at 70 msec. The onset of VT is marked by the *arrow* and a *dashed vertical line.*

The cycle length of VT induced with single VES is usually longer than that induced with double or triple extrastimuli or rapid pacing (Fig. 11-60, Table 11-12).[177] Occasionally, rapid VT can also be induced with a single extrastimulus (Fig. 11-61). This usually occurs in the rare patient presenting with cardiac arrest in whom a single extrastimulus can initiate VT. Fast or slow tachycardias can be induced by double extrastimuli. When the same VT is induced from multiple sites it has a similar cycle length (Figs. 11-62 and 11-63). The cycle length of VTs requiring ≥3 extrastimuli for induction is comparable to that induced by two extrastimuli. These VT cycle lengths are usually shorter than those induced with single extrastimuli. An example of a rapid VT induced by triple extrastimuli is shown in Figure 11-64. Nonetheless, exceptions to this general pattern are not uncommon. We have seen a patient whose VT required four extrastimuli from the left ventricle during sinus rhythm for initiation that had a cycle length of 360 msec (Fig. 11-65). Moreover, even when rapid pacing is used, there is usually no relation between the PCL initiating the VT and the interval to the first complex of the tachycardia, the cycle length of early beats of the tachycardia, or the minimum rate of the tachycardia. Rapid pacing produces the same tachycardia that is induced with less aggressive measures of stimulation (Fig. 11-66).

Thus, the reproducibility of initiation by single, double, or triple extrastimuli delivered during sinus rhythm or eight-beat PCLs, the low yield of rapid pacing-induced initiation, the lack of requirement for a period of quiescence between inductions, and the failure to demonstrate a linear relationship of the PCL to the interval to the first complex and initial cycle length of the tachycardia all suggest reentry rather than triggered activity as the mechanism of the arrhythmia. Moreover, the relationship of the ease of inducibility (single extrastimuli vs. double or triple extrastimuli) and the VT cycle length to abnormalities of conduction are further support of reentry, because such abnormalities should not affect triggered activity.

Isoproterenol infusion, which markedly facilitates the induction of triggered activity, has a limited effect on inducing sustained VT, particularly that which is due to coronary artery disease. As mentioned earlier, although some investigators have noted facilitation of induction of VT by isoproterenol infusion of up to 20%,[161] in our experience, it is significantly lower, usually in the range of 5%. This is opposite of what would be expected if the sustained uniform VT were due to triggered activity. Exercise-related VT is a specific type of VT in which rapid pacing and/or isoproterenol are the most efficacious methods of initiation. It can be terminated by carotid sinus pressure and adenosine which is diagnostic of triggered activity due to DADs.[163,178] Typically, these have an LBBB right inferior axis and arise from the right ventricular outflow tract. An example of such a tachycardia in which atrial and ventricular pacing and isoproterenol initiated the tachycardia at approximately the

**TABLE 11-12 Mode of Initiation of VT Compared with Cycle Length of the 126 Morphologically Distinct Tachycardias in 104 Patients**

| Mode of Initiation of VT | Cycle | VT Length (msec) |
|---|---|---|
| Single | 27 | 342 ± 72[a] |
| Double | 55 | 295 ± 60 |
| Triple | 35 | 282 ± 56 |
| Rapid Pacing | 9 | 293 ± 40 |

Values are mean ± standard deviation. Numbers in parentheses indicate number of morphologically distinct tachycardias initiated with each modality.

[a] $p < 0.05$.

From Doherty JU, Kienzle MG, Waxman HL, et al. Relation of mode of induction and cycle length of ventricular tachycardia: Analysis of 104 patients. *Am J Cardiol* 1963;52:60.

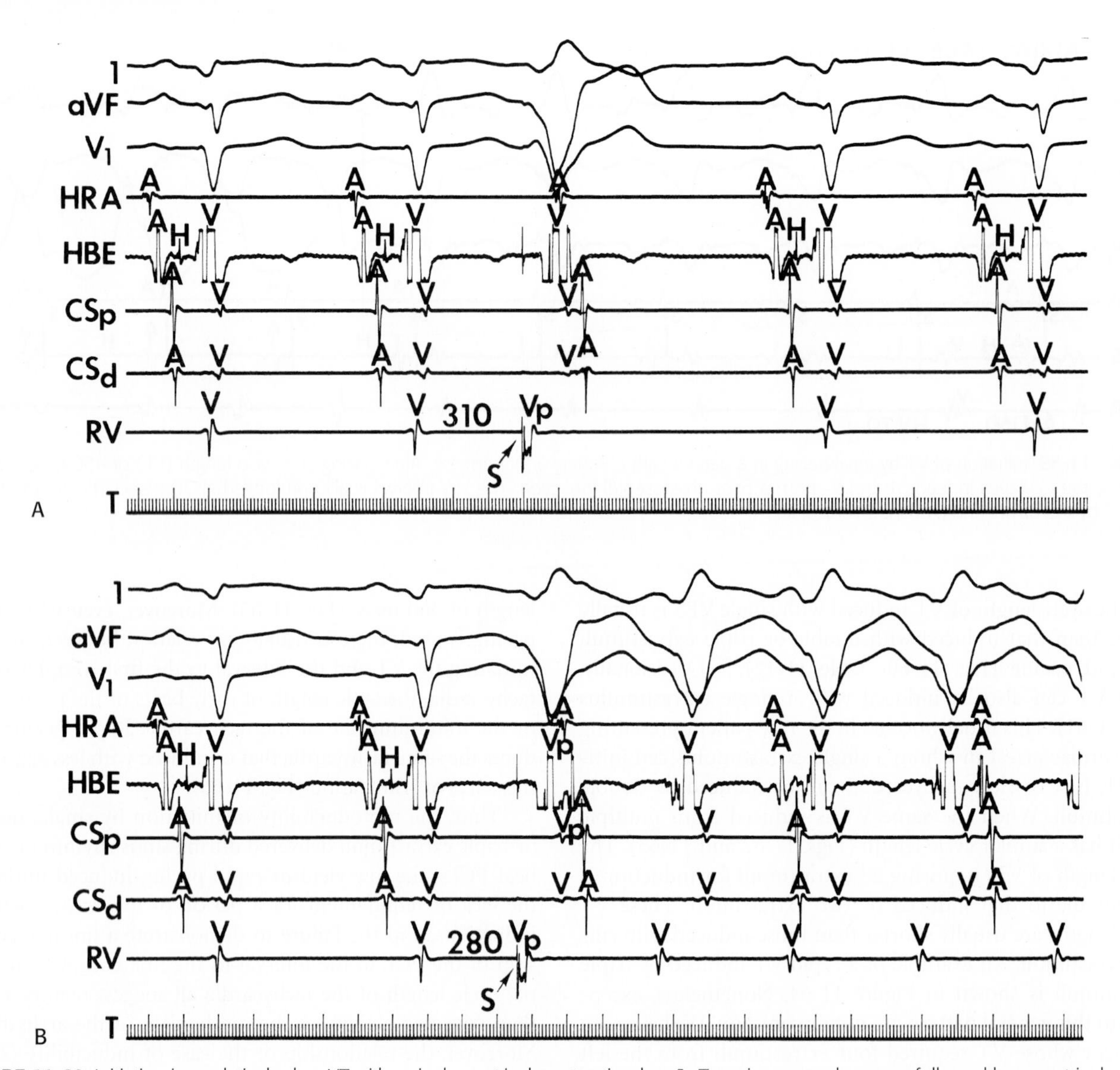


**FIGURE 11-60** Initiation in a relatively slow VT with a single ventricular extrastimulus. **A:** Two sinus complexes are followed by a ventricular extrastimulus ($V_p$) delivered at 310 msec, which fails to initiate a tachycardia. **B:** When the coupling interval of the ventricular stimulus is decreased to 280 msec, VT with left bundle branch block morphology is induced. Note the relatively long VT CL of 370 msec. See text for discussion. $CS_d$, distal CS; $CS_p$, proximal CS.

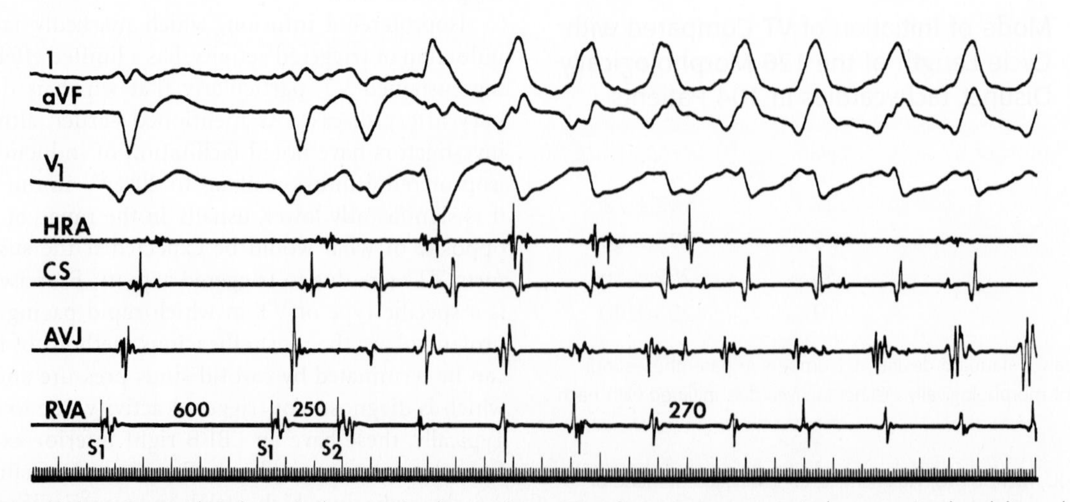


**FIGURE 11-61** Initiation of a rapid VT by a single extrastimulus. During a BCL of 600 msec, a ventricular extrastimulus delivered at a coupling interval ($S_1$-$S_2$) of 250 msec initiates a rapid VT with a cycle length of 270 msec. See text for discussion.

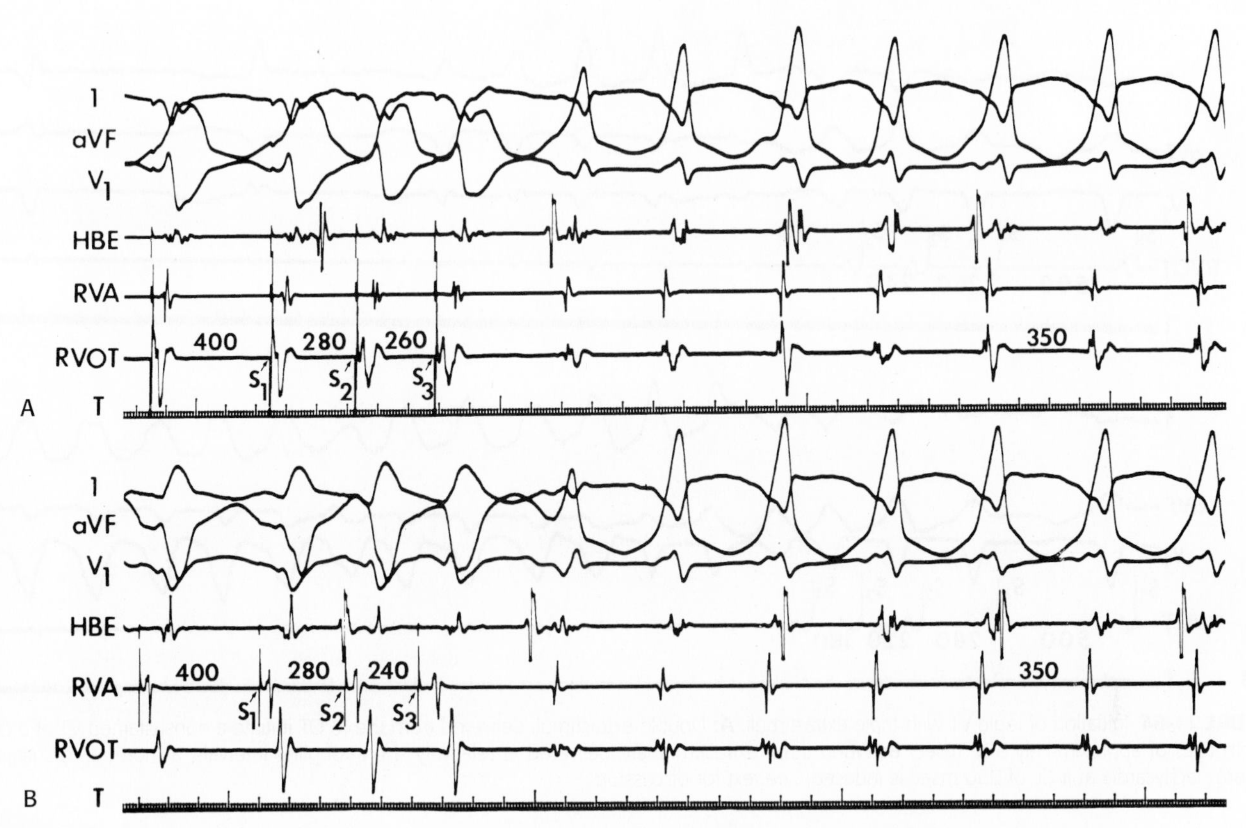


**FIGURE 11-62** Initiation of the same VT from two right ventricular sites. VT with a left bundle branch block right inferior axis and a CL of 350 msec is induced by double VES delivered at the same coupling intervals from **(A)** the RVOT and **(B)** the RVA.

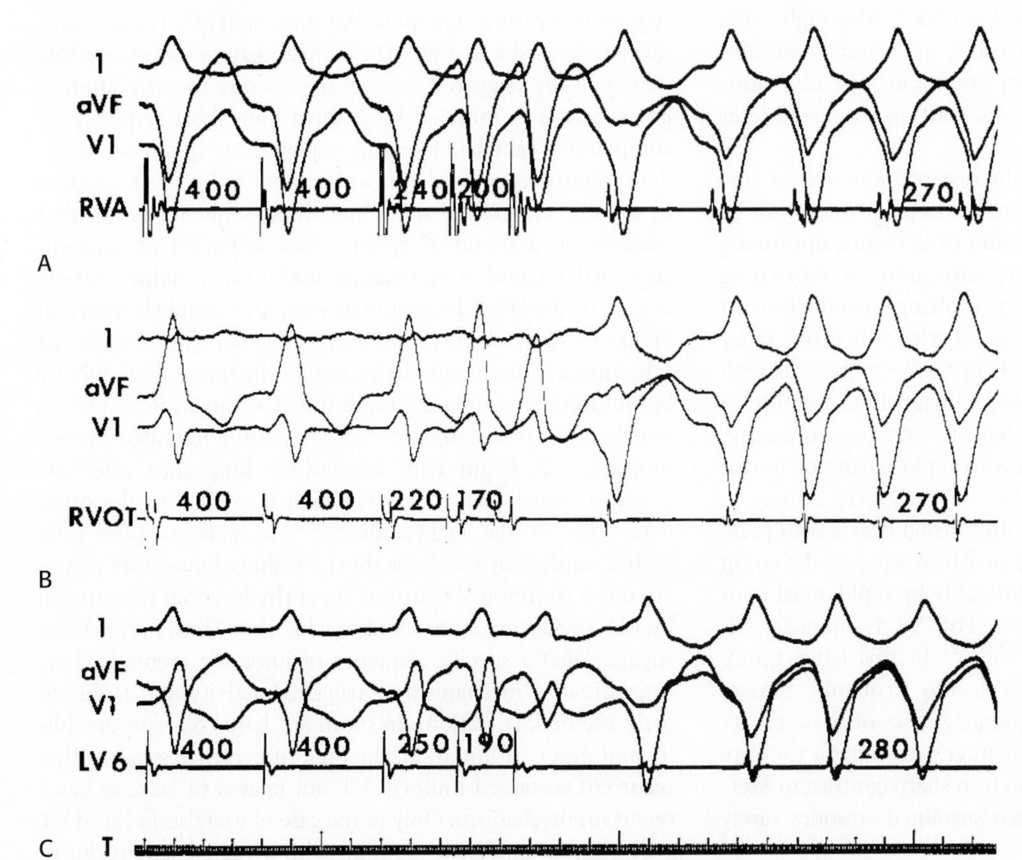


**FIGURE 11-63** Initiation of VT with the same morphology and cycle length by right or left ventricular stimulation. Double extrastimuli delivered at 400 msec from **(A)** the RVA, **(B)** RVOT, and **(C)** inferobasal LV initiate a left bundle branch block VT with a similar cycle length. See text for discussion.

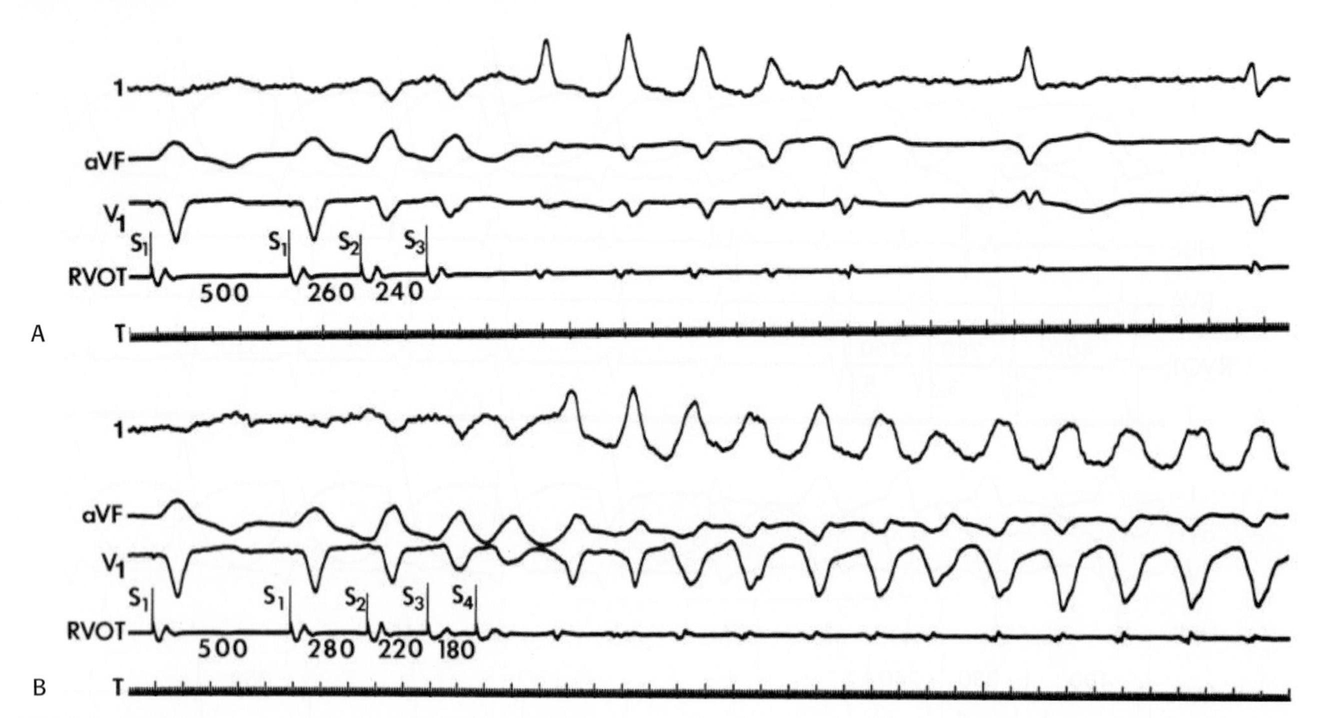


**FIGURE 11-64** Initiation of rapid VT with triple extrastimuli. **A:** Double extrastimuli delivered from the RVOT initiate a nonsustained VT at a cycle length (CL) of approximately 300 msec. **B:** When three extrastimuli are delivered at relatively short coupling intervals, a more rapid sustained uniform tachycardia at a CL of 250 msec is induced. See text for discussion.

same cycle length is shown in Figure 11-67. Similar tachycardias can arise in the left ventricle outflow tract (right and left coronary cusps, aortomitral continuity, or subjacent myocardium).[183–186] or from the fascicles[187] Although these catecholamine-mediated tachycardias occasionally present as sustained VT, more often, they present as repetitive nonsustained tachycardia. This specific entity is discussed later in this chapter.

Possible mechanisms for facilitation of induction of sustained monomorphic VT associated with prior infarction by isoproterenol include the production of ischemia, improving ventricular conduction by hyperpolarization, or shortening ventricular refractoriness, thereby allowing introduction of VES of greater prematurity. In my experience it is this latter mechanism that is most commonly operative in patients with coronary artery disease (Fig. 11-68). Obviously, facilitation of initiation would occur if the mechanism were triggered activity. One would expect initiation with rapid pacing or longer coupling intervals if the mechanism were triggered activity.

Paroxysmal VT in patients with normal hearts who present with paroxysmal VT having an RBBB left axis deviation configuration can also be induced easily by rapid atrial and/or ventricular pacing (Fig. 11-69). This VT is characteristically sensitive to verapamil.[169–173,188,189] In this latter group of patients, single and double VES also frequently initiate arrhythmia. In addition, other characteristics of these tachycardias, discussed in subsequent paragraphs, suggest they are more consistent with reentry. This is in sharp contrast to exercise-related tachycardias, in which sustained episodes rarely can be initiated with VES.

Although torsade de pointes is a rhythm that some investigators say is compatible with early afterdepolarizations (described later in this chapter). Cranefield and Aronson[126,130] suggest that early afterdepolarizations could give rise to a uniform tachycardia as well. These investigators have suggested that typically triggered activity that is due to early afterdepolarizations is initiated by a short-long-short sequence of complexes. Cranefield uses this sequence to explain why standard electrophysiologic protocols do not induce tachycardias. In my experience, the short-long-short sequence is not that uncommon a mode of spontaneous initiation of uniform sustained VT and is particularly useful for initiating bundle branch reentry (see discussion below). An example is shown in Figure 11-70 in which a short-long-short sequence is observed initiating a spontaneous arrhythmia, which can subsequently be induced by standard programmed stimulation. Approximately 50% of sustained hemodynamically tolerated monomorphic VTs begin with a relatively long (just after the T wave) ventricular complex, which is similar to the other complexes of the tachycardia.[190,191] In patients presenting with a cardiac arrest, long-short or short-long-short onsets are more common.[192] Most of these rhythms can be initiated by PES suggesting a reentrant mechanism. Thus, no evidence suggests that a specific sequence of initiating events is characteristic of a mechanism of triggered activity that is due to early afterdepolarizations. In summary, based on reproducibility and mode of initiation, the bulk of evidence suggests that recurrent sustained uniform VT not related to exercise has a reentrant mechanism. Only in the case of exercise-induced VT are the initiation data compatible with triggered activity due to

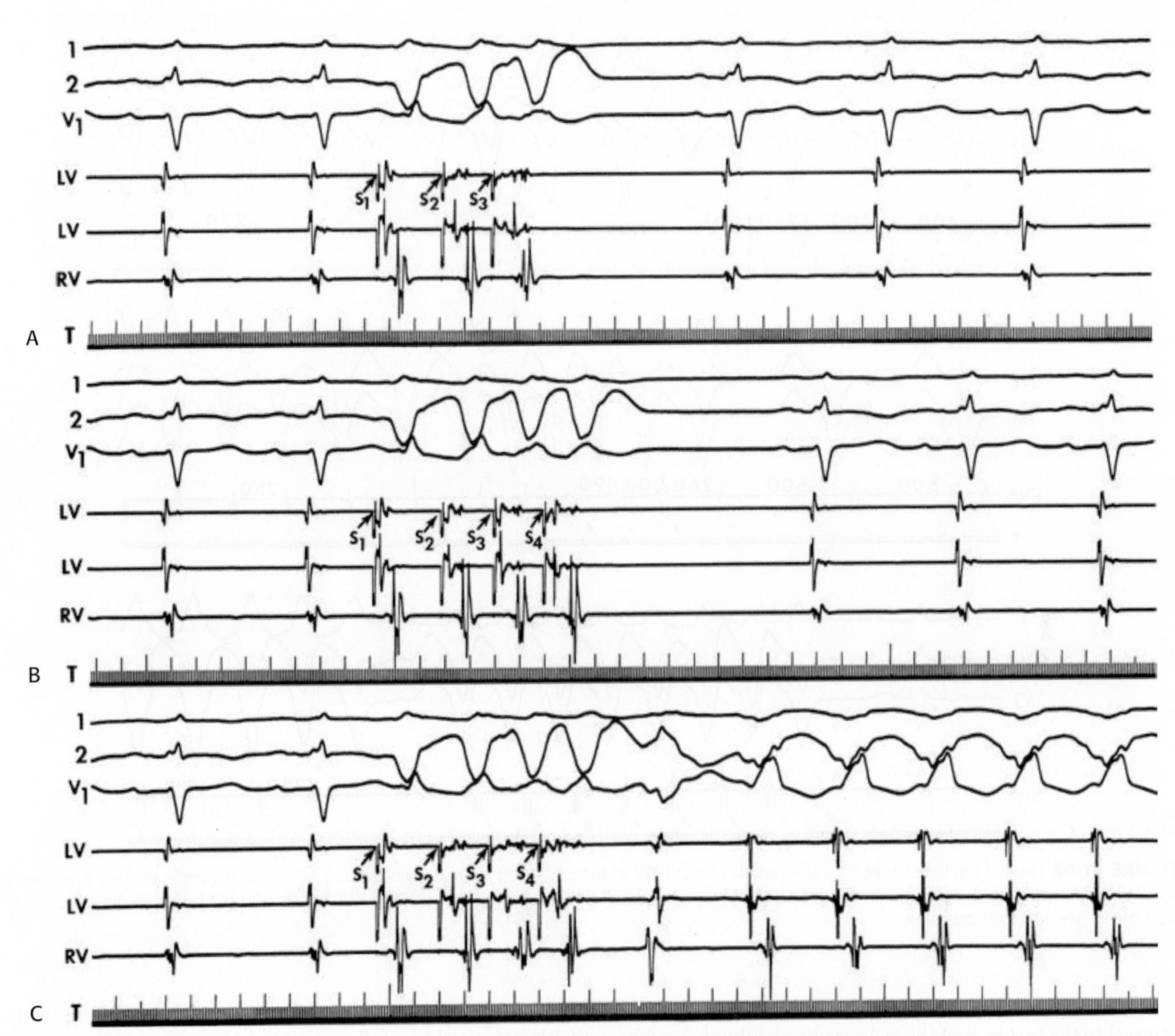


**FIGURE 11-65** Initiation of a slow VT by four ventricular extrastimuli. **A** and **B:** Triple (**top**) and **(C)** quadruple extrastimuli delivered from the LV during sinus rhythm fail to initiate VT. When the coupling intervals of the third and fourth extrastimuli are shortened slightly, S-UVT with a CL of 360 msec is initiated. This was the only mode of induction of VT in this patient. See text for discussion.

DADs. No stimulation protocol has been studied which initiates tachycardias due to early afterdepolarizations in humans.

### *Relationship of Coupling Intervals and Cycle Length Initiating Tachycardia to the Onset of Ventricular Tachycardia and the Initial Ventricular Tachycardia Cycle Length*

Conduction delay is required for the initiation of reentrant rhythms (see following discussion). Therefore, an inverse relationship between the coupling interval of the extrastimulus initiating the tachycardia and the interval from the stimulus to the first complex of the tachycardia favors reentry. Similarly, an inverse relationship between the drive cycle length during which extrastimuli at the same coupling interval initiate the tachycardia, and the interval to the onset of the tachycardia, would also favor reentry. When multiple VES are used, it is difficult to evaluate this relationship. In either case, if a reentrant rhythm is present, the initial cycle length would reflect conduction through the tachycardia circuit, which, in the absence of exit block, should demonstrate the same or longer cycle length as the remaining tachycardia cycles, depending on whether any conduction delay is produced in the circuit on initiation.

These findings are in contrast to those observed in triggered rhythms due to DADs in ventricular tissue that often exhibit a direct relationship to the PCL or to the coupling intervals of the extrastimuli that initiate them. Typically, in tachycardias due to DADs the initial cycle of the tachycardia usually bears a direct relationship to the PCL, with or without a direct relationship to the coupling interval of extrastimuli delivered.[180] Thus, the shorter the PCL, with or without

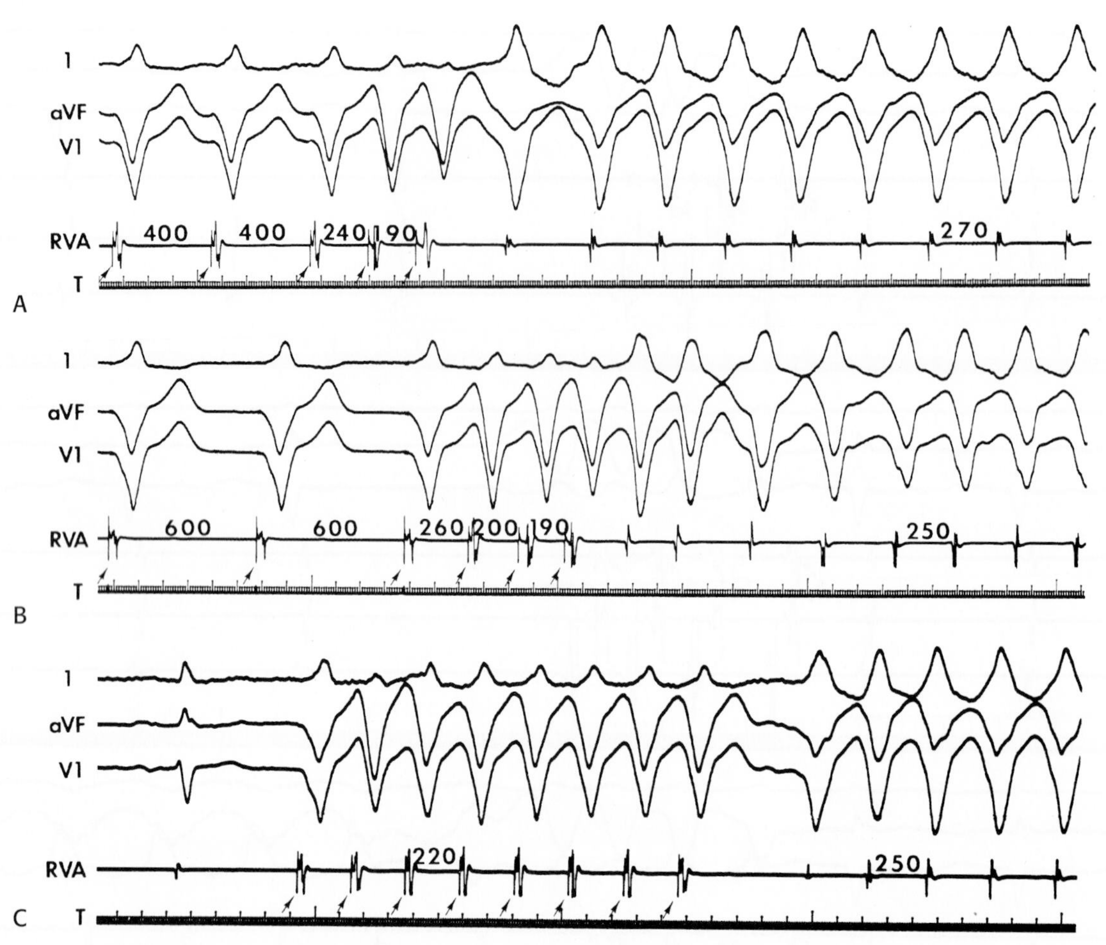


**FIGURE 11-66** Lack of relationship of VT cycle length to mode of induction. A left bundle branch block VT of similar cycle lengths is induced by **(A)** double extrastimuli delivered at 400 msec; **(B)** triple extrastimuli delivered at a basic drive of 600 msec; and **(C)** bursts of rapid pacing at 220 msec. See text for discussion.

extrastimuli, that initiates the tachycardia, the shorter the interval to the first beat of the tachycardia and the shorter the initial cycle length of the tachycardia. Occasionally, with early extrastimuli in digitalis-intoxicated preparations, a jump in the interval to the onset of the triggered rhythm occurs such that it is approximately double the interval to the onset of the tachycardia initiated by later coupled extrastimuli. This has been explained by failure of the initial DAD to reach threshold while the second reaches threshold. Thus, in triggered activity due to DADs in ventricular tissue, the coupling interval of the initial complex of the tachycardia either shortens or suddenly increases in response to progressively premature extrastimuli. It never demonstrates an inverse or gradually increasing relationship. It must be reiterated that, in response to drive cycle length, the onset of the tachycardia always has a direct relationship with the drive cycle length, regardless of the tissue used. Only with the addition of very early extrastimuli or occasionally very rapid pacing (<300 msec), the sudden jump in the interval to the first complex of the tachycardia may be observed. We have never noted a direct relationship between PCL and the interval to the onset of the tachycardia or early tachycardia cycles in the case of paroxysmal, nonexercise-related, sustained monomorphic VT in humans with structural heart disease.

When single extrastimuli are delivered, and one can assess the relationship between coupling interval and the interval to the first VT complex, one sees an inverse relationship in approximately 40% of patients (Figs. 11-71 and 11-72).[1,122,193–195] Sometimes one initially sees an isolated repetitive response followed by initiation of the tachycardia (Fig. 11-71), while at other times, the first extrastimulus initiates a sustained VT (Fig. 11-72). When the drive cycle length is short and tachycardia can be initiated by extrastimuli delivered at the same coupling interval, an inverse relationship is also seen (Fig. 11-73). Most often, particularly when multiple extrastimuli and/or rapid pacing initiate a tachycardia, there is no direct relationship or measurable relationship to the onset of the tachycardia or tachycardia cycle length (Fig. 11-66). In many patients, the coupling interval to the first complex of the tachycardia as well as the initial tachycardia cycle length are unaffected by the mode of stimulation. Thus, as shown in Figure 11-74, atrial pacing at a cycle length of 320 msec, ventricular pacing at 360 msec, and a single extrastimulus delivered at a PCL of 400 msec initiate VT with identical intervals to the onset of the tachycardia and initial cycle lengths

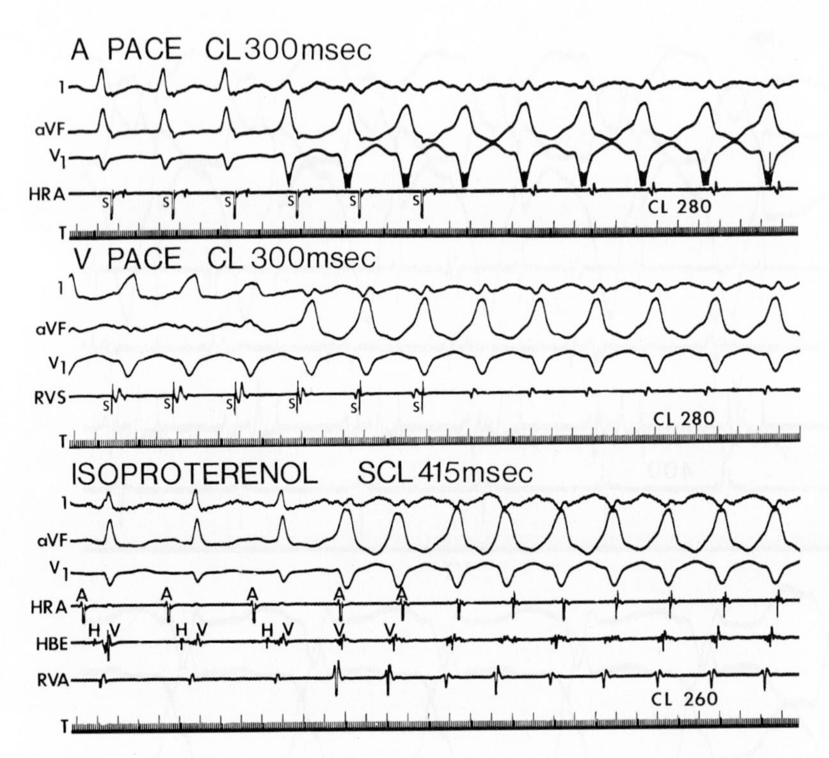


**FIGURE 11-67** Initiation of exercise-induced VT by programmed stimulation and isoproterenol infusion. In the top two panels, atrial pacing and ventricular pacing at CLs of 300 msec initiate VT with a left bundle branch block right inferior axis configuration and a CL of 280 msec. Following isoproterenol infusion, which shortened the sinus cycle length (SCL) to 415 msec, VT occurs spontaneously. See text for discussion.

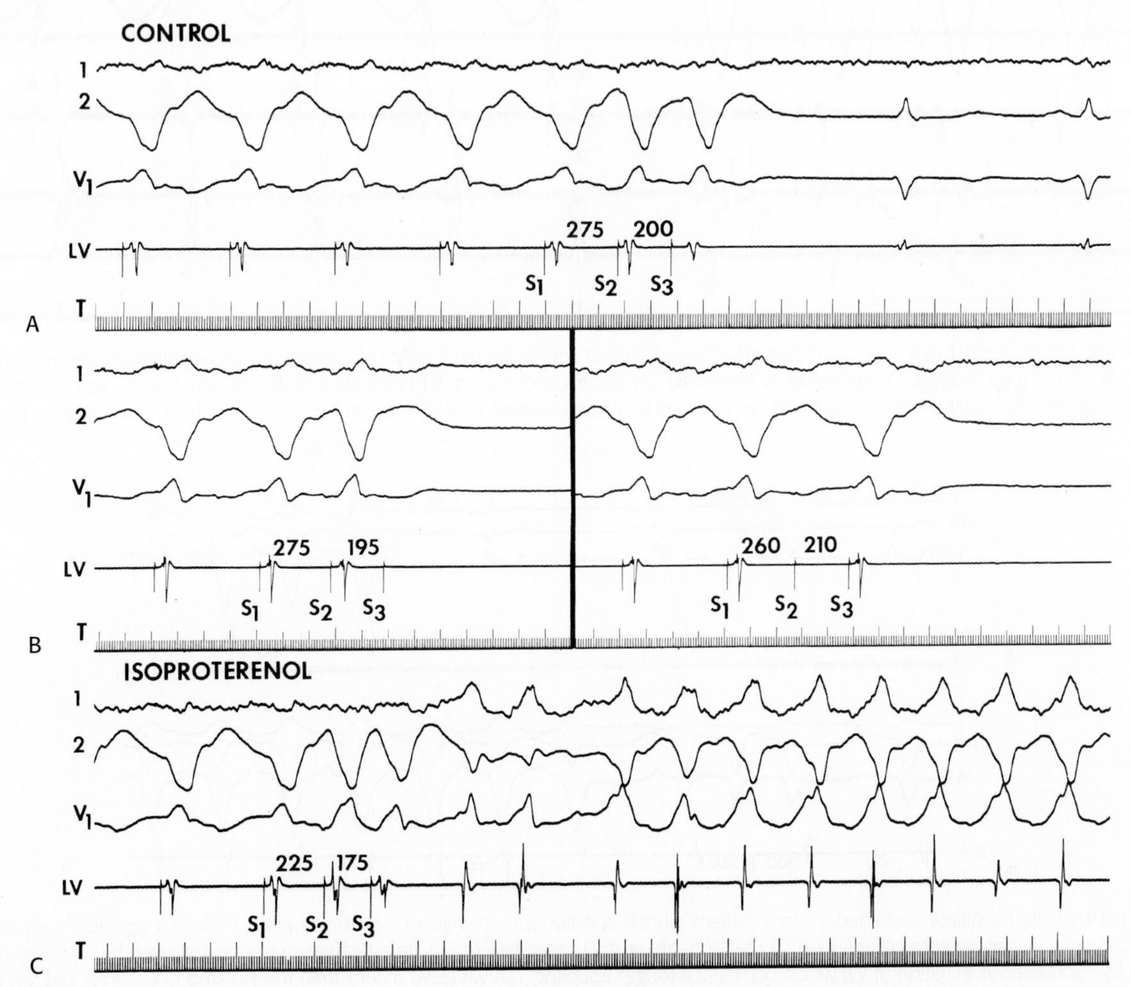


**FIGURE 11-68** Facilitation of induction of VT by isoproterenol in a patient with coronary artery disease. **A–C.** Double extrastimuli fail to initiate VT. Following isoproterenol, the local refractory period at the stimulation site is shortened and closer coupled premature stimuli can capture the ventricle and initiate VT. This rapid VT was identical to that spontaneously occurring in a patient that caused cardiac arrest.

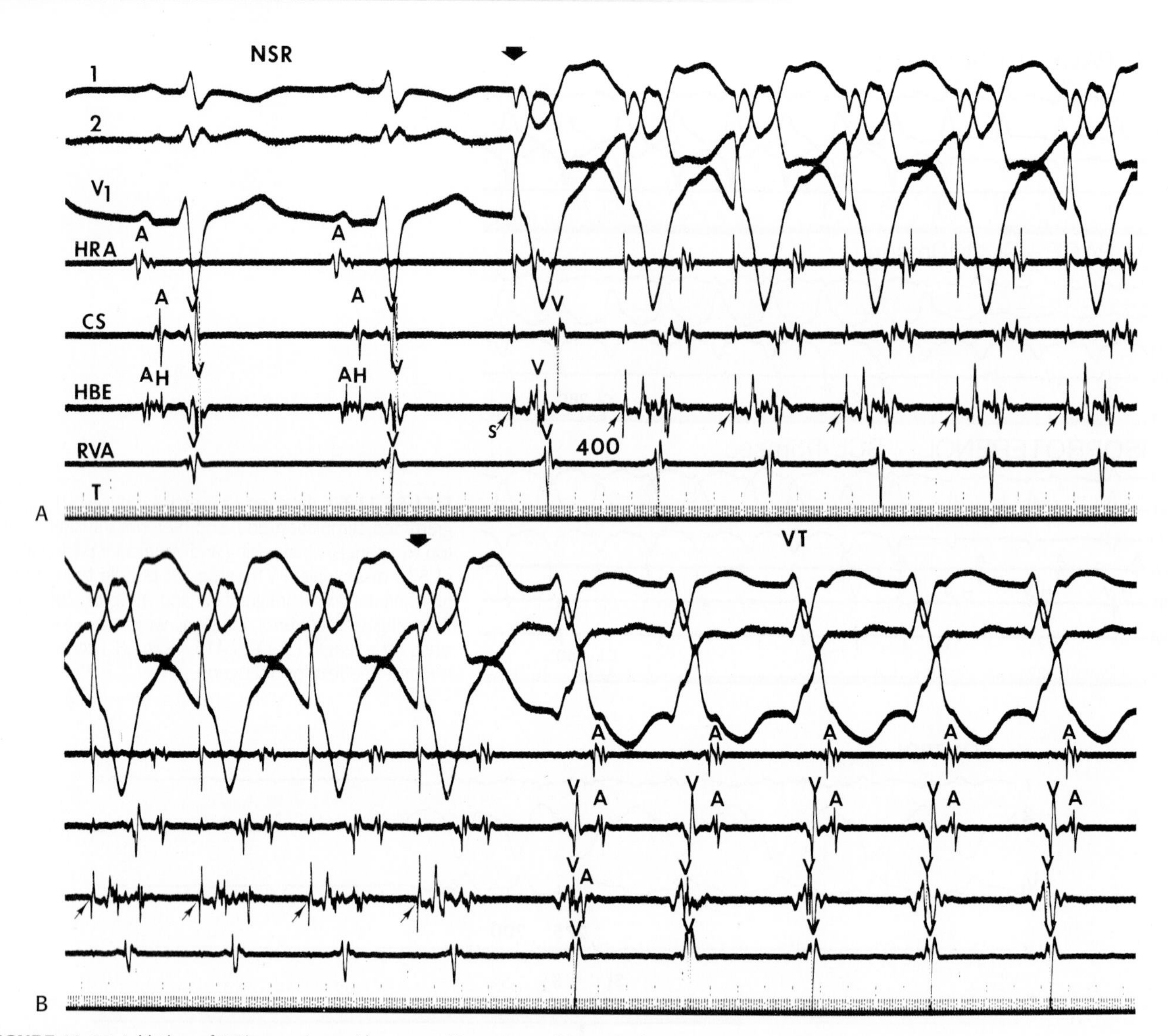


FIGURE 11-69 Initiation of VT in a patient with a normal heart by rapid ventricular pacing. **A:** Following two sinus complexes, stimulation from the RVOT (not shown) at a cycle length of 400 msec is begun. **B:** On cessation of pacing, VT is initiated. Note the right bundle branch block superior axis morphology, which is characteristic of patients with idiopathic VT and normal hearts. See text for discussion. NSR, normal sinus rhythm.

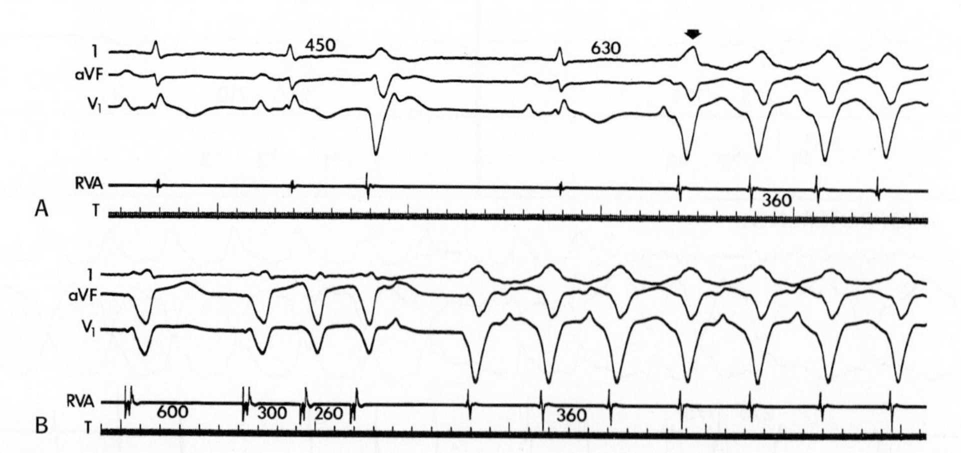


FIGURE 11-70 Ability to initiate sustained VT in a patient whose spontaneous tachycardia occurred after a "short-long-short" sequence. **A:** A spontaneous ventricular premature complex (VPC) that appears at 450 msec fails to initiate a tachycardia but is followed by a pause. This pause is followed by spontaneous initiation of VT, which occurs at a longer coupling interval (630 msec) than the isolated VPC, which did not initiate an arrhythmia. **B:** The same tachycardia can be initiated by double extrastimuli from the RVA. Thus, the spontaneous initiation of VT by "short-long-short" CLs does not imply a specific mechanism of the tachycardia. See text for discussion.

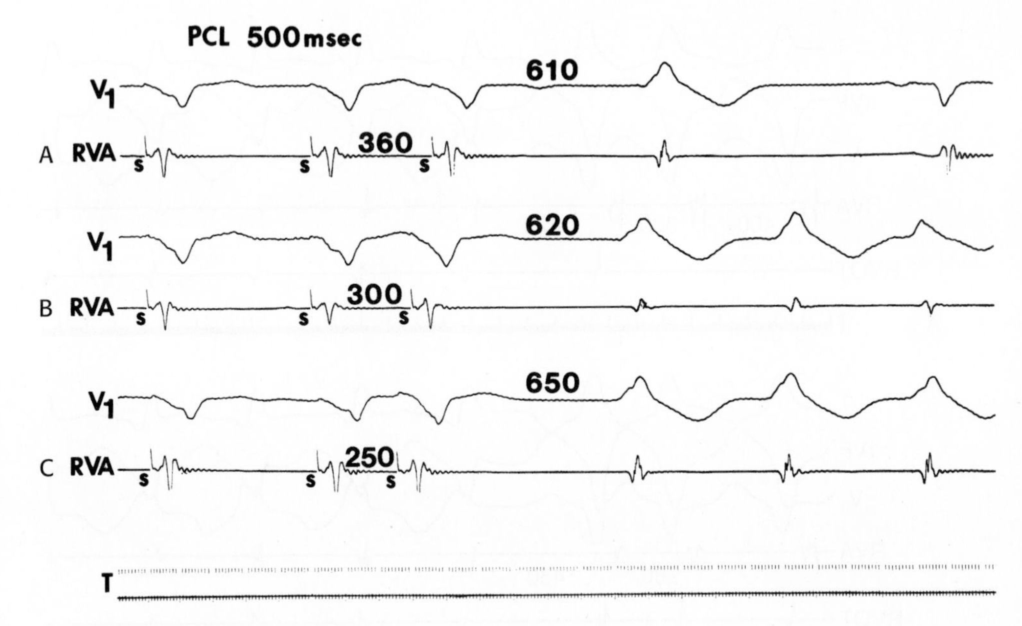


**FIGURE 11-71** Initiation of VT with an inverse relationship of coupling intervals to the interval preceding the onset of the tachycardia. A single ECG lead, $V_1$, and an electrogram from the RVA are shown in three panels. **A:** At a coupling interval of 360 msec, a single repetitive ventricular response is noted with a coupling interval of 610 msec. **B:** At a closer coupling interval of 300 msec, VT begins after a pause of 620 msec. **C:** Finally, at an even shorter coupling interval of 250 msec, VT is again initiated, with an even longer pause of 650 msec. This inverse relationship is compatible with a reentrant mechanism. See text for discussion.

of the tachycardia. We have never seen a direct relationship of PCLs to onset intervals of tachycardias in patients with sustained uniform VT associated with coronary artery disease. Although we have not studied tachycardias associated with digitalis intoxication, Gorgels et al.[196] demonstrated a direct relationship of such rhythms in experimental canine models of digitalis intoxication. Whether a human VT associated with digitalis intoxication behaves the same way has not yet been evaluated. When multiple VES and/or rapid pacing are used to initiate the tachycardia, no consistent relationship has been observed between the initiating sequence (number and coupling interval of extrastimuli, paced drive cycle lengths, or cycle lengths of burst pacing) and the initial characteristics of the tachycardia (the interval to the onset of the tachycardia or early tachycardia cycle length).

### *Relationship of Stimulation Site to Initiation of Ventricular Tachycardia*

With triggered rhythms, the site of stimulation should have no effect on initiating a tachycardia as long as the impulse reaches the site of triggered activity. This is not so for reentrant arrhythmias, where wavefront of activation may be important in developing block and slow conduction. Unpublished observations from our laboratory have shown that single and double extrastimuli delivered at PCLs of 600 or 400 msec always reach the "site of origin" of left VTs, even in the presence of markedly abnormal conduction manifested by abnormal electrograms. One can usually demonstrate changes in local abnormal electrograms at arrhythmogenic sites in response to different sites of stimulation. This observation supports the role of tissue anisotropy in creating conduction delays and/or block associated with initiation of VT. Thus, failure to reach the site of tachycardia origin cannot be used to explain differences in incidence of inducibility by the site of stimulation. As stated earlier, although in most patients, the same tachycardia can be initiated from both the right ventricular outflow tract and right ventricular apex (Figs. 11-50 and 11-62), this is most often true when single extrastimuli (Fig. 11-75) initiate the tachycardia. The site of stimulation may be an extremely important factor in initiating VT in humans if only the right ventricular apex is used. Twenty to 30% of patients will require stimulation from a second right ventricular site if two extrastimuli delivered at two PCLs are employed. If three extrastimuli are employed, 10% to 25% of patients will require a second right ventricular site.[140,156] As noted earlier, we have found that if three extrastimuli fail to initiate sustained uniform VT from the right ventricular apex, 22% of tachycardias can be initiated from the right ventricular outflow tract (Fig. 11-76).[156] If only two extrastimuli are involved, nearly 10% of patients will require stimulation from the left ventricle (Fig. 11-77).[157] If a protocol including three extrastimuli delivered at two right ventricular sites and at multiple drive cycle lengths is used, the incidence for requirement of left ventricular stimulation to initiate a sustained VT is <5% (Fig. 11-78).[1,42,122,149]

Because the incidence of inducing nonspecific polymorphic tachycardias increases with the use of increasing numbers of extrastimuli, one should employ a protocol that allows testing from multiple sites with the least number of stimuli before using more aggressive protocols. Using the protocol shown in Table 11-11, we have found that in approximately 20% of people sustained monomorphic VT can be initiated with less extrastimuli at one site than at another. This is an important observation, if one wants to limit the potential for developing polymorphic VT and VF. A dramatic example is shown in Figure 11-79 in which triple extrastimuli from the right ventricular apex could initiate only a polymorphic VT in a patient with spontaneous sustained monomorphic VT. Stimulation from the right ventricular outflow tract at longer coupling intervals induced two different sustained monomorphic VTs, which were identical to those spontaneously occurring in the

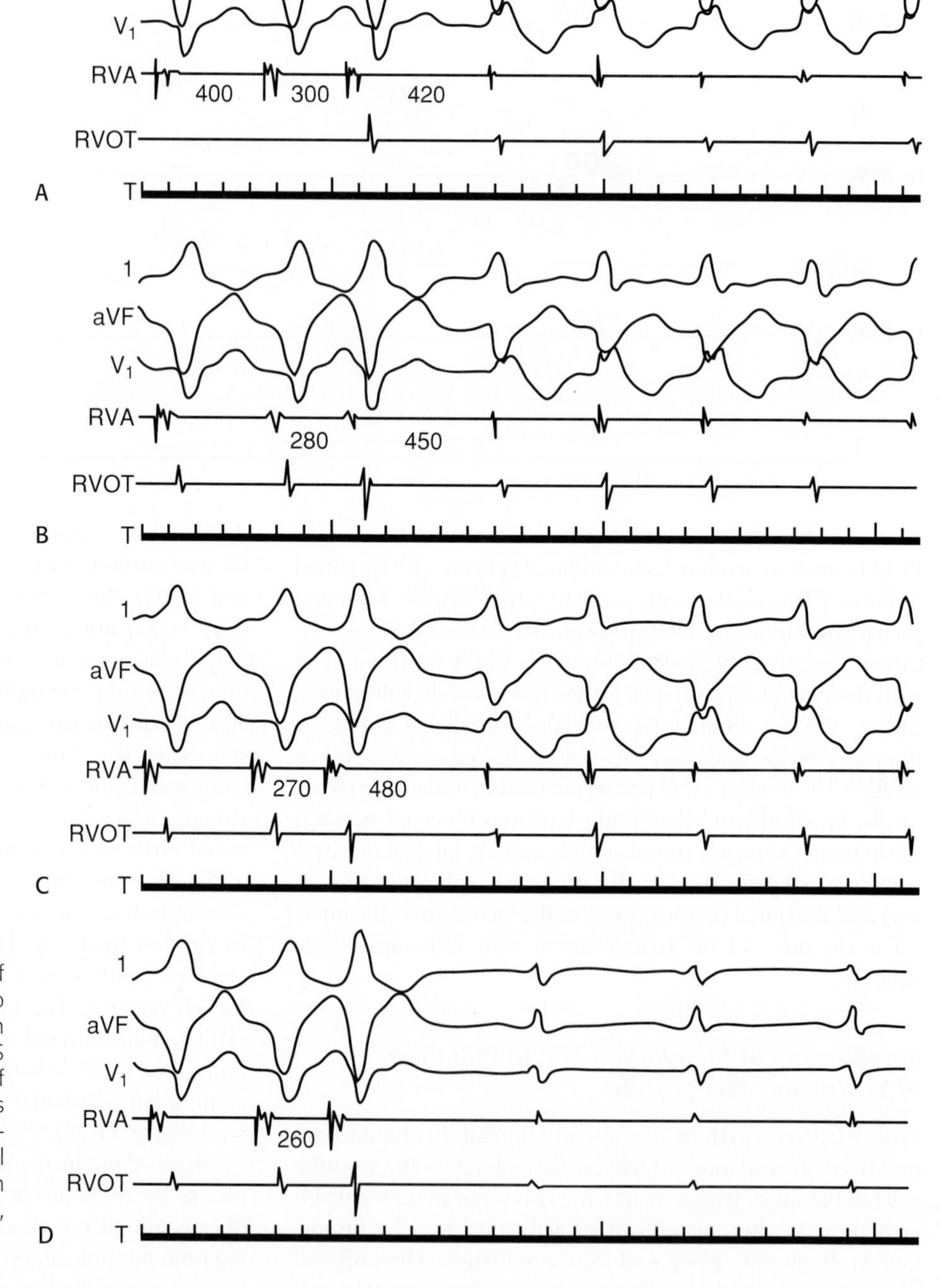


**FIGURE 11-72** Inverse relationship of coupling interval of premature stimuli to the interval at onset of initiation of VT in a patient with no heart disease. **A–D:** VES are delivered from the RVA at a BCL of 400 msec. **A–C:** As the coupling interval is reduced from 300 to 270 msec, VT is initiated but with a progressively longer interval to the onset of the tachycardia. **D:** At an even shorter coupling interval of 260 msec, no VT is initiated. See text for discussion.

patient. An even more dramatic example of the influence of inducibility is shown in Figure 11-80. Here, triple extrastimuli from the right ventricular apex failed to initiate any VT, but a single extrastimulus delivered from the right ventricular outflow tract initiated a well-tolerated sustained monomorphic VT. Thus, a second right or left ventricular site may be required for initiation or may make initiation possible with a fewer number of stimuli in 30% to 40% of patients. As noted earlier, patients with sustained uniform VT who present with a cardiac arrest more frequently require left ventricular stimulation than patients presenting with tolerated uniform VT.[42] The reasons for this are unclear, but may be related to a lesser amount of conduction abnormalities and/or greater extent of homogeneous refractoriness produced by a broad wavefront from the RV compared to that produced by a more narrow wavefront initiated in the LV. In sum, the demonstration of absolute or relative site specificity for initiation of VT, using standard stimulation protocols that have been demonstrated to reach the site of tachycardia origin, favors a reentrant mechanism for VT. Rhythms related to DADs should show no evidence of site specificity as long as comparable coupling intervals can reach the site of DADs.

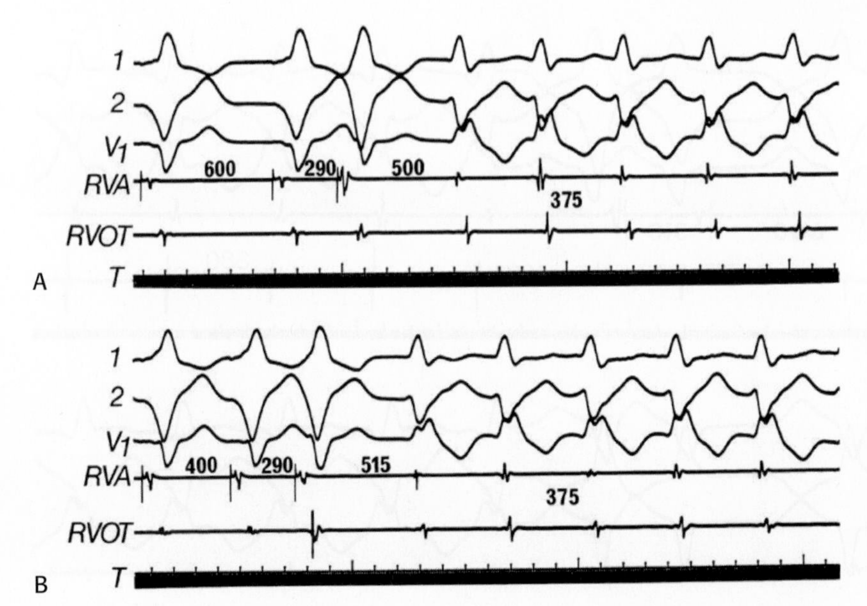


**FIGURE 11-73** Inverse relationship of basic drive cycle length and interval to onset of induced VT. **A:** At a BCL of 600 msec, a premature stimulus delivered at 290 msec initiates VT, which begins after a delay of 500 msec. **B:** When the basic drive cycle length is reduced to 400 msec, a single extrastimulus induced at an identical coupling interval of 290 msec initiates the same VT but after a longer delay of 515 msec. This inverse relationship at a BCL is supportive of a reentrant mechanism. See text for discussion.

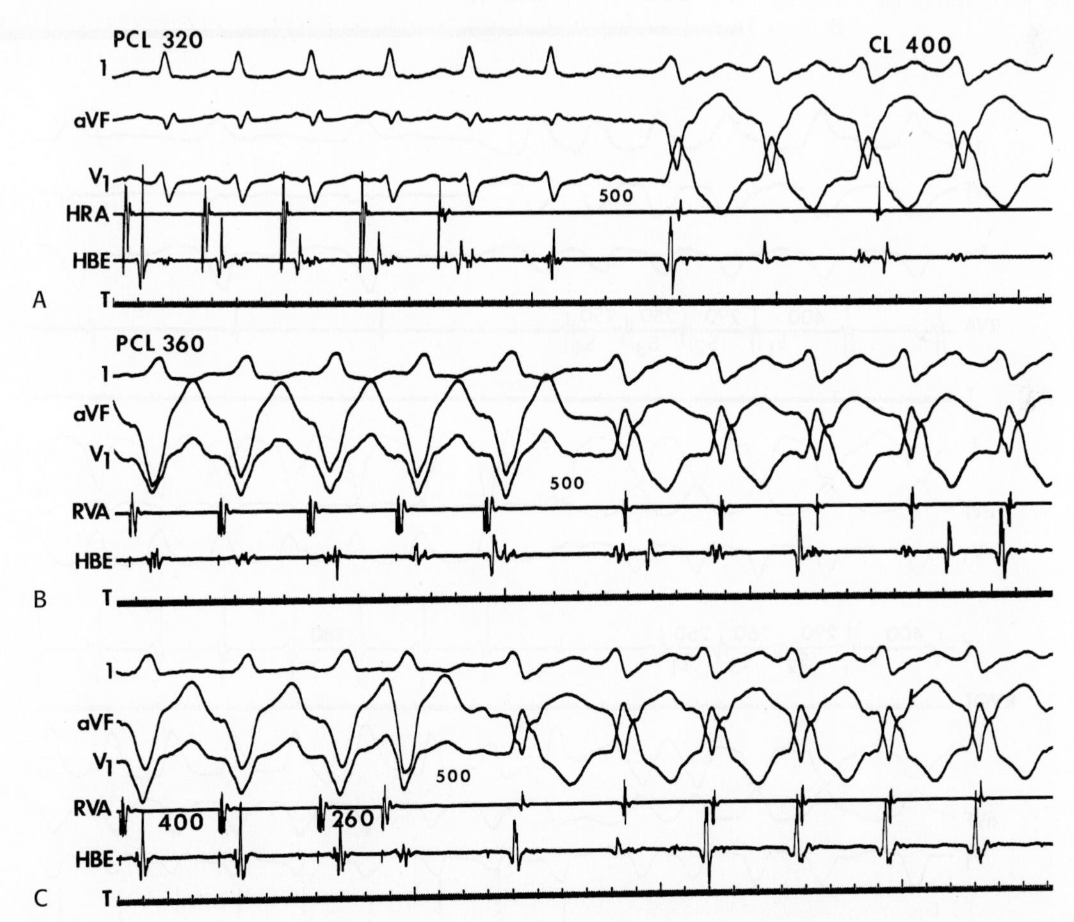


**FIGURE 11-74** Lack of effect of basic drive cycle length (CL) or mode of stimulation on coupling interval to onset of induced VT. **A:** VT is initiated by atrial pacing at a CL of 320 msec. The tachycardia begins after an interval of 500 msec from the last ventricular depolarization. **B:** Pacing from the RVA at a CL of 360 msec initiates the identical VT, which begins after the same delay as observed in **(A)** when the drive CL was shorter. **C:** At an even longer drive CL of 400 msec, a single extrastimulus delivered from the RVA again initiates the same tachycardia with the same delay to the onset of the tachycardia as noted in **(A)** and **(B)**. The failure of paced cycle length or mode or initiation to influence either the coupling interval to the onset of VT or the early cycles of VT are incompatible with triggered activity. See text for discussion.

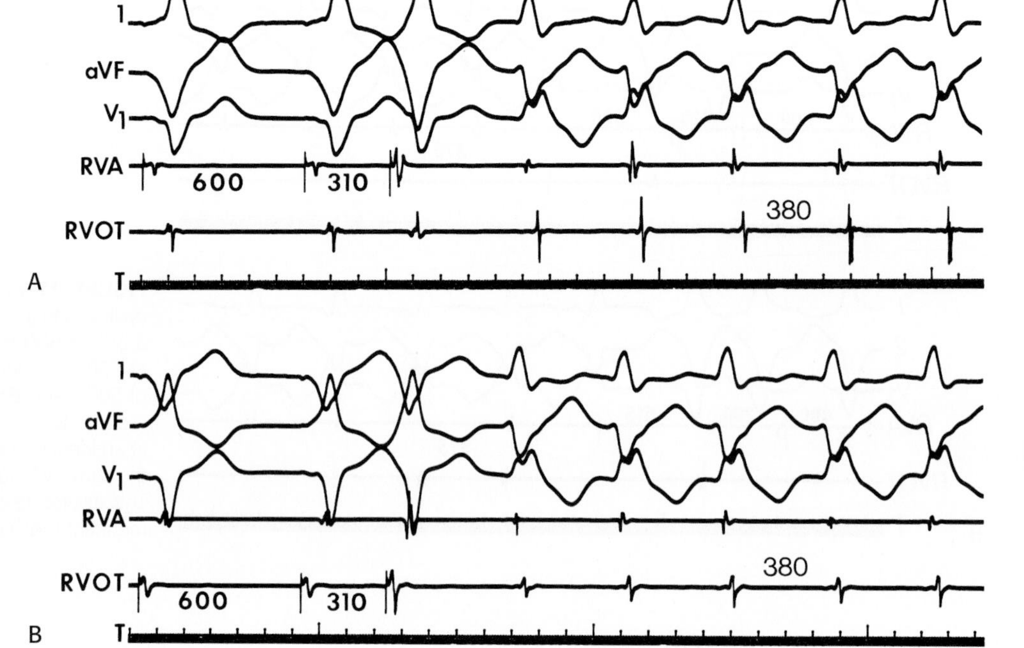


**FIGURE 11-75** Initiation of the same morphologically distinct tachycardia by stimulation at the right ventricular apex and outflow tract. **A** and **B:** Programmed stimulation is performed at a basic drive cycle length of 600 msec, and premature stimuli are delivered at 310 msec. Stimulation from **(A)** the RVA and **(B)** the RVOT initiates the identical tachycardia.

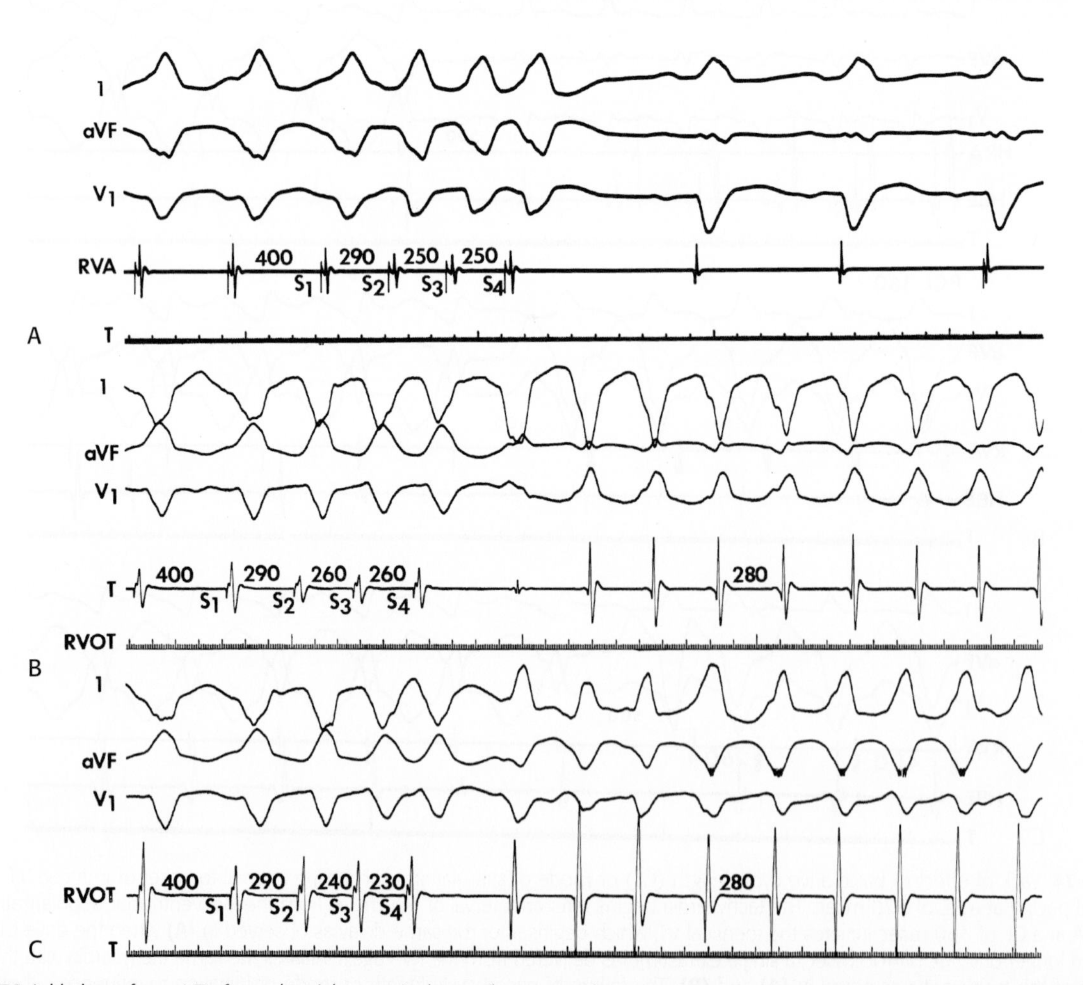


**FIGURE 11-76** Initiation of two VTs from the right ventricular outflow tract when stimulation from the right ventricular apex failed to initiate a tachycardia. **A:** Triple ventricular extrastimuli delivered at a paced cycle length of 400 msec from the RVA failed to initiate VT. **B** and **C:** Pacing from the RVOT at a comparable drive cycle length and coupling intervals of extrastimuli initiates two morphologically distinct tachycardias. This observation may be seen in ≈20% of patients. See text for discussion.

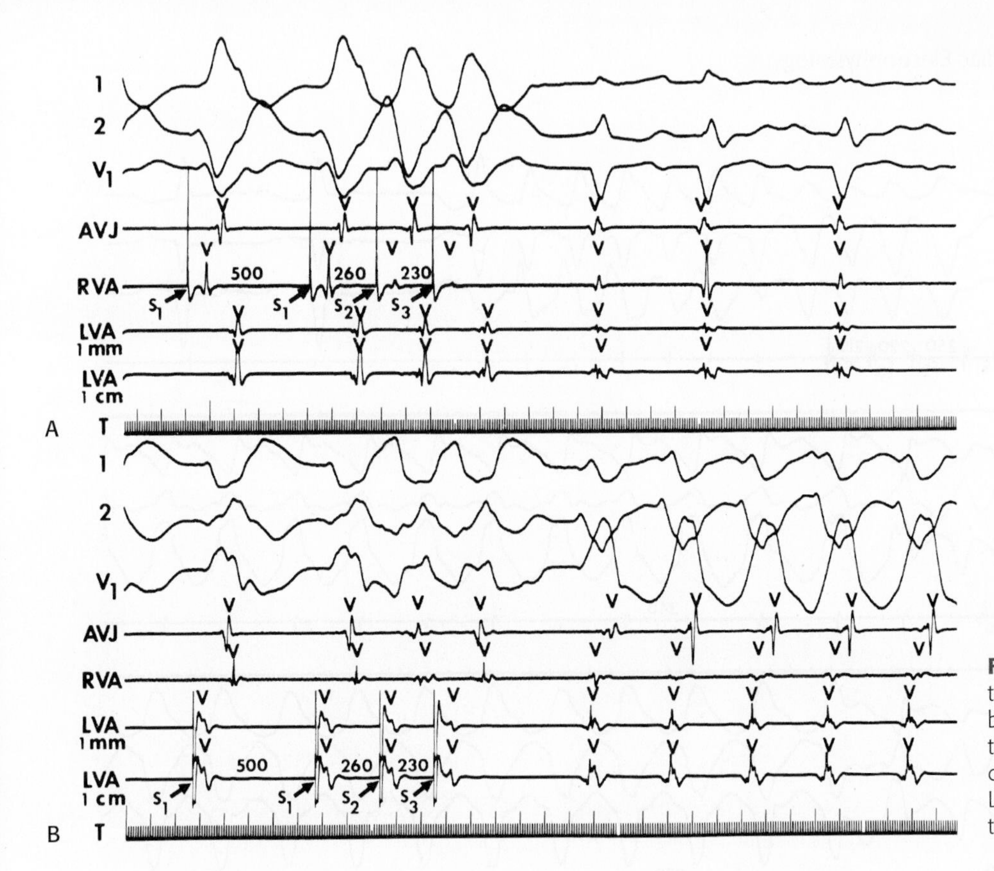


**FIGURE 11-77** Requirement of left ventricular stimulation to initiate VT. **A:** Double VES delivered from the RVA fail to initiate VT. **B:** When double VES at identical coupling intervals are introduced at the LVA, sustained uniform VT is initiated. See text for discussion.

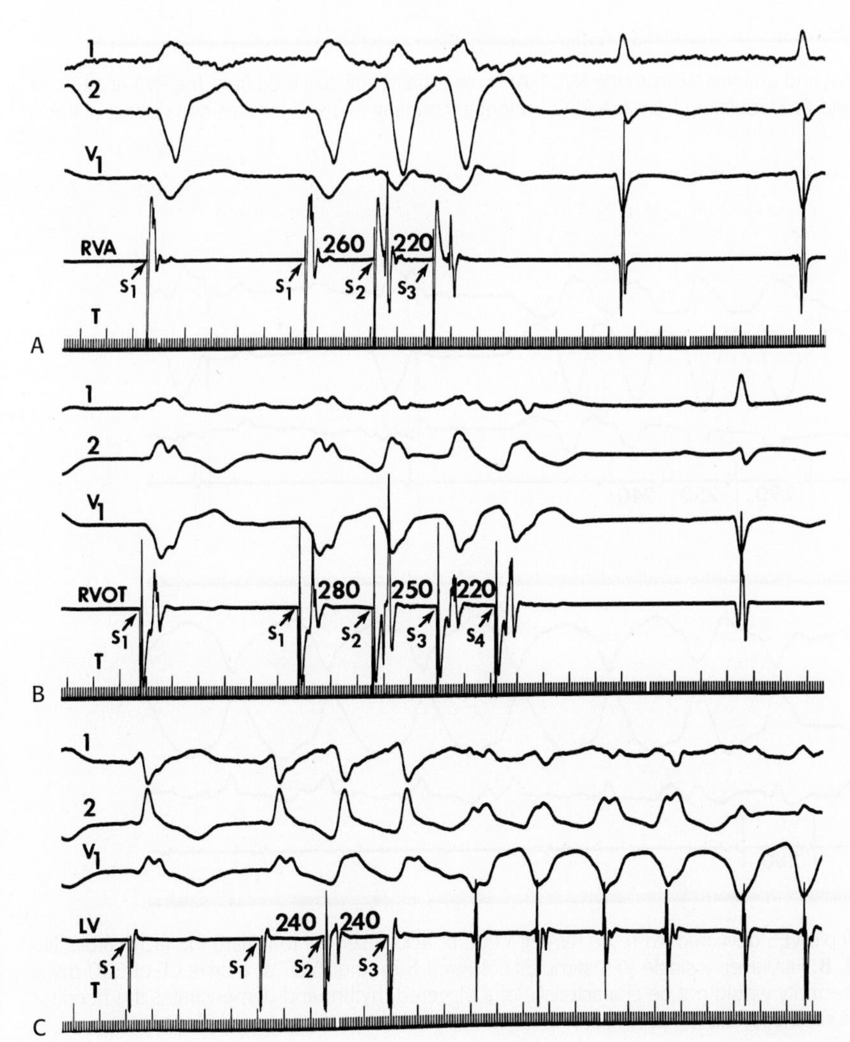


**FIGURE 11-78** Initiation of VT from the LV after failure of initiation from the RV. **A** and **B:** Stimulation from the RVA (double extrastimuli) and RVOT (triple extrastimuli) fail to initiate VT. **C:** Double extrastimuli from the LV initiate sustained VT. See text for discussion.

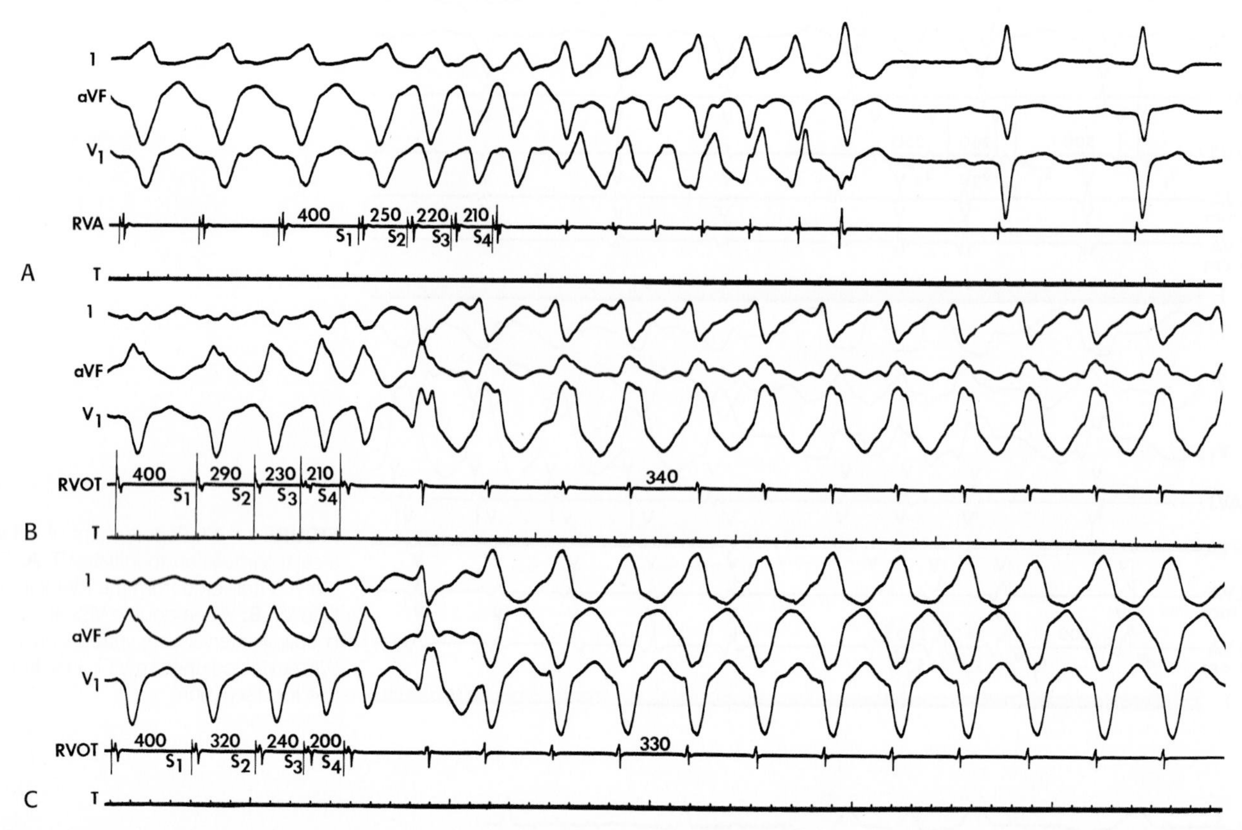


**FIGURE 11-79** Initiation of polymorphic VT from the RVA and uniform VT from the RVOT. **A:** Triple extrastimuli delivered from the RVA at a PCL of 400 msec initiates a nonsustained polymorphic VT. **B** and **C:** Stimulation from the RVOT at longer coupling intervals initiates two distinct uniform VTs. See text for clinical significance.

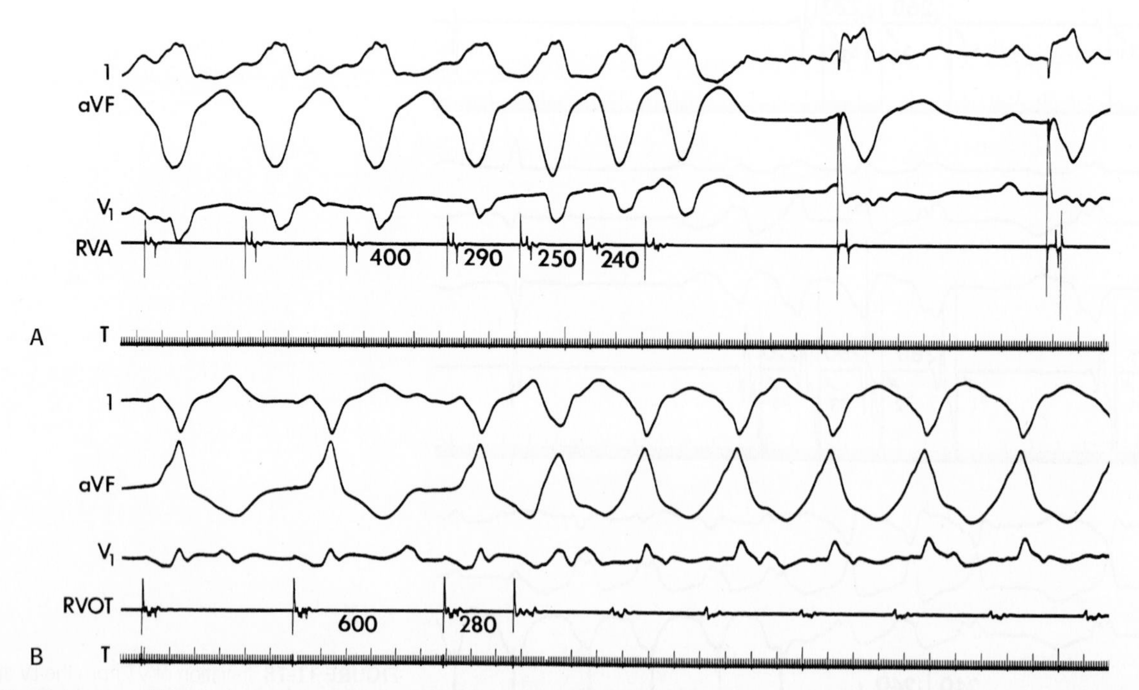


**FIGURE 11-80** Site specificity for induction of VT. **A:** Triple VES delivered from the RVA at a PCL of 400 msec fail to initiate the tachycardia. No form of stimulation from the RVA initiated sustained VT. **B:** However, a single VES stimulus delivered from the RVOT at a drive CL of 600 msec initiates a sustained uniform VT. This remarkable site specificity would not be characteristic of a triggered rhythm and demonstrates the need for a protocol using at least two right ventricular stimulation sites. See text for discussion.

### *Relationship of Initiation of VT to Conduction Delay, Block, and/or Continuous Activity*

Rhythms that are due to automaticity or triggered activity do not require associated conduction delay and/or block for initiation while classically, reentry requires conduction delay with or without the development of block, which may be present at baseline. As discussed earlier, evidence of conduction abnormalities is virtually universal in patients with cardiac disease (primarily coronary artery disease) during sinus rhythm, manifested by abnormal electrograms during endocardial mapping (see earlier discussion on Substrate), or positive SAECGs, in patients in whom inducible tachycardias are present. Theoretically, if reentry was the mechanism of the tachycardia, electrical activity should occur throughout the tachycardia cycle. Thus, during diastole, conduction must be extremely slow and in a small enough area such that it is not recorded on the surface ECG. The demonstration that initiation of the tachycardia depended on a critical degree of slow conduction, manifested by fragmented electrograms spanning diastole, and that maintenance of the tachycardia was associated with repetitive continuous activity, would be compatible with reentry.[197] The initiation of tachycardias associated with continuous activity was initially recorded in acute ischemic arrhythmias in an experimental canine model by Boineau and Cox[198] and Waldo and Kaiser[199] and subsequently by El-Sherif et al.[200] in a canine model of infarction with inducible sustained VT. We have found similar, continuous repetitive activity in local areas of the endocardium, which was required to initiate and maintain the tachycardia in humans in 5% of patients during catheter mapping[197] and in 10% of patients using intraoperative mapping. Although some have questioned continuous activity as potentially being due to motion artifact,[44,201,202] in vitro tissue studies[43,44] have shown that such fragmented electrograms are not due to motion artifact. In humans, Waxman and Sung[203] and Brugada et al.[204] claimed that continuous activity is not related to the tachycardia mechanism, but the examples that they proposed demonstrating continuous activity showed inconsistent electrograms lasting only two cardiac cycles. This clearly would not meet our definition of continuous activity, which is required to maintain the tachycardia. Electrical signals that come and go throughout diastole should not be considered continuous.

This is not to say that all fragmented electrical activity noted at the onset and during VT represents reentrant activity. Such activity may represent artifacts, dead-end pathways, or electrical activity otherwise unrelated to the genesis and maintenance of the tachycardia. For continuous activity to be consistent with reentry, the following must be demonstrated: (a) The initiation of VT depends on broadening of electrograms that span diastole, as in Figures 11-81 and 11-82. (b) The tachycardia maintenance depends on continuous activity, such that termination of the continuous activity, either spontaneously or following stimulation, without affecting the tachycardia would exclude such "continuous" activity as requisite for sustaining the tachycardia (Figs. 11-83 and 11-84). (c) Pacing at a cycle length comparable to VT does not produce a broadening of electrogram to span the cardiac cycle and appear continuous, that is, create an electrogram whose duration equals the PCL. (d) Motion artifact is excluded (this is easiest because such electrograms are recorded only in infarcted ventricle, and never from moving contractile normal ventricle. (e) The continuous activity is recorded from a circumscribed area (Figs. 11-81 to 11-84). (f) Finally, if possible, ablation of the area from which continuous activity is recorded will terminate the tachycardia. Thus, the mere presence of "continuous activity" at the onset and during VT does not automatically imply that this electrical activity is related to the genesis and maintenance of the tachycardia. One must stimulate during VT to prove that the presence of such electrical activity is requisite for the arrhythmia. Persistent changes in the repetitive continuous waveform produced by stimulation should be associated either with termination of the arrhythmia or with changing it to a different tachycardia. A change in the electrogram on the stimulated beat may reflect antidromic capture by the stimulated wavefront of part of the tissue from which the continuous activity is recorded. The tachycardia would either be reset or terminated if the electrical signals were recorded from the reentrant circuit (see subsequent discussion on Resetting and Entrainment).

Conduction delay that is not quite continuous can also be seen at initiation of tachycardia in an additional 5% of patients (Fig. 11-85). Conduction delays producing nearly continuous activity may critically depend on rate. They may only be seen when extrastimuli are delivered during a short-paced drive cycle length (Fig. 11-85) or during a burst of ventricular pacing (Fig. 11-86). If the recording electrode is not recording the entire circuit, one may see broadening of the electrogram such that the delayed late component becomes the early component during the tachycardia (Figs. 11-86 and 11-87). Proof that this late potential in fact becomes an early potential (as far as the tachycardia circuit is concerned) requires demonstration that this potential bears a fixed relationship to the subsequent QRS despite changes in cycle length observed spontaneously or during pacing. This is discussed further in the section regarding methods of localizing VT. It is imperative that such validation be attempted so that dead-end pathways, which are late and unrelated to the tachycardia, are not mistaken for early activity. Failure to demonstrate continuous activity in all cases suggests that the tachycardia circuit is larger than the recording area of the catheter and/or that the catheter is not covering the entire circuit. Because catheter and intraoperative mapping of VT associated with prior infarction suggests that most tachycardias exit a diastolic pathway 1 to 3 cm long and a few millimeters to 1 cm wide, with a circuit area probably in excess of 4 $cm^2$, failure to record continuous activity is not surprising (see later section on activation mapping during VT). Continuous activity, when observed, is always found at sites that demonstrate a markedly abnormal electrogram in sinus rhythm (Fig. 11-88; also see Figs. 11-81 to 11-84). Evidence supporting the significance of fractionated electrograms and continuous activity has been reviewed by Josephson and Wit.[43]

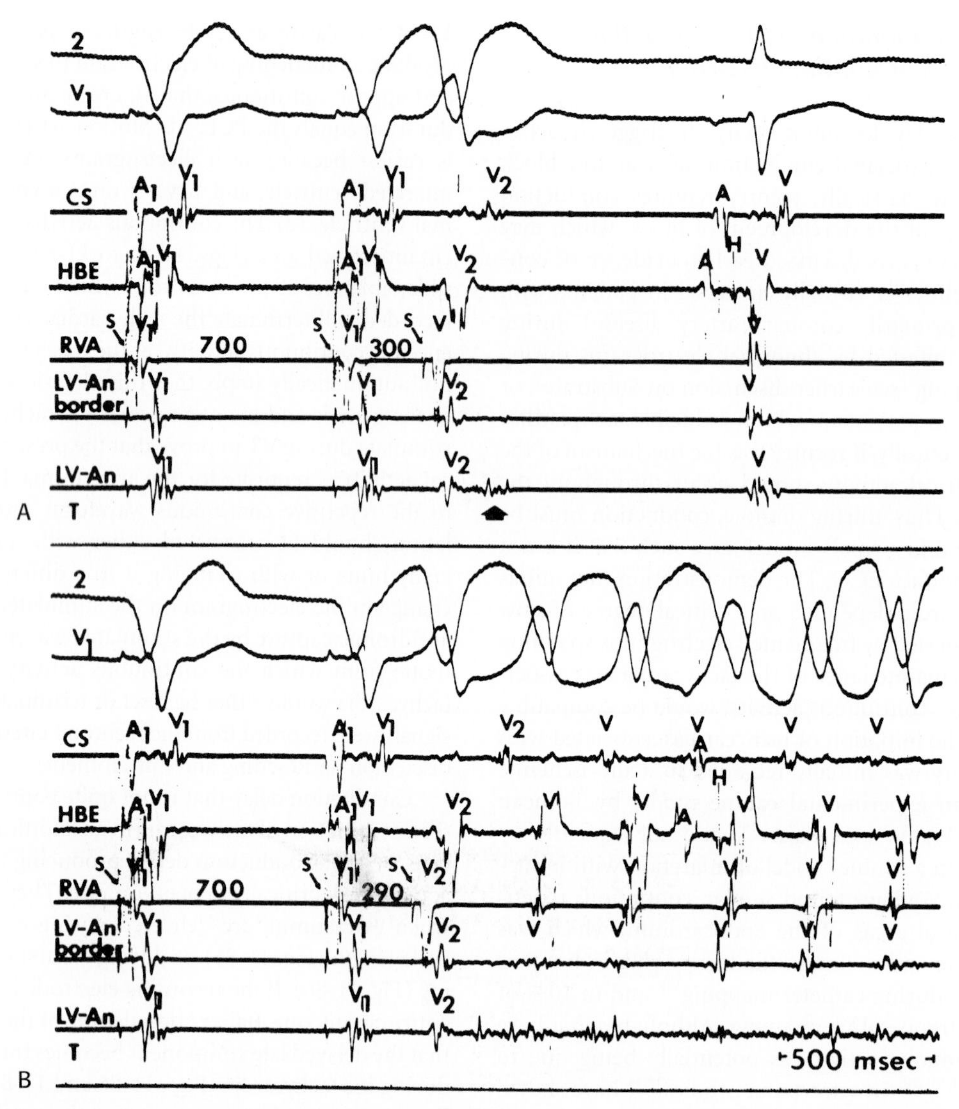


**FIGURE 11-81** Initiation of VT associated with the development of continuous activity in a patient with coronary artery disease. Surface leads 2 and $V_1$ are shown with electrograms from the CS, HBE, RVA, and at the border of left ventricular aneurysm (LV-An) and just inside the LV-An. **A** and **B:** Ventricular pacing is carried out from the RVA at a CL of 700 msec. **A:** A ventricular extrastimulus delivered at 300 msec produces marked prolongation of duration of the electrogram in the LV-An (*arrow*). This is not followed by VT. Note in the ensuing sinus complex that the electrogram recorded from the LV-An has multiple components, is of low amplitude, and long duration. **B:** When the coupling interval is reduced to 290 msec, $V_2$ in the LV-An is associated with prolonged continuous electrical activity, which spans diastole and is associated with initiation of VT. Note that during VT, continuous electrical activity remains in the electrogram from the LV-An, yet the electrogram recorded from a proximal pair of electrodes, 1 cm away, at the border of the LV-An, does not show continuous activity. See text for discussion.

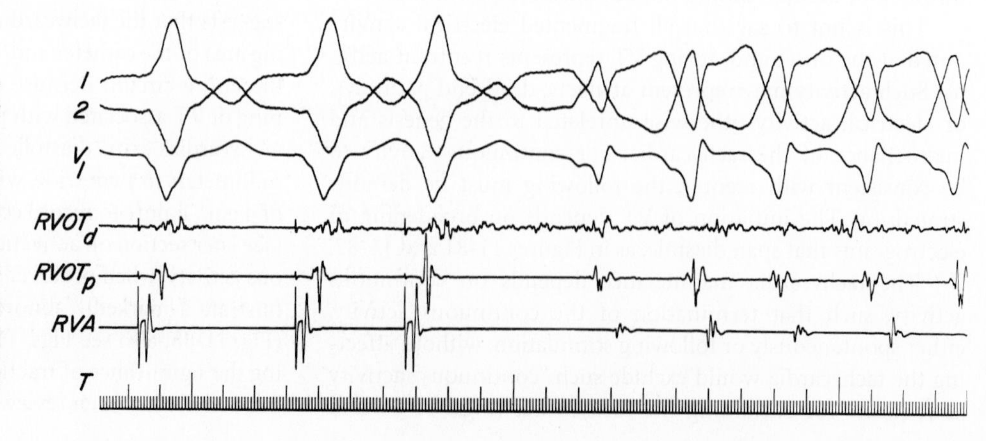


**FIGURE 11-82** Initiation of VT associated with continuous activity in a patient status post repair of tetralogy of Fallot. Three ECG leads and electrograms from the distal RVOT ($RVOT_d$) at the site of a prior infundibulotomy scar, the proximal RVOT ($RVOT_p$) and the RVA are shown. A single extrastimulus delivered from the RVA initiates VT. Note the initiation is associated with fragmentation and delay of the electrogram in the distal RVOT, which remains continuous during the tachycardia. See text for discussion.

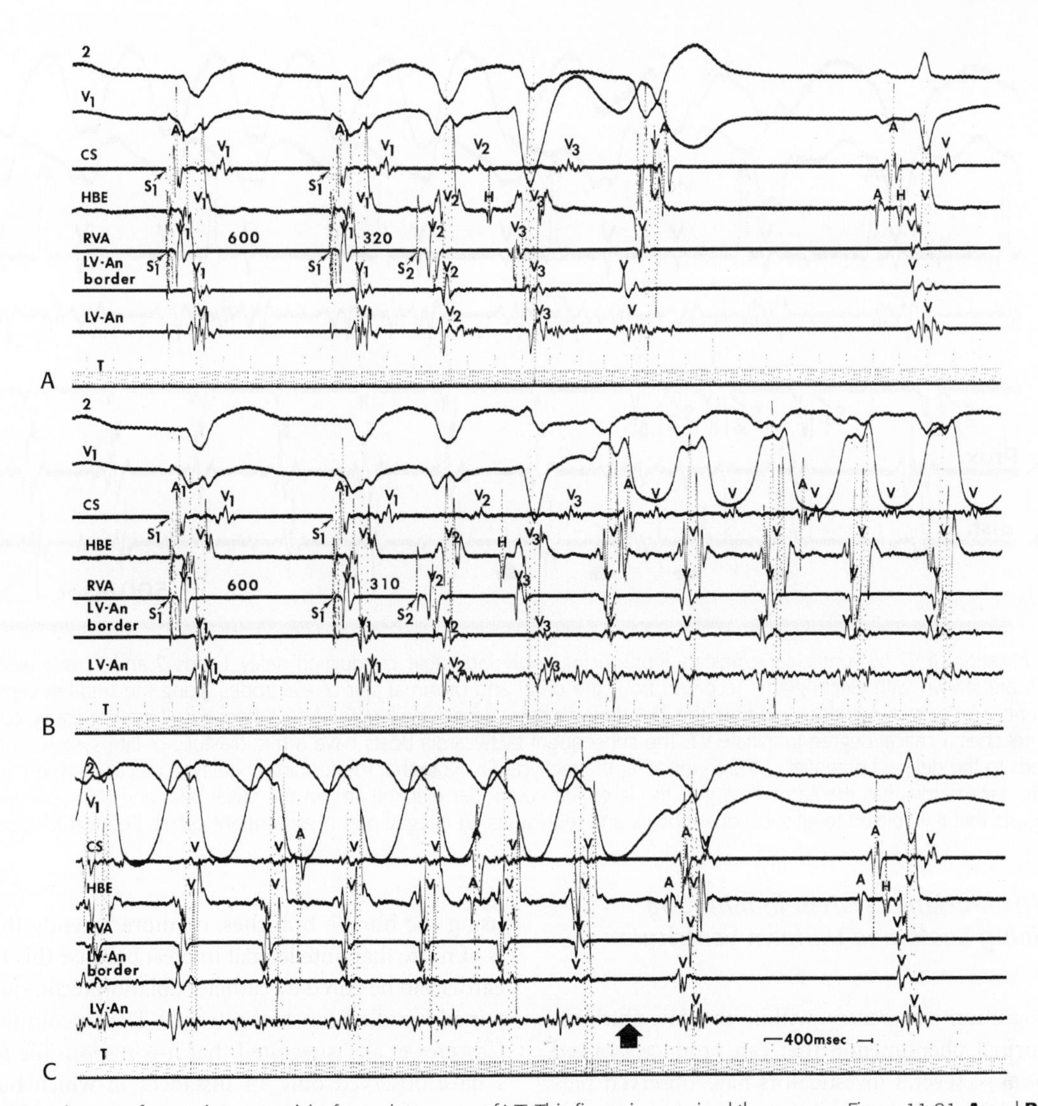

**FIGURE 11-83** Requirement for continuous activity for maintenance of VT. This figure is organized the same as Figure 11-81. **A** and **B:** Ventricular pacing and extrastimuli are delivered during a cycle length of 600 msec. **A:** An extrastimulus from the RVA at 320 msec initiates a bundle branch reentrant complex followed by a single repetitive response. **B:** When the coupling interval is reduced to 310 msec, continuous electrical activity is produced in the electrogram from the LV-An, and VT is initiated. **C:** When continuous activity stops (*broad arrow*), the tachycardia terminates. See text for discussion.

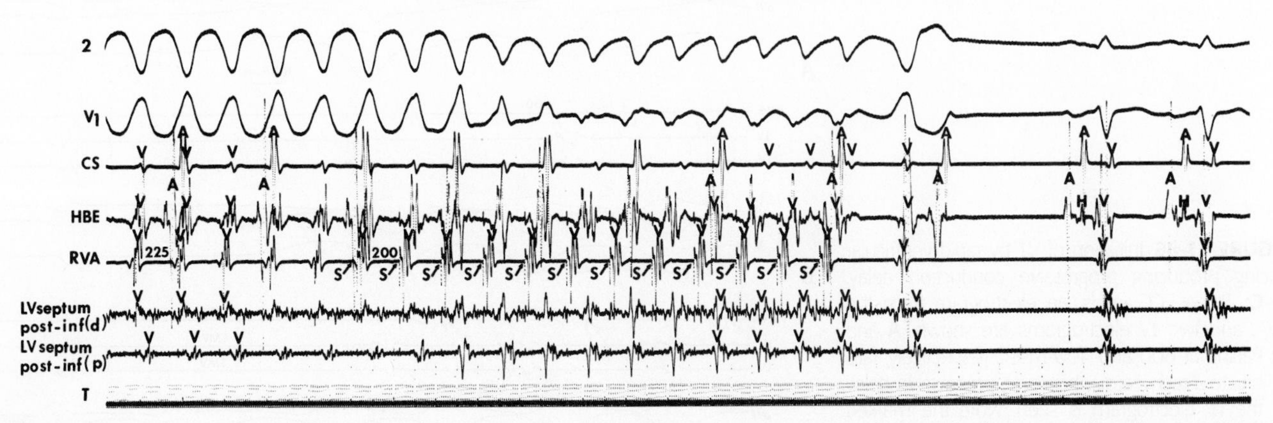

**FIGURE 11-84** Termination of VT with termination of continuous activity. Surface leads 2 and $V_1$ are shown with electrograms from the CS, HBE, RVA, and electrograms along the posterior-inferior left ventricular septum from the distal pair (d) and proximal (p) pair of electrodes on the same catheter. Continuous electrical activity is observed during VT in the distal LV septal electrogram. Following a burst of ventricular pacing at 200 msec, continuous activity is disrupted and tachycardia terminates. Note the flat baseline following termination. The electrogram from the distal LV is markedly abnormal, with multiple components, long duration, and low amplitude during the two sinus beats that follow termination of the tachycardia. See text for discussion. (From Josephson ME, Horowitz LN, Farshidi A. Continuous local electrical activity: a mechanism of recurrent ventricular tachycardia. *Circulation* 1978;57:659.)

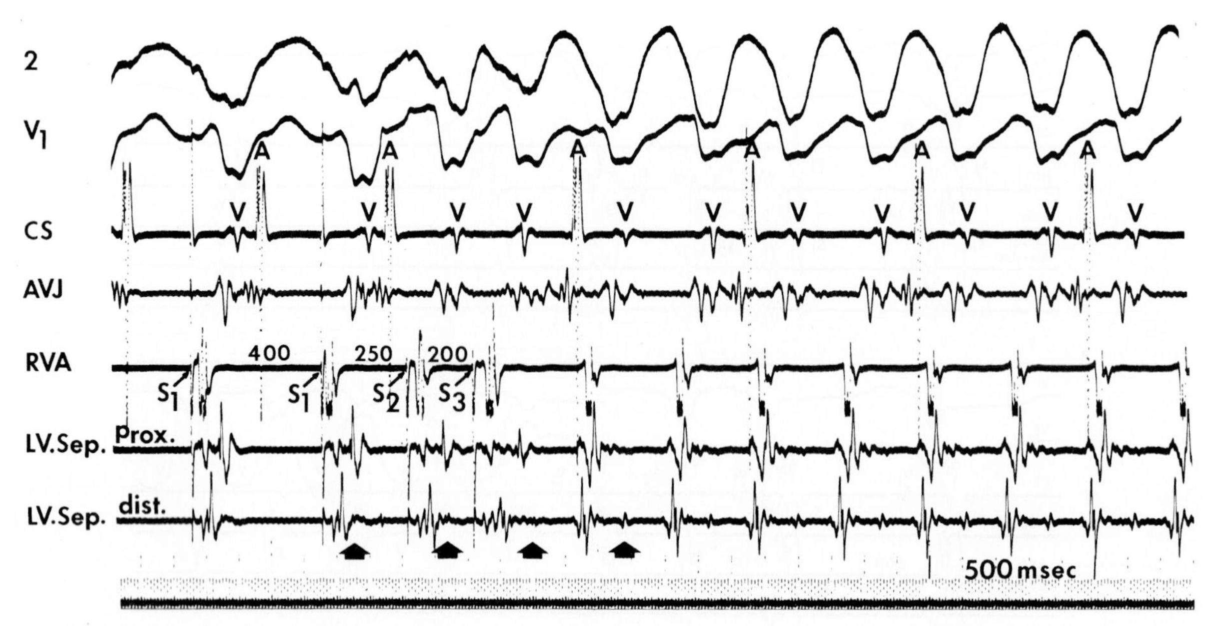


**FIGURE 11-85** Initiation of VT by ventricular extrastimuli producing nonholodiastolic conduction delay. Leads 2 and $V_1$ and electrograms from CS, AVJ, and RVA are shown with electrograms recorded from the distal and proximal pair of electrodes along the mid-left ventricular septum (LV Sep.). Two ventricular extrastimuli delivered from the RVA during a basic drive cycle length of 400 msec result in progressive conduction delay (*arrows*), which reaches a critical degree to initiate VT. The subsequent tachycardia beats have a mid-diastolic or late systolic potential (*arrow*), which corresponds to the delayed potential of the $S_3$ initiating the tachycardia. Note that the terminally delayed electrogram on $S_3$ (*third arrow*), which initiates the tachycardia, has the same timing to the large left ventricular electrogram on the initial beat and on subsequent beats. This relationship suggests that it is related to all subsequent beats and represents an integral part of a reentrant circuit. See text for discussion.

### *Role of the His–Purkinje System in Initiating and Maintaining Sustained Uniform Ventricular Tachycardia*

Since the recognition of reentry within the His–Purkinje system as a normal phenomenon that can produce isolated repetitive responses, several investigators have observed persistent His–Purkinje reentry try as a form of macroreentrant VT.[18,19,205] The demonstration of a macroreentrant circuit using the bundle branches, or more recently the fascicles,[206] is of more than intellectual interest because this type of tachycardia can be cured by catheter ablation techniques.[205–208] Sustained bundle branch reentrant VT is uncommon. Although Casceres et al.[19] suggested that it is responsible for 6% of VT, I have observed only 14 instances in which bundle branch reentry was the ***sole*** inducible, and presumed clinical, monomorphic VT out of approximately 1650 consecutively studied

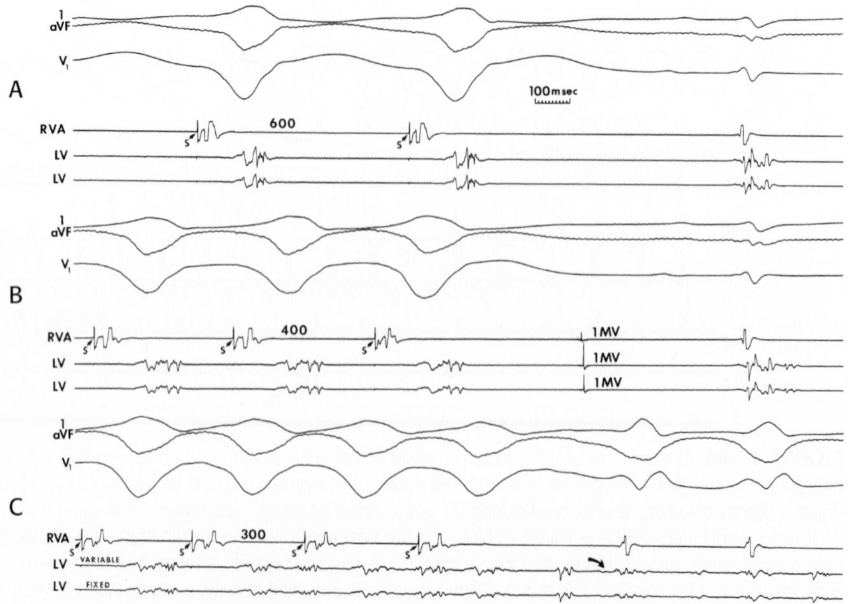


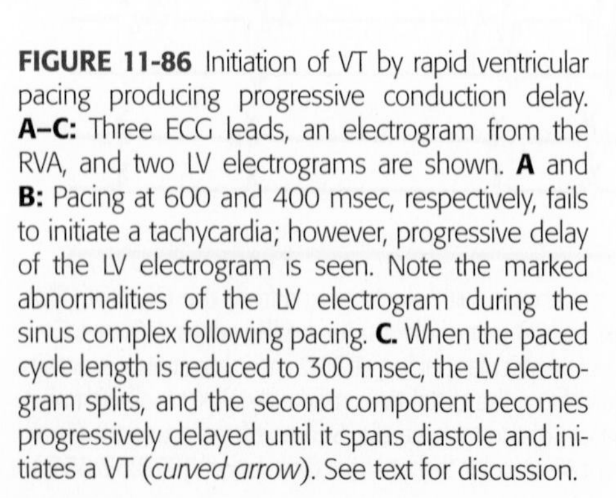
**FIGURE 11-86** Initiation of VT by rapid ventricular pacing producing progressive conduction delay. **A–C:** Three ECG leads, an electrogram from the RVA, and two LV electrograms are shown. **A** and **B:** Pacing at 600 and 400 msec, respectively, fails to initiate a tachycardia; however, progressive delay of the LV electrogram is seen. Note the marked abnormalities of the LV electrogram during the sinus complex following pacing. **C.** When the paced cycle length is reduced to 300 msec, the LV electrogram splits, and the second component becomes progressively delayed until it spans diastole and initiates a VT (*curved arrow*). See text for discussion.

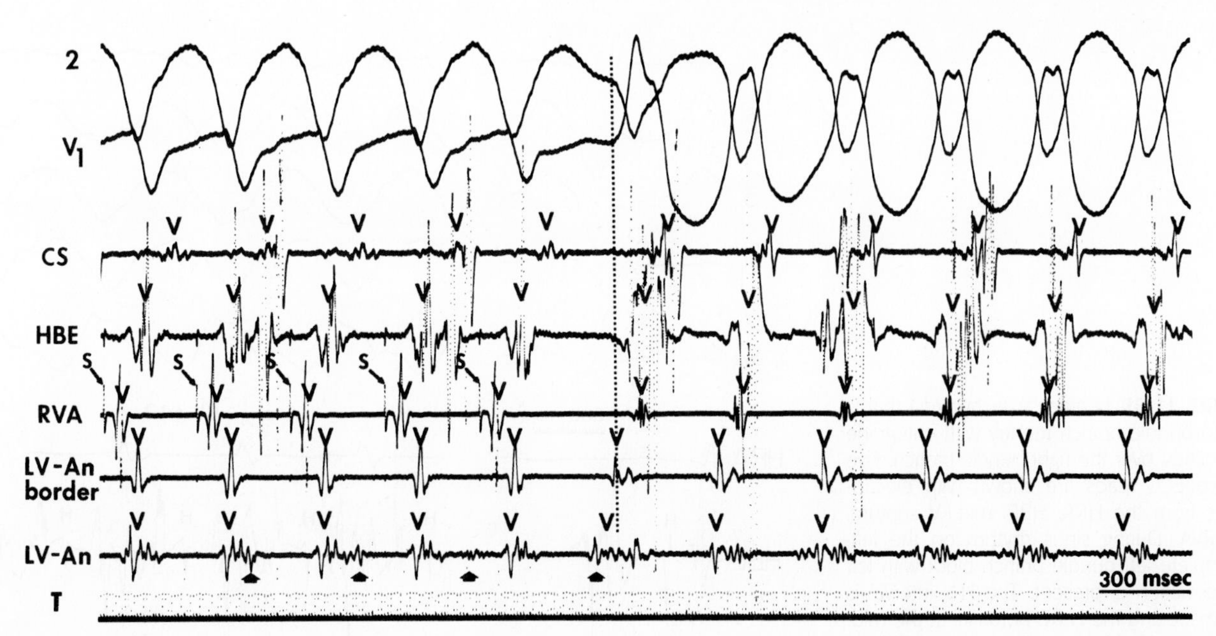


**FIGURE 11-87** Ventricular tachycardia induced by ventricular pacing associated with local left ventricular conduction delay. This figure is organized identically to Figures 11-81 and 11-88. The catheter, however, has moved slightly. During ventricular pacing from the RVA at 300 msec, progressive fractionation and conduction delay in the LV-An recording (*broad arrows*) result in initiation of VT. See text for discussion. (From Josephson ME, Horowitz LN, Farshidi A. Continuous local electrical activity: a mechanism of recurrent ventricular tachycardia. *Circulation* 1978;57:659.)

cases. None of our 14 cases had a prior infarction: 10 had cardiomyopathy, 2 had aortic valve disease, and 2 had myotonic dystrophy. All but 2 of our patients and the vast majority reported in the literature[18,19,205–207] had either complete or incomplete LBBB pattern and H-V intervals ≥65 msec in sinus rhythm. They all had bundle branch reentry with an LBBB pattern (see Chapter 2; Fig. 11-89). Two patients had incomplete RBBB, and had bundle branch reentry with a RBBB pattern. In contrast, in patients with prior infarction (virtually always a large anterior infarction complicated by bifascicular block) interfascicular reentry (using anterior and posterior fascicle) is the only macroreentrant rhythm observed requiring the His–Purkinje system (see Chapter 2). Moreover, I have never seen interfascicular reentry as the sole arrhythmia in these patients; they invariably have multiple intramyocardial VTs as well. I have never seen bundle branch reentry using the right and left bundle branches in this patient population. This is consistent with our observation that when RBBB occurs and persists following anteroseptal infarction, complete bidirectional RBBB is present. Interfascicular reentry may also be seen in

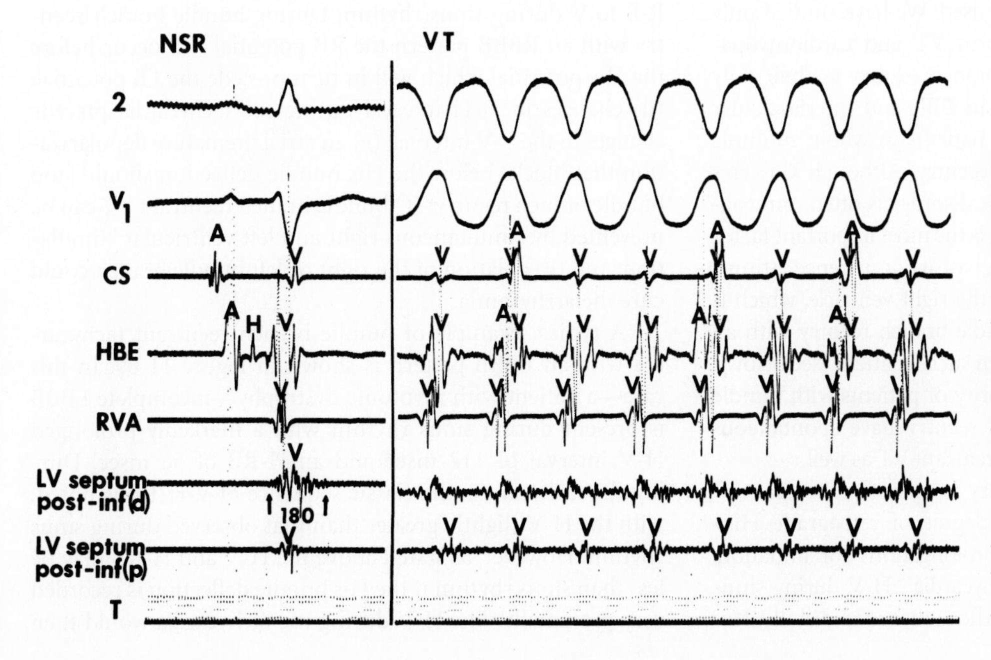


**FIGURE 11-88** Relationship of electrogram demonstrating continuous activity during VT to sinus rhythm. This figure is organized the same as Figure 11-76. During VT on the right, continuous electrical activity is present in the distal posteroinferior septal recording. During sinus rhythm on the left, the same electrogram demonstrates a multicomponent low-amplitude signal, 180 msec in duration, which extends well beyond the end of the QRS. Such abnormal electrograms are typical of sites from which continuous electrical activity is observed. (From Josephson ME, Horowitz LN, Farshidi A. Continuous local electrical activity: a mechanism of recurrent ventricular tachycardia. *Circulation* 1978;57:659.)

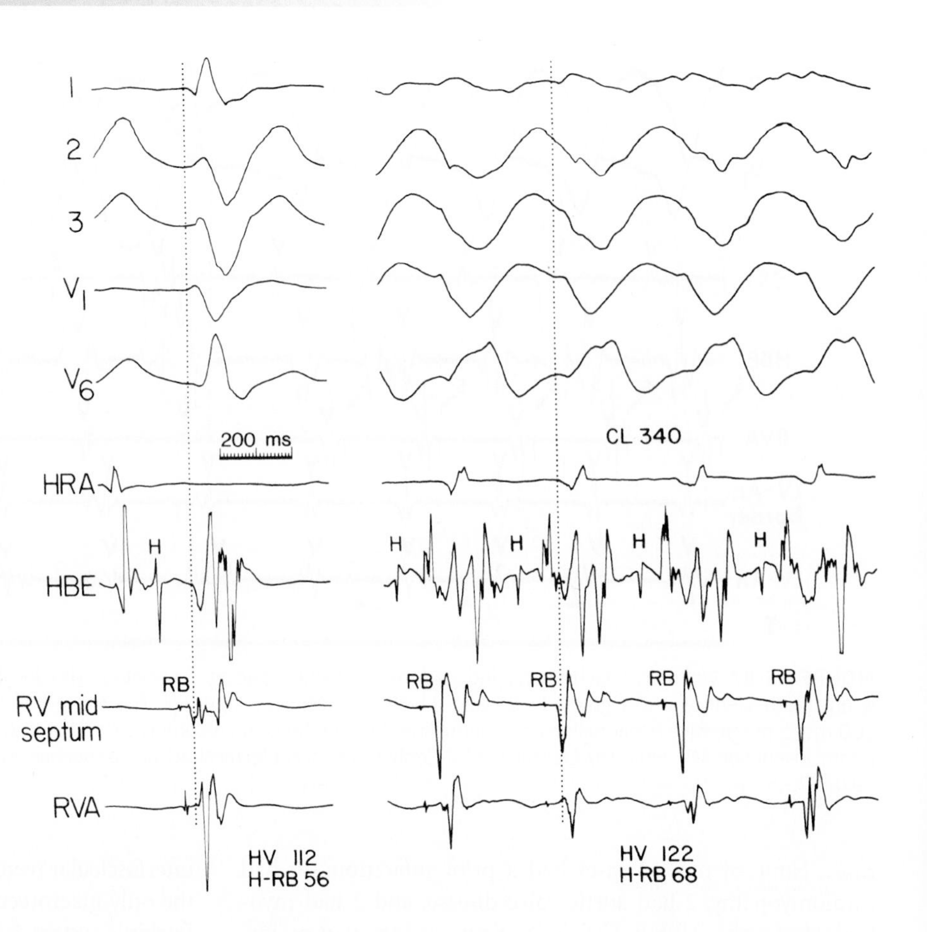


**FIGURE 11-89** Ventricular tachycardia that is due to bundle branch reentry with antegrade conduction over the right bundle branch. Five surface ECG leads are shown with electrograms from the HRA, HBE, mid-RV septum, and RVA. During sinus rhythm on the left, incomplete left bundle branch block with left axis deviation is present. The H-V interval is 112 msec and the H-RB potential at the mid-septum is 56 msec. A distal RB potential is observed in the RVA electrogram. During VT, the HV is slightly prolonged to 122 msec and the His precedes the RB by 68 msec. The RB also precedes the distal RB recording in the RVA, as in sinus rhythm. Note the presence of 1:1 retrograde conduction. The VT has a left bundle branch block left axis deviation configuration. See text for discussion.

patients without infarction, including patients with bifascicular block due to degenerative disease of the conducting system. I have seen 2 patients with both BBR with an LBBB pattern and interfascicular reentry. During their BBR a changing axis was observed. In both cases, interfascicular reentry occurred after ablation of the RBB (Fig. 11-90A–C). Our failure to observe a higher incidence of sustained bundle branch reentry may be directly related to the patient population studied and, to a lesser degree, to the stimulation protocol used. We have studied only 112 patients with sustained uniform VT and cardiomyopathy, only 8 of whom had bundle branch reentry as their only arrhythmia and an additional 2 had BBR and interfascicular reentry. I have seen another seven patients in whom multiple VTs accompanied bundle branch reentry. Although Casceres et al.[19] suggest, and I agree, that this disorder is often unrecognized, I think the patient population is the most important factor in trying to determine the frequency of its occurrence. Stimulation is generally performed from the right ventricle, which is much less likely to give rise to bundle branch reentry with an RBBB pattern, although we have seen such a patient (see below). Moreover, as noted above the majority of patients with bundle branch reentry and interfascicular reentry have spontaneous and/or inducible intramyocardial reentrant VT as well.

To prove bundle branch reentry is operative, several criteria should be met: (a) critical degree of retrograde His–Purkinje conduction delay (V-H prolongation) for initiation; (b) an H-V interval during the tachycardia ≥H-V during sinus rhythm can be seen if the His bundle is recorded distally. It is also possible to see a shorter H-V interval during the tachycardia than sinus rhythm if a very proximal His bundle (far from the turnaround site) is recorded; (c) during bundle branch reentry with an LBBB pattern, the His deflection occurs before the right bundle deflection (the H-RB during VT can be greater or less than the H-RB in sinus rhythm, depending on the recording site of the His bundle relative to the turnaround site). The RB to V should be greater than or equal to the R-B to V during sinus rhythm. During bundle branch reentry with an RBBB pattern the RB potential will occur before the His potential which will in turn precede the LB potential; (d) changes in H-H interval during the tachycardia precede changes in the V-V interval; (e) an atrial premature depolarization that blocks below the His bundle deflection should stop bundle branch reentry; (f) bundle branch reentrant VT can be prevented by simultaneous right and left ventricular stimulation; and (g) ablation of the right or left bundle branch could cure the arrhythmia.

A typical example of bundle branch reentrant tachycardia with an LBBB pattern is shown in Figure 11-89. In this case—a patient with myotonic dystrophy—incomplete LBBB is present during sinus rhythm with a markedly prolonged H-V interval of 112 msec and an H-RB of 56 msec. During the tachycardia, the classic sequence of V-H-RB is noted, with the H-V slightly greater than that observed during sinus rhythm. However, as stated above the H-V and H-RB may be less than sinus rhythm if the His bundle deflection is recorded very proximally. The H-V during the tachycardia would then

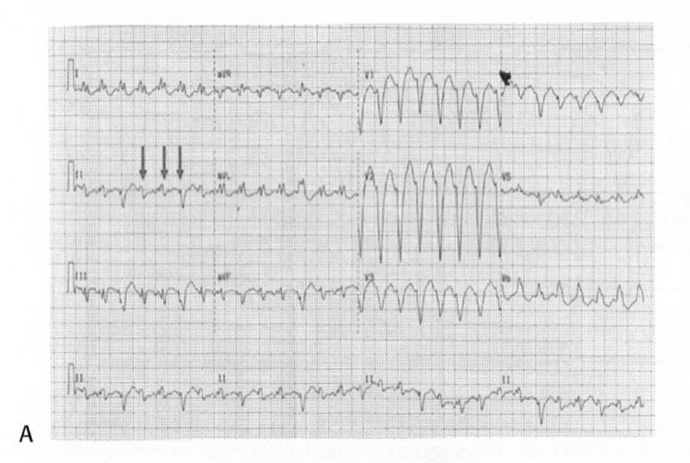

A

During Ablation

B

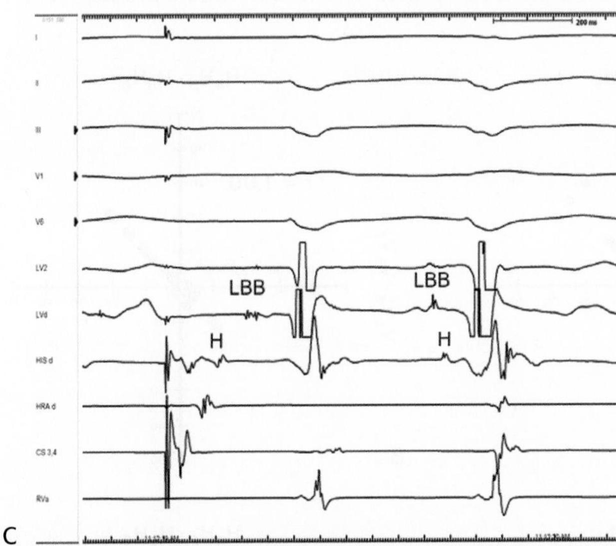


C

**FIGURE 11-90** Intrafascicular reentry and bundle branch reentry in the same patient. **A:** A 12-lead ECG showing VT with a typical LBBB morphology but a changing axis consistent with Wenckebach in the left anterior fascicle. **B:** During ablation of the RBB, marked left axis deviation and RBBB appear. **C:** Pacing the CS initiates intrafascicular reentry which is characterized by an RBBBB/LAH morphology (the same as in **B**) and reversal of the His and LBB potential. See text for explanation.

represent the difference between retrograde conduction to the proximal His bundle and antegrade conduction to the right bundle. I have not seen an H-V in VT more than 15 msec shorter than sinus in either a single bundle branch reentrant complex or sustained bundle branch reentry. A much shorter H-V during tachycardia than sinus rhythm is the rule in interfascicular reentry (see below).

Unfortunately, right and/or left bundle branch potentials are not always recorded so that the typical activation sequences (LB-H-RB-V or RB-H-LB-V) are not available for analysis. As noted earlier in the chapter, even if either sequence is present, the His–Purkinje system (usually, the left bundle branch) could be activated passively in the retrograde fashion to produce a His-RB-V sequence during a tachycardia with an LBBB pattern without reentry requiring the bundle branches. This was pointed out earlier in the chapter, in Figure 11-12, in which a wide-complex tachycardia with left bundle and left axis deviation was induced by ventricular stimulation and V-H prolongation, with an H-V interval during the tachycardia greater than that during sinus rhythm. This tachycardia, although meeting initiation criteria and H-V interval criteria, was not due to bundle branch reentry because left ventricular mapping demonstrated earliest activity at the apex of the left ventricle. For documentation of bundle branch reentry using the right bundle branch antegradely and the left bundle branch retrogradely, right ventricular excitation must precede the left ventricular excitation. If left ventricular mapping cannot be done, other critical and essential elements for the diagnosis of bundle branch reentry must be tested. The most important of these is the demonstration that changes in the H-H and RB-RB and/or LB-LB interval during the tachycardia precede changes in the V-V interval. These changes can be initiated by ventricular stimulation during the tachycardia or may occur spontaneously following initiation. This observation, shown in Figure 11-91, is essential in proving that a macroreentrant circuit using the proximal His–Purkinje system is operative. Casceres et al.[19] have shown this elegantly by linear regression analysis (Fig. 11-92). As stated earlier, the vast majority of bundle branch reentrant tachycardias have had LBBB morphology and have used the left bundle conducting system retrogradely and the right bundle branch system antegradely. Although the reverse situation—an RBBB reentrant tachycardia (using left bundle system antegradely and right bundle branch system retrogradely)—has been reported, the same criteria used for typical bundle branch reentry are more difficult to document without obtaining an LB recording. Although the RB-H-V sequence may be noted, this may be a passive phenomenon. Tachycardia oscillations with V-V intervals dependent on prior RB-H intervals should be looked for, but are difficult to see because the RB is usually activated during the QRS. Thus, an LB potential is mandatory to confirm the diagnosis. It is of interest that of the cases reported to be bundle branch reentry with an RBBB pattern, an incomplete RBBB with a long H-V was seen during sinus rhythm. This was the case in one of the two right bundle branch reentrant VT I have seen (Figs. 11-93 and 11-94).

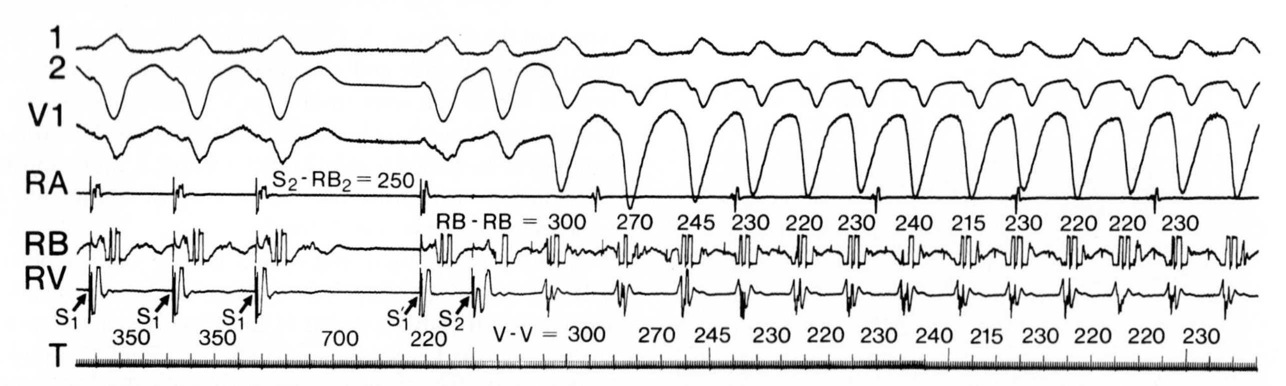


**FIGURE 11-91** Relationship of VT CL to changes in His–Purkinje activation. Three surface ECG leads and electrograms from the right atrium (RA), the right bundle (RB), and the RV are shown. A short-long-short sequence (350, 700, 220) initiates VT. RB potentials can be seen before each QRS. Note that the change in RB-RB intervals precedes an identical change in V-V intervals. This suggests a causal relationship of the RV potential to the subsequent QRS. See text for discussion. (From Casceres J, Jazayeri M, McKinnie J, et al. Sustained bundle branch reentry as a mechanism of clinical tachycardia. *Circulation* 1989;79:256.)

Why is bundle branch reentrant VT as rare as an isolated form of VT if single bundle branch reentrant complexes can be seen in 50% of normal patients?[18,205,209] The reason lies in the underlying substrate of conduction delay in the left or right bundle branch system. True complete bundle branch block of either type would make bundle branch reentry impossible. Therefore, conduction delay, manifested by H-V prolongation, but not true block must be present in both the left and right bundle systems for typical bundle branch reentry to occur. Although the mode of induction of bundle branch reentry usually is by single extrastimuli, Casceres et al.[19] have reported that sudden short-to-long change in cycle length before the introduction of extrastimuli facilitates induction of bundle branch reentry. This is related to the previously demonstrated effect of altered cycle length on His–Purkinje refractoriness.[151]

Bundle branch reentry not infrequently is observed at the initiation of monomorphic intramyocardial VT but is not necessary either to initiate or maintain the tachycardia). This can be proven by the demonstration that the tachycardia can be initiated with or without bundle branch reentry

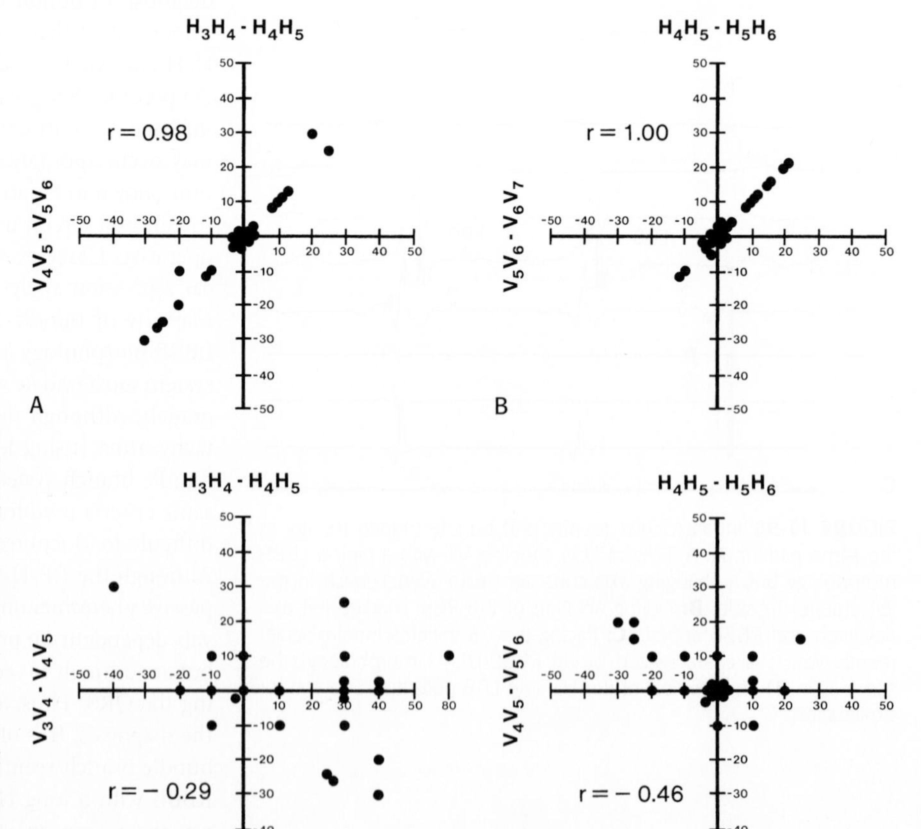


**FIGURE 11-92** Linear regression analysis of H-H and V-V intervals. **A:** The $H_3H_4$–$H_4H_5$ intervals are plotted against the subsequent V-V intervals ($V_4V_5$-$V_5V_6$) and a linear result is observed. **B:** The same finding is shown if $H_4H_5$–$H_5H_6$ is plotted against $V_5V_6$–$V_6V_7$. This suggests a causal relationship of the H to the subsequent V. **C** and **D:** Analysis of the preceding V-V intervals to the subsequent H-H intervals (i.e., to assess whether the V-V interval was causally related to the H-H interval) shows no relationship. This analysis confirms a causal role of the His–Purkinje system in the development of this tachycardia. See text for discussion. (From Casceres J, Jazayeri M, McKinnie J, et al. Sustained bundle branch reentry as a mechanism of clinical tachycardia. *Circulation* 1989;79:256.)

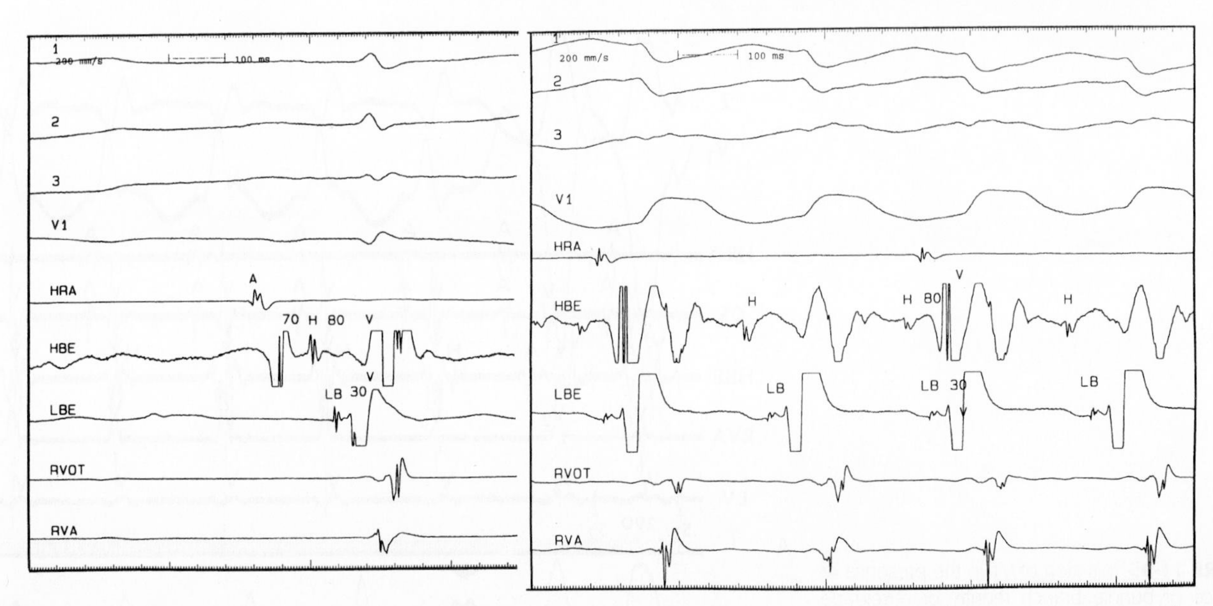


**FIGURE 11-93** Bundle branch reentry with antegrade conduction over the left bundle branch. Surface ECG leads 1, 2, 3, and $V_1$ are shown with electrograms from the HRA, HBE, left bundle branch (LBE), RVOT, and RVA. On the left is a sinus beat. The HV is 80 msec and LB-V is 30 msec. Incomplete RBBB is present. On the right bundle branch reentry with a complete RBBB pattern is shown. Note that the HV and LB-V are identical to that seen in sinus rhythm. See text for discussion.

(Fig. 11-95) and the failure to demonstrate His deflections with a normal or greater than normal H-V interval or a dependence of VT cycle length on prior H-H intervals.

Because His bundle deflections may be observed in approximately 80% of VTs,[16] does this imply that the fascicles are an integral component of the tachycardia circuit? I believe that in patients who have diseased hearts incorporation of a fascicle in the tachycardia circuit is not necessary to explain the presence of a His deflection before or just following the onset of the QRS. The lack of requirement for the more proximal His–Purkinje system has been demonstrated by intermittent His deflections (Fig. 11-96). These are typically in a 2:1 fashion but may also be seen in a 3:2 pattern or, less commonly, in a Wenckebach periodicity (Fig. 11-97). In patients with chronic coronary disease, the relative timing of the retrograde His deflection in the QRS depends on how

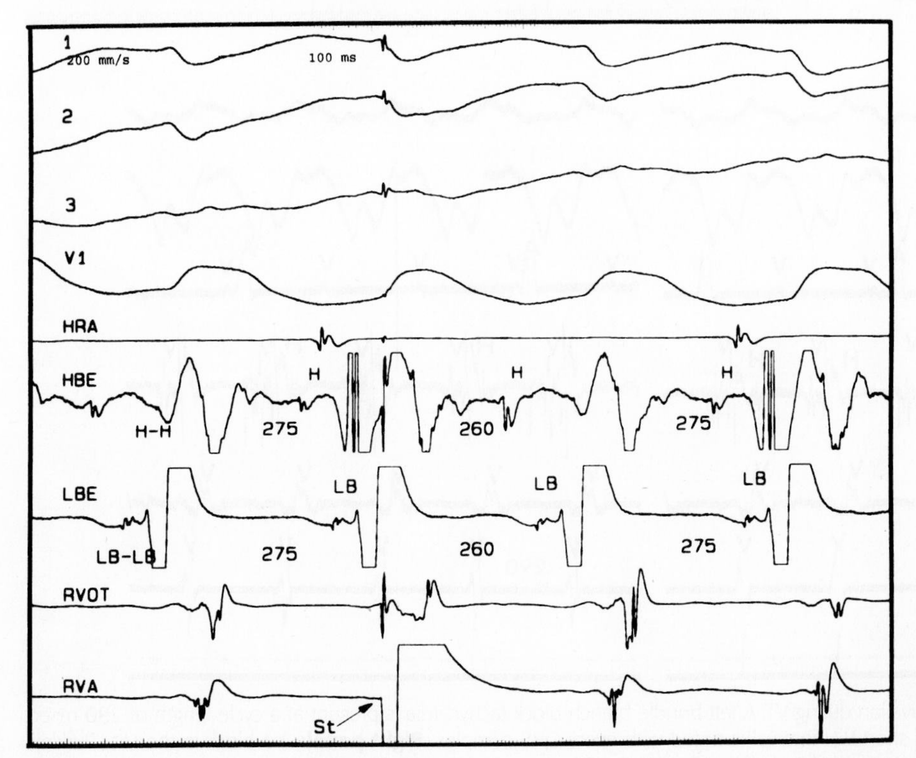


**FIGURE 11-94** Proof of bundle branch reentry. This is the same patient as in Figure 11-93. During the tachycardia a VPC is delivered from the RVA. This VPC advances the subsequent H, LB, and V without altering their relationship confirming role of the His–Purkinje system in the tachycardia. See text for discussion.

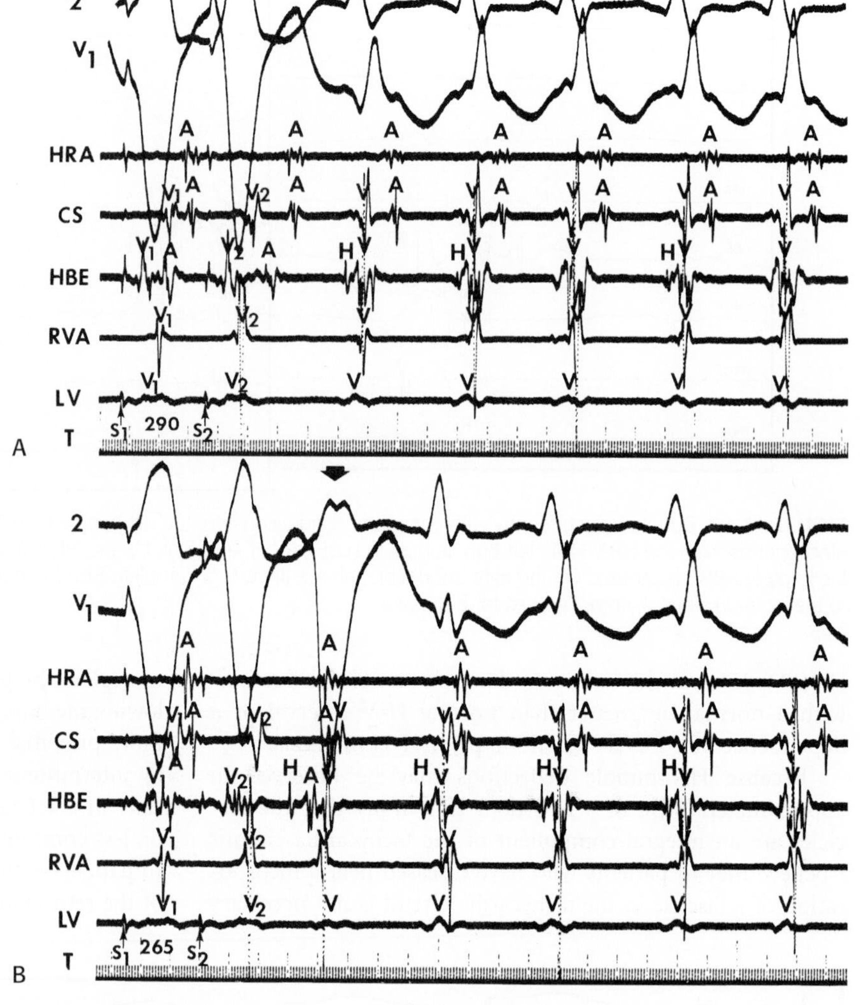


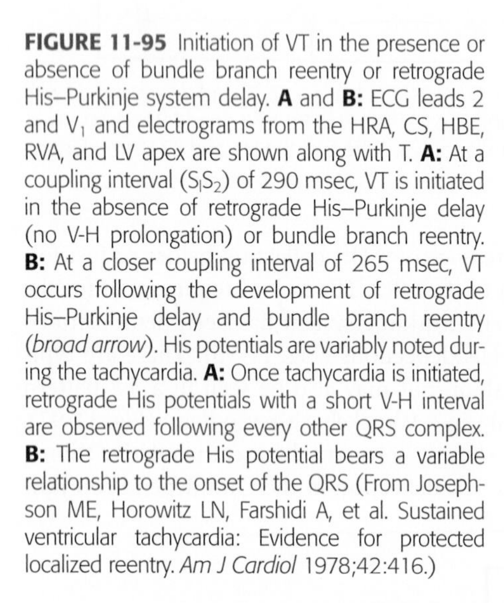

**FIGURE 11-95** Initiation of VT in the presence or absence of bundle branch reentry or retrograde His–Purkinje system delay. **A** and **B:** ECG leads 2 and $V_1$ and electrograms from the HRA, CS, HBE, RVA, and LV apex are shown along with T. **A:** At a coupling interval ($S_1S_2$) of 290 msec, VT is initiated in the absence of retrograde His–Purkinje delay (no V-H prolongation) or bundle branch reentry. **B:** At a closer coupling interval of 265 msec, VT occurs following the development of retrograde His–Purkinje delay and bundle branch reentry (*broad arrow*). His potentials are variably noted during the tachycardia. **A:** Once tachycardia is initiated, retrograde His potentials with a short V-H interval are observed following every other QRS complex. **B:** The retrograde His potential bears a variable relationship to the onset of the QRS (From Josephson ME, Horowitz LN, Farshidi A, et al. Sustained ventricular tachycardia: Evidence for protected localized reentry. *Am J Cardiol* 1978;42:416.)

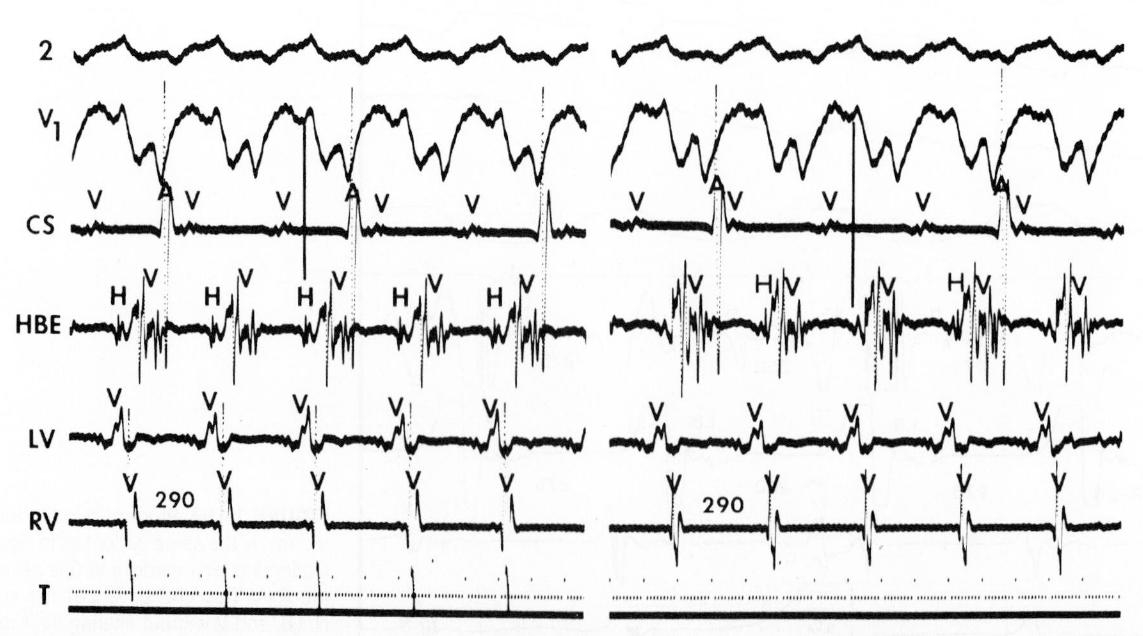


**FIGURE 11-96** Relationship of His bundle activation during VT. A left bundle branch block tachycardia is present at a cycle length of 290 msec. **Left panel:** A retrograde His deflection with a short V-H interval is noted with every QRS complex. **Right panel:** 2:1 block in the His–Purkinje system is observed; that is, a His deflection is seen, associated with every other QRS.

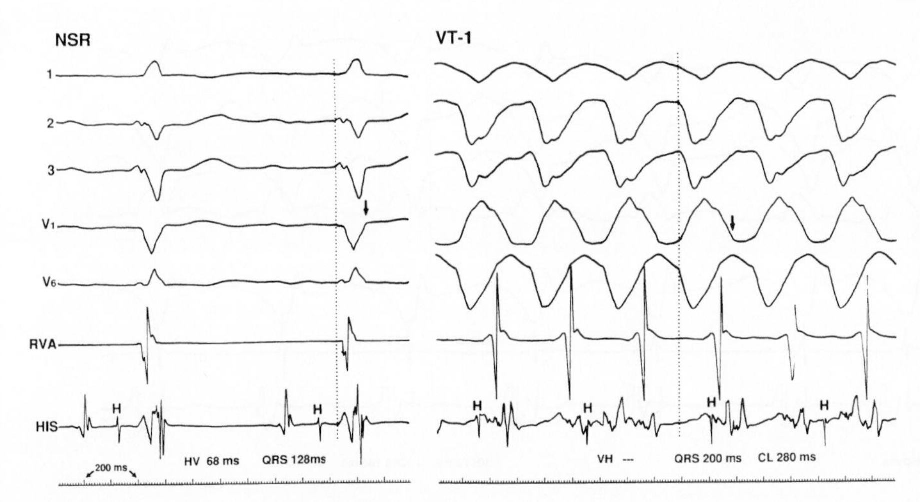


**FIGURE 11-97** Retrograde Wenckebach periodicity in the His–Purkinje system during VT. During sinus rhythm (NSR), an incomplete left bundle branch block pattern is seen. The H-V interval is prolonged at 68 msec. During induced VT (VT-l), retrograde His–Purkinje Wenckebach is seen. The V-H interval in the first three QRS complexes demonstrates prolongation, then block, thereby demonstrating 3:2 Wenckebach in the His–Purkinje system. The beat following the block in the His–Purkinje system (*vertical dotted line*) restarts the sequence.

quickly the His–Purkinje system is engaged and how slowly the impulse reaches the ventricular myocardium to begin to produce the QRS. Thus, retrograde His potentials can actually precede the QRS or follow it. The retrograde His deflection appears to reflect passive activation of the His–Purkinje system and not involvement of the His–Purkinje system in the reentrant circuit. The bases for this conclusion are threefold: (a) His–Purkinje deflections may appear intermittently, as noted. (b) The changing V-H interval can occur without a change in cycle length (Fig. 11-98). If the His–Purkinje system were involved, a change in V-H interval should be mirrored by a change in tachycardia cycle length. (c) Marked changes in tachycardia cycle length can be present with no change in V-H interval (Fig. 11-99). These data suggest two things. First, the His–Purkinje system is passively activated in VT associated with coronary artery disease and is not related to the reentrant circuit per se. Second, engagement of the His–Purkinje system allows for more rapid activation of the myocardium, which in turn results in a narrower QRS. Our data analyzing the relationship between the V-H interval and QRS duration in VTs of similar morphology in the same patient demonstrate a direct relationship between the V-H interval and the QRS (Fig. 11-100).[16] Thus, the His–Purkinje system is important for global ventricular activation, but at least the more

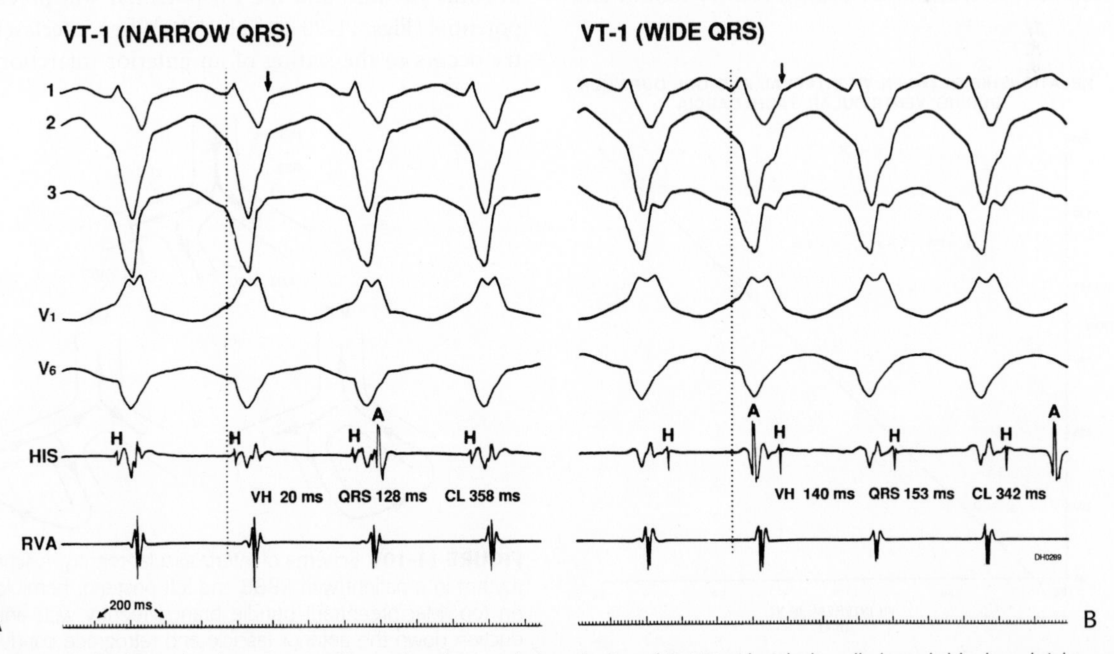


**FIGURE 11-98** Lack of relationship between V-H interval and VT cycle length. **A** and **B:** VT with right bundle branch block and right superior axis is shown. **A:** The V-T1 is relatively narrow (QRS = 128 msec). **B:** The QRS morphology is identical, but the QRS is wider, at 153 msec. In the panel on the left (**A**, the narrow QRS VT), the V-H interval is 20 msec, and the tachycardia cycle length is 358 msec. In the panel on the right (**B**, the wide QRS), the V-H interval is 140 msec, and the tachycardia cycle length is slightly shorter, at 342 msec. The prolongation in V-H conduction is therefore unrelated to the tachycardia cycle length. This confirms a lack of participation of the His–Purkinje system in the tachycardia mechanism. See text for discussion.

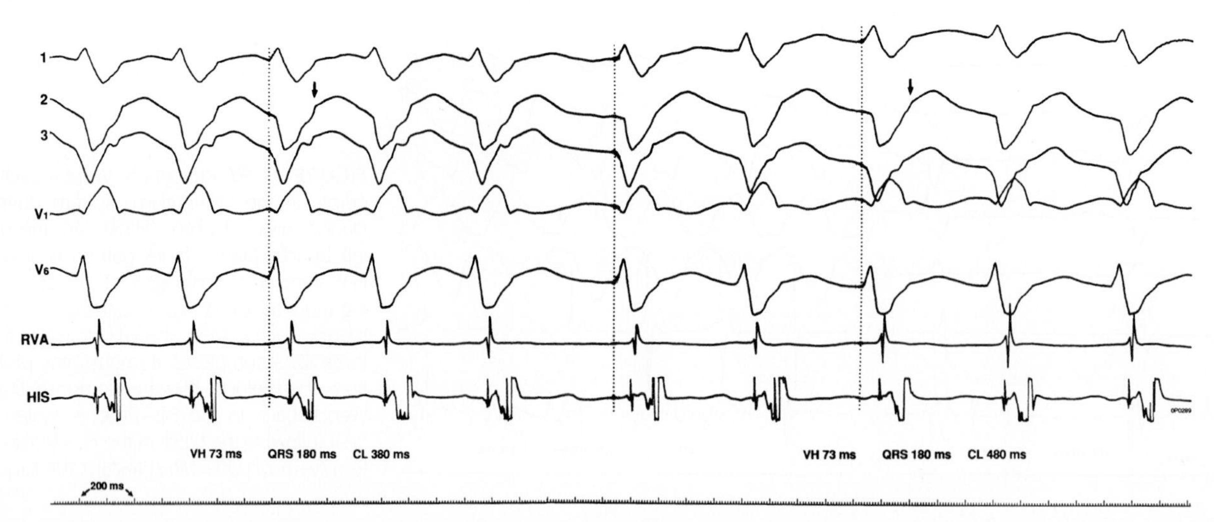


**FIGURE 11-99** Change in cycle length of VT without a change in retrograde His–Purkinje activation. VT is present with a right bundle right superior axis morphology. **Left:** The tachycardia CL is 380 msec and is associated with a QRS of 180 msec and a V-H interval of 73 msec. **Middle:** Tachycardia cycle length suddenly prolongs to 480 msec without any change in the QRS duration or V-H interval. The failure of tachycardia cycle length changes to be associated with changes in V-H interval suggests lack of involvement of the His–Purkinje system in the tachycardia mechanism. See text for discussion.

proximal areas do not seem to participate in the tachycardia mechanism. Whether the same is true in patients with normal ventricles and sustained VT has not been evaluated.

VT due to interfascicular reentry, in contrast to bundle branch reentry, is most commonly seen in patients with coronary artery disease, specifically those with an anterior infarction and either left anterior or posterior hemiblock. A schema is shown in Figure 11-101. In these patients RBBB is complete and bidirectional, so true bundle branch reentry cannot take place. In such cases there is slow conduction in the "apparently blocked" fascicle. Initiation of interfascicular reentry occurs when an APD, increase in heart rate, or a VPD produces transient block in the slowly conducting fascicle. The impulse conducts over the "healthy" fascicle, giving rise to a QRS identical to that in sinus rhythm, and then reenters the blocked fascicle to induce reentrant VT. In this instance the H-V interval will always be >40 msec shorter than the H-V in sinus rhythm, and the LB potential will precede the His potential (Figs. 11-90 and 11-102). When interfascicular reentry occurs in the setting of an anterior infarction, "cure" by

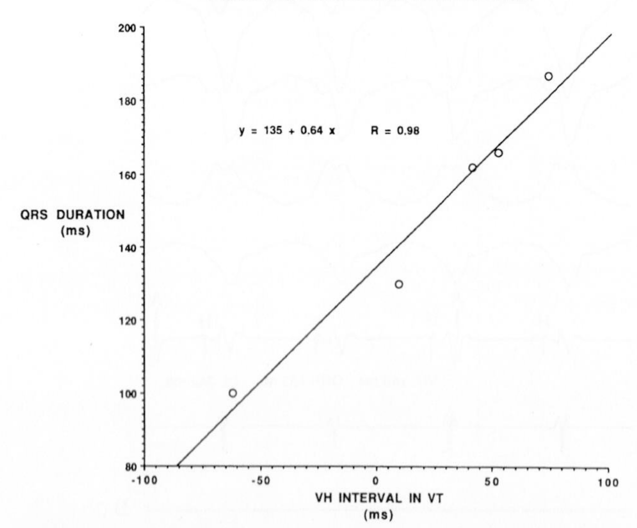


**FIGURE 11-100** Relationship between V-H interval and QRS duration during VT. A V-H interval of five tachycardias in the same individual is plotted against the QRS duration of each of the tachycardias. Note the remarkable linear relationship between QRS duration and V-H interval. This suggests the potential role of the His–Purkinje system in overall ventricular activation. See text for discussion.

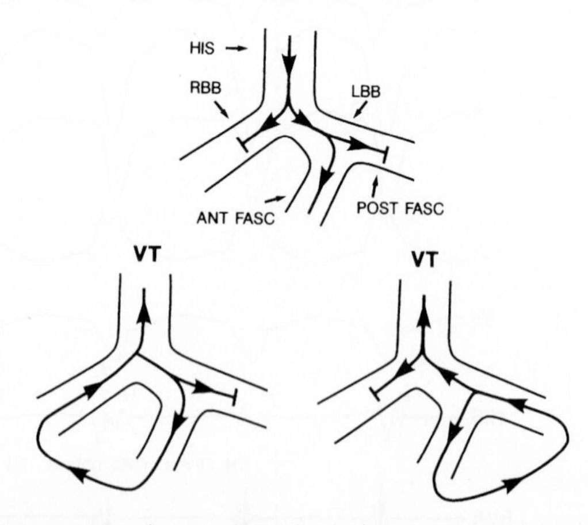


**FIGURE 11-101** Schema of interfascicular reentry. A schema of sinus rhythm in a patient with RBBB and left posterior hemiblock is shown on top. Macroreentrant bundle branch reentry with antegrade conduction down the anterior fascicle and retrograde conduction up the right bundle is shown on the lower left. Interfascicular reentrant VT is shown on the lower right. Antegrade conduction is over the anterior fascicle and retrograde conduction up the posterior fascicle. The His bundle is activated retrogradely during antegrade conduction over the posterior fascicle giving rise to a shorter "H-V" than during sinus. See text for discussion.

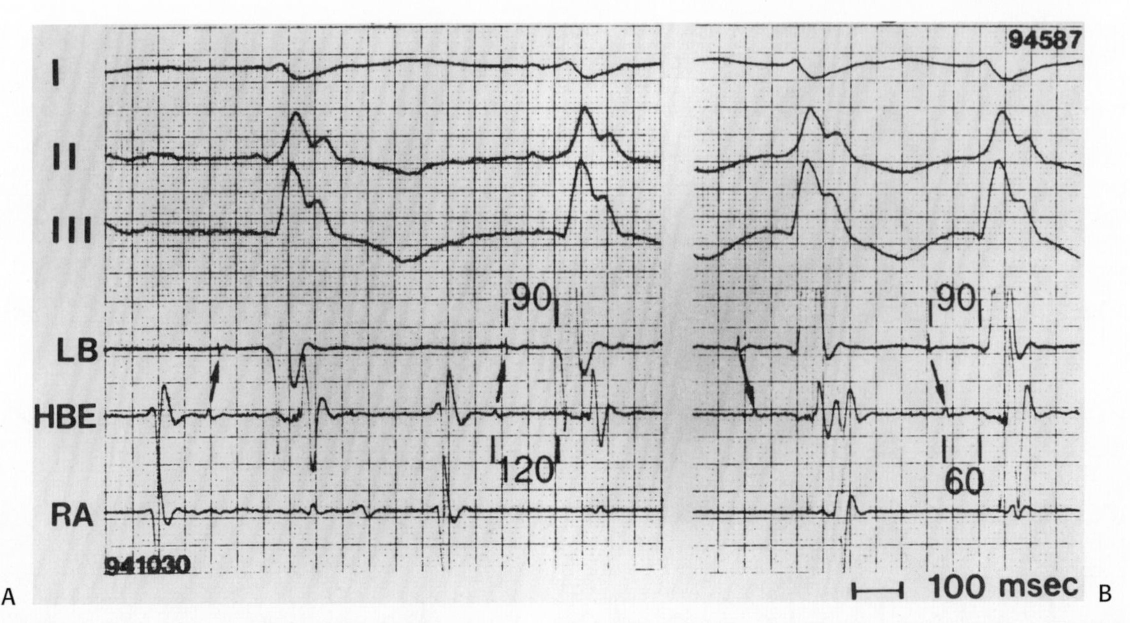


**FIGURE 11-102** Intracardiac recordings during interfascicular reentrant VT. Both panels have ECG leads I, II, III, and recordings from the left bundle branch (LB), HBE, and RA. **A:** Sinus rhythm is present with an H-V interval of 120 msec and an LB-V of 90 msec. During interfascicular tachycardia **(B)**, retrograde activation of the LB precedes the HBE leading to an apparent "H-V" of 60 msec. See text for discussion.

ablation is not possible because other myocardial VTs are, in my experience, always present and the ejection fractions are usually below 30%, thereby mandating a defibrillator to improve survival. This is not the case in the occasional patient with interfascicular reentry in the setting of degenerative conducting system disease with preserved ventricular function. In such a patient cure of the VT is possible by ablation of the diseased fascicle, although a pacemaker would likely be required.

## Initiation of Polymorphic Ventricular Tachycardia-Ventricular Fibrillation

As noted earlier, patients presenting with cardiac arrest may have sustained uniform VT or polymorphic VT leading to VF (Figs. 11-52 and 11-53).[6,22,23,43,190–198] In addition, patients may have nonsustained polymorphic VT, which may be symptomatic or may result in syncope. Polymorphic VT, with or without degeneration to VF, is most commonly observed in ischemic heart disease followed by other forms of structural heart disease. Another group of patients in whom there is much interest are those with apparently normal hearts and primary inherited arrhythmic syndromes.[210] This latter group includes those with congenital long QT syndromes and those with normal or short QT intervals, including the syndromes of idiopathic ventricular fibrillation,[211–219] Brugada syndrome,[112,113,220–222] and catecholaminergic PMVT.[115,116,118,119]

The Brugada syndrome is genetically determined and is characterized by labile ST elevation and T-wave inversion in the right precordial leads (Fig. 11-103).[112,113,223] Currently the classic coved ST segment elevation of >2 mm and terminal T-wave inversion only has to be present in only one right precordial lead, regardless of the interspace in which it is recorded, to make the diagnosis of Brugada syndrome.[210] Savastano et al.[224] recently reviewed the electrocardiographic, molecular, and echocardiographic features of Brugada syndrome. It was initially described as caused by early inactivation of the Na channel leading to early epicardial repolarization, which produces the characteristic ST elevation.[112,113,223] More recently genetic defects producing early inactivation of the L-type calcium channel have also been shown to produce the syndrome.[209,225] At least 9 genes have now been implicated in the Brugada syndrome. The major problem appears to be in the transient outward current ($I_{to}$) which, if it drives the membrane potential below opening of the L-type calcium channel, produces an early shortening of the action potential leading to ST elevation. Sodium channel–blocking drugs accentuate this finding, as does vagal stimulation, while exercise decreases it. Quinidine, at low doses, by virtue of $I_{to}$ blocking properties, can diminish ST elevation and may prevent spontaneous arrhythmia episodes.[214,215,226] At higher doses at which sodium cannel blocking effects are prominent, it can increase ST elevation and theoretically, facilitate arrhythmia occurrence. The current thinking of the pathophysiology of this syndrome has been recently reviewed.[112–114,227] Controversy exists that the Brugada syndrome is related to conduction delay in the RVOT epicardium and not due to repolarization abnormalities.[121] Ablation of high frequency, fractionated electrograms and late potentials recorded on the epicardium of the RVOT have cured the syndrome.[121] Regardless of the controversy, the Brugada syndrome, idiopathic VF, and the short QT syndromes are now being lumped under the rubric of "Early Repolarization Syndromes."[228] All of these disorders have very short-coupled VPCs initiating polymorphic VT. In one study the mean coupling interval of initiating VPCs in the idiopathic VF syndrome was 302 ± 52 msec.[214] The prematurity index of the initiating VPCs was 0.4, with the VPCs occurring within 40 msec of

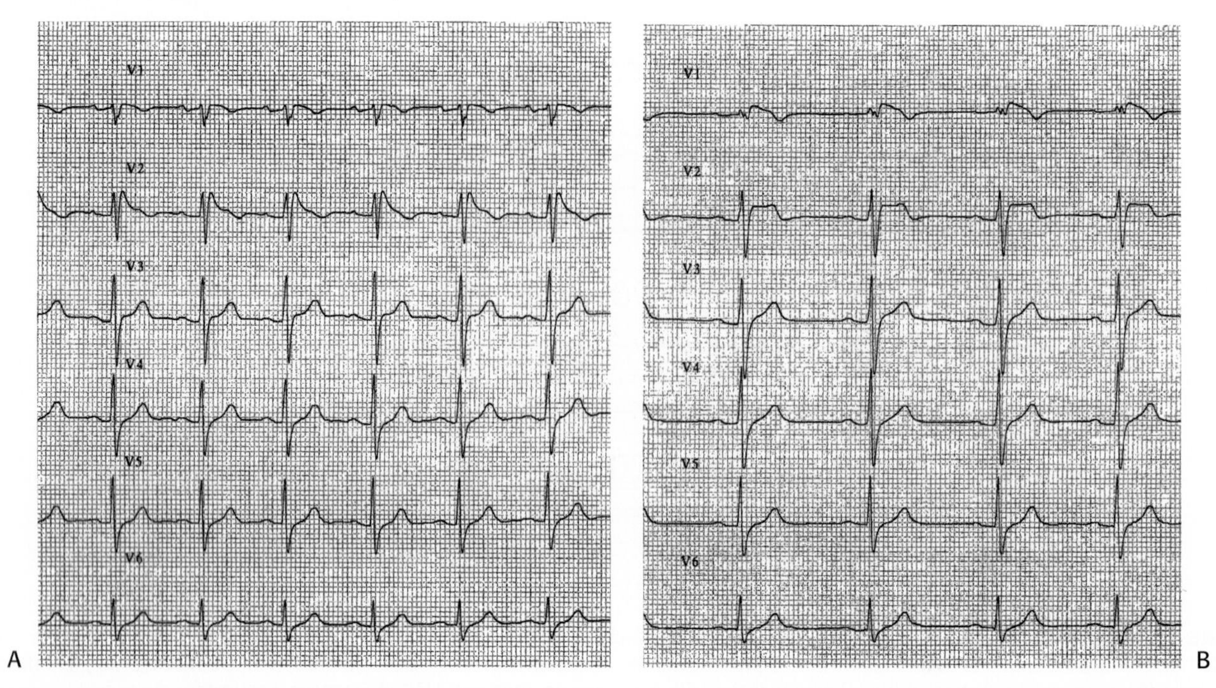


**FIGURE 11-103** ECG in Brugada syndrome. Characteristic precordial S-T segment changes in Brugada syndrome. ECGs from two patients in a family with Brugada syndrome are shown **(A, B)**.

the peak of the T wave. In the idiopathic VF group 50% have increasing J point elevation that is pause dependent.[229] The mechanism of the sustained arrhythmia associated with early repolarization is believed to be due to Phase 2 reentry.[227,230]

Haissaguerre and colleagues recently described a series of patients with various types of electrical disorders (Brugada syndrome, LQTS, idiopathic VF and postmyocardial infarction), in which uniform, reproducible and early-coupled PVCs initiated ventricular fibrillation.[231–233] These patients were recognized by frequent PVCs with an identical morphology being consistently present at the onset of episodes of PMVT. In his series these PVCs appeared originate from the RV outflow tract or the Purkinje system. Of note, the normal RVOT does not contain Purkinje fibers. Mapping and ablation of the PVC triggers appeared to reduce or even eliminate subsequent episodes of PMVT in small, selected patients series over short-term follow-up. An example of a PVC from the moderator band initiating VF is shown in Figure 11-104; ablation of the PVC eliminated VF.[234]

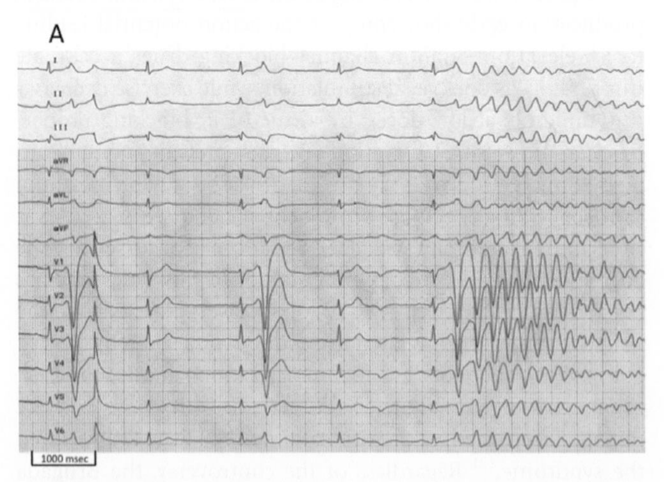


**FIGURE 11-104** Ventricular fibrillation initiated by VPC from moderator band. **A:** 12-lead ECG showing 3 spontaneous VPCs, the latter of which initiates VF. The VPCs have characteristic morphology of activity exiting the RBBB at the moderator band anterior papillary muscle junction. **B:** Purkinje potential in NSR and VPC initiating VF. See text for discussion.

Catecholaminergic polymorphic VT is a familial disorder manifest by adrenergic-mediated bidirectional tachycardia and polymorphic VT.[115,116,118,119,210] The typical presentation is frequent PVCs, syncope or sudden death in children and adolescents precipitated by physical or emotional stress. The resting ECG is normal, and structural heart disease is typically absent. Two genetic forms of this condition have been recognized, an autosomal dominant form caused by mutations in the RyR2 gene encoding the cardiac isoform of the ryanodine receptor, and an autosomal recessive form caused by mutations in the calsequestrin-2 gene. Because both of these proteins are essential for control of intracellular calcium release, the mechanism of this arrhythmia is thought due to triggered activity caused by DADs. When untreated, cPMVT results in a high mortality, estimated at 30% to50% by the age of 30 years. Treatment of the polymorphic VT consists of high-dose beta blockers (nadolol 1 to 2 mg/kg/day) and an implantable defibrillator therapy. Recent experimental evidence in a mouse model of catecholaminergic VT suggests Flecainide might also be useful,[235] and several small clinical series support flecainide's salutary effect in this disorder.[236–238] Videoscopic stellectomy has also recently been employed with great success.[239,240]

Division of patients with polymorphic VT into those with normal, short, and long QT intervals is important from both mechanistic and therapeutic standpoints. The former are described in earlier paragraphs. Patients with polymorphic VT-VF and long QT intervals may be subdivided into those with congenital long QT syndrome[108,111,112,241–244] and those with acquired long QT syndrome.[4,5,111,245–249] The congenital and acquired forms of the long QT syndrome are quite distinct. The acquired form is usually bradycardia dependent and short-long-short sequences are frequently observed at arrhythmia onset.[4,5,111,130,245–249] The acquired form has a whole host of causes including exposure to certain drugs (Table 11-13) (i.e., antiarrhythmic agents, antihistamines, antifungal drugs, phenothiazines, tricyclic antidepressants, and organophosphates); electrolyte abnormalities (i.e., hypokalemia and hypomagnesemia); altered nutritional states (particularly those associated with a liquid protein diet); and bradyarrhythmias either sinus bradycardia or A-V block.[4,5,111,245–249] These are all situations in which $IK_r$ is reduced or blocked by. Catecholamine agonists tend to improve this disorder, as do other methods that increase rate and shorten refractoriness, such as pacing.[111,249] In the absence of acceleration of rate (e.g., in the setting of complete heart block), catecholamines may actually worsen the arrhythmia. This acquired form was initially described by Dessertenne as torsade de pointes.[4] Many patients experiencing secondary long QT syndrome have genetic variants in the gene controlling this ion channel, which is responsible for long QT syndrome 2.[117]

There are several genetically determined long QT syndromes based on specific ion channel defects; at present, at least 13 different genes have been implicated, all of which affect cardiac repolarization.[117,117,244,250–252] In addition to inherited forms, acquired forms may be caused by less profound genetic abnormalities that reduce the degree of "repolarization reserve" to the point that challenges by drugs or conditions that prolong repolarization may result in ventricular arrhythmias.[253] It is important to realize that (a) there may be many different point mutations on the same gene and (b) phenotypic expressions of the same genotype can differ. Thus QT prolongation and/or arrhythmias may be absent or present in patients with the same genotype. This suggests that an interaction with environmental factors is necessary in addition to genotype in order to manifest the phenotype and clinical syndrome and/or the potential for modification of the effect of a given gene by promoters or modifiers that may be independently inherited, resulting in differential penetrance.

Early observations suggested that the congenital long QT syndrome was remarkably adrenergic dependent, with emotional or physical stress being the most important triggers.[111,112,241,244,254,255] As such, many investigators described the congenital long QT syndrome as "adrenergic dependent" and the acquired form as "bradycardic or pause dependent."[111] This has been shown to be too simplistic. At least three well-characterized autosomal dominant genetic abnormalities have been described, each of which appears to have a different

TABLE 11-13 Relationship of Mode of Termination of VT with VT Cycle Length (139 Patients)

| Mode of Termination | VT Cycle Length (msec) | | | | Number of VTs |
|---|---|---|---|---|---|
| | 400–500 | 350–400 | 300–350 | <300 | |
| 1 VPD | 16 | 5 | 2 | | 23 |
| 2 VPDs | 12 | 15 | 8 | 4 | 39 |
| 3 VPDs | 3 | 3 | 1 | 7 | |
| RVP | 1 | 5 | 15 | 20 | 41 |
| Cardioversion | 2 | 2 | 25 | 29 | |
| Number of VTs | 29 | 30 | 30 | 50 | 139 |

VT, ventricular tachycardia; RVP, rapid ventricular pacing; VPD, ventricular premature depolarization.

phenotypic expression and clinical pattern.[112,256,257] The first long QT syndrome (LQTS1) described a defect on chromosome 11 in the gene (KVLQT1) controlling the slowly inactivating potassium channel (IKs). This syndrome appears to be variably influenced by catecholamines. The second long QT syndrome (LQTS2) was found to be associated with a defect in a gene (HERG) on chromosome 7, which controls the rapidly inactivating potassium channel ($Ik_r$). The syndrome associated with this defect appears to be adrenergically dependent. The third long QT syndrome (LQTS3) is associated with a defect in the gene controlling the sodium channel (SCN5A) located on chromosome 5. People with this syndrome have arrhythmias during slow heart rates and experience sudden death during sleep. There may also be overlap in primary arrhythmic syndromes; that is, the recognized genetic cause of Brugada syndrome, mutations in the SCN5A gene, are also associated with LQTS3.[258] That differences in genotype can produce a similar phenotype (long QT) suggests, but does not prove, that different therapies may be required to treat specific syndromes. For example, empiric beta blocker therapy may worsen LQT3, as arrhythmias are facilitated by bradycardia; sodium channel blocking agents may be helpful in this disorder and would not expected to have any significant effect on LQT1 or LQT2. Sympathectomy has been useful in long QT 1 and 2.[240]

As noted earlier in the chapter, patients with congenital long QT syndromes have marked abnormalities of repolarization, with prolonged dispersion of refractoriness and total recovery time of the whole left ventricle and/or adjacent sites.[107] Their ventricular activation is normal. Patients with acquired long QT intervals have not been studied during their episodes, because they are symptomatic and efforts to treat the arrhythmia are made before investigation. Thus, no data are available concerning dispersion of refractoriness.

### *Initiation of Polymorphic Ventricular Tachycardia-Ventricular Fibrillation with Normal QT Intervals*

In patients with normal QT intervals and coronary disease, who have polymorphic tachycardia and/or ventricular fibrillation, a similar tachycardia can be induced perhaps 75% to 85% of the time by programmed stimulation using the standard protocol described previously (Figs. 11-52 and 11-53).[6,22,23,42,164,259–263] The induction of nonsustained polymorphic tachycardia and polymorphic VT-VF by two extrastimuli are shown in Figures 11-105 and 11-106. One must remember that polymorphic VT-VF may be a nonspecific response to aggressive stimulation,[42,134,138,139,141,264] such that occasionally (≈30%) patients with normal hearts and normal QT intervals will have

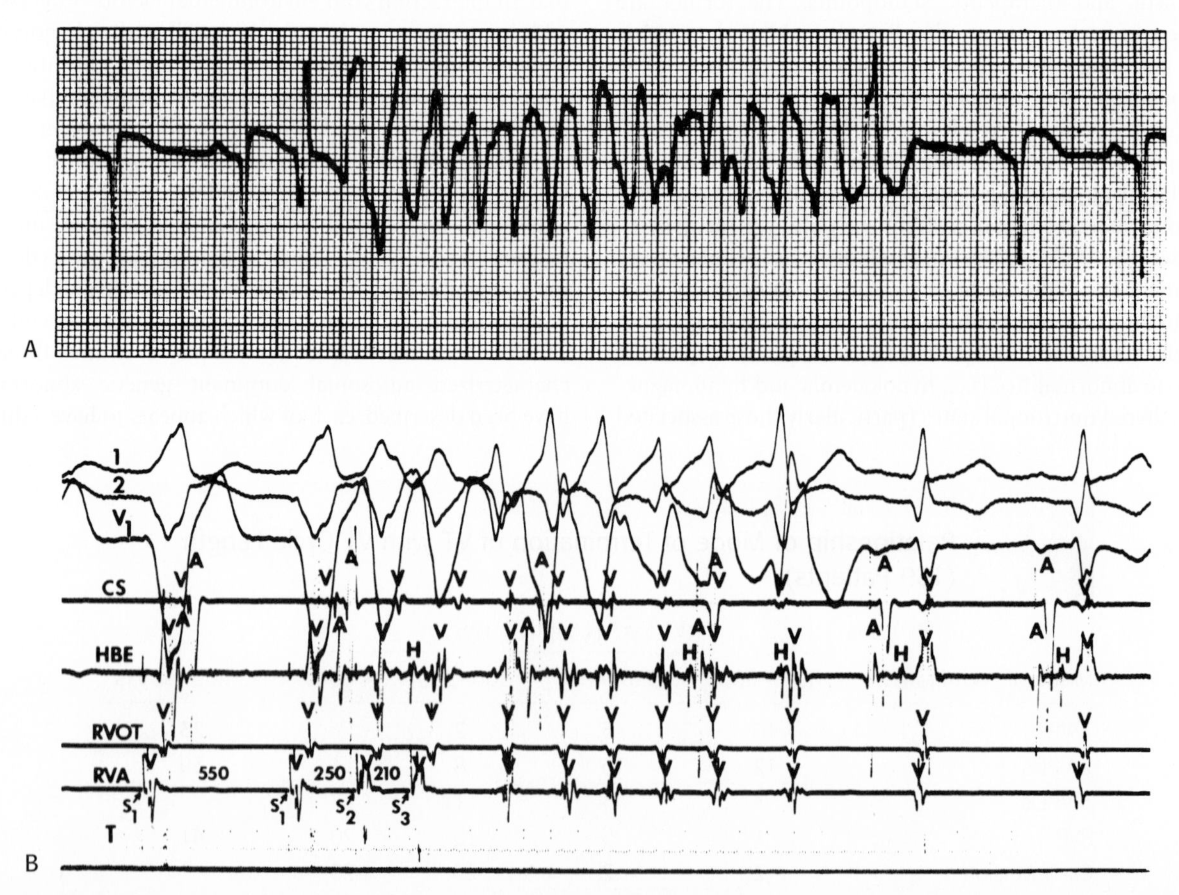


**FIGURE 11-105** Initiation of nonsustained polymorphic VT by double extrastimuli. **A:** A rhythm strip of a monitor lead $V_2$ is shown. Spontaneous nonsustained polymorphic tachycardia is observed. **B:** Double ventricular extrastimuli at coupling intervals of 250 and 210 msec, respectively, delivered at a drive CL of 550 msec from the RVA initiate a polymorphic tachycardia, whose termination appears similar to that of the spontaneous episode.

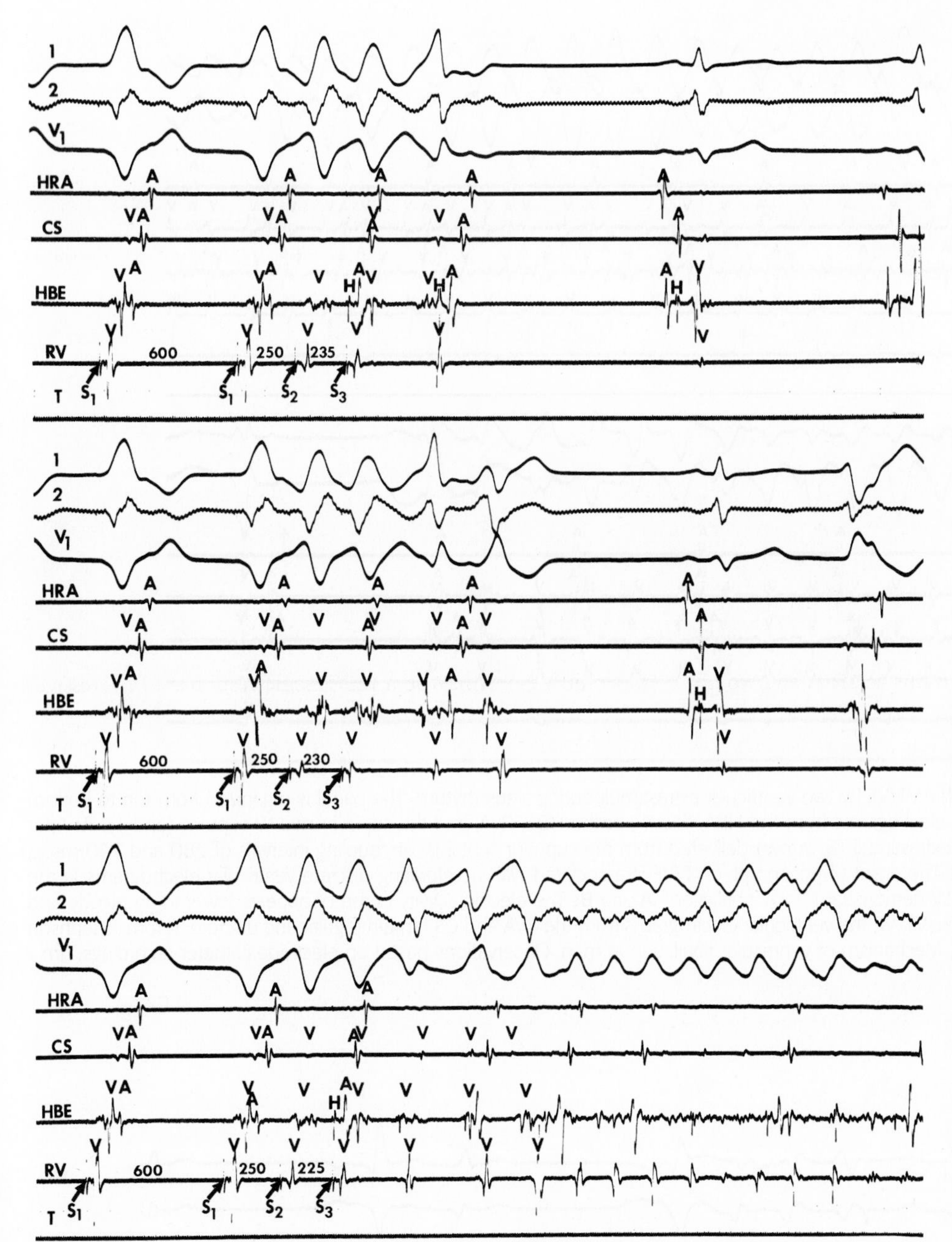


**FIGURE 11-106** Initiation of ventricular fibrillation by two ventricular extrastimuli during ventricular pacing. The recordings are organized from top to bottom as ECG leads 1, 2, and $V_1$ and intracardiac electrograms from the HRA, CS, HBE, and RVA (and T). During a basic ventricular drive of 600 msec ($S_1$, *arrows*) two VES delivered from the RVA at progressively premature complex intervals initiate VF. The onset of VF is associated with progressive acceleration and fragmentation of the intracardiac ventricular electrograms, which occurs initially in the HBE, which is distant from the site of stimulation. Fractionation occurs last in the RVA, which was the site of stimulation. (From Josephson ME, Spielman SR, Greenspan AM, et al. Mechanism of ventricular fibrillation in man. Observations based on electrode catheter recordings. *Am J Cardiol* 1979;44:623.)

a polymorphic VT induced with triple extrastimuli delivered at twice diastolic threshold.[265] This should not be taken as having significance with respect to their clinical disorder. Most nonspecific responses are associated with very short coupling intervals (≤180 msec) and are far more frequent with triple extrastimuli than with double extrastimuli.[42,138,140,141,149,264] In my experience, in survivors of cardiac arrest with prior myocardial infarction, reproducible induction of polymorphic VT by two or three extrastimuli is associated with coupling intervals that are usually >180 msec. This is no different from those coupling intervals inducing sustained uniform VT in these patients. However, the coupling intervals that initiate polymorphic VT-VF should not, per se, be used to establish the clinical significance of the induced rhythm. The reproducible initiation of polymorphic VT with the same "template" of changing QRS, despite changes in pacing site and/or cycle length, suggests some structural basis (functional or anatomic) for the induced rhythm. In such instances, I believe the induced rhythm is meaningful.

Rarely, polymorphic VT or VT-VF is induced with single or double VES during sinus rhythm (Fig. 11-107). In our experience, this is extremely rare in the absence of a clinical history of syncope and/or cardiac arrest. Induction of polymorphic VT-VF may be site dependent (Fig. 11-108). Refractory periods at the right ventricular apex and outflow tract do not distinguish the sites from which they may be induced.[42] In some patients, left ventricular stimulation may be necessary to induce polymorphic VT-VF (Fig. 11-109).

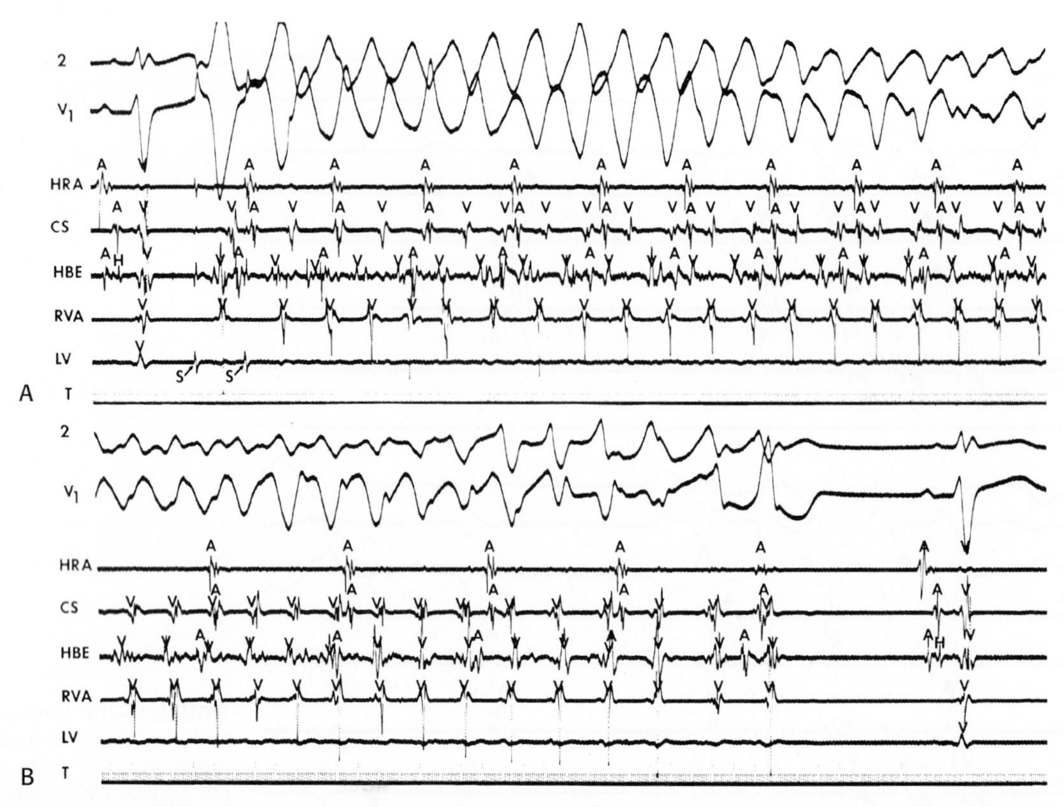


**FIGURE 11-107** Initiation of polymorphic VT/VF by two ventricular extrastimuli during sinus rhythm. The panel is organized from top to bottom as electrocardiographic leads 2 and $V_1$, electrograms from the HRA, CS, AVJ at the HBE, RVA, and the superior mid-LV septum (and T). **A:** After the first sinus complex, two ventricular extrastimuli (S, *arrow*) delivered from the superior septal LV at coupling intervals of 280 and 240 msec, respectively, initiate polymorphic VT/VF. The onset of polymorphic VT/VF is associated with accelerating discrete ventricular electrograms in the CS and RVA, while the His bundle and LV demonstrate "local fibrillation." **A** and **B:** The electric activity in the LV appears lower in amplitude and irregularly undulating. During polymorphic VT/VF, the ventricular electrograms from the RVA and CS remain regular and discrete. (From Josephson ME, Spielman SR, Greenspan AM, et al. Mechanism of ventricular fibrillation in man. Observations based on electrode catheter recordings. *Am J Cardiol* 1979;44:623.)

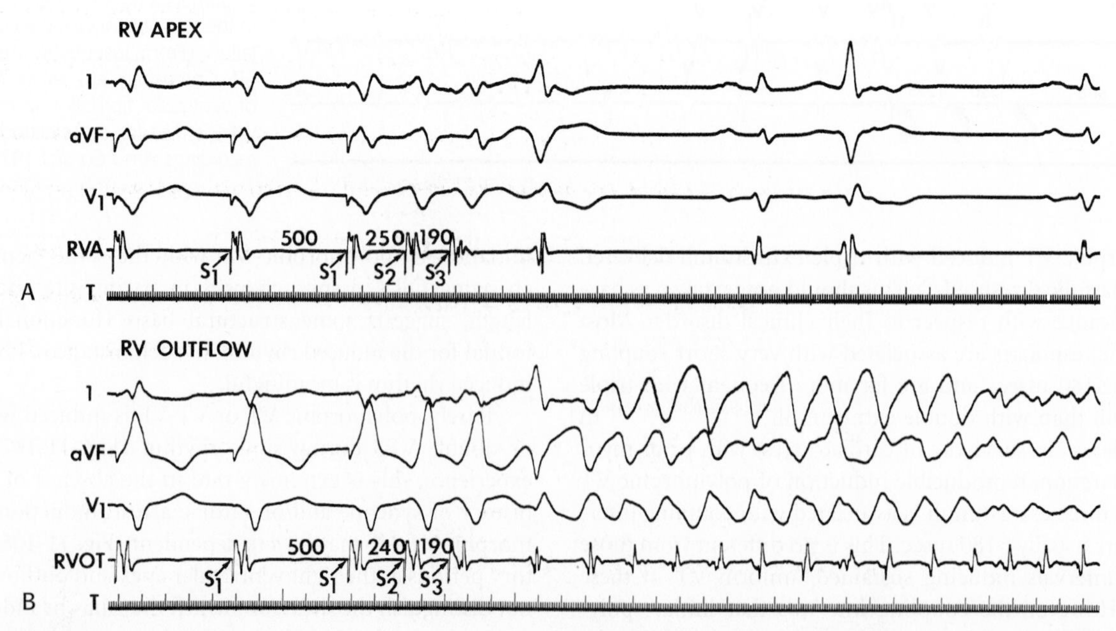


**FIGURE 11-108** Site dependency of initiation of ventricular fibrillation. **A:** Double extrastimuli from the RVA fail to initiate VF. **B:** Double ventricular extrastimuli delivered at similar coupling intervals from the RVOT initiate sustained polymorphic VT-VF.

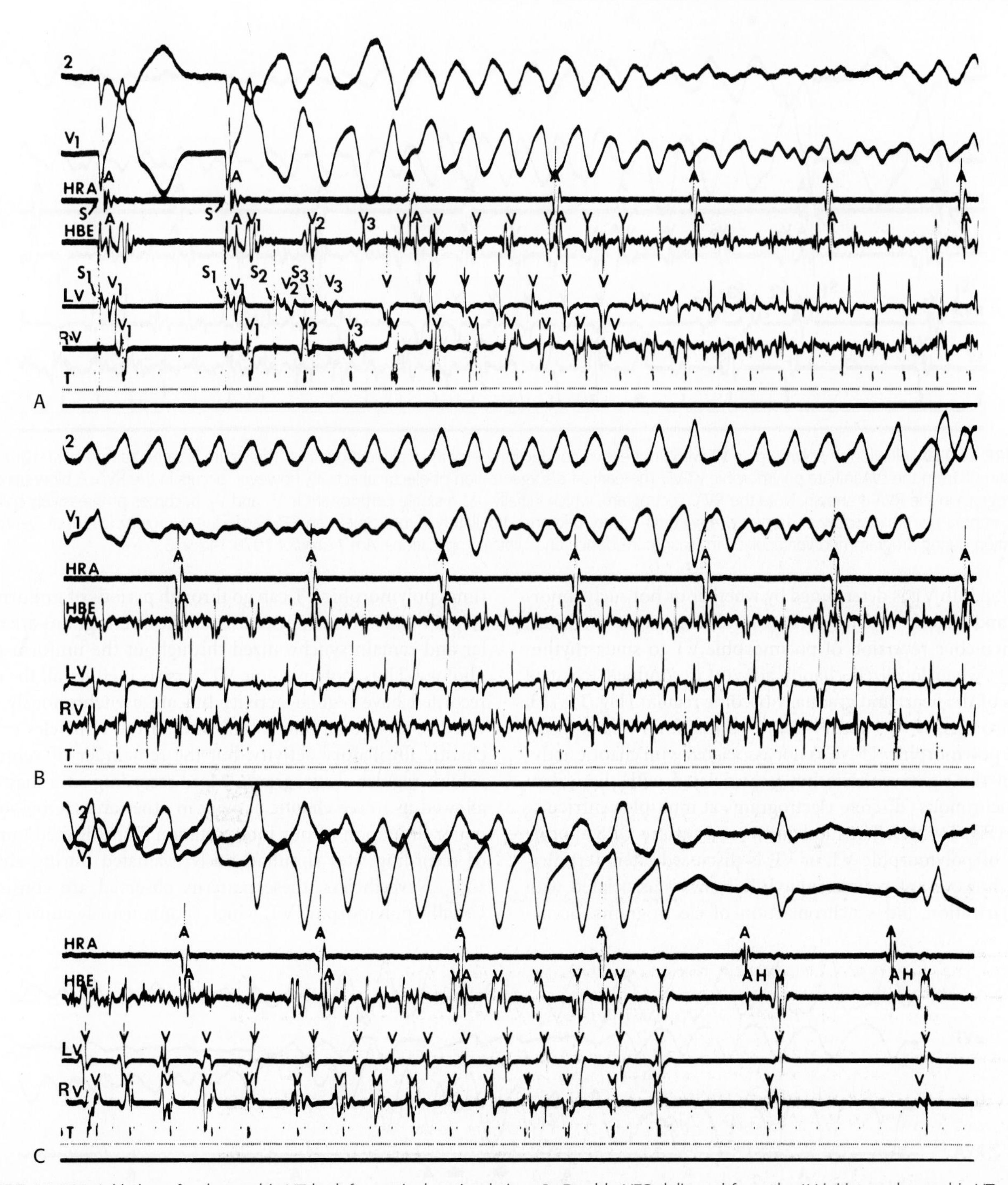


**FIGURE 11-109** Initiation of polymorphic VT by left ventricular stimulation. **A:** Double VES delivered from the LV initiate polymorphic VT, which resembles VF. Note the chaotic activity in all three ventricular recording sites. **B:** The chaotic irregular activity continues in the HBE and RV, but intermittent organization of the electrogram is noted in the LV. **C:** Spontaneous termination occurs as electrical activity at all three ventricular sites becomes organized. See text for discussion.

Why some patients have self-terminating polymorphic VT and some go on to VF is not well understood. In those who develop VF, an accelerated phase of VT occurs. Progressive conduction delay in local electrograms is observed until total fractionation and irregular activity is noted in all electrograms throughout the heart (Fig. 11-110).[266] Ventricular fibrillation can arise by spontaneous degeneration from VT (Fig. 11-111) or stimulation during VT (Fig. 11-112). Saumarez et al.[84] suggest that fractionation of electrograms occurs at longer coupling intervals in patients with a history of idiopathic VF and should be evaluated as a risk stratifier. Regardless of the initiating mechanism, VF usually begins with an accelerating VT with either breakdown and fragmentation of a local electrogram in one lead, which gradually spreads to the remainder of the heart, or the simultaneous appearance of chaotic activity in multiple areas. Whether or not the polymorphic VT will

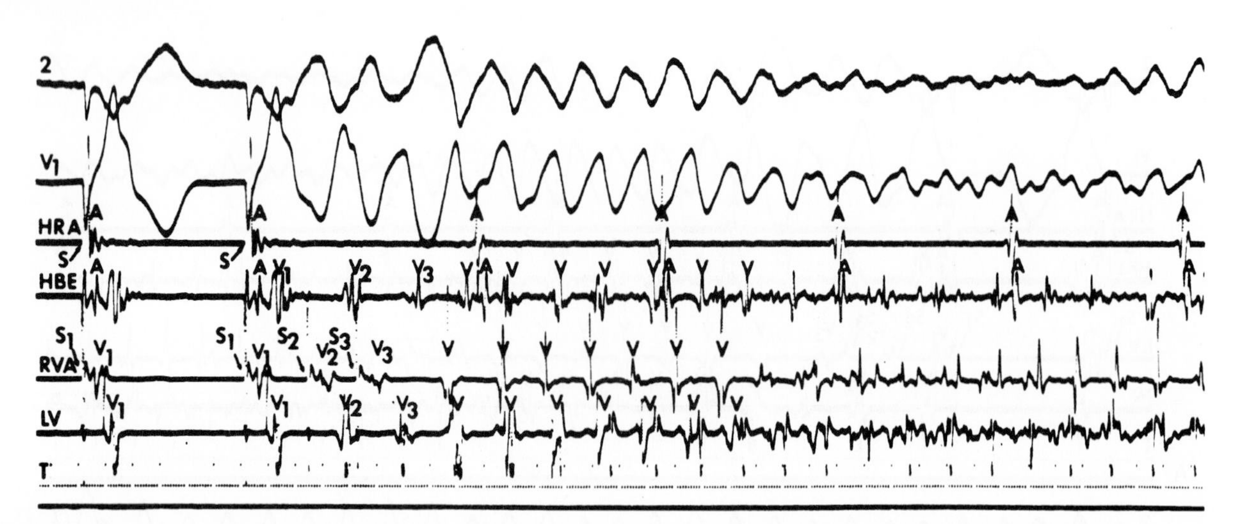


**FIGURE 11-110** Initiation of polymorphic VT with progressive conduction delay in local electrograms. This figure is same as Figure 11-109A. Two extrastimuli from the LVA initiate polymorphic VT-VF. The earliest disorganization of electrical activity, however, occurs in the RVA. A blow-up of the electrogram in the RVA is shown. Note the RVA electrogram, which initially has a single component in $V_2$ and $V_3$, becomes progressively split into two components (*solid arrow* and *open arrow*) until activity becomes fibrillatory (From Spielman SR, Farshidi A, Horowitz LN, et al. Ventricular fibrillation during programmed ventricular stimulation: Incidence and clinical implications. *Am J Cardiol* 1978;142:913.)

develop into VF is determined by whether or not such abnormal and chaotic activity persists in all regions of the heart. Spontaneous reversion of polymorphic VT to sinus rhythm occurs when localized chaotic activity is confined to small areas of the heart and gradually become regular (Fig. 11-113; see also Figs. 11-109 and 11-102).[266] Sometimes what appears to be polymorphic VT-VF is not associated with chaotic activity in the right ventricle but is associated with discordant (asynchronous) discrete electrograms at multiple ventricular sites (Fig. 11-114). The mechanism of a surface QRS appearance of polymorphic VT or VF is discussed later. Termination, however, of polymorphic VT is always associated with regularization and synchronization of electrograms. Sometimes polymorphic VT can go through periods of uniform VT (Fig. 11-115). In such instances, all the electrograms are regular and remain synchronized throughout the uniform morphology. Thus, polymorphic VT persists if either all the areas recorded have regular activity but are asynchronously activated or if several, but not all, sites in the ventricles exhibit chaotic fibrillatory activity, but the remainder of ventricles exhibit regular electrograms. More recording sites may have allowed us to see chaotic activity in other areas. Obviously a major limitation of our interpretation is the limited number of recording sites simultaneously evaluated during an episode. Nevertheless, these patterns observed are consistent. Usually, polymorphic VT, which spontaneously converts, has

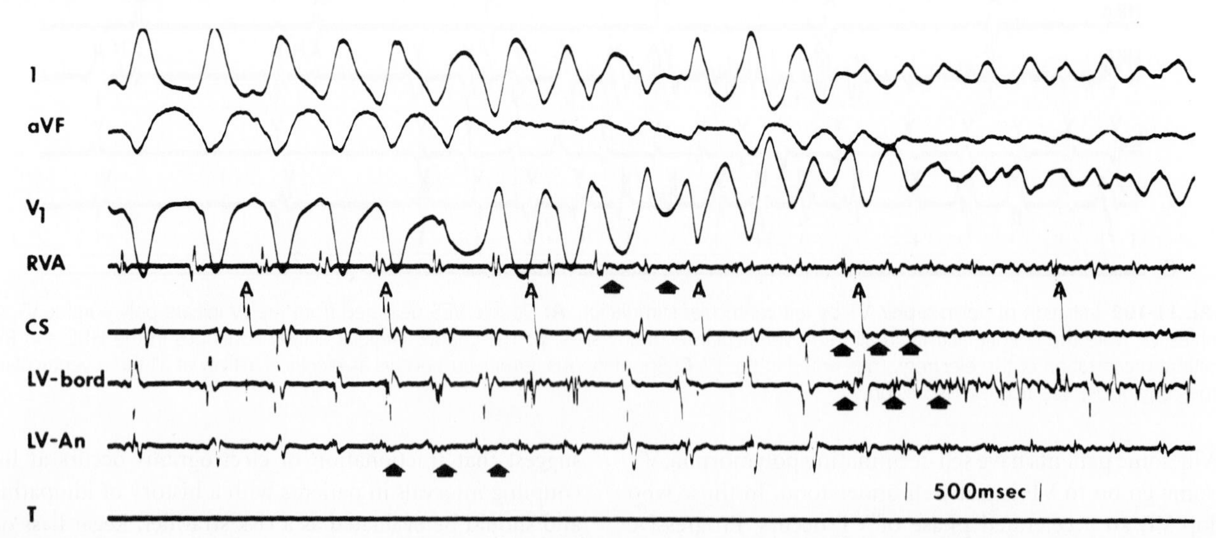


**FIGURE 11-111** Spontaneous degeneration of VT to ventricular fibrillation. The panel is arranged from top to bottom as ECG leads 1, aVF, and $V_1$ and electrograms from the RVA, CS, border of an apical left ventricular aneurysm (LV-bord), and from within the aneurysm (LV-An) (and T). Before the development of VF (right) there is sudden acceleration of VT with the development of pleomorphic forms. The intracardiac electrograms also demonstrate acceleration with the noncontiguous development of fractionation of each electrogram (*arrows*). The fractionation was initially transient in the LV-An but then became persistent. (From Josephson ME, Spielman SR, Greenspan AM, et al. Mechanism of ventricular fibrillation in man. Observations based on electrode catheter recordings. *Am J Cardiol* 1979;44:623.)

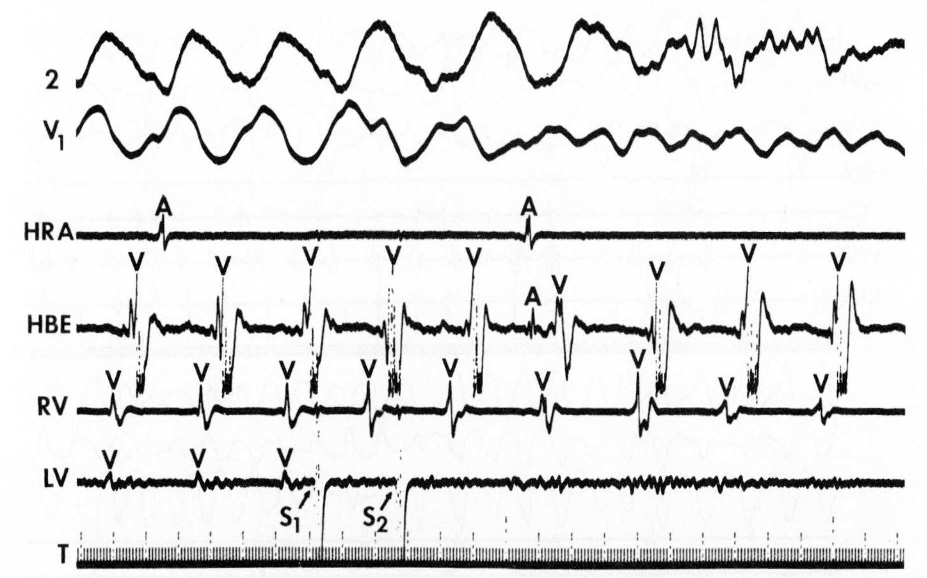


**FIGURE 11-112** Initiation of ventricular fibrillation by double ventricular extrastimuli during VT. From top to bottom are ECG leads 2 and $V_1$ and electrograms from the HRA, HBE, RV, and LV (and T; 10 and 100 msec). Initially, VT is present at a CL of 270 msec. Double ventricular extrastimuli delivered from the mid-right ventricular septum (not shown), at coupling intervals of 190 and 240 msec, initiate VF. Disorganized activity is confined to the left ventricular electrogram. (From Spielman SR, Farshidi A, Horowitz LN, et al. Ventricular fibrillation during programmed ventricular stimulation: Incidence and clinical implications. *Am J Cardiol* 1978;142:913.)

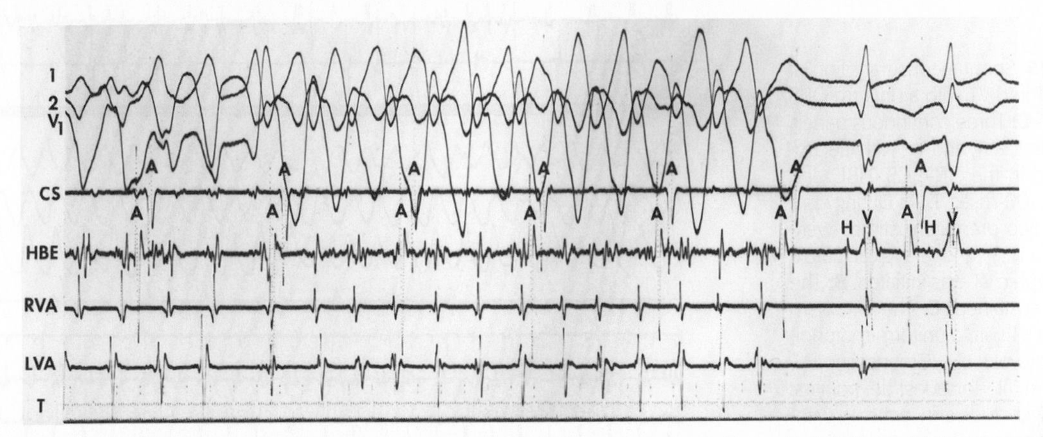


**FIGURE 11-113** Spontaneous conversion of polymorphic VT to sinus rhythm. In this patient with a prior inferior wall infarction, polymorphic VT is present on the left. Note that spontaneous termination of the tachycardia occurs when the grossly chaotic ventricular activity in the HBE becomes suddenly organized with the remainder of the ventricular electrograms.

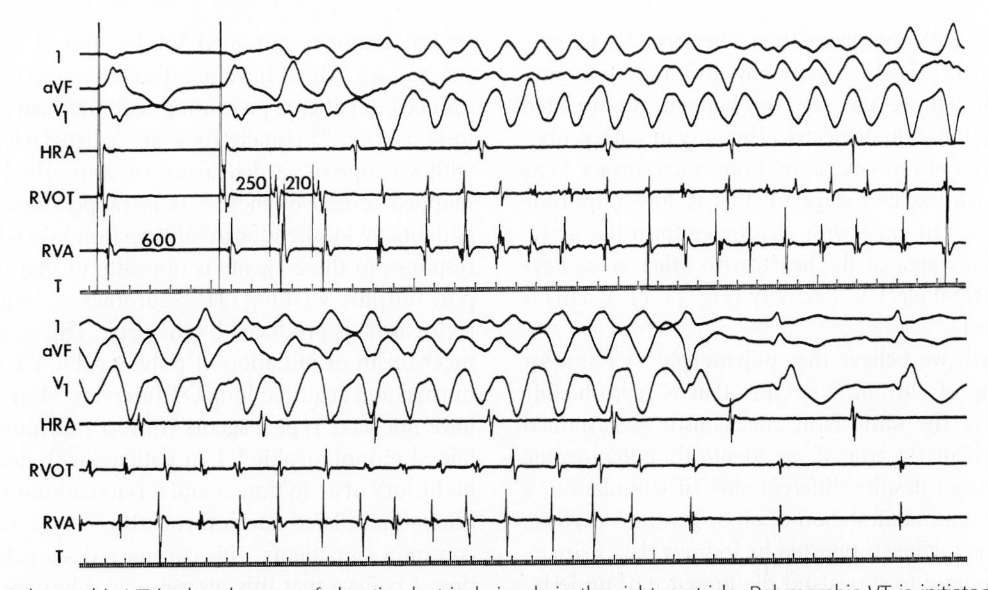


**FIGURE 11-114** Polymorphic VT in the absence of chaotic electrical signals in the right ventricle. Polymorphic VT is initiated with double ventricular extrastimuli delivered at the RVOT. Note that the electrograms in both RVA and RVOT remain discrete, yet the tachycardia is polymorphic. Polymorphism results because of the changing relationship of RVOT and RVA electrograms. The tachycardia terminates (**bottom panel**) after the last four complexes become uniform. See text for discussion.

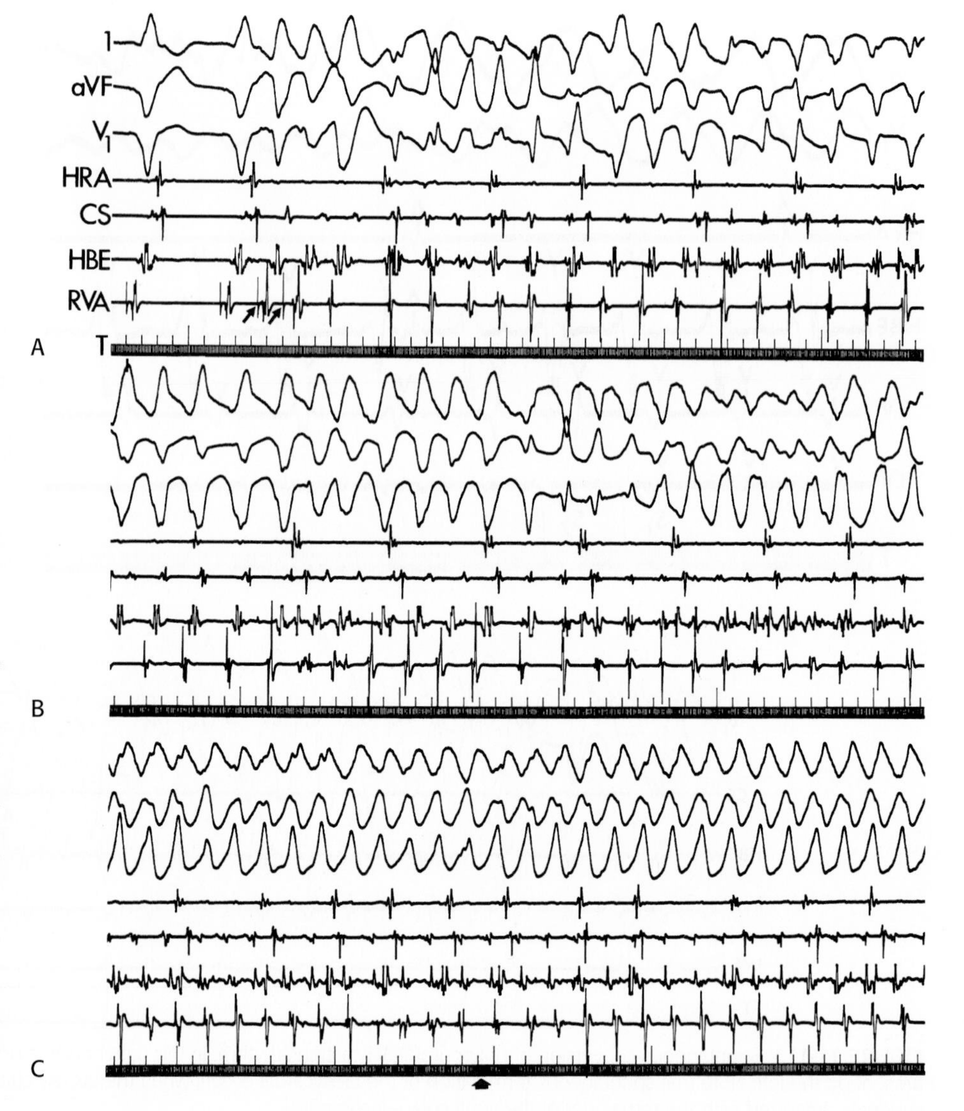


**FIGURE 11-115** Spontaneous transition of polymorphic VT into VT with a uniform QRS morphology. **A–C:** Three continuous panels show ECG leads 1, aVF, and $V_1$; with electrograms recorded in the HRA, CS, HBE, and RVA; and with 100-msec T. **A:** During ventricular pacing, two premature stimuli were introduced (*arrows*), and a typical paroxysm of polymorphic VT was initiated. **B:** The paroxysm was sustained. **C:** The paroxysm stabilized into a VT with a uniform morphology. (From Horowitz LN, Greenspan AM, Spielman SR, et al. Torsades de pointes: Electrophysiologic studies in patients without transient pharmacologic or metabolic abnormalities. *Circulation* 1981;63:1120.)

higher amplitude QRS complexes than when true VF is present. As mentioned, VF, which generally does not spontaneously revert (although we have seen this happen) is associated with chaotic fractionation of electrical activity in both ventricles (Fig. 11-116). On rare occasions, however, a surface ECG looking very much like end-stage VF, that is, low-amplitude fibrillatory waves, can exist with chaotic endocardial activity localized to one area of the heart, with other areas having relatively normal electrical activity (Fig. 11-117). This is extremely unusual.

As mentioned, we believe that polymorphic VT and/or VF in the setting of chronic infarction that is reproducibly initiated can have the same basic mechanism as sustained VT. This is particularly true if an identical "polymorphic template" is induced despite different sites of stimulation, a finding I believe is a manifestation of an "organized" rhythm. This hypothesis is further supported by indirect data primarily related to response to drugs and the presence of underlying conduction disturbances. We have observed that many polymorphic VTs, and occasionally VF, can be changed to a typical uniform sustained VT by Type I agents (e.g., procainamide), which have identical characteristics as those VT induced in patients presenting with uniform VT (Figs. 11-118 to 11-120).[164,165] Usually, these are patients who have presented with syncope or cardiac arrest on antiarrhythmic agents. We mapped several of these VTs intraoperatively and cured the patients by local endocardial resection (see Chapter 13). This response to these agents is opposite to that in drug-induced polymorphic VT long QT syndromes in which polymorphic tachycardia is produced by the drug. This suggests a different mechanism of initiation of polymorphic VT in patients with normal and acquired long QT intervals. More importantly, we have not seen Type I agents convert polymorphic VT to sustained monomorphic VT in patients with normal hearts and no history of arrhythmias and it is uncommon in patients with idiopathic dilated cardiomyopathy.[165] This response is most common in patients with coronary disease and prior infarction. I believe that this response, in addition to reproducible initiation of template of polymorphic VT from different sites of stimulation, may be useful methods of distinguishing a

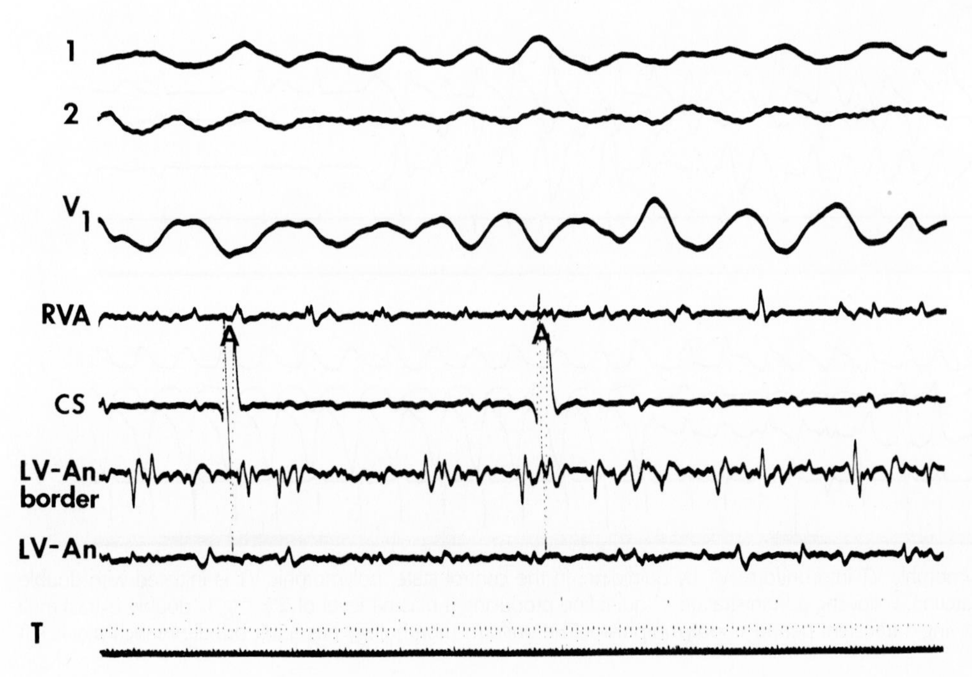


**FIGURE 11-116** Relation of intracardiac electrograms to QRS configuration during ventricular fibrillation. During VF, all ventricular electrograms show chaotic activity. Note low amplitude of QRS complexes. (From Josephson ME, Spielman SR, Greenspan AM, et al. Mechanism of ventricular fibrillation in man. Observations based on electrode catheter recordings. *Am J Cardiol* 1979;44:623.)

nonspecific polymorphic VT from one that may have clinical import.

Again, I must stress that polymorphic VT and/or VF can be induced in normal patients as well as in patients with cardiac disease but without prior history of syncope or cardiac arrest.[42,136,138,139,141,264] These nonspecific responses are morphologically identical to those seen in patients who present with cardiac arrest. Thus, it is difficult to be absolutely certain of the clinical significance of induced polymorphic VT. However, in the presence of a prior myocardial infarction, positive SAECG, or endocardial mapping demonstrating marked abnormalities of conduction, especially with a history of syncope, cardiac arrest, or documented polymorphic VT, these arrhythmias—especially if reproducibly initiated with relatively long-coupled extrastimuli—may have clinical significance. In the absence of these findings, in my opinion, the comparably induced arrhythmias should be considered nonspecific responses and not treated.

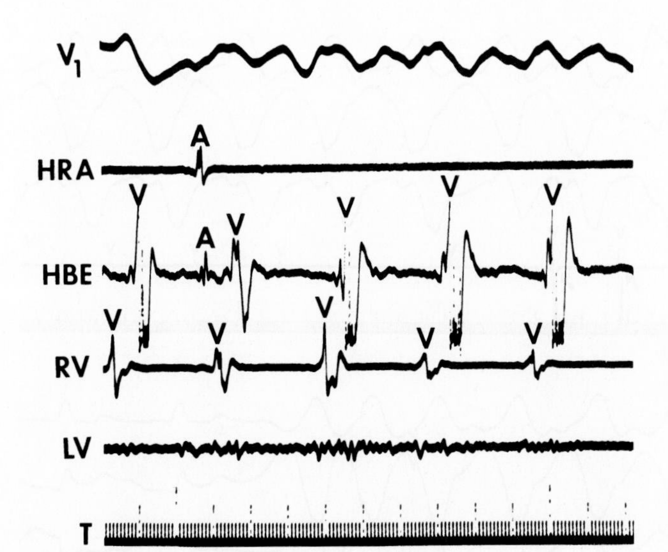


**FIGURE 11-117** Atypical ventricular fibrillation. The surface ECG of $V_1$ looks like classic VF; however, the bulk of the heart demonstrates regular discrete ventricular activity. Fragmented, asynchronous activity is only seen in an area of large infarction in the LV.

In summary, at least for coronary artery disease, reproducible initiation of polymorphic VT-VF that can be converted to uniform VT by antiarrhythmic agents which slow conduction, that demonstrates site specificity for initiation and/or has a "polymorphic template" regardless of the site of stimulation, and that is associated with abnormalities of conduction during sinus rhythm suggests that reentry is the most compatible mechanism of these arrhythmias.

Neither rapid pacing nor isoproterenol facilitates induction of polymorphic VT associated with normal QT intervals. The rarity with which these arrhythmias can be induced with single extrastimuli does not allow assessment of the relationship of coupling interval to onset of the tachycardia or early tachycardia cycle length. The drive cycle length, however, does not influence the early cycles of the tachycardia. The absence of bradycardic-dependence or the requirement of short-long-short sequences and failure to have a tachycardia induced by rapid pacing or facilitated by catecholamines militates against triggered activity that is due to early or late afterdepolarizations of the underlying mechanism.

### *Initiation of Polymorphic Ventricular Tachycardia-Ventricular Fibrillation in the Presence of Long QT Intervals*

Polymorphic VT-VF associated with acquired or congenital long QT syndromes cannot be reproducibly initiated.[111,265–267] Although in 25% to 50% of such patients polymorphic VTs

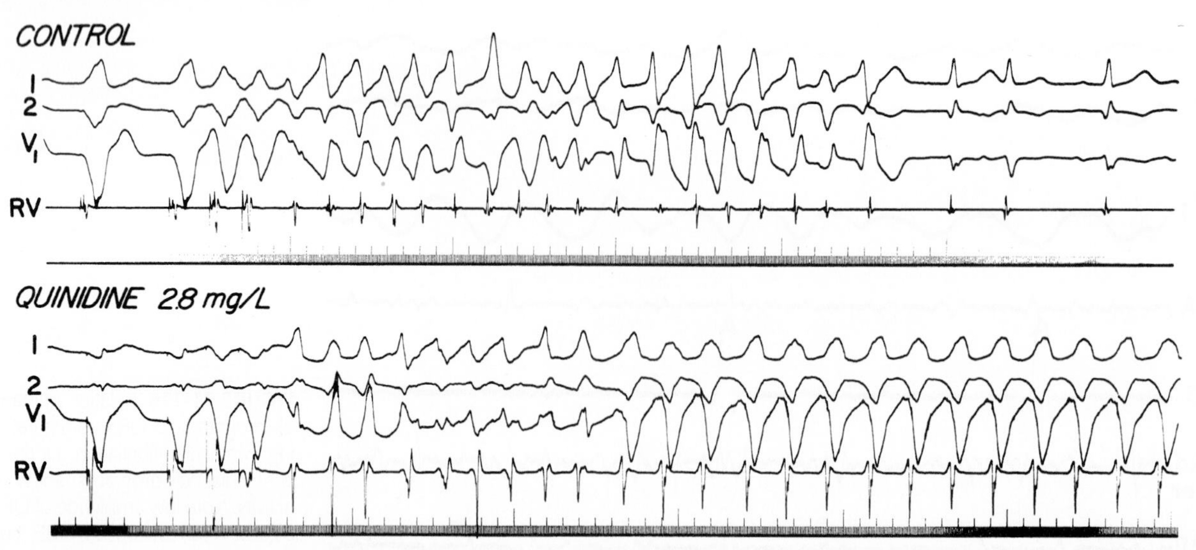


**FIGURE 11-118** Transformation of polymorphic VT into uniform VT by quinidine. In the control state, polymorphic VT is initiated with double VES in a patient with an inferior wall infarction. Following administration of quinidine producing a plasma level of 2.8 mg/L, double extrastimuli initiate VT, which becomes uniform following a transient period of polymorphism. The uniform morphology has a left bundle branch block, left axis morphology.

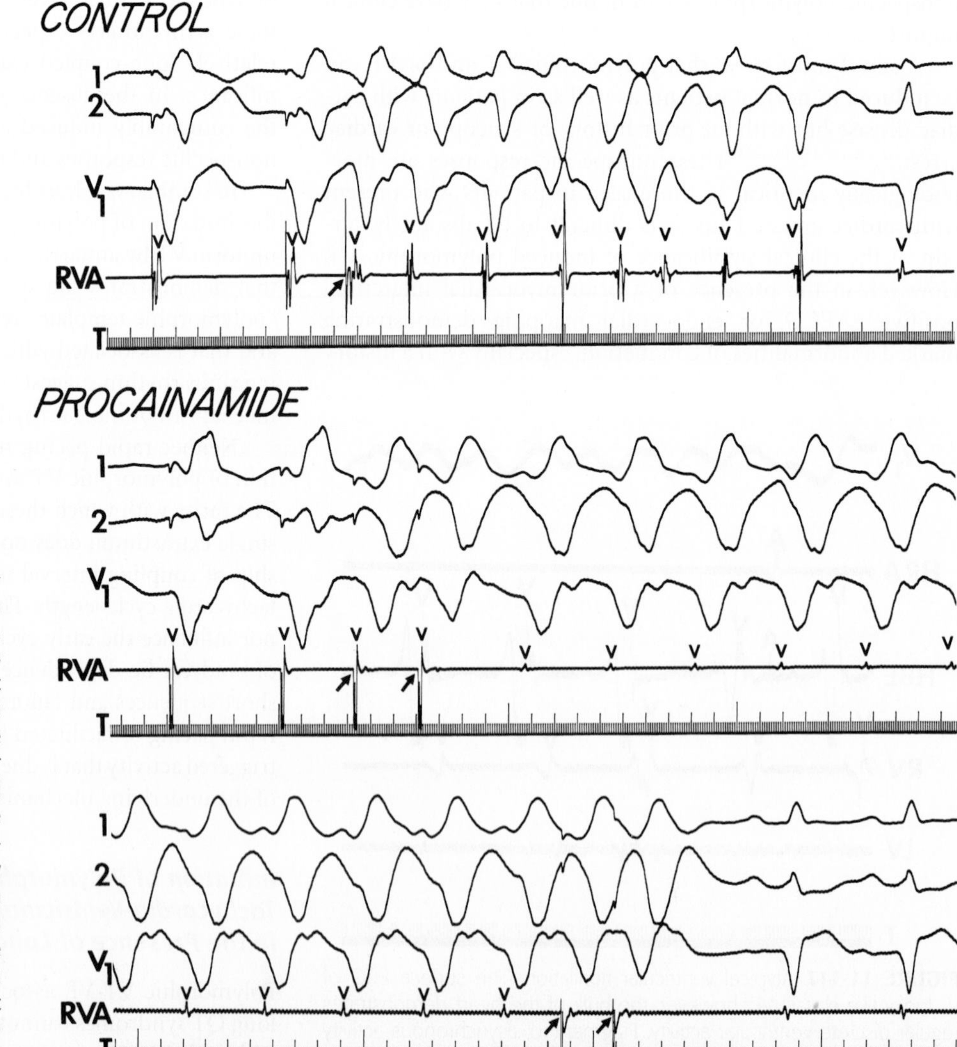


**FIGURE 11-119** Conversion of polymorphic VT to typical sustained uniform VT by procainamide. In the control state, a single right ventricular extrastimulus initiates a nonsustained polymorphic VT. No other ventricular arrhythmia could be initiated by single or double extrastimuli in the control state. After 1,500 mg of procainamide, a sustained uniform VT was initiated with double extrastimuli. The tachycardia was reproducibly initiated as well as reproducibly terminated, as shown in the **bottom panel**. (From Horowitz LN, Greenspan AM, Spielman SR, et al. Torsades de pointes: Electrophysiologic studies in patients without transient pharmacologic or metabolic abnormalities. *Circulation* 1981;63:1120.)

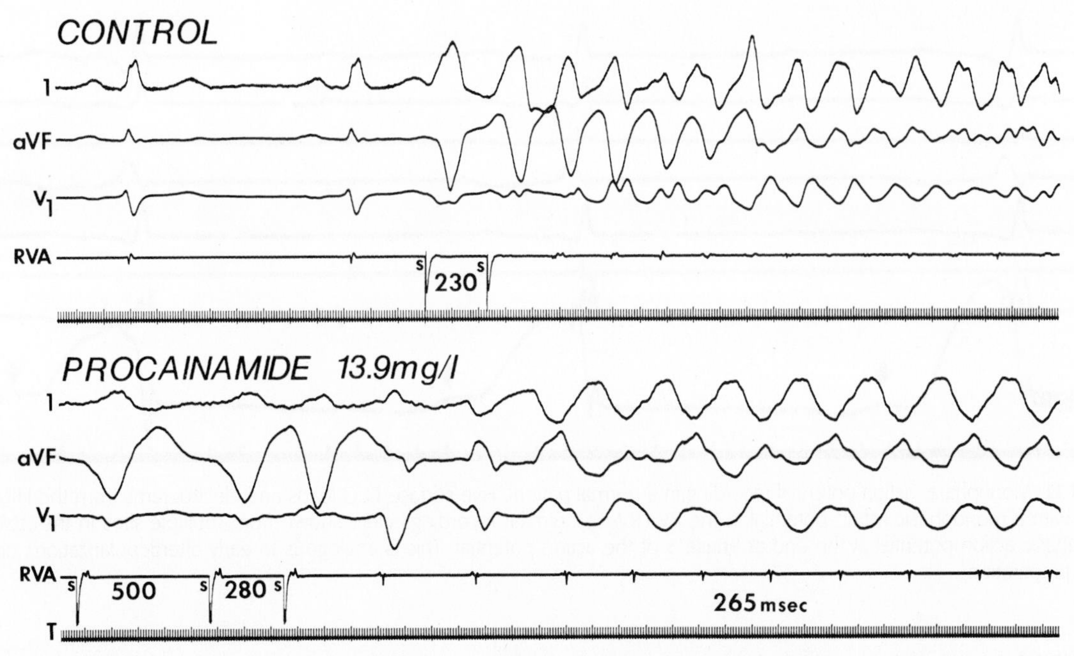


**FIGURE 11-120** Change from induction of VF to induction of sustained uniform VT by procainamide. In the control state, double ventricular extrastimuli during sinus rhythm initiate VF. Following 1,200 mg of procainamide producing a plasma level of 13.9 mg/L, a single extrastimulus delivered during right ventricular pacing initiates a uniform sustained VT. See text for discussion.

may be initiated with rigorous stimulation protocols, this is not significantly different from the response to comparable stimulation in patients with no history of ventricular tachyarrhythmias. These VT may be sustained or nonsustained and most likely represent nonspecific responses unrelated to the clinical arrhythmia. Therefore, the goal of programmed stimulation should not be to induce these arrhythmias.

The infusion of isoproterenol in patients with hereditary long QT syndrome may initiate a polymorphic tachycardia.[111,241,255] It may also induce polymorphic VT in patients with normal QT intervals who have a clinical history of adrenergically mediated polymorphic VT. Some of these adrenergically mediated polymorphic VT with normal QT intervals may represent ryanodine receptor defects responsible for catecholaminergic polymorphic VT, such patients could represent a genotypic congenital long QT1 syndrome but are phenotypically normal due to incomplete penetrance. It may also represent an overlap syndrome. Resolution of this question requires further study. Clearly, it will be necessary to develop different types of stimulation protocols if one is to use programmed stimulation to initiate **clinically relevant polymorphic VT** in congenital or acquired bradycardic-dependent long QT syndromes.

Cranefield and Aronson[130] suggested that the short-long-short sequence that characterizes torsade de pointes (i.e., bradycardic-dependent arrhythmias) would not be induced with typical stimulation protocols. Denker et al.[151] however, employed short-long-short sequence protocols to facilitate initiation of typical sustained uniform VT. Its use in studying arrhythmias in the bradycardic-dependent long QT syndromes has not been reported. In my experience, this stimulation protocol has not been able to initiate VT other than those that we would consider nonspecific responses in this patient population. Perhaps a stimulation protocol could be developed that mimics bigeminal sequences during which VES can be delivered to initiate the bradycardic-dependent polymorphic VT associated with long QT syndromes. We have tried such a stimulation protocol in a few patients and have not been successful in initiating any type of tachycardia with any more frequency than those in patients with normal QT intervals and no arrhythmias. These are very preliminary data, however; further work is necessary to devise a protocol that may specifically induce arrhythmias in these patients.

Failure to initiate specific polymorphic VTs in patients with long QT interval syndromes is consistent with an automatic mechanism or an initiating mechanism that is due to triggered activity secondary to early afterdepolarizations. This theory has been proposed for the bradycardic-dependent long QT interval syndromes (classic torsade de pointes).[111,130] The experimental data concerning early afterdepolarizations are certainly consistent with this mechanism.[111,129,130,267–269] Most of the experimental studies have used cesium chloride to initiate early afterdepolarizations and triggered activity. Vos et al.[270] have developed a model of "inducible" torsades de pointes by creating heart block and administering sotalol. Beta-adrenergic stimulation and left stellate stimulation may also facilitate early afterdepolarizations and arrhythmias.[111,271,272] Monophasic action potential recordings in experimental studies and in humans[111,269,273,274] purport to show afterdepolarizations in cesium-induced torsade de pointes or in patients with long QT syndromes. We have used monophasic action potentials in an attempt to assess the specificity of such findings. Unfortunately, we have seen potentials that would be classically defined as early afterdepolarizations in virtually all normal subjects (Fig. 11-121) that look quite similar to those

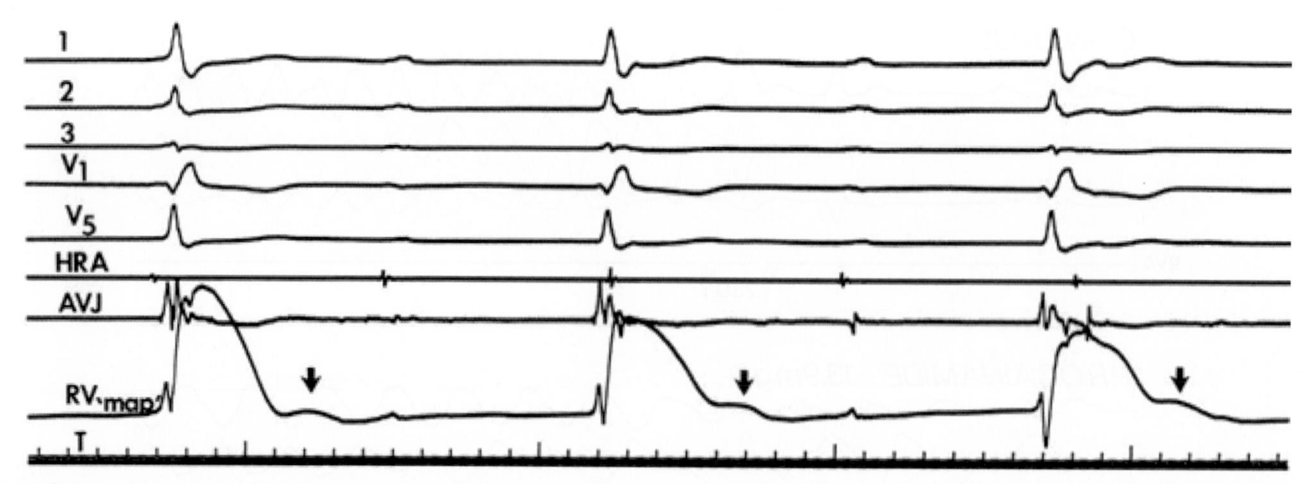


**FIGURE 11-121** Monophasic action potential recording in a normal patient. Five surface ECG leads and electrograms from the HRA and AVJ are shown along with a monophasic action potential in the RV ($RV_{'map'}$). Similar recordings were shown from multiple sites in the LV. Note a hump in the monophasic action potential at the end of Phase 3 of the action potential. This is analogous to early afterdepolarizations observed in an experimental preparation.

reported by Levine et al.[269] in cesium-induced polymorphic VT (Fig. 11-122). Thus, caution must be given to interpretation of these abnormal deflections. They may reflect electrotonic influence of heterogeneity of refractoriness of adjacent cells or bear some relationship to aftercontractions. To rule out the former, it would be necessary to record from microelectrodes in tissues around the area from which monophasic potentials are recorded to ensure that dispersion of action potentials does not produce these "humps" on monophasic action potentials recorded from the center of the tissue. This obviously cannot be done in humans. Similar humps with timing consistent with DADs can also be recorded in normal humans.

Thus, at this time I urge caution in interpreting abnormal potentials observed from the right or left ventricle in

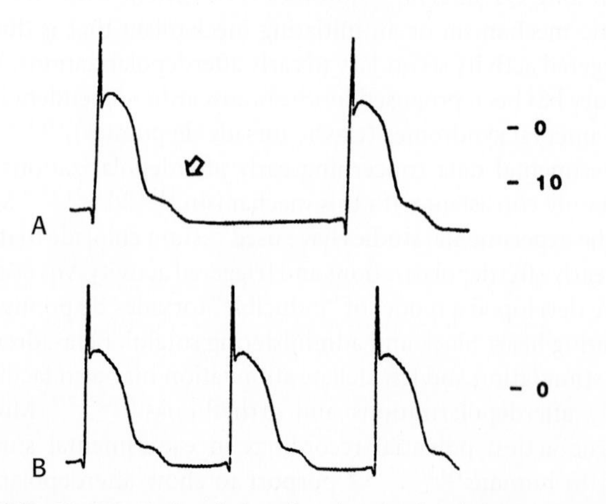


**FIGURE 11-122** Cesium-induced early afterdepolarizations. **A** and **B:** Early afterdepolarizations (*arrow*) associated with cesium-induced polymorphic VT are shown. Atrial overdrive pacing in **(B)** leads to a progressive attenuation of the afterdepolarizations (*arrow*) at the shorter cycle length. (Adapted from Levine JH, Spear JP, Guarnieri T, et al. Cesium chloride-induced long QT syndrome: demonstration of afterdepolarizations and triggered activity in vivo. *Circulation* 1985;72:1092.)

patients with polymorphic VT. Even if one can demonstrate that such humps are not a manifestation of electrotonic interaction of dispersion of refractoriness and were due to a local or diffuse abnormality delaying repolarization currents, this does not mean that these abnormalities are causally related to the arrhythmias. Moreover, investigators of cesium-mediated early afterdepolarization have questioned whether the sustained arrhythmias that occur following the initial afterdepolarization are not due to enhanced abnormal automaticity.[129] Although bradycardic-dependent and adrenergic-dependent long QT syndromes differ in clinical presentation and in setting factors, the electrocardiographic abnormalities of the T waves and U waves and the morphologic similarity of arrhythmias have led some investigators to suggest that both are related to early afterdepolarizations.[111] Substantiation of this proposal is required; so far none exists. Regardless of whether or not early afterdepolarizations initiate these arrhythmias, most investigators believe the sustained arrhythmia is due to reentry.[108,275,276]

In my opinion, long QT intervals that are congenital and adrenergic dependent (LQTS1 and some LQTS2) should be considered distinct from those secondary to transient abnormalities that are bradycardic dependent. The marked adrenergic dependency of these congenital syndromes, which are usually associated with normal or rapid heart rates, suggests a different mechanism of arrhythmogenesis may be operative. Certainly, catecholamines can facilitate early afterdepolarizations if the rate of the ventricular rhythm can be controlled by producing heart block.[270] In the clinical situation, adrenergic stimulation (by isoproterenol infusion) produces a tachycardia that abolishes early afterdepolarizations yet can facilitate initiation of polymorphic VT in some patients with congenital long QT syndromes. As noted earlier in the chapter, marked heterogeneity of refractory periods has been observed in these patients. In this instance, local differences in APD may lead to electrotonically mediated afterdepolarizations, reflected reentry, or fibrillation analogous to that in acute myocardial infarction, which seems to proceed down voltage gradients.[108,112,277] Recent experimental evidence suggests reentry due to disparate action potentials in the wall of the myocardium is responsible for arrhythmias in the LQTS.[108,112,274–276] If this were true in humans, polymorphic VT should be more reproducibly initiated in a higher percent of patients. Whether both potassium channel or sodium channel–based LQTS have the same mechanism of initiation (or maintenance) is unresolved.

Abnormalities of the autonomic nervous system have been considered responsible for some of the LQTS, particularly LQTS1 and LQTS2.[244] Certainly, stimulation of the left stellate ganglion has produced QT–T-wave changes and arrhythmias analogous to that seen in the congenital long QT syndrome.[244,278,279] Early use of cervical stellectomy proved useful in treating these patients, although not universally so.[244,280–283] More recent use of videoscopic stellectomy to the level of T1-T4 has been more successful without producing Horner syndrome.[240,276] Beta-adrenergic blockers alone or in combination with sedative or antiepileptic drugs may also be useful.[244] Whether these are specific for any genotype of LQTS is not known. Demonstration of abnormal sympathetic innervation of the human heart in patients with congenital long QT syndromes has not been extensively evaluated. We and others[244] have used meta-iodo benzylguanidine (MIBG, which is an analog of guanethidine and norepinephrine) scanning to evaluate patients with arrhythmias. Using this technique, we have demonstrated marked heterogeneity of MIBG uptake in patients with hereditary long QT interval syndromes whether or not they are on beta-blockade therapy. These preliminary data are exciting and support the hypothesis that the clinical arrhythmias associated with at least some LQTS patients may be primarily related to an imbalance of sympathetic activity. All of our patients with heterogeneity of MIBG had catecholamine-mediated LQTS. Additional studies are necessary to document these abnormalities in a larger group of patients with different LQTS as well as to show their functional significance, perhaps by correlating them with changes in refractoriness and genotype.

One of the major issues still to be addressed is whether or not the QT interval is related to, or just a marker of, these arrhythmias. In patients with congenital long QT syndrome successful therapy with beta-blocking drugs or stellectomy, the QT intervals may remain long in the absence of recurrent tachycardias.[111,244,281–284] Thus, more work is necessary to relate the abnormalities of the QT interval to the genesis of arrhythmias. The exact mechanisms for initiation and maintenance of the polymorphic VTs in the LQTS remain elusive. It is likely that multiple mechanisms are operative.

### *Mechanism of QRS Morphology in Polymorphic Ventricular Tachycardia*

Although the mechanisms of polymorphic VT associated with a normal or prolonged (congenital or acquired) QT interval are probably different, the morphologic characteristics of the tachycardia are surprisingly similar. In analyzing intracardiac recordings during polymorphic VT in patients with normal QT intervals, we have noted that chaotic electrical activity usually follows a period of rapid VT, and either spreads from one area through the entire heart or appears simultaneously in several parts of the heart (Figs. 11-109 to 11-111).[266] Moreover, similar polymorphic VT could be associated with discrete electrograms that were asynchronous (Fig. 11-114). These observations suggested that regardless of the exact mechanism generating the primary arrhythmia, multiple simultaneous wavefronts on the heart were necessary for the surface QRS to look polymorphic. Ideker et al.,[285] recording from multiple simultaneous sites in a canine model of VF, observed that during the early cycles of VF (which are identical to polymorphic VT) repetitive focal excitation could lead to multiple wavefronts on the heart before completion of global cardiac activation.

These investigators suggested that the early QRS complexes of polymorphic VT or VF could be due to an accelerating single VT focus regardless of mechanism. This was analogous to our previously described findings in humans.[266] Recently, two canine models of quinidine-related torsade de pointes have been reported.[286,287] One required additional ischemia and programmed stimulation[286] while the other required at least two sites of aconitine-induced early afterdepolarizations.[287] Both suggested that at least two simultaneous epicardial wavefronts were required to produce the ECG characteristics of polymorphic VT associated with torsade de pointes. In one of these studies,[286] simultaneous pacing from two epicardial sites asynchronously at slightly different rates induced polymorphic VT. These data suggest that regardless of the mechanism of polymorphic VT (i.e., enhanced automaticity, triggered activity that is due to early afterdepolarizations or focal reentry), the pattern of ventricular activation is responsible for the ECG manifestations. Therefore, ECG characteristics alone should not be used to imply a specific mechanism for the arrhythmia. As such, one must continue to think of polymorphic VT-VF associated with normal QT intervals, congenitally long QT intervals, acquired long QT intervals, and catecholaminergic PMVT as distinct disorders, each having a specific mechanism whose ultimate electrocardiographic expression is polymorphic VT.

## Initiation of Monomorphic Nonsustained Ventricular Tachycardia

Although electrophysiologic studies have been performed in patients with nonsustained monomorphic VT, it is difficult to evaluate the electrophysiologic characteristics of this arrhythmia. This is a consequence of the heterogeneity of the patient population and the mixing of patients with nonsustained and sustained monomorphic and polymorphic VT. Thus, limited information is available concerning initiation of nonsustained monomorphic VT other than in RVOT and other VTs caused by cyclic AMP–mediated triggered activity due to DADs (see below). Even those few studies that specifically address nonsustained VT often fail to distinguish between monomorphic and polymorphic VT.[40,41,162,288–292] The disease states in which this arrhythmia occurred were so diffuse that none of the studies are comparable. Thus, the differences in morphologic characteristics of VT and the diverse populations in which they occurred have been largely responsible for widely varied reported incidence of inducibility in patients with nonsustained VT. In a large study of nonsustained VT, Buxton et al.[289,291] attempted to consider these multiple factors. These investigators found that the number of daily episodes of spontaneous nonsustained VT and the number of complexes of VT during the spontaneous episodes did not influence inducibility. They observed that the highest rate of inducibility of nonsustained VT was in patients with coronary artery disease, prior infarction, and low ejection fraction. Those patients with cardiomyopathy and other cardiac disorders or without heart disease had a much lower incidence of reproducibly initiated nonsustained VT. A similar conclusion was reached by Naccarelli et al.[162] although these authors failed to distinguish between polymorphic and monomorphic nonsustained VT. Because it may be difficult to distinguish monomorphic from polymorphic VT owing to the limited number of leads recorded during spontaneous episodes, potential misclassification is a limitation of all studies. For example, if a monitor lead equivalent to a $V_1$ or $V_2$ demonstrates the uniform, RBBB pattern, this does not mean that changes in axis could not be occurring. In such cases, a tachycardia may be considered monomorphic when it is actually polymorphic. Given this limitation, however, we analyzed 88 patients with coronary artery disease, prior infarction and nonsustained VT and demonstrated an inducibility rate (any ventricular tachyarrhythmia) of nearly 75% in this highly selected group (Fig. 11-53). An example of a spontaneous nonsustained VT with only a $V_1$ monitor and the induced arrhythmia is shown in Figure 11-123. Induced VTs may be short-lived, >5 to 10 beats, or may last for >15 beats (Fig. 11-124). Although the duration of induced VT initiated by single or double extrastimuli may roughly correlate with that of the spontaneous nonsustained VT, in >30% of patients with spontaneous nonsustained VT, a sustained VT may be initiated in the laboratory, usually by triple extrastimuli.

The induction of sustained monomorphic VT in patients who present with nonsustained uniform VT is primarily limited to patients with coronary artery disease, prior infarction, and depressed ejection fraction. Sustained polymorphic VT may be initiated in any patient, but as mentioned earlier in the chapter, this may be a nonspecific response. Sustained monomorphic VT can be initiated in approximately 30% of patients with nonsustained VT and prior infarction and reduced ejection fractions. This has been confirmed in the MUSTT.[293] If one analyzes **hospitalized** patients with prior infarction, nonsustained monomorphic VT and ejection fractions <40%, the rate of inducible sustained uniform VT approaches 50%. The factors related to induction of sustained monomorphic VT are the presence of a prior infarction, low ejection fraction, and left ventricular aneurysms.[40] Of note, two-thirds of the patients in whom sustained monomorphic VT is induced required triple extrastimuli. Nonsustained VT is usually induced in the same patient with a lesser number of VES (Fig. 11-125). We have evaluated the role of the SAECG in predicting those patients with uniform nonsustained VT in

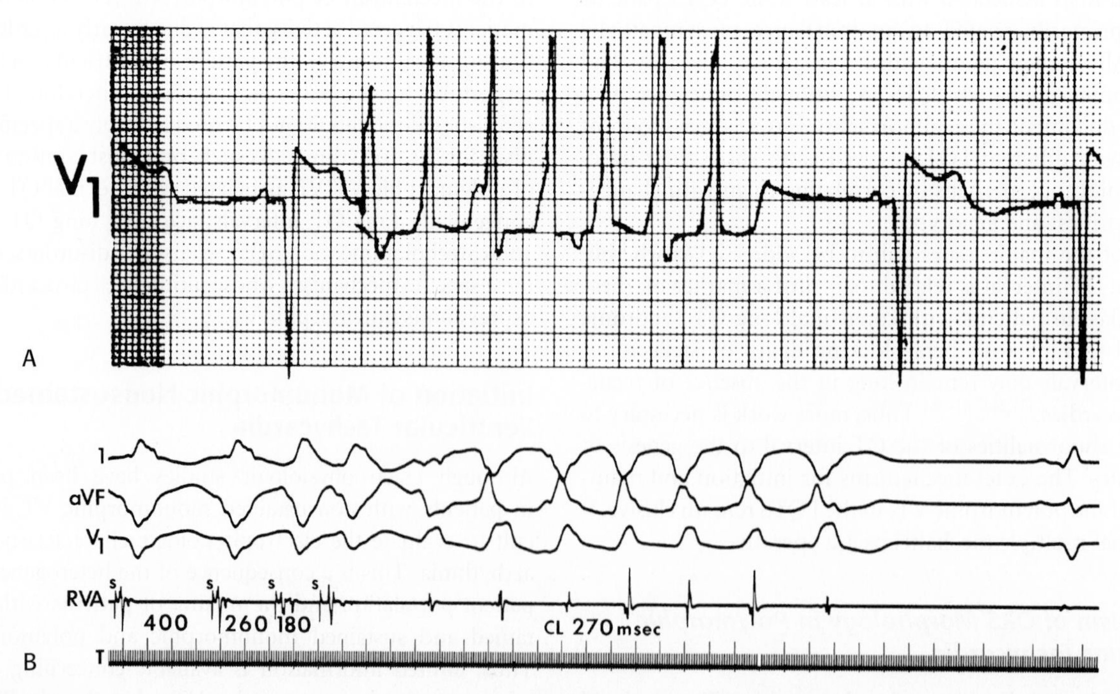


**FIGURE 11-123** Initiation of nonsustained VT. **A:** A rhythm strip demonstrating a seven-beat run of NS-VT with a right bundle branch block morphology. **B:** Double extrastimuli during a basic drive cycle length of 400 msec induces a seven-beat run of nonsustained VT in the same patient.

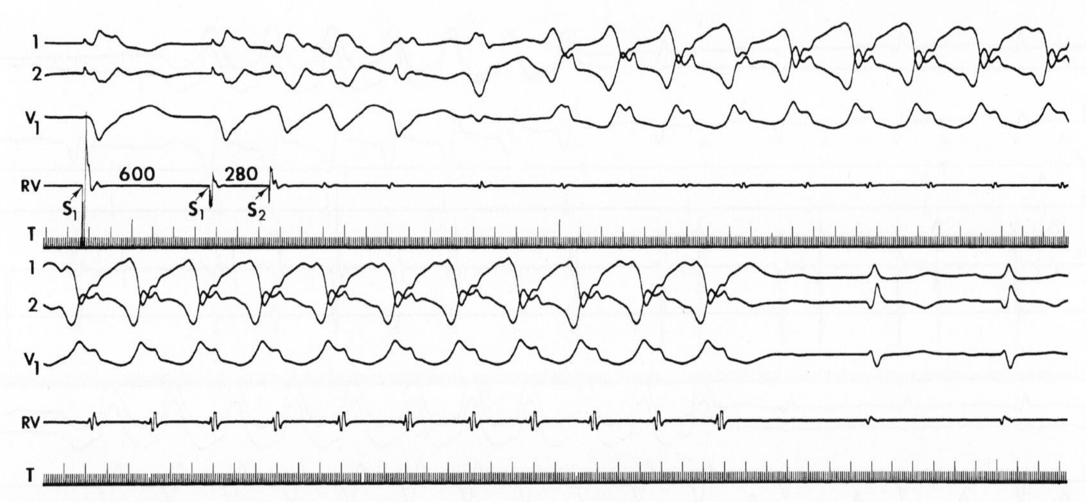


**FIGURE 11-124** Initiation of a prolonged run of VT. A single extrastimulus delivered from the VA during a drive cycle length of 600 msec initiates a 20-beat run of nonsustained VT. The patient has a prior inferior wall myocardial infarction.

whom sustained VT could be induced.[96–98,294] Although this technique is sensitive (i.e., >80% of patients with inducible sustained VT will have a positive SAECG, usually a prolonged duration of the ECG), it has a positive predictive value of only approximately 60%, and in the MUSTT study was not of value in predicting which patients would have inducible sustained monomorphic VT. This may be a consequence of the fact that patients with nonsustained VT and anterior infarction have a much lower incidence of positive SAECG than those with inferior infarction. This may relate to the observation that infarction-related conduction delay at the base of the heart further extends electrograms that are already activated late in the QRS, thereby facilitating the appearance of a late potential. Infarction of the apex or anterior wall is associated with conduction delay that begins within the QRS and is less likely to be seen as an extension beyond the end of the QRS unless the conduction delay is marked. It is my impression that such conduction delay in anterior infarction is usually associated with spontaneous sustained VT. Patients with lesser amounts of conduction delay and anterior infarction frequently present with cardiac arrest. Thus, I believe the patients who are studied with nonsustained VT and coronary artery disease are a selected population, usually composed of a higher number of patients with prior inferior infarction.

As noted, in most patients with coronary artery disease and prior infarction, single or double VES can initiate nonsustained VT. Rapid pacing rarely improves the inducibility rate. This is not true, however, in patients with normal hearts, particularly those with exercise-related tachycardias, which account for a significant component of the so-called repetitive monomorphic tachycardias.[96,163,295–299] Although the majority of these tachycardias arise from the right or left ventricular outflow tract, they can arise from essentially anywhere in the myocardium and are thought due to the same

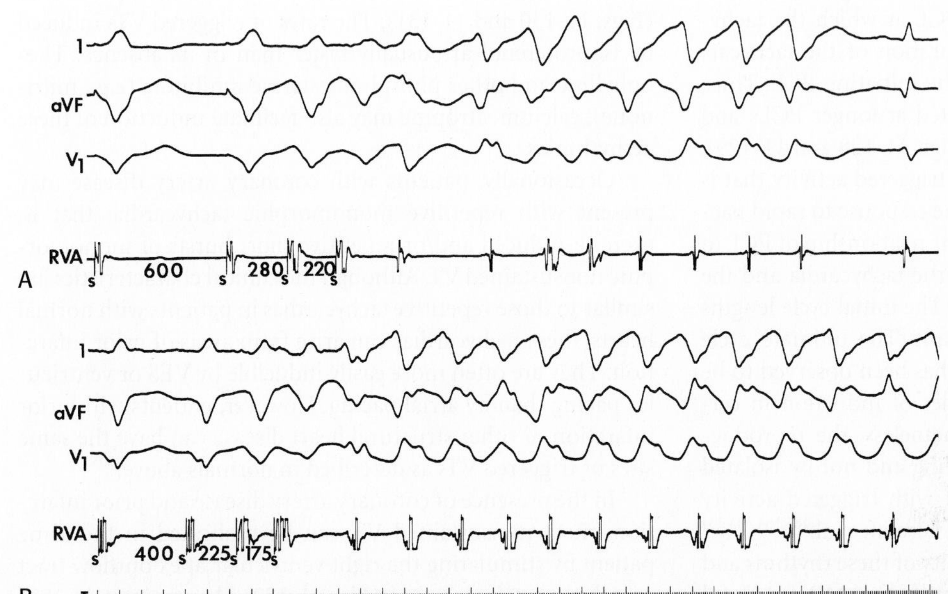


**FIGURE 11-125** Initiation of nonsustained and sustained VT in a patient with coronary artery disease. **A:** Double extrastimuli delivered from the RVA initiate nonsustained VT with a right bundle right superior axis morphology. **B:** When a shorter drive cycle length is used and close-coupled extrastimuli are delivered, sustained uniform VT is initiated. Note that the sustained VT has a similar morphology to the terminal four complexes of the NSVT. See text for discussion.

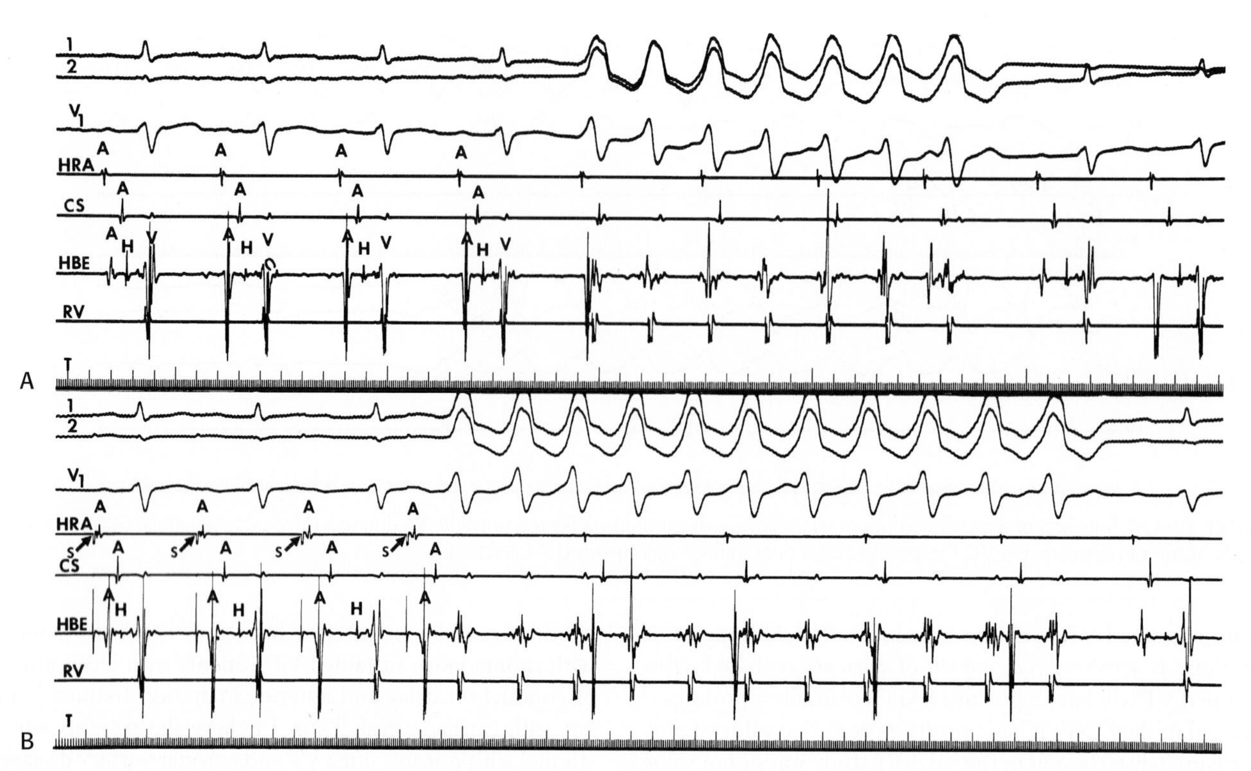


**FIGURE 11-126** Induction of nonsustained ventricular tachycardia by atrial pacing. **A:** A spontaneous episode of NSVT lasting seven beats is observed. The morphology is left bundle left inferior axis. **B:** HRA pacing at 500 msec initiates nonsustained VT with the same morphology and cycle length as the spontaneous episode. This patient had no organic heart disease.

mechanism, cyclic AMP–mediated DADs.[300] In addition to the RV outflow tract, there are other sites that frequently give rise to idiopathic VT, including the left and right sinuses of Valsalva, the tricuspid and mitral annulae, and the LV anterior epicardium.[184,301,302] In these patients atrial or ventricular pacing are the most common methods of tachycardia initiation. Although VES can initiate these tachycardias, the vast majority can be initiated by atrial or ventricular pacing alone or following the administration of isoproterenol (Figs. 11-126 and 11-127). Usually, there is a critical PCL at which the tachycardia is initiated. Frequently, the duration of the tachycardia bears an inverse relationship to the initiating PCL. Thus, nonsustained episodes may be initiated at longer PCLs and sustained episodes at shorter PCLs (Figs. 11-128 and 11-129). Unlike most experimental models of triggered activity that is due to DADs,[125,126,128,180] in humans the response to rapid pacing uncommonly demonstrates a linear relationship of PCL to the coupling interval to the onset of the tachycardia and the early cycles (Figs. 11-127 to 11-129). The initial cycle lengths of the tachycardia are usually constant. The ultimate cycle length of sustained triggered activity has been observed to be constant in response to various modes of induction in certain experimental preparations. Nonetheless, the reproducible initiation primarily by rapid pacing and not by isolated extrastimuli appears more consistent with triggered activity that is due to DADs than with reentry. Lerman et al.[163,164,303,304] have demonstrated adenosine sensitivity of these rhythms and suggested that the response supports a cyclic AMP–mediated triggered activity mechanism. Such rhythms can also be terminated by carotid sinus pressure and other vagal maneuvers as well as by beta blockers and calcium channel blockers.

As noted, exercise frequently precipitates these arrhythmias spontaneously. Not surprisingly, therefore, the administration of isoproterenol facilitates the induction of the arrhythmia by VES or the development of spontaneous nonsustained or sustained arrhythmias when stimulation was required to produce nonsustained VT before the administration of isoproterenol (Figs. 11-130 and 11-131). The rates of triggered VTs induced by isoproterenol are usually faster than in its absence. Theophylline and other phosphodiesterase inhibitors (e.g., milrinone), calcium, atropine may also facilitate induction of these arrhythmias.

Occasionally, patients with coronary artery disease may present with repetitive monomorphic tachycardia; that is, exercise-induced and/or repetitive short bursts of monomorphic nonsustained VT. Although the clinical characteristics are similar to those repetitive tachycardias in patients with normal hearts, these tachycardias can arise from areas of prior infarction. They are often more easily inducible by VES or ventricular pacing than by atrial pacing. However, patients with prior infarction or other structural heart disease can have the same sites of triggered VTs as described in normals above.[305]

In the presence of coronary artery disease and prior infarction, most nonsustained VT can be replicated in the same patient by stimulating the right ventricular apex outflow tract or other ventricular sites (Fig. 11-132). Approximately 15%

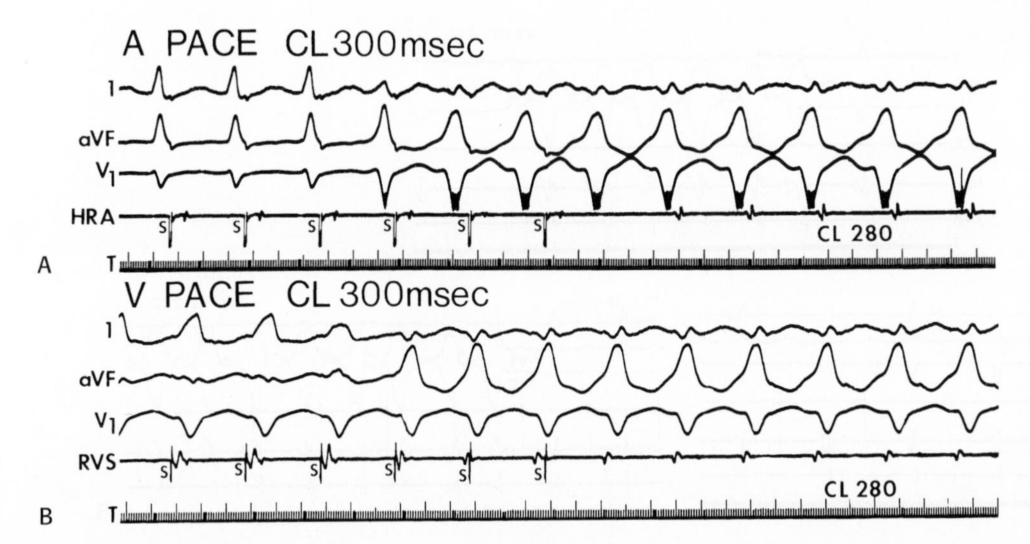


**FIGURE 11-127** Initiation of monomorphic tachycardia by atrial and ventricular pacing. **A:** VT with a left bundle right inferior axis is induced by atrial pacing at a cycle length of 300 msec. **B:** Ventricular posing at the same cycle length induces an identical tachycardia. See text for discussion.

of patients with nonsustained uniform VT will require a second site to induce VT. The vast majority will be subsequently initiated from the right ventricular outflow tract. In approximately 10% of cases, left ventricular stimulation is required (Fig. 11-133). Most of the nonsustained VT that is initiated is initiated by one or two VES but 15% to 20% require triple extrastimuli.

Heretofore, it has not been possible to demonstrate prolonged conduction delay and/or block associated with initiation of the tachycardia so that that criterion for reentry cannot be evaluated. This is due to our inability to map nonsustained VT. Newer technologies that allow for simultaneous multisite mapping may provide this capability. Indirect evidence supports reentry as the mechanism of most nonsustained VT associated with coronary artery disease. Class I agents such as procainamide can change nonsustained VT to sustained VT (Fig 11-134). This is usually associated with increased ease of induction of the tachycardia (i.e., initiation using longer coupling intervals or at longer drive cycle lengths) and a prolongation of the tachycardia cycle length. Facilitation of induction of sustained VT by drugs that slow conduction almost only occurs in the presence of coronary disease. It may therefore suggest a reentrant mechanism because this situation is analogous to that described earlier in the discussion of sustained VT. Such patients may give a history of syncope associated with rapid palpitations following the empiric administration of such agents. Thus, we believe initiation of sustained uniform VT following administration of a drug in a patient who has never had symptoms in the absence of a drug, but in whom symptomatic arrhythmias occurred following administration of the drug, suggests a proarrhythmic effect of the drug. The induction of sustained VT in the absence of drugs also has

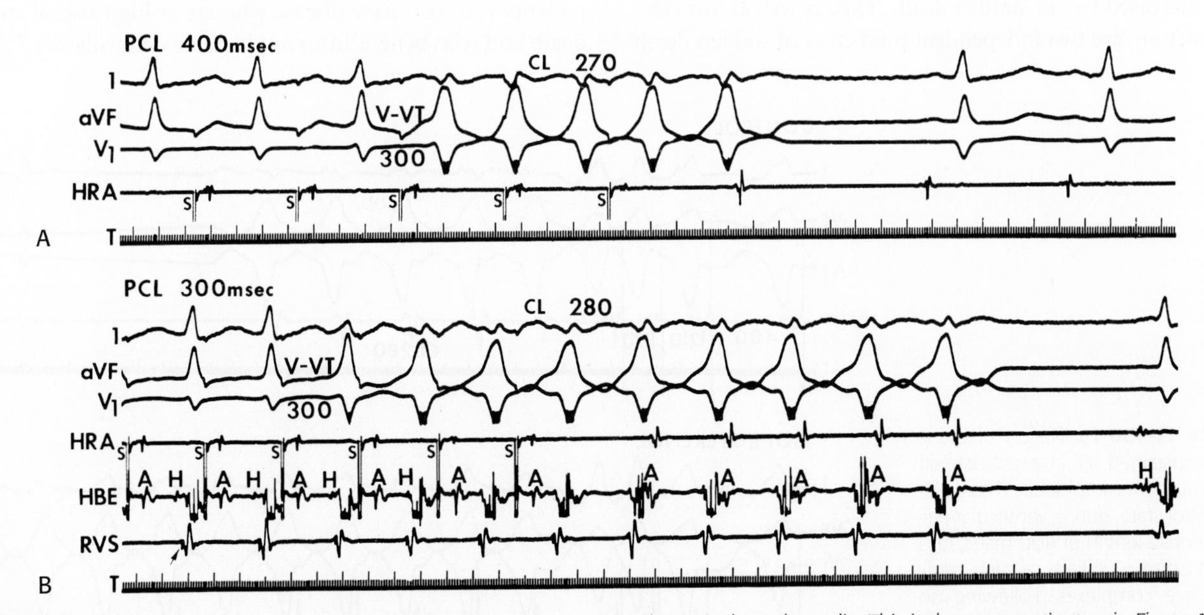


**FIGURE 11-128** Effect of drive cycle length on the duration of nonsustained ventricular tachycardia. This is the same patient as in Figure 11-127. **A:** During atrial pacing at a cycle length of 400 msec, nonsustained VT is induced and lasts five complexes. **B:** When the paced cycle length is reduced to 300 msec, a longer run of nonsustained VT is induced.

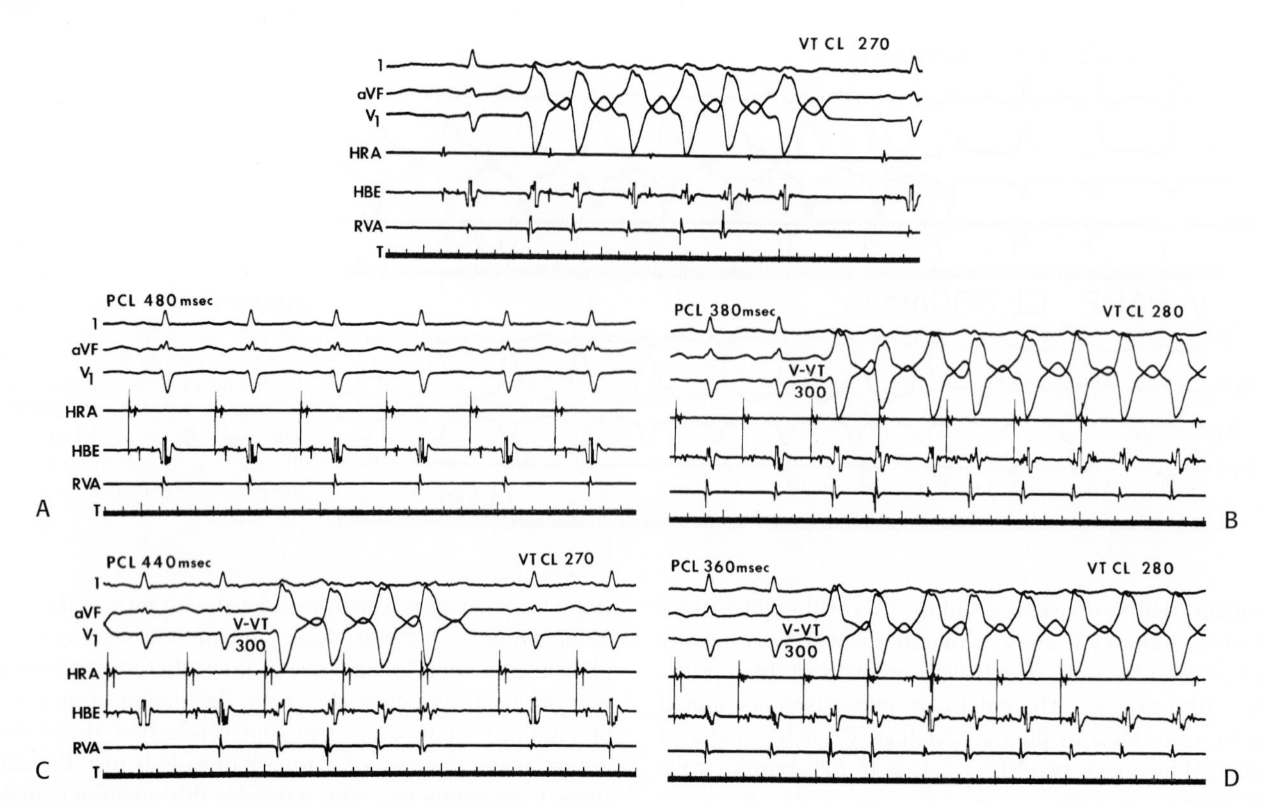


**FIGURE 11-129** Critical role of cycle length on induction of nonsustained ventricular tachycardia. In the top, a spontaneous episode of VT is seen. **A–D:** Atrial pacing at progressively shorter CLs is shown. **A:** When the paced cycle length is 480 msec, no VT is induced. **B:** At a paced cycle length of 440 msec, a four-beat run of VT is induced. **C:** When the paced cycle length is reduced to 380 msec, a prolonged run of nonsustained VT is present. **D:** When the cycle length is further decreased to 360 msec, a prolonged episode is again induced. Note that the interval from the last paced complex to the onset of the VT is constant, regardless of the paced cycle length, and that the cycle length of the tachycardia (VT CL) remains constant, regardless of the paced cycle length. See text for discussion.

clinical significance.[291,293] We have demonstrated that those patients who present with spontaneous nonsustained VT and coronary artery disease and in whom sustained VT is induced are at increased risk of sudden death. This, as well as low ejection fraction, are two independent predictors of sudden death that are additive. We and others have recently demonstrated that programmed stimulation in patients with nonsustained VT and ejection fractions <40% may identify a group of patients with coronary disease who are at high risk of sudden death and who benefit from implantable defibrillators.[291,293,306]

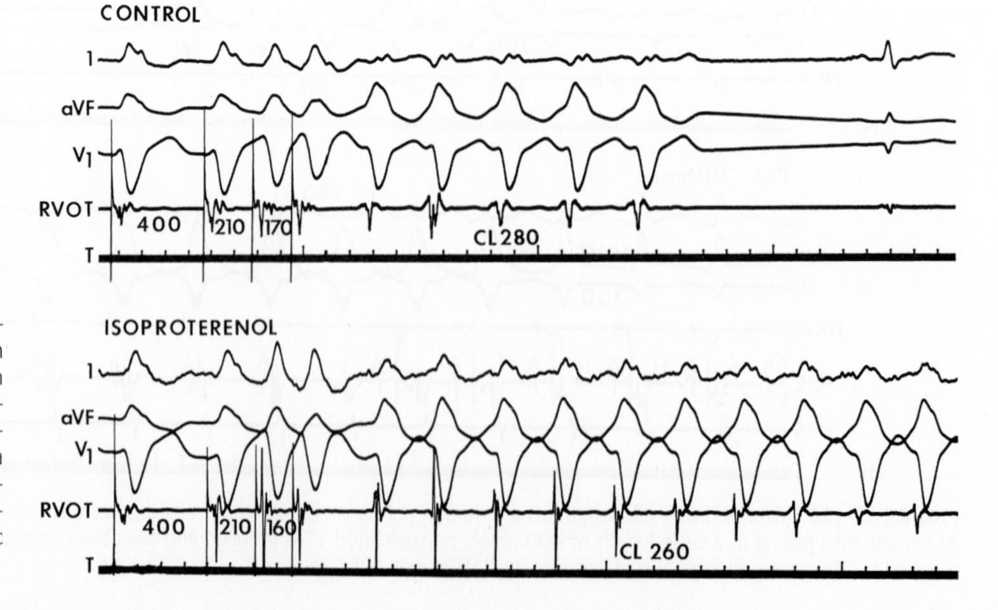


**FIGURE 11-130** Facilitation of induction of sustained VT in a patient with repetitive monomorphic tachycardia. In the control state, during ventricular pacing at a cycle length of 400 msec, double extrastimuli initiate a tachycardia lasting five complexes. Following isoproterenol, ventricular stimuli of comparable prematurity at the same basic cycle length initiate a sustained VT.

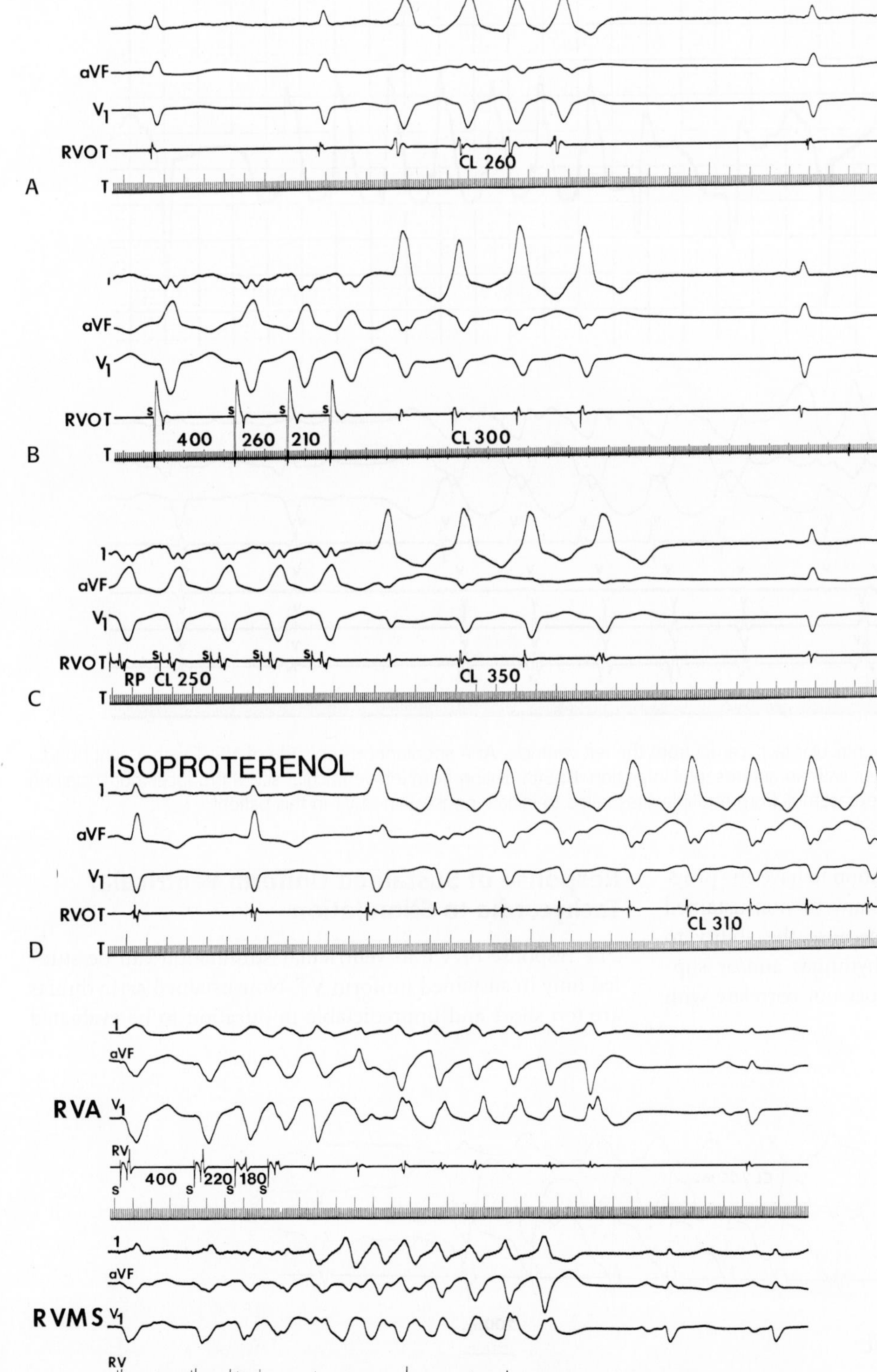


**FIGURE 11-131** Spontaneous initiation of VT following isoproterenol administration. **A:** A spontaneous four-beat episode of VT is shown. **B:** Double extrastimuli at a drive CL of 400 msec induces a four-beat run of VT. **C:** Rapid ventricular pacing also produces a four-beat run of VT. Note the cycle length of the VT is slower during burst pacing than it is following the introduction of double extrastimuli. **D:** Following a small dose of isoproterenol, which shortened the sinus CL from 840 msec to 560 msec, the spontaneous initiation of a sustained episode of VT occurs. Note that the cycle length of 310 msec is shorter than that following programmed stimulation.

**FIGURE 11-132** Induction of nonsustained ventricular tachycardia from multiple sites in the right ventricle. Double extrastimuli from the RVA, the right ventricular midseptum (RVMS), and RVOT initiate the same nonsustained VT.

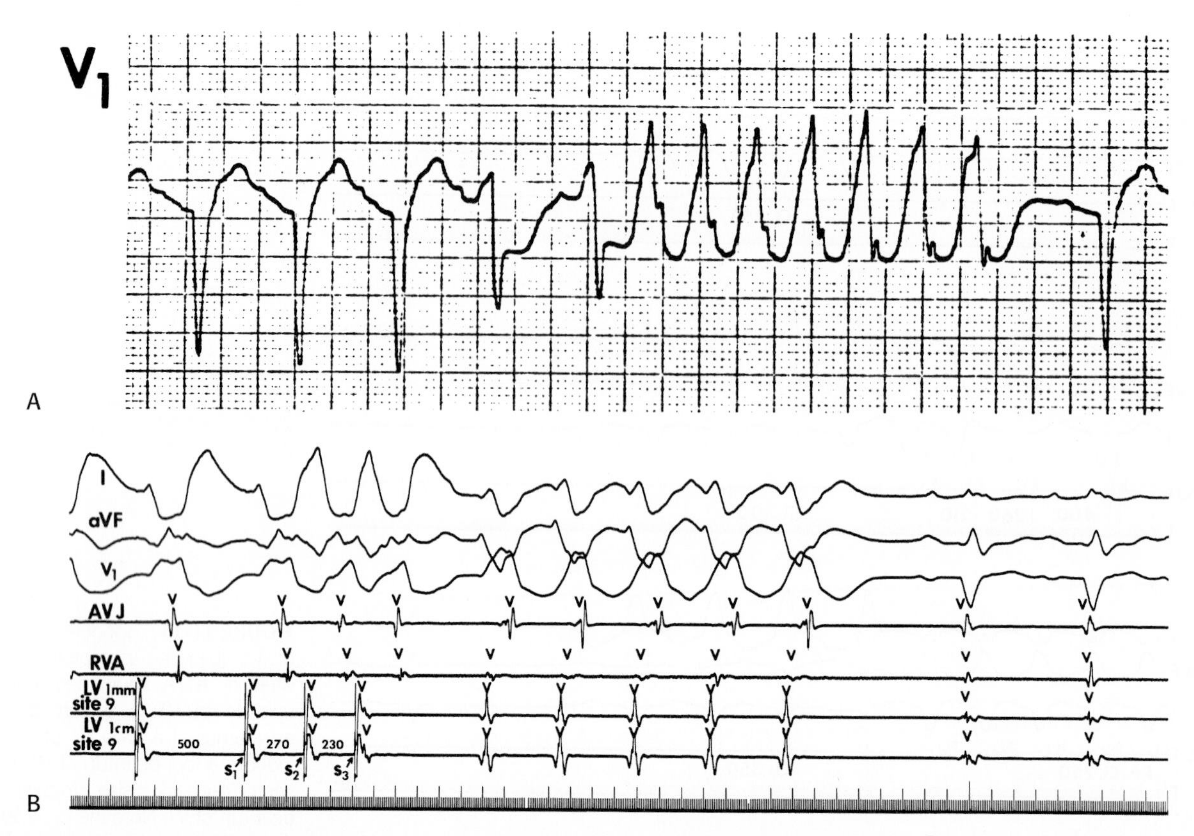


**FIGURE 11-133** Initiation of nonsustained ventricular tachycardia from the left ventricle. **A:** A spontaneous episode of NSVT with a right bundle branch block morphology is shown in a patient with an anteroseptal infarction. **B:** Stimulation from left ventricular site 9 produces nonsustained VT. Right ventricular stimulation with double extrastimuli from multiple sites failed to initiate nonsustained VT in this patient.

We have not found programmed stimulation to have any prognostic value in the evaluation and therapy of nonsustained VT associated with cardiomyopathy, because the ability to initiate nonsustained or sustained arrhythmias and/or suppress them by antiarrhythmic agents does not correlate with outcome.

## Response of Sustained Uniform Ventricular Tachycardia to Stimulation

The response of VT to ventricular stimulation can be studied only in sustained uniform VT. Nonsustained arrhythmias are too short and unpredictable in duration to be evaluated

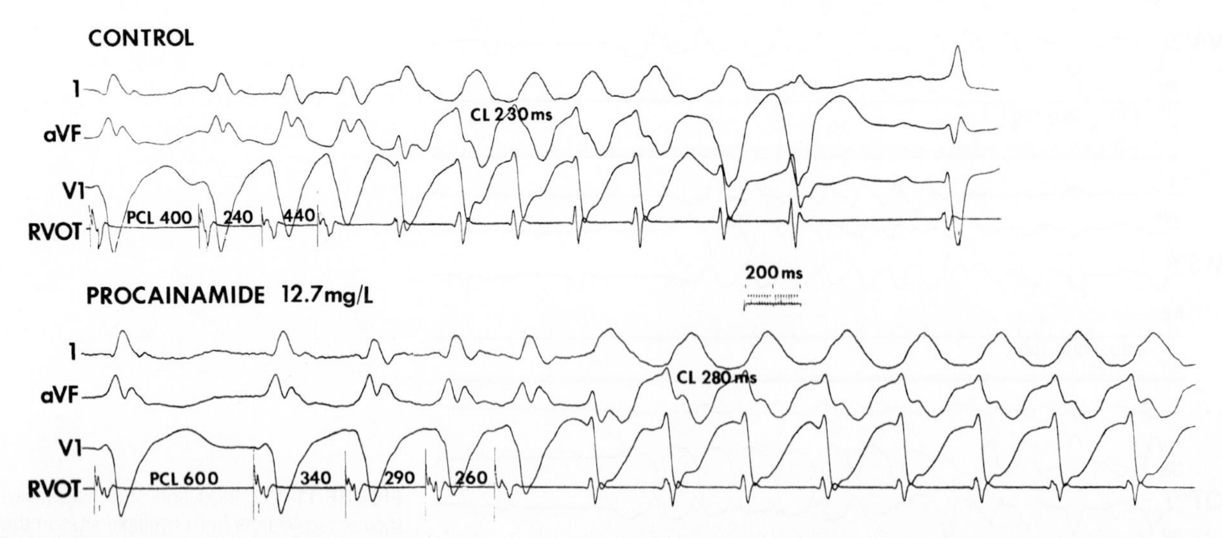


**FIGURE 11-134** Conversion of nonsustained ventricular tachycardia to sustained VT by procainamide. In the control state, double extrastimuli from the RVOT initiate NSVT with a left bundle branch block left axis deviation morphology. This was the same as the patient's spontaneous nonsustained VT. Following a loading dose of procainamide, triple extrastimuli initiate S-UVT with the same QRS morphology. See text for discussion.

meaningfully, and sustained polymorphic VT is invariably associated with rapid hemodynamic collapse. Sustained uniform VT is the only ventricular tachyarrhythmia to which programmed stimulation can be employed in an attempt to characterize its mechanism and potential therapy. Several responses to programmed extrastimuli and overdrive pacing during VT are possible, including the following: (a) no effect on the tachycardia (manifest and concealed perpetuation of VT); (b) resetting of the tachycardia by single, double, or multiple extrastimuli or continuous resetting of the tachycardia circuit by rapid pacing (i.e., entrainment); (c) overdrive suppression of the arrhythmia without termination; (d) overdrive acceleration of the tachycardia, with or without a change in morphology; and (e) termination. The evaluation of the effect of both programmed extrastimuli and overdrive pacing on sustained VT can provide insight into the underlying mechanism, the amount of ventricle required for that mechanism, defining critical sites for ablation, analyzing the effects of drugs on VT cycle length, and the potential role of ATP as a form of therapy.

As mentioned earlier in the chapter, experimental studies have been performed to assess the effects of single extrastimuli and overdrive pacing on automatic (normal and abnormal) and triggered rhythms.[125–128,180] Although those experiments used a variety of atrial and ventricular tissues in vitro, no comparable data are available from excised human tissues in which spontaneously occurring or induced sustained arrhythmias were similarly studied. Nonetheless, one can compare the response of human sustained VT to programmed stimulation with the responses of experimental arrhythmias of known mechanism. Automatic rhythms, which can be neither initiated nor terminated by programmed stimulation, can be reset by single extrastimuli and can demonstrate overdrive suppression.[51,126,127] Resetting of rhythms that are due to both normal and abnormal automaticity has been observed with a flat response curve having a return cycle approximating the rate of the automatic rhythm plus the time it takes the stimulated impulse to reach and return from the focus. This is analogous to resetting of the sinus node (see Chapter 3), but the stimulation site is usually farther from the automatic focus than high right atrial stimulation is from the sinus node. Overdrive suppression is voltage dependent and is thus primarily observed in cells exhibiting normal resting potentials (i.e., normal automaticity), while the absence of overdrive suppression, or the appearance of overdrive acceleration, is noted with automatic rhythms at lower resting membrane potentials (abnormal automaticity).[51,52,125,127]

Triggered activity that is due to DADs, particularly that which is caused by enhanced catecholamines, consistently demonstrates overdrive acceleration in response to rapid pacing. Thus, these rhythms demonstrate a positive correlation between the cycle length of overdrive pacing and the interval to the first complex of the resumed triggered rhythm and the initial cycle lengths of the triggered rhythm.[52,125–128,180] Once accelerated, these rhythms may gradually resume their original cycle length or may slow and terminate.[51,52,125–128] Termination of all nondigitalis-induced triggered activity caused by DADs is preceded by gradual slowing.[51,125,126,128] This is believed to be due to activation of the Na/K pump, which hyperpolarizes the cells so that threshold for DAD firing is not reached. The response of triggered activity caused by DADs to programmed extrastimuli is more variable and can demonstrate a flat resetting response with the return cycle 100% to 110% of the cycle length of the original triggered activity (plus the time to and from the stimulus site to the site of the triggered activity), a shortening of the return cycle in response to increasingly premature extrastimuli (i.e., a direct relationship to coupling interval), or termination. Termination by either extrastimuli or overdrive pacing can be abrupt but is often preceded by several afterdepolarizations of increasing cycle length. Digitalis-induced triggered activity producing VT has been studied in the conscious canine model; a direct relationship of the return cycle to coupling interval of single extrastimuli and to overdrive pacing at rapid rates was demonstrated.[196] Of note, the duration of the first postpacing interval in response to either single extrastimuli or overdrive pacing was independent of the site of stimulation although the QRS morphology of the return cycle was dependent on the site of stimulation. In isolated tissues, the response of digitalis-induced triggered activity is somewhat more complex with regard to extrastimuli. Resetting with a flat response approximating 110% of the triggered cycle length is usually observed at long coupling intervals with single extrastimuli. A decrease in the return cycle may be observed with closely coupled double extrastimuli. Occasionally, an acute doubling of the return cycle may be seen if the first afterdepolarization fails to reach threshold.[129] A gradual increase in return cycle over a long range of decreasing coupling intervals has not been observed in any triggered rhythm. Rhythms that are due to early afterdepolarizations are less well studied, and some investigators believe that the sustained rhythms associated with early afterdepolarizations recorded by microelectrodes actually represent abnormal automaticity, because they do not typically demonstrate overdrive suppression and may occasionally demonstrate overdrive acceleration.[97,105]

The response of experimental reentrant arrhythmias to extrastimuli and overdrive pacing has been less well studied. Canine models of VT demonstrating reentrant excitation by activation mapping have been able to be terminated by overdrive pacing or extrastimuli.[29,307–309] The specific response patterns of the reentrant circuit to single extrastimuli and overdrive pacing (including entrainment) have been reported.[309–312] Peters et al.[311] recently characterized the spatial and temporal excitable gap of the canine model of **anisotropic reentrant VT** using high-density mapping. These investigators found a remarkable effect of anisotropy on the response to extrastimuli and on the characteristics of the resetting response curves. Complex resetting patterns were seen dependant on the relationship of the wavefront of activation and the reentrant circuit. Frame and Simson[313] described reentry in an anatomically determined reentrant circuit. They studied an in vitro preparation of canine atrial tissue surrounding the tricuspid valve having a fixed pathway but an incomplete recovery of excitability of the involved tissue. Although they observed resetting, complex response patterns were noted that were due to the effects of APD, conduction velocity, and diastolic intervals in different regions of the reentrant circuit. The complex relationships produced oscillations within the circuit that could predict and localize the site of termination. Relating the results of these models to human arrhythmias, in which only the output of the reentrant circuit is observed, is not possible.

The best documented reentrant arrhythmias in humans (i.e., those associated with the Wolff–Parkinson–White syndrome) have been studied in detail and have demonstrated resetting in response to single or multiple extrastimuli or rapid pacing and abrupt termination but have not demonstrated reproducible overdrive acceleration (see Chapter 10).[314]

Thus, the patterns of responses to single and multiple extrastimuli and overdrive pacing (analyzing resetting responses, overdrive suppression versus acceleration, entrainment, and/or termination), together with the knowledge of whether or not the rhythm is reproducibly initiated, can help distinguish automatic, triggered, or reentrant mechanisms. Evaluation of the response of a tachycardia to programmed stimulation is only possible in sustained, hemodynamically tolerated tachycardias. Thus, only in sustained monomorphic tachycardia can the response to programmed stimulation and overdrive pacing be assessed. Although nonsustained VT (regardless of morphology), or polymorphic VT/VF cannot be studied, in those patients in whom these arrhythmias can be changed to sustained uniform VT by drugs or stimulation techniques, evaluation of the response to overdrive stimulation and/or extrastimuli may be possible. In such cases, the response parallels that seen with uniform sustained VT.

## Protocol for Stimulation During Sustained VT

To evaluate the effects of stimulation on sustained uniform VT, the tachycardia must be well tolerated hemodynamically and must have a stable cycle length. Therefore, the response to programmed stimulation can be evaluated only in a selected group of patients with relatively slow VTs (cycle lengths usually ≥280 msec). This necessitates the inclusion of patients with monomorphic sustained VT slowed by antiarrhythmic agents. Stimulation protocols have varied among laboratories. Few studies have been performed using a carefully designed and systematic stimulation protocol; as a result, interpretation of responses with regard to underlying mechanism is limited. The major problem has been the immediate reaction of the investigator to try to terminate the tachycardia, thus limiting a systematic approach to understanding the response of the tachycardia to a specific mode of stimulation. In some instances, regardless of whether or not a systematic protocol is used, the appearance of a poorly tolerated tachycardia will necessitate abbreviating the protocol to safely and rapidly terminate the rhythm. Another limitation is that stimulation may change one tachycardia to another or accelerate it to VF. Nonetheless, use of a systematic approach is imperative if one is to interpret the response to programmed stimulation. Several factors influence the ability of extrastimuli and/or rapid pacing to interact with the tachycardia. These include VT cycle length (which is probably the most important); the refractory period at the stimulation site and at the site of impulse formation or the reentrant circuit; the conduction time from the site of stimulation to the site of impulse formation or reentrant circuit; and, in the case of reentrant arrhythmias, the duration of the excitable gap. These must be taken into account to properly interpret the significance of responses of VT to stimulation.

We use the following protocol to investigate the mechanism of sustained uniform VT.[1,315–320] Initially, single VES are delivered from the right ventricular apex with the use of an electrogram recorded from that catheter to synchronize the stimulation. Stimulation from other right and/or left ventricular sites may be carried out in a comparable manner to gain information relative to site specificity of a given response.[318,321] Stimulation at sites believed to be in the reentrant circuit is critical in delineating critical diastolic pathways to which one can target ablative energy to cure VT (see Mapping of VT later in this chapter and Chapter 13). It is essential that stimulation at these additional sites be performed systematically as will be described for the right ventricular apex. Initially, extrastimuli are delivered at coupling intervals just shorter than the VT cycle length. The coupling interval is decreased in 5- to 10-msec decrements until local refractoriness is reached. Analysis of the return cycle is necessary to evaluate whether or not the extrastimulus has influenced the tachycardia. If resetting or termination of the tachycardia is not observed with single extrastimuli, double extrastimuli should be delivered.

The most common reason for single extrastimuli to fail to terminate or influence the tachycardia is that the tachycardia cycle length is too short and/or local refractoriness too long to permit the stimulated impulse to reach the excitable gap of a reentrant tachycardia circuit or site of impulse formation in a focal tachycardia. In such instances, the use of two or more extrastimuli will usually succeed. The first extrastimulus acts as a conditioning extrastimulus and will shorten refractoriness at the stimulation site and alter the wavefront of activation from the stimulus site which reverses the wavefront of activation in the intervening tissue between the pacing site and the tachycardia. This will allow delivery of a second extrastimulus at a longer coupling interval, which can reach the tachycardia circuit (or focus) in time to affect it (Fig. 11-135). The first extrastimulus ($S_1$) is introduced at a coupling interval 20 msec greater than the longest coupling interval at which $S_1$ resets the tachycardia or 20 msec above refractoriness if $S_1$ failed to interact with the tachycardia. $S_2$ is then delivered at a coupling interval equal to the VT cycle length, and the $S_1$-$S_2$ interval is progressively decreased in 5- to 10-msec decrements. This method enables $S_1$-$S_2$ intervals to influence the tachycardia at comparable, or longer, coupling intervals than VT-$S_1$ intervals that failed to influence the VT (Fig. 11-135). Moreover, this

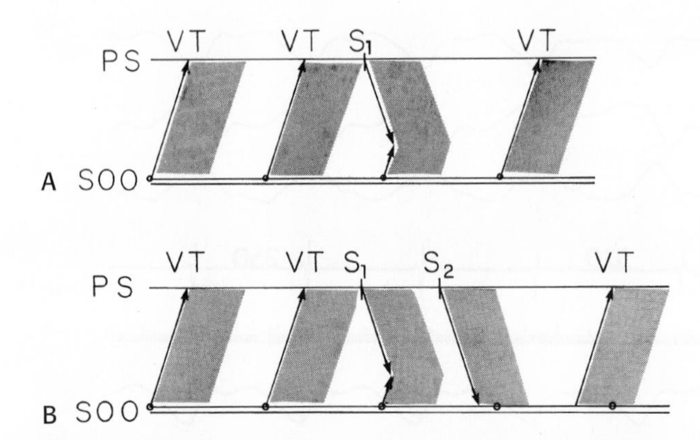


**FIGURE 11-135** Mechanism by which double extrastimuli facilitate reaching the site of origin during VT. The VT circuit or focus is shown at the **bottom** of the panel, and the wavefront of activation propagating toward the pacing site (PS) is shown at the top of each panel. A single extrastimulus in the **top panel** is limited by local refractoriness and cannot reach the site of the VT circuit or focus, colliding with it in the intervening tissue. In the **bottom panel** during the delivery of double extrastimuli, the first extrastimulus again fails to reach the site of origin of the VT; however, it peels back intervening tissue refractoriness and decreases local refractoriness which allow the second extrastimulus to reach and reset the VT circuit. (From Stamato NJ, Rosenthal ME, Almendral JM, et al. The resetting response of ventricular tachycardia to single and double extrastimuli: implications for an excitable gap. *Am J Cardiol* 1987;60:596.)

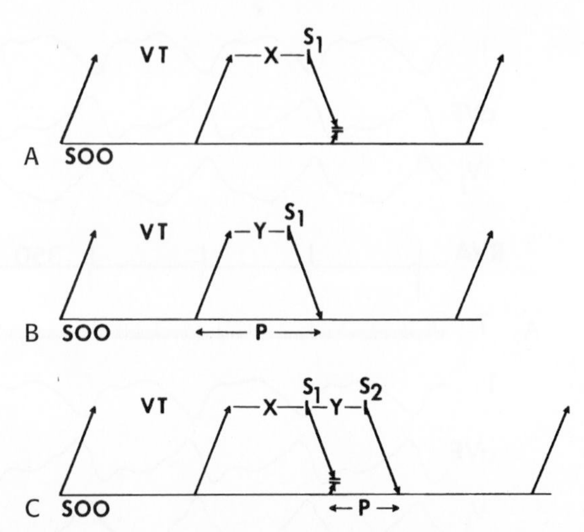


**FIGURE 11-136** Diagram showing how double extrastimuli, with the first extrastimulus set outside of the resetting zone determined with single extrastimuli, can achieve greater prematurity relative to the VT origin than can single extrastimuli with similar coupling intervals. **A–C:** Ventricular activation is represented by *arrows.* The ventricular activation of VT beats is represented as spreading from a site of origin SOD, whereas the activation of paced beats is represented in the opposite direction **A:** The activation wavefront generated by a single extrastimulus ($S_1$) with a coupling interval of X msec does not reach the site of origin, because of collision with the next VT wavefront. **B:** An earlier $S_1$ (coupling interval of Y msec) reaches the site of origin and resets the VT. **C:** However, if an extrastimulus ($S_2$) with the same coupling interval (Y) is preceded by an $S_1$ outside of the resetting zone (coupling interval of X msec), it achieves greater prematurity (P in **B** and **C**) relative to the site of origin of the VT. $S_1$, first extrastimulus; $S_2$, second extrastimulus. (From Almendral JM, Gottlieb CD, Rosenthal ME, et al. Entrainment of ventricular tachycardia: explanation for surface electrocardiographic phenomena by analysis of electrograms recorded within the tachycardia circuit. *Circulation* 1986;77:569.)

method allows comparable coupling intervals to reach the circuit at a greater relative degree of prematurity than if that same coupling interval were used for the first extrastimulus (Fig. 11-136). By this methodology, only a single extrastimulus interacts with the circuit.

This method also permits examination of the effect of single extrastimuli on a VT over a greater range of coupling intervals by minimizing or eliminating electrophysiologic factors at the stimulation site or intervening tissue that could influence the ability to influence the VT. An example of this methodology is shown in Figure 11-137, in which single extrastimuli delivered up to local refractoriness (170 msec) failed to influence the tachycardia. When the first extrastimulus is delivered 20 msec above refractoriness (VT-$S_1$ = 190 msec), a second extrastimulus ($S_2$) delivered 10 msec shorter than the VT cycle length produces resetting. The ability to use relatively long $S_1$-$S_2$ intervals to interact with the VT eliminates the introduction of local conduction delays (at the stimulus site or between the stimulus site and reentrant circuit), which can influence the absolute value of the return cycle, leading to misinterpretation of the response. Double or triple extrastimuli can also be delivered such that each extrastimulus interacts with the site of impulse formation to varying degrees before termination. However, without controlling the degree to which each impulse interacts with the tachycardia circuit, it becomes difficult to interpret (particularly quantitatively) the significance of the response aside from whether or not the tachycardia was terminated. As such, this form of stimulation may be useful in evaluating the potential of antitachycardia pacemakers using scanning or decremental extrastimuli as a method of termination but provides little information that can be used to understand the mechanism of VT. We therefore recommend a stimulation protocol that will permit assessment of the effect of a single extrastimulus on the VT to evaluate the mechanism of the tachycardia and characteristics of the reentrant circuit, if present. For example, if three extrastimuli are used, the first two extrastimuli should be delivered at coupling intervals above those that induce resetting, and the third can be used to interact with the tachycardia. In this case, only the third extrastimulus would interact with the tachycardia as a single perturbation. In this instance, the initial coupling interval of the third extrastimulus should be greater than or the same as the VT cycle length.

Rapid pacing should be performed, particularly if two or three extrastimuli fail to influence the tachycardia or if the VT is poorly tolerated. It is critical to synchronize the initiation of pacing to the electrogram at the pacing site because absence of synchronization will lead to a variable coupling interval of the first impulse of the burst to the VT. This assumes import because many investigators immediately turn to "burst" pacing to terminate tachycardias (even if the patient is hemodynamically stable), and the initial stimulus is delivered at various coupling intervals from the tachycardia for each burst.

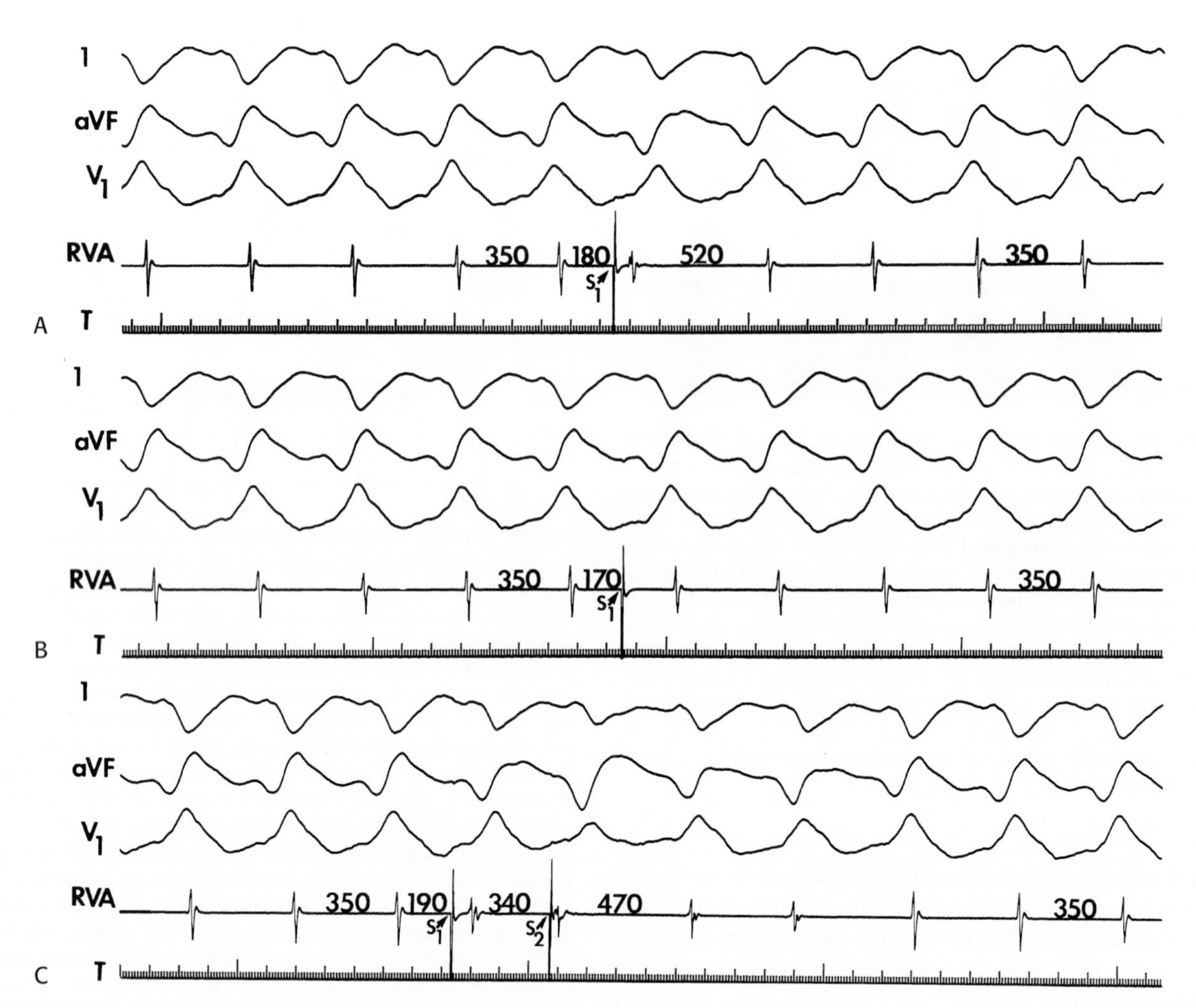


**FIGURE 11-137** Use of double extrastimuli to produce resetting. VT with a right bundle inferior axis is present in all three panels. **A:** An extrastimulus delivered at the RVA at 180 msec failed to reset the tachycardia. **B:** An extrastimulus delivered at 170 msec finds the ventricle refractory. **C:** When the first extrastimulus is placed at 190 msec, an interval when no resetting occurred, and a second extrastimulus is then placed at 340 msec, resetting of the tachycardia is produced. The sum of the coupling intervals of the two extrastimuli and the return cycle is 1,000 msec. This is 50 msec earlier than expected, thereby confirming that the tachycardia was reset.

Moreover, most investigators do not control the number of extrastimuli delivered. In many instances, pacing is given for a variable duration (e.g., 3 to 30 seconds), which compounds interpretive problems. These factors can lead to a situation in which tachycardias may be reset, terminated, and reinitiated without the investigator knowing it. They may also increase the incidence of acceleration of VT to a faster VT or VF. These two factors make data from the literature difficult to interpret and apply to the VT being studied.

Once ensuring synchronization, the investigator should employ a series of paced beats delivered at cycle lengths beginning just shorter than the tachycardia cycle length, then decreasing the cycle length until the tachycardia is terminated. At each cycle length, the response to a variable number of extrastimuli should be assessed (i.e., 1, 2, 3, 4, 5, 6, etc.).[1,122,123,315,317,320] The use of a controlled and increasing number of extrastimuli is necessary to assure the investigat or that the tachycardia was not reset, terminated, and then reinitiated at the PCL used. By using these techniques, the ability to reset, entrain, and/or demonstrate overdrive acceleration, suppression, or termination can be assessed and evaluated and compared to the respective responses of known triggered and reentrant rhythms. Because at least 95% of all sustained monomorphic VT is reproducibly initiated, it is assumed normal or abnormal automaticity is not operative in those cases.

For VTs that are not stable enough to allow completion of an entire protocol, synchronized bursts of pacing of variable cycle lengths and for a specified, but variable, number of beats can usually be performed and can provide information about resetting or entrainment, overdrive acceleration and suppression, and termination. However, approximately 25% of tachycardias (particularly those with cycle lengths <300 msec) will not be able to be terminated by rapid pacing and/or will be accelerated to different tachycardias and will require cardioversion.[322–325] The faster the VT and the more vigorous the stimulation, the more likely acceleration will result.[322–325] In such patients, the response to stimulation cannot be used to define the underlying mechanism. Thus, patients with very rapid tachycardias producing rapid hemodynamic collapse, VT degenerating to VF, or nonsustained VT are not suitable candidates for detailed study. In patients with hemodynamically tolerated, stable, sustained monomorphic VT, the responses to programmed stimulation that should be assessed are the following: (a) the resetting response to single or double extrastimuli;[1,122,123,315–319] (b) continuous resetting (i.e., entrainment), overdrive acceleration, or overdrive suppression in response to rapid pacing;[1,122,123,315,318–320,326,327,328] (c) the ability of stimulation techniques to terminate the tachycardia and the pattern of termination;[1,122,123,193,194,315,322–325,329–334] and (d) the site specifically for stimuli affecting the tachycardia.[1,122,123,194,195,318,321,335]

### *Manifest and Concealed Perpetuation of Ventricular Tachycardia*

Programmed extrastimuli and occasionally even short bursts of overdrive pacing may fail to influence the tachycardia. This results in fully compensatory pauses surrounding the delivery of single or multiple extrastimuli. The tachycardia cycle length, the presence of and duration of an excitable gap in the VT circuit, the time it takes the stimulated impulse to reach the tachycardia circuit, and the refractoriness at the local site of stimulation are the major factors that influence the ability of stimuli to interact with the VT. The tachycardia circuit or the site of origin is "relatively" protected by these physiologic factors, which are unrelated to the tachycardia mechanism. This in no way implies protection of the tachycardia mechanism from responding to an increased number of extrastimuli or extrastimuli delivered at a shorter cycle length and/or closer to the tachycardia origin. In our experience, VT associated with coronary artery disease and prior infarction with cycle lengths <300 msec are almost never terminated with single extrastimuli,[322] and, in most cases, cannot even be reset by single extrastimuli delivered at twice threshold from the right ventricle. This is not surprising in view of the fact that these VTs usually arise from areas of prior infarction in the left ventricle, which limits the ability of an extrastimulus delivered from the right ventricle to reach the site of tachycardia before refractoriness is reached at the stimulus site. An example of the inability of right or left ventricular stimulation to reach and influence VT is shown in Figure 11-138. Occasionally, simultaneous stimulation from both right and left ventricles fails to influence the tachycardia (Fig. 11-139).[336] This suggests that the tachycardia circuit is relatively protected by external factors that limit access of stimulated impulses to the tachycardia, particularly if it occurs in an area of a large aneurysm. The term concealed perpetuation is used when extrastimuli not only fail to influence the tachycardia but are followed by pauses that exceed the tachycardia cycle length or that occasionally are interrupted by sinus captures before the next tachycardia beat (Fig. 11-140).[336] In Figure 11-141, one can observe that the presystolic electrogram, which is in the reentrant circuit, continues undisturbed by two right VES. The long pause following the second extrastimulus is due to the inability of the impulse from the reentrant circuit to depolarize the remainder of the ventricles, which have been just activated and captured by the second extrastimulus. This could be considered a form of functional exit block.

The significance of manifest and/or concealed perpetuation is that its presence can be used to demonstrate the extent of ventricular myocardium not required for the tachycardia. Thus, the ability to capture (i.e., depolarize) significant portions of the ventricle by ventricular premature depolarizations without affecting the tachycardia suggests that those captured areas are not required for the tachycardia. In most patients with recurrent sustained VT that is due to coronary artery disease, right ventricular stimulation late in diastole can capture the ventricle ipsilateral to the stimulus site and part of the contralateral ventricle without influencing the tachycardia. As shown in Figure 11-139, occasionally this can be observed with simultaneous stimulation in both ventricles. This phenomenon suggests that the tachycardia mechanism requires only a small area of the ventricle. In a similar fashion, intermittent capture of the His–Purkinje system during the tachycardia suggests that it, too, is not necessary to maintain the arrhythmia, regardless of where the His deflection is located during the tachycardia (Figs. 11-4 to 11-7).

Occasionally, one may observe continuous ventricular capture by ventricular pacing that does not influence the tachycardia (Fig. 11-142). In most instances, ventricular pacing is begun late in diastole at a rate slightly different from the tachycardia rate. In all such cases, one must demonstrate that ventricular pacing at this cycle length did not terminate and reinitiate the tachycardia. In these cases, ventricular pacing—because its cycle length is close to that of the VT and the distance of stimulus site is far from the tachycardia—fails to reach the tachycardia at a time to influence it. This must be distinguished from continuous resetting of the tachycardia circuit, which will be described subsequently. As noted earlier, sinus captures, occurring either spontaneously or in response to atrial stimulation, can occur without influencing tachycardia. The demonstration that neither the proximal His–Purkinje system nor the majority of ventricles are required to sustain the tachycardia, and that supraventricular captures can occur without influencing the tachycardia, suggests that the tachycardia must occupy a relatively small and electrocardiographically silent area of the heart.

### *Resetting of Ventricular Tachycardia*

Resetting of a sustained rhythm is the interaction of a premature wavefront with the tachycardia resulting in advancement or delay of the original rhythm. The first return VT complexes must have the same morphology and cycle length as the VT before delivery of the extrastimulus regardless of whether single or multiple extrastimuli are used. As noted in the preceding paragraphs, extrastimuli delivered at long coupling intervals and/or pacing at slow heart rates approximating those of the tachycardia may fail to interact with the tachycardia, resulting in a fully compensatory pause producing manifest or

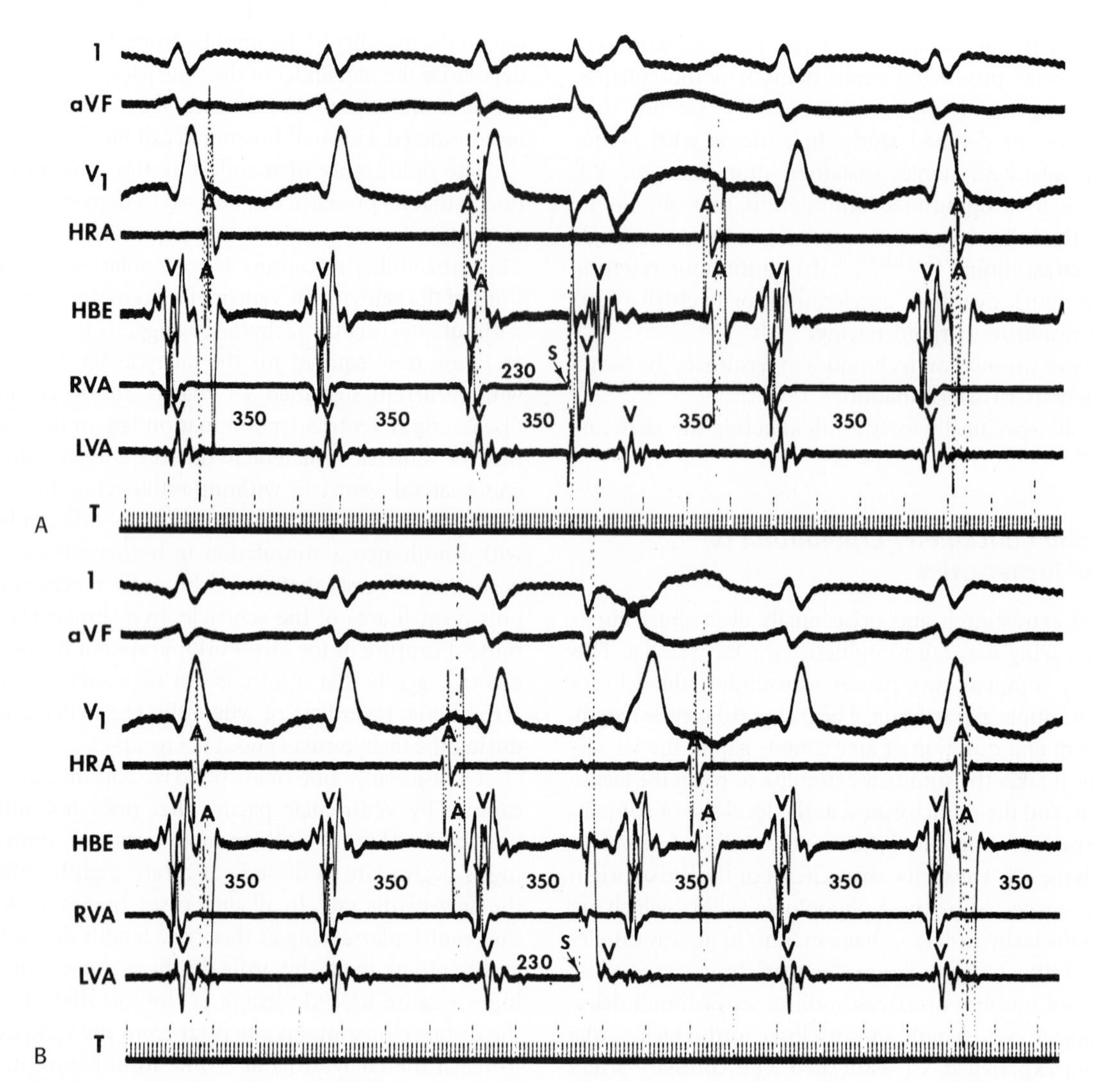


**FIGURE 11-138** Failure of right and left ventricular stimulation to affect VT. **A** and **B:** From top to bottom are leads 1, a VF, and $V_1$ and electrograms from the HRA, HBE, RVA, and LVA (and T). VT is present at a CL of 350 msec. **A:** A right ventricular extrastimulus (S, *arrow*) results in capture of the RVA and HBE and changes the QRS configuration. The tachycardia is not affected, because the LVA electrogram is unaltered. **B:** A left ventricular stimulus captures the LVA and changes the QRS complex but fails to affect the tachycardia. See text for discussion. (From Josephson ME, Horowitz LN, Farshidi A, et al. Sustained ventricular tachycardia: Evidence for protected localized reentry. *Am J Cardiol* 1978;42:416.)

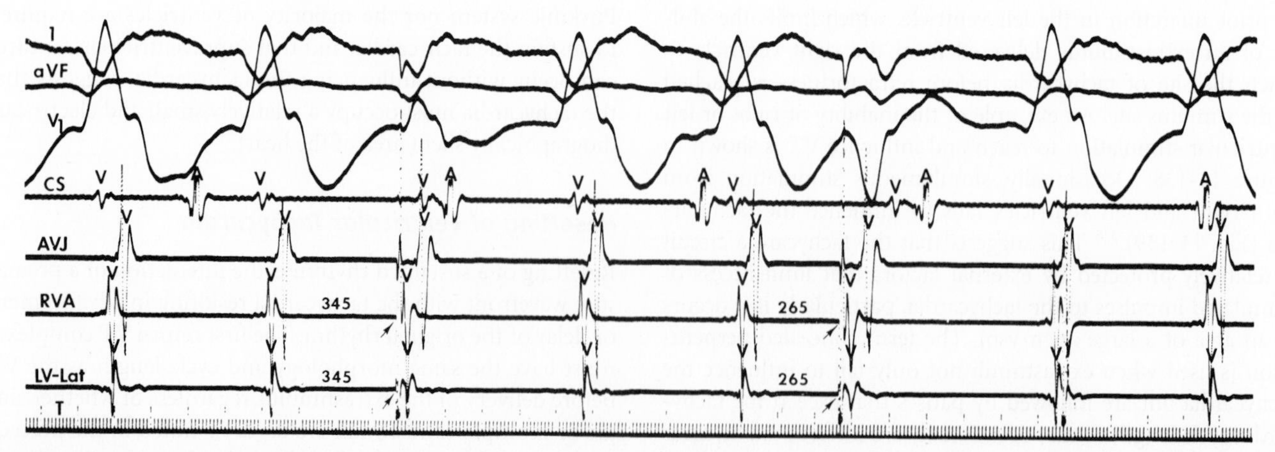


**FIGURE 11-139** Biventricular stimulation during VT. From top to bottom are ECG leads 1, aVF, $V_1$, and electrograms from the CS, AVJ, RVA, and the lateral edge of a left ventricular apical aneurysm (LV-Lat) (and T). After two beats of VT, stimuli (*arrow*) from both the RVA and LV-Lat are delivered at a coupling interval of 345 msec, without effect on the tachycardia. After two more VT complexes, simultaneous biventricular extrastimuli are delivered at a coupling interval of 265 msec. A full compensatory pause follows the extrastimuli, suggesting they have not influenced the VT. (From Josephson ME, Horowitz LN, Farshidi A, et al. Sustained ventricular tachycardia: evidence for protected localized reentry. *Am J Cardiol* 1978;42:416.)

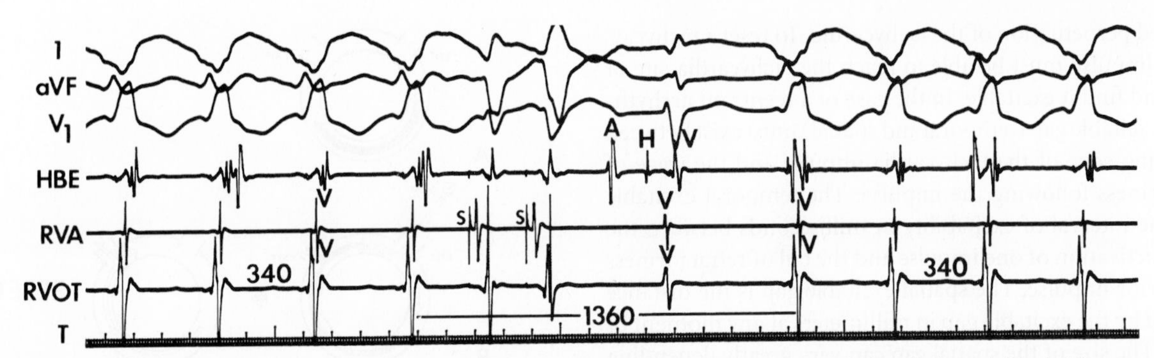


**FIGURE 11-140** Concealed perpetuation of VT following double ventricular extrastimuli. VT with a right bundle branch block right superior axis is present at a cycle length of 340 msec. Following the fourth VT complex, two VT extrastimuli are delivered from the RVA. This results in a pause, during which a sinus capture occurs subsequently followed by resumption of the tachycardia. The return of the tachycardia is an exact multiple of four VT cycle lengths, suggesting the absence of effect of the extrastimuli or the sinus capture on the VT cycle length. The presence of pauses in excess of the tachycardia cycle length and the sinus capture without influencing the tachycardia defines concealed perpetuation. See text for discussion.

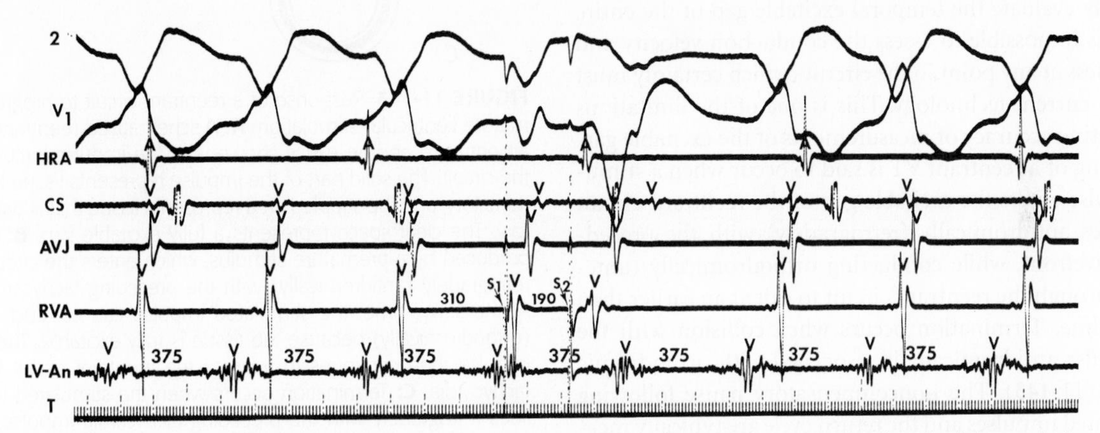


**FIGURE 11-141** Mechanism of protection during VT. The panel is organized as in Figure 11-122 except that the left ventricular catheter has been moved to within the aneurysm (LV-An) and the ECG leads are 2 and $V_1$. An HRA electrogram is also shown. During VT, two right ventricular extrastimuli are delivered, resulting in capture (note the changed QRS complex) without termination of the tachycardia. Continuing activity at the site of origin within the aneurysm is seen despite biventricular capture. (From Josephson ME, Horowitz LN, Farshidi A, et al. Sustained ventricular tachycardia: evidence for protected localized reentry. *Am J Cardiol* 1978;42:416.)

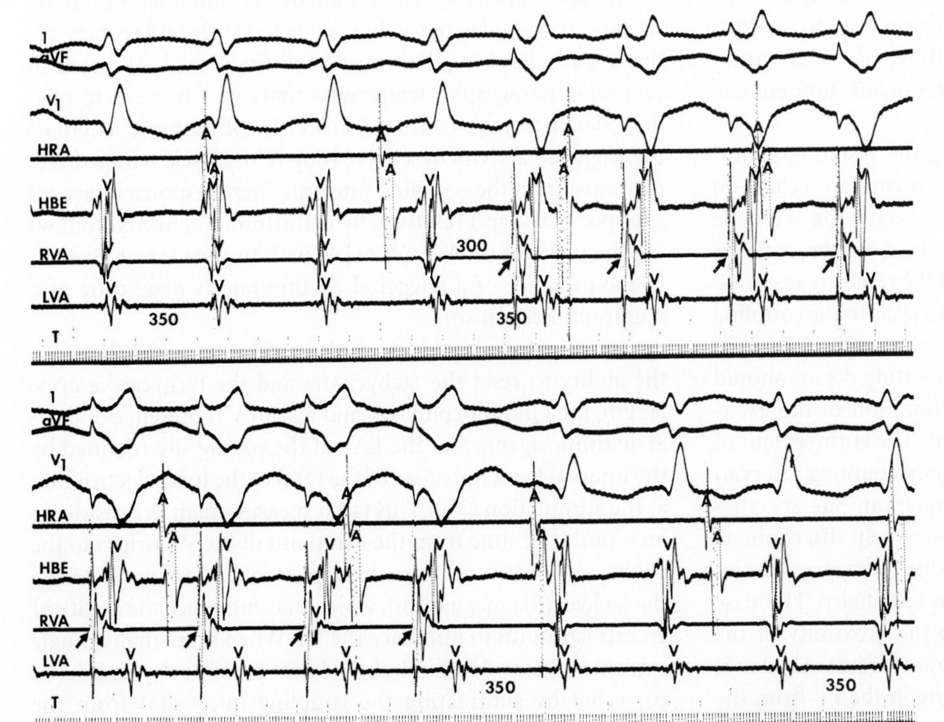


**FIGURE 11-142** Failure of ventricular pacing to alter VT. The panel is organized as in Figure 11-1. VT is present at a CL of 350 msec. Right ventricular pacing (*arrows*) is begun after the fourth complex (**top panel**), resulting in ventricular capture (change in QRS complex). When pacing is discontinued (**bottom panel**), the tachycardia is still present. Note that during right ventricular pacing the electrogram from the LVA remains unaffected. (From Josephson ME, Horowitz LN, Farshidi A, et al. Sustained ventricular tachycardia: evidence for protected localized reentry. *Am J Cardiol* 1978;42:416.)

concealed perpetuation of the tachycardia. To reset a tachycardia, the impulse must be able to reach the tachycardia site of origin and find it excitable. In the case of a reentrant arrhythmia, an excitable gap (temporal and spatial) must exist between the leading edge of the tachycardia impulse and the wave of refractoriness following the impulse. The temporal excitable gap is the interval of excitability in milliseconds between the head of activation of one impulse and the tail of refractoriness of the prior impulse. The spatial excitable gap is the distance occupied by the excitable gap in millimeters at any moment of time.[311] The size of the spatial gap can vary greatly depending on the conduction velocity and refractoriness that determine the length of the excitable gap. This results because the wavelength (conduction velocity × refractory period) of the VT impulse changes in different parts of the circuit. In humans we can only evaluate the temporal excitable gap of the entire circuit. It is impossible to assess the conduction velocity and refractoriness at any point in the circuit (which certainly must vary) with current technology. This is one of the limitations in interpreting accuracy of measurements of the excitable gap.

Resetting of a reentrant VT is said to occur when a stimulated impulse enters the excitable gap of the reentrant circuit and collides antidromically (retrogradely) with the preceding VT wavefront, while conducting orthodromically (antegradely) through the reentrant circuit to exit at an earlier than expected time. Termination occurs when collision with the prior impulse antidromically is associated with orthodromic block (Fig. 11-143). The noncompensatory pause following the stimulated impulses and the return cycle are typically measured at the pacing site; however, they may also be measured to the onset of the VT QRS complex or at a left ventricular site. In the case of a reentrant arrhythmia, the range of coupling intervals over which resetting occurs can be considered a measure of the duration of the temporal excitable gap existing in the reentrant circuit. Overdrive pacing can be used to produce entrainment (or continuous resetting) of the reentrant circuit.[1,123,315,319,320,326–328,334,335,336] Features of entrainment will be discussed subsequently.

Data that must be analyzed during the resetting protocol and that are critical in evaluating tachycardia mechanism include the duration of the return cycle versus the VT cycle length, the ability to reset the tachycardia in the presence of surface ECG or intracardiac fusion, and the resetting response pattern (i.e., the relationship of the return cycle to the coupling interval of the extrastimulus producing resetting). The entire zone of coupling intervals over which resetting occurs should also be evaluated as a measure of the duration of the excitable gap in the case of reentrant rhythms. The entire extent of the fully excitable gap would be the zone of coupling intervals from the onset of resetting until termination. Site specificity for resetting is another factor that may help discriminate mechanisms because rhythms that are due to triggered activity or automaticity do not exhibit site specificity. The ease of resetting a reentrant VT depend on the proximity of the pacing site to the entrance of the reentrant circuit. As such it should be easier to reset a VT originating in the LV from the

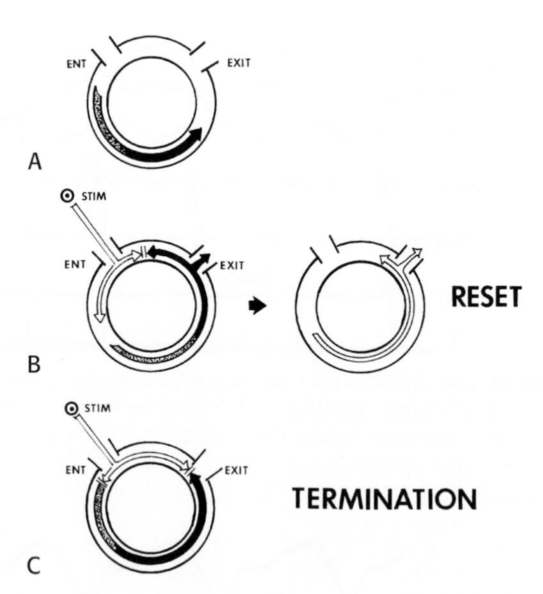


**FIGURE 11-143** Response of a reentrant circuit to progressively premature ventricular stimulation. **A:** A schematized reentrant circuit with an entrance and an exit is shown with the impulse circulating within the circuit. The solid part of the impulse represents tissue that is totally refractory, and the stippled area represents tissue that is partially refractory. The clear space represents a fully excitable gap. **B:** Resetting is produced by a premature stimulus, which enters the circuit to collide retrogradely (antidromically) with the preceding tachycardia impulse. At the same time, the stimulated impulse can conduct antegradely (orthodromically) because the tissue is fully excitable. The stimulated impulse then continues to traverse the reentrant circuit to reset the tachycardia. **C:** Termination occurs when the stimulated impulse collides retrogradely with the preceding tachycardia impulse and blocks antegradely owing to encroachment on the refractory period of the preceding wavefront.

LV. In view of the fact that >95% of sustained monomorphic VT is reproducibly initiated, thereby excluding an automatic rhythm, triggered activity that is due to DADs and reentry are the two mechanisms that must be distinguished. As stated in preceding paragraphs, triggered activity may be reset to produce flat return cycles at 100% to 110% of the cycle length of the triggered activity or a decreasing return cycle with a direct relationship to the coupling interval. These responses have no site specificity, and resetting by extrastimuli delivered following the onset of the VT QRS (i.e., with fusion) is not possible in the presence of a triggered rhythm and is diagnostic of a reentrant mechanism.

Investigators should also evaluate the relationship between the ability to reset the tachycardia and the tachycardia cycle length, the QRS morphology and axis of VT, presence of antiarrhythmic agents and the LAT at the pacing site (defined by the interval from the onset of the QRS to the local electrogram at the stimulation site). This latter measurement is considered an estimate of time from the exit point of the VT origin to the pacing site. These data are descriptors of factors unrelated to the tachycardia mechanism, which may influence the ability of an extrastimulus to influence the VT. When more than a single extrastimulus is delivered, the relative prematurity should be corrected by subtracting the coupling interval(s) from the

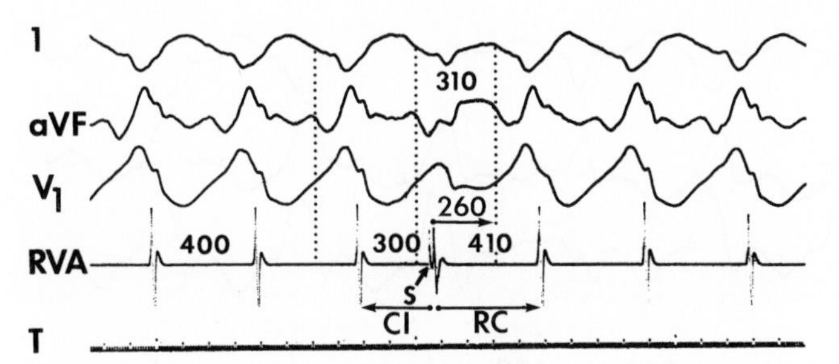


**FIGURE 11-144** Example of resetting of a uniform VT by a single ventricular extrastimulus introduced at the right ventricular apex. Surface ECG leads 1, aVF, and $V_1$ are displayed with an intracardiac recording from the RVA as well as T. Paper speed is 100 mm/min. The CL of the VT is 400 msec. A premature ventricular extrastimulus (S) is introduced with a coupling interval of 300 msec. The return cycle, as measured at the RVA, is 410 msec, resulting in a less than compensatory pause. Note that there is fusion of the QRS on the surface ECG and that the stimulus artifact occurs after the onset of the QRS. The resumption of tachycardia after the premature paced beat occurs on the surface ECG 310 msec after the onset of the fused beat, and after this, the VT resumes with its prior configuration and cycle length. (From Almendral JM, Rosenthal ME, Stamato NJ, et al. Analysis of the resetting phenomenon in sustained uniform ventricular tachycardia: incidence and relation to termination. *J Am Coll Cardiol* 1986;8:294.)

spontaneous VT cycles when the extrastimuli are delivered. To account for any cycle length oscillation we require at least a 20-msec shortening of the return cycle to demonstrate resetting (Fig. 11-144). Resetting of VT with RBBB and LBBB patterns is shown in Figures 11-144 and 11-145. The measurement of the LAT at the pacing site is shown in Figure 11-144.

We have systematically studied the resetting phenomenon using single or multiple extrastimuli during ≈375 sustained monomorphic VTs. All VTs in which we tested single and double extrastimuli were hemodynamically well tolerated and had a stable cycle length (<20 msec variation over 20 consecutive complexes). The mean cycle length of all tachycardias studied with single and double extrastimuli was approximately 365 msec. As noted earlier, when we used double extrastimuli, we set the first at a coupling interval that did not influence the tachycardia, so that only the second impulse affected the tachycardia. Using the protocol described in the preceding paragraphs, we reset ≈60% of VTs with single extrastimuli and ≈85% with double extrastimuli using **RV** stimulation. Those tachycardias requiring double extrastimuli to demonstrate resetting had somewhat shorter cycle lengths (355 vs. 375 msec) than those that could be reset by single extrastimuli, but this did not reach statistical significance. VTs with LBBB morphology were less likely to require double extrastimuli to demonstrate resetting than those with RBBB morphology, regardless of axis. Neither local ventricular refractoriness nor LAT (assumed to reflect the distance of the stimulation site from the VT) influenced the number of extrastimuli required for resetting. The resetting interval or zone (i.e., zone of coupling intervals over which resetting occurred, reflecting size of excitable gap) was 70 msec for all VTs studied, but was significantly longer in those tachycardias reset with both single and double extrastimuli than in those requiring double extrastimuli from the same stimulation site. Moreover, in tachycardias that could be reset with both single and double extrastimuli, the total reset zone measured was much greater using double extrastimuli (95 vs. 55 msec). These data are similar to those previously reported by Stamato et al.[317] Resetting zones in response to single extrastimuli usually occupy 10% to 20% of the cardiac cycle. This increases to ≈25% in response to double extrastimuli, but occasionally can exceed 30% even in response to single extrastimuli. In patients in whom both single and double extrastimuli reset the tachycardia, the shortest return cycles seen by both methods were identical (Figs. 11-146 and 11-147). The same is true if one compares the shortest return cycle in tachycardias reset by single or triple extrastimuli (with only the third extrastimulus interacting with VT) (Fig. 11-148).

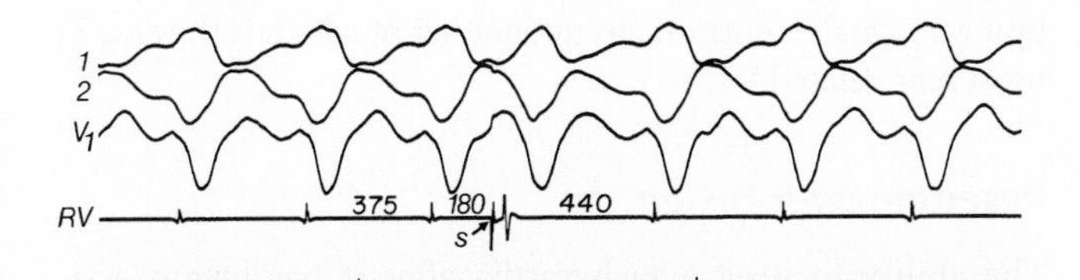


**FIGURE 11-145** Analog tracing demonstrating resetting of a left bundle branch type VT by a single premature stimulus. The tachycardia cycle length is 375 msec; the premature stimulus is delivered from the RV at a coupling interval of 180 msec. The return cycle, the cycle of the first tachycardia beat following the extrastimulus, measured at the pacing site, is 440 msec. Resetting is recognized because the same VT immediately resumes and because the return cycle is 130 msec less than fully compensatory. (From Almendral JM, Stamato NJ, Rosenthal ME, et al. Resetting response patterns during sustained ventricular tachycardia: relationship to the excitable gap. *Circulation* 1986;74:722.)

### *Return Cycle Versus Ventricular Tachycardia Cycle Length*

If the return cycle is measured from the extrastimulus producing resetting to the onset of the QRS of the first return VT complex, the shortest return cycle will be **less** than the VT cycle length in 40% to 45% of sustained VT. Because stimulation is carried out from the right ventricle, conduction time to the tachycardia circuit and through the circuit determines the return cycle measure to the onset of the QRS. If one considers conduction time between the pacing site and the site at which it interacts with the tachycardia circuit or focus to be equal to conduction time from the circuit to the stimulation site (so-called LAT), and subtracts this number from the return cycle as measured to the QRS, the resultant value for the return cycle is less than the VT cycle length >80% of VTs. The return cycle is dependent on the presence QRS fusion during resetting (see subsequent discussion on Resetting with Fusion). Of note, the time from the RV stimulus site to a presystolic electrogram in the tachycardia circuit during pacing in sinus rhythm is frequently less than the conduction time from the QRS to the LAT (at the site of stimulation). This reflects antidromic capture of the exit site in response to pacing in sinus

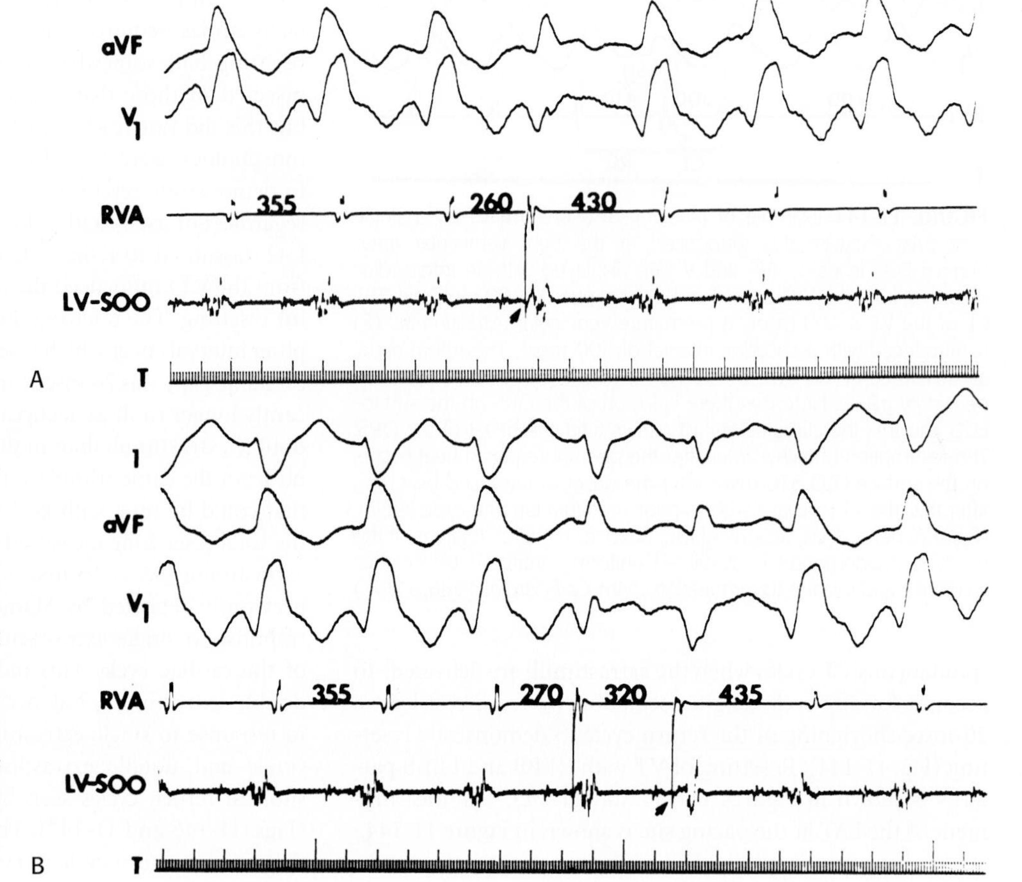


**FIGURE 11-146** Resetting of VT with single and double extrastimuli. **A** and **B:** ECG leads 1, aVF, and $V_1$ are shown with electrograms from the RVA and an electrogram from the left ventricle at the site of origin LV-SOO. The tachycardia has a right bundle right inferior axis and a cycle length of approximately 355 msec. **A:** A single extrastimulus delivered at 260 msec resets the tachycardia and exhibits a return cycle of 430 msec. **B:** Double extrastimuli are delivered, which produce resetting with a similar return cycle. See text for discussion.

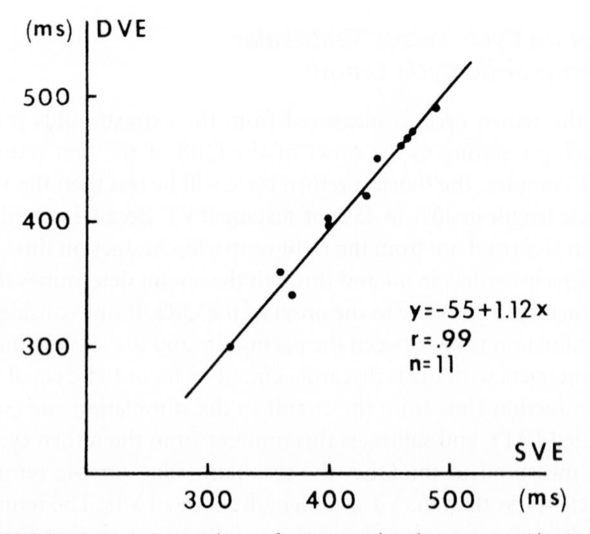


**FIGURE 11-147** Comparison of return cycle of VT reset with single and double extrastimuli. The shortest return cycle in response to both single ventricular extrastimuli (SVE) and double ventricular extrastimuli (DVE) in 11 VT are shown. The shortest return cycles seen with each method were correlated with an $r = 0.99$. (From Almendral JM, Stamato NJ, Rosenthal ME, et al. Resetting response patterns during sustained ventricular tachycardia: relationship to the excitable gap. *Circulation* 1986;74:722.)

rhythm. This difference depends on the site of stimulation, the VT-QRS morphology and axis, and the VT site of origin. There are, however, no data to support an equal conduction time to and from the VT circuit. The return cycle would be expected to be slightly longer (by the conduction time to the site of origin of the tachycardia) than the tachycardias cycle length in a focal tachycardia or if the tachycardia was caused by a very small reentrant circuit, neither of which is the case in most scar-related VT.

### Resetting with Fusion

The ability to reset a tachycardia after it has begun activating ventricular myocardium makes any mechanism of arrhythmia involving a single focus (whether automatic or triggered) untenable. By definition, fusion implies two wavefronts of activation occurring simultaneously in the heart, in this case, one from the tachycardia and one from the site of stimulation. Fusion of the stimulated impulse can be observed on the ECG if the stimulated impulse is intermediate in morphology between a fully paced complex and the VT complex or if resetting is produced by an extrastimulus delivered after the onset of the tachycardia QRS complex

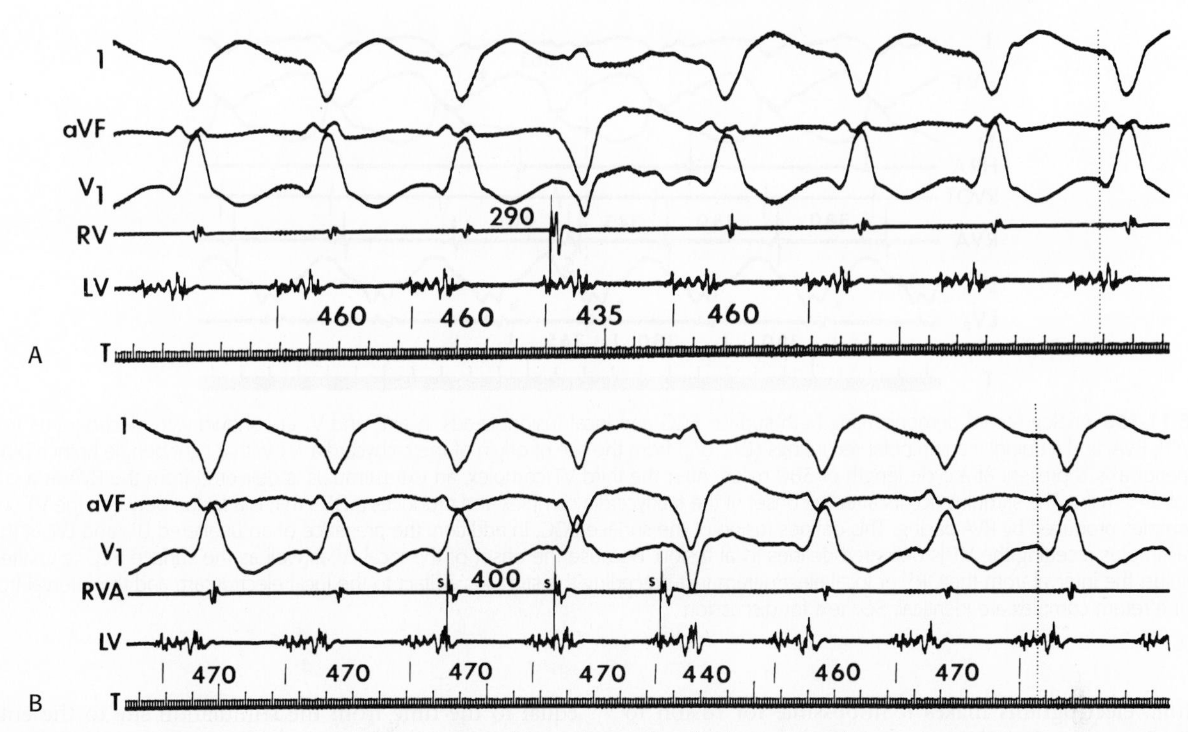


**FIGURE 11-148** Resetting of VT by one and three extrastimuli. **A** and **B:** Surface leads 1, aVF, and $V_1$ are shown with electrograms from the RV and LV site of origin. The tachycardia has a right bundle branch block right inferior axis morphology and a cycle length of 460 to 470 msec. **A:** A single extrastimulus delivered at 290 msec produces resetting with tachycardia. **B:** When three extrastimuli are delivered at 400 msec, the first two do not reset the tachycardia but alter the wavefront of activation so that the third extrastimulus resets the tachycardia. Note that the return cycle measured at the site of origin is similar when resetting is produced by a single extrastimulus or following three extrastimuli.

(*prestimulus fusion*). However, the ability to recognize ECG fusion requires a significant mass of ventricular muscle to be depolarized by both the tachycardia and the pacing stimulus. If presystolic activity in the VT reentrant circuit is present before delivery of an extrastimulus that resets the tachycardia, one must consider this to represent "local fusion." The time from the stimulus site to such presystolic activity is virtually always shorter than the VT cycle length. A schema demonstrating both local and surface ECG fusion is shown in Figure 11-149. A site recorded by a catheter, which demonstrates local fusion usually, but not necessarily, demonstrates presystolic activity depending on how long after the onset of the tachycardia QRS the stimulus that resets the VT is delivered (see the discussion of mapping of VT later in this chapter and Chapter 13). Thus, an extrastimulus that is delivered after the onset of the QRS, which enters the circuit and resets the tachycardia, will always demonstrate local fusion. An analog record of resetting with both ECG and local fusion is shown in Figure 11-150 where the extrastimulus is delivered after the onset of the QRS. The resultant QRS is a hybrid morphology between that of right ventricular pacing and of the VT. The presystolic activity in the reentrant circuit is recorded before the stimulated impulse (local fusion). The determinants of surface fusion include: (1) the site of pacing relative to the VT circuit: if the stimulation site is distant from the VT circuit exit, fusion is more likely (as the stimulation site and the exit site capture different parts of the myocardium; (2) antidromic capture of the exit site and

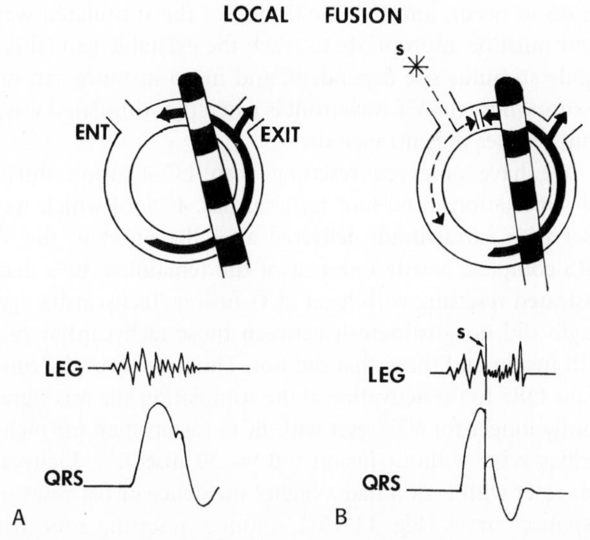


**FIGURE 11-149** Schema of local and surface ECG fusion. **A** and **B:** The relationship between the recording electrode catheter and the reentrant circuit is shown. **A:** The local presystolic electrogram (LEG) is shown as a low-amplitude fractionated signal preceding the onset of the QRS. **B:** Resetting with local (as well as ECG) fusion is shown. The extrastimulus is delivered and collides antidromically with the prior VT wavefront and then conducts orthodromically. The stimulus is delivered after the onset of the QRS; thus, ECG fusion is present. However, local fusion is defined by the presence of an unaltered LEG (specifically, the onset of the LEG) when the extrastimulus is delivered. See text for discussion. (From Rosenthal ME, Stamato NJ, Almendral JM, et al. Resetting of ventricular tachycardia with electrocardiographic fusion: incidence and significance. *Circulation* 1988;77:581.)

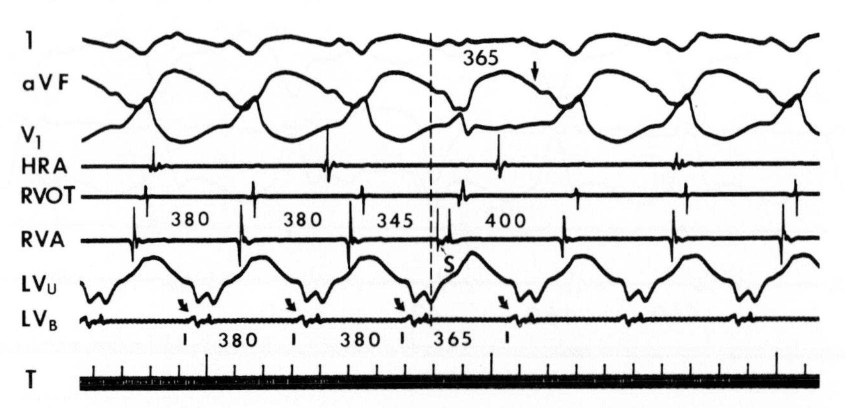


**FIGURE 11-150** Analog record demonstrating both surface ECG and local fusion. Leads 1, aVF, and $V_1$ are shown with electrograms from the HRA, RVOT, RVA, and a unipolar and bipolar recordings ($LV_U$, $LV_B$) from the site of origin of the tachycardia. VT with a right bundle branch block and right superior axis is present at a cycle length of 380 msec. After the third VT complex, an extrastimulus is delivered from the RVA at a coupling interval of 345 msec. The stimulus occurs after the onset of the tachycardia complex and produces a QRS that is a fusion between the VT complex and a complex produced by RVA pacing. This defines fusion of the surface EGG. In addition, the presence of an unaltered $LV_U$ and $LV_B$ at the time the extrastimulus resetting the VT is delivered defines local fusion. Because the onset of the local LV as well as the surface ECG is unaltered by the stimulus, the interval from the QRS or local electrogram just preceding the stimulus artifact to the local electrogram and the interval from the QRS of the return complex are identical. See text for discussion.

presystolic electrograms makes it impossible for fusion to occur because the prior VT wave front cannot reach the exit site: (3) distance between entrance and exit sites; if entrance and exit are widely separated, entry into the circuit can occur at a distance from the exit site producing the VT QRS; (4) the size of the excitable gap; a large excitable gap facilitates the ability to see fusion, but is, in and of itself, not required for fusion to occur; and (5), the timing of the stimulated wave front must be appropriate to reach the excitable gap (this is highly stimulus site dependent, and in no instance can one be sure where the VT wavefront is when the stimulated wavefront reaches the entrance site).

We have observed resetting with ECG fusion during RV stimulation in 60% of tachycardias, 40% of which were reset with extrastimuli delivered after the onset of the VT QRS complex. Nearly one-half of the remaining 40% demonstrated resetting with local ECG fusion. Tachycardia cycle length did not distinguish between those tachycardias reset with fusion and those that did not. The time from the onset of the QRS to the activation at the stimulation site was significantly longer for VTs reset with ECG fusion than for tachycardias reset without fusion (90 vs. 30 msec).[337] Tachycardias reset with fusion had a higher incidence of flat resetting response curves (Fig. 11-151), a longer resetting zone with double extrastimuli (see Resetting Response Curves below), and a significantly shorter return cycle measured from the stimulus to the onset of the VT QRS (325 vs. 420 msec) than tachycardias not reset with fusion. Moreover, the return cycle corrected for VT cycle length was shorter with VT reset with fusion than those without fusion (0.89 vs. 1.12). In 80% of tachycardias reset with fusion, the return cycle was less than the VT cycle length measured to the onset of the QRS. This finding was present in only 4% of those without fusion. If one subtracted the time from the onset of QRS to the local activation at the stimulus site (and we assume it is approximately equal to the time from the stimulation site to the entrance of the circuit) from the return cycle length, the remaining interval equals the time for the wave to traverse the distance from the entrance to the exit of the circuit. This interval is less than the VT cycle length in 100% of VTs that are reset with fusion, as one would expect. These findings are compatible with widely separate (in time and/or distance) entrance and exit sites of the tachycardia circuit. This is schematized in Figure 11-152 and explains why the return cycles are short in tachycardias demonstrating resetting with fusion. In essence, this results because more of the circuit can be "short circuited" by the premature stimulus. Although proximity of the pacing site to the entrance of the reentrant circuit may influence the return cycle and the ability to see ECG fusion during resetting, the longest coupling interval causing resetting did not differ significantly between VTs reset with and without ECG fusion. The longest coupling interval at which resetting occurs reflects ease of reaching the excitable gap and proximity to an entrance to the circuit. Resetting with ECG fusion requires wide separation of entrance and exit with the stimulated wavefront preferentially engaging the entrance. As noted earlier, the site of stimulation may in fact have been farther from the exit site (if it was defined by the time from the onset of the VT QRS to the electrogram at the pacing site) in tachycardias reset with fusion.

Resetting with local fusion and a totally "paced" QRS complex provides further evidence that the reentrant circuit in VT is electrocardiographically small. Sinus capture beats with total normalization of the QRS and H-V intervals that produce resetting without affecting the local presystolic ventricular electrograms associated with VT are the most dramatic example of how small the reentrant circuit is (Fig. 11-153). The ability to normalize the QRS, yet still produce resetting, suggests that the VT circuit is small and/or electrocardiographically silent.

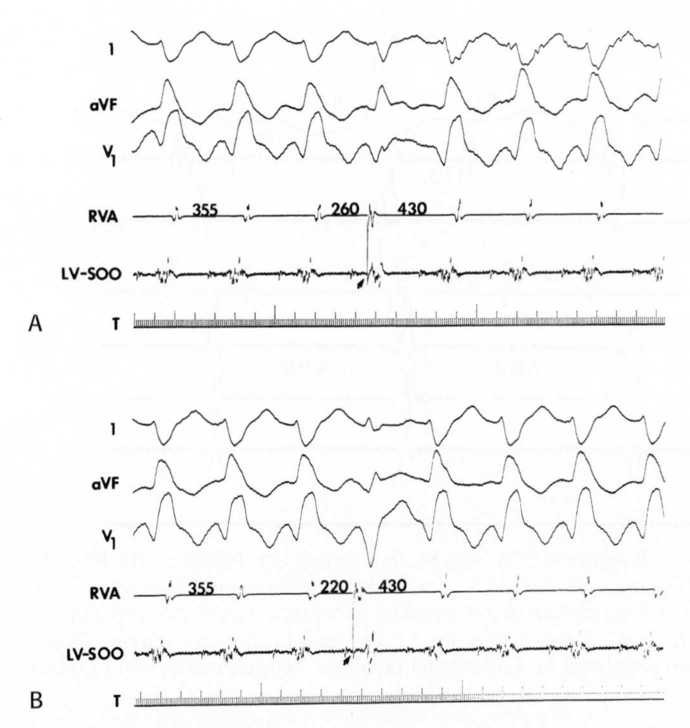


**FIGURE 11-151** Resetting of sustained VT with concomitant ECG fusion by single ventricular extrastimulus. **A** and **B:** Surface ECG leads 1, aVF, and $V_1$ are displayed with the intracardiac electrogram from the RVA, and an electrogram from the left ventricular site of origin LV-SOO. **A:** A single ventricular extrastimulus with a coupling interval of 260 msec resets VT, with a return cycle of 430 msec measured at the RVA. A fully compensatory pause would have yielded a return cycle of 450 msec. Note that the QRS morphology of the VT beat coincident with the extrastimulus is intermediate in morphology between a fully paced beat and a native VT QRS; surface ECG fusion is therefore present. The extrastimulus follows the onset of the electrogram recorded at the site of VT origin and does not alter the morphology of the initial portion of this electrogram compared with baseline. By definition, there is local fusion as well. **B:** A more premature ventricular extrastimulus (coupling interval 220 msec) results in a less than compensatory pause with concomitant surface ECG and local fusion. Note that the QRS coincident with the premature beat more closely resembles the fully paced QRS complex as opposed to the native VT beat. (From Rosenthal ME, Stamato NJ, Almendral JM, et al. Resetting of ventricular tachycardia with electrocardiographic fusion: incidence and significance. *Circulation* 1988;77:581.)

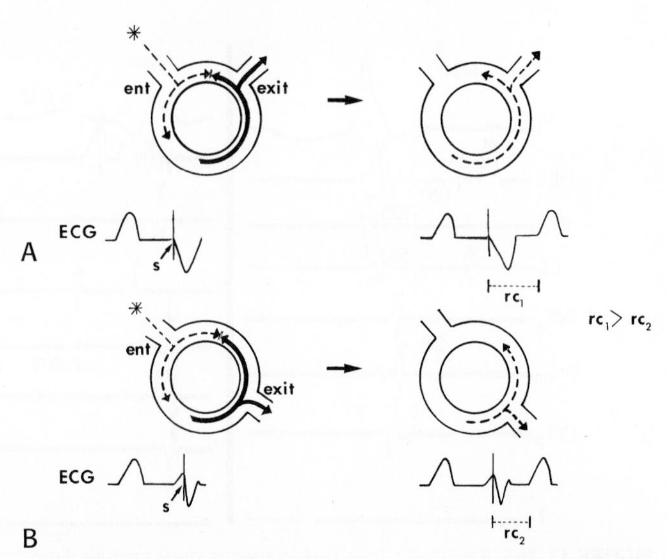


**FIGURE 11-152** Schematic representation of the relationship of the return cycle during resetting of VT to **(A)** absence or **(B)** presence of ECG fusion. **A:** A premature extrastimulus (*asterisk*) propagates toward the reentrant circle (*dotted line*) and enters the circuit to collide retrogradely with the already circulating wavefront in the circuit (*solid line*). The premature wavefront propagates around the circuit and exits to cause inscription of a VT QRS complex. The QRS produced by the premature extrastimulus appears fully paced and does not show ECG fusion. The return cycle is measured from the stimulus artifact to the onset of the following VT complex and is labeled $rc_1$. **B:** The same phenomenon is pictured with more widely separated entrance (ent) and exit sites in the same-size circuit. In this instance, the premature extrastimulus resetting the VT occurs after the VT QRS, resulting in ECG fusion. Because of the shorter conduction time between entrance and exit sites in the circuit, the return cycle in this case, $rc_2$, is shorter than in the example in **(A)**. (From Rosenthal ME, Stamato NJ, Almendral JM, et al. Resetting of ventricular tachycardia with electrocardiographic fusion: incidence and significance. *Circulation* 1988;77:581.)

### *Site Specificity of Resetting*

Although most VT characteristics, aside from the tachycardia cycle length, and QRS morphology, do not appear to influence the ability to reset tachycardia, the site of RV stimulation may. Although it has not been studied systematically, LV stimulation at selected sites can always reset reentrant VT arising in the LV. To address the question of site specificity of resetting, stimulation should be attempted from different RV sites of stimulation. We have compared the ability to reset 75 VTs from the right ventricular apex and right ventricular outflow tract. The mean cycle length of these VTs was ≈365 msec, with an approximately equal distribution of RBBB and LBBB morphologies. Twice as many tachycardias had superior axis as inferior axis. Overall, ≈65% of tachycardias were reset by single VES. Of those that were reset, ≈70% were reset by extrastimuli delivered at both the right ventricular apex and right ventricular outflow tract (Fig. 11-154). Eighteen percent were reset from only the right ventricular apex and 12% were reset from only the right ventricular outflow tract. Only the presence of LBBB was associated with a higher resetting from both sites. The site of origin of VT (defined as either the most presystolic electrogram closest to mid-diastole or a site of successful ablation; see Localization of VT in this chapter and Chapter 13) did not influence the ability to reset tachycardia from a specific right ventricular site (Fig. 11-155). When we employed double or multiple extrastimuli in the same patients, the site specificity for resetting diminished. Overall, 85% of tachycardias were reset, 80% of which could be reset from both right ventricular sites (Fig 11-156). As stated above, although we have not studied the influence of left ventricular stimulation in detail, we were always able to find a site in the LV at which resetting by a single extrastimulus was possible. As a consequence, it is not uncommon for a single VES from the left ventricle to reset a tachycardia that could not be reset

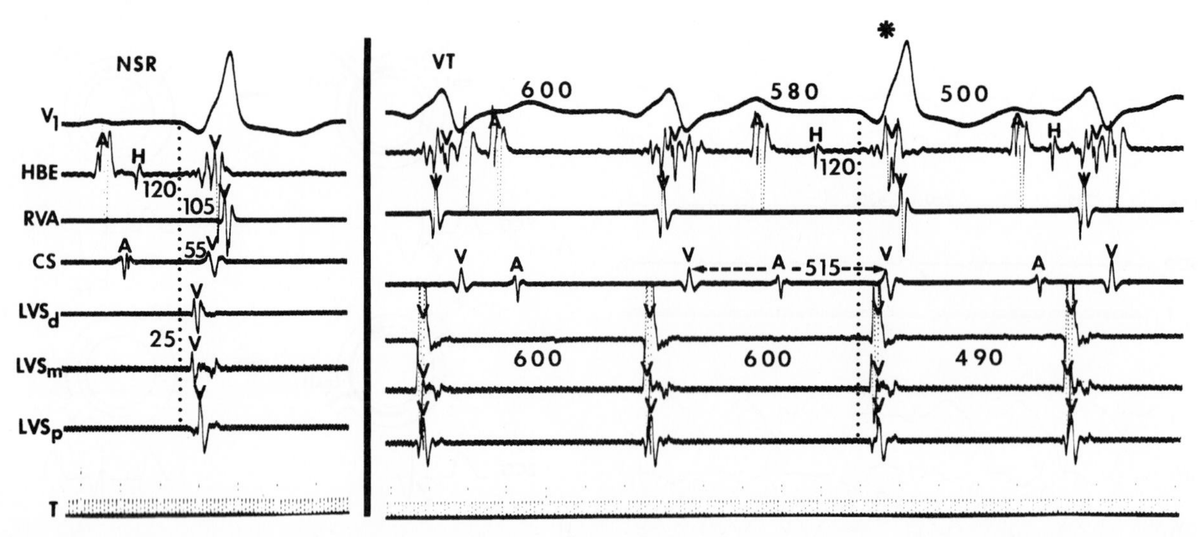


**FIGURE 11-153** Resetting VT by a spontaneous sinus capture. From top to bottom are ECG leads $V_1$ and electrograms from the HBE, RVA, CS, and distal, mid, and proximal left ventricular septum ($LVS_d$), $LVS_m$, and $LVS_p$, respectively (and T). On the left is a sinus complex (NSR); on the right VT with A-V dissociation is present. After the second complex of VT, a sinus capture occurs, resulting in normalization of the QRS and H-V intervals without interruption of the tachycardia. The subsequent VT complex is advanced; thus, the VT was reset by the sinus capture. (Modified from Josephson ME, Horowitz LN, Farshidi A, et al. Sustained ventricular tachycardia: Evidence for protected localized reentry. *Am J Cardiol* 1978;42:416.)

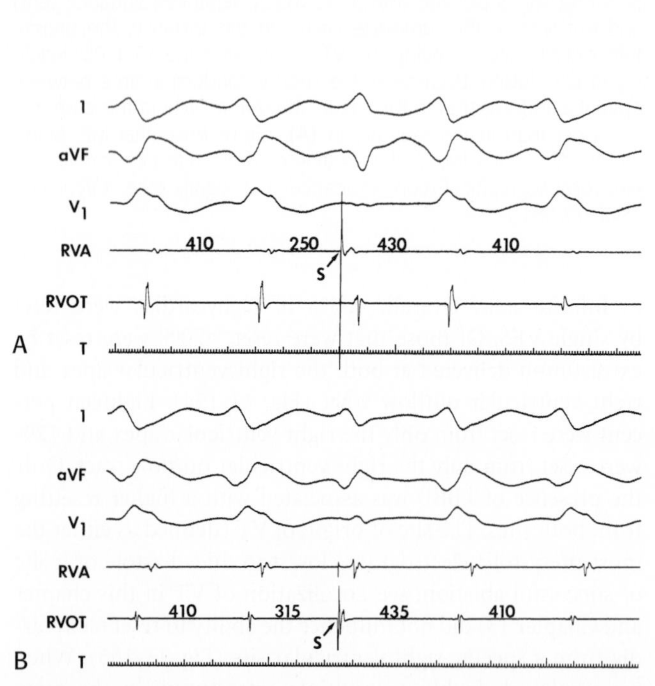


**FIGURE 11-154** Analog recordings of the same VT reset with single ventricular extrastimuli delivered at **(A)** the right ventricular apex and **(B)** the outflow tract. Surface ECG leads 1, aVF, and $V_1$ are shown with the intracardiac recordings from the RVA and RVOT. Recordings are made at a paper speed of 100 mm/sec. **A** and **B.** The pause after each premature extrastimulus, as measured at the site of stimulation, is less than fully compensatory. S, stimulus artifact. (From Rosenthal ME, Stamato NJ, Almendral JM, et al. Influence of the site of stimulation on the resetting phenomenon in ventricular tachycardia. *Am J Cardiol* 1986;58:970.)

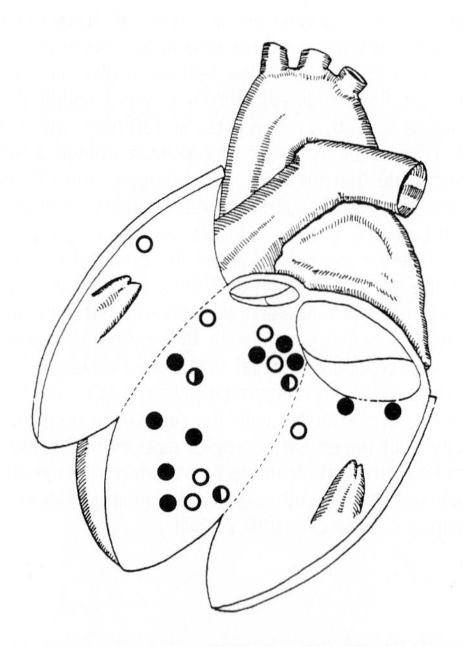


**FIGURE 11-155** Distribution of site-dependent resetting responses for 19 VTs in which the site of origin was determined by catheter mapping. The LV is shown with the endocardial surface of the anterior wall, ventricular septum, and inferior wall exposed. The site of origin of each VT is designated by a circle. The degree of shading within each circle represents the site-dependent response to single ventricular extrastimuli during each VT. Note the scatter of responses seen at the different left ventricular sites. (From Rosenthal ME, Stamato NJ, Almendral JM, et al. Influence of the site of stimulation on the resetting phenomenon in ventricular tachycardia. *Am J Cardiol* 1986;58:970.)

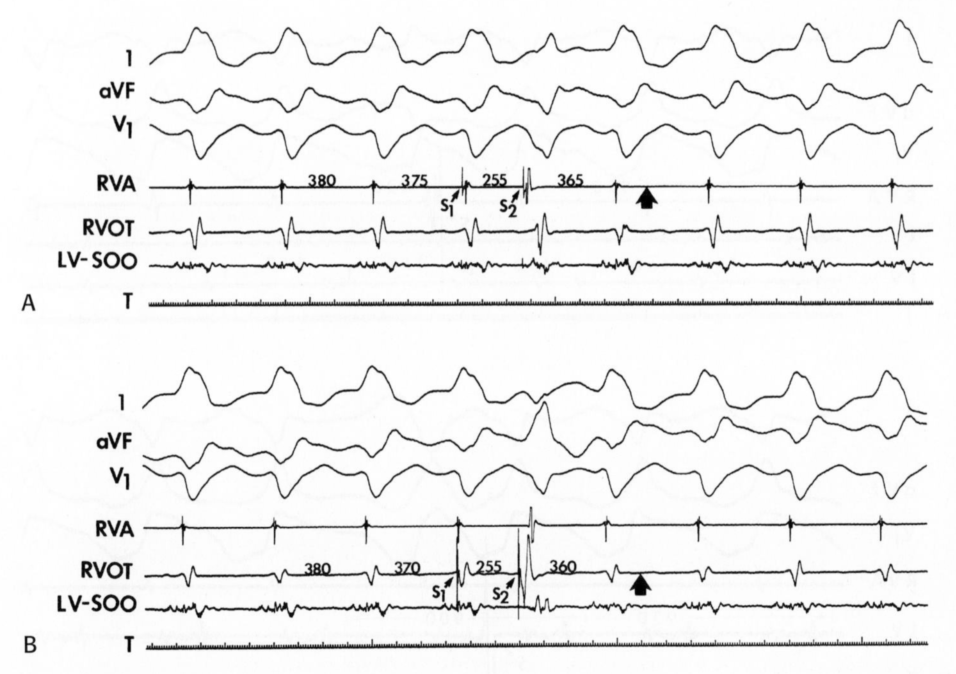


**FIGURE 11-156** Resetting of the same VT in Figure 11-154 with double ventricular extrastimuli ($S_1S_2$) delivered at both **(A)** the right ventricular apex and **(B)** the right ventricular outflow tract. **A** and **B:** Surface ECG leads 1, aVF, and $V_1$ are displayed with intracardiac recordings from the RVA, RVOT, and a presystolic left ventricular site(LV). $S_1$ is delivered with a coupling interval that did not reset the tachycardia during delivery of single ventricular extrastimuli. $S_2$ yields a less than compensatory pause. The *large arrow* designates where the local electrogram at the pacing site would have occurred if the tachycardia had not been reset. (From Rosenthal ME, Stamato NJ, Almendral JM, et al. Influence of the site of stimulation on the resetting phenomenon in ventricular tachycardia. *Am J Cardiol* 1986;58:970.)

by single extrastimuli from the right ventricle (Fig. 11-157). In these patients, the use of double extrastimuli from the right ventricle could usually overcome the influence of electrophysiologic characteristics of the intervening tissue and permit the second extrastimulus to reset the tachycardia (Fig. 11-157). It is of interest that when tachycardias were reset by extrastimuli from both the right ventricular apex and right ventricular outflow tract, the shortest return cycle was often similar (Figs. 11-154 and 11-156), suggesting comparable conduction times to and from the circuit in these VTs. In other instances they could differ markedly. Importantly, the longest coupling interval at which resetting could be observed was longer from LV sites than RV sites, particularly with VT arising on the LV-free wall. Although the total reset zone and resetting response curves were usually similar, we occasionally noted marked differences, even from two RV sites. These observations, and their significance, are discussed in the following section.

### Resetting Response Curves

Response patterns during resetting are characterized by plotting the return cycle versus the coupling intervals of the extrastimuli producing resetting measured at the site of stimulation. Qualitatively similar but quantitatively different return cycles are obtained if the return cycle is measured to the onset of the QRS of the first VT complex following stimulation. To document resetting, the VT-VT interval encompassing the stimulus should be at least 20 msec earlier than the expected compensatory pause following a single extrastimulus and at least 20 msec less than three VT cycle lengths when double VES are used. Four possible response patterns are schematically shown in Figure 11-158. A flat response is defined by the presence of a return cycle that is constant (<10 msec difference) over a 30-msec or greater range of coupling intervals. Thus, if resetting occurred over only a 20-msec period, a curve could not be characterized as flat. An increasing response pattern is defined as an increase in the return cycle as the coupling interval of the extrastimulus is decreased. A decreasing curve demonstrates the opposite: a decrease in the return cycle in response to a decrease in coupling interval of VES. A flat or decreasing response is what would be expected of triggered activity that is due to DADs. A mixed response is one that meets criteria for a flat response at long coupling intervals and an increasing response at shorter coupling intervals. Occasionally, a response pattern to single extrastimuli cannot be characterized because resetting occurs over too narrow a range of coupling intervals or because of variability in the return cycle. In such instances, one should attempt to use double extrastimuli or pacing (see following discussion) to characterize the mechanism of the arrhythmia.

All VTs reset by single VES can be reset by double VES. Double extrastimuli produce resetting over a longer range of coupling intervals and should therefore be used to more fully characterize the excitable gap of the VT. Only if single or double extrastimuli result in termination, can one conclude that the entire excitable gap was scanned. Given this limitation, for each VT the difference between the longest and shortest coupling intervals resulting in resetting is defined as the resetting interval, or reset zone. If termination occurs, the resetting zone would approximate the temporal excitable gap. Thus, when one analyzes the percentage of the VT cycle length occupied by the reset zone (i.e., the excitable gap), single VES markedly underestimate it. Double extrastimuli, in the absence of termination, also underestimate the excitable gap, but to a lesser degree.

As noted previously, during RV stimulation the mean reset interval for all tachycardias, including those reset with single

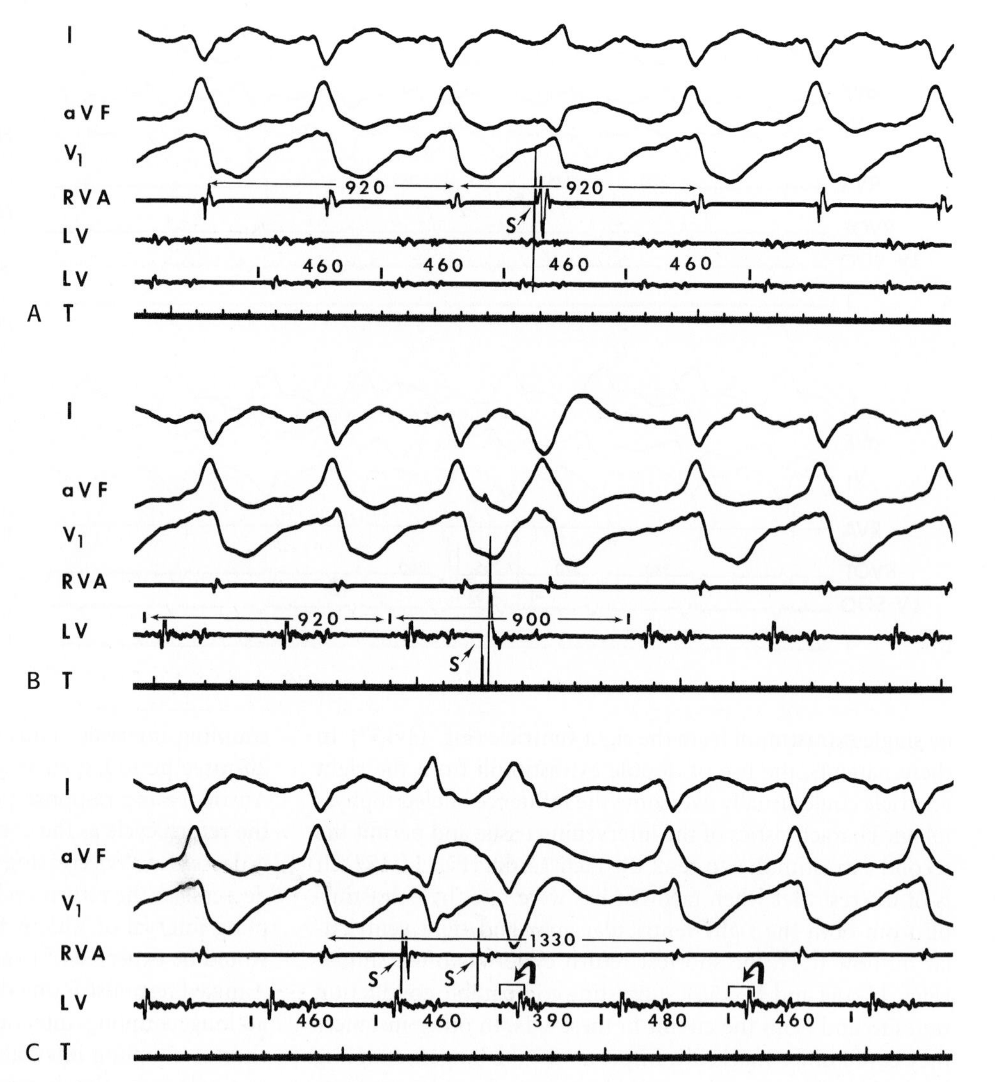


**FIGURE 11-157** Resetting VT from the left ventricle. **A–C:** Organized similarly, although two LV electrograms at the site of origin are shown in **(A)**. In all panels, VT with a right bundle branch block right inferior axis morphology is present with a cycle length of 460 msec. **A:** RVA extrastimulus at 310 msec fails to reset the tachycardia. **B:** LV stimulation at a slightly longer coupling interval produces resetting of the tachycardia. **C:** Double ventricular extrastimuli from the RVA produce resetting of the tachycardia. See text for discussion.

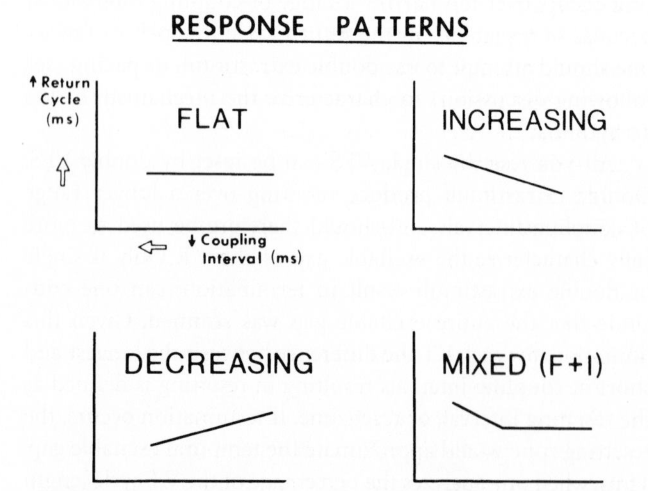


**FIGURE 11-158** Possible resetting response patterns of VT. The coupling interval of the extrastimulus is shown along the abscissa, and the return cycle is shown along the ordinate. Only flat, increasing, and mixed patterns have been observed in paroxysmal sustained VT. A decreasing pattern has not been seen. (From Almendral JM, Stamato NJ, Rosenthal ME, et al. Resetting response patterns during sustained ventricular tachycardia: relationship to the excitable gap. *Circulation* 1986;74:722.)

and/or double extrastimuli, was approximately 20% of the VT cycle length (excluding those in whom the reset pattern could not be defined). When only VTs reset by single and double extrastimuli were assessed, the mean resetting zone was nearly 100 msec, which was just under 30% of the VT cycle length. There will always be some underestimation of the total excitable gap because one cannot predict where the VT wavefront will be when the stimulated impulse enters the circuit. Stimulation within the circuit would be the only way to fully characterize the entire excitable gap. We have not systematically studied the reset zone in response to LV stimulation; however, when resetting is performed to identify a protected isthmus in the reentrant circuit, termination is commonly observed and the full excitable gap determined (see subsequent section on mapping of VT).

In an early study we observed a flat response curve in one-third of VTs (Fig. 11-159). The mean duration of the flat portion of the curve was 52 msec and was greater in response to two extrastimuli than with a single extrastimulus (65 vs. 45 msec).[316,317] In certain tachycardias as in Figure 11-159, this zone was ≥100 msec with single extrastimuli. Although a flat response curve may be seen in automatic, triggered, or

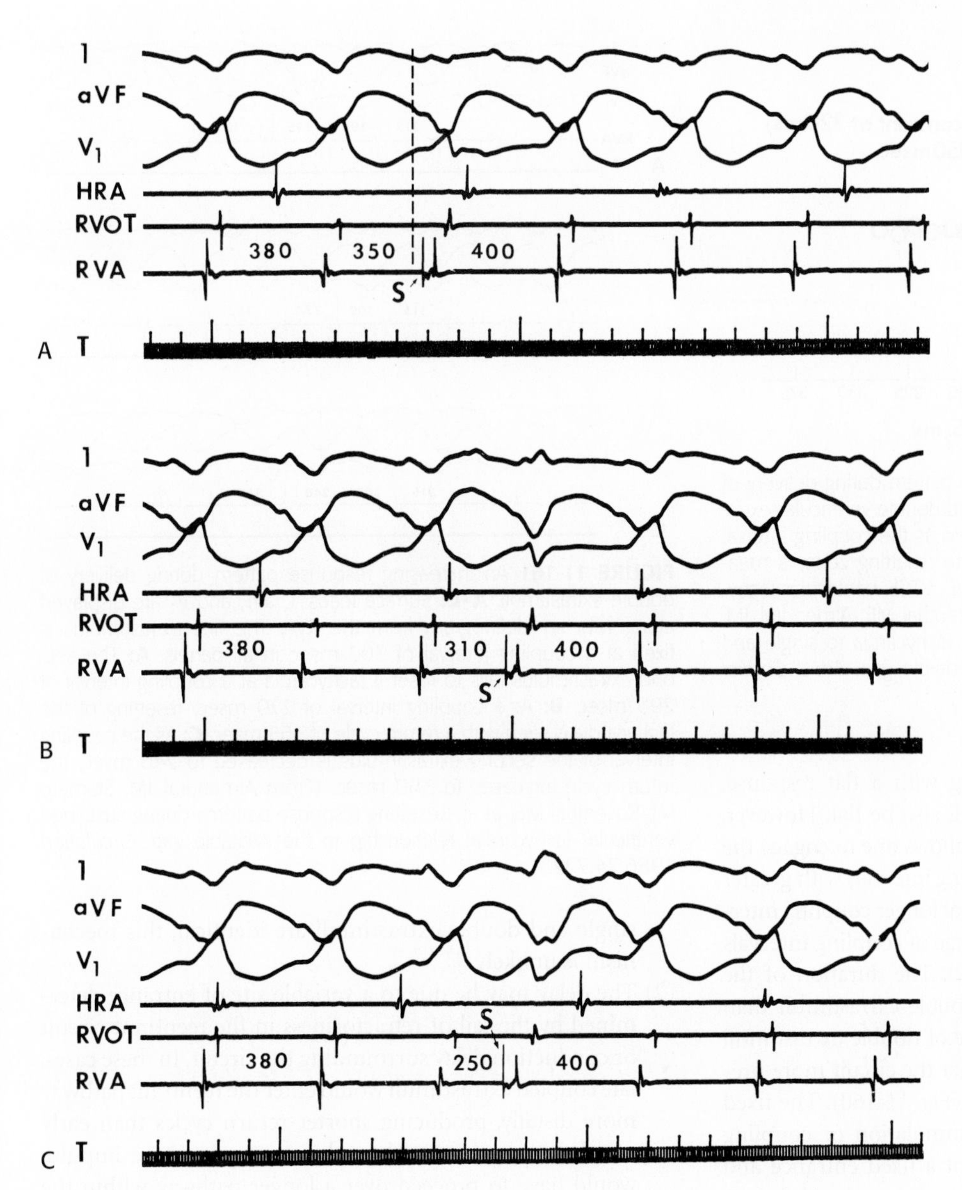


**FIGURE 11-159** A flat response pattern during the resetting of a VT with single extrastimuli. **A–C:** Surface leads 1, aVF, and $V_1$, and intracardiac electrograms from the HRA, RVOT, and RVA are recorded simultaneously. The cycle length of tachycardia is 380 msec. Single extrastimuli are delivered from the RVA with coupling intervals of **(A)** 350 msec, **(B)** 310 msec, and **(C)** 250 msec. The return cycle remains fixed at 400 msec. (From Almendral JM, Stamato NJ, Rosenthal ME, et al. Resetting response patterns during sustained ventricular tachycardia: relationship to the excitable gap. *Circulation* 1986;74:722.)

reentrant rhythms, responses of human VT were most compatible with reentry. First, automatic rhythms (which are basically excluded by the fact that all tachycardias were induced by programmed stimulation) as well as triggered rhythms have return cycles longer than or equal in length to the tachycardia cycle length. As noted, if one measures the return cycle from the stimulus at the longest coupling interval to reset VT to the onset of the QRS and subtracts the LAT, the return cycle will be less than the VT cycle length in ≈80% of VTs. In triggered activity, the return cycle is less than the tachycardia cycle length only when a decreasing curve is observed.

Assuming a reentrant arrhythmia mechanism, the ***temporal excitable gap*** can be evaluated by analyzing resetting response curves.[314,316,319,330,333,338–340] A resetting response demonstrating a flat curve indicates that there is no decremental conduction of the stimulated impulse in the VT circuit over a wide range of coupling intervals. The characteristics of a reentrant circuit in which a flat resetting response is observed suggest the following: (a) A fully excitable gap exists over the range of coupling intervals reaching the reentrant circuit during the flat part of the curve. The total duration of the excitable gap should exceed the range of coupling intervals producing resetting with a flat response. (b) Fixed sites of entrance and exit from the circuit are present. Because by definition the QRS morphology of the first return VT was identical to that of the VT before the extrastimulus, a fixed exit site from the VT circuit is suggested. The flat return cycle suggests a fixed conduction time from the stimulus site through the reentrant circuit over a wide range of coupling intervals. Because return cycles measured to the onset of the QRS (assumed to be near the exit site) remained fixed over a wide range of coupling intervals, a fixed pathway of propagation is likely present, at least as the circuit is entered and traversed by stimuli from a given site. If one assumes that the time from the stimulus site to the circuit is not changing, one must conclude that there is a fixed interval from the site of entrance to the circuit to the site of exit from the circuit.

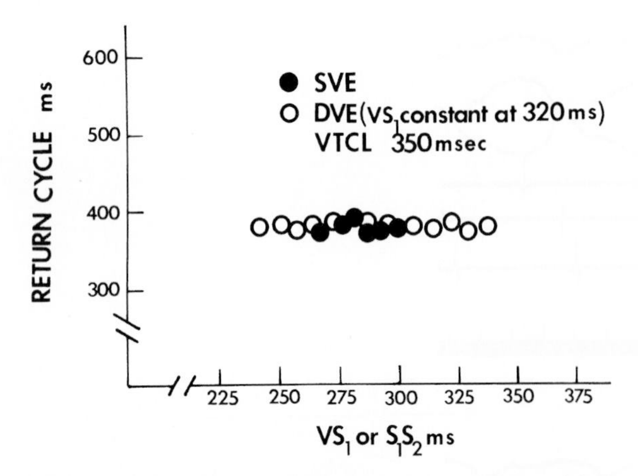


**FIGURE 11-160** A VT with a flat response pattern during delivery of both single ventricular extrastimuli (SVE) and double ventricular extrastimuli (DVE). The return cycle remains fixed as the coupling interval of the extrastimuli are decreased, while the resetting zone, a measure of the excitable gap, is longer with DVE. VTCL, ventricular tachycardia cycle length. (From Stamato NJ, Rosenthal ME, Almendral JM, et al. The resetting response of ventricular tachycardia to single and double extrastimuli: implications for an excitable gap. *Am J Cardiol* 1987;60:596.)

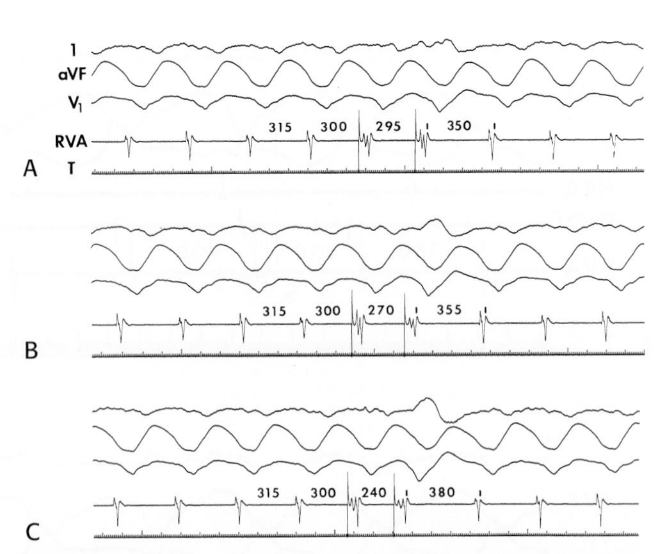


**FIGURE 11-161** An increasing response pattern during delivery of double extrastimuli. **A–C:** Surface leads 1, aVF, and $V_1$ are displayed along with an electrogram from the RVA. The first extrastimulus is fixed at a coupling interval of 300 msec in all panels. **A:** The second extrastimulus fails to reset a tachycardia at a coupling interval of 295 msec. **B:** At a coupling interval of 270 msec, resetting of the tachycardia is seen with a return cycle of 355 msec. **C:** As the coupling interval of the second extrastimulus is decreased to 240 msec, the return cycle increases to 380 msec. (From Almendral JM, Stamato NJ, Rosenthal ME, et al. Resetting response patterns during sustained ventricular tachycardia: relationship to the excitable gap. *Circulation* 1986;74:722.)

If a single VES produced resetting with a flat response, the response to double extrastimuli will also be flat. However, because the use of double extrastimuli allows one to engage the reentrant circuit at relatively long coupling intervals with greater relative prematurity, resetting will begin at longer coupling intervals and will continue over a greater range of coupling intervals than observed using single extrastimuli. The duration of the resetting curve will be longer using double extrastimuli than with single extrastimuli because the use of double extrastimuli enables the stimulated wavefront to enter the circuit more prematurely than with single extrastimuli (Fig. 11-160). The fixed return cycles, regardless of mode of stimulation or coupling interval, further support the concept of a fixed entrance and exit site for the tachycardia circuit, at least as analyzed from a single site. Theoretically, double extrastimuli, because they allow impulses to reach the circuit earlier, may produce a flat then an increasing curve (see following discussion).

We have observed a pure, increasing curve in approximately one-third of VTs studied (Figs. 11-161 and 11-162).[1,122,123,316] Three mechanisms for an increasing curve are possible:

(1) The increasing curve may represent progressive conduction delay of the paced impulse between the pacing site and the reentrant circuit. This is highly unlikely because the shortest return cycles are virtually identical when the response to single and double extrastimuli from the same site are compared. Moreover, because resetting with double VES is achieved at longer coupling intervals than with single extrastimuli, conduction delays at the stimulus site and/or in intervening myocardium in response to single extrastimuli (if they occur) should be abolished or decreased, resulting in shorter return cycles with double extrastimuli. Because shortest return cycles in response to single and double extrastimuli are identical, this mechanism is unlikely.[315–317]

(2) The delay may be due to a variable site of entrance determined by the tail of refractoriness in the reentrant circuit or conduction delay surrounding the circuit. In these cases, late coupled extrastimuli would enter the reentrant pathway more distally, producing shorter return cycles than early coupled extrastimuli. Thus, the more premature impulse would have to proceed over a longer pathway within the reentrant circuit, resulting in a longer return cycle and an increasing response. Because double extrastimuli, which are relatively more premature at the site of the reentrant

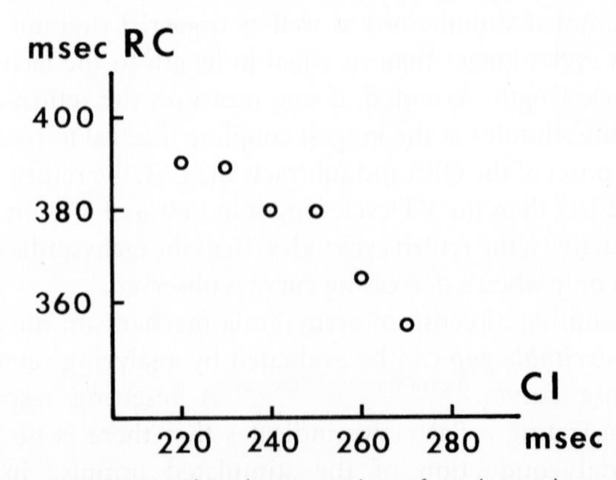


**FIGURE 11-162** Graphic demonstration of an increasing resetting response curve. The return cycle (RC) is plotted on the ordinate, and the coupling interval ($C_1$) of ventricular extrastimuli is on the abscissa. A purely increasing curve is shown.

circuit than single extrastimuli, produce the same response, a changing entrance site and pathway is excluded.

(3) An increasing curve may be due to the VES encroaching on partial refractory tissue in the circuit. In this case, progressively more premature stimuli encounter increasingly refractory tissue producing increasing conduction delays and longer return cycles at shorter coupling intervals. This interval-dependent conduction delay may be due to either encroachment on Phase 3 of the action potential or caused by nonuniform anisotropic conduction. The resetting zones exhibiting only increasing patterns are shorter than those with flat or mixed patterns even though VT cycle lengths in both cases are comparable.[315,330,331] This suggests that the increasing curve is due to a property of the reentrant circuit itself and is most likely related to encroachment on refractoriness in the orthodromic direction.

In a mixed response curve, the initial coupling intervals demonstrate a flat portion of the curve of variable duration (but always exceeding 30 msec) followed by a zone during which the return cycle increases. As shown in Figure 11-163, in some cases a flat curve may be seen with single extrastimuli, and it is only by using double extrastimuli that an increasing component of the resetting response curve can be observed. This further demonstrates that double extrastimuli more fully characterize the excitable gap than single extrastimuli. A comparison of the response of VT to single and double extrastimuli from the RV apex is shown in Figure 11-164. In this example, single extrastimuli produce a flat response, while double extrastimuli produce a flat response followed by an increasing response, and finally, termination of the tachycardia. The entire excitable gap demonstrated in Figure 11-164 was 155 msec and occupied 35% of the tachycardia cycle length.

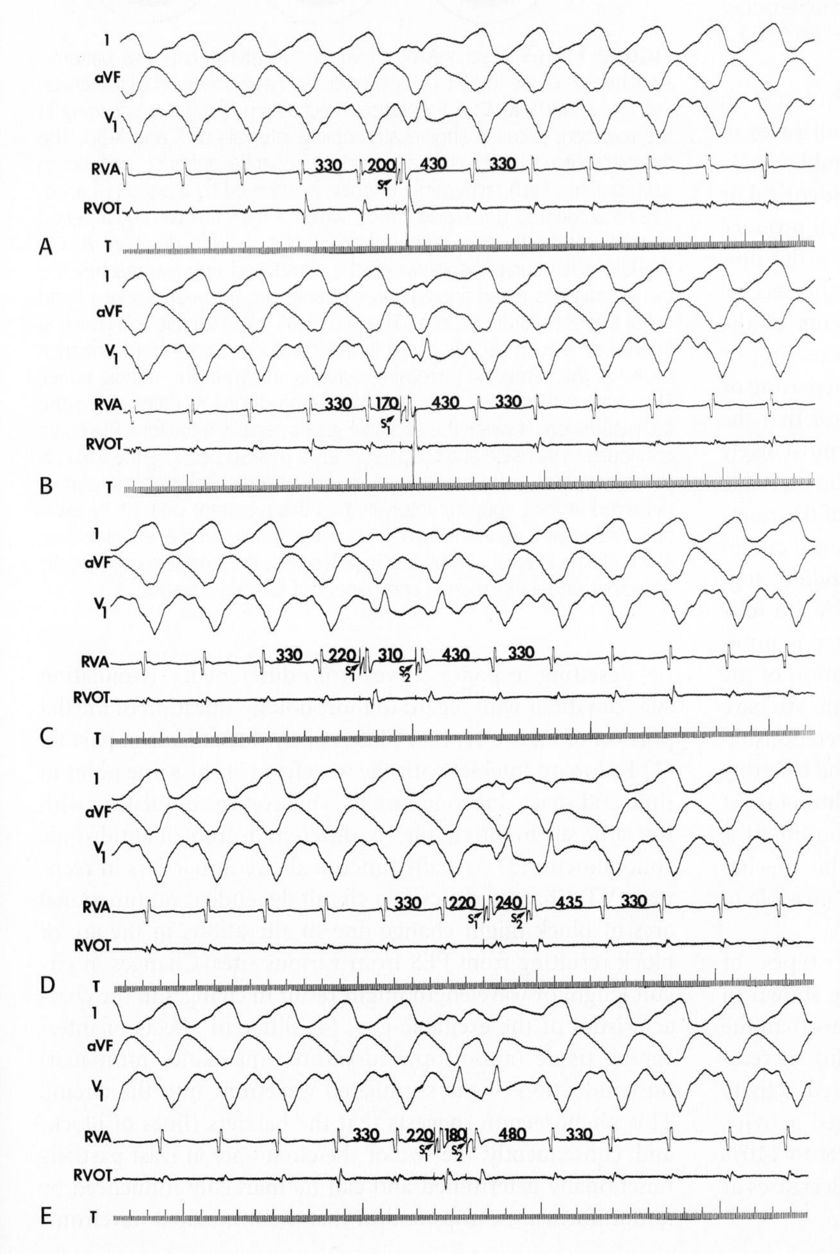


**FIGURE 11-163** Analog recordings of a VT that has a flat response during the delivery of single ventricular extrastimuli and a flat plus increasing response pattern during the delivery of double ventricular extrastimuli. **A:** The VT cycle length is 330 msec. Single extrastimuli delivered at a coupling interval of 200 msec reset the VT with a return cycle being less than fully compensatory at 430 msec. **B:** As the coupling interval of the extrastimulus is decreased to 170 msec, the return cycle remains fixed at 430 msec. At a coupling interval of 160 msec, the effective refractory period was reached. Therefore, a flat response pattern having a duration of 30 msec was demonstrated with single extrastimuli. **C:** Double extrastimuli are delivered with the coupling interval of the first extrastimulus fixed at 220 msec, 20 msec above that which caused resetting with single extrastimuli. Beginning at an $S_1$ and $S_2$ interval of 310 msec, resetting is seen with a return cycle of 430 msec. **D:** The return cycle remains essentially fixed as the $S_1S_2$ is decreased to 240 msec. **E:** As the $S_1S_2$ is further decremented below 240 msec, the return cycle increases until, at an $S_1S_2$ of 180 msec, the return cycle had increased to 480 msec. Thus, the VT demonstrated a flat plus increasing response pattern to double extrastimuli. (From Stamato NJ, Rosenthal ME, Almendral JM, et al. The resetting response of ventricular tachycardia to single and double extrastimuli: implications for an excitable gap. *Am J Cardiol* 1987;60:596.)

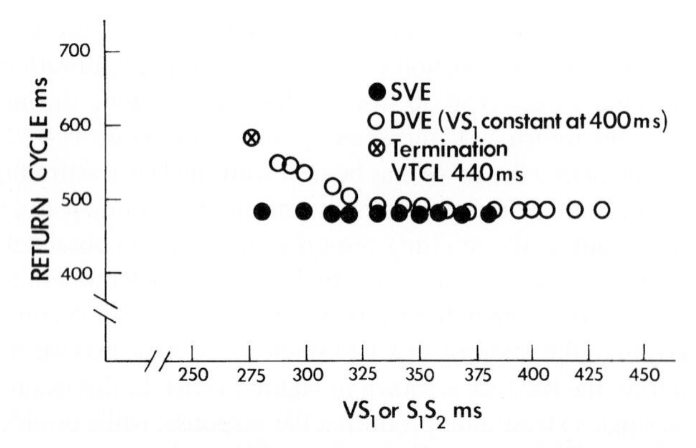


**FIGURE 11-164** Response pattern of a VT to both single ventricular extrastimuli (SVE) and double ventricular extrastimuli (DVE). During the delivery of SVE, a flat response pattern is seen, while during the delivery of DVE, a flat plus increasing response pattern is seen followed by the termination of the VT with DVE. VTCL-VT cycle length. See text for discussion. (From Stamato NJ, Rosenthal ME, Almendral JM, et al. The resetting response of ventricular tachycardia to single and double extrastimuli: implications for an excitable gap. *Am J Cardiol* 1987;60:596.)

We have never observed a decreasing return cycle in response to single or double VES. Moreover, in all cases in which single extrastimuli reset the tachycardia, double extrastimuli delivered from the same site produced an identical or expected resetting curve. Thus, if single extrastimuli produce a flat curve, double extrastimuli produce a flat or a flat plus increasing curve, depending on whether or not the second extrastimulus encroaches on refractory components of the excitable gap. If single extrastimuli exhibit an increasing or mixed curve, double extrastimuli also exhibit an increasing or mixed curve, respectively. These findings all suggest that the resetting response curves and resetting zone are most likely related to functional properties and duration of the excitable gap in the VT reentrant circuit. A flat component of the resetting response curve (either a totally flat curve or mixed curve) was observed in two-thirds of the VT we have studied, suggesting that, at least in this selected population of VT, a fully excitable gap is present. Although the type of curve is unrelated to tachycardia cycle length, the absolute duration of the curve does seem to relate to tachycardia cycle length. We have observed a weak but significant ($p = 0.03$) direct relationship between the VT cycle length and the duration of the resetting interval. These data suggest that sustained VT in humans (at least those studied using the preceding protocol outlined) is not due to a leading circle-type mechanism.[341] This mechanism has no fully excitable gap and would not be possible to reset by stimulation performed at a distant site.[341]

The proposed mechanisms for the three types of curves observed in our patients are schematically shown in Figure 11-165. The flat curves with return cycles less than the tachycardia cycle length and the mixed or smoothly increasing curve have never been documented in triggered activity that is due to late afterdepolarizations. In triggered activity, extrastimuli produce either a return cycle at 100% to 110% of tachycardia cycle length or a return cycle that decreases as stimuli become more premature.

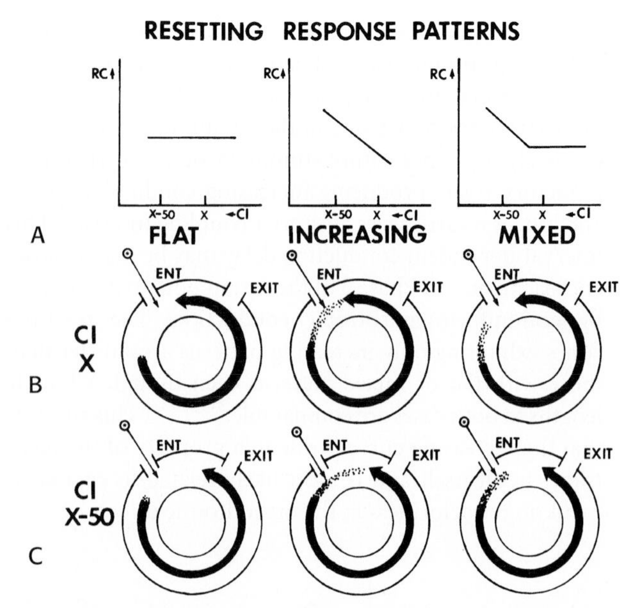


**FIGURE 11-165** Mechanisms of various resetting response patterns. **A:** Schemas of the three types of curves we have observed (flat, increasing, and mixed). **B, C:** A theoretical mechanism of what is occurring in the reentrant circuit is shown at coupling intervals of X and X-50. The reentrant circuit is depicted as having a separate entrance and exit in each pattern. Each tachycardia impulse is followed by a period of absolute refractoriness (*thick dark area*), which is then followed by a period of relative refractoriness (*stippled area*) of a variable duration. **A:** On the left, a flat curve results when the stimulated impulse reaches the tachycardia circuit and finds a fully excitable gap between the head and tail of the tachycardia impulse. The gap is still fully excitable at a coupling interval of X-50 msec. As a result, the conduction time from entrance to exit is the same. An increasing curve is shown in the middle panel. This curve results when the initial impulse producing resetting enters the tachycardia circuit when the excitable gap is partially refractory. The curve continues to increase at a coupling interval of X-50 because the tissue is still in a relatively refractory state. A mixed curve results when extrastimuli delivered at long coupling intervals find the reentrant circuit fully excitable and reset it, as in the typical flat curve shown on the left. However, at a coupling interval of X-50 the impulse finds the excitable gap partially refractory, and an increasing component of the curve results.

Resetting response curves from different RV stimulation sites can differ with regard to morphology, duration of the flat portion of Figure 11-166. This is likely due at least in part to: (1) Failure to interact with the wavefront at the same point in time and space due to failure to synchronize stimulation with the same site in the circuit; (2) different degrees of antidromic concealment; (3) partially functional circuit barriers in reentrant VT. Characteristics of a circuit dependent on functional arcs of block might change due to alterations in the arc of block resulting from PES from various sites. Changes in circuit length or wavelength might result in changes in the characteristics of the excitable gap; (4) different effects of intervening tissue (anisotropy, curvature, impedance mismatch) on conduction of the stimulated wavefront into the circuit. This phenomenon suggests that the barriers (lines of block) and, consequently, the size of the circuit are at least partially functionally determined and can be markedly influenced by nonuniform anisotropy and/or that the stimulated wavefronts

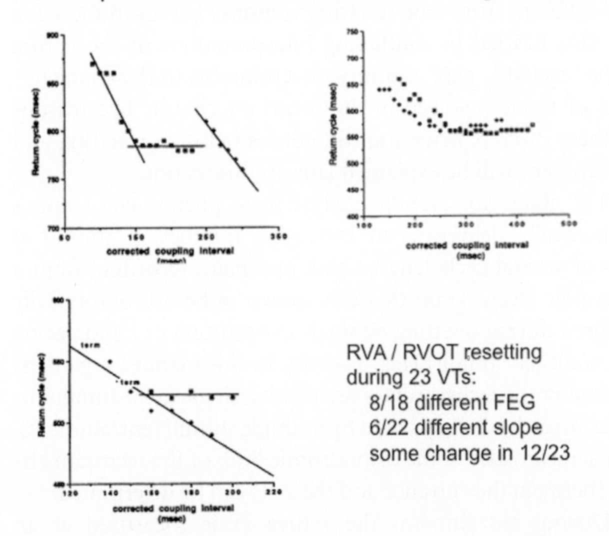
Site Dependent Differences in Resetting Curves
corrected coupling interval
RVA / RVOT resetting
during 23 VTs:
8/18 different FEG
6/22 different slope
some change in 12/23
Callans et al JACC 1996

**FIGURE 11-166** Different resetting responses depending upon site of stimulation. Resetting responses from RV apical stimulation (*squares*) are compared to responses from RV outflow tract stimulation (*diamonds*) in three tachycardias. Corrected coupling intervals of extrastimuli are shown on the X axis and the return cycles on the Y axis. In the VT at the upper left the resetting pattern in response to RV apical stimulation showed a flat (80 msec) and increasing pattern. Resetting from the RV outflow tract resulted in a purely increasing response pattern. Note that the slopes of the increasing component of the resetting curves from both sites is similar. In the VT at the lower left resetting from the RV apex results in a flat response pattern for 50 msec followed by abrupt termination at a coupling interval of 155 msec. Stimulation from the RV outflow tract results in a purely increasing resetting pattern for 100 msec until termination occurs. In the VT at the upper right the curves are similar. FEG, fully excitable gap; slope, slope of the increasing curve. See text for discussion. (From Callans DJ, Zardini M, Gottleib CD, et al. The variable contribution of functional and anatomic barriers in human ventricular tachycardia. An analysis with resetting from two sites. *J Am Coll Cardiol* 1996;27:1106–1111.)

from the different sites engage different sites in the reentrant circuit that are in different states of excitability or refractoriness. It is highly likely that all tissue in the reentrant circuit is not the same and that conduction velocity, excitability, and refractoriness vary at different sites along the reentrant pathway. The variable directions of the incoming wavefronts, due to the different sites of stimulation, will necessarily be associated with different conduction velocities dependent on the arrangement of fibers that the wavefront encounters.[29,51,52,311]

## Response of Ventricular Tachycardia to Overdrive Pacing—Continuous Resetting (Entrainment)

Although most VTs can be reset with single or double extrastimuli, 15% to 20% cannot. In these cases, the use of multiple extrastimuli, more commonly overdrive pacing, can demonstrate resetting. The use of overdrive pacing at decreasing cycle lengths with the addition of an incremental number of extrastimuli to each train of pacing at each cycle length can allow one to recognize (a) how many extrastimuli are required before the tachycardia is first reset and (b) the phenomenon of continuous resetting (entrainment). As noted earlier, the requirement for multiple extrastimuli to influence the tachycardia depends on the tachycardia cycle length, the duration of the excitable gap of that tachycardia, refractoriness at the stimulation site, and conduction time from the stimulation site to the tachycardia circuit. With overdrive pacing, a variable number of extrastimuli in the train are used to allow a single extrastimulus to reach the circuit in time to interact with the tachycardia. We refer to the first stimulus in a train that resets the circuit as the *n*th stimulus. If pacing were stopped at that point, one would assess the influence of a single extrastimulus on the tachycardia circuit. If pacing at that cycle length is continued, continuous resetting of the reset (by the *n*th stimulus) tachycardia circuit is observed. Entrainment is defined as a specific response to overdrive pacing: Following the first beat of a train of stimuli that penetrates and resets the tachycardia (*n*th stimulus), subsequent stimuli interact with the reset circuit. Depending on the degree that the excitable gap is pre-excited by the *n*th stimulus, the subsequent stimuli will fall on either fully excitable or partially excitable tissue. ***Entrainment is said to be present when two consecutive stimuli conduct orthodromically through the circuit with the same conduction time while colliding antidromically with the preceding paced wavefront.***

The number of extrastimuli required before the *n*th resets the tachycardia is cycle length dependent (both the VT and PCL). The relative prematurity with which the *n*th stimulus resets the VT is therefore not controllable, as it is with resetting. At shorter drive cycle lengths, fewer extrastimuli will be necessary before one resets the tachycardia. Regardless of cycle length used, we have found that the return cycle following the *n*th stimulus is identical to that during resetting at comparably premature coupling intervals. The influence of the drive cycle length on number of extrastimuli required to reset of the tachycardia (i.e., the *n*th stimulus) can be studied only by using the protocol described earlier in the chapter. Although the initial impulse that resets the tachycardia (*n*th) does so as described earlier (see the discussion of resetting), if pacing is continued, the reset tachycardia circuit is continuously reset. It is important that the investigator realize that continuous resetting of the circuit (i.e., entrainment) is not acceleration of the tachycardia to the PCL. Only the first extrastimulus that resets the tachycardia (*n*th stimulus) interacts with the tachycardia. All subsequent stimuli during entrainment produce antidromic collision with the last stimulated impulse while simultaneously propagating in the orthodromic direction, that is, in the same direction as the VT impulse. Consequently, all stimuli following the *n*th stimulus interact with the "reset circuit," which has an excitable gap that has been foreshortened by the degree of prematurity with which it was reset. Just as the cycle length chosen influences the number of extrastimuli required to produce resetting, it also affects the number of extrastimuli required to produce entrainment. This

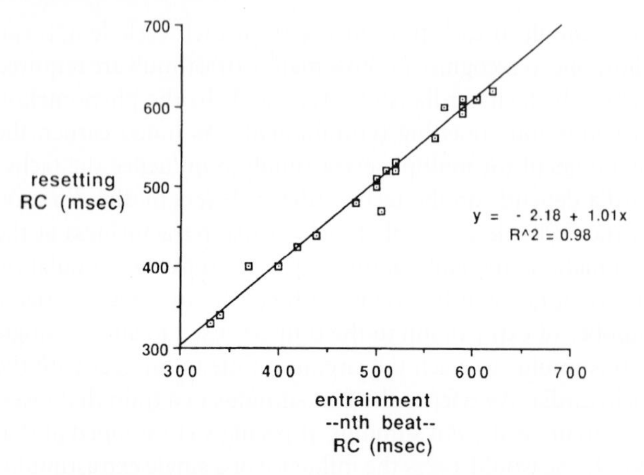


**FIGURE 11-167** Relationship of return cycle during resetting to that following the *n*th beat during entrainment. The return cycle (RC) during resetting (ordinate) is compared to that following the *n*th beat during entrainment at comparable coupling intervals. They are nearly identical. See text for discussion.

number equals that required for resetting ($n$) plus one ($n + 1$) or more until a fixed, stable situation of orthodromic conduction and antidromic collision are present. The characteristics of the excitable gap of VT are best determined by resetting of the tachycardia with a single extrastimulus (regardless of the preceding number of extrastimuli used to allow the single extrastimulus to reset the VT). Once entrainment of the circuit occurs, not only are subsequent stimuli interacting with a reset circuit with a smaller gap, but the characteristics of the reentrant circuit may be altered by the frequency-dependent effects on refractoriness, excitability, and nonuniform anisotropic conduction. Thus, the responses to resetting of the VT by a single extrastimulus may not resemble those responses to entrainment. However, as stated previously, if one compares the first impulse of a train that resets the VT (*n*th beat), it has an identical return cycle to that produced by a single extrastimulus delivered at comparable prematurity (Fig. 11-167).

During entrainment each impulse following the first to reset the VT propagates in both an antidromic and orthodromic direction around the circuit. The antidromic impulse of the last introduced stimulus collides with the orthodromic impulse of the preceding stimulus. The orthodromic impulse of the last introduced stimulus propagates around the circuit to become the first complex of the resumed VT. The conduction time of this impulse to the exit site or QRS is termed the last entrained interval and characterizes the properties of the reset circuit during entrainment. Measurement of the interval from the last stimulus to the first nonpaced VT QRS complex (or the presystolic electrogram) during entrainment at progressively shorter cycle lengths could characterize an "entrainment response curve" analogous (but not identical) to plotting the return cycle versus the coupling interval of single extrastimuli producing resetting described earlier. This return cycle depends critically on the number of extrastimuli delivered that reset the tachycardia circuit before the return cycle is measured, because following the first extrastimulus producing resetting, the subsequent stimuli are relatively more premature and can lead to a different return cycle. Such curves can be very different from true resetting response curves in the same VT. This has led to conflicting interpretations of the nature of the "excitable gap" and misconceptions as to the characteristics of tissue involved in the reentrant circuit. The reasons for these discrepancies and differences between resetting and entrainment will be explained later in this section.

The ability to carefully analyze these phenomena requires methodically delivering an increasing number of stimuli at each of several cycle lengths and, optimally, recording from a presystolic electrogram that was shown to be orthodromically captured during resetting by single extrastimuli or rapid pacing (i.e., multiple stimuli) (Fig. 11-148). In this manner, regardless of whether the tachycardia is reset with a single extrastimulus or the tachycardia circuit is reset by multiple stimuli (entrainment), the characteristics of the orthodromic limb of the reentrant circuit (between the entrance and the exit) can be determined.

During entrainment the return cycle measured at an orthodromically captured presystolic electrogram should equal the PCL (Figs. 11-168 and 11-169). The return cycle length measured at the presystolic electrogram will equal the paced cycle regardless of the site of pacing as long as the presystolic electrogram is orthodromically activated at a fixed stimulus to electrogram interval (i.e., with a fixed orthodromic conduction time) (Fig. 11-170). This would not be seen if the electrogram were captured antidromically (see subsequent paragraphs).

If the time from the orthodromically activated electrogram during VT to the onset of the return cycle QRS remains constant (this is a requirement to prove the electrogram is within or attached to the reentrant circuit proximal to exit of the impulse from the circuit), then the stimulus to QRS will also remain constant at different cycle lengths. The same is true of the electrogram measured at the stimulation site. In the absence of recording a presystolic electrogram, other measurements may be used to characterize the last entrained interval at any PCL. All these measurements are shown in Figure 11-171. Therefore, during entrainment, "curves" relating the PCL to the last entrained interval can be measured from the stimulus to the orthodromic presystolic electrogram, the onset of the QRS of the first VT (nonpaced) complex or local electrogram time (LAT) at the pacing site of the first VT complex. These measurements will be qualitatively identical but have different absolute values. Only sites captured orthodromically during entrainment will occur at the PCL. These intervals must be measured only after entrainment is documented, that is, identical postpacing intervals in response to two consecutive (increasing number) stimuli. Obviously, if continuous resetting of the circuit is present, VT termination will not occur. Thus the expression "termination by entrainment" is an oxymoron, since, by definition, if entrainment is present termination cannot occur. In view of the fact that rapid pacing may influence some of the characteristics of the reentrant circuit, and multiple extrastimuli may engage the tachycardia circuit with different relative prematurity, response curves during entrainment differ from those noted

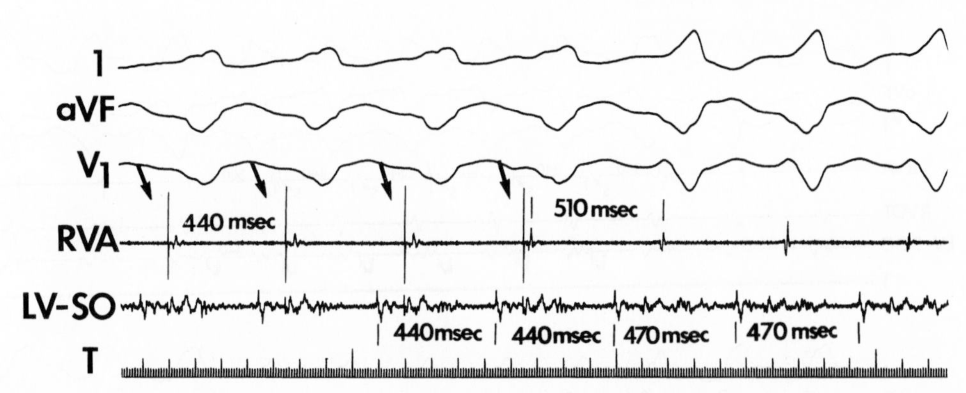


**FIGURE 11-168** Continuous resetting (entrainment) with a return cycle equal to the paced cycle length. Leads 1, aVF, and $V_1$ are shown with electrograms from the RVA and the LV. Overdrive pacing of the tachycardia is shown at a paced cycle length of 440 msec during which the LV is captured orthodromically. Following termination of pacing, the tachycardia returns. The interval between the LV during the last paced interval and the LV of the first nonpaced impulse is 440 msec and equals the paced cycle length. Note that the return cycle measured in the RVA is 510 msec. The presence of an unaltered LV, before the stimulus in the RVA demonstrates local fusion.

with single extrastimuli. These differences are based on the fact that resetting describes characteristics of the VT while the responses to entrainment reflect the influences of multiple extrastimuli on a "reset" circuit that has different electrophysiologic characteristics from the VT circuit itself.

Nearly 70% of VTs reset by single or double extrastimuli have flat or mixed response curves. Overdrive pacing at long cycle lengths (e.g., VTCL 10 msec) can almost always entrain those VTs with large flat resetting curves with a postpacing interval equal to the return cycle observed during the flat part of the resetting curve. During overdrive pacing once the *n*th stimulus of the pacing train resets the tachycardia, the next extrastimulus $(n + 1)$th will reach the reentrant circuit relatively more prematurely. Depending on how premature it is, this $(n + 1)$th extrastimulus may produce no change in return cycle (compared to that in response to the *n*th stimulus), progressive conduction delay—until a fixed, longer return cycle occurs—or termination of the tachycardia. The larger the flat curve observed during resetting and/or the longer the PCL, the more likely the return cycle of the *n*th and $(n + 1)$th stimulus will be the same.[320] In this instance, no matter how many subsequent stimuli are delivered, that return cycle will be the same and equal to that observed during the flat portion of the resetting response curve. However, if the flat portion of the curve is small and/or the PCL is short, the $(n + 1)$th stimulus will fall on partially refractory tissue and the return cycle will

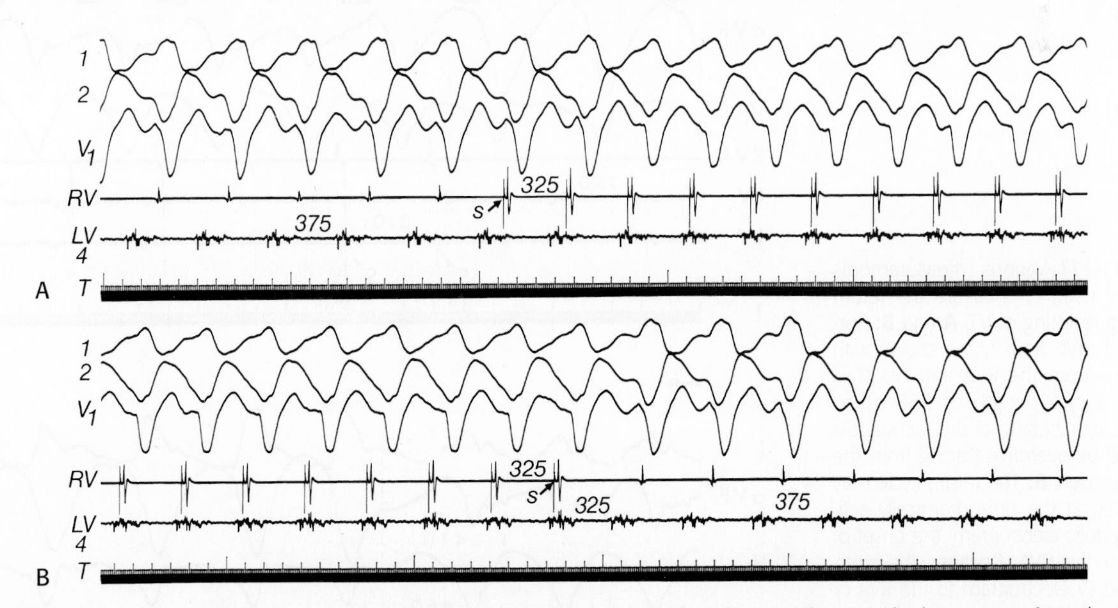


**FIGURE 11-169** Entrainment of VT by right ventricular pacing. **A** and **B:** Leads 1, aVF, and $V_1$, are shown with electrograms from the RV and site 4 in the LV, which was near the exit from the VT circuit. The tachycardia is present at a cycle length of 375 msec. **A:** Right ventricular pacing is begun in the middle of the panel, demonstrating capture of the local electrogram. A fusion complex is seen, which remains fixed during pacing at 325 msec. The RV apical electrogram is captured at the same time that the presystolic electrogram from the VT circuit is recorded. **B:** Each stimulated electrical apical electrogram advances the subsequent site of origin to the cycle length of the pacing. When the pacing is terminated, the first beat of the resumed tachycardia occurs at the time cycle length of the pacing. Thus, pacing entrained the tachycardia. Note an abrupt change from the fused complex on the left in the **bottom panel** to the tachycardia complex on the right of the panel. See text for discussion.

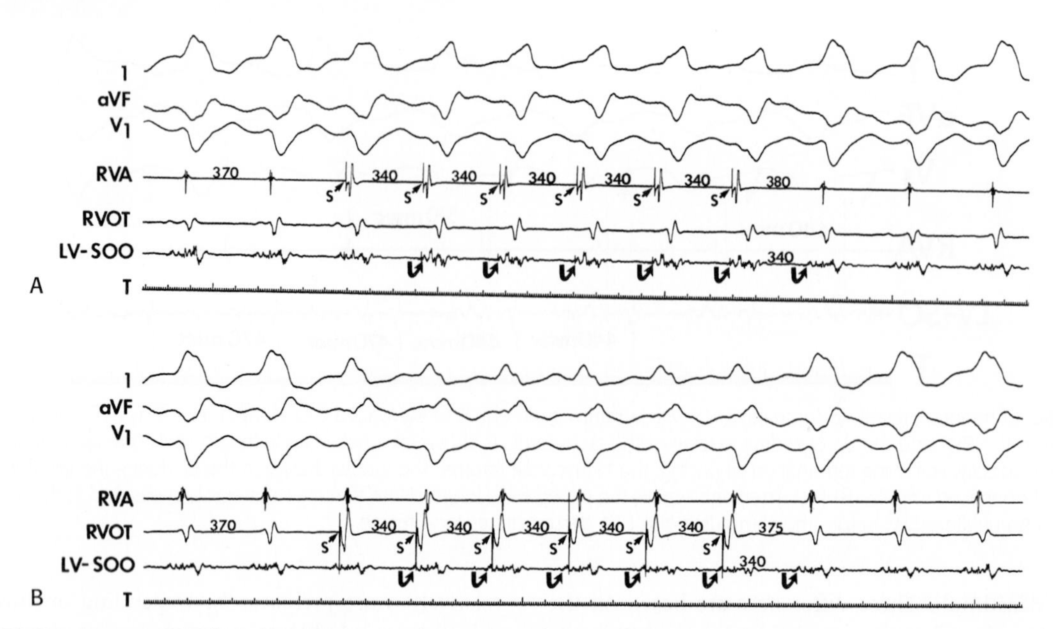


**FIGURE 11-170** Entrainment of VT from both the RVA and RVOT. **A** and **B:** Leads 1, aVF, and $V_1$ are shown with electrograms from the RVA, RVOT, and LV. Tachycardia cycle length is 370 msec. **A:** Overdrive pacing from the RVA at 340 msec entrains VT. Each LV electrogram is advanced by the preceding stimulus artifact; thus, the LV returns at the paced cycle length of 340 msec. The return cycle measured in the RVA is 380 msec. **B:** The same response is noted. Continuous resetting of the tachycardia with a fixed conduction time of the orthodromically captured LV (*curved arrows*) will always result in a return cycle equal to the paced cycle length when measured at the LV. See text for discussion.

increase (Fig. 11-172). Continued pacing at this cycle length will result in a stable but longer return cycle (Fig. 11-172) than the $n$th beat or termination of VT. This occurs because the $(n + 1)$th stimulus falls on the relative refractory period of the $n$th stimulus. A schema explaining these responses is shown in Figure 11-173. Thus, the last entrained interval and the return cycle in response to resetting with single can markedly differ. Consequently, VTs with large fully excitable gaps (flat resetting

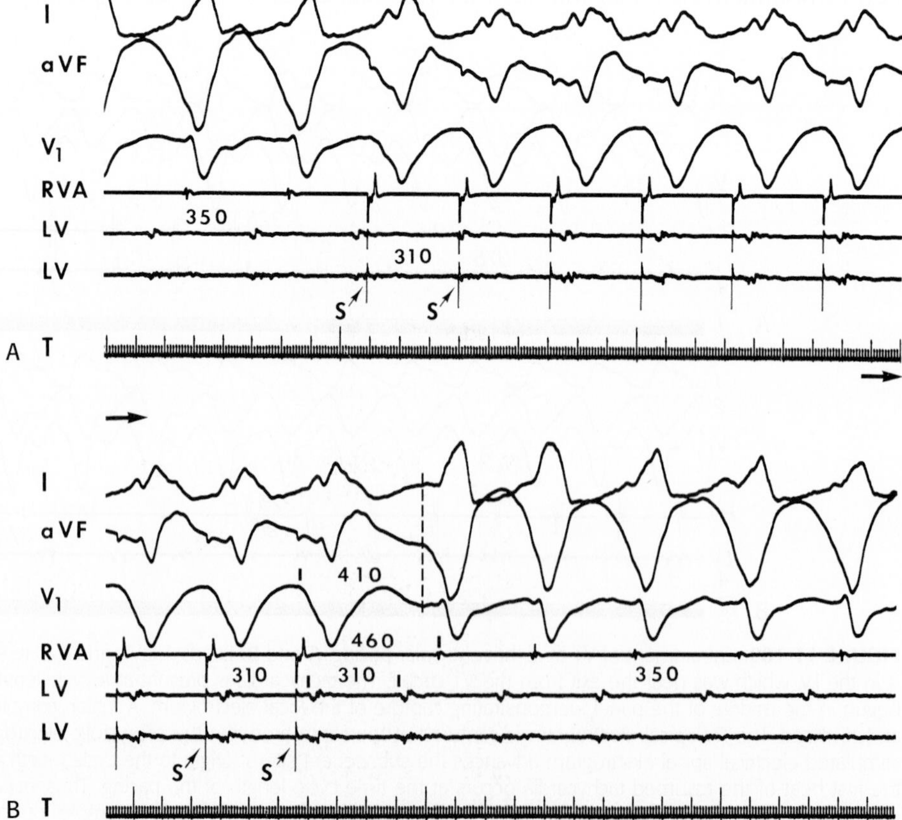


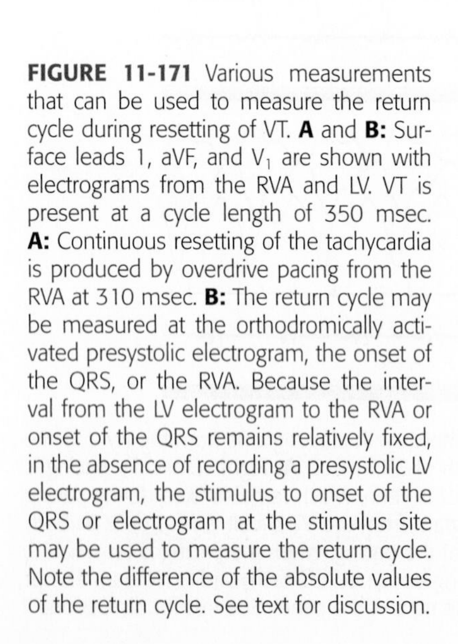
**FIGURE 11-171** Various measurements that can be used to measure the return cycle during resetting of VT. **A** and **B:** Surface leads 1, aVF, and $V_1$ are shown with electrograms from the RVA and LV. VT is present at a cycle length of 350 msec. **A:** Continuous resetting of the tachycardia is produced by overdrive pacing from the RVA at 310 msec. **B:** The return cycle may be measured at the orthodromically activated presystolic electrogram, the onset of the QRS, or the RVA. Because the interval from the LV electrogram to the RVA or onset of the QRS remains relatively fixed, in the absence of recording a presystolic LV electrogram, the stimulus to onset of the QRS or electrogram at the stimulus site may be used to measure the return cycle. Note the difference of the absolute values of the return cycle. See text for discussion.

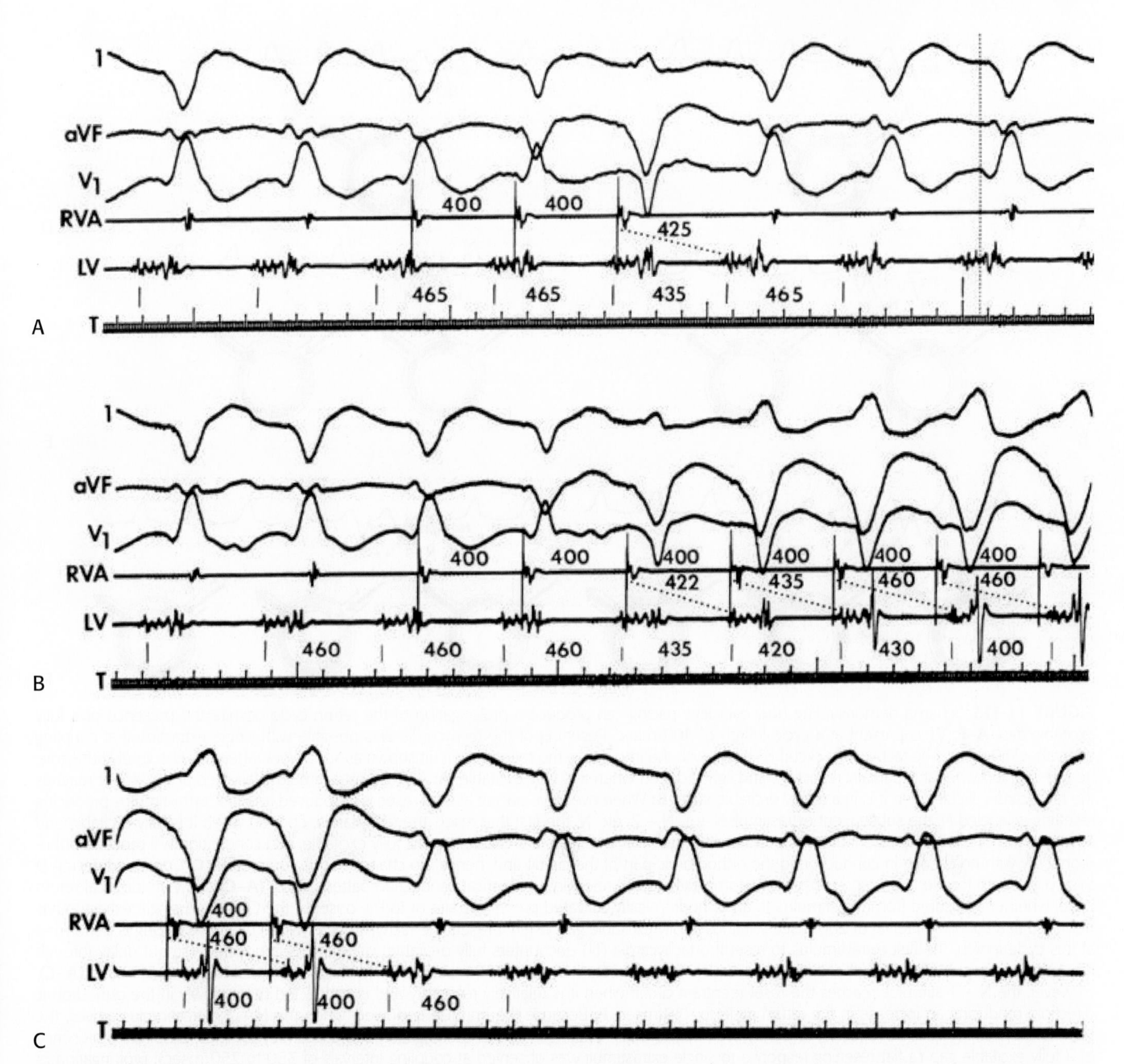


**FIGURE 11-172** Prolongation of conduction time from the stimulus to the orthodromically activated LV site of origin during entrainment in a tachycardia with a known fully excitable gap. **Panels A–C** are arranged similarly. A presystolic electrogram from the VT circuit is shown. VT is present at a cycle length of 460 to 465 msec. **A:** The earliest ventricular extrastimulus that reset the VT during the flat part of the resetting curve (full excitable gap from 420–300 msec) conducts to the LV electrogram in 425 msec. **B–C:** Overdrive pacing is begun at a cycle length of 400 msec. Neither the first nor the second impulse resets the tachycardia, but the third-paced impulse produces resetting manifested by a less than compensatory pause **(B)**. The conduction time from the stimulus to the orthodromically activated LV electrogram is 425 msec. **C:** Pacing at 400 msec is continued. Again, the third impulse is the first to produce resetting of the tachycardia and has a conduction time similar to that in the top panel (422 msec). However, the subsequent extrastimuli fall on the relative refractory period of the reset reentrant circuit, producing a prolongation of the stimulus to orthodromically activated presystolic LV electrogram. As pacing continues, the conduction time prolongs further and then stabilizes at 460 msec. Because the stimulus to orthodromically activated LV electrogram remains fixed at 460 msec, on cessation of pacing, the return cycle, as measured in the LV, will equal the paced cycle length, that is, 400 msec. Thus, even though this tachycardia was shown to have a fully excitable gap by single extrastimuli, overdrive pacing produced a prolongation of conduction of the impulse in the orthodromic direction. See text for discussion.

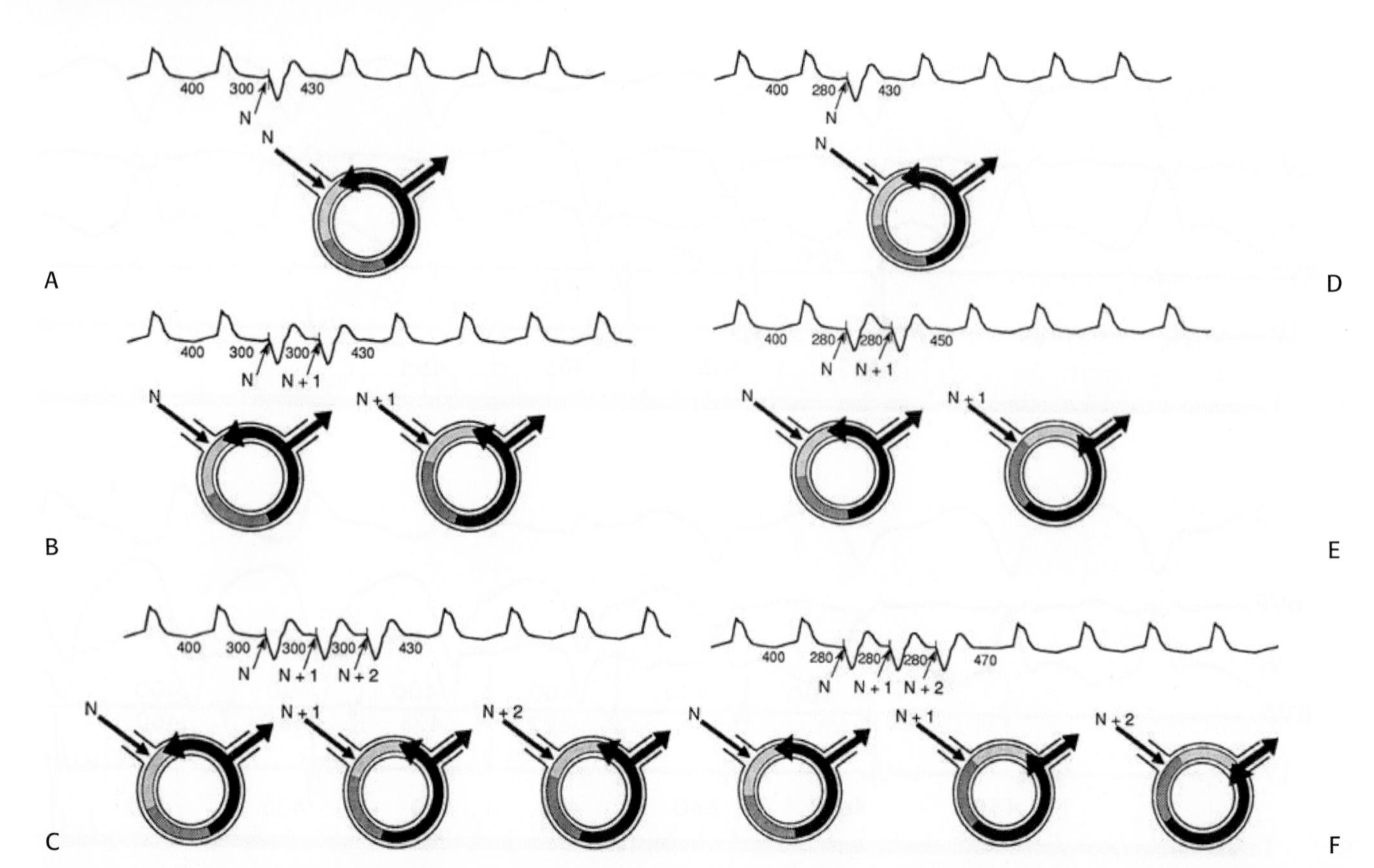


**FIGURE 11-173** Schema demonstrating how overdrive pacing can produce a prolongation of the return cycle despite the presence of a fully excitable gap. **A–F:** VT is present at a cycle length of 400 msec. Resetting of the tachycardia was possible with single extrastimuli at coupling intervals <350 msec. The tachycardia circuit is shown with the impulse in the reentrant circuit shown as *solid black* when it is absolutely refractory, heavily stippled when it is partially refractory, and lightly dotted when it is fully excitable. **A:** A single extrastimulus delivered at 300 msec reaches the tachycardia circuit when it is in a totally excitable state. **B:** When overdrive pacing at 300 msec is introduced, the first extrastimulus producing resetting is labeled N, the subsequent extrastimuli N + 1, N + 2, etc. N, the first that resets the tachycardia, does so when it is fully excitable and advances the circuit by the extent that it is premature. When N + 1 reaches the circuit, it is still fully excitable, and conduction will proceed orthodromically with no change in conduction in the orthodromic part of the circuit and, hence, no change in the return cycle. **C:** Continued pacing at this cycle length for the N + 2 and subsequent complexes would result in an identical conduction pattern. Thus, **(A–C)** show an identical return cycle, whether measured from the stimulus to an orthodromically activated presystolic site or to the onset of the QRS. **D:** A single extrastimulus delivered at a coupling interval of 280 msec still finds a fully excitable gap when it resets the tachycardia. **E:** When overdrive pacing is performed at this cycle length, the first extrastimulus to reset the tachycardia (N) encounters fully excitable tissue and is conducted without delay through the orthodromic part of the circuit and would have given rise to a return cycle of 430 msec (see D), which is identical to that observed in **(A–C)**. However, the N + 1 stimulus reaches the reset reentrant circuit when it is relatively refractory and is conducted more slowly in the orthodromic direction, producing an increase in the return cycle to 450 msec. **F:** Because the impulse is slowed, when the N + 2 extrastimulus arrives, the tachycardia circuit will still be refractory and may even be more so, resulting in further prolongation of the return cycle. Thus, despite the presence of a fully excitable gap (a flat resetting response to single extrastimuli was observed at coupling intervals of 350 to 250 msec), prolongation of conduction in the orthodromic direction by N + 2 and subsequent extrastimuli produce an increased return cycle on cessation of pacing. Thus, during entrainment, the return cycle is not necessarily an accurate reflection of the extent of the excitable gap as determined by single extrastimuli. It is, in fact, the response to the (N + 1)th stimulus that determines the ultimate conduction time through the reentrant circuit during overdrive pacing. If the (N + 1)th stimulus arrives at the circuit when it is still relatively refractory, prolongation of the return cycle or termination will occur, regardless of whether use of a single extrastimulus (N) demonstrated a flat curve. See text for discussion.

response curves) can demonstrate prolonged return cycles, or even termination, at PCLs equal to coupling intervals of single extrastimuli demonstrating a fully excitable gap.[320]

It is not surprising, therefore, that termination is the usual response of VT to overdrive pacing of VT that demonstrated an increasing curve to a single extrastimulus. However, if the number of stimuli following the *n*th complex producing resetting is limited to one or two, particularly at long cycle lengths, termination may not be observed, although the return cycle will be progressively longer following each stimulus. Entrainment is not present until two consecutive postpacing intervals are identical. In such cases, when termination does not occur, the return cycle, as measured from the stimulus to the presystolic electrogram, to the onset of the QRS, or to the LAT will be longer than that observed if pacing were discontinued following the first impulse of the train producing resetting of the tachycardia (*n*th stimulus) at that PCL (Fig. 11-172). In general, the return cycle measured from the stimulus that first produces resetting will be less than the return cycle following cessation of pacing after 10 additional cycles when pacing is carried out at short cycle lengths relative to the VT cycle length. Continued pacing at that cycle length usually produces either a fixed first post-pacing interval with a return cycle longer than that observed following resetting of the tachycardia by a single extrastimulus (Fig. 11-172, entrainment present) or termination of VT. Thus, if only the return cycle following entrainment is used to analyze the "excitable gap," an increasing curve suggesting decremental conduction may result, even though a flat response is observed with single and/or double extrastimuli. Analog recording of this phenomenon and graphs of the return cycles in response to overdrive pacing are shown in Figures 11-174 and 11-175 This has led to conflicting interpretation of the nature of the excitable gap.[1,122,123,316,317,319,326,342,343] We believe that only resetting phenomena describe the characteristics of the VT circuit. Entrainment analyzes a reset circuit that has a shorter excitable gap. It is not surprising that return cycles measured during entrainment might exceed those during resetting, leading to the misconception that the VT circuit is composed of decrementally conducting tissues. This is obviously not the case when VT exhibits a flat resetting response curve. Although flat, flat and increasing, and increasing curves can be seen during entrainment of reentrant VT associated with structural abnormalities (i.e., prior myocardial infarction), increasing curves are virtually always observed during entrainment of idiopathic, verapamil sensitive, left ventricular VT.

When "entrainment" was first described, certain criteria were used to recognize its presence.[1,122,319,326,327] These included (a) fixed fusion of the paced complexes at any cycle length; (b) progressive fusion (i.e., the QRS complex progresses from looking more like the VT complex to looking more like a purely paced complex as pacing cycle length decreases), which is still fixed at any given PCL; and (c) resumption of the tachycardia following pacing with a nonfused complex at a return cycle equal to the PCL. The interpretation of the results of these studies are limited by their failure to use a protocol that allowed analysis of the response to a progressive finite number of extrastimuli at each PCL (pacing was carried out for 3 to 30 seconds). Thus, these studies failed to eliminate the possibility of stopping and starting the tachycardia during the pacing train as well as distorting the characteristics of the excitable gap of the VT itself. Nonetheless, I generally agree with the conclusion of these studies, which held that the presence of any of these findings suggests a reentrant mechanism. The basic physiology of what occurs during entrainment (i.e., resetting of the tachycardia circuit) was not stressed as much as its use to determine the mechanism of the tachycardia as reentry. This has unfortunately led to many misconceptions about what entrainment means and a lack of understanding of the differences between entrainment and resetting by many cardiologists.

None of the initially proposed criteria to recognize entrainment are required to demonstrate resetting of the tachycardia circuit, which is the physiologic basis for entrainment. The demonstration of each of these criteria depends critically on the cycle length of the tachycardia, the characteristics of the excitable gap, and the PCL used. If one studied only the

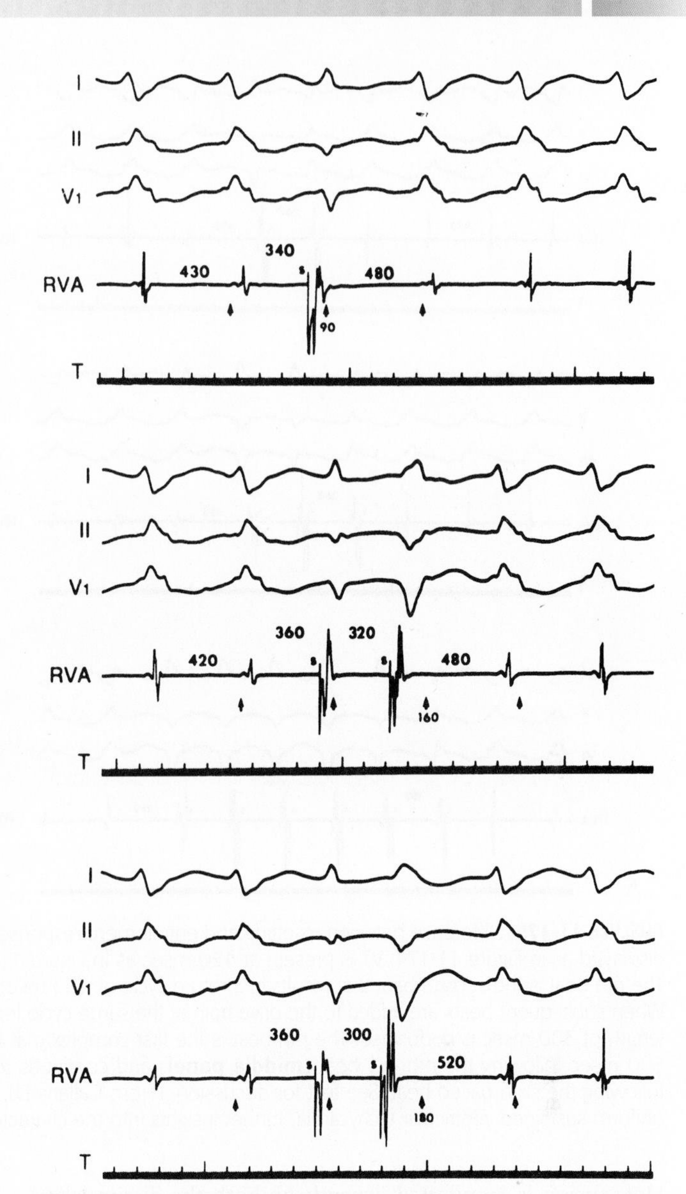


**FIGURE 11-174** Difference between resetting and entrainment-influence of resetting response on subsequent responses to overdrive pacing. ECG leads I, II, and $V_1$ are shown with an electrogram from the RVA. VT is present at a cycle length of 430 msec. **Top panel:** A single extrastimulus is delivered at a coupling interval of 340 msec which arrives 90 msec ahead of the next expected VT complex (*arrow*) and resets the VT with a return cycle of 480 msec. **Middle panel:** Using double extrastimuli (the first being a conditioning stimulus) the second extrastimulus (delivered 320 msec after the first) arrives 160 msec prior to the expected VT complex but has the identical return cycle as single extrastimuli. A flat response of at least 160 msec is present. **Bottom panel:** When the second extrastimulus is delivered 180 msec prior to the expected VT complex an increase in the return cycle is observed (520 msec). Thus a flat and increasing curve is present. See text for discussion. (From Callans DJ, Hook BG, Josephson ME. Comparison of resetting and entrainment of uniform sustained ventricular tachycardia; further insights into the characteristics of the excitable gap. *Circulation* 1993;87:1229–1238.)

response to single extrastimuli during slow tachycardias that demonstrated long flat portions of their resetting response curves and used an initial PCL 20 msec shorter than the tachycardia, all VT would demonstrate the first two characteristics.

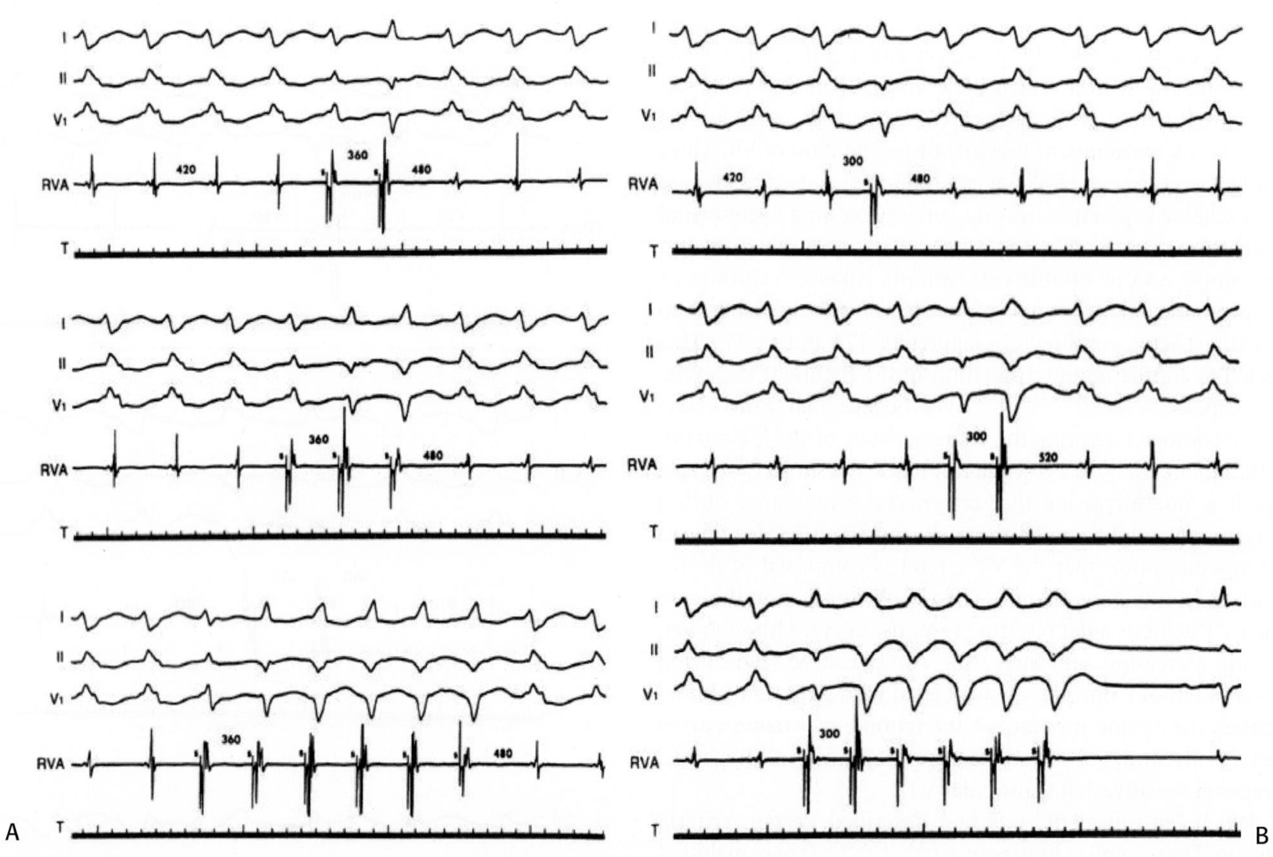


**FIGURE 11-175** Difference between resetting and entrainment-response to overdrive pacing in patient shown in Figure 11-174. Both panels are displayed as in Figure 11-174. VT is present at 420 msec as in Figure 11-174. **A:** Overdrive pacing at a cycle length of 360 msec is performed. The *n*th beat is the second beat that results in a return cycle of 480 msec. The *n*th + 1 beat (**third complex**) results in an identical return cycle. When subsequent beats are added to the drive train at the same cycle length, no increase in return cycle is noted. **B:** Overdrive pacing at a cycle length of 300 msec is performed. The *n*th beat is the first complex that has a return cycle of 480 msec. However, the return cycle increases to 520 msec following the *n*th + 1 beat (**middle panel**) and continues to increase with each incremental beat until the tachycardia terminates following the sixth paced beat. See text for discussion. (From Callans DJ, Hook BG, Josephson ME. Comparison of resetting and entrainment of uniform sustained ventricular tachycardia; further insights into the characteristics of the excitable gap. *Circulation* 1993;87:1229–1238.)

How fusion is manifested depends on both the dissimilarity in morphology between the paced beats and VT as well as the PCL necessary to demonstrate continuous resetting. Surface ECG fusion would be very difficult to recognize for tachycardias having a similar QRS morphology to that produced by pacing from the right ventricular apex, even if fusion were present. If rapid pacing producing a totally "paced QRS" were required to produce resetting, no fusion would be seen. As a result, the criteria for entrainment are less frequently demonstrable than the phenomenon of continuous resetting. Thus, although the presence of any of these criteria always means continuous resetting is occurring, it is important to recognize that resetting occurs in their absence more commonly than in their presence.

To analyze the relationship between the resetting phenomenon and the criteria for "entrainment," we analyzed the response to overdrive pacing of VT in which presystolic electrograms, assumed to arise at or just proximal to the exit site from the reentrant circuit of VT (see following discussion of endocardial mapping of VT), were also orthodromically recorded during resetting of the VT.

The ability to demonstrate surface electrocardiographic fusion and thus fulfill two of the proposed criteria for "entrainment" depends on enough of the ventricular myocardium being depolarized by both the stimulated and tachycardia wavefronts so that the presence of both wavefronts can be recognized (i.e., a QRS complex intermediate between a purely paced QRS and a tachycardia QRS). Because fusion between the stimulated wavefront and that emanating from the tachycardia circuit (the orthodromic wavefront) may be restricted to a small area and not produce a "fused QRS," the basic resetting phenomenon of "entrainment" may not be recognized on the surface ECG. Presystolic electrograms in the VT circuit that are activated orthodromically can be used to demonstrate the presence of fusion when the ECG is insufficiently sensitive. Specifically, using this electrogram one may (a) evaluate the relationship between electrocardiographic and endocardial correlates of fusion, (b) evaluate the mechanisms for inapparent electrocardiographic fusion, and (c) explain why the first postpacing interval measured from the ECG is rarely exactly equal to the PCL.

To have electrocardiographic fusion, the QRS must be composed of a portion of ventricular myocardium activated

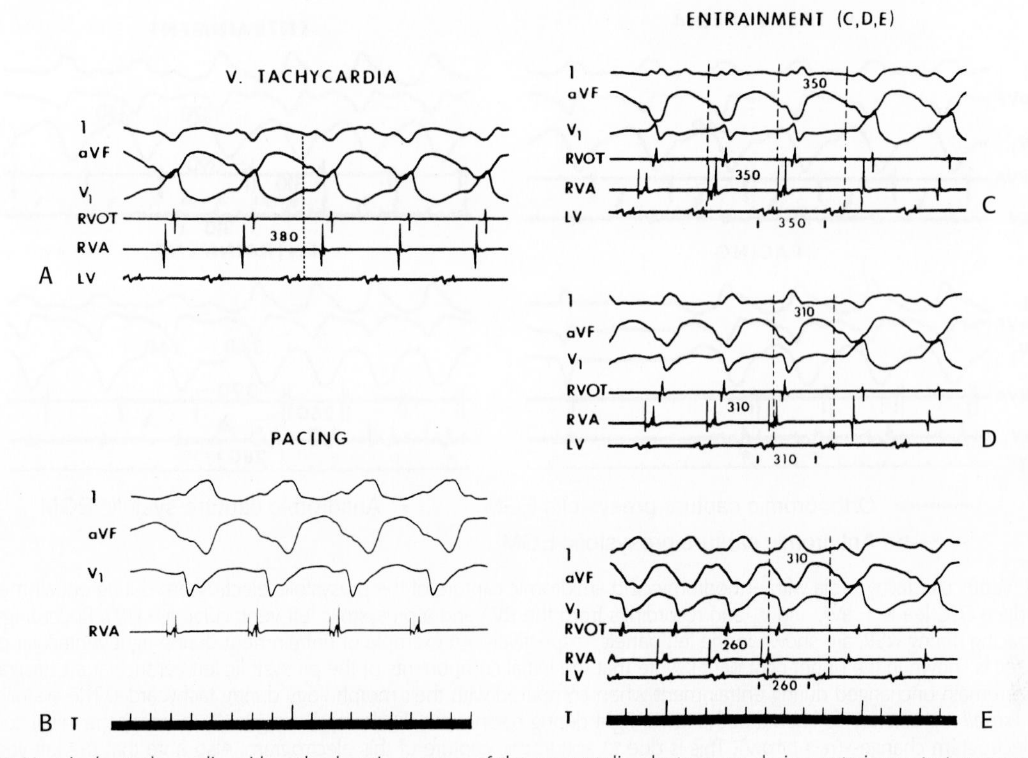


**FIGURE 11-176** Ventricular tachycardia with orthodromic capture of the presystolic electrogram during entrainment at any paced cycle length. **A–E:** Three surface ECG leads (I, aVF, and $V_1$) are shown with intracardiac recordings from the RVA and from the LV at the site of origin of tachycardia (LV). **A:** Uniform sustained VT. **B:** Pacing during NSR. **C–E:** Examples of pacing during VT at cycle lengths of 350, 310, and 260 msec, respectively. The surface ECG and all intracardiac recordings are accelerated to the pacing rate, with immediate resumption of the original VT on cessation of pacing. The QRS morphology in **(C–E)** is intermediate between that of **(A)** and **(B)** (fixed fusion) and displays different degrees of fusion (progressive fusion) The first postpacing interval, as measured at the surface ECG, is equal to the paced cycle in **(C)** and **(D)** but exceeds the paced cycle length in **(E)**. Note that the configuration of the LV presystolic electrogram remains unchanged, with a constant stimulus to LV electrogram interval, at all paced cycle lengths, confirming orthodromic activation and no decremental conduction. (From Almendral JM, Gottlieb CD, Rosenthal ME, et al. Entrainment of ventricular tachycardia: explanation for surface electrocardiographic phenomena by analysis of electrograms recorded within the tachycardia circuit. *Circulation* 1988;77:569.)

from the impulse exiting the tachycardia circuit as well as from the stimulation site. As such, whenever fusion is present, there must be orthodromic activation of the presystolic electrogram in the circuit, which is believed to represent activity at or proximal to the exit from the circuit which has been arbitrarily defined by the onset of the VT QRS. As noted earlier in this section, orthodromic capture of the presystolic electrogram at multiple cycle lengths results in a steady state in which the return cycle equals the PCL when measured at the local presystolic electrogram. This is shown in Figure 11-176, in which PCLs from 350 to 260 msec result in entrainment of the tachycardia. Pacing at cycle lengths of 350 to 310 msec results in a fused QRS complex. Pacing at 260 msec results in the appearance of a fully paced surface QRS complex; however, the phenomenon of entrainment is still present, as demonstrated by the fact that during pacing the local presystolic electrogram is continuously activated in an orthodromic direction so that its configuration is identical to that during the tachycardia. As such, fusion occurs within the circuit at the level of the local electrogram even at the fastest PCL during which the QRS resembles a fully paced QRS, but the stimulus is delivered after the beginning of the orthodromically activated left ventricular electrogram. This is an identical situation to that described earlier (see the section entitled Resetting with Fusion). Surface electrocardiographic fusion is, therefore, not necessary to define the presence of entrainment.

Conversely, if the paced impulse results in antidromic activation (or the so-called "retrograde capture") of the presystolic electrogram before the time at which the tachycardia wavefront would exit to activate the mass of myocardium, then fusion not would be possible. The surface ECG would appear entirely paced. The stimulated impulse would also conduct orthodromically; thus, resumption of the tachycardia would occur with the presystolic electrogram orthodromically activated. Therefore, the last stimulus of the train activates the presystolic electrogram antidromically to produce retrograde capture and simultaneously conducts orthodromically through the circuit. When antidromic or retrograde capture of the local presystolic electrogram occurs, the return cycle, even measured at the site of the presystolic electrogram, will exceed the PCL by the difference in time between when the electrogram is activated retrogradely (i.e., pre-excited antidromically) and when it would have been activated orthodromically (Figs. 11-177 to 11-179). Local fusion and, hence, the possibility of fusion (albeit nonrecognized) outside the circuit can only occur if the presystolic electrogram is activated orthodromically. Collision with

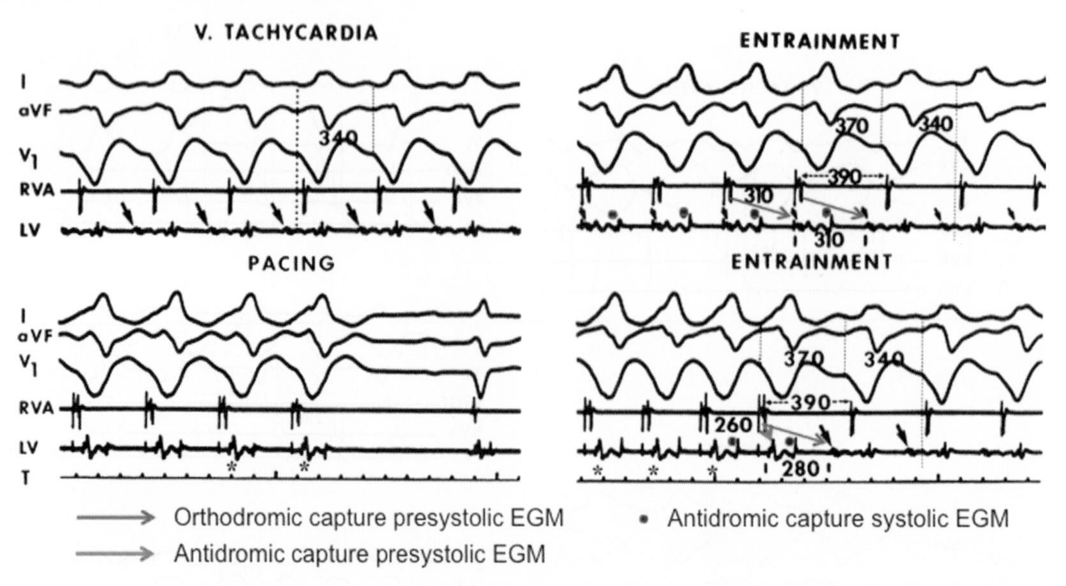


**FIGURE 11-177** Ventricular tachycardia with orthodromic and antidromic capture of the presystolic electrogram during entrainment. Recorded in all panels are surface ECG leads 1, aVF, and $V_1$ and recordings from the RVA and a presystolic left ventricular site (LV). Recordings during VT and right ventricular pacing during NSR, are shown in the left panels, respectively. An example of entrainment during right ventricular pacing at a cycle length of 310 msec is shown in the upper right panel. Note that the initial components of the presystolic left ventricular electrogram (denoted by the *black arrows*) remain unchanged during entrainment when compared with their morphology during tachycardia. The systolic component of this electrogram (*small red asterisk*) is altered at the lower right during pacing at a shorter cycle length (260 msec) the initial component of the left ventricular electrogram changes (*red arrow*). This is due to antidromic capture of this electrogram. Also note that the left ventricular electrogram recorded during entrainment is almost identical to the electrogram recorded during right ventricular pacing in sinus rhythm (*lower left*). The orthodromic activation time to the presystolic electrogram (*green arrow*) remains unchanged. See text for discussion. (Modified from Almendral JM, Gottlieb CD, Rosenthal ME, et al. Entrainment of ventricular tachycardia: explanation for surface electrocardiographic phenomena by analysis of electrograms recorded within the tachycardia circuit. *Circulation* 1988;77:569.)

the last stimulated impulse must occur distal to the presystolic electrogram, either at exit from or outside the circuit. In all such cases, the return cycle measured at this local electrogram will equal the paced cycle. If pacing is performed at a shorter cycle length, then the paced impulse can penetrate the circuit antidromically and retrogradely capture the presystolic electrogram so that no exit from the tachycardia circuit is possible. When pacing is stopped, the impulse that conducts antidromically also conducts orthodromically to reset the reentrant circuit with orthodromic activation of the presystolic electrogram. In Figure 11-177 orthodromic activation time to the presystolic electrogram of the first unpaced QRS is the same as during fusion (green arrow), implying recovery of that presystolic site and a very large fully excitable gap.

Failure to recognize ECG fusion during entrainment by RV pacing during an LV tachycardia, therefore, has two possible explanations. A fully paced QRS (no apparent ECG fusion) can result even when the tachycardia impulse exits the circuit (orthodromic activation of the presystolic electrogram present), if not enough of the ventricular myocardium is activated to alter the QRS. This should be classified inapparent fusion and is depicted in the right-hand panel of Figure 11-178. Absence of ECG fusion is definitely present when retrograde activation of the presystolic impulse occurs (Figs. 11-177 and 11-178). Obviously, the PCL influences the ability to see fusion; pacing at longer cycle lengths can produce inapparent fusion, and shorter cycle lengths can produce absence of fusion. This can be detected only by analyzing whether or not the presystolic electrogram is orthodromically or antidromically activated.

We analyzed the relationship between change in presystolic left ventricular electrogram morphology during entrainment and the presence or absence of surface ECG fusion during 59 pacing events in 18 VT.[319] Retrograde capture had a 100% predictive accuracy for the absence of surface ECG fusion. However, the absence of a change of morphology (i.e., orthodromic activation maintained) did not always predict the presence of ECG fusion. These data are shown in Figures 11-179 and 11-180.

The criterion that the first postpacing interval equals the PCL is obviously not necessary and, in fact, is absent 95% of the time when measured at the surface QRS and 100% of the time when measured at the right ventricular pacing site.[319] This is clearly shown in Figures 11-171, 11-176, and 11-177 The return cycle can equal the paced cycle when measured at the surface ECG if the stimulation site is carried out at the exit site or within a protected isthmus proximal to the exit site from tachycardia circuit or if the stimulus is delivered after the onset of the VT-QRS. When pacing is carried out from the right ventricle and gives rise to the initial (or total) paced QRS complex, the return cycle will be longer than the PCL by the amount of time it takes to begin generating a QRS complex following the presystolic electrogram. Even when measured at the local presystolic electrogram, the return cycle need not equal the PCL.

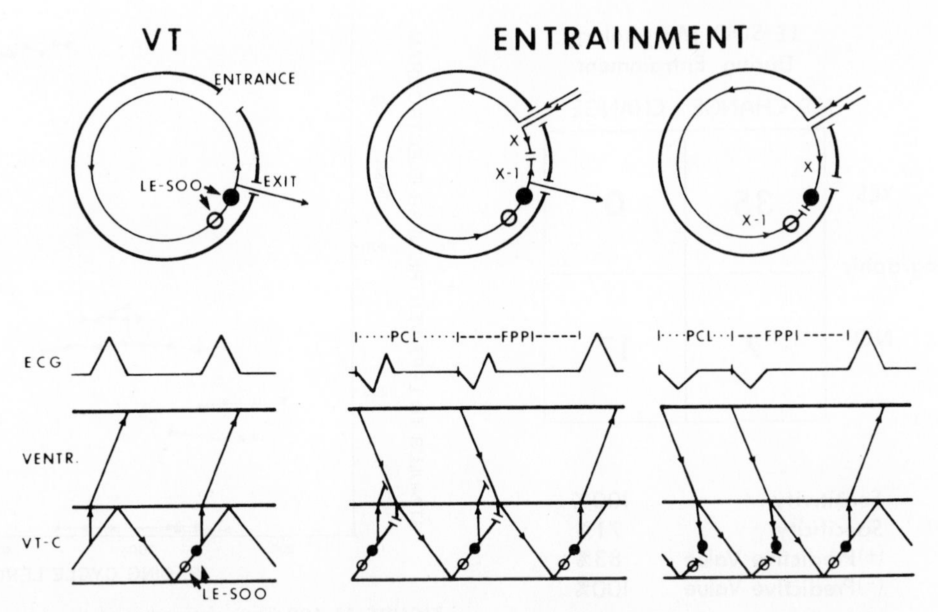


**FIGURE 11-178** Continuous resetting of VT with and without ECG fusion. The *circles* represent sites within the reentrant circuit just proximal to the exit site from the presystolic electrogram is recorded. The *open circles* represent recordings from VTs demonstrating fusion during entrainment, while the *closed circles* represent recordings in VTs in which entrainment in the absence of fusion was also documented. A ladder diagram displaying the VT circuit (VT-C) and the mass of the ventricular myocardium (VENTR) is shown. The panel on the left diagrammatically represents sustained VT. The panel in the middle represents entrainment at a long-paced cycle length. Note the premature penetration of the stimulus into the entrance of the tachycardia circuit so that the tachycardia is advanced to the paced cycle length. During entrainment, collision occurs between the entrance and exit of the tachycardia circuit. Because the impulse exited the circuit before the collision, fusion is present on the surface ECG. The presystolic electrogram is activated by the wavefront entering the circuit and propagating antegradely (orthodromically). Thus, the initial morphology of this electrogram does not change during pacing, and the impulse can exit to produce a fusion complex. However, as depicted in the panel on the right, during pacing at a shorter cycle length, retrograde collision between the stimulated wavefront and the previous tachycardia (or stimulated wavefront) occurs before the point at which the tachycardia can exit the reentrant circuit. The solid electrogram recorded from the reentrant circuit is now activated in a retrograde fashion and is therefore changed in morphology. The open electrogram, however, is still activated in an antegrade fashion (with no change in its initial morphology). Because the presystolic solid electrogram is captured retrogradely, the preceding impulse with which it collides can never exit the circuit; therefore, fusion is impossible during entrainment with retrograde capture of the presystolic electrogram. See text for discussion. FPPI, first postpacing impulse. (From Almendral JM, Gottlieb CD, Rosenthal ME, et al. Entrainment of ventricular tachycardia: explanation for surface electrocardiographic phenomena by analysis of electrograms recorded within the tachycardia circuit. *Circulation* 1988;77:569.)

As mentioned earlier and as demonstrated in Figure 11-177, if antidromic (i.e., retrograde) capture of the presystolic electrogram is observed during pacing, the return cycle will never equal the PCL even at the local presystolic electrogram. It will exceed the PCL by the amount of time that the antidromically **activated** electrogram is pre-excited (i.e., prior to the time it would have been activated orthodromically). Thus, one can demonstrate two pathways of conduction to the presystolic electrogram: one that has a more prolonged conduction time—that is, the orthodromic pathway in the circuit—and one that results in antidromic capture of that electrogram. Thus, stimulation from the same site in the heart can manifest two activation times to the same point in the reentrant circuit. This has led to the concept that the orthodromic limb of the circuit exhibits a long conduction time.[1,122,319,326,327,337,342,343] This can be easily demonstrated with progressively rapid pacing. At longer PCLs, orthodromic capture of the presystolic electrogram occurs, and at a critical shorter cycle length, antidromic capture occurs. During orthodromic activation, the stimulus to local electrogram interval is greater than during antidromic capture (Fig. 11-180). Note that in Figure 11-180 the interval from the stimulus to local presystolic electrogram remains flat over a period of cycle lengths during both orthodromic and antidromic activation, suggesting that no decremental conduction was present. Although others have "demonstrated" the so-called "decremental properties" in the orthodromic limb,[326,327,335,342,343] this concept is misleading. Slowing is secondary to interval-dependent conduction delay through tissue that has only partially recovered excitability when the $(n + 1)$th stimulus reached the circuit. As noted earlier one can observe a flat resetting curve in response to single extrastimuli, yet when rapid pacing is initiated, following the first extrastimulus producing resetting ($n$th stimulus) the subsequent stimuli can occur during the relative refractory period of the excitable gap and prolong the return cycle. This prolonged stimulus to presystolic electrogram compared to a single extrastimulus does not imply decremental properties analogous to that of the A-V node (Fig. 11-175 for explanation). Whether or not the stimulus to local presystolic electrogram increases with decreased PCL depends on whether the $(n + 1)$th stimulus (stimulus following the first that produces resetting of the tachycardia) arrives at the circuit in a fully excitable, partially excitable, or

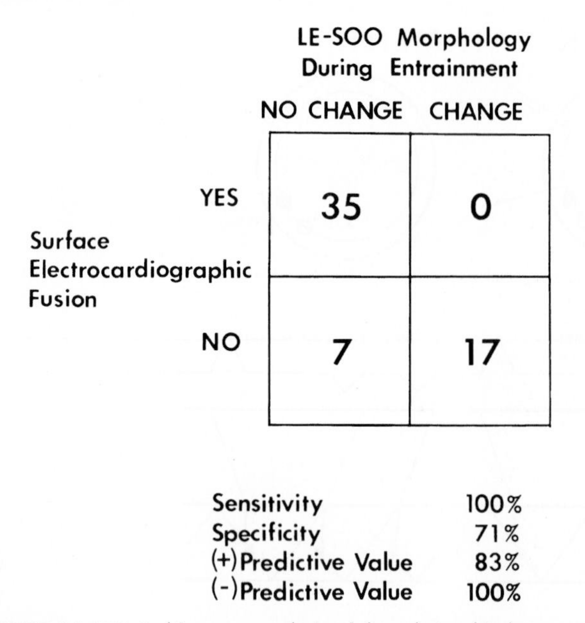


**FIGURE 11-179** A chi-square analysis of the relationship between a change in the presystolic left ventricular electrogram during entrainment and the presence or absence of surface ECG fusion during resetting by overdrive pacing at 59 drive cycle lengths. Of particular note is the absence of surface ECG fusion being correctly predicted (100%) by a change in the morphology of the initial component of the presystolic electrogram. Conversely, however, the absence of a change in morphology of the presystolic electrogram recorded from the tachycardia circuit did not always predict the presence of surface electrocardiographic fusion. (From Almendral JM, Gottlieb CD, Rosenthal ME, et al. Entrainment of ventricular tachycardia: explanation for surface electrocardiographic phenomena by analysis of electrograms recorded within the tachycardia circuit. *Circulation* 1988;77:569.)

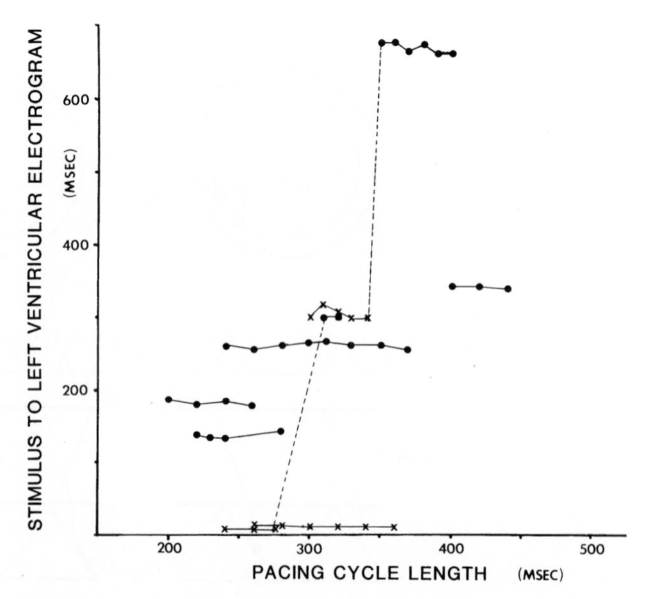


**FIGURE 11-180** The relationship of the conduction time from the stimulus to the presystolic left ventricular electrogram as a function of the paced cycle length in seven sustained VTs. The *closed circles* represent the conduction time in the absence of a change in the morphology of the initial component of the LE-SOO. The Xs represent the conduction time from the stimulus to the left ventricular electrogram in the presence of a change in the initial component of this electrogram. Note that there is no significant change in conduction time over a range of cycle lengths when the morphology of the electrogram is preserved. Although there is dramatic change in conduction time from the stimulus to the left ventricular electrogram at the site of origin when there is a change in the morphology of this electrogram, once the electrogram has changed in morphology, the conduction time remains stable over a wide range of paced cycle lengths. (From Almendral JM, Gottlieb CD, Rosenthal ME, et al. Entrainment of ventricular tachycardia: explanation for surface electrocardiographic phenomena by analysis of electrograms recorded within the tachycardia circuit. *Circulation* 1988;77:569.)

unexcitable state.[320] If it arrives at a fully excitable state, the stimulus to local electrogram will be the same as observed using a single extrastimulus regardless of the cycle length of pacing. This is demonstrated in analog records in Figure 11-176 and in graphic representation in Figure 11-180. The prolongation of the stimulus to local electrogram interval at shorter cycle length means that the $(n + 1)$th stimulus has encountered partially excitable tissue in the reentrant circuit. It does not mean that the circuit does not have a fully excitable gap. The presence of a flat response curve in response to single extrastimuli (regardless of the number of preceding stimuli) during VT at cycle lengths <400 msec suggests that no "decremental" properties analogous to the A-V node were present in the VT circuit.

During entrainment, when the initial components of the paced QRS result from pacing, the first return cycle, as measured from the stimulus to the onset of the QRS of the return VT complex, will be fixed. A fixed postpacing interval greater than the PCL following two consecutive stimuli is another criterion suggesting that entrainment is present. This obviously requires a constant stimulus to local presystolic electrocardiogram conduction time in the orthodromic direction (e.g., the return cycle of $n + 2$ = that following $n + 3$). This is demonstrated in Figures 11-176 and 11-177, where the first postpacing cycle measured at the onset of the QRS of the return cycle is constant and not necessarily equal to the PCL. If the postpacing interval were made at the local presystolic electrogram, the interval will vary depending on whether the presystolic electrogram is orthodromically or antidromically captured during pacing, which in turn will depend on the PCL.

The conduction time in the orthodromic limb is the determinant of whether or not a fixed first postpacing interval occurs, regardless of where it is measured. If the conduction time from the stimulus to the local presystolic electrogram prolongs, then the return cycle, as measured to the onset of the QRS, will also be prolonged. To reiterate, when an increase in orthodromic conduction is observed during overdrive pacing resetting of the reentrant circuit is taking place. It is only when a stable state of orthodromic conduction follows an incremental number of paced complexes that entrainment is said to be present. However, at any PCL, once a steady state of orthodromic activation time is reached, and entrainment is achieved, the first postpacing will remain constant.

Entrainment of VT by atrial pacing has been observed in reentrant VT due to coronary artery disease and idiopathic

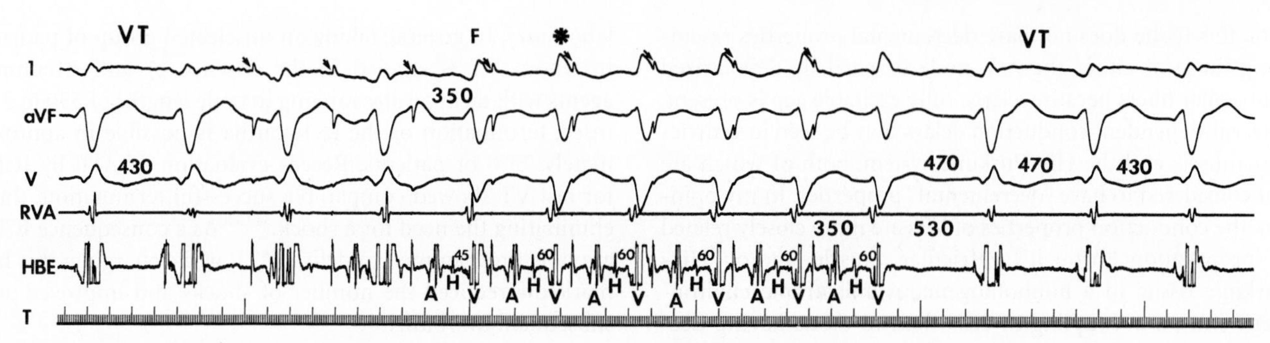


**FIGURE 11-181** Entrainment of VT by atrial pacing. VT is present at a cycle length of 430 msec. Atrial pacing is begun at a cycle length of 350 msec. This ultimately results in total supraventricular capture with appropriate A-H and H-V intervals. Following termination of pacing, the tachycardia resumes with a prolonged return cycle. See text for discussion. (From Almendral JM, Gottlieb C, Marchlinski FE, et al. Entrainment of ventricular tachycardia by atrial depolarizations. *Am J Cardiol* 1985;56:298.)

verapamil–sensitive VT, and in bundle branch reentry.[326,328,344–346] Entrainment of VT from multiple ventricular sites can always be demonstrated in such cases; continuous resetting during atrial pacing merely reflects ventricular activation initiated at the same site of earliest activation as during normal sinus rhythm. Examples of atrial pacing entraining tachycardias are shown in Figures 11-181 and 11-182. As in tachycardias entrained by overdrive ventricular pacing, those demonstrating similar phenomena in response to atrial pacing can have relatively short return cycles equal to the PCL or prolonged return cycles greater than the tachycardia cycle length. The ability to entrain the tachycardia and maintain a supraventricular QRS complex is further support that the tachycardia circuit must be small and electrocardiographically silent.

All studies using overdrive pacing as well as single extrastimuli suggest that the conduction time through the tachycardia circuit in the orthodromic direction is relatively long. The site(s) and mechanism of this slow conduction is unclear, but in view of the fact that nearly 70% of VT demonstrate a flat resetting curve to single or double extrastimuli, representing a fully excitable gap for >15% of the tachycardia cycle, the mechanism of this slow conduction must differ from that of the A-V node. Flat return cycle curves can also be observed during overdrive pacing (Fig. 11-180). If the decremental conduction observed with premature impulses and shortened PCLs were due to decremental conduction in slow response fibers analogous to those of the A-V node; a flat return cycle should not be observed. But a flat resetting response is the rule. Thus, I believe that slow conduction in the orthodromic direction is likely due to the nonuniform anisotropic characteristics and abnormalities of gap junctions of the circuit. Although depolarized fibers using partially inactivated sodium channels are associated with slow conduction, such fibers also demonstrate decremental properties. As noted earlier in the chapter, the response of the arrhythmogenic substrate to pharmacologic agents is most consistent with normally polarized myocardial fibers.[54] It is also theoretically possible that the prolonged conduction time reflects a longer pathway of activation in the orthodromic direction and is unrelated to conduction velocity per se. Nonetheless, based on available

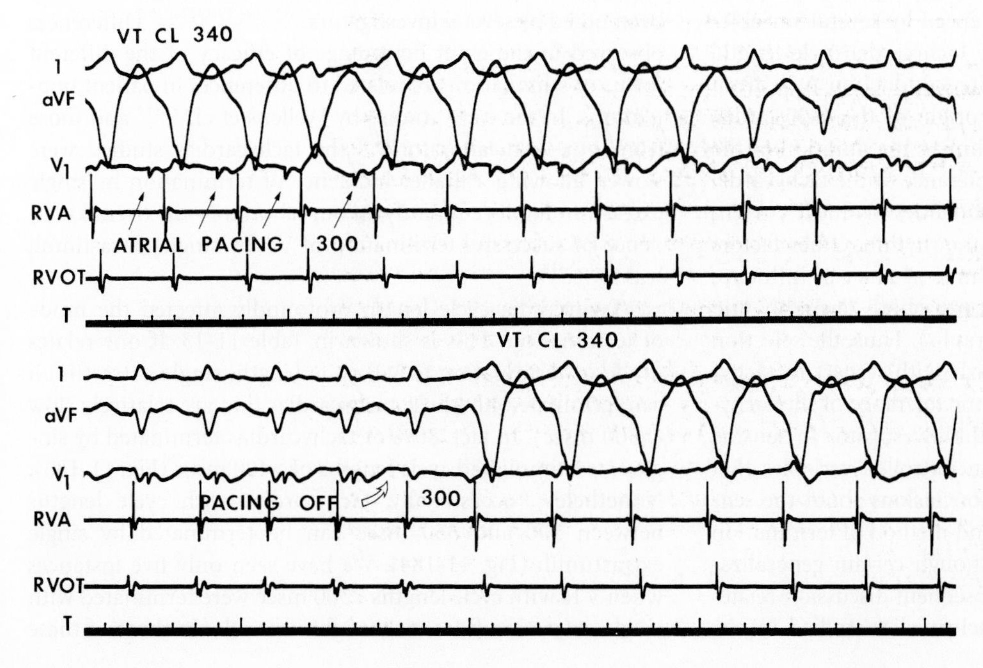


**FIGURE 11-182** Entrainment of VT by atrial pacing with orthodromic capture of the right ventricular apex. Three surface ECG leads and electrograms from the RVA and RVOT are shown. VT is present at a cycle length of 340 msec when atrial pacing is begun. Eventually, supraventricular capture occurs, during which time there is a fixed relationship of the RVA and RVOT that differs from that during VT. On cessation of pacing, the first return cycle measured in the RVA equals the paced cycle length, suggesting that it was orthodromically captured during right atrial pacing. This is not the case of the RVOT. See text for discussion. (From Almendral JM, Gottlieb C, Marchlinski FE, et al. Entrainment of ventricular tachycardia by atrial depolarizations. *Am J Cardiol* 1985;56:298.)

data, this tissue does not have decremental properties resembling those of either the A-V node or partially depolarized ventricular fibers because a large fully excitable gap is present. Interval-dependent conduction delays may be seen in ventricular muscle and the His–Purkinje system, both of which are not considered to have "decremental" properties. In my opinion, the conduction properties of VTs are more closely related to propagation through ventricular muscle and/or His–Purkinje tissue in a nonhomogeneous anisotropic environment and poor coupling of cells than to tissue having decremental properties. Detailed mapping of the reentrant circuit of VT in experimental models and in humans has shown abnormalities of gap junctions and nonuniform anisotropic conduction in areas of the VT circuit.[29,47,48,51,347,348]

We have not noted overdrive acceleration analogous to that seen in triggered rhythms (i.e., linear relation of PCL to early acceleration of the cycle length) in patients with VT that is due to coronary artery disease or with idiopathic VTs. Overdrive acceleration has been observed during rapid pacing, but in this instance, a more rapid rhythm ensues on cessation of rapid pacing without acceleration or deceleration during that tachycardia. In this instance, it is as if the rapid pacing decreases the size of the reentrant circuit or produces double wave reentry. The ability to terminate these rapid tachycardias by pacing from distant sites favors a functional shortening of the VT circuit since it is difficult to penetrate double wave reentry. It is also consonant with the functional nature of barriers as demonstrated by different resetting curves from different sites of stimulation.[320] Overdrive suppression analogous to that seen in automatic fibers has not been observed in sustained VTs although prolonged return cycles are seen at rapid paced rates.

### *Termination of Sustained Ventricular Tachycardia*

The ability to terminate sustained VT by programmed stimulation and/or rapid pacing is influenced by several variables previously discussed. They include tachycardia cycle length, refractoriness at the stimulation site, conduction time from the stimulation site to the site of origin of the tachycardia, and in the case of reentrant arrhythmias, the duration of the excitable gap. The hemodynamic tolerance of the tachycardia also determines whether pacing modalities or direct current cardioversion is used to terminate the rhythm. Other factors such as the presence of antiarrhythmic agents can influence the ability to terminate the tachycardia both favorably and unfavorably (see subsequent paragraphs). Thus, the selection of patients to be studied, particularly with respect to tachycardia cycle length and hemodynamic tolerance of the tachycardia as well as the "anxiety" of the investigator in sensing the urgency of termination, are uncontrolled variables that make it impossible to reach firm conclusions about the sensitivity of the ability to terminate and method of termination of VT based on the literature. Although certain generalizations can be made, much of the subsequent discussion relates to personal experience with the tachycardias studied in our laboratory. In general, taking an unselected group of patients in whom VT is studied in the absence of antiarrhythmic agents with tachycardias ranging in cycle lengths of 550 to 220 msec, termination of the tachycardia is possible in approximately 75% of patients. Recent evaluation of ATP by ICDs for fast VT showed comparable successful termination; thus, eliminating the need for a shock.[349,350]As a consequence ICDs are now programmed to deliver ATP while charging; this has markedly reduced the number of shocks and improved and subsequent morbidity.

The tachycardia cycle length seems to be the main determinant of whether the tachycardia can be terminated by some form of programmed stimulation or pacing or will require cardioversion.[322–325] Thus, as shown in Table 11-13, of 139 consecutively studied patients one-half the tachycardias having cycle lengths <300 msec required cardioversion.[322–325] This was due to a combination of factors including rapid collapse of the patient and, therefore, inability to test programmed stimulation, acceleration of the tachycardia with subsequent necessity for cardioversion, or failure of several pacing modalities optional to cardioversion.[322–325] It should be noted that some VT with short cycle lengths can be converted by pacing. Although 50% of VTs with cycle lengths <300 msec required cardioversion, at other times the same VT could be terminated by pacing. Nonetheless, the vast majority of VT can be reproducibly terminated by some pacing method. Regardless of the mode of stimulation used, termination is usually abrupt, which distinguishes it from termination of triggered activity. The tachycardia cycle length has the most marked influence on the mode of termination.

In a consecutive series of patients, we found that rapid ventricular pacing was the most efficacious way of terminating the tachycardia (Table 11-14).[322] Although we did not compare the use of single, double, or triple extrastimuli and/or rapid pacing in each patient, the success of termination was directly related to the number of extrastimuli used. This has been noted by several investigators.[1,122,194,195,322–325] Differences observed in the exact percentage of efficacy of the different forms of stimulation are related to differences in patient populations. In the early studies by Wellens et al.[193,194] and those from our own laboratory,[195] the tachycardias studied were slower, allowing a higher incidence of termination by single extrastimuli. More recently, in our laboratory the overall incidence of successful termination of VT by single extrastimuli was 27%.[319]

Tachycardia cycle length profoundly affected the mode of termination. This is shown in Table 11-13. If one relates mode of termination to VT cycle length, single extrastimuli can terminate only those tachycardias that are relatively slow (>300 msec). In fact, 80% of tachycardias terminated by single extrastimuli had cycle lengths of >400 msec (Fig. 11-183). Nonetheless, occasionally, tachycardias with cycle lengths between 300 and 350 msec can be terminated by single extrastimuli (Fig. 11-184). We have seen only five instances when VTs with cycle lengths <300 msec were terminated with single extrastimuli from the right ventricle. In three of these

TABLE 11-14 Effects of Programmed Ventricular Stimulation (PVS) During VT (123 Patients)

| Mode oF PVS | Patients (N) | Termination | | Acceleration | |
|---|---|---|---|---|---|
| | | n | % | n | % |
| 1 VES | 85 | 23 | 27 | 1 | 1.2 |
| 2 VES | 62 | 39 | 63 | 2 | 3.2 |
| 3 VES | 16 | 7 | 44 | 2 | 13 |
| RVP | 54 | 41 | 76 | 19 | 35 |

VT, ventricular tachycardia; VES, ventricular extrastimuli; RVP, rapid ventricular pacing.
From Roy D, Waxman HL, Buxton AE, et al. Termination of ventricular tachycardia: Role of tachycardia cycle length. *Am J Cardiol* 1982;50:1346.

instances, this was nonreproducible. Two or more RV extrastimuli are often required for termination when tachycardias have cycle lengths shorter than 400 msec or occur in the setting of a large ventricular aneurysm associated with marked abnormalities of conduction between the stimulation site and the site of the tachycardia. This is usually manifested by the intervening tissue having markedly abnormal electrograms during sinus rhythm,[31–33] and/or by a bizarre, wide QRS during VT (Fig. 11-185). Occasionally two extrastimuli are required to terminate tachycardias that are not too rapid

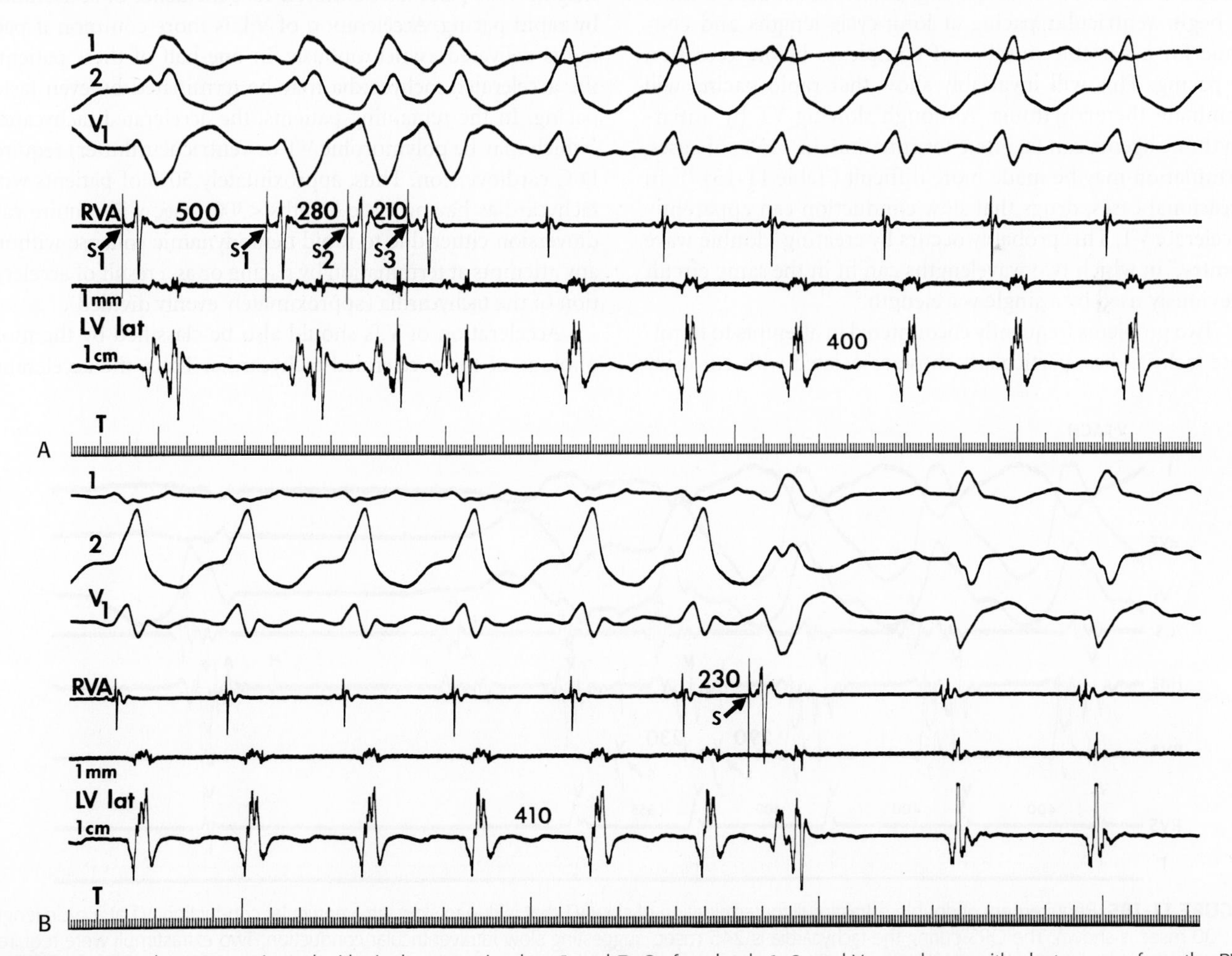


**FIGURE 11-183** Slow VT terminated with single extra stimulus. **A** and **B:** Surface leads 1, 2, and $V_1$ are shown with electrograms from the RVA and LV lateral wall (LV lot) using a 1-mm and 1-cm interelectrode distance. **A:** Sustained uniform VT is initiated with double extrastimuli. The tachycardia has a cycle length of 400 msec. **B:** A single extrastimulus at 230 msec terminates the tachycardia.

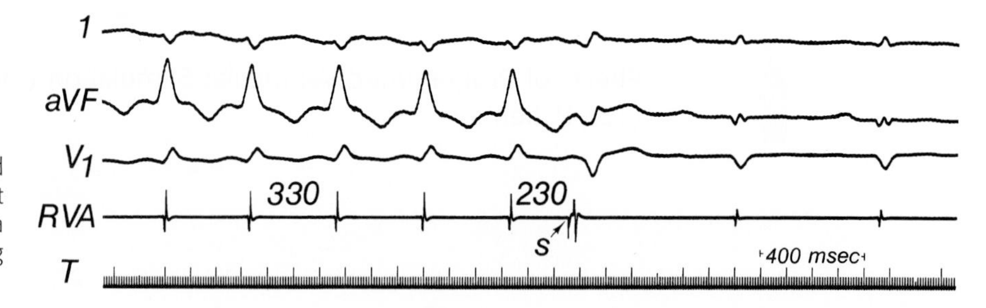


**FIGURE 11-184** Termination of relatively rapid VT with a single ventricular extrastimulus. VT at a cycle length of 330 msec is terminated by a single extrastimulus from the RVA at a coupling interval of 230 msec.

or have relatively "narrow" QRS complexes, regardless of the site of stimulation (Fig. 11-186). In contrast to the use of "double" extrastimuli during resetting, these studies used double extrastimuli such that the coupling intervals of both were reduced until refractoriness was reached or VT termination occurred. Rapid pacing is the most effective form of termination, regardless of tachycardia cycle length (Fig. 11-187). In fact, all tachycardias that are terminable by single or double extrastimuli can be terminated by rapid pacing. Failure of rapid pacing to terminate an arrhythmia that has previously been shown to be terminated by single or double extrastimuli suggests that the tachycardia was terminated then reinitiated before discontinuation of pacing. Thus, care must be taken to begin ventricular pacing at long cycle lengths and continue for a variable number of complexes before cessation of pacing. This will invariably show that rapid pacing will terminate the arrhythmia. Although slowing VT by antiarrhythmic agents can facilitate termination, in ≈25% of cases, termination may be made more difficult (Table 11-15).[322] In occasional cases, drugs that slow conduction can apparently accelerate VT. This probably occurs by creating "double wave reentry," in which two wavelengths can fit in the same circuit previously used by a single wavelength.[51,351]

Two problems frequently encountered in attempts to terminate tachycardias, particularly those associated with coronary artery disease, are acceleration of the arrhythmia by overdrive pacing or the appearance of multiple distinct uniform VT morphologies. We have arbitrarily defined acceleration of a tachycardia as a sustained shortening of the tachycardia cycle length by >30 msec following cessation of pacing. In our experience, this occurs in approximately 25% of tachycardias.[322–325] The frequency of acceleration is related to the mode of stimulation, which in turn is related to the tachycardia cycle length. Acceleration is rare, using single or double extrastimuli (<5%) but approaches 35% during rapid pacing.[322–325] Because rapid pacing is required to terminate fast tachycardias, these VT have a higher incidence of acceleration: tachycardias with cycle lengths <300 msec have almost a 40% incidence of acceleration by rapid pacing. Acceleration of VT is more common if pacing is delivered asynchronously. In one-half of these patients, the accelerated tachycardia may be terminated by even faster pacing. In the remaining patients, the accelerated tachycardia (which may be polymorphic VT or ventricular flutter) requires D/C cardioversion. Thus, approximately 50% of patients with tachycardias having cycle lengths <300 msec will require cardioversion either due to rapid hemodynamic collapse without any attempts at termination by pacing or as a result of acceleration of the tachycardia (approximately evenly divided).

Acceleration of VTs should also be classified by the morphology of the accelerated tachycardia. Thus, the accelerated

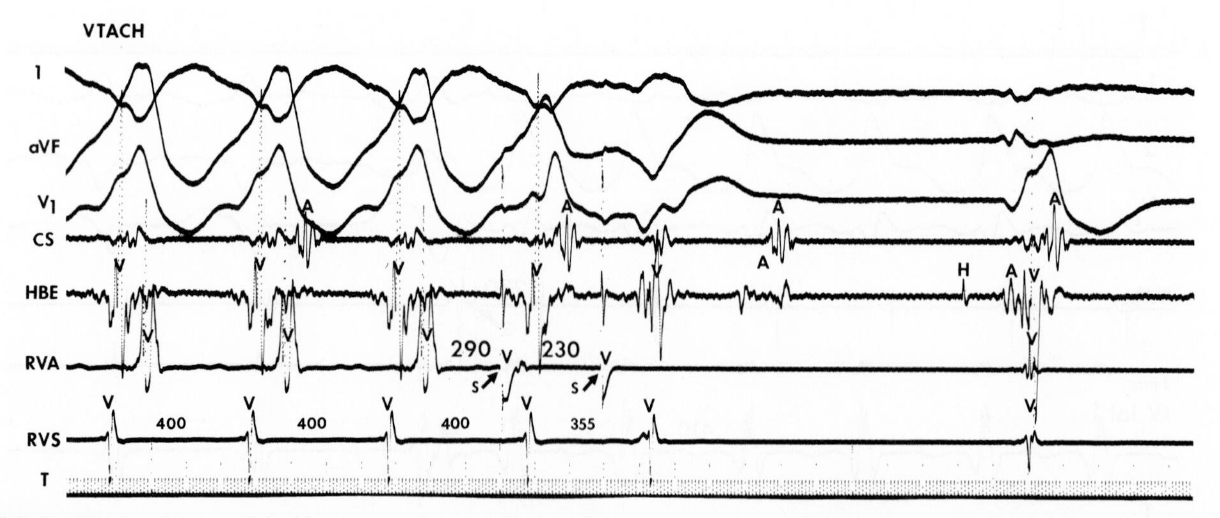


**FIGURE 11-185** Requirement of double extrastimuli for termination of slow VT that is due to slow intraventricular conduction. VT at a cycle length of 200 msec is shown. The QRS during the tachycardia is 245 msec, suggesting slow intraventricular conduction. Two extrastimuli were required to terminate this relatively slow tachycardia. The first extrastimulus delivered at 290 msec fails to influence the tachycardia but changes the path of ventricular activation and shortens local ventricular refractoriness so that a second extrastimulus delivered at 230 msec penetrates the reentrant circuit and terminates the tachycardia.

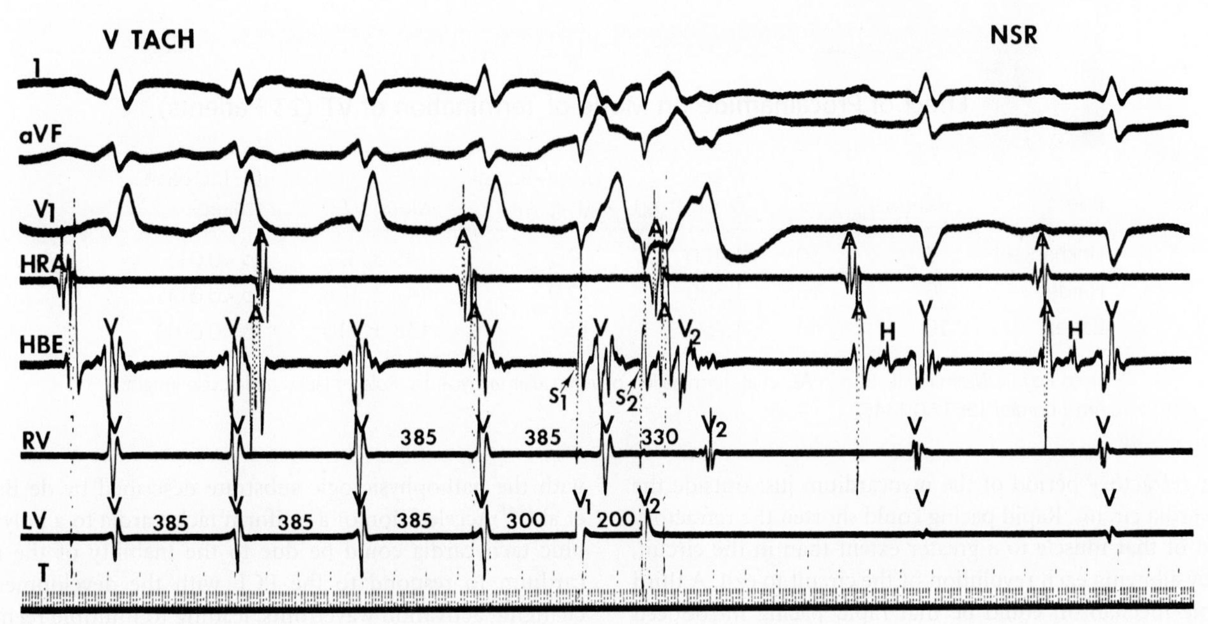


FIGURE 11-186 Termination of relatively narrow VT by two ventricular extrastimuli. Leads 1, aVF, and $V_1$ are shown with electrograms from the HRA, HBE, RV, and LV. The QRS is relatively narrow at 110 msec because the site of origin was shown to be intraseptal. The cycle length of the tachycardia is 385 msec. After the fourth VT complex, two ventricular extrastimuli ($S_1S_2$) are introduced to the LV coupling intervals of 300 msec and 200 msec, respectively. $S_1$ captures the LV but fails to capture the RV and the ventricular electrogram in the HBE, both of which occur on time. However, $S_1$ shortens the refractoriness of the intervening tissues so that $S_2$ can depolarize the reentrant circuit and terminate the arrhythmia.

tachycardia could have an identical morphology to the original VT, could have a different uniform morphology, or could be changed to a polymorphic VT, with or without degeneration to VF. The mechanisms of the different forms of acceleration probably differ, but documentation would require detailed study with multisite mapping of the reentrant circuit. Therefore, the following proposed mechanisms should be considered hypothetical. When the morphology of the accelerated tachycardia is identical to that of the original tachycardia, one must assume that the exit from the tachycardia circuit is the same. As such, four explanations are possible. First, it is possible that pacing could somehow increase conduction velocity in the circuit. This could probably only occur by pacing induced shortening of refractoriness in a VT circuit whose cycle length was refractoriness-dependent. In such tachycardias there would be little or no excitable gap. As stated earlier in this chapter, the vast majority of stable, monomorphic VTs have a significant fully excitable gap. In this circumstance the proposed mechanism of acceleration could not be operative. Second, the apparent original tachycardia cycle length is in fact double the true tachycardia cycle length owing to exit block from the circuit. This could result from a relatively

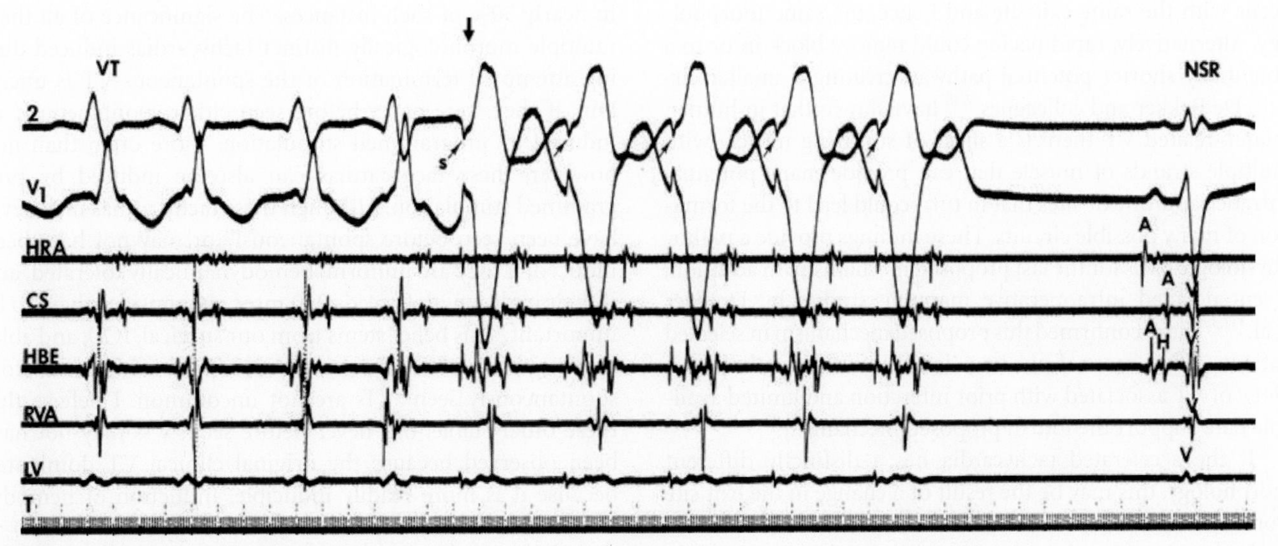


FIGURE 11-187 Ventricular tachycardia terminated by overdrive pacing. VT is present at a cycle length of 420 msec. Overdrive pacing at a cycle length of 400 msec terminates the arrhythmia.

TABLE 11-15 Effect of Procainamide on Mode of Termination of VT (23 Patients)

| Effect | Patients | % | Mean Dose (mg) | Mean Level (mg/mL) | Mean VT | CL Increase (msec) |
|---|---|---|---|---|---|---|
| Unchanged | 7 | 30 | 1,460 | 7.5 | 49 ± 42 | ($p$ <0.01) |
| Harder | 6 | 26 | 1,500 | 12.9 | 142 ± 108 | ($p$ <0.01) |
| Easier | 10 | 44 | 1,750 | 13.7 | 138 ± 110 | ($p$ <0.001) |

From Roy D, Waxman HL, Buxton AE, et al. Termination of ventricular tachycardia: Role of tachycardia cycle length. *Am J Cardiol* 1982;50:1346.

longer refractory period of the myocardium just outside the tachycardia circuit. Rapid pacing could shorten the refractory period of that muscle to a greater extent than in the circuit, thereby allowing each revolution of the circuit to exit. A third possible mechanism could be that rapid pacing introduced two wavelengths within a reentrant circuit that had a very wide excitable gap. Depending on whether a fully excitable gap still existed between these two wavelengths (something never observed in experimental double wave reentry[351] or whether each wavelength encroached on the tail of refractoriness of the other, the accelerated tachycardia cycle length is usually somewhat less than twice the rate (≈2/3 the VT cycle length) owing to a slowing of conduction secondary to impingement on refractoriness. In such a mechanism, the head of one wavelength would encroach on the tail of refractoriness of the second wavelength, so there is virtually no excitable gap remaining. A fourth explanation, which I believe is most plausible, is that an area of block that determines the size of the reentrant circuit is determined, to some extent, by refractoriness. Rapid pacing could shorten the refractoriness in a proximal region of the arc of block, which would in turn shorten the length of the reentrant pathway. If the distal component of the arc of block remained unchanged, acceleration of the tachycardia would occur with the same exit site and hence, the same morphology. Alternatively, rapid pacing could remove block in or to a potentially shorter potential pathway, creating a smaller circuit. De Bakker and colleagues[47,48] have shown that in human infarct–related VT there is a sheet of surviving muscle with multiple strands of muscle that can provide many potential entrance and/or exit sites that in turn could lead to the formation of many possible circuits. These findings provide a pathophysiologic basis for the last proposed mechanism. In addition, recent detailed intraoperative mapping studies by Downer et al.[352,353] have confirmed this proposed mechanism in selected patients. Thus, most of our knowledge about the pathophysiology of VT associated with prior infarction and limited available data support the fourth proposed mechanism.

If the accelerated tachycardia has a distinctly different morphology, this may be the result of a change in the exit site from the reentrant circuit, a reversal of the reentrant circuit, or the termination of the initial tachycardia and reinitiation of a different tachycardia elsewhere. This is also consistent with the pathophysiologic substrate described by de Bakker et al.[47,48] Acceleration of a uniform tachycardia to a polymorphic tachycardia could be due to the inability of the myocardium to respond to the PCL with the development of changing activation wavefronts, leading to multiple reentrant wavelets that may degenerate to VF. There is no way to predict which type of acceleration will occur. However, in the presence of antiarrhythmic drugs, acceleration to different morphologically distinct tachycardias is common. Acceleration of tachycardia by attempts at termination is a major limitation of ATP without a defibrillator backup.

The other problem frequently encountered, particularly in VTs associated with coronary disease treated with medication, is the occurrence of multiple uniform VTs either spontaneously and/or in response to pacing. In such patients, it is not infrequent for stimulation during one tachycardia to induce another VT of different morphology and cycle length, only to be changed to a third or fourth morphologically distinct VT by continued stimulation. If one is lucky, the changed tachycardias will have a longer cycle length and be more readily terminated (Fig. 11-188). However, as noted, acceleration of tachycardia is frequent, and failure to terminate the accelerated tachycardia, thereby necessitating cardioversion, occurs in nearly 50% of such instances. The significance of all these multiple morphologically distinct tachycardias induced during attempted termination of the spontaneous VT is uncertain, if they were never before seen either spontaneously or induced by programmed stimulation. More often than not, however, these tachycardias can also be induced by programmed stimulation. Although these tachycardias may never have been seen before spontaneously or may not have been induced, if they are uniform, hemodynamically tolerated, and if their cycle length exceeds 250 msec, we consider them to be important. This belief stems from our surgical, ICD, and ablation experience in which recurrences of these "never before spontaneously seen" VTs are not uncommon. I believe that these other stable, but never before seen, VTs may not have been observed because the original clinical VT dominates, because it is more readily inducible. Induction of hemodynamically unstable, rapid VTs (cycle lengths <250 msec) in patients who have presented with only stable VT, does not, in my experience, have prognostic value. The electrophysiologic

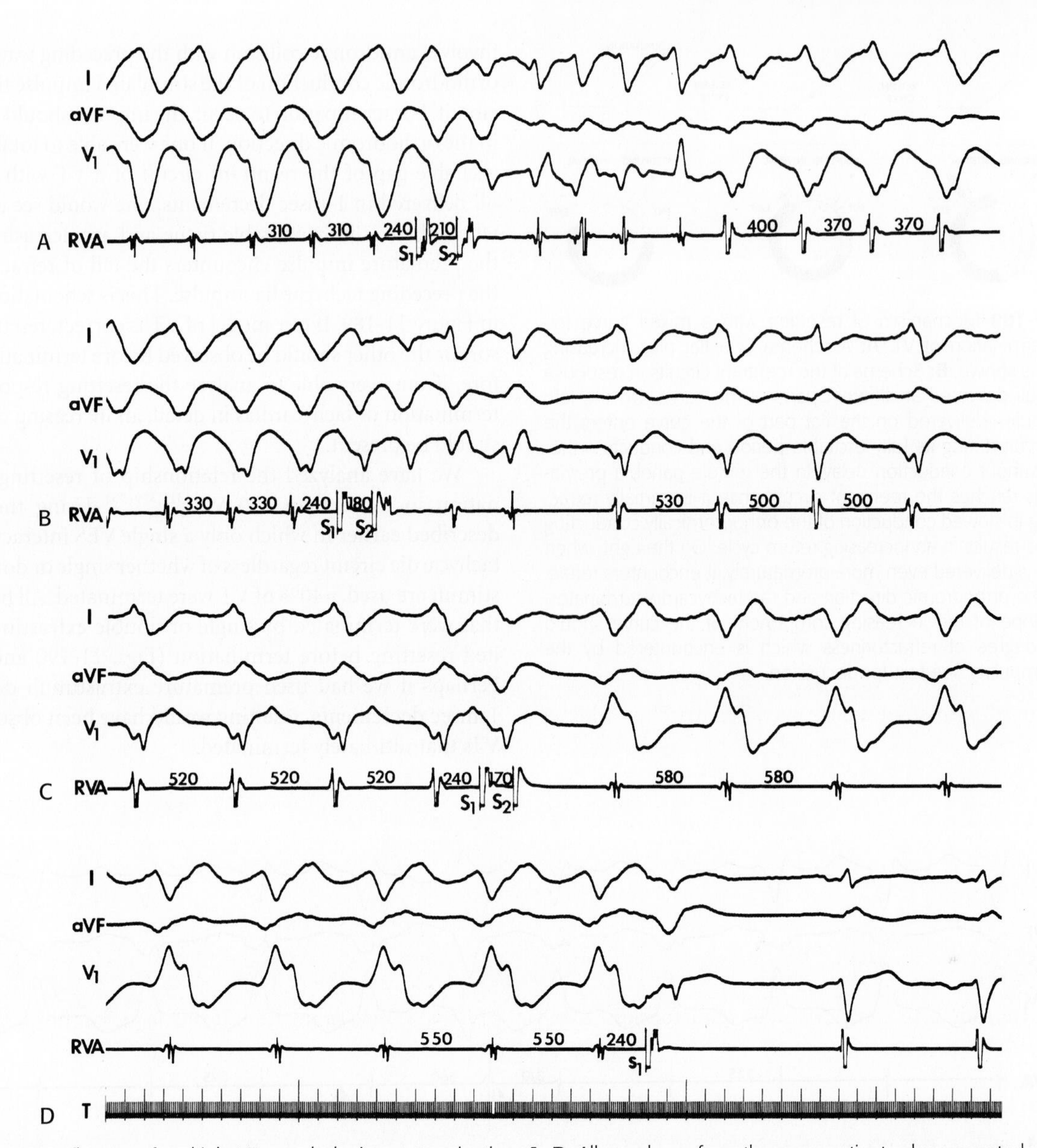


**FIGURE 11-188** Influence of multiple VT morphologies on termination. **A–D:** All panels are from the same patient, who presented with multiple VTs on different occasions. **A:** VT with a left bundle branch block and right superior axis is initially present. In an attempt to terminate the tachycardia, we introduced double ventricular extrastimuli which induced a slow left bundle tachycardia after an initial period of polymorphic tachycardia. **B:** Subsequently, this tachycardia spontaneously accelerated to 330 msec. We again introduced double ventricular extrastimuli which changed this tachycardia to a slow tachycardia having a slightly different morphology. **C:** We delivered double extrastimuli during this slow tachycardia, which changed it to a slightly slower tachycardia with a different morphology. **D:** Finally a single extrastimulus terminated this slow tachycardia with a right bundle branch block morphology. See text for discussion.

properties of potential arrhythmic sites determine which VT is induced by stimulation from a given site. The use of drugs in these patients can change these properties and, hence, frequently brings out these other latent morphologically distinct tachycardias, which may originate from a similar region or disparate areas of the heart. The potential to have such varying distinct tachycardias suggests that any ATP modality should use an adaptive mode in which the PCL used for termination is determined by the cycle length of the tachycardia to be terminated by that burst. The ability to change from one VT to another with a different cycle length using single or double extrastimuli is infrequent during triggered rhythms (other than those due to digitalis) and is another observation that is most compatible with reentrant excitation.

### *Mechanism of Termination and Relationship to Resetting Phenomena*

The reproducible initiation of VT and the responses to stimulation, particularly resetting and entrainment, as well as abrupt termination, all favor reentry as the mechanism for sustained VT. If sustained VT is due to reentry, then termination of the arrhythmia must occur when an impulse penetrates the circuit and blocks in both directions. As previously described, resetting

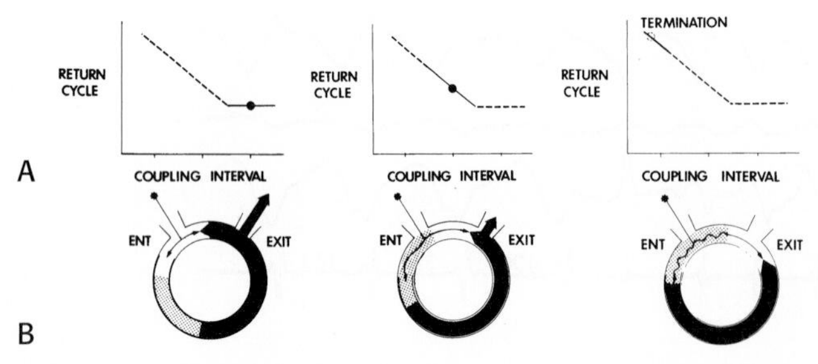


**FIGURE 11-189** Mechanism of resetting with a mixed curve followed by termination of VT. **A:** A schema of a flat plus increasing return cycle is shown. **B:** Schema of the reentrant circuits in response to extrastimuli delivered at different parts of the curve. On the left, an extrastimulus delivered on the flat part of the curve enters the reentrant circuit during its fully excitable period and conducts orthodromically without conduction delay. In the middle panel, a premature stimulus reaches the reentrant circuit while it is partially refractory resulting in slowed conduction of the orthodromically conducting impulse. This results in an increasing return cycle. On the right, when the impulse is delivered even more prematurely, it encounters refractoriness in the orthodromic direction and the tachycardia terminates. Thus, the slope of the increasing component of the curve should reflect the degree of refractoriness which is encountered by the premature impulse. See text for discussion.

involves antidromic collision with the preceding wavefront and orthodromic conduction of the stimulated impulse through the circuit. For termination to occur, the impulse should be blocked in the orthodromic direction. If one were able to totally scan the excitable gap of the reentrant circuit of a VT with extrastimuli delivered in 1-msec decrements, one would see a flat curve where there is fully excitable tissue and an increasing curve as the premature impulse encounters the tail of refractoriness of the preceding tachycardia impulse. This is schematically shown in Figure 11-189. If our model of VT is correct, resetting of one sort or the other should be observed before termination. Therefore, if one were able to analyze the resetting response before termination of tachycardias in detail, an increasing component should be present.

We have analyzed the relationship of resetting to termination in more than 100 VTs.[315,329–331] Using the protocol described earlier in which only a single VES interacts with the tachycardia circuit regardless of whether single or double extrastimuli are used, ≈40% of VT were terminated. All but five VTs that were terminated by single or double extrastimuli exhibited resetting before termination (Figs. 11-190 and 11-191). Perhaps if we had used premature extrastimuli delivered in 1-msec decrements, resetting would have been observed in all VTs that ultimately terminated.

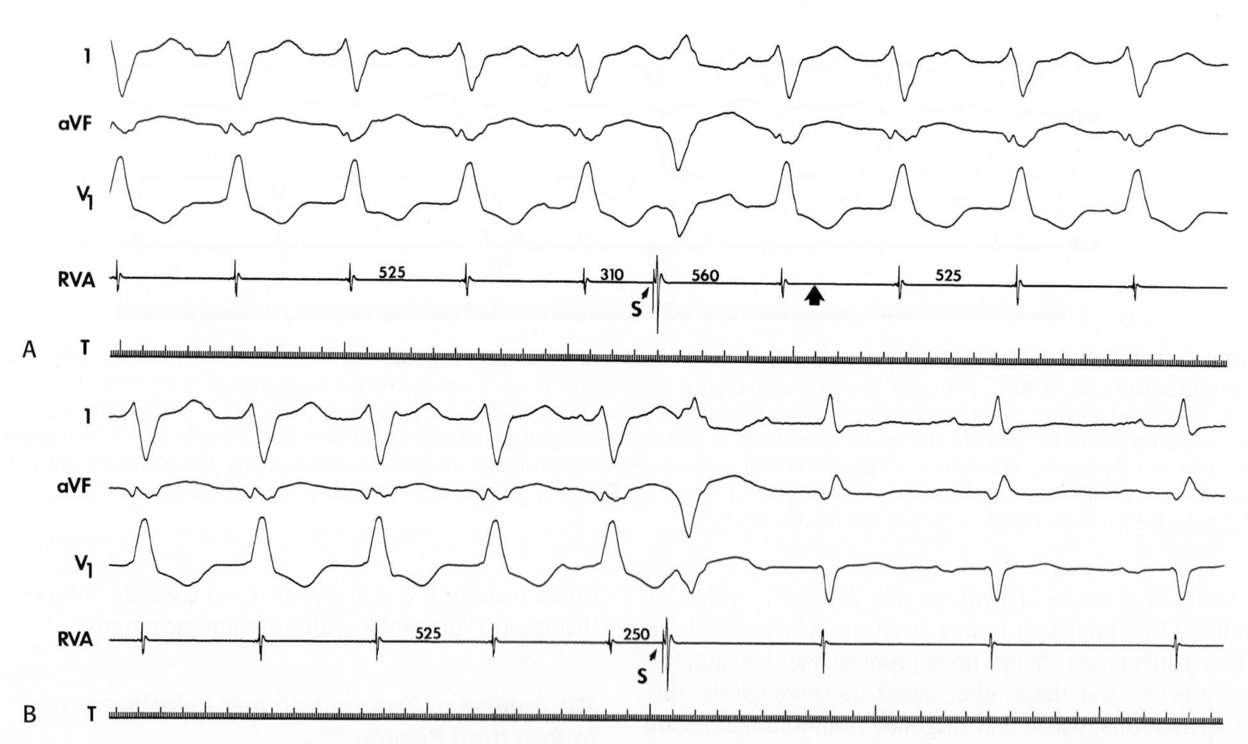


**FIGURE 11-190** Resetting and termination of uniform, sustained VT with increasingly premature single ventricular extrastimuli. Surface ECG leads 1, aVF, and $V_1$ are displayed with an intracardiac recording from the RVA. **A:** A single ventricular extrastimulus (S) is delivered with a coupling interval to the prior tachycardia beat of 310 msec. The resulting pause of 560 msec, measured at the RVA, is less than fully compensatory; the tachycardia is therefore reset. The bold upright *arrow* indicates where a fully compensatory right ventricular apical electrogram would occur. Note that after the premature extrastimulus, the tachycardia resumes without a change in morphology or cycle length. **B:** A single extrastimulus (S) delivered at the RVA with a coupling interval of 250 msec terminates the tachycardia. (From Rosenthal ME, Stamato NJ, Almendral JM, et al. Coupling intervals of ventricular extrastimuli causing resetting of sustained ventricular tachycardia secondary to coronary artery disease: relation to subsequent termination. *Am J Cardiol* 1988;61:770.)

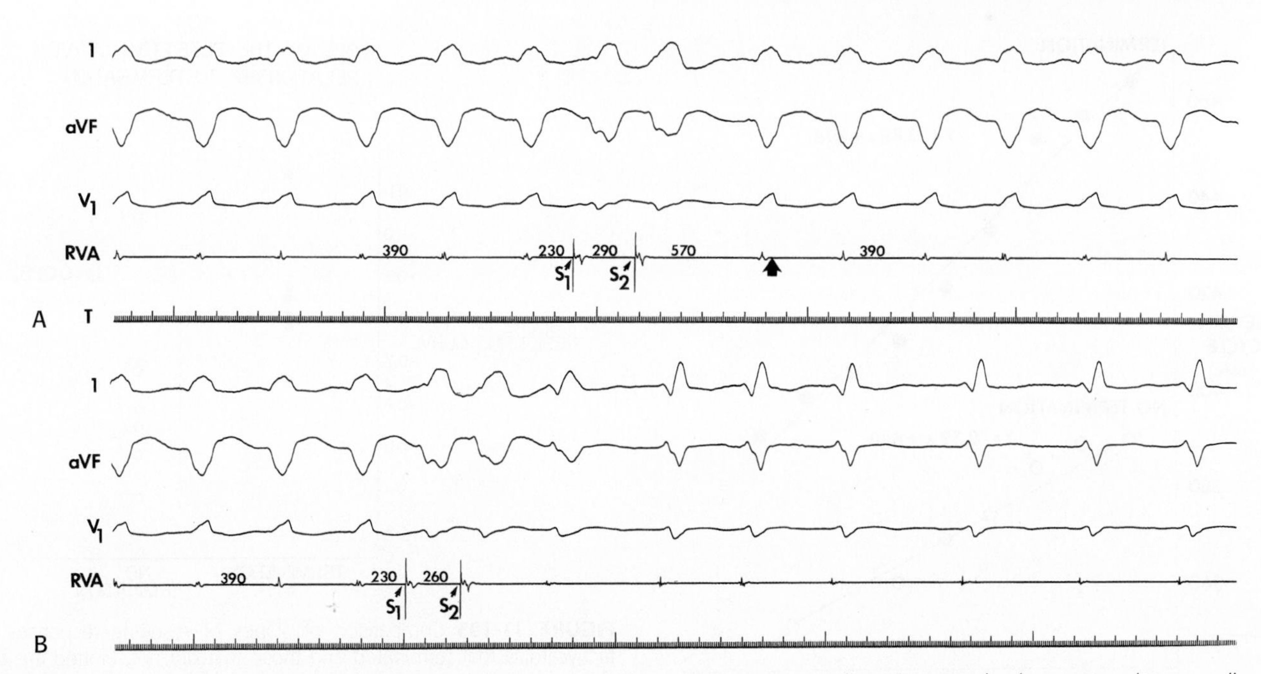


**FIGURE 11-191** Resetting and termination of sustained VT with double ventricular extrastimuli. Surface ECG leads 1, aVF, and $V_1$ as well as an intracardiac recording from the RVA are displayed. Single extrastimuli did not reset this tachycardia, and therefore the coupling interval of the first extrastimulus ($S_1$) is set at 230 msec, 20 msec greater than the effective refractory period during VT. **A:** The interval between $S_1$ and the second extrastimulus ($S_2$) was set at 290 msec and resulted in a pause of 570 msec. This is less than fully compensatory (*bold arrow* demonstrates the timing of a fully compensatory electrogram), and therefore the tachycardia is reset. **B:** The $S_1$-$S_2$ interval is 260 msec, and termination of VT occurs with the resumption of the baseline rhythm and atrial fibrillation. (From Rosenthal ME, Stamato NJ, Almendral JM, et al. Coupling intervals of ventricular extrastimuli causing resetting of sustained ventricular tachycardia secondary to coronary artery disease: relation to subsequent termination. *Am J Cardiol* 1988;61:770.)

We also noted that if resetting did not occur with a VES delivered with a prematurity index (VT-$S_1$/VT-CL or VT-$S_2$/2VT-CL) >0.75 (i.e., 75% of the next expected VT complex), only 2% of VTs were terminated by this method of stimulation. When tachycardias were reset at coupling intervals >75% of the expected VT cycle length, 21% were terminated with single extrastimuli and 42% with double extrastimuli. In those VTs that were terminated by this protocol, termination was observed at a corrected coupling interval of approximately 0.70 of the VT cycle length, while resetting was observed at approximately 0.85 of the VT cycle length. This study confirmed our hypothesis that resetting should occur before termination. We also identified critical coupling intervals at which failure of extrastimuli to produce resetting predicted failure of termination by this pacing modality.[315,329] These data could have potential for developing algorithms by which single or double premature extrastimuli (delivered as in our protocol) could be used in ATP. This would be advantageous because the incidence of acceleration is negligible when a single extrastimulus interacts with the circuit.

Although the failure to reset the tachycardia with single or double extrastimuli predicted failure of termination by these modalities, resetting occurring at coupling intervals exceeding 0.75 did not predict termination with great accuracy. Approximately 20% of those VT reset with single extrastimuli, and 40% of those reset with double extrastimuli at corrected coupling intervals ≥0.75 terminated at shorter coupling intervals. We therefore sought to define what factors determine whether or not termination will occur. We hypothesized that termination was related to the orthodromically conducting impulse encroaching on the refractory period of the last VT wavelength and blocking. If this were the case, as the premature impulse first encroached on the relative refractory period of the prior tachycardia wavefront, an increasing resetting curve should be observed. We postulated that the degree of interval-dependent conduction delay (i.e., slope of the increasing resetting curve) should be related to the degree of encroachment on the refractory period of the prior cycle and, hence, the ability to terminate the tachycardia. Thus, a steeper slope would be noted if more refractory tissues were encountered. To test our hypothesis, we calculated the slope of the increasing limb of the resetting response curve to double extrastimuli and related it to termination.[330,331] The slope of the resetting response in VTs that were terminated was significantly steeper than those that did not terminate. A comparison of the increasing component of the resetting curve in a VT that was terminated and in one that was not is shown in Figure 11-192. A comparison of the slopes of the resetting curves of those tachycardias that terminated and those that did not is shown in Figure 11-193. Six of seven VTs that terminated with programmed extrastimuli had a slope steeper than –0.75, while only 1 of 10 VTs that did not terminate exceeded this value. There was no difference in the tachycardia cycle length in the two groups; thus, one must conclude that the slope of the increasing portion of the resetting curve is a property unique to the tachycardia circuit, which can be used to predict which tachycardias

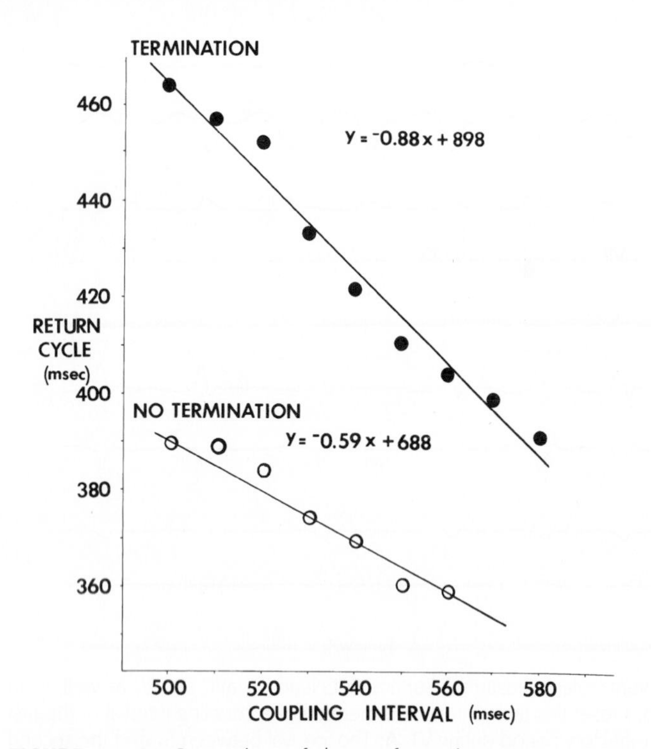


**FIGURE 11-192** Comparison of slopes of resetting response curves in VTs terminated and not terminated. The coupling interval of the second extrastimuli is displayed on the abscissa, and the resultant return cycle is on the ordinate. Note that with progressively premature extrastimuli, conduction delay occurs within the tachycardia circuit. This is demonstrated by the progressive prolongation of the return cycle in response to a decrement in extrastimulus coupling interval. The slope of the resetting response curve was −0.59 in VT not terminated and −0.88 in those that did terminate. The coefficient of correlation was 0.95. (From Gottlieb CD, Rosenthal ME, Stamato NJ, et al. A quantitative evaluation of refractoriness within a reentrant circuit during ventricular tachycardia: relationship to termination. *Circulation* 1990;82: 1289–1295.)

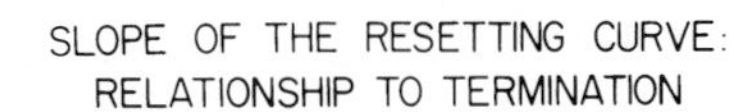


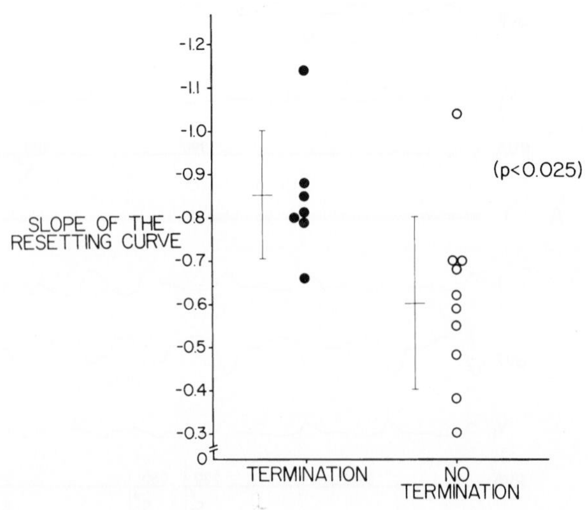


**FIGURE 11-193** Comparison of slopes of resetting responses in tachycardias that terminated and those that did not. Plotted are the slopes of the resetting response curves for the 10 tachycardias that did not terminate in response to double extrastimuli and seven tachycardias that did terminate. The mean slope of the tachycardias that did not terminate in response to double ventricular extrastimuli was −0.61 ± 0.21. The mean slope of those tachycardias that terminated in response to extrastimuli were significantly steeper, −0.85 ± 0.15. (From Gottlieb CD, Rosenthal ME, Stamato NJ, et al. A quantitative evaluation of refractoriness within a reentrant circuit during ventricular tachycardia: relationship to termination. *Circulation* 1990;82:1289–1295.)

can be terminated by this protocol. Whether the differences in curves reflect a different mechanism for interval-dependent conduction delay (i.e., refractoriness or nonuniform anisotropic conduction) is not known and requires further study. Similar conduction delay prior to termination in response to overdrive pacing was observed by Callans et al.[334]

The fact that termination of VT may be site dependent (see subsequent discussion) suggests that nonuniform anisotropy may have an important role in determining the type of slope of the curve. I hypothesize that termination requires block that is due to encroachment on refractoriness in the circuit while interval-dependent conduction delay proximal to that site, by whatever mechanism, can prevent block from occurring. The difference in slopes noted in response to extrastimuli introduced in tachycardias that terminated versus those that did not may reflect whether the site of block required for termination is proximal or distal to the site of conduction delay in the orthodromic limb of the circuit. Proof of this hypothesis requires high-density multisite mapping of the reentrant circuit during programmed stimulation. Experimental studies in a canine model of postinfarction anisotropic reentry showed that spontaneous block occurred orthodromically in the central common pathway of a figure-of-eight reentrant circuit.[310] Block was sometimes preceded by a shortening of barrier length leading to earlier penetration of the central common pathway (isthmus). Hanna et al.[312] showed several mechanisms by which stimulation could reset and terminate VT in the canine anisotropic reentrant model. The most common mechanism of termination was orthodromic block in the isthmus, but antidromic invasion and collapse of the circuit was also noted. How these observations in a functional reentrant model relate to postinfarction human VT is uncertain. Intraoperative detailed mapping of postinfarction VT has demonstrated spontaneous block at the entrance, center, or exit from the isthmus (diastolic central pathway) in the orthodromic direction.[353] This can be markedly influenced by the site of stimulation. These data provide information that can be applied in an algorithm for ATP. Thus, analysis of the slope of the increasing portion of the resetting curve may be useful to determine during the electrophysiologic study in patients in whom antitachycardia pacemakers are considered a therapeutic option.

Demonstration that block occurs in the orthodromic component of the reentrant circuit, as depicted in Figure 11-189, can be obtained by recording orthodromically activated presystolic activity from the reentrant circuit during a delivery of extrastimuli or rapid pacing. Examples of this are shown in Figures 11-194 and 11-195. In Figure 11-194,

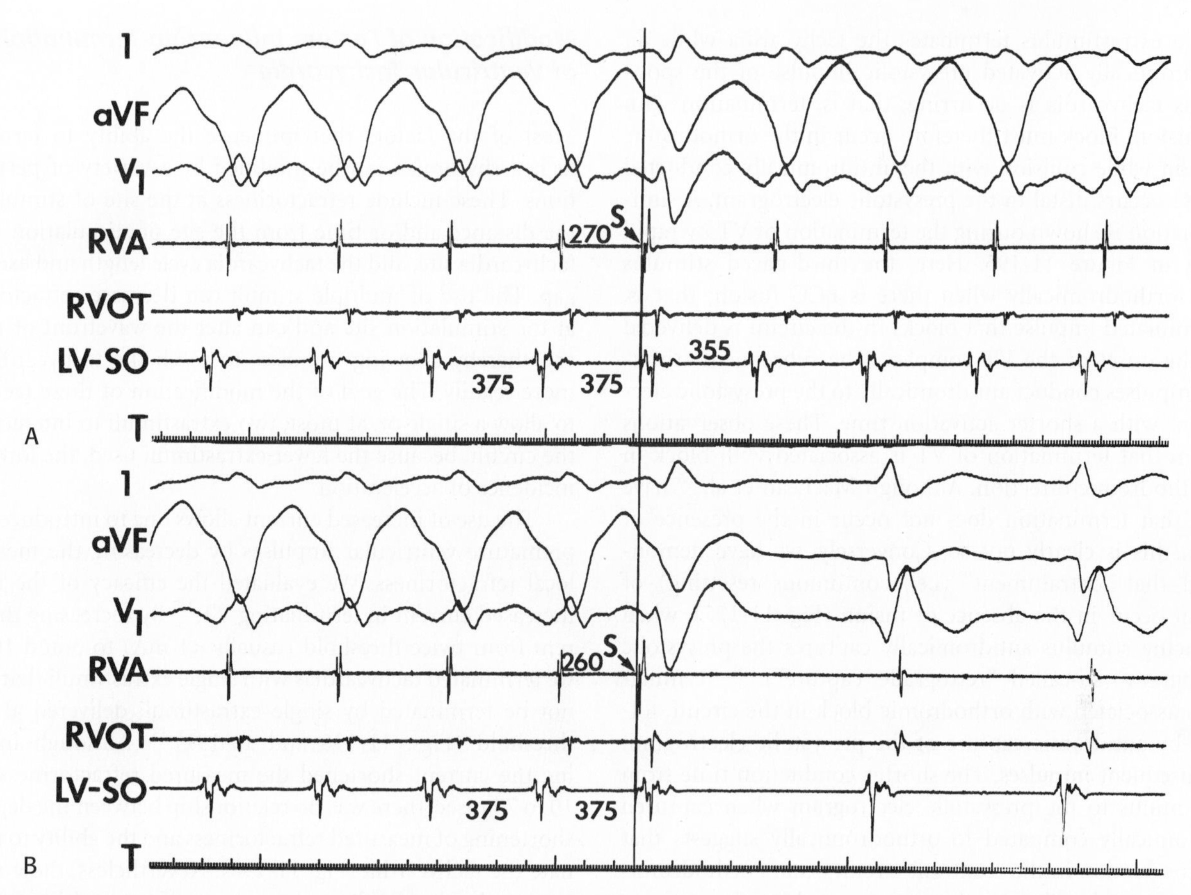


**FIGURE 11-194** Termination of VT by a single extrastimulus with local fusion. **A** and **B:** Leads 1, aVF, and $V_1$ and electrograms from the RVA, RVOT, and the presystolic electrogram arbitrarily defined as the "site of origin" (LV-SO) are shown. VT is present at a cycle length of 375 msec. **A:** An extrastimulus delivered at 270 msec resets the tachycardia with local fusion and surface ECG fusion. **B:** When the extrastimulus is delivered 10 msec earlier (coupling interval 260 msec), the tachycardia is terminated abruptly in the orthodromic direction. Note the local electrogram at the LV-SO occurs on time; therefore, local fusion is present at the time of termination. See text for discussion.

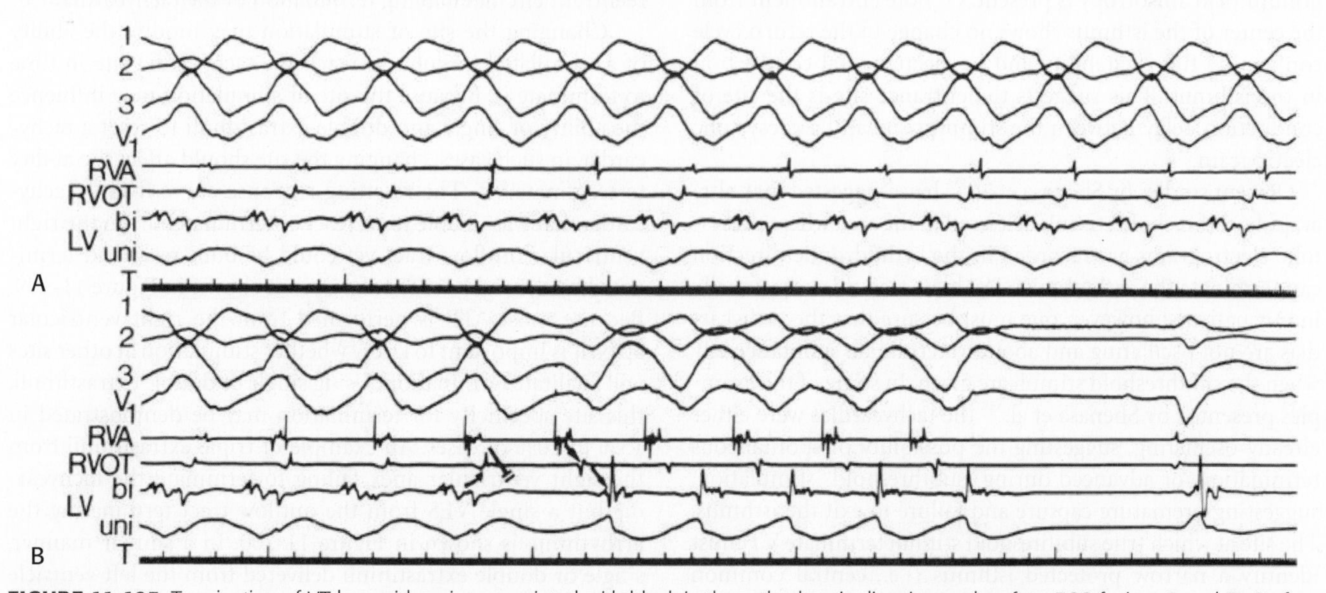


**FIGURE 11-195** Termination of VT by rapid pacing associated with block in the orthodromic direction and surface ECG fusion. **A** and **B:** Surface leads 1, 2, 3, and $V_1$ are shown along with electrograms from the RVA, RVOT, and LV at the site of origin. Uni- and bipolar LV recordings are present. **A:** VT is present at a cycle length of 380 msec. **B:** Overdrive pacing is begun. The first two extrastimuli fail to influence the tachycardia, and the electrogram from the RVOT occurs as a consequence of the tachycardia. Following the third ventricular extrastimulus (which is delivered after the onset of the third VT complex; i.e., surface ECG fusion), block occurs in the orthodromic direction, despite the presence of the orthodromically activated LV electrogram and the RVOT electrogram, which occur on time. Subsequent to the block in the orthodromic direction, conduction occurs antidromically in the circuit. On cessation of pacing, the tachycardia is no longer present. See text for discussion.

a single extrastimulus terminates the tachycardia while an orthodromically activated presystolic impulse of the spontaneous tachycardia is occurring, that is, termination with local fusion. Block must therefore occur in the orthodromic direction while collision with the antidromically conducted impulse occurs distal to the presystolic electrogram. A similar situation is shown during the termination of VT by rapid pacing in Figure 11-195. Here, the third-paced stimulus blocks orthodromically when there is ECG fusion; that is, the stimulated impulse that blocks in the circuit is delivered after the onset of the VT complex. The subsequent stimulated impulses conduct antidromically to the presystolic electrogram with a shorter activation time. These observations confirm that termination of VT is associated with block in the orthodromic direction. Although MacLean et al.[326] have stated that termination does not occur in the presence of fusion, this is clearly not so. Conversely, we have demonstrated that "entrainment" (i.e., continuous resetting) of VT can occur in the absence of fusion (Fig. 11-177), when the pacing stimulus antidromically captures the presystolic electrogram (so-called "retrograde capture").[319] Termination is associated with orthodromic block in the circuit, followed by antidromic capture of the presystolic electrogram on subsequent impulses. The shorter conduction time from the stimulus to the presystolic electrogram when captured antidromically compared to orthodromically suggests that slow conduction in the reentrant circuit occurs orthodromically between the stimulated wavefront reaching the entrance and the exit sites.[319,326,342,343] Without detailed mapping of the entire circuit, particularly at entrance and exit sites, it will be impossible to tell whether the slowing is in the isthmus itself or at turning points at which high curvature and/or marked nonuniform anisotropy is present. Of note entrainment from the center of the isthmus shows no change in the return cycle confirming full excitability and no decremental conduction in the isthmus. This suggests the entrance site is the site of conduction delay between the stimulus site and a presystolic electrogram.

Recent studies by Shenasa et al.[354] have suggested that ultrarapid subthreshold stimuli delivered in the area where presystolic electrograms are recorded in the orthodromic direction can terminate the arrhythmias. We have seen this occasionally in our patients; however, one must be sure that the tachycardias are not oscillating and about to terminate spontaneously when the subthreshold stimuli are given. In some of the examples presented by Shenasa et al.[354] the tachycardias were either already oscillating, suggesting the possibility of spontaneous termination, or advanced during "subthreshold" stimulation, suggesting premature capture and failure to exit the isthmus. The site at which true subthreshold stimuli terminate VT must identify a narrow protected isthmus (i.e., central common pathway). Nonetheless, this area including and in between the entrance and exit of a central common appears to be the site at which tachycardia termination in the orthodromic direction occurs.

### *Modification of Factors Influencing Termination of Ventricular Tachycardia*

Most of the factors that influence the ability to terminate tachyarrhythmias can be modified by a variety of perturbations. These include refractoriness at the site of stimulation, the distance and/or time from the site of stimulation to the tachycardia site, and the tachycardia cycle length and excitable gap. The use of multiple stimuli can decrease refractoriness at the stimulation site and can alter the wavefront of recovery, thereby allowing impulses to reach the tachycardia site more readily. The goal of the modification of these factors is to allow a single or, at most, two extrastimuli to interact with the circuit, because the fewer extrastimuli used, the lower the incidence of acceleration.

The use of increased current allows one to introduce more premature ventricular impulses by decreasing the measured local refractoriness. We evaluated the efficacy of the use of increased current in terminating VT.[355] By increasing the current from twice threshold (usually <1 mA) to 5 and 10 mA, we terminated tachycardias with single extrastimuli that could not be terminated by single extrastimuli delivered at twice threshold (Figs. 11-196 and 11-197).[355] Although increasing the current shortened the measured refractoriness from 10 to 70 msec, there was no relationship between the degree of shortening of measured refractoriness and the ability to terminate the tachycardia (Fig. 11-198). Nevertheless, these results suggest that local refractoriness by itself is a limiting factor in a portion of the cases that can be terminated by single extrastimuli. The increase in current, if produced by increasing voltage, produces a larger virtual electrode which may capture more "distant" tissue such that it takes less time to reach the reentrant circuit enabling termination of the tachycardia.

Changing the site of stimulation may modify the ability of a stimulated impulse to reach the tachycardia site in time to terminate it. Because the site of stimulation may influence the ability of single and double extrastimuli to reset a tachycardia, in such cases, changing the site should affect the ability to terminate VT. The resetting response curve from a tachycardia that was unable to be reset or terminated from the right ventricular outflow tract yet could be both reset and terminated by the right ventricular apex is shown in Figure 11-199. Because most ATP is performed from the right ventricular apex, it is important to know whether stimulation at other sites will facilitate termination. Using single or double extrastimuli, this site specificity for termination may be demonstrated in 15% to 20% of cases. An example of triple extrastimuli from the right ventricular apex failing to terminate the tachycardia but a single VES from the outflow tract terminating the arrhythmia is shown in Figure 11-200. In a similar manner, single or double extrastimuli delivered from the left ventricle may terminate a tachycardia where comparable stimulation from the right ventricle failed (Figs. 11-201 and 11-202). We have not been able to predict which tachycardias will demonstrate site specificity for facilitation of termination aside from

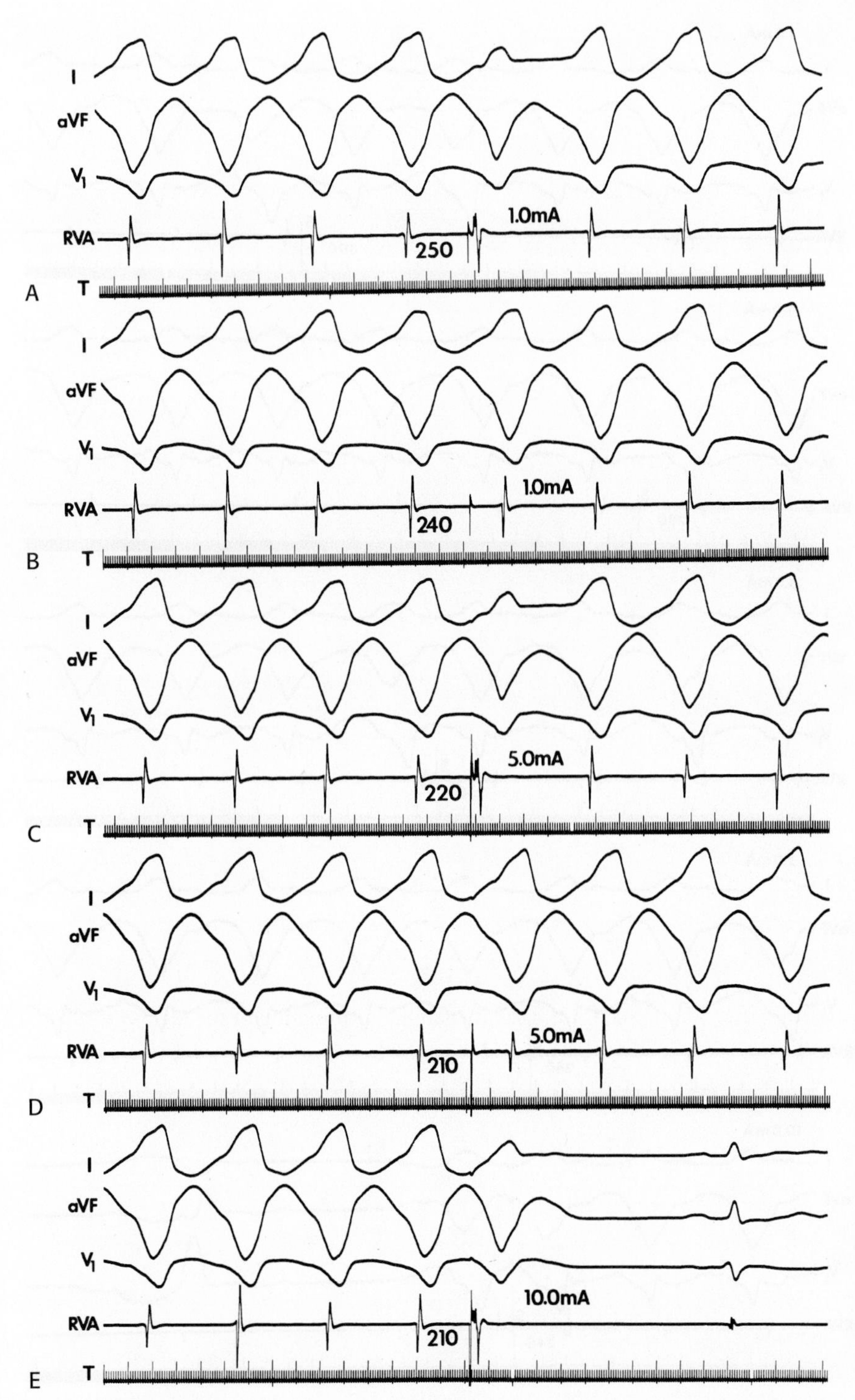


**FIGURE 11-196** Facilitation of termination of VT by increased current. Leads 1, aVF, and $V_1$ and electrograms from the RVA are shown (with T). VT is present at a CL of 390 msec. **A:** A premature stimulus is introduced from the RVA at a coupling interval of 250 msec using twice diastolic threshold stimulation (1 mA). **B:** Premature stimulus at twice threshold fails to capture the ventricle at a coupling interval of 240 msec. **C:** The stimulating current is increased to 5 mA, and the coupling interval is shortened in 10-msec decrements, with ventricular capture maintained at 220 msec. VT, however, is not terminated. **D:** A 210-msec stimulus fails to capture the ventricle at 5 mA. **E:** When the stimulus current is increased at 10 mA, ventricular capture is possible at a coupling interval of 210 msec and the tachycardia is terminated. (From Waxman HL, Cain ME, Greenspan AM, et al. Termination of ventricular tachycardia with ventricular stimulation: Salutary effect of increased current strength. *Circulation* 1982;65:800.)

noting the resetting responses (presence or absence and slope) described earlier. As stated previously, more than 40% of VTs will demonstrate different resetting responses when stimulation from the RV apex and RV outflow tract are compared, yet the incidence of site specificity for termination is less frequent. The lack of relationship between site specificity for resetting and termination may have to do with the relationship of the site of entry in the excitable gap and the site of termination.

Although the influence of stimulation site on termination of VT has been recognized for many years,[1,122,123,193–195] it has never been taken into account in the placement of ICDs. This is most likely because burst of pacing are programmed for ATP, which diminish the role of site specificity. Perhaps with the new active fixation pacing leads, knowledge of site specificity for termination can be taken advantage of. As stated earlier, site specificity for either resetting or termination is not a

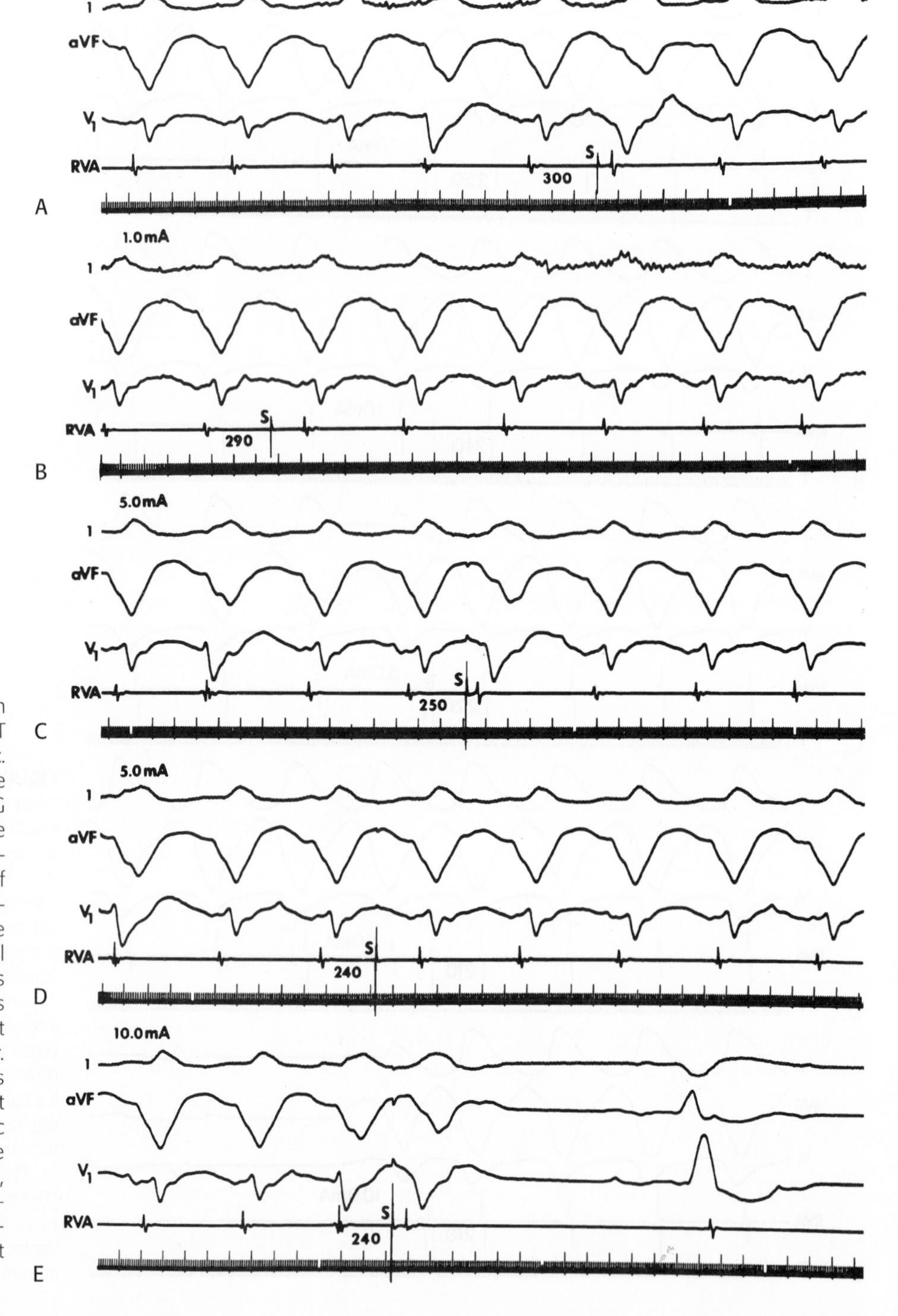


**FIGURE 11-197** Facilitation of termination of tachycardia with increased current. VT is present at a cycle length of 440 msec. The stimulating current is shown in the upper left corner of each panel. Three ECG leads and an electrogram from the RVA are shown in each panel. **A:** A ventricular extrastimulus delivered at a coupling interval of 300 msec at twice diastolic threshold captures the ventricles but fails to terminate the tachycardia. **B:** At a coupling interval of 290 msec, ventricular refractoriness is encountered. **C:** When the current is increased to 5 mA, capture is possible at 250 msec, but termination does not occur. **D:** At 240 msec, ventricular refractoriness is again reached. **E:** Finally, when the current is increased at 10 mA, capture at 240 msec is possible and results in termination of the tachycardia. (From Waxman HL, Cain ME, Greenspan AM, et al. Termination of ventricular tachycardia with ventricular stimulation: Salutary effect of increased current strength. *Circulation* 1982;65:800.)

feature of triggered activity and further supports both reentrant excitation and the role of anisotropic conduction in the genesis of the arrhythmia.

Because tachycardia cycle length appears to be a major determinant of the ability to terminate the arrhythmia, prolongation of the cycle length by antiarrhythmic agents could theoretically facilitate termination. Unfortunately, the response is not predictable. Although slowing of VT is the rule in response to Class I agents or amiodarone,[325,356–358] this does not necessarily facilitate termination. Although in 40% to 50% of tachycardias, facilitation of termination does occur following procainamide (Fig. 11-203), in up to 25% of patients, termination is more difficult (Fig. 11-204).[322] Neither the plasma level of procainamide nor the prolongation of tachycardia cycle length could predict which tachycardia would be more difficult to terminate. In fact, we have noted an increased incidence of acceleration to polymorphic VT and VF when multiple extrastimuli and/or very rapid pacing is used in the presence of drugs that markedly slow conduction and prolong the tachycardia cycle length (Table 11-15). These observations suggest that these

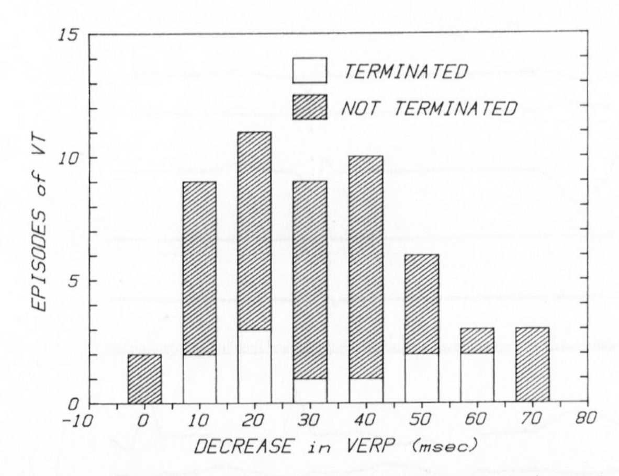


**FIGURE 11-198** Relationship of decrease in measured ventricular refractory period produced by increasing current to ability to terminate the tachycardia. The decrease in ventricular effective refractory period (VERP) when measured at twice threshold and 10 mA is plotted on the horizontal axis. The VERP was not measured in episodes of VT that were terminated but the change in refractory period up to that point is plotted. As much as 70 msec of shortening in the ERP was not associated with termination of VT, whereas in others, only 10 msec of shortening preceded termination. (From Waxman HL, Cain ME, Greenspan AM, et al. Termination of ventricular tachycardia with ventricular stimulation: Salutary effect of increased current strength. *Circulation* 1982;65:800.)

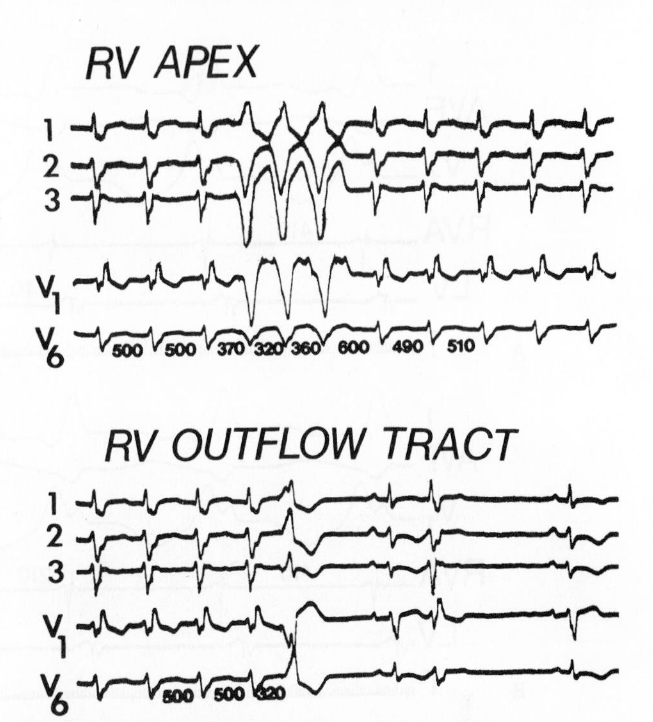


**FIGURE 11-200** Effect of site of stimulation on tachycardia termination. Stimulation from the RV apex and RV outflow tract are shown. Surface leads 1, 2, 3, $V_1$, and $V_6$ are shown in each panel, with VT present on the left of each panel. On the top, three extrastimuli delivered from the right ventricular apex fail to terminate VT; however, a single ventricular extrastimulus delivered from the right ventricular outflow tract terminates the arrhythmia abruptly. Such site specificity favors reentry. See text for discussion. (From Josephson ME, Marchlinski FE, Cassidy DM, et al. Sustained ventricular tachycardia in coronary artery disease—Evidence for reentrant mechanism. In: Zipes DP, Jalife J, eds. *Cardiac electrophysiology and arrhythmias*. Orlando, FL: Grune & Stratton, 1985:409.)

drugs, while slowing the tachycardia, simultaneously increased the excitable gap, and therefore, the window during which stimuli could interact with the circuit, also prolonged conduction between the stimulation site and the circuit. If this prolongation of conduction through intervening tissue is marked, termination of the tachycardia may be more difficult. Similarly if the excitable gap is large, more stimuli will be needed to encroach on the refractory period of the VT impulse. Finally, these drugs can produce block and slow conduction elsewhere in the heart, which may be responsible for initiation of multiple reentrant circuits elsewhere and/or acceleration of the initial VT in response to overdrive pacing.

Based on our understanding of resetting and entrainment, we developed a method that gives easier access to the excitable gap and facilitates termination, particularly of those tachycardias for which antiarrhythmic agents have made VT more difficult to terminate by standard and pacing techniques.[333] This technique requires that the VT can be entrained by overdrive pacing and reset by single extrastimuli. Although neither single extrastimuli nor the PCL of overdrive pacing used can terminate the arrhythmia, the combination does. The technique works because overdrive pacing ensures stable resetting of the VT circuit, allowing the single premature stimulus to interact with the circuit much more prematurely than it could in the absence of entrainment. The overdrive pacing also shortens the excitable gap of tissue in the reset circuit, making it possible for the single stimulus to terminate the VT. This technique results in termination without the need for multiple VES, which may increase the heterogeneity of conduction and refractoriness in the intervening tissue and produce polymorphic VT, or rapid pacing, which might induce acceleration of the tachycardia. We have found this method particularly useful in VTs that were accelerated by rapid pacing and especially in tachycardias that were resistant to standard techniques of pacing in the presence of antiarrhythmic agents.[333] The mechanism of this method and examples of its effectiveness

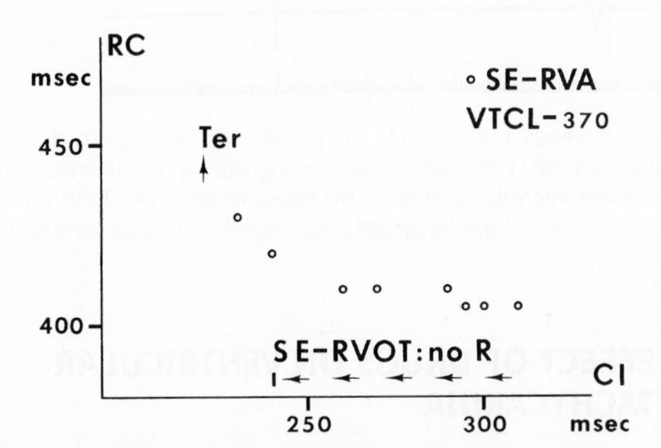


**FIGURE 11-199** Site specificity for termination. The coupling intervals (CI) of ventricular extrastimuli are shown on the horizontal axis, and the return cycle (RC) is shown on the vertical axis. Single extrastimuli (SE) as delivered from the RVOT produce no resetting. However, SE from the RVA produce resetting with a mixed curve, ultimately resulting in termination of the tachycardia (Ter). See text for discussion.

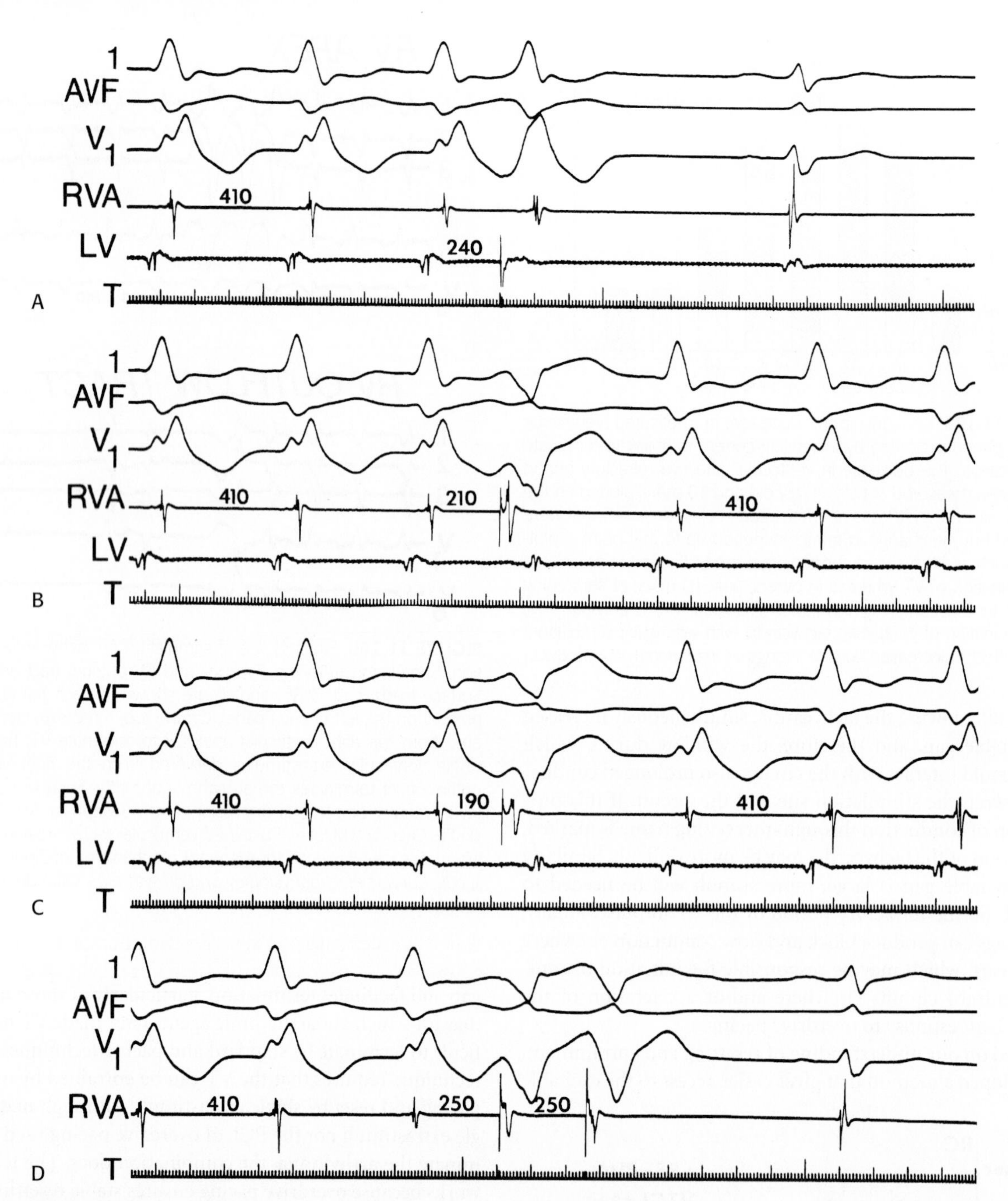


**FIGURE 11-201** Facilitation of tachycardia termination by left ventricular stimulation. Leads 1, AVF, and $V_1$ are shown with electrograms from the RVA and LV. **A:** During VT with a cycle length of 410 msec, a single extrastimulus from the LV delivered at a coupling interval of 240 msec terminates the tachycardia. **B** and **C:** Single extrastimuli delivered at much closer coupling intervals (210 and 190 msec, respectively) from the RVA fail to terminate the tachycardia. **D:** Only when double extrastimuli are used is termination of the tachycardia accomplished by RVA stimulation.

are shown in Figures 11-205 to 11-207. This method of pacing, which takes advantage of our understanding of resetting phenomena, can be used to design an algorithm that can be employed in antitachycardia pacemakers. The risk of acceleration of tachycardias always exists whenever pacing modalities are used in an attempt to terminate VT, regardless of tachycardia cycle length or pacing modality. Therefore, if an ATP is to be used as a primary therapy, it must be used as a component of defibrillator system.

## EFFECT OF DRUGS ON VENTRICULAR TACHYCARDIA

Unfortunately, aside from adenosine, we do not have antiarrhythmic agents that are effective for a specific type of tachycardia mechanism. If we did, one could theoretically separate reentry from triggered activity, or automaticity, based on the response of the tachycardia to the drug and

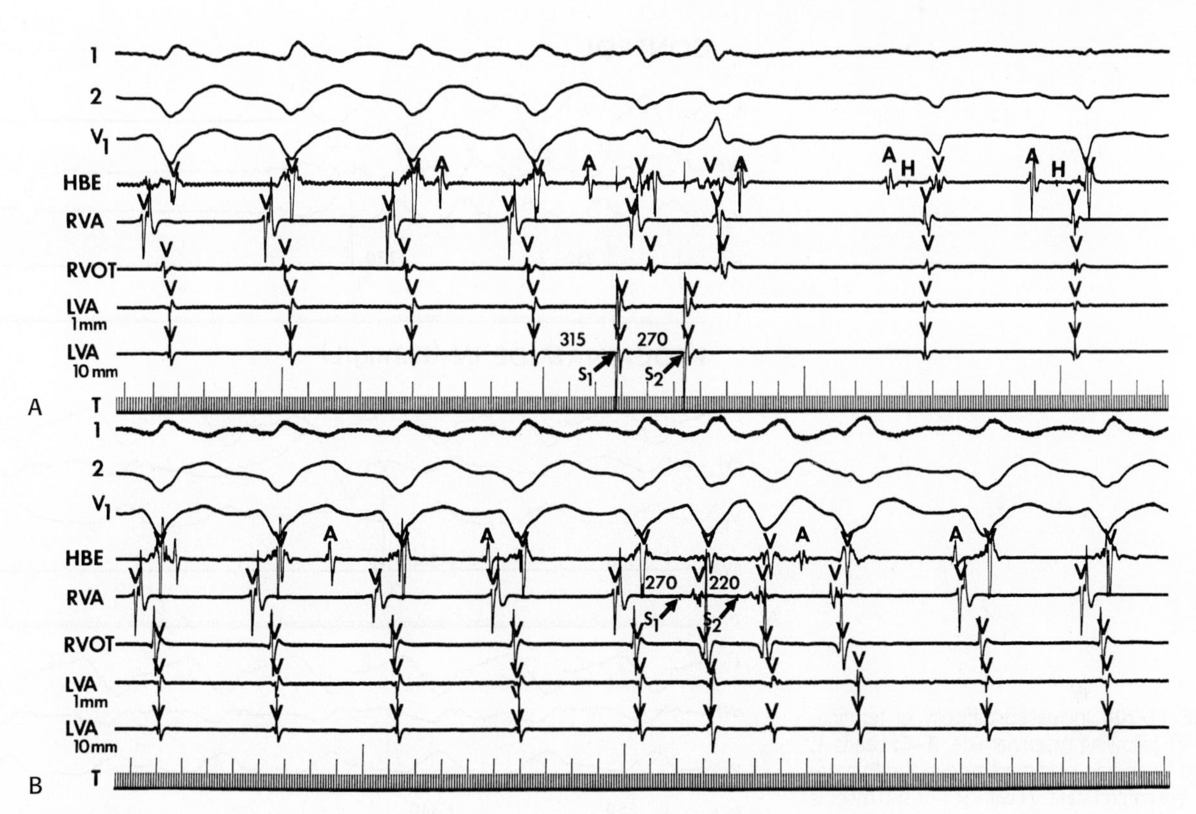


**FIGURE 11-202** Effect of stimulation site on ability to terminate VT. **A** and **B:** ECG leads 1, 2, and $V_1$ are shown with electrograms from the HBE, RVA, RVOT, and LVA recorded from electrodes 1 mm and 10 mm apart. **A:** Two ventricular extrastimuli from the LVA terminate VT. **B:** Two ventricular extrastimuli from the RVA do not terminate VT. No coupling intervals of RVA stimulation terminated VT.

on the drug's ability to prevent the initiation of the tachycardia. In the case of VT, in contrast to atrial tachycardia, in which adenosine can terminate both reentrant and triggered rhythms, termination of the VT by adenosine appears fairly specific for adenyl cyclase–mediated triggered activity due to DADs. However I do not believe adenosine should be used in patients with significant coronary artery disease because it can produce a "coronary steal" and result in ventricular fibrillation. Nevertheless, one can relate the effectiveness of a drug against VT in humans to the known effect of that drug on documented experimental arrhythmia mechanisms. For example, triggered activity, whether or not associated with digitalis intoxication, can be abolished by verapamil or lidocaine, and when triggered activity is catecholamine

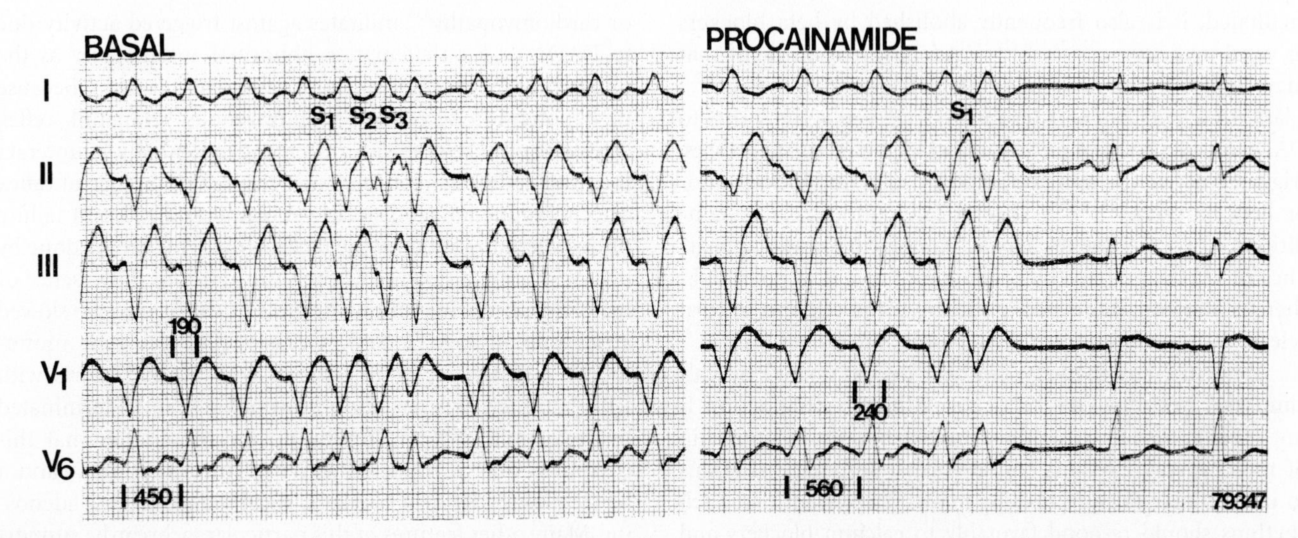


**FIGURE 11-203** Facilitation of tachycardia termination by procainamide. Leads I, II, III, $V_1$, and $V_6$ are shown of a patient with VT having a left bundle branch block configuration. In the basal state, three right ventricular extrastimuli ($S_1S_2S_3$) fail to terminate VT. The cycle length of VT in the basal state is 450 msec, and the QRS width is 190 msec. Following procainamide, the tachycardia is slowed to 560 msec and is associated with a QRS of 240 msec. This slower tachycardia is now readily terminated by a single right ventricular extrastimulus.

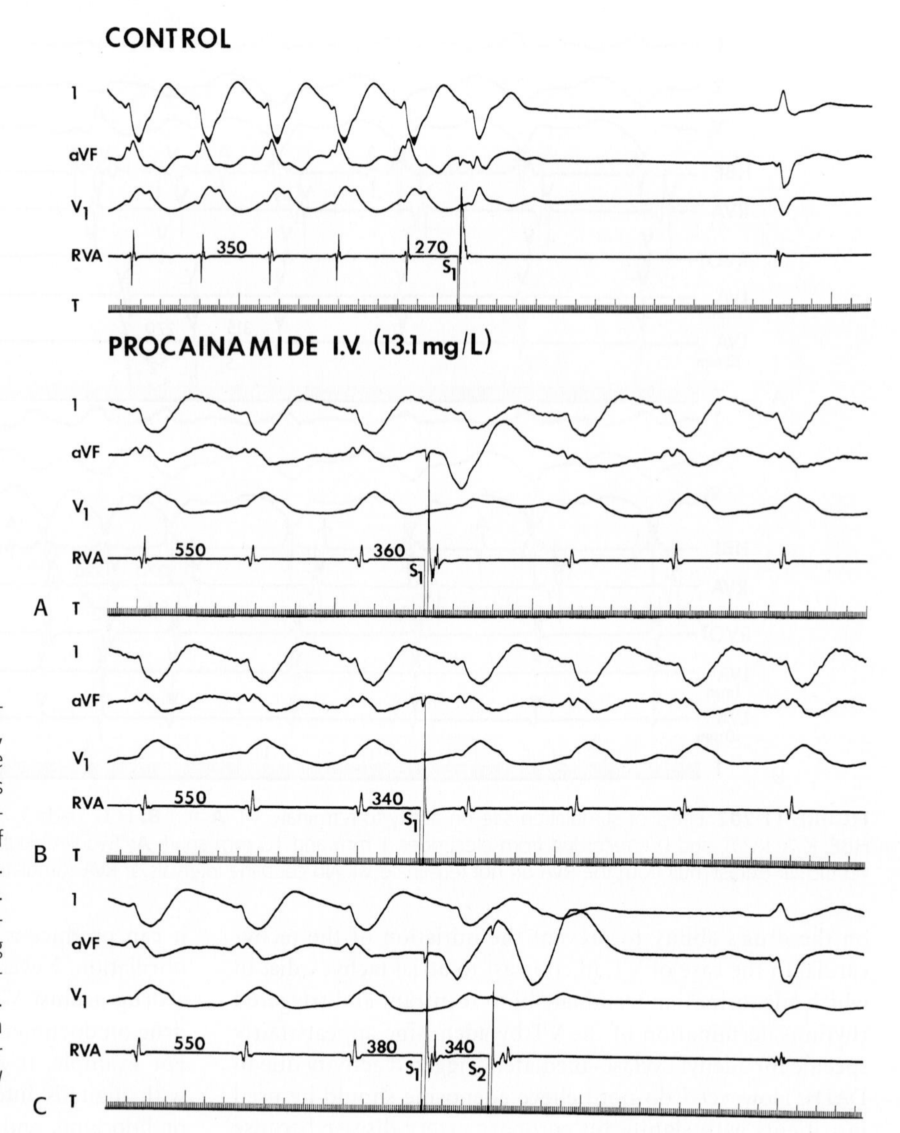


**FIGURE 11-204** Increased difficulty of termination of VT following procainamide. **A–C:** Leads 1, aVF, and $V_1$ and an electrogram from the RVA are shown. In a control state, VT with a CL of 350 msec is terminated by a single RVA stimulus. Following infusion of procainamide producing a plasma level of 13.1 mg/L, the tachycardia is slowed to 550 msec. However, this increases ventricular refractoriness. **A** and **B:** This results in the ability of single extrastimuli to depolarize the ventricles at coupling intervals <360 msec. **C.** As a result, double extrastimuli are required to terminate the tachycardia. See text for discussion. (From Roy D, Waxman HL, Buxton AE, et al. Termination of ventricular tachycardia: Role of tachycardia cycle length. *Am J Cardiol* 1982;50:1346.)

facilitated, it is also frequently abolished by beta blockers or vagal maneuvers.[51,125,126,128,359] Adenosine is an agent that may abolish cyclic AMP–dependent triggered activity.[163,299] Class IA agents can also terminate triggered activity due to DADs in the presence or absence of digitalis. In such cases, triggered activity is also abolished by calcium blockers and/or beta blockers.[125,126,359] Theoretically, under certain conditions, Class IA agents may actually facilitate the appearance of DADs, perhaps by prolonging the action potentials, thereby allowing more calcium to enter the cell and in turn release more calcium from the sarcoplasmic reticulum.[126]

Abnormal automaticity can also be terminated by calcium and beta blockers.[51,126] Thus, although drug action is not specific for an arrhythmia mechanism, the relationship of the triggered rhythms and abnormal automatic rhythms to intracellular calcium loading makes it apparent that such rhythms should respond favorably to calcium blockers and beta blockers. Thus, the fact that verapamil, beta blockers, or adenosine fail to terminate >95% of paroxysmal sustained monomorphic VT associated with coronary artery disease or cardiomyopathy[356] militates against triggered activity due to DADs, or for that matter, abnormal automaticity as the underlying mechanism in those cases (Fig. 11-208). Because of hypotension secondary to intravenous verapamil, reflex catecholamine release can occur and potentially counteract the drug's effectiveness, one must ensure the absence of reflex catecholamine antagonism to verapamil as a cause of failure of this agent to influence the tachycardia. This can be done by demonstrating a slowing of the sinus rate and the absence of hypotension during administration of the agent (see slowed atrial rate in Fig 11-208). Occasionally, recurrent monomorphic sustained VT in patients with normal hearts with RBBB and left axis deviation morphology can be terminated by verapamil.[163,168–173] This by no means signifies that this rhythm is due to triggered activity. This arrhythmia cannot be terminated by beta blockers, vagal maneuvers, or adenosine. Many other features of this particular tachycardia support reentry, including an inverse relationship of a coupling interval of the extrastimuli inducing the arrhythmia and the onset of the tachycardia, the ability of a variety of Class I agents to

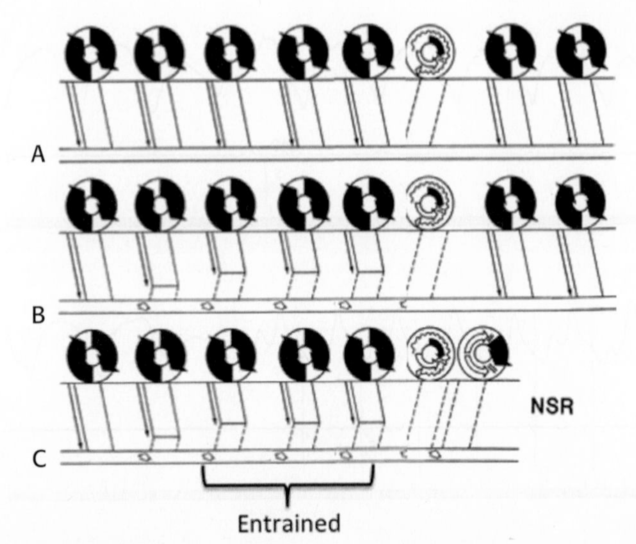


**FIGURE 11-205** Mechanism of combination method for termination of VT. **A–C:** The assumed reentrant circuit is schematically shown as the circle. The long, thin *arrow* and adjacent enclosed area represent the activation wavefront of the VT and from the pacing site and the accompanying refractory period. **A:** A very early VES reaches the circuit but can produce block only in one direction and therefore resets the circuit. **B:** Rapid pacing is shown to reverse the wavefront of activation and refractoriness until a stable collision of both wavefronts occur during fixed fusion (entrainment),but still only resets the tachycardia. **C:** With the combination method, the VT circuit is entrained by pacing to allow the premature stimulus to engage the circuit early enough to produce bidirectional block and terminate tachycardia. While the extrastimulus was delivered at the same coupling interval as in **(A)** it reaches the tachycardia circuit relatively earlier than in **(A)**. In addition, the reset circuit has a smaller excitable gap by the degree of prematurity with which it was reset. (From Gardner MJ, Waxman HL, Buxton AE, et al. Termination of ventricular tachycardia. Evaluation of a new pacing method. *Am J Cardiol* 1982;50:1338.)

also terminate the arrhythmia, and importantly, the ability of VPCs or overdrive stimulation to reset and/or entrain the VT with fusion.

In contrast, Class I agents are the most uniformly successful drugs in prolonging the tachycardia cycle length or terminating sustained monomorphic VT (Fig. 11-209) (see Chapter 12).[356–358,360,361–364] Marchlinski et al.[357,358] have also demonstrated a direct relationship between slowing of the tachycardia cycle length and prolongation of the QRS, thereby suggesting a relationship of a slowing of these tachycardias to slowing of conduction. Such a relationship would not be expected if other mechanisms were operative. We have further demonstrated that the prolongation of VT cycle length is due to slowing conduction within the reentrant circuit by demonstrating a persistent flat portion of the excitable gap during procainamide-induced slowing of VT.[365] As noted by Schmitt et al.[54] procainamide produces a prolongation of the abnormal electrograms recorded from the tachycardia sites of origin without any effect of lidocaine on these electrograms, which suggests that tissues responsible for the tachycardia have normal action potential characteristics.

As noted earlier in the chapter, Class I agents can also facilitate the induction of sustained monomorphic VT in patients in whom it cannot be induced by routine stimulation (Fig. 11-51), and these agents can occasionally produce sustained monomorphic VT in patients with coronary disease who present with nonsustained tachycardia spontaneously. Whenever monomorphic sustained VTs were slowed by Class I agents, the interval to the onset of the tachycardia was prolonged. Moreover, Horowitz et al.[164] and Buxton et al.[165,366] have demonstrated conversion of polymorphic tachycardia

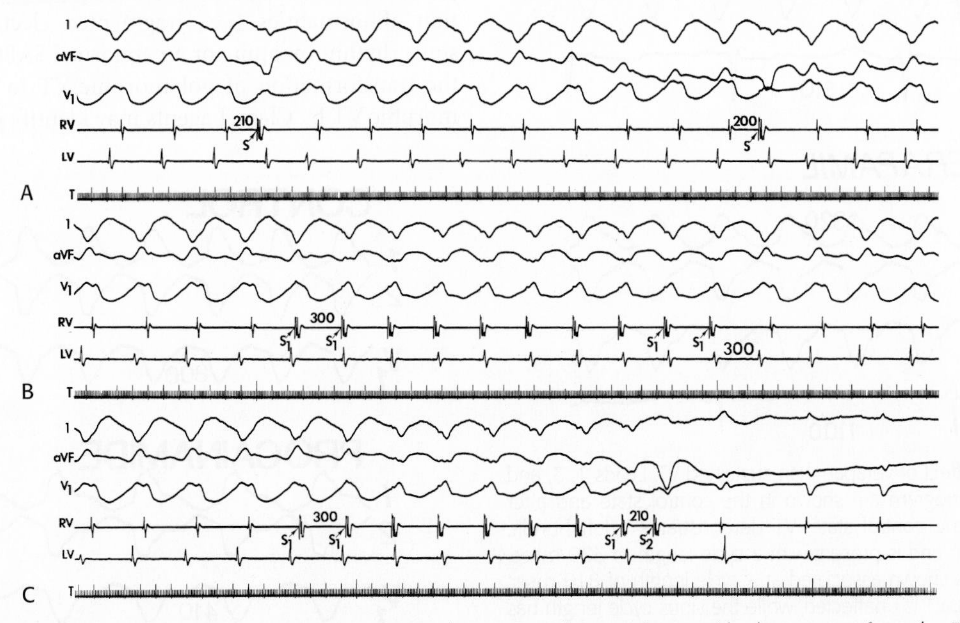


**FIGURE 11-206** Combination method of terminating VT. **A–C:** Leads 1, aVF, and $V_1$ are shown with electrograms from the RV and LV. **A:** During VT, single extrastimuli delivered at 210 and 200 msec reset the VT. **B:** Overdrive pacing at 300 msec produces entrainment of VT with fixed fusion of the QRS which resets the tachycardia on cessation of pacing. **C:** The combination of entrainment of the VT and the introduction of a premature stimulus terminates the tachycardia, where previously pacing alone or extrastimuli alone at the same cycle lengths and coupling intervals, respectively, failed to do so. See text for discussion.

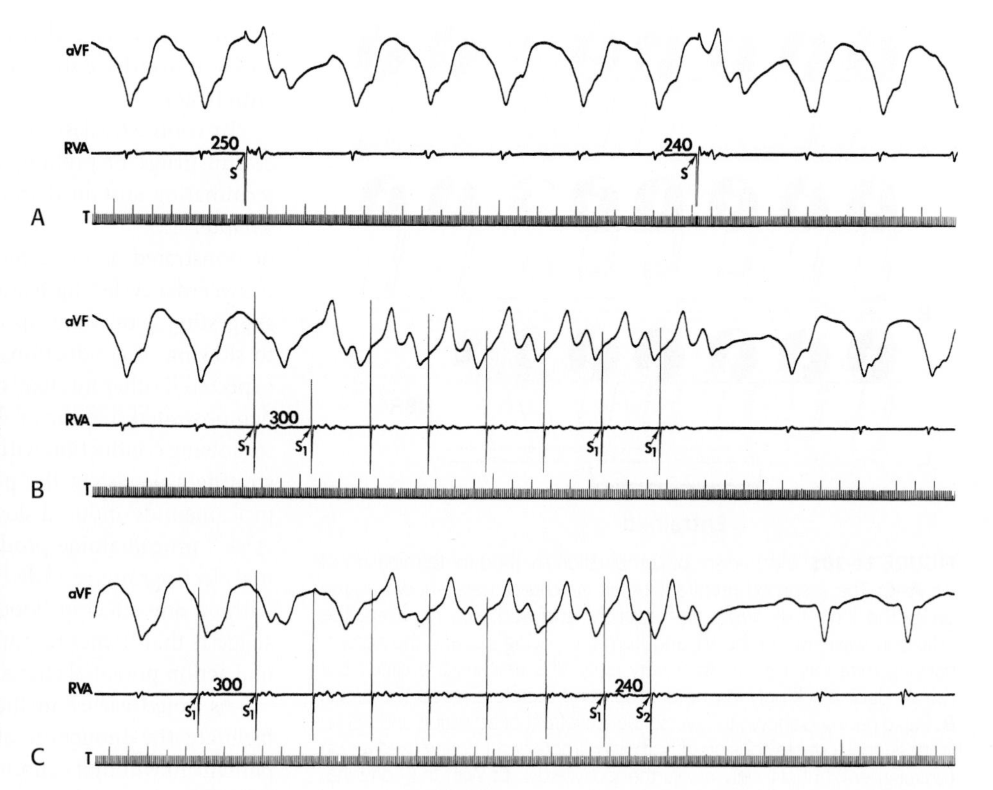


**FIGURE 11-207** Combination method of terminating VT. **A–D:** Recordings of lead aVF and the RVA are shown. **A:** A single premature stimulus (S) fails to terminate VT. **B:** Overdrive ventricular pacing at a paced cycle length to 300 msec ($S_1$-$S_1$) is also unsuccessful. **C:** Overdrive ventricular pacing at a paced cycle length of 250 msec results in acceleration of VT from a cycle length of 360 to 260 msec. (From Gardner MJ, Waxman HL, Buxton AE, et al. Termination of ventricular tachycardia. Evaluation of a new pacing method. *Am J Cardiol* 1982;50:1338.)

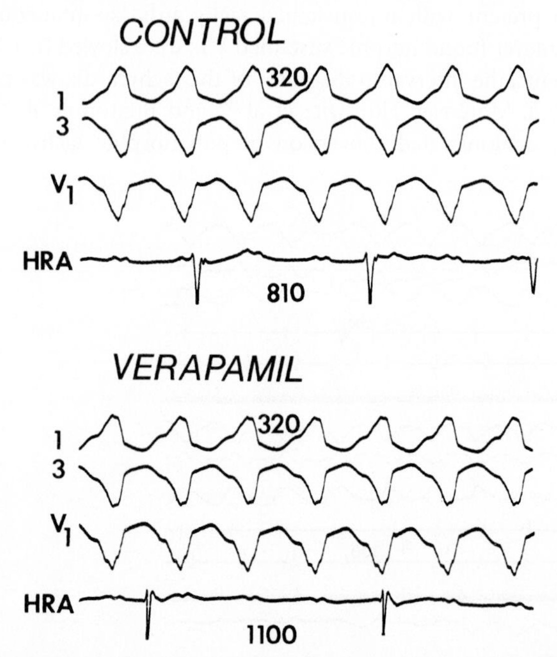


**FIGURE 11-208** Effect of verapamil on sustained VT. Leads 1, 3, and $V_1$ and a HRA electrogram are shown in the control state and after verapamil. During the control state, VT demonstrates a left bundle branch block pattern and is present with a cycle length of 320 msec, and sinus rhythm is shown associated at a cycle length of 810 msec Following verapamil, VT is unaffected, while the sinus cycle length has increased to 1100 msec. See text for discussion. (From Josephson ME, Marchlinski FE, Cassidy DM, et al. Sustained ventricular tachycardia in coronary artery disease—Evidence for reentrant mechanism. In: Zipes DP, Jalife J, eds. *Cardiac electrophysiology and arrhythmias.* Orlando, FL: Grune & Stratton, 1985:409.)

to a uniform tachycardia by Class I agents (Figs. 11-118 to 11-120, and Fig. 11-210). This response of polymorphic VT to procainamide occurs almost exclusively in patients with coronary artery disease and prior myocardial infarction. These patients can be distinguished from those in whom polymorphic VT cannot be made uniform by the presence of conduction abnormalities (i.e., fragmented electrograms) during sinus rhythm mapping or an abnormal SAECG. I believe that the transformation of polymorphic VT to uniform, monomorphic VT by Class I agents may identify patients in whom

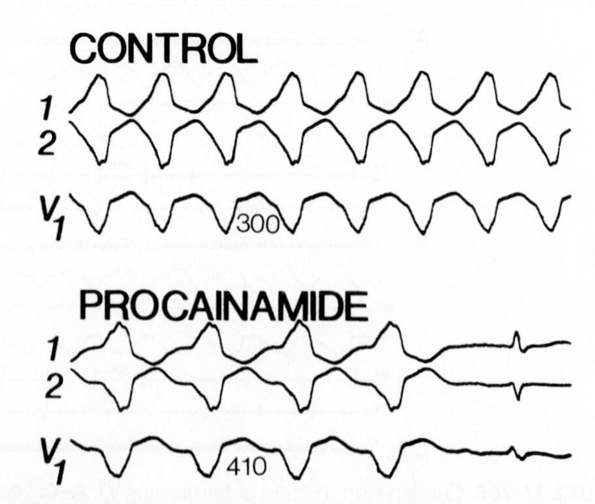


**FIGURE 11-209** Response of VT to procainamide. Leads 1, 2, and $V_1$ are shown during VT in the control state and following procainamide. In the control state, the cycle length of the tachycardia is 300 msec. Following procainamide, the tachycardia slows and then terminates.

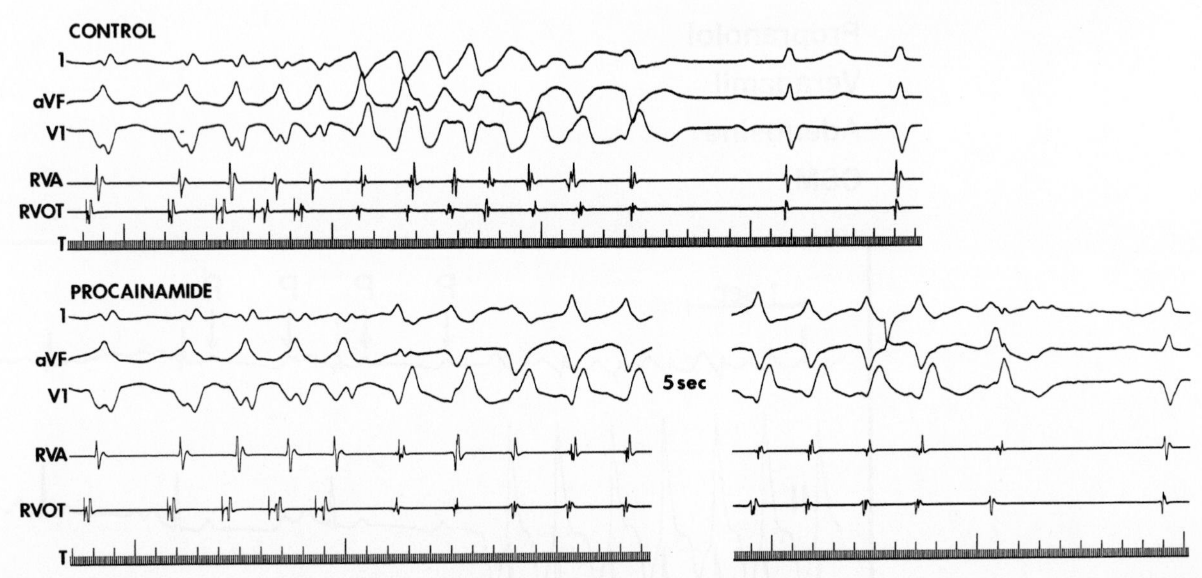


**FIGURE 11-210** Change of nonsustained polymorphic VT to uniform nonsustained VT following procainamide. In the control state, triple extrastimuli delivered from the RVOT produce a nonsustained polymorphic VT. Following procainamide, triple extrastimuli from the RVOT produce a uniform nonsustained VT of longer duration. See text for discussion.

induction of polymorphic VT may be a manifestation of an underlying arrhythmogenic substrate and not an artifact of stimulation.

Buxton et al.,[367] evaluating the electropharmacology of nonsustained VT associated with coronary artery disease, demonstrated that neither verapamil nor propranolol prevented or altered the mode of induction of VT by premature stimulation, nor did they slow the rate of the induced tachycardias. Occasionally, verapamil shortened the cycle length and prolonged the duration of the tachycardias (Fig. 11-211).

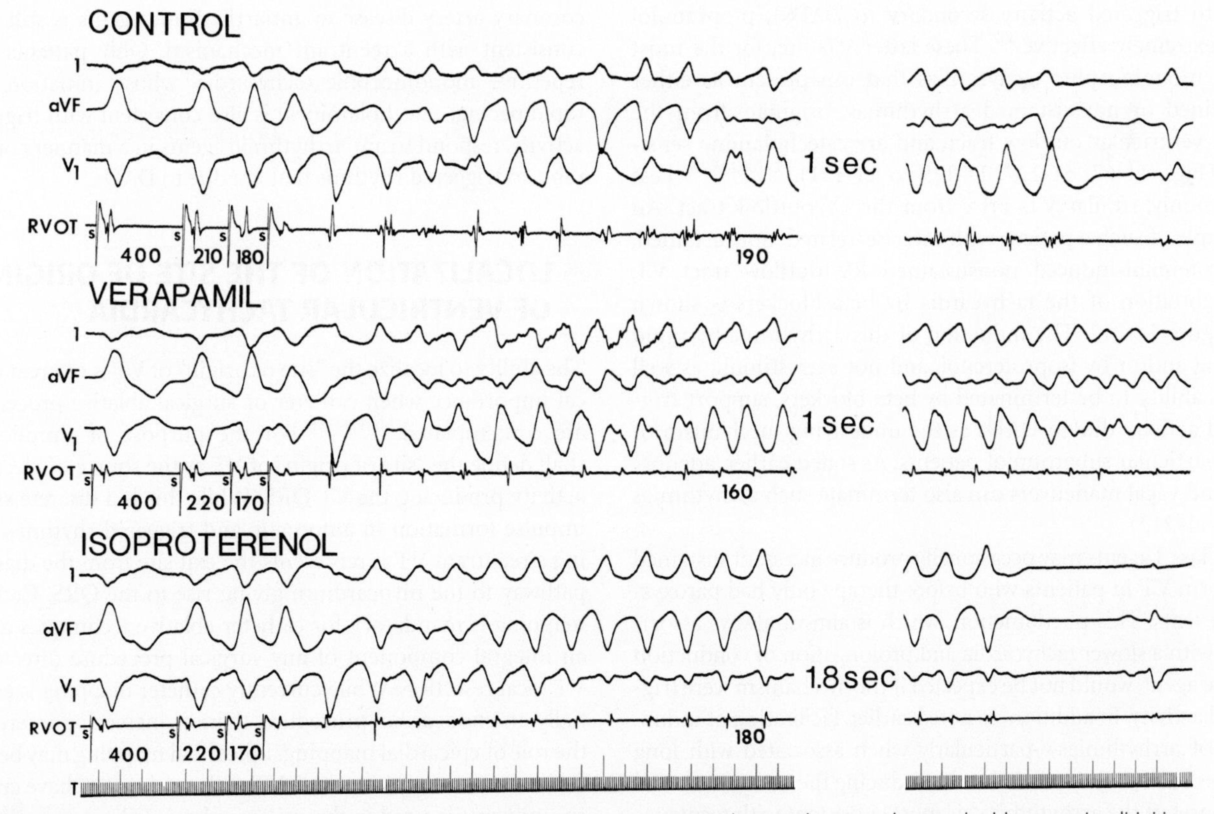


**FIGURE 11-211** Effect of verapamil and isoproterenol on polymorphic nonsustained VT. In the control state, double extrastimuli initiate a polymorphic VT. Following verapamil using similar coupling intervals, polymorphic tachycardia is induced, which degenerates to sustained polymorphic VT, which degenerates to VF. Isoproterenol, on the other hand, has no significant effect on the induction or duration of polymorphic VT.

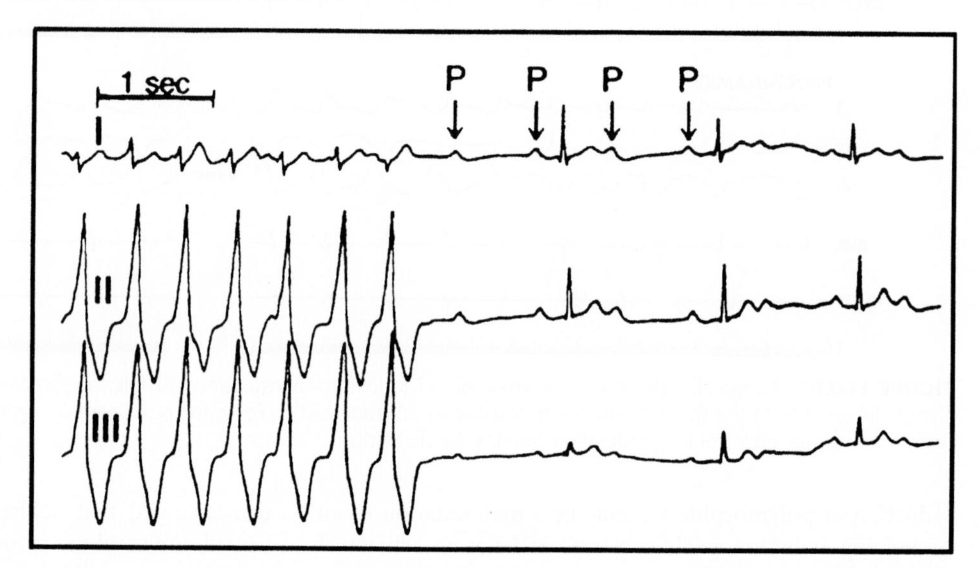


**FIGURE 11-212** Termination of catecholamine-mediated idiopathic right ventricular outflow tract VT by beta blockers, carotid sinus pressure, and adenosine. See text for discussion.

As noted earlier Class I agents either abolished the tachycardias or slowed them (Figs. 11-209 and 11-210). In nonsustained arrhythmias induced by isoproterenol (i.e., those due to triggered activity secondary to DADs), propranolol was extremely effective.[367] These latter VTs are, for the most part, monomorphic tachycardias that can present as either sustained or nonsustained arrhythmias, originate from the right ventricular outflow tract, and are catecholamine sensitive (Figs. 11-67, 11-127, 11-129 to 11-131).[163,168,295,296] Less commonly, similar VTs arise from the LV outflow tract. An example of such a patient with exercise-related, nonsustained, isoproterenol-induced nonsustained RV outflow tract VT, and abolition of the tachycardia by beta blockers is shown in Figure 11-212. The induction of this arrhythmia by rapid pacing and/or by isoproterenol, and not extrastimuli, as well as its ability to be terminated by beta blockers, support triggered activity due to DADs as the underlying mechanism of this particular subgroup of patients. As stated earlier, adenosine and vagal maneuvers can also terminate such arrhythmias (Fig. 11-212).

Class I agents may occasionally produce incessant sustained uniform VT in patients who before therapy only had paroxysmal events. This phenomenon, which is almost always associated with a slower tachycardia and prolongation of conduction by the agent, would not be expected if the mechanism were triggered activity. In addition, as noted earlier, facilitation of induction of arrhythmias—particularly when associated with long pauses between the extrastimulus inducing the arrhythmia and the onset of the arrhythmia—is most consistent with reentry.

In summary, although antiarrhythmic agents are not mechanism specific, the pattern of response of VT to these drugs can provide indirect evidence favoring one mechanism. Thus, the response of sustained uniform VT, nonsustained uniform or polymorphic VT, or even polymorphic VT/VF in the setting of coronary artery disease to antiarrhythmic agents is still most consistent with a reentrant mechanism. Only patients with repetitive monomorphic tachycardia, whose initiation (i.e., rapid pacing, catecholamines) is also consistent with triggered activity, respond to antiarrhythmic agents in a manner comparable to triggered rhythms that are due to DADs.

## LOCALIZATION OF THE SITE OF ORIGIN OF VENTRICULAR TACHYCARDIA

The ability to localize the "site of origin" of VT is of great clinical importance when catheter or surgical ablative procedures are contemplated.[148,368–381] For the purpose of simplicity, I shall define the "site of origin" of VT as the source of electrical activity producing the VT QRS. While this is a discrete site of impulse formation in automatic and triggered rhythms, during a reentrant VT it represents the exit site from the diastolic pathway to the myocardium giving rise to the QRS. Catheter mapping is mandatory for catheter ablative techniques and is an integral component of any surgical procedure directed at VT local resection. While currently catheter mapping is essentially an endocardial procedure, there is increasing interest in the role of epicardial mapping. Epicardial mapping may be useful in circumstances in which VTs either arise at or have critical components located in the epi- or subepicardium.[75,382,383] This may become an important technique for the ablation of VTs associated with certain cardiomyopathies.[382,383] The ablative procedures and associated studies are discussed in more detail in Chapter 13.

In addition to its clinical utility, mapping provides information about the mechanism of the tachycardia. This is particularly true if reentrant excitation can be demonstrated. The demonstration of a complete reentrant circuit has been nearly impossible in the catheterization laboratory using standard catheters and point-by-point mapping and, in the past, required detailed intraoperative mapping.[46,352,353,371,374–376] Recent technologic advances in mapping allowing acquisition of multiple simultaneous sites can provide a great deal of activation mapping information on a single beat. The noncontact mapping system (Endocardial Solutions, Inc.) can display several thousand mathematically derived electrograms using the inverse solution.[69,384,385] These electrograms correlate reasonably well with those recorded simultaneously by direct contact, but have limited accuracy in very large ventricles. Currently the system is cumbersome and expensive. Future enhancements to ascertain stability of the intracavitary balloon and facilitate more uniformly accurate spatial localization of the electrogram and separate ablation catheter may make this system more useful, particularly in ablating unstable rhythms. The ability to display several thousand derived electrograms can allow for the demonstration of complete reentrant circuits,[386] realizing that much of the data is interpolated from the 64 "recording poles." More recently noninvasive electrocardiographic imaging (ECGI) has been developed .[387–389] This system uses 250 body surface leads integrated with cardiac CT or MRI images using inverse solution methodology. It appears useful for focal tachycardias and can give the impression of reentrant excitation but is limited to the epicardium and cannot follow activity in the intraventricular septum or the endocardium in densely infarcted areas. Further work is needed to define its role in scar related reentrant VTs.

Occasionally, detailed mapping using the Carto system (Biosense, Inc.) has demonstrated reentrant excitation. There are, in addition observations, using standard catheters and recording equipment that suggest reentry. These include mapping a diastolic pathway or demonstrating diastolic bridging or continuous electrical activity, which is requisite to maintain the tachycardia.[1,43,44,197,200,369] Analysis of the response of electrograms to programmed stimulation helps demonstrate the requirement of the recorded electrical signal for the genesis of the arrhythmia and can distinguish between early or late electrograms.[1,122,148,315,316,319,377–381] Recently Carto, Navix (St Jude), and Rhythmia (Boston Scientific) have enabled multisite "contact mapping" using multipolar electrode catheters. These can take the form of 10 to 12 pole standard catheters with standard ring electrodes (1- to 2-mm circumferential electrodes with 2- to 4-mm inter(mid)-electrode distance), the PentArray catheter from Biosense Webster (20 very small electrodes 2 to 5 mm apart), and the Rhythmia 64 pole (smallest electrodes at very low impedance) small basket (see figures of catheters in Chapter 1). These systems allow for the collection of large amounts of data in much shorter period of time. While this mass of information can theoretically provide

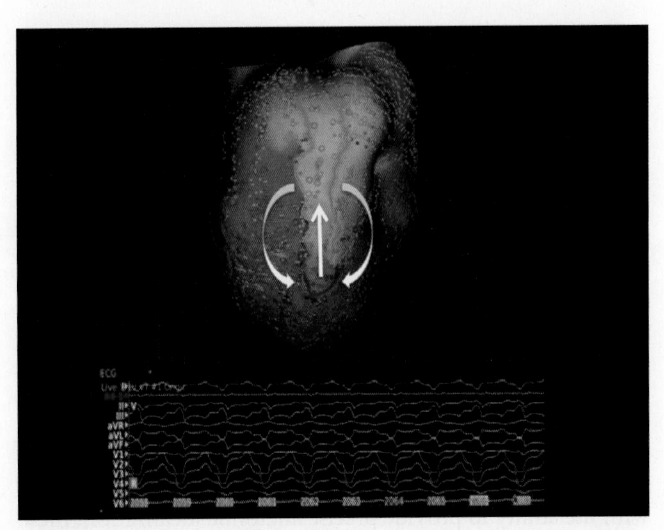

**FIGURE 11-213** High-density mapping of infarct-related VT with Rhythmia System. A 12 lead ECG of VT is displayed below an activation map derived from 18,000 points in an 8-week-old porcine anterior infarction. The anterior view is shown. A figure-of-eight pattern of reentrant excitation is demonstrated. Color code: red early, purple late.

more accurate information, the automated annotation algorithms for unipolar and bipolar recordings need more refining to make them accurate. Furthermore, variable contact of the multipolar electrodes detract from their accuracy. Methods to assess contact are currently being developed to enhance the accuracy of the findings. An example of an 18,000 point map demonstrating a reentrant VT circuit using the Rhythmia system is shown in Figure 11-213.

When activation mapping of the tachycardia per se cannot be accomplished because of hemodynamic instability, indirect methods of tachycardia localization can be employed (e.g., sinus rhythm mapping, pace mapping, and analysis of the 12-lead ECG) and may be helpful in making clinical decisions.[9,10,31–36,38,61,390–395] These latter techniques, however, provide little information regarding mechanism, although as noted earlier in the chapter, sinus rhythm mapping can define abnormalities that correlate with a substrate conducive to reentry.[31–36,38,61]

Recently there has been an interest in using hemodynamic support (e.g., ECMO, Impella, Tandem Heart) to allow for activation mapping during poorly tolerated VT.

## General Methods of Catheter Mapping

Activation mapping of VT requires either the presence of the arrhythmia at the time of the procedure or that it can be initiated. Optimally, the patient should be hemodynamically stable during the tachycardia so that the map may be completed. If a sustained arrhythmia is hemodynamically unstable, mapping can still be accomplished by starting and stopping the tachycardia after data acquisition at each site. In unusual circumstances an intraaortic balloon pump or LV support (Impella, ECMO) can provide the hemodynamic stability required to map the VT. More often, rapid tachycardias that are poorly tolerated can be slowed by antiarrhythmic agents to allow for mapping. Slowing of the tachycardia is also useful to distinguish between electrical systole and diastole when confusion is present during the rapid untreated VT. The administration of an antiarrhythmic agent does not alter the sequence of activation despite slowing of the tachycardia and widening of the QRS morphology. While the electrogram at the "site of origin" may widen, its relationship to the onset of the QRS remains unchanged.[396] Development of newer technologies, such as large and small basket catheters (circumferential splines with multiple electrodes on each spline) and noncontact mapping (mathematical derivation of thousands of electrograms based on the inverse solution) with an invasive balloon (ESI)[384] or ECGI can provide activation mapping data of nonsustained or unstable arrhythmias. Coupled with the ability to provide precise anatomic localization, these technologies are critical to developing ablative techniques for transient or hemodynamically unstable VT. If more than one morphologically distinct tachycardia is induced, it should also be completely mapped. Obviously, the development of these multisite data acquisition systems may make analysis of multiple morphologically distinct VT, particularly those that constantly change, possible. A schema of the left ventricle, which we use for mapping, has been previously shown in Figure 11-16. Because VT can arise from either ventricle, a schema of both ventricles is used (Fig. 11-214). This schema remains useful in defining the ECG patterns arising from different regions. Obviously one of several 3D electroanatomic systems can be used to define the location of each recorded electrogram in space and correlate it to an anatomic shell.

Using standard equipment, 15 to 20 regions are mapped during VT. The numbered sites in Figure 11-214 represent segmental areas of the heart of approximately 5 to 10 $cm^2$. Mapping is also performed in subdivisions of these standard sites. The number of sites mapped depends on the goals of mapping. For example, a map to define abnormalities of activation during sinus rhythm usually requires 80 to 200 sites taken using a point-to-point. Use of the Carto system for this endeavor provides information about electrogram amplitude (voltage map), activation time, and allows for the creation of electrogram duration and late potential maps. The small roving basket catheter from Rhythmia can record 64 simultaneous electrograms and more than 10,000 points can be acquired in 15 to 20 minutes. While software is becoming available to provide automated maps of activation, voltage, duration, and late potential , currently these must be manually annotated. Similarly, while the noncontact mapping system and ECGI can provide "thousands" of electrograms and an activation map, software are under development to allow display of voltage, duration and/or late potential maps. The accuracy of the ESI system will always be questioned since all data are ***interpolated*** from the 64 recording electrodes, which must remain absolutely fixed in relation to the wall of the chamber being map. The ECGI system will be limited because of its inability to show accurate activation of the septum or within dense endocardial scar. Thus, in my mind it is not more accurate than a detailed contact map. To map a single monomorphic VT, a more focused map may be all that is needed to guide ablation (see Chapter13). The number of sites mapped is based on the investigator's ability to regionalize the mapping sites of interest from the morphology of the VT on the ECG. Usually only 20 to 40 mapping points are required for a single, stable VT. For most of the remainder of this discussion I shall describe data gathered by point-by-point mapping with a roving catheter. In the absence of a 3D electroanatomic each position must be verified with fluoroscopy in multiple planes. Currently the Carto and Navix systems are widely used for electroanatomic mapping. The Rhythmia system will become widely available in the next year. These systems allow accurate and reproducible localization without requiring excessive, and in some cases, any fluoroscopy. The validity of the mapping technique depends on stability, reproducibility, and verification of catheter position for each site; thus, the activation time at each site should have a beat-to-beat variation of <5 msec. Attempts to reposition the catheter to previously recorded sites are of value in demonstrating one's ability to record from specific areas of the heart. The site(s) of origin (or the isthmus of a reentrant circuit) should be reproducibly mappable to an area of approximately 2 $cm^2$. Using the Carto system the location of each recorded site is stored with an anatomic localizing accuracy of ≈1 mm. The Navix system has somewhat less accuracy because it uses impedance from the body surface to localize position, a method that is associated with significant catheter motion on respiration. The ability to get back to any desired site is facilitated by the 3D guidance provided by the system. Any acquired electrogram can provide a target that will be within 1 mm of the position displayed by the system. A skillful operator is needed to maneuver the catheter precisely back to the target site provided by the system. A complete left ventricular map of a single VT that is due to coronary disease usually takes <20 minutes if only passive recordings are obtained. Mapping additional tachycardias[369,370,396] and evaluating the response of electrograms to programmed stimulation[148,314,315,318,376,377,377–380,390] significantly prolongs the procedure. Programmed stimulation is necessary to define

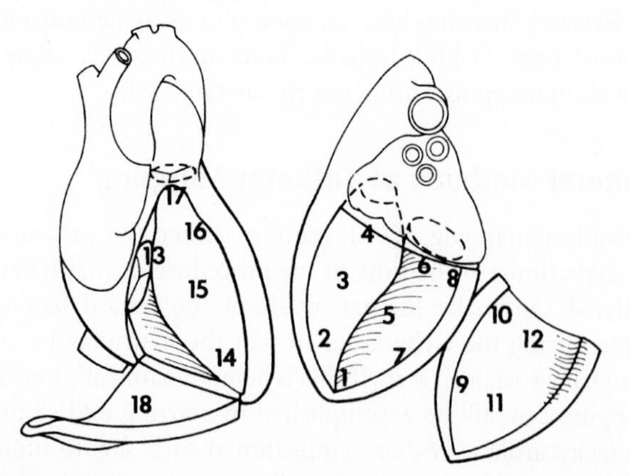


**FIGURE 11-214** Schema of mapping sites in the right and left ventricles. Sites 1 through 12 are segments of the LV and 13 through 17 are segments of the RV.

critical parts of a reentrant circuit amenable to ablation but is not necessary for focal mechanisms. In the future, mapping technologies may be refined to demonstrate critical diastolic pathways and eliminate the need for programmed stimulation.

Point-by-point endocardial mapping usually requires the use of three or more catheters. We usually use catheters placed at the right ventricular apex and outflow tract to serve both as reference electrograms and as an anatomic guide to the position of the right ventricular side of the septum. In addition, we do not infrequently use a coronary sinus catheter to provide an anatomic reference for the base of the heart. The RV catheters are also used for induction of VT and the CS or another atrial catheter is used for synchronized atrial pacing, which is sometimes necessary to assure stable drive trains (i.e., prevent capture beats) as well as to provide an "atrial kick" during VT that helps maintain hemodynamic stability. We usually use a standard #6 or #7 French quadripolar ablation catheter (4-mm tip electrode) with a 2-5-2 or 2-2-2 mm interelectrode distance for left ventricular mapping in most instances (see Chapter 1). Special catheters with close-spaced electrodes at the tip (e.g., split tip) and of smaller French size are occasionally useful. All catheters have deflectable tips to facilitate positioning. Deflection may be possible in one or two directions with different size curves in each direction (EPT, Boston Scientific). Some catheters also have lateral rotation capabilities. Nevertheless, the ability to perform good maps using these tools depends more on the investigator than on the catheters or recording equipment. The use of multisite data acquisition systems (the Rhythmia basket catheter, the PentArray, or simple multipolar catheters) can provide more information more quickly. Until the automated annotation capabilities improve, either manual editing of activation data or use of additional localizing methods are needed to guide the ablation catheter to the critical site required for ablation. Hopefully, combinations of technologies will be developed and employed in the next five years. While the costs of these systems will be great, it is hoped (but not yet proven) that they will facilitate mapping of heretofore unmappable arrhythmias (transient or hemodynamically untolerated) and provide a cost advantage for their acquisition.

In the typical patient with hemodynamically stable monomorphic VT and coronary artery disease, initially only a left ventricular catheter is used for mapping. Once mapping of the left ventricle is accomplished, one of the reference RV electrode catheters can be used to assess the need to map the RV in detail. For VT unassociated with coronary artery disease, or when LV mapping does not reveal a "site of origin," or when a right sided exit of a coronary VT is suggested by the RV reference catheter, we undertake detailed mapping of the RV using a separate RV mapping catheter. Fluoroscopy in multiple views is required to assess the position of the catheters. Biplane fluoroscopy has obvious advantages, but it is expensive. Use of any of the electroanatomic mapping systems may eliminate the need for biplane fluoroscopy systems and prevent complications from excessive radiation exposure and save hundreds of thousands of dollars. Optimally, one should have the capability of recording the catheter positions on cineradiographic film or on videotape for subsequent review.

We perform arterial catheterization via the Seldinger technique percutaneously from the femoral artery. In the presence of severe peripheral vascular disease or abdominal aneurysms, or in patients who have had previous vascular surgery on their aorta or femoral arteries, a brachial arteriotomy or puncture can be used for the left ventricular mapping catheter. The radial artery approach, while safer, may be impractical because use of the large size of catheters used for ablation. The transseptal approach can be used in such cases, although, in my experience with current catheter technology, accessing the entire ventricle is more difficult than by the retrograde approach. The use of steerable sheathes (e.g., Agillis, from St Jude) facilitates LV mapping via this approach, and in my opinion, is necessary to acquire complete data with good contact. The use of noncontact mapping catheters may require a transseptal approach for their placement. A transseptal puncture is necessary to place the ablation catheter if the retrograde approach is not feasible. In all instances, we use full heparinization with 5,000 to 10,000 U as a bolus and 1,200 to 3,000 U/h drip, adjusted to maintain an activated clotting time of 250 to 350 seconds. Greater anticoagulation may be required when using the basket catheters.

During the spontaneous or induced tachycardia, we record bipolar and unipolar electrograms (poles 1 and 2) as the catheter is positioned at each new mapping site. The unipolar electrograms are open filtered (0.05 to 500 Hz) when we are studying patients with normal hearts, and are filtered at a comparable setting (between 30 and 500 Hz) to those used with the acquisition of bipolar electrograms using standard catheters, when dealing with scar-related VTs (i.e., CAD, RV dysplasia, etc.). Filtering is used to eliminate far field activity and maximize local activity. In patients with large scars unfiltered unipolar signals are dominated by cavity potentials making it difficult/impossible to see small, local activity. If possible we record at variable and fixed (1 cm = 1 mV) gains to be able to standardize duration measurements. Unfortunately this is not possible on most laboratory systems. This is important for substrate mapping as described earlier in this chapter. Out of the box filtering of standardized bipolar recordings with Carto system have varied with the model: in Carto XP filtering was set at 10 to 300 Hz, and Carto 3 it was set at 16 to 240 Hz. These differ from what had been used in the original mapping data and can affect electrogram amplitude and shape (see discussion of VT substrate earlier in this chapter). Normal values for voltage need to be ascertained for each electrode catheter because electrogram amplitude and duration are affected by electrode size (the tip is the largest) and interelectrode distance, as well as the relation of the distal and proximal poles to the site of contact and wavefront of activation (see discussion below). This is very important if one tries to compare substrate voltage using very small electrodes and small interelectrode distance (Rhythmia and PentArray catheters). For most standard catheters, the tip electrode is the major source of the recorded EGM because it is the electrode that is in best contact. If catheters have a 2-5-2 or greater interelectrode distance, we obtain distal and proximal bipolar electrograms by recording from the tip and the third electrode (distal pair) of the quadripolar catheter and use the second and fourth poles to record electrical activity adjacent to or overlapping the site of origin (proximal pair) when we use stimulation from the distal and third poles. Thus, recording and stimulation occur over a shared area, which electrophysiologically is "large" in terms of source of recorded signal. If we use a catheter with a 2-mm interelectrode distance, poles 1 and 2 are used as the distal pair and 3 and 4 as the proximal pair. The advantage of using catheters with smaller interelectrode distances (i.e., 1 mm) is somewhat offset by the inability to precisely reposition the catheter to the smaller area from which such electrodes record. Recording from multiple bipolar pairs from a multipolar electrode catheter in the left ventricle (particularly if bipolar pairs are >1 cm apart) is inappropriate, because one has no control over the degree of contact of the proximal electrode pairs and/or their distance from the ventricular wall. This can lead to very inaccurate recordings and misinterpretation of the data. The only accurate data are from electrograms recorded from electrodes in contact with the endocardium. One should therefore use only electrograms recorded from a bipolar pair that includes the **tip** electrode, because it is almost always in contact with the endocardium. A proximal electrode pair is useful for analyzing events during pacing since polarization of the distal electrodes makes simultaneous recording and pacing not possible in most available laboratory systems. Contact is critical when a standard quadripolar, decapolar, or basket catheters are used. The degree of contact can be assessed by pacing thresholds or impedance measurements at each electrode pair. The noncontact mapping system (Endocardial solutions, Inc.[115]) generates mathematically derived electrograms and places them on an LV or RV chamber defined by a second, roving catheter which is dragged along the ventricular walls. This "chamber" is limited by the absence of direct confirmation of contact of the roving catheter. The electrical/anatomic accuracy (i.e., the relationship of the electrogram and the 3D site from which it was truly generated) is further limited by the distance of the noncontact electrode from the ventricular wall and movement of the noncontact probe following generation of the electrograms due to "bumping" by the roving catheter. Newer technology is being incorporated into this system, which has improved and will continue to improve its anatomic localizing capability. However as noted above, the activation times are interpolated on the basis of the inverse solution for 64 poles. The ECGI system also uses inverse solution technology, but the heart is assess using 250 body surface electrodes projected on a CT or MRI image. Its weaknesses are its limited view of the septum und endocardium.

Either unfiltered or filtered unipolar and filtered bipolar electrograms are used; however, we prefer filtered electrograms in scar-related VTs. The advantages of unipolar electrograms are that they provide a more precise measure of local activation, because the maximum negative dV/dt corresponds to the maximum Na+ conductance. They also provide information about the direction of impulse propagation. The disadvantages of unipolar recordings are that they have a poor signal-to-noise ratio and distant activity can be difficult to separate from local activity. This is particularly true when recording from areas of prior infarct. In such instances, QS potentials are ubiquitous, and it is often impossible to select a rapid negative dV/dt when the entire negative QS potential is slowly inscribed (i.e., cavity potential). On the other hand, bipolar recording techniques provide an improved signal-to-noise ratio and reduce the effect of distant activity on the local electrogram (Fig. 11-13). While local activation is less precisely defined, the peak amplitude of a filtered (30 to 500 Hz) close (2 to 5mm) bipolar recording of a "normal" electrogram corresponds to the maximum negative dV/dt of the unipolar recording. Variable low- and/or high-pass filters can give different amplitudes, duration, shape, etc. Although a bipolar electrode pair, positioned perpendicular to the direction of propagation of the wavefront, should theoretically result in the absence of an electrical signal, this is rarely a problem. Nevertheless, the electrogram amplitude may be diminished when propagation is relatively perpendicular to the recording electrodes. Thus normal values will differ if they have been acquired with the catheter perpendicular to the LV wall versus if acquired parallel to the wall. Use of very small electrodes and interelectrode distance (1 mm) overcomes many of the limitations that standard mapping/ablation catheters have because their tip is 3.5 to 4 mm and capped with 2-mm ring electrode 2 mm from the tip (≈4.75- to 5-mm mid-electrode to mid-electrode distance). One therefore cannot obtain directional information from an isolated bipolar electrogram recorded from a standard mapping/ablation catheter. Filtering is useful to eliminate noise and distant activity.

Defining the site of origin (or exit from a protected isthmus in a reentrant circuit) and the overall pattern of activation of impulse propagation requires detailed recordings from multiple sites. Despite the limitations of bipolar recordings, we prefer them in scar-related VTs because extraneous noise is removed, and with appropriate filtering, the high-frequency components are more accurately seen. However, as stated above, unfiltered unipolar recordings are extremely useful in mapping VT in patients with normal hearts. Filtered or unfiltered unipolar recordings are valuable in determining the relative contributions of the distal and second pole of the bipolar pair. Clear demonstration that the distal pole is earliest is necessary to assure the highest success of ablation (see Chapter 13). As stated in earlier paragraphs, several factors affect electrogram amplitude and width, including (a) conduction velocity (the greater the velocity the higher the peak amplitude of the unfiltered and filtered bipolar electrogram); (b) the mass of activated tissue; (c) the distance between the electrodes and the propagating wavefront; (d) the direction of the propagation relative to the bipoles (Figs. 11-215 and 11-216; Anter and Josephson, unpublished observations); (e) the interelectrode distance (Fig. 11-217; Anter and Josephson, unpublished observations); (f) the electrode surface

Bipolar Amplitude Depends on Bipolar Orientation and Wavefront of Activation

*Small changes in orientation can affect voltage*

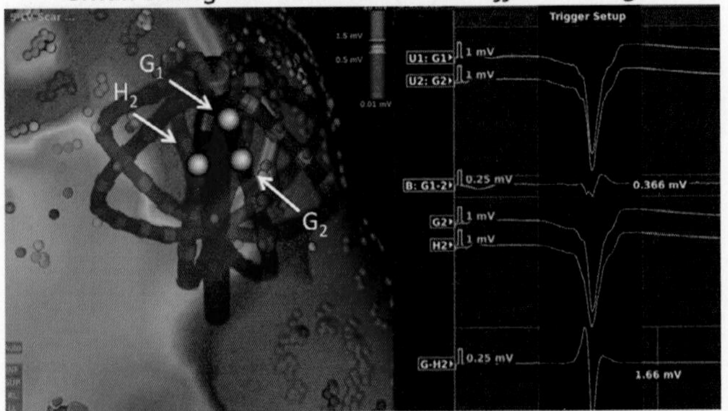


**FIGURE 11-215** Effect of bipolar orientation and wavefront of activation on bipolar voltage. Unipolar and derived bipolar recordings are shown from electrodes $G_1$, $G_2$, and $H_2$ which are each 0.4 $mm^2$ and ≈2 mm apart. The bipoles are oriented at 90 degrees from each other. The unipolar signals show $G_1$ and $G_2$ are activated nearly simultaneously producing a bipolar signal of 0.366 mV. When the bipolar signal is recorded between $G_2$ and $H_2$, there is a slight difference in local activation and the recorded electrogram has a normal voltage of 1.66 mV. See text for discussion.

**Dependence of bipolar voltage on angle of contact (i.e. parallel vs perpendicular)**

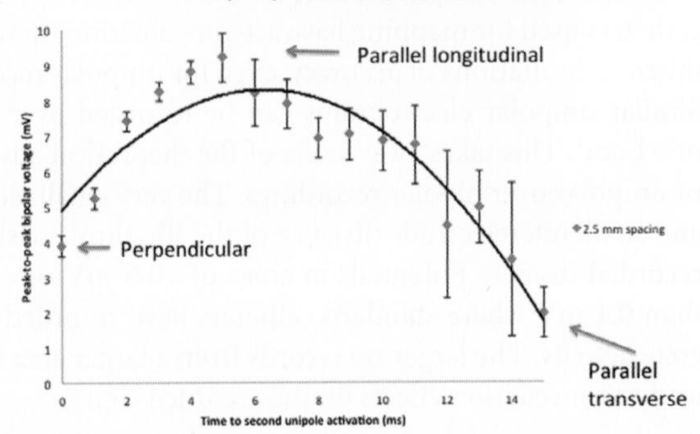


- Each diamond represents the average of the mean bipolar voltages from 9 sinus studies at the appropriate unipolar delay.
- The black line is a quadratic fit of the data.

**FIGURE 11-216** Dependence of bipolar voltage on angle of contact. Peak-to-peak bipolar voltage is shown on the ordinate and activation time between the two unipolar signals from which the bipolar electrogram is derived. When the poles are perpendicular to the surface, the difference between the unipolar activation is close to 0 and the bipolar voltage is low. When the electrodes are parallel to the surface the bipolar amplitude depends on the activation times between the electrodes. See text for discussion.

The relationship between interelectrode spacing and bipolar voltage

Sinus rhythm

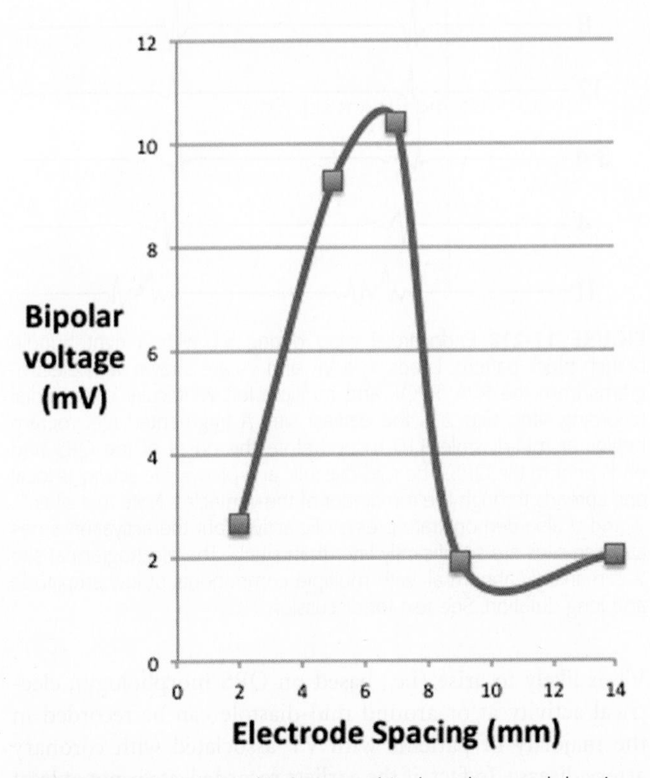


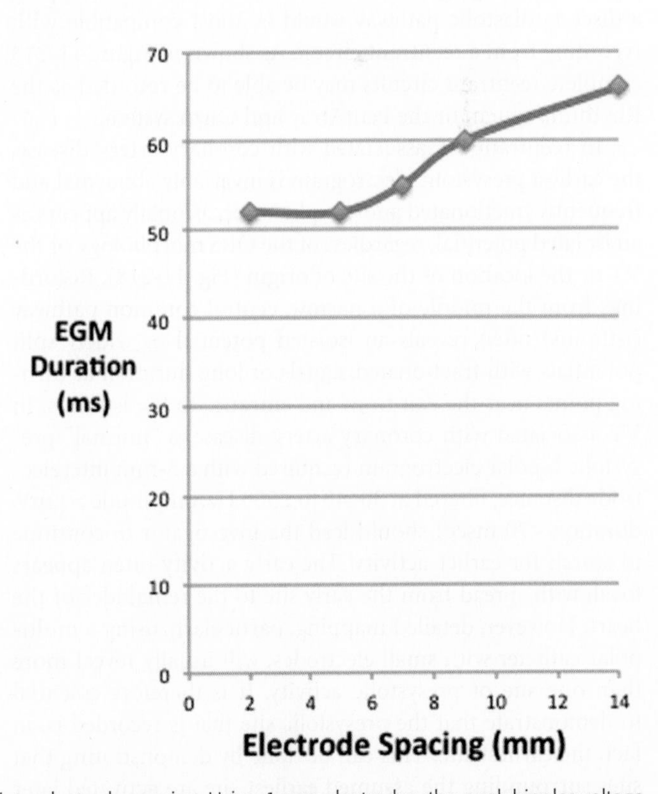


**FIGURE 11-217** Relationship between bipolar voltage and duration and interelectrode spacing. Using 1-mm electrodes, the peak bipolar voltage is recorded with 6 mm, but gradually decreases at wider interelectrode distances. The electrogram duration appears directly related to the interelectrode distance. See text for discussion.

areas; (g) the amplifier gain; and (h) other signal-processing techniques that may introduce artifacts. The fact that most catheters used for mapping have a 4-mm ablation tip results in inherent limitations of accuracy, even for unipolar recordings. Similar unipolar electrograms can be recorded over an area of ≈1 cm². This takes away some of the theoretical advantages of unipolar over bipolar recordings. The very small electrodes and small interelectrode distance of the Rhythmia basket have recorded discrete potentials in areas of <0.5 mV or even less than 0.1 mV where standard catheters have recorded no discrete activity. The larger tip records from a larger area that can lead to cancellation effects on the recorded signal.

### *Acquisition and Interpretation of Activation Mapping During Ventricular Tachycardia*

The "site of origin" of a tachycardia is determined by locating the earliest recorded discrete or fractionated ventricular electrogram closest to mid-diastole. In this section the discussion will be based on recordings from standard ablation catheters. Because we uncommonly can record the activation of an entire reentrant circuit using standard "ablation" catheters for mapping, we have arbitrarily defined mid-diastole (50% of the VT cycle length) as the earliest point, recognizing that if a reentrant arrhythmia is present, activity should be recorded throughout diastole. Thus, while the earliest presystolic electrogram closest to mid-diastole is the most commonly used definition for the "site of origin," continuous diastolic activity and/or bridging of diastole at adjacent sites or mapping a discrete diastolic pathway would be most compatible with recording from a reentrant circuit. As shown in Figure 11-213 complete reentrant circuits may be able to be recorded as the Rhythmia system or the PentArray and Carto system.

In reentrant VT associated with coronary artery disease, the earliest presystolic electrogram is invariably abnormal and frequently fractionated and/or split, or occasionally appears as an isolated potential, regardless of the QRS morphology of the VT or the location of the site of origin (Fig. 11-218). Recordings from the middle of a narrow, central common pathway (isthmus) often reveals an isolated potential or widely split potentials with fractionated signals of long duration at turning points near the exit from and entrance to the isthmus. In VT associated with coronary artery disease, a "normal" presystolic bipolar electrogram (acquired with a 5-mm interelectrode distance, filtered at 30–40 to ≤500 Hz, amplitude >3 mV, duration <70 msec) should lead the investigator to continue to search for earlier activity. The early activity often appears focal, with spread from the early site to the remainder of the heart. However, detailed mapping, particularly using a multipolar catheter with small electrodes, will usually reveal more than one site of presystolic activity. It is therefore essential to demonstrate that the presystolic site that is recorded is, in fact, the earliest site. This can be done by demonstrating that sites surrounding the assumed earliest site are activated later than that site, even though they may be presystolic in timing. With careful mapping, particularly in regions from which the

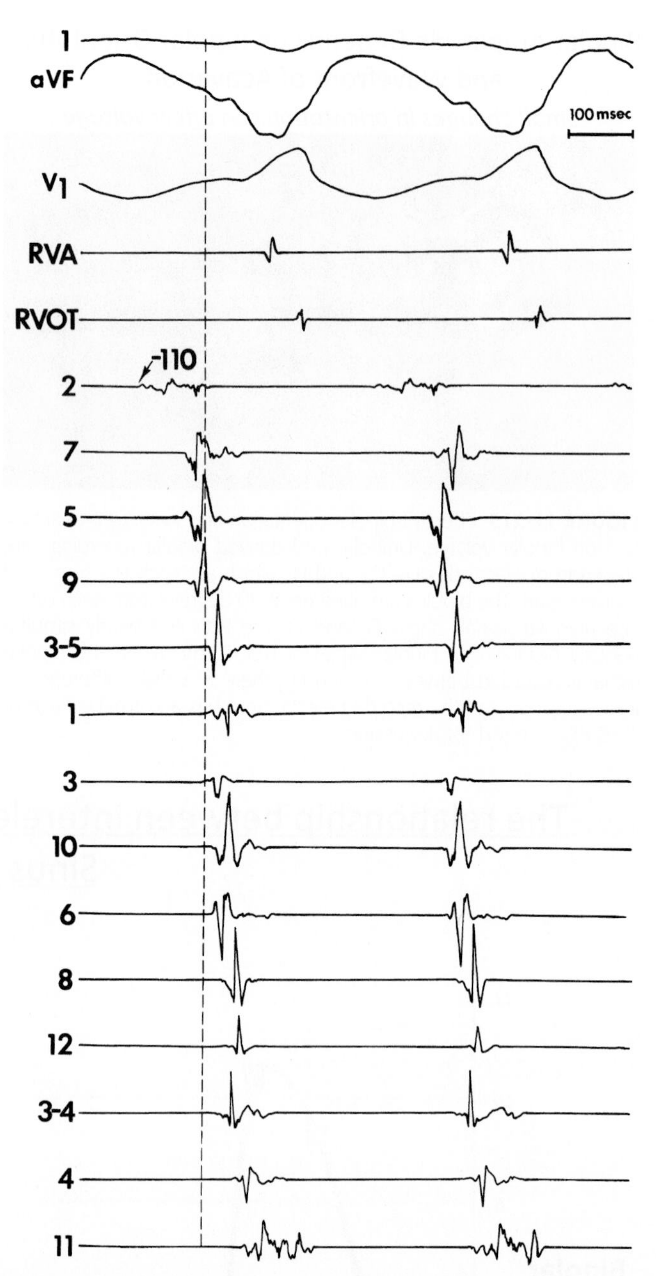


**FIGURE 11-218** Endocardial map during VT with a right bundle branch block pattern. Leads 1, a VF, and $V_1$ are shown with electrograms from the RVA, RVOT, and multiple left ventricular endocardial recording sites. Site 2 is the earliest site. A fragmented electrogram begins at mid-diastole 110 msec before the onset of the QRS and ends prior to the QRS. The mid-diastolic and presystolic activity is focal and spreads through the remainder of the ventricles. Note that sites 5, 7, and 9 also demonstrate presystolic activity but the activation times at these sites are significantly later than site 2. The electrogram at site 2 is markedly abnormal, with multiple components of low amplitude and long duration. See text for discussion.

VT is likely to arise (i.e., based on QRS morphology), electrical activity at or around mid-diastole can be recorded in the majority of patients with VT associated with coronary artery disease. In fact, if the earliest recorded site is not at least 50 to 80 msec presystolic, this suggests either that the map is inadequate or that the tachycardia arises deeper than the subendocardium, in the midmyocardium, or even incorporating the subepicardium. An inadequate map is probably the most common reason for such a finding in VT due to coronary disease, although in the presence of other disease states, VT arising from the midmyocardium or the subepicardium is more likely.

As stated above, in the setting of VT due to prior infarction, unfiltered unipolar recordings have not been useful in helping to demonstrate that a presystolic site is the "earliest" because the major is a far field cavity potential which obscure very small local activation. This is shown in Figure 11-219, in which electrical activity is recorded 90 msec before the onset of the QRS at site inferior-2 in the bipolar recording. The unipolar recording at that site shows a slow-moving negative intrinsicoid deflection, which occurs well after the onset of the bipolar signal. It is extremely difficult to define the most rapid negative deflection in a unipolar recording in which the negative components of the electrogram are slowly inscribed and/or reflect a cavity potential. This is particularly true when the electrical signal is recorded from a large aneurysm using a large tip electrode. Magnification of unipolar signals to look for discrete potentials is difficult due to amplifier saturation, offset problems, and swamping of these tiny signals by irrelevant waveforms. Filtering unipolar signals eliminates far field signals, but the signals are often so small that there is often a problem with signal-to-noise ratio. Activation times are therefore taken using the filtered bipolar electrogram.

In my opinion, the activation time that is most meaningful, reproducible, and interpretable in VT associated with coronary artery disease is taken from the onset of the bipolar electrogram as it leaves the baseline. We use these low-amplitude high-frequency signals because these events appear to represent "local" activity recorded from the bipolar pair.[34,44,50] Use of the peak deflection or the point where the most rapid deflection crosses the baseline is of less value in multicomponent, fractionated electrograms than the onset of the electrogram. Some investigators[397] have called these components local abnormal ventricular activation (LAVA) and have suggested they are meaningful targets for ablation; I totally disagree (see Chapter 13). Since in coronary disease, the vast majority of early sites are abnormal and have multiple components, we use the onset of the electrogram for activation time. Each peak deflection could also be measured because each represents a "local" activation, but for practical purposes, because the bipolar electrogram gives little directional information, the onset is all that is required, particularly in view of the fact that all of the components are generated from the same small area.[44,50] However one must be sure that the earliest signal used to target an ablation is recorded from the distal electrode; hence we prefer to simultaneously record filtered unipolar signals from the distal and proximal poles. For simplicity's sake, all signals whose maximum amplitude is below 50 μV are considered no local activity because this amplitude is typically are lower than ambient noise. It is important to know whether the local activity is recorded by the tip electrode or the second pole, especially if ablation is contemplated. In this situation filtered unipolar recordings

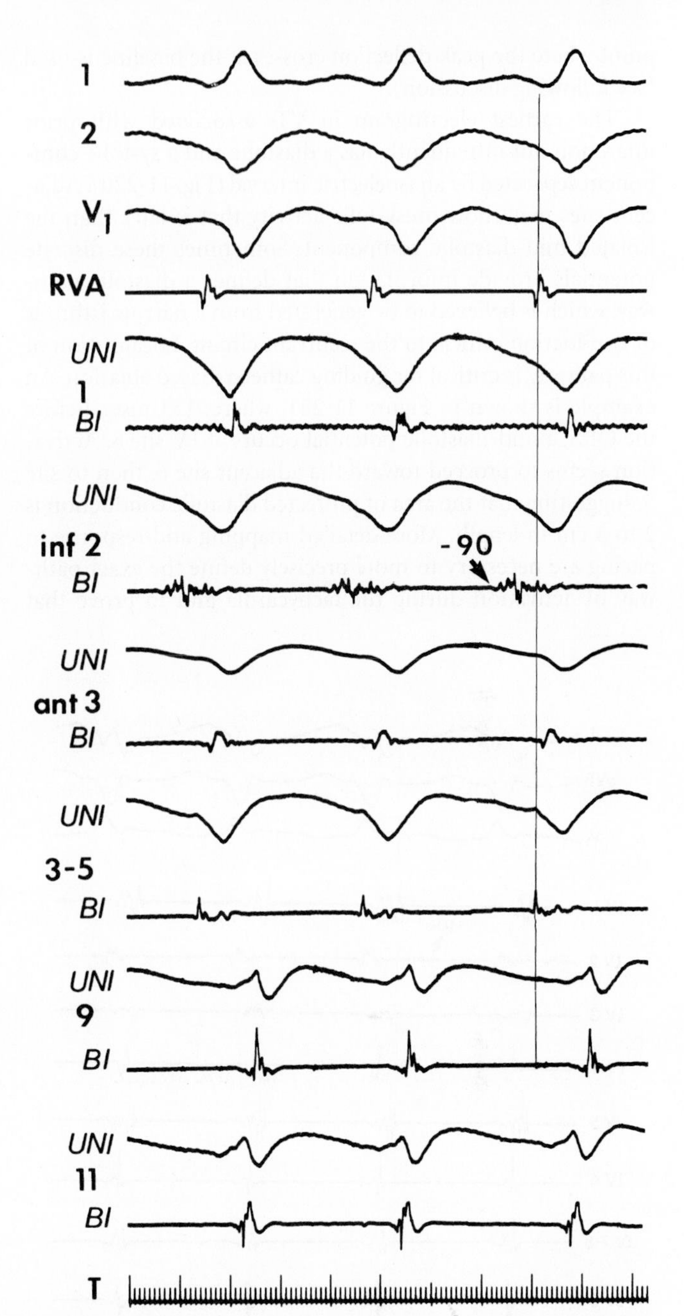


**FIGURE 11-219** Comparison of unipolar and bipolar electrograms during map of left bundle branch block tachycardia. VT with left bundle branch block left axis deviation in a patient with an anteroseptal infarction is shown. Leads 1, 2, and $V_1$ are shown along with a reference electrogram from the RVA. Uni- and bipolar signals are recorded from multiple left ventricular sites. The earliest site is at the interior left ventricular septum at site 2. Electrical activity begins near mid-diastole, 90 msec before the QRS. Note that at this site there is no rapid negative deflection in the unipolar electrogram and all negative dV/dts are seen well after the onset of electrical activity in the bipolar electrogram. Many of the unipolar electrograms exhibit QS complexes with slow, negative deflections. These QS complexes most likely represent cavity potentials. See text for discussion.

can be useful. The electrograms in VTs associated with normal hearts, particularly those due to triggered activity or enhanced automaticity, are usually normal at the earliest site, and there is little difference whether the onset, the peak deflection, or the point where the peak deflection crosses at the baseline is used (see following discussion).

The earliest electrogram in VTs associated with prior infarction not infrequently has a diastolic and a systolic component separated by an isoelectric interval (Fig. 11-220). Adjacent sites may show presystolic activity that is later than the isolated mid-diastolic component. Sometimes these discrete potentials provide information that defines a diastolic pathway, which is believed to be generated from a narrow isthmus of conduction critical to the reentrant circuit. Localization of this pathway is critical for guiding catheter-based ablation. An example is shown in Figure 11-221, where, 153 msec before the QRS, a mid-diastolic potential occurs at LV site 8. Activation seems to proceed toward the adjacent site 6, then to site 5, suggesting that the area of protected diastolic conduction is 2 to 3 cm in length. More detailed mapping and response to pacing are necessary to more precisely define the exact pathway of activation during the tachycardia and to prove that these and/or other diastolic sites are requisite components of a reentrant circuit. Occasionally complete reentrant circuits can be recorded with standard catheters but not with the detail of such recordings acquired with very small electrodes and narrow interelectrode distance (Fig. 11-213). This may appear as a figure-of-eight or single loop reentry (Figs. 11-222 and 11-223). Mid-diastolic sites can be very focal and part of a reentrant pathway (Fig. 11-224) or may be part of a larger area of abnormal, slow conduction unrelated to the VT reentrant circuit (i.e., a dead-end pathway). Unfiltered unipolar electrograms using standard ablation catheters are also inadequate in this situation; the electrical signals in mid-diastole are too small because they are generated by only a few fibers. This results in the absence of deflections on the unfiltered unipolar electrogram at the site of bipolar mid-diastolic potentials, again pointing out how limited the use of unfiltered unipolar recordings is in this particular situation (Fig. 11-224). Filtering the unipolar signal, particularly if the ground electrode is in the inferior vena cava, gives reasonably clean signals that help define the relative components of the distal bipole. The signal, however, is often of very low amplitude. Unipolar signals (filtered or unfiltered) may be recorded using very small electrodes on newer multipolar catheters (Fig. 11-13). As noted earlier, filtered and unfiltered unipolar electrograms are particularly useful in mapping automatic and triggered VTs, particularly in normal hearts (Fig. 11-225). However, the large distal tip electrode (4 mm) records similar complexes over an area of ≈1 $cm^2$. Thus, the advantage of unipolar versus bipolar recordings (2-mm interelectrode distance) is diminished.

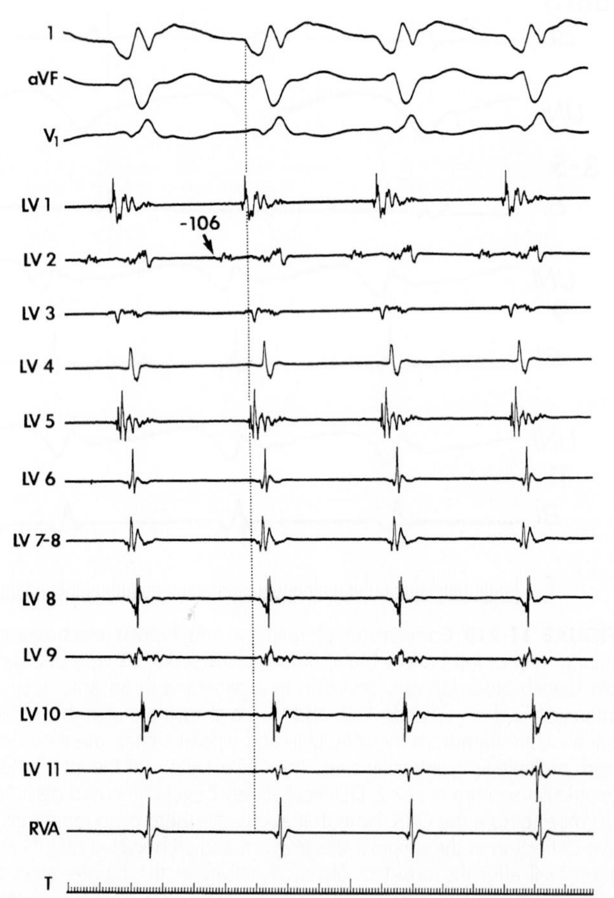


**FIGURE 11-220** Endocardial catheter map of VT demonstrating discrete mid-diastolic and systolic activity at the "site of origin." VT with right bundle branch block right superior axis is shown along with electrograms from multiple left ventricular sites and a reference electrogram from the RVA. The earliest activity is recorded at LV 2, where a discrete mid-diastolic component is observed along with a systolic component. The mid-diastolic component is 106 msec before the onset of the QRS. No presystolic activity is observed.

### *Continuous Activity and Diastolic Bridging*

Continuous diastolic activity can be recorded in 5% to 10% of VTs associated with coronary artery disease with detailed mapping using standard equipment (Fig. 11-226). Even when continuous diastolic activity is recorded on a single electrogram, substantial data exist demonstrating that this electrical pattern is not an artifact but reflects very slow, saltatory conduction through poorly coupled fibers.[43,44,50] One must demonstrate that such electrical activity is required for initiation and maintenance of the VT to suggest that this represents recording from a reentrant circuit.[43,44,197] One must also demonstrate that an electrogram that extends through diastole is not just a broad electrogram whose duration equals the tachycardia cycle length. This can be done by analyzing the local electrogram during pacing at the tachycardia cycle length. If pacing produces a "continuous" diastolic electrogram in the absence of VT, the continuous electrogram has no mechanistic significance. Such activity should also be recorded only from a circumscribed area. This is discussed in more detail earlier (Figs. 11-81 to 11-84). Continuous activity invariably occurs at sites that demonstrate markedly abnormal electrograms during sinus rhythm. If one uses the first and third and second and fourth electrodes as two bipolar pairs to record overlapping areas, in many instances both show continuous activity, but accentuation of different components will be

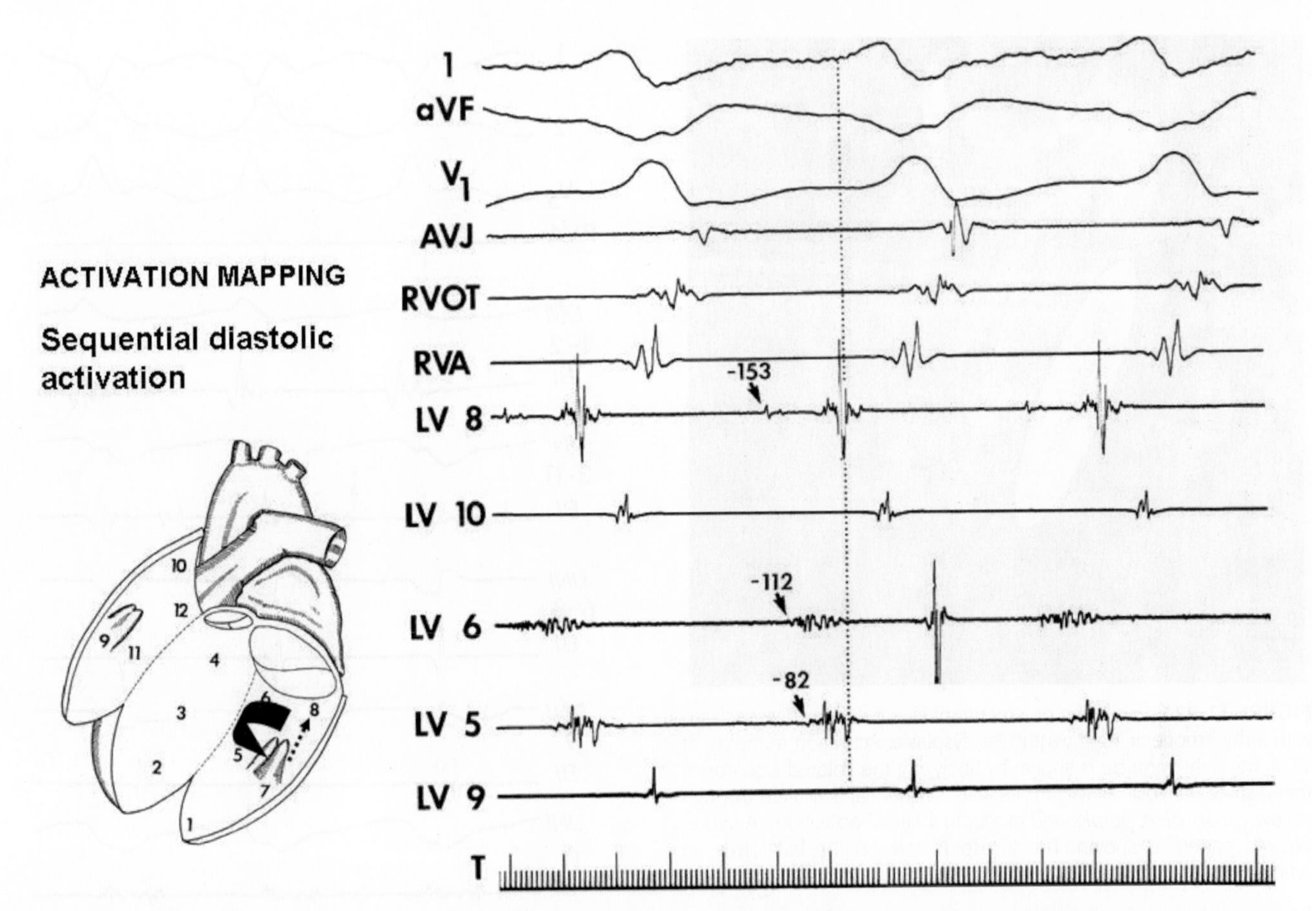


**FIGURE 11-221** Endocardial catheter map with multiple sites of marked presystolic activity suggestive of recording a diastolic pathway in the reentrant circuit. Leads 1, aVF, and $V_1$ are shown with electrograms from the AVJ, RVOT, RVA, and several left ventricular sites. The earliest site of activation is at LV 8, where a discrete mid-diastolic potential is seen 153 msec before the QRS. Presystolic activity is also observed at adjacent sites LV 6 and LV 5, suggesting activation of a diastolic pathway from LV 8 to LV 6 and LV 5. See text for discussion.

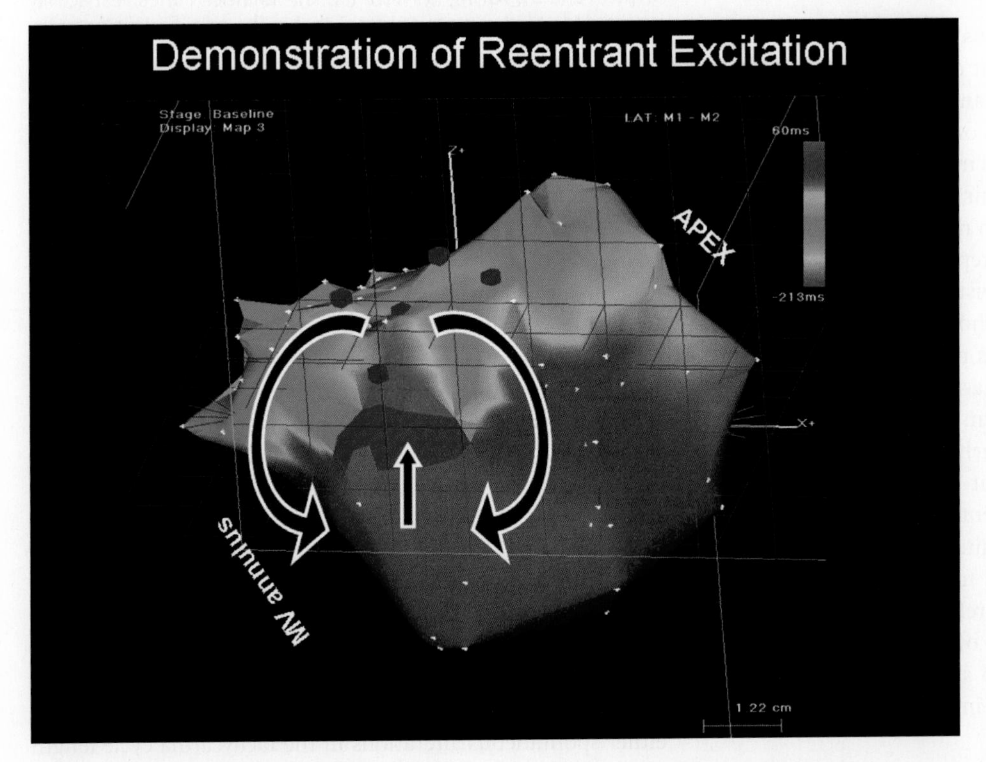


**FIGURE 11-222** Recording of a reentrant circuit during VT associated with coronary artery disease. Activation map of VT using the Carto system in a patient with an inferoposterior infarction. VT arose from the basal septum. The activation map is displayed in the posterolateral view. The VT circuit is demonstrated by analyzing the colored isochrones that display "earliest" activity in *red,* with sequential activation through *yellow, green, blue, purple,* and *magenta* ("latest" activation). Color scale is shown on the right. The magenta zone is the region at "earliest" and "latest" activation abut. *Arrows* depict the figure-of-eight circuit.

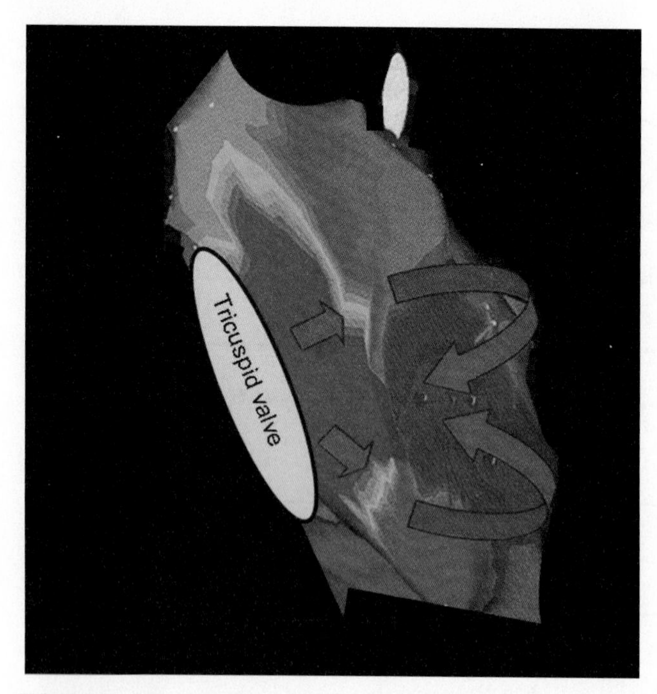


**FIGURE 11-223** Recording of a reentrant circuit during VT associated with arrhythmogenic right ventricular dysplasia. Activation mapping of VT in the right ventricle is shown by analyzing the colored isochrones that display "earliest" activity in *red,* with sequential activation through *yellow, green, blue, purple,* and *magenta* ("latest" activation). A figure-of-eight pattern is shown. The tricuspid valve on the left forms an anatomic barrier for the circuit.

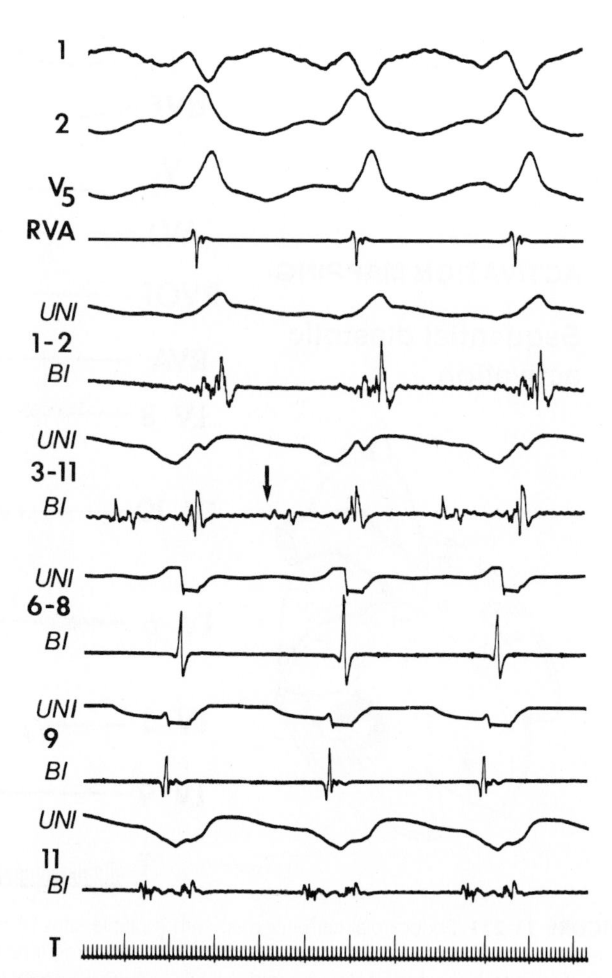


**FIGURE 11-224** Failure of unipolar electrograms to record mid-diastolic potentials. VT with a right bundle branch block inferior axis is seen. A reference electrogram from the RVA is shown with multiple unipolar and bipolar signals from the left ventricle. The earliest activity is recorded at left ventricular sites 3 to 11. The mid-diastolic potential clearly observed in the bipolar electrogram (*arrow*) has no counterpart in the unipolar recording. In fact, no discrete diastolic intrinsicoid deflection can be observed in the unipolar recordings.

observed in the two recordings (Fig. 11-227). As stated earlier in the chapter, if continuous activity is meaningful, termination of continuous activity must result in termination of the tachycardia.

The ability to record continuous activity depends on the spatial and geometric arrangement of the involved tissue as well as the position of the catheter and the interelectrode distance. Thus, continuous activity is only likely to be recorded if the bipolar pair records a small circuit. If the circuit is too large to record from the bipolar pair, nonholodiastolic activity will be recorded. In VT in which nonholodiastolic activity is recorded at a "site of origin," repositioning of the catheter to adjacent sites may allow visualization of "bridging" of diastole. An example of this is shown in Figure 11-228, in which a catheter at site 11 records near holodiastolic activity that is most apparent as mid-diastolic activity continuing into systole. At a site less than 1 cm away, electrical activity is more clearly observed in the early half of diastole. Thus, electrical activity in these adjacent sites spans diastole. We believe that such activity represents a recording within a critical area of a reentrant circuit. All areas from which diastolic activity are recorded are not necessarily part of a reentrant circuit. Such sites may reflect late activation and may not be related to the VT site of origin. Analysis of the response of these electrograms to spontaneous or induced changes in cycle length are critical in deciding their relationship to the VT mechanism.

### *Role of Programmed Stimulation in Identifying the Critical Sites in a Reentrant Circuit*

As noted previously, presystolic activity may represent late activity or activity unrelated to a reentrant circuit or tachycardia mechanism. The ideal map therefore would require the demonstration that such electrograms are critically related to the reentrant circuit. Some investigators suggest that the appearance of such presystolic electrograms at the initiation of a tachycardia suggests their relevance to the tachycardia mechanism.[379] I disagree; this finding may be necessary but not sufficient to assume significance. Regardless of where in diastole the electrogram occurs—early, mid, or late—its position on initiation does not confirm its importance for the tachycardia mechanism. As stated in the discussion of continuous activity,[43,44,197] one must also show that the electrogram is required to maintain the tachycardia. Thus, during either spontaneous alterations in the tachycardia cycle length

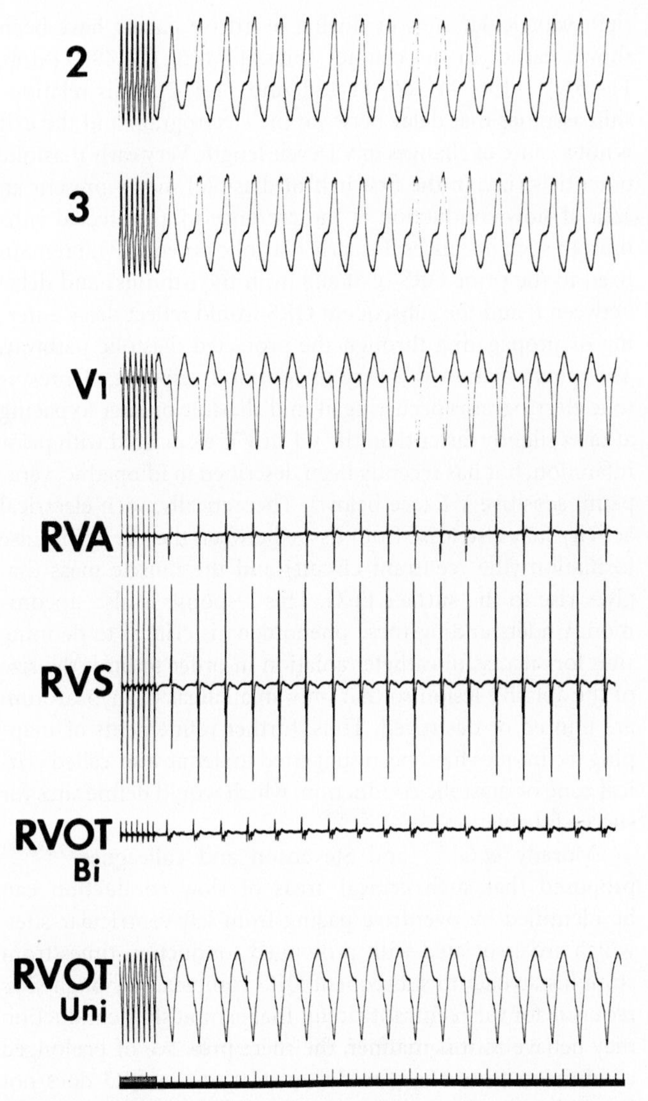


**FIGURE 11-225** Value of unfiltered unipolar recordings for mapping VT in a patient with a normal ventricle. Leads 2, 3, and $V_1$ are shown with bipolar recordings from the RVA, RV septum (RVS), and RVOT. A unipolar recording from the earliest bipolar site in the RVOT ($RVOT_{uni}$) shows a QS morphology. Ablation at this site was successful.

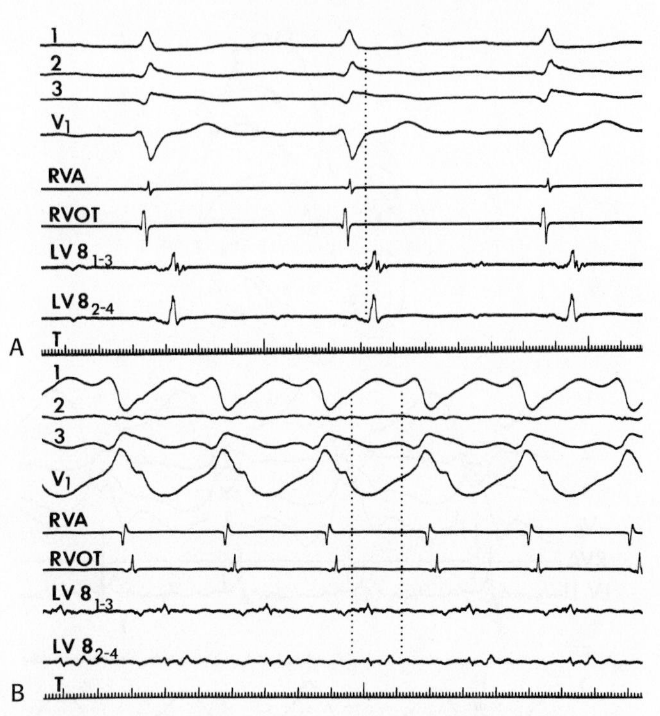


**FIGURE 11-227** Ability to record late potentials and continuous electrical activity with overlapping bipolar electrodes. **A** and **B:** Leads 1, 2, 3, and $V_1$ are shown with electrograms from the RVA and RVOT and recordings from LV site 8 from electrodes 1 to 3 and 2 to 4. **A.** During sinus rhythm, a late potential is observed. Note the similar timing of both bipolar recordings. **B:** During VT, continuous electrical activity is observed in both electrode pairs. However, different components are exaggerated in the two bipolar pairs.

or those produced by extrastimuli or pacing, the electrogram (regardless of its position in diastole) should show a fixed relationship to the subsequent QRS.[315–319,398] An example of spontaneous oscillations during which the early presystolic electrogram remains fixed in timing to the subsequent QRS is shown in Figure 11-229. Resetting of VT with persistent relationship of multiple presystolic electrograms to the subsequent QRS is shown in Figure 11-230. The mechanism by which overdrive

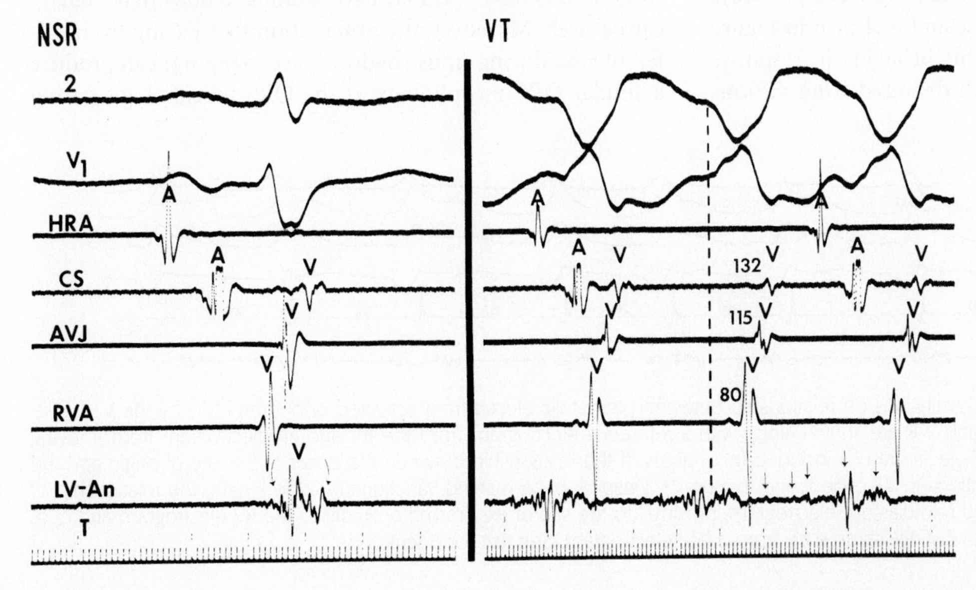


**FIGURE 11-226** Electrogram during NSR and VT. An electrogram just inside the LV-An demonstrates continuous electrical activity during sustained VT (**right**). Small inverted *arrows* mark low repetitive electrical activations during the tachycardia During NSR (**left**), this electrogram is markedly abnormal. It is 500 mV in amplitude, 100 msec in duration, and extends beyond the end of the surface ECG.

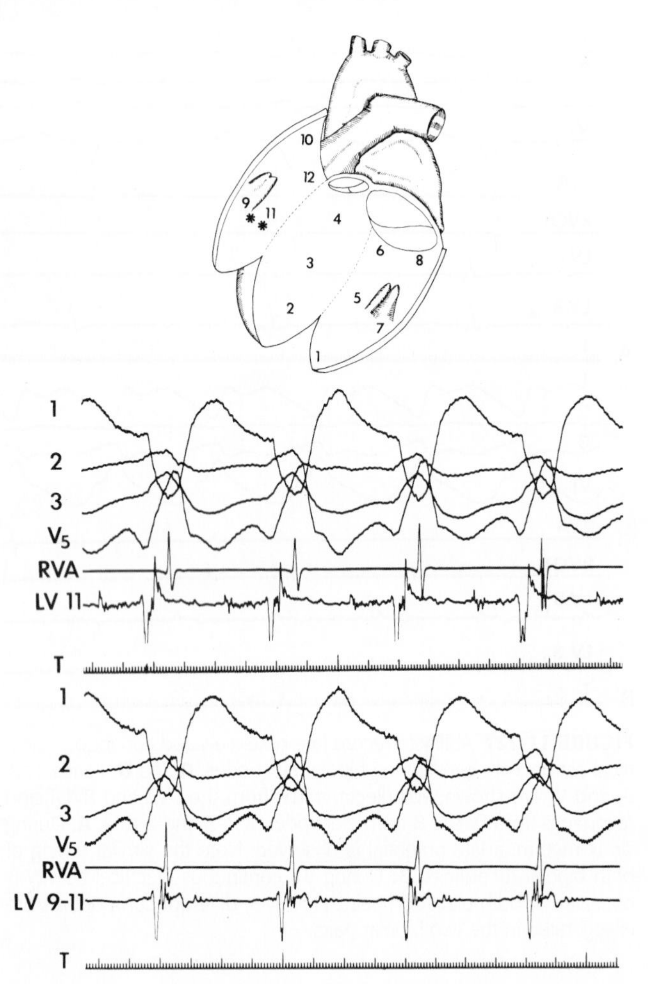


**FIGURE 11-228** Endocardial map during VT demonstrating bridging of diastole at adjacent left ventricular sites. A schema of the LV is shown along with recordings from LV site 11 and adjacent sites 9 to 11, which is <1 cm away. At site LV 11, electrical activity is almost holodiastolic but is most obvious in the second half of diastole. At the adjacent site, LV 9 to 11, early diastolic activity is recorded. Bridging of diastole between adjacent sites suggests recording of a solely conducting impulse of a reentrant circuit. See text for discussion.

pacing can distinguish early sites from late dead-end pathways depends on this physiologic response and is shown in Figure 11-231. Many other examples of this behavior in response to single and/or double extrastimuli delivered from various right ventricular sites or during overdrive pacing have been shown earlier in the chapter (Figs. 11-146, 11-148, 11-150, 11-151, 11-156, 11-168, 11-172, and 11-177). This relationship assumes that delay between the electrogram and the exit is not a cause of changes in VT cycle length. Very early diastolic potentials (i.e., in the first half of diastole) may represent an area of slow conduction at the entrance to a protected isthmus. In such instances the early diastolic potential will remain fixed to the prior QRS (exit site from the isthmus) and delay between it and the subsequent QRS would reflect delay entering or propagating through the protected diastolic pathway. This phenomenon is a very uncommon response of presystolic electrograms occurring at mid-diastole or later to pacing at rates slightly faster than the VT in VTs associated with prior infarction, but has recently been described in idiopathic, verapamil sensitive VT (see below). Theoretically, such electrical activity may also arise from tissue between the site of impulse formation (the reentrant circuit) and the muscle mass that gives rise to the surface ECG. This response is also uncommon. Understanding these phenomena is critical to defining sites for successful catheter ablation in order to limit the size of the ablative lesion so that only small areas of myocardium are injured or destroyed. Thus, further refinements of mapping techniques have been suggested to define a so-called critical zone of diastolic conduction, which would define sites for successful ablation.[148,375–381,398]

Morady et al.[378] and Stevenson and colleagues[377,380,381] proposed that such critical areas of slow conduction can be identified by overdrive pacing from left ventricular sites, which are associated with prolonged conduction times from stimulus artifact to subsequent QRS complex. Although sites requisite for the reentrant circuit that exhibit slow conduction may behave in this manner, the mere presence of prolonged conduction from the stimulus artifact to the QRS does not prove that the slow conduction was part of a reentrant pathway. Multiple areas within myocardial infarction can exhibit fractionated or abnormal electrograms[31–33] and reduced excitability,[106] which are associated with prolongation of stimulus-to-QRS intervals[390] yet may have nothing to do with the tachycardia itself. Moreover, the observation that pacing from different sites during sinus rhythm (pace mapping) can produce a similar QRS morphology as the QRS morphology during

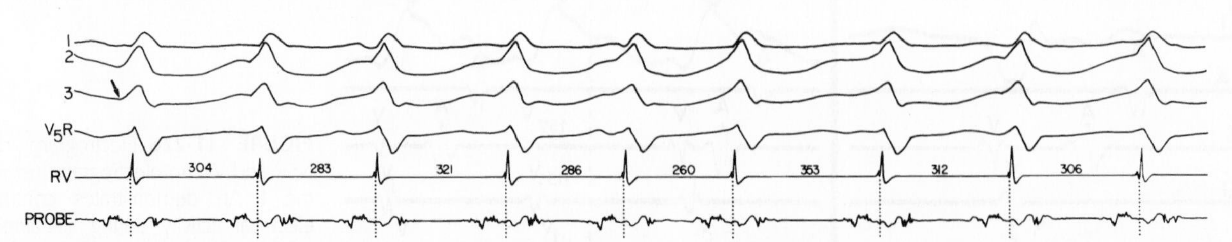


**FIGURE 11-229** Effect of spontaneous oscillations on relationship between presystolic electrogram activated orthodromically by the VT wavefront and onset of QRS. Leads 1, 2, 3, and $V_5R$ are shown along with a reference electrogram from the RV and an electrogram from a roving probe. A vertical *dotted line* from the RV electrogram is included for analysis of the relationship between the onset of the site of origin and the RV electrogram. Note the marked oscillations in VT cycle length during VT. Despite these marked variations in cycle length, the relationship of the onset of the orthodromically activated mid-diastolic electrogram, proximal to the site of exit from the circuit, to the RV electrogram and QRS remains fixed. This is one of the criteria to distinguish an early from a late electrogram. See text for discussion.

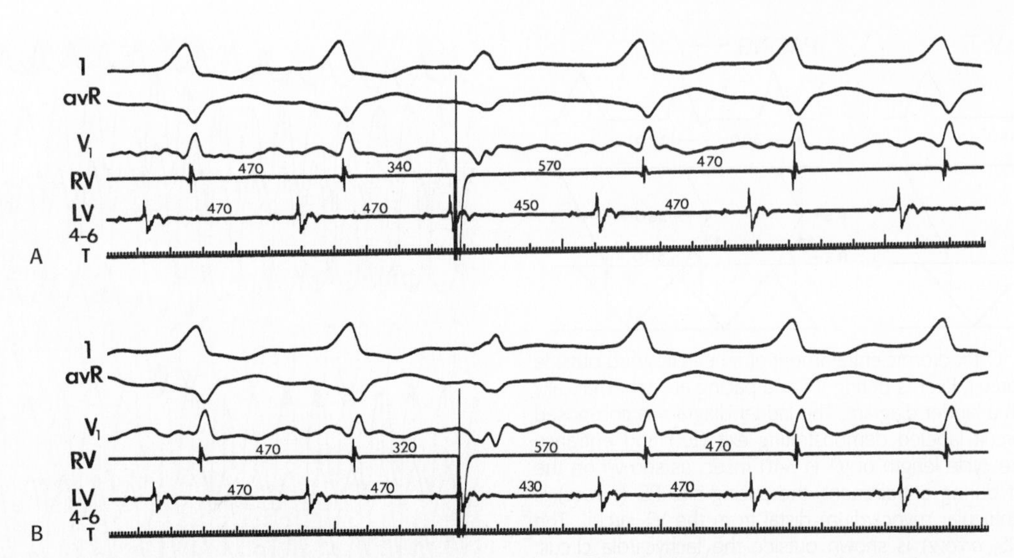


**FIGURE 11-230** Use of programmed stimulation to demonstrate that a presystolic electrogram is early. Surface leads 1, avR, and $V_1$ are shown during VT with a reference electrogram from the RV and an electrogram from the site of origin of LV sites 4 to 6. VT has a CL of 470 msec. At LV 4 to 6, two presystolic signals are recorded. A smaller mid-diastolic potential is observed 156 msec before the onset of the QRS, and a larger signal is recorded 92 msec before the onset of the QRS. During VT, right ventricular stimuli are delivered at coupling intervals of **(A)** 340 and **(B)** 320 msec. Both result in resetting of the tachycardia. The return cycle following each extrastimulus demonstrates a consistent relationship of both presystolic components of LV 4 to 6 to the onset of the ORS. This confirms that it is an early site, not a dead-end late pathway. See text for discussion.

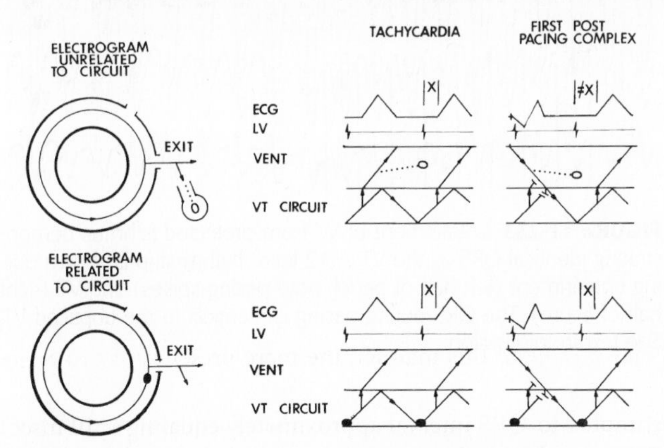


**FIGURE 11-231** Distinguishing a late electrogram unrelated to the tachycardia circuit from a presystolic electrogram that is a component of the reentrant circuit. A late unrelated electrogram (**top**) and a presystolic electrogram related to the circuit (**bottom**) are shown schematically on the left. On the right are an ECG and a presystolic electrogram as well as ladder diagrams demonstrating the position of the electrogram during the tachycardia and following pacing, which is associated with resetting. In each of the panels, there is a region of the intervening ventricular myocardium and a VT circuit. Exit from the ventricular myocardium is shown by upward *arrows,* and an entrance into the circuit from the pacing site is shown by diagonal inferiorly directed *arrow.* During the tachycardia, an unrelated electrogram or an electrogram within the circuit can have the same relationship (X) to the onset of the VT QRS complex. Following pacing, however, the unrelated dead-end pathway is associated with the pacing stimulus and on cessation of pacing will have a different relationship to the onset of the return cycle QRS (i.e., the interval between the electrogram at the unrelated site to the QRS will not be equal to X). On the other hand, if the tachycardia is related to the circuit, pacing will produce orthodromic activation of that site, and following cessation of pacing, the orthodromically activated electrogram will have a fixed relationship to the onset of the QRS equal to X. See text for discussion. (From Almendral JM, Gottlieb CD, Rosenthal ME, et al. Entrainment of ventricular tachycardia: explanation for surface electrocardiographic phenomena by analysis of electrograms recorded within the tachycardia circuit. *Circulation* 1986;77:569.)

VT is not surprising, because many sites in the region of the tachycardia origin or exit , but not related to the tachycardia, may give rise to similar QRS morphologies.[392] The role and limitations of pace mapping in localizing the origin of reentrant and nonreentrant VTs are discussed later in this chapter.

Others have used a prolonged stimulus-to-local electrogram time during continuous resetting (i.e., entrainment) to identify pathways containing slow conduction.[319,342,343] This again does not prove that the electrogram at the recording site has anything to do with the tachycardia, because the slow conduction involved in the orthodromic capture of this electrogram may occur in or outside of the circuit. In fact, whenever ECG fusion occurs, some electrograms outside the circuit (i.e., those activated after leaving the "exit" that are part of the "VT" wavefront) will be orthodromically activated and will **fulfill the requirements for entrainment. This is schematically shown in** Figure 11-232. For the same reason, termination with block before this orthodromically entrained electrogram does not mean it was a critical component of the reentrant circuit, as suggested by Waldo and his colleagues.[326,342,343]

How can one then recognize when a diastolic electrogram is part of a reentrant pathway? In the absence of recording the entire diastolic reentrant pathway, I believe that stimulation at the presumed "sites of origin" during the tachycardia is extremely useful. The sites at which stimulation should be performed are those that demonstrate a diastolic electrogram that can be orthodromically entrained (from the RV) at one or more cycle lengths (regardless of whether it is antidromically captured at a shorter coupling interval or drive cycle length). Stimulation from that site can provide evidence of its relationship to the reentrant circuit. If that electrogram was a requisite

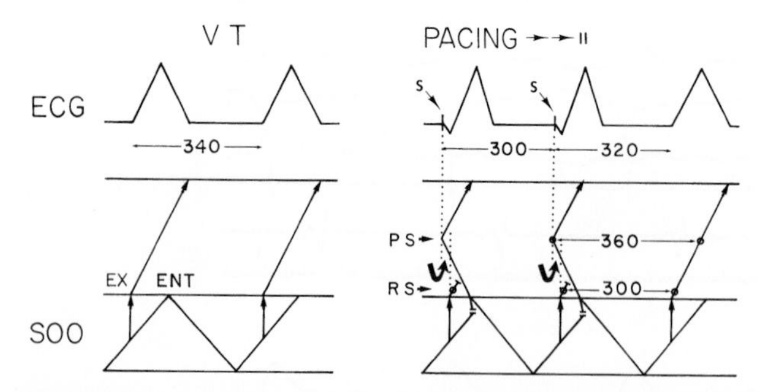


**FIGURE 11-232** Orthodromic entrainment of an electrogram outside the tachycardia circuit. Events during VT and pacing are schematically shown along with a ladder diagram. The ladder diagram is composed of tachycardia circuit labeled demonstrating exit (EX) and entrance (ENT) region. The cycle length of VT is 340 msec, as shown on the left. On the right during entrainment, the pacing site PS (*arrow*) is shown in the ventricular myocardium distal from the VT circuit. The recording site (RS, *arrow*) is shown outside the tachycardia circuit. During pacing, a stimulated impulse enters the circuit at the same time that the prior stimulated impulse exits the circuit to depolarize the RS. This produces fusion of the QRS. The RS is orthodromically captured following each stimulated impulse, thus when pacing is discontinued, the electrogram will return at the paced cycle length. On the other hand, the return cycle as measured from the PS far exceeds the paced cycle length. Thus, sites outside of the reentrant circuit may exhibit return cycles equal to or different from the paced cycle length. See text for discussion.

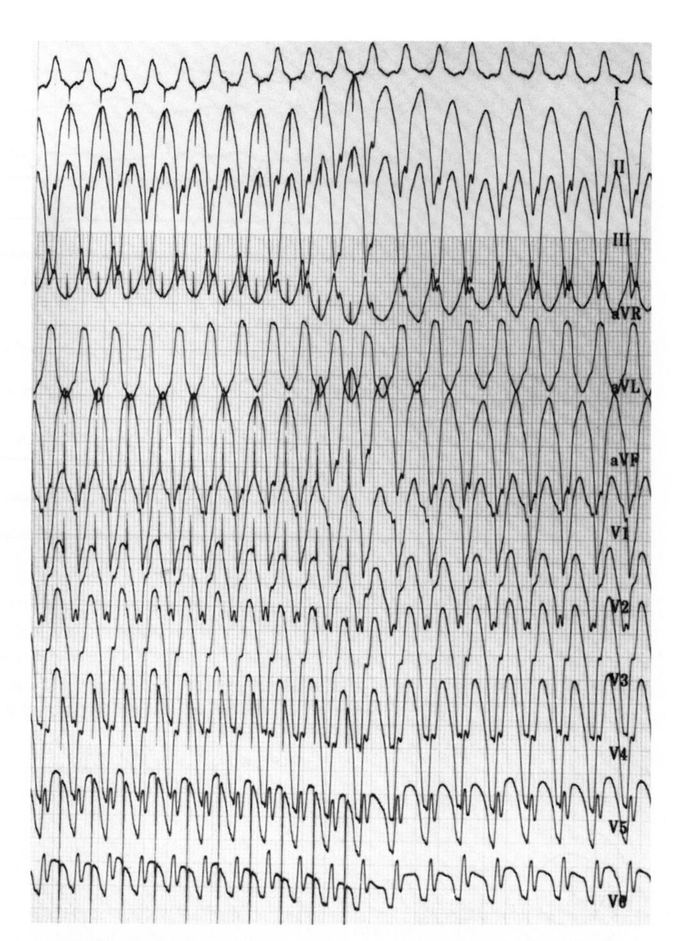


**FIGURE 11-233** Entrainment of VT from protected isthmus demonstrating identical QRS as the VT. A 12-lead rhythm strip is shown during entrainment (left half of panel, note pacing spikes) and VT (right half of figure). The QRS during pacing is identical to the unpaced VT. See text for discussion.

component of the reentrant circuit, stimulation from that site during the tachycardia should produce a return cycle that is equal to the VT cycle length (as long as no slowing of conduction is produced by the stimulation). If the orthodromically entrained electrogram is outside the circuit, then following cessation pacing at that site, the return cycle should exceed the tachycardia cycle length. These studies can only be done if one records and stimulates from the same area. If one could record and stimulate from the same pole (tip and 2), it would be ideal, but standard systems are not able to do this. If catheters with a tip-2-5-2 configuration are used, recording from the second and fourth pole of a catheter and stimulation from the first and third pole of the same catheter ensure that the site of stimulation is as close as possible to the site of recording. If all electrodes are 2 mm apart, stimulation from the tip and pole 2 and recording from poles 3 and 4 are reasonable. If the electrogram were in the reentrant circuit, the stimulus-to-QRS interval should approximate the interval of the recorded electrogram to the QRS. Finally, since we are trying to define a site that can be targeted to successfully ablate VT, it should be within a protected isthmus. Pacing from such a site at a cycle length 10 to 20 msec shorter than the VT cycle length should produce an identical QRS to that of the VT. Thus, we suggest a form of entrainment mapping be used to confirm the relationship of an electrogram to a reentrant circuit.

Thus, once a potential electrogram has been identified as possibly in the isthmus, entrainment or resetting from this site is performed and responses noted. The criteria that identify a site as being in a protected isthmus critical to the reentrant circuit include (a) an identical QRS to the VT QRS, (b) pacing from close to the recording site should produce a stimulus-to-QRS interval approximately equaling (±10 msec) the interval from the onset of the recorded electrogram to the onset of the QRS, and (c) pacing at that site should produce a return cycle measured in the LV recording approximating the VT cycle length (±10 msec). In our laboratory, only if all these three criteria are met is concealed entrainment said to be present. An entrained QRS that is identical to the VT QRS (Fig. 11-233) suggests that the site is in, attached to, or at the entrance to a protected isthmus that forms the diastolic pathway of the reentrant circuit. A stimulus to QRS that equals the electrogram to QRS suggests the site is not a dead-end pathway attached to the circuit (i.e., innocent bystander). A return cycle equal to the VT cycle length suggests that the site is part of the reentrant circuit. Examples of these latter two criteria are shown in Figures 11-234 and 11-235. A site demonstrating all these criteria is shown in Figure 11-236. Stimulation from an innocent bystander attached to the isthmus will give rise to an identical QRS as the VT, but the stimulus to QRS will exceed the electrogram to QRS interval and the return cycle will exceed the VT cycle length (Fig. 11-237).

There are limitations to this technique that include (a) differences (albeit slight) of the area from which the second

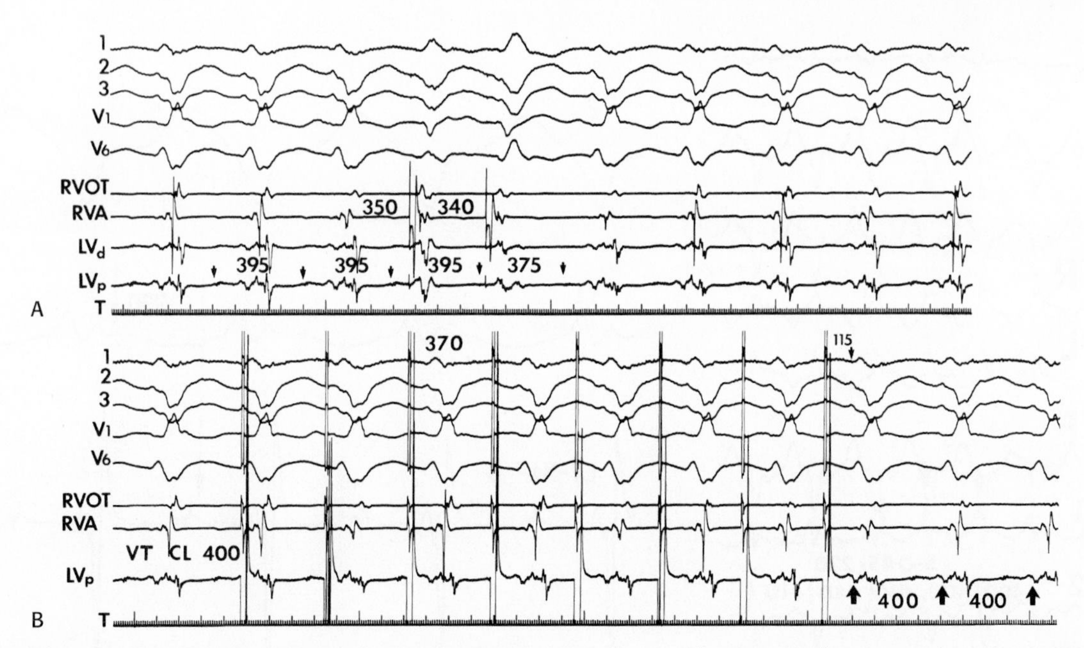


**FIGURE 11-234** Entrainment mapping of VT. Leads 1, 2, 3, $V_1$, and $V_6$ are shown with reference electrograms from the RVOT and RVA and electrograms from the distal LV ($LV_d$) and proximal LV ($LV_p$) in the protected isthmus of the reentrant circuit responsible for VT. The earliest electrical activity during VT is shown by the *inverted arrow* at the low-amplitude signal in mid-diastole. VT is present at a cycle length of 395 msec. **A:** Double extrastimuli are delivered from the RVA, the second of which resets the tachycardia with the mid-diastolic electrogram maintaining a fixed relationship to the subsequent QRS. Thus, the electrogram at the LV is orthodromically captured. **B:** Pacing from the $LV_d$ at a cycle length of 370 msec produces capture of the $LV_p$ at a QRS interval of 115 msec, which is virtually identical to the interval from the mid-diastolic electrogram to the onset of the QRS during tachycardia. Moreover, the return cycle following cessation of pacing equals the VT cycle length. See text for discussion.

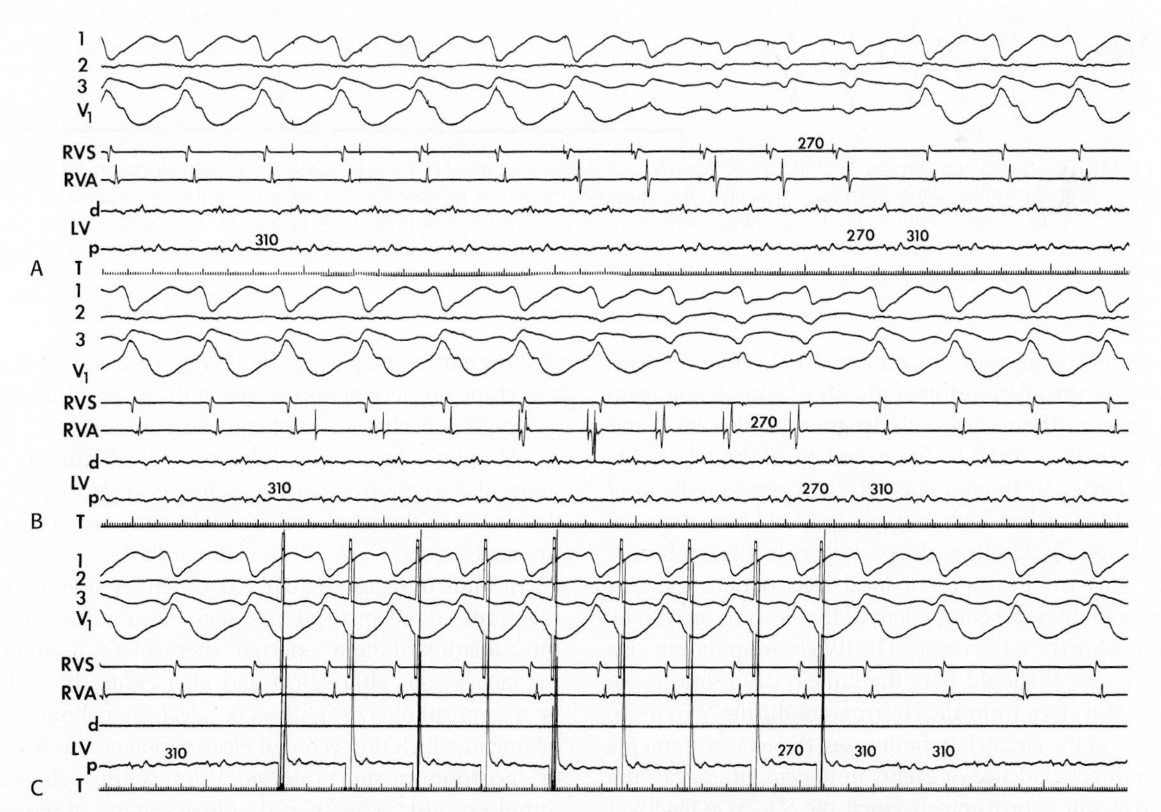


**FIGURE 11-235** Entrainment mapping of VT. **A–C**. All panels are arranged similarly to Figure 11-234. **A:** Entrainment from the right ventricular septum (RVS) is shown at a PCL of 270 msec. The $LV_d$ and $LV_p$ electrograms are orthodromically entrained. **B:** Orthodromic entrainment of the LV electrograms is produced by pacing the RVA. **C**. Stimulation from the $LV_d$ at 270 msec captures the ventricle with a long stimulus-to-QRS interval. When pacing is discontinued, the return cycle equals the tachycardia cycle as measured from a comparable component of the LV electrogram or from the RV electrogram, which is captured in a manner during pacing identical to that during the tachycardia. The return cycle, which is equal to the tachycardia cycle length, confirms that the recorded electrogram is within the reentrant circuit. See text for discussion.

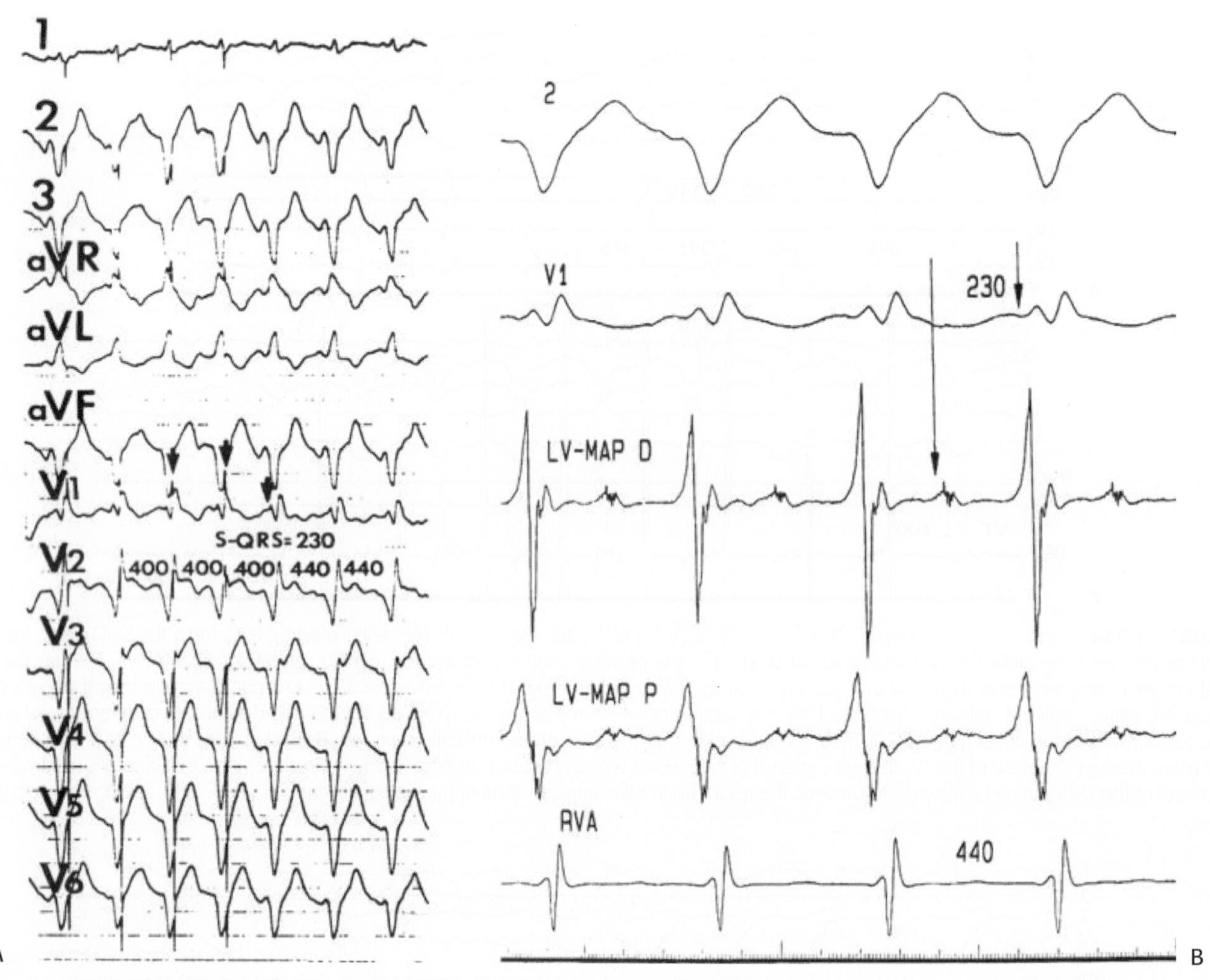


**FIGURE 11-236** Concealed entrainment of VT. **A:** Leads 2 and $V_1$ are shown with distal (D) and proximal (P) bipolar electrograms recorded from a presumed protected isthmus of the VT circuit. An isolated mid-diastolic potential is recorded 230 msec prior to the QRS during VT with a cycle length of 440 msec. **B:** 12-lead rhythm strip during entrainment from the LV-MAPD. During pacing the 12-lead ECG is identical to the unpaced VT and the stimulus to QRS is 230 msec. The return cycle is identical to the VT cycle length. All three criteria are met, therefore concealed entrainment is present. See text for discussion.

and fourth electrodes record as compared to the first and third electrodes; (b) the relationship of the site of stimulation from poles 1 and 3 to the recorded electrogram from poles 2 and 4 (i.e., proximal or distal to the recording site); and (c) the total area affected by the stimulus, which may exceed the local area, particularly when high currents (>10 mA) are required for stimulation. In addition, the pacing artifact may obscure the early part of the captured local electrogram. In such instances, a comparable component of the electrogram can be used to measure the return cycle. The RV electrogram can also be used because it should have the same relationship to the paced site as it does from the electrogram during VT (if the paced site is in the circuit). In both cases, these measurements provide indirect evidence of events in the circuit, that is, the return cycle will approximately equal the VT cycle length if the stimulation site is in the reentrant circuit. In cases where it is still not clear Soejima et al.[399] proposed a method using the last stimulus to a measurable point in the return QRS; apply that interval to the next (N + 1) complex to identify what the electrogram at the pacing site is (Fig. 11-238). Unfortunately sometime no electrogram is seen at the St-N + 1 interval, suggesting that pacing was capturing far field tissue.

Although the proposed methods of identifying components of a reentrant circuit is useful, focal ablation of all sites defined as in the reentrant circuit may not result in a cure of the tachycardia. Cure of the tachycardia requires ablation of an isthmus bordered by barriers on either side. Because the reentrant circuit incorporates sites outside this critical isthmus, ablation of these "external" sites will not result in cure of the tachycardia, although it may alter either the cycle length or the morphology slightly. The ideal map should therefore be one in which the recorded electrogram comes from within or incorporates the protected isthmus through which the impulses must circulate. If the three criteria proposed above are met, the electrogram most likely is recorded from this zone. We have shown that use of these criteria identifies successful and unsuccessful ablation sites with high predictive accuracy.[148] Although Wit and his colleagues[44,51,308] suggest

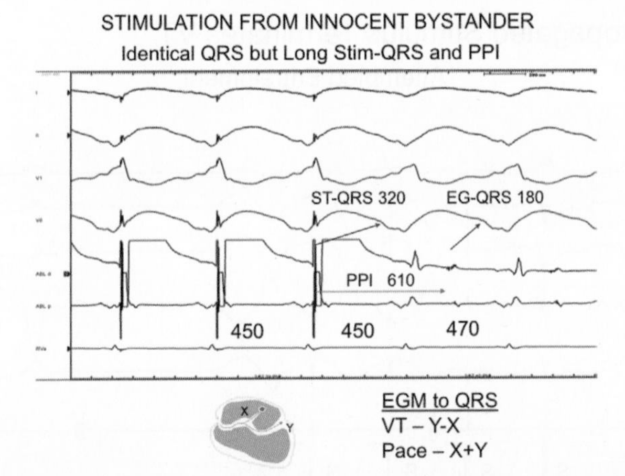


**FIGURE 11-237** Stimulation from an innocent bystander attached to the isthmus. Leads 1, II, $V_1$, and $V_6$ are shown with bipolar signals from the distal and proximal electrode pairs on the ablation catheter ($Abl_d$ and $Abl_p$) and a catheter in the RV apex (RVA). Pacing during VT demonstrates an identical QRS, but longer postpacing interval (PPI) and longer stimulus to QRS (ST-QRS) than the electrogram to QRS (EG-QRS) during the VT. This is diagnostic of recording from an innocent bystander. An explanation for the findings is shown in the schema below. See text for discussion.

that fractionated electrograms represent slow propagation around and/or through areas of "pseudo"-block, which may define components of the barriers of the isthmus,[51,308] this does not mean that all presystolic fragmented activity involves these barriers. Proof of localization within this isthmus would require alteration of the tachycardia cycle length and termination by a perturbation at that site. If this could be done by the delivery of subthreshold stimuli, as suggested by Shenasa et al.,[354] the ideal site map would have been identified. Termination of VT by a nonpropagated stimulus identifies the isthmus by defining an area that produce block without exiting the isthmus event though the stimulus is supra threshold (Fig. 11-239). See Chapter 13 for further discussion. Similarly, termination by transient application of cryothermia would suggest an isthmus location. There are many limitations to accomplishing all of these components of mapping, not the least of which is patient tolerance. Nevertheless, if one could fulfill all these mapping criteria, one should identify the critical zone of the reentrant pathway, which, if ablated, should cure the arrhythmia. Limitations of catheter position and recording electrodes as well as the inability to predict the amount of current delivered to the reentrant pathway may obviously result in responses that would not meet all the requirements of the ideal ablation site.

## Relationship of Mapping Data to Heart Disease

Although the vast majority of VTs are associated with coronary artery disease, VT can occur in cardiomyopathies (either dilated, infiltrative, or hypertrophic), right ventricular dysplasia, or even normal hearts. The principles of catheter mapping also apply to these patients. As noted earlier in this chapter, patients with either dilated or hypertrophic cardiomyopathy demonstrate reasonably normal endocardial electrograms and activation patterns (Figs. 11-26 and 11-29).[32,73] Even in those patients with sustained uniform VT, the incidence of abnormal endocardial electrograms is lower, and the electrograms are less abnormal, than those in patients with VT and myocardial infarction.[32,73] Some investigators use unipolar recordings to suggest an intramural or subepicardial substrate, although it is unclear what decreased unipolar voltage actually means (see earlier discussion on Substrate).[77] In an analogous fashion, the endocardial electrograms are also often normal during VT including the earliest site and presumed "site of origin." This is in contrast to that observed at the so-called "site of origin" of a postinfarction VT. The vast majority of tachycardias associated with coronary artery disease and prior infarction arise from the left ventricular endocardial or subendocardial areas. Occasionally VTs associated with blotchy infarcts (particularly, inferior infarcts) can have an intramural or subepicardial critical component of their VT circuit and can be ablated from the epicardium (Fig. 11-240) (see Chapter 13).

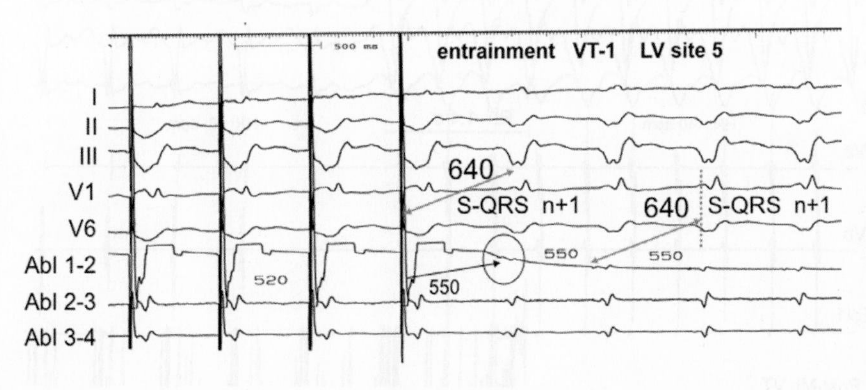


**FIGURE 11-238** Use of N + 1 to assess electrogram from which entrainment is attempted. Five ECG leads and three bipolar pair of electrograms from a quadripolar ablation catheter are shown. If on measure the stimulus to a fixed point in the first unpaced beat during entrainment, measuring back from the same portion the subsequent QRS will identify what signal is recorded at the site of stimulation. See text for discussion. (Modified from Soejima K, Stevenson WG, Maisel WH, et al. The N + 1 difference: a new measure for entrainment mapping. *J Am Coll Cardiol* 2001;37:1386–1394.)

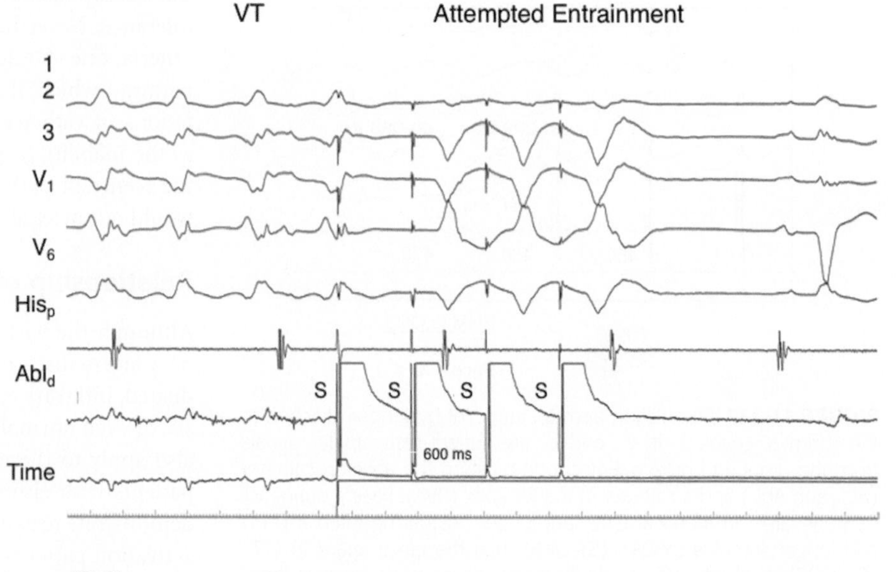


**FIGURE 11-239** Termination by a nonpropagated stimulus during attempted entrainment at a site with a mid-diastolic potential. Five ECG leads a proximal His electrogram ($His_p$) and distal pair of electrodes on the ablation catheter ($Abl_d$) are shown. A mid-diastolic potential is seen in the ablation catheter. Ventricular pacing is initiated. The first spike terminates the VT without a propagated response and is followed by a completely paced QRS. See text for discussion.

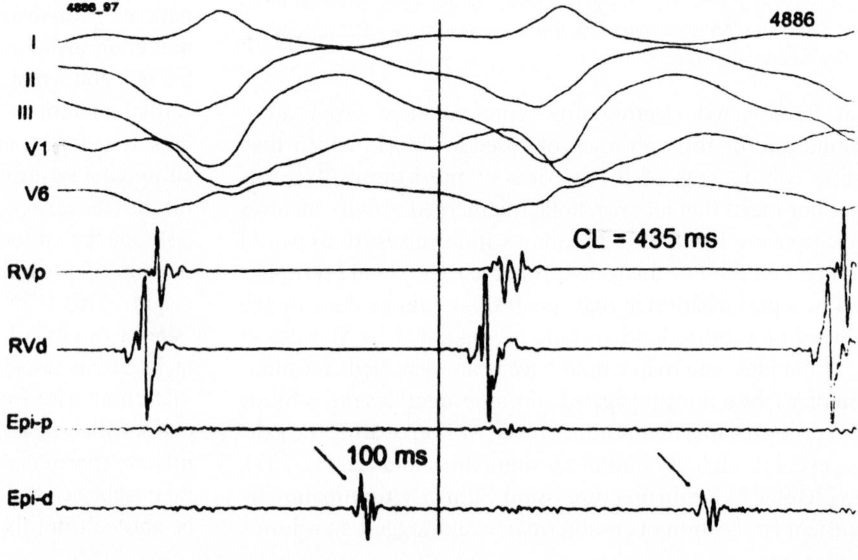


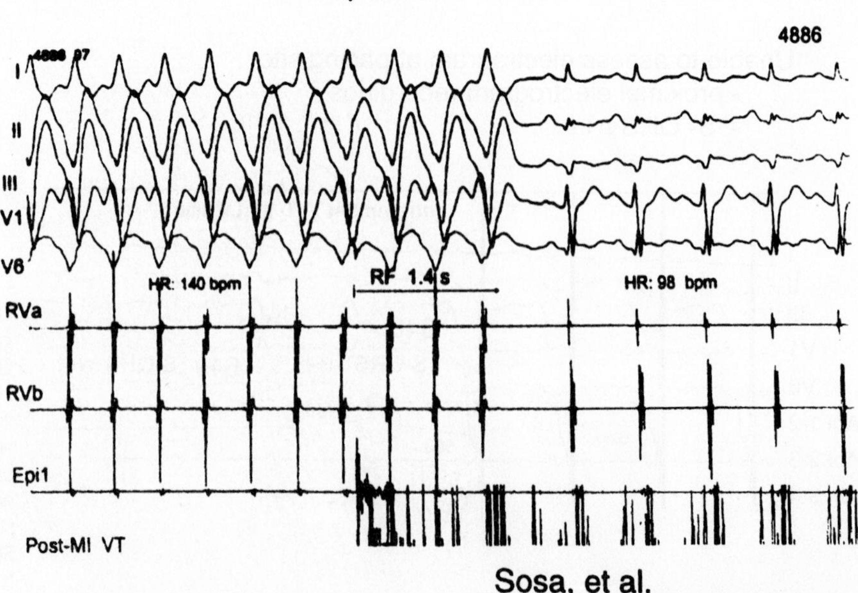


**FIGURE 11-240** Epicardial "origin" of VT associated with inferior myocardial infarction. ECG leads I, II, III, $V_1$, and $V_6$ are shown with proximal and distal RV endocardial and LV epicardial electrograms. **Top panel:** VT is present at a cycle length of 435 msec. Epicardial mapping revealed a mid-diastolic potential (*arrows*) 100 msec prior to the QRS. Although entrainment mapping was not performed, delivery of radiofrequency energy at this site terminated the VT (**bottom panel**) suggest an epicardial or subepicardial component of the reentrant circuit. (From Sosa E, Scanavacca M, d'Avila A, et al. Nonsurgical transthoracic epicardial catheter ablation to treat recurrent ventricular tachycardia occurring late after myocardial infarction. *J Amer Coll Cardiol* 2000;35:1442–1449.)

Such tachycardia locations may become more frequent with early reperfusion of acute infarction. In contrast those VT associated with cardiomyopathy can arise anywhere in the heart—in either right or left ventricle and from endocardium to epicardium. Because the bipolar electrogram records endocardial and subendocardial activity, the electrograms can be normal if the tachycardia has an intramural or epicardial origin (see earlier discussion). Therefore, in the presence of VT associated with cardiomyopathy, one may only be able to demonstrate focal activity because the bulk of electrical activity related to the tachycardia mechanism may be midmyocardial or even epicardial. An example is shown in Figure 11-241 in which an LBBB-type VT appears to arise in the anterior right ventricular wall ($RV_{18}$). Note that the earliest electrogram is perfectly normal and precedes the QRS complex by only 25 msec. Sosa et al.[75,382] have developed the technique of epicardial mapping using an intrapericardial approach. Using this technique they have demonstrated early activation on the epicardium in patients with Chagas disease and in highly selected patients with inferior infarction, which they targeted for ablation. Several investigators have confirmed the utility of epicardial mapping to guide ablation of VT in ARVD and other nonischemic cardiomyopathies (see Chapter 13).[80,400–402] In such patients epicardial mapping via the pericardium and entrainment mapping as described above can define critical sites of a reentrant circuit that can guide successful ablation. While epicardial mapping and ablation via the pericardium may be useful in selective cases, there are special factors that must be considered. Significant epicardial fat may lead to inaccurate activation times and reduction of bipolar voltage due to the recording of far field signals. Radiofrequency ablation in the pericardial space is less effective, given poor contact force, the lack of electrode cooling because of absent blood flow (although "cool tip" catheters can be used), and the presence of insulating epicardial fat.[403] In addition, the possibility of damage to the immediately contiguous epicardial coronary arteries, the left phrenic nerve, and the lungs need to be appreciated and avoided. Epicardial ablation is discussed in detail in Chapter 13.

Repetitive monomorphic tachycardias occurring in normal hearts that may be nonsustained or sustained[163,295] most commonly arise in the right ventricular outflow tract. This tachycardia, which is due to DADs that are characteristically facilitated by enhanced adenyl cyclase-dependent cyclic

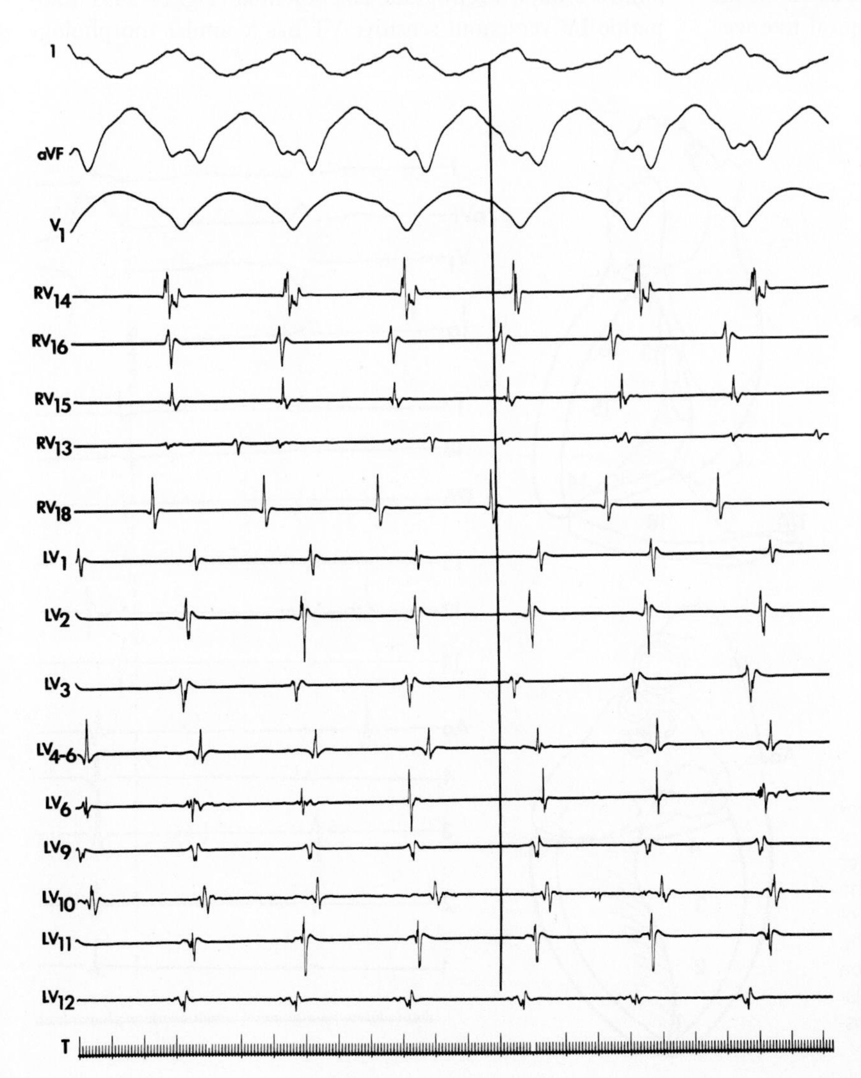


**FIGURE 11-241** Endocardial map in a patient with an idiopathic dilated cardiomyopathy and right ventricular VT. VT with a left bundle branch block left axis deviation morphology is present. The earliest site of endocardial activity is the midanterior wall of the right ventricle ($RV_{18}$). Note that the electrogram is a normal electrogram and occurs 25 msec before the onset of the QRS. See text for discussion.

AMP activity, has an LV counterpart that usually arises at the superior-basal aspect of the LV near the mitral annulus, or within the sinuses of Valsalva. Occasionally similar VTs due to DADs arise high in the interventricular septum, the epicardium, or even within a prior. Obviously these triggered VTs can also occur in the presence of structural heart disease,[305] and really should be named for the underlying mechanism (i.e., triggered VT) rather than be placed under the rubric of "idiopathic VT." Epicardial or deep intramural locations are suggested by slurred upstrokes of the QRS. The earliest electrograms (unipolar or bipolar) at the earliest sites are usually but not always normal, and are recorded, on the average, 30 to 50 msec prior to the QRS (Figs. 11-242 and 11-243). If the electrogram is severely abnormal in an apparent RV outflow tract VT, and the catheter is positioned over the free wall of the outflow tract, one must consider the possibility that the patient has an early form of right ventricular dysplasia or sarcoidosis. In such patients, sites of origin are typically abnormal. Typically, VT that is due to right ventricular dysplasia exits from isthmuses on the free wall at the outflow tract, near the apex of the heart, or in the inferobasal portion of the right ventricle.[170] The inferobasal portion of the right ventricle which uses the tricuspid annulus as a fixed barrier is the most common site of an isthmus, while the apical free wall is the least common. These are reentrant VTs, and the same mapping techniques used to localize VT in CAD should be employed, although epicardial mapping is more useful than in VT due to a prior infarct. In fact the appearance of a VT with an LBBB pattern and superior axis in someone with an apparently normal heart should suggest the possibility of right ventricular dysplasia (Fig. 11-223). The extent of the disease is paralleled by the extent of abnormalities of electrograms in sinus rhythm (see following section entitled Sinus Rhythm Mapping).

Another group of patients in whom reentrant activity is certainly likely are patients with VT after repair of tetralogy of Fallot. In such cases, the scar in the right ventricular outflow tract appears to provide at least one potential barrier around which the impulse may circulate.[157,160] In such cases continuous activity reflecting the activation around the scar can be recorded (Fig. 11-244). A critical isthmus is often found in the conotruncal septum (see Chapter 13).

Finally, some fascicular tachycardias can be caused by DADs (digitalis-induced or adenyl cyclase–dependent cyclic AMP–mediated). These have characteristic fascicular morphologies and are preceded by a fascicular spike in the LV and, almost always, a retrograde His potential (Fig. 11-245). Idiopathic LV verapamil sensitive VT has a similar morphology

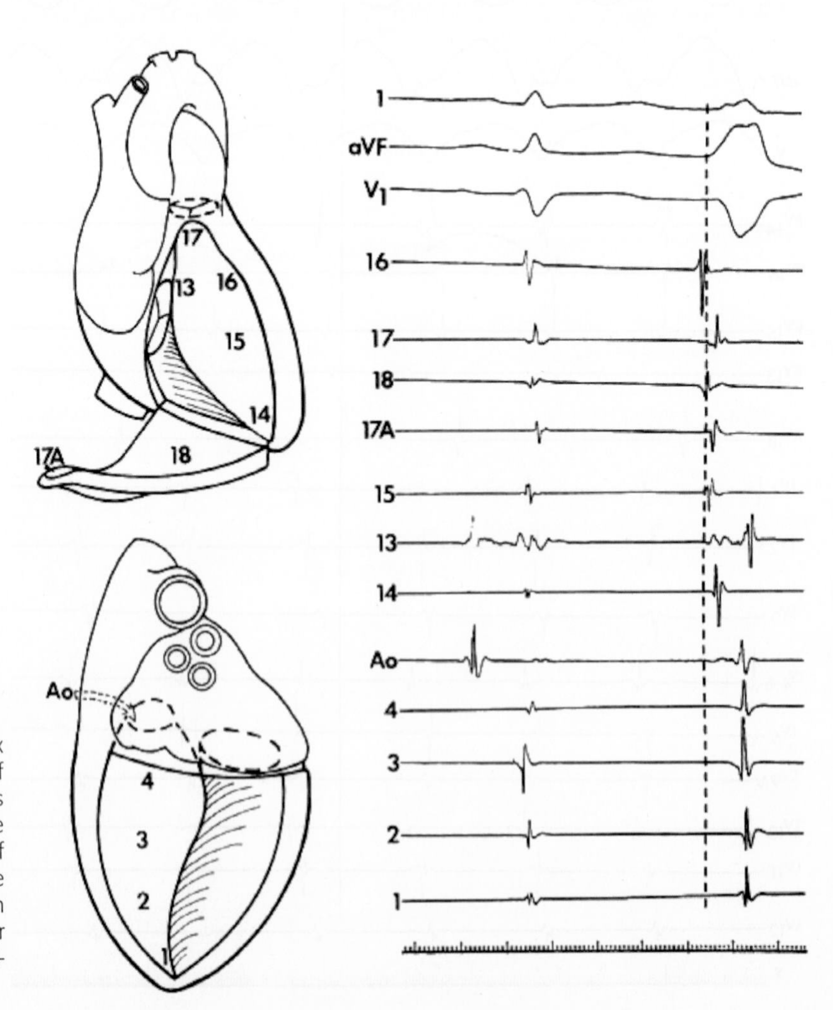


**FIGURE 11-242** Endocardial mapping of a VT complex during repetitive monomorphic tachycardia. Schema of the RV and LV are shown along with analog recordings during a sinus complex and a ventricular complex. The earliest ventricular activity occurs at the infundibulum of the RVOT and is a normal electrogram. It precedes the QRS by 22 msec. See text for discussion. (From Buxton AE, Waxman HL, Marchlinski FE, et al. Right ventricular tachycardia: clinical and electrophysiologic characteristics. *Circulation* 1983;68:917.)

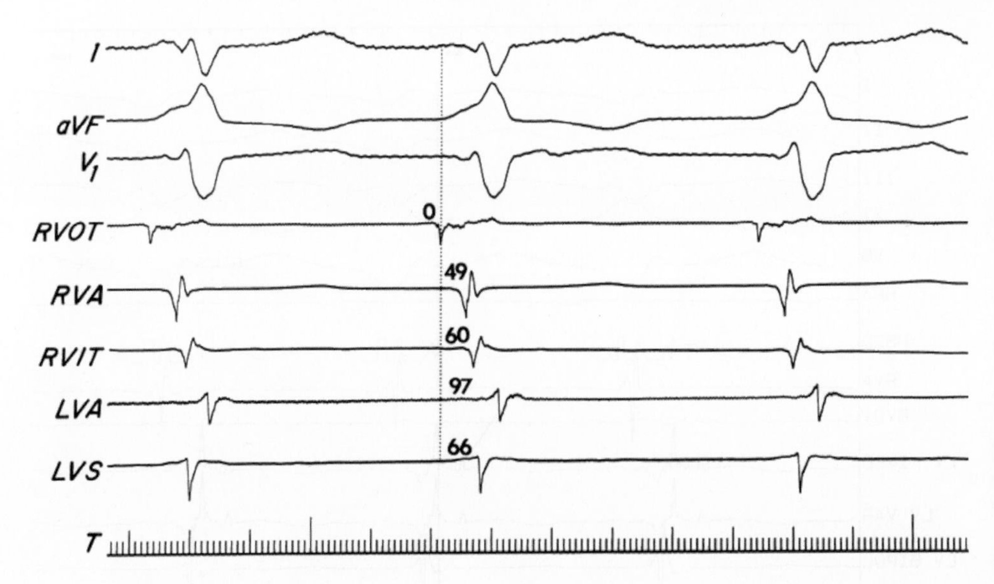


**FIGURE 11-243** Endocardial map from an adolescent with possible right ventricular outflow tract VT from the epicardium. Leads 1, aVF, and $V_1$ are shown with electrograms from the RVOT, RVA, right ventricular inflow tract (RVIT), left ventricular apex (LVA), and mid-left ventricular septum (mid-LVS). The tachycardia has a left bundle right inferior axis morphology. Earliest activity occurs at the RVOT and is associated with a broad low-amplitude electrogram. The markedly slurred upstroke of the QRS suggests an epicardial or deep septal location.

to posterior fascicular rhythms, but has a reentrant mechanism.[168–173,212,344,345] These VTs often have a Purkinje spike preceding the QRS, which has suggested to many that it is fascicular in origin. For various reasons discussed earlier in this chapter, I do not believe the fascicles have been proven to be part of the reentrant circuit. These VT can be entrained from the RV or right atrium, and in rare instances, concealed entrainment is possible, usually from on the mid to lower LV septum. These tachycardias frequently demonstrate diastolic potentials on the septum leading to a zone of slow conduction,[345] but such potentials have not been universally found. An example of such late potentials and proposed mechanism of the VT is shown in Figure 11-246.

Regardless of the cause of the tachycardia, proof that the earliest endocardial or epicardial electrogram is in fact earliest requires the same procedures described in the preceding paragraphs. The mode of initiation, response to stimulation, and effect of drugs on such tachycardias will also provide indirect evidence for the type of mechanism for the arrhythmia. Of importance, however, is the recognition that because tachycardias in cardiomyopathy may be midmyocardial or even subepicardial, the earliest site of activation on the endocardium

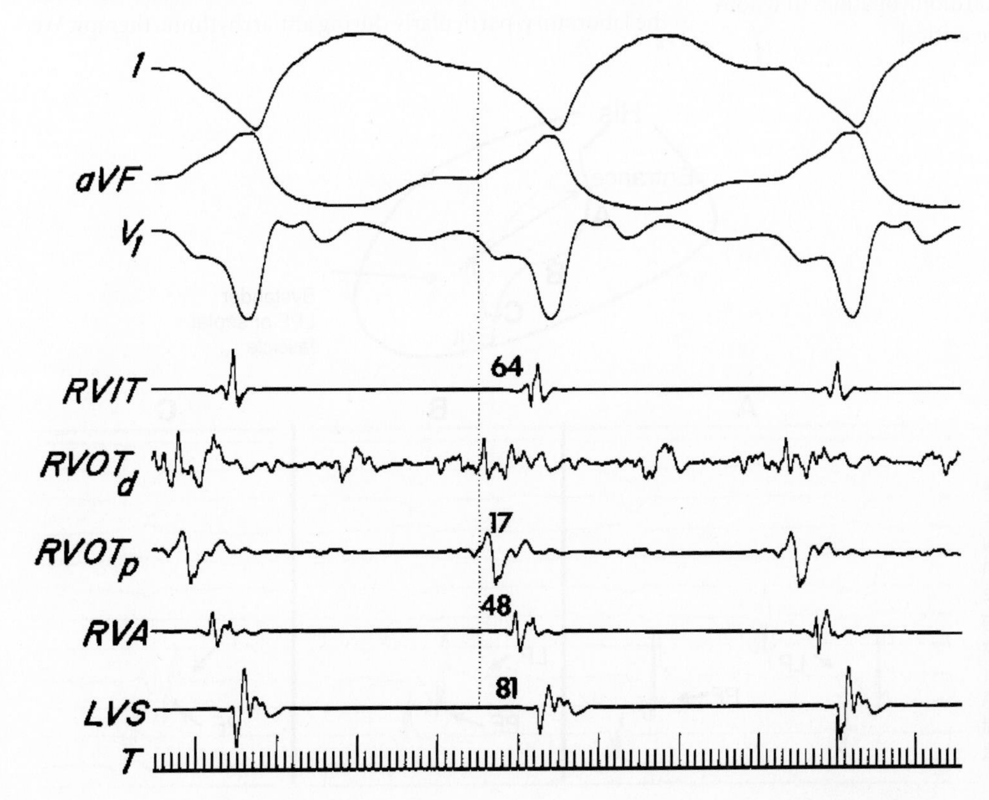


**FIGURE 11-244** Endocardial map in a patient with VT status postrepair of tetralogy of Fallot. Leads 1, aVF, and $V_1$ are shown with electrograms from the RVIT, $RVOT_d$, $RVOT_p$, RVA, and the mid-left ventricular septum LVS. The $RVOT_d$ demonstrates continuous electrical activity, while the adjacent $RVOT_p$ has a diastolic potential in the first third of diastole. The widely separate potentials are recorded from opposite sides of the ventriculotomy scar. See text for discussion. (From Horowitz LN, Vetter VL, Harken AH, et al. Electrophysiologic characteristics of sustained ventricular tachycardia occurring after repair of tetralogy of Fallot. *Am J Cardiol* 1980; 46:446.)

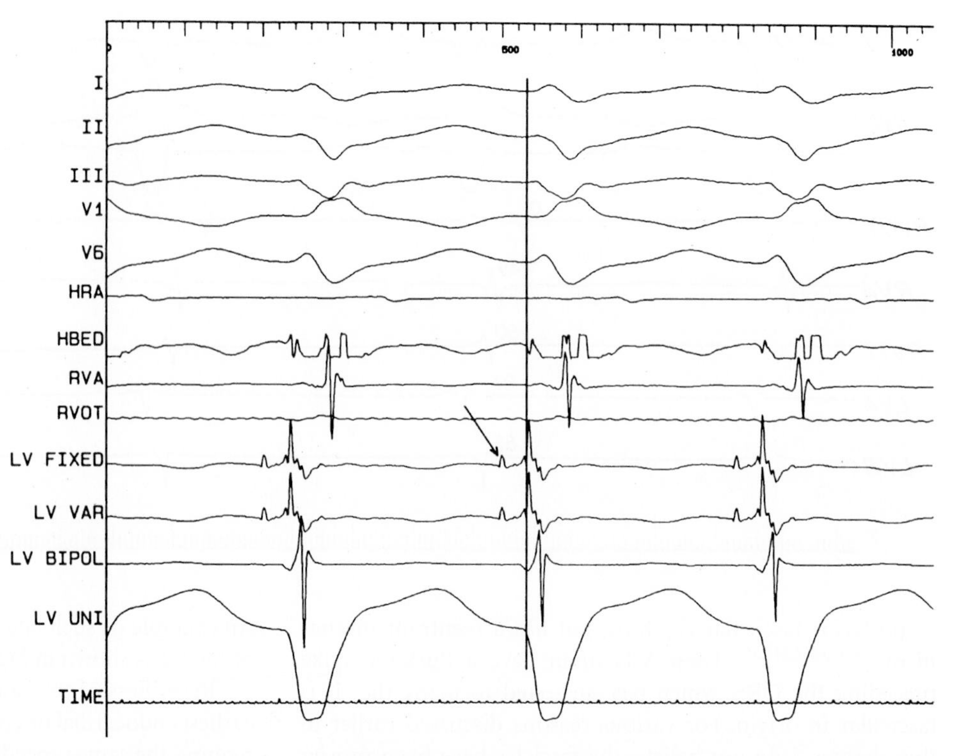


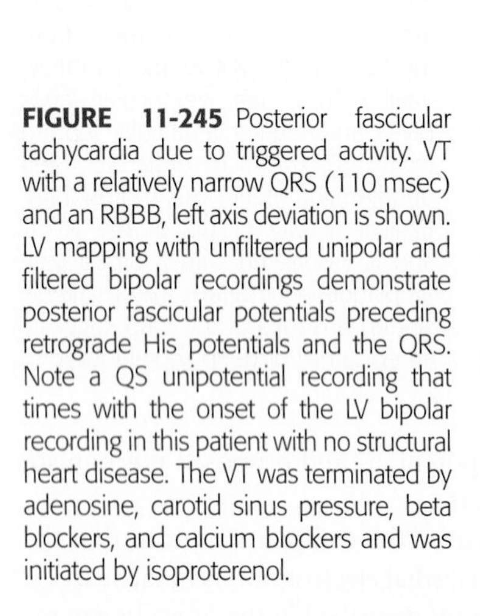

**FIGURE 11-245** Posterior fascicular tachycardia due to triggered activity. VT with a relatively narrow QRS (110 msec) and an RBBB, left axis deviation is shown. LV mapping with unfiltered unipolar and filtered bipolar recordings demonstrate posterior fascicular potentials preceding retrograde His potentials and the QRS. Note a QS unipotential recording that times with the onset of the LV bipolar recording in this patient with no structural heart disease. The VT was terminated by adenosine, carotid sinus pressure, beta blockers, and calcium blockers and was initiated by isoproterenol.

may not provide a precise enough marker for the origin of the tachycardia to use for catheter ablative techniques. This is important because most standard radiofrequency catheter ablation techniques result in a lesion <2 to 5 mm in depth and could therefore fail to ablate a tachycardia that is subepicardial. Epicardial mapping or use of newer technologies may be necessary to define critical sites for ablation in patients with nonreentrant mechanisms and/or cardiomyopathies in whom intramural or subepicardial sites are critical.

### *Multiple Ventricular Tachycardia Morphologies: Relationship to Site of Origin*

It is now widely recognized that patients with sustained monomorphic VT due to reentry, associated with prior infarction, frequently have more than one morphology of VT. In our experience, even in patients presenting with a single uniform sustained VT, multiple distinct uniform VT may be induced in the laboratory, particularly during antiarrhythmic therapy. We

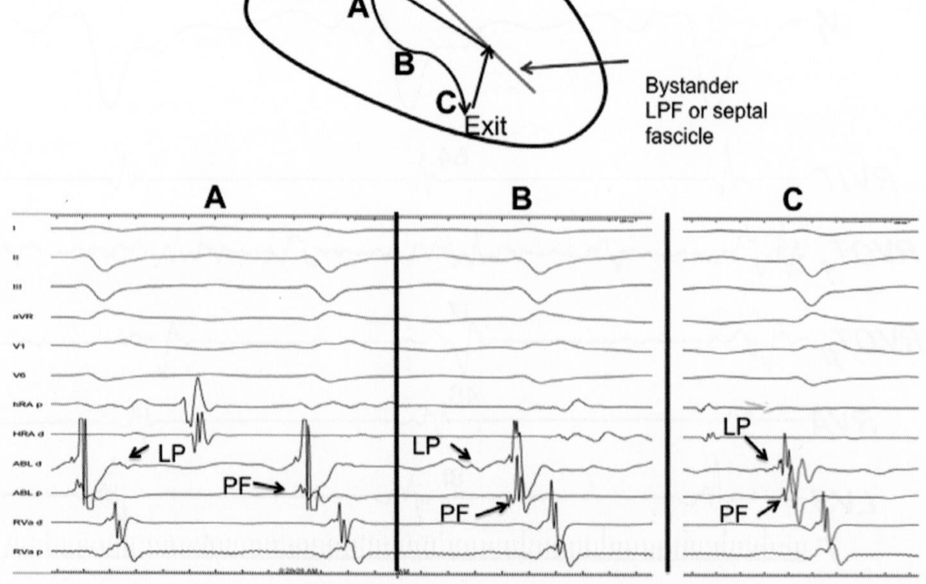


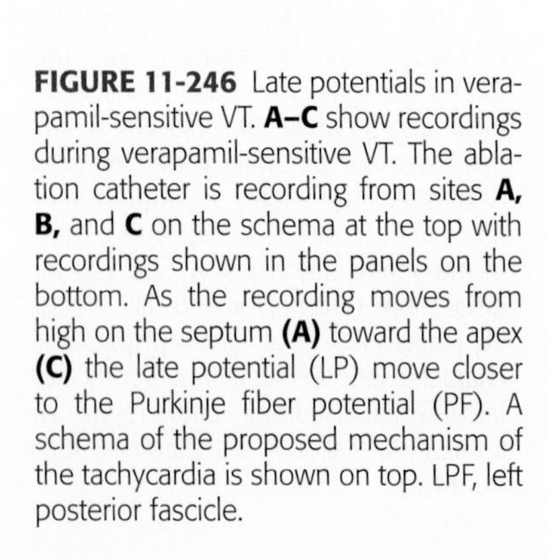

**FIGURE 11-246** Late potentials in verapamil-sensitive VT. **A–C** show recordings during verapamil-sensitive VT. The ablation catheter is recording from sites **A, B,** and **C** on the schema at the top with recordings shown in the panels on the bottom. As the recording moves from high on the septum **(A)** toward the apex **(C)** the late potential (LP) move closer to the Purkinje fiber potential (PF). A schema of the proposed mechanism of the tachycardia is shown on top. LPF, left posterior fascicle.

now rarely see among the patient population in our laboratory an individual with a single morphologic type of sustained VT. We believe that these uniform VTs are of clinical significance for the following reasons: (a) If 12-lead ECGs are obtained during multiple spontaneous episodes on a variety of different antiarrhythmic agents, different morphologic types of VT will frequently be seen. The use of single-lead rhythm strips to record VT has been a major misleading factor suggesting that there is only "one" VT. (b) Inducible tachycardias that were never seen spontaneously in the preablation state occasionally occur spontaneously following the surgical or catheter ablation of another induced arrhythmia. In fact, virtually all of the VT recurrences noted in our ablation patients are those VT that were never seen spontaneously before ablation and in which no attempt was made to ablate them, if they were induced.

Multiple morphologic types of reentrant VTs include those that have different bundle branch block patterns and/or manifest variations of axis or pericardial R-wave progression of a given bundle branch block pattern (Figs. 11-247 and 11-248). In our experience, 85% of multiple, morphologically distinct monomorphic VTs arise from the same region of the heart (i.e., they have closely located exit sites or shared components of an isthmus or diastolic pathway), which we arbitrarily have defined to include an area of 5 to 10 $cm^2$. This occurs because many potential channels can go through the scar leading to many different tachycardia circuits. In the remaining 15% of tachycardias, reentrant circuits and/or exit sites are more disparate.[368–370] Obviously, detailed mapping is necessary to determine the sites of origin or critical isthmus of each tachycardia, because the success of catheter ablation or surgery can be markedly influenced by the locations of these

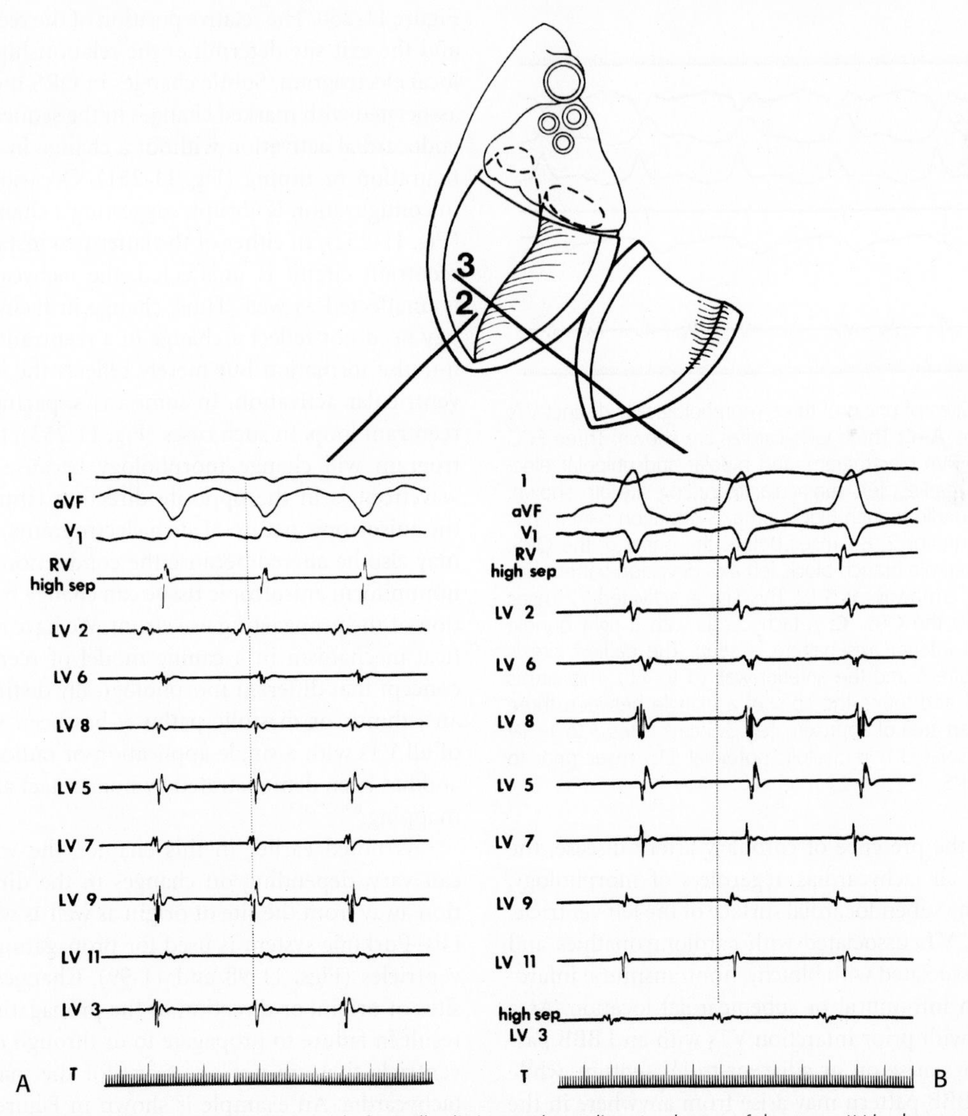


**FIGURE 11-247** Endocardial catheter map in two morphologically distinct tachycardias. A schema of the open LV is shown with analog records of two morphologically distinct VTs. **A:** VT with a right bundle branch block right superior axis is shown. A reference RV high septal electrogram is shown along with multiple ventricular recordings. The earliest electrogram is recorded at mid LV 2, 70 msec before the onset of the QRS. **B:** VT with a left bundle branch block right inferior axis is shown. The earliest electrical activity in this tachycardia arises from the high septum near LV 3, 2 cm from the right bundle branch block tachycardia. These are considered as a similar region. See text for discussion.

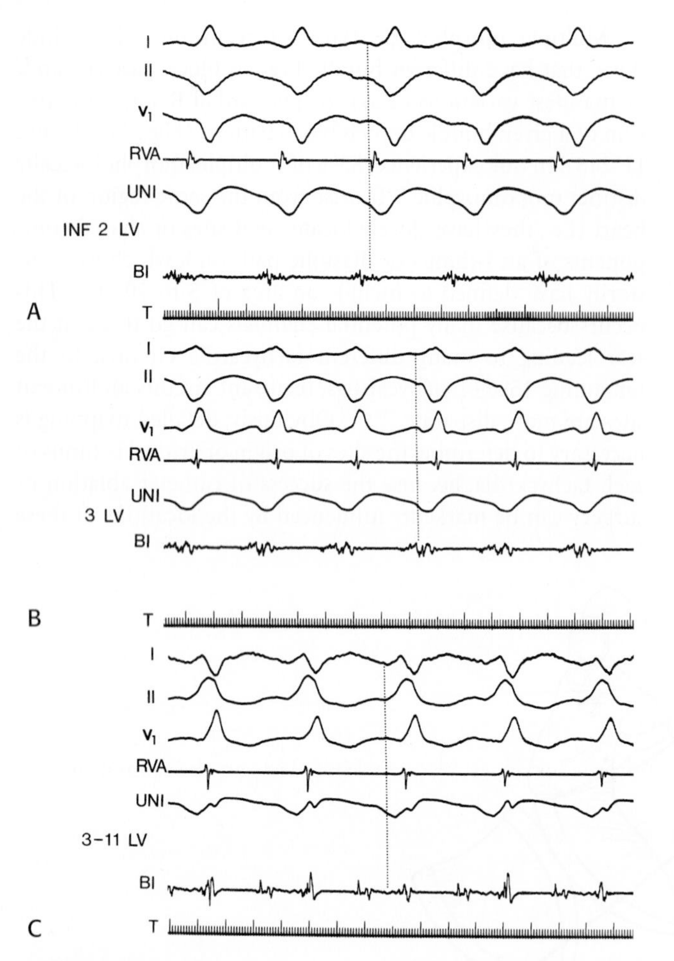


**FIGURE 11-248** Sites of origin of three morphologically distinct VTs in the same patient. **A–C:** Three tachycardias are shown. Three ECG leads, a reference RVA electrogram, and bipolar and unipolar electrograms from the earliest left ventricular recording site are shown. **A:** VT with a left bundle branch block, left axis deviation pattern has its earliest site at inferior 2, 85 msec before the onset of the QRS. **B:** VT with a right bundle branch block, left axis deviation pattern has its earliest site 1.5 cm away, at 3 LV. This site is activated 72 msec before the onset of the QRS. **C:** A tachycardia with a right bundle branch block, right inferior axis pattern is seen. The earliest site is at the junction of site 3 and the anterior wall (3 to 11). This site is 2 cm above site 3 and forms the apex of a triangle between three sites, which cover an area of approximately 3.5 $cm^2$. Sites 3 to 11 LV demonstrates an isolated mid-diastolic potential 115 msec prior to the onset of the QRS.

tachycardias. In the presence of coronary artery disease, the vast majority of all tachycardias, regardless of morphology, arise in or near the subendocardial surface of the left ventricle. As noted earlier, VTs associated with cardiomyopathies and occasional VTs associated with blotchy, nontransmural infarction can have an intramural or subepicardial location. As a rule, in patients with prior infarction VTs with an LBBB pattern almost always arise on or adjacent to LV septum, while those with an RBBB pattern may arise from anywhere in the LV. I have only seen four VTs with LBBB patterns associated with inferior infarction and one with anterior infarction with RV septal breakthroughs. In the presence of normal hearts or cardiomyopathies, tachycardias with an LBBB pattern can arise from either the right or left ventricle. Mapping and programmed stimulation are necessary to determine the site of the isthmus or exit from reentrant VTs. The 12-lead ECG can be used in some cases as a guide to segmental localization but is not precise enough to direct ablative therapy.

Although individual tachycardia morphologies can be initiated at different times, not infrequently one tachycardia changes to another in response to programmed stimulation (Fig. 11-249). In such instances, if one is recording a site in an isthmus, it is not infrequent to see the electrogram at that site remain relatively constant despite the changing QRS (Fig. 11-249). In such cases, we believe that stimulation either causes a change in location or direction of activation from the site of exit from the reentrant circuit or a change in the activation sequence in the ventricular tissue surrounding the exit site by altering the electrophysiologic properties of this tissue. The former explanation is schematically shown in Figure 11-250. The relative position of the recording electrodes and the exit site determines the relationship of the QRS and local electrogram. Subtle changes in QRS morphology can be associated with marked changes in the sequence of ventricular endocardial activation without a change in electrogram configuration or timing (Fig. 11-251). Occasionally, the change in configuration is abrupt, suggesting a change in exit pattern (Fig. 11-252). In either of the latter two instances, because the reentrant circuit is unaffected, the tachycardia cycle length is unaffected as well. Thus, change in tachycardia morphology need not reflect a change in a reentrant circuit or site of impulse formation but merely reflects the overall pattern of ventricular activation. In some cases, pacing can reverse the reentrant loop. In such cases (Fig. 11-253), the recorded electrogram will change morphology because the propagating wavefront is in the opposite direction (thus, demonstrating the anisotropic nature of such electrograms). The cycle length may also be altered because the conduction velocity through nonuniform anisotropic tissue can change based on the direction of the propagating wavefront. We have observed an identical mechanism in a canine model of reentrant VT.[404] The concept that different morphologically distinct VTs can share an isthmus or diastolic pathway has been validated by cure of all VTs with a single application of radiofrequency energy and has been demonstrated by noncontact and intraoperative mapping.[69,352,353]

As noted earlier in this chapter, the width of the QRS can vary, depending on changes in the direction of activation away from the site of origin as well as whether or not the His–Purkinje system is used for propagation throughout the ventricles (Figs. 11-98 and 11-99). Changes in cycle length, sites of origin, or direction of the propagating wavefront can result in failure to propagate to or through other areas of the ventricle that are not necessary for the maintenance of the tachycardia. An example is shown in Figure 11-254; an area of a left ventricular aneurysm is activated by every cycle of a tachycardia with a cycle length of 350 msec but suddenly fails to be activated during every other complex of a new tachycardia with a shorter cycle length. Such local failure of

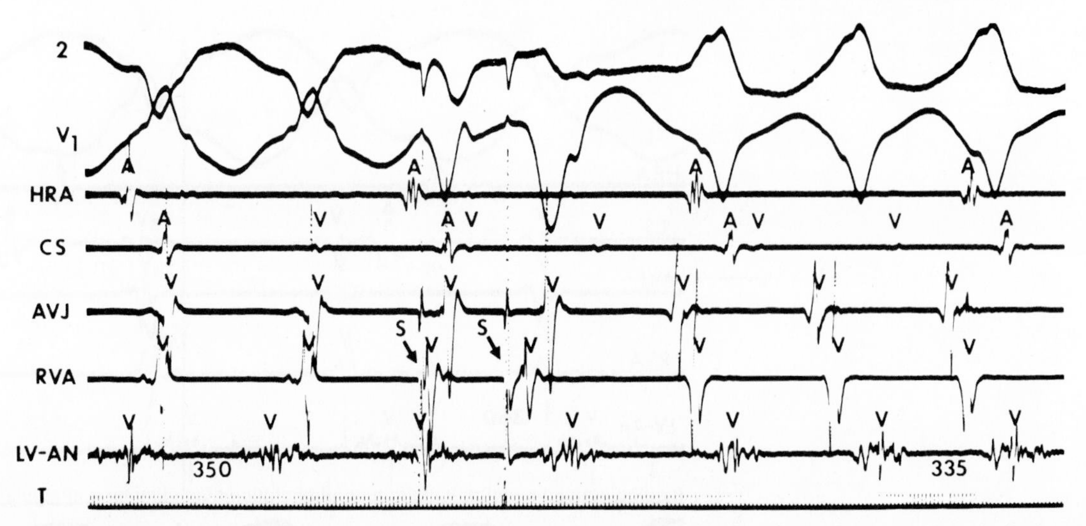


**FIGURE 11-249** Change in QRS morphology of VT produced by ventricular extrastimuli. Leads 2 and $V_1$ are shown with electrograms from the HRA, CS, AVJ, RVA, and inside a left ventricular aneurysm (LV-AN). VT with right bundle branch block morphology is present in the first two complexes. The site of origin in the LV-AN demonstrates diastolic and systolic fragmented activity. Two ventricular extrastimuli delivered from the RVA change the ventricular activation sequence and the QRS morphology to a left bundle branch block pattern without significantly altering configuration of the electrogram in the LV-AN. However, the relationship of the electrogram in the LV-AN to the QRS changes markedly. (From Josephson ME, Horowitz LN, Farshidi A, et al. Recurrent sustained ventricular tachycardia. 4. Pleomorphism. *Circulation* 1979;59:459.)

propagation has also been observed during intraoperative mapping and may reflect the influence of nonuniform anisotropy in the diseased tissue in addition to nonuniform "refractoriness".[374] Of interest, as shown by Miller et al.[374] such local failure of conduction usually occurs at or near exit sites of reentrant VTs, suggesting this finding may be characteristic of arrhythmogenic tissue.

Intraoperative mapping has demonstrated that most sustained uniform VTs exit from a "focal" circumscribed area in the ventricle in the majority of cases.[46,48,122,123,352,353,371–373,375,376]

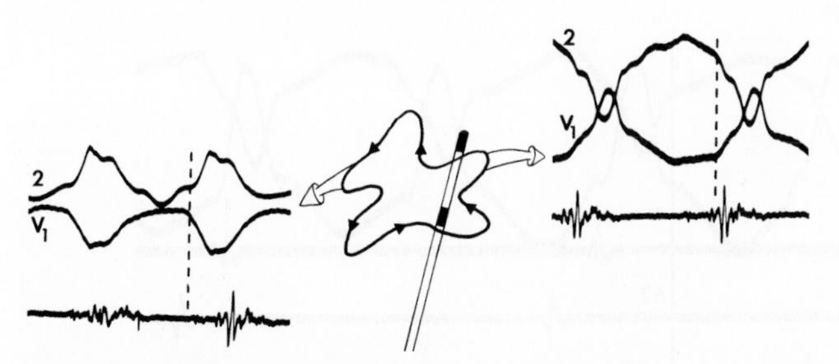


**FIGURE 11-250** Proposed mechanism for change in morphology of VT by extrastimuli shown in Figure 11-249. A bipolar catheter is schematically positioned over part of the reentrant circuit and records a local fragmented activity during different parts of the cardiac cycle, depending on the relationship of the exiting wavefront to the catheter recording site. If the ventricles are depolarized by a wavefront that exits after passing the electrode (tachycardia on the right), fragmented activity will be recorded before the QRS. If ventricular activation occurs before reaching the area of the catheter recording, the fragmented activity will appear during and after the QRS (tachycardia on the left). Thus, the right and left bundle branch block morphologies shown here come from the same reentrant circuit, despite a change in relationship of the fractionated electrogram to the onset of the QRS. See text for discussion. (From Josephson ME, Horowitz LN, Farshidi A, et al. Recurrent sustained ventricular tachycardia. 4. Pleomorphism. *Circulation* 1979;59:459.)

In some instances this probably reflects an exit from a subendocardial sheet of surviving muscle as suggested by de Bakker et al.[46,48] and Downar et al.[352] In other instances, a larger macroreentrant figure-of-eight reentrant pathway has been desc ribed.[46,352,353,371,374–376] These studies also confirmed that the QRS morphology reflects global ventricular activation and closely parallels that of the epicardial activation sequence.

### Validation of Catheter Mapping

Validation of the catheter map requires demonstration that application of radiofrequency energy at the site of origin of focal VTs or the center or exit from a protected isthmus in reentrant VTs terminates VT. However, the successful outcome of a catheter ablation to define the accuracy of mapping is often unjustified because multiple radiofrequency applications at different sites are frequently used, prohibiting analysis of the importance of any single local electrogram. In my experience, the use of the various steps suggested for proving that an electrogram is at a critical site in the reentrant circuit or is at the "site of origin" results in successful termination of VT.[148] For reentrant VT associated with prior infarction, all three entrainment criteria must be met. Use of the postpacing interval alone is inadequate, but contrary to the suggestion of Bogun et al.,[405] the postpacing interval is extremely useful. It is necessary, but not sufficient. Obviously, thickness of scar, presence of endocardial clot, a wide isthmus or no isthmus (single loop reentry), intramural or subepicardial location, and inadequate lesion make 100% success an unrealistic goal. However, for focal mechanisms and most VT associated with prior infarction, the ability to terminate VT approaches this lofty goal. Access issues and inability to induce the targeted clinical VT are other limitations.

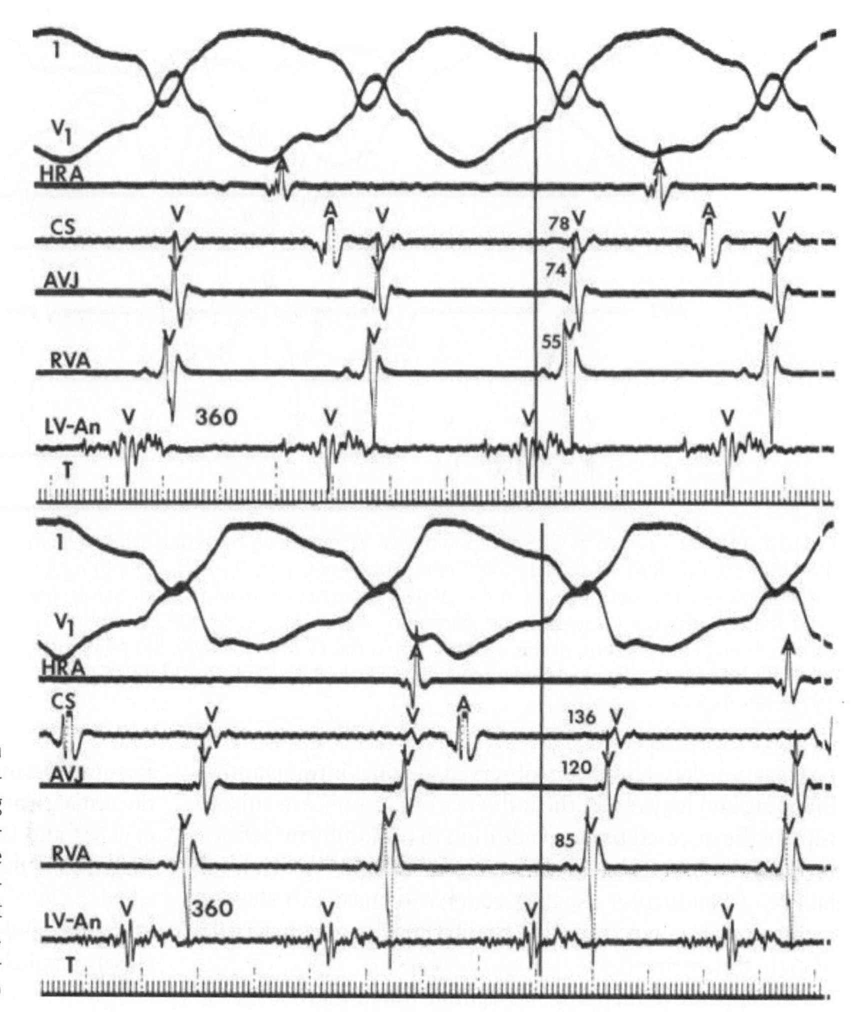


**FIGURE 11-251** Subtle change in QRS configuration during VT associated with a marked change in ventricular activation. The two QRS configurations during VT shown in the panels are similar, but the ventricular activation sequences are markedly different. Note that the rate of the tachycardia and the local electrogram from the LV-An remain unchanged. See text for discussion. (From Josephson ME, Horowitz LN, Farshidi A, et al. Recurrent sustained ventricular tachycardia. 4. Pleomorphism. *Circulation* 1979;59:459.)

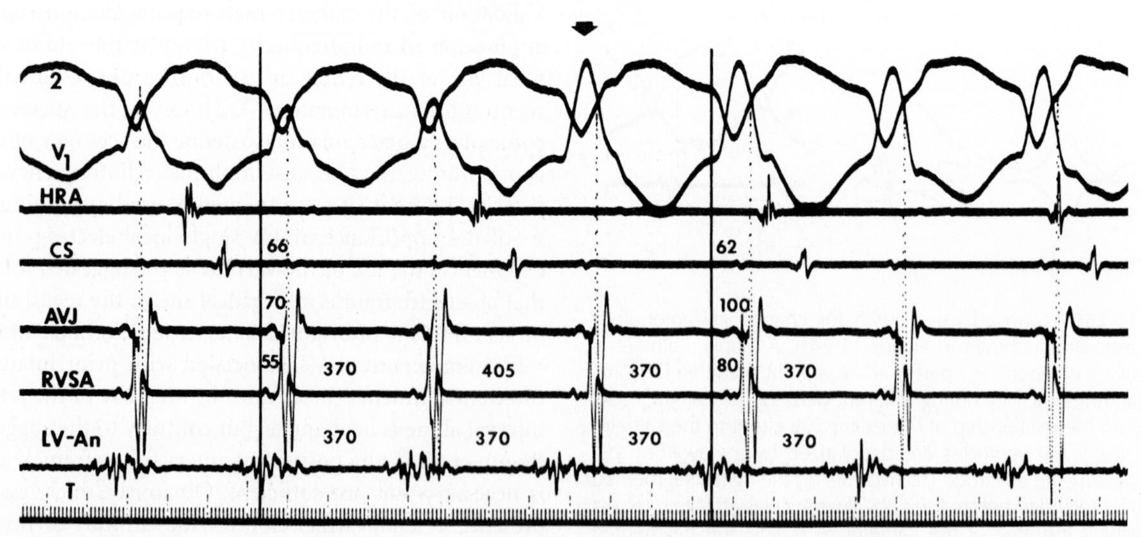


**FIGURE 11-252** Abrupt change in QRS morphology and endocardial activation sequence during VT. The tachycardia as recorded in the LV-An is unaltered by the sudden change in QRS noted by the inverted *broad arrow.* However, the morphologic change in the QRS is associated with a one-cycle delay (370 to 405 msec) in the electrogram recorded at the right ventricular apex along the septum (RVSA) and subsequent change in ventricular activation recorded in the CS and AVJ and RVSA (*vertical lines*). This suggests that a change in exit site has occurred in the absence of any change in the underlying tachycardia mechanism. (From Josephson ME, Horowitz LN, Farshidi A, et al. Recurrent sustained ventricular tachycardia. 4. Pleomorphism. *Circulation* 1979;59:459.)

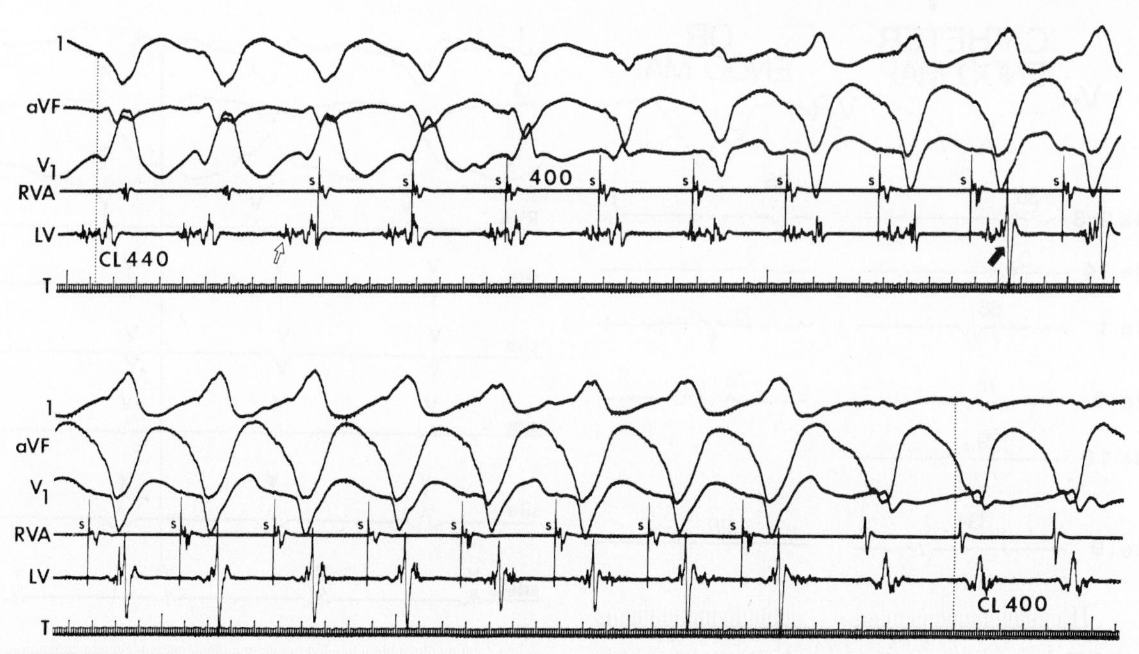


FIGURE 11-253 Change in morphology of VT by overdrive pacing and reversal of activation through the reentrant circuit. Leads 1, aVF, and $V_1$ are shown with electrograms from the RVA and the LV site of origin (i.e., presystolic, orthodromically activated site within the VT circuit). VT with a right bundle branch block right superior axis is present with a cycle length of 440 msec. Pacing from the RVA at 400 msec produces a total change in the LV electrogram, suggesting antidromic capture. On cessation of pacing, the tachycardia morphology has reversed itself to a left bundle branch block pattern. This suggests that overdrive pacing stopped the tachycardia and reinitiated in the opposite direction. See text for discussion.

We have performed both catheter and intraoperative maps on several hundred tachycardias to date and have found an excellent correlation between the catheter map and the intraoperative map. Our catheter map corresponds within 2 cm (i.e., an area of 4 $cm^2$) to the earliest site recorded intraoperatively (Figs. 11-255 and 11-256). We have shown that endocardial catheter mapping is far more accurate than intraoperative epicardial mapping for localizing the origin of VT associated with coronary artery disease.[94,369,371] Examples are shown in Figures 11-256 and 11-257, where the endocardial site of activation precedes the QRS while the earliest epicardial activation occurs after the QRS. This is particularly true in LBBB VT (Fig. 11-257) in which epicardial activation almost always reveals early right ventricular activation followed by left ventricular activation; yet, the earliest site is on the septal endocardium. Thus, while there is active interest in epicardial approaches to VT associated with infarction, in my experience, the overwhelming majority of VTs have critical sites located in the subendocardium. Early intervention of acute infarction may change this; however, I believe the change in substrate is more likely to change the type of tachycardia to one that is more unstable. Mapping such tachycardias will require the use of newer technologies as suggested earlier in the chapter. The less frequently encountered stable monomorphic VTs are still likely to be subendocardial.

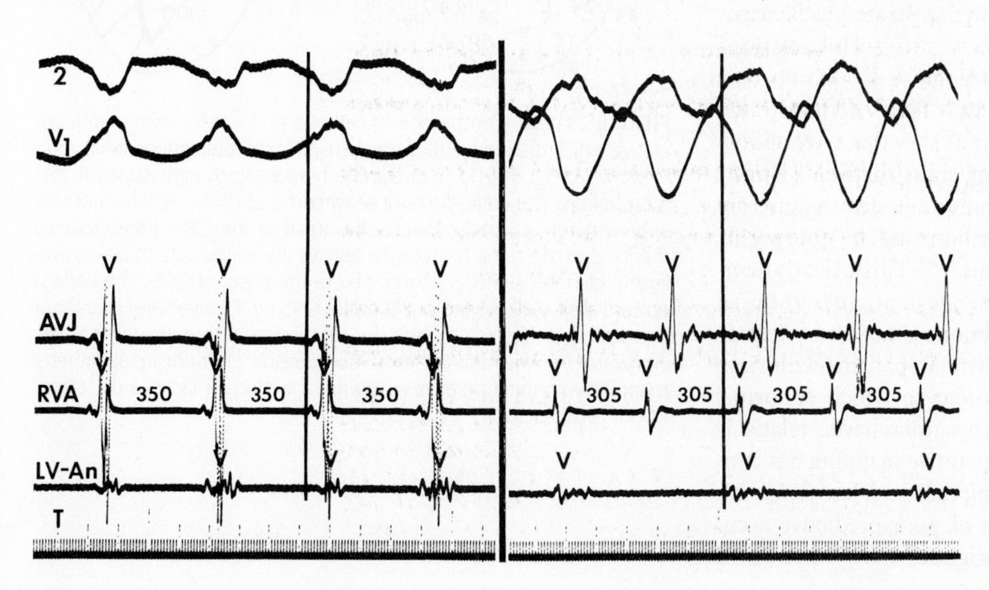


FIGURE 11-254 Two-to-one conduction to a left ventricular aneurysm during VT. ECG leads 2 and $V_1$ are shown with electrograms from the AVJ and RVA along with an electrogram from within an LV-An. During VT with a right bundle branch block morphology and a cycle length of 350 msec, there is 1:1 activation at all ventricular sites. With a switch in tachycardia morphology and a decrease in the tachycardia cycle length electrical activity in the LV-An electrogram appears following every other complex. (From Josephson ME, Horowitz LN, Farshidi A, et al. Recurrent sustained ventricular tachycardia. 4. Pleomorphism. *Circulation* 1979;59:459.)

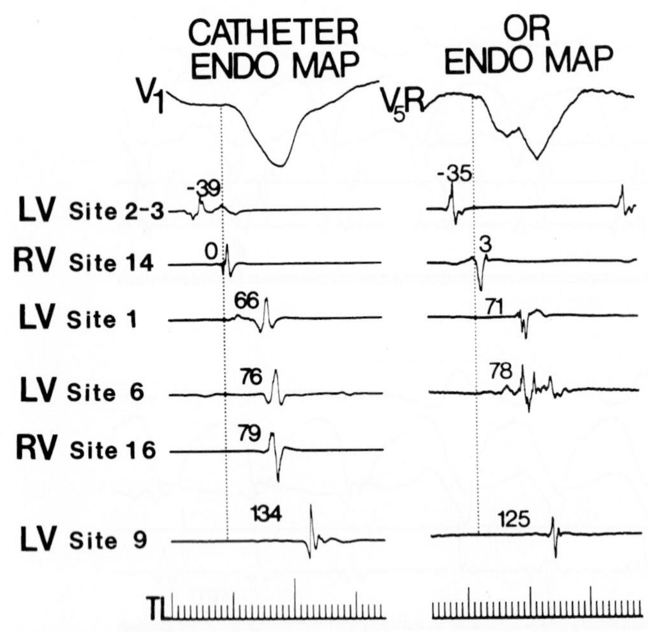


**FIGURE 11-255** Comparison of catheter and intraoperative (OR) endocardial (ENDO) maps. The activation times obtained during catheter mapping closely correspond to data obtained intraoperatively. (From Josephson ME, Horowitz LN, Spielman SR, et al. Role of catheter mapping in the preoperative evaluation of ventricular tachycardia. *Am J Cardiol* 1982;49:207.)

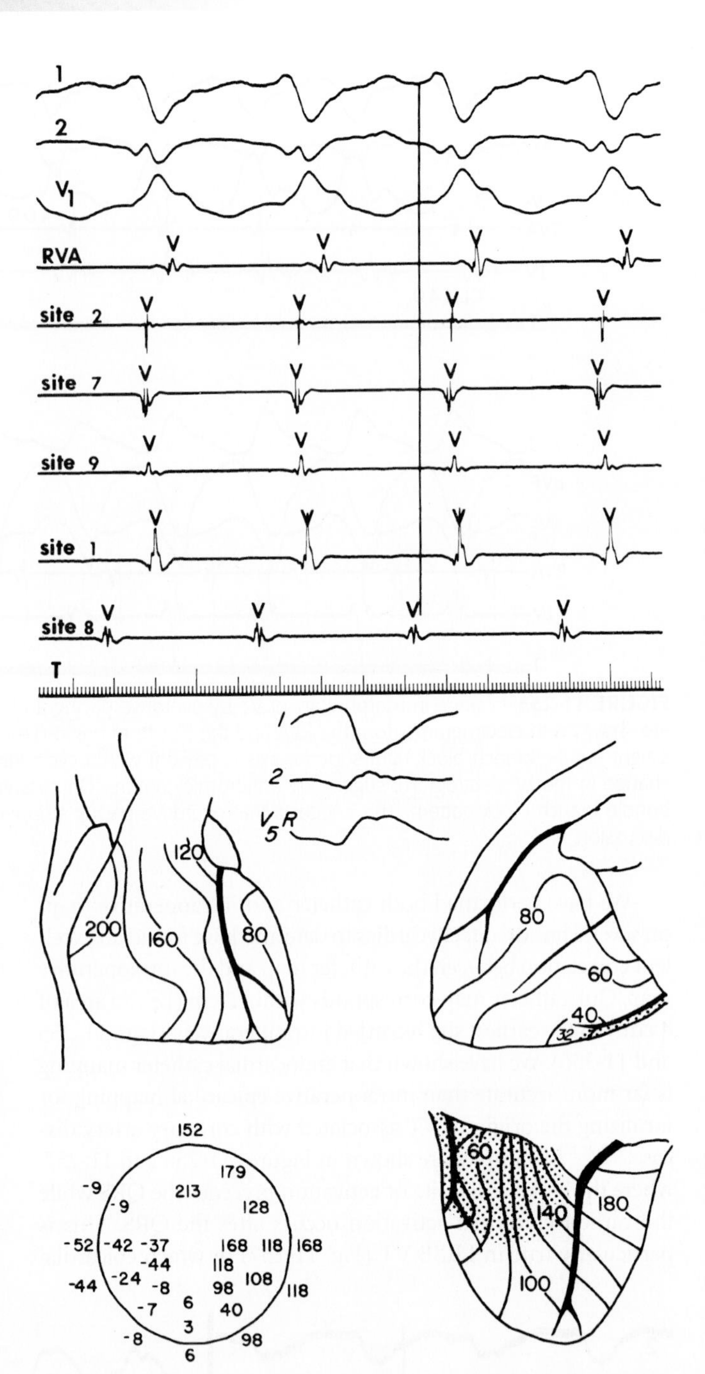


**FIGURE 11-256** Comparison of catheter endocardial map in intraoperative epicardial and endocardial map. A catheter endocardial map is shown of VT with a right bundle branch block right superior axis morphology. The earliest site of activation is at LV site 8, which occurs approximately 45 msec before the onset of the QRS. Intraoperative mapping of the same tachycardia reveals the earliest site to be equivalent to catheter site 8, 52 msec before the onset of QRS. The earliest epicardial site follows the onset of the QRS by 32 msec and is anterior and lateral to site 8. See text for discussion. (From Josephson ME, Horowitz LN, Spielman SR, et al. Comparison of endocardial catheter mapping with intraoperative mapping of ventricular tachycardia. *Circulation* 1980;61:395.)

## Sinus Rhythm Mapping

Occasionally, activation mapping cannot be performed in the catheterization laboratory because of hemodynamic intolerance. While new technologies may be useful in acquiring single beat maps or placing patients on left ventricular assist devices or on extracorporeal membrane oxygenation (ECMO) or on full cardiopulmonary bypass can allow for standard mapping techniques, sinus rhythm mapping may be of value in ablating these untolerated arrhythmias (see Chapter 13). In such instances, potential arrhythmogenic areas can be identified in the presence of abnormal and/or late electrograms, which we and others have demonstrated to be **associated** with arrhythmogenic tissue.[31–36,38,39,61] This relationship led to the use of SAECGs to recognize arrhythmogenic substrates.[84–90,98–100,102,103] Mapping of VTs has demonstrated that the vast majority (≈85%) occur at sites that have abnormal and/or late electrograms during sinus rhythm.[31] Unfortunately, abnormal, fractionated, and/or late electrograms are found throughout infarcted myocardium and are nonspecific for the site of **origin or critical isthmus**.[31,385] This is clearly demonstrated in Figure 11-258, where the site of origin is "focal" at site 2, which has neither the most abnormal nor latest electrogram in sinus rhythm. This is also true in patients with right ventricular dysplasia, another disorder in which abnormal electrograms are widespread yet tachycardias have a relatively focal isthmus (Fig. 11-259). Intraoperative mapping has confirmed these findings, demonstrating that such late potentials and/or abnormal electrograms are of poor predictive accuracy for documenting the site of origin of VT.[35,94] Use of the

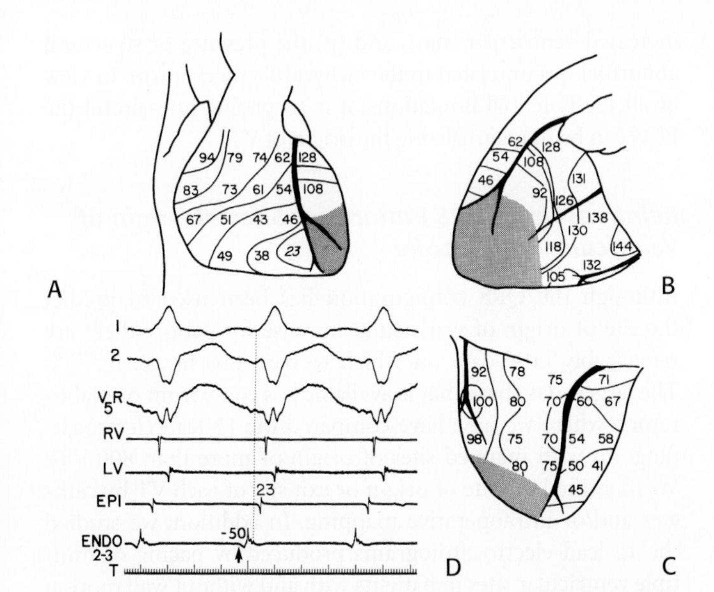


**FIGURE 11-257** Relationship of endocardial and epicardial mapping in VT with a left bundle branch block morphology. Isochronic maps of a VT with a left bundle branch block are shown in **(A)**, the anterior **(B)**, left lateral, and **(C)** inferior (bottom right) views. The stippled area represents the site of a prior infarction and LV-An. During the tachycardia, the earliest ventricular activation breaks through at the apex of the right ventricle. Right ventricular activation is completed before left ventricular activation. **D:** Three ECG leads, RV and LV references, and the earliest epicardial site (EPI) and endocardial site are shown. The earliest epicardial site is at the RV apex while the site recorded during the tachycardia was on the midapical third of the left ventricular septum See text for discussion.

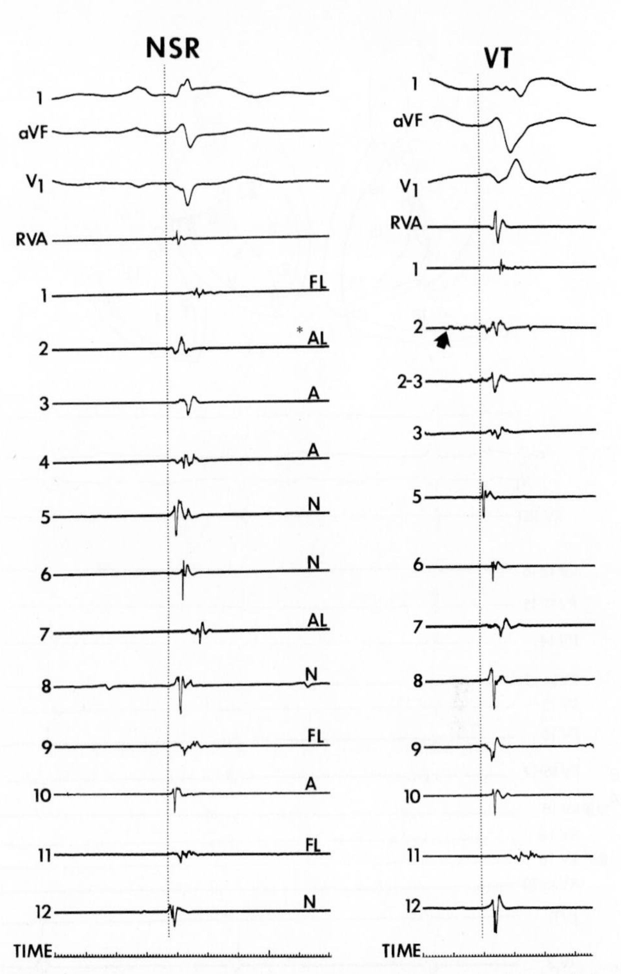


**FIGURE 11-258** Analog map from a patient in sinus rhythm and during VT. Three surface ECG leads (I, aVF, and $V_1$) are shown with one electrogram from the RVA and electrograms from the 12 standard left ventricular sites. The dotted vertical lines define the onset of the surface QRS activity. During sinus rhythm, eight sites demonstrate abnormal (A), fractionated (F), or late (L) electrical activity. Only four sites were normal. During VT, the site of earliest activity is at site 2. In sinus rhythm, however, site 2 is neither the most abnormal nor the latest. See text for discussion. (From Cassidy DM, Vassallo JA, Buxton AE, et al. The value of catheter mapping during sinus rhythm to localize site of origin of ventricular tachycardia. *Circulation* 1984;69:1103.)

Biosense, Carto system (and more recently, Navix and Rhythmia) allows for voltage mapping, late potential and duration mapping, which supports our earlier work in identifying arrhythmogenic tissue. An example of such maps and the relationship of abnormalities recorded during sinus rhythm to the site of successful ablation at an entrainment map defined protected isthmus is shown in Figure 11-260. Because these electrograms probably represent **potential** arrhythmogenic sites (i.e., a specific anatomic substrate), when one cannot map a tachycardia, the use of such abnormal and/or late electrograms to develop and guide ablation lesions is reasonable. Preliminary studies suggest these areas can be bisected or encircled by radiofrequency lesions and successfully eliminate VTs.[61] Some investigators suggest homogenization of the endocardial and epicardial area of low-voltage and abnormal electrograms[406] (see Chapter 13 for discussion). In view of the limitations of voltage mapping related to catheter electrode size and orientation as well as the effects of the wavefront of activation described earlier, this approach clearly destroys tissue that does not need destruction and may miss tissue that does.

Approximately 15% of tachycardias, however, will arise at sites that appear normal during sinus rhythm.[31] Currently, there is no way to identify which normal sites are potentially arrhythmogenic; however, evaluating the response of such electrograms to ventricular pacing and extrastimuli might provide some insight into this question (Fig. 11-261). Preliminary data in our laboratory suggest that normal electrograms that ultimately turn out to be sites of origin of VTs demonstrate diminution in amplitude, fractionation, and a prolongation of duration that is significantly greater than normal electrograms that do not turn out to be sites of origin. Further work is necessary to see whether this would be of predictive value and hence can be used clinically.

## Relationship of QRS Morphologies to Sites of Origin of Tachycardias

To evaluate whether or not the QRS morphology of VT can be used to localize sites of origin, three questions must be addressed. The first two address the issue of whether specific QRS patterns are associated with specific sites of impulse formation in the ventricle. We have compared the QRS morphologies and sites of

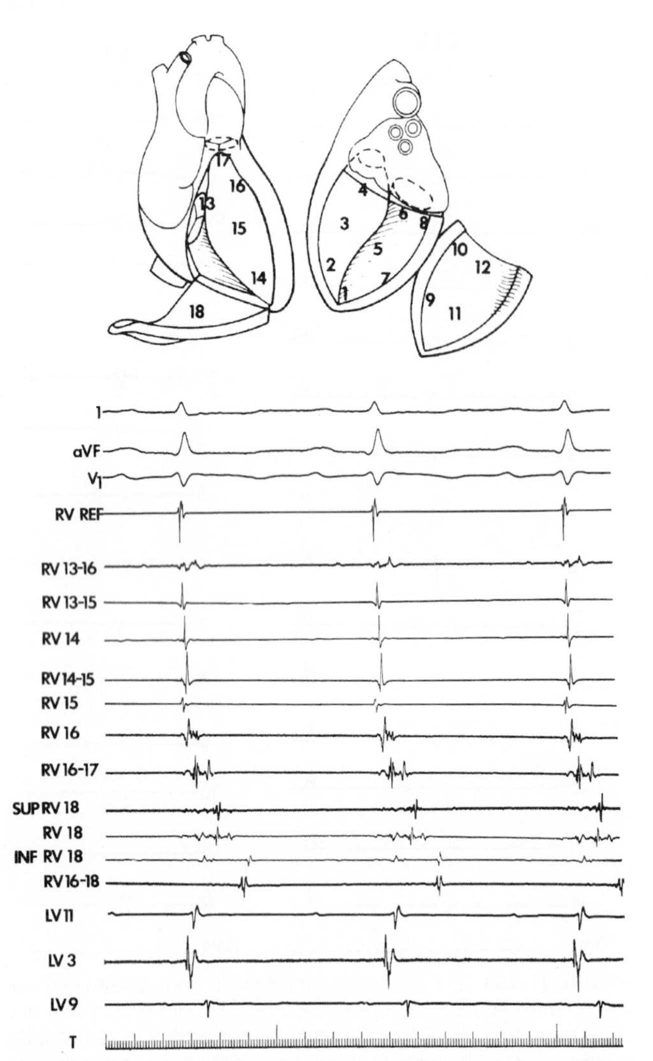


**FIGURE 11-259** Sinus rhythm map in a patient with right ventricular dysplasia. ECG leads and an RV reference are shown along with multiple sites from the RV and LV. Note the marked abnormality of electrograms in the right ventricular free wall. Electrical activity extending nearly 200 msec beyond the end of the QRS is seen at site 18 and sites 16 to 18. Note that the LV electrograms are normal. See text for discussion.

origin or exit sites of tachycardias in patients undergoing endocardial mapping.[9,10] We also analyzed the QRS morphologies of pacing specific endocardial sites in patients without tachycardias.[393] The third question to address is the hypothesis that a paced QRS morphology (during sinus rhythm) that matches that of spontaneous tachycardia would identify the pacing site as the origin of a focal VT or the exit site of a reentrant VT of the tachycardia.[392] We have performed these studies, which have demonstrated both the usefulness and limitations of the QRS morphology to identify sites of origin and of pace mapping to localize site of origin of VT. Factors influencing the ability of QRS patterns to localize VT origin include (a) the presence and size of infarction, (b) the degree of fibrosis, the shape of the heart in the chest cavity, (c) the site and mechanism of VT within an infarct or scarred area, (d) the effect of nonuniform anisotropy and propagation from the site of origin, (e) the effects of acute ischemia and/or electrolyte abnormalities, (f) the presence of increased ventricular mass, and (g) the presence of structural abnormalities unrelated to the tachycardia mechanism. In view of all the potential limitations, it is surprising how useful the ECG can be in regionalizing the origin of VT.

### *Relationship of QRS Patterns of Sites of Origin of Ventricular Tachycardia*

Although the QRS configuration has been used to predict the site of origin of ventricular impulse formation, there are remarkably little data on which to base this usage.[9,10,391–395] The largest data base that is available has come from our laboratory, where we now have compared the 12-lead electrocardiogram with mapped sites of origin of more than 800 VTs. We identified the site of origin or exit site of each VT by catheter and/or intraoperative mapping. In addition, we studied the 12-lead electrocardiograms produced by pacing of multiple ventricular sites in patients with and without wall motion abnormalities.[393] Similar studies analyzing the 12-lead electrocardiographic patterns and response to left ventricular pacing have been used by others to develop algorithms to identify "sites of origin" of VT.[394,395] Although QS complexes in leads expected to have a small R wave due to endo to epi activation suggest epicardial origin in normal hearts or in those with cardiomyopathy (in the latter case, this is an inherent bias because of the more common origin of VT in the epicardium and subepicardium), similar QS complexes may be seen in VTs with endocardial origins in the presence of prior infarction.

In general, QRS patterns are less accurate predictors of the exit sites or protected isthmuses of reentrant VTs in patients with prior infarction and wall motion abnormalities than they are for focal VTs in patients with normal ventricles. The pattern of ventricular activation and hence, resultant QRS, depends on how the wavefront propagates from the site of origin to the remainder of the heart; this may be totally different during the tachycardia than during pacing from the same site in sinus rhythm. In fact pacing during sinus rhythm in the center of an isthmus during reentrant VT would be expected to produce a different QRS than the VT since the paced wavefront spreads centrifugally to the heart while the VT wavefront moves in one direction (i.e., orthodromic). This latter observation is one of the important limitations of the use of pace mapping to identify the "site of origin" of VT. While there may be a better relationship of the paced QRS to the VT QRS in VTs with focal mechanisms in normal hearts, there is an inherent physical limitation of mapping or stimulation techniques to identify the site of origin of the tachycardia such that reproducible catheter placement in the ventricle can only be accomplished in an area of a few square centimeters. Furthermore bipolar pacing stimulates an area of $\approx 1\ cm^2$, further limiting the accuracy of this technique. In the presence of infarction this limitation is exaggerated since high currents are often used.

Our initial studies demonstrated that it was possible to separate apical from basal sites based on comparisons of 12-lead ECGs and mapped exit sites of reentrant VTs or analyzing the

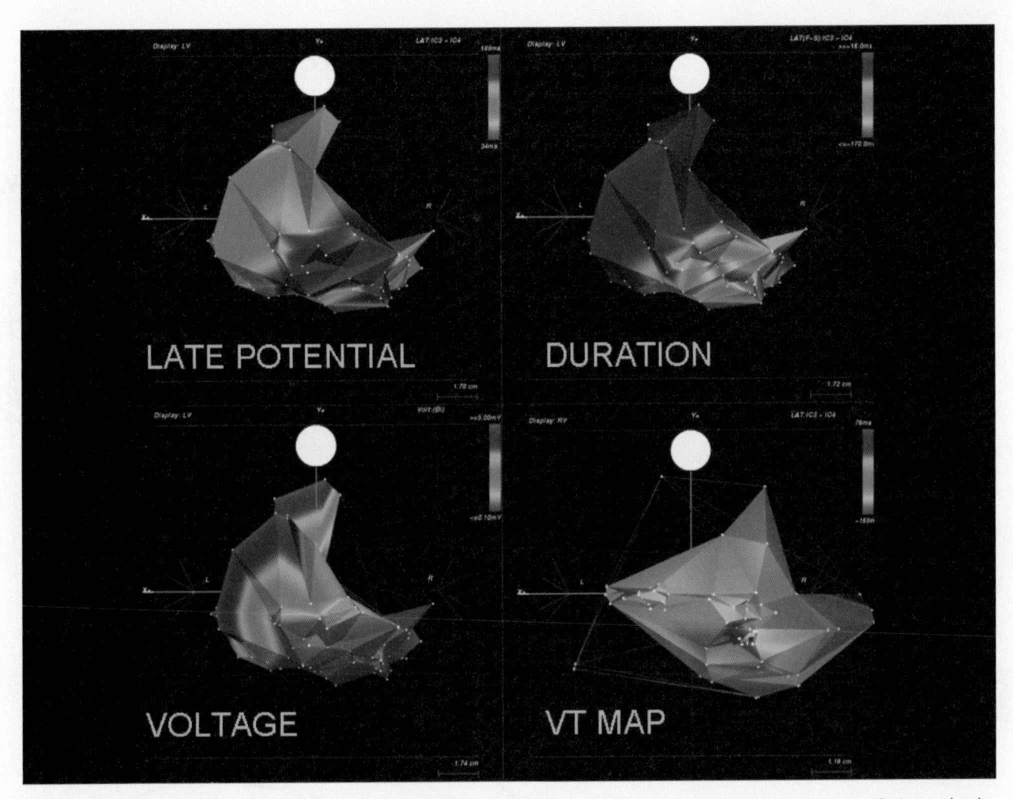


**FIGURE 11-260** Substrate mapping in a patient with VT associated with coronary artery disease. Comparison of sinus rhythm mapping and VT mapping in a patient with VT and old inferior infarction. Clockwise from upper left. Late potential, duration, VT, and voltage maps recorded using the Carto system. The heart is viewed in the PA position. Electrograms of latest activation (*purple*), longest duration (*red*), lowest voltage (*red*), correlate with the critical isthmus of VT (*red*).

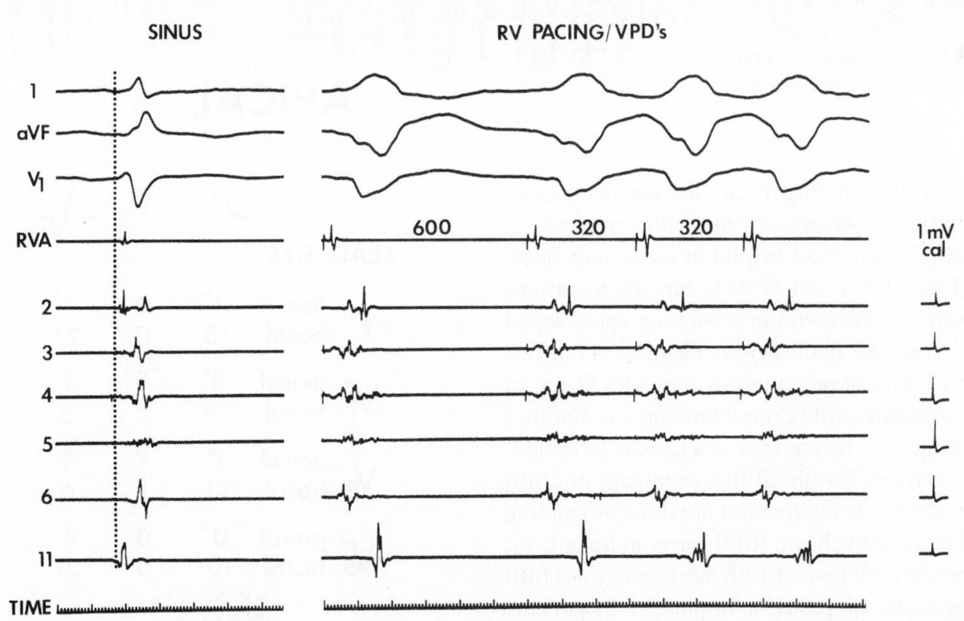


**FIGURE 11-261** Response of normal and abnormal electrograms to ventricular pacing and extrastimuli. Electrograms from multiple left ventricular sites are shown during sinus rhythm and during right ventricular pacing with two ventricular premature depolarizations (VPDs). Electrograms from sites 2, 3, 4, and 5 are abnormal in sinus rhythm, while those from sites 6 and 11 are normal. In response to ventricular pacing, only modest changes are seen in site 6, and site 11 remains totally normal. Following double extrastimuli, however, site 6 remains mildly changed, but there is a marked change in site 11. Note that site 2, which had a split potential during sinus rhythm, remained almost unchanged during both pacing and ventricular extrastimuli with a reversal of the early and late components of the electrogram. Sites 3, 4, and 5 became progressively more abnormal. See text for discussion.

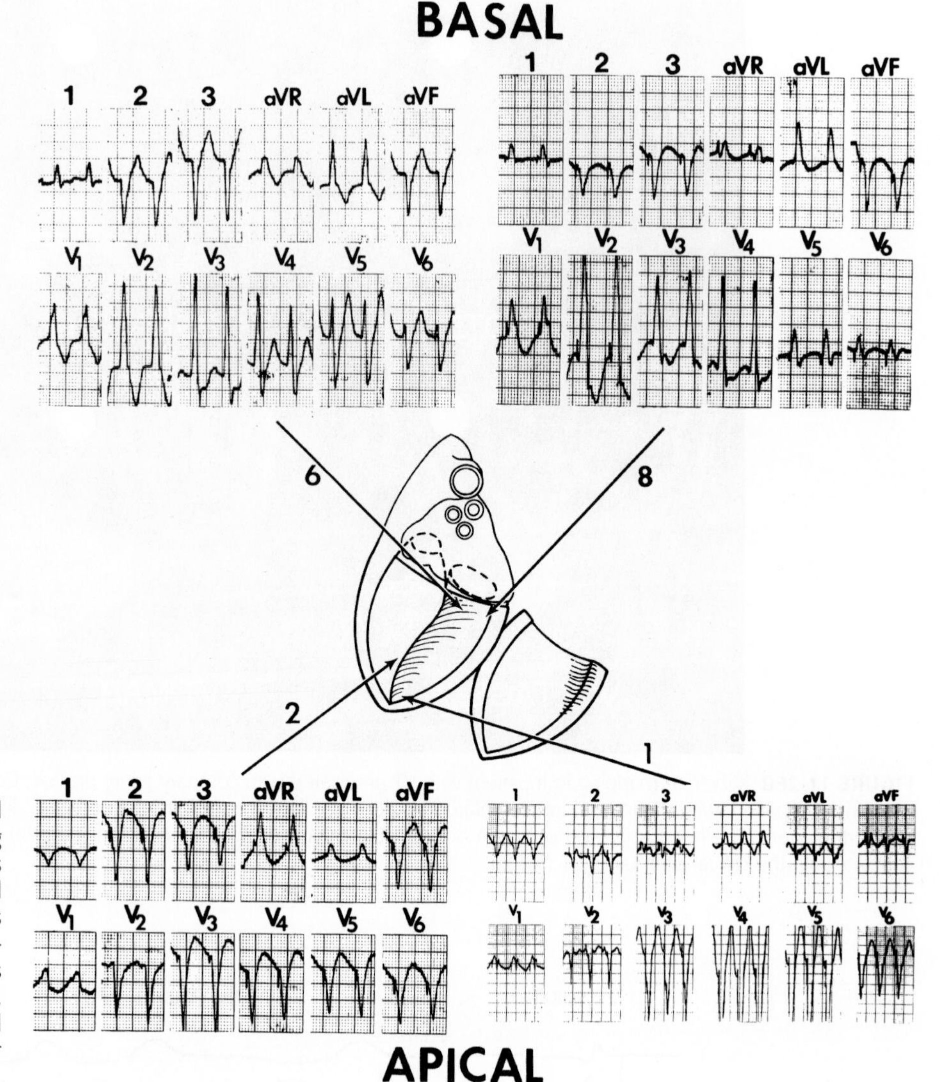


**FIGURE 11-262** Representative 12-lead ECGs recorded during endocardial pacing at basal and apical sites. Twelve-lead ECGs from basal sites 6 and 8 are shown and from apical sites 1 and 2. All four examples manifest right bundle branch block configuration. Note that basal sites have R waves in leads 1 and VE as well as in $V_1$ and $V_2$, whereas apical sites have Q waves in 1 and $V_6$ and a loss of R wave in $V_2$. See text for discussion.

resultant 12-lead ECG from pacing specific left ventricular sites during sinus rhythm.[392,393] Analyses of the QRS complexes in leads 1, $V_1$, $V_2$, and $V_6$ were most helpful in separating apical from basal sites (Figs. 11-262 and 11-263), but configurations in similar leads were far less useful in separating apical septal from apical lateral sites. Our findings were identical in our initial correlation of VT sites of origin or exit sites with ECGs. In summary, for VTs associated with prior infarction, our findings revealed the following: (a) The presence of a Q wave in leads 1, $V_1$, $V_2$, and $V_6$ was seen in VTs with RBBB morphology or LBBB morphology originating near the apex but not those originating in the inferobasal parts of the heart. (b) R waves in leads 1, $V_1$, $V_2$, and $V_6$ were specific for VT with RBBB morphology or LBBB morphology, respectively, of posterior origin. (c) In patients with LBBB morphology, the presence of a Q wave in leads 1 and $V_6$ was associated with an apical septal location, while the presence of an R wave in 1 and $V_6$ was associated with inferobasal septal origin. When ECGs showed both right and LBBB patterns from the same exit area of origin, their morphologies were characteristic of apical or basal locations (Figs. 11-264 and 11-265).

| LEAD | SITE | | | | | |
|---|---|---|---|---|---|---|
| $I^{\circ}$ | apical | $1^{ns}$ | 0 | $4^{\bullet}$ | $5^{ns}$ | $18^{\circ}$ |
| | basal | 13 | 0 | 25 | 0 | 8 |
| $V_1^{\bullet}$ | apical | $8^{\bullet}$ | $5^{ns}$ | $1^{ns}$ | $11^{ns}$ | $3^{ns}$ |
| | basal | 29 | 2 | 3 | 12 | 0 |
| $V_2^{\circ}$ | apical | $1^{\circ}$ | $1^{ns}$ | $3^{ns}$ | $4^{ns}$ | $19^{\circ}$ |
| | basal | 33 | 1 | 6 | 6 | 0 |
| $V_6^{\circ}$ | apical | $0^{ns}$ | 0 | $4^{\circ}$ | 0 | $24^{\circ}$ |
| | basal | 10 | 0 | 31 | 0 | 5 |

ns P = NS
• P < 0.01
° P < 0.001

**FIGURE 11-263** Frequency of QRS configurations observed in ECG leads I, $V_1$, $V_2$, and $V_6$ during pacing at apical (sites 1 and 2) compared with that at basal (sites 4, 6, 8, 10, and 72) locations. (From Waxman HL, Josephson ME. Ventricular activation during ventricular endocardial pacing. I. Electrocardiographic patterns related to the site of pacing. *Am J Cardiol* 1982;50:1.)

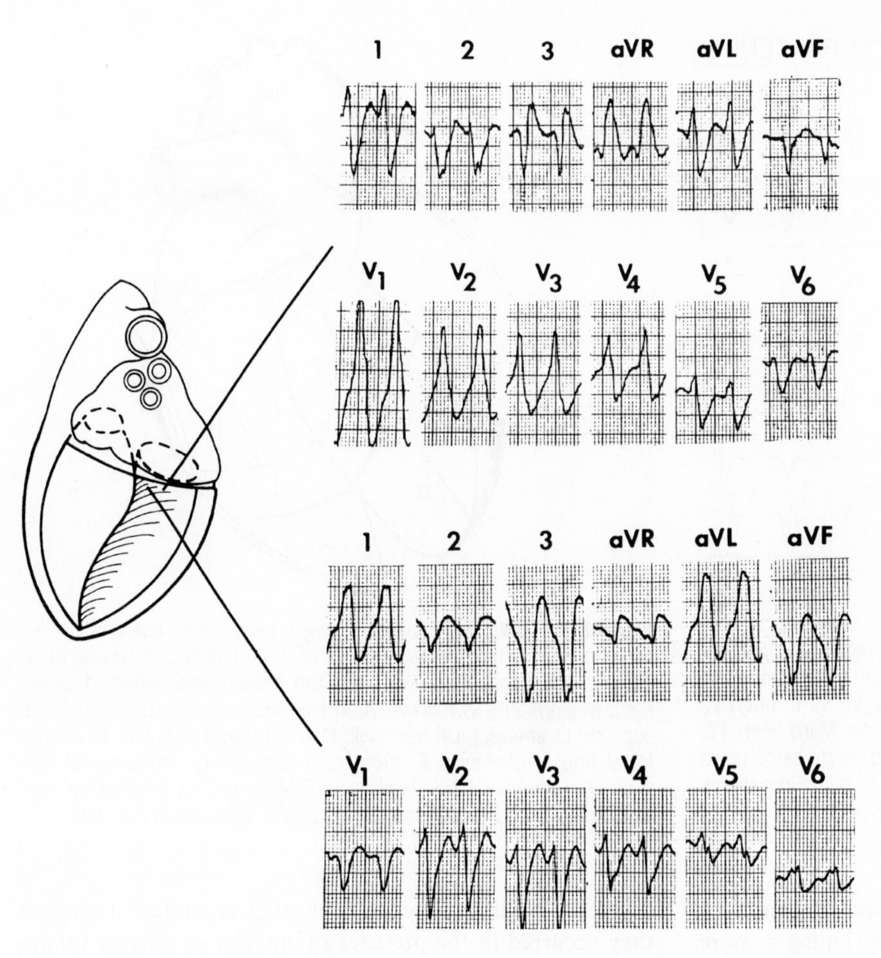


**FIGURE 11-264** Ventricular tachycardia with right and left bundle branch block morphologies originating at the same posterobasal site. A schematized LV is shown with two tachycardias arising from site 6 at the inferior wall. On top is a right bundle branch block and on the bottom is a left bundle branch block. Both morphologically distinct tachycardias rose from the same area. (From Josephson ME, Horowitz LN, Waxman HL, et al. Sustained ventricular tachycardia: role of the 12-lead electrocardiogram in localizing site of origin. *Circulation* 1981;64:257.)

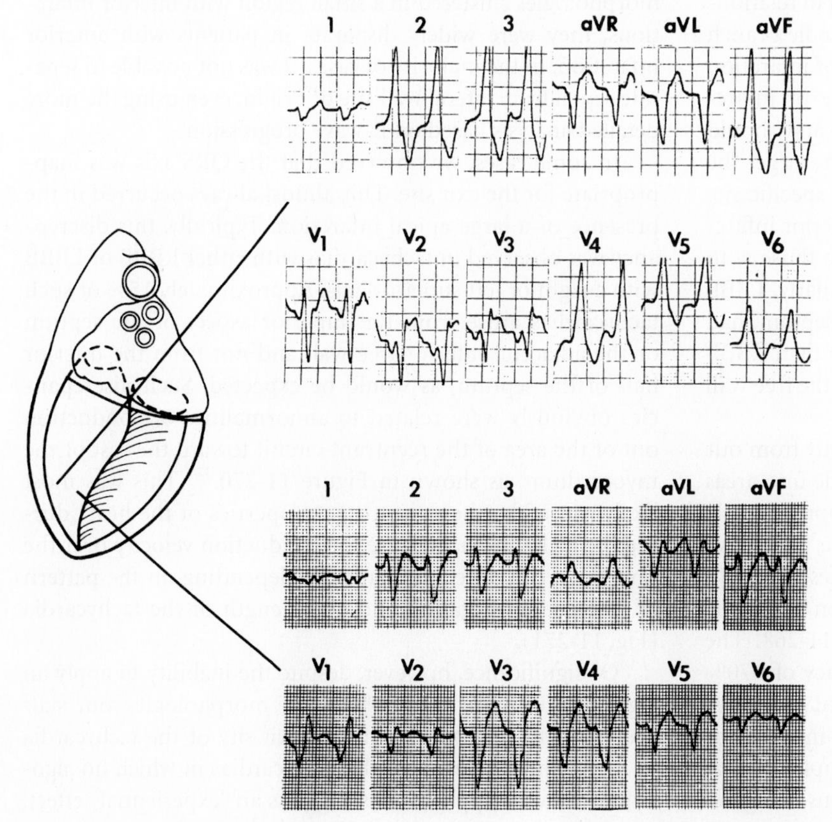


**FIGURE 11-265** Ventricular tachycardias with right and left bundle branch block morphologies arising at similar anteroseptal sites. The LV is schematically shown. Left bundle branch block with inferior axis (**top**) and a right bundle branch block, right superior axis (**bottom**) originate within 1 cm of each other. (From Josephson ME, Horowitz LN, Waxman HL, et al. Sustained ventricular tachycardia: role of the 12-lead electrocardiogram in localizing site of origin. *Circulation* 1981;64:257.)

PRECORDIAL R–WAVE PROGRESSION PATTERNS

| PATTERN (NO.) | $V_1$ | $V_2$ | $V_3$ | $V_4$ | $V_5$ | $V_6$ |
|---|---|---|---|---|---|---|
| INCREASING (30) | | | | | | |
| NONE OR LATE (27) | | | | | | |
| REGRESSION/GROWTH (NOT QS) (18) | | | | | | |
| REGRESSION/GROWTH (QS) (15) | | | | | | |
| DOMINANT (15) | | | | | | |
| ABRUPT LOSS (20) | | | | | | |
| LATE REVERSE (41) | | | | | | |
| EARLY REVERSE (16) | | | | | | |

**FIGURE 11-266** Precordial R-wave progression patterns. Eight different R-wave progression patterns are listed, with the number of examples in parentheses. Typical R-wave patterns for $V_1$ through $V_6$ are shown. See text for discussion. (From Miller JM, Marchlinski FE, Buxton AE, et al. Relationship between the 12-lead electrocardiogram during ventricular tachycardia and endocardial site of origin in patients with coronary artery disease. *Circulation* 1988;77:759.)

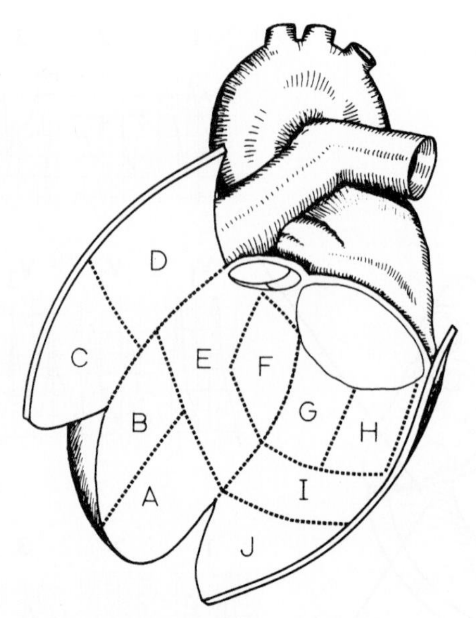


**FIGURE 11-267** Regions of VT origin used to assess the predictive accuracy of the 12-lead EGG. The LV is depicted as having been opened along the lateral wall with the anterior wall reflected to the right. Regions are as follows: A, inferoapical septum; B, anteroapical septum; C, anteroapical free wall; D, anterobasal free wall; E, anterobasal and midseptum; F, inferobasal septum; G, inferomedial free wall; H, inferolateral free wall; I, midinferior wall; J, inferoapical free wall. Areas G and H together constitute the inferobasal free wall.

We more recently tried to enhance the specificity and predictive accuracy of the 12-lead ECG by developing a more "sophisticated" algorithm using eight different patterns of R-wave progression in the precordium in addition to relationship with prior infarction, axis deviation, and bundle branch block morphology (Fig. 11-266).[10] Although site of infarction is not an electrocardiographic criterion, the site of infarction can significantly influence the ECG pattern and should be taken into consideration for any algorithm. The larger the infarct, the less predictive are ECG patterns for a specific site of origin. Thus, ECG patterns associated with anterior infarction were less likely to predict sites of origin than those with inferior patterns (37% vs. 74%, $p$ <0.001).[10] Similarly, LBBB patterns, which all cluster on or adjacent to the septum, had a higher predictive accuracy for exit site of origin than RBBB morphology, which could be septal or located on the free wall (73% vs. 31%, $p$ <0.001).[10]

Using a schema of the heart that differed slightly from our mapping schema but that divided the left ventricle into areas of approximately 15 cm$^2$ (Fig. 11-267), only approximately one-half of the tachycardia morphologies were predictive for a specific site of origin. The mapped exit sites and QRS morphologies of 182 consecutive reentrant VTs on which the algorithm was developed are shown in Figure 11-268. The algorithms we developed had a predictive accuracy of >70% for a specific QRS morphology to identify an exit site. They are shown in Figure 11-269. We did not include in the algorithm VT morphologies with less than five examples of that pattern. LBBB left superior or inferior axis patterns had good predictive accuracy for exit site of origin regardless of whether they occurred in the presence of anterior or inferior infarction. On the other hand, although the vast majority of RBBB morphologies clustered in a small region with inferior infarctions, they were widely disparate in patients with anterior infarction. In the majority of cases, it was not possible to separate septal from lateral wall site of origin, even using the more detailed analysis based on R-wave progression.

In some cases, we observed that the QRS axis was inappropriate for the exit site. This almost always occurred in the presence of a large apical infarction. Typically, this discrepancy was observed in tachycardias with either RBBB or LBBB with a right or left superior axis. Approximately 15% of such tachycardias arose from the superior aspect of the septum or the adjacent anterior free wall and not from the inferior half of the septum, as would be expected. Such discrepancies obviously were related to abnormalities of conduction out of the area of the reentrant circuit toward the rest of the myocardium, as shown in Figure 11-270.[374] This was most likely caused by the anisotropic properties of the heart during the tachycardia, because the conduction velocity over the same area can differ dramatically, depending on the pattern of impulse propagation and cycle length of the tachycardia (Fig. 11-271).

Of significance, however, despite the inability to apply an algorithm to more than 50% of VT morphologies, our staff was correctly able to identify the exit site of the tachycardia in nearly three quarters of the tachycardias in which no algorithm could be applied. This suggests an "experiential" effect,

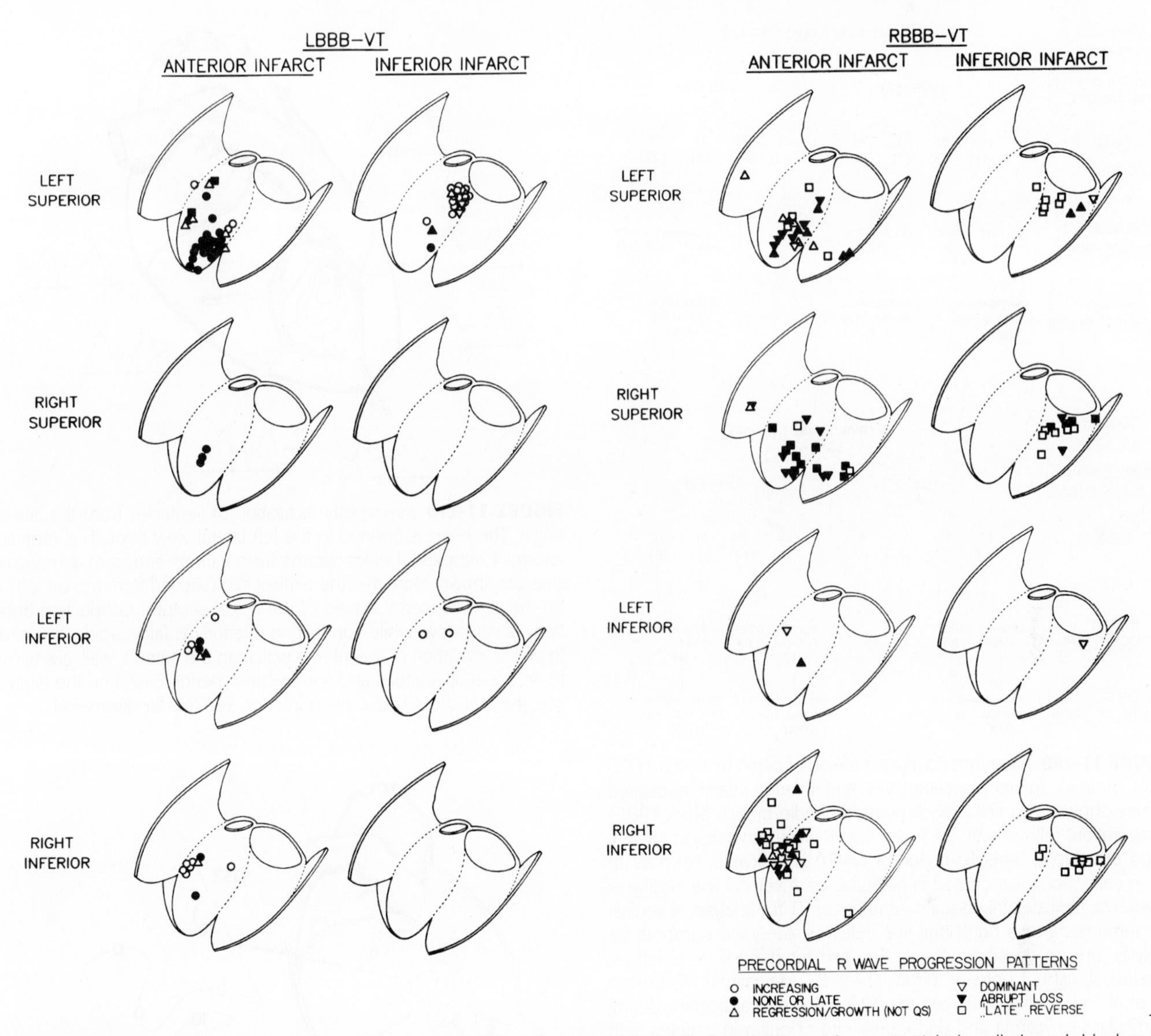


**FIGURE 11-268** Mapped sites of origin for 182 VTs. **A.** Left bundle branch block VTs (LBBB-VT) are shown. B. Right bundle branch block tachycardias (RBBB-VT). **A** and **B:** Among each bundle branch block type, anterior infarcts are shown on the left and inferior on the right. QRS axis is segregated by infarct and morphology. The left ventricular endocardium is displayed as in Figure 11-267. Each characteristic morphology is plotted according to the key. (From Miller JM, Marchlinski FE, Buxton AE, et al. Relationship between the 12-lead electrocardiogram during ventricular tachycardia and endocardial site of origin in patients with coronary artery disease. *Circulation* 1988;77:759.)

which we have been heretofore unable to characterize and develop into an algorithm. Regardless of the limitations of the ECG, in the majority of cases, an exit area from which a tachycardia is likely to arise can be determined by the 12-lead ECG. A lack of precision in identifying the precise exit site is expected; however, the ability to regionalize a tachycardia can facilitate mapping of that tachycardia by allowing the investigator to focus on a specific region.

## Role of Pace Mapping in Determining the Site of Origin of Ventricular Tachycardia

Because it may not be possible to map all VTs that occur either spontaneously or are initiated in the laboratory, pace mapping has been suggested as a means to identify the site of origin of tachycardias that are not mapped. By this technique, the site from which pacing produces the same QRS morphology as VT would identify the exit site of origin of that tachycardia.[394] However, we have previously shown, particularly for anterior infarction, that the QRS morphology may not correlate with a specific site of origin[392,393] regardless of whether that site of origin is determined by mapping during VT or by pacing from a specific site. Thus, it is not surprising that pace mapping suffers from the same limitations. Although it is not uncommon to have a similar or even nearly identical morphology result when pacing a known site of origin or exit site determined by mapping (Figs. 11-272 and 11-273), pacing various sites within the ventricle and producing a QRS morphologic pattern identical to the tachycardia in the absence of a known site of origin is extremely difficult. Even when one knows the general

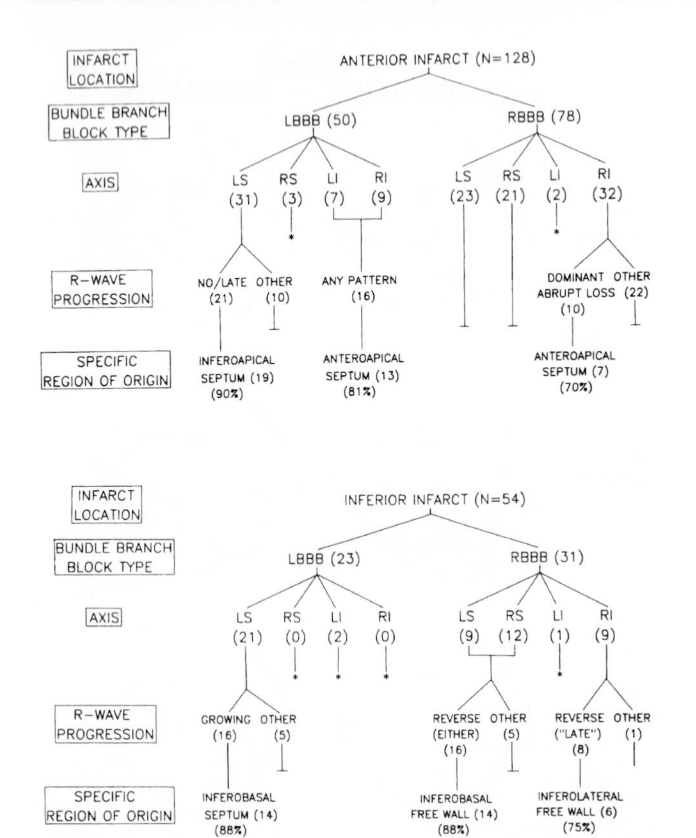


**FIGURE 11-269** Algorithm correlating region of origin to 12-lead ECG of VT. Anterior infarct-associated VTs and inferior infarct-associated VTs are shown. The first branch point is bundle branch block (BBE) configuration, followed by QRS axis, and R-wave progression (RWP). When possible, a "specific region of origin" is indicated. Number of VTs in each group is indicated in parentheses. A vertical line ending in an asterisk indicates inadequate numbers of VT for analysis; a vertical line terminating in a horizontal line indicates adequate numbers for analysis, but no specific patterns. See text for discussion. L, left; S, superior; fl, right, 1, inferior. (From Miller JM, Marchlinski FE, Buxton AE, et al. Relationship between the 12-lead electrocardiogram during ventricular tachycardia and endocardial site of origin in patients with coronary artery disease. *Circulation* 1988;77:759.)

region from which the tachycardia must originate, because of limitations described earlier, pacing within 2 cm can result in morphologies of different axes or on occasion even different bundle branch block configurations (Fig. 11-274). This may be explained by the fact that the most similar paced morphologies to the VT should be near the exit while pacing from the area of the entrance should give rise to a totally different QRS. DeChilou et al.[407] have taken advantage of these findings to define the isthmus of reentrant VT and bisect it be a aline of ablation in the area where the pace map goes from good to bad. This will be discussed further in Chapter 13. A prospective study is needed to confirm these findings. The presence of multiple morphologies ornon-inducible arrhythmias limits this approach.

The angle of contact of the catheter to the ventricular wall and the area over which the current is delivered (particularly where high current is required for relatively inexcitable tissue) can influence the pattern of subsequent ventricular activation.

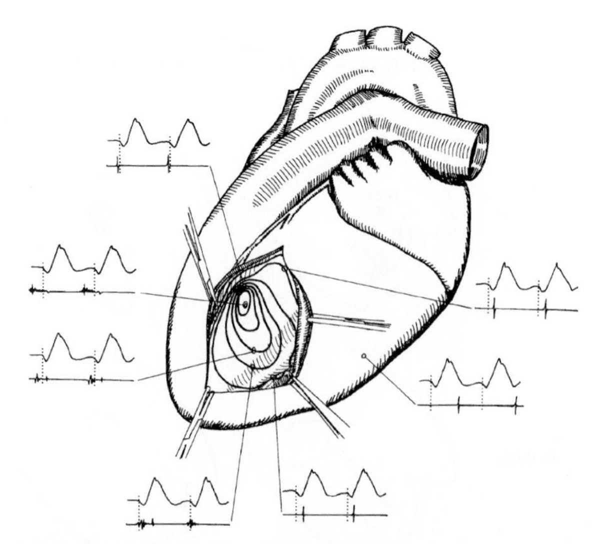

**FIGURE 11-270** Asymmetric activation of ventricles from the site of origin. The heart is opened in the left lateral view through a ventriculotomy. Examples of electrograms from various endocardial mapping sites are shown. Note that the earliest site (second from top on left) is on the anterosuperior aspect of the apical septum. Conduction anteriorly is very slow, while conduction inferiorly is fairly rapid. This leads to earlier activation of the inferior wall than the anterior wall, giving rise to an axis that is lateral and somewhat superior. Based on the earliest site, the axis should have been inferior. See text for discussion.

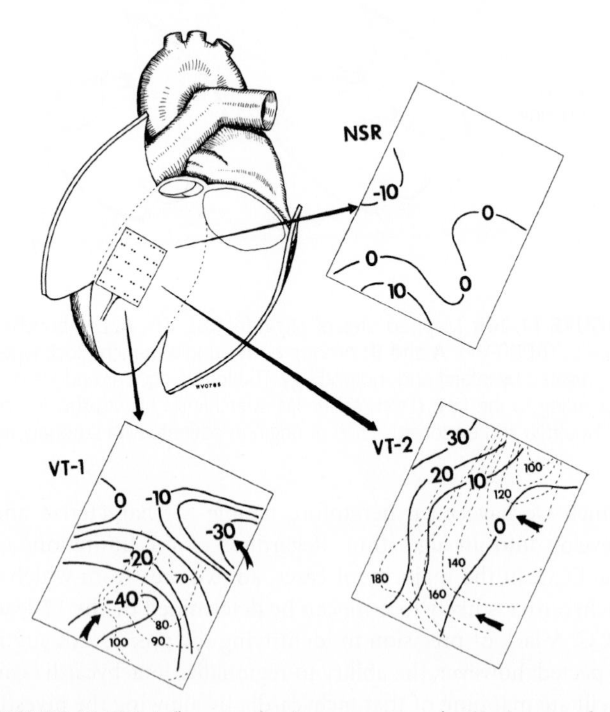


**FIGURE 11-271** Influence of anisotropy on conduction in area of origin. A schema of the heart is shown with a 20 bipolar plaque placed over the site of origin of tachycardia $V_1$. Two tachycardias arose from areas underneath this plaque, which had an area of approximately 4 cm$^2$. Note that conduction parameters in VT-1 are totally different from those in VT-2. Moreover, conduction during NSR is much more rapid than in both tachycardias. This demonstrates the functional nature of conduction disturbances, which influence the rapidity of propagation and the wave of propagation of impulses in the same area. See text for discussion.

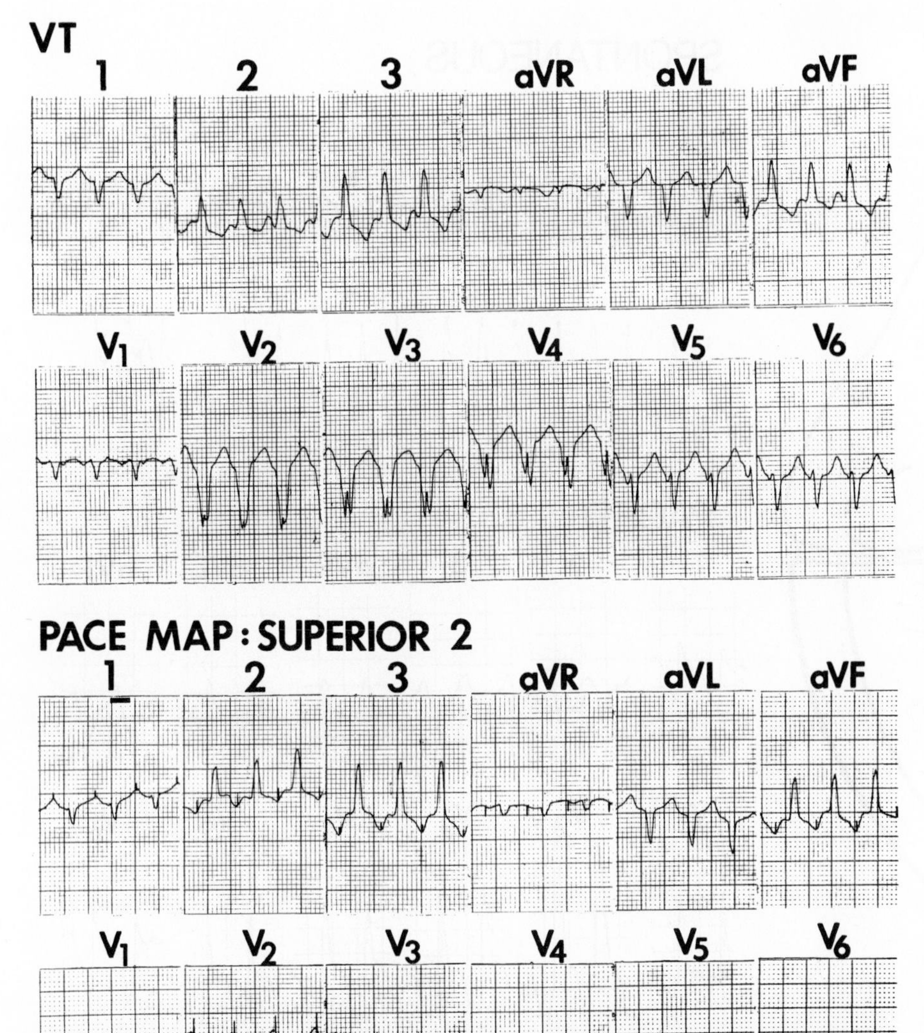


**FIGURE 11-272** Pace mapping of a tachycardia originating at the superior apical septum. VT is shown with a left bundle branch block inferior axis morphology. Pacing from that site produces a similar, but not identical, QRS as the tachycardia morphology. Note the long stimulus-to-QRS interval of approximately 140 msec. This was similar to the degree of presystolic activity at that site. See text for discussion.

Because the QRS morphology depends on global activation, and is centrifugal in response to pacing in sinus rhythm, pacing will most frequently result in a different (to a greater or lesser degree) QRS morphology than during the tachycardia. This is a major limitation of the use of pace mapping in absence of an inducible VT. Although an "exact" match usually means that the pacing site is close to the exit site of the tachycardia, exact matches are rare. Conversely, if one paces during the tachycardia, and entrains the VT, it may be possible to replicate the VT morphology by pacing sites distant from exit site, because the tachycardia wavefront will influence the pattern of activation of the stimulated wavefront. The stimulated wavefront is "physiologically forced" to follow the same route of activation as the tachycardia during entrainment such that the resultant QRS will mimic the tachycardia QRS as long as pacing is carried out between the entrance and exit of the protected isthmus. This can be accomplished over an area of several centimeters and provides one of the diagnostic features of entrainment mapping.

A method by which pace mapping can be further refined is to demonstrate that activation to different sites, such as the RV reference electrogram, is the same during pacing as during the tachycardia (Fig. 11-275). This would further corroborate that the stimulation site is near the tachycardia exit site and that the wave of activation from this site is similar to that during VT. However, differences in conduction during pacing in sinus rhythm and VT originating or exiting at the same site can lead to different patterns of ventricular activation. An identical match is useful, but absence of a match does not mean one is not at or near the site of origin or exit site. Thus, I believe that pace mapping remains at best a corroborative method of localizing tachycardias. Pacing during a tachycardia in combination with activation mapping of VT and resetting provide the optimal method of identifying the

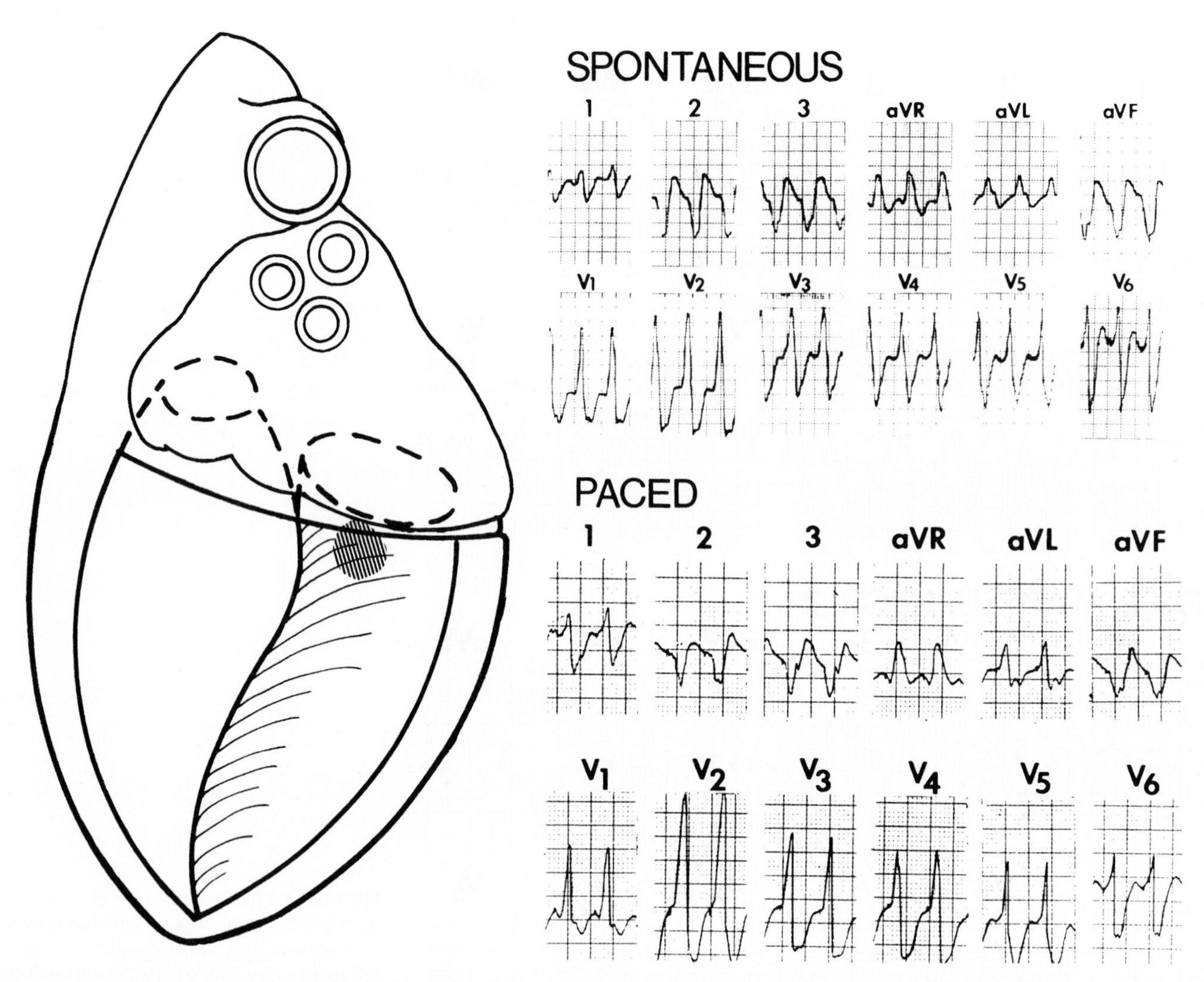


**FIGURE 11-273** Pace mapping of a tachycardia from the inferobasal part of the heart. The heart is opened up on the left, with the shaded area identifying the site of origin. Spontaneous tachycardia is shown with a right bundle, right superior axis morphology. Pacing from the site almost reproduces the tachycardia morphology. (From Josephson ME, Waxman HL, Cain ME, et al. Ventricular activation during ventricular endocardial pacing II. Role of pace-mapping to localize origin of ventricular tachycardia. *Am J Cardiol* 1982;50:11.)

site of origin. If one cannot map tachycardias using the methods outlined earlier in the chapter, pace mapping coupled with substrate mapping (i.e., abnormalities of electrograms that identify potential arrhythmogenic substrates) may provide information upon which ablation can be directed. This will be discussed further in Chapter 13.

## VENTRICULAR STIMULATION IN MISCELLANEOUS DISORDERS

Although sustained and nonsustained VT are arrhythmias for which electrophysiologic studies may provide useful information concerning both mechanism and therapy, there is less agreement about the use of electrophysiologic studies in other situations. The use of programmed stimulation in patients with isolated VPCs should be regarded as highly experimental. The use of programmed stimulation following myocardial infarction to identify patients at high/low risk is controversial. Recent studies from Australia have confirmed the utility of programed stimulation for risk stratification postinfarction.[28,143,144] The results of the MADIT[306] and MUSTT[293] trials suggested that, in the presence of a diminished ejection fraction (<40%) and nonsustained VT in patients with coronary artery disease, induction of sustained monomorphic VT predicts increased risk of sudden death and total mortality, both of which are reduced by ICDs. Although we clearly need better methods to identify patients at high risk for the development of sustained arrhythmias and/or sudden death, at this date recommendation of electrophysiologic studies for this purpose is limited to the aforementioned highly selected group. In the future, programmed stimulation and/or other noninvasive tests may be used to identify high-risk patients. Until such combined data can

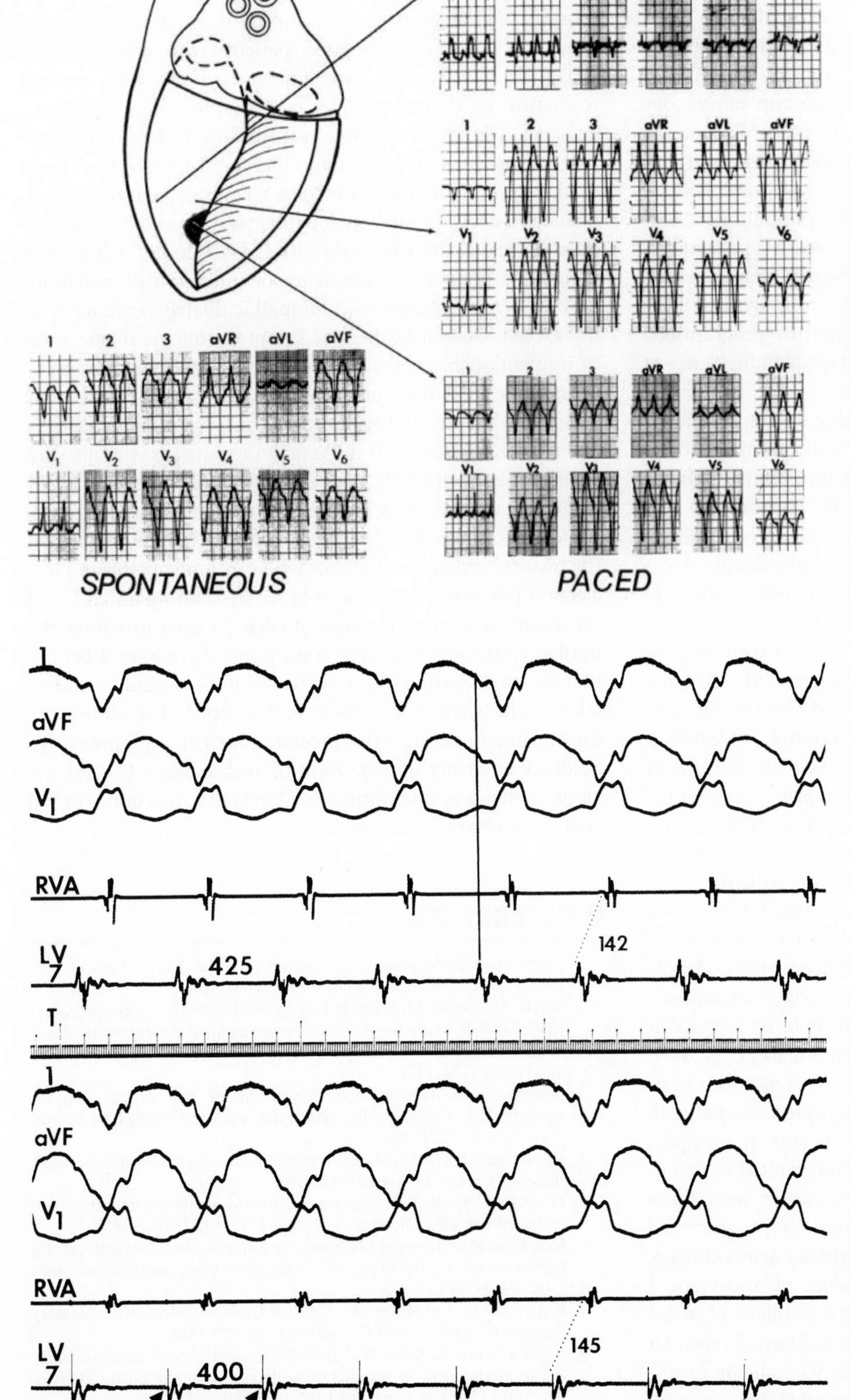


**FIGURE 11-274** Pace mapping from the same and adjacent sites. The heart is schematically shown with the shaded area indicating the site of origin of the spontaneous tachycardia (**bottom left**). Pacing from that site (**bottom right**) replicates the tachycardia. Pacing 1 cm away on the septum produces either a similar morphology (**middle right**) or a totally different morphology with an inferior axis (**top right**). See text for discussion. (From Josephson ME, Waxman HL, Cain ME, et al. Ventricular activation during ventricular endocardial pacing II. Role of pace-mapping to localize origin of ventricular tachycardia. *Am J Cardiol* 1982;50:11.)

**FIGURE 11-275** Comparison of ECG morphology and interventricular conduction time during VT and pacing. ECG leads 1, aVF, and $V_1$ are shown with a reference electrogram from the RVA and from site 1 in the LV. Site 1 was the site from which the earliest presystolic activity could be recorded. Conduction time from site 1 to the RVA recording was 142 msec during the tachycardia. Pacing at this site during sinus rhythm at a rate similar to that during tachycardia resulted in an identical QRS pattern and an interventricular conduction time similar to that during VT. (Adapted from Josephson ME, Horowitz LN, Spielman SR, et al. Comparison of endocardial catheter mapping with intraoperative mapping of ventricular tachycardia. *Circulation* 1980;61:395.)

identify a high-risk group, it is inappropriate to recommend the use of electrophysiologic studies as a routine method for "risk stratification."

One area where programmed ventricular stimulation has been useful is in the evaluation of patients with syncope.[408–416] Syncope is an extremely common disorder for which in many instances one cannot determine the cause. This is particularly true in patients without organic heart disease. After a careful history and physical exam, the workup of syncope should obviously include a workup for neurocardiac causes, sinus node dysfunction, A-V conduction disorders (particularly when bundle branch block is present), supraventricular tachyarrhythmias, and most importantly, programmed ventricular stimulation when organic heart disease is present. We have found that nearly 50% of patients with cardiac disease, particularly prior infarction, who suffer from syncope have sustained and/or symptomatic VT induced by programmed stimulation.[410,415] Others have confirmed the high incidence of ventricular arrhythmias in such patients.[409,411–415] The risk of cardiac death is high in patients with cardiac disease presenting with syncope and is highest in patients with syncope who are being treated for prior documented life-threatening arrhythmias. We have been able to demonstrate that treatment of syncope, particularly that associated with induction of sustained ventricular arrhythmias, based on electrophysiologic techniques, has led to an outcome comparable to those patients in whom nothing was found at EPS.[415] Link et al.[417] have demonstrated appropriate ICD therapies in patients with syncope and inducible VT in whom ICDs were implanted. Although the utility of electrophysiologically guided therapy for syncope has not been documented in a double-blind, randomized, controlled trial, the demonstration that effective control of arrhythmias portends a good prognosis, suggests that (a) the results of the electrophysiologic study are clinically significant and (b) treatment of the responses induced by programmed stimulation provides therapeutic benefit to the patient.

How stringent should programmed stimulation be in patients without documented sustained ventricular arrhythmias who have syncope? In patients with syncope and normal hearts, we have refrained from using triple extrastimuli because, in our experience, all that is likely to be induced is polymorphic VT, with or without degeneration to VF. As noted earlier in this chapter, in normal hearts this is usually a nonspecific response that can be found in asymptomatic patients. Thus, in patients with normal hearts and syncope, in my opinion, polymorphic VT/VF should not be interpreted as meaningful. Even in patients with heart disease, controversy exists concerning the appropriate aggressiveness of programmed stimulation. In patients with chronic coronary artery disease, prior infarction, especially in the presence of aneurysm, I believe that the investigator should use a standard protocol because sustained uniform VT may be induced. I consider the induction of sustained monomorphic VT as being meaningful. This is particularly true when an aneurysm is present. Polymorphic VT/VF should not be considered meaningful in such patients although the change of polymorphic VT by type I agents to uniform VT appears to identify a subgroup in which the induced arrhythmia is meaningful.[164,165] Failure of a type I agent to transform the arrhythmia to uniform VT should not, however, be interpreted as a good response.

In patients with cardiomyopathy, the induction of polymorphic VT/VF by triple extrastimuli is so common that its induction does not distinguish patients with syncope from those without syncope. Therefore, in patients with cardiomyopathy, we do not consider polymorphic VT/VF, particularly when induced by triple extrastimuli, to be a meaningful response. It is my impression that many investigators have used the induction of polymorphic VT/VF as a marker for risk of sudden death in cardiomyopathic patients and have subsequently treated these patients with ICDs. I do not believe this is justified because the incidence of induction of polymorphic VT/VF in patients with idiopathic dilated cardiomyopathy exceeds 50% regardless of symptomatology. If one were to implant such devices in all patients with inducible polymorphic VT/VF, it would subject an enormous number of patients to the morbidity, mortality, and cost of such devices and would not deal with the remaining patients who also are at risk for sudden death. We need better predictors for risk of sudden death before such devices may be implanted prophylactically. Recently Knight et al.[418] suggested that unexplained (by history) syncope in patients with cardiomyopathy and low ejection fractions (<40%) should have ICDs implanted based on results of a small number of such patients in whom the implanted devices exhibited appropriate discharges. I believe that the implantation of prophylactive ICDs should be undertaken only when a data base is developed that allows the investigator to define a risk profile of high enough predictive accuracy to justify implantation of such devices. Several trials are under way attempting to address this question, but the results are several years away.

## REFERENCES


1. Josephson ME, Almendral JM, Buxton AE, et al. Mechanisms of ventricular tachycardia. *Circulation* 1987;75:III41–III47.
2. Waldo AL, Akhtar M, Brugada P, et al. The minimally appropriate electrophysiologic study for the initial assessment of patients with documented sustained monomorphic ventricular tachycardia. *J Am Coll Cardiol* 1985;6:1174–1177.
3. Josephson ME. Programmed stimulation for risk stratification for postinfarction sudden cardiac arrest: why and how? *Pacing Clin Electrophysiol* 2014;37:791–794.
4. Dessertenne F. [Ventricular tachycardia with 2 variable opposing foci]. *Arch Mal Coeur Vaiss* 1966;59:263–272.
5. Fontaine G, Frank R, Grosgogeat Y. Torsades de poites: definition and management. *Mod Concepts Cardiovasc Dis* 1982;51:103–108.
6. Josephson ME, Horowitz LN, Spielman SR, et al. Electrophysiologic and hemodynamic studies in patients resuscitated from cardiac arrest. *Am J Cardiol* 1980;46:948–955.
7. Kempf FC Jr., Josephson ME. Cardiac arrest recorded on ambulatory electrocardiograms. *Am J Cardiol* 1984;53:1577–1582.
8. Bayes de Luna A, Coumel P, Leclercq JF. Ambulatory sudden cardiac death: mechanisms of production of fatal arrhythmia on the basis of data from 157 cases. *Am Heart J* 1989;117:151–159.
9. Josephson ME, Horowitz LN, Waxman HL, et al. Sustained ventricular tachycardia: role of the 12-lead electrocardiogram in localizing site of origin. *Circulation* 1981;64:257–272.

10. Miller JM, Marchlinski FE, Buxton AE, et al. Relationship between the 12-lead electrocardiogram during ventricular tachycardia and endocardial site of origin in patients with coronary artery disease. *Circulation* 1988;77:759–766.
11. Miller JM, Hsia H, Rothman SA, et al., eds. *Ventricular tachycardia versus supraventricular tachycardia with aberration: Electrocardiographic distinctions.* Philadelphia, PA: WB Saunders, 2000.
12. Sandler IA, Marriott HJ. The differential morphology of anomalous ventricular complexes of Rbbb-type in lead V; ventricular ectopy versus aberration. *Circulation* 1965;31:551–556.
13. Wellens HJ, Bar FW, Lie KI. The value of the electrocardiogram in the differential diagnosis of a tachycardia with a widened QRS complex. *Am J Med* 1978;64:27–33.
14. Kindwall KE, Brown J, Josephson ME. Electrocardiographic criteria for ventricular tachycardia in wide complex left bundle branch block morphology tachycardias. *Am J Cardiol* 1988;61:1279–1283.
15. Vereckei A, Duray G, Szenasi G, et al. New algorithm using only lead aVR for differential diagnosis of wide QRS complex tachycardia. *Heart Rhythm* 2008;5:89–98.
16. Miller JM, Gottlieb CD, Lesh MD, et al. His-Purkinje activation during ventricular tachycardia: a determinant of QRS duration. *J Am Coll Cardiol* 1989;13:21A.
17. Cohen HC, Gozo EG Jr, Pick A. Ventricular tachycardia with narrow QRS complexes (left posterior fascicular tachycardia). *Circulation* 1972;45:1035–1043.
18. Akhtar M, Denker S, Lehmann MH, et al. Macro-reentry within the His Purkinje system. *Pacing Clin Electrophysiol* 1983;6:1010–1028.
19. Caceres J, Jazayeri M, McKinnie J, et al. Sustained bundle branch reentry as a mechanism of clinical tachycardia. *Circulation* 1989;79:256–270.
20. Spielman SR, Schwartz JS, Untereker WJ, et al., eds. *Chronic recurrent sustained ventricular tachycardia: anatomic, hemodynamic and electrophysiologic substrates.* Mt Kisco, NY: Futura Publishing, 1982.
21. Bolick DR, Hackel DB, Reimer KA, et al. Quantitative analysis of myocardial infarct structure in patients with ventricular tachycardia. *Circulation* 1986;74:1266–1279.
22. Adhar GC, Larson LW, Bardy GH, et al. Sustained ventricular arrhythmias: differences between survivors of cardiac arrest and patients with recurrent sustained ventricular tachycardia. *J Am Coll Cardiol* 1988; 12:159–165.
23. Stevenson WG, Brugada P, Waldecker B, et al. Clinical, angiographic, and electrophysiologic findings in patients with aborted sudden death as compared with patients with sustained ventricular tachycardia after myocardial infarction. *Circulation* 1985;71:1146–1152.
24. Cohen M, Wiener I, Pichard A, et al. Determinants of ventricular tachycardia in patients with coronary artery disease and ventricular aneurysm. Clinical, hemodynamic, and angiographic factors. *Am J Cardiol* 1983;51:61–64.
25. Marchlinski FE, Waxman HL, Buxton AE, et al. Sustained ventricular tachyarrhythmias during the early postinfarction period: electrophysiologic findings and prognosis for survival. *J Am Coll Cardiol* 1983;2:240–250.
26. Roy D, Marchand E, Theroux P, et al. Long-term reproducibility and significance of provokable ventricular arrhythmias after myocardial infarction. *J Am Coll Cardiol* 1986;8:32–39.
27. Hsieh CH, Chia EM, Huang K, et al. Evolution of ventricular tachycardia and its electrophysiological substrate early after myocardial infarction: an ovine model. *Circ Arrhythm Electrophysiol* 2013;6:1010–1017.
28. Zaman S, Narayan A, Thiagalingam A, et al. Significance of repeat programmed ventricular stimulation at electrophysiology study for arrhythmia prediction after acute myocardial infarction. *Pacing Clin Electrophysiol* 2014;37(7):795–802.
29. Peters NS, Wit AL. Myocardial architecture and ventricular arrhythmogenesis. *Circulation* 1998;97:1746–1754.
30. Cassidy DM, Vassallo JA, Marchlinski FE, et al. Endocardial mapping in humans in sinus rhythm with normal left ventricles: activation patterns and characteristics of electrograms. *Circulation* 1984;70:37–42.
31. Cassidy DM, Vassallo JA, Buxton AE, et al. The value of catheter mapping during sinus rhythm to localize site of origin of ventricular tachycardia. *Circulation* 1984;69:1103–1110.
32. Cassidy DM, Vassallo JA, Miller JM, et al. Endocardial catheter mapping in patients in sinus rhythm: relationship to underlying heart disease and ventricular arrhythmias. *Circulation* 1986;73:645–652.
33. Cassidy DM, Vassallo JA, Buxton AE, et al. Catheter mapping during sinus rhythm: relation of local electrogram duration to ventricular tachycardia cycle length. *Am J Cardiol* 1985;55:713–716.
34. Untereker WJ, Spielman SR, Waxman HL, et al. Ventricular activation in normal sinus rhythm: abnormalities with recurrent sustained tachycardia and a history of myocardial infarction. *Am J Cardiol* 1985;55:974–979.
35. Kienzle MG, Miller J, Falcone RA, et al. Intraoperative endocardial mapping during sinus rhythm: relationship to site of origin of ventricular tachycardia. *Circulation* 1984;70:957–965.
36. Vassallo JA, Cassidy DM, Marchlinski FE, et al. Abnormalities of endocardial activation pattern in patients with previous healed myocardial infarction and ventricular tachycardia. *Am J Cardiol* 1986;58:479–484.
37. Miller JM, Tyson GS, Hargrove WC 3rd, et al. Effect of subendocardial resection on sinus rhythm endocardial electrogram abnormalities. *Circulation* 1995;91:2385–2391.
38. Wiener I, Mindich B, Pitchon R. Endocardial activation in patients with coronary artery disease: effects of regional contraction abnormalities. *Am Heart J* 1984;107:1146–1152.
39. Wiener I, Mindich B, Pitchon R, et al. Epicardial activation in patients with coronary artery disease: effects of regional contraction abnormalities. *Circulation* 1982;65:154–160.
40. Buxton AE, Hafley GE, Lehmann MH, et al. Prediction of sustained ventricular tachycardia inducible by programmed stimulation in patients with coronary artery disease. Utility of clinical variables. *Circulation* 1999;99:1843–1850.
41. Buxton AE, Lee KL, DiCarlo L, et al. Nonsustained ventricular tachycardia in coronary artery disease: relation to inducible sustained ventricular tachycardia. MUSTT Investigators. *Ann Intern Med* 1996;125:35–39.
42. Buxton AE, Waxman HL, Marchlinski FE, et al. Role of triple extrastimuli during electrophysiologic study of patients with documented sustained ventricular tachyarrhythmias. *Circulation* 1984;69:532–540.
43. Josephson ME, Wit AL. Fractionated electrical activity and continuous electrical activity: fact or artifact? *Circulation* 1984;70:529–532.
44. Wit AL, Josephson ME, eds. *Fractionated Electrograms and continuous electrical activity: fact or artifact.* Orlando, FL: Grune & Stratton, 1985.
45. Fenoglio JJ Jr., Pham TD, Harken AH, et al. Recurrent sustained ventricular tachycardia: structure and ultrastructure of subendocardial regions in which tachycardia originates. *Circulation* 1983;68:518–533.
46. de Bakker JM, van Capelle FJ, Janse MJ, et al. Reentry as a cause of ventricular tachycardia in patients with chronic ischemic heart disease: electrophysiologic and anatomic correlation. *Circulation* 1988;77:589–606.
47. de Bakker JM, van Capelle FJ, Janse MJ, et al. Slow conduction in the infarcted human heart. 'Zigzag' course of activation. *Circulation* 1993; 88:915–926.
48. de Bakker JMT, Janse MJ, eds. *Pathophysiological correlates of ventricular tachycardia in hearts with a healed infarct* (Chapter 47). Philadelphia, PA: WB Saunders, 2000.
49. Peters NS, Green CR, Poole-Wilson PA, et al. Reduced content of connexin43 gap junctions in ventricular myocardium from hypertrophied and ischemic human hearts. *Circulation* 1993;88:864–875.
50. Gardner PI, Ursell PC, Fenoglio JJ Jr., et al. Electrophysiologic and anatomic basis for fractionated electrograms recorded from healed myocardial infarcts. *Circulation* 1985;72:596–611.
51. Peters NS, Cabo C, Wit AL, eds. *Arrhythmogenic mechanisms: automaticity, triggered activity, and reentry* (Chapter 40). Philadelphia, PA: WB Saunders, 2000.
52. Spach MS, Dolber PC. Relating extracellular potentials and their derivatives to anisotropic propagation at a microscopic level in human cardiac muscle. Evidence for electrical uncoupling of side-to-side fiber connections with increasing age. *Circ Res* 1986;58:356–371.
53. Cardinal R, Vermeulen M, Shenasa M, et al. Anisotropic conduction and functional dissociation of ischemic tissue during reentrant ventricular tachycardia in canine myocardial infarction. *Circulation* 1988;77:1162–1176.
54. Schmitt CG, Kadish AH, Marchlinski FE, et al. Effects of lidocaine and procainamide on normal and abnormal intraventricular electrograms during sinus rhythm. *Circulation* 1988;77:1030–1037.
55. Josephson ME. Lidocaine and sustained monomorphic ventricular tachycardia: fact or fiction. *Am J Cardiol* 1996;78:82–83.
56. Spear JF, Michelson EL, Moore EN. Reduced space constant in slowly conducting regions of chronically infarcted canine myocardium. *Circ Res* 1983;53:176–185.
57. Lesh MD, Spear JF, Balke CW, et al. Fractionated electrograms can be produced by regional changes in conduction velocity. *Circulation* 1987;76:241.
58. Lesh MD, Spear JF, Simson MB. A computer model of the electrogram: what causes fractionation? *J Electrocardiol* 1988;21(Suppl):S69–S73.

59. Lesh MD, Pring M, Spear JF. Cellular uncoupling can unmask dispersion of action potential duration in ventricular myocardium. A computer modeling study. *Circ Res* 1989;65:1426–1440.
60. Balke CW, Lesh MD, Spear JF, et al. Effects of cellular uncoupling on conduction in anisotropic canine ventricular myocardium. *Circ Res* 1988;63:879–892.
61. Marchlinski FE, Callans DJ, Gottlieb CD, et al. Linear ablation lesions for control of unmappable ventricular tachycardia in patients with ischemic and nonischemic cardiomyopathy. *Circulation* 2000;101:1288–1296.
62. Callans DJ, Ren JF, Michele J, et al. Electroanatomic left ventricular mapping in the porcine model of healed anterior myocardial infarction. Correlation with intracardiac echocardiography and pathological analysis. *Circulation* 1999;100:1744–1750.
63. Wrobleski D, Houghtaling C, Josephson ME, et al. Use of electrogram characteristics during sinus rhythm to delineate the endocardial scar in a porcine model of healed myocardial infarction. *J Cardiovasc Electrophysiol* 2003;14:524–529.
64. Soejima K, Stevenson WG, Maisel WH, et al. Electrically unexcitable scar mapping based on pacing threshold for identification of the reentry circuit isthmus: feasibility for guiding ventricular tachycardia ablation. *Circulation* 2002;106:1678–1683.
65. Reddy VY, Neuzil P, Taborsky M, et al. Short-term results of substrate mapping and radiofrequency ablation of ischemic ventricular tachycardia using a saline-irrigated catheter. *J Am Coll Cardiol* 2003;41:2228–2236.
66. Arenal A, del Castillo S, Gonzalez-Torrecilla E, et al. Tachycardia related channel in the scar tissue in patients with sustained monomorphic ventricular tachycardias. Influence of the voltage scar definition. *Circulation* 2004;110(17):2568–2574.
67. Hsia HH, Lin D, Sauer WH, et al. Anatomic characterization of endocardial substrate for hemodynamically stable reentrant ventricular tachycardia: identification of endocardial conducting channels. *Heart Rhythm* 2006;3:503–512.
68. Tung R, Nakahara S, Ramirez R, et al. Accuracy of combined endocardial and epicardial electroanatomic mapping of a reperfused porcine infarct model: a comparison of electrofield and magnetic systems with histopathologic correlation. *Heart Rhythm* 2011;8:439–447.
69. Schilling RJ, Peters NS, Davies DW. Feasibility of a noncontact catheter for endocardial mapping of human ventricular tachycardia. *Circulation* 1999;99:2543–2552.
70. Jacobson JT, Afonso VX, Eisenman G, et al. Characterization of the infarct substrate and ventricular tachycardia circuits with noncontact unipolar mapping in a porcine model of myocardial infarction. *Heart Rhythm* 2006;3:189–197.
71. Vassallo JA, Cassidy DM, Marchlinski FE, et al. Endocardial activation of left bundle branch block. *Circulation* 1984;69:914–923.
72. Vassallo JA, Cassidy DM, Miller JM, et al. Left ventricular endocardial activation during right ventricular pacing: effect of underlying heart disease. *J Am Coll Cardiol* 1986;7:1228–1233.
73. Hsia HH, Callans DJ, Marchlinski FE. Characterization of endocardial electrophysiological substrate in patients with nonischemic cardiomyopathy and monomorphic ventricular tachycardia. *Circulation* 2003;108:704–710.
74. Soejima K, Stevenson WG, Sapp JL, et al. Endocardial and epicardial radiofrequency ablation of ventricular tachycardia associated with dilated cardiomyopathy: the importance of low-voltage scars. *J Am Coll Cardiol* 2004;43:1834–1842.
75. Sosa E, Scanavacca M, d'Avila A, et al. A new technique to perform epicardial mapping in the electrophysiology laboratory. *J Cardiovasc Electrophysiol* 1996;7:531–536.
76. Giniger AG, Retyk EO, Laino RA, et al. Ventricular tachycardia in Chagas' disease. *Am J Cardiol* 1992;70:459–462.
77. Hutchinson MD, Gerstenfeld EP, Desjardins B, et al. Endocardial unipolar voltage mapping to detect epicardial ventricular tachycardia substrate in patients with nonischemic left ventricular cardiomyopathy. *Circ Arrhythm Electrophysiol* 2011;4:49–55.
78. Spears DA, Suszko AM, Dalvi R, et al. Relationship of bipolar and unipolar electrogram voltage to scar transmurality and composition derived by magnetic resonance imaging in patients with nonischemic cardiomyopathy undergoing VT ablation. *Heart Rhythm* 2012;9:1837–1846.
79. Chopra N, Tokuda M, Ng J, et al. Relation of the unipolar low-voltage penumbra surrounding the endocardial low-voltage scar to ventricular tachycardia circuit sites and ablation outcomes in ischemic cardiomyopathy. *J Cardiovasc Electrophysiol* 2014;25:602–608.
80. Marchlinski FE, Zado E, Dixit S, et al. Electroanatomic substrate and outcome of catheter ablative therapy for ventricular tachycardia in the setting of right ventricular cardiomyopathy. *Circulation* 2004;110:2293–2298.
81. Marcus FI, Fontaine GH, Guiraudon G, et al. Right ventricular dysplasia: a report of 24 adult cases. *Circulation* 1982;65:384–398.
82. Polin GM, Haqqani H, Tzou W, et al. Endocardial unipolar voltage mapping to identify epicardial substrate in arrhythmogenic right ventricular cardiomyopathy/dysplasia. *Heart Rhythm* 2011;8:76–83.
83. Watson RM, Schwartz JL, Maron BJ, et al. Inducible polymorphic ventricular tachycardia and ventricular fibrillation in a subgroup of patients with hypertrophic cardiomyopathy at high risk for sudden death. *J Am Coll Cardiol* 1987;10:761–774.
84. Saumarez RC, Camm AJ, Panagos A, et al. Ventricular fibrillation in hypertrophic cardiomyopathy is associated with increased fractionation of paced right ventricular electrograms. *Circulation* 1992;86:467–474.
85. McKenna WJ, Elliott PM, eds. *Arrhythmia, sudden death, and clinical risk stratification in hypertrophic cardiomyopathy* (Chapter 63). Philadelphia, PA: WB Saunders, 2000.
86. Simson MB. Use of signals in the terminal QRS complex to identify patients with ventricular tachycardia after myocardial infarction. *Circulation* 1981;64:235–242.
87. Denes P, Santarelli P, Hauser RG, et al. Quantitative analysis of the high-frequency components of the terminal portion of the body surface QRS in normal subjects and in patients with ventricular tachycardia. *Circulation* 1983;67:1129–1138.
88. Kuchar DL, Thorburn CW, Sammel NL. Late potentials detected after myocardial infarction: natural history and prognostic significance. *Circulation* 1986;74:1280–1289.
89. Breithardt G, Borggrefe M. Pathophysiological mechanisms and clinical significance of ventricular late potentials. *Eur Heart J* 1986;7:364–385.
90. Steinberg JS, Berbari EJ. The signal-averaged electrocardiogram: update on clinical applications. *J Cardiovasc Electrophysiol* 1996;7:972–988.
91. Berbari EJ, ed. *High-resolution electrocardiography* (Chapter 81). Philadelphia, PA: WB Saunders, 2000.
92. Vassallo JA, Cassidy D, Simson MB, et al. Relation of late potentials to site of origin of ventricular tachycardia associated with coronary heart disease. *Am J Cardiol* 1985;55:985–989.
93. Simson MB, Untereker WJ, Spielman SR, et al. Relation between late potentials on the body surface and directly recorded fragmented electrograms in patients with ventricular tachycardia. *Am J Cardiol* 1983;51:105–112.
94. Josephson ME, Simson MB, Harken AH, et al. The incidence and clinical significance of epicardial late potentials in patients with recurrent sustained ventricular tachycardia and coronary artery disease. *Circulation* 1982;66:1199–1204.
95. Freedman RA, Gillis AM, Keren A, et al. Signal-averaged electrocardiographic late potentials in patients with ventricular fibrillation or ventricular tachycardia: correlation with clinical arrhythmia and electrophysiologic study. *Am J Cardiol* 1985;55:1350–1353.
96. Buxton AE, Simson MB, Falcone RA, et al. Results of signal-averaged electrocardiography and electrophysiologic study in patients with nonsustained ventricular tachycardia after healing of acute myocardial infarction. *Am J Cardiol* 1987;60:80–85.
97. Cain ME, Anderson JL, Arnsdorf MF, et al. American college of cardiology consensus document on signal-averaged electrocardiography. *J Am Coll Cardiol* 1996;27:238–249.
98. Kuchar DL, Thorburn CW, Sammel NL. Signal-averaged electrocardiogram for evaluation of recurrent syncope. *Am J Cardiol* 1986;58:949–953.
99. Gang ES, Peter T, Rosenthal ME, et al. Detection of late potentials on the surface electrocardiogram in unexplained syncope. *Am J Cardiol* 1986;58:1014–1020.
100. Winters SL, Stewart D, Gomes JA. Signal averaging of the surface QRS complex predicts inducibility of ventricular tachycardia in patients with syncope of unknown origin: a prospective study. *J Am Coll Cardiol* 1987;10:775–781.
101. Cain ME, Anderson JL, Arnsdorf MF, et al. American college of cardiology consensus document on signal-averaged electrocardiography. *J Am Coll Cardiol* 1996;27:238–249.
102. McGuire M, Kuchar D, Ganis J, et al. Natural history of late potentials in the first ten days after acute myocardial infarction and relation to early ventricular arrhythmias. *Am J Cardiol* 1988;61:1187–1190.
103. Poll DS, Marchlinski FE, Falcone RA, et al. Abnormal signal-averaged electrocardiograms in patients with nonischemic congestive cardiomyopathy: relationship to sustained ventricular tachyarrhythmias. *Circulation* 1985;72:1308–1313.
104. Middlekauff HR, Stevenson WG, Woo MA, et al. Comparison of frequency of late potentials in idiopathic dilated cardiomyopathy and

ischemic cardiomyopathy with advanced congestive heart failure and their usefulness in predicting sudden death. *Am J Cardiol* 1990;66:1113–1117.
105. Mancini DM, Wong KL, Simson MB. Prognostic value of an abnormal signal-averaged electrocardiogram in patients with nonischemic congestive cardiomyopathy. *Circulation* 1993;87:1083–1092.
106. Kienzle MG, Doherty JU, Cassidy D, et al. Electrophysiologic sequelae of chronic myocardial infarction: local refractoriness and electrographic characteristics of the left ventricle. *Am J Cardiol* 1986;58:63–69.
107. Vassallo JA, Cassidy DM, Kindwall KE, et al. Nonuniform recovery of excitability in the left ventricle. *Circulation* 1988;78:1365–1372.
108. El-Sherif N, Caref EB, Yin H, et al. The electrophysiological mechanism of ventricular arrhythmias in the long QT syndrome. Tridimensional mapping of activation and recovery patterns. *Circ Res* 1996;79:474–492.
109. Schwartz PJ, Priori SG, Locati EH, et al. Long QT syndrome patients with mutations of the SCN5A and HERG genes have differential responses to Na+ channel blockade and to increases in heart rate. Implications for gene-specific therapy. *Circulation* 1995;92:3381–3386.
110. Krishnan SC, Antzelevitch C. Flecainide-induced arrhythmia in canine ventricular epicardium. Phase 2 reentry? *Circulation* 1993;87:562–572.
111. Jackman WM, Friday KJ, Anderson JL, et al. The long QT syndromes: a critical review, new clinical observations and a unifying hypothesis. *Prog Cardiovasc Dis* 1988;31:115–172.
112. Antzelevitch C, Yan GX, Shimuzu W, et al., eds. *Electrical heterogeneity, the ECG, and cardiac arrrhythmias* (Chapter 26). Philadelphia, PA: WB Saunders, 2000.
113. Antzelevitch C. The Brugada syndrome. *J Cardiovasc Electrophysiol* 1998;9:513–516.
114. Antzelevitch C, Brugada P, Brugada J, et al. Brugada syndrome: a decade of progress. *Circ Res* 2002;91:1114–1118.
115. Priori SG, Napolitano C, Memmi M, et al. Clinical and molecular characterization of patients with catecholaminergic polymorphic ventricular tachycardia. *Circulation* 2002;106:69–74.
116. Sumitomo N, Harada K, Nagashima M, et al. Catecholaminergic polymorphic ventricular tachycardia: electrocardiographic characteristics and optimal therapeutic strategies to prevent sudden death. *Heart* 2003;89:66–70.
117. Roden DM, Viswanathan PC. Genetics of acquired long QT syndrome. *J Clin Invest* 2005;115:2025–2032.
118. Kontulaa K, Paivi PJ, Laitinena A, et al. Catecholaminergic polymorphic ventricular tachycardia: recent mechanistic insights. *Cardiovasc Res* 2005;67:379–387.
119. di Barletta MR, Viatchenko-Karpinski S, Nori A, et al. Clinical phenotype and functional characterization of CASQ2 mutations associated with catecholaminergic polymorphic ventricular tachycardia. *Circulation* 2006;114:1012–1019.
120. Veerakul G, Nademanee K. Brugada syndrome: two decades of progress. *Circ J* 2012;76:2713–2722.
121. Nademanee K, Veerakul G, Chandanamattha P, et al. Prevention of ventricular fibrillation episodes in Brugada syndrome by catheter ablation over the anterior right ventricular outflow tract epicardium. *Circulation* 2011;123:1270–1279.
122. Josephson ME, Marchlinski FE, Cassidy DM, et al., eds. *Sustained ventricular tachycardia in coronary artery disease-evidence for reentrant mechanism.* Orlando, FL: Grune & Stratton, 1985.
123. Callans DJ, Josephson ME, eds. *Ventricular tachycardia in patients with coronary artery disease.* Philadelphia, PA: WB Saunders, 2000.
124. Wellens HJ. Value and limitations of programmed electrical stimulation of the heart in the study and treatment of tachycardias. *Circulation* 1978;57:845–853.
125. Johnson NJ, Rosen MR, eds. *The distinction between triggered activity and other cardiac arrhythmias.* Mount Kisco, NY: Futura Publishing, 1987.
126. Cranefield PF, Aronson RS. *Cardiac arrhythmias: the role of triggered activity and other mechanisms.* Mount Kisco, NY: Futura Publishing, 1988.
127. le Marec H, Dangman KH, Danilo P Jr., et al. An evaluation of automaticity and triggered activity in the canine heart one to four days after myocardial infarction. *Circulation* 1985;71:1224–1236.
128. Johnson N, Danilo P Jr, Wit AL, et al. Characteristics of initiation and termination of catecholamine-induced triggered activity in atrial fibers of the coronary sinus. *Circulation* 1986;74:1168–1179.
129. Damiano BP, Rosen MR. Effects of pacing on triggered activity induced by early afterdepolarizations. *Circulation* 1984;69:1013–1025.
130. Cranefield PF, Aronson RS. Torsade de pointes and other pause-induced ventricular tachycardias: the short-long-short sequence and early afterdepolarizations. *Pacing Clin Electrophysiol* 1988;11:670–678.
131. Bigger JT Jr, Reiffel JA, Livelli FD Jr, et al. Sensitivity, specificity, and reproducibility of programmed ventricular stimulation. *Circulation* 1986; 73:II73–II78.
132. McPherson CA, Rosenfeld LE, Batsford WP. Day-to-day reproducibility of responses to right ventricular programmed electrical stimulation: implications for serial drug testing. *Am J Cardiol* 1985;55:689–695.
133. DiCarlo LA Jr, Morady F, Schwartz AB, et al. Clinical significance of ventricular fibrillation-flutter induced by ventricular programmed stimulation. *Am Heart J* 1985;109:959–963.
134. Cooper MJ, Hunt LJ, Richards DA, et al. Effect of repetition of extrastimuli on sensitivity and reproducibility of mode of induction of ventricular tachycardia by programmed stimulation. *J Am Coll Cardiol* 1988;11:1260–1267.
135. Schoenfeld MH, McGovern B, Garan H, et al. Long-term reproducibility of responses to programmed cardiac stimulation in spontaneous ventricular tachyarrhythmias. *Am J Cardiol* 1984;54:564–568.
136. Morady F, Shapiro W, Shen E, et al. Programmed ventricular stimulation in patients without spontaneous ventricular tachycardia. *Am Heart J* 1984;107:875–882.
137. Hummel JD, Strickberger SA, Daoud E, et al. Results and efficiency of programmed ventricular stimulation with four extrastimuli compared with one, two, and three extrastimuli. *Circulation* 1994;90:2827–2832.
138. Brugada P, Abdollah H, Heddle B, et al. Results of a ventricular stimulation protocol using a maximum of 4 premature stimuli in patients without documented or suspected ventricular arrhythmias. *Am J Cardiol* 1983;52:1214–1218.
139. Brugada P, Green M, Abdollah H, et al. Significance of ventricular arrhythmias initiated by programmed ventricular stimulation: the importance of the type of ventricular arrhythmia induced and the number of premature stimuli required. *Circulation* 1984;69:87–92.
140. Herre JM, Mann DE, Luck JC, et al. Effect of increased current, multiple pacing sites and number of extrastimuli on induction of ventricular tachycardia. *Am J Cardiol* 1986;57:102–107.
141. Morady F, DiCarlo L, Winston S, et al. A prospective comparison of triple extrastimuli and left ventricular stimulation in studies of ventricular tachycardia induction. *Circulation* 1984;70:52–57.
142. Martinez-Rubio A, Shenasa M, Borggrefe M, et al. Electrophysiologic variables characterizing the induction of ventricular tachycardia versus ventricular fibrillation after myocardial infarction: relation between ventricular late potentials and coupling intervals for the induction of sustained ventricular tachyarrhythmias. *J Am Coll Cardiol* 1993;21:1624–1631.
143. Zaman S, Kumar S, Sullivan J, et al. Significance of inducible very fast ventricular tachycardia (cycle length 200-230 ms) after early reperfusion for ST-segment-elevation myocardial infarction. *Circ Arrhythm Electrophysiol* 2013;6:884–890.
144. Zaman S, Narayan A, Thiagalingam A, et al. Long-term arrhythmia-free survival in patients with severe left ventricular dysfunction and no inducible ventricular tachycardia after myocardial infarction. *Circulation* 2014;129:848–854.
145. Buxton AE. Programmed ventricular stimulation: not dead. *Circulation* 2014;129:831–833.
146. Buxton AE. Risk stratification for sudden death in patients with coronary artery disease. *Heart Rhythm* 2009;6:836–847.
147. Belhassen B, Ohayon-Tsioni T, Glick A, et al. An "aggressive" protocol of programmed ventricular stimulation for selecting post-myocardial infarction patients with a low ejection fraction who may not require implantation of an automatic defibrillator. *Isr Med Assoc J* 2009;11:520–524, 526, 528.
148. El-Shalakany A, Hadjis T, Papageorgiou P, et al. Entrainment/mapping criteria for the prediction of termination of ventricular tachycardia by single radiofrequency lesion in patients with coronary artery disease. *Circulation* 1999;99:2283–2289.
149. Brugada P, Wellens HJ. Comparison in the same patient of two programmed ventricular stimulation protocols to induce ventricular tachycardia. *Am J Cardiol* 1985;55:380–383.
150. Cain ME, Martin TC, Marchlinski FE, et al. Changes in ventricular refractoriness after an extrastimulus: effects of prematurity, cycle length and procainamide. *Am J Cardiol* 1983;52:996–1001.
151. Denker S, Lehmann M, Mahmud R, et al. Facilitation of ventricular tachycardia induction with abrupt changes in ventricular cycle length. *Am J Cardiol* 1984;53:508–515.
152. Estes NA 3rd, Garan H, McGovern B, et al. Influence of drive cycle length during programmed stimulation on induction of ventricular arrhythmias: analysis of 403 patients. *Am J Cardiol* 1986;57:108–112.
153. Gillis AM, Winkle RA, Echt DS. Role of extrastimulus prematurity and intraventricular conduction time in inducing ventricular tachycardia

or ventricular fibrillation secondary to coronary artery disease. *Am J Cardiol* 1987;60:590–595.
154. Rosenfeld LE, McPherson CA, Kennedy EE, et al. Ventricular tachycardia induction: comparison of triple extrastimuli with an abrupt change in ventricular drive cycle length. *Am Heart J* 1986;111:868–874.
155. Vassallo JA, Marchlinski FE, Cassidy DM, et al. Shortening of ventricular refractoriness with extrastimuli: role of the degree of prematurity and number of extrastimuli. *J Electrophysiol* 1988;2:227–236.
156. Doherty JU, Kienzle MG, Waxman HL, et al. Programmed ventricular stimulation at a second right ventricular site: an analysis of 100 patients, with special reference to sensitivity, specificity and characteristics of patients with induced ventricular tachycardia. *Am J Cardiol* 1983; 52:1184–1189.
157. Robertson JF, Cain ME, Horowitz LN, et al. Anatomic and electrophysiologic correlates of ventricular tachycardia requiring left ventricular stimulation. *Am J Cardiol* 1981;48:263–268.
158. Morady F, Dicarlo LA Jr, Liem LB, et al. Effects of high stimulation current on the induction of ventricular tachycardia. *Am J Cardiol* 1985;56:73–78.
159. Akhtar M. Clinical application of rapid ventricular burst pacing versus extrastimulation for induction of ventricular tachycardia. *J Am Coll Cardiol* 1984;4:305–307.
160. Reddy CP, Gettes LS. Use of isoproterenol as an aid to electric induction of chronic recurrent ventricular tachycardia. *Am J Cardiol* 1979;44: 705–713.
161. Freedman RA, Swerdlow CD, Echt DS, et al. Facilitation of ventricular tachyarrhythmia induction by isoproterenol. *Am J Cardiol* 1984;54: 765–770.
162. Naccarelli GV, Prystowsky EN, Jackman WM, et al. Role of electrophysiologic testing in managing patients who have ventricular tachycardia unrelated to coronary artery disease. *Am J Cardiol* 1982;50:165–171.
163. Lerman BB, Stein KM, Markowitz SM, et al., eds. *Ventricular tachycardia in patients with structurally normal hearts* (Chapter 70). Philadelphia, PA: WB Saunders, 2000.
164. Horowitz LN, Greenspan AM, Spielman SR, et al. Torsades de pointes: electrophysiologic studies in patients without transient pharmacologic or metabolic abnormalities. *Circulation* 1981;63:1120–1128.
165. Buxton AE, Josephson ME, Marchlinski FE, et al. Polymorphic ventricular tachycardia induced by programmed stimulation: response to procainamide. *J Am Coll Cardiol* 1993;21:90–98.
166. Poll DS, Marchlinski FE, Buxton AE, et al. Sustained ventricular tachycardia in patients with idiopathic dilated cardiomyopathy: electrophysiologic testing and lack of response to antiarrhythmic drug therapy. *Circulation* 1984;70:451–456.
167. Poll DS, Marchlinski FE, Buxton AE, et al. Usefulness of programmed stimulation in idiopathic dilated cardiomyopathy. *Am J Cardiol* 1986;58: 992–997.
168. Lemery R, Brugada P, Bella PD, et al. Nonischemic ventricular tachycardia. Clinical course and long-term follow-up in patients without clinically overt heart disease. *Circulation* 1989;79:990–999.
169. Klein GJ, Millman PJ, Yee R. Recurrent ventricular tachycardia responsive to verapamil. *Pacing Clin Electrophysiol* 1984;7:938–948.
170. German LD, Packer DL, Bardy GH, et al. Ventricular tachycardia induced by atrial stimulation in patients without symptomatic cardiac disease. *Am J Cardiol* 1983;52:1202–1207.
171. Lin FC, Finley CD, Rahimtoola SH, et al. Idiopathic paroxysmal ventricular tachycardia with a QRS pattern of right bundle branch block and left axis deviation: a unique clinical entity with specific properties. *Am J Cardiol* 1983;52:95–100.
172. Ohe T, Shimomura K, Aihara N, et al. Idiopathic sustained left ventricular tachycardia: clinical and electrophysiologic characteristics. *Circulation* 1988;77:560–568.
173. Lee KL, Lauer MR, Young C, et al. Spectrum of electrophysiologic and electropharmacologic characteristics of verapamil-sensitive ventricular tachycardia in patients without structural heart disease. *Am J Cardiol* 1996;77:967–973.
174. Horowitz LN, Vetter VL, Harken AH, et al. Electrophysiologic characteristics of sustained ventricular tachycardia occurring after repair of tetralogy of fallot. *Am J Cardiol* 1980;46:446–452.
175. Kugler JD, Pinsky WW, Cheatham JP, et al. Sustained ventricular tachycardia after repair of tetralogy of Fallot: new electrophysiologic findings. *Am J Cardiol* 1983;51:1137–1143.
176. Kudenchuk PJ, Kron J, Walance CG, et al. Reproducibility of arrhythmia induction with intracardiac electrophysiologic testing: patients with clinical sustained ventricular tachyarrhythmias. *J Am Coll Cardiol* 1986;7:819–828.
177. Doherty JU, Kienzle MG, Waxman HL, et al. Relation of mode of induction and cycle length of ventricular tachycardia: analysis of 104 patients. *Am J Cardiol* 1983;52:60–64.
178. Lerman BB, Stein KM, Markowitz SM, et al., eds. *Ventricular tachycardia in patients with structurally normal hearts* (Chapter 72). 4th ed. Philadelphia, PA: WB Saunders, 2004.
179. Dangman KH, Danilo P Jr., Hordof AJ, et al. Electrophysiologic characteristics of human ventricular and Purkinje fibers. *Circulation* 1982;65: 362–368.
180. Moak JP, Rosen MR. Induction and termination of triggered activity by pacing in isolated canine Purkinje fibers. *Circulation* 1984;69: 149–162.
181. Wellens HJ, Bar FW, Farre J, et al. Initiation and termination of ventricular tachycardia by supraventricular stimuli. Incidence and electrophysiologic determinants as observed during programmed stimulation of the heart. *Am J Cardiol* 1980;46:576–582.
182. Roy D, Brugada P, Wellens HJ. Atrial tachycardia facilitating initiation of ventricular tachycardia. *Pacing Clin Electrophysiol* 1983;6:47–52.
183. Callans DJ, Menz V, Schwartzman D, et al. Repetitive monomorphic tachycardia from the left ventricular outflow tract: electrocardiographic patterns consistent with a left ventricular site of origin. *J Am Coll Cardiol* 1997;29:1023–1027.
184. Ouyang F, Fotuhi P, Ho SY, et al. Repetitive monomorphic ventricular tachycardia originating from the aortic sinus cusp: electrocardiographic characterization for guiding catheter ablation. *J Am Coll Cardiol* 2002;39:500–508.
185. Chun KR, Satomi K, Kuck KH, et al. Left ventricular outflow tract tachycardia including ventricular tachycardia from the aortic cusps and epicardial ventricular tachycardia. *Herz* 2007;32:226–232.
186. Ouyang F, Mathew S, Wu S, et al. Ventricular arrhythmias arising from the left ventricular outflow tract below the aortic sinus cusps: mapping and catheter ablation via transseptal approach and electrocardiographic characteristics. *Circ Arrhythm Electrophysiol* 2014;7:445–455.
187. Anselme F, Boyle N, Josephson M. Incessant fascicular tachycardia: a cause of arrhythmia induced cardiomyopathy. *Pacing Clin Electrophysiol* 1998;21:760–763.
188. Nogami A. Purkinje-related arrhythmias part I: monomorphic ventricular tachycardias. *Pacing Clin Electrophysiol* 2011;34:624–650.
189. Nogami A, Naito S, Tada H, et al. Demonstration of diastolic and presystolic Purkinje potentials as critical potentials in a macroreentry circuit of verapamil-sensitive idiopathic left ventricular tachycardia. *J Am Coll Cardiol* 2000;36:811–823.
190. Berger MD, Waxman HL, Buxton AE, et al. Spontaneous compared with induced onset of sustained ventricular tachycardia. *Circulation* 1988;78: 885–892.
191. Marchlinski FE, Callans DJ, Gottlieb CD, et al. Benefits and lessons learned from stored electrogram information in implantable defibrillators. *J Cardiovasc Electrophysiol* 1995;6:832–851.
192. Bardy GH, Olson WH, eds. *Clinical characteristics of spontaneous onset of sustained ventricular tachycardia and ventricular fibrillation in survivors of cardiac arrest.* Philadelphia, PA: WB Saunders, 1990.
193. Wellens HJ, Lie KI, Durrer D. Further observations on ventricular tachycardia as studied by electrical stimulation of the heart. Chronic recurrent ventricular tachycardia and ventricular tachycardia during acute myocardial infarction. *Circulation* 1974;49:647–653.
194. Wellens HJ, Duren DR, Lie KI. Observations on mechanisms of ventricular tachycardia in man. *Circulation* 1976;54:237–244.
195. Josephson ME, Horowitz LN, Farshidi A, et al. Recurrent sustained ventricular tachycardia. 1. Mechanisms. *Circulation* 1978;57:431–440.
196. Gorgels AP, Beekman HD, Brugada P, et al. Extrastimulus-related shortening of the first postpacing interval in digitalis-induced ventricular tachycardia: observations during programmed electrical stimulation in the conscious dog. *J Am Coll Cardiol* 1983;1:840–857.
197. Josephson ME, Horowitz LN, Farshidi A. Continuous local electrical activity. A mechanism of recurrent ventricular tachycardia. *Circulation* 1978;57:659–665.
198. Boineau JP, Cox JL. Slow ventricular activation in acute myocardial infarction. A source of re-entrant premature ventricular contractions. *Circulation* 1973;48:702–713.
199. Waldo AL, Kaiser GA. A study of ventricular arrhythmias associated with acute myocardial infarction in the canine heart. *Circulation* 1973;47:1222–1228.
200. El-Sherif N, Hope RR, Scherlag BJ, et al. Re-entrant ventricular arrhythmias in the late myocardial infarction period. 2. Patterns of initiation and termination of re-entry. *Circulation* 1977;55:702–719.

201. Ideker RE, Lofland GK, Bardy GH, et al. Late fractionated potentials and continuous electrical activity caused by electrode motion. *Pacing Clin Electrophysiol* 1983;6:908–914.
202. Gallagher JJ, Kasell JH, Cox JL, et al. Techniques of intraoperative electrophysiologic mapping. *Am J Cardiol* 1982;49:221–240.
203. Waxman HL, Sung RJ. Significance of fragmented ventricular electrograms observed using intracardiac recording techniques in man. *Circulation* 1980;62:1349–1356.
204. Brugada P, Abdollah H, Wellens HJ. Continuous electrical activity during sustained monomorphic ventricular tachycardia. Observations on its dynamic behavior during the arrhythmia. *Am J Cardiol* 1985;55:402–411.
205. Blanck Z, Sra J, Dhala A, et al., eds. *Bundle branch reentry: mechanisms, diagnosis, and treatment* (Chapter 71). Philadelphia, PA: WB Saunders, 2000.
206. Crijns HJ, Smeets JL, Rodriguez LM, et al. Cure of interfascicular reentrant ventricular tachycardia by ablation of the anterior fascicle of the left bundle branch. *J Cardiovasc Electrophysiol* 1995;6:486–492.
207. Touboul P, Kirkorian G, Atallah G, et al. Bundle branch reentrant tachycardia treated by electrical ablation of the right bundle branch. *J Am Coll Cardiol* 1986;7:1404–1409.
208. Tchou P, Jazayeri M, Denker S, et al. Transcatheter electrical ablation of right bundle branch. A method of treating macroreentrant ventricular tachycardia attributed to bundle branch reentry. *Circulation* 1988; 78:246–257.
209. Farshidi A, Michelson EL, Greenspan AM, et al. Repetitive responses to ventricular extrastimuli: incidence, mechanism, and significance. *Am Heart J* 1980;100:59–68.
210. Priori SG, Wilde AA, Horie M, et al. Executive summary: HRS/EHRA/APHRS expert consensus statement on the diagnosis and management of patients with inherited primary arrhythmia syndromes. *Heart Rhythm* 2013;10:e85–e108.
211. Aizawa Y, Naitoh N, Washizuka T, et al. Electrophysiological findings in idiopathic recurrent ventricular fibrillation: special reference to mode of induction, drug testing, and long-term outcomes. *Pacing Clin Electrophysiol* 1996;19:929–939.
212. Belhassen B, Viskin S. Idiopathic ventricular tachycardia and fibrillation. *J Cardiovasc Electrophysiol* 1993;4:356–368.
213. Viskin S, Belhassen B. Idiopathic ventricular fibrillation. *Am Heart J* 1990;120:661–671.
214. Viskin S, Lesh MD, Eldar M, et al. Mode of onset of malignant ventricular arrhythmias in idiopathic ventricular fibrillation. *J Cardiovasc Electrophysiol* 1997;8:1115–1120.
215. Haissaguerre M, Chatel S, Sacher F, et al. Ventricular fibrillation with prominent early repolarization associated with a rare variant of KCNJ8/KATP channel. *J Cardiovasc Electrophysiol* 2009;20:93–98.
216. Haissaguerre M, Derval N, Sacher F, et al. Sudden cardiac arrest associated with early repolarization. *N Engl J Med* 2008;358:2016–2023.
217. Aizawa Y, Chinushi M, Hasegawa K, et al. Electrical storm in idiopathic ventricular fibrillation is associated with early repolarization. *J Am Coll Cardiol* 2013;62:1015–1019.
218. Antzelevitch C, Barajas-Martinez H. A gain-of-function I (K-ATP) mutation and its role in sudden cardiac death associated with J-wave syndromes. *Heart Rhythm* 2010;7:1472–1474.
219. Wilde AA. "J-wave syndromes" bring the ATP-sensitive potassium channel back in the spotlight. *Heart Rhythm* 2012;9:556–557.
220. Brugada P, Brugada J. Right bundle branch block, persistent ST segment elevation and sudden cardiac death: a distinct clinical and electrocardiographic syndrome. A multicenter report. *J Am Coll Cardiol* 1992; 20:1391–1396.
221. Miyazaki T, Mitamura H, Miyoshi S, et al. Autonomic and antiarrhythmic drug modulation of ST segment elevation in patients with Brugada syndrome. *J Am Coll Cardiol* 1996;27:1061–1070.
222. Aizawa Y, Tamura M, Chinushi M, et al. Idiopathic ventricular fibrillation and bradycardia-dependent intraventricular block. *Am Heart J* 1993;126:1473–1474.
223. Chen Q, Kirsch GE, Zhang D, et al. Genetic basis and molecular mechanism for idiopathic ventricular fibrillation. *Nature* 1998;392:293–296.
224. Savastano S, Rordorf R, Vicentini A, et al. A comprehensive electrocardiographic, molecular, and echocardiographic study of Brugada syndrome: validation of the 2013 diagnostic criteria. *Heart Rhythm* 2014; 11:1176–1183.
225. Burashnikov E, Pfeiffer R, Barajas-Martinez H, et al. Mutations in the cardiac L-type calcium channel associated with inherited J-wave syndromes and sudden cardiac death. *Heart Rhythm* 2010;7:1872–1882.
226. Belhassen B, Glick A, Viskin S. Efficacy of quinidine in high-risk patients with Brugada syndrome. *Circulation* 2004;110:1731–1737.
227. Antzelevitch C, Brugada P, Borggrefe M, et al. Brugada syndrome: report of the second consensus conference: endorsed by the Heart Rhythm Society and the European Heart Rhythm Association. *Circulation* 2005; 111:659–670.
228. Gussak I, Antzelevitch C. Early repolarization syndrome: a decade of progress. *J Electrocardiol* 2013;46:110–113.
229. Aizawa Y, Sato A, Watanabe H, et al. Dynamicity of the J-wave in idiopathic ventricular fibrillation with a special reference to pause-dependent augmentation of the J-wave. *J Am Coll Cardiol* 2012;59:1948–1953.
230. Koncz I, Gurabi Z, Patocskai B, et al. Mechanisms underlying the development of the electrocardiographic and arrhythmic manifestations of early repolarization syndrome. *J Mol Cell Cardiol* 2014;68:20–28.
231. Haissaguerre M, Extramiana F, Hocini M, et al. Mapping and ablation of ventricular fibrillation associated with long-QT and brugada syndromes. *Circulation* 2003;108:925–928.
232. Haissaguerre M, Shoda M, Jais P, et al. Mapping and ablation of idiopathic ventricular fibrillation. *Circulation* 2002;106:962–967.
233. Szumowski L, Sanders P, Walczak F, et al. Mapping and ablation of polymorphic ventricular tachycardia after myocardial infarction. *J Am Coll Cardiol* 2004;44:1700–1706.
234. Anter E, Buxton AE, Silverstein JR, et al. Idiopathic ventricular fibrillation originating from the moderator band. *J Cardiovasc Electrophysiol* 2013;24:97–100.
235. Liu N, Denegri M, Ruan Y, et al. Short communication: flecainide exerts an antiarrhythmic effect in a mouse model of catecholaminergic polymorphic ventricular tachycardia by increasing the threshold for triggered activity. *Circ Res* 2011;109:291–295.
236. Hong RA, Rivera KK, Jittirat A, et al. Flecainide suppresses defibrillator-induced storming in catecholaminergic polymorphic ventricular tachycardia. *Pacing Clin Electrophysiol* 2012;35:794–797.
237. Khoury A, Marai I, Suleiman M, et al. Flecainide therapy suppresses exercise-induced ventricular arrhythmias in patients with CASQ2-associated catecholaminergic polymorphic ventricular tachycardia. *Heart Rhythm* 2013;10:1671–1675.
238. Pott C, Dechering DG, Reinke F, et al. Successful treatment of catecholaminergic polymorphic ventricular tachycardia with flecainide: a case report and review of the current literature. *Europace* 2011;13:897–901.
239. Kenyon CA, Flick R, Moir C, et al. Anesthesia for videoscopic left cardiac sympathetic denervation in children with congenital long QT syndrome and catecholaminergic polymorphic ventricular tachycardia–a case series. *Paediatr Anaesth* 2010;20:465–470.
240. Collura CA, Johnson JN, Moir C, et al. Left cardiac sympathetic denervation for the treatment of long QT syndrome and catecholaminergic polymorphic ventricular tachycardia using video-assisted thoracic surgery. *Heart Rhythm* 2009;6:752–759.
241. Jervell A, Lange-Nielsen F. Congenital deaf-mutism, functional heart disease with prolongation of the Q-T interval and sudden death. *Am Heart J* 1957;54:59–68.
242. Jervell A, Thingstad R, Endsjo TO. The surdo-cardiac syndrome: three new cases of congenital deafness with syncopal attacks and Q-T prolongation in the electrocardiogram. *Am Heart J* 1966;72:582–593.
243. Levine SA, Woodworth CR. Congenital deaf-mutism, prolonged QT interval, syncopal attacks and sudden death. *N Engl J Med* 1958;259: 412–417.
244. Schwartz PJ, Priori SG, Napolitano C, eds. *The long QT syndrome* (Chapter 68). Philadelphia, PA: WB Saunders, 2000.
245. Keren A, Tzivoni D, Gavish D, et al. Etiology, warning signs and therapy of torsade de pointes. A study of 10 patients. *Circulation* 1981;64:1167–1174.
246. Kay GN, Plumb VJ, Arciniegas JG, et al. Torsade de pointes: the long-short initiating sequence and other clinical features: observations in 32 patients. *J Am Coll Cardiol* 1983;2:806–817.
247. Bauman JL, Bauernfeind RA, Hoff JV, et al. Torsade de pointes due to quinidine: observations in 31 patients. *Am Heart J* 1984;107:425–430.
248. Roden DM, Woosley RL, Primm RK. Incidence and clinical features of the quinidine-associated long QT syndrome: implications for patient care. *Am Heart J* 1986;111:1088–1093.
249. El-Sherif N, Turitto G, eds. *Torsades de pointes* (Chapter 72). Philadelphia, PA: WB Saunders, 2000.
250. Roberts R. Genomics and cardiac arrhythmias. *J Am Coll Cardiol* 2006; 47:9–21.
251. Ackerman MJ, Priori SG, Willems S, et al. HRS/EHRA expert consensus statement on the state of genetic testing for the channelopathies and

cardiomyopathies this document was developed as a partnership between the Heart Rhythm Society (HRS) and the European Heart Rhythm Association (EHRA). *Heart Rhythm* 2011;8:1308–1339.
252. Morita H, Wu J, Zipes DP. The QT syndromes: long and short. *Lancet* 2008;372:750–763.
253. Roden DM. Long QT syndrome: reduced repolarization reserve and the genetic link. *J Intern Med* 2006;259:59–69.
254. Wellens HJ, Vermeulen A, Durrer D. Ventricular fibrillation occurring on arousal from sleep by auditory stimuli. *Circulation* 1972;46:661–665.
255. Coumel P, Fidelle J, Lacer V, et al. Catecholamine-induced severe ventricular arrhythmias with Adams-Stokes syndrome in children: report of four cases. *Br Heart J* 1978;40:28.
256. Moss AJ, Zareba W, Benhorin J, et al. ECG T-wave patterns in genetically distinct forms of the hereditary long QT syndrome. *Circulation* 1995;92:2929–2934.
257. Priori SG, Schwartz PJ, Napolitano C, et al. Risk stratification in the long-QT syndrome. *N Engl J Med* 2003;348:1866–1874.
258. Rivolta I, Abriel H, Tateyama M, et al. Inherited Brugada and long QT-3 syndrome mutations of a single residue of the cardiac sodium channel confer distinct channel and clinical phenotypes. *J Biol Chem* 2001; 276:30623–30630.
259. Freedman RA, Swerdlow CD, Soderholm-Difatte V, et al. Prognostic significance of arrhythmias induced at electrophysiologic study in cardiac arrest survivors. *Circulation* 1985;72:III45.
260. Ruskin JN, DiMarco JP, Garan H. Out-of-hospital cardiac arrest: electrophysiologic observations and selection of long-term antiarrhythmic therapy. *N Engl J Med* 1980;303:607–613.
261. Schoenfeld MH, McGovern B, Garan H, et al. Determinants of the outcome of electrophysiologic study in patients with ventricular tachyarrhythmias. *J Am Coll Cardiol* 1985;6:298–306.
262. Spielman SR, Farshidi A, Horowitz LN, et al. Ventricular fibrillation during programmed ventricular stimulation: incidence and clinical implications. *Am J Cardiol* 1978;42:913–918.
263. Swerdlow CD, Bardy GH, McAnulty J, et al. Determinants of induced sustained arrhythmias in survivors of out-of-hospital ventricular fibrillation. *Circulation* 1987;76:1053–1060.
264. Mann DE, Luck JC, Griffin JC, et al. Induction of clinical ventricular tachycardia using programmed stimulation: value of third and fourth extrastimuli. *Am J Cardiol* 1983;52:501–506.
265. Wellens HJ, Brugada P, Stevenson WG. Programmed electrical stimulation of the heart in patients with life-threatening ventricular arrhythmias: what is the significance of induced arrhythmias and what is the correct stimulation protocol? *Circulation* 1985;72:1–7.
266. Josephson ME, Spielman SR, Greenspan AM, et al. Mechanism of ventricular fibrillation in man. Observations based on electrode catheter recordings. *Am J Cardiol* 1979;44:623–631.
267. Bhandari AK, Shapiro WA, Morady F, et al. Electrophysiologic testing in patients with the long QT syndrome. *Circulation* 1985;71:63–71.
268. Schechter E, Freeman CC, Lazzara R. Afterdepolarizations as a mechanism for the long QT syndrome: electrophysiologic studies of a case. *J Am Coll Cardiol* 1984;3:1556–1561.
269. Levine JH, Spear JF, Guarnieri T, et al. Cesium chloride-induced long QT syndrome: demonstration of afterdepolarizations and triggered activity in vivo. *Circulation* 1985;72:1092–1103.
270. Vos MA, Verduyn SC, Gorgels AP, et al. Reproducible induction of early afterdepolarizations and torsade de pointes arrhythmias by d-sotalol and pacing in dogs with chronic atrioventricular block. *Circulation* 1995;91:864–872.
271. Hanich RF, Levine JH, Spear JF, et al. Autonomic modulation of ventricular arrhythmia in cesium chloride-induced long QT syndrome. *Circulation* 1988;77:1149–1161.
272. Ben-David J, Gerbig NR, Zipes DP. Differential response of early afterdepolarizations and ventricular tachycardia during right and left stellate stimulation in the dog treated with cesium. *J Am Coll Cardiol* 1988; 11:254A.
273. Bonatti V, Rolli A, Botti G. Recording of monophasic action potentials of the right ventricle in long QT syndromes complicated by severe ventricular arrhythmias. *Eur Heart J* 1983;4:168–179.
274. Bonatti V, Rolli A, Botti G. Monophasic action potential studies in human subjects with prolonged ventricular repolarization and long QT syndromes. *Eur Heart J* 1985;6(Suppl D):131–143.
275. El-Sherif N. Mechanism of ventricular arrhythmias in the long QT syndrome: on hermeneutics. *J Cardiovasc Electrophysiol* 2001;12:973–976.
276. Restivo M, Caref EB, Kozhevnikov DO, et al. Spatial dispersion of repolarization is a key factor in the arrhythmogenicity of long QT syndrome. *J Cardiovasc Electrophysiol* 2004;15:323–331.
277. Janse MJ, Kleber AG. Electrophysiological changes and ventricular arrhythmias in the early phase of regional myocardial ischemia. *Circ Res* 1981;49:1069–1081.
278. Crampton R. Preeminence of the left stellate ganglion in the long Q-T syndrome. *Circulation* 1979;59:769–778.
279. Abildskov JA. Neural mechanisms involved in the regulation of ventricular repolarization. *Eur Heart J* 1985;6(Suppl D):31–39.
280. Schwartz PJ, Malliani A. Electrical alternation of the T-wave: clinical and experimental evidence of its relationship with the sympathetic nervous system and with the long Q-T syndrome. *Am Heart J* 1975;89:45–50.
281. Moss AJ, McDonald J. Unilateral cervicothoracic sympathetic ganglionectomy for the treatment of long QT interval syndrome. *N Engl J Med* 1971;285:903–904.
282. Bhandari AK, Scheinman MM, Morady F, et al. Efficacy of left cardiac sympathectomy in the treatment of patients with the long QT syndrome. *Circulation* 1984;70:1018–1023.
283. Coyer BH, Pryor R, Kirsch WM, et al. Left stellectomy in the long QT syndrome. *Chest* 1978;74:584–586.
284. Surawicz B, Knoebel SB. Long QT: good, bad or indifferent? *J Am Coll Cardiol* 1984;4:398–413.
285. Ideker RE, Bardy VH, Worley SJ, et al., eds. *Patterns of activation during ventricular fibrillation.* Philadelphia, PA: Lea & Febiger, 1984.
286. Bardy GH, Ungerleider RM, Smith WM, et al. A mechanism of torsades de pointes in a canine model. *Circulation* 1983;67:52–59.
287. Leichter D, Danilo P Jr., Boyden P, et al. A canine model of torsades de pointes. *Pacing Clin Electrophysiol* 1988;11:2235–2245.
288. Vandepol CJ, Farshidi A, Spielman SR, et al. Incidence and clinical significance of induced ventricular tachycardia. *Am J Cardiol* 1980;45:725–731.
289. Buxton AE, Waxman HL, Marchlinski FE, et al. Electrophysiologic studies in nonsustained ventricular tachycardia: relation to underlying heart disease. *Am J Cardiol* 1983;52:985–991.
290. Veltri EP, Platia EV, Griffith LS, et al. Programmed electrical stimulation and long-term follow-up in asymptomatic, nonsustained ventricular tachycardia. *Am J Cardiol* 1985;56:309–314.
291. Buxton AE, Marchlinski FE, Waxman HL, et al. Prognostic factors in nonsustained ventricular tachycardia. *Am J Cardiol* 1984;53:1275–1279.
292. Wilber DJ, Kopp D, Olshansky B, et al. Nonsustained ventricular tachycardia and other high-risk predictors following myocardial infarction: implications for prophylactic automatic implantable cardioverter-defibrillator use. *Prog Cardiovasc Dis* 1993;36:179–194.
293. Buxton AE, Lee KL, Fisher JD, et al. A randomized study of the prevention of sudden death in patients with coronary artery disease. Multicenter Unsustained Tachycardia Trial Investigators. *N Engl J Med* 1999;341:1882–1890.
294. Buxton AE, Britton N, Simson MB. Application of the signal-averaged electrocardiogram in patients with nonsustained ventricular tachycardia after myocardial infarction: implications for prediction of sudden cardiac death risk. *J Electrocardiol* 1988;21(Suppl):S40–S45.
295. Buxton AE, Waxman HL, Marchlinski FE, et al. Right ventricular tachycardia: clinical and electrophysiologic characteristics. *Circulation* 1983;68:917–927.
296. Buxton AE, Marchlinski FE, Doherty JU, et al. Repetitive, monomorphic ventricular tachycardia: clinical and electrophysiologic characteristics in patients with and patients without organic heart disease. *Am J Cardiol* 1984;54:997–1002.
297. Sung RJ, Shen EN, Morady F, et al. Electrophysiologic mechanism of exercise-induced sustained ventricular tachycardia. *Am J Cardiol* 1983; 51:525–530.
298. Fleg JL, Lakatta EG. Prevalence and prognosis of exercise-induced nonsustained ventricular tachycardia in apparently healthy volunteers. *Am J Cardiol* 1984;54:762–764.
299. Lerman BB, Belardinelli L, West GA, et al. Adenosine-sensitive ventricular tachycardia: evidence suggesting cyclic AMP-mediated triggered activity. *Circulation* 1986;74:270–280.
300. Iwai S, Cantillon DJ, Kim RJ, et al. Right and left ventricular outflow tract tachycardias: evidence for a common electrophysiologic mechanism. *JCardiovasc Electrophysiol* 2006;17:1052–1058.
301. Kanagaratnam L, Tomassoni G, Schweikert R, et al. Ventricular tachycardias arising from the aortic sinus of valsalva: an under-recognized variant of left outflow tract ventricular tachycardia. *J Am Coll Cardiol* 2001;37:1408–1414.
302. Tanner H, Hindricks G, Schirdewahn P, et al. Outflow tract tachycardia with R/S transition in lead V3: six different anatomic approaches for successful ablation. *J Am Coll Cardiol* 2005;45:418–423.

303. Lerman BB, Ip JE, Shah BK, et al. Mechanism-specific effects of adenosine on ventricular tachycardia. *J Cardiovasc Electrophysiol* 2014;25(12):1350–1358.
304. Ip JE, Liu CF, Thomas G, et al. Unifying mechanism of sustained idiopathic atrial and ventricular annular tachycardia. *Circ Arrhythm Electrophysiol* 2014;7:436–444.
305. Ellis ER, Shvilkin A, Josephson ME. Nonreentrant ventricular arrhythmias in patients with structural heart disease unrelated to abnormal myocardial substrate. *Heart Rhythm* 2014;11:946–952.
306. Moss AJ, Hall WJ, Cannom DS, et al. Improved survival with an implanted defibrillator in patients with coronary disease at high risk for ventricular arrhythmia. Multicenter Automatic Defibrillator Implantation Trial Investigators. *N Engl J Med* 1996;335:1933–1940.
307. Wit AL, Allessie MA, Bonke FI, et al. Electrophysiologic mapping to determine the mechanism of experimental ventricular tachycardia initiated by premature impulses. Experimental approach and initial results demonstrating reentrant excitation. *Am J Cardiol* 1982;49:166–185.
308. Wit AL, Dillons S, Ursell PC, eds. *Influences of anisotropic tissue structure of ventricular tachycardia.* Mount Kisco, NY: Futura Publishing, 1987.
309. El-Sherif N, Gough WB, Restivo M. Reentrant ventricular arrhythmias in the late myocardial infarction period: 14. Mechanisms of resetting, entrainment, acceleration, or termination of reentrant tachycardia by programmed electrical stimulation. *Pacing Clin Electrophysiol* 1987;10:341–371.
310. Waldecker B, Coromilas J, Saltman AE, et al. Overdrive stimulation of functional reentrant circuits causing ventricular tachycardia in the infarcted canine heart. Resetting and entrainment. *Circulation* 1993;87:1286–12305.
311. Peters NS, Coromilas J, Hanna MS, et al. Characteristics of the temporal and spatial excitable gap in anisotropic reentrant circuits causing sustained ventricular tachycardia. *Circ Res* 1998;82:279–293.
312. Hanna MS, Coromilas J, Josephson ME, et al. Mechanisms of resetting reentrant circuits in canine ventricular tachycardia. *Circulation* 2001;103:1148–1156.
313. Frame LH, Simson MB. Oscillations of conduction, action potential duration, and refractoriness. A mechanism for spontaneous termination of reentrant tachycardias. *Circulation* 1988;78:1277–1287.
314. Waldo AL, Plumb VJ, Arciniegas JG, et al. Transient entrainment and interruption of the atrioventricular bypass pathway type of paroxysmal atrial tachycardia. A model for understanding and identifying reentrant arrhythmias. *Circulation* 1983;67:73–83.
315. Almendral JM, Rosenthal ME, Stamato NJ, et al. Analysis of the resetting phenomenon in sustained uniform ventricular tachycardia: incidence and relation to termination. *J Am Coll Cardiol* 1986;8:294–300.
316. Almendral JM, Stamato NJ, Rosenthal ME, et al. Resetting response patterns during sustained ventricular tachycardia: relationship to the excitable gap. *Circulation* 1986;74:722–730.
317. Stamato NJ, Rosenthal ME, Almendral JM, et al. The resetting response of ventricular tachycardia to single and double extrastimuli: implications for an excitable gap. *Am J Cardiol* 1987;60:596–601.
318. Rosenthal ME, Stamato NJ, Almendral JM, et al. Influence of the site of stimulation on the resetting phenomenon in ventricular tachycardia. *Am J Cardiol* 1986;58:970–976.
319. Almendral JM, Gottlieb CD, Rosenthal ME, et al. Entrainment of ventricular tachycardia: explanation for surface electrocardiographic phenomena by analysis of electrograms recorded within the tachycardia circuit. *Circulation* 1988;77:569–580.
320. Callans DJ, Hook BG, Josephson ME. Comparison of resetting and entrainment of uniform sustained ventricular tachycardia. Further insights into the characteristics of the excitable gap. *Circulation* 1993;87:1229–1238.
321. Callans DJ, Zardini M, Gottlieb CD, et al. The variable contribution of functional and anatomic barriers in human ventricular tachycardia: an analysis with resetting from two sites. *J Am Coll Cardiol* 1996;27:1106–1111.
322. Roy D, Waxman HL, Buxton AE, et al. Termination of ventricular tachycardia: role of tachycardia cycle length. *Am J Cardiol* 1982;50:1346–1350.
323. Fisher JD, Kim SG, Matos JA, et al. Comparative effectiveness of pacing techniques for termination of well-tolerated sustained ventricular tachycardia. *Pacing Clin Electrophysiol* 1983;6:915–922.
324. Waldecker B, Brugada P, Zehender M, et al. Importance of modes of electrical termination of ventricular tachycardia for the selection of implantable antitachycardia devices. *Am J Cardiol* 1986;57:150–155.
325. Naccarelli GV, Zipes DP, Rahilly GT, et al. Influence of tachycardia cycle length and antiarrhythmic drugs on pacing termination and acceleration of ventricular tachycardia. *Am Heart J* 1983;105:1–5.
326. MacLean WA, Plumb VJ, Waldo AL. Transient entrainment and interruption of ventricular tachycardia. *Pacing Clin Electrophysiol* 1981;4:358–366.
327. Waldo AL, Henthorn RW, Plumb VJ, et al. Demonstration of the mechanism of transient entrainment and interruption of ventricular tachycardia with rapid atrial pacing. *J Am Coll Cardiol* 1984;3:422–430.
328. Almendral JM, Gottlieb C, Marchlinski FE, et al. Entrainment of ventricular tachycardia by atrial depolarizations. *Am J Cardiol* 1985;56:298–304.
329. Rosenthal ME, Stamato NJ, Almendral JM, et al. Coupling intervals of ventricular extrastimuli causing resetting of sustained ventricular tachycardia secondary to coronary artery disease: relation to subsequent termination. *Am J Cardiol* 1988;61:770–774.
330. Gottlieb CD, Rosenthal ME, Stamato NJ, et al. The slope of the resetting response curve predicts termination with extrastimuli in ventricular tachycardia. *Circulation* 1987;76:219.
331. Gottlieb CD, Rosenthal ME, Stamato NJ, et al. A quantitative evaluation of refractoriness within a reentrant circuit during ventricular tachycardia. Relation to termination. *Circulation* 1990;82:1289–1295.
332. Fisher JD, Kim SG, Waspe LE, et al. Mechanisms for the success and failure of pacing for termination of ventricular tachycardia: clinical and hypothetical considerations. *Pacing Clin Electrophysiol* 1983;6:1094–1105.
333. Gardner MJ, Waxman HL, Buxton AE, et al. Termination of ventricular tachycardia. Evaluation of a new pacing method. *Am J Cardiol* 1982;50:1338–1345.
334. Callans DJ, Hook BG, Mitra RL, et al. Characterization of return cycle responses predictive of successful pacing-mediated termination of ventricular tachycardia. *J Am Coll Cardiol* 1995;25:47–53.
335. Mann DE, Lawrie GM, Luck JC, et al. Importance of pacing site in entrainment of ventricular tachycardia. *J Am Coll Cardiol* 1985;5:781–787.
336. Josephson ME, Horowitz LN, Farshidi A, et al. Sustained ventricular tachycardia: evidence for protected localized reentry. *Am J Cardiol* 1978;42:416–424.
337. Rosenthal ME, Stamato NJ, Almendral JM, et al. Resetting of ventricular tachycardia with electrocardiographic fusion: incidence and significance. *Circulation* 1988;77:581–588.
338. Almendral J. Resetting and entrainment of reentrant arrhythmias: part II: informative content and practical use of these responses. *Pacing Clin Electrophysiol* 2013;36:641–661.
339. Almendral J, Caulier-Cisterna R, Rojo-Alvarez JL. Resetting and entrainment of reentrant arrhythmias: part I: concepts, recognition, and protocol for evaluation: surface ECG versus intracardiac recordings. *Pacing-Clin Electrophysiol* 2013;36:508–532.
340. Josephson ME, Almendral J, Callans DJ. Resetting and entrainment of reentrant ventricular tachycardia associated with myocardial infarction. *Heart Rhythm* 2014;11:1239–1249.
341. Allessie MA, Bonke FI, Schopman FJ. Circus movement in rabbit atrial muscle as a mechanism of tachycardia. III. The "leading circle" concept: a new model of circus movement in cardiac tissue without the involvement of an anatomical obstacle. *Circ Res* 1977;41:9–18.
342. Okumura K, Olshansky B, Henthorn RW, et al. Demonstration of the presence of slow conduction during sustained ventricular tachycardia in man: use of transient entrainment of the tachycardia. *Circulation* 1987;75:369–378.
343. Kay GN, Epstein AE, Plumb VJ. Region of slow conduction in sustained ventricular tachycardia: direct endocardial recordings and functional characterization in humans. *J Am Coll Cardiol* 1988;11:109–116.
344. Okumura K, Matsuyama K, Miyagi H, et al. Entrainment of idiopathic ventricular tachycardia of left ventricular origin with evidence for reentry with an area of slow conduction and effect of verapamil. *Am J Cardiol* 1988;62:727–732.
345. Okumura K, Yamabe H, Tsuchiya T, et al. Characteristics of slow conduction zone demonstrated during entrainment of idiopathic ventricular tachycardia of left ventricular origin. *Am J Cardiol* 1996;77:379–383.
346. Merino JL, Peinado R, Fernandez-Lozano I, et al. Transient entrainment of bundle-branch reentry by atrial and ventricular stimulation: elucidation of the tachycardia mechanism through analysis of the surface ECG. *Circulation* 1999;100:1784–1790.
347. Spach MS. Changes in the topology of gap junctions as an adaptive structural response of the myocardium. *Circulation* 1994;90:1103–1106.
348. Peters NS, Coromilas J, Severs NJ, et al. Disturbed connexin43 gap junction distribution correlates with the location of reentrant circuits in the epicardial border zone of healing canine infarcts that cause ventricular tachycardia. *Circulation* 1997;95:988–996.

349. Schoels W, Steinhaus D, Johnson WB, et al. Optimizing implantable cardioverter-defibrillator treatment of rapid ventricular tachycardia: antitachycardia pacing therapy during charging. *Heart Rhythm* 2007;4:879–885.
350. Sweeney MO, Sherfesee L, DeGroot PJ, et al. Differences in effects of electrical therapy type for ventricular arrhythmias on mortality in implantable cardioverter-defibrillator patients. *Heart Rhythm* 2010;7:353–360.
351. Boersma L, Brugada J, Abdollah H, et al. Effects of heptanol, class Ic, and class III drugs on reentrant ventricular tachycardia. Importance of the excitable gap for the inducibility of double-wave reentry. *Circulation* 1994;90:1012–1022.
352. Downar E, Kimber S, Harris L, et al. Endocardial mapping of ventricular tachycardia in the intact human heart. II. Evidence for multiuse reentry in a functional sheet of surviving myocardium. *J Am Coll Cardiol* 1992;20:869–878.
353. Downar E, Saito J, Doig JC, et al. Endocardial mapping of ventricular tachycardia in the intact human ventricle. III. Evidence of multiuse reentry with spontaneous and induced block in portions of reentrant path complex. *J Am Coll Cardiol* 1995;25:1591–1600.
354. Shenasa M, Cardinal R, Kus T, et al. Termination of sustained ventricular tachycardia by ultrarapid subthreshold stimulation in humans. *Circulation* 1988;78:1135–1143.
355. Waxman HL, Cain ME, Greenspan AM, et al. Termination of ventricular tachycardia with ventricular stimulation: salutary effect of increased current strength. *Circulation* 1982;65:800–804.
356. Wellens HJ, Bar FW, Lie KI, et al. Effect of procainamide, propranolol and verapamil on mechanism of tachycardia in patients with chronic recurrent ventricular tachycardia. *Am J Cardiol* 1977;40:579–585.
357. Marchlinski FE, Buxton AE, Josephson ME, et al. Predicting ventricular tachycardia cycle length after procainamide by assessing cycle length-dependent changes in paced QRS duration. *Circulation* 1989;79:39–46.
358. Marchlinski FE, Buxton AE, Kindwall KE, et al. Comparison of individual and combined effects of procainamide and amiodarone in patients with sustained ventricular tachyarrhythmias. *Circulation* 1988;78:583–591.
359. Rosen MR, Danilo P Jr. Effects of tetrodotoxin, lidocaine, verapamil, and AHR-2666 on Ouabain-induced delayed afterdepolarizations in canine Purkinje fibers. *Circ Res* 1980;46:117–724.
360. Horowitz LN, Josephson ME, Farshidi A, et al. Recurrent sustained ventricular tachycardia 3. Role of the electrophysiologic study in selection of antiarrhythmic regimens. *Circulation* 1978;58:986–997.
361. Mason JW, Winkle RA. Electrode-catheter arrhythmia induction in the selection and assessment of antiarrhythmic drug therapy for recurrent ventricular tachycardia. *Circulation* 1978;58:971–985.
362. Josephson ME, Horowitz LN. Electrophysiologic approach to therapy of recurrent sustained ventricular tachycardia. *Am J Cardiol* 1979;43:631–642.
363. Horowitz LN, Josephson ME, Kastor JA. Intracardiac electrophysiologic studies as a method for the optimization of drug therapy in chronic ventricular arrhythmia. *Prog Cardiovasc Dis* 1980;23:81–98.
364. Fisher JD, Cohen HL, Mehra R, et al. Cardiac pacing and pacemakers II. Serial electrophysiologic-pharmacologic testing for control of recurrent tachyarrhythmias. *Am Heart J* 1977;93:658–668.
365. Stamato NJ, Frame LH, Rosenthal ME, et al. Procainamide-induced slowing of ventricular tachycardia with insights from analysis of resetting response patterns. *Am J Cardiol* 1989;63:1455–1461.
366. Buxton AE, Marchlinski FE, Miller JM, et al. Role of procainamide in identifying clinically relevant polymorphic tachycardias. *Circulation* 1988;78:II71.
367. Buxton AE, Waxman HL, Marchlinski FE, et al. Electropharmacology of nonsustained ventricular tachycardia: effects of class I antiarrhythmic agents, verapamil and propranolol. *Am J Cardiol* 1984;53:738–744.
368. Josephson ME, Horowitz LN, Farshidi A, et al. Recurrent sustained ventricular tachycardia. 2. Endocardial mapping. *Circulation* 1978;57:440–447.
369. Josephson ME, Horowitz LN, Spielman SR, et al. Role of catheter mapping in the preoperative evaluation of ventricular tachycardia. *Am J Cardiol* 1982;49:207–220.
370. Waspe LE, Brodman R, Kim SG, et al. Activation mapping in patients with coronary artery disease with multiple ventricular tachycardia configurations: occurrence and therapeutic implications of widely separate apparent sites of origin. *J Am Coll Cardiol* 1985;5:1075–1086.
371. Horowitz LN, Josephson ME, Harken AH. Epicardial and endocardial activation during sustained ventricular tachycardia in man. *Circulation* 1980;61:1227–1238.
372. Josephson ME, Horowitz LN, Spielman SR, et al. Comparison of endocardial catheter mapping with intraoperative mapping of ventricular tachycardia. *Circulation* 1980;61:395–404.
373. de Bakker JM, Janse MJ, Van Capelle FJ, et al. Endocardial mapping by simultaneous recording of endocardial electrograms during cardiac surgery for ventricular aneurysm. *J Am Coll Cardiol* 1983;2:947–953.
374. Miller JM, Harken AH, Hargrove WC, et al. Pattern of endocardial activation during sustained ventricular tachycardia. *J Am Coll Cardiol* 1985;6:1280–1287.
375. Harris L, Downar E, Mickleborough L, et al. Activation sequence of ventricular tachycardia: endocardial and epicardial mapping studies in the human ventricle. *J Am Coll Cardiol* 1987;10:1040–1047.
376. Downar E, Harris L, Mickleborough LL, et al. Endocardial mapping of ventricular tachycardia in the intact human ventricle: evidence for reentrant mechanisms. *J Am Coll Cardiol* 1988;11:783–791.
377. Stevenson WG, Weiss JN, Wiener I, et al. Resetting of ventricular tachycardia: implications for localizing the area of slow conduction. *J Am Coll Cardiol* 1988;11:522–529.
378. Morady F, Frank R, Kou WH, et al. Identification and catheter ablation of a zone of slow conduction in the reentrant circuit of ventricular tachycardia in humans. *J Am CollCardiol* 1988;11:775–782.
379. Fitzgerald DM, Friday KJ, Wah JA, et al. Electrogram patterns predicting successful catheter ablation of ventricular tachycardia. *Circulation* 1988;77:806–814.
380. Stevenson WG, Khan H, Sager P, et al. Identification of reentry circuit sites during catheter mapping and radiofrequency ablation of ventricular tachycardia late after myocardial infarction. *Circulation* 1993;88:1647–1670.
381. Stevenson WG, Friedman PL, Sager PT, et al. Exploring postinfarction reentrant ventricular tachycardia with entrainment mapping. *J Am Coll Cardiol* 1997;29:1180–1189.
382. Sosa E, Scanavacca M, d'Avila A, et al. Nonsurgical transthoracic epicardial catheter ablation to treat recurrent ventricular tachycardia occurring late after myocardial infarction. *J Am Coll Cardiol* 2000;35:1442–1449.
383. Josephson ME. Epicardial approach to the ablation of ventricular tachycardia in coronary artery disease: an alternative or ancillary approach. *J Am Coll Cardiol* 2000;35:1450–1452.
384. Khoury DS, Taccardi B, Lux RL, et al. Reconstruction of endocardial potentials and activation sequences from intracavitary probe measurements. Localization of pacing sites and effects of myocardial structure. *Circulation* 1995;91:845–863.
385. Schilling RJ, Peters NS, Davies DW. Simultaneous endocardial mapping in the human left ventricle using a noncontact catheter: comparison of contact and reconstructed electrograms during sinus rhythm. *Circulation* 1998;98:887–898.
386. Chow AW, Schilling RJ, Davies DW, et al. Characteristics of wavefront propagation in reentrant circuits causing human ventricular tachycardia. *Circulation* 2002;105:2172–2178.
387. Rudy Y. Noninvasive electrocardiographic imaging of arrhythmogenic substrates in humans. *Circ Res* 2013;112:863–874.
388. Ghanem RN, Jia P, Ramanathan C, et al. Noninvasive electrocardiographic imaging (ECGI): comparison to intraoperative mapping in patients. *Heart Rhythm* 2005;2:339–354.
389. Intini A, Goldstein RN, Jia P, et al. Electrocardiographic imaging (ECGI), a novel diagnostic modality used for mapping of focal left ventricular tachycardia in a young athlete. *Heart Rhythm* 2005;2:1250–1252.
390. Stevenson WG, Weiss JN, Wiener I, et al. Fractionated endocardial electrograms are associated with slow conduction in humans: evidence from pace-mapping. *J Am Coll Cardiol* 1989;13:369–376.
391. Josephson ME. The origin of premature ventricular complexes–role and limitations of the 12-lead electrocardiogram. *Int J Cardiol* 1982;2:87–90.
392. Josephson ME, Waxman HL, Cain ME, et al. Ventricular activation during ventricular endocardial pacing. II. Role of pace-mapping to localize origin of ventricular tachycardia. *Am J Cardiol* 1982;50:11–22.
393. Waxman HL, Josephson ME. Ventricular activation during ventricular endocardial pacing: I. Electrocardiographic patterns related to the site of pacing. *Am J Cardiol* 1982;50:1–10.
394. Holt PM, Smallpeice C, Deverall PB, et al. Ventricular arrhythmias. A guide to their localisation. *Br Heart J* 1985;53:417–430.
395. Kuchar DL, Ruskin JN, Garan H. Electrocardiographic localization of the site of origin of ventricular tachycardia in patients with prior myocardial infarction. *J Am Coll Cardiol* 1989;13:893–903.
396. Josephson ME, Horowitz LN, Farshidi A, et al. Recurrent sustained ventricular tachycardia. 4. Pleomorphism. *Circulation* 1979;59:459–468.
397. Jais P, Maury P, Khairy P, et al. Elimination of local abnormal ventricular activities: a new end point for substrate modification in patients with scar-related ventricular tachycardia. *Circulation* 2012;125:2184–2196.
398. Fisher JD. Stimulation as a key to tachycardia localization and ablation. *J Am Coll Cardiol* 1988;11:889–893.

399. Soejima K, Stevenson WG, Maisel WH, et al. The N + 1 difference: a new measure for entrainment mapping. *J Am Coll Cardiol* 2001;37:1386–1394.
400. Tedrow U, Stevenson WG. Strategies for epicardial mapping and ablation of ventricular tachycardia. *J Cardiovasc Electrophysiol* 2009;20:710–713.
401. Liuba I, Marchlinski FE. The substrate and ablation of ventricular tachycardia in patients with nonischemic cardiomyopathy. *Circ J* 2013;77:1957–1966.
402. Zei PC, Stevenson WG. Epicardial catheter mapping and ablation of ventricular tachycardia. *Heart Rhythm* 2006;3:360–363.
403. d'Avila A, Houghtaling C, Gutierrez P, et al. Catheter ablation of ventricular epicardial tissue: a comparison of standard and cooled-tip radiofrequency energy. *Circulation* 2004;109:2363–2369.
404. Frame LH, Rhee EK, Bernstein RC, et al. Reversal of reentry and acceleration due to double-wave reentry: two mechanisms for failure to terminate tachycardias by rapid pacing. *J Am Coll Cardiol* 1996;28:137–145.
405. Bogun F, Knight B, Goyal R, et al. Clinical value of the postpacing interval for mapping of ventricular tachycardia in patients with prior myocardial infarction. *J Cardiovasc Electrophysiol* 1999;10:43–51.
406. Di Biase L, Santangeli P, Burkhardt DJ, et al. Endo-epicardial homogenization of the scar versus limited substrate ablation for the treatment of electrical storms in patients with ischemic cardiomyopathy. *J Am Coll Cardiol* 2012;60:132–141.
407. de Chillou C, Groben L, Magnin-Poull I, et al. Localizing the critical isthmus of postinfarct ventricular tachycardia: the value of pace-mapping during sinus rhythm. *Heart Rhythm* 2014;11:175–181.
408. DiMarco JP, Garan H, Harthorne JW, et al. Intracardiac electrophysiologic techniques in recurrent syncope of unknown case. *Ann Intern Med* 1981;95:542–548.
409. Hess DS, Morady F, Scheinman MM. Electrophysiologic testing in the evaluation of patients with syncope of undetermined origin. *Am J Cardiol* 1982;50:1309–1315.
410. Ezri M, Lerman BB, Marchlinski FE, et al. Electrophysiologic evaluation of syncope in patients with bifascicular block. *Am Heart J* 1983;106:693–697.
411. Akhtar M, Shenasa M, Denker S, et al. Role of cardiac electrophysiologic studies in patients with unexplained recurrent syncope. *Pacing Clin Electrophysiol* 1983;6:192–201.
412. Morady F, Shen E, Schwartz A, et al. Long-term follow-up of patients with recurrent unexplained syncope evaluated by electrophysiologic testing. *J Am Coll Cardiol* 1983;2:1053–1059.
413. Morady F, Higgins J, Peters RW, et al. Electrophysiologic testing in bundle branch block and unexplained syncope. *Am J Cardiol* 1984;54:587–591.
414. Olshansky B, Mazuz M, Martins JB. Significance of inducible tachycardia in patients with syncope of unknown origin: a long-term follow-up. *J Am Coll Cardiol* 1985;5:216–223.
415. Doherty JU, Pembrook-Rogers D, Grogan EW, et al. Electrophysiologic evaluation and follow-up characteristics of patients with recurrent unexplained syncope and presyncope. *Am J Cardiol* 1985;55:703–708.
416. Krol RB, Morady F, Flaker GC, et al. Electrophysiologic testing in patients with unexplained syncope: clinical and noninvasive predictors of outcome. *J Am Coll Cardiol* 1987;10:358–363.
417. Link MS, Costeas XF, Griffith JL, et al. High incidence of appropriate implantable cardioverter-defibrillator therapy in patients with syncope of unknown etiology and inducible ventricular arrhythmias. *J Am Coll Cardiol* 1997;29:370–375.
418. Knight BP, Goyal R, Pelosi F, et al. Outcome of patients with nonischemic dilated cardiomyopathy and unexplained syncope treated with an implantable defibrillator. *J Am Coll Cardiol* 1999;33:1964–1970.

CHAPTER

# 12 Evaluation of Antiarrhythmic Agents

The application of recording and stimulation techniques has made it possible to evaluate the electrophysiologic effects and preferential sites of action of the entire spectrum of antiarrhythmic agents. Knowledge of major sites and characteristics of drug action may provide a database for the selection of safe and effective agents for acute and chronic therapy. The reproducible initiation and termination of paroxysmal supraventricular and ventricular tachyarrhythmias allow the electrophysiologist to develop pharmacologic means to predict successful drug therapy. This chapter presents a discussion of the current classification and action of antiarrhythmic agents and how they relate to clinical effects in humans as well as their value as antiarrhythmic agents. The use of programmed stimulation to develop therapy for tachyarrhythmias will also be outlined in detail.

## CLASSIFICATION OF ANTIARRHYTHMIC AGENTS

Theoretically, the choice of an antiarrhythmic agent should be based on the drug's known electrophysiologic effects and the relationship of such effects to the arrhythmia in question. Thus, drugs having potent electrophysiologic effects on specific cardiac tissues should be chosen to treat arrhythmias arising from those tissues. The ideal situation would be the ability to select an antiarrhythmic agent that had specific activity against arrhythmia mechanisms (i.e., automaticity, triggered activity, or reentry) involving particular cardiac tissues. In other words, the pharmacologic therapy of an arrhythmia would depend on both the mechanism and the site of the arrhythmia. Unfortunately, this is not the case. As such, choice of the antiarrhythmic agent is dictated solely on the ability of a drug to produce electrophysiologic changes in specific arrhythmogenic tissue. Such empiricism is a consequence of (a) a limited understanding of drug action in vivo and (b) the reliance on in vitro drug classifications, which are based on how drugs affect ionic currents and not on how they influence particular arrhythmias. Therefore, we need a better understanding of how individual drugs work on specific arrhythmogenic tissues in vivo to learn why a given antiarrhythmic agent can behave in either an antiarrhythmic or proarrhythmic manner. This will ultimately provide clinicians with an improved ability to tailor antiarrhythmic drug therapy for particular indications.

### In Vitro Classification of Antiarrhythmic Agents

The most commonly used classification of antiarrhythmic drugs is based on the ability of a drug to block specific ionic currents (e.g., sodium, potassium, or calcium), as well as those that block beta-adrenergic receptors.[1–3] Thus, Class 1 agents are those that primarily block the fast sodium channel. These agents have been further subdivided into lA, lB, and lC agents. Class lA agents include quinidine, procainamide, and disopyramide, all of which are characterized by slowing the maximum rate of rise of the action potential as well as by increasing action potential duration. Class lB drugs are those that allegedly have little effect on the maximum rate of rise of the action potential and tend to shorten action potential duration. Included in this group are lidocaine, phenytoin, mexiletine, and tocainide. Finally, Class lC drugs, which include flecainide, encainide, moricizine, and propafenone, are those that primarily slow conduction by depression of the maximum rate of rise of depolarization of the action potential with minimal prolongation of refractoriness. Class 2 drugs fall under the general heading of beta blockers. Propranolol and metoprolol are the paradigms of this class of agents, but also includes nadolol, timolol, acebutolol, atenolol, and pindolol. Class 3 agents are those that block repolarization currents (i.e., potassium channels) and prolong action potential duration. Included in this group are amiodarone, dofetilide, bretylium, sotalol (also with beta-blocker effects), azimilide, ibutilide (IV only), dronedarone, tedisimil and the major metabolite of procainamide, n-acetyl procainamide. Class 4 agents are those agents that block the calcium channel. These primarily include nondihydropyridine agents verapamil and diltiazem, but also include dihydropyridine agents including amlodipine, felodipine, nifedipine, etc.

In my opinion, this classification suffers many limitations and has little value in assessing the choice of antiarrhythmics for a given arrhythmia. Some of these limitations follow: (a) The classification is based on in vitro studies of isolated cell types, usually the normal Purkinje fiber or, in some instances, on A-V nodal fibers. The failure to consider other tissue types and, more importantly, abnormal tissues (e.g., ischemic fibers) leads to inadequate, and often misleading, information. For example, ischemic fibers are composed of cells that have lower resting membrane potentials and depressed fast sodium channel activity and, in addition, demonstrate abnormal intercellular coupling.[4,5] Such fibers exhibit slow conduction and postrepolarization refractoriness; that is, the refractory period extends beyond completion of repolarization. In such fibers, even Class IB agents readily produce block. (b) Drugs have complex actions. Drugs may affect multiple channels (i.e., sodium channels to depress $V_{max}$ and potassium channels to prolong repolarization), and/or may affect both the autonomic nervous system as well as ionic channels (i.e., Class IA agents all have vagolytic activity, and both amiodarone and propafenone have beta-blocking activity). Moreover, antiarrhythmic agents can depress myocardial function, resulting in altered hemodynamics and autonomic reflex activity, which in turn can affect antiarrhythmic drug action. Finally, some drugs have metabolites, which may be more active and/or have different pharmacokinetics than the parent drug, neither of which is tested in vitro (i.e., procainamide and its metabolite n-acetyl procainamide). (c) Drugs exert greater electrophysiologic effects at different rates of stimulation and after prolonged periods of stimulation (i.e., use-dependence).[6–10] The ability to bind and dissociate rapidly from channels is highly variable. For example, Class IB drugs have rapid kinetics (i.e., rapid binding and dissociation), while IC drugs have slow kinetics. Class IA drugs are intermediate. Thus, IB agents will demonstrate minimal effects at relatively slow rates, while IC agents will demonstrate significant effects at comparable or even slower rates. In addition, cells that are partially depolarized (e.g., secondary to ischemia) are associated with much slower binding kinetics of antiarrhythmics than those at more negative membrane potentials. This is one of the causes of postrepolarization refractoriness noted in such fibers. (d) Related to use-dependence is a model proposed by Hondeghem and Katzung[11–13] termed the "modulated receptor hypothesis." By this hypothesis, antiarrhythmic agents interact with receptors in the membrane in either the resting, activated, or inactivated state. These interactions are voltage and time dependent and appear operative for both sodium and calcium channels. Some drugs are bound primarily in the active state (i.e., Class IA agents), while others are primarily bound in the inactive state (i.e., amiodarone),[14] and some (e.g., lidocaine) are bound in both active and inactive states. Use-dependence and the modulated receptor hypothesis are interactive and may lead to totally different conclusions about the electrophysiologic effects of a given agent than if the agent was evaluated on a normal isolated Purkinje fiber at a slow rate. (e) Alterations in cellular metabolism and the intra- and extracellular ionic milieu can affect a drug's actions. Changes in extracellular potassium, intracellular calcium, and pH can affect active membrane currents through ionic channels and may induce nonspecific ionic channels.[5,15–18] In addition, increased intracellular calcium decreases intercellular coupling and impairs propagation of impulses. The inhibition of the sodium/potassium pump by digitalis and the sodium/calcium pump during ischemia may also affect the action of antiarrhythmic agents. (f) Alterations in circulating catecholamines and in autonomic tone can alter electrophysiologic drug action. Many of the effects on sodium, potassium, and calcium channels can be reversed by enhanced sympathetic tone or circulating catecholamines.[19] (g) Little attention has been paid to the influence of drugs on passive membrane properties, in particular, their effects on the coupling of cells and propagation through anisotropic (particularly nonuniform anisotropic) tissues. The effects on passive membrane properties may differ among agents of the same class.[20] Preliminary data suggest that an agent may affect conduction longitudinal to fiber orientation differently than that transverse to fiber orientation.[21] (h) There are major differences in drug metabolism between subjects, which may greatly affect efficacy and toxicity of antiarrhythmic agents, particularly those with active metabolites.[22] One important example of this phenomenon is fast/slow acetylator status for flecainide and propafenone. The developing field of pharmacogenomics will no doubt revolutionize our understanding of antiarrhythmic drug effects. (i) A major new focus for drug development is hoping to take advantage of antiarrhythmic effects that are specific to a particular tissue. Atrial specific Class 3 drugs in development (e.g., AZD 7009, AVE 0118) may be useful in treating atrial fibrillation by blockade of the ultrarapid delayed rectifying current ($I_{Kur}$), which is not present in ventricular tissue. The Vaughan Williams classification has no contingencies to take this sort of specificity into account.

It is clear, therefore, that the simple classification of antiarrhythmic agents that is most widely used provides insufficient information relative to electrophysiologic action in vivo and even less information relative to a drug's actual antiarrhythmic effects. The "classic" mechanism of action of these antiarrhythmic agents is shown in Table 12-1. One must remember that these "actions," which are based on data from single-cell microelectrode recordings, whole-cell voltage clamping, and patch clamping, simply reveal how these drugs modify ionic conductance in normal tissues. To better understand how drugs may act in humans, it is important to study the electrophysiologic effects of these agents on the human in vivo so that one might understand a drug's action on that tissue.

## EVALUATION OF ELECTROPHYSIOLOGIC EFFECTS OF DRUGS IN HUMANS

Using standard intracardiac recording and stimulation techniques, one can determine the effects of individual drugs on specific cardiac tissue. As noted in Chapters 2 and 3, measurements of sinoatrial conduction time and automaticity, as well as conduction and refractoriness in the atrium, A-V node, His–Purkinje system, and ventricle during sinus and paced rhythms are readily obtainable and generally reproducible. A summary of the electrophysiologic properties of various currently available and some promising experimental antiarrhythmic agents in humans is shown in Tables 12-2 and

TABLE 12-1 In Vitro Electrophysiologic Characteristics

| Drug | Phase | | | | | Conduction Velocity | Sinus Node Automaticity | Phase 4 | Membrane Responsiveness |
|---|---|---|---|---|---|---|---|---|---|
| | APA | APD | 0 | MDP | ERP | | | | |
| Quinidine | ↓ | ↑ | ↓ | ↔ | ↑ | ↓ | ↔ | ↓ | ↓ |
| Procainamide | ↓ | ↑ | ↓ | ↔ | ↑ | ↓ | ↔ | ↓ | ↓ |
| Disopyramide | ↓ | ↑ | ↓ | ↔ | ↑ | ↓ | ↑↔↓ | ↓ | ↓ |
| Lidocaine | ↓ | ↓ | ↔↓ | ↔ | ↓ | ↔↓ | ↔ | ↓ | ↔↓ |
| Phenytoin | ↔ | ↓ | ↔↓ | ↔ | ↓ | ↔ | ↔ | ↓ | ↔↑ |
| Mexiletine | ↔ | ↓ | ↔↓ | ↔ | ↓ | ↓ | ↔ | ↓ | ↓ |
| Tocainide | ↔ | ↓ | ↔↓ | ↔ | ↓ | ↓ | ↔ | ↓ | ↓ |
| Flecainide | ↓ | ↑ | ↓ | ↔ | ↑ | ↓ | ↔ | ↓ | ↓ |
| Encainide | ↓ | ↔↓ | ↓ | ↔ | ↑ | ↓ | ↔ | ↓ | ↓ |
| Lorcainide | ↓ | ↑ | ↓ | ↔ | ↑ | ↓ | ↔ | ↓ | ↓ |
| Propafenone | ↓ | ↔↑ | ↓ | ↔ | ↔↑ | ↓ | ↓ | ↓ | ↓ |
| Moricizine | ↓ | ↓ | ↓ | ↔ | ↔↑ | ↓ | ↔ | ↔ | ↓ |
| Propranolol | ↔↓ | ↔↑* | ↔↓ | ↔ | ↔↓* | ↔ | ↓ | ↓* | ↔↑ |
| Ibutilide | ↔ | ↑↓ | ↔↓ | ↔ | ↑ | ↔ | ↓ | ↓ | ↔ |
| Dofetilide | ↔ | ↑ | ↔ | ↔ | ↑ | ↔ | ↓ | ↓ | ↔ |
| Azimilide | ↔ | ↑ | ↔ | ↔ | ↑ | ↔ | ↓ | ↓ | ↔ |
| Tedisimil | ↔ | ↑ | ↔ | ↔ | ↑ | ↔ | ↓ | ↓ | ↔ |
| Sotalol | ↔ | ↑ | ↔ | ↔ | ↑ | ↔ | ↓ | ↓ | ↔ |
| Amiodarone | ↔ | ↑ | ↔↓ | ↔ | ↑ | ↓ | ↓ | ↓ | ↓ |
| Dronedarone | ↔ | ↑ | ↔↓ | ↔ | ↑ | ↓ | ↓ | ↓ | ↓ |
| Bretylium | ↔ | ↑ | ↔ | ↔ | ↑ | ↔ | ↔↓ | ↔↓* | ↔ |
| Verapamil | ↔ | ↓ | ↔ | ↔ | ↔ | ↔ | ↓ | ↓* | ↔ |
| Ranolazine | ↔ | ↑ | ↔ | ↔ | ↑ | ↔ | ↔ | ↓ | ↔ |

APA, action potential amplitude; APD, action potential duration; ERP, effective refractory period; MDP, maximum diastolic potential; ↑, increase; ↓, decrease; ↔, no change; ↔↑ or ↔↓, slight inconsistent increase or decrease.
*With a background of sympathetic activity.

12-3.[23–113] Data used in Table 12-2 apply to the effects of these agents on nonischemic, normal tissues measured in sinus rhythm or during pacing from standard right atrial and right ventricular sites (see Chapter 2). Limitations of such measurements and suggestions for other parameters to be studied are discussed in subsequent paragraphs.

Besides evaluating the effect of antiarrhythmic agents on conduction (intra-atrial, A-V nodal, His–Purkinje, and intraventricular) and refractoriness, measurements of threshold of excitability and strength-interval curves[114,115] should also be performed. The frequency-dependent effects of these drugs should be evaluated by assessing the effects of different drive cycle lengths on these parameters. Several investigators have demonstrated use-dependent effects in vivo using canine models as well as in humans.[94,114,116–119] The effects of procainamide on cycle length–induced changes in threshold of excitability of the human atrium as well as on strength-interval curves in the human ventricle are shown in Figures 12-1 and 12-2.[114,119] Propafenone caused pronounced cycle length–dependent changes in threshold of excitability in 25% of the patients studied that were associated with marked prolongation of refractoriness and clinical efficacy.[120] The effects of procainamide and other agents on cycle length–dependent changes in refractoriness and/or strength-interval curves may therefore be clinically meaningful. For example, the blunting or reversal of cycle length–dependent shortening of refractoriness by an antiarrhythmic agent may signify an important electrophysiologic response that predicts clinical efficacy.[7,8] The effect of agents on interval-dependent conduction delay in response to extrastimuli may also provide clinically useful data in the management of certain arrhythmias.[119,121] More data are required relating efficacy and frequency or

## TABLE 12-2 In Vivo Electrophysiologic Characteristics of Antiarrhythmic Drugs Electrophysiologic Effects

| Drug | ERP AVN | ERP HPS | ERP A | ERP V | ERP AP |
|---|---|---|---|---|---|
| Quinidine | ↓↔↑ | ↑ | ↑ | ↑ | ↑ |
| Procainamide | ↔↑ | ↑ | ↑ | ↑ | ↑ |
| Disopyramide | ↔↓ | ↑ | ↑ | ↑ | ↑ |
| Lidocaine | ↔↓ | ↔↓ | ↔ | ↔ | ↔ |
| Phenytoin | ↔↓ | ↓ | ↔ | ↔ | ↔ |
| Mexiletine | ↔↑ | ↔↑ | ↔ | ↔ | ↔ |
| Tocainide | ↓ | ↔ | ↔↓ | ↔↓ | ↔↑ |
| Flecainide | ↑ | ↑ | ↑ | ↑ | ↑ |
| Encainide | ↑ | ↑ | ↑ | ↑ | ↑ |
| Propafenone | ↔↑ | ↔ | ↔↑ | ↑ | ↑ |
| Moricizine | ↔ | ↔↑ | ↔↑ | ↔↑ | ↑ |
| Propranolol | ↑ | ↔ | ↔ | ↔ | ↔ |
| Sotalol | ↑ | ↑ | ↑ | ↑ | ↑ |
| Dofetilide | ↔ | ↔ | ↑ | ↑ | ↑ |
| Ibutilide | ↑ | ↑ | ↑ | ↑ | ↑ |
| Amiodarone | ↑ | ↑ | ↑ | ↑ | ↑ |
| Bretylium | ↔↑ | ↑ | ↑ | ↑ | ↔ |
| Verapamil | ↑ | ↔ | ↔ | ↔ | ↔ |
| Ranolazine | ↔ | ↔ | ↑ | ↑ | ? |

Results presented may vary according to tissue type, experimental conditions, and drug concentration.
↑, increase; ↓, decrease; ↔, no change; ↔↑ or ↔↓, slight inconsistent increase or decrease; A, atrium; AVN, AV node; HPS, His–Purkinje system; V, ventricle; AP, accessory pathway (WPW); ERP, effective refractory period—longest $S_1$–$S_2$ interval at which $S_2$ fails to produce a response.

## TABLE 12-3 In Vivo Electrophysiologic Characteristics of Antiarrhythmic Drugs Electrocardiographic Effects

| Drug | Sinus Rate | P-R | QRS | Q-T | A-H | H-V |
|---|---|---|---|---|---|---|
| Quinidine | ↔↑ | ↓↔↑ | ↑ | ↑ | ↓↔↑ | ↔↑ |
| Procainamide | ↔ | ↔↑ | ↑ | ↑ | ↔↑ | ↔↑ |
| Disopyramide | ↔↑ | ↔ | ↔↑ | ↔↑ | ↔ | ↔↑ |
| Lidocaine | ↔ | ↔ | ↔ | ↔ | ↓↔ | ↓↔ |
| Phenytoin | ↔ | ↔ | ↔ | ↔↓ | ↔↓ | ↔ |
| Mexiletine | ↔ | ↔ | ↔ | ↔ | ↔↑ | ↔↑ |
| Tocainide | ↔↓ | ↔ | ↔ | ↔↓ | ↔↑ | ↔ |
| Flecainide | ↔↓ | ↑ | ↑ | ↑ | ↑ | ↑ |
| Propafenone | ↔↓ | ↑ | ↑ | ↑ | ↑ | ↑ |
| Moricizine | ↔↓ | ↔↑ | ↔↑ | ↔ | ↑ | ↑ |
| Propranolol | ↓ | ↔↑ | ↔ | ↔↓ | ↔ | ↔ |
| Sotalol | ↓ | ↔↑ | ↔ | ↔↑ | ↑ | ↔ |
| Ibutilide | ↔ | ↔ | ↔ | ↑ | ↑ | ↔ |
| Dofetilide | ↔↓ | ↔ | ↔ | ↑ | ↔ | ↔ |
| Amiodarone | ↓ | ↔↑ | ↑ | ↑ | ↑ | ↔↓ |
| Bretylium | ↔↓ | ↔↑ | ↔ | ↔↑ | ? | ? |
| Verapamil | ↔↓ | ↑ | ↔ | ↔ | ↑ | ↔ |
| Ranolazine | ↔ | ↔ | ↔ | ↑ | ↔ | ↔ |

Results presented may vary according to tissue type, experimental conditions, and drug concentration.
↑, increase; ↓, decrease; ↔, no change; ↔↑ or ↔↓, slight inconsistent increase or decrease.

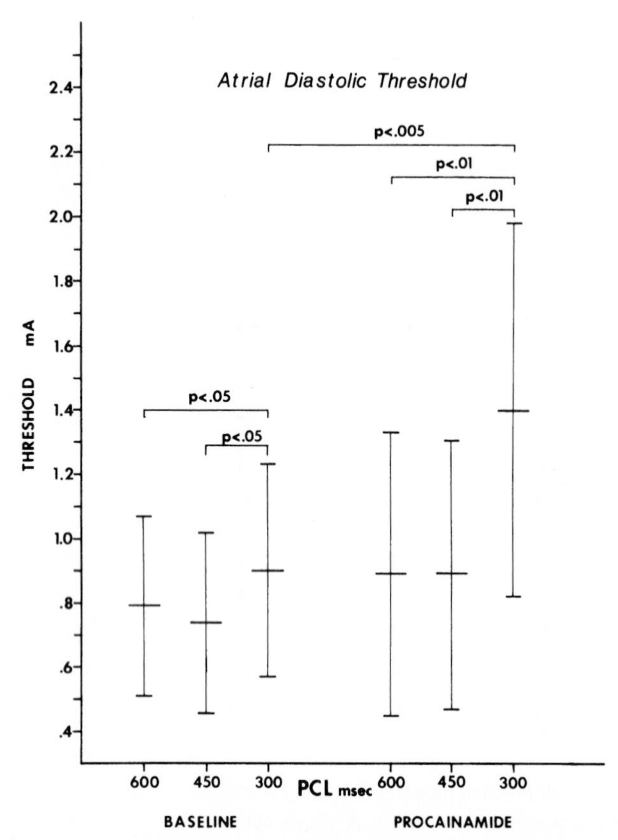


**FIGURE 12-1** *Effect of procainamide on threshold of excitability.* The threshold of excitability is shown on the vertical axis and paced cycle length (PCL) during baseline and following procainamide infusion. During baseline there is no change in excitability as the PCL decreases from 600 to 450 msec; however, at 300 msec the threshold of excitability significantly rises. Following procainamide the threshold of excitability is slightly increased at a PCL of 600 and 450 msec compared to control, but they are not different from each other. At 300 msec there is a marked increase of the threshold of excitability, which is statistically significant from the other PCLs during procainamide infusion and at a PCL of 300 msec before procainamide. (From Buxton AE, Marchlinski FE, Miller JM, et al. The human atrial strength-interval relation. Influence of cycle length and procainamide. *Circulation* 1989; 79:271–280.)

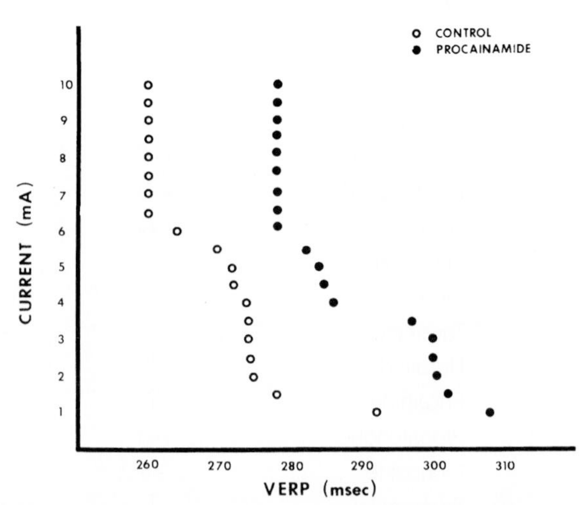


**FIGURE 12-2** *The effect of procainamide on strength-interval curves.* The stimulation strength is shown on the vertical axis and the measured ventricular effect of refractory period (VERP) on the horizontal axis. Following procainamide the curve is shifted somewhat upward and to the right compared to the control. See text for discussion. (From Camardo JS, Greenspan AM, Horowitz LN, et al. Strength-interval relation in the human ventricle: Effect of procainamide. *Am J Cardiol* 1980;45:856–860.)

interval-dependent effects of agents on threshold of excitability, conduction, and refractoriness.

As noted previously, the presence of disease states can markedly influence the effect of a drug on conduction or refractoriness. An example is shown in Figure 12-3, in which lidocaine, a drug that is supposed to have no significant effect on A-V nodal or His-Purkinje conduction, produces ventricular asystole in a patient with left bundle branch block and prolonged H-V conduction. Block is produced in the A-V node, as is marked depression of conduction in the His–Purkinje system (H-V increased from 50 to 95 msec on conducted beats). Thus, the presence of abnormal A-V nodal function and His–Purkinje function (manifested by left bundle branch block) can provide a substrate in which lidocaine is able to markedly impair conduction. One must be cognizant of such potential responses when using drugs in patients with diseased conducting systems.

In addition to the limitations of measurements and conduction and refractoriness, discussed previously here and in Chapter 2, other methodologic problems must be considered and understood by the investigator. These problems include the following:

1. Conduction and refractory period measurements (both of which are based on the ability to record propagated impulses) are generally reproducible (±10 msec) over a period of several hours for the atria, His–Purkinje system, and ventricles. However, they are not nearly as consistent for measurements of electrophysiologic characteristics of the sinus and A-V nodes.[119] This discrepancy is due to the important autonomic influence on function of the sinus and A-V nodes that can vary from moment to moment. Such changes in autonomic tone can alter sinoatrial conduction and recovery times, A-H intervals, and A-V nodal refractory periods by as much as 20% during a single study. While there is an influence of the autonomic nervous system on the atrium, His–Purkinje system, and ventricle,[67] in most cases it is not significant enough to affect the reproducibility of measurements. However, unless the patient is in a truly basal state throughout the study, the effects of drugs on the sinus and A-V nodes, in particular, must be interpreted with caution.
2. Refractory period measurements should be performed at comparable stimulus strengths before and after administration of an antiarrhythmic agent. Generally, refractory period measurements are performed using stimuli at twice the diastolic threshold. The current needs to be checked before and after drug administration to ensure that stimulation is carried out at comparable current strengths

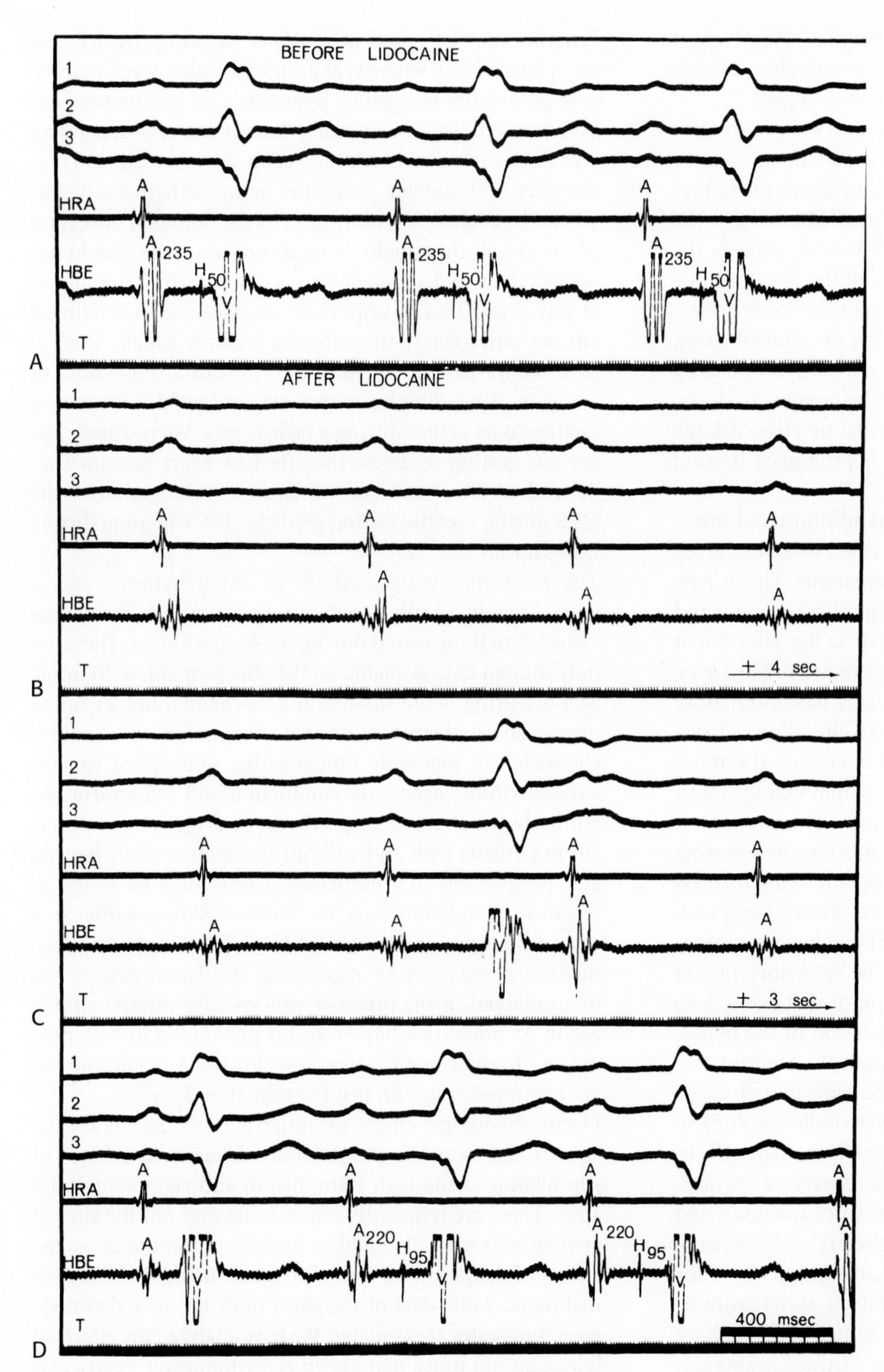


**FIGURE 12-3** *Effect of lidocaine on abnormal tissue.* **A to D:** Top to bottom, leads 1, 2, 3, high right atrial (HRA), His bundle electrogram (HBE), and time lines (T). Before lidocaine administration, left bundle branch block with prolonged (A-V) conduction is observed. The A-H interval is 235 msec and H-V is 50 msec. Following lidocaine complete A-V block is produced with failure of conduction localized to the A-V node. Conduction resumes in 3 seconds, at which time the H-V is markedly increased to 95 msec. See text for discussion.

relative to threshold. This also provides information about the drug's effect on threshold of excitability, which as stated above, may be clinically relevant. In the performance of strength-interval curves, as the current used is increased from threshold to 10 mA, we have observed a decrease in the measured refractory period of 20 to 100 msec (mean ≈40 msec) in the atrium and ventricle.[115] Of interest is the fact that once the absolute value of current exceeds 5 to 6 mA (using 1-msec pulse width), there is little change in the measured refractoriness; that is, the steep portion of the strength-interval curve has been reached. Thus, while most laboratories use twice diastolic threshold to measure refractoriness, strength-interval curves, or the use of 10 mA routinely may provide more reliable information since the steep portion of the strength-interval curve appears to always be reached by 10 mA. Whether use of this measurement has clinical significance is uncertain; it would, however, ensure that local tissue refractoriness is not the limiting factor in induction of arrhythmias. This has to be weighed against the induction of atrial or ventricular fibrillation using these current strengths. However, it is important that investigators use comparable current strengths before and after an antiarrhythmic agent.

3. Assessment of refractory periods of the A-V node or His–Purkinje system is impossible if the functional and/or effective refractory period of the atrium exceeds the refractory period of these subatrial structures. Similarly, if the functional refractory period of the A-V node exceeds the relative and effective refractory period of the His–Purkinje system, the latter measurement cannot be determined. Difficulties may be encountered during the control study, or they may be produced following antiarrhythmic drug administration. Therefore, it may not be possible to determine the effect of a drug on A-V nodal or His–Purkinje refractoriness if atrial refractoriness is prolonged beyond the A-V nodal refractory period.
4. The effect of an antiarrhythmic agent administered intravenously may not be the same as the effect of a drug given orally, even when blood levels are comparable. This is particularly true of an antiarrhythmic drug's effect on sinus and A-V nodal function, especially if the drug has effects that are mediated via the autonomic nervous system. Moreover, if the diluent in which the drug is prepared has vasodilatory properties, or if the drug itself induces alterations in systemic blood pressure, this may result in enhanced sympathetic tone, producing a different electrophysiologic effect than when the drug is administered orally. This was shown by Klein et al.[91] to be particularly important in assessing the effect of verapamil on the anterograde refractoriness of an A-V bypass tract. Whereas intravenous verapamil produces hypotension, and secondarily enhances sympathetic tone producing a decrease in the refractory period of the bypass tract, oral administration of that agent does not significantly affect the refractory period of the bypass tract.[91] Moreover, hypotension may limit the amount of a drug that can be administered intravenously; in such cases, higher doses of these agents can be given orally, resulting in higher plasma levels and greater electrophysiologic effects. In our experience, electrophysiologic effects of intravenously administered Group lA drugs (procainamide and quinidine) are similar to the effects ascertained following oral administration.[41] This is remarkable, particularly for procainamide, since its major metabolite, n-acetyl procainamide, has electrophysiologic effects. Nonetheless, we have demonstrated that the clinical efficacy of these agents can be predicted if administered acutely, as long as hypotension and myocardial depression do not take place. In view of the fact that the rate of administration can markedly influence the hemodynamic response, we recommend that Class 3 studies always be determined on chronic oral doses of various agents. This observation suggests limited clinical antiarrhythmic efficacy of n-acetyl procainamide.
5. A single dose of a given agent may be inadequate to assess its range of effects; therefore, multiple incremental doses should be evaluated, particularly if no effects are noted initially. For example, minimal effects on His–Purkinje function may be noted in response to Group lA drugs at one plasma level, whereas at a slightly higher level, marked and potentially dangerous depression of conduction can be observed. This is especially true if the use-dependent effects of the antiarrhythmic agents are assessed.[117] Thus, the electrophysiologic properties of antiarrhythmic agents should be evaluated with respect to the potential doses and plasma levels that might be used clinically. One should not neglect the use-dependent effects of antiarrhythmic agents at any dose. This is important in assessing their clinical efficacy and toxicity since these agents are usually used to treat tachyarrhythmias; thus, the effect of a single dose of an agent at baseline heart rate may not yield information relative to its action during a tachycardia. We routinely use exercise testing to assess the effect of heart rate on use-dependent effect of Class 1C agents. Prolongation of the QRS during exercise testing predicts QRS widening during tachycardias.[122]
6. The electrophysiologic effects of antiarrhythmic agents may differ if administered during acute ischemic states rather than if measured during stable conditions. There are only limited data available on the effects of antiarrhythmic agents during acute infarction or ischemia, but as noted previously, ischemia-associated depression of sodium channels can markedly influence the potency of various antiarrhythmic agents on conduction and refractoriness.[5] Similarly, the effects of antiarrhythmic drugs may be different in patients with and without conduction disturbances, and progression of conduction defects may be noted in response to individual agents. This was shown earlier in a case of lidocaine-induced heart block. Thus, apparent conduction defects can be aggravated, and latent defects can be unmasked in the presence of a specific antiarrhythmic agent. As noted in Chapter 4, this phenomenon may provide a pharmacologic "stress test" for the A-V conduction system in patients with prior conduction defects.
7. Electrophysiologic effects of antiarrhythmic agents on the atrium and ventricle are generally determined at sites of stimulation in the high right atrium and right ventricular apex. These are frequently normal sites and not the sites of arrhythmogenesis. It would be more important to assess the effects of drugs on the arrhythmogenic tissue than on normal tissue. Little data of the effect of drugs on arrhythmogenic substrates are available. We have analyzed the effects of lidocaine and procainamide on arrhythmogenic ventricular tissue, that is, tissue manifesting abnormal fractionated electrical activity (see Chapters 2 and 11). These areas of fractionated electrical activity in the left ventricle occur as a result of infarction, which leads to separation of viable muscle fibers by scar tissue. We have shown that these are areas from which ventricular tachycardias (VTs) arise. We have studied the effect of lidocaine and procainamide on these fractionated and abnormal electrograms and compared their effects to that on normal electrograms from the right ventricle (Tables 12-4 to 12-6).[123] These studies reveal lidocaine had little effect on electrogram duration from both normal and

TABLE 12-4 Effects of Lidocaine on QRS Width and Electrogram Duration (msec)

| | QRS | | RVA | | RVOT | | LV | |
|---|---|---|---|---|---|---|---|---|
| | C | L | C | L | C | L | C | L |
| NSR | 122 ± 48 | 124 ± 48 | 37 ± 16 | 40 ± 17 | 54 ± 24 | 55 ± 23 | 94 ± 26 | 97 ± 24 |
| 600 | 197 ± 19 | 198 ± 23 | 30 ± 7 | 31 ± 5 | 49 ± 29 | 52 ± 31 | 102 ± 30 | 108 ± 30 |

C, control; L, lidocaine; LV, left ventricle; NSR, normal sinus rhythm; RVA, right ventricular apex; RVOT, right ventricular outflow tract; 600, pacing at a cycle length of 600 msec from the EVA.
From Schmitt CG, Kadish AH, Marchlinski FE, et al. Effects of lidocaine and procainamide on normal and abnormal intraventricular electrograms during sinus rhythm. *Circulation* 1988;77:1030–1037.

TABLE 12-5 Effects of Procainamide on QRS Width and Electrogram Duration (msec)

| | QRS | | RVA | | RVOT | | LV | |
|---|---|---|---|---|---|---|---|---|
| | C | P | C | P | C | P | C | P |
| NSR | | | | | | | | |
| Mean ± SD | 110 ± 31 | 127 ± 33 | 32 ± 11 | 36 ± 13 | 37 ± 12 | 44 ± 15 | 84 ± 17 | 101 ± 23 |
| p value (paired t test) | <0.0001 | | <0.0001 | | <0.001 | | <0.001 | |
| % change | +16± | | +19 ± 8 | | +19 ± 11 | | +20 ± 9 | |
| 600 | | | | | | | | |
| Mean ± SD | 194 ± 28 | 226 ± 45 | 32 ± 9 | 36 ± 14 | 34 ± 11 | 39 ± 13 | 86 ± 26 | 108 ± 31 |
| p value (paired t test) | <0.001 | | <0.05 | | <0.01 | | <0.001 | |
| % change | +16 ± 8 | | +13 ± 20 | | +18 ± 16 | | +27 ± 22 | |

C, control; NSR, normal sinus rhythm; P, procainamide.
From Schmitt CG, Kadish AH, Marchlinski FE, et al. Effects of lidocaine and procainamide on normal and abnormal intraventricular electrograms during sinus rhythm. *Circulation* 1988;77:1030–1037.

TABLE 12-6 Amplitude (in mV)

| | RVA | | RVOT | | LV | |
|---|---|---|---|---|---|---|
| | C | Drug[a] | C | Drug[a] | C | Drug[a] |
| Procainamide | | | | | | |
| NSR | 6.9 ± 3.1 | 6.7 ± 4.8 | 5.0 ± 2.6 | 4.6 ± 2.2 | 1.6 ± 0.9 | 1.4 ± 0.8 |
| 600 | 8.5 ± 7.5 | 8.0 ± 8.8 | 8.8 ± 4.2 | 8.7 ± 8.4 | 1.6 ± 0.8 | 1.7 ± 1.8 |
| Lidocaine | | | | | | |
| NSR | 4.8 ± 1.5 | 4.4 ± 0.8 | 6.7 ± 3.0 | 6.2 ± 3.2 | 1.2 ± 0.6 | 1.3 ± 0.8 |
| 600 | 11.3 ± 2.8 | 10.3 ± 1.9 | 6.8 ± 3.2 | 6.7 ± 3.2 | 2.1 ± 1.1 | 2.0 ± 1.5 |

C, control.
[a]p, NS for all comparisons (controls vs. drug).
From Schmitt CG, Kadish AH, Marchlinski FE, et al. Effects of lidocaine and procainamide on normal and abnormal intraventricular electrograms during sinus rhythm. *Circulation* 1988;77:1030–1037.

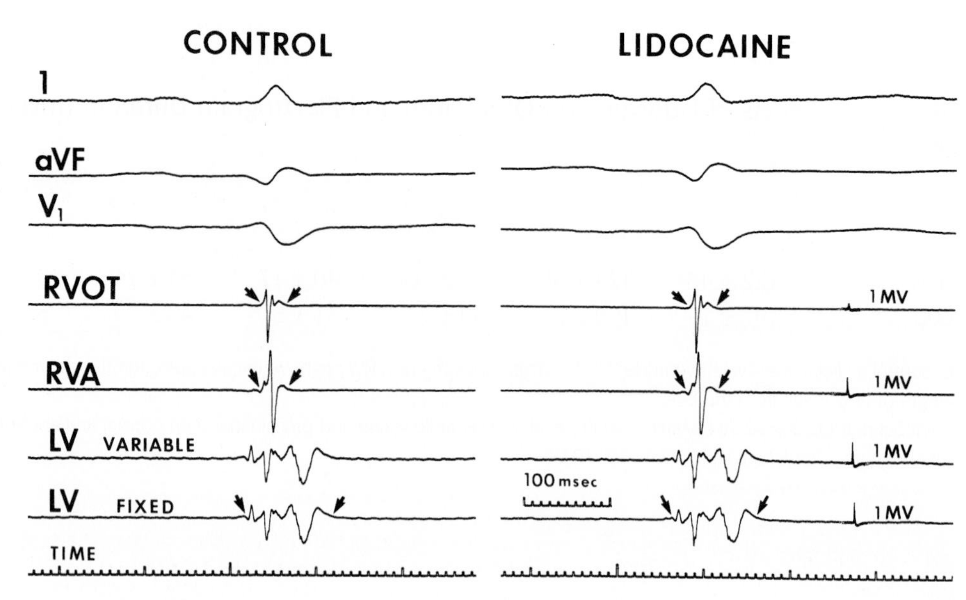


**FIGURE 12-4** *Effect of lidocaine on normal and fragmented electrograms.* Leads 1, aVF, and $V_1$ are shown with electrograms from the right ventricular outflow tract (RVOT), right ventricular apex (RVA), and the left ventricle (LV) at variable and fixed gains. Time lines and calibration signals are shown. The small *arrows* denote the sites of measurement of electrograms. Note that the normal electrograms from the RV and markedly abnormal electrogram from the LV are unaffected by lidocaine. See text for discussion. (From Schmitt CG, Kadish AH, Marchlinski FE, et al. Effects of lidocaine and procainamide on normal and abnormal intraventricular electrograms during sinus rhythm. *Circulation* 1988;77:1030–1037.)

abnormal sites during sinus rhythm or ventricular pacing at 600 msec (Fig. 12-4). On the other hand, procainamide had a similar effect on the duration of normal and abnormal electrograms (Fig. 12-5). These findings suggest that the tissue from which the electrograms arise is composed of nearly normal ventricular myocytes. If the arrhythmogenic myocardium was composed of fibers exhibiting depressed sodium channels or slow response fibers, lidocaine would have affected them markedly, and procainamide would have not affected them had they been associated with calcium-mediated slow responses. In fact, in a few patients we have been able to study the effect of verapamil on such abnormal electrograms and, indeed, no effect of the drug on fragmented electrograms was noted (Fig. 12-6). Of note, the QRS duration in sinus rhythm and during ventricular pacing increased following procainamide but not following lidocaine (Tables 12-4 and 12-5). All of these observations support the belief that the arrhythmogenic substrate is in fact composed of normally polarized fibers, but the fractionated electrograms are due to saltatory conduction produced by poor coupling of cells and nonuniform anisotropy. While Kadish et al.[21] have suggested that procainamide may affect conduction parallel to longitudinal orientation slightly more than conduction transverse to fiber orientation tissues in relatively uniform anisotropic canine tissue at paced rates of 1,000 to 400 msec, no data are available concerning the directional effects of propagation in nonuniform anisotropic tissue. A study from our laboratory[124] demonstrated that procainamide had a greater effect on conduction through the abnormal arrhythmogenic substrate than a normal tissue at fast paced rates, that is, cycle lengths of 300 msec (Figs. 12-7 and 12-8). While pacing at 600 and 400 msec showed no significant change in electrogram duration in normal and abnormal sites, when the paced cycle length was reduced to 300 msec, a significant increase in electrogram duration at abnormal sites was noted following procainamide. While there was a small increase in electrogram duration at normal sites produced by procainamide at all cycle lengths, which was comparable to the increase in electrogram duration in abnormal sites at 600 and 400 msec, at paced cycle lengths of 300 msec, the increase in electrogram duration was significantly greater in abnormal sites

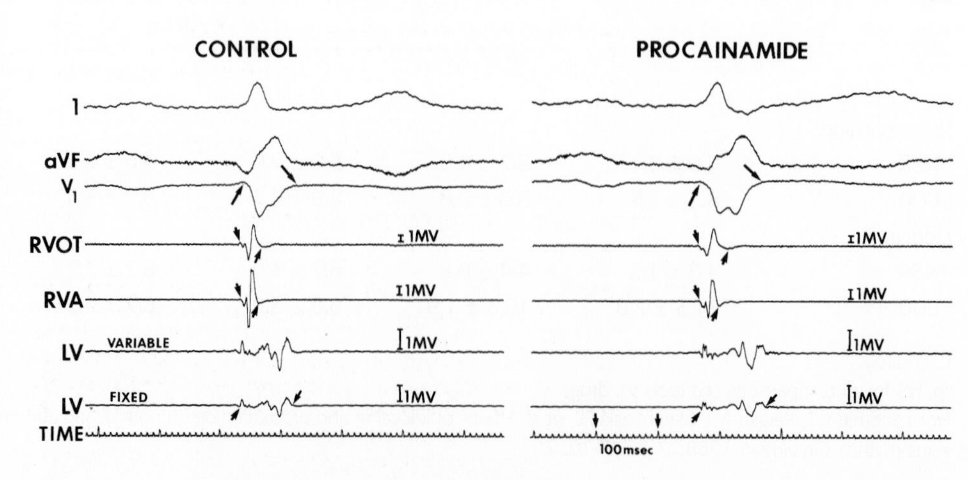


**FIGURE 12-5** *Effect of procainamide on normal and abnormal electrograms.* This tracing is organized the same as Figure 12-4. The small *arrows* denote width of electrogram. Following procainamide, the QRS width, electrograms from the RV, and LV all prolong. A relatively similar increase of normal and abnormal electrograms in response to procainamide suggests that the fibers responsible for their generation are not associated with slow potentials. See text for discussion. (From Schmitt CG, Kadish AH, Marchlinski FE, et al. Effects of lidocaine and procainamide on normal and abnormal intraventricular electrograms during sinus rhythm. *Circulation* 1988;77:1030–1037.)

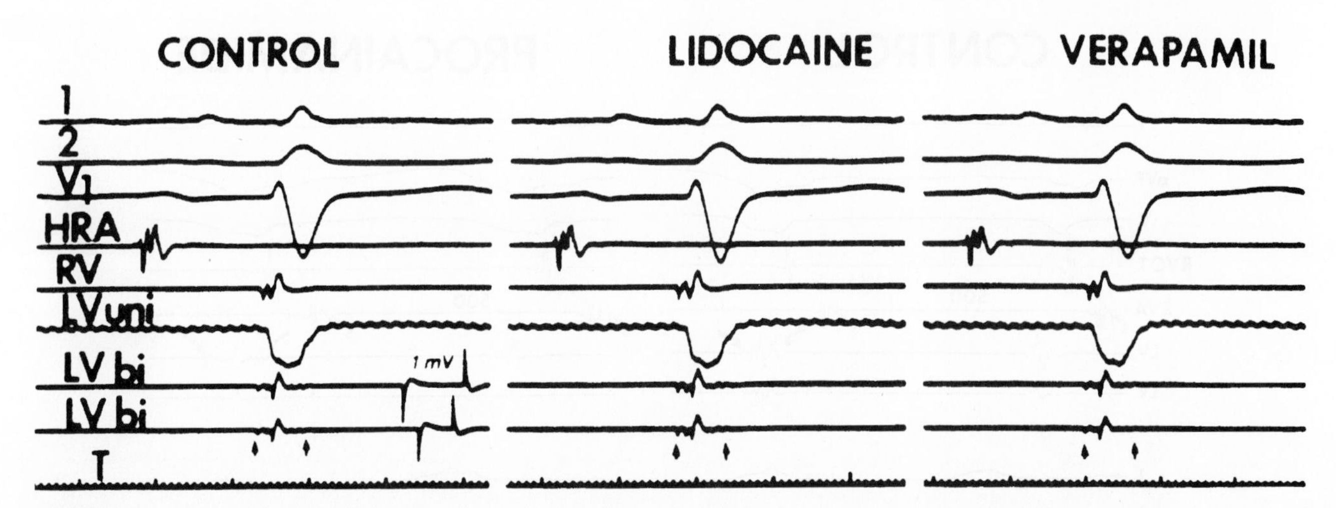


**FIGURE 12-6** *Comparison of lidocaine and verapamil on abnormal electrograms.* Leads 1, 2, and $V_1$ are shown with electrograms from the HRA, RV, and unipolar and two bipolar electrograms from an abnormal LV site. The small *arrows* denote the width of the abnormal electrogram. Following lidocaine and verapamil, there is no significant change in electrogram configuration or duration. See text for discussion.

(Fig. 12-7). Occasionally, loss of a component of an electrogram could be noted and, in some instances, progressive prolongation of the electrogram led to initiation of VT (see Chapter 11). These findings suggest that in arrhythmogenic ventricular tissue procainamide produces a cycle length–dependent effect on saltatory conduction that is beyond its use-dependent effects. More research is mandatory to study the effects of antiarrhythmic agents on arrhythmogenic tissue. It is only through such studies that one may begin to understand the antiarrhythmic effects of antiarrhythmic agents. This last point is one of the major limitations in evaluating antiarrhythmic efficacy and mechanism. To summarize, drug effects are not generally measured at the arrhythmogenic site. Thus, extrapolation of measurements from either the right atrium or right ventricle to arrhythmogenic sites in either the atria or left ventricle is not necessarily valid; that is, tissue other than at sites of atrial and right ventricular stimulation (e.g., left atrium and left ventricle) may differ in active and passive electrophysiologic properties. Further discussion on evaluation of antiarrhythmic drug action will be discussed later in this chapter.

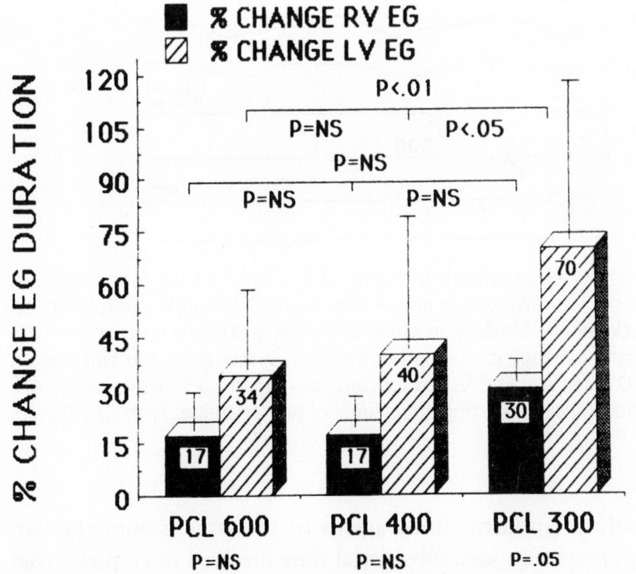


**FIGURE 12-7** *Effect of procainamide on electrogram duration at various paced cycle lengths.* The percentage (%) of change in electrogram (EG) duration is shown on the vertical axis, and the paced cycle lengths (PCL) at which electrogram durations were measured are shown on the horizontal axis. Following procainamide, there is a significant increase in both normal and abnormal electrograms at a PCL of 300 msec. While the difference in effect on normal and abnormal electrograms at a PCL of 600 and 400 msec is not significantly different, the marked increase in electrogram duration at abnormal sites following procainamide at a PCL of 300 msec is significantly different from abnormal electrograms at other PCLs. See text for discussion. (From Schmitt C, Kadish AH, Balke WC, et al. Cycle length–dependent effects on normal and abnormal intraventricular electrograms: effect of procainamide. *J Am Coll Cardiol* 1988;12:395–403.)

Limitations of studying the electrophysiologic properties of antiarrhythmic agents in humans are summarized in Table 12-7.

**TABLE 12-7 Limitations in Evaluating Antiarrhythmic Drug Action**

1. In humans, all electrophysiologic measurements depend on impulse propagation.
2. Impulse propagation depends on active and passive membrane properties.
3. Failure to consider use-dependence and the binding characteristics of antiarrhythmic agents in different states of activation of the channel (modulated receptor hypothesis).
4. There is little available knowledge of drug actions on passive properties.
5. Many factors can influence these properties and effect antiarrhythmic drug action, that is, ischemia, changes in autonomic tone, electrolytes, etc.

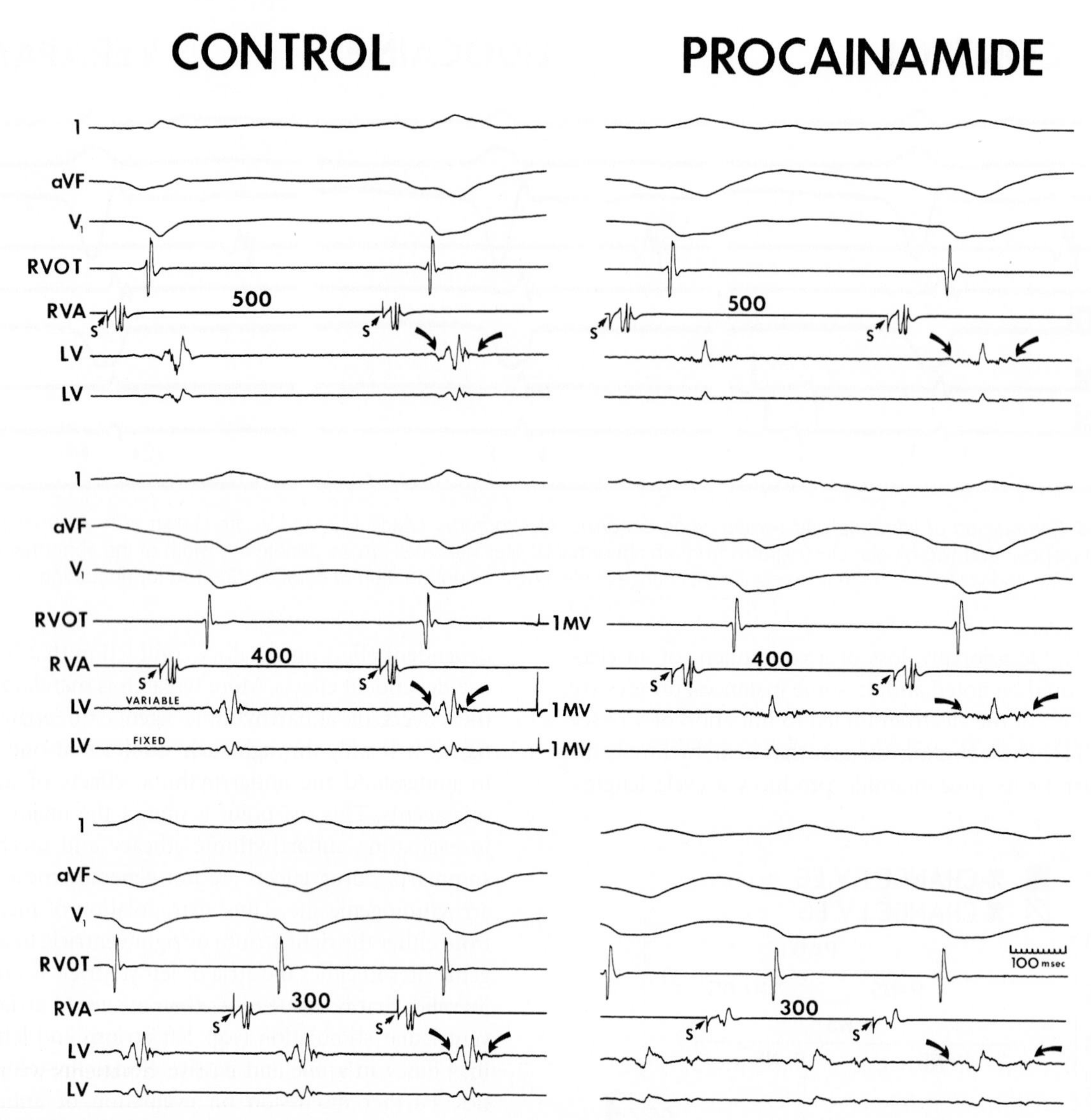


**FIGURE 12-8** *Effect of procainamide on fractionated electrograms.* This tracing is set up similarly to Figure 12-5. Curved *arrows* denote width of LV electrogram. Pacing from the RVA at cycle lengths of 500, 400, and 300 msec is shown before and after procainamide. In the control state no significant change in the fractionated electrogram is shown at each paced cycle length. Similarly, in a qualitative sense, there is no change in the electrogram from the RVOT. Following procainamide, although there is a minimal change in duration of the RVOT electrogram, the electrogram from the LV becomes markedly splintered and at a paced cycle length of 300 msec is split. See text for discussion. (From Schmitt C, Kadish AH, Balke WC, et al. Cycle length-dependent effects on normal and abnormal intraventricular electrograms: effect of procainamide. *J Am Coll Cardiol* 1988;12:395–403.)

## SELECTION OF ANTIARRHYTHMIC DRUG THERAPY FOR REENTRANT TACHYCARDIAS

### Use of Programmed Stimulation

The ability to reproducibly initiate a tachycardia provides an objective method by which the efficacy of an antiarrhythmic agent in preventing the arrhythmia can be tested. The use of electrophysiologic testing to analyze the effects of different drugs, singly or in combination, can provide a relatively rapid and rational method of selecting drug therapy.[125–143] Support for this method has evolved because of the realization that patients with the same arrhythmia can respond quite differently to antiarrhythmic agents of the same group. Such an approach can save substantial time involved in empiric "trial and error therapy," the efficacy of which must be based on the frequency of symptoms, the ability of ambulatory monitoring to record such events, and in the case of malignant ventricular arrhythmias, sudden death. The paroxysmal nature of most reentrant arrhythmias makes the use of Holter monitoring less reliable as an indicator of effective therapy. The limitations of Holter monitoring for the management of such arrhythmias are (a) the infrequent nature of spontaneous ectopy, (b) the spontaneous variability of such activity, and (c) the inability of suppression of ambient ectopy to predict prevention of the sustained arrhythmias for which the therapy is given. This is particularly true in the case of ventricular

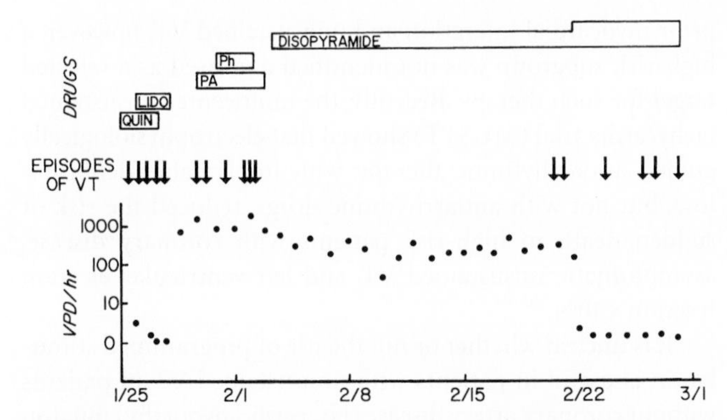


**FIGURE 12-9** *A lack of correlation of spontaneous ectopy with recurrences of ventricular tachycardia (VT).* The number of ventricular premature depolarizations (VPD) per hour is shown on the vertical axis in a logarithmic scale, and the dates over which recordings were made are shown on the horizontal axis. Episodes of spontaneous sustained VT are shown with the inverted *vertical arrows.* The timing of administration of various antiarrhythmic agents is shown in rectangular boxes. An increase in the box width represents an increase in the dose. Note that recurrent episodes of sustained VT occur following all antiarrhythmic agents and there is no relationship to the presence or absence of spontaneous ectopy. (From Horowitz LN, Josephson ME, Kastor JA. Intracardiac electrophysiologic studies as a method for the optimization of drug therapy in chronic ventricular arrhythmia. *Prog Cardiovasc Dis* 1980;23:81–98.)

arrhythmias (Fig. 12-9). The ease of placement and safety of insertable cardiac monitors have helped to overcome some of these limitations.

The use of an electrophysiologic protocol for drug selection is based on two assumptions: (a) The tachycardia initiated in the laboratory by programmed stimulation is identical to that occurring spontaneously, and (b) the response of antiarrhythmic agents in the laboratory predicts the clinical response. Both of these assumptions appear well established in the case of paroxysmal supraventricular tachycardias and sustained uniform VT (as long as a 12-lead electrogram during the spontaneous episode is available to compare to the induced arrhythmia). While it is rarely possible to record the rhythm initiating cardiac arrest, as has been discussed in detail in Chapter 11, most episodes appear to be initiated by either a uniform VT, which produces hemodynamic collapse or degenerates into ventricular fibrillation, or a rapidly accelerating VT, uniform or polymorphic, degenerating into ventricular fibrillation after a variable amount of time. Our experience and that of many institutions have supported the clinical utility of programmed stimulation for developing drug therapy for these arrhythmias.[130–143] While pharmacologic therapy has assumed a secondary role for the treatment of malignant ventricular arrhythmias because of the demonstrated superiority of ICDs in preventing sudden death, pharmacologic therapy is still required to (a) prevent recurrences resulting in multiple ICD discharges and (b) slow the VT cycle length to facilitate antitachycardia pace termination (see Chapter 13).

Grayboys et al.[144] suggested that noninvasive methods (Holter monitoring and exercise testing) yield a similar outcome to programmed stimulation. Several small studies suggested that programmed stimulation more accurately predicts success of pharmacologic therapy than Holter monitoring in the case of sustained ventricular tachyarrhythmias.[139,145,146] The electrophysiologic versus electrocardiographic monitoring (EVSEM) trial was a prospective multicenter trial that compared the outcome of patients in whom antiarrhythmic therapy with Class 1 agents or sotalol was guided by serial electrophysiologic study with the outcome of patients in whom therapy was guided by ambulatory ECG monitoring. The 486 patients in this trial had documented sustained ventricular arrhythmias (85%) or resuscitated sudden death that were inducible during electrophysiologic study (EPS) and had significant, measurable ectopy (>10 PVCs/hr) on Holter monitoring. Two-thirds had failed "standard" Class 1 agents. The patients were randomized to electrophysiologic testing or Holter monitoring to predict drug efficacy and received up to six drugs in random order until one was predicted to be effective.[147,148]

This trial showed that Holter monitoring and electrophysiologic testing had similar accuracy in predicting antiarrhythmic drug efficacy.[147–149] Drug efficacy, predicted by Holter or electrophysiologic testing, was associated with improved mortality.[150] Sotalol was shown to have greater efficacy and lower cost when compared to Class 1 agents, but the patient population was biased against Class 1 agents.[147,148,151,152] The study had many flaws which were never addressed. Sotalol had to be tolerated in high enough doses to be effective which preselects patients without CHF and/or significantly reduce ejection fraction. Two-thirds of patients had previously failed Class 1 agents, an observation which selects patients likely to fail other Class 1 agents. The stimulation protocol was inadequate in both number of extrastimuli and sites of stimulation. Finally, I believe the incidence of such patients with frequent enough ectopy on Holter monitoring to allow evaluation of drug suppression was significantly exaggerated. In my experience less than 15% of our patients with sustained VT of VF have such frequent ectopy.

A trial conducted by Steinbeck et al.[153,154] prospectively looked at beta-blocker monotherapy compared to EPS-guided antiarrhythmic drug therapy plus beta-blocker therapy in 170 patients. The patient population included those with sustained VT, resuscitated sudden death, or syncope presumed to be due to VT. All patients underwent EPS. Those who were noninducible received metoprolol. Those who were inducible were randomized to receive metoprolol or serial EPS-guided antiarrhythmic drug therapy with propafenone, flecainide, disopyramide, sotalol, or amiodarone. Drugs were assigned randomly, but amiodarone was used last. All patients received metoprolol as well except those who were taking amiodarone or sotalol. Surprisingly, the left ventricular ejection fraction was >40% in the average patient enrolled in this study.

Using a combined endpoint of symptomatic arrhythmia recurrence or arrhythmic death, outcome was better in those who at baseline were noninducible when compared to those who were inducible. There was no significant difference between the two groups who were inducible and received beta blockers or beta blockers and antiarrhythmic medication. However, when stratified on the basis of the results of EP testing, those who were inducible but suppressed by antiarrhythmic therapy fared best even when compared to those who were noninducible at outset.[154] Outcome was not stratified by drugs in this study, but others showed, as was the case with Class 1 agents in the ESVEM trial, that EPS-guided suppression of arrhythmia by amiodarone administration confers a favorable prognosis.[155]

High-risk survivors of cardiac arrest were evaluated in the CASADE study.[156] Empiric therapy with amiodarone was compared to EPS-guided therapy with antiarrhythmic agents (generally Class 1 agents) in patients resuscitated from out-of-hospital sudden death with poor LV function. Those who were inducible at EPS had antiarrhythmic therapy guided by serial study. At 6 years, survival free of cardiac death and sustained VT was higher in those taking amiodarone compared to those on Class 1 agents (41% vs. 21%; $p < 0.001$). When amiodarone-treated patients were compared to those whose arrhythmias were suppressed on Class 1 agents at 2 years, there was a trend toward superiority with amiodarone (83% vs. 60%; $p < 0.09$). Again, it should be recognized that in this population with coronary disease and prior infarction, beta-blocker use was extremely low (5% to 6%), particularly in those treated with Class 1 agents, and may have modified the findings. This trial was the first to suggest greater efficacy of amiodarone, but did not address the utility of programmed stimulation.

When interpreting data presented in the preceding paragraphs, it is critical to recognize the differing baseline risk of arrhythmic death within the heterogeneous populations enrolled in these trials when comparing results within and between these studies. For instance, people who are noninducible at EPS or have normal left ventricular ejection fractions have better survival when compared to those with impaired left ventricular function and who remain inducible despite serial drug testing. In addition, drug failure end points should be different in patients with sustained uniform, tolerated VT, and those with cardiac arrest. Sudden death should be an end point for patients presenting with cardiac arrest, but it should not be used for someone who presents with sustained, tolerated uniform VT, since sudden death is uncommon in these patients. In such patients, recurrent sustained VT is the appropriate end point. Finally patients with different disease substrates (e.g., coronary artery disease with prior infarction, dilated or hypertrophic cardiomyopathy, or no overt organic heart disease) behave differently to programmed stimulation (see Chapter 11) and antiarrhythmic agents.

The use of electrophysiologic testing to guide pharmacologic therapy for nonsustained ventricular arrhythmias is controversial. Prior studies suggested that EPS-guided therapy was superior to other forms of therapy for the management of nonsustained VT associated with coronary artery disease in whom the left ventricular ejection fraction is <40% and in whom sustained uniform VT is inducible.[157–160] One study[161] did not find electrophysiologic testing of value in patients with prior myocardial infarction and nonsustained VT; however, a high-risk subgroup was not identified and used as a selected target for such therapy. Recently, the multicenter unsustained tachycardia trial (MUSTT) showed that electrophysiologically guided antiarrhythmic therapy with implantable defibrillators, but not with antiarrhythmic drugs, reduced the risk of sudden death in high-risk patients with coronary disease, asymptomatic unsustained VT, and left ventricular ejection fraction <40%.[162]

It is unclear whether or not the use of programmed stimulation is useful in patients with nonsustained VT in patients without coronary artery disease (i.e., cardiomyopathy). Buxton et al.[160] did not find programmed stimulation useful in identifying a high-risk subgroup of patients with cardiomyopathy and nonsustained VT, and therefore, we do not believe that the technique can or should be used to effectively assess therapy in such patients.

Other investigators[163,164] have suggested the use of signal-averaged electrocardiography to identify the high-risk subgroup of patients with coronary artery disease and low ejection fractions in whom nonsustained VT should be treated by programmed stimulation.[163–167] We, however, have not found the signal-averaged electrocardiogram to be of independent value in selecting patients with prior infarction and nonsustained VT who are at high risk for developing sustained VT or sudden cardiac death.[168] At least for sustained ventricular arrhythmias, the electrophysiologic approach appears to be cost effective.[169]

Some generalizations can be made based on these data regarding the role of EP testing for the evaluation of antiarrhythmic efficacy for ventricular tachyarrhythmias: (a) Patient population (disease state and left ventricular function) markedly affect outcomes and predictability of EP testing. (b) Drug efficacy demonstrated by EPS or Holter monitoring is associated with better outcomes than if the arrhythmias continue to remain inducible or are spontaneously present. (c) Survival is improved in those with sustained ventricular arrhythmias with regimens that include beta blockade compared to antiarrhythmic agents without beta blockade. (d) Empiric amiodarone therapy is better than Class 1 agents given without beta blockade. (e) The ability to predict recurrence based on the results of EP testing is imperfect. (f) EPS-guided therapy with ICDs is superior to EPS-guided antiarrhythmic therapy. (g) There has been a decrease in use of EPS-guided and non–EPS-guided drug therapy for both supraventricular and ventricular arrhythmias as a result of the development and success of nonpharmacologic approaches.

## Study Protocol

Electrophysiologic testing may be done following acute intravenous administration of an agent or following oral therapy once a steady state has been reached for both the parent drug and its active metabolites. Although theoretically limitations may exist in comparing the response to intravenous therapy with that of oral therapy, at least for some of the Class 1 agents, this has not been a problem.[35] Thus, we continue to use an intravenous infusion of procainamide to initially evaluate its efficacy. The same is true for beta blockers and calcium channel blockers, which are almost exclusively used for supraventricular arrhythmias. We rarely test the efficacy of other agents following intravenous administration, although intravenous administration may be used for acute therapy. Regardless of whether or not intravenous drug testing is done, we always test the efficacy of antiarrhythmic agents following oral administration. This allows one to assess the patient's tolerance of the drug, to observe any hemodynamic, hematologic, gastrointestinal, or proarrhythmic side effects of the drug, and allows for the assessment of both the parent drug and active metabolites of the parent drug. Obviously, the length of time of oral administration of an agent required to achieve a steady state varies. As such, a single hospitalization to undergo study with multiple agents with long half-lives is unacceptable. We will study in a single hospitalization only agents that have short half-lives in which steady states can be achieved, and the study will be done within a week. Currently, in those patients with supraventricular tachyarrhythmias the patients will be placed on a drug and discharged with an event recorder to monitor rhythm, rate, and intervals. They are then re-evaluated as outpatients. In the case of amiodarone, which has a half-life of almost a month, depending on the severity of the arrhythmia, we use two different approaches. For sustained VT/fibrillation, we initiate therapy in the hospital. We administer 1,000 to 1,400 mg daily for a week followed by a maintenance dose of 400 mg/day as an outpatient with event recorder monitoring. After 2 weeks of maintenance therapy, an EPS is repeated. As with other antiarrhythmic drugs, we administer beta blockers concomitantly with amiodarone. When amiodarone is considered as an agent for supraventricular arrhythmias, the oral dosing can be entirely done as an outpatient with event recorder monitoring.

I recommend starting Class 1C agents at the lower dose range because of fear of the proarrhythmic effects of these agents. Incremental increases of these drugs are done slowly, as outpatients, during which time the ECG is monitored at rest and following exercise testing because of the known enhancement of conduction abnormalities and potential proarrhythmic effects by increased heart rates. I believe exercise testing to be a critical component of assessing drug tolerance and potential toxicity, particularly in lC agents because of their marked use-dependent effects.[170] Efforts at cost containment by reducing the number of studies and/or days in the hospital will likely be mandated in the future.

Before testing antiarrhythmic therapy, if possible, a control study is performed in the absence of all antiarrhythmic agents. The stimulation protocols described in Chapters 8 to 11 for supraventricular tachycardias in the presence or absence of pre-excitation, atrial flutter and fibrillation, and VT are employed. In an occasional patient, isoproterenol infusion may be necessary to enhance induction of the arrhythmia (be it supraventricular or ventricular); in such cases, the antiarrhythmic drug–efficacy test must be done in the presence of isoproterenol. As noted previously, all stimulation must be performed at twice diastolic threshold during the control period and again after administration of the drugs. Whether the use of higher current strengths will be more useful is uncertain and will be discussed later in this chapter. As noted earlier in this chapter, the effect of an antiarrhythmic agent on threshold of excitability, particularly at faster paced rates, as well as the normal direct relationship of refractoriness to changes in cycle length, may have clinical value, but this has not been established in well-controlled studies. Unfortunately, a limitation in assessing the effects of orally administered drugs on these specific parameters is that the patient will have the catheter placed at two widely separate dates. The variation in catheter placement may result in minor changes in refractoriness unrelated to the drug. In our laboratory, for both supraventricular and ventricular arrhythmias, at least one intravenous antiarrhythmic agent is assessed on the same day as the initial study. For ventricular arrhythmias, this is almost always procainamide, while for supraventricular arrhythmias, it may be either procainamide or calcium blockers or beta blockers. This will be discussed in subsequent paragraphs.

For ventricular tachyarrhythmias, the response of intravenous procainamide can be useful in assessing the likelihood of responding to other Class 1 agents alone or in combination and, therefore, is a useful part of a decision-making branch point in the selection of antiarrhythmic drugs. Although an indwelling catheter may be left in place, we have moved away from this approach and remove all catheters following the initial study. Patients can return 7 to 14 days later for a repeat study, depending on the drug and indication for the study. The presence of heart failure, diuretics, electrical abnormalities, and/or hepatic renal disease affects the drugs selected and, hence, affects the timing of the studies.

Drug levels are used for two purposes. First is to evaluate the electrophysiologic response to a drug at a given level. Second is to demonstrate that chronic therapy is associated with a plasma level shown to be effective in the laboratory; this provides assurance that the patient has taken the medicine at the prescribed dosage and that the metabolism and excretion of the drug in the outpatient have not affected the plasma level. We do not use drug levels as targets to be achieved. The investigator must be able to assess the effect of multiple drug levels since comparable levels of any agent demonstrate totally different efficacy in different patients. Furthermore, this method will allow the investigator to select a lower effective dose of the drug, thereby eliminating some dose-dependent toxicity. Table 12-8 demonstrates the normal loading and maintenance doses of several antiarrhythmic agents. The methodologies, efficacy of specific drugs, results, and determinants for success, particularly for VTs, will be discussed in the following paragraphs.

## Selection of Pharmacologic Therapy for Ventricular Tachyarrhythmias

EPS-guided pharmacologic therapies are perhaps most valuable in the management of sustained VT and in patients resuscitated from cardiac arrest associated with coronary

TABLE 12-8 Dosage and Therapeutic Serum Concentrations for Antiarrhythmic Agents

| Drug | Intravenous | | Oral (mg) |
|---|---|---|---|
| | Intravenous (mg) | Maintenance[c] | |
| Quinidine | 8–12 mg/kg at 0.3–0.5 mg/kg/min | | 800–2,400 |
| Procainamide | 10–15 mg/kg at 0.3–0.15 mg/kg/min | 0.5–1 mg/kg/min | 3,000–6,000 |
| Disopyramide[a] | 1–2 mg/kg over 15 min | 1 mg/kg/h | 300–1,200 |
| Lidocaine | 3–5 mg/kg at 25–50 mg/min | 1–4 mg/min | NA |
| Phenytoin | 1,000-mg IV infusion at 25 mg/min | | 300 |
| Mexilitine[a] | 500 mg | 0.5–1 g/24 h | 300–600 |
| Tocainide[a] | 750 mg | | 1,600–2,400 |
| Flecainide[a] | 2 mg/kg | | 200–400 |
| Encainide | 0.6–0.9 mg/kg | | 75–225 |
| Lorcainide[b] | 1–2 mg/kg | | 200–300 |
| Propafenone | 1–2 mg/kg | | 300–900 |
| Moricizine[a] | 1–2 mg/kg over 45 min | | 300–1200 |
| Propranolol | 0.1–0.2 mg/kg at 0.5–1 mg/min | | 40–720 |
| d,l-Sotalol[a] | 1.5–3.0 mg/kg over 30 min (d-Sotalol) | | 80–640 |
| Ibutilide | 0.01–0.02 mg/kg over 10 min | | NA |
| Dofetilide[a] | 8 μg/kg over 30 min | | 250–100 (μg) |
| Amiodarone | 5–10 mg/kg over 20–30 min, then 1g/24 h | | 200–400 |
| Bretylium | 5–10 mg/kg at 1–2 mg/kg/min | 0.5–2 mg/min | 4 mg/kg/day |
| Verapamil | 10 mg over 1–2 min | 0.005 mg/kg/min | 120–160 |

[a]Intravenous administration; investigational only.
[b]Investigational.
[c]Total dose; schedule depends on whether preparation is sustained release or not.

artery disease and other scar-related substrates. The use of EP testing in patients with cardiomyopathy, valvular disease, or in normal hearts (e.g., idiopathic VF, Brugada syndrome, long QT syndrome) has not been validated.[171,172] However, there are single center series that have demonstrated the efficacy of quinidine in the Brugada syndrome and idiopathic ventricular fibrillation using programmed stimulation.[173–176] In contrast numerous studies[130,133–143] have attested to the utility of programmed stimulation in selecting drugs that are likely to prevent spontaneous recurrence as well as to predict those patients with a high likelihood of recurrence in individuals with **prior infarctions.** The criteria of drug efficacy as determined by programmed stimulation have varied. Some have suggested narrowing of the tachycardia zone (i.e., the coupling intervals of extrastimuli over which the tachycardia is initiated); more vigorous stimulation required to initiate the tachycardia (i.e., a greater number of extrastimuli); prevention of induction of VT less than a certain number of beats; or prevention of induction of the sustained ventricular tachyarrhythmia that one is trying to prevent. In my opinion, prevention of sustained VT is the most appropriate end point.

Swerdlow et al. suggested that the induction of 15 or less beats was predictive of good outcome[177] while others have not found this to be true.[178,179] Unfortunately, these studies mixed patient populations (i.e., those with sustained uniform VT and those with cardiac arrest), as well as the induced rhythm (uniform VT and polymorphic VT). I do not believe that studies looking at these admixed variables can be accurately interpreted. Moreover, if one uses induction of sustained tachyarrhythmias as an end point, then the induction of a nonsustained tachycardia would meet our laboratory's criterion for successful therapy. Thus, for example, if a patient presented with spontaneous sustained VT, and only a nonsustained tachycardia was induced following an antiarrhythmic drug, whether it was 5 complexes or 15 complexes, it would be considered a successful study. While 15 complexes should not be considered a magical number, it is uncommon for an arrhythmia to last more than 15 or 20 complexes without being sustained. Therefore, the use of 15 complexes merely represents a statistical likelihood that any spontaneous nonsustained arrhythmia will not exceed 15 complexes.

I do not believe either the absolute number of extrastimuli used or the relative ease of induction of sustained VT can be

**VT: PES AND OUTCOME OF VT**
**MODE OF INDUCTION**

| Recurrence | 1 VES | 2 VES | RP | 3 VES |
|---|---|---|---|---|
| No | 20 | 42 | 3 | 19 |
| Yes | 8 | 16 | 4 | 5 |

**FIGURE 12-10** *Relationship of mode of induction of initiation of VT and outcome.* The presence or absence of recurrences is shown on the vertical axis and the mode of initiation of VT is shown on the horizontal axis. Note there is no difference in recurrence rate whether the tachycardia was initiated with one ventricular extrastimulus (VES), two VES, rapid pacing (RP), or three VES. PES, programmed electrical stimulation.

**PES AND OUTCOME OF VT: AMIODARONE**
**MODE OF INDUCIBILITY**

| Recurrence | SINGLES | DOUBLES | RAPID PACING | TRIPLES |
|---|---|---|---|---|
| No | 17 | 31 | 3 | 10 |
| Yes | 6 | 11 | 3 | 2 |

**FIGURE 12-12** *Effect of mode of induction of VT on amiodarone to outcome.* The figure is organized identically to Figure 12-10. Note that the mode of induction does not influence the recurrence rate.

used to predict outcome of Class 1 (A, B, or C) agents, sotalol, or amiodarone. This is shown in Figures 12-10 to 12-13. These data are derived from studies from 211 patients taking Class 1 agents and 106 patients on amiodarone in our laboratory. While these data are in contrast to data presented by other investigators,[77,179] these latter investigators either used a different stimulation protocol or included patients with inducible sustained uniform VT and sustained polymorphic VT in the same group. It is conceivable that a change in difficulty of at least two extrastimuli may be useful, but this is an uncommon observation in patients having sustained monomorphic VT and is extremely rare in patients with cardiac arrest.

Inducibility of the clinical arrhythmia (sustained monomorphic VTs) remains the most useful end point using a full protocol incorporating three ventricular extrastimuli, at least two pace cycle lengths, from at least two right ventricular pacing sites. The significance of induction of polymorphic VT/VF, even in patients with cardiac arrest, remains uncertain. For this reason, I do not believe the results of the ESVEM study to be clinically useful since a complete, control protocol was not performed (only the stimulation required to initiate one VT was used) and the stimulation protocol on antiarrhythmic agents never exceeded the number of extrastimuli needed to induce the single baseline VT in the control state.

Examples of the development of successful antiarrhythmic therapy for sustained uniform VT on a Class 1 agent are shown in Figures 12-14 and 12-15. In our experience, Class 1 agents have also been effective in uniform VT associated with recent myocardial infarction (Fig. 12-16) and in patients with cardiac arrest, regardless of whether sustained uniform VT or sustained polymorphic VT is initiated (Fig. 12-17).

The relative efficacy of antiarrhythmic agents in suppressing VT inducibility or changing the relative mode of initiation is not really known. For example, amiodarone only prevents initiation of VT in 10% to 15% of our patients, whether studied at 2 weeks or 3 months (Fig. 12-18). However, amiodarone is often only used after several drugs have failed. The same is true for other drugs (i.e., the Class lC agents). If each of these drugs had been tried as a first-line agent, the relative efficacy might have been different. As such, the relative efficacy of antiarrhythmic agents is shown in Figure 12-19. It can be seen that the Class lA agents are most likely to prevent induction of sustained VT with a success rate ranging between 26% and 38%. Since these data are compiled from many laboratories, however, the order in which a given laboratory selects antiarrhythmic agents to be tested also can influence relative success rate of a given agent. Of note is the fact that suppression of inducibility of VT by sotalol is lower in our experience than reported in ESVEM.

**VT: PES AND OUTCOME OF VT**
**RELATIVE EASE OF INITIATION**

| Recurrence | EASIER | HARDER | NO CHANGE |
|---|---|---|---|
| No | 22 | 27 | 38 |
| Yes | 10 | 10 | 11 |

**FIGURE 12-11** *Relationship of VT recurrence to relative change in mode of initiation produced by antiarrhythmic agents.* The presence of recurrence is shown on the vertical axis, and the relative ease of initiation produced by an antiarrhythmic is shown on the horizontal axis. Note that the recurrence rate is unaffected by whether the antiarrhythmic agent makes VT initiation easier, harder, or unchanged.

**PES AND OUTCOME OF VT: AMIODARONE**
**RELATIVE EASE OF INDUCTION**

| Recurrence | EASIER | HARDER | NO CHANGE |
|---|---|---|---|
| No | 18 | 20 | 25 |
| Yes | 6 | 8 | 9 |

**FIGURE 12-13** *Relationship of effect of amiodarone on ease of induction and clinical outcome.* This figure is organized identically to Figure 12-11. The relative ease of initiation of VT following amiodarone does not correlate with recurrence rate.

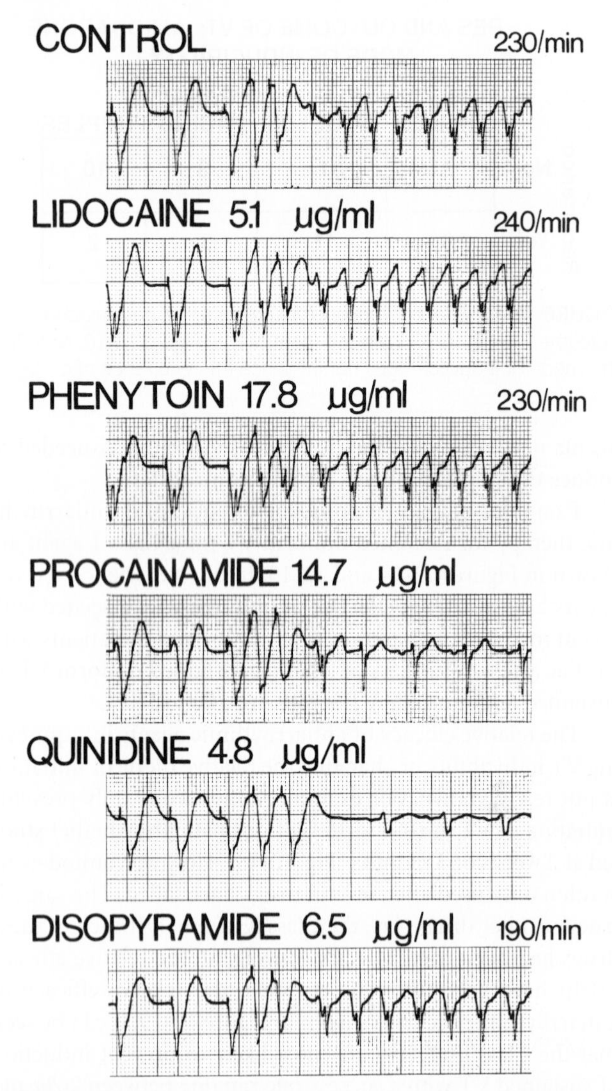


**FIGURE 12-14** *Serial drug testing in a patient with sustained uniform VT.* In the control tracing, sustained uniform VT at a heart rate of 230 beats per minute is induced by two extrastimuli. In subsequent panels, the effect of lidocaine, phenytoin, procainamide, quinidine, and disopyramide on initiation of the tachycardia is shown. Note that procainamide and quinidine both prevent induction of the tachycardia See text for discussion. (From Kastor JA, Horowitz LN, Harken AH, Josephson ME. Clinical electrophysiology of ventricular tachycardia. *New Engl J Med* 1981;304:1004.)

Beta blockers and calcium blockers are rarely effective in preventing sustained uniform VT. There is, however, one group of patients in whom calcium blockers appear to be useful. These are the patients with apparently normal hearts, usually male, who have sustained uniform VT characterized by a right bundle branch block, left superior axis morphology. As commented on in Chapter 11, these patients have tachycardias that can frequently be initiated by atrial pacing as well as by ventricular extrastimuli and can be entrained; thereby establishing a reentrant mechanism. In this group of patients, verapamil frequently produces a dose-dependent slowing and termination of the tachycardia (Fig. 12-20). In our experience,

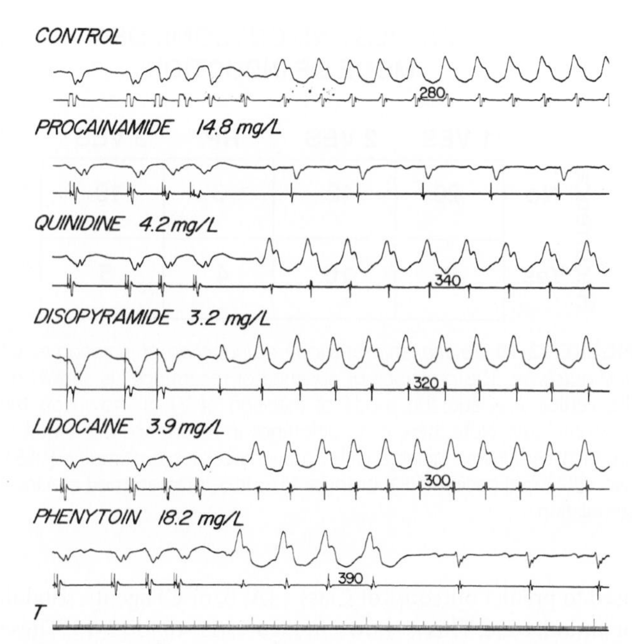


**FIGURE 12-15** *Serial drug testing for recurrent sustained VT.* The figure includes an ECG lead $V_1$ and an electrogram from the RVA. During the control, state VT at a cycle length of 280 msec is initiated. Following procainamide and phenytoin, no sustained arrhythmias can be induced. Quinidine, disopyramide, and lidocaine all failed to prevent induction of VT. See text for discussion. (From Horowitz LN, Josephson ME, Kastor JA. Intracardiac electrophysiologic studies as a method for the optimization of drug therapy in chronic ventricular arrhythmia. *Prog Cardiovasc Dis* 1980;23:81–98.)

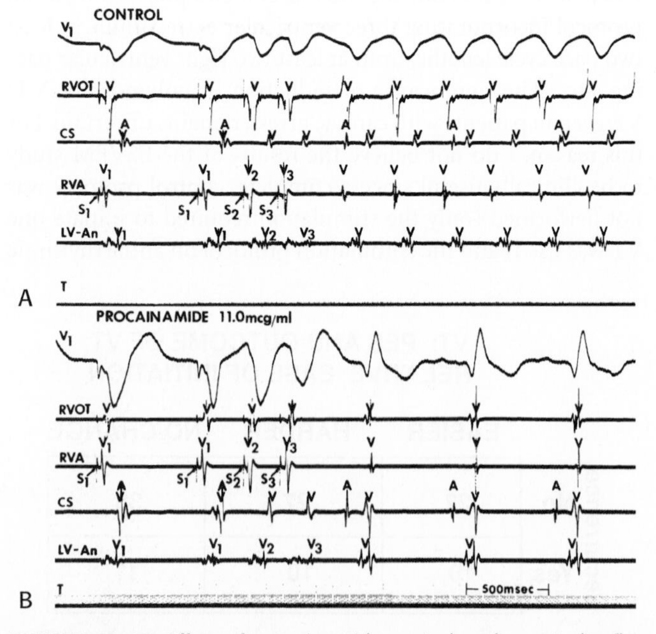


**FIGURE 12-16** *Effect of procainamide on induced ventricular flutter.* **A** and **B:** Top to bottom, surface lead $V_1$ and electrograms from the RVOT, coronary sinus (CS), RVA, and a left ventricular aneurysm (LV–An). A sine wave–like ventricular flutter is initiated by two ventricular extrastimuli from the RVA. **B:** Following procainamide, producing a plasma level of 11 µg/mL, no VT is initiated.

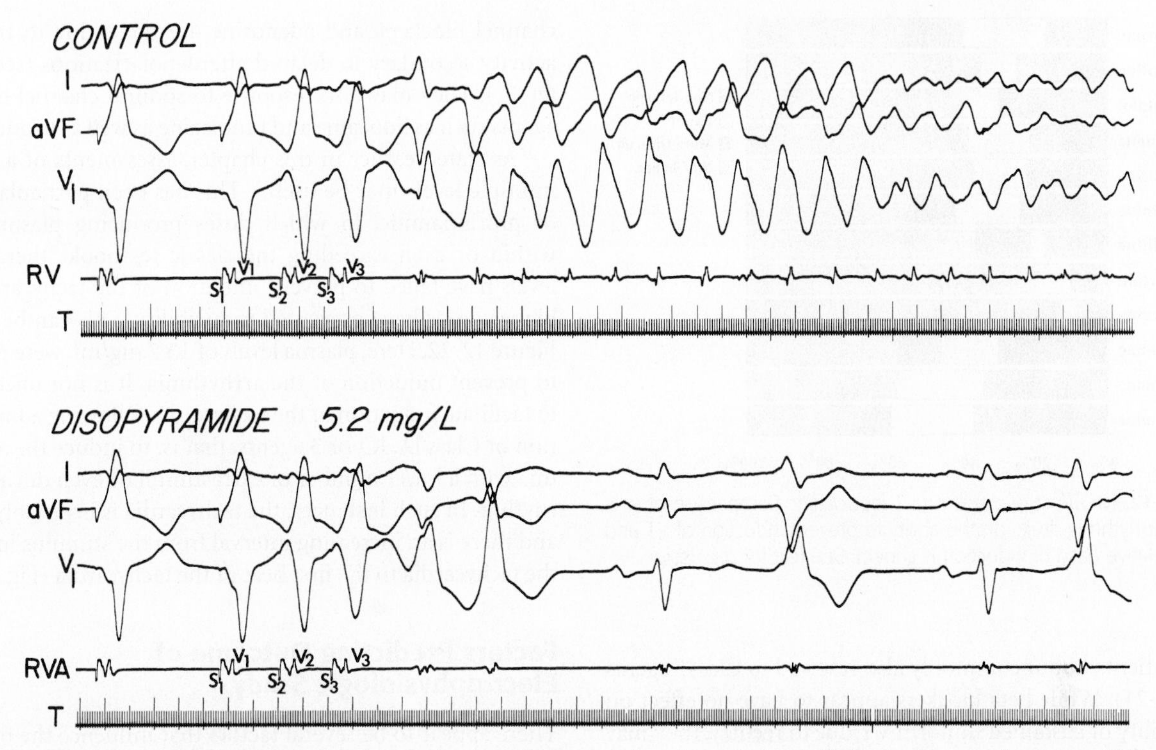


**FIGURE 12-17** *Use of programmed stimulation to detect drug efficacy in induced ventricular fibrillation.* In the control state, two VESs from the RV initiate polymorphic VT, which degenerates into ventricular fibrillation. Following 3 days of oral disopyramide, no sustained arrhythmia can be induced.

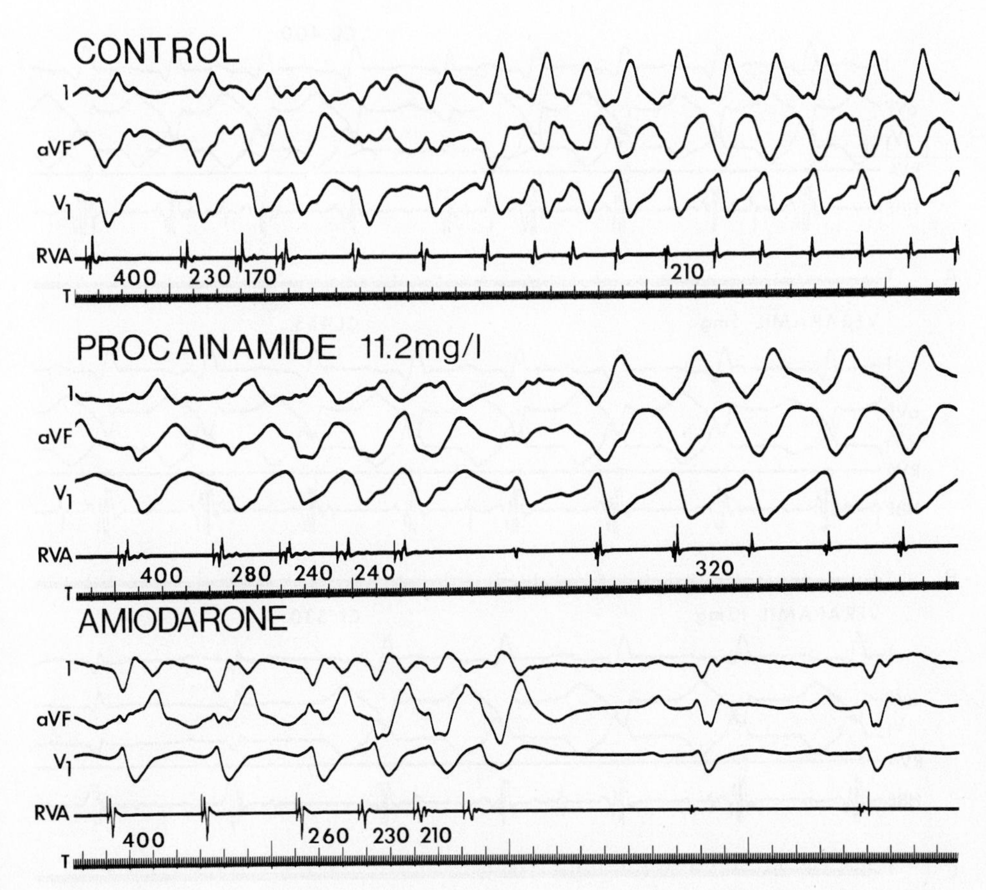


**FIGURE 12-18** *Prevention of VT by amiodarone.* In the control panel, two extrastimuli initiate a rapid VT with a cycle length of 210 msec. Procainamide fails to prevent induction of the tachycardia but slows the VT markedly. However, following 2 weeks of amiodarone loading, no ventricular arrhythmia is induced.

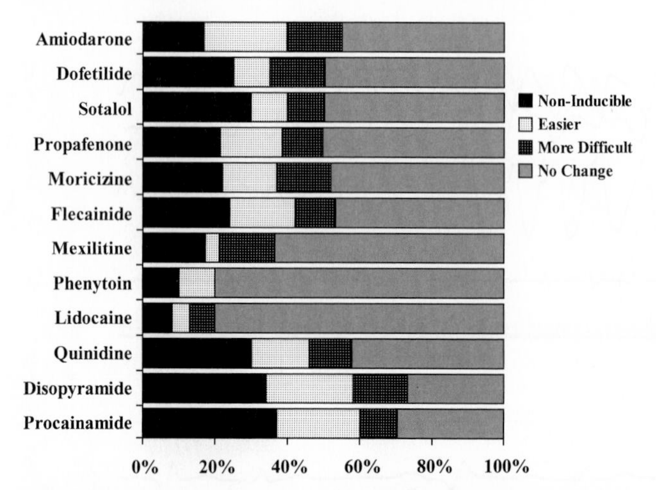


**FIGURE 12-19** *Effect of drugs on VT inducibility.* Comparison of several antiarrhythmic drugs on the ability to prevent induction of VT and on the relative ease of induction is shown. See text for discussion.

these patients not uncommonly also respond to Class1 agents (Fig. 12-21). While beta blockers appear to have no effect on inducibility of sustained uniform VT due to reentry, they may be a useful adjunct, since enhanced sympathetic tone may either counteract an antiarrhythmic agent's effect directly or produce ischemia as an initial trigger to the event.[180] A group of arrhythmias that may respond to beta blockers, calcium channel blockers, and adenosine are those due to triggered activity secondary to delayed afterdepolarizations (see Chapter 11). They may also response to sodium channel blocking agents such as lidocaine and ranolazine as well as to adenosine.

As stated earlier in this chapter, assessments of a drug at multiple levels may be useful. This has been particularly true of procainamide, in which doses producing plasma levels within or even exceeding the classic textbook "therapeutic" levels have failed to prevent initiation of the tachycardia, but higher doses have prevented inducibility. This can be seen in Figure 12-22. Here, plasma levels of 15.7 mg/mL were required to prevent induction of the arrhythmia. It is not uncommon to facilitate induction of the tachycardia following administration of Class lA, lC, or 3 agents, that is, to induce the arrhythmia with a lower number of extrastimuli or even during sinus rhythm. In such instances, the tachycardia is invariably slower and there is an increasing interval from the stimulus initiating the tachycardia to the first beat of the tachycardia (Fig. 12-23).

## Factors Predicting Outcome of Electrophysiologic Study

There appear to be several factors that influence the outcome of electrophysiologic testing. In general, patients presenting with sustained uniform VT are less likely to have their arrhythmia rendered noninducible by an antiarrhythmic agent than patients presenting with a cardiac arrest. This is particularly

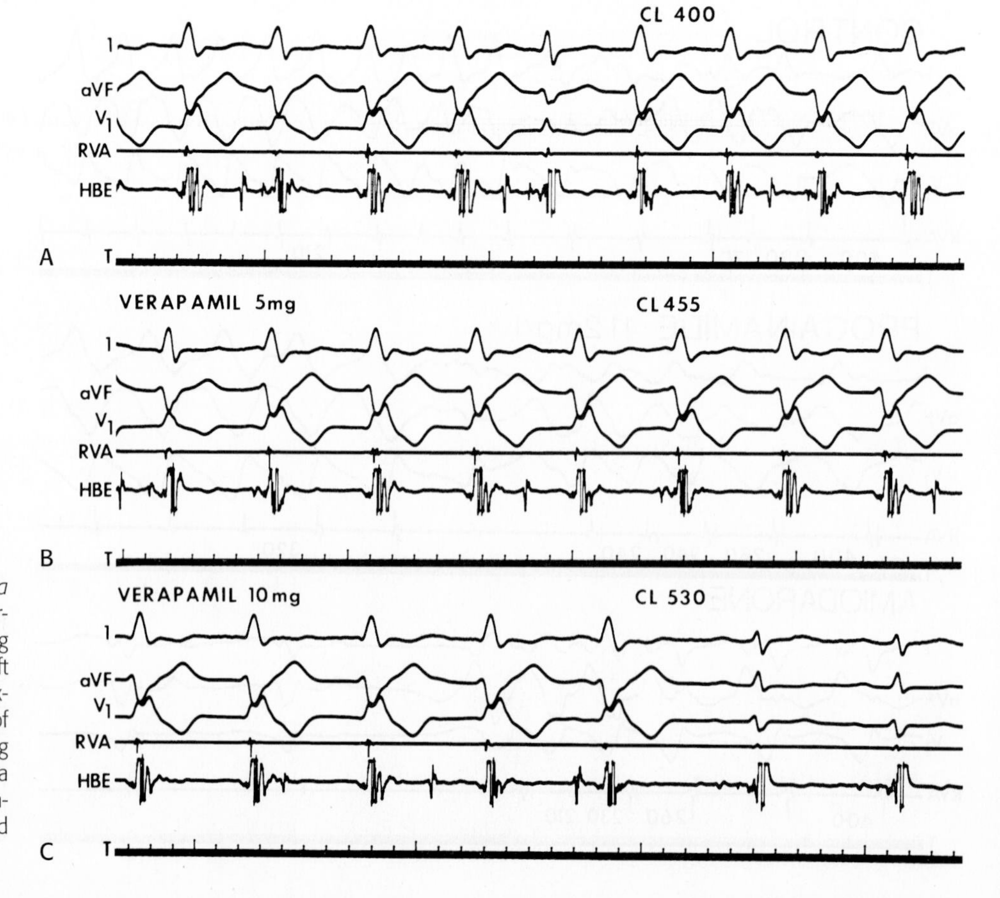


**FIGURE 12-20** *Effect of verapamil in a patient with VT associated with a normal heart.* **A:** A control tracing showing VT with a right bundle branch block left axis deviation at a cycle length of approximately 400 msec. Note the presence of fusions and capture beats. **B:** Following 5 mg of IV verapamil, the tachycardia is slowed. **C:** Following 10 mg of verapamil, the tachycardia slows further and then stops. See text for discussion.

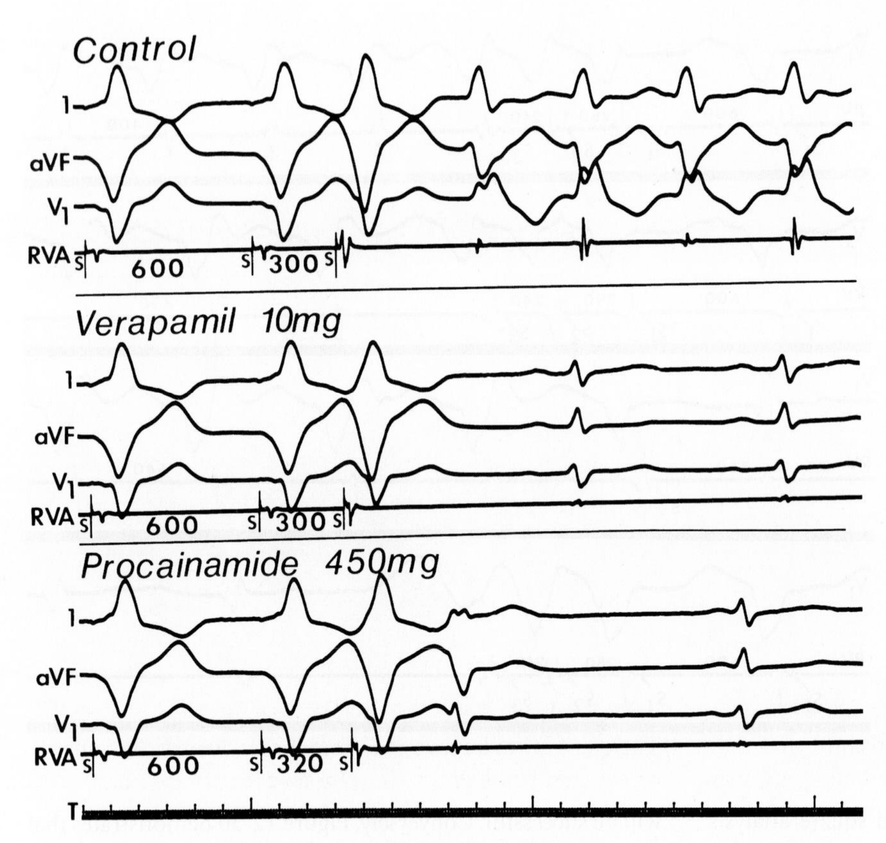


**FIGURE 12-21** *Sensitivity of VT in normal hearts to multiple agents.* This is the same patient as in Figure 12-20. In the control study, a single (VPC) initiates VT. The tachycardia induction is prevented by both verapamil and procainamide.

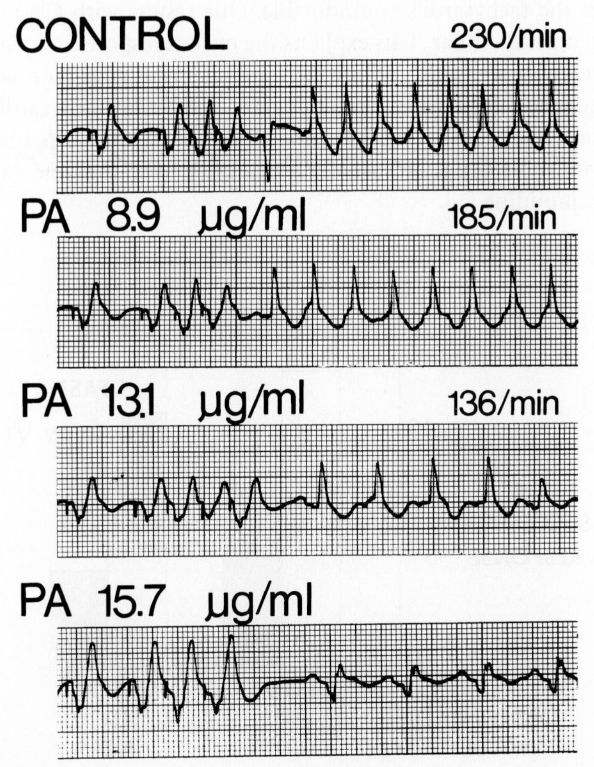


**FIGURE 12-22** *Effect of increasing doses of procainamide on VT induction.* During the control state, two extrastimuli initiate a rapid VT. Following procainamide (PA) at increasing plasma levels, the tachycardia is initially still inducible but slower. When a procainamide plasma level of 15.7 mg/mL is reached, no VT is inducible.

true if they had already failed prior antiarrhythmic therapy, whether it was administered empirically or chosen by electrophysiologic testing.[181] We retrospectively evaluated the ability of Class lA and lB agents to prevent induction of sustained VT and correlated the results with the VT cycle lengths. We found that Class 1A drugs are more likely to prevent initiation of fast VT (defined by cycle lengths <270 msec) than slow VT (defined by cycle lengths >270 msec) (Fig. 12-24). We noted that tachycardia cycle length had little influence on the ability of Class lB agents (mexiletine, lidocaine, phenytoin, tocainide) to prevent induction of these arrhythmias (Fig. 12-25). Tachycardias with cycle lengths <270 msec had a nearly 50% response rate to Type lA drugs, while slow tachycardias had a success rate of slightly more than 20%. The response to each of the Class lA drugs tested was comparable (Fig. 12-26). These findings are in accord with our clinical observations of ability to find an effective drug in patients resuscitated from cardiac arrest versus those with uniform sustained VT.

Since Class lA drugs individually had comparable efficacy, we analyzed whether the response to procainamide, which could be given intravenously in the laboratory, could predict the effect of other Class 1 drugs. In a study of 129 patients, Waxman et al.[182] found that if a tachycardia was rendered noninducible by procainamide, it was likely to be noninducible on other Type 1 drugs singly and/or in combination, although one would not predict which drug or combination of drugs would work (Fig. 12-27). Conversely, if a VT was still inducible on procainamide, it was likely to

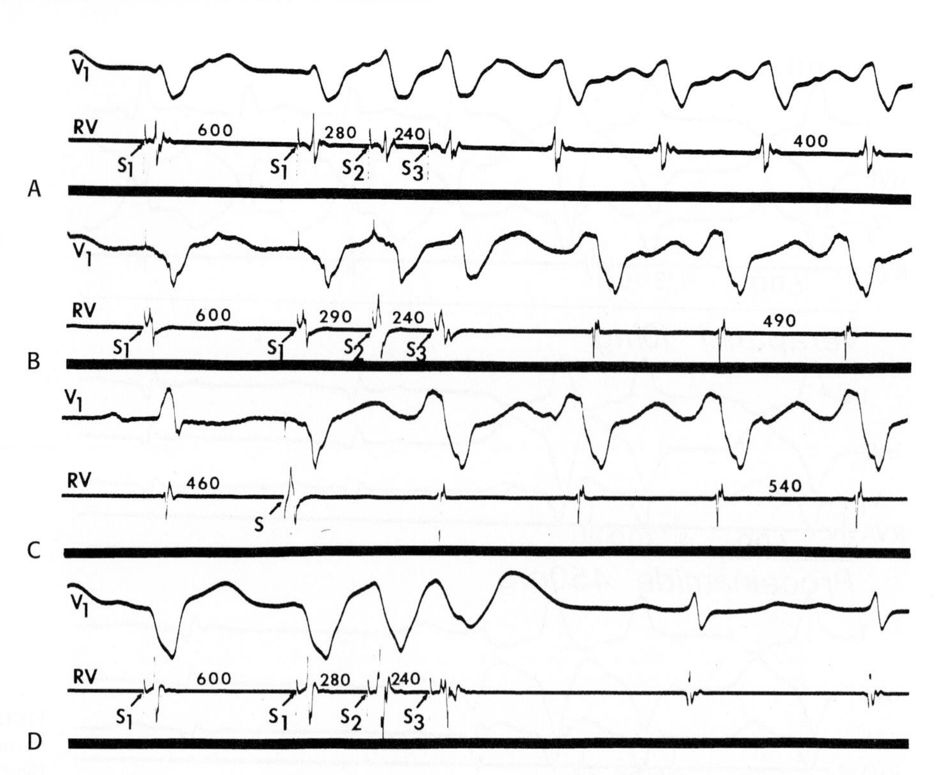


**FIGURE 12-23** *Effect of increasing the plasma procainamide concentration on VT inducibility.* **A** to **D:** ECG lead $V_1$ and a right ventricular electrogram are shown. **A:** The control study; VT was induced by two extrastimuli, and the cycle length was 400 msec. **B:** Following intravenous administration of 1,000 mg of procainamide (9.5 mg/mL), VT was induced at longer coupling intervals and the cycle length was increased to 490 msec. **C:** After an additional 250 mg of procainamide (12.8 mg/mL), VT could be induced by a single ventricular extrastimulus, but it has a longer cycle length (540 msec). **D:** After an additional 250 mg of procainamide (15.2 mg/mL), VT was not inducible S1, paced cycle length; S2, S3, premature extrastimuli. See text for discussion. (From Josephson ME, Horowitz LN. Electrophysiologic approach to therapy of recurrent sustained ventricular tachycardia. *Am J Cardiol* 1979;43:631.)

be inducible on other Type 1 agents.[182] Chi-square analysis of these data (Fig. 12-28) revealed that the predictive value for noninducibility (negative predictive value) was 83%, and for inducibility (positive predictive value) was 87%. Analog tracings from patients demonstrating both these predictive values are shown in Figures 12-29 and 12-30. In Figure 12-29, procainamide at a plasma level of 4.5 mg/mL prevented induction of VT. Quinidine and lidocaine were also successful in preventing initiation. Similarly, Figures 12-14 and 12-15 showed that procainamide was effective, and at least one other Class 1 agent was effective. However, not all Class 1 agents were effective. Thus, the negative predictive value would suggest that there is an 83% chance that another Class 1 drug would be successful. Unfortunately, it is not possible to predict which other drug or combination of drugs will be successful. Conversely, Figure 12-30 demonstrates that the failure of procainamide to prevent induction is associated with a 90% likelihood of failure of other Class 1 agents to render the tachycardia noninducible. Our results with Class lC agents are similar. This explains the overall response to drugs shown in Figure 12-19 in which propafenone, encainide, and flecainide each have a frequency of rendering tachycardias noninducible between 18% and 22% This is not surprising, since these drugs are usually tested after procainamide and/ or quinidine fail.

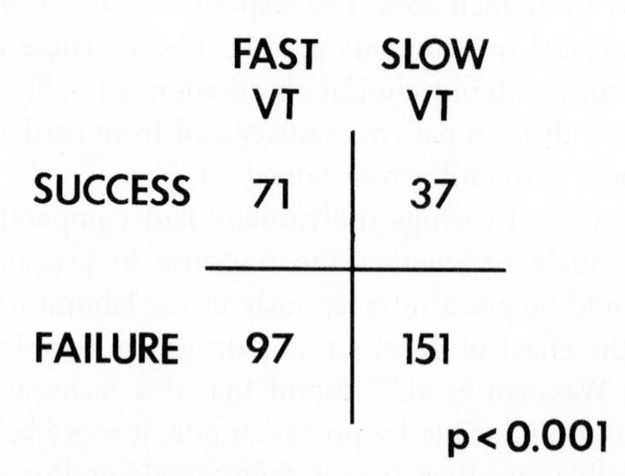

| | FAST VT | SLOW VT |
|---|---|---|
| SUCCESS | 71 | 37 |
| FAILURE | 97 | 151 |

p < 0.001

**FIGURE 12-24** *Relationship of tachycardia cycle length on prevention of VT induction.* Antiarrhythmic agents are more likely to prevent induction of fast VT (cycle lengths ≤270 msec) than slow VT (>270 msec). See text for discussion.

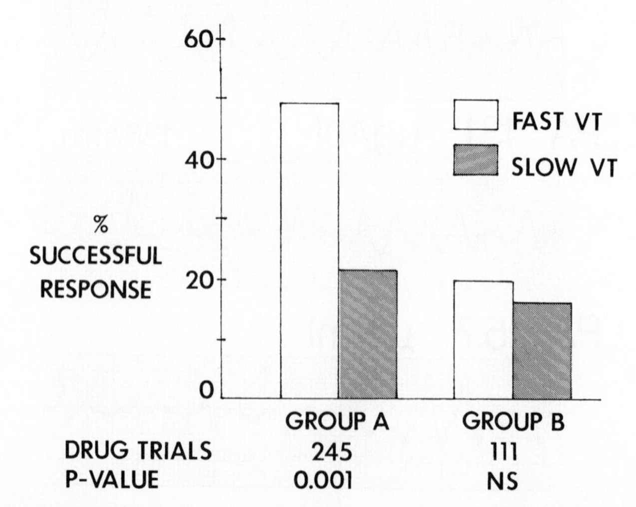


**FIGURE 12-25** *Effect of tachycardia cycle length on response to Type 1A or Type 1B agent.* The response to Class 1A (Group A) agents is markedly cycle length dependent, whereas the response to Type 1B agents (Group B) is not influenced by tachycardia cycle lengths. See text for discussion.

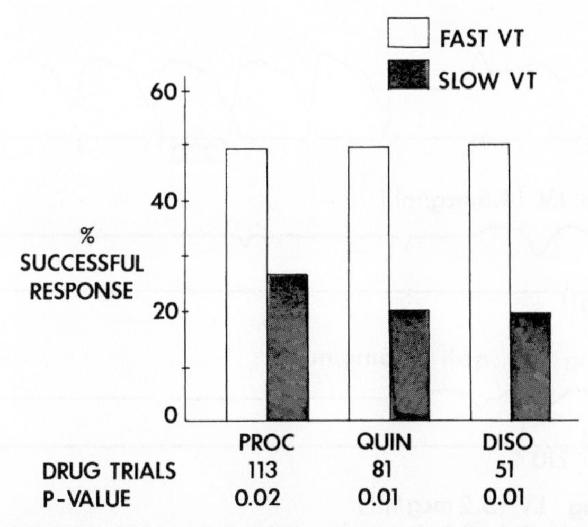


**FIGURE 12-26** *Effect of VT cycle length on inducibility following Type 1A agents.* The response of tachycardias to procainamide (PROC), quinidine (QUIN), and disopyramide (DISO) is similar. All show greater effect on tachycardias with short cycle lengths.

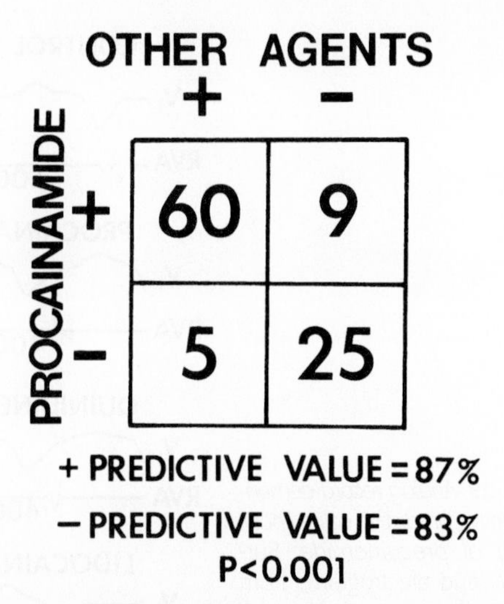


**FIGURE 12-28** *Chi-square analysis of procainamide's predictive value for efficacy of other antiarrhythmic agents.* See text for discussion. (From Waxman HL, Buxton AE, Sadowski LM, Josephson ME. The response to procainamide during electrophysiologic study for sustained ventricular tachyarrhythmias predicts the response to other medications. *Circulation* 1983;67:30–37.)

Combination drug therapy does not appear more useful in preventing initiation of ventricular tachyarrhythmia than single drugs,[183,184] but may decrease the side effects of high doses of an individual agent.[184–186] One drug combination that we have found to be occasionally successful in several patients has been quinidine and mexiletine. Another is sotalol and mexiletine. The addition of Class 1 drugs to amiodarone has likewise not led to an increase in noninducibility but has resulted in slowing of both the induced tachycardia and of spontaneous recurrences.[187]

Some of the discrepancies in relative efficacy of various agents include (a) failure to compare inducibility and cycle length of the same VT and (b) the induction of VTs that were not observed before antiarrhythmic administration. Regardless of drugs used, we have found that noninducibility has a 90% predictive accuracy for freedom of recurrences

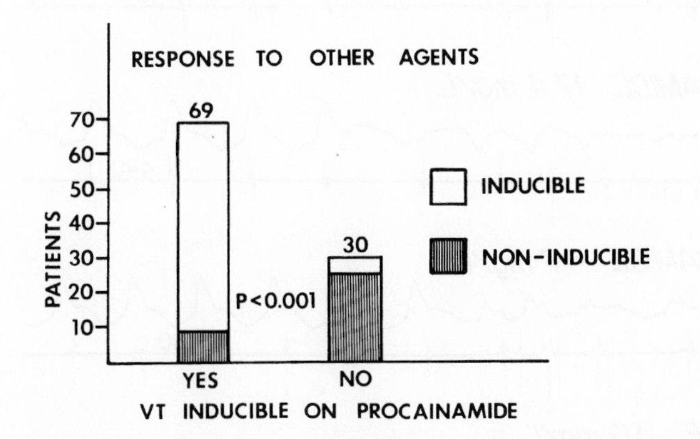


**FIGURE 12-27** *Relationship of response to procainamide and to other Type 1A agents.* The diagrams demonstrate that when VT is inducible on procainamide it is likely to be inducible on other antiarrhythmic agents and, conversely, if VT is not inducible on procainamide, it is likely to be noninducible on other agents.

(Figs. 12-31 and 12-32) and a 30% to 40% predictive accuracy for recurrences. The inducibility rate is higher and the predicted clinical failures slightly lower for amiodarone than Type 1 agents. Of importance in evaluating efficacy is the natural history of VT in which there is only a 30% to 50% recurrence over 2 years. Thus, all VTs that are inducible would not be expected to recur.

## Effect of Drugs on VT Cycle Length

Another potentially beneficial response of antiarrhythmics is to slow the VT and make it hemodynamically tolerated. Studies by Waller et al.[188] and Kadish et al.[74] suggest that making a tachycardia slower and well tolerated is beneficial. By this, one means that patients in whom VT is slowed and hemodynamically tolerated following antiarrhythmic agents have a low risk of sudden death, while those in whom VT is not slowed and/or is poorly tolerated have a significantly higher incidence of sudden death (Fig. 12-33). However, the recurrence rate is not different from those patients in whom a rapid VT is still inducible (Fig. 12-34). Unfortunately, the presenting arrhythmia is also important.[74,189] For those patients presenting with cardiac arrest, we have found that ≈25% of recurrences will be a cardiac arrest even if the VT was slowed. This is especially critical with amiodarone, for which recurrence cannot be predicted among inducible VTs. In these patients we have found a 15% to 30% incidence of recurrent cardiac arrest in patients with slowed VT (Figs. 12-35 and 12-36).[189] Thus, patients with spontaneously well-tolerated VT have a low incidence of sudden death and those presenting with cardiac arrest have a high incidence of cardiac arrest regardless of what is induced in the laboratory.

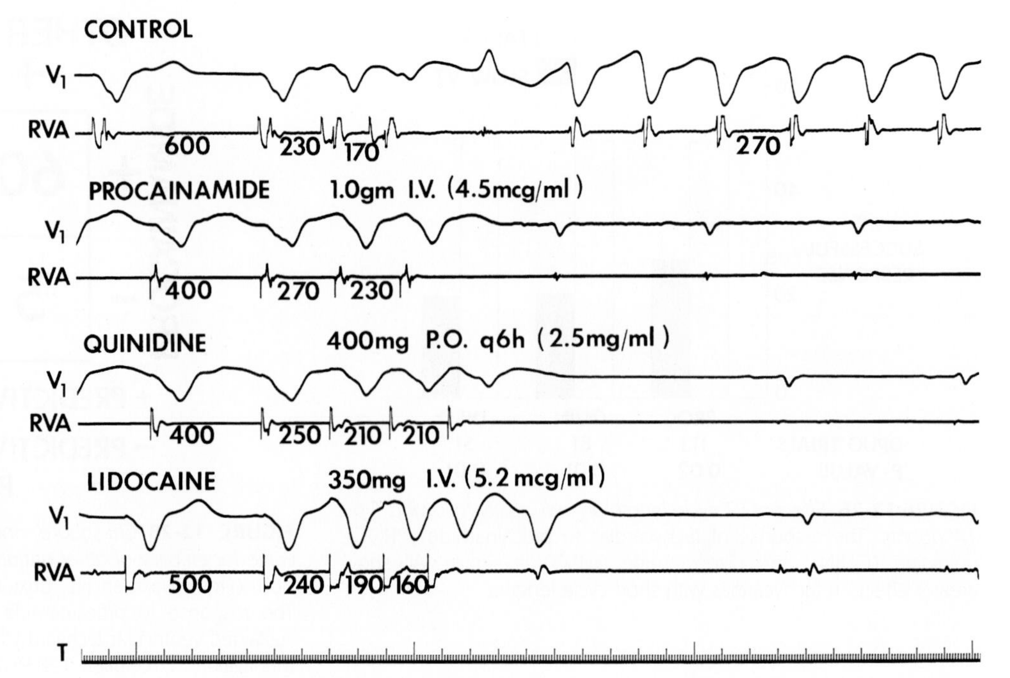


**FIGURE 12-29** *Analog record demonstrating negative predictive value (noninducibility) of procainamide.* Surface lead $V_1$ and electrograms from the RVA are shown in each panel. In the control state, two ventricular extrastimuli initiate VT. Following procainamide no VT is inducible. Similarly, quinidine and lidocaine prevent induction of VT.

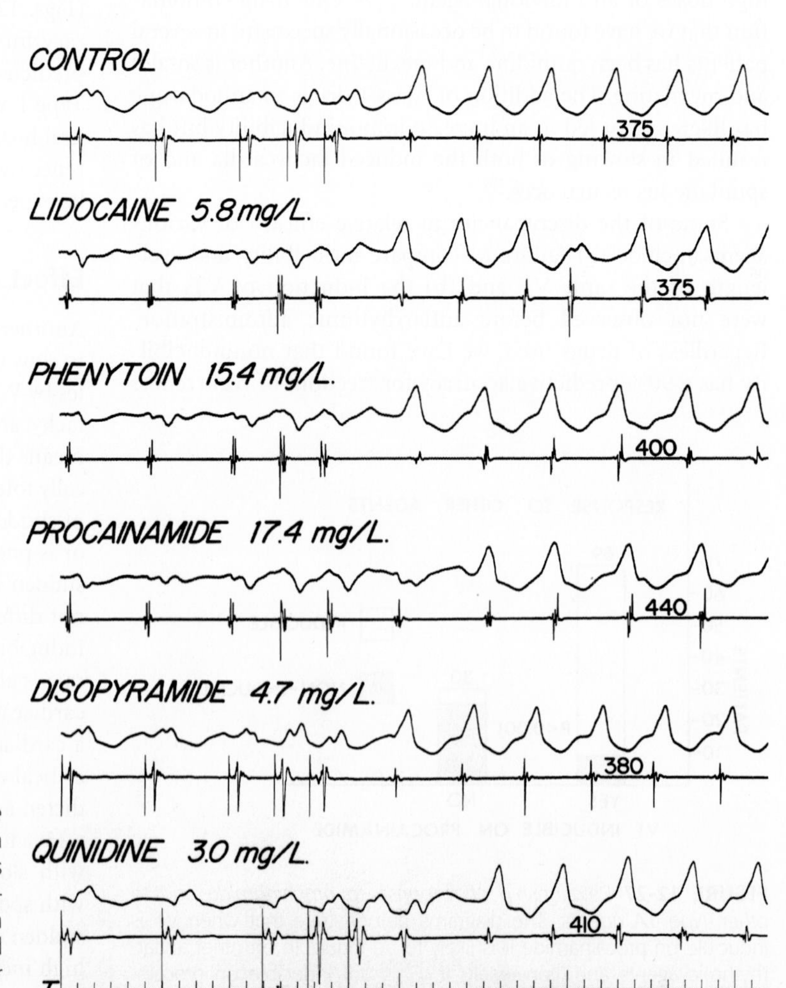


**FIGURE 12-30** *Analog records demonstrating positive predictive value (positive inducibility) of procainamide.* In the control tracing, VT with a cycle length of 375 msec is induced. Procainamide at a level of 17.4 mg/L fails to prevent induction of VT, although it makes the VT slower. On separate occasions lidocaine, phenytoin, disopyramide and quinidine also failed to prevent induction of VT. See text for discussion.

**INDUCIBILITY AND OUTCOME**
**211 PTS**

| Recurrence | NI | I |
|---|---|---|
| No | 89 | 78 |
| Yes | 9 | 35 |

**FIGURE 12-31** *Relationship of inducibility to outcome in patients on Type 1 agents.* The recurrence rate in 211 patients on Type 1 agents is related to whether they were noninducible (NI) or inducible (I) on the agent. Noninducibility predicted a 90% freedom from recurrence rate while persistent inducibility was associated with the 33% recurrence rate. See text for discussion.

**INDUCIBILITY AND OUTCOME**
**AMIODARONE 106 PTS**

| Recurrence | NI | I |
|---|---|---|
| No | 18 | 62 |
| Yes | 2 | 24 |

**FIGURE 12-32** *Effect of amiodarone on inducibility and recurrences.* The figure is organized like Figure 12-31. One hundred and six patients were treated with amiodarone. Noninducibility predicted a 90% freedom from recurrence rate of persistent inducibility and was associated with a 28% recurrence rate. See text for discussion.

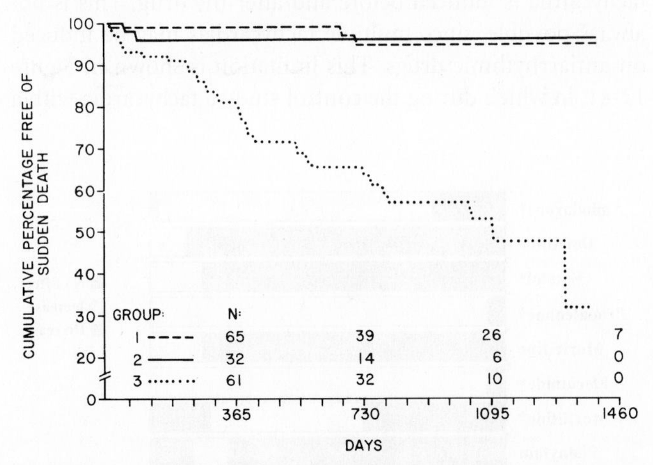


**FIGURE 12-33** *Relationship of tolerated and nontolerated tachycardias to subsequent outcome.* The survival of patients with induced but hemodynamically tolerated and slow tachycardias (*solid line*) is shown together with survival curves of patients with induced nontolerated tachycardia (*dotted line*). Those with induced tachycardias that were slower and better tolerated had a low incidence of sudden cardiac death comparable to those with no inducible VT (*dashed line*), while those whose tachycardias remained nontolerated had a significantly higher incidence of death. (From Waller TJ, Kay HR, Spielman SR, et al. Reduction in sudden death and total mortality by antiarrhythmic therapy evaluated by electrophysiologic drug testing: criteria of efficacy in patients with sustained ventricular tachyarrhythmia. *J Am Coll Cardiol* 1987;10:83–89.)

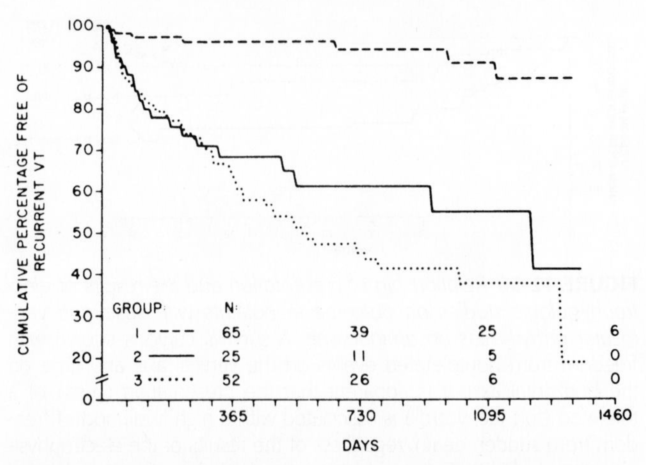


**FIGURE 12-34** *Relationship of recurrence of VT to inducibility and cycle length of induced tachycardia.* The cumulative percentage free of recurrent VT is shown on the vertical axis, and time is on the horizontal axis. Group 1 (*dashed line*) are patients in whom the drugs made the tachycardia not inducible. Group 2 (*solid line*) are those patients with inducible VT which was slowed and was hemodynamically tolerated. Group 3 (*dotted line*) were those in whom antiarrhythmic agents failed to slow the tachycardia. Patients with no inducible arrhythmias had a 90% likelihood of no recurrences in 3 years. Those patients with inducible arrhythmias, regardless of cycle length or hemodynamic tolerance, had comparable recurrence rates. (From Waller TJ, Kay HR, Spielman SR, et al. Reduction in sudden death and total mortality by antiarrhythmic therapy evaluated by electrophysiologic drug testing: criteria of efficacy in patients with sustained ventricular tachyarrhythmia. *J Am Coll Cardiol* 1987;10:83–89.)

One of the major limitations of published studies, with regard to outcome, is the combining of patients with cardiac arrest and those with sustained, hemodynamically stable VT. As seen in Figures 12-37 and 12–38, in patients treated with amiodarone, both the tolerance of the tachycardia induced in the laboratory on amiodarone and the presenting arrhythmia were highly significant determinants of nontolerated recurrences. Waller et al.[188] did not address this latter observation.

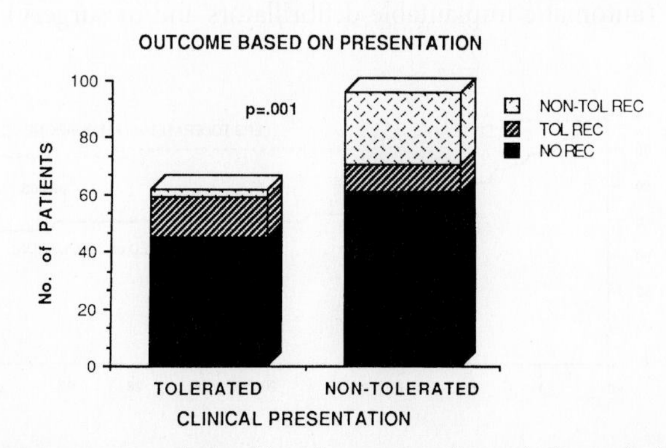


**FIGURE 12-35** *Relationship of outcome of ventricular arrhythmia based on presentation in patients taking amiodarone.* The clinical presentation of the arrhythmia is shown on the horizontal axis and the number of patients on the vertical axis. Patients presenting with tolerated tachycardias tend to have tolerated recurrences, while those presenting with nontolerated tachycardia tend to have nontolerated recurrences. See text for discussion.

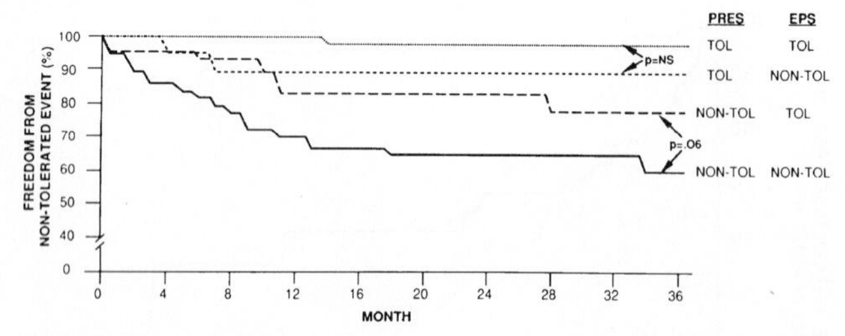


**FIGURE 12-36** *Relationship of presentation and the results of electrophysiologic studies on outcome in patients with sustained ventricular arrhythmias on amiodarone.* A survival curve is shown with freedom from nontolerated events on the vertical axis and time on the horizontal axis. It is apparent that the presentation (pres) of a tolerated (tol) tachycardia is associated with a high likelihood of freedom from sudden death, regardless of the results of the electrophysiologic study (EPS). Conversely, patients presenting with nontolerated (non-tol) tachycardias have a 20% to 40% incidence of nontolerated recurrences regardless of whether or not the induced arrhythmia was tolerated. See text for discussion.

However, Kadish et al.[74] and the study by Gottlieb et al.[189] demonstrated that patients with tolerated tachycardias generally have tolerated recurrences, and those with nontolerated tachycardias tend to have nontolerated recurrences. This appears to be true regardless of what is induced in the laboratory. As shown graphically in Figure 12-36, regardless of the tolerance of the laboratory-induced arrhythmia on amiodarone, spontaneously tolerated tachycardias do extremely well, while nontolerated tachycardias do significantly worse. In this particular study, 22% of patients who presented with a cardiac arrest and who had a tolerated tachycardia or no tachycardia induced in the laboratory still had recurrent cardiac arrest over a 36-month follow-up. This has made us cautious in using amiodarone alone to treat patients with cardiac arrest. Although noninducibility usually predicts a good outcome, VT is uncommonly made noninducible by amiodarone. Thus, in the 80% to 90% of patients in whom VT remains inducible on amiodarone, the inability to predict who will have a recurrence has led us to use more aggressive modes of therapy (automatic implantable defibrillators and/or surgery) in

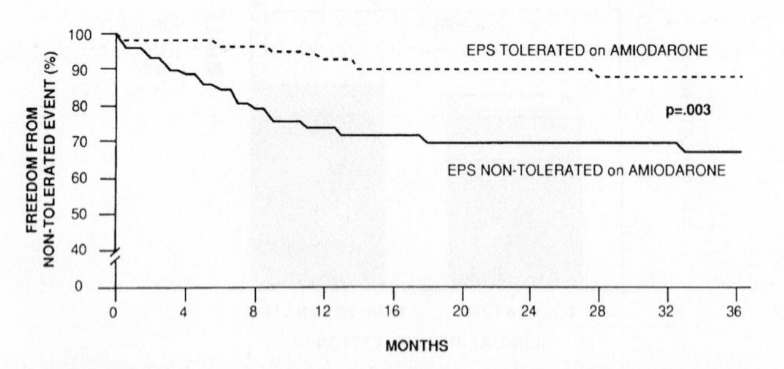


**FIGURE 12-37** *Comparison of effective electrophysiologic results on clinical outcome in patients with both tolerated and nontolerated tachycardias spontaneously.* For the group with sustained ventricular arrhythmia as a whole, patients in whom the induced tachycardia was slow and tolerated on amiodarone had a lower incidence of nontolerated recurrence than those patients in whom nontolerated tachycardias were induced on amiodarone. See text for discussion.

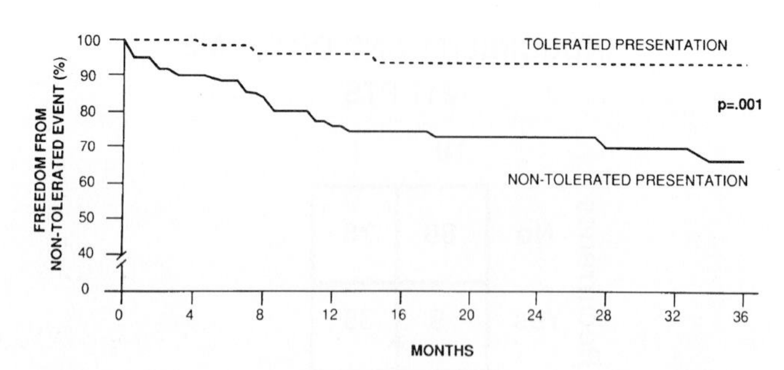


**FIGURE 12-38** *Relationship of clinical presentation to clinical outcome regardless of electrophysiologic studies.* Tolerated tachycardias (*dashed line*) had an extremely low incidence of nontolerated recurrent events. This was highly significant and different from patients presenting with nontolerated tachycardias who had a 35% incidence of recurrent nontolerated events. See text for discussion.

such patients, since their incidence of recurrent cardiac arrest exceeds 20%.

The effect of various antiarrhythmic agents on VT cycle length is predictable. As can be seen in Figure 12-39, Class IA and IC agents all almost invariably slow VT rate. The same is true for amiodarone. Examples are shown in Figures 12-40 to 12-42. On the other hand, phenytoin and lidocaine rarely have any effect on tachycardia cycle length and, in some instances, may even shorten it (Fig. 12-43). Mexiletine's effects on VT cycle length are variable, ranging from no effect to a slight increase or decrease. Sotalol and the Class 3 agents have minimal effect on VT cycle length and appear to affect VT initiation rather than cycle length. An accurate assessment of a drug's influence on VT cycle length can only be made if the same tachycardia is induced before and after the drug. This is not always possible, since multiple tachycardias may be induced on antiarrhythmic drugs. This limitation is shown in Figure 12-41, in which during the control study a tachycardia with a

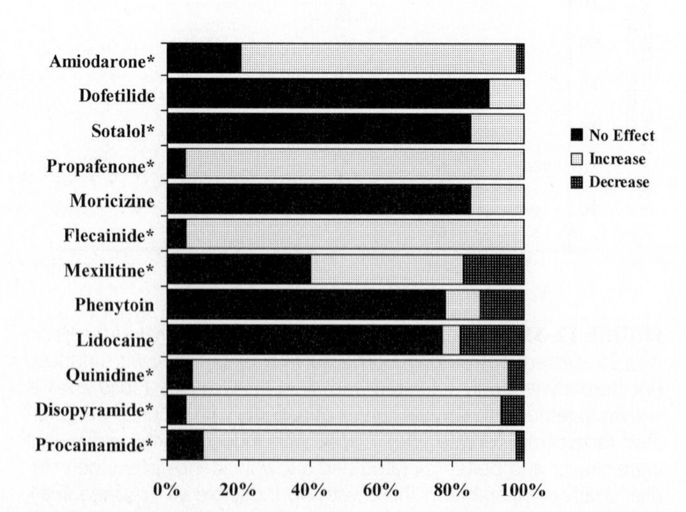


**FIGURE 12-39** *Effect of drugs on VT cycle length.* Class IA and IC agents as well as amiodarone generally prolong tachycardia cycle lengths, whereas phenytoin and lidocaine usually have no effect and mexiletine's effect is unpredictable. See text for discussion.

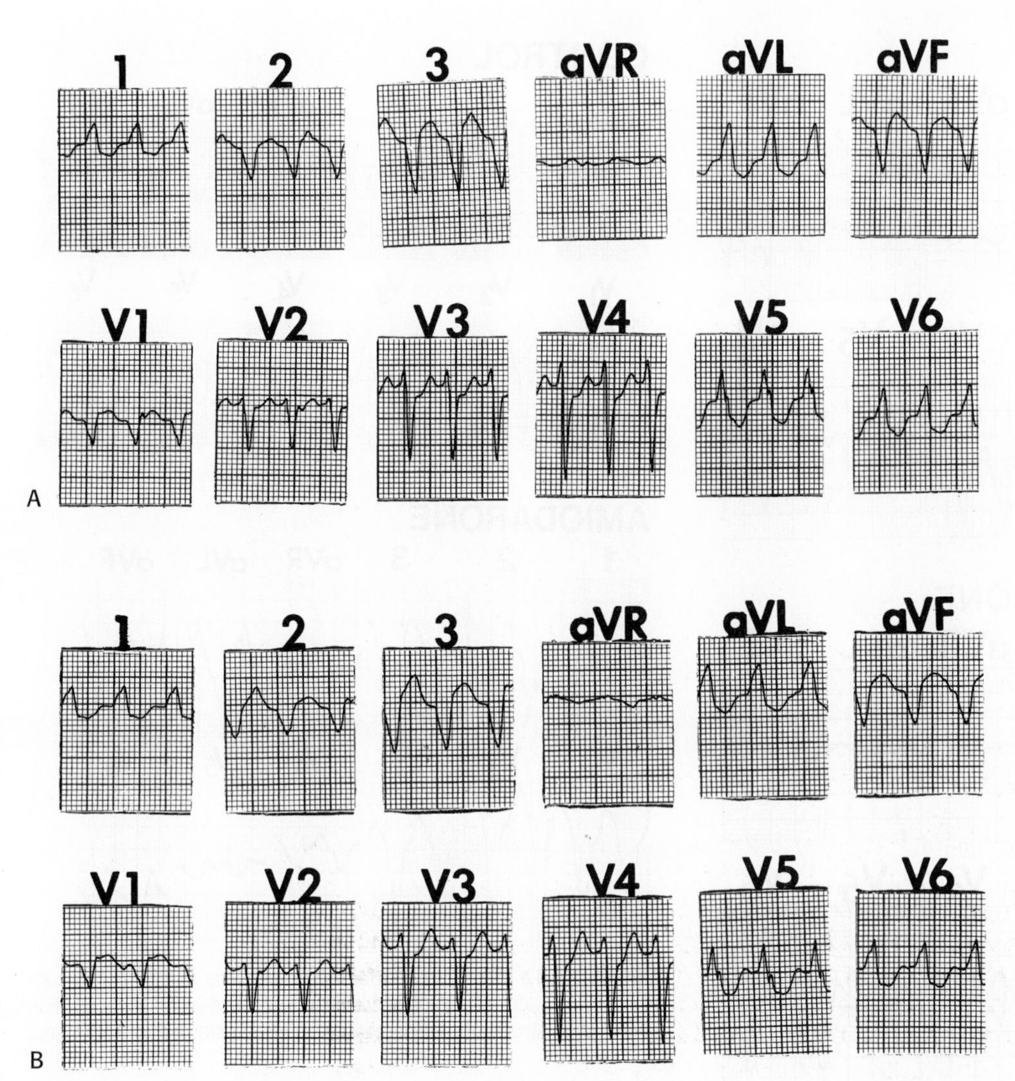


**FIGURE 12-40** *Effect of procainamide on tachycardia cycle length.* **A:** In the control state, VT with a left bundle branch block morphology has a cycle length of 320 msec. **B:** Following procainamide, the tachycardia morphology is the same but the cycle length has increased to 400 msec.

right bundle branch block, left superior axis morphology at a cycle length of 340 msec was induced. Following propafenone, the only tachycardia that could be induced had a left bundle, left superior axis at a cycle length of 520 msec. A similar circumstance following amiodarone administration is shown in Figure 12-42. In such instances, all one can state is that if the only tachycardias that are inducible while on the drug were slow, it suggests a good outcome.

## Empiric Use of Antiarrhythmic Drugs in the Setting of Concurrent ICD Therapy

Antiarrhythmic drugs are often chosen empirically (i.e., without formal electrophysiologic testing, or with cursory noninvasive testing through the defibrillator) in patients with ICDs with the hope of decreasing the frequency of ventricular arrhythmia episodes. Pacifico and coworkers demonstrated that sotalol therapy reduced all cause mortality and reduced the risk of first defibrillator shock by 48%.[190] The Optimal Pharmacologic Therapy in Cardioverter Defibrillator Patients (OPTIC) trial, randomized 412 patients with standard ICD indications to amiodarone + beta blockers, sotalol, or beta blockers alone.[191] They found that the occurrence of ICD shocks was reduced in the groups receiving amiodarone + beta blockers and sotalol, compared to those taking beta blockers alone. The 1-year incidence of ICD shock was 38.5%, 24.3%, and 10.3% in the beta blocker, sotalol, and amiodarone + beta-blocker groups, respectively ($p < 0.001$). Unfortunately drug discontinuation because of side effects was rather high in this trial, even despite its short follow-up duration; rates of discontinuation were 18.2%, 23.5%, and 5.3% for amiodarone, sotalol, and beta blocker, respectively. The use of antiarrhythmic drugs to reduce the frequency of ICD therapy after a patient has received a shock is less well studied.

## Predictability of Drug Effect on Tachycardia Cycle Length

It would be useful to be able to predict the effect of a drug on tachycardia cycle length without requiring induction of the tachycardia. We evaluated whether the effect of procainamide on the duration of sinus rhythm or paced QRS complexes could be

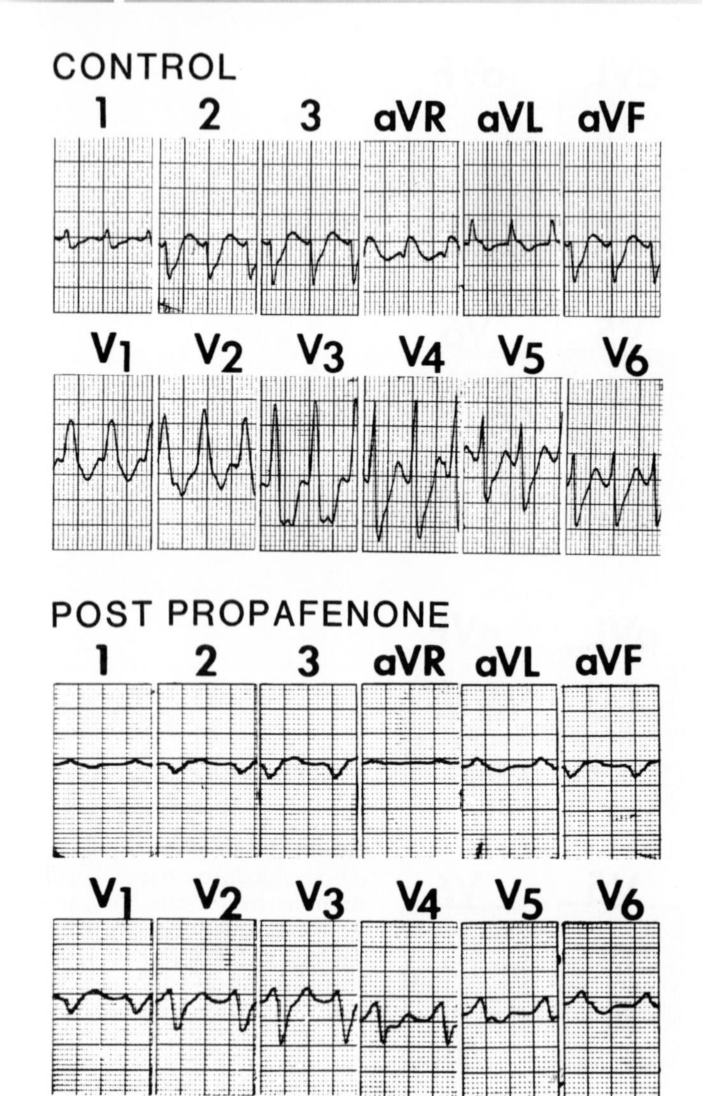


**FIGURE 12-41** *Effects of propafenone on induced VT cycle length.* In the control state panel, VT with a right bundle branch block left axis deviation was induced. The cycle length of that tachycardia was 340 msec. Following propafenone administration, only a left bundle branch block tachycardia was induced, which was extremely slow, having a cycle length of 520 msec.

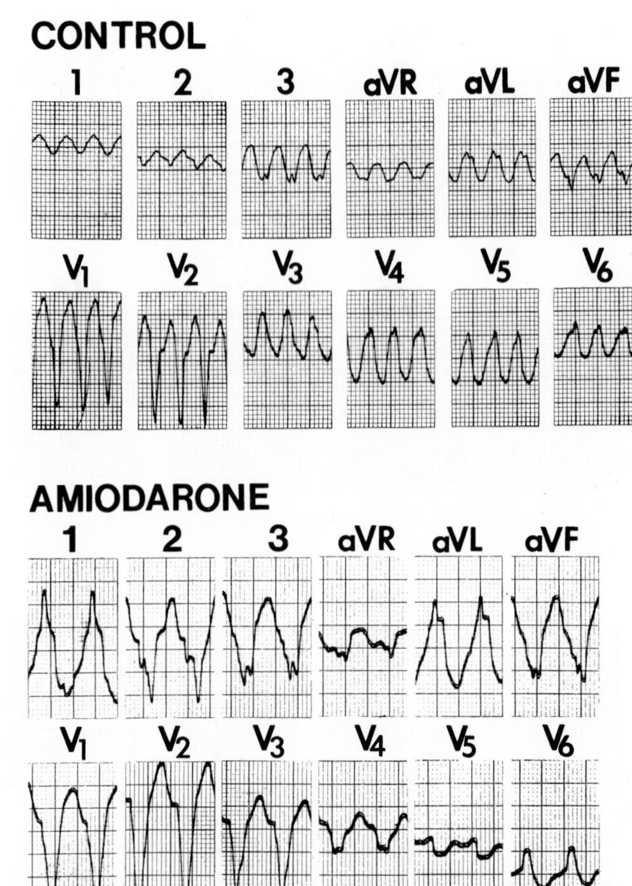


**FIGURE 12-42** *Effect of amiodarone on VT cycle length.* In the control tracing, a left VT at a cycle length of 240 msec is induced. Following amiodarone, the tachycardia is markedly slowed to 430 msec.

used to predict the effect of procainamide on tachycardia cycle length. In a group of patients in whom procainamide prolonged the tachycardia cycle length approximately 29%, Marchlinski et al.[192] compared the change in VT cycle length with the change in QRS duration observed during sinus rhythm and paced cycle lengths of 600 and 300 msec. Mean QRS duration during sinus rhythm, slow ventricular pacing, and fast ventricular pacing are shown in Figure 12-44, and an analog record of a single case is shown in Figure 12-45. It can be seen that following procainamide, the faster one paces, the more prolonged the QRS. When the change in VT cycle length was compared to the change in QRS duration during sinus rhythm and ventricular pacing, we found the change in VT cycle length (29%) approximated that associated with rapid pacing (27%) (Fig. 12-46). The change in QRS duration during sinus rhythm or slow pacing did not

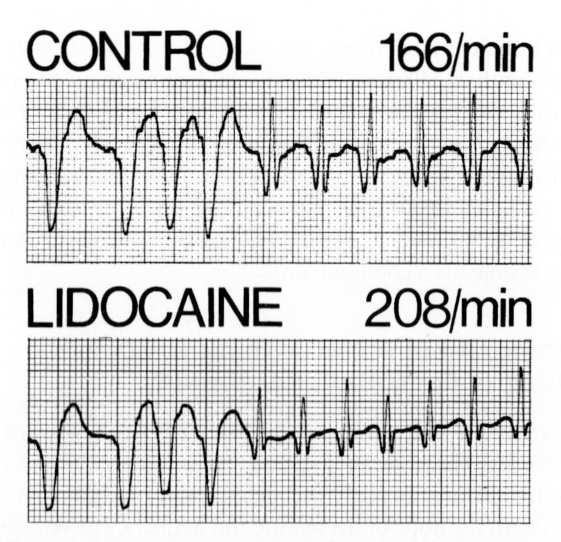


**FIGURE 12-43** *Shortening of VT cycle length by lidocaine.* In the control tracing, VT with a rate of 166 beats per minute was induced. Following lidocaine, the tachycardia, which was induced at a cycle length of 208 beats per minute, was identical in morphology. Administration of lidocaine in the clinical setting also resulted in acceleration of the tachycardia.

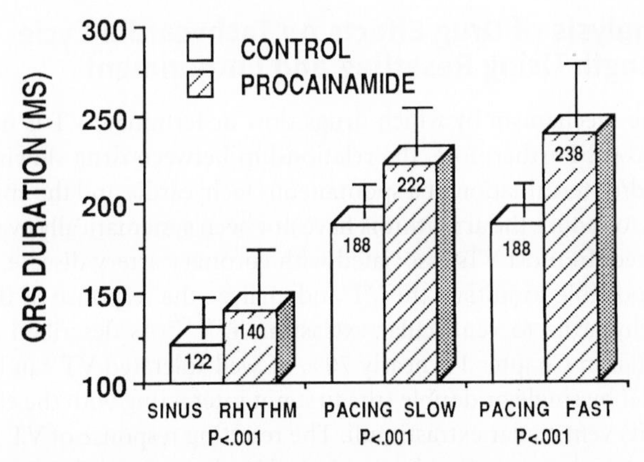


**FIGURE 12-44** *Effect of procainamide on QRS.* The effect of procainamide on the QRS width during sinus rhythm slow pacing (500 to 600 msec) or fast pacing (300 msec) is shown. While procainamide increases QRS duration at any rate, the greatest increase is during fast pacing. (From Marchlinski FE, Buxton AE, Josephson ME, Schmitt C. Predicting ventricular tachycardia cycle length after procainamide by assessing cycle length-dependent changes in paced QRS duration. *Circ* 1989;79:39–46.)

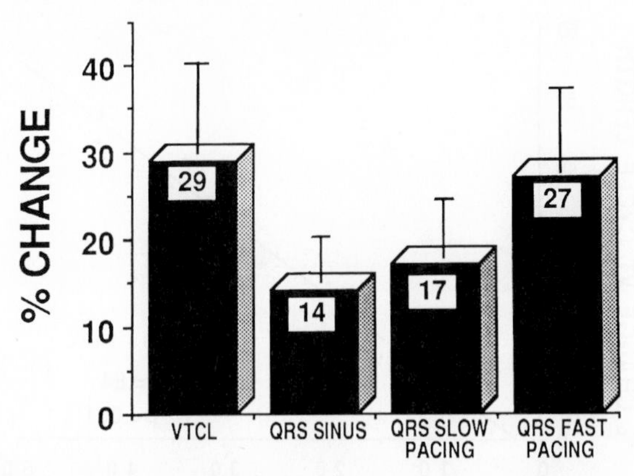


**FIGURE 12-46** *Relationship of change in VT cycle length and change in QRS duration produced by procainamide.* The percentage (%) of change in VT cycle length (VTCL) and QRS during rapid pacing was comparable (29% vs. 27%). The changes in QRS duration during sinus rhythm or slow pacing (14% and 17%) were not as great as the change in VT cycle length. (From Marchlinski FE, Buxton AE, Josephson ME, Schmitt C. Predicting ventricular tachycardia cycle length after procainamide by assessing cycle length-dependent changes in paced QRS duration. *Circulation* 1989;79:39–46.)

correlate with the change in VT cycle length as well. Linear regression relating change in QRS during rapid pacing and change in VT cycle length showed an r value of 0.84, which was highly significant at the $p < 0.001$ level (Fig. 12-47).

We have shown that the effects of amiodarone on VT cycle length are similar to those of procainamide[193] and that it may be possible to use the response to procainamide to predict that of amiodarone. Despite the generally good relationship between the change in VT cycle length on amiodarone and procainamide, approximately 20% of patients had longer tachycardia cycle lengths on amiodarone than on procainamide, and the converse was also true. Nonetheless, the response of the QRS during rapid pacing to procainamide might provide a reasonable predictor of what the response of amiodarone might be. Moreover, the response of procainamide alone and amiodarone can be used to predict the response of the combination using the formula 0.67 of sum of the individual effects on cycle lengths plus 40 msec.[193]

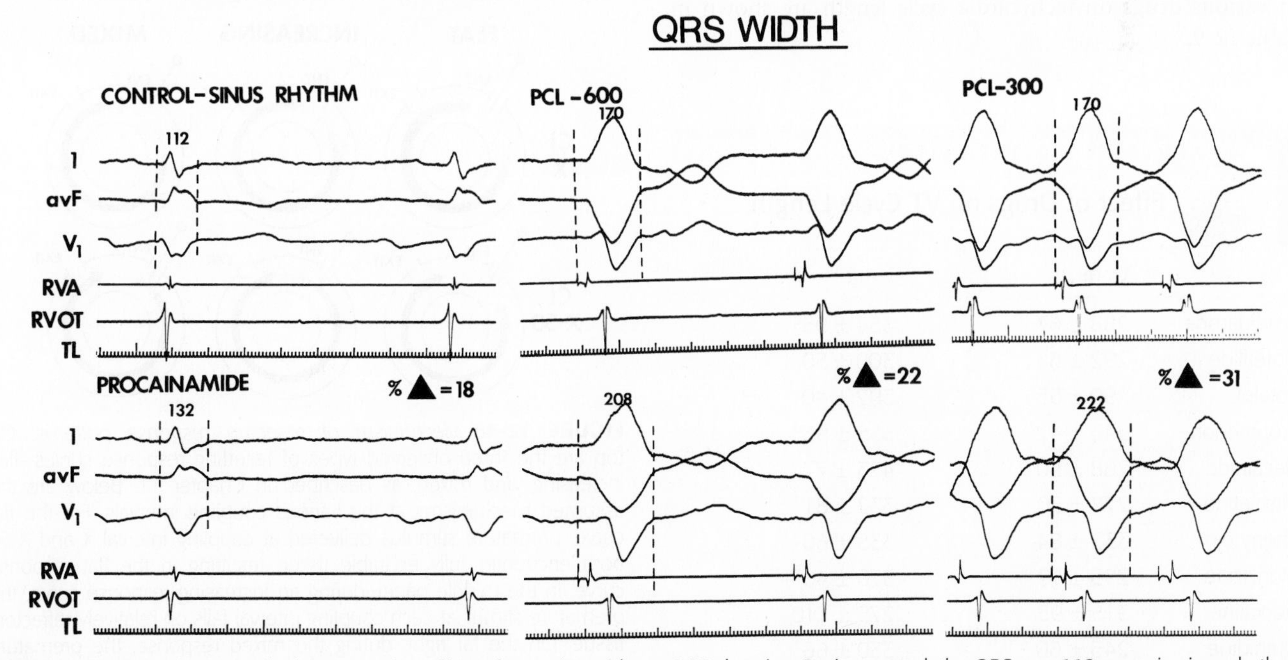


**FIGURE 12-45** *Analog records demonstrating effect of procainamide on QRS duration.* During control, the QRS was 112 msec in sinus rhythm, 170 msec during RV apical pacing at 600 msec, and 170 msec at RV pacing at 300 msec. Following procainamide, the QRS duration increased 18%, 22%, and 31%, respectively, during sinus rhythm, pacing at 600 msec, and pacing at 300 msec. (From Marchlinski FE, Buxton AE, Josephson ME, Schmitt C. Predicting ventricular tachycardia cycle length after procainamide by assessing cycle length-dependent changes in paced QRS duration. *Circulation* 1989;79:39–46.)

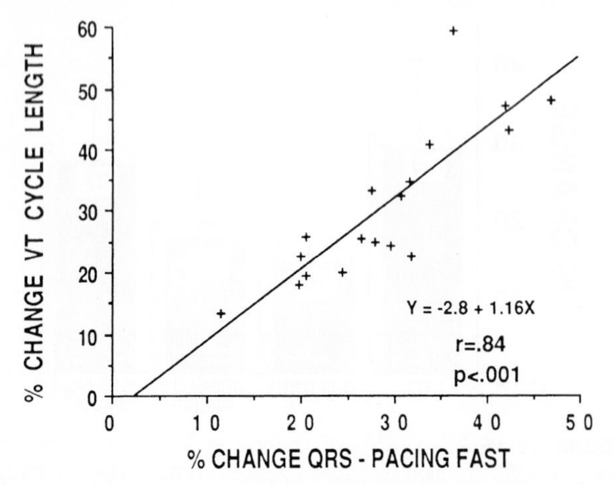


**FIGURE 12-47** *Linear regression relating change in QRS during fast pacing with change in VT cycle length produced by procainamide.* An r value of 0.84 demonstrates a high correlation between change in QRS at fast pacing and change in VT cycle length produced by procainamide. See text for discussion. (From: Marchlinski FE, Buxton AE, Josephson ME, Schmitt C. Predicting ventricular tachycardia cycle length after procainamide by assessing cycle length-dependent changes in paced QRS duration. *Circulation* 1989;79:39–46.)

Of interest, analysis of the effects of Class IA and IC agents on VT cycle length from several laboratories[33,38,39,41–44,50–54,60–62] shows them to be quite similar. I again stress the point that accurate analyses of such data require the same tachycardia being induced before and after the drug. Unfortunately, much of the literature concerning the effect of these drugs on tachycardia cycle length does not state whether the same tachycardia was evaluated before and after the drug. The effects of various drugs on tachycardia cycle length are shown in Table 12-9.

**TABLE 12-9 Effect of Drugs on VT Cycle Length**

| | Control | Drug |
|---|---|---|
| Amiodarone | 288 ± 67 | 354 ± 95$^a$ |
| Dofetilide | 292 ± 65 | 300 ± 50 |
| Sotalol | 290 ± 55 | 302 ± 40 |
| Propafenone | 246 ± 42 | 355 ± 96$^a$ |
| Flecainide | 268 ± 50 | 423 ± 77$^a$ |
| Mexiletine | 278 ± 50 | 332 ± 81$^a$ |
| Phenytoin | 332 ± 84 | 335 ± 60 |
| Moricizine | 295 ± 72 | 370 ± 40$^a$ |
| Lidocaine | 315 ± 95 | 275 ± 110 |
| Quinidine | 245 ± 60 | 330 ± 66$^a$ |
| Disopyramide | 281 ± 70 | 347 ± 64$^a$ |
| Procainamide | 285 ± 62 | 368 ± 70$^a$ |

$^a p < 0.05$.

## Analysis of Drug Effects on Tachycardia Cycle Length Using Resetting and Entrainment

The mechanism by which drugs slow or terminate VT is not known. Furthermore, the relationship between drug slowing and/or termination of a spontaneous tachycardia and the ability to induce the arrhythmia have not been systematically evaluated. In most VTs associated with coronary artery disease, it is possible to initiate the VT and analyze the response of the tachycardia to ventricular extrastimuli.[194,195] As described in detail in Chapter 11, nearly 70% of well-tolerated VT can be reset by single or double (the first not interacting with the circuit) ventricular extrastimuli. The resetting response of VT to ventricular extrastimuli can be used to characterize the extent of the fully or partially excitable gap in the reentrant circuit of VT (see Chapter 11).[194,196] Resetting response curves are constructed by plotting the return cycles in response to extrastimuli delivered during VT. The response curves may be flat, increasing, or mixed (flat and increasing). These curves are felt to represent the extrastimuli encountering fully excitable tissue (flat curve), partially excitable tissue (increasing curve), or fully excitable tissue at long coupling intervals and partially excitable tissue at close coupling intervals (mixed curve). These curves are schematically depicted in Figure 12-48.

RESETTING RESPONSE PATTERNS

RC | X-50 X ←CI | FLAT | INCREASING | MIXED | ENT | EXIT | CI X | CI X-50

**FIGURE 12-48** *Mechanism of resetting response patterns.* On top are the three observed types of resetting response curves—flat, increasing, and mixed, as described in Chapter 11. Below are the assumed mechanisms at the various coupling intervals. For the flat curve, premature stimulus delivered at coupling interval X and X-50 both encounter fully excitable tissue resulting in the flat response curve. In the middle panel, during an increasing response curve, the premature stimuli at each coupling interval falls on relatively refractory tissue. On the far right, during the mixed response, the premature stimulus delivered at coupling interval X falls on fully excitable tissue and on X-50 falls on partially excitable tissue. See text for discussion. (From Stamato NJ, Frame LH, Rosenthal ME, et al. Procainamide-induced slowing of ventricular tachycardia with insights from analysis of resetting response patterns. *Am J Cardiol* 1989;63:1455–1461.)

Theoretically, the VT cycle length could be slowed by a drug as a result of (a) slowing of conduction at one or more areas in the circuit, (b) prolongation of refractoriness in the circuit such that the head of the circulating impulse encroaches on the tail of refractoriness of the prior impulse, or (c) an increase in length of the reentrant pathway (Fig. 12-49). If a drug produced slowing of the VT cycle length as a result of a primary effect on conduction or lengthening of the pathway, it should produce an increase in the fully excitable gap; that is, an increase in flat portion of the curve would be observed. On the other hand, if slowing of the tachycardia was produced by prolonging the refractoriness such that the head of the impulse encroached on the tail of refractoriness of the prior wavelength, there would be no fully excitable gap, and no flat portion would be seen. For a flat portion to be seen, all tissues within the circuit must be fully recovered and excitable. This obviously would not be the case if a prolongation of refractoriness were responsible for slowing of the tachycardia. Even if a drug produced slowing of conduction and increased refractoriness, the presence of a flat curve suggests the circuit still had a fully excitable gap.

It is difficult to directly demonstrate an increase in path length during clinical EPSs. However, if the morphology of the slowed tachycardia is identical to that of the control tachycardia, the exit site is assumed to be unchanged. In such cases if a drug-induced lengthening of the pathway occurred, it would require lengthening of the proximal arc of block or "pseudoblock" around which the impulse circulates.[197–199] While slowing of VT associated with an increased length of the arc of "block" has been observed in experimental models of reentrant VT,[200] it has never been recorded in the absence of a marked slowing of conduction. Perhaps the use of high-resolution mapping using Carto and the PentArray or the Rhythmia mapping system can address this possibility. While currently we are studying this in a porcine infarction model, it is unlikely that this study will be performed in human VT.

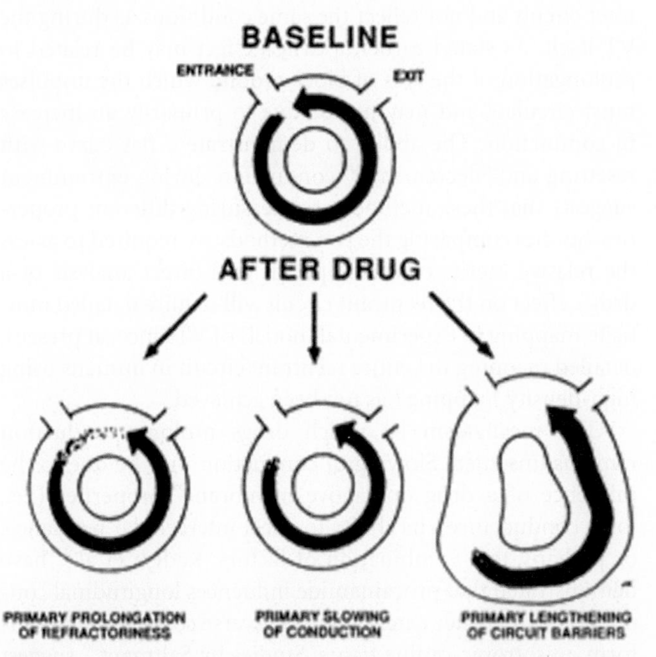


**FIGURE 12-49** *Possible mechanisms of drug-induced increase in VT cycle length.* A hypothetical tachycardia in the baseline state is shown on top with a wavelength of full refractory and partially refractory tissue in minimal excitable gap. After a drug, the tachycardia can slow because of slowing of conduction, which would be associated with an increase in the fully excitable gap, primary prolongation of refractoriness where the head of the circulating wavefront would encounter the refractory period of the preceding impulse producing an increasing curve, or an increase in path length, which would also produce a fully excitable gap. See text for discussion.

If a complete resetting curve can be defined before and following drug administration, the relative effects of a drug on conduction and refractoriness can be evaluated. A complete resetting curve extends from the initial coupling interval of the ventricular extrastimulus, which first results in resetting, to the coupling interval at which the ventricular extrastimulus terminates the tachycardia. The inability to fully measure the entire gap with single extrastimuli (with or without prior conditioning extrastimuli) is a major limitation of this technique and has led to the use of continuous resetting (i.e., entrainment) by some investigators to assess drug effects.[201] The uses and limitations of that technique will be described in subsequent paragraphs.

If one could perform a complete resetting curve, the extent of the flat portion and increasing portion of the curve could be determined, allowing calculation of the total duration of the fully excitable and partially excitable (relative refractoriness) gap, respectively. Thus, the effect of a drug on conduction and refractoriness in the VT circuit can be assessed. However, the site in the circuit responsible for interval-dependent conduction delay producing the onset of the increasing curve will not be able to be determined in the catheterization laboratory. Since the flat portion of the curve signifies that all tissues in the circuit are fully excitable, focal delays at any site should not give rise to a "pseudo-flat curve," due to accelerated conduction distal to the delay, since the impulse would already be propagating through fully excitable tissue at its maximal rate.

If the change in duration of the flat portion of the curve does not equal the change in VT cycle length, the difference must be due to change in refractoriness in some part of the VT pathway. Thus, these indirect measurements can be used to evaluate the electrophysiologic effect of a drug on the reentrant circuit responsible for VT. Unfortunately, as noted in Chapter 11, termination of VT by a single extrastimulus interacting with the circuit is uncommon—15% to 20% with one extrastimulus and 30% to 50% with two extrastimuli, when the first is a conditioning impulse. The use of two or more conditioning extrastimuli may increase the ability to analyze the excitable gap. Moreover, it is obvious that the selection of tachycardias studied can influence these results. Studies as those just described form the major thrust of our laboratory's attempt to understand the mechanism of drug action during VT.

At present, results with procainamide[196] and amiodarone[202–204] have demonstrated a persistent flat portion of the curve in tachycardias slowed by either of these drugs. Similar results have been observed in preliminary studies of quinidine, propafenone, and flecainide (unpublished observation). These data are consistent with a primary slowing of conduction within the circuit, with or without a change in pathway length, as a mechanism of prolongation of tachycardia cycle length. A fixed increase in refractoriness at any point in the circuit is unlikely to account for the increase in VT cycle length seen with these agents since a flat portion of the curve persists. However, a marked change in refractoriness greater than a change in conduction time could produce a decrease in the flat part of the resulting curve. Nevertheless, since a flat portion is still present, the change in cycle length cannot be attributed to the change in refractoriness. Using our model of resetting, one would postulate that the inability of lidocaine to slow VT is compatible with its known lack of effect on conduction in normally polarized tissue. Shortening of VT cycle length, which is occasionally seen, may be due to a decrease in the length of the arc of block around which the impulse must circulate, thereby decreasing the length of the pathway. Such studies, which are currently under way in our laboratories, are necessary to explain the response of tachycardias to antiarrhythmic drugs.

In view of the limited capability of single extrastimuli to determine the entire excitable gap, continuous resetting (entrainment) of the tachycardia has been used to evaluate the effects of antiarrhythmic drugs on the VT circuit.[201] Kay et al.[201] used this technique to study the mechanism of procainamide-induced prolongation of VT cycle length in five patients. They used left ventricular mapping to demonstrate orthodromic capture of left ventricular sites in response to right ventricular pacing during VT. They then compared the effect of procainamide on orthodromic and antidromic activation to a local left ventricular site. The orthodromic activation time was measured from the stimulated right ventricular impulse to the orthodromically "entrained" electrogram in the left ventricle. The antidromic activation time was measured from the right ventricular electrogram to the same left ventricular electrogram recorded during ventricular pacing initiated during sinus rhythm. The assumption made by these investigators was that a greater effect on orthodromic activation time would reflect a drug's effect on the area of "slow conduction" in the reentrant circuit. These investigators demonstrated that an increase in tachycardia cycle length of 27% was associated with a 28% increase in the orthodromic activation time, compared to an increase of only 9% in the antidromic activation time. The difference between the change in orthodromic and antidromic activation time was 40%. These investigators concluded that these findings supported a primary effect of procainamide on conduction in the "slow limb" of the reentrant circuit.

There are, however, several limitations to their study.[201] First, the recorded left ventricular electrograms were not presystolic and, therefore, may not have been in the tachycardia circuit. Since orthodromic activation of such sites includes the time to the circuit, through the circuit, and to this potentially noncritical or distant (from the circuit) electrogram, it seems to be a giant leap of faith to suggest any changes in activation time in either antidromic or orthodromic direction reflect a change in the circuit alone. Moreover, during their entrainment protocol, 15 beats of pacing were used before assessing the return cycle. As discussed in Chapter 11 and demonstrated in Figures 11-173 and 11-174, the response to "entrainment" may yield misleading information with respect to the excitable gap. As discussed in Chapter 11, of a train of 15 stimuli, the *n*th stimulus resets the VT circuit and subsequent extrastimuli reset the reset circuit. If the $n + 1$th stimulus falls on the relative refractory period of the *n*th stimulus, prolongation of return cycle or termination will be observed. Obviously, in this situation, prolongation of the orthodromic activation time would be a result of a combination of impingement of successive extrastimuli on the refractory period of the prior resetting stimulus and a primary effect on conduction velocity. This prolonged conduction time, in fact, may be unrelated to a primary effect of the drug on conduction velocity within the tachycardia circuit but may simply represent impingement of the $n + 1$th and subsequent extrastimuli on the refractory period of the preceding reset circuit. It is only possible to avoid this confounding response by analyzing the results of the interaction of a single ventricular extrastimulus with the VT circuit itself. Unfortunately, as mentioned in prior paragraphs, this cannot be done completely in most tachycardias.

Moreover, continuous stimulation at rapid rates may alter the properties of refractoriness and conduction within the reset circuit and not reflect the same conditions as during the VT itself. As stated earlier, a drug's effect may be related to prolongation of the arcs of block around which the impulses must circulate and may not be due to primarily an increase in conduction. The ability to demonstrate a flat curve with resetting and "decremental" conduction during entrainment suggests that these methods are measuring different properties. Studies comparing the two methods are required to assess the relative merits of each. Specific and direct analysis of a drug's effect on the reentrant circuit will require detailed multisite mapping in experimental models of VT since, at present, detailed mapping the entire reentrant circuit in humans using high-density mapping has not been achieved.

The mechanism by which drugs prolong conduction remains unsettled. Slowing of conduction may be due to the influence of a drug on "active membrane" properties (i.e., ionic conductance), its ability to affect intercellular resistance, or perhaps, to a combination of factors. Kadish et al.[21] have demonstrated that procainamide influences longitudinal conduction to a greater extent than transverse conduction in uniform anisotropic canine tissue. Studies by Saltman[200] suggest that following infarction, significant nonuniform anisotropy must exist because the areas of block and slow conduction do not relate to fiber orientation.

We have demonstrated that the effect of procainamide on infarcted tissue with nonuniform anisotropic characteristics (i.e., that tissue associated with fragmented electrograms) is more marked than on uniform anisotropic tissue (Fig. 12-8).[124] This suggests that areas of fragmented electrograms, which appear to be caused by nonuniform anisotropy and poor intercellular coupling, may be the primary sites of antiarrhythmic drug action. Experimental studies using multisite mapping will hopefully resolve these issues in the next decade.

## Mechanism of Drug Effect on Inducibility and Termination of VT

The mechanism by which drugs prevent induction of VT or terminate VT remains unresolved despite much speculation.[199,205–207] Theoretically, in given circumstances, drugs that prolong refractoriness and slow conduction can be either proarrhythmic or antiarrhythmic, and drugs that facilitate conduction can increase the rate of a tachycardia or terminate it. Moreover, the same drug can have different effects on a reentrant VT in different people. If one assumes that sustained uniform VT is reentrant, as it most likely is in coronary disease, there must be different electrophysiologic characteristics of the myocardium in which the potential circuit is formed in individual patients to explain the variability of drug effect on the same arrhythmia mechanism. Furthermore, the mechanism by which drugs terminate VT may not be related to the way they prevent inducibility of VT. In fact, we have studied 20 patients immediately following termination of VT by procainamide, and in 13 the VT was still inducible, although slower.[202] Thus, noninducibility and termination need not be coupled.

If one thinks about it, drugs that slow conduction should not be expected to terminate VT but to perpetuate it. In fact, Saltman[200] found that flecainide was unable to terminate reentrant VT in a canine model of reentrant VT. On the other hand, Spinelli and Hoffman have shown drug-induced block in their reentrant model of atrial flutter around a fixed obstacle without a change in wavelength and without eliminating the excitable gap.[207] As stated in preceding paragraphs, procainamide, which can terminate reentrant VT, tends to increase the excitable gap. Therefore, the mechanism by which termination occurs requires explanation.

Since termination of VT requires failure of conduction through some common isthmus, how would procainamide or other drugs that slow conduction terminate VT? Several possibilities exist including (a) selected depression of conduction or cellular uncoupling in the narrow isthmus such that propagation through it is not possible; (b) prolongation of refractoriness in the isthmus causing block of the impulse; (c) creating an increase in the wavelength of the cardiac impulse so that it cannot fit within the circuit;[208,209] (d) slow conduction around the arc of block slowing the proximal part of the refractory-determined arc of block to recover excitability, resulting in earlier entrance of the impulse into the isthmus at a time when it is refractory; or (e) slow conduction of the impulse allowing further saltatory slow conduction in the region of "pseudoblock" leading to narrowing of the isthmus such that it becomes inexcitable by the electrotonic influence of the arc of "pseudoblock".[197,199]

There are no experimental data suggesting that procainamide can terminate VT by selective conduction block in the isthmus. The marked slowing of conduction should not be totally selective, and other evidence of significant slowing of conduction should be present, for example, broadening of the QRS. Nonetheless, we have demonstrated that procainamide can produce conduction delay and/or block in areas of fractionated electrograms at a time when propagation through normal tissue is only slightly altered (Figs. 12-4 and 12-8).[123,124] This suggests that procainamide can produce selective block in certain types of tissue. If conduction through the isthmus was saltatory and associated with such electrograms, procainamide might be able to terminate the arrhythmia. Unfortunately, high-density mapping in experimental reentrant VT in a canine model has shown that such electrograms are usually recorded along the arcs of block and are more pronounced at the turning points.[197–200] In fact, in tachycardias in which the arcs of block are long, conduction time through the isthmus is frequently rapid.[200] We have found relative normal conduction velocity in a porcine postinfarction model of reentrant VT (see Chapter 11). Procainamide may not be expected to work in the first case but theoretically could work in the latter instance. However, block at the turning point entering the isthmus might terminate the VT.

Prolongation of refractoriness seems unlikely as a mechanism of termination of stable uniform VT. A change in the effective refractory period in the right ventricle and changes at abnormal sites in the left ventricular electrogram rarely exceed 40 msec. This does not seem sufficient to produce block in VTs with cycle lengths >300 msec. In such tachycardias, the excitable gap usually significantly exceeds such a change in refractoriness. The excitable gaps in such tachycardias are typically in the range of 50 to 100 msec in the control state. The excitable gap is even less likely to be "closed" by the prolongation of refractoriness by procainamide since the drug slows conduction, which tends to increase the excitable gap. However, in rapid VTs with short excitable gaps, it is possible for the gap to be closed by prolongation of refractoriness by procainamide. Clinical data suggest that tachycardias with short cycle lengths are more responsive to antiarrhythmic therapy.[210]

For a similar reason, the concept of increasing the wavelength of the cardiac impulse being antiarrhythmic generally does not appear applicable, particularly in cases with large excitable gaps. Although the model of the cardiac wavelength, which incorporates both refractoriness and conduction velocity, may be useful in assessing the effects of drugs in tachycardias with short cycle lengths and no excitable gap (i.e., those that appear to be due to a leading circle type of arrhythmia)[208,209] in most VTs, a large excitable gap exceeds the change in wavelength that drugs might produce. Furthermore, the study by Spinelli and Hoffman[207] demonstrated termination of tachycardia without any effect on the wavelength of that tissue. While I believe that wavelength is an important determinant of the initiation of reentry, it does not seem to be applicable to mechanism of drug termination in anatomically or anisotropically determined reentrant models.

In my opinion, the latter two potential mechanisms may be applicable, that is, slow conduction allowing proximal parts of a refractory determined block to recover excitability, leading to a short circuit of the impulse into the isthmus of block, or slow conduction allowing convergence of the arcs of blocks producing an electrotonic drag causing inexcitability in the isthmus. A shift in the arc of block has been observed in nonsustained tachycardias[199,200] altering the pathway length, and Lesh et al.[211] have demonstrated the potential for electronic "drag" of the arc of block on conduction parameters through the isthmus using a computer model. Thus, both of these latter mechanisms are possible. Block I believe primarily occurs at or near the proximal entrance to the isthmus, by whatever mechanism. Detailed multisite mapping of infarction-related canine models of VT as well as those VT in humans may provide an answer.

As for the mechanism of prevention of initiation of arrhythmia, this may be totally different from the mechanism of termination of the arrhythmia. For example, the wavelength of the stimulated impulse may be a critical determinant of the ability to initiate an arrhythmia. However, I do not think this is predictable since drugs that prolong refractoriness may make it easier or more difficult to initiate the arrhythmia by either facilitating the development of block or extending the refractory period beyond the wavelength of the stimulated impulse. On the other hand, drugs that shorten refractoriness have been shown to facilitate some arrhythmias.[208,209] We have not found any relationship of drug-induced change in local right ventricular refractory periods or QT intervals on the ability to initiate arrhythmias unless the change in refractoriness is due to a reduction in excitability (Table 12-10).[210]

We have evaluated whether noninducibility of an arrhythmia in response to a drug signifies an effect of the drug on the reentrant circuit itself or an effect of the drug that limits the ability of premature stimuli to develop a reentrant circuit. In this study we used extrastimuli at increased current strength to overcome the drug's effect on local conduction and refractoriness, which might prevent the initiation of block and reentry. Although we did not use simultaneous left ventricular mapping, we found that in more than one-half of the patients in whom a tachycardia was not inducible during the standard protocol, a tachycardia could be initiated when the current was increased to 10 mA.[202] The induced tachycardias were usually slower than the control VT. These findings suggested that in many instances a drug's primary effect might be to prevent initiation of the circuit by altering properties of propagating impulses that could produce the requisite degree of block and/or slow conduction. However, if block could be produced by facilitation of capture at earlier coupling intervals by increased current, enough slow conduction would be present to initiate and maintain the arrhythmia. The ability to achieve ventricular premature beats at closer coupling intervals by using high current overcame the limitations imposed by the drug on intervening tissue properties.

Similarly, Jazayeri et al.[212] demonstrated a 60% reinducibility rate following isoproterenol. The mechanism of isoproterenol facilitation of reinduction was similar to that of increased current. Local refractoriness was shortened, which allowed more premature impulses to be delivered, which were then able to initiate VT. Isoproterenol-induced shortening of refractoriness was unable to overcome the efficacy of the antiarrhythmic agent in 40% of their patients. Follow-up of their patients suggested that reversal of noninducibility by isoproterenol was associated with recurrences in 3 of 10 patients, all of which occurred during periods of a heightened sympathetic tone.

These latter two studies[202,212] suggest that drugs may primarily work to prevent initiation by prolonging refractoriness to exceed the wavelength of the premature impulses. Catecholamines, which shorten refractoriness more than they improve conduction, would therefore facilitate initiation of VT. Alternatively, the drugs in both studies were Class 1 agents, which can produce marked slowing of conduction from the stimulation site, preventing these impulses from arriving early enough to produce block. Failure to produce unidirectional block could also prohibit initiation of VT. Proof of this concept will require recording and stimulation from both the right and left ventricles, the latter being "site of origin" of the arrhythmia. This would allow one to determine if the stimulated beats reached the site of origin early enough to produce block. The study of Jazayeri et al.[212] suggested that the potential role of spontaneous fluxes in catecholamine activity may facilitate reentry in some patients

**TABLE 12-10 Correlation Between Efficacy and Magnitude of Change in $QT_C$ and ERP by Type IA Drugs**

| Change in Parameter (msec) | <0 | 0–19 | 20–39 | 40–59 | 60–79 | 80–99 | >100 | Total Group |
|---|---|---|---|---|---|---|---|---|
| For change in ERP | | | | | | | | |
| % Efficacy | 11 | 48 | 49 | 53 | 37 | 0 | | 46 |
| n | 9 | 50 | 51 | 38 | 11 | 3 | | 159 |
| For change in $QT_C$ | | | | | | | | |
| % Efficacy | 46 | 52 | 56 | 39 | 54 | 29 | 38 | 45 |
| n | 26 | 21 | 25 | 33 | 39 | 11 | 45 | 212 |

and suggests a role for beta blockers in combination with Class 1 agents.

## Selection of Antiarrhythmic Agents for Supraventricular Tachyarrhythmias

In view of the high success rate of catheter ablation to cure atrial flutter, A-V nodal tachycardias, and tachycardias associated with bypass tracts (see Chapter 13) the role of EP testing to guide antiarrhythmic therapy for these disorders is minimal. In those patients who do not wish to undergo catheter ablation, physicians often successfully use empiric antiarrhythmic therapy for mildly symptomatic patients with supraventricular arrhythmias including A-V nodal reentry, A-V reentry using a concealed or manifest bypass tract, intra-atrial and sinus node reentry, and paroxysmal atrial flutter and fibrillation. Automatic tachycardias, which by definition cannot be reproducibly initiated or terminated, do not lend themselves to EPS-guided drug therapy, and are primarily treated by catheter ablation or empiric drug therapy. It is of interest that the first published paper suggesting a role for programmed stimulation in developing drug therapy was for paroxysmal atrial fibrillation.[125,126] Currently, the major indication for EPS-guided antiarrhythmic therapy is for those patients who refuse catheter ablation or have failed catheter ablation.

In this latter group of patients the EPSs that are most useful are those with paroxysmal arrhythmias that are frequent and/or symptomatic (dizziness, syncope, angina, dyspnea, or heart failure). The special case of the Wolff—Parkinson–White syndrome with atrial fibrillation having a rapid ventricular response that may be life threatening has been discussed in detail in Chapter 10. All such patients should undergo EPSs to define the number and sites of origin of their bypass tracts as a guide to ablation, the preferred treatment for such patients at this time. The EPS may also assess the effects of antiarrhythmic agents on circus movement tachycardia, which often initiates atrial fibrillation, as well as on the antegrade effective refractory period of the bypass tract, which is the determinant of the ventricular response during atrial fibrillation.[40,47,58,59,63,79–81] It is obvious, therefore, that patients with overt pre-excitation and tachyarrhythmias are usually studied, and pharmacologic therapy is tested as part of the overall decision of choice of therapy (pharmacologic or ablative).

The need to perform EPSs of A-V nodal reentrant tachycardias or tachycardias using concealed A-V bypass tracts is less urgent, primarily because they usually are not life threatening, particularly in patients with normal hearts. Nonetheless, an electrophysiologic evaluation to evaluate the role for pharmacologic or ablative therapy is reasonable when empiric therapy has not been effective or if the patient remains symptomatic. Currently, most electrophysiologists consider ablation the therapy of choice since it is curative (see Chapter 13), an opinion I share. Patients, however, may wish to try pharmacologic therapy first because of the potential risk of ablation-induced heart block necessitating a pacemaker.

Although the role of EPS-guided pharmacologic therapy is limited, the following information about drug effects on these arrhythmias provides a better understanding of the properties of the reentrant circuit as well as therapeutically useful information. The most commonly evaluated SVTs are A-V nodal reentry and reentry using concealed A-V bypass tracts. The stimulation protocols used to study these patients are detailed in Chapter 8. As described in Chapter 8, with A-V nodal reentry, beta blockers, calcium blockers, and digitalis primarily affect the antegrade slow pathway, while Class lA drugs usually primarily affect the retrograde fast pathway.[34,35] Class lC drugs can affect either pathway,[49] as can amiodarone and sotalol. Typical examples of the effect of beta blockers, calcium blockers, or procainamide on induced A-V nodal reentry are shown in Figure 12-50. In each of these tachycardias, the drug has rendered the arrhythmia nonsustained, where it had previously been always sustained. Termination in the antegrade slow pathway is produced by propranolol and verapamil, while termination in the retrograde fast pathway is produced by procainamide. Propranolol, and occasionally verapamil, can produce retrograde block in the fast pathway, but this is always accompanied by slowing in the antegrade slow pathway (Fig. 12-51). In my opinion, block in the retrograde fast pathway has the highest correlation with good long-term outcome. Thus, if drug therapy is to be undertaken, Class lA or lC agents, which primarily block the retrograde fast pathway, would be most effective. The proarrhythmic potentials of these agents, while extremely low in patients with normal hearts, are potentially lethal. As such they are not usually used unless beta blockers, calcium blockers, or even digoxin have failed empirically. In that case, catheter ablation should be encouraged. Nonetheless, some patients refuse the risk of heart block and desire antiarrhythmic therapy. An easy way to test the potential effect of Class 1A or 1C agents on retrograde fast pathway conduction is to compare the response of the retrograde fast pathway to ventricular pacing before and after the drug. If one can demonstrate that block occurs retrogradely in the A-V node (i.e., a retrograde His potential can be observed), at longer cycle lengths than during control, this suggests a potent effect on the retrograde fast pathway (Fig. 12-52). While this usually signifies a good result, we prefer to assess a drug's ability on induction of the arrhythmia rather than just to characterize its effect on the antegrade and retrograde conduction. In some instances, retrograde conduction can be slowed, but antegrade conduction may be slowed to a greater degree, and reentry may still occur, albeit more slowly. Another limitation of this technique is that unless a retrograde His deflection is seen, one cannot conclude that block is in the retrograde fast pathway, since it could be in the His–Purkinje system. Thus, complete V-A dissociation may mean block in the His–Purkinje system, and there would be no method of assessing any effect on the retrograde fast pathway. It is even theoretically possible to produce V-A block in a lower final common pathway in the A-V node and still have A-V nodal reentry occur, if the turnaround is above the lower final common pathway (see Chapter 8). As noted earlier, amiodarone and sotalol may prevent induction of sustained A-V nodal reentry by block in either the antegrade slow or retrograde fast pathway (Fig. 12-53). The effects

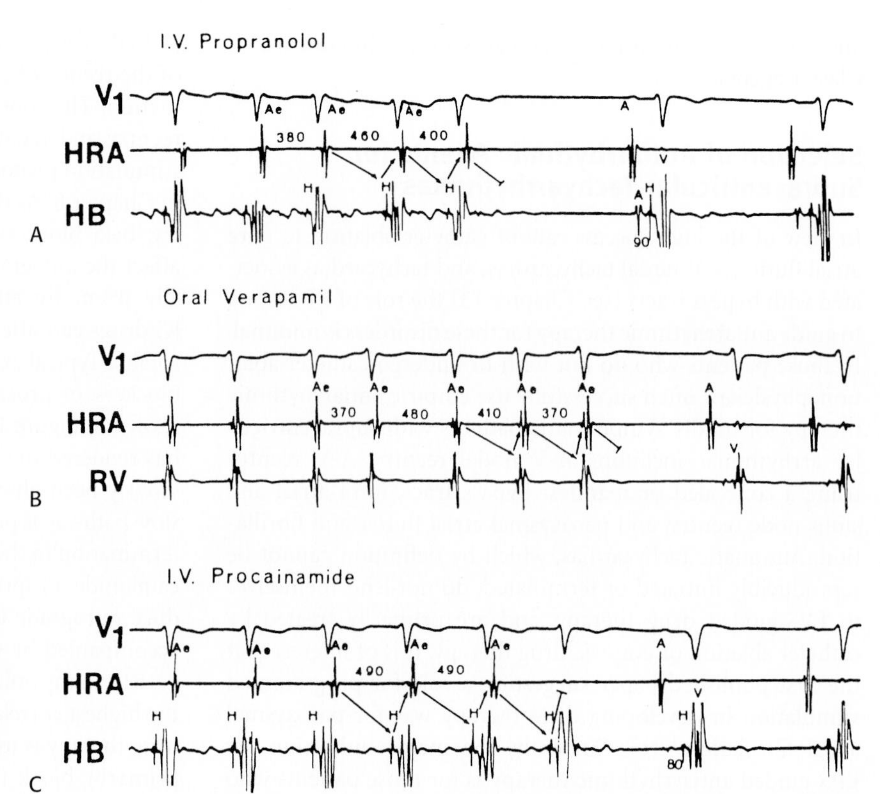


**FIGURE 12-50** *Effect of beta-blockers, calcium-blockers, and Class 1A agents on A-V nodal reentry.* **A** and **B:** Both propranolol and verapamil prevent sustained A-V nodal reentry by antegrade block in the slow pathway **C.** In contrast, procainamide results in nonsustained A-V nodal reentry by blocking retrograde conduction in the fast pathway. HB, His bundle electrogram.

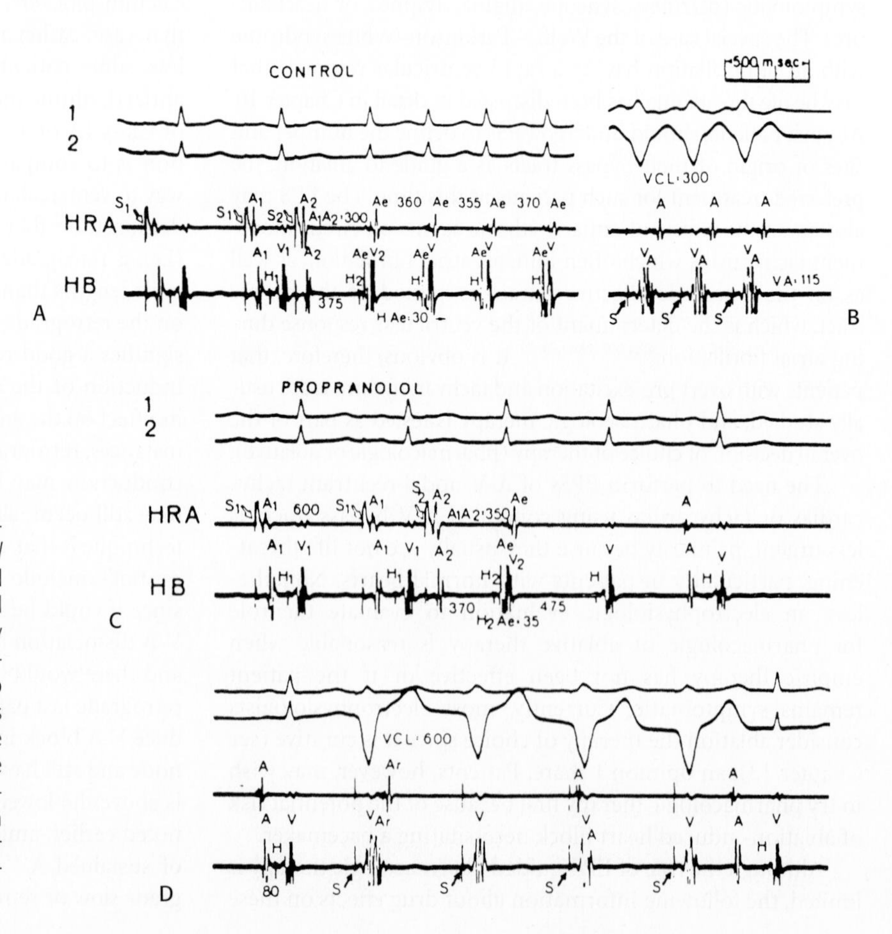


**FIGURE 12-51** *Propranolol producing retrograde block in the fast pathway during A-V nodal reentry.* **A:** Sustained A-V nodal reentry is initiated with an atrial premature beat. **B:** In the control state, 1:1 V-A conduction over the fast pathway is shown at a cycle length of 300 msec. **C:** Following administration of propranolol, only two echo beats are seen. The second echo terminates with retrograde block in the fast pathway. Note that there is a marked increase in the antegrade slow pathway conduction before block in the retrograde fast pathway. **D:** Following administration of propranolol, retrograde conduction is no longer possible. See text for discussion. VCL, ventricular paced cycle length.

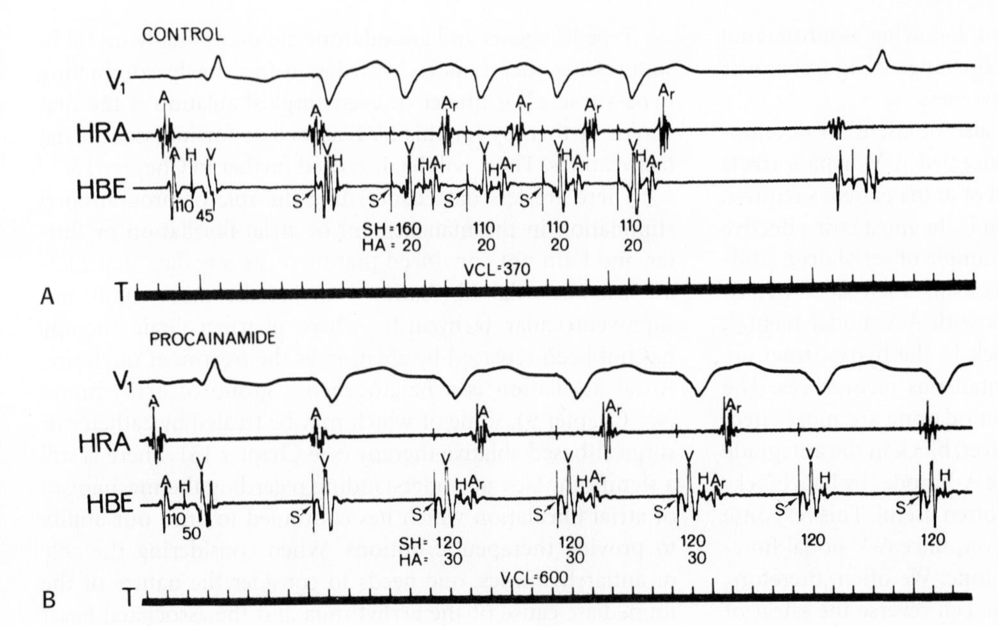


**FIGURE 12-52** *Use of response to ventricular pacing to assess retrograde fast pathway function.* **A:** In the control tracing in a patient with A-V nodal reentry, retrograde conduction over the fast pathway was maintained at a ventricular paced cycle length (VCL) of 370 msec. The H-A interval is 20 msec. **B:** Following procainamide, there is a minimal increase in the H-A interval representing prolongation in retrograde conduction through the fast pathway. Following the fifth stimulated ventricular impulse at a VCL of 600 msec, retrograde block in the A-V node is seen. While this may correlate with retrograde block in the fast pathway, retrograde block may also occur in the lower final common pathway. See text for discussion.

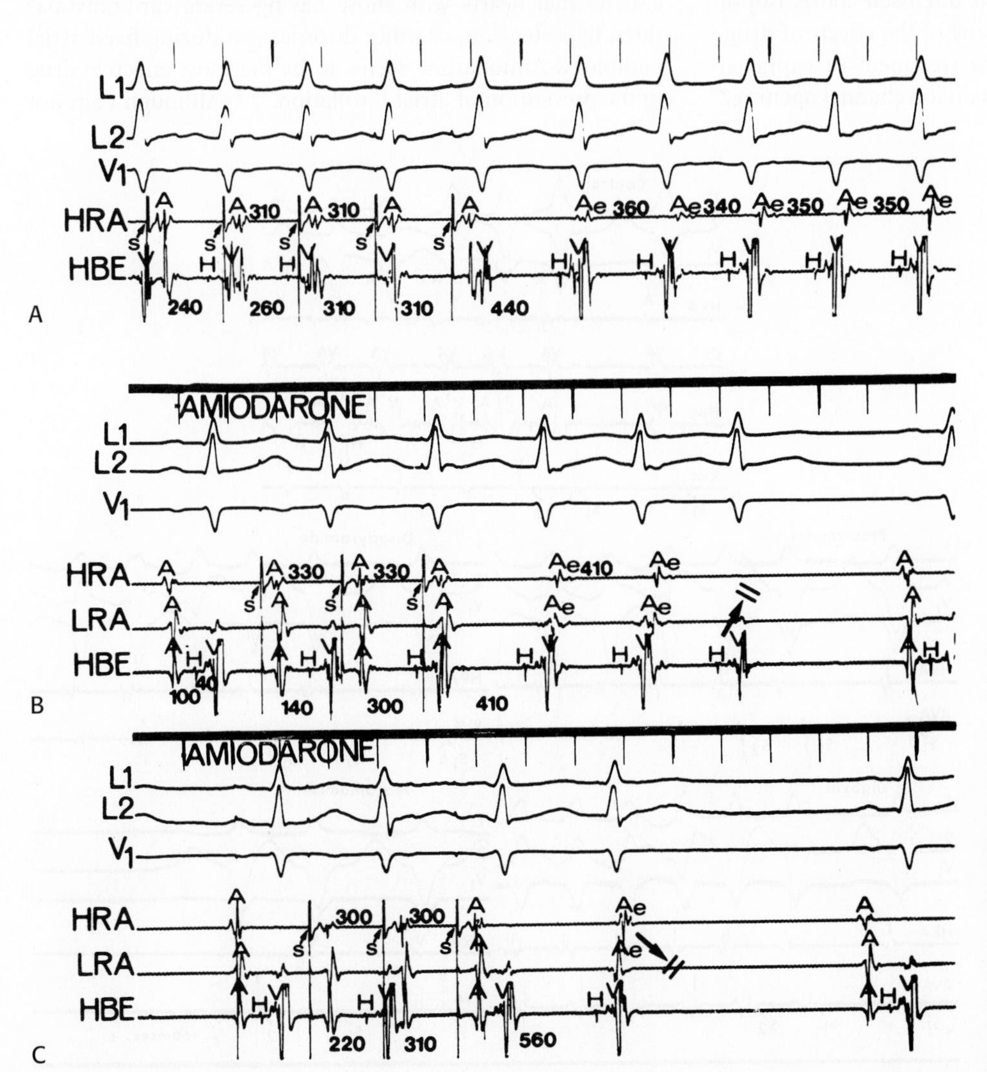


**FIGURE 12-53** *Effects of amiodarone on A-V nodal reentry.* **A:** Rapid atrial pacing at a cycle length of 310 msec initiates A-V nodal reentry. The cycle length of A-V nodal reentry is approximately 350 msec. **B:** Following amiodarone, only nonsustained A-V nodal reentry is induced and terminates spontaneously by block retrogradely in the fast pathway (*arrow*). **C:** When induction of A-V nodal reentry is attempted at a shorter drive cycle length, nonsustained A-V nodal reentry also results, but on this occasion termination results because of block in the antegrade slow pathway (*arrow*). See text for discussion.

of these drugs should be evaluated following isoproterenol since catecholamines increase the openings of ion channels and can antagonize the drugs' effectiveness.

Electrophysiologic testing may also be useful in developing antiarrhythmic therapy for concealed A-V bypass tracts for which empiric therapy has failed or at the patient's request. As discussed in Chapter 13, ablation is the most cost-effective therapy of these arrhythmias. An example of serial drug studies on circus movement tachycardia using a left-sided bypass tract is shown in Figure 12-54. As with A-V nodal reentry, drugs that produce retrograde block in the bypass tract are most effective in suppressing spontaneous recurrences. The Class IC agents and occasionally amiodarone are most effective in doing this.[47–49,58,59,77,80] However, block in the antegrade limb of the reentrant circuit (i.e., the A-V node) by beta blockers, calcium blockers, or digitalis is often useful. This response is not as accurate a predictor, however, since A-V nodal function can be altered by autonomic tone. We often, therefore, use isoproterenol to see whether we can reverse the effect of antiarrhythmic agents to prevent induction of the arrhythmia to assess the potential influence of change in autonomic tone (i.e., primarily enhanced sympathetic tone) on the drug's effect to prevent the arrhythmia. As discussed above, isoproterenol and exercise can reverse many of the effects of drugs, including amiodarone, used in the treatment of supraventricular arrhythmias by their effects on ion channel opening.[80]

Type IC agents and amiodarone are occasionally useful in suppressing incessant tachycardias using slowly conducting bypass tracts.[48] Catheter or even surgical ablation is the first choice of therapy for this SVT as well as for incessant atrial tachycardias. These will be discussed further in Chapter 13.

There are less data concerning the role of programmed stimulation in the management of atrial fibrillation or flutter, and I am not convinced that there are any data that EPSs are useful. Atrial fibrillation remains the most significant supraventricular tachycardia where pharmacologic therapy has not been replaced by ablation as the treatment of choice. Atrial fibrillation is a heterogeneous group of arrhythmias (see Chapter 9), some of which may be treated by catheter or surgical-based ablative therapy (see Chapter 13). There is still a significant lack of understanding regarding the mechanism of atrial fibrillation which has continued to limit our ability to provide therapeutic options. When considering the role of antiarrhythmics, one needs to consider the nature of the immediate cause of the arrhythmia and the associated heart disease as far as likelihood of drug efficacy. I do not believe one can compare efficacy of antiarrhythmic therapy (empirically administered or EPS guided) in patients with atrial fibrillation and normal hearts with those having severe cardiomyopathies, hypertension, or other disorders producing fixed atrial pathology. Amiodarone seems to be the most effective drug in the prevention of atrial fibrillation.[66,213] Although I am not

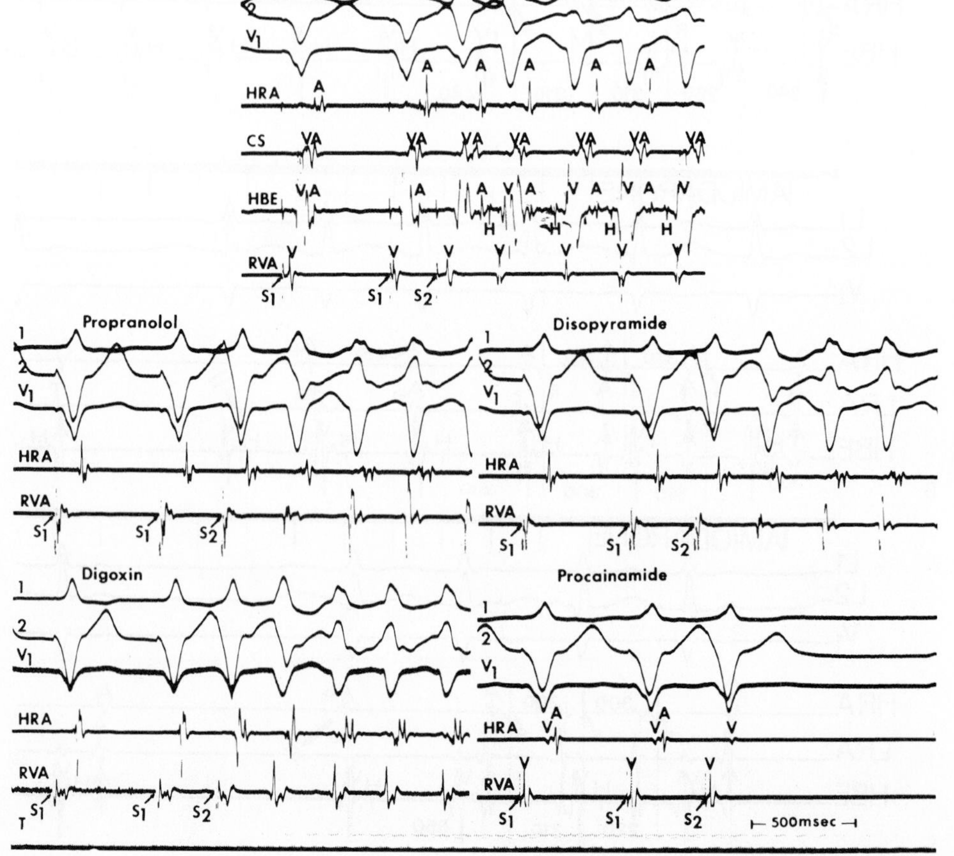


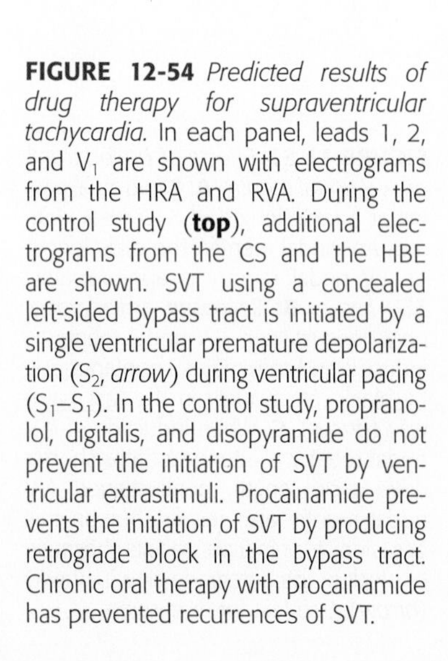
**FIGURE 12-54** *Predicted results of drug therapy for supraventricular tachycardia.* In each panel, leads 1, 2, and $V_1$ are shown with electrograms from the HRA and RVA. During the control study (**top**), additional electrograms from the CS and the HBE are shown. SVT using a concealed left-sided bypass tract is initiated by a single ventricular premature depolarization ($S_2$, *arrow*) during ventricular pacing ($S_1$–$S_1$). In the control study, propranolol, digitalis, and disopyramide do not prevent the initiation of SVT by ventricular extrastimuli. Procainamide prevents the initiation of SVT by producing retrograde block in the bypass tract. Chronic oral therapy with procainamide has prevented recurrences of SVT.

convinced that EPSs are useful in assessing its efficacy, preliminary data from our laboratory have suggested that amiodarone is not likely to be successful if changes in the atrial refractory period produced by amiodarone are either initially less than 10 msec or diminish over time to 10 msec or less. In such cases, EPSs appear to have reasonable negative predictive value, that is, predicting failure.

In regard to empiric therapy for atrial fibrillation amiodarone has certainly seemed to be fairly efficacious. In terms of Class 1 agents for atrial fibrillation, only quinidine and disopyramide are commercially available orally in the United States. I prefer to use quinidine and have found it to be more efficacious than other Class 1 agents if the side effect profile is tolerable. There are two trials in Europe that showed comparable efficacy of quinidine and verapamil compared to sotalol. I have found sotalol to be less effective and only for prevention of atrial fibrillation. Dronedarone is less useful and may precipitate heart failure.

It is of interest that the mechanism of antiarrhythmic drugs to terminate atrial flutter or fibrillation bears no relationship to the class action of the agent. Class 1A, 1C, and 3 agents always selectively block in the isthmus of atrial flutter (see Chapter 9) or areas of fractionated electrograms. Since the action of these agents on ion channels is so different, this observation confirms our ignorance of the mechanisms by which drugs are antiarrhythmic. The Sicilian Gambit[214,215] proposes to attack the "weak link" of arrhythmias with antiarrhythmic agents, but defining the weak link and relating it to the ion channel effects of these drugs is problematic.

In summary, programmed stimulation can be a useful technique to assess the efficacy of therapy of SVT, particularly in A-V nodal reentry and reentry incorporating an atrioventricular bypass tract, either manifest or concealed. Although the efficacy of programmed stimulation for other supraventricular arrhythmias is suggested, it is not established. In such instances, however, programmed stimulation may predict the likelihood of failure of antiarrhythmic therapy; this, in fact, may be useful in developing an alternative mode of therapy.

## Proarrhythmic Effects of Antiarrhythmic Agents

It is commonly held that antiarrhythmic agents may facilitate arrhythmias as well as prevent them. Since we have little understanding as to the mechanism by which drugs are therapeutic (i.e., prevent arrhythmias), it follows that we are equally ignorant of the mechanisms by which antiarrhythmic agents are proarrhythmic.

The definition of proarrhythmia is a problem. One must distinguish between a proarrhythmic drug effect versus drug failure or spontaneous variability of the arrhythmia.[170,216–228] One, therefore, is required to know the natural history of arrhythmias to make any sense out of this problem. Several reviews[216–218] have not considered this aspect of arrhythmogenesis. The natural history of disease may be influenced by the underlying etiology (coronary vs. noncoronary) or the arrhythmia itself (sustained uniform VT vs. cardiac arrest following myocardial infarction).

Two generally accepted examples of proarrhythmia are torsades de pointes and the development of incessant VT. Dessertenne[219] initially described torsades de pointes as a polymorphic VT associated with long QT intervals and with transient abnormalities. One of those abnormalities was the use of drugs such as quinidine. At approximately the same time, Selzer and Wray[229] described quinidine syncope during treatment for atrial arrhythmias (Fig. 12-55). Torsades de pointes was believed to be due to triggered activity produced by early afterdepolarizations.[220–224] Currently the role

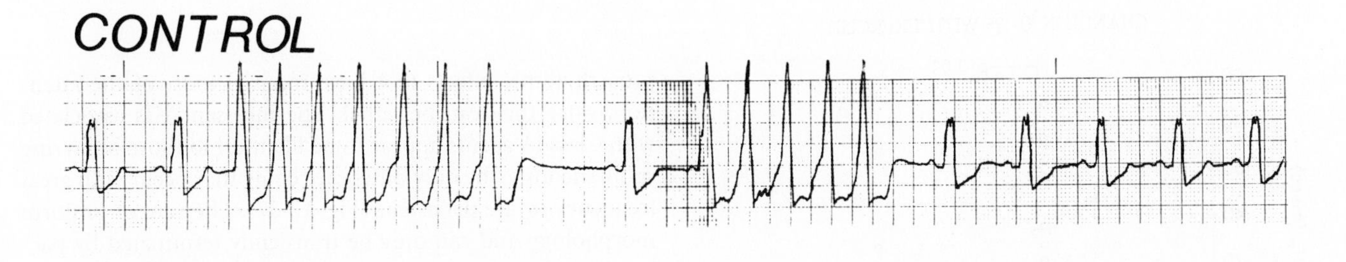


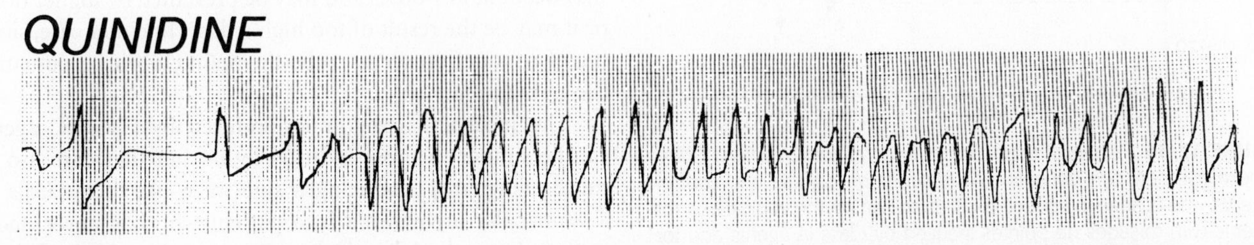


**FIGURE 12-55** *Quinidine syncope.* **Top:** Nonsustained asymptomatic ventricular arrhythmias are present in the control state. **Bottom:** Attempted suppression of these arrhythmias by quinidine resulted in prolongation of the QT interval and classic torsades de pointes with syncope and cardiac arrest.

of early afterdepolarizations has been more as an initiator of torsades. Whether the early afterdepolarizations then result in continuous triggered activity or, more likely, the sustained tachycardia is produced by abnormal automaticity or reentry has not yet been established.[221,224,230] This arrhythmia can be produced by Class lA agents and Class 3 agents, but I have also seen mexiletine-induced torsades de pointes. Despite its effect on the QT interval, amiodarone has a low incidence of torsades de pointes, although it does occur. I have seen only 11 examples of torsades de pointes attributable to amiodarone among more than 1,400 patients in whom this drug has been used over the past 25 years. Eight had renal failure, and all had marked suppression of sinus node function and junctional rhythm as well as significant structural heart disease. Hypokalemia tends to precipitate this arrhythmia, consistent with experimental data.[223] Kadish et al.[231] noted that patients who developed torsades de pointes on Class lA drugs exhibited an increase in the corrected QT interval on exercise (Fig. 12-56). This was significantly different from controls. This suggests that response of the $QT_C$ during exercise might be a useful screening procedure for patients in whom therapy with Class lA agents is considered. Further data are necessary to confirm this observation and to address the predictive value of an abnormal response. Women more frequently get torsades de pointes than men (except with amiodarone). Torsades de pointes frequently occurs at low doses of Class 1A agents and is dose-dependent for Class 3 agents.

The development of incessant VT is invariably produced by antiarrhythmic agents that slow ventricular conduction. Thus, incessant uniform tachycardia can be produced by Class lA and lC agents as well as by amiodarone. Incessant supraventricular arrhythmias, particularly the Wolff–Parkinson–White syndrome, may also be produced by drugs that are associated with antegrade block in the bypass tract and slow conduction down the A-V node. However, it is the ventricular proarrhythmic effects that have received most of the attention, since they can be lethal. The incessant VTs associated with Class lA agents appear to be identical to those occurring spontaneously, the only difference being they occur with great frequency or are persistent (Fig. 12-57). They are of uniform morphology and can only be transiently terminated by pacing. This may or may not be a dose-related response, since it may occur at low doses and may be prevented by higher doses or it may be the result of too high a dose. In either case, slowing of conduction seems to be the main culprit perpetuating the arrhythmia.

The incessant arrhythmias induced by Class lC agents can be similar to those induced by lA, but they can also be more malignant, producing a sine wave–like tachycardia or a ventricular arrhythmia in a patient who has never had a ventricular arrhythmia before. These tachyarrhythmias are almost invariably associated with hemodynamic embarrassment, with or without cardiovascular collapse. Moreover, they

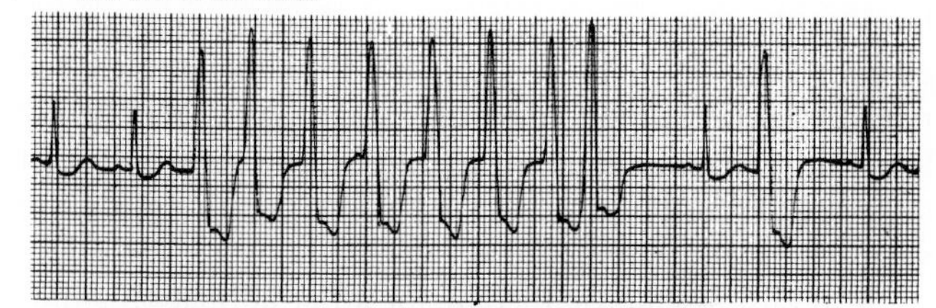


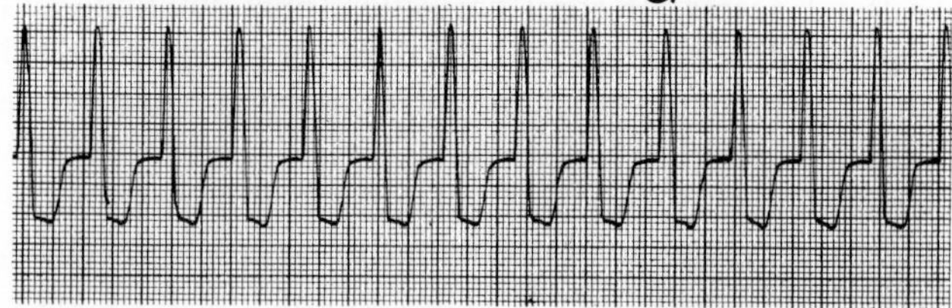


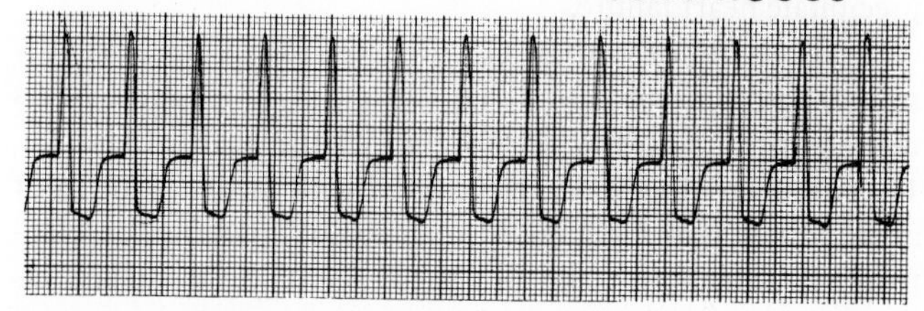


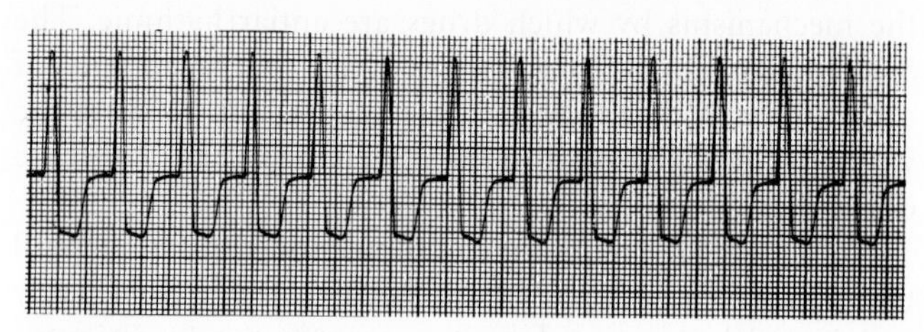

**FIGURE 12-57** *Induction of incessant tachycardia by procainamide.* In the baseline study (**top**), nonsustained VTs associated with exercise are observed. Following attempted suppression of these arrhythmias by procainamide, sustained incessant VT is seen.

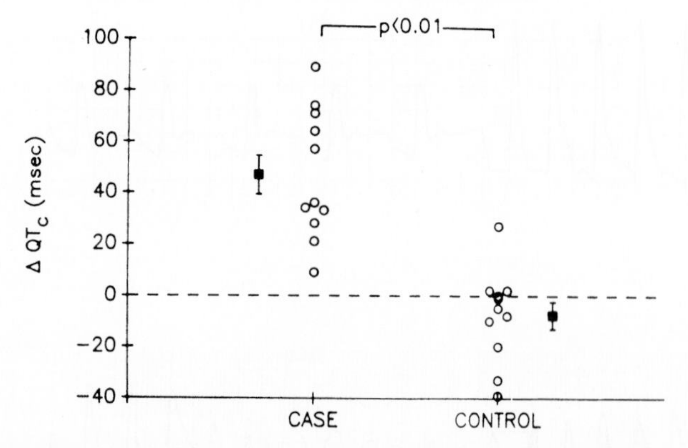


**FIGURE 12-56** *Relationship of change in corrected QT interval during exercise between patients with torsades de pointes and control patients.* The change in corrected $QT_C$ is shown on the vertical axis for patients with torsades de pointes induced by Class lA agents and for control patients. The patients with drug-induced torsades de pointes have an increase in their corrected QT interval to exercise, while controls have a decrease. See text for discussion.

are often difficult to cardiovert. The latter group of arrhythmias is most commonly seen in patients with pre-existent heart disease and prior ventricular arrhythmias who have received too high dose or doses that have been increased too rapidly.[170,216–218,225,226] Occasionally, exercise testing brings on these disastrous events,[170,226] most likely due to marked use-dependent effects of these drugs (Fig. 12-58A,B). This can also be seen with slowing of atrial flutter resulting in one-to-one

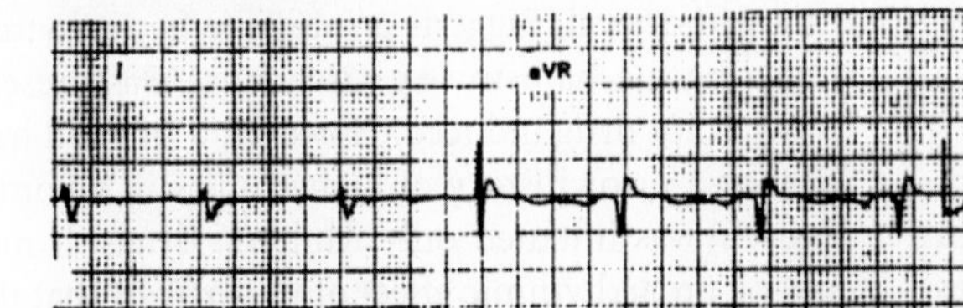
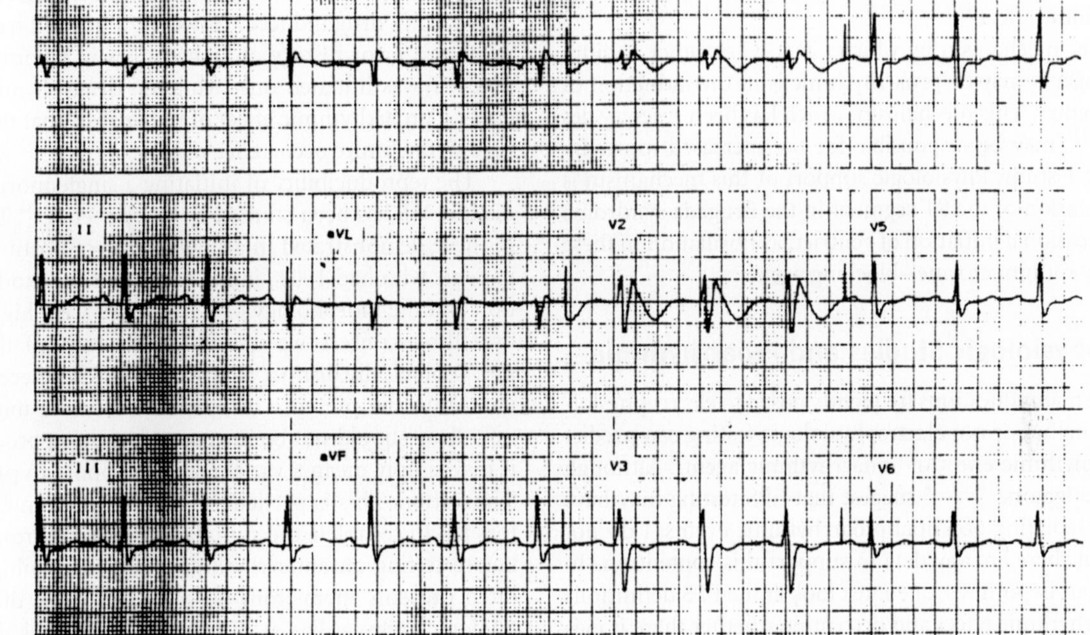


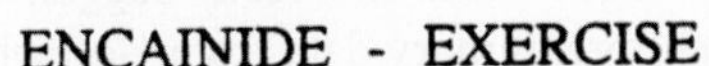


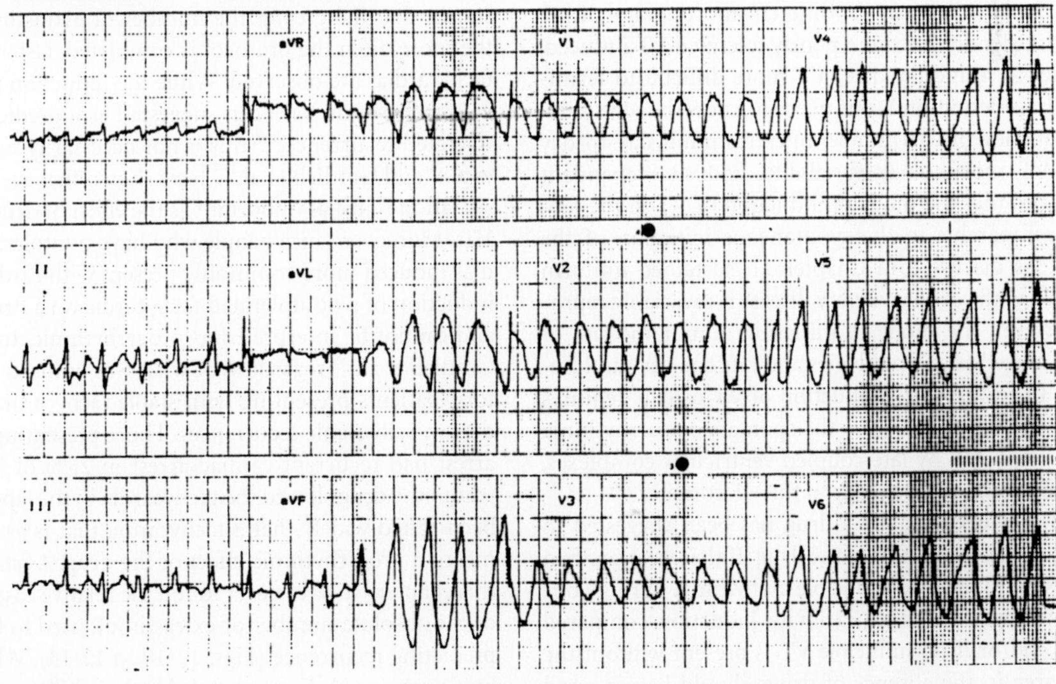


**FIGURE 12-58** *Proarrhythmic effect of Class 1C agents.* **A:** Prolongation of the QRS is seen in sinus rhythm. **B:** During exercise testing, a wide, sine wave–like tachycardia is induced. The patient, who had a cardiomyopathy, never had sustained arrhythmias. Note the ST elevation in $V_1$ and $V_2$ mimicking a Brugada syndrome ECG. There was no family history of sudden death and the patient always had a normal ECG before the Class 1C was administered.

conduction. As such, I always recommend beta blockers with Class 1C agents. More difficult to establish as having proarrhythmia are patients who develop a sustained arrhythmia for the first time while on an antiarrhythmic drug, whether this presents as syncope or cardiac arrest, or just as a VT of new morphology. Similarly, the appearance of a spontaneous sustained tachycardia in a patient who has only had asymptomatic nonsustained arrhythmias need not represent a proarrhythmic effect.[216,218,227,228]

Another mechanism by which Class IC or other sodium blocking agents may be proarrhythmic is in the induction of Phase 2 reentry. This mechanism, which has been recently described,[232–236] may be responsible for the increased mortality in the CAST study. Physiologic support of this mechanism is the exaggeration of the ST segment in the Brugada syndrome and the occasional initiation of ventricular fibrillation in these patients by sodium channel–blocking agents.

## Electrophysiologic Studies and Proarrhythmia

One of the major questions frequently posed to electrophysiologists is whether or not electrophysiologic testing can predict the proarrhythmic effect of antiarrhythmic agents. Although some investigators[216,227,228] suggest that EPS testing may have a role in predicting potential proarrhythmic events, I do not believe that there are any data to support this contention. To validate their hypothesis, one must look at the EPS definitions of a proarrhythmic effect and determine whether there is evidence to support their definition. Definitions commonly used by electrophysiologists suggesting a proarrhythmic effect of a drug include the following: compared to baseline study, (a) inducible VT only on drug, (b) different morphology of VT induced, (c) faster and/or more poorly tolerated VT induced, (d) VT easier to induce, and (e) VT more difficult to terminate. To address definition 1, one needs to know the reproducibility of induction of VT (number of extrastimuli, day-to-day variability, VT morphology variability, and site-dependent variability) and that the mode of induction of VT in the laboratory is comparable to the spontaneous initiation of the arrhythmia. As discussed in Chapter 11, sustained uniform VT associated with coronary artery disease is invariably reproducible; however, the mode of initiation and/or the site of stimulation as well as morphologies and rate can vary and frequently do. In addition, the induction of VT usually requires two or more extrastimuli where the spontaneous arrhythmia is frequently initiated by late-coupled ventricular complexes, which is of a similar morphology to the VT complex.[237]

VT that first occurred on a drug has been suggested to reflect a proarrhythmic effect of the drug. If that were so, then the patient should have no inducible arrhythmia during control studies; the drug should facilitate induction compared to baseline, and/or if no inducible VT is present without the drug, discharge in the absence of drugs should have a good outcome. Preliminary data from our institution suggest that in most patients none of these is in fact true. We have evaluated the patients resuscitated from cardiac arrest who had the arrest while taking Class IA antiarrhythmic agents. Drug therapy was discontinued, yet most patients still had inducible VT (70%). Of the 30% without inducible VTs who were discharged in the absence of medicine, four have had recurrent cardiac arrests. Thus, cardiac arrest while on a Class 1 agent, even if no inducible arrhythmia is present following drug withdrawal, suggests a substrate for arrhythmias and/or triggering mechanism (e.g., ischemia) was present, and that this was not drug induced. However, if one did have a patient without a prior history of arrhythmias in whom monomorphic VT was initiated only while on drugs, it might suggest either a proarrhythmic effect of the drug or that the drug may predict the future occurrence of VT.

The reproducibility of initiating a single morphologically distinct VT has been studied by Cooper et al.[238] These workers have demonstrated in a small group of postinfarction VT patients who had 100% inducibility that the mode of induction and the morphology of VT induced were highly variable over three consecutive studies.[238] The rates of the different morphologically distinct tachycardias are not necessarily similar. Thus, the presence of a new tachycardia induced while on a drug should not be interpreted as being proarrhythmic; it may simply mean a variability of response to programmed stimulation. This is particularly true because most investigators fail to complete the stimulation protocol from both sites before testing an antiarrhythmic drug. The failure to do so often prevents them from observing multiple distinct morphologic tachycardias at different cycle lengths during control. Having a faster poorly tolerated tachycardia while on an antiarrhythmic agent does not really suggest a proarrhythmic effect. First, preliminary data from Gottlieb et al.[239] have shown that the greater the number of extrastimuli used and the more often the protocol is completed, faster nontolerated tachycardias are observed. While the induction of a nontolerated tachycardia has been suggested as a predictor of a nontolerated recurrence,[188] this is not necessarily so. Both Kadish et al.[74] and Gottlieb et al.[189] have shown that the mode of presentation is just as important as the effect of drugs on induced VTs. Moreover, since people who have nontolerated tachycardias induced more commonly present with cardiac arrest, the induction of a nontolerated tachycardia on a drug should not and cannot be interpreted as proarrhythmic. In the study by Gottlieb et al.[189] regardless of what was induced in the laboratory, patients presenting with stable tachycardias had hemodynamically stable recurrences. Those presenting with cardiac arrest had recurrent cardiac arrest in 25% of individuals in whom the drug slowed the tachycardia in the laboratory. It has been stated widely that a tachycardia that is easier to induce means a proarrhythmic effect of the drug. As stated earlier in this chapter, we have never found the relative ease of induction or the absolute number of extrastimuli used to be of value in predicting recurrence (Figs. 12-10 to 12-13). While the study by Cooper et al.[238] suggested that variability of induction is usually two extrastimuli or less, the predictive accuracy of a change in inducibility of at least two grades of stimulation (e.g., from three extrastimuli to one extrastimulus) has not been assessed. Thus, I believe that there are no hard data to support that the relative ease of induction or number of extrastimuli has any role in predicting a proarrhythmic effect.

Finally, inducing a tachycardia that is harder to terminate has nothing to do with proarrhythmia. That may have something to do with termination of the arrhythmia, but it has nothing to do with the development of an arrhythmia. As previously discussed in Chapter 11, it is well known that drugs that slow conduction can make it more difficult to terminate an arrhythmia, either by preventing extrastimuli from reaching the circuit at an appropriate time interval or by accelerating arrhythmias by less clearly defined mechanisms.

Therefore, in my opinion, electrophysiologic testing cannot be used to predict the type of recurrence or the frequency of recurrence. While slow tachycardias that are induced in the laboratory appear to be associated with slow recurrences, the spontaneous presentation of a slow tachycardia is a more important predictor of type of recurrence. As Gottlieb et al.[189] have shown, patients having cardiac arrest frequently have recurrent cardiac arrests despite the fact of having a tolerated tachycardia induced in the laboratory. As such, assessment of the proarrhythmic effect of antiarrhythmic agents cannot be considered an indication for an EPS.

## ■ REFERENCES


1. Vaughan Williams EM. A classification of antiarrhythmic actions reassessed after a decade of new drugs. *J Clin Pharmacol* 1984;24:129–147.
2. Harrison DC. Antiarrhythmic drug classification: new science and practical applications. *Am J Cardiol* 1985;56:185–187.
3. Zipes DP. A consideration of antiarrhythmic therapy. *Circulation* 1985;72: 949–956.
4. Fozzard HA, Makielski JC. The electrophysiology of acute myocardial ischemia. *Annu Rev Med* 1985;36:275–284.
5. Lazzara R, Scherlag BJ. Generation of arrhythmias in myocardial ischemia and infarction. *Am J Cardiol* 1988;61:20A–26A.
6. Johnson EA, Mc KM. The differential effect of quinidine and pyrilamine on the myocardial action potential at various rates of stimulation. *J Pharmacol Exp Ther* 1957;120:460–468.
7. Chen CM, Gettes LS, Katzung BG. Effect of lidocaine and quinidine on steady-state characteristics and recovery kinetics of (dV/dt)max in guinea pig ventricular myocardium. *Circ Res* 1975;37:20–29.
8. Courtney KR. Interval-dependent effects of small antiarrhythmic drugs on excitability of guinea-pig myocardium. *J Mol Cell Cardiol* 1980; 12:1273–1286.
9. Campbell TJ. Importance of physico-chemical properties in determining the kinetics of the effects of Class I antiarrhythmic drugs on maximum rate of depolarization in guinea-pig ventricle. *Br J Pharmacol* 1983;80: 33–40.
10. Campbell TJ. Kinetics of onset of rate-dependent effects of Class I antiarrhythmic drugs are important in determining their effects on refractoriness in guinea-pig ventricle, and provide a theoretical basis for their subclassification. *Cardiovasc Res* 1983;17:344–352.
11. Hondeghem LM, Katzung BG. Time- and voltage-dependent interactions of antiarrhythmic drugs with cardiac sodium channels. *Biochim Biophys Acta* 1977;472:373–398.
12. Hondeghem LM, Katzung BG. Antiarrhythmic agents: the modulated receptor mechanism of action of sodium and calcium channel-blocking drugs. *Annu Rev Pharmacol Toxicol* 1984;24:387–423.
13. Hondeghem L, Katzung BG. Test of a model of antiarrhythmic drug action. Effects of quinidine and lidocaine on myocardial conduction. *Circulation* 1980;61:1217–1224.
14. Mason JW, Hondeghem LM, Katzung BG. Block of inactivated sodium channels and of depolarization-induced automaticity in guinea pig papillary muscle by amiodarone. *Circ Res* 1984;55:278–285.
15. Buchanan JW, Jr., Saito T, Gettes LS. The effects of antiarrhythmic drugs, stimulation frequency, and potassium-induced resting membrane potential changes on conduction velocity and dV/dtmax in guinea pig myocardium. *Circ Res* 1985;56:696–703.
16. Sada H, Kojima M, Ban T. Effect of procainamide on transmembrane action potentials in guinea-pig papillary muscles as affected by external potassium concentration. *Naunyn Schmiedebergs Arch Pharmacol* 1979; 309:179–190.
17. Grant AO, Strauss LJ, Wallace AG, et al. The influence of pH on the electrophysiological effects of lidocaine in guinea pig ventricular myocardium. *Circ Res* 1980;47:542–550.
18. Grant AO, Trantham JL, Brown KK, et al. PH-Dependent effects of quinidine on the kinetics of dV/dtmax in guinea pig ventricular myocardium. *Circ Res* 1982;50:210–7.
19. Gilmour RF, Jr., Morrical DG, Ertel PJ, et al. Depressant effects of fast sodium channel blockade on the electrical activity of ischaemic canine ventricle: mediation by the sympathetic nervous system. *Cardiovasc Res* 1984;18:405–413.
20. Arnsdorf MF, Bigger JT, Jr. The effect of procaine amide on components of excitability in long mammalian cardiac Purkinje fibers. *Circ Res* 1976;38:115–122.
21. Kadish AH, Spear JF, Levine JH, et al. The effects of procainamide on conduction in anisotropic canine ventricular myocardium. *Circulation* 1986;74:616–625.
22. Darbar D, Roden DM. Pharmacogenetics of antiarrhythmic therapy. *Expert Opinion on Pharmacotherapy* 2006;7:1583–1590.
23. Prystowsky EN, Lloyd EA, Fineberg N, et al., eds. *A comparison of electrophysiologic effects of antiarrhythmic agents in humans.* Mount Kisco, NY: Futura Publishing, 1987.
24. Gomes JA, Kang PS, El-Sherif N. Effects of digitalis on the human sick sinus node after pharmacologic autonomic blockade. *Am J Cardiol* 1981; 48:783–788.
25. Alboni P, Shantha N, Filippi L, et al. Clinical effects of digoxin on sinus node and atrioventricular node function after pharmacologic autonomic blockade. *Am Heart J* 1984;108:1255–1261.
26. Bexton RS, Hellestrand KJ, Cory-Pearce R, et al. The direct electrophysiologic effects of disopyramide phosphate in the transplanted human heart. *Circulation* 1983;67:38–45.
27. Shenasa M, Gilbert CJ, Schmidt DH, et al. Procainamide and retrograde atrioventricular nodal conduction in man. *Circulation* 1982;65:355–362.
28. Josephson ME, Caracta AR, Ricciutti MA, et al. Electrophysiologic properties of procainamide in man. *Am J Cardiol* 1974;33:596–603.
29. Shechter JA, Caine R, Friehling T, et al. Effect of procainamide on dispersion of ventricular refractoriness. *Am J Cardiol* 1983;52:279–282.
30. Josephson ME, Seides SF, Batsford WP, et al. The electrophysiological effects of intramuscular guinidine on the atrioventricular conducting system in man. *Am Heart J* 1974;87:55–64.
31. Josephson ME, Caracta AR, Lau SH, et al. Effects of lidocaine on refractory periods in man. *Am Heart J* 1972;84:778–786.
32. Josephson ME, Caracta AR, Lau SH, et al. Electrophysiological evaluation of disopyramide in man. *Am Heart J* 1973;86:771–780.
33. Breithardt G, Seipel L, Abendroth RR. Comparison of the antiarrhythmic efficacy of disopyramide and mexiletine against stimulus-induced ventricular tachycardia. *J Cardiovasc Pharmacol* 1981;3:1026–1037.
34. Brugada P, Wellens HJ. Effects of intravenous and oral disopyramide on paroxysmal atrioventricular nodal tachycardia. *Am J Cardiol* 1984;53:88–92.
35. DiMarco JP, Garan H, Ruskin JN. Quinidine for ventricular arrhythmias: value of electrophysiologic testing. *Am J Cardiol* 1983;51:90–95.
36. Denniss AR, Ross DL, Waywood JA, et al. Effect of procainamide, mexilitine, and propranolol on ventricular activation time recorded at cardiac mapping in chronic canine myocardial infarction. *J Electrophysiol* 1988;2:3.
37. Goldberg D, Reiffel JA, Davis JC, et al. Electrophysiologic effects of procainamide on sinus function in patients with and without sinus node disease. *Am Heart J* 1982;103:75–79.
38. Greenspan AM, Horowitz LN, Spielman SR, et al. Large dose procainamide therapy for ventricular tachyarrhythmia. *Am J Cardiol* 1980;46:453–462.
39. Heger JJ, Nattel S, Rinkenberger RL, et al. Mexiletine therapy in 15 patients with drug-resistant ventricular tachycardia. *Am J Cardiol* 1980;45:627–632.
40. Kerr CR, Prystowsky EN, Smith WM, et al. Electrophysiologic effects of disopyramide phosphate in patients with Wolff-Parkinson-White syndrome. *Circulation* 1982;65:869–878.
41. Marchlinski FE, Buxton AE, Vassallo JA, et al. Comparative electrophysiologic effects of intravenous and oral procainamide in patients with sustained ventricular arrhythmias. *J Am Coll Cardiol* 1984;4:1247–1254.

42. Mason JW, Hondeghem LM. Quinidine. *Ann N Y Acad Sci* 1984;432: 162–176.
43. Morady F, Scheinman MM, Desai J. Disopyramide. *Ann Intern Med* 1982; 96:337–343.
44. Nattel S, Zipes DP. Clinical pharmacology of old and new antiarrhythmic drugs. *Cardiovasc Clin* 1980;11:221–248.
45. Wu D, Hung JS, Kuo CT, et al. Effects of quinidine on atrioventricular nodal reentrant paroxysmal tachycardia. *Circulation* 1981;64:823–831.
46. Wu KM, Hoffman BF. Effect of procainamide and N-acetylprocainamide on atrial flutter: studies in vivo and in vitro. *Circulation* 1987;76:1397–1408.
47. Breithardt G, Borggrefe M, Wiebringhaus E, et al. Effect of propafenone in the Wolff-Parkinson-White syndrome: electrophysiologic findings and long-term follow-up. *Am J Cardiol* 1984;54:29D–39D.
48. Brugada P, Abdollah H, Wellens HJ. Suppression of incessant supraventricular tachycardia by intravenous and oral encainide. *J Am Coll Cardiol* 1984;4:1255–1260.
49. Camm AJ, Hellestrand KJ, Nathan AW, et al. Clinical usefulness of flecainide acetate in the treatment of paroxysmal supraventricular arrhythmias. *Drugs* 1985;29(Suppl 4):7–13.
50. Carey EL, Jr., Duff HJ, Roden DM, et al. Encainide and its metabolites. Comparative effects in man on ventricular arrhythmia and electrocardiographic intervals. *J Clin Invest* 1984;73:539–547.
51. Chilson DA, Heger JJ, Zipes DP, et al. Electrophysiologic effects and clinical efficacy of oral propafenone therapy in patients with ventricular tachycardia. *J Am Coll Cardiol* 1985;5:1407–1413.
52. Duff HJ, Dawson AK, Roden DM, et al. Electrophysiologic actions of O-demethyl encainide: an active metabolite. *Circulation* 1983;68:385–391.
53. Echt DS, Shapiro M, Trusso J, et al. Treatment with oral lorcainide in patients with sustained ventricular tachycardia and fibrillation. *Am Heart J* 1985;109:28–33.
54. Guehler J, Gornick CC, Tobler HG, et al. Electrophysiologic effects of flecainide acetate and its major metabolites in the canine heart. *Am J Cardiol* 1985;55:807–812.
55. Hellestrand KJ, Bexton RS, Nathan AW, et al. Acute electrophysiological effects of flecainide acetate on cardiac conduction and refractoriness in man. *Br Heart J* 1982;48:140–148.
56. Horowitz LN, Spielman SR, Webb CR, et al. The clinical electrophysiology of intravenous indecainide. *Am Heart J* 1985;110:784–788.
57. Jackman WM, Zipes DP, Naccarelli GV, Rinkenberger RL, Heger JJ, Prystowsky EN. Electrophysiology of oral encainide. *Am J Cardiol* 1982; 49:1270–1278.
58. Prystowsky EN, Klein GJ, Rinkenberger RL, et al. Clinical efficacy and electrophysiologic effects of encainide in patients with Wolff-Parkinson-White syndrome. *Circulation* 1984;69:278–287.
59. Kunze KP, Kuck KH, Schluter M, et al. Electrophysiologic and clinical effects of intravenous and oral encainide in accessory atrioventricular pathway. *Am J Cardiol* 1984;54:323–329.
60. Mann DE, Luck JC, Herre JM, et al. Electrophysiologic effects of ethmozin in patients with ventricular tachycardia. *Am Heart J* 1984;107: 674–679.
61. Naccarella F, Bracchetti D, Palmieri M, et al. Propafenone for refractory ventricular arrhythmias: correlation with drug plasma levels during long-term treatment. *Am J Cardiol* 1984;54:1008–1014.
62. Naccarelli GV, Rinkenberger RL, Dougherty AH, et al. Encainide: a review of its electrophysiology, pharmacology and clinical efficacy. *Clin Prog Electrophysiol Pacing* 1985;3:268.
63. Singh BN. Mechanism of action of antiarrhythmic agents: focus on propafenone. *J Electrophysiol* 1987;1:503.
64. Touboul P, Atallah G, Kirkorian G, et al. Electrophysiologic effects of cibenzoline in humans related to dose and plasma concentration. *Am Heart J* 1986;112:333–339.
65. Seides SF, Josephson ME, Batsford WP, et al. The electrophysiology of propranolol in man. *Am Heart J* 1974;88:733–741.
66. Marchlinski FE, Buxton AE, Waxman HL, et al. Electrophysiologic effects of intravenous metoprolol. *Am Heart J* 1984;107:1125–1131.
67. Prystowsky EN, Jackman WM, Rinkenberger RL, et al. Effect of autonomic blockade on ventricular refractoriness and atrioventricular nodal conduction in humans. Evidence supporting a direct cholinergic action on ventricular muscle refractoriness. *Circ Res* 1981;49:511–518.
68. Zipes DP, Prystowsky EN, Heger JJ. Amiodarone: electrophysiologic actions, pharmacokinetics and clinical effects. *J Am Coll Cardiol* 1984; 3:1059–1071.
69. Waxman HL, Groh WC, Marchlinski FE, et al. Amiodarone for control of sustained ventricular tachyarrhythmia: clinical and electrophysiologic effects in 51 patients. *Am J Cardiol* 1982;50:1066–1074.
70. Singh BN, Nademanee K, Josephson MA, et al. The electrophysiology and pharmacology of verapamil, flecainide, and amiodarone: correlations with clinical effects and antiarrhythmic actions. *Ann N Y Acad Sci* 1984;432:210–235.
71. Shenasa M, Denker S, Mahmud R, et al. Effect of amiodarone on conduction and refractoriness of the His-Purkinje system in the human heart. *J Am Coll Cardiol.* 1984;4:105–110.
72. Morady F, DiCarlo LA, Jr., Krol RB, et al. Acute and chronic effects of amiodarone on ventricular refractoriness, intraventricular conduction and ventricular tachycardia induction. *J Am Coll Cardiol* 1986;7:148–157.
73. Kappenberger LJ, Fromer MA, Steinbrunn W, et al. Efficacy of amiodarone in the Wolff-Parkinson-White syndrome with rapid ventricular response via accessory pathway during atrial fibrillation. *Am J Cardiol* 1984;54:330–335.
74. Kadish AH, Buxton AE, Waxman HL, Flores B, Josephson ME, Marchlinski FE. Usefulness of electrophysiologic study to determine the clinical tolerance of arrhythmia recurrences during amiodarone therapy. *J Am Coll Cardiol*1987;10:90–96.
75. Ikeda N, Nademanee K, Kannan R, et al. Electrophysiologic effects of amiodarone: experimental and clinical observation relative to serum and tissue drug concentrations. *Am Heart J* 1984;108:890–898.
76. Horowitz LN, Spielman SR, Greenspan AM, et al. Use of amiodarone in the treatment of persistent and paroxysmal atrial fibrillation resistant to quinidine therapy. *J Am Coll Cardiol* 1985;6:1402–1407.
77. Heger JJ, Prystowsky EN, Jackman WM, et al. Clinical efficacy and electrophysiology during long-term therapy for recurrent ventricular tachycardia or ventricular fibrillation. *N Engl J Med* 1981;305:539–545.
78. Ezri MD, Shima MA, Denes P. Amiodarone: a review of its clinical and electrophysiologic effects. *Clin Prog Electrophysiol Pacing* 1983;1:20.
79. Brugada P, Wellens HJ. Effects of oral amiodarone on rate-dependent changes in refractoriness in patients with Wolff-Parkinson-White syndrome. *Am J Cardiol* 1985;56:863–866.
80. Brugada P, Facchini M, Wellens HJ. Effects of isoproterenol and amiodarone and the role of exercise in initiation of circus movement tachycardia in the accessory atrioventricular pathway. *Am J Cardiol* 1986;57: 146–149.
81. Feld GK, Nademanee K, Weiss J, Stevenson W, Singh BN. Electrophysiologic basis for the suppression by amiodarone of orthodromic supraventricular tachycardias complicating pre-excitation syndromes. *J Am Coll Cardiol* 1984;3:1298–1307.
82. Mitchell LB, Wyse DG, Duff HJ. Electropharmacology of sotalol in patients with Wolff-Parkinson-White syndrome. *Circulation* 1987;76: 810–818.
83. Sung RJ, Juma Z, Saksena S. Electrophysiologic properties and antiarrhythmic mechanisms of intravenous N-acetylprocainamide in patients with ventricular dysrhythmias. *Am Heart J* 1983;105:811–819.
84. Touboul P, Atallah G, Kirkorian G, et al. Clinical electrophysiology of intravenous sotalol, a beta-blocking drug with class III antiarrhythmic properties. *Am Heart J* 1984;107:888–895.
85. Wellens HJ, Brugada P, Abdollah H, et al. A comparison of the electrophysiologic effects of intravenous and oral amiodarone in the same patient. *Circulation* 1984;69:120–124.
86. Wynn J, Miura DS, Torres V, et al. Electrophysiologic evaluation of the antiarrhythmic effects of N-acetylprocainamide for ventricular tachycardia secondary to coronary artery disease. *Am J Cardiol* 1985;56:877–881.
87. Wu D, Kou HC, Yeh SJ, et al. Effects of oral verapamil in patients with atrioventricular reentrant tachycardia incorporating an accessory pathway. *Circulation* 1983;67:426–433.
88. Waxman HL, Myerburg RJ, Appel R, et al. Verapamil for control of ventricular rate in paroxysmal supraventricular tachycardia and atrial fibrillation or flutter: a double-blind randomized cross-over study. *Ann Intern Med* 1981;94:1–6.
89. Sung RJ, Shapiro WA, Shen EN, et al. Effects of verapamil on ventricular tachycardias possibly caused by reentry, automaticity, and triggered activity. *J Clin Invest* 1983;72:350–360.
90. Prystowsky EN. Electrophysiologic and antiarrhythmic properties of bepridil. *Am J Cardiol* 1985;55:59C–62C.
91. Klein GJ, Gulamhusein S, Prystowsky EN, et al. Comparison of the electrophysiologic effects of intravenous and oral verapamil in patients with paroxysmal supraventricular tachycardia. *Am J Cardiol* 1982;49: 117–124.
92. Harper RW, Whitford E, Middlebrook K, et al. Effects of verapamil on the electrophysiologic properties of the accessory pathway in patients with the Wolff-Parkinson-White syndrome. *Am J Cardiol* 1982;50:1323–1330.

93. Gulamhusein S, Ko P, Carruthers SG, et al. Acceleration of the ventricular response during atrial fibrillation in the Wolff-Parkinson-White syndrome after verapamil. *Circulation* 1982;65:348–354.
94. Ellenbogen KA, German LD, O'Callaghan WG, et al. Frequency-dependent effects of verapamil on atrioventricular nodal conduction in man. *Circulation* 1985;72:344–352.
95. DiMarco JP, Sellers TD, Berne RM, et al. Adenosine: electrophysiologic effects and therapeutic use for terminating paroxysmal supraventricular tachycardia. *Circulation* 1983;68:1254–1263.
96. Nademanee K, Noll HE, Feld GK. Effects of Sotalol on His-Purkinje Conduction and Refractoriness in Humans. *J Cardiovasc Pharmacol Ther* 1996;1:9–16.
97. Inama G, Furlanello F, Vergara G, et al. [Sotalol in the Wolff-Parkinson-White syndrome: an electrophysiological and clinical study]. *G Ital Cardiol* 1992;22:701–713.
98. Nademanee K, Feld G, Hendrickson J, et al. Electrophysiologic and antiarrhythmic effects of sotalol in patients with life-threatening ventricular tachyarrhythmias. *Circulation* 1985;72:555–564.
99. Kopelman HA, Woosley RL, Lee JT, et al. Electrophysiologic effects of intravenous and oral sotalol for sustained ventricular tachycardia secondary to coronary artery disease. *Am J Cardiol* 1988;61:1006–1011.
100. Naccarelli GV, Lee KS, Gibson JK, et al. Electrophysiology and pharmacology of ibutilide. *Am J Cardiol* 1996;78:12–16.
101. Kobayashi Y, Atarashi H, Ino T, et al. Clinical and electrophysiologic effects of dofetilide in patients with supraventricular tachyarrhythmias. *J Cardiovasc Pharmacol* 1997;30:367–373.
102. Feld GK, Cha Y. Electrophysiologic Effects of the New Class III Antiarrhythmic Drug Dofetilide in an Experimental Canine Model of Pacing-induced Atrial Fibrillation. *J Cardiovasc Pharmacol Ther* 1997;2:195–203.
103. Echt DS, Lee JT, Murray KT, et al. A randomized, double-blind, placebo-controlled, dose-ranging study of dofetilide in patients with inducible sustained ventricular tachyarrhythmias. *J Cardiovasc Electrophysiol* 1995; 6:687–699.
104. Bashir Y, Thomsen PE, Kingma JH, et al. Electrophysiologic profile and efficacy of intravenous dofetilide (UK-68,798), a new class III antiarrhythmic drug, in patients with sustained monomorphic ventricular tachycardia. Dofetilide Arrhythmia Study Group. *Am J Cardiol* 1995;76: 1040–1044.
105. Sedgwick ML, Dalrymple I, Rae AP, et al. Effects of the new class III antiarrhythmic drug dofetilide on the atrial and ventricular intracardiac monophasic action potential in patients with angina pectoris. *Eur Heart J* 1995;16:1641–1646.
106. Sedgwick ML, Rasmussen HS, Cobbe SM. Clinical and electrophysiologic effects of intravenous dofetilide (UK-68,798), a new class III antiarrhythmic drug, in patients with angina pectoris. *Am J Cardiol* 1992;69: 513–517.
107. Antzelevitch C, Belardinelli L, Zygmunt AC, et al. Electrophysiological effects of ranolazine, a novel antianginal agent with antiarrhythmic properties. *Circulation* 2004;110:904–910.
108. Antzelevitch C, Burashnikov A, Sicouri S, et al. Electrophysiologic basis for the antiarrhythmic actions of ranolazine. *Heart Rhythm* 2011; 8:1281–1290.
109. Wu L, Shryock JC, Song Y, et al. Antiarrhythmic effects of ranolazine in a guinea pig in vitro model of long-QT syndrome. *J Pharmacol Exp Ther* 2004;310:599–605.
110. Zygmunt AC, Nesterenko VV, Rajamani S, et al. Mechanisms of atrial-selective block of Na(+) channels by ranolazine: I. Experimental analysis of the use-dependent block. *Am J Physiol Heart Circ Physiol* 2011;301:H1606–H1614.
111. Sicouri S, Blazek J, Belardinelli L, et al. Electrophysiological characteristics of canine superior vena cava sleeve preparations: effect of ranolazine. *Circ Arrhythm Electrophysiol* 2012;5:371–379.
112. Sicouri S, Burashnikov A, Belardinelli L, et al. Synergistic electrophysiologic and antiarrhythmic effects of the combination of ranolazine and chronic amiodarone in canine atria. *Circ Arrhythm Electrophysiol* 2010;3: 88–95.
113. Sicouri S, Glass A, Belardinelli L, et al. Antiarrhythmic effects of ranolazine in canine pulmonary vein sleeve preparations. *Heart Rhythm* 2008;5: 1019–1026.
114. Camardo JS, Greenspan AM, Horowitz LN, et al. Strength-interval relation in the human ventricle: effect of procainamide. *Am J Cardiol* 1980;45:856–860.
115. Greenspan AM, Camardo JS, Horowitz LN, et al. Human ventricular refractoriness: effects of increasing current. *Am J Cardiol* 1981;47: 244–250.
116. Davis J, Matsubara T, Scheinman MM, et al. Use-dependent effects of lidocaine on conduction in canine myocardium: application of the modulated receptor hypothesis in vivo. *Circulation* 1986;74:205–214.
117. Gang ES, Denton TA, Oseran DS, et al. Rate-dependent effects of procainamide on His-Purkinje conduction in man. *Am J Cardiol* 1985;55: 1525–1529.
118. Morady F, DiCarlo LA, Jr., Baerman JM, et al. Rate-dependent effects of intravenous lidocaine, procainamide and amiodarone on intraventricular conduction. *J Am Coll Cardiol* 1985;6:179–185.
119. Buxton AE, Marchlinski FE, Miller JM, et al. The human atrial strength-interval relation. Influence of cycle length and procainamide. *Circulation* 1989;79:271–280.
120. Soriano J, Almendral J, Arenal A, et al. Rate-dependent failure of ventricular capture in patients treated with oral propafenone. *Eur Heart J* 1992;13: 269–274.
121. Gossinger HD, Siostrzonek P, Jung M, et al. Electrophysiologic determinants of recurrent atrial flutter after successful termination by overdrive pacing. *Am J Cardiol* 1990;65:463–466.
122. Ranger S, Talajic M, Lemery R, Roy D, Nattel S. Amplification of flecainide-induced ventricular conduction slowing by exercise. A potentially significant clinical consequence of use-dependent sodium channel blockade. *Circulation* 1989;79:1000–1006.
123. Schmitt CG, Kadish AH, Marchlinski FE, et al. Effects of lidocaine and procainamide on normal and abnormal intraventricular electrograms during sinus rhythm. *Circulation* 1988;77:1030–1037.
124. Schmitt C, Kadish AH, Balke WC, et al. Cycle length-dependent effects on normal and abnormal intraventricular electrograms: effect of procainamide. *J Am Coll Cardiol* 1988;12:395–403.
125. Bauernfeind RA, Wyndham CR, Dhingra RC, et al. Serial electrophysiologic testing of multiple drugs in patients with atrioventricular nodal reentrant paroxysmal tachycardia. *Circulation* 1980;62:1341–1349.
126. Bauernfeind RA, Swiryn SP, Strasberg B, et al. Electrophysiologic drug testing in prophylaxis of sporadic paroxysmal atrial fibrillation: technique, application, and efficacy in severely symptomatic preexcitation patients. *Am Heart J* 1982;103:941–949.
127. Horowitz LN, Josephson ME, Kastor JA. Intracardiac electrophysiologic studies as a method for the optimization of drug therapy in chronic ventricular arrhythmia. *Prog Cardiovasc Dis* 1980;23:81–98.
128. DiMarco JP, Lerman BB. Role of invasive electrophysiologic studies in the evaluation and treatment of supraventricular tachycardia. *Pacing Clin Electrophysiol* 1985;8:132–139.
129. Klein GJ, Sharma AD, Yee R. An approach to therapy for paroxysmal supraventricular tachycardia. *Am J Cardiol* 1988;61:77A–82A.
130. Fisher JD, Cohen HL, Mehra R, et al. Cardiac pacing and pacemakers II. Serial electrophysiologic-pharmacologic testing for control of recurrent tachyarrhythmias. *Am Heart J* 1977;93:658–668.
131. Mason JW, Winkle RA. Electrode-catheter arrhythmia induction in the selection and assessment of antiarrhythmic drug therapy for recurrent ventricular tachycardia. *Circulation* 1978;58:971–985.
132. Doherty JU, Josephson ME. Role of electrophysiologic testing in the therapy of ventricular arrhythmias. *Pacing Clin Electrophysiol* 1983; 6:1070–1083.
133. Swerdlow CD, Winkle RA, Mason JW. Determinants of survival in patients with ventricular tachyarrhythmias. *N Engl J Med* 1983;308:1436–1442.
134. Breithardt G, Borggrefe M, Seipel L. Selection of optimal drug treatment of ventricular tachycardia by programmed electrical stimulation of the heart. *Ann N Y Acad Sci* 1984;427:49–66.
135. Rae AP, Greenspan AM, Spielman SR, et al. Antiarrhythmic drug efficacy for ventricular tachyarrhythmias associated with coronary artery disease as assessed by electrophysiologic studies. *Am J Cardiol* 1985;55:1494–1499.
136. Reddy CP, Chen TJ, Guillory WR. Electrophysiologic studies in selection of antiarrhythmic agents: use with ventricular tachycardia. *Pacing Clin Electrophysiol* 1986;9:756–763.
137. Gottlieb C, Josephson ME. Programmed stimulation in the evaluation of life-threatening or potentially life-threatening ventricular arrhythmias. *Cardiovasc Drugs Ther* 1987;1:155–159.
138. Gottlieb CD, Josephson ME, eds. *The preference of programmed stimulation-guided therapy for sustained ventricular arrhythmias.* Mount Kisco, NY: Futura Publishing, 1987.
139. Swerdlow CD, Peterson J. Prospective comparison of Holter monitoring and electrophysiologic study in patients with coronary artery disease and sustained ventricular tachyarrhythmias. *Am J Cardiol* 1985;56:577–580.

140. Ruskin JN, DiMarco JP, Garan H. Out-of-hospital cardiac arrest: electrophysiologic observations and selection of long-term antiarrhythmic therapy. *N Engl J Med* 1980;303:607–613.
141. Morady F, Scheinman MM, Hess DS, et al. Electrophysiologic testing in the management of survivors of out-of-hospital cardiac arrest. *Am J Cardiol* 1983;51:85–89.
142. Skale BT, Miles WM, Heger JJ, et al. Survivors of cardiac arrest: prevention of recurrence by drug therapy as predicted by electrophysiologic testing or electrocardiographic monitoring. *Am J Cardiol* 1986;57:113–119.
143. Kim SG, Seiden SW, Matos JA, et al. Discordance between ambulatory monitoring and programmed stimulation in assessing efficacy of mexiletine in patients with ventricular tachycardia. *Am Heart J* 1986;112:14–19.
144. Graboys TB, Lown B, Podrid PJ, et al. Long-term survival of patients with malignant ventricular arrhythmia treated with antiarrhythmic drugs. *Am J Cardiol* 1982;50:437–443.
145. Mitchell LB, Duff HJ, Manyari DE, et al. A randomized clinical trial of the noninvasive and invasive approaches to drug therapy of ventricular tachycardia. *N Engl J Med* 1987;317:1681–1687.
146. Platia EV, Reid PR. Comparison of programmed electrical stimulation and ambulatory electrocardiographic (Holter) monitoring in the management of ventricular tachycardia and ventricular fibrillation. *J Am Coll Cardiol* 1984;4:493–500.
147. Mason JW. A comparison of electrophysiologic testing with Holter monitoring to predict antiarrhythmic-drug efficacy for ventricular tachyarrhythmias. Electrophysiologic Study versus Electrocardiographic Monitoring Investigators. *N Engl J Med* 1993;329:445–451.
148. Mason JW. A comparison of seven antiarrhythmic drugs in patients with ventricular tachyarrhythmias. Electrophysiologic Study versus Electrocardiographic Monitoring Investigators. *N Engl J Med* 1993;329:452–458.
149. Omoigui NA, Marcus FI, Mason JW, et al. Cost of initial therapy in the Electrophysiological Study Versus ECG Monitoring trial (ESVEM). *Circulation* 1995;91:1070–1076.
150. Mason JW, Marcus FI, Bigger JT, et al. A summary and assessment of the findings and conclusions of the ESVEM trial. *Prog Cardiovasc Dis* 1996;38:347–358.
151. Klein RC. Comparative efficacy of sotalol and class I antiarrhythmic agents in patients with ventricular tachycardia or fibrillation: results of the Electrophysiology Study Versus Electrocardiographic Monitoring (ESVEM) Trial. *Eur Heart J* 1993;14(Suppl H):78–84.
152. Reiffel JA, Hahn E, Hartz V, et al. Sotalol for ventricular tachyarrhythmias: beta-blocking and class III contributions, and relative efficacy versus class I drugs after prior drug failure. ESVEM Investigators. Electrophysiologic Study Versus Electrocardiographic Monitoring. *Am J Cardiol* 1997;79:1048–1053.
153. Steinbeck G, Greene HL. Management of patients with life-threatening sustained ventricular tachyarrhythmias–the role of guided antiarrhythmic drug therapy. *Prog Cardiovasc Dis* 1996;38:419–428.
154. Steinbeck G, Andresen D, Bach P, et al. A comparison of electrophysiologically guided antiarrhythmic drug therapy with beta-blocker therapy in patients with symptomatic, sustained ventricular tachyarrhythmias. *N Engl J Med* 1992;327:987–992.
155. Roberts SA, Viana MA, Nazari J, et al. Invasive and noninvasive methods to predict the long-term efficacy of amiodarone: a compilation of clinical observations using meta-analysis. *Pacing Clin Electrophysiol* 1994;17:1590–1602.
156. Randomized antiarrhythmic drug therapy in survivors of cardiac arrest (the CASCADE Study). The CASCADE Investigators. *Am J Cardiol* 1993; 72:280–287.
157. Buxton AE, Marchlinski FE, Flores BT, et al. Nonsustained ventricular tachycardia in patients with coronary artery disease: role of electrophysiologic study. *Circulation* 1987;75:1178–1185.
158. Klein RC, Machell C. Use of electrophysiologic testing in patients with nonsustained ventricular tachycardia: prognostic and therapeutic implications. *J Am Coll Cardiol* 1989;14:155–161; discussion 62–63.
159. Manolis AS, Estes NA, 3rd. Value of programmed ventricular stimulation in the evaluation and management of patients with nonsustained ventricular tachycardia associated with coronary artery disease. *Am J Cardiol* 1990;65:201–205.
160. Buxton AE, Waxman HL, Marchlinski FE, et al. Electrophysiologic studies in nonsustained ventricular tachycardia: relation to underlying heart disease. *Am J Cardiol* 1983;52:985–991.
161. Kowey PR, Waxman HL, Greenspon A, et al. Value of electrophysiologic testing in patients with previous myocardial infarction and nonsustained ventricular tachycardia. Philadelphia Arrhythmia Group. *Am J Cardiol* 1990;65:594–598.
162. Buxton AE, Lee KL, Fisher JD, et al. A randomized study of the prevention of sudden death in patients with coronary artery disease. Multicenter Unsustained Tachycardia Trial Investigators. *N Engl J Med* 1999;341:1882–1890.
163. Winters SL, Stewart D, Targonski A, et al. Role of signal averaging of the surface QRS complex in selecting patients with nonsustained ventricular tachycardia and high grade ventricular arrhythmias for programmed ventricular stimulation. *J Am Coll Cardiol* 1988;12:1481–1487.
164. Turitto G, Fontaine JM, Ursell S, et al. Risk stratification and management of patients with organic heart disease and nonsustained ventricular tachycardia: role of programmed stimulation, left ventricular ejection fraction, and the signal-averaged electrocardiogram. *Am J Med* 1990;88:35N–41N.
165. Steinberg JS, Regan A, Sciacca RR, et al. Predicting arrhythmic events after acute myocardial infarction using the signal-averaged electrocardiogram. *Am J Cardiol* 1992;69:13–21.
166. Kuchar DL, Thorburn CW, Sammel NL. Prediction of serious arrhythmic events after myocardial infarction: signal-averaged electrocardiogram, Holter monitoring and radionuclide ventriculography. *J Am Coll Cardiol* 1987;9:531–538.
167. Farrell TG, Bashir Y, Cripps T, et al. Risk stratification for arrhythmic events in postinfarction patients based on heart rate variability, ambulatory electrocardiographic variables and the signal-averaged electrocardiogram. *J Am Coll Cardiol* 1991;18:687–697.
168. Buxton AE, Simson MB, Falcone RA, et al. Results of signal-averaged electrocardiography and electrophysiologic study in patients with nonsustained ventricular tachycardia after healing of acute myocardial infarction. *Am J Cardiol* 1987;60:80–85.
169. Saksena S, Greenberg E, Ferguson D. Prospective reimbursement for state-of-the-art medical practice: the case for invasive electrophysiologic evaluation. *Am J Cardiol* 1985;55:963–967.
170. Josephson ME. Antiarrhythmic agents and the danger of proarrhythmic events. *Ann Intern Med* 1989;111:101–103.
171. Poll DS, Marchlinski FE, Buxton AE, et al. Sustained ventricular tachycardia in patients with idiopathic dilated cardiomyopathy: electrophysiologic testing and lack of response to antiarrhythmic drug therapy. *Circulation* 1984;70:451–456.
172. Poll DS, Marchlinski FE, Buxton AE, et al. Usefulness of programmed stimulation in idiopathic dilated cardiomyopathy. *Am J Cardiol* 1986;58:992–997.
173. Belhassen B. Is quinidine the ideal drug for brugada syndrome? *Heart Rhythm* 2012;9:2001–2002.
174. Belhassen B, Glick A, Viskin S. Efficacy of quinidine in high-risk patients with Brugada syndrome. *Circulation* 2004;110:1731–1737.
175. Belhassen B, Glick A, Viskin S. Excellent long-term reproducibility of the electrophysiologic efficacy of quinidine in patients with idiopathic ventricular fibrillation and Brugada syndrome. *Pacing Clin Electrophysiol* 2009;32:294–301.
176. Viskin S, Antzelevitch C, Marquez MF, Belhassen B. Quinidine: a valuable medication joins the list of 'endangered species'. *Europace* 2007; 9:1105–1106.
177. Swerdlow CD, Winkle RA, Mason JW. Prognostic significance of the number of induced ventricular complexes during assessment of therapy for ventricular tachyarrhythmias. *Circulation* 1983;68:400–405.
178. Platia EV, Reid PR. Nonsustained ventricular tachycardia during programmed ventricular stimulation: criteria for a positive test. *Am J Cardiol* 1985;56:79–83.
179. Borggrefe M, Trampisch HJ, Breithardt G. Reappraisal of criteria for assessing drug efficacy in patients with ventricular tachyarrhythmias: complete versus partial suppression of inducible arrhythmias. *J Am Coll Cardiol* 1988;12:140–149.
180. Huikuri HV, Cox M, Interian A, Jr., et al. Efficacy of intravenous propranolol for suppression of inducibility of ventricular tachyarrhythmias with different electrophysiologic characteristics in coronary artery disease. *Am J Cardiol* 1989;64:1305–1309.
181. Schoenfeld MH, McGovern B, Garan H, et al. Determinants of the outcome of electrophysiologic study in patients with ventricular tachyarrhythmias. *J Am Coll Cardiol* 1985;6:298–306.
182. Waxman HL, Buxton AE, Sadowski LM, et al. The response to procainamide during electrophysiologic study for sustained ventricular tachyarrhythmias predicts the response to other medications. *Circulation* 1983; 67:30–37.
183. Ross DL, Sze DY, Keefe DL, et al. Antiarrhythmic drug combinations in the treatment of ventricular tachycardia. *Circulation* 1982;66:1205–1210.

184. Duffy CE, Swiryn S, Bauernfeind RA, et al. Inducible sustained ventricular tachycardia refractory to individual class I drugs: effect of adding a second class I drug. *Am Heart J* 1983;106:450–458.
185. Kim SG, Seiden SW, Matos JA, et al. Combination of procainamide and quinidine for better tolerance and additive effects for ventricular arrhythmias. *Am J Cardiol* 1985;56:84–88.
186. Kim SG, Mercando AD, Tam S, et al. Combination of disopyramide and mexiletine for better tolerance and additive effects for treatment of ventricular arrhythmias. *J Am Coll Cardiol* 1989;13:659–664.
187. Marchlinski FE, Buxton AE, Miller JM, et al. Amiodarone versus amiodarone and a type IA agent for treatment of patients with rapid ventricular tachycardia. *Circulation* 1986;74:1037–1043.
188. Waller TJ, Kay HR, Spielman SR, et al. Reduction in sudden death and total mortality by antiarrhythmic therapy evaluated by electrophysiologic drug testing: criteria of efficacy in patients with sustained ventricular tachyarrhythmia. *J Am Coll Cardiol* 1987;10:83–89.
189. Gottlieb C, Berger MD, Miller JM, et al. What is acceptable risk for cardiac arrest patients treated with amiodarone [abstract]. *Circ* 1988;78:500.
190. Pacifico A, Hohnloser SH, Williams JH, et al. Prevention of Implantable-Defibrillator Shocks by Treatment with Sotalol. *N Engl J Med* 1999;340:1855–1862.
191. Connolly SJ, Dorian P, Roberts RS, et al. Comparison of {beta}-Blockers, Amiodarone Plus {beta}-Blockers, or Sotalol for Prevention of Shocks From Implantable Cardioverter Defibrillators: The OPTIC Study: A Randomized Trial. *JAMA* 2006;295:165–171.
192. Marchlinski FE, Buxton AE, Josephson ME, et al. Predicting ventricular tachycardia cycle length after procainamide by assessing cycle length-dependent changes in paced QRS duration. *Circulation* 1989;79:39–46.
193. Marchlinski FE, Buxton AE, Kindwall KE, et al. Comparison of individual and combined effects of procainamide and amiodarone in patients with sustained ventricular tachyarrhythmias. *Circulation* 1988;78:583–591.
194. Almendral JM, Stamato NJ, Rosenthal ME, et al. Resetting response patterns during sustained ventricular tachycardia: relationship to the excitable gap. *Circulation* 1986;74:722–730.
195. Almendral JM, Rosenthal ME, Stamato NJ, et al. Analysis of the resetting phenomenon in sustained uniform ventricular tachycardia: incidence and relation to termination. *J Am Coll Cardiol* 1986;8:294–300.
196. Stamato NJ, Frame LH, Rosenthal ME, et al. Procainamide-induced slowing of ventricular tachycardia with insights from analysis of resetting response patterns. *Am J Cardiol* 1989;63:1455–1461.
197. Wit AL, Dillons S, Ursell PC, eds. *Influences of anisotropic tissue structure of ventricular tachycardia.* Mount Kisco, NY: Futura Publishing, 1987.
198. Dillon SM, Allessie MA, Ursell PC, et al. Influences of anisotropic tissue structure on reentrant circuits in the epicardial border zone of subacute canine infarcts. *Circ Res* 1988;63:182–206.
199. Janse MJ, Wit AL. Electrophysiological mechanisms of ventricular arrhythmias resulting from myocardial ischemia and infarction. *Physiol Rev* 1989;69:1049–1169.
200. Saltman AE. *Anisotropic conduction in the infarcted canine ventricle: conduction characteristics of stimulated and reentrant beats and the influence of the antiarrhythmic drug flecainide.* New York, NY: Columbia University, 1990.
201. Kay GN, Epstein AE, Plumb VJ. Preferential effect of procainamide on the reentrant circuit of ventricular tachycardia. *J Am Coll Cardiol* 1989;14:382–390.
202. Hook BG, Buxton AE, Marchlinski FE, et al. Reversal of antiarrhythmic drug-induced suppression of sustained ventricular tachycardia by increased pacing current strength during programmed stimulation [abstract]. *Circ* 1990;82:82.
203. Stamato NJ, Rosenthal ME, Almendral JM, Gottlieb CD, Josephson ME. Amiodarone induced slowing of ventricular tachycardia: insights from analysis of resetting patterns. *J Am Coll Cardiol* 1987;9:48A.
204. Lorca M, Almendral JM, Pastor A, et al. Comparative effects of quinidine and amiodarone in monomorphic ventricular tachycardia. *Circ* 1989;80:652.
205. Wellens HJ, Brugada P, Farre J. Ventricular arrhythmias: mechanisms and actions of antiarrhythmic drugs. *Am Heart J* 1984;107:1053–1057.
206. Rosen MR, Spinelli W. Some recent concepts concerning the mechanisms of action of antiarrhythmic drugs. *Pacing Clin Electrophysiol* 1988;11:1485–1498.
207. Spinelli W, Hoffman BF. Mechanisms of termination of reentrant atrial arrhythmias by class I and class III antiarrhythmic agents. *Circ Res* 1989;65:1565–1579.
208. Smeets JL, Allessie MA, Lammers WJ, et al. The wavelength of the cardiac impulse and reentrant arrhythmias in isolated rabbit atrium. The role of heart rate, autonomic transmitters, temperature, and potassium. *Circ Res* 1986;58:96–108.
209. Rensma PL, Allessie MA, Lammers WJ, et al. Length of excitation wave and susceptibility to reentrant atrial arrhythmias in normal conscious dogs. *Circ Res* 1988;62:395–410.
210. Vassallo JA, Cassidy DM, Frame LH, et al. Prevention of ventricular tachycardia induction: frequency-dependent effects of Type I drugs [abstract]. *Circ* 1983;68:381.
211. Lesh MD, Pring M, Spear JF. Cellular uncoupling can unmask dispersion of action potential duration in ventricular myocardium. A computer modeling study. *Circ Res* 1989;65:1426–1440.
212. Jazayeri MR, Van Wyhe G, Avitall B, McKinnie J, Tchou P, Akhtar M. Isoproterenol reversal of antiarrhythmic effects in patients with inducible sustained ventricular tachyarrhythmias. *J Am Coll Cardiol* 1989;14:705–711; discussion 12–14.
213. Roy D, Talajic M, Dorian P, et al. Amiodarone to prevent recurrence of atrial fibrillation. Canadian Trial of Atrial Fibrillation Investigators. *N Engl J Med* 2000;342:913–920.
214. The search for novel antiarrhythmic strategies. Sicilian Gambit. *Eur Heart J* 1998;19:1178–1196.
215. The Sicilian gambit. A new approach to the classification of antiarrhythmic drugs based on their actions on arrhythmogenic mechanisms. Task Force of the Working Group on Arrhythmias of the European Society of Cardiology. *Circulation* 1991;84:1831–1851.
216. Zipes DP. Proarrhythmic events. *Am J Cardiol* 1988;61:70A-76A.
217. Bigger JT, Jr., Sahar DI. Clinical types of proarrhythmic response to antiarrhythmic drugs. *Am J Cardiol* 1987;59:2E–9E.
218. Horowitz LN, Zipes DP, Bigger JT, Jr., et al. Proarrhythmia, arrhythmogenesis or aggravation of arrhythmia–a status report, 1987. *Am J Cardiol* 1987;59:54E–56E.
219. Dessertenne F. [Ventricular tachycardia with 2 variable opposing foci]. *Arch Mal Coeur Vaiss* 1966;59:263–272.
220. Jackman WM, Friday KJ, Anderson JL, et al. The long QT syndromes: a critical review, new clinical observations and a unifying hypothesis. *Prog Cardiovasc Dis* 1988;31:115–172.
221. Roden DM, Hoffman BF. Action potential prolongation and induction of abnormal automaticity by low quinidine concentrations in canine Purkinje fibers. Relationship to potassium and cycle length. *Circ Res* 1985;56:857–867.
222. Brachmann J, Scherlag BJ, Rosenshtraukh LV, et al. Bradycardia-dependent triggered activity: relevance to drug-induced multiform ventricular tachycardia. *Circulation* 1983;68:846–856.
223. Davidenko JM, Cohen L, Goodrow R, et al. Quinidine-induced action potential prolongation, early afterdepolarizations, and triggered activity in canine Purkinje fibers. Effects of stimulation rate, potassium, and magnesium. *Circulation* 1989;79:674–686.
224. Damiano BP, Rosen MR. Effects of pacing on triggered activity induced by early afterdepolarizations. *Circulation* 1984;69:1013–1025.
225. Morganroth J. Risk factors for the development of proarrhythmic events. *Am J Cardiol* 1987;59:32E–37E.
226. Falk RH. Flecainide-induced ventricular tachycardia and fibrillation in patients treated for atrial fibrillation. *Ann Intern Med* 1989;111:107–111.
227. Horowitz LN, Greenspan AM, Rae AP, et al. Proarrhythmic responses during electrophysiologic testing. *Am J Cardiol* 1987;59:45E–48E.
228. Buxton AE, Rosenthal ME, Marchlinski FE, al. e. Ventricular arrhythmias in patients on antiarrhythmic drugs-Proarrhythmia or drug failure [abstract]. *J Am Coll Cardiol* 1988;111:182A.
229. Selzer A, Wray HW. Quinidine syncope. paroxysmal ventricular fibrillation occurring during treatment of chronic atrial arrhythmias. *Circulation* 1964;30:17–26.
230. El-Sherif N, Turitto G. The long QT syndrome and torsade de pointes. *Pacing Clin Electrophysiol* 1999;22:91–110.
231. Kadish AH, Weisman HF, Veltri EP, et al. Paradoxical effects of exercise on the QT interval in patients with polymorphic ventricular tachycardia receiving type Ia antiarrhythmic agents. *Circulation* 1990;81:14–19.
232. Yan GX, Antzelevitch C. Cellular basis for the Brugada syndrome and other mechanisms of arrhythmogenesis associated with ST-segment elevation. *Circulation* 1999;100:1660–1666.

233. Antzelevitch C. Ion channels and ventricular arrhythmias: cellular and ionic mechanisms underlying the Brugada syndrome. *Curr Opin Cardiol* 1999;14:274–279.
234. Antzelevitch C. Transmural dispersion of repolarization and the T wave. *Cardiovasc Res* 2001;50:426–431.
235. Krishnan SC, Antzelevitch C. Sodium channel block produces opposite electrophysiological effects in canine ventricular epicardium and endocardium. *Circ Res* 1991;69:277–291.
236. Krishnan SC, Antzelevitch C. Flecainide-induced arrhythmia in canine ventricular epicardium. Phase 2 reentry? *Circulation* 1993;87:562–572.
237. Berger MD, Waxman HL, Buxton AE, et al. Spontaneous compared with induced onset of sustained ventricular tachycardia. *Circulation* 1988;78:885–892.
238. Cooper MJ, Hunt LJ, Palmer KJ, et al. Quantitation of day to day variability in mode of induction of ventricular tachyarrhythmias by programmed stimulation. *J Am Coll Cardiol* 1988;11:101–108.
239. Gottlieb C, Marchlinski FE, Miller JM, et al. Drug testing for sustained ventricular tachycardia: Is completion of stimulation protocol necessary [abstract]. *Pacing Clin Electrophysiol* 1986;11:515.

CHAPTER 13

# Catheter and Surgical Ablation in the Therapy of Arrhythmias

Experience over the last decade has demonstrated that pharmacologic therapy for the management of paroxysmal ventricular and supraventricular arrhythmias may not be adequate and/or may be associated with significant proarrhythmic effects. The development of antitachycardia pacing techniques and, in particular, the recent development of implantable devices with antitachycardia pacing, cardioversion, and defibrillation capabilities at both an atrial and ventricular level have added a new dimension to our therapeutic armamentarium. These electronic devices are expensive, but more importantly, they are a treatment, not a cure of the disorder. Ideally, the preferred therapy for all arrhythmias would be to prevent their occurrence by either destroying or removing the tissue responsible for the arrhythmia. If that were not possible, indirect approaches such as isolating arrhythmogenic tissue from the remainder of the myocardium or modifying tissue passively involved, but contributing to the symptoms related to the arrhythmia (e.g., the A-V node in patients with atrial fibrillation and a rapid ventricular response), would be an alternative approach.

Over the past four decades, we have observed a rapid expansion of our knowledge of the pathophysiologic basis for arrhythmogenesis and have developed and refined electrophysiologic tools to localize the site of origin of such arrhythmias. The ability to identify the mechanism and/or site of origin of an arrhythmia provides the rationale for surgical or catheter-based ablative techniques to treat the arrhythmias. The use of the electrophysiologic techniques of programmed stimulation and catheter based as well as intraoperative mapping led to the evolution of electrophysiologically guided surgical techniques to deal with specific arrhythmias, the first of which was the Wolff–Parkinson–White syndrome.[1,2] This was followed by the development of new surgical approaches for the management of a variety of supraventricular and ventricular arrhythmias.[3–16] Subsequently, catheter-based methods of ablating myocardial tissue were developed to control and/or cure many tachyarrhythmias for which surgery had become the only mode of therapy.[17–20] Today catheter ablation has replaced surgery as a first-line therapy to "cure" most supraventricular and ventricular tachycardias. Techniques using electric, thermal (hot or cold), light (laser), mechanical (ultrasound), and chemical methods of ablation have been developed, some of which are already being used clinically. The exact mechanisms of damage of any given technique are complex and involve multiple biophysical and/or chemical factors, depending on the method employed. Although our knowledge of the biophysical factors responsible for producing electrophysiologic changes in arrhythmogenic tissue is limited, the experimental basis for tissue injury by these various techniques has been studied and reviewed.[17–23]

Several steps must be taken for catheter ablation techniques to be successful. These steps include (a) accurate localization of the arrhythmogenic tissue; (b) delivery of the ablative electric field, heat, cold, light, or chemicals to the appropriate site in the heart; (c) transfer of the ablative factors from the interface of the catheter and the tissue to the arrhythmic site, which may be deep in the myocardium; (d) production of damage to arrhythmogenic tissue; which (e) results in electrophysiologic changes in the arrhythmogenic tissue, which render it nonarrhythmogenic. All of these factors require a better understanding if successful and accurate catheter ablation techniques are to be developed. The catheter-based ablative techniques that have been employed clinically or are currently under clinical investigation include (a) electrical deflagratory shocks (fulguration)—damage done by electrical current disruption of membranes, barotrauma, and thermal injury; (b) nonarcing electrical shocks (electroporation)—damage done by current to disrupt membranes and thermal injury;[24–26] (c) laser—thermal damage resulting in either surface vaporization (argon laser) or photocoagulation (neodymium:YAG laser); (d) radiofrequency (RF)—thermal injury and desiccation;[21,27] (e) microwave—thermal injury and desiccation; (f) chemical destruction of tissue; (g) focused ultrasound; and (h) cryothermal ablation. While some of these techniques have been used during surgery (i.e., laser, cryoablation, and electric shocks), there has been an increasing interest in their use in catheter delivery systems. Catheter-delivered DC ablation (arcing and nonarcing) was the initial method used but has largely been replaced by RF ablation, which will be the basis for discussion in this chapter. It is impossible and impractical to discuss the biophysical basis of all these techniques, which will continue to evolve over the next decade.

The main focus of this chapter is the role of the electrophysiologist in the management of arrhythmias by surgical and catheter-based ablation. The electrophysiologist must select the appropriate patients, choose the technique available that offers the highest rate of success with lowest morbidity to that patient, and most importantly, accurately localize the tissue to be ablated. The most important and critical job of the electrophysiologist is to accurately identify the arrhythmogenic tissue to be removed or destroyed through the use of catheter or intraoperative mapping, or both. Success of any ablative technique depends on accurate localization of the source of the arrhythmia. As such, this chapter will mainly concentrate on how one defines arrhythmogenic tissue and how one can approach destruction or removal of this tissue by catheter-based or surgical techniques. Brief descriptions of the specific ablative techniques used are given in the following paragraphs.

## BIOPHYSICS OF CURRENT ABLATION TECHNIQUES

Catheter ablation techniques have been so successful in treating a variety of arrhythmias that they have almost totally replaced operative approaches to the management of supraventricular and ventricular arrhythmias. Of the several modes of ablation available, RF ablation is by far the most commonly used, having replaced DC ablation for more than two decades because of improved efficacy and safety. Nevertheless DC ablation remains in use at some institutions. Our understanding of the biophysics of lesion creation is almost completely based on studies using energy delivery in model systems with normal myocardium. Unfortunately there is little data or understanding of how energy delivery changes in the presence of myocardial scar.

### DC Ablation

With DC ablation, the electrical energy is delivered through either a catheter or a hand-held probe in the operating room. The energy delivered is from a standard defibrillator/cardioverter in most cases. Most standard defibrillator/cardioverters deliver between 1 and 3 kV to a specific electrode to which the device is connected. Although a variety of waveforms are used in different defibrillators, most commonly peak voltage is achieved in 1 to 2 msec, which is associated with a peak current flow of 40 to 60 amperes shortly thereafter. In most instances, a single electrode (usually the tip of a catheter) is used as the cathode, and an indifferent backplate serves as an anode sink for the discharge. This technique allows the delivery of high-energy shocks in the range of 100 to 400 J per shock. When DC catheter ablation is performed using a standard defibrillator, a vapor globe is initially formed as a result of electrolysis. This globe subsequently expands and becomes ionized, ultimately resulting in arcing. The arcing is associated with extremely high temperatures and a veritable concussive explosion in the heat. The explosion can be thought of in terms of a compressive shock that is due to the formation of a vapor globe within noncompressible blood, followed by rebound shocks with the collapse of the globe. High-speed cinematography has shown dramatic changes in cardiac shape during this "explosion." The arcing explosion has led to the widespread use of the term fulguration for this type of catheterization. According to Fontaine et al.,[28] a shock energy of 40 to 160 J produces pressure waves of 2.5 to 7.5 atmospheres.

If one measures current and voltage during the delivery of the discharge, there will be a sudden increase in voltage and decrease in current as the vapor globe forms, as a result of a rise in impedance. The high temperature of the electrical arc, which may approach several thousand degrees, results in pitting of the distal and occasionally more proximal electrodes of the catheter. Despite the high temperature associated with the arc, there is insignificant heating of the tissue, suggesting that thermal damage is not the primary mechanism by which the fulguration works. There is still debate as to the relative role of barotrauma and the effects of the high-energy electrical field of the DC shock as the cause of the ultimate pathologic damage and electrophysiologic sequelae. Most investigators believe that it is the direct electrical effect that disrupts myocardial membranes, resulting from either dielectrical breakdown, change in membrane lipids, or physical compression and mechanical disruption of the membrane.[29] Using cultured myocytes, Jones et al.[30] demonstrated that the delivery of 200 V/cm can affect membrane depolarization, which may represent membrane breakdown with higher-energy discharges.

Barotrauma is undesirable, despite the fact that it may play a role disrupting and/or separating myocardial fibers in some types of ablation. Barotrauma associated with fulguration has consistently caused rupture of the coronary sinus when energy is delivered there and has been associated with rupture of other cardiac structures, myocardial dysfunction, and arrhythmias.[28–32] Experimental studies have shown that the extent of damage that is produced by DC shocks is directly related to the amount of energy delivered.[19,28,31–36] The integrity of catheters is frequently disrupted in the caring process, which is due to the transient high temperatures.[28,33,37] Arcing not only affects the distal tip but can also result in damage to more proximal electrodes, since a high-voltage gradient is formed between the distal electrode and more proximal ring electrodes by the expanding vapor globe. Bardy et al.[37] have shown that following the first large shock the dielectric strength of catheters was reduced. A greater disruption is seen when proximal electrodes are used to deliver the energy instead of the distal tip. Thus, there is reasonable evidence that most electrode catheters demonstrate some current leakage, particularly when multiple shocks are delivered. This may lead to misdirected shocks and clinical failures, as well as to unnecessary barotrauma. No catheter has ever been FDA-approved for DC ablation. More work is necessary to develop catheters capable of withstanding fulguration-type shocks if this technique is going to be used in the future. This is unlikely to occur.

Pathologically, fulguration shocks produce a somewhat patchy contraction band necrosis. The volume of damage done generally correlates with the amount of energy delivered and is relegated to the electric field.[31,32,34] Perhaps it is the patchiness of the damage that apparently makes the tissue more arrhythmogenic than the homogeneous necrosis associated with cryothermal or RF injury.

Irreversible electroporation is a new variation of electrical ablation. In this technique, cell membranes are exposed to high-voltage electrical fields, resulting in nonthermal, nonbaratraumatic damage to the cell membrane resulting in cell death. In experimental ablation studies, this technique appears to be relatively specific for myocardial tissue damage. du Pre and coworkers delivered electroporation discharges (50 to 360 J, using a standard monophasic defibrillator) to the epicardium intentionally over the left anterior descending coronary artery. At 3 weeks, intimal hyperplasia was not detected and coronary angiography demonstrated no stenosis.[38] Neven and colleagues delivered catheter-based electroporation discharges (50 to 200 J) to the epicardium using a percutaneous subxyphoid approach which resulted in transmural lesions without acute effects on coronary arteries.[25] Obviously, additional research is necessary, but this may result in a powerful new ablation technique.

## Radiofrequency Energy

RF energy is generated as an alternating current at a frequency of 300 to 750 kHz (range 100 to 2,000 kHz) delivered between the tip of an ablation catheter and a cutaneous patch.[39] The sinusoidal waveform creates a potential difference between the cutaneous patch and the catheter tip, which alternates in polarity. Because of the small surface area of the tip of the catheter relative to the cutaneous patch, the current density will be high at the tip and low at the patch. During RF application electrical energy is converted to thermal energy by resistive heating. The heat that is generated is transferred to the subjacent cardiac tissue primarily by conduction and to a minor extent by radiation, which decreases by the fourth power of the distance from the catheter tip. Heat is simultaneously dissipated by convection into the blood pool. Since the catheter tip–myocardial interface is the major resistor in this AC circuit, current density and heat are greatest at the catheter tip and minimal at the cutaneous patch. Effective heating of the myocardium is critically dependent on catheter contact and stability as well as on the surface area of the catheter tip. Poor contact or stability will lead to heat loss to the blood pool and failure to generate adequate myocardial temperatures despite application of high voltage/power. Although a larger surface area (length of the catheter tip electrode) can lead to greater lesion size, it will require delivery of greater power, since the greater surface area will be subjected to greater convective heat loss to the blood pool to which it has greater exposure. Thus maximum lesion size using a 4- to 5-mm ablation tip can be accomplished using a maximum power of 50 W while up to 100 W may be required to achieve maximal lesion size using an 8- to 10-mm catheter tip. Electrodes of 4 to 5 mm through which the RF energy is delivered provide the best control and most reasonably sized lesion to accomplish the tasks of catheter ablation for most paroxysmal supraventricular arrhythmias.[40–43] The size of the lesions produced by RF are smaller than those associated with fulguration; moreover, scar tissue limits the ability to transfer thermal energy, making RF ablation of ventricular arrhythmias associated with scarred endocardium more difficult. A variety of deflectable catheters are available that can have different arcs of curvature, bidirectional deflecting capabilities (with similar or different lengths of deflection), rotational capability, or magnetic sensors (Biosense) that allow for precise localization in three dimensions (Fig. 13-1).

RF ablation results in thermal injury with coagulation necrosis and desiccation when tissue heating exceeds approximately 50°C for at least 10 seconds.[20–23,39,40] Application of RF energy results in a lesion with a volume half-time of ≈8 seconds and maximum volume achieved in 30 to 40 seconds. As heat is produced at the catheter-myocardial interface the impedance drops. A drop of impedance of 5 to 10 Ω is a sign of conductive heating to the subjacent tissue. The lesion is smaller than that seen with DC ablation and is more homogeneous. If the temperature at the electrode-myocardial interface increases excessively, a rise in impedance develops because of gas formation caused by vaporization of the blood around the catheter tip. A drop in current necessarily occurs with an impedance rise. Impedance rise also causes formation of coagulum on the catheter tip, and it is mandatory to remove the catheter and wipe off the coagulum, which is a potential source of emboli. If the tissue is heated to >100°C, steam will be generated as a consequence of boiling within the myocardium. This often can be detected as an audible popping sound, which will just precede a marked rise in impedance. The steam can produce myocardial rupture and subsequent tamponade. Smaller tears may also occur. Various catheter modifications have been evaluated to optimize the size of the lesions and control the lesions produced by the RF.

The initial modification of ablation catheters was use of thermocouples or thermistors imbedded near the catheter tip

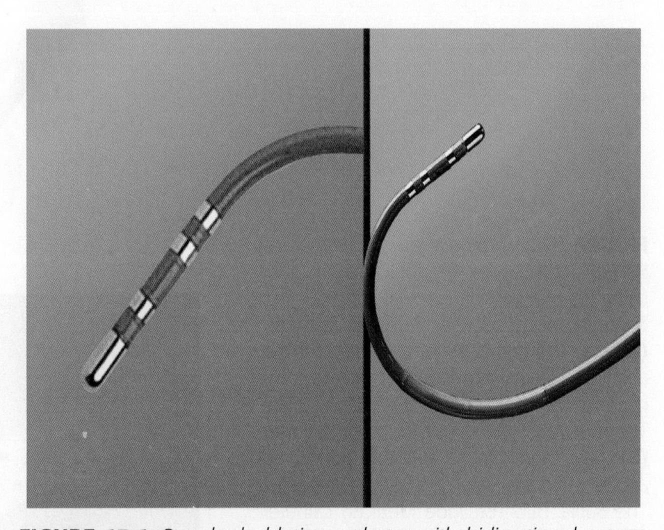

**FIGURE 13-1** *Standard ablation catheter with bidirectional curves.* Ablation catheters typically have 4- to 5-mm tips and can be deflected in a variety of different manners. This particular catheter has deflection capabilities in two directions with different curves in each direction.

to provide information as to the temperature generated at the tip of the catheter at any given power. This modification was deemed necessary because of the inability to relate the power used to tissue heating. These are closed loop-temperature control systems such that the power is automatically adjusted to maintain a desired temperature. Such a system allows for the maintenance of electrode temperature despite changes in catheter contact produced by respiration or unstable catheter position. Such control of temperature largely (but not entirely) avoids the formation of coagulum. Unfortunately, the thermistor or thermocouple does not accurately provide information about tissue temperature. Due to convective heat loss to the blood the temperature recorded at the catheter tip may give a falsely low reading relative to tissue temperatures achieved if inadequate catheter contact is present. This might result in intramyocardial tissue boiling and steam production (see above). Thus, to assure that excessive intramural heating does not take place, target temperatures should be set at 55° to 65°C.

Another modification to increase lesion size has been the development of irrigated catheters (Fig. 13-2). As discussed above, delivery of heat energy is limited because interface temperatures cannot exceed 100°C. By cooling the catheter tip more voltage can be applied without a rise in temperature at the catheter-myocardial interface. This results in a greater current density at the catheter-tissue interface, which results in a larger volume (and depth) of tissue heated by conduction.[27] While cool-tip catheters can produce larger lesions, one cannot control the lesion size by assessing catheter tip temperature, since it is constantly being cooled. Excessive tissue heating, steam formation, and myocardial rupture can easily occur if the tip temperature is allowed to get too high. As a result, I recommend using impedance as the main method of assessing lesion formation. A 10-Ω drop in impedance is ideal, and this occurs despite maintaining catheter tip temperature at <42°C. The method of cooling varies from an internal counter-current system to catheters in which the saline is flushed through a lumen at the tip of the catheter or through pores at the tip of the catheter. Experimental data suggest the cool-tip saline spray catheter may produce less char and thrombus than the internally cooled catheter.[44] Whether this has clinical relevance is untested. The latter two methods necessarily result in introducing a variable amount of saline into the circulation blood volume depending on the number of and time over which the lesions are given. Recently, several companies have redesigned irrigation catheters to have more irrigation ports which allow effective ablation at lower rates of saline flow (Thermocool SF Biosense, Sapphire St. Jude Medical).

Phased RF energy delivery is an old idea that has been recently rediscovered. Multipolar catheters can be configured to deliver duty-cycled unipolar and bipolar (between adjacent electrodes) RF energy. At present, two companies manufacture phased RF catheters designed for ablation of atrial fibrillation (PVAC Medtronic, EnMARQ Biosense), and clinical trials are ongoing. Early trials of one device demonstrated more frequent development of asymptomatic cerebral lesions detected on diffusion weighted magnetic resonance imaging (MRI) of the brain, as compared to other ablation energy systems.[45–47] Clinical trials continue to determine if catheter redesign and/or irrigation with moderate risk.

A

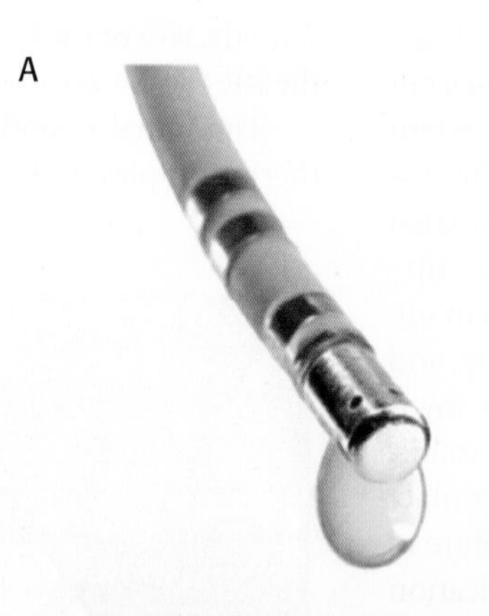

B

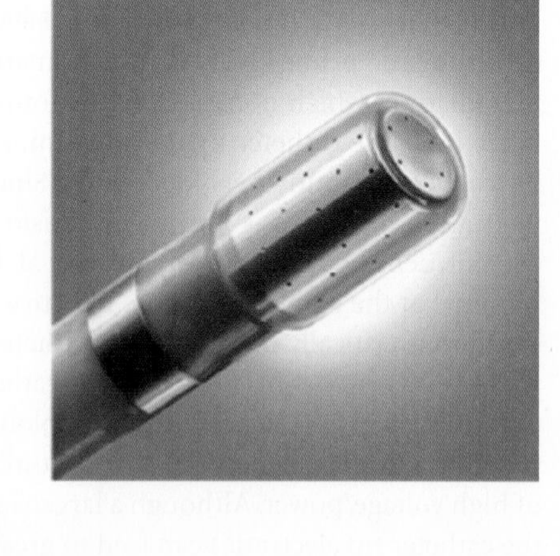

C

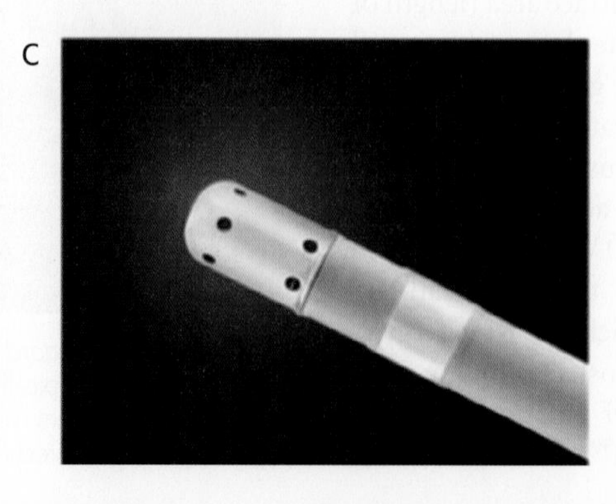

**FIGURE 13-2** *Externally irrigated catheters.* Several companies manufacture ablation catheters that provide external irrigation. The Thermocool (Biosense Webster) catheter **(A)**, was the first catheter approved for the ablation of atrial fibrillation; it uses six irrigation ports at the tip of the catheter. The Thermocool SF (Biosense Webster) catheter **(B)** has many more delivery ports and allows a smaller volume of saline irrigation. The Safire BLU (St. Jude Medical) catheter **(C)** has six irrigation ports at the tip of the catheter. (Images A and B courtesy of Biosense Webster; image C courtesy of St. Jude Medical.)

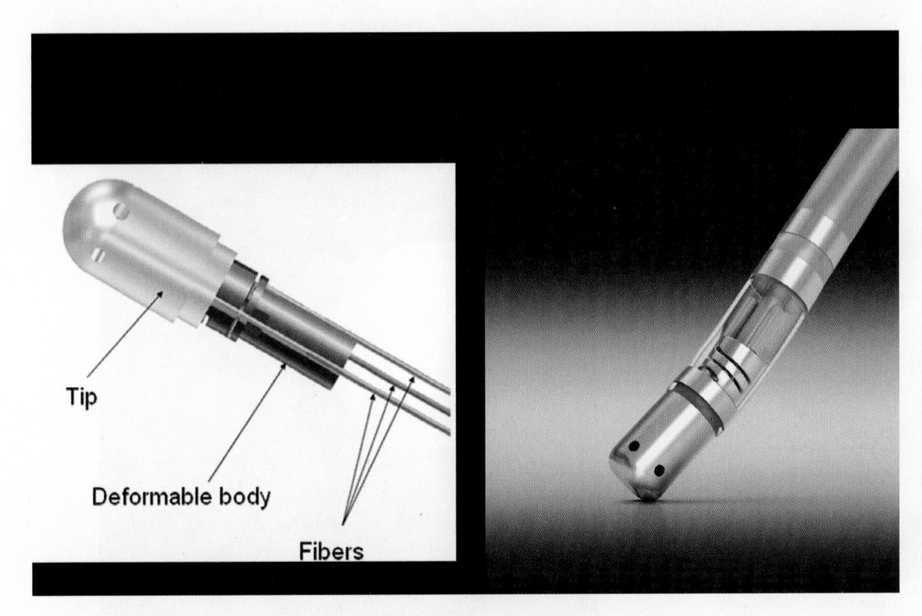


**FIGURE 13-3** *Force sensing catheters.* The TactiCath Quartz ablation catheter (St. Jude Medical) provides real-time contact force and vector measurements based on light interferometry. The SmartTouch catheter (Biosense Webster) utilizes a precision spring in the catheter tip; spring displacement proportional to tip contact force/vector. (Images courtesy of St. Jude Medical and Biosense Webster, respectively.)

The major advantages of RF energy are absence of barotrauma, lack of requirement of general anesthesia, lack of muscle stimulation, and the ability to control very focal injury. It is because of these factors that RF ablation has supplanted fulguration as the method of ablation in most centers. Another advantage of RF ablation is the fact that intracardiac electrograms may still be recorded throughout the procedure; and following delivery of RF energy, the catheter electrodes function perfectly to record and stimulate. Nevertheless, RF techniques remain limited by the requirement of good contact to achieve appropriate damage and by the fact that the extent of tissue damage is not predictable.

Recently the limitation of contact has been addressed by real-time measurement of contact force (Fig. 13-3). Clinical trials of force sensing catheters for ablation of atrial fibrillation showed that unblinded access to real-time data produced meaningful improvements in freedom from atrial fibrillation in short-term follow-up.[48–52] Theoretically, lesions are formed by the intersection of contact force, power, and time and new dosing strategies are being developed to try to make lesion delivery more uniform and permanent.

## Laser Ablation

Lasers have been used in surgery for many years. In the past decade, there has been interest in using lasers intraoperatively for the management of ventricular arrhythmias or the creation of A-V block.[53–57] There has also been an interest, however, in the development of catheter delivery of laser light.[58] The mechanism by which laser ablation works is based on heat generation within tissue by the conversion of light energy into thermal energy. Depending on the laser used, the distribution of light within the tissue and the degree and site of destruction are quite variable and highly dependent on the wavelength. The two major laser systems used are argon laser light, which has a wavelength of 500 nM, and the ND:YAG laser, which has a wavelength of 1,060 nM. With the argon laser, the light energy is absorbed rapidly in the first few millimeters of tissue, resulting in surface vaporization with crater formation. In contrast, the ND:YAG laser is associated with significant scatter in tissue, causing more diffuse and deeper tissue injury resulting in photocoagulation necrosis. Lee et al.[59] compared the electrophysiologic effects of the ND:YAG laser with DC shock in normal canine left ventricular endocardium. While the pathologic responses were similar qualitatively, the laser lesions were associated with less ventricular arrhythmias. The gross lesions produced by 40 to 80 J of laser energy were comparable to lesions produced by 100 to 200 J of DC shock in volume; however, lesions produced by the ND:YAG laser are homogeneous and well circumscribed (Fig. 13-4). The advantages of laser-delivered energy are that it takes a short period of time to deliver and the amount of energy delivered can be easily controlled. However, if catheter delivery systems are to be developed, contact issues with the endocardium, the site in the heart at which ablation is to take place (e.g., venous and arterial blood absorb laser energy to different degrees), and the ability to focus the laser on the specific target are issues that need further resolution. A laser balloon delivery system (Cardiofocus) which could allow tissue visualization (to ensure contact) is currently under investigation (Fig. 13-5).[60] A recent multicenter study reported pulmonary vein isolation using this system in 200 patients with paroxysmal atrial fibrillation. Acute isolation was obtained in 98.8% of PVs with reasonable procedural times (200 ± 54 minutes); complications included a 2% incidence of tamponade and a 2.5% incidence of phrenic nerve palsy. Freedom from AF at 12 months off antiarrhythmic drugs was 60.2%.[61] Cost may be a limitation to laser therapy.

## Cryoablation

Cryoablation has been used in the surgical treatment of a variety of arrhythmias for over 30 years. Well-demarcated, homogeneous lesions produced by endocardial or epicardial

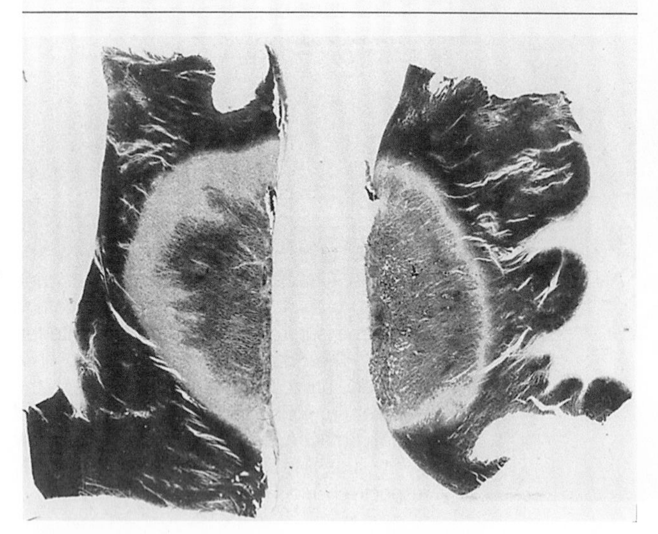


**FIGURE 13-4** *Comparison of lesions produced by cryoablation and ND:YAG photocoagulation.* Both cryoablation and ND:YAG laser photocoagulation produce circumscribed, homogeneous necrosis. (From Svenson RH, Gallagher JJ, Selle JG, et al. Neodymium:YAG laser photocoagulation of ventricular tachycardia: rationale, method of application, and results in 17 patients. In: Breithardt G, Borggrefe M, Zipes DP, eds. *Nonpharmacological therapy of tachyarrhythmias*. Mt. Kisco, NY: Futura Publishing, 1987:181, with permission.)

application are similar to those produced by the ND:YAG laser (Fig. 13-4). The lesions produced preserve the underlying fibrous structure, so they are inherently stronger and less likely to rupture than RF lesions. They were also apparently nonthrombogenic (e.g., no emboli in the absence of anticoagulation). While near transmural lesions can be produced intraoperatively using temperatures of –60°C in the presence of cold cardioplegia, achievement of such lesions with a catheter-based delivery system has not been definitively established at this time. However, several companies have developed catheter-based

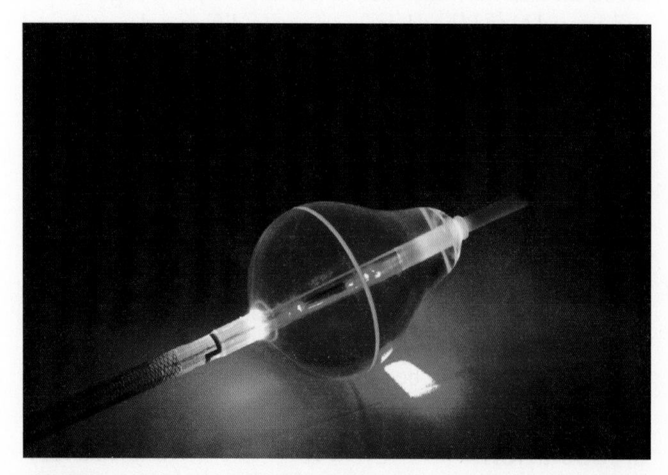

**FIGURE 13-5** The Endoscopic Ablation System (HeartLight, CardioFocus) is a compliant balloon–based laser delivery system, equipped with a 500 micron endoscope to allow lesion visualization. (Image courtesy of CardioFocus.)

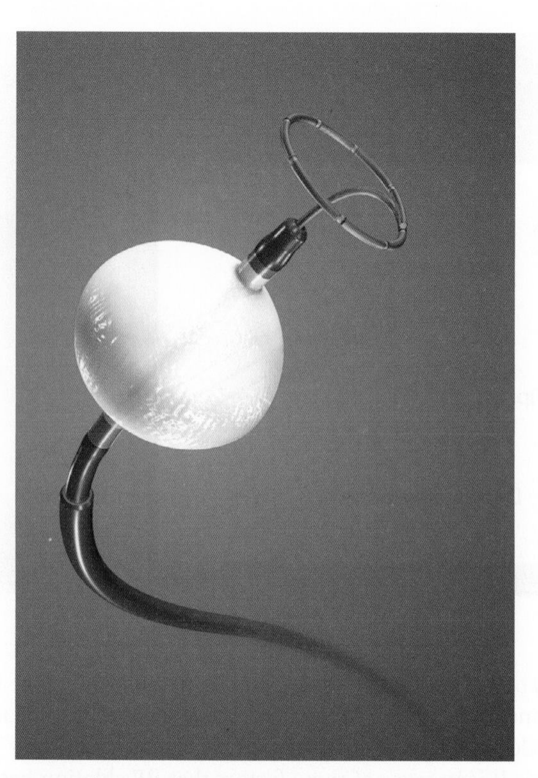

**FIGURE 13-6** The cryoballoon catheter (Artic Front Advance, Medtronic) which can be deployed to the pulmonary veins over a wire or utilizing a multielectrode circular catheter (Achieve, as shown). (Image courtesy of Medtronic, Inc.)

cryodelivery systems, which improved energy delivery based on phase change (liquid nitrogen to gas) within the catheter tip.[62] The blood pool is a major impediment to achieving temperatures necessary to create permanent lesions that are adequate in size using cryothermia. Catheter-based delivery systems are used for ablation of A-V nodal tachycardia and paraseptal bypass tracts, particularly in children. Cryoablation has the advantage of cryoadherence once energy is delivered, which eliminates unwanted catheter movement; however, recurrence rates with cryoablation have been higher than with RF energy.[63] A cryoballoon catheter has been developed for pulmonary vein isolation (Artic Front Medtronic) (Fig. 13-6). This design obviates some of the difficulty with local blood flow as the balloon structure occludes the pulmonary vein being ablated. A randomized trial in 245 patients with atrial fibrillation (78% paroxysmal) demonstrated superior efficacy of cryoablation compared to antiarrhythmic drug treatment, with similar success rates as would have been expected with RF energy ablation; however, phrenic nerve palsy, which is typically temporary, was observed in 11% of patients.[64] A second-generation catheter (Artic Front Advance Medtronic as well as improved cryoablation "dosing" are expected to improve efficacy and reduce phrenic nerve damage.

## Ultrasound

Ultrasound energy converts mechanical energy to heat. The frequency required to produce destructive lesions ranges from

4 to 9 MHz. Ultrasound can be focused, and therefore has the unique property of not requiring tissue contact. Preliminary studies have applied ultrasound to the ablation of focal triggers by isolating the pulmonary vein from the atrial myocardium using ultrasound delivered via a balloon placed in a pulmonary vein.[65] Experience with this first-generation device was not favorable, both in terms of poor efficacy and an unacceptable rate of pulmonary vein stenosis. A second-generation forward firing device which delivered high-intensity focused ultrasound (Prorhythm) was removed from clinical use because of a high incidence of procedural complications, particularly atrioesophageal fistula.[66] Directional focused ultrasound delivery systems (Epicor St. Jude Medical) are still utilized in surgical ablation of atrial fibrillation.

## CONTROL OF SUPRAVENTRICULAR ARRHYTHMIAS BY ABLATIVE TECHNIQUES

The development of surgical techniques to cure arrhythmias began with the first successful electrophysiologically directed cure of the Wolff–Parkinson–White syndrome. This took place in 1968, when Dr. Will Sealy successfully divided an A-V bypass tract localized to the right lateral A-V groove by epicardial mapping.[1,2] This event initiated the development of surgical techniques to manage the Wolff–Parkinson–White syndrome,[3–9] and subsequently, led to the development of innovative surgical interventions for the treatment of A-V nodal reentrant tachycardia, atrial tachycardias, and atrial flutter/fibrillation.[5,10–13,67–74] Cryothermal injury, electrical shock, and lasers have also been used intraoperatively to manage these arrhythmias.[28,33,75–79] In the past three decades, catheter-delivered ablative techniques have been developed to manage arrhythmias that had previously required surgical intervention. In fact, the widespread use of catheter ablation techniques has virtually eliminated the need for surgery to manage drug-resistant supraventricular tachycardias that are due to the Wolff–Parkinson–White syndrome and A-V nodal reentry, and A-V junctional ablation, which represents of course an indirect treatment of atrial fibrillation in terms of control of the ventricular response.[80–100]

Localization of the arrhythmogenic substrate and defining the mechanism of arrhythmias has led to the development of these techniques and will be the focus of the discussion in this and subsequent sections. The major role of surgery today is for the "cure" of atrial fibrillation as a primary procedure or as an adjunct to valvular surgery (see below).

### Ablation of Atrioventricular Bypass Tracts and Variants of Pre-excitation

Successful ablation of atrioventricular bypass tracts requires precise localization of the atrial and/or ventricular insertion site of the bypass tract. As noted in Chapter 10, A-V bypass tracts may occur anywhere around the tricuspid and mitral annulae except for the region of aortomitral continuity, at which no ventricular myocardium lies below the atrium. The anatomy of right-sided and left-sided bypass tracts differs somewhat (Fig. 13-7). The tricuspid annulus has a greater circumference (approximately 12 cm) than the mitral annulus (approximately 10 cm) and is not a complete fibrous ring, but may have many regions of discontinuity. This obviously

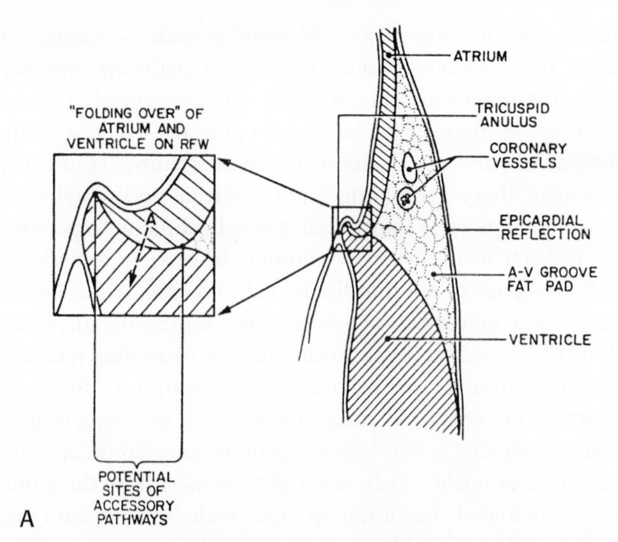


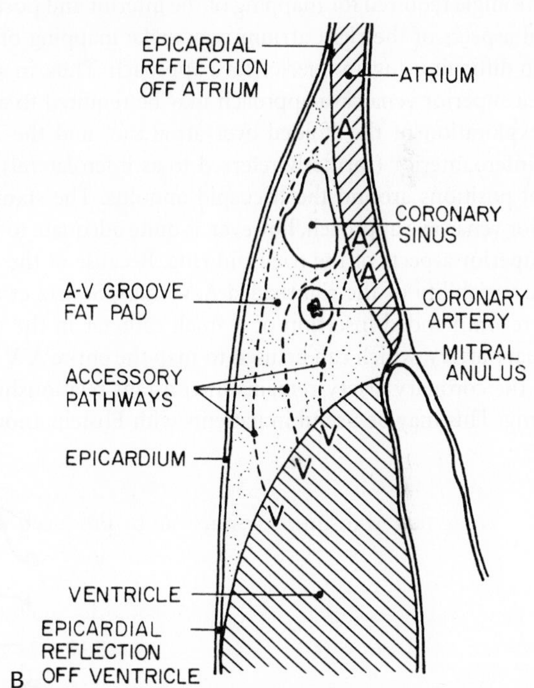


**FIGURE 13-7** *Anatomy of the right and left A-V rings.* **A:** The right atrioventricular (A-V) ring is schematically shown with a blow-up of the annular region. The ring is incomplete and the atrium "folds" over the ventricle producing a sack. **B:** The left A-V ring is solid, and the relationship of the coronary sinus, coronary artery, and potential bypass tracts are shown. The anatomy of both A-V rings differs and has led to different ablation approaches for right- and left-sided bypass tracts. See text for discussion. (From Ferguson TB Jr, Cox JL, Surgical treatment for the Wolff–Parkinson–White syndrome: the endocardial approach. In: Zipes DP, Jalife J, eds. *Cardiac electrophysiology: from cell to bedside.* Philadelphia, PA: WB Saunders, 1990:697–907.)

means that the entire tricuspid annulus must be mapped in detail to accurately located right-sided pathways, whereas only approximately three-fourths of the mitral annulus needs to be mapped for left-sided pathways, because of the absence of pathways in the region of aortomitral continuity. Moreover, there is a folding over the atrium and ventricle, as shown in Figure 13-7, such that it may be difficult to position the catheter at the tricuspid annulus because of a tendency of the catheter to fall into the folded over "sac." Since bypass tracts can connect between atrium and ventricular anywhere along the folded sac, bypass tracts may be somewhat removed from the annulus: making accurate localization of the atrial insertion site critical to successful ablation. An annular ablation at a site that is nearly at the annulus may fail because the atrial insertion site may be as far as 1 cm away from the annulus in the folded-over atrial sac. This folded-over atrium and bizarre angle required for mapping of the inferior and posterolateral aspects of the right atrium may make mapping of this region difficult using an inferior cava approach. Thus, in some cases a superior vena cava approach may be required to allow full exploration of the "folded-over atrial sac" and the inferior, inferoanterior (formerly referred to as inferolateral) and lateral positions around the tricuspid annulus. The standard inferior vena cava approach, however, is quite adequate to map the superior aspects of the tricuspid ring. Because of the anatomic variability of the right-sided A-V rings, Swartz et al.[101] have recommended insertion of a small catheter in the right coronary artery, which can be used to map the entire A-V ring since the coronary artery remains in constant relationship to the ring. This may be useful in patients with Ebstein anomaly in which the triscupid valve is displaced into the ventricle or in patients who have had multiple unsuccessful attempts at ablation of right-sided pathways. I do not believe a right coronary catheterization should be used routinely, and in fact should be discouraged, since it has potential disastrous consequences. There has been no long-term follow-up of coronary arteries in patients in whom this procedure has been performed, and there should be serious concern regarding endothelial abrasion by such a catheter, resulting in initiation of an atherogenic process. In my opinion, careful and detailed mapping with standard ablation catheters is adequate. A guiding sheath is particularly useful when an inferior vena cava approach to an inferoanterior bypass tract is utilized. Use of a halo catheter or a multipolar catheter positioned around the tricuspid annulus can provide very good regional localization capabilities to guide the roving ablation catheter (Fig. 13-8). These multipolar catheters are used in an analogous fashion to coronary sinus catheterization for left-sided pathways (see below).

On the left side of the heart, there is no significant folding over of the atrium and ventricle on each other, and a mitral annulus is a continuous fibrous structure. Initial mapping of the left atrial insertion sites of bypass tracts can be accomplished via the coronary sinus with standard 10 to 20 pole catheters with 2- to 5-mm interelectrode spacing. One must recognize that the coronary sinus has a variable relationship to the mitral annulus. Since the mitral valve is a posterior structure (i.e., relative to the tricuspid valve), the appropriate nomenclature for left-sided pathways is superior, inferior, superoposterior, posterior, and inferoposterior. Attempts at reforming electrophysiologists' anatomical descriptions have

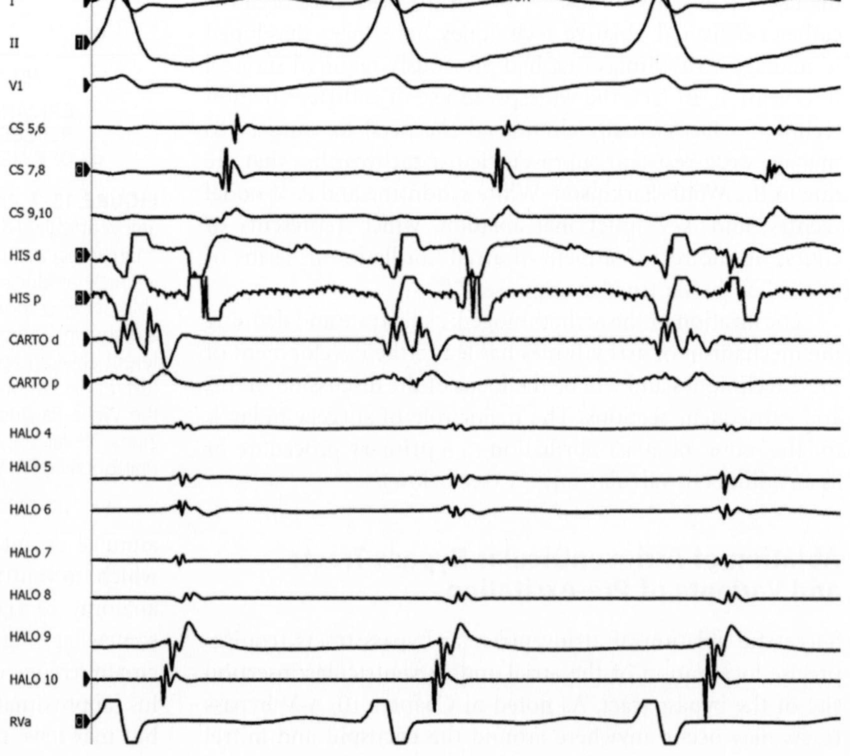


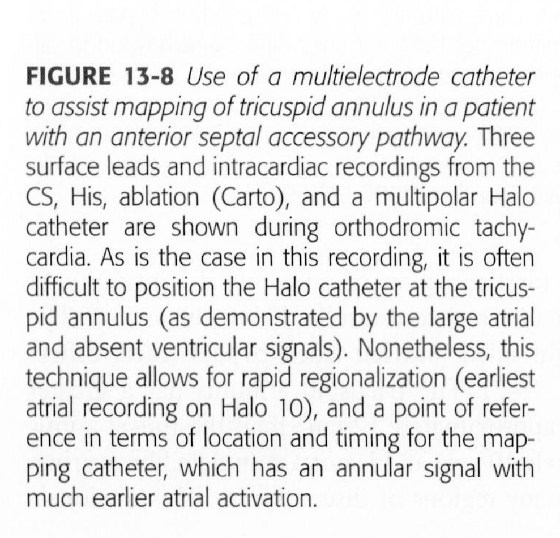

**FIGURE 13-8** *Use of a multielectrode catheter to assist mapping of tricuspid annulus in a patient with an anterior septal accessory pathway.* Three surface leads and intracardiac recordings from the CS, His, ablation (Carto), and a multipolar Halo catheter are shown during orthodromic tachycardia. As is the case in this recording, it is often difficult to position the Halo catheter at the tricuspid annulus (as demonstrated by the large atrial and absent ventricular signals). Nonetheless, this technique allows for rapid regionalization (earliest atrial recording on Halo 10), and a point of reference in terms of location and timing for the mapping catheter, which has an annular signal with much earlier atrial activation.

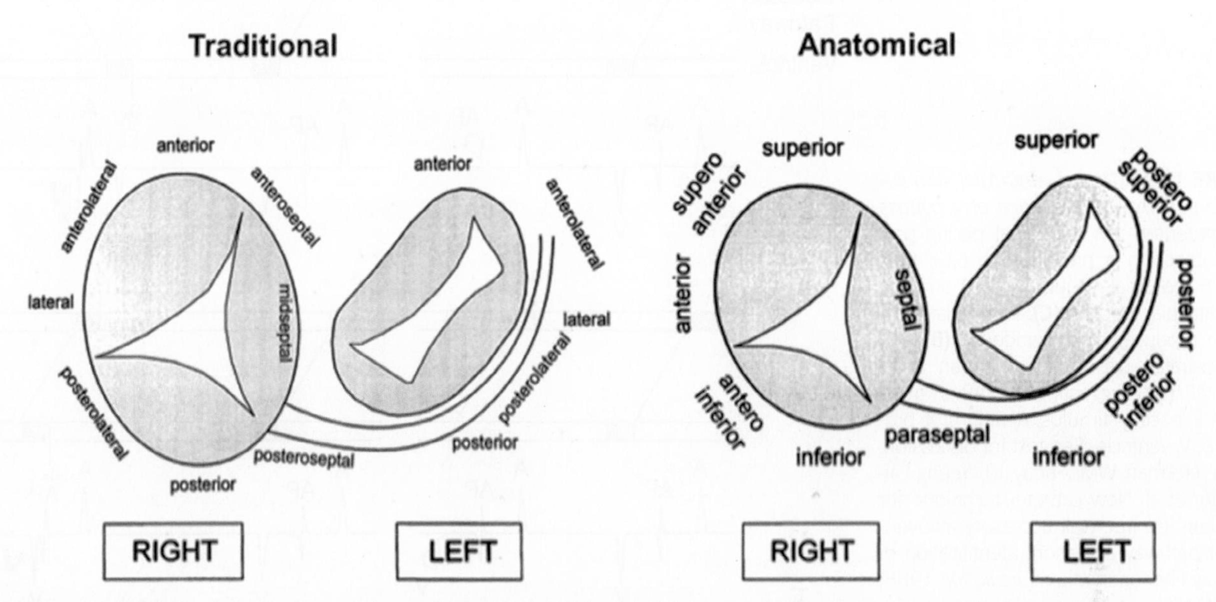


**FIGURE 13-9** Schematic representation of the traditional (electrophysiologic) versus true anatomic characterization of bypass tract locations along the A-V annulae. (Adapted from Cosio FG, Anderson RH, Kuck KH, et al. Living anatomy of the atrioventricular junctions. A guide to electrophysiologic mapping. A consensus statement from the cardiac nomenclature study group, working group of arrhythmias, european society of cardiology, and the task force on cardiac nomenclature from NASPE. *Circulation* 1999;100:e31–e37.)

not been well accepted, however (Fig. 13-9).[102] In all patients the proximal portion of the coronary sinus lies at least 2 cm superior to the annulus as it crosses the right to left atrium producing a pyramid-shaped space between the coronary sinus (base of the pyramid), the right and left atrium (sides of the pyramid), and central fibrous trigone (apex of the pyramid). Superiorposteriorly (formerly called anterolaterally), it frequently overrides the left ventricle, although there is significant variability of the relationship between the coronary sinus and the mitral annulus from the posterior portion to the anterior portion (see Chapter 10). Thus the coronary sinus may lie above the annulus and be associated with the left atrium itself, or may cross over to the ventricular side of the annulus. Thus, electrograms recorded from coronary sinus only can provide a reference for the atrial and/or ventricular (in the case of overt pre-excitation) insertion sites of the bypass tract. As such, these electrograms can only be used to guide the ablation catheter to areas in which more detailed mapping can be performed. In addition, there are occasional anomalies of the coronary sinus, such as diverticuli, which may form the conduit for bypass tracts. In such cases, the bypass tract is epicardial and the ablation may need to be carried out in the coronary sinus, in which the earliest atrial activity during circus movement tachycardia or bypass tract potentials is found (see subsequent discussion on mapping). Conduction at the insertion sites of bypass tracts is markedly anisotropic, which is due to the nearly horizontal orientation of atrial and ventricular fibers as they insert into the mitral annulus. In addition, the atrial fibers run parallel to the annulus giving rise to rapid conduction away from the insertion site, parallel to the annulus, and slow conduction to the free wall of the atrium, perpendicular to the annulus. This has been demonstrated by Smeets et al.[103] using high-density intraoperative computerized mapping. Irregular waveforms associated with fragmented electrograms may begin as either broad (approximately 2 cm) or narrow onsets of activation. This frequently leads to the recording of multicomponent atrial electrograms of various shapes and durations when recorded from the coronary sinus, left atrium, or left ventricle. It is my opinion that many so-called "bypass tract" potentials may actually represent "fragmented" atrial or ventricular electrograms (see subsequent discussion).

## Localization of Bypass Tracts

The mapping techniques that are used to localize the origin of the atrial and ventricular insertion sites bypass tracts have been detailed in Chapter 10. Nevertheless, it is important to reiterate that the earliest site of ventricular activation during antegrade pre-excitation and the earliest site of retrograde atrial activation during circus movement tachycardia remain the most important markers for ventricular and atrial insertion sites of the bypass tract, respectively. The presence of bypass tract potentials should be sought and are occasionally present (see Chapter 10, Figs. 10-72 and 10-73). In my opinion, activity recorded from a bypass tract should be recorded as a sharp, narrow spike in both unipolar and bipolar electrograms, and not just as one part of a multicomponent bipolar

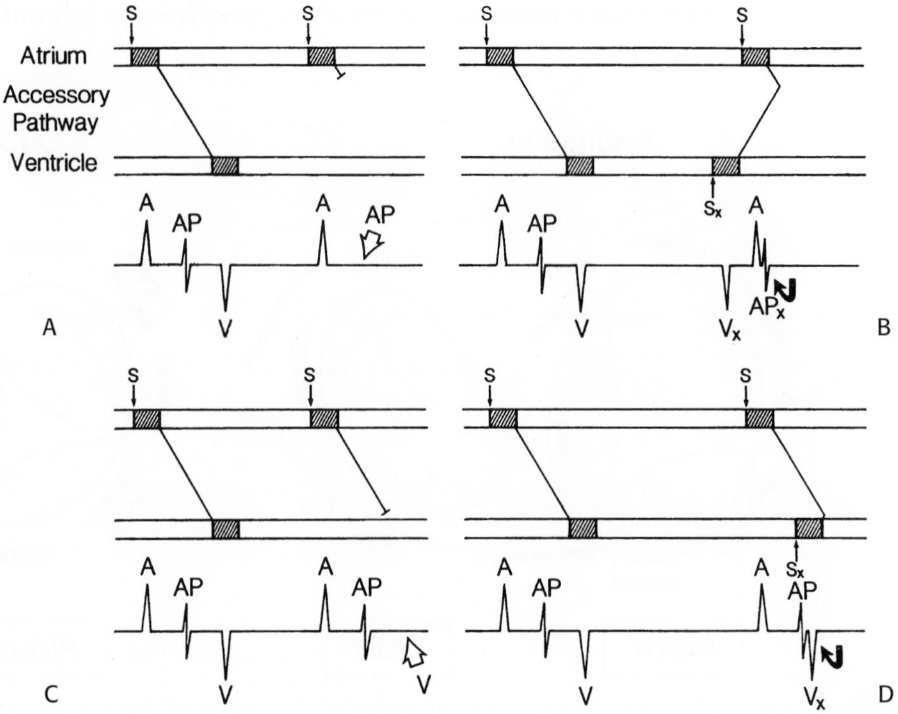

**FIGURE 13-10** *Use of ventricular stimulation to confirm the presence of a bypass tract potential.* On top, atrial pacing produces block in a presumed bypass tract (AP) at the atrial-AP junction **(A)** and the AP-ventricular junction **(C)**. Ventricular stimulation produces a retrograde AP **(B)** and demonstrates dissociation with an antegrade AP **(D)**, suggesting that AP is "truly" an AP. S, pacing stimulus; A, atrium; X, premature; V, ventricle. See text for discussion. (From Jackman WM, Friday KJ, Yeung-Lai-Wah JA, et al. New catheter technique for recording left free-wall accessory atrioventricular pathway activation: identification of pathway fiber orientation. *Circulation* 1988; 78:598.)

signal. Jackman et al.[104] have proposed methods of atrial and ventricular stimulations to validate the presence of a bypass tract potential (Figs. 13-10 and 13-11). V-A conduction over a bypass tract with the accessory pathway (AP) potential noted between the ventricular and atrial electrograms is schematically shown in Figure 13-11. V-A block could theoretically be noted either proximal to (loss of potential) or distal to (persistence of a potential) the AP. Proof that this AP is related to the ventricle requires demonstration of the inability of a premature atrial complex to alter the AP. Conversely, if during V-A block the middle potential is absent, the appearance of this potential in response to a premature atrial extrastimulus suggests that the "AP potential" is related to the atrial signal and is not part of ventricular activity.

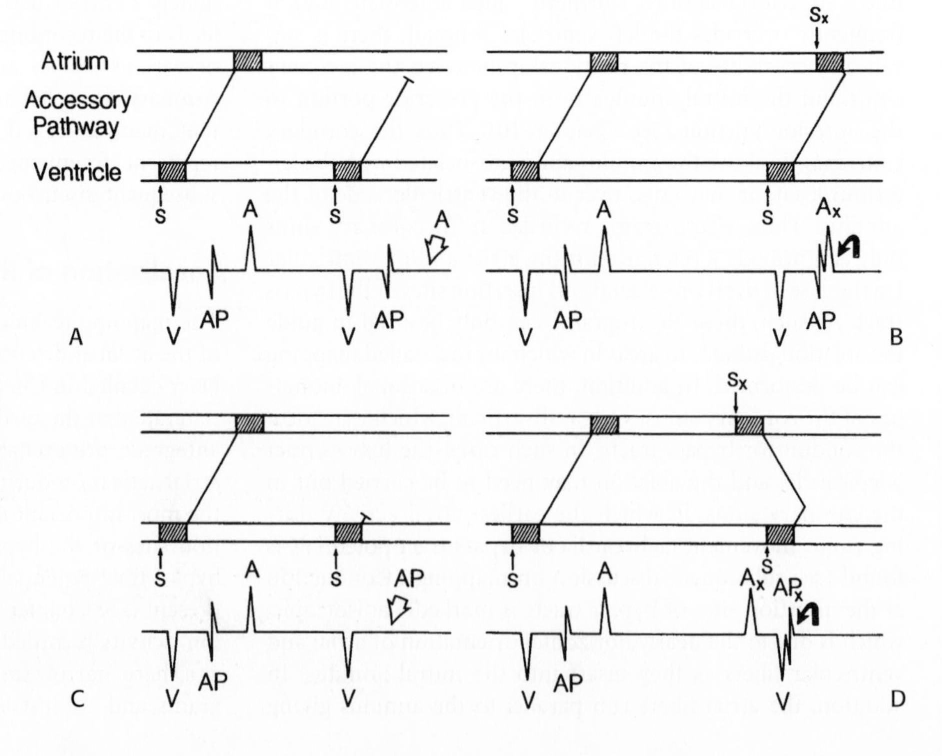


**FIGURE 13-11** *Use of atrial stimulation to validate the presence of a bypass tract potential in which retrograde block had occurred.* On bottom, atrial stimulation is used to confirm that AP is truly an AP. Retrograde block is produced at the AP-atrial junction **(A)** and the ventricular-AP junction **(C)**. Atrial stimulation does not affect AP **(B)** and produces an AP **(D)**, allegedly validating the "AP" potential. S, pacing stimulus; X, premature; A, atrium; V, ventricle. See text for discussion. (From Jackman WM, Friday KJ, Yeung-Lai-Wah JA, et al. New catheter technique for recording left free-wall accessory atrioventricular pathway activation: identification of pathway fiber orientation. *Circulation* 1988;78:598.)

During pacing-induced antegrade block in the bypass tract (Fig. 13-10), premature stimulation of the ventricle can demonstrate separation of the bypass tract from atrial tissue or a definite association with ventricular tissue. However, unless there is discordance between the results of the AP response to atrial or ventricular stimulation, these responses do not distinguish the AP from a component of either the atrial or ventricular electrogram. Furthermore, since retrograde block is not frequently seen in the bypass tract, the methodology suggested by Jackman et al.[104] in Figure 13-11 is not generally applicable. Finally, while AP potentials should appear as sharp spikes, most examples of AP potentials are rarely sharp deflections. In my opinion, the proposed stimulation protocols should only be applied when a sharp spike between atrial ventricular electrograms is present in both unipolar and bipolar recordings. One must remember that the use of filtering of bipolar signals can create a multicomponent electrogram that can be mistaken as a bypass tract. Even the presence of a spike does not necessarily distinguish that signal from one component of a multicomponent atrial or ventricular signal. I personally have never seen an "AP" potential that could be dissociated from both A and V electrogram by these stimulation techniques. Thus, in my opinion most of what have been labeled as AP potentials merely reflect one component of a multicomponent electrogram. Neibauer et al.[105] evaluated the criteria proposed by Jackman et al.[104] to validate accessory pathway potential (see Chapter 10, Figs. 10-74 and 10-78). They used atrial electrograms that simulated accessory pathway potentials (i.e., atrial electrograms manifesting a split potential separated by at least 30 msec) and assessed the response of these potentials to atrial and ventricular extrastimuli. All but one of the proposed criteria was seen in response to atrial and ventricular stimulations, despite the fact that none of these patients had bypass tracts present. The only observation that they never saw was block between the first and the second component of the atrial electrogram simulating block between the atrium and the bypass tract. This latter observation has never been convincingly demonstrated in our laboratory in any patient with pre-excitation. Although bypass tract recordings can be obtained, and may serve as a marker for catheter ablation of the bypass tract, proof that the electrical signal interpreted as a bypass tract potential is a bypass tract potential, in my opinion, is rarely achieved. More often it is not possible to distinguish a component of the atrial or ventricular electrogram from a true bypass tract potential. In the coronary sinus many, so-called, bypass tract potentials represent signals from muscle sleeves around the coronary sinus.

I do not personally believe the use of an orthogonal electrode enhances one's ability to record accessory pathway potentials. In contrast to Jackman et al.[84,94,104,106,107] I believe that true bypass tract potentials are only recorded in 5% to 15% of patients with pre-excitation syndromes. It is, however, frequent to find abnormal, fragmented atrial signals at sites of early activation during orthodromic tachycardia and ventricular pacing. I think this reflects the marked anisotropic activation in the insertion sites of the bypass tracts or coronary sinus musculature. In our experience, such signals are often associated with the site of earliest activity. It is important to recognize that conduction delays of up to 100 msec or more, including split potentials, may be observed in very small regions of only a few millimeters due to nonuniform anisotropic conduction.[108–110] Thus, what in some investigator's opinion is a bypass tract potential, our laboratory would frequently define as the earliest site of atrial activation; hence, in both cases that site would be appropriately ablated by either catheter or surgical technique.

In summary, to validate the presence of an accessory pathway potential, one must be able to dissociate it from both the local atrial and local ventricular electrogram. Most of the examples reporting to demonstrate proof of a bypass tract have not accomplished this. This is also true in some of the examples published attempting to demonstrate the differences between antegrade and retrograde sites of block in accessory pathways during programmed stimulation.[111] In my opinion, most electrograms that have been described as accessory pathway potentials represent one component of a fragmented atrial electrogram. Often, the choice of component designated as an accessory pathway potential can vary, depending on whether the investigator is looking at block in the antegrade or retrograde direction. This confusion is readily seen in Figure 13-12 in which the rapid component of a fragmented atrial electrogram is marked as an accessory pathway when block occurs during antegrade stimulation and is considered an atrial deflection during ventricular stimulation.[111,112]

The multicomponent characteristics of both unipolar and bipolar electrograms recorded during the retrograde conduction of a bypass tract may reflect many factors including (a) fiber orientation of the accessory pathway relative to that of the insertion site in the atrial and ventricular myocardium; (b) the orientation of atrial fibers relative to the recording electrodes (these are usually nearly horizontal at the point of attachment to the annulae); (c) the geometric/spatial relationship of the recording electrode and the site of insertion of the accessory pathway, which is related to; (d) the anatomic location (endocardial vs. epicardial) and physical characteristics (length, width, single trunk vs. "twig-like" insertion) of the bypass tract; and (e) coronary sinus musculature.

More important than trying to decide whether or not a multiple component signal contains an accessory pathway potential is the recognition of the presence of multiple bypass tracts. While this was discussed in Chapter 10, it needs to be reiterated, because a single ablative procedure may fail to cure symptomatic arrhythmias if the presence of an additional bypass tract or another source of arrhythmias, such as A-V nodal reentry, is not diagnosed at the time of the electrophysiology study. Thus, the concept of "single catheter" approaches to ablation of arrhythmias should be abandoned since at least 10% of patients who have multiple arrhythmias and another 10% to 20% (depending on the patient population at the institution performing the

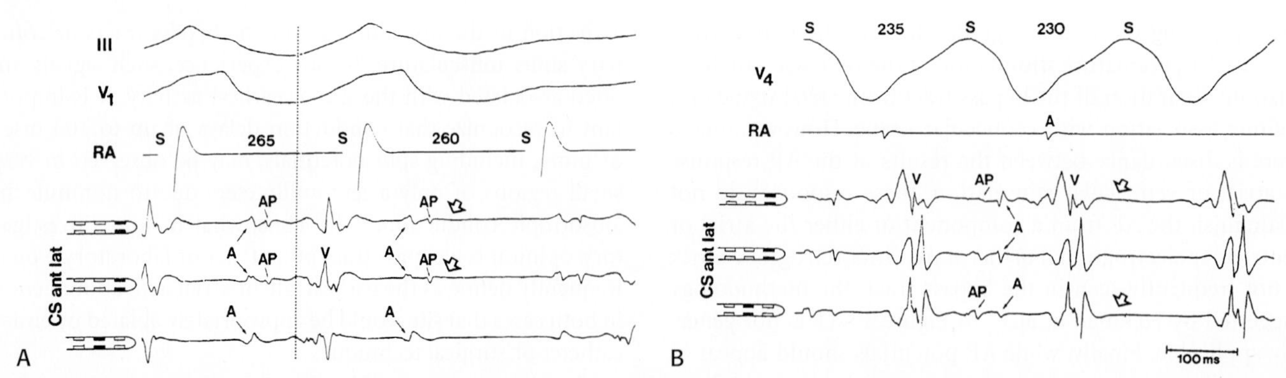


**FIGURE 13-12** *Example of arbitrary and inconsistent definition of accessory pathway potential.* **A** and **B:** Purported demonstration of antegrade **(A)** and retrograde **(B)** block at the junction of the accessory pathway (AP)-ventricular junction. Close inspection of the electrograms suggests that two components of a fragmented atrial electrogram are arbitrarily labeled AP and A. This is best seen in the middle CS recording in which the slowly inscribed deflection and sharp deflection are called A and AP, respectively, during antegrade block and AP and A, respectively, during retrograde block. (From Kuck KH, Friday KJ, Kunze KP, et al. Sites of conduction block in accessory atrioventricular pathways: basis for concealed accessory pathways. *Circulation* 1990;82:407.)

studies) will have multiple bypass tracts. Signs of multiple bypass tracts include:

- Multiple atrial breakthrough sites during orthodromic tachycardia (Fig. 13-13),
- Eccentric atrial activation during circus movement pre-excited tachycardias,
- Tachycardia showing fusion between fully pre-excited and narrow QRS complexes, can also be observed with during AVNRT with variable conduction over a bypass tract acting as a bystander,
- Different retrograde atrial activation sequences that are present during different tachycardia types (Fig. 13-14),
- A mismatch between the earliest site of antegrade ventricular pre-excitation and retrograde atrial activation during circus movement tachycardia, which actually defines multiple pathways, and
- The observation of a changing relationship of the His potential to the ventricular electrogram, without any change in the cycle length or atrial activation sequence during a pre-excited tachycardia. This finding suggests the presence of multiple bypass tracts because the His–Purkinje system cannot be a component of the reentrant circuit (Fig. 13-15).

One must also determine whether or not the bypass tract is an innocent bystander during an unrelated arrhythmia. As discussed previously in Chapter 10, atrioventricular, atriofascicular, or nodofascicular bypass tracts may be innocent bystanders during A-V nodal reentry or orthodromic circus

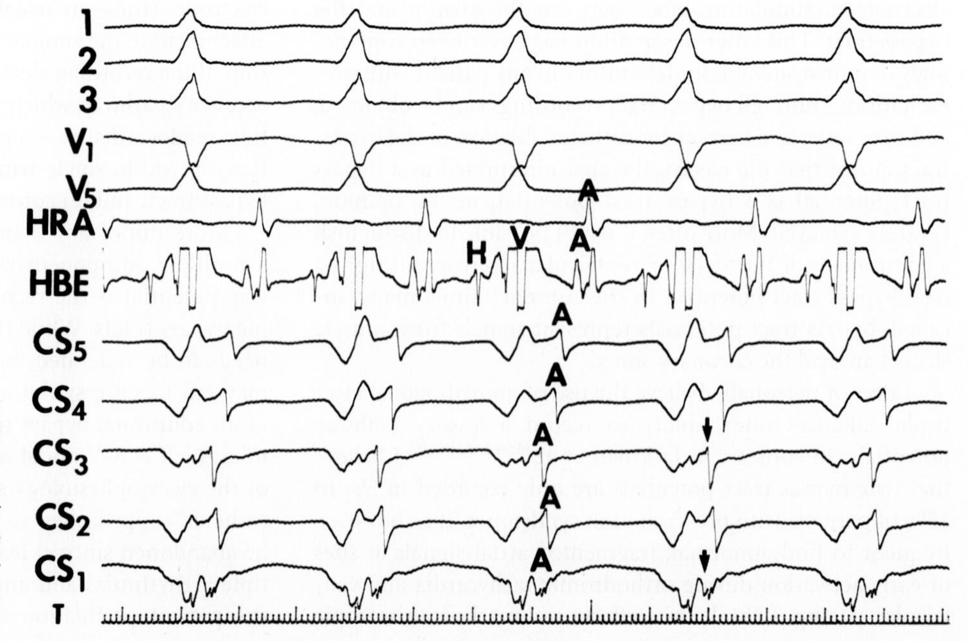


**FIGURE 13-13** *Multiple bypass tracts recognized by two atrial breakthrough sites.* Five surface ECG leads are shown with bipolar, filtered electrograms from the HRA and HBE, and five unipolar (0.05 to 400 Hz) recordings from the CS. $CS_1$ and $CS_3$ show early breakthrough separated by later activation, suggesting two pathways.

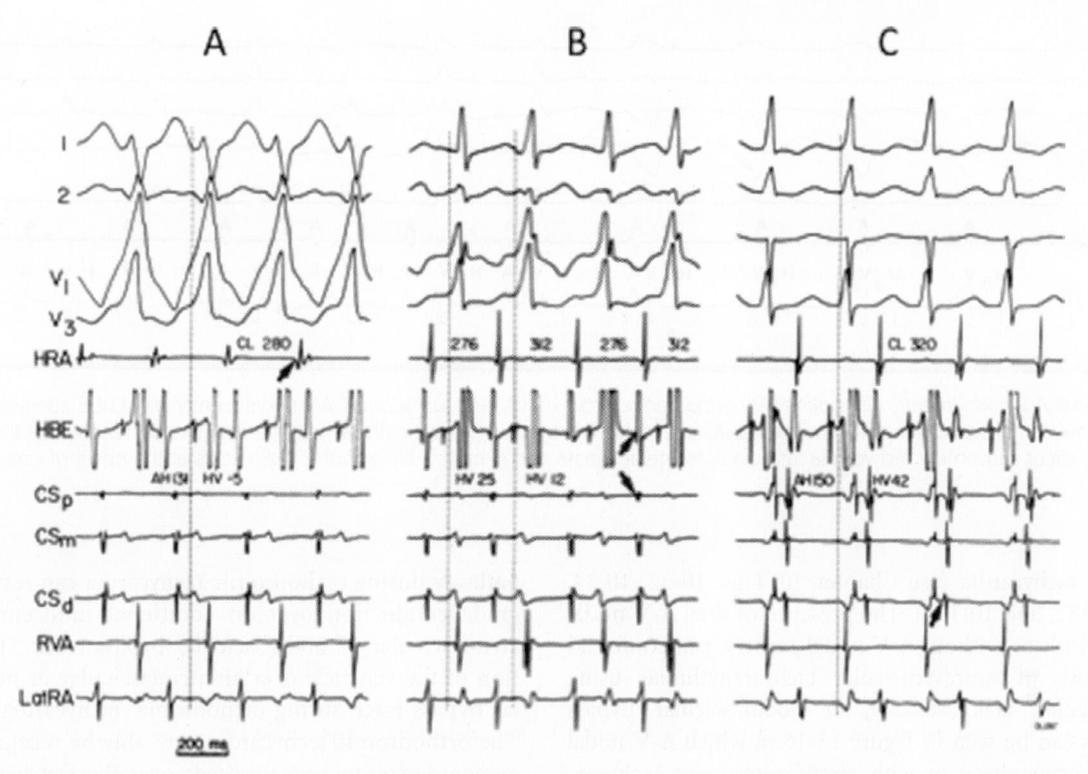


**FIGURE 13-14** *Multiple bypass tract manifested by fusion during pre-excited tachycardia and different routes of retrograde atrial activation.* Three tachycardias are shown. A totally pre-excited tachycardia using a left lateral bypass tract antegradely **(A)**, narrow QRS orthodromic tachycardia **(C)**, and a wide complex tachycardia, which is a fusion of antegrade conduction over a left lateral bypass tract and the A-V node **(B)**. Retrograde atrial activation shows a right anterolateral bypass tract **(A)**, a septal bypass tract **(B)**, and a left lateral bypass tract **(C)**.

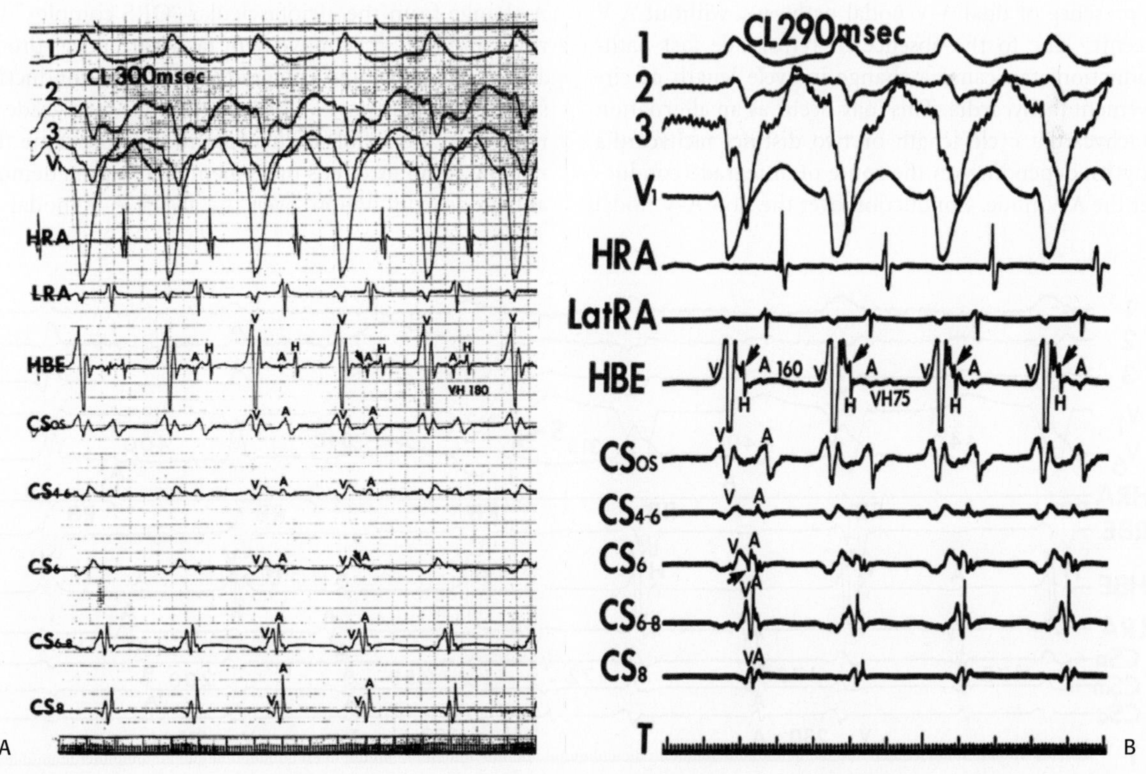


**FIGURE 13-15** Pre-excited tachycardia with eccentric atrial activation and changing His bundle activation. **A** and **B:** A pre-excited tachycardia is present with retrograde activation over a left posterior free wall bypass tract (retrograde activation earliest in CS site 6). An additional posteroseptal bypass may be present because the atrial activation **(A)** in the HBE is earlier than the CS os. The His bundle is activated retrogradely by two routes left bundle branch **(A)** and right bundle branch **(B)**, giving rise to two V-H intervals. The lack of effect of V-H on tachycardia cycle length suggests no role for the normal A-V conducting system in the tachycardia. CL, cycle length; LRA, low right atrium.

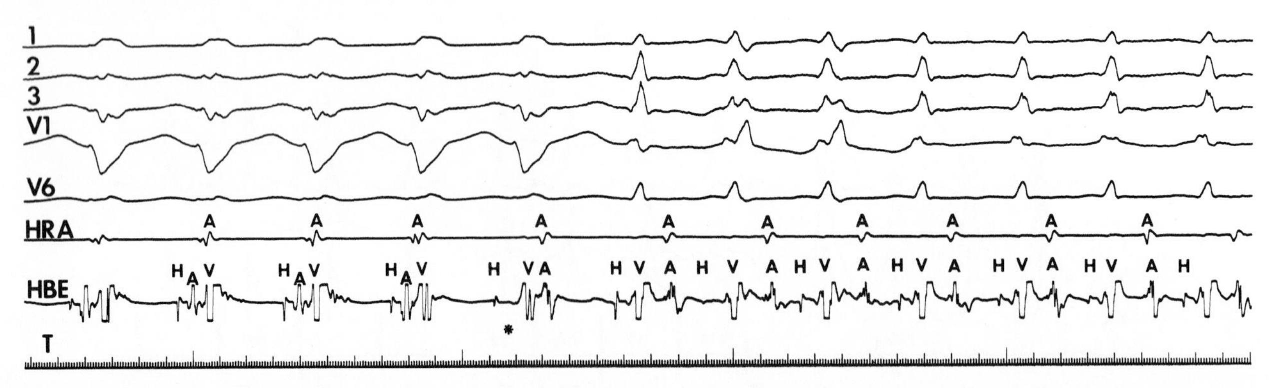


**FIGURE 13-16** *A-V nodal reentry alternating with orthodromic circus movement tachycardia.* A-V nodal reentry with LBBE aberration is present for the first four complexes. On the fifth complex (*asterisk*), retrograde block in the fast pathway terminates A-V nodal reentry, but the tachycardia continues as circus movement tachycardia, using a right lateral bypass tract. Phase 3 block in the RBE occurs at the onset of circus movement tachycardia.

movement tachycardia (see Chapter 10, Figs. 10-32, 10-34, 10-35, 10-132, and 10-136). The presence of dual A-V nodal pathways, with or without A-V nodal reentry, can confound the diagnosis of supraventricular tachyarrhythmias using atrioventricular, atriofascicular, or nodofascicular bypass tracts. This can be seen in Figure 13-16 in which A-V nodal tachycardia can alternate with circus movement tachycardia resulting in variable heart rates and QRS configurations. Detailed analysis of retrograde atrial activation is necessary to delineate both mechanisms so that they may both be appropriately treated during any ablative procedure.

The presence of dual A-V nodal pathways, without A-V nodal reentry due to the absence of retrograde fast pathway conduction, can cause a change in cycle length of circus movement tachycardia. This may occur as an alternation of the tachycardia cycle length or two distinct tachycardia cycle lengths, depending on the route of antegrade conduction over the A-V node. Conduction over the slow A-V nodal pathway during orthodromic tachycardia can result in antegrade conduction over an additional innocent bystander atriofascicular or nodofascicular bypass tract. Thus, activation of the ventricle over an atriofascicular or nodofascicular bypass tract during orthodromic tachycardia can occur. The orthodromic tachycardia may only be recognized when antegrade conduction proceeds over the fast pathway. This latter situation is demonstrated in Figure 13-17, in which an atriofascicular bypass tract functions passively to produce an apparent atriofascicular circus movement tachycardia when antegrade conduction uses a slow A-V nodal pathway. A change from the atriofascicular "QRS complex" to a narrow complex circus movement tachycardia was produced by a VPC, which shifted antegrade A-V nodal conduction from slow to fast pathway. This could produce retrograde concealment into the atriofascicular pathway at the same time. The narrow complex circus movement tachycardia demonstrated antegrade conduction over the faster A-V nodal pathway

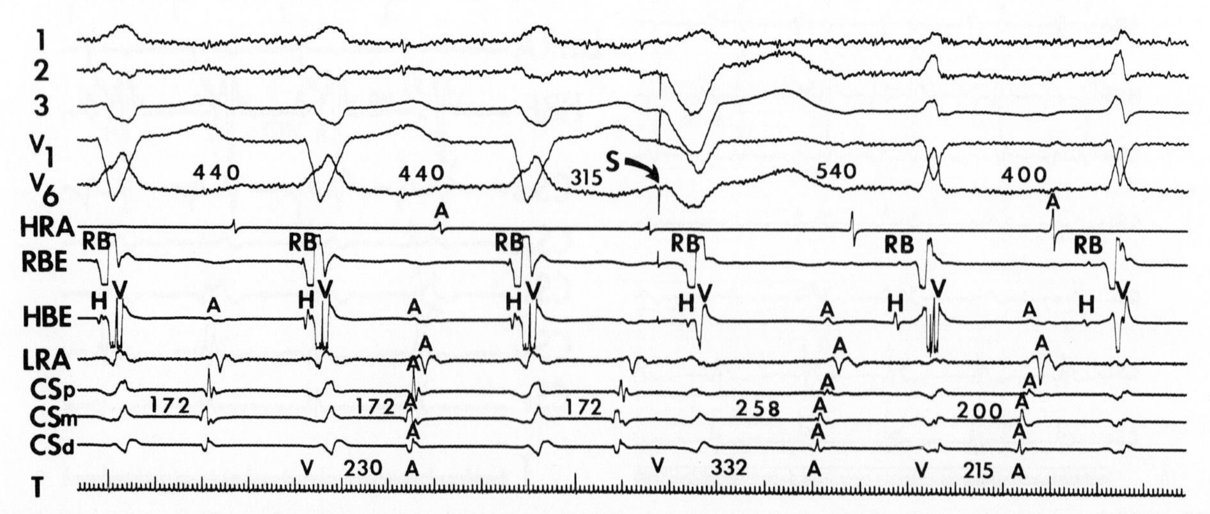


**FIGURE 13-17** *Atriofasicular reentry during circus movement tachycardia.* Five ECG leads are shown with electrograms from the HRA, right bundle (RBE), HBE, lateral right atrium (LRA), and proximal, mid- and distal coronary sinus (CS, at lateral left atrium). Antegrade conduction initially occurs over an atriofasicular bypass tract (note RB precedes H), and retrograde conduction over a slowly conducting left lateral bypass tract. A VPC penetrates the A-V node, shifting conduction to a fast A-V nodal pathway and the tachycardia continues as a narrow QRS. See text for discussion.

with retrograde conduction over a slowly conducting left lateral bypass tract. Alternatively one could suggest that this is a nodofascicular pathway arising from the slow A-V nodal pathway. In this instance the VPC would change the QRS complex solely due to the shift to "fast pathway" conduction due to a marked delay in retrograde atrial conduction over the slowly conducting left lateral bypass tract. The longer A-A interval allows the fast pathway to recover. The His timing from the onset of ventricular activation to the right bundle potential is much shorter during the "Mahaim" tachycardia (V-RB = 10 msec) than during the VPD delivered at the right ventricular apex (V-RB = 65 msec) suggesting a close physical relationship of the origin of the Mahaim fiber to the proximal right bundle branch. In this instance, during sinus rhythm right atrial pacing produced pre-excitation and left atrial pacing did not, confirming the presence of an atriofascicular pathway at the anterolateral tricuspid annulus. Thus, a systematic approach must be undertaken to delineate the necessary components of reentrant tachycardias so that catheter-based or surgical ablative procedures will not destroy tissues unrelated to the tachyarrhythmia, leading to unnecessary adverse, long-term sequelae.

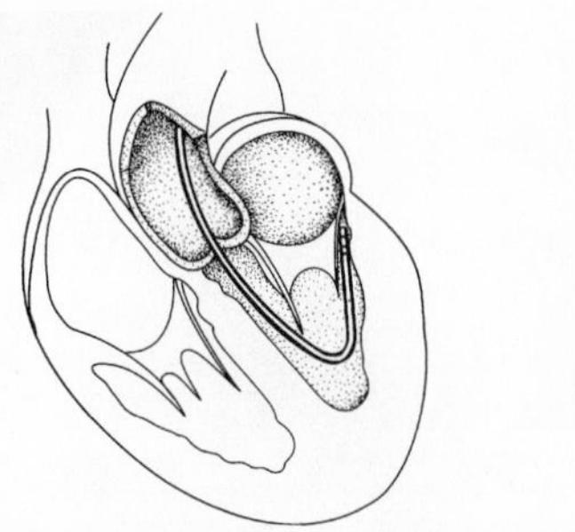

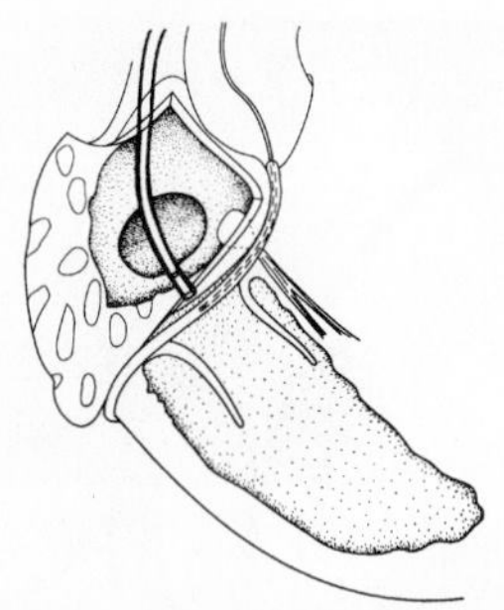

**FIGURE 13-18** Methods of catheter ablation of bypass tracts. Ablation of left-sided bypass tracts is most commonly performed from a ventricular approach in which the electrode through which energy is delivered is placed at the mitral annulus under the mitral valve. (**Left**) For right-sided bypass tracts, we use an atrial approach with the ablating electrode placed on the A-V ring. (**Right**) A guiding mapping catheter in the right coronary artery has been suggested by some.

## Catheter Ablation of Bypass Tracts

The indications for catheter ablation of bypass tracts have been markedly liberalized with the development and refinement of catheter technology and newer mapping data acquisition systems, both of which have led to an extremely high success rate for curing arrhythmias associated with bypass tracts. Multicenter experience reports acute success rates averaging 95% with a recurrence rate of 3% to 10%.[113–117] More importantly, cost-effectiveness of this procedure has been established.[118] As such, virtually all patients with symptomatic arrhythmias due to accessory pathways should undergo catheter ablation as a primary therapy. However, as stated in Chapter 10, I do not believe that the asymptomatic patient with manifest pre-excitation, regardless of the refractory period of the bypass tract or the ventricular response during induced atrial fibrillation, should undergo ablation. This concept has been recently reviewed in the literature.[119–122] There is no evidence that such patients develop life-threatening arrhythmias. For patients with symptomatic arrhythmias due to accessory pathways RF, catheter ablation, with its high success rate and low morbidity, is the standard of care.

Ablation of bypass tracts may be accomplished using an atrial or ventricular approach, as schematically depicted in Figure 13-18. Simultaneous recordings from both approaches are shown in Figure 13-19. In our laboratory, we prefer a left ventricular approach for left-sided bypass tracts and a right atrial approach for right-sided and septal bypass tracts. A transseptal approach for ablating left-sided bypass tracts on the atrial side has also been used and shown to be equally effective to the retrograde aortic approach.[123,124] We use a retrograde aortic approach to the left ventricular approach in order to avoid the potential complications of transseptal catheterization. Severe aortic or femoral atherosclerotic disease would be another indication for a transseptal approach. Others prefer a transseptal approach for all left-sided bypass tracts. In my experience, contact and stability are generally better with a retrograde approach and ablation on the ventricular side of the mitral annulus. As such, the power needed to achieve adequate temperatures or impedance changes is less using the retrograde approach than during a transseptal approach. I believe this decreases the incidence of coagulum formation and potential for stroke. Left posteroseptal bypass tracts can be ablated from either the left ventricle or transseptal left atrium at the medial aspect of the mitral annulus, but in my opinion, the retrograde approach is easier. Finally, some cases of posteroseptal bypass tracts, particularly those that are epicardial and that are associated with abnormality in the coronary sinus (e.g., coronary sinus diverticulum) must be ablated from within the coronary sinus. In the presence of overt pre-excitation, an epicardial location of the bypass tract is suggested if the earliest site of endocardial ventricular activation does not precede the onset of the delta wave. In my experience, such bypass tracts are almost always in the left posterior paraseptal space or associated with a coronary vein in which the bypass tract is located.

Left-sided bypass tracts (manifest or concealed) are the most common types of atrioventricular bypass tracts. They make up approximately 60% of all bypass tracts that we have studied. Regardless of whether a transseptal or a retrograde aortic left ventricular approach is used, an initial attempt at localization is made using a multipolar coronary sinus catheter. The recordings from the coronary sinus catheter are usually made in the bipolar configuration, but it is often helpful to include unipolar as well as bipolar signals. Unipolar signals are used to more precisely localize the sites of atrial or ventricular insertion of the bypass tract. In the coronary sinus, an atrial or ventricular unipolar electrogram with a QS complex demonstrating a rapid intrinsicoid deflection

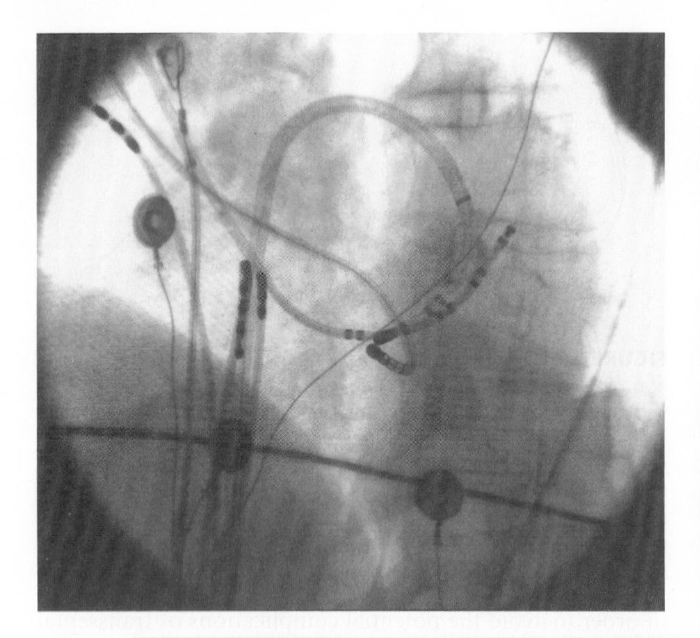

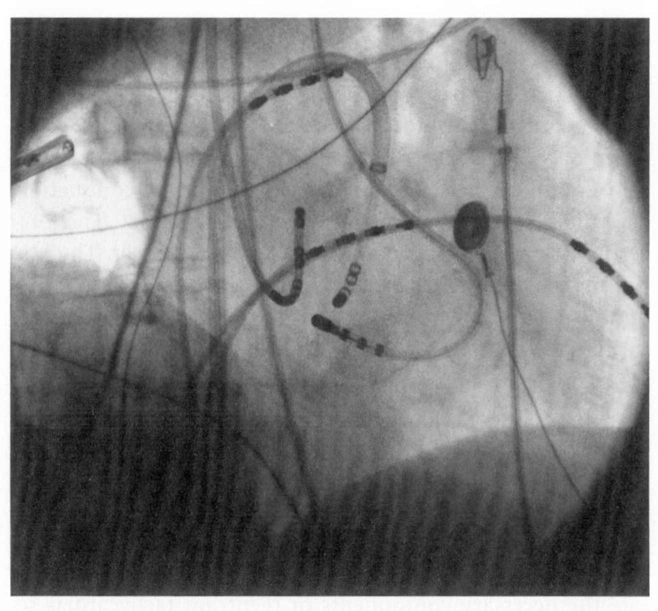

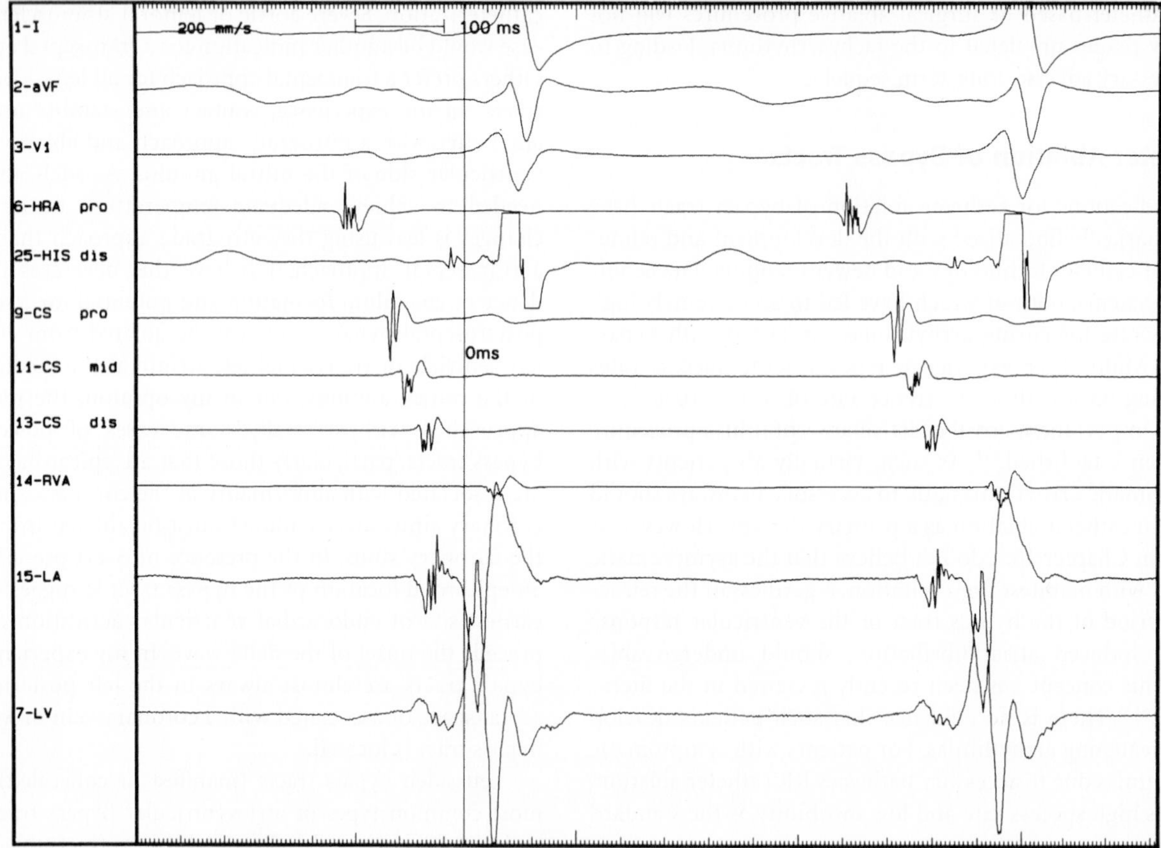


**FIGURE 13-19** Atrial (transseptal) and ventricular (retrograde aortic) approaches to the ablation of left posterior bypass tract. Left anterior oblique (**left**) and right anterior oblique (**right**) are shown with analog recordings of atrial and ventricular activation at the site of earliest ventricular activation recorded from either the left atrium or left ventricle (**bottom**). Both demonstrate ventricular activation prior to the delta wave, but the ventricular electrogram recorded from the left ventricle begins slightly earlier than that recorded from the left atrium.

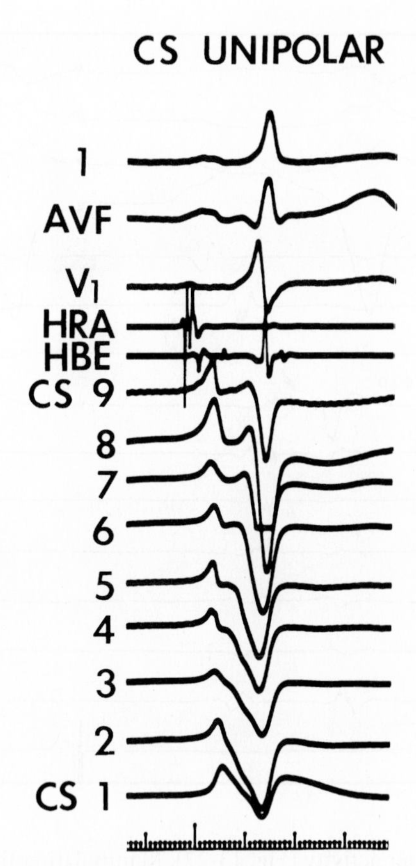


**FIGURE 13-20** *Unipolar electrograms from the coronary sinus in a patient with a left-sided bypass tract.* Nine unipolar electrograms from a decapolar catheter are shown with ECG leads and electrograms from the HRA and HBE. Pole 2 shows the earliest intrinsicoid deflection. Note the P-QS configuration. See text for discussion.

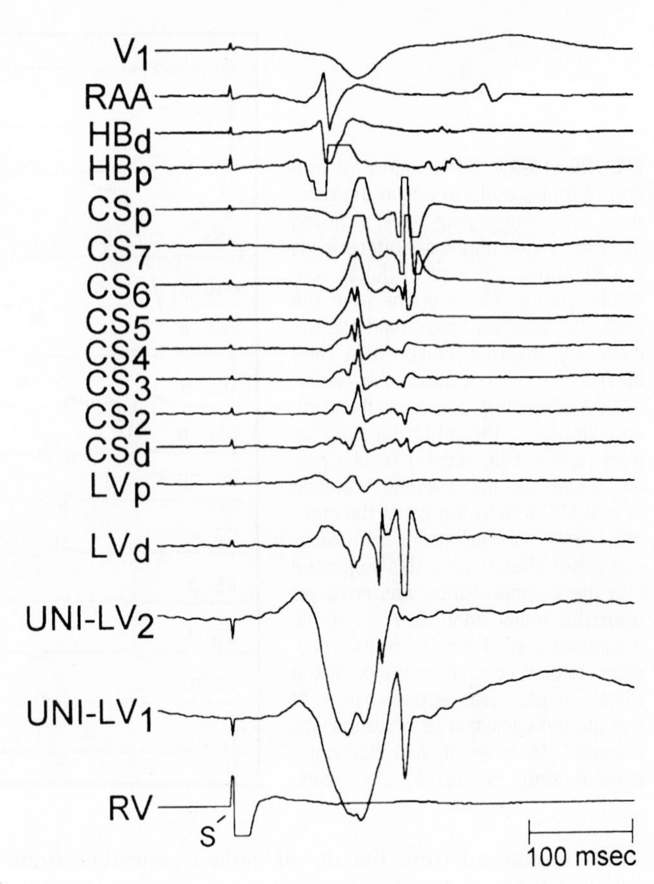


**FIGURE 13-21** *Use of unipolar recordings to demonstrate the source of the different components of a bipolar electrogram.* Surface ECG lead $V_1$ is shown with electrograms from the right atrial appendage (RAA), His bundle (HB), and eight electrograms from the proximal (p) to distal (d) coronary sinus (CS). Left ventricular distal and proximal bipolar electrograms are shown following that, and underneath that, unipolar signals from the distal electrode and second pole. The left ventricular distal electrogram shows the earliest recorded atrial activity during ventricular pacing. The atrial electrogram is made up of two components. Using the unipolar signals, one can see that the second pole ($LV_2$) is responsible for the earliest component of the distal LV electrogram while the tip electrode is responsible for the second component. This suggests that this is an inappropriate site for ablation since the tip electrode was not recording from the site of earliest atrial activation. See text for discussion.

is believed to represent the site of insertion of an epicardially positioned bypass tract (Fig. 13-20). A ventricular electrogram with an rS morphology recorded from the coronary sinus may be the earliest activation of an endocardially located bypass tract.[93,125] Alternatively, the rS may represent a recording that is somewhat removed from the site of atrial and/or ventricular insertion. Both atrial and ventricular components may exhibit normal smooth contours or may be polyphasic or fragmented. Fragmentation of unipolar signals is always associated with fragmented bipolar signals and, in my opinion, reflects either anisotropic conduction from the site of insertion of the bypass tract or potentials from the CS musculature, or both. Examples of QS and rS atrial signals, which are smooth or fragmented, are demonstrated earlier in Figure 13-13. Use of unipolar signals is also critical in order to demonstrate that the distal electrode, which is used for RF delivery, is actually the electrode recording the earliest activity. If only bipolar recordings are utilized, one does not know which of the two poles is responsible for the earliest component of the bipolar electrogram. Figure 13-21 demonstrates how the use of unipolar electrograms demonstrates that the second (proximal) pole of the distal bipolar electrogram was responsible for the earliest activity in that bipolar electrogram. Delivery of RF energy at this site through unipolar lead 1 would not have resulted in elimination of the bypass tract. Thus, the use of unipolar electrograms cannot be overstated. They provide directional information and importantly provide critical information that is necessary to demonstrate that the distal pole through which the RF energy is delivered is at the site of earliest activation. This is true regardless of whether one is accessing the earliest site of ventricular activation in a pre-excited complex or the earliest atrial activation during retrograde activation over the bypass tracts.

There are additional features in the coronary sinus recordings that should make one expect an epicardial location requiring manipulation of the catheter down one of the cardiac veins. First is the appearance of the early, near-simultaneous activation along at least three bipolar pairs of the coronary sinus catheter. This suggests that the coronary

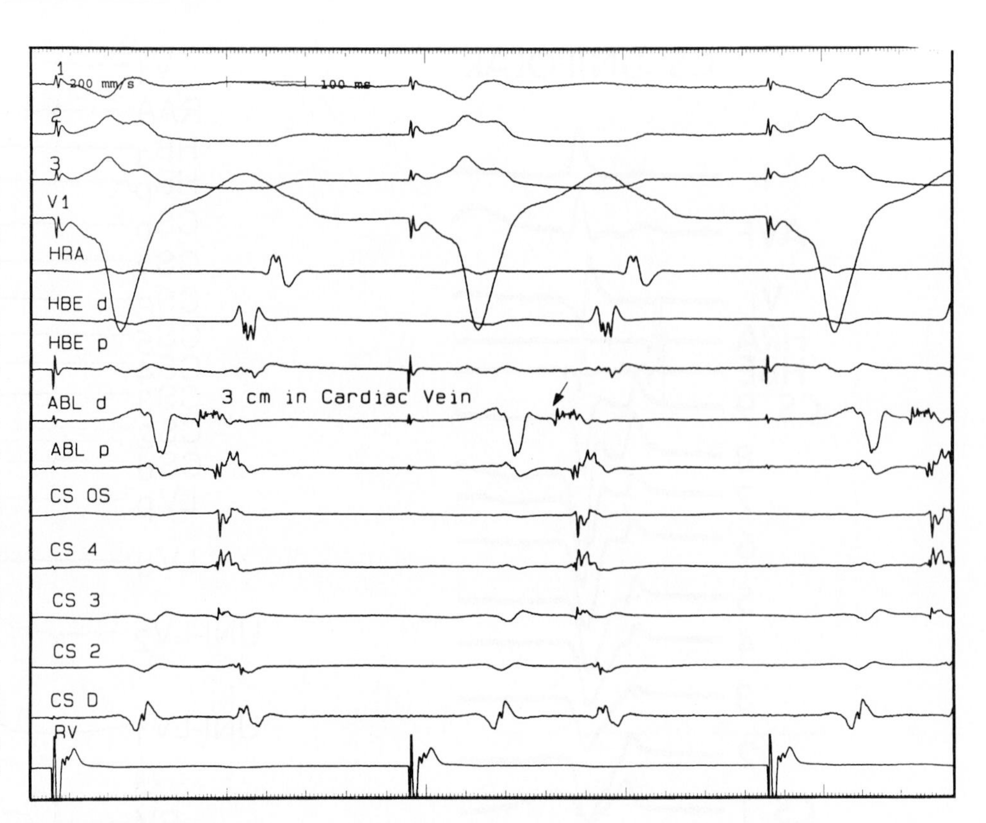


**FIGURE 13-22** Simultaneous activation of multiple electrodes in the coronary sinus suggesting it is removed from the mitral annulus. Surface leads I, II, III, and $V_1$ are shown during ventricular pacing. Electrograms from the HRA, the distal and proximal HBE, the distal and proximal ablation (ABL catheter) located 3 cm inside the cardiac drain and electrograms from the coronary sinus OS, the fourth bipolar pair, third bipolar pair, second bipolar pair, and distal pair and the RV. Activation in poles 3, 4, and the os of the coronary sinus showed nearly simultaneous onset of activation. This suggested that the coronary sinus was removed from the mitral annulus. As a result, a catheter was placed 3 cm in a posterior cardiac vein, at which point the mitral annulus was approximated. At this site the earliest atrial activation was recorded, 35 msec prior to that in the coronary sinus. See text for discussion.

sinus is removed from the site of earliest activation from which radial spread approaches the coronary sinus catheter in a broad wavefront and that the coronary sinus is remote from the mitral annulus. In such an instance, one should attempt to manipulate catheters in various cardiac veins in an attempt to find earlier activity (Fig. 13-22). Manipulating the catheter in the cardiac vein located an early potential 3 cm down the vein closer to the mitral annulus and the ventricular epicardium. Delivery of RF energy at this site resulted in block in the bypass tract (Fig. 13-23). These pathways are also able to

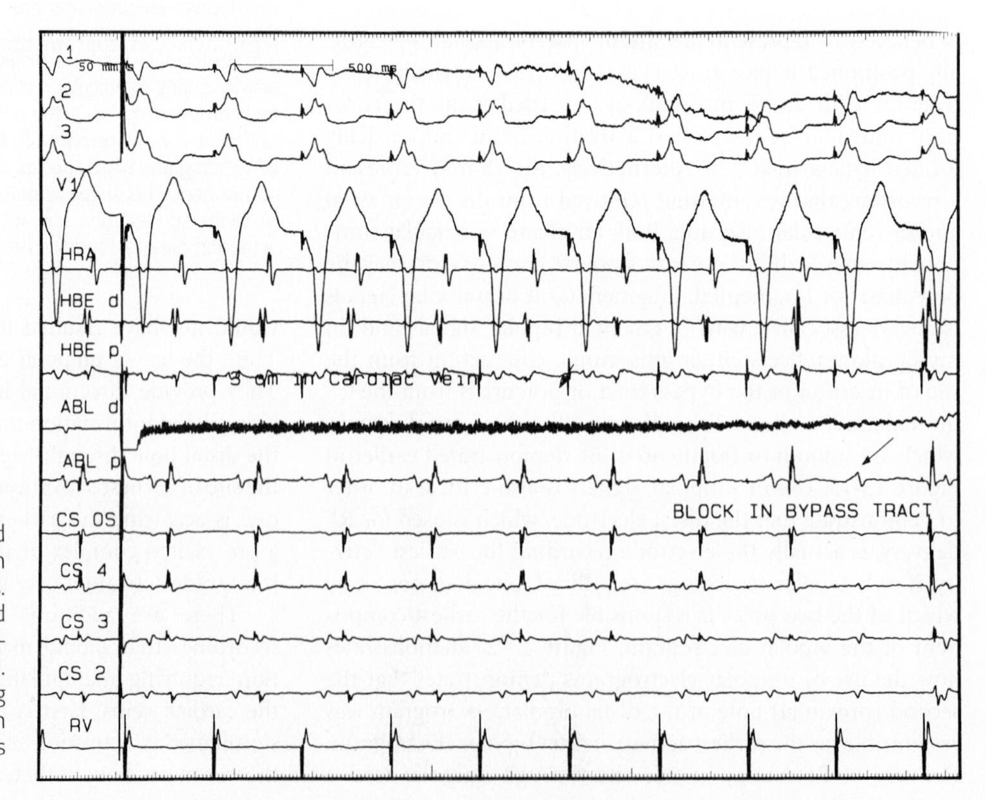


**FIGURE 13-23** Ablation of concealed bypass tract in a posterior cardiac vein 3 cm from the os of the coronary sinus. This is the same patient as recorded in Figure 13-16 in whom earliest activation was recorded in a cardiac vein. Ablation in that cardiac vein during ventricular pacing resulted in block in the bypass tract in less than 3 seconds (see *arrow*).

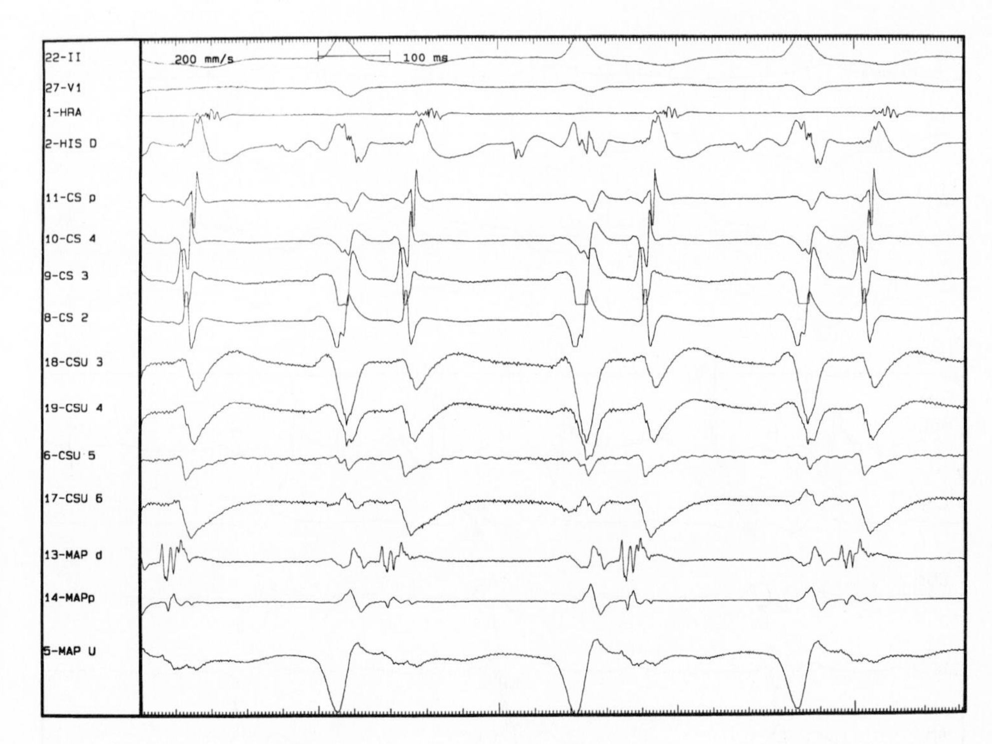


**FIGURE 13-24** *Local coronary sinus with V-A conduction times exceeding 50 msec suggest the presence of a bypass tract removed from the coronary sinus.* In this figure, during circus movement tachycardia bipolar recordings are shown from four coronary sinus pairs (CS2-CSP) and unipolar coronary sinus recordings from poles 2 to 6. These poles were chosen since the earliest bipolar recording was in CS3 (poles 5 and 6). The earliest activation time locally was nearly 75 msec in pole 5, which had a small R-deep S wave. This suggested that the coronary sinus was removed from the mitral annulus and earliest site. A catheter (mapd) inserted in the vein proximate to pole 3 revealed the earliest bipolar and unipolar recording some 30 msec at the head of the earliest bipolar recording (in the coronary sinus). This was the target site for successful ablation. See text for discussion.

be ablated by the retrograde approach in which a catheter can be placed at the mitral annulus. In this case ablation can be performed without concern of perforating the coronary sinus. Another important observation shown in this tracing is the finding of a local V-A time exceeding 50 msec in the coronary sinus in the presence of a rapidly conducting bypass tract. Even if the earliest CS recording is bracketed, as shown in Figure 13-24, this long, local V-A time at the earliest site suggests that exploration of a cardiac vein be undertaken and that the coronary sinus is far away from the site of earliest activation. Unipolar electrograms from the electrodes surrounding the early bipolar sites usually show a small R wave (Fig. 13-24). Exploration of the cardiac vein proximal to CS bipolar pair 3 yielded an earlier atrial electrogram with a V-A interval of 30 msec at a site adjacent to the mitral annulus. This electrogram preceded the earliest recorded in the coronary sinus by 35 msec. Successful ablation of the bypass tract was accomplished at this site.

If at all possible, ablation should be carried out in sinus rhythm or preferably during atrial or ventricular pacing. Application of RF energy during a tachycardia is often associated with catheter instability, particularly if there is abrupt loss of conduction over the bypass tract. Block in a bypass tract results in immediate termination of the tachycardia, which is often associated with displacement of the catheter from its critical position. Since there will be no conduction for a variable period of time one cannot find a suitable target to complete the RF lesion. One can only hope for return of conduction over the bypass tract in a short period of time so that it can again be targeted. Unfortunately, on some occasions the bypass tract conduction will not return until the patient leaves the hospital and the tachycardia recurs. Ablation during continuous ventricular pacing either during sinus rhythm (as long as eccentric activation is seen) or while entraining the SVT prevents this problem. Use of mapping system may obviate this problem by tagging the initial site of ablation, allowing the investigator to return with great precision to that site.

Selection of a good site during ventricular pacing may sometimes be difficult because of diminution of the amplitude of the atrial electrogram and merging of the atrial electrogram with the ventricular electrogram because of the influence of slanted bypass tracts. Rapid ventricular pacing to produce V-A block can demonstrate what component of the ablation electrogram is ventricular and what is atrial (Fig. 13-25). Another maneuver is to alternatively pace the atrium and ventricle and the ventricle separately (Fig. 13-26). In this way, V-A conduction over the bypass tract will only be evident with ventricular pacing only; electrograms present only during ventricular pacing represent atrial activity. As mentioned above, as well as in Chapter 10, bypass tracts are frequently slanted (see Figs. 10-48 and 10-49).[126,127] If one uses a ventricular approach to ablate a concealed bypass tract, the ventricular insertion site can be identified as that site that maintains a constant V-A interval on the mapping catheter, despite differences in the direction of activation to the ventricular site and differences in the coronary sinus recordings. This is schematically shown in Figure 13-27. The local V-A time measured on the ablation catheter must remain constant if activation occurs over the bypass tract, regardless of which direction the ventricular wavefront engaging a bypass tract is traveling. Sites that may have a shorter V-A interval in response to retrograde conduction over bypass tract activation during a ventricular activation from one direction may have a markedly different V-A

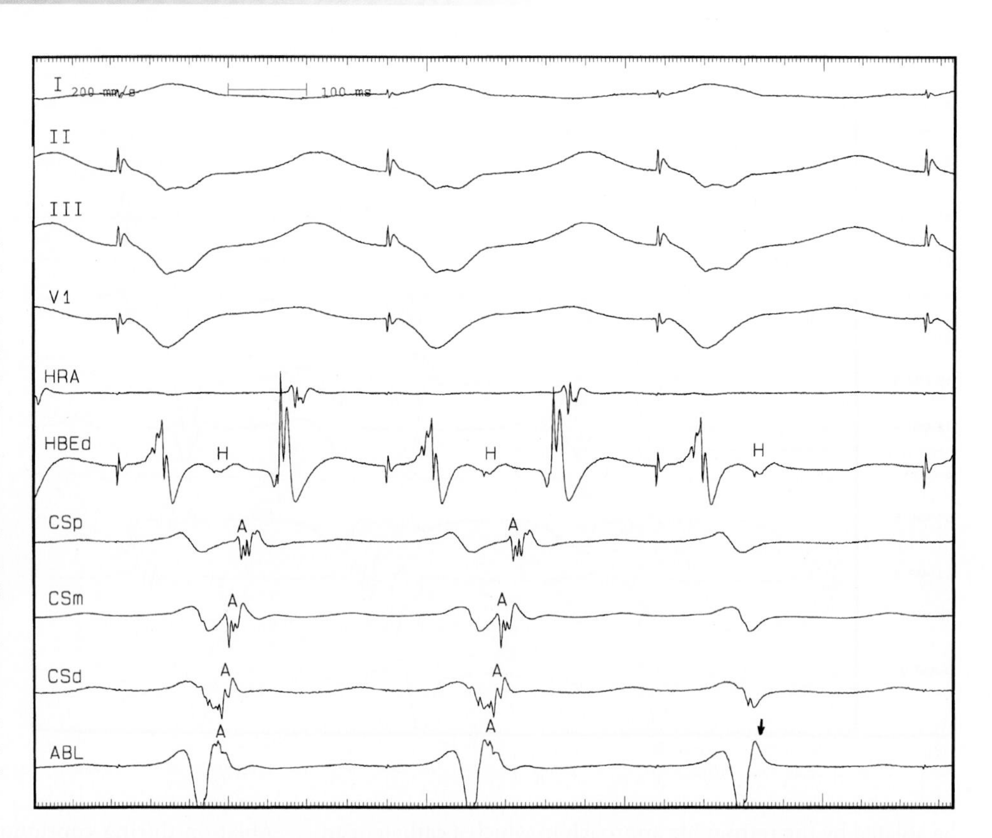


**FIGURE 13-25** *Use of rapid ventricular pacing to ascertain where the atrial deflection is located during circus movement tachycardia or ventricular pacing.* Ventricular pacing with a cycle length of 350 msec is shown with surface lead II, III, and $V_1$ and recordings from the HRA, HBE 3, CS leads and an ablation catheter. The first two pace complexes are a search of the atrial deflections, the beginning of which are hard to see in the distal coronary sinus and the ablation catheter. This third ventricular paced complex is not associated with atrial electrograms and allows one to see where the atrial electrogram began. V-A block during rapid pacing is therefore a good method to assess the exact location of atrial activity during circus movement tachycardia or ventricular pacing. See text for discussion.

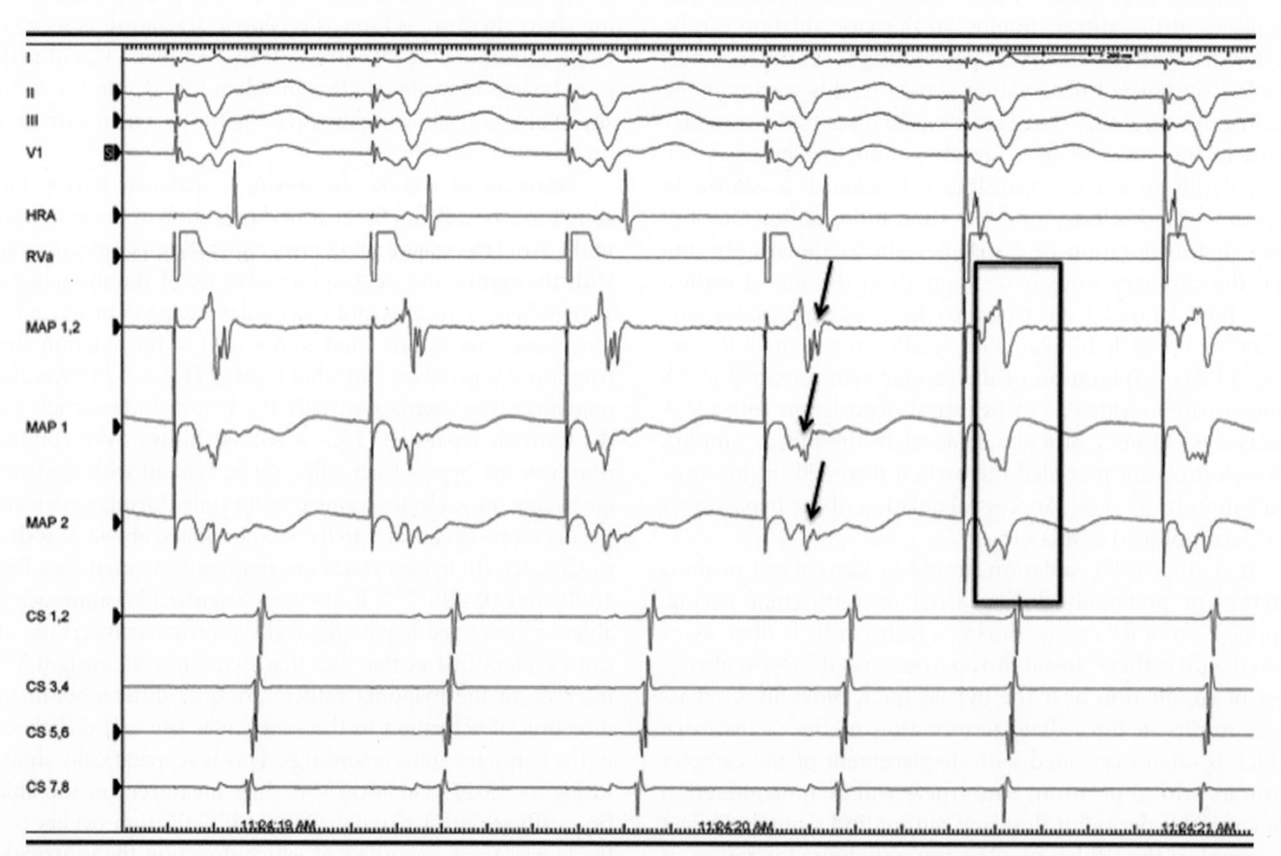


**FIGURE 13-26** *Use of differential atrial and ventricular pacing to understand the onset of the atrial electrogram.* Three surface leads and intracardiac recordings from the HRA, RV, mapping catheter (MAP 1,2 bipolar recording, MAP1 and MAP, unipolar recordings) and CS are shown in a patient with a right-sided accessory pathway during ventricular pacing (**left**) and simultaneous atrial and ventricular pacing (**right**). Simultaneous pacing captures the local atrial electrogram; its absence helps to determine the onset of the atrial activation during ventricular pacing (*arrows*). (Courtesy of Peter Low, MD.)

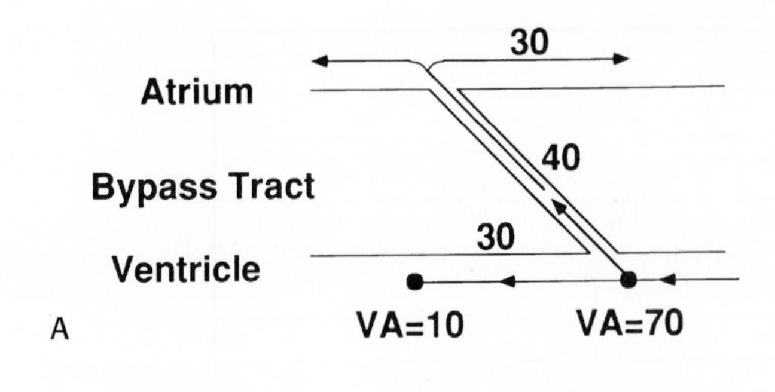


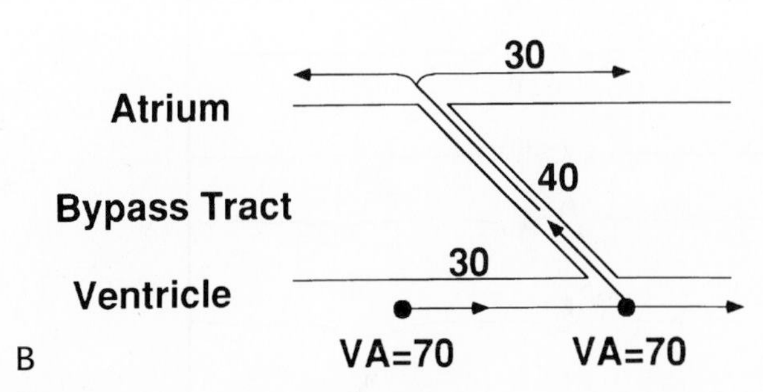


**FIGURE 13-27** *Locating the ventricular site of insertion of a concealed bypass tract.* A bypass tract is shown to connect the atrium and ventricle at an angle. The effect of a paced wavefront from right to left **(A)** and left to right **(B)** on local V-A times is shown. The ventricular site of insertion should have a constant (V-A) interval regardless of the direction of activation. See text for discussion.

interval when the ventricle and bypass tract are activated in the opposite direction.

Using the ventricular approach the catheter is positioned just underneath the mitral annulus as depicted in Figures 13-18 and 13-19, to record a ventricular electrogram and an atrial electrogram. At the appropriate position (near the ventricular insertion site) the atrial deflection is usually one-fourth the size of the ventricular deflection and during ventricular pacing the atrial deflection gets even smaller and sometimes becomes lost in the ventricular electrogram. The maneuvers discussed above can help define the onset of atrial activation during conduction over the bypass tract. During ventricular pacing, retrograde atrial activation is usually earlier than that recorded in the coronary sinus. Once this site is recorded and is stable, RF is delivered during ventricular pacing (Fig. 13-28).

During antegrade pre-excitation the site of earliest ventricular activation usually precedes the delta waves by 10 to 30 msec and is associated with a QS or rS morphology depending on whether it is endocardial, intramural, or subepicardial in location. In rare cases, a left lateral bypass tract with a long A-V conduction time (which may or may not be decremental) is present. In such cases, no overt pre-excitation is obvious in sinus rhythm, but may only be manifest by pacing at the left atrium or via the coronary sinus. In such cases, successful ablation of the bypass tract may cause a change of the mid or terminal components of the QRS, which is associated with an abrupt increase in the local A-V interval at the site of the bypass tract (Fig. 13-29).

When using the ventricular approach, because the contact is usually good, we aim for a temperature of 55° to 65°C with temperature control catheters, or the lowest power, which results in a 10-Ω drop in lead impedance. This is typically easily achievable. If one is at the appropriate site, loss of conduction over the bypass tract is accomplished in less than 10 seconds (Figs. 13-30 and 13-31). If the transseptal approach is used, catheter stability is not as reliable, and a sheath is invariably required to maintain stable contact. The sheath is usually positioned in the lateral left atrium through which the catheter is passed toward the medial aspect of the mitral annulus. The catheter can then be withdrawn slowly to map the mitral annulus until the earliest retrograde atrial activation is recorded during the tachycardia or ventricular pacing. Achievement of appropriate temperatures, or, more importantly, drops in impedance are more difficult from the transseptal approach due to the loss of temperature via convective cooling of the blood. Finally, if the ablation is carried out within the coronary sinus, and a standard 4- to 5-mm tip catheter is used, I recommend keeping temperatures ≤55°C, and use impedance drops to determine how much energy is delivered. I generally use the lowest energy, which results in a 10-Ω drop in impedance, regardless of the temperature. Use of a cool-tip catheter decreases the risk of char and, as stated above, temperature cannot be used and a decrease in impedance demonstrates effective energy delivery. Usually, epicardial pathways are eliminated quickly, but I try to maintain delivery of energy for a minute since I believe many of these bypass tracts insert as multiple twigs or broad bands in the muscular sheath of the coronary vein. Using such precautions, ablation from within the coronary sinus appears safe,[128] although I usually attempt ablation from the LV or LA first. The safety parameters of ablation in the CS using larger tip (8 to 10 mm) or cool-tip catheters are not known, but experimental studies and clinical experiences have demonstrated some potential for inadvertent damage to adjacent coronary arteries.[129]

For ablation of bypass tracts located around the tricuspid annulus, one may need to use a superior vena cava approach. The vast majority of bypass tracts around the tricuspid valve can be reached through catheters introduced via the inferior vena cava, although occasionally the catheter must be placed via the superior vena cava when the bypass tract is located inferolaterally (i.e., inferoanterior). As stated earlier in the chapter, although some investigators have suggested using a small catheter placed in the right coronary artery to guide mapping of right-sided bypass tracts, we believe this should not be done routinely and that regionalization of the bypass tract can be readily accomplished using a Halo catheter or a multipolar catheter positioned around the tricuspid annulus. When pre-excitation is present, the earliest onset of ventricular activation recorded on the ablation catheter should precede the delta wave by at least 25 msec using either unipolar or bipolar electrograms. Examples of mapping and ablation of a right anterior manifest, anterogradely conducting and a concealed right lateral bypass tract

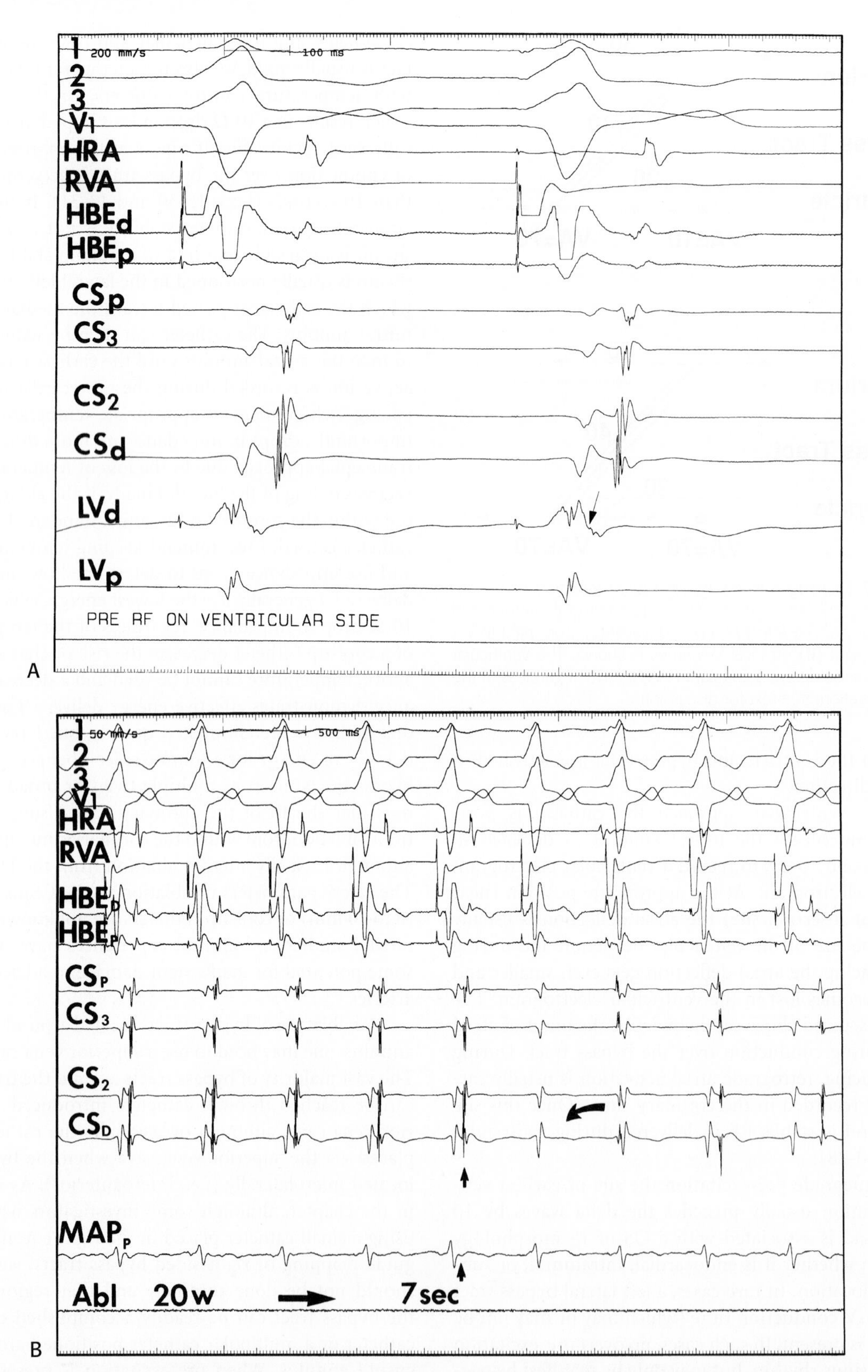


**FIGURE 13-28** *Ventricular approach to mapping and ablation of a concealed bypass tract.* Surface ECG leads I, II, III, $V_1$, and electrograms from the HRA, HBE, 4, CS recordings and left ventricular mapping recordings from the ablation catheter are shown. In **(A)**, during ventricular pacing, the earliest activity recorded in the left ventricular mapping catheter was seen to be opposite the recording in the distal CS. Note the small atrial deflection which is 30 msec earlier than the earliest recording in the CS. Rapid ventricular pacing is often necessary to discern the onset of atrial activity (Fig. 13-25). In **(B)** application of RF energy during pacing produces loss of activation over the bypass tract and atrioventricular dissociation after 7 seconds.

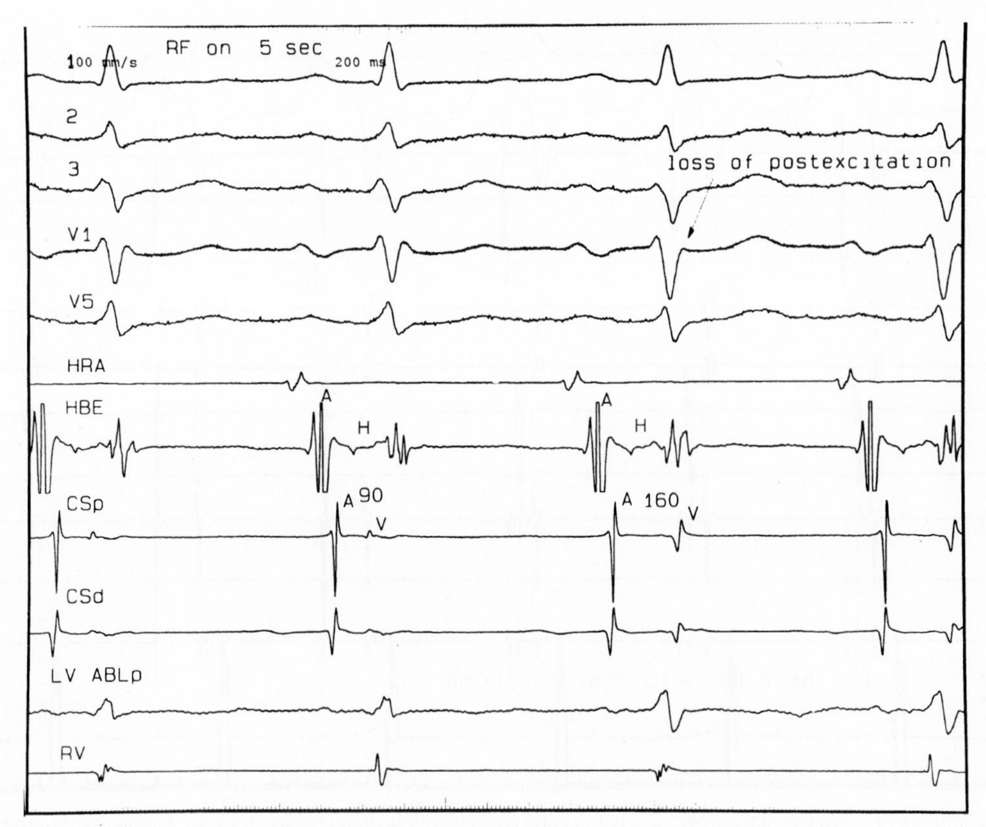


**FIGURE 13-29** *Effect of ablation of a bypass tract with "post excitation."* ECG leads I, II, III, $V_1$, and $V_5$ are shown with electrograms from the HRA, HBE, CS, and left ventricular ablation catheter and RV. A left lateral bypass tract is present with a long conduction time, which was associated with a local A-V interval of 90 msec. No overt pre-excitation is present because the area of the ventricle that is "pre-excited" occurs after the onset of normal activation. With radiofrequency application one can see a loss of the terminal forces in the QRS and a lengthening of the local A-V interval. Thus, successful ablation of an antegradely conducting bypass tract with a long conduction time may produce changes in the mid and terminal parts of the QRS since a delta wave may not be seen. See text for discussion.

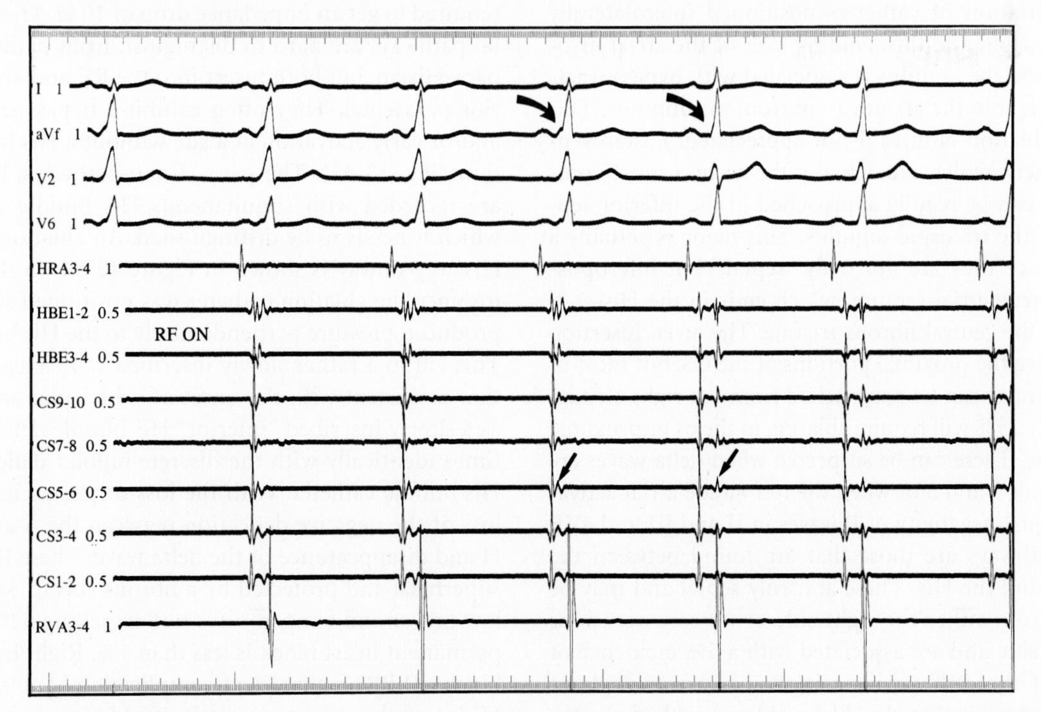


**FIGURE 13-30** *Ablation of left lateral bypass tract from the sinus rhythm.* Surface ECG leads I, AVF, $V_2$, and $V_6$ are shown with intracardiac recordings. The earliest site of ventricular activation is opposite CS bipolar electrogram 5 to 6. Radiofrequency energy abolishes antegrade conduction over the bypass tract (*arrows*), which is clearly seen on both the surface ECG and the intracardiac recording from $CS_{5-6}$.

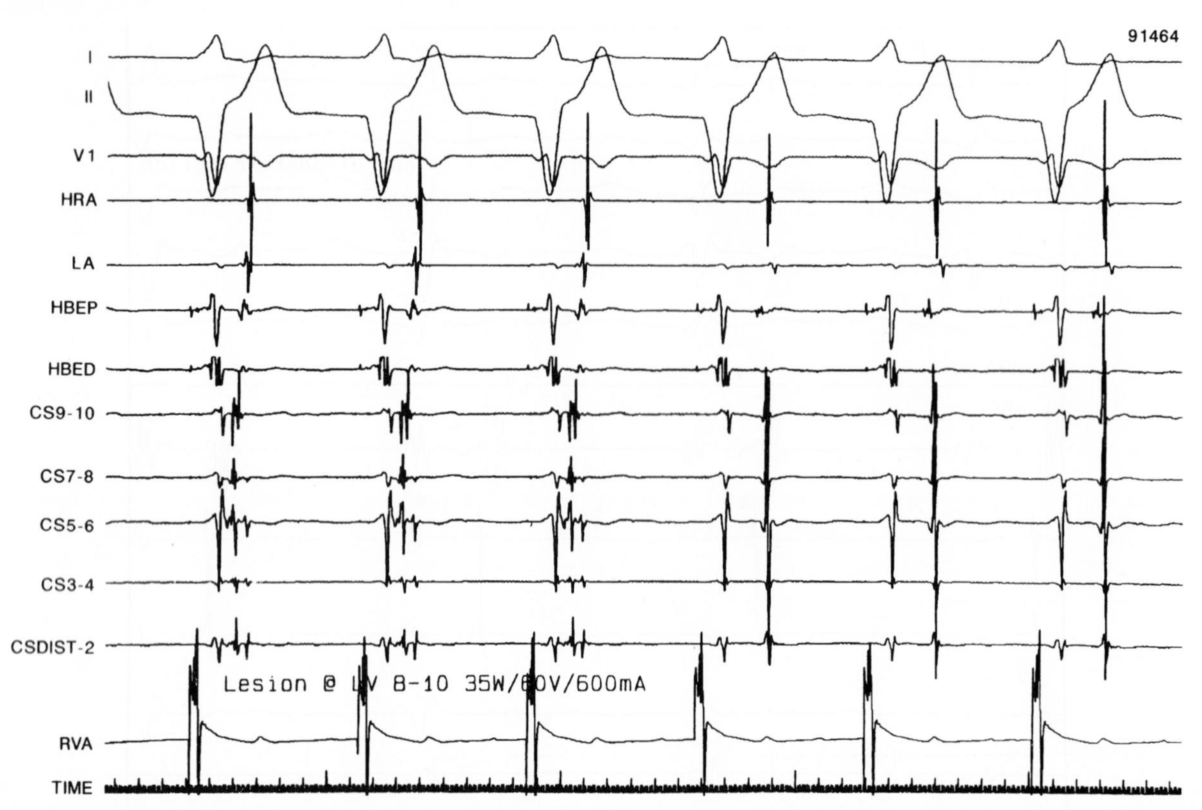


**FIGURE 13-31** Radiofrequency ablation of a retrogradely conducting concealed left lateral bypass tract. RF energy is delivered during ventricular pacing in a patient with a concealed left-sided bypass tract. The earliest atrial activation is recorded with the ventricular approach opposite CS 5 to 6 during ventricular pacing. Note the remarkable fractionation in the CS electrograms. There is an abrupt block of retrograde conduction in the bypass tract 4 seconds after the onset of 35 W of RF energy.

are shown in Figure 13-32. Sheaths are available and helpful for the stabilization of catheters positioned inferolaterally along the tricuspid annulus. Folding over of the atrial myocardium around the annulus is associated with bypass tracts that may insert into the atrium 1 cm from the annulus. This can lead to ablation failures if not appreciated. Posteroseptal bypass tracts, which are actually the second most common, usually can be readily approached in the inferior septal regions of the tricuspid annulus. This name is actually a misnomer, since they are not truly "septal," but inferoposterior to the true atrial septum, which ends in the His–A-V node area, at the central fibrous trigone. The atrial insertion site may involve the proximal portions of the CS, but most of these bypass tracts can be approached from the right atrium. Approximately 25% will require ablation in the os or proximal coronary sinus. These can be suspected when delta waves are negative in leads 2 and 3 or when the retrograde atrial activation shows equal negativity of P waves in II and III and aVF. Midseptal pathways are those that are found between the os of the CS and the His. These are truly septal and may be approached from either the right side or on rare occasions from the left side and are associated with a 5% incidence of heart block if the catheter is positioned in the triangle of Koch. Such bypass tracts should be ablated with the catheter on the tricuspid annulus or on the ventricular side of the tricuspid annulus to decrease the incidence of A-V block. Safety will further be enhanced by using the lowest power required to get an impedance drop of 10 Ω. The anterior septal pathways are hard to distinguish from pathways that are para-Hisian, but both insert into the RV and are really superior paraseptal. They often exhibit a bypass tract potential and/or early activation at a site without a His bundle deflection (Fig. 13-33). The para-Hisian pathways, by definition, are recorded with simultaneous His bundle activity from which it needs to be distinguished. An ablation of the para-Hisian pathway is shown in Figure 13-34. In this particular instance the ablation catheter was positioned so that the tip produced pressure perpendicularly to the His bundle region. This led to a rather slowly inscribed ventricular depolarization consistent with the onset of ventricular activity as well as a slowly inscribed "inferior" His bundle deflection, which times identically with the discrete bipolar deflection on the His bundle catheter. With the loss of pre-excitation there is loss of the negative deflection between the A and the broad H and disappearance of the delta wave. These fibers are very superficial and protected by a fibrous sheath, so with use of low power and temperatures not exceeding 52°C the risk of permanent heart block is less than 1%. Right bundle branch block (RBBB) is a frequent complication of ablation of para-Hisian pathways (particularly if ablation is performed on the ventricular side of the annulus) since the right bundle is often injured as it emerges from the central fibrous trigone.

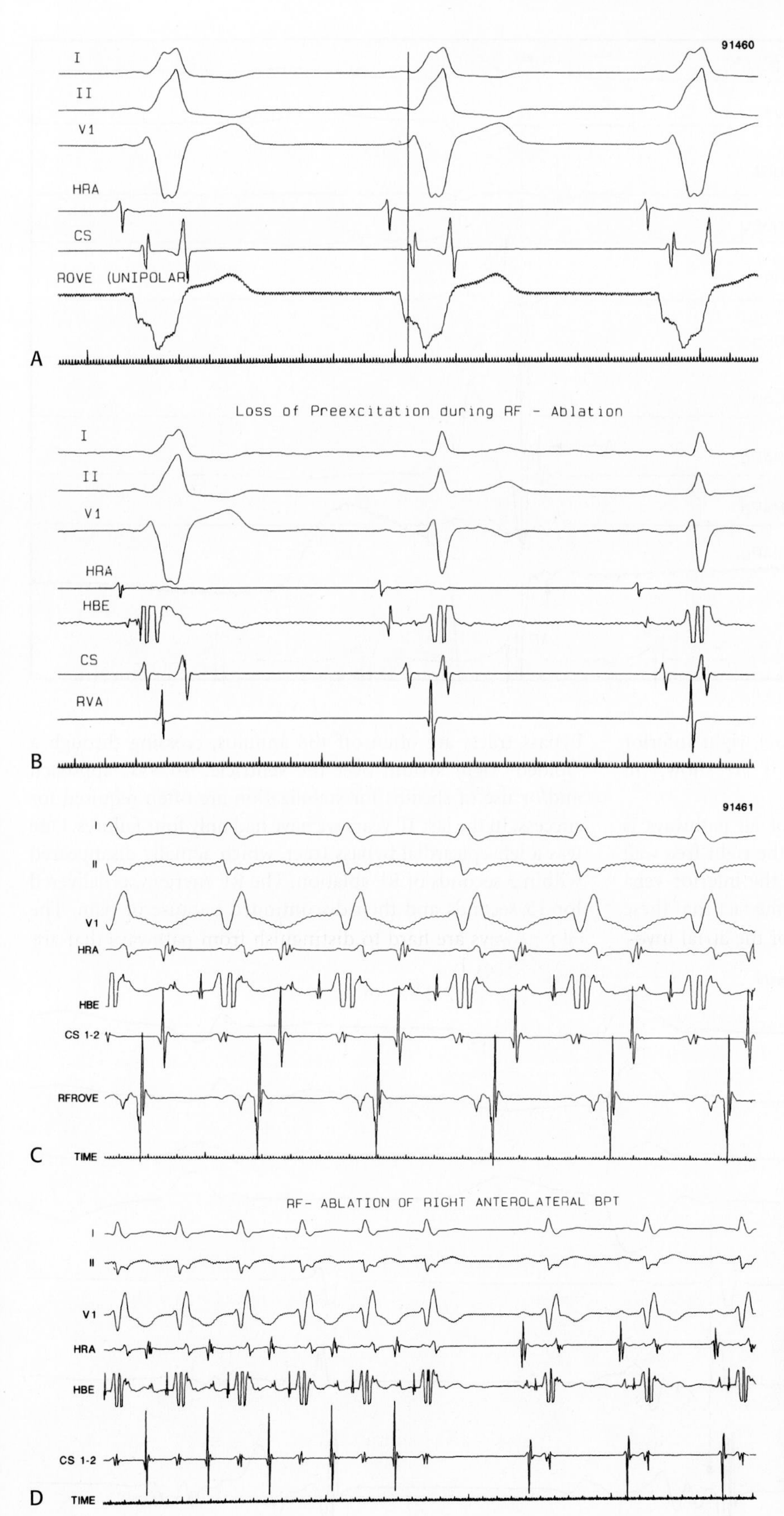


**FIGURE 13-32** *Radiofrequency ablation of right-sided bypass tracts.* **A and B:** Ventricular pre-excitation is recorded from a unipolar rove electrode as an intrinsicoid deflection 25 msec before the delta wave during sinus rhythm. RF energy delivered at this site abruptly causes loss of pre-excitation over this anteroseptal bypass tract. **C** and **D:** SVT using a right anterolateral bypass tract is present **(C)**. The RF rove catheter records earliest bipolar activity on the atrial side of the tricuspid valve. RF energy delivered during SVT produces block in the bypass tract with immediate return to sinus rhythm and no evidence of pre-excitation.

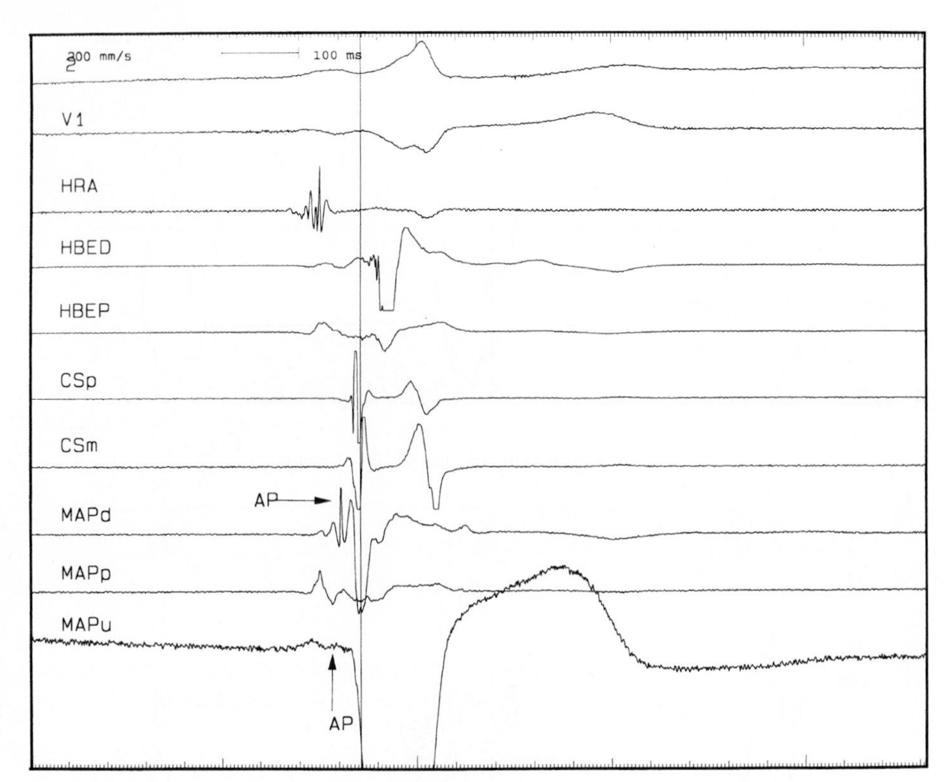


**FIGURE 13-33** *Anteroseptal bypass tract.* Anteroseptal bypass tracts are characterized by the presence of a bypass tract potential and the absence of a His bundle potential in the apex of the triangle of Koch. Note that the mapping catheter ($MAP_D$) has an accessory pathway potential in the bipolar and perhaps in the unipolar ($MAP_U$) recordings. Note that the HBE does not show a clear His deflection. See text for discussion.

Catheter positions for left lateral (posterior), right inferior paraseptal and right anterior bypass tracts are shown in Figures 13-35 to 13-37.

Our overall success rate for ablation of all pathways is 97%. The most difficult for me have been the right free wall pathways, particularly if approached from the inferior vena cava. This is due to both poor contact and the fact that these bypass tracts are often off the annulus, crossing through a "folded" right atrium over the ventricle. An SVC approach and/or use of sheaths for stabilization are often required for success. In the last 10 years we have had only four failures. One was a left epicardial bypass tract, which actually disappeared within 3 seconds of RF ablation. The RF energy was delivered for 15 seconds and then discontinued because of pain. The

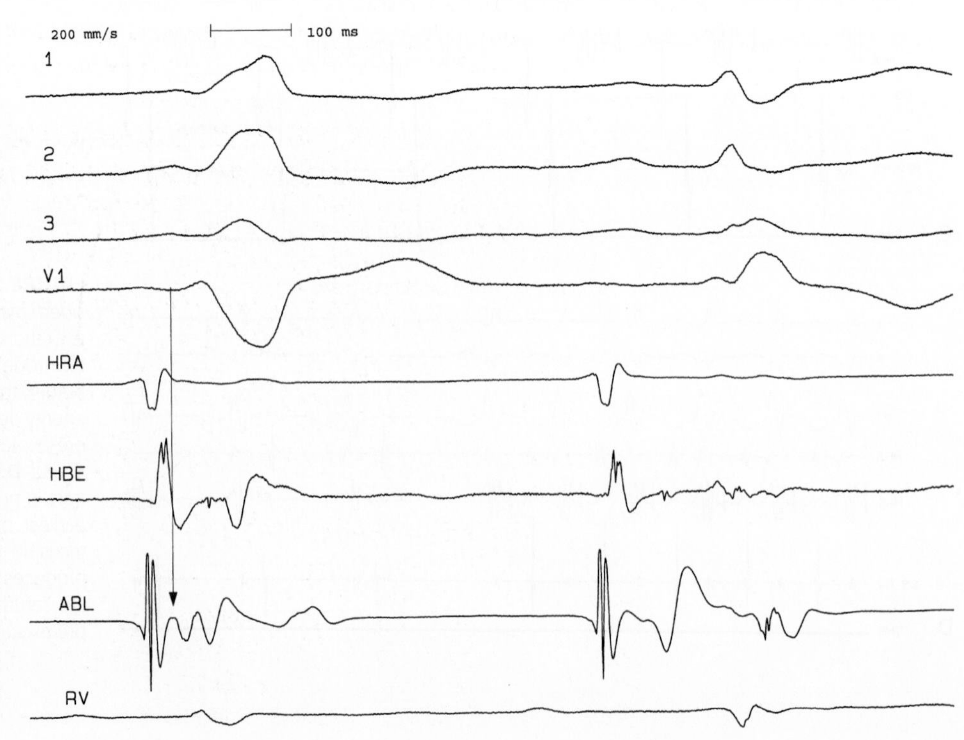


**FIGURE 13-34** *Para-Hisian bypass tract.* This tracing compares the electrograms recorded in the His bundle recording and the ablation catheter before (**left**) and after (**right**) catheter pressure caused temporary bypass tract block. The ABL electrogram recording shows a slowly inscribed potential at the onset of ventricular activation (*arrow*) which is simultaneous with a similar deflection in the His catheter recording (which represents activation over the bypass tract). There is a similar slowly inscribed potential in the ABL signal that is simultaneous with His activation. This is validated with loss of pre-excitation demonstrating consistent positioning of the His bundle potential associated with the slowly inscribed second potential in the first complex and loss of the pre-excitation in the first negative potential in the first complex. Right bundle branch block is present, which facilitates the observation of a broad slowly inscribed His deflection from the ventricular myocardium. See text for discussion.

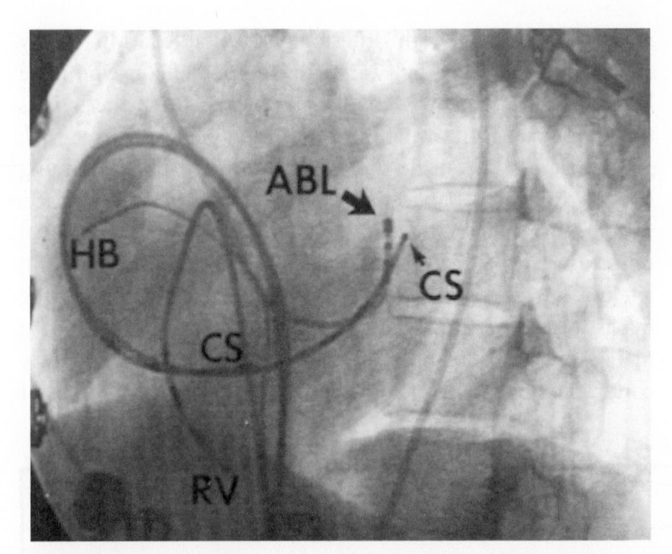


**FIGURE 13-35** *Catheter position for left-sided bypass tract ablation.* Two catheters are placed in the CS (one at the os and the other at the lateral wall). An RV catheter and a His bundle (HB) catheter are also shown. The (ABL) catheter was passed retrogradely to the LV, and the tip (*large arrow*) was placed opposite the distal pole of the CS catheter, from which the earliest retrograde activity was recorded (*small arrow*).

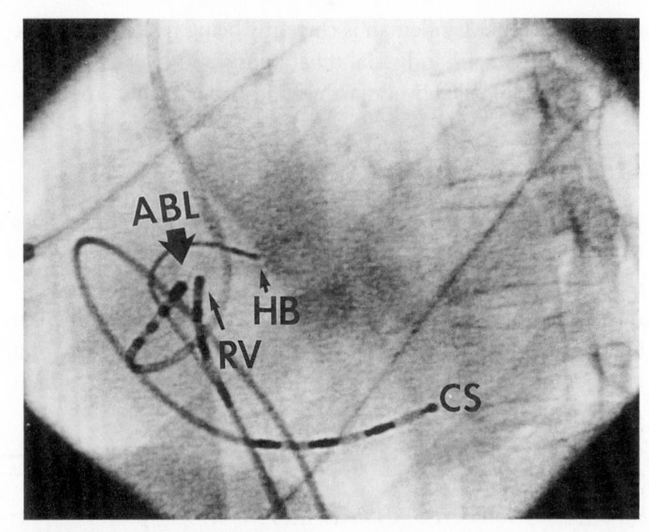


**FIGURE 13-37** *Catheter position for ablation of a right anterior bypass tract.* Catheters are shown in the 45-degree LAO view. The His bundle catheter (*small arrow,* HB) is medial to the ablation catheter (ABL, *heavy solid arrow*), which is on the atrial side of the anterolateral aspect of the tricuspid valve. A roving catheter is placed just across the valve in the RV adjacent to the ABL catheter (*thin arrow*).

procedure was terminated at that time at the patient's request. Bypass tract conduction returned several hours later. The second failure was in an intermediate pathway. Initial attempts at ablation from the right side produced transient success but the arrhythmia recurred 6 hours later. On the following day a second ablation was successful using the retrograde aortic approach. The third was right free wall pathway that disappeared in 10 seconds after the onset of ablation, only to recover 2 weeks later; repeat ablation resulted in subsequent durable success. The fourth was in right-sided accessory pathway in a patient with Ebstein anomaly. Bypass tract conduction blocked in less than 10 seconds with ablation, but recurred within 2 weeks; a recurrent ablation attempt resulted in the same sequence of events. At surgery, a 1.5-cm wide A-V band was observed with scar from RF lesion delivery in the center. Extensive cryoablation was performed but pathway conduction and SVT returned by 1 month.

In general, the greater the experience of the operator, the higher the success rate and the fewer lesions used. While success rates in many laboratories exceed 95%, the use of multisite "insurance lesions" to achieve these results should be discouraged. The use of two or less sites should be a goal and requires attention to careful mapping to achieve. We have had only two recurrences, both in two patients in whom we failed initially. One of these underwent a second successful ablation as described

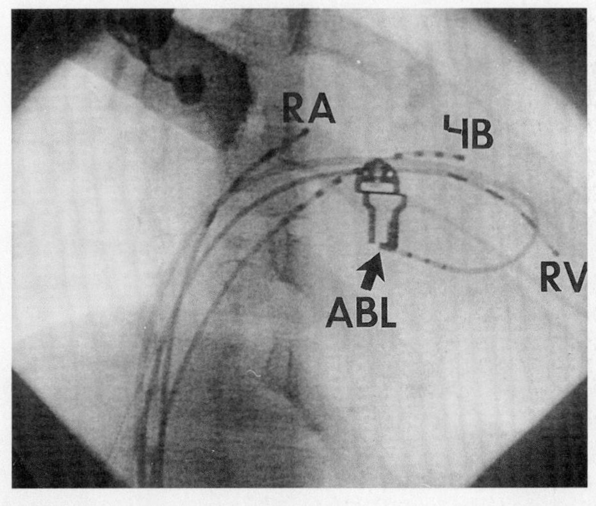


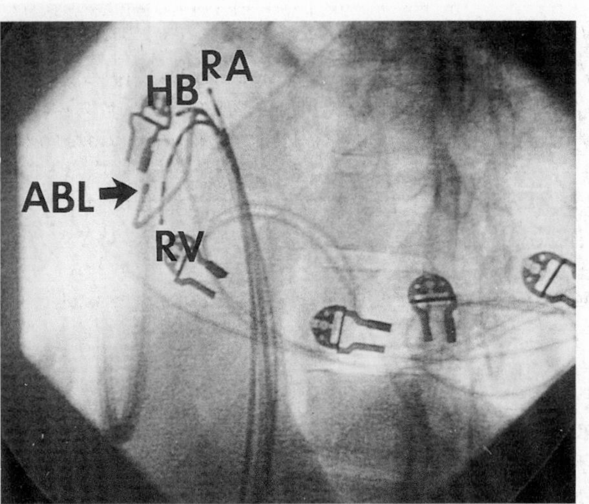


**FIGURE 13-36** Catheter position for the ablation of a right inferior paraseptal bypass tract. **A:** A right anterior oblique (RAO) view is shown in which the ablation (ABL) catheter is looped in the right atrium (RA) and positioned at the ventricular side of the A-V ring (*arrow,* ABL). **B:** A left anterior oblique (LAO) view of the same catheter is shown (*arrow,* ABL). Quadripolar catheters are also seen in the RA and RV as well as a decapolar catheter in the His bundle-A-V junction catheter.

above. The other gentleman is currently being treated for active hepatic pulmonary and renal tuberculosis and his tachycardias are readily controlled by antiarrhythmic drugs at this time.

## Ablation of Pre-excitation Variants

The two major variants of pre-excitation that lend themselves to catheter ablation are slowly conducting concealed bypass tracts and atriofascicular bypass tracts. The recognition, diagnosis, and characteristics of both these variants are detailed in Chapter 10. The permanent form of reciprocating tachycardia is generally caused by a slowly conducting bypass tract, which is commonly in the right inferior paraseptal location. In my experience, in almost half (45%) of the patients in whom we have diagnosed a slowly conducting bypass tract, the bypass tract was located in the left inferior or left posterior (free wall, greater than 4 cm inside the coronary sinus). The remaining half were located between the base of the pyramidal space, which is formed by the points of contact of the pericardial reflection with the posterior right and left atrium (right and left inferior paraseptal). An example of a slowly conducting bypass tract inserting 4 cm inside the coronary sinus is shown in Figure 13-38. In most series the majority of these slowly conducting bypass tracts occur around the region of the os of

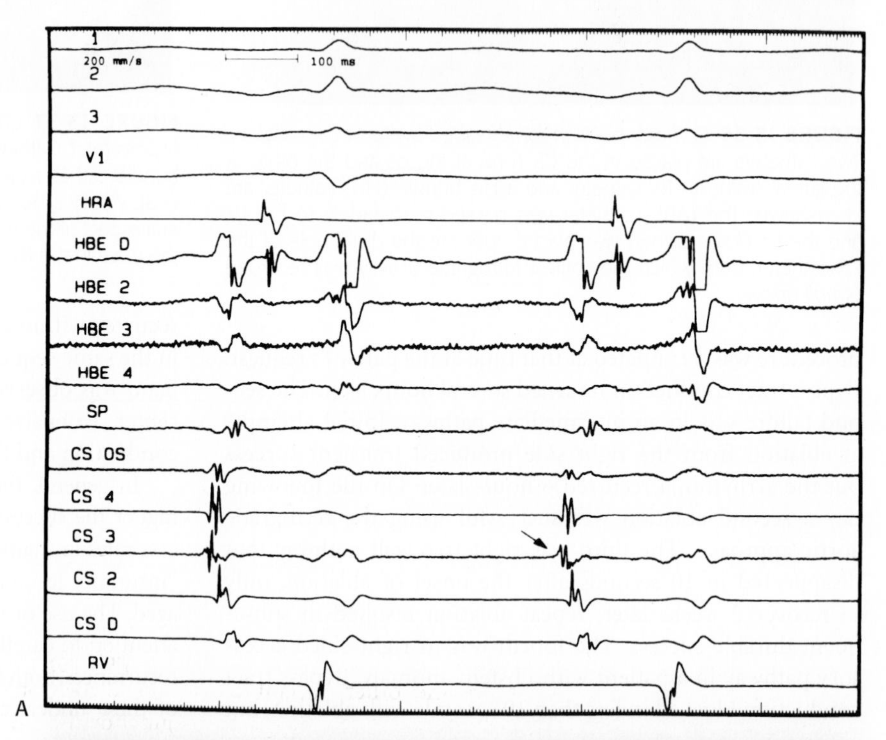


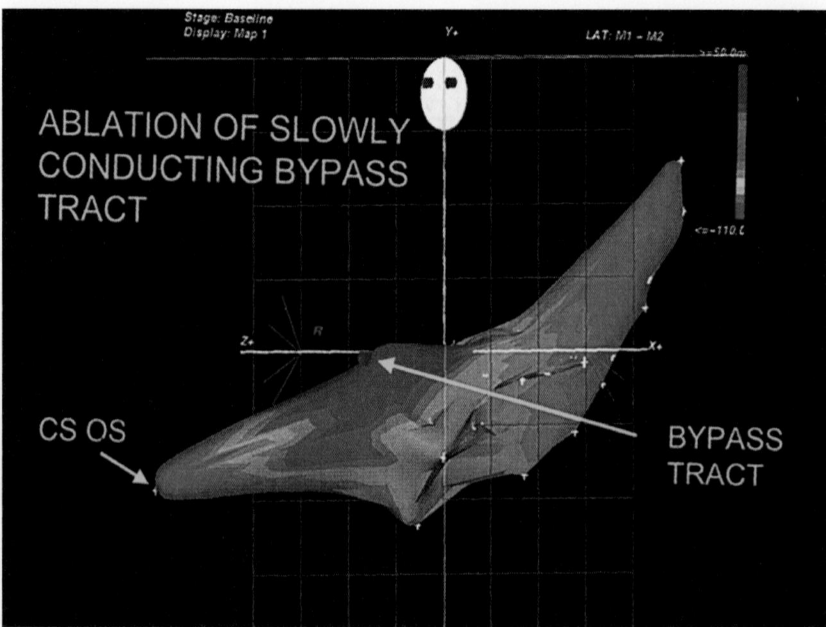


**FIGURE 13-38** Ablation of a slowly conducting left posterior bypass tract. In **(A)**, circus movement tachycardia in a slowly conducting bypass tract is present. Note that the earliest activation is seen in CS bipolar pair 3 (*arrow*). This corresponds to a site 4 cm inside the os of the CS where successful ablation was accomplished guided by electroanatomic mapping **(B)**.

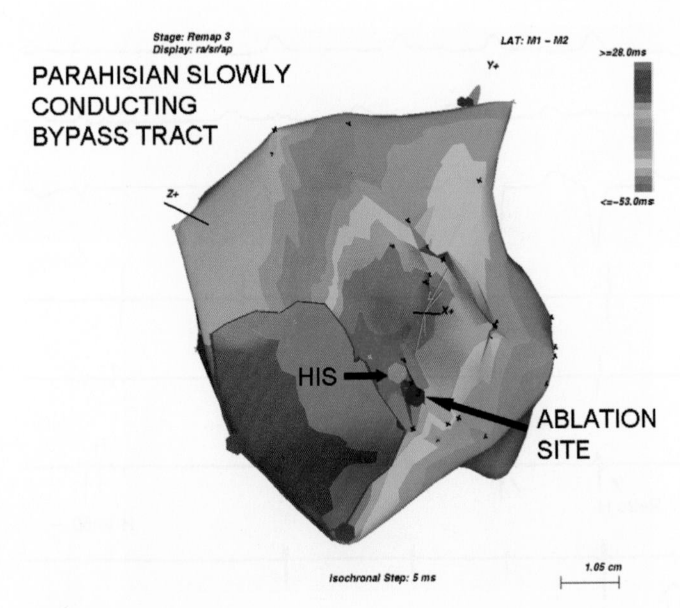


**FIGURE 13-39** Ablation of a slowly conducting para-Hisian bypass tract. Atrial activation is color coded in the electroanatomical map during circus movement tachycardia. The His bundle is marked by the orange circle and the ablation sites adjacent to it are shown. The earliest atrial activation is shown in *dark red* with subsequent activation in *lighter red, orange, yellow, green,* etc. This bypass tract was successfully ablated without producing heart block.

the coronary sinus, although others have recognized the variability of location of such bypass tracts.[130] Although unusual, I have encountered two patients with slowly conducting para-Hisian bypass tracts (Fig. 13-39). The atrial insertion sites of these slowly conducting bypass tracts usually demonstrate multicomponent electrograms. Successful ablation of these bypass tracts exceeds 90% but often requires lesions delivered in the coronary sinus.

Atriofascicular bypass tracts are the other variant of pre-excitation in which ablative techniques have been useful. Although it was originally thought that these pathways were nodofascicular, it is clear that the vast majority of these pathways originate in the anterolateral right atrial tricuspid annulus and act as a secondary conducting system inserting into the distal right bundle branch. While insertion into the myocardium adjacent to the right bundle branch is possible in some cases, the presence of a retrograde V-H interval of less than 25 msec suggests a direct insertion into the right bundle branch itself. These patients suffer from wide complex tachycardias with a left bundle branch block (LBBB) morphology and usually leftward axis, although the axis is variable (see discussion in Chapter 10). While much has been made of the precordial transition point in these tachycardias, it should not be any different from LBBB of any cause, during which ventricular activation proceeds only over the right bundle branch. Direct recordings of this pathway at the anterolateral tricuspid annulus look like a typical A-V junctional recording with an atrial deflection, a sharp spike, and a ventricular deflection. The sharp spike is believed to represent the "Mahaim" fiber, and may indeed represent an equivalent to a His potential in an auxiliary conduction system.[131] This bypass tract can be traced along the free wall of the right ventricle to insert into the right bundle branch. Details of the mapping techniques used to prove the presence of an atriofascicular bypass tract were given in Chapter 10. The approach to this bypass tract is via the inferior vena cava and may or may not require a sheath for catheter stability. Most of these bypass tracts can be located along the lateral tricuspid annulus from which the atrial and "Mahaim" potential can be recorded. Catheter positions are shown in Figure 13-40. These bypass tracts are all susceptible to mechanical interruption of conduction and some have used this to guide ablative therapy. When gentle catheter positioning is used, ablation at the lateral tricuspid annulus often gives rise to an accelerated rhythm with a left bundle branch morphology and a retrograde His activation prior to successful ablation (Fig. 13-41). This is analogous to accelerated junctional rhythm observed during A-V nodal modification for A-V nodal reentry (see subsequent section on A-V nodal tachycardia).

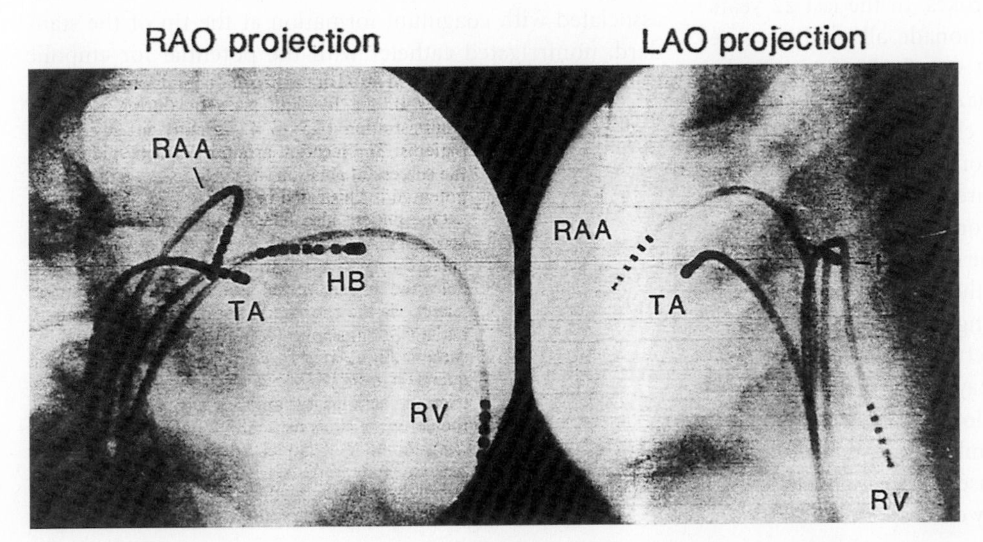


**FIGURE 13-40** Catheter position for the ablation of an atriofascicular bypass tract. RAO and LAO projections are shown with the ablation catheter at 10 o'clock on the tricuspid annulus. This is the usual site for the atrial insertion of the atriofascicular bypass tract. See text for discussion.

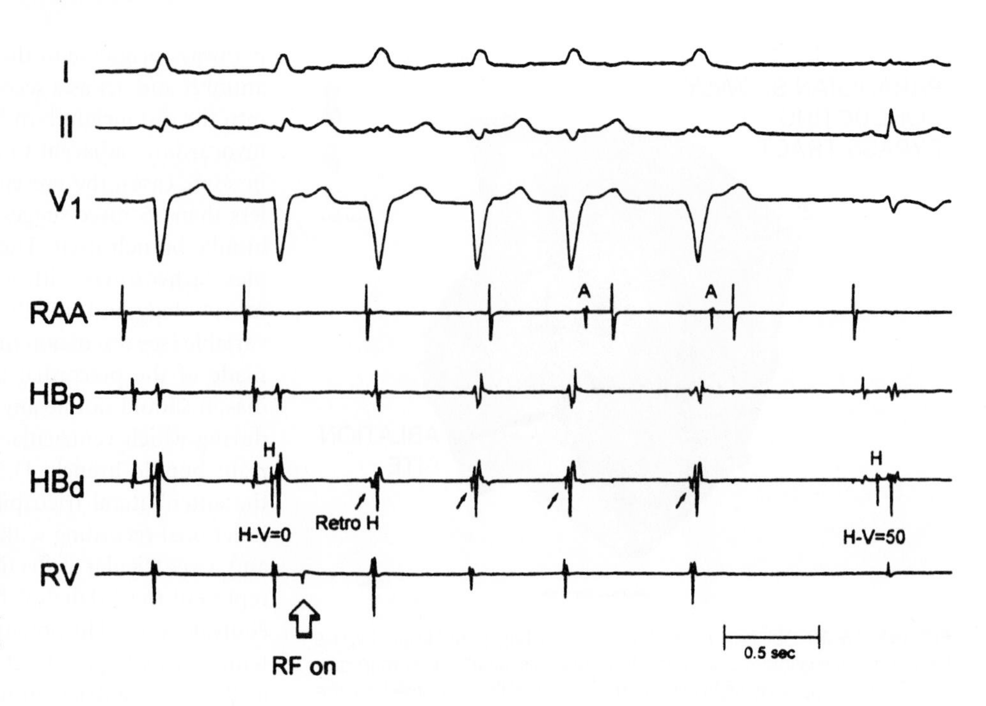


**FIGURE 13-41** Catheter ablation of an atriofascicular bypass tract. During sinus rhythm, a retrograde His bundle potential is seen with an H-V interval of 0. During RF application an accelerated rhythm from the atriofascicular bypass tract appears, which is manifested at an accelerated rhythm with the same morphology as the pre-excited rhythm but without an atrial deflection preceding it, yet with a fixed retrograde His preceding it. This then slows and is followed abruptly by loss of pre-excitation and normalization of the QRS with normal AH and H-V intervals. Note the negative T wave in lead $V_1$, which is due to cardiac memory.

## Complications of Procedures

A variety of studies have evaluated procedure-related complications. It is clear that complications are higher in older patients, but are not insignificant in all patients. In the Multicenter European Radiofrequency Survey (MERFS) death occurred in 0.13%, embolic stroke in 0.49% (most of which were reversible), myocardial perforation with pericardial tamponade requiring drainage in nearly 0.8%, complete heart block in 0.6%, arterial or venous thrombosis in 0.36%, and pulmonary embolism in 0.09%.[132] A total of 4.4% complication rate was reported. While this seems high I believe it is probably an underestimate since this was a voluntary registry, which is subject to marked bias. With greater experience complication rates go down but still exist. A more recent single center experience demonstrated major complications in 0.8% of SVT ablation procedures.[133] In our own laboratory, we have had no deaths or strokes. In the last 22 years we have had only four cases of tamponade, all of which were caused by perforation of the right ventricular pacing catheter, and one arterial-venous fistula. While we routinely use heparin for all ablations, activated clotting times (ACTs) are only followed for left-sided ablations that take longer than 15 minutes in which case they are maintained at 250 to 300 seconds. The majority ablations using the retrograde approach are accomplished after the initial bolus and prior to assessment of the ACT. This is not the case for the transseptal approach, which typically takes longer. Of note, a report by Zhou et al.[134] from the Massachusetts General Hospital suggests that heparinization alone may be inadequate to prevent thromboembolism. The development and use of other energy sources, which are less thrombogenic, such as cryoablation, cool-tip RF ablation, and use of direct antithrombin or antiplatelet agents will hopefully decrease this risk. In our laboratory, all patients are routinely heparinized during the acute study, but not following these studies. Patients having right-sided ablation receive a bolus of 2,500 units of heparin and an infusion of 1,000 units per hour. When the left side of the heart is entered for ablation (either transeptally or retrogradely) a 5,000 to 10,000 unit bolus is given, followed by a 1,000 units per hour infusion adjusted to maintain an ACT of 250 to 300 seconds. Following this procedure, heparin is discontinued. In patients who have had left-sided ablations most laboratories anticoagulate patients with warfarin or newer oral anticoagulants for 1 to 3 months. We have used aspirin and have not observed evidence of systemic or pulmonary emboli during or following the procedures. Perhaps this is due to the short procedure time and limited number of lesions delivered. Another feature that may help decrease our embolic rate is the abrupt cessation of delivery of RF energy if there is an impedance rise at all. This is universally associated with coagulum formation at the tip of the standard, nonirrigated catheter with the potential for embolic phenomenon. Another finding associated with coagulum formation is loss of power (<10 W) associated with a rise in temperature, and usually, a minimal change in impedance. These findings suggest poor contact. While we have heretofore escaped any embolic phenomenon with our precautions, the use of cool-tip catheters or cryothermal catheters probably will reduce the incidence of coagulum formation and embolization.

## Intraoperative Mapping and Surgical Ablation of Accessory Pathways

With the development of epicardial mapping by Durrer and Roos[135] localization of bypass tracts became possible and led to the first successful surgical ablation of the Wolff–Parkinson–White syndrome by Dr. Will Sealy at Duke University.[1,2] This event in fact initiated the concept that arrhythmias could be cured by surgery. While this initially precipitated an explosion of it stimulated the interest of electrophysiologists to develop both surgical and nonsurgical methods to treat a variety of other arrhythmias. With the advent of catheter ablation the surgical approach to the management of Wolff–Parkinson–White syndrome has been relegated to a minor role, only being employed following failure of RF ablation. Since the success rates for RF ablation are greater than 95%, and the remainder of patients are frequently treatable by antiarrhythmic agents, surgical correction of pre-excitation syndromes is a rare event. Nevertheless, in selected patients surgery for failed RF ablation can provide improved quality of life without the need of long-term antiarrhythmic agents. Surgical approaches to Wolff–Parkinson–White syndrome involve the use of both epicardial and endocardial approaches with the adjunctive use of cryosurgery.[7–10] Using these techniques surgical correction of pre-excitation syndromes approaches 100% with an operative mortality of less than 1%. Most cases currently undergoing surgery involve right-sided pathways, multiple pathways, and those associated with congenital abnormalities including Ebstein anomaly, transposition of the great vessels and congenital diverticulae of the coronary venous system. The rarity of the need for surgical intervention is exemplified by the fact that only 15 patients were operated on at Washington University for unsuccessful RF catheter ablation for tachycardias due to accessory pathways in the period between 1990 and 1993.[136] Most of the patients were failures because of complex anatomical abnormalities associated with the presence of bypass tracts. One of the important lessons to be learned was that excessive use of RF ablation can obliterate tissue planes in the A-V groove and/or render the tissues in these areas too friable to prohibit safe surgical correction. This further stresses my belief that catheter ablation should be limited to a few sites based on careful mapping and that the use of "insurance" burns as a result of poor mapping techniques should be abandoned. We have had one patient with Ebstein anomaly in whom ablation failed and surgery was undertaken to cure her SVTs and the CONE procedure was performed to repair her tricuspid valve. A 2-cm wide A-V muscular connection was found during intraoperative mapping and the region was treated with extensive cryoablation. One month later intermittent pre-excitation and SVT recurred. Encircling ablation of the atrial breakthrough with a cool-tip catheter was performed and in short-term follow-up she is doing well.

## Ablation of the A-V Junction for Ventricular Rate Control during Atrial Tachyarrhythmias

Although cure of atrial fibrillation is a goal, and one that will be discussed subsequently, it is not possible in most people and rate control is considered a reasonable option. Unfortunately, pharmacologic rate control is difficult to achieve and/or is associated with side effects leading to poor patient compliance. As such, ablation and/or modification of the A-V junction with subsequent pacemaker implantation is a reasonable alternative in selected patients. The first use of catheter ablation was for the creation of A-V block using high-energy DC shocks.[80,81] This technique was the mainstay of creation of A-V block and the primary indication for catheter ablation until the advent and refinement of RF ablative techniques. Since that time RF ablation has replaced high-energy shocks to create A-V block. While data[137–139] suggested that DC ablation was as effective as RF energy in creating heart block, DC ablation required general anesthesia and was associated with greater morbidity and mortality than RF ablation. DC ablative techniques were associated with subsequent sudden deaths that were related to polymorphic ventricular tachycardia associated with long QT syndromes[29,138] typically in patients with severely compromised ventricular function. Several of these patients had polymorphic VT prior to ablation and were placed on type I agents after ablation. The causative role of drugs versus ablation in these patients was not clarified. Sudden death has also been observed after RF A-V node ablation. The cause of this appears to be prolongation in ventricular refractoriness secondary to acute change in ventricular rate, leading to torsade des pointes. As a result most laboratories implant pacemakers programmed to pace at rates of 80 beats/minute or more for a month ablation with gradual reduction in the lower rate afterward.

The major advantage of RF energy is the ability to precisely block the A-V node and leave a junctional escape pacemaker. While this does not obviate the need for permanent pacing it provides reassurance in case of pacemaker failure. Moreover, even if heart block is not created by an attempted A-V nodal ablation one has the alternative of ablating the His bundle directly or accepting a modified A-V node that can conduct, albeit more slowly. Another problem with the DC ablation approach was the lack of control of the delivered energy and associated atrial injury. Most importantly, it was hard to precisely ablate the A-V node so that a junctional escape rhythm would be maintained. Even when A-V nodal block was induced, an RBBB pattern during His bundle escape rhythms was noted suggesting a distal effect of the ablative procedure. Just as frequent was the presence of a fascicular escape rhythm. The reason for the high incidence of His bundle lesions was the requirement for a good His bundle recording on the ablation catheter to assure block of any type appeared. Gallagher et al.[82] demonstrated the requirement for specific amplitudes of His bundle recordings to achieve A-V nodal block. Examples of DC catheter ablation–induced intranodal block with a normal and intranodal block with an RBBB are shown in Figures 13-42 and 13-43.

RF ablation has become the dominant mode of achieving A-V block. This technique does not require general anesthesia, and one can more precisely achieve A-V nodal block with it. The method I generally use to achieve A-V nodal block requires secure positioning of a His bundle catheter. The ablation catheter is positioned 2 cm below the third and fourth poles of His bundle catheter (Fig. 13-44). At this site, a very small His deflection may be recorded in approximately half of the cases.

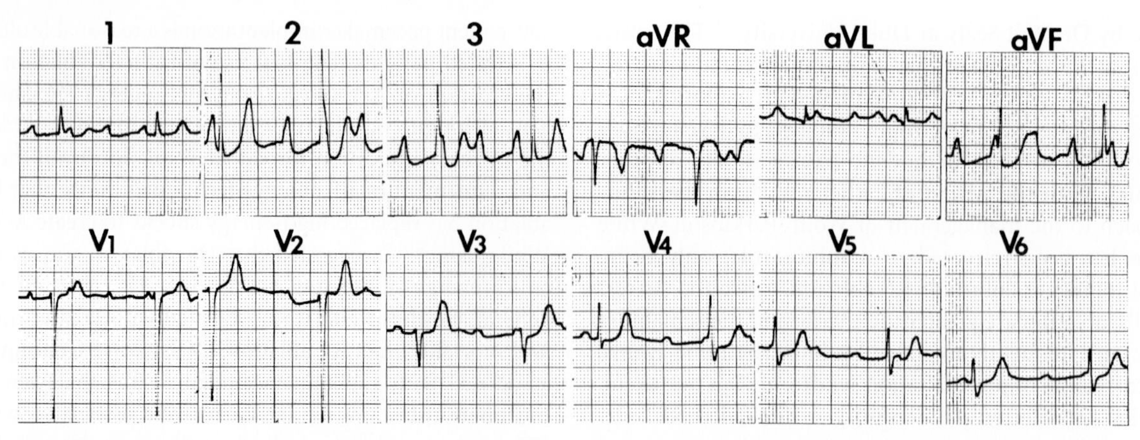


**FIGURE 13-42** Twelve-lead ECG following optimal DC His ablation. A narrow QRS complex with complete A-V block is shown. Note the reasonable escape rate.

Using temperature control catheters, a target temperature of 65°C is used and with nontemperature control catheters, any energy producing a 10 Ω decrease in impedance is accepted. I believe that regardless of whether temperature or impedance is used as a target, RF energy should begin at 10 W and gradually increased. Sometimes block appears almost immediately and at other times it takes several lesions to produce block. Typically, when one is at a good site to ablate, a junctional rhythm is induced with delivery of RF energy. Occasionally, following the development of complete heart block transient resumption of A-V conduction can be observed, which is subsequently followed by late heart block. The recognition of a potential for late development of A-V block after early resumption of a conduction following ablation-induced transient A-V block, mandates use of a pacemaker in whom transient A-V block is produced. We arbitrarily use 3 to 5 minutes of complete A-V block as a time frame for consideration of a permanent pacemaker. Patients with otherwise normal hearts have a 95% success rate. Patients who are most difficult to ablate are those with longstanding heart failure, hypertension, or other disorders in which atrial enlargement or hypertrophy is noted. On occasion, one has to ablate the His bundle either on the right side, or even on rare occasion on the left side to achieve A-V block. Our success rate in achieving A-V nodal block in such cases is approximately 85%. The vast majority of these patients maintain an escape rhythm in follow-up. An example of a patient with a cardiomyopathy and uncontrolled atrial fibrillation who underwent A-V nodal ablation is shown in Figure 13-45. In the 1998 NASPE Registry[116] the acute success rate for achieving complete heart block was 97.6% with only a 3% risk of recurrence of A-V conduction. Randomized comparisons of ablation versus medical therapy for rate control demonstrate better rate control improvement in left ventricular function, and improved quality of life with ablation.[140–142]

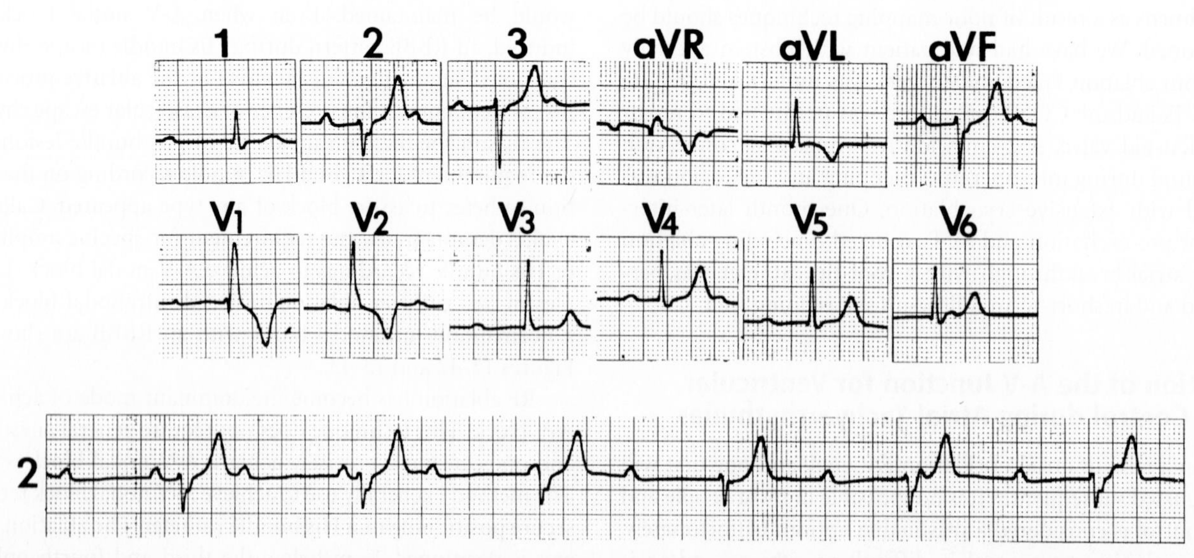


**FIGURE 13-43** Escape rhythm with RBBB following DC ablation of the A-V junction. If ablation is performed too distally, right bundle branch block frequently develops. This is most likely a fascicular rhythm because of the relatively "narrow" QRS. Note the presence of left axis deviation. See text for discussion.

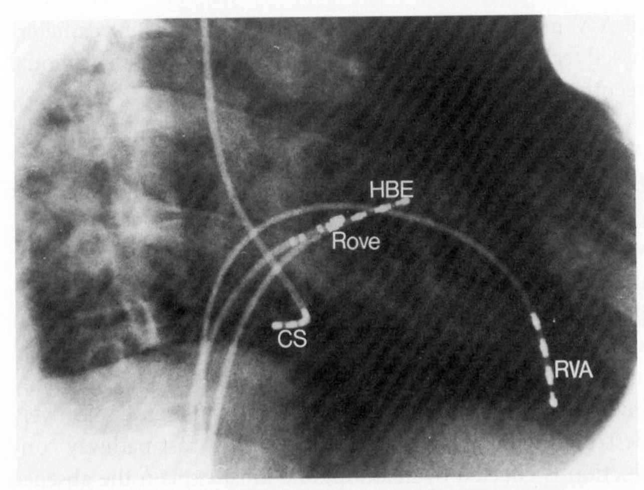


**FIGURE 13-44** Appropriate catheter position for the production of A-V nodal block. In the RAO projection, the ablation catheter is moved just subjacent to the proximal poles of the His bundle catheter. A small His deflection may or may not be seen in this position at which site block when produced is almost always in the A-V node with a good junctional escape rhythm.

Because the requirement for a pacemaker, several groups attempted to develop a strategy of A-V nodal modification to reduce the rate response during atrial fibrillation without producing heart block.[100,143] This procedure is a hit and miss attempt to injure the A-V node without producing A-V block. There are several limitations to this approach. First, it is only applicable to patients who do not have symptoms due to an irregular heart rhythm. Second, at least 25% of the patients in whom it is attempted develop inadvertent complete A-V block. Third, its long-term success is uncertain.[144] Fourth, an irregular rhythm may be hemodynamically less efficient than a regular rhythm. As such, it is our approach to attempt to achieve complete A-V nodal block. Implantation of a pacemaker in fact is well received by most of our patients.

Several studies have been performed with the hypothesis that biventricular pacing would be superior to RV pacing following A-V junction ablation.[145,146] Although the level of evidence is not extraordinary, biventricular pacing is commonly used in this setting, particularly in the setting of pre-existing structural heart disease. Conversely, in patients with atrial fibrillation in whom cardiac resynchronization therapy is used for the treatment of heart failure, many advocate A-V junction ablation, particularly in nonresponders, to reduce the percentage of conducted (and therefore nonbiventricularly paced) beats.[147]

## Catheter Ablation Techniques to Treat A-V Nodal Tachycardia

A-V nodal reentrant tachycardia is the most common form of supraventricular tachycardia, being responsible for more than half of the cases. The exact pathophysiologic substrate for A-V nodal reentrant tachycardia is still uncertain and remains under appropriate active investigation. My own personal research of the interpretation of the data concerning the pathophysiology of A-V nodal reentry is detailed in Chapter 8. Basically a few points should be made that are generally agreed upon. First, there are no anatomic specific pathways that have

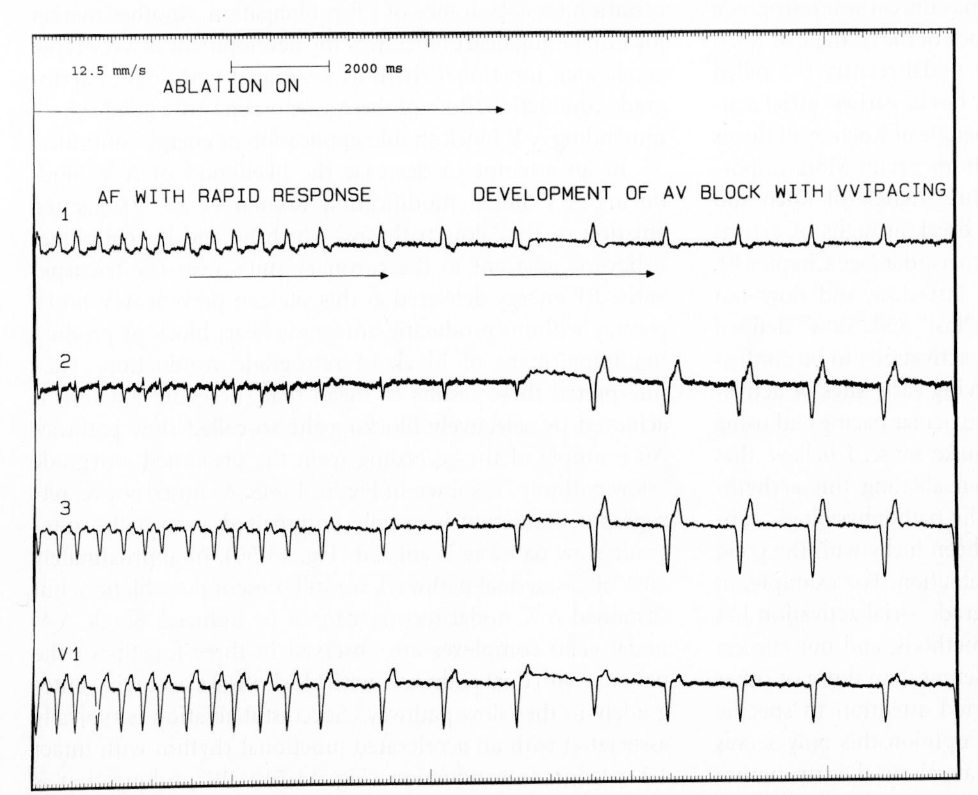


**FIGURE 13-45** *Demonstration of radiofrequency-induced A-V block to control ventricular response and atrial fibrillation.* Atrial fibrillation with a rapid response is present in the patient with cardiomyopathy despite beta blockers and digoxin. Radiofrequency ablation with the catheter positioned as shown in Figure 13-44 produced A-V nodal block almost immediately with a good junctional escape. VVI pacing at a rate of 60 (junctional rate 50) takes over on the right-hand side of the tracing.

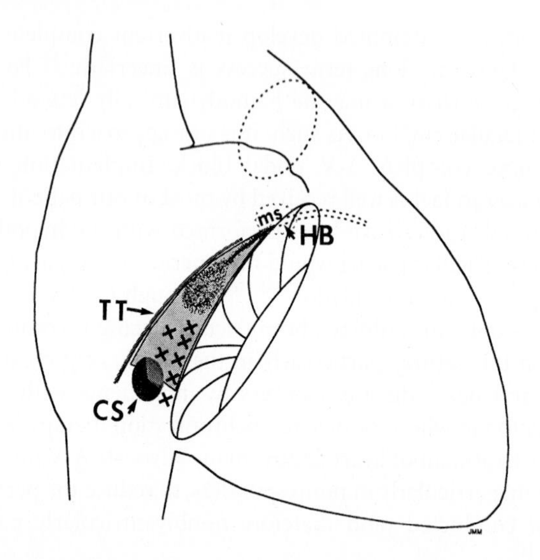


**FIGURE 13-46** *Location of "slow pathway" potentials.* A schema of the triangle of Koch is shown. Hatched areas are those over which multicomponent potentials that are believed by some to represent slow pathway potentials are seen. TT, tendon of Todaro; CS, coronary sinus; MS, membranous system.

been described that correlate with the fast and slow A-V nodal pathways. Second, slow pathway potentials as described by Jackman et al.[148] and Haissaguerre et al.[149] are nonspecific electrograms that may be found in all individuals and represent composite electrograms of superficial and deep atrial and/or nodal tissues that can be found in the midtriangle of Koch.[150] This is schematically shown in Figure 13-46. Third, although A-V nodal reentry with short retrograde conduction times (typical A-V nodal reentry) usually has the earliest retrograde atrial activation recorded near the apex of the triangle of Koch and the uncommon variety of A-V nodal reentry (so called fast-slow A-V nodal reentry) usually has its earliest atrial activation recorded at the base of the triangle of Koch or in the os of the coronary sinus, many exceptions occur. More importantly, detailed mapping of the entire triangle of Koch and the coronary sinus shows multiple breakthroughs of activation during A-V nodal reentrant tachycardia (see Chapter 8). Fourth, I believe use of slow–slow, fast–slow, and slow–fast A-V nodal reentry (with the terms "fast" and "slow" defined by apical or basal breakthroughs of activation) to be confusing. As such, the concept of identifying early sites of activation during A-V nodal reentry or ventricular pacing and using them to guide ablation does not make sense. I believe that we as electrophysiologists have been ablating this arrhythmia without precise knowledge of the pathophysiologic substrate for the arrhythmia and have been lucky with the good outcomes that have resulted from ablation. For example, in our laboratory the pattern of retrograde atrial activation has not at all influenced our ablation methods, and our success rates, which exceed 97%, are no different than those of other laboratories in which alleged directed attention to specific electrograms has been used. In my opinion this only serves as testimony as to how ignorant we are about the true nature of A-V nodal tachycardia. That being said, current catheter-based techniques to modify the A-V node and cure A-V nodal reentry are highly successful.

Initially high-energy DC shocks were used to modify the A-V node. This form of energy has totally been replaced by the use of RF energy sources.[96–100,148–154] Ablation at the apex of the triangle of Koch in the region where earliest atrial activation over the "fast" pathway was highly successful (greater than 90%) but was associated with an unacceptably high incidence of development of A-V block of nearly 10%. Even with successful ablation there was lengthening of the PR interval and retrograde conduction block (Fig. 13-47). This led many investigators to conclude that ablation in this region selectively destroys the fast pathway. However, if only fast pathway conduction is effected by ablation, one must explain the absence of retrograde conduction over the slow pathway. The fact that antegrade fast pathway conduction is present but slower, and the absence of V-A conduction, suggests the possibility that the area in which the fast and slow pathway are joined distally and that part of the lower final common pathway were involved in the ablation injury. This could account for the failure of retrograde fast pathway conduction in the presence of even slower antegrade slow pathway conduction (i.e., the absence of A-V nodal tachycardia episodes). Although approximately 50% of the patients with successful ablation at this site demonstrate the absence of dual pathways, in occasional cases, dual A-V nodal pathways are still present, and in some V-A conduction remains intact, and even unimpaired. An example of "retrograde fast pathway" ablation is shown in Figure 13-48. In an attempt to decrease the incidence of A-V block some investigators suggested using lower energies with the immediate cessation on appearance of PR prolongation. Another marker for impending heart block was the development of very rapid accelerated junctional rhythms associated with loss of retrograde conduction. Both of these phenomena are a good sign of impending A-V block should application of energy continue.

In an attempt to decrease the likelihood of A-V block during A-V nodal modification Roman et al.[154] suggested ablation of the "slow pathway," which he and his colleagues believe is adjacent to the coronary sinus near the tricuspid valve. RF energy delivered at this site can prevent A-V nodal reentry without producing antegrade heart block or producing impairment of block of retrograde conduction. They interpreted these results to mean that successful ablation is achieved by selectively blocking the so-called slow pathway. An example of the recording from the presumed antegrade "slow pathway" is shown in Figure 13-49. As noted above, retrograde conduction is usually unimpaired, even if the antegrade slow pathway is ablated (Fig. 13-50). In approximately 40% of cases, dual pathways are still present postablation, but sustained A-V nodal reentry cannot be induced. Single A-V nodal echo complexes are observed in three-fourths of the patients with dual pathways, with block always occurring antegradely in the "slow pathway." Successful ablation is typically associated with an accelerated junctional rhythm with intact 1:1 retrograde conduction (Fig. 13-51). PR prolongation is

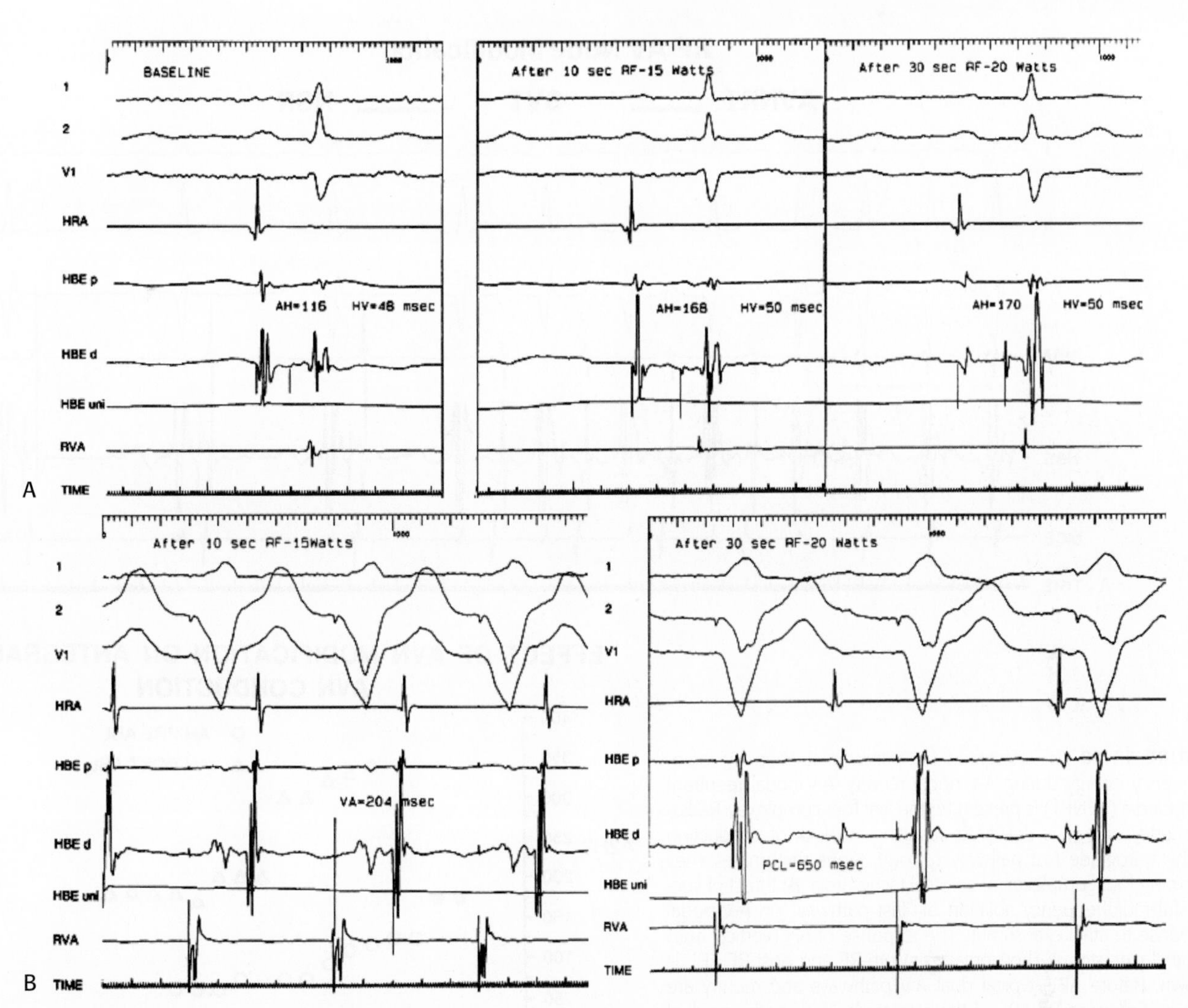


**FIGURE 13-47** *Modification of "fast pathway" with radiofrequency energy to "cure" typical A-V nodal reentry.* **A:** Three panels are shown during sinus rhythm in a patient with typical A-V nodal reentry. **Left:** The control AH is 116 msec. Following 10 seconds of RF energy using 15 W, the AH increases to 168 msec without significant change in H-V. Following 30 seconds of 20 W, the AH remains at 170 msec. **B:** V-A conduction is shown during pacing at 650 msec in the control state and following delivery of RF energy. Good V-A conduction was present in control (not shown). V-A conduction prolongs to 204 msec following 10 seconds of 15 W (**top**), and V-A block is produced following 30 seconds at 20 W (**bottom**). PCL, paced cycle length.

generally not noted. However, on occasion we have seen patients in whom ablation in the inferior part of the triangle of Koch has produced loss of retrograde (V-A) conduction, and we have also demonstrated the absence of retrograde conduction over the fast pathway with the maintenance of dual A-V nodal pathways antegradely. We have occasionally noted development of transient complete heart block with ablation at the inferior portion of the triangle of Koch, at the level of the os of the coronary sinus. One such patient developed block in the lower final common pathway with persistence of A-V nodal tachycardia during the first delivery of RF energy. Retrograde fast pathway block followed the second application of RF energy (Fig. 13-52). Of note, despite retrograde block in the "fast" pathway, antegrade conduction over the "fast" pathway remains unaffected in the sinus beat following termination of SVT. This further supports the functional nature of conduction through the A-V node, and certainly demonstrates that antegrade and retrograde conduction over the "fast" pathway are not necessarily the same. In general, higher RF energies can be delivered in the region of the so-called "slow" pathway without fear of producing A-V block. Unfortunately, exceptions are not rare. We have encountered the least transient block of the retrograde fast pathway in ~20% of cases in which RF energy was delivered between the os of the coronary sinus at its ***superior*** aspect and the tricuspid valve. The reason for this is uncertain, but likely results from proximity to the posterior extension of the A-V node at the superior aspect of the CS os (which is often large in patients with AVNRT).

As described in Chapter 8, detailed mapping of the triangle of Koch and coronary sinus has revealed heterogeneous atrial activation during A-V nodal reentry (Fig. 13-53).[155] These data are consistent with experimental studies using hundreds of simultaneous recording sites[156] and intraoperative mapping in humans[157] which fails to demonstrate reentrant excitation. A

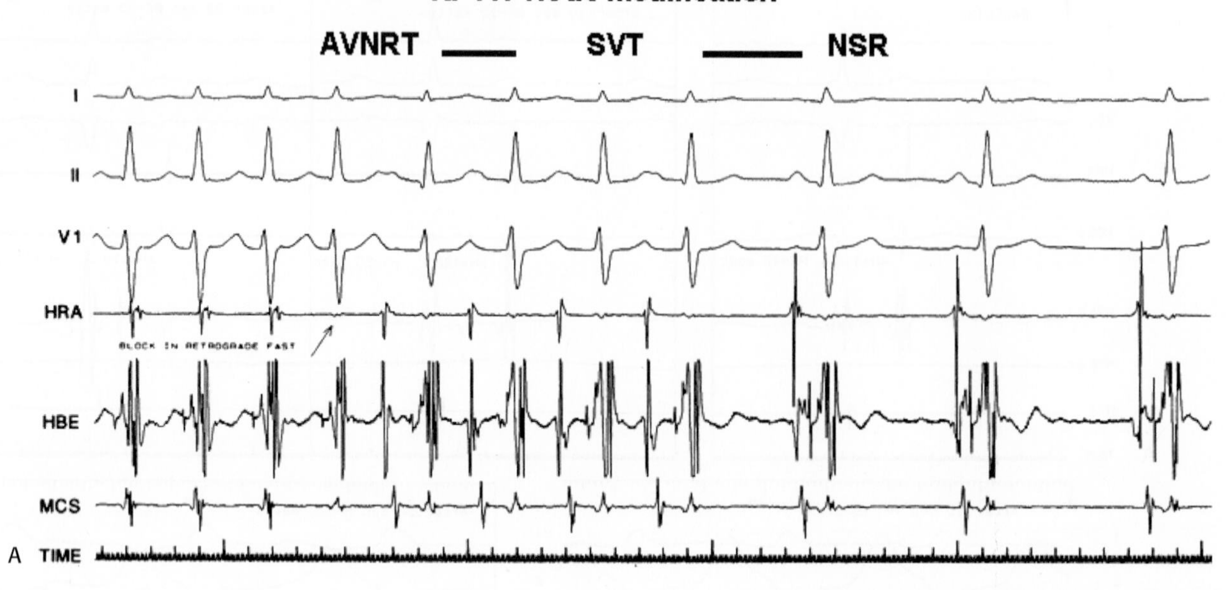


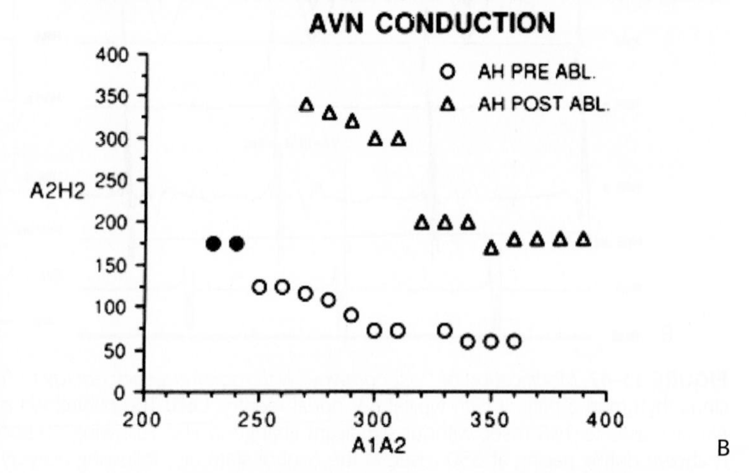


**FIGURE 13-48 A:** Retrograde fast-pathway ablation by radiofrequency energy during A-V nodal reentry. A-V nodal reentrant tachycardia (AVNRT) is present for the first four complexes. Radiofrequency energy is delivered, resulting in block of conduction in the retrograde fast pathway (*arrow*). Sinus rhythm resumes following four complexes of an atrial tachycardia. **B:** Effect of successful radiofrequency ablation of "fast pathway" on A-V nodal response to atrial extrastimuli. The response of AH (vertical axis) to atrial extrastimuli (horizontal axis) pre-RF and post-RF ABL is shown. Before ABL, typical dual A-V pathways and reentry are shown. Following RF ABL of the retrograde "fast" pathway, dual A-V nodal pathways persist. Conduction time and refractoriness of both fast and slow pathways are increased, and no A-V nodal reentry was observed. See text for discussion.

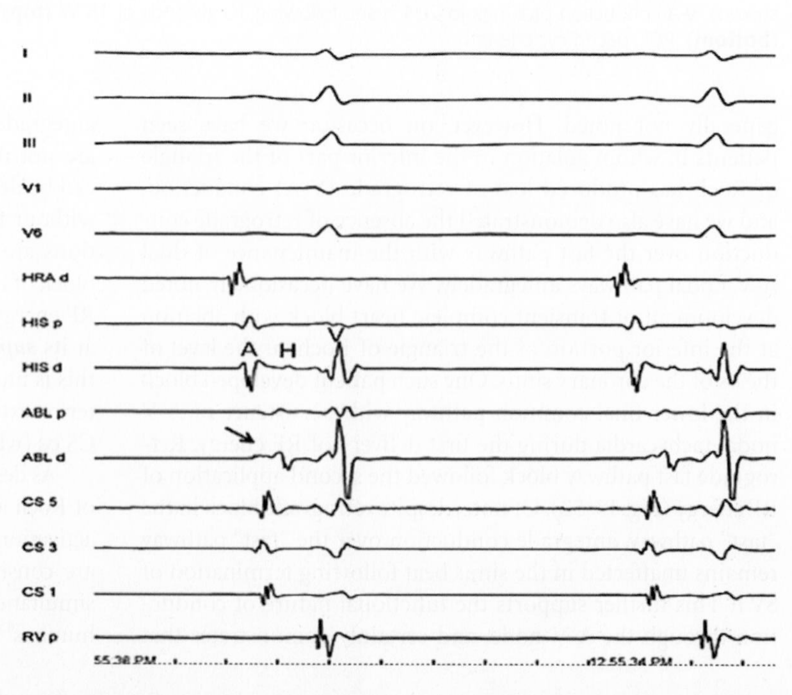


**FIGURE 13-49** *Recording from site targeted for "slow pathway" ablation.* Five surface leads are shown with HBE and CS recordings. The ablation catheter is positioned at a site targeted for slow pathway ablation. Note the ablation site ($ABL_d$) demonstrates a low-amplitude slow component followed by a high-frequency component, both of which occur significantly later than atrial activity in the HBE.

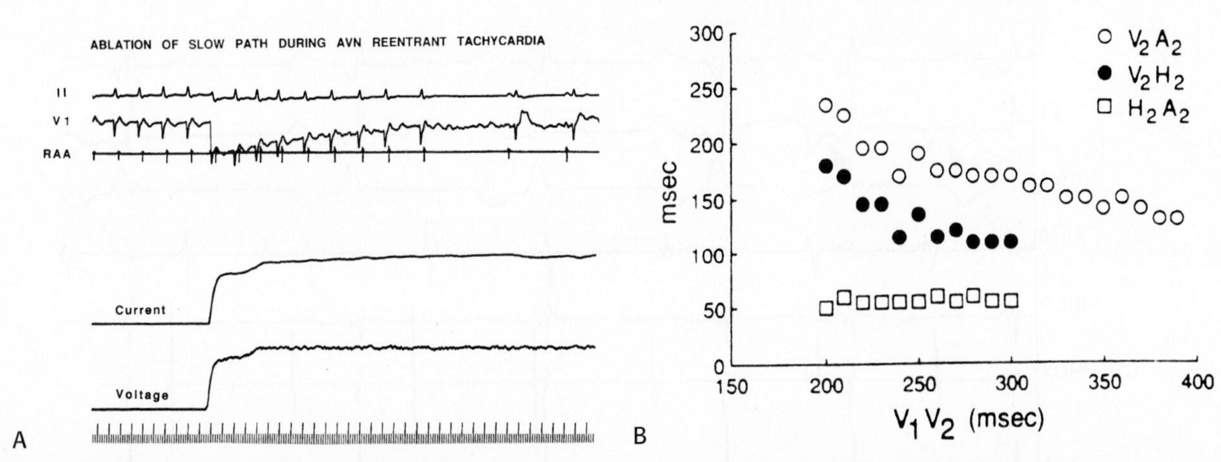


**FIGURE 13-50 A:** Anterograde "slow-pathway" ablation during SVT. ECG lead II and $V_1$ and electrograms from the RAA are shown. During typical AVNRT SVT, RF energy slows, then terminates SVT by block in the slow pathway. **B:** Retrograde conduction following ablation of the "slow pathway." Retrograde conduction in response to VPCs is slow. Conduction times are plotted on the vertical axis, and coupling intervals of VPCs are on the horizontal axis. Note the constant H-A interval with parallel VH and V-A curves—a normal response.

number of patients were noted to have nearly simultaneous activation of the apex and base of the triangle of Koch (the so-called slow pathway region) as well as additional breakthroughs in the coronary sinus. Patients in whom such activation patterns are noted appear to be at higher risk for the development of transient and/or permanent A-V block. As such, we always carefully map the apex and base of the triangle of Koch and coronary sinus. If atrial activation at the apex and base of the triangle of Koch occur within 5 msec of one another, we use temperatures initially set at 55°C beginning at the *inferior* border of the coronary sinus os at the tricuspid annulus. During the accelerated junctional rhythm at such sites atrial pacing is often performed to assure maintenance of 1:1 antegrade conduction. The optimal response to RF ablation should be: (a) loss of conduction over the slow pathway, (b) an increase in Wenckebach cycle length, (c) an increase in the effective refractory and functional refractory period of the A-V node, (d) no effect or shortening of the A-H interval in sinus rhythm, and (e) preservation without change in retrograde conduction. The mechanism of producing junctional rhythms is unclear. While some believe this is due to thermal injury of the "slow" pathway, studies in our laboratory[158] suggest that this may be produced by either uncoupling of the superficial atrium from the underlying transitional cells or A-V node, and/or nonspecific heating of the subatrial transitional nodal cells, which in both instances can result in automatic firing. Change in detailed retrograde activation during junctional rhythms when compared to A-V nodal reentry is more consistent with the latter hypothesis. An example of subtle but definite qualitative and quantitative changes in retrograde conduction during

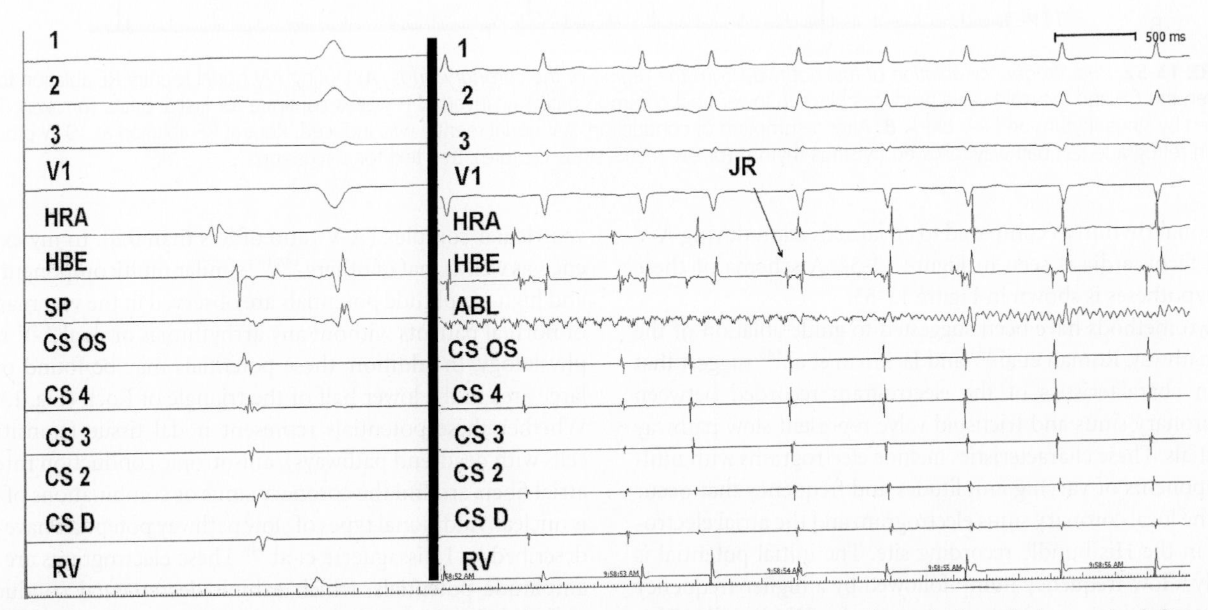


**FIGURE 13-51** *Junctional rhythm associated with successful RF application.* The site of ablation is shown in sinus rhythm on the **left**. Note the "late" local atrial electrogram at the SP. RF energy applied at this site produces an accelerated junctional rhythm (**right**).

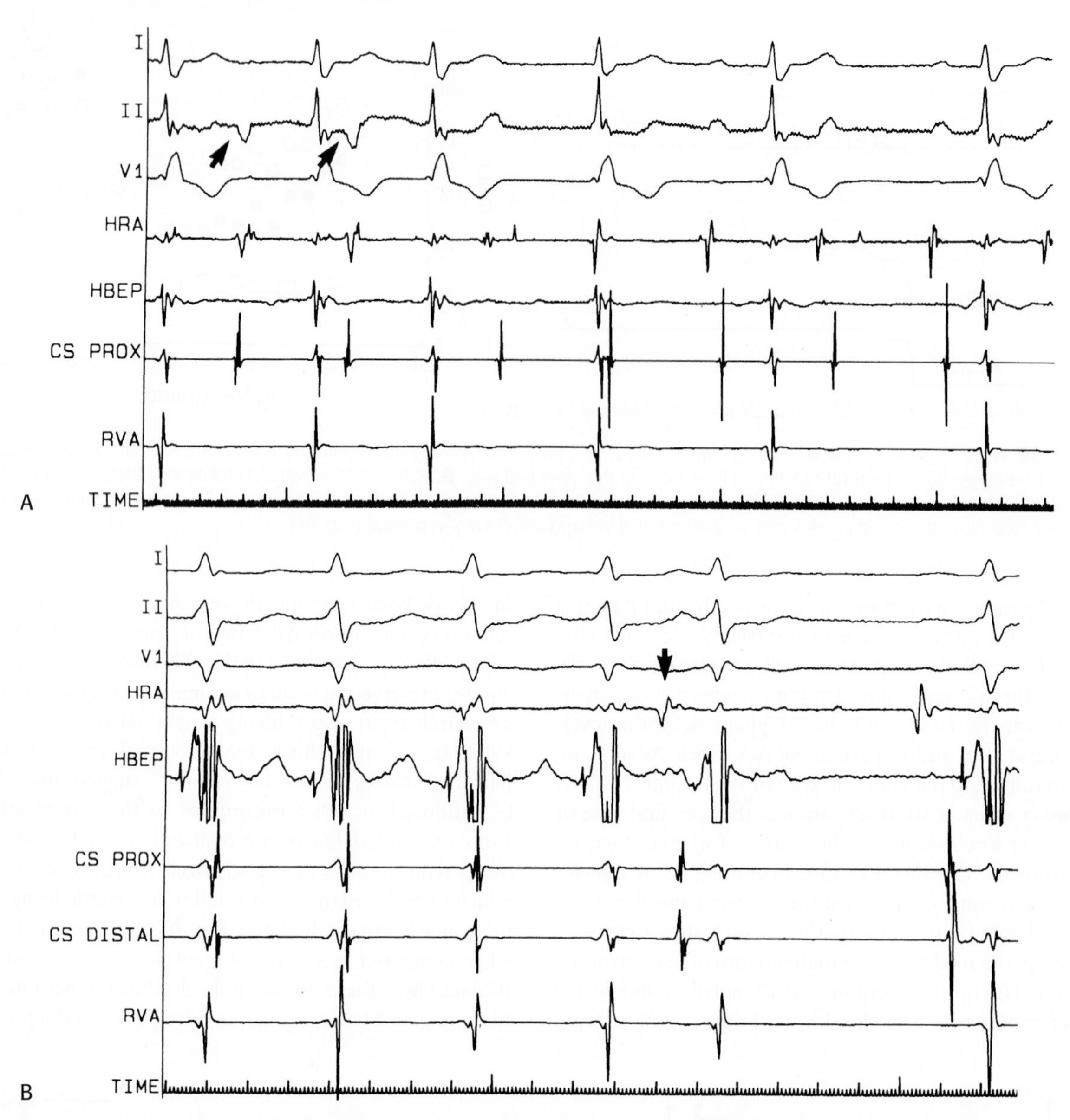


**FIGURE 13-52** *Radiofrequency ablation of fast pathway from the region of the coronary sinus.* **A:** During A-V nodal reentry RF ablation to area between the CS and tricuspid valve produces block in lower final common pathway; inverted P waves continue for first 2 beats (*arrows*). This is followed by sinus rhythm and A-V block. **B:** After resumption of conduction, A-V nodal reentry was induced. Repeat RF ablation at 10 W produces block in retrograde fast pathway followed by sinus rhythm (*arrow* marks sinus capture). See text for discussion.

junctional rhythm as compared to atrial activation during A-V nodal tachycardia is seen in Figure 13-54. A schema of these two hypotheses is shown in Figure 13-55.

Two methods have been suggested to guide ablation of the slow pathway. Roman et al.[154] and Jackman et al.[148] suggest that certain characteristics of the electrogram recorded between the coronary sinus and tricuspid valve represent slow pathway potentials. These characteristics include electrograms with multicomponents of varying amplitudes and frequency that occur after the local coronary sinus electrogram and the atrial electrogram in the His bundle recording site. The initial potential is usually a low-frequency hump followed by a higher-frequency component that may occur as late as the His bundle. This so-called slow pathway electrogram is associated with a large ventricular complex (A-V ratio of less than 0.3). In my experience, as well as that of others,[148,150] similar multicomponent low- and high-amplitude potentials are observed in the vast majority of normal patients without any arrhythmias or dual A-V nodal physiology. In addition, these potentials may be found over a large area in the lower half of the triangle of Koch (Fig. 13-56). Whether these potentials represent nodal tissue (transitional cells with dead-end pathways), anisotropic conduction through atrial fibers around the coronary sinus or combinations of both is unclear. Additional types of slow pathway potentials have been described by Haissaguerre et al.[149] These electrograms are low-amplitude potentials, which exhibit decremental conduction and are believed to represent nodal cells. As with the potentials described by Jackman et al.[123] these potentials are also found in

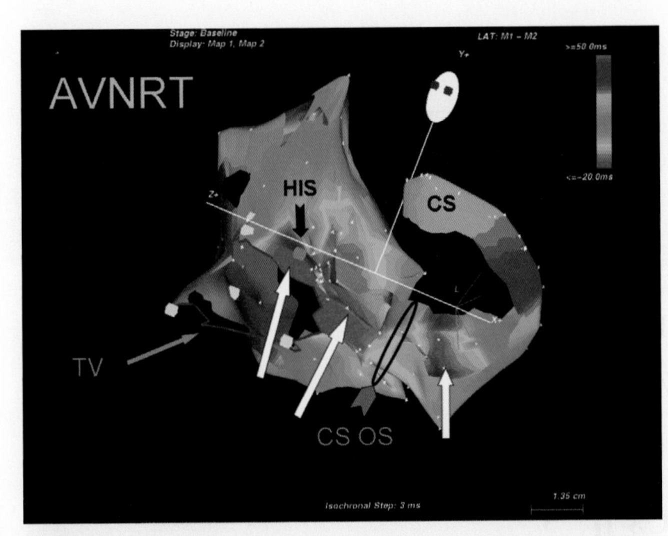


**FIGURE 13-53** *Heterogeneous activation of the triangle of Koch and coronary sinus in AVNRT.* Electroanatomic mapping of AVNRT is shown in a tilted LAO (**top**) view. Some of the wall has been removed to allow visualization of the triangle of Koch. This is an isochronal map with 3 msec isochrones from *red* (earliest) to *purple* (latest).The entire triangle of Koch is activated nearly simultaneously (*white arrows*). An additional early breakthrough is seen in the CS (*white arrow*). The His, CS os and tricuspid valve (TV) are marked. No evidence of reentrant excitation is seen.

patients without A-V nodal tachycardia or dual pathway physiology. In both instances experimental work has demonstrated that these types of "slow pathway potentials" are actually composite electrograms reflecting electrical activity both near and distant, from different tissues. As such they do not represent any specific pathophysiologic substrate but merely an anatomic site in which these tissues overlie one another. The second method that has been more widely employed is an anatomic approach in which there is a stepwise positioning of the ablation catheter from low in the triangle of Koch to more superior areas.[151] The catheter is first placed at the base of the triangle of Koch at the level of the inferior portion of the os of the coronary sinus with the tip at the tricuspid annulus to record a large ventricular electrogram and a small atrial electrogram. RF energy is delivered, and if no junctional rhythm is produced the catheter is moved superiorly by a few millimeters. Repeated delivery of RF energy is applied until an accelerated junctional rhythm is noted. RF energy is maintained for approximately 1 minute, after which stimulation is performed to assess the effect of ablation. The most successful sites of ablation are just at the anterior aspect of the os of the coronary sinus at the tricuspid valve. According to these investigators, approximately one-third of patients require ablation superior to the os. Although ablation above the level of the "ceiling" of the coronary sinus can be effective for ablation of A-V nodal tachycardia, these would be considered midseptal sites, and the risk of heart block is much higher. Care must be taken to assure that the distal ablation pair is recording a very large ventricular electrogram with only a small atrial electrogram. Delivery of energy to a more posterior position in which the atrial and ventricular electrograms are equal in amplitude may result in A-V block. In our laboratory we use a combination of approaches. We generally start with an ablation lesion delivered at the level of the CS of the coronary sinus adjacent to the tricuspid valve where a multicomponent delayed atrial electrogram is observed. RF energy is delivered with a temperature of 60° to 65°C. The atrial EGM is often activated 30 to 40 msec later than the atrial electrogram recorded on the HBE. The

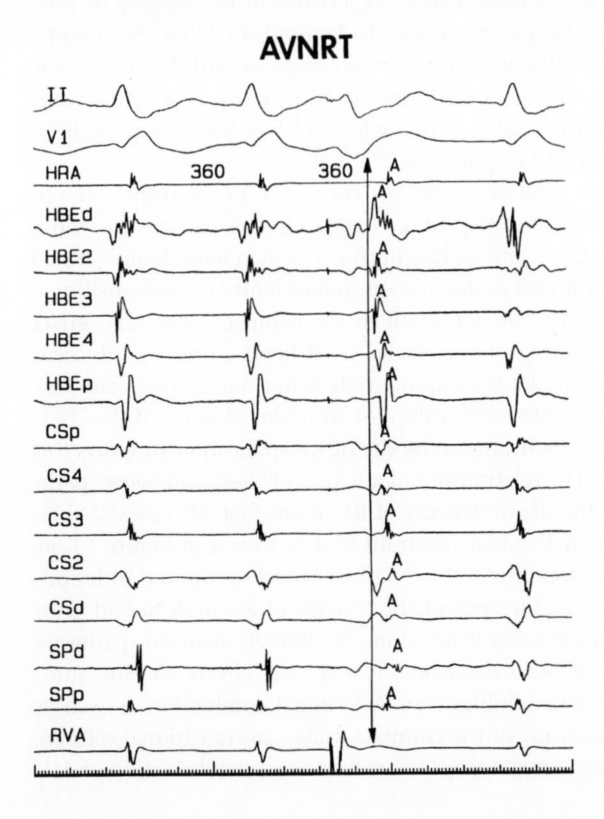


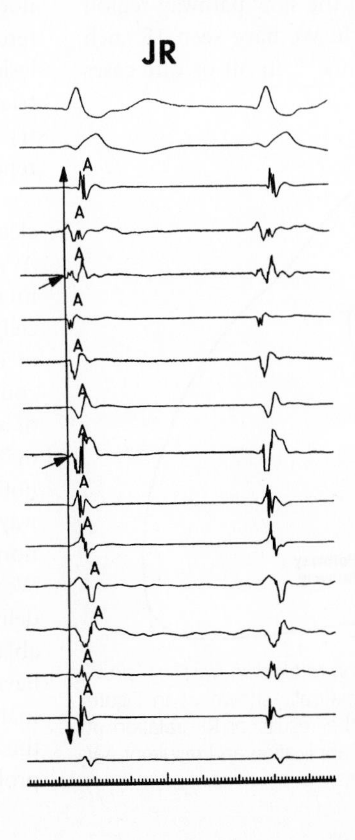


**FIGURE 13-54** *Subtle differences in atrial activation during AVNRT and junctional rhythm.* AVNRT on the left and junctional rhythm on the right demonstrate subtly different qualitative and quantitative atrial activation patterns (see text and Chapter 8).

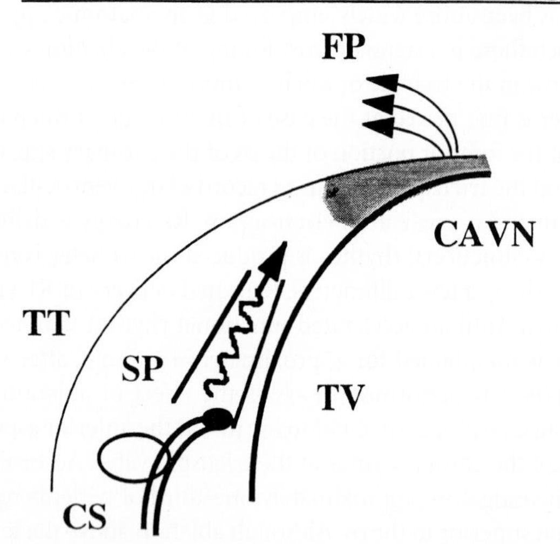


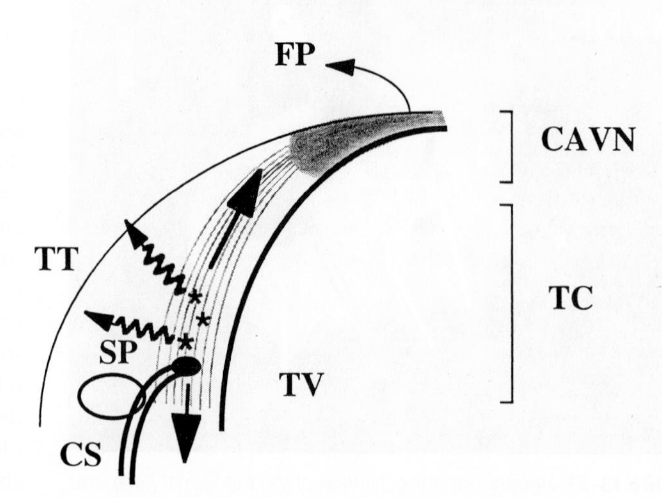


**FIGURE 13-55** *Proposed mechanism for junctional rhythm during RF ablation.* The conventional hypothesis (**left**) suggests that the slow pathway is stimulated, producing the identical activation pattern as AVNRT. Our hypothesis is that the tissue ablated is both stimulated and uncoupled (atrium from the transitional cells, and possibly the posterior extension of the compact A-V node) to produce a variable pattern of atrial activation. See Chapter 8 for detailed discussion.

development of a rapid junctional rhythm or loss of retrograde conduction, or increase in the PR interval of conducted beats mandates immediate cessation of RF delivery. Using this technique we have had success in 320 out of 325 consecutive cases, and only one incidence of complete A-V block. Block occurred almost instantly when energy was delivered at the level of the CS at the tricuspid valve. Such events are humbling and make one realize how little we know about the A-V junction.

In occasional patients earliest retrograde atrial activation is in the CS with later activation in the slow pathway region or the apex of the triangle of Koch. We have seen 18 such examples in 222 consecutive patients.[159] In all of our cases successful ablation has been accomplished with the standard approach described above. Others, however, have noted occasional incidences in which ablation in the coronary sinus or even the left side of the heart may be necessary.[126,160–162] The mechanism by which ablation works in these cases is unclear. Anatomically one must remember the A-V node is a subepicardial cardiac structure lying between the two atria just anterior to the CS OS. It is not surprising therefore that ablation in the CS os can injure the A-V node itself and terminate A-V nodal tachycardia. Earlier experience in the surgery of posteroseptal bypass tracts clearly demonstrated that cryothermal lesions underneath the coronary sinus toward the apex of the triangle of Koch could produce heart block. A-V nodal reentry requiring ablation in the lateral CS or left atrium has been reported, but is quite rare.[126,163]

**FIGURE 13-56** *Relation of site of ablation to block in "fast" or "slow" pathway.* The triangle of Koch is schematically shown as in Figure 13-46. Three regions are shown with the results of RF ablation at these sites. There is overlap in site of RF application and resultant A-V nodal conduction. See text for discussion.

How ablation works to "cure" A-V nodal reentry is not clear. While a few postmortem studies of patients in whom A-V nodal ablations had been performed have demonstrated intact compact nodes, the amount of injury to the transitional cells, injury but not death to the compact node, and effect of uncoupling of superficial atrial fibers from the subjacent compact nodal transitional cells is not understood. The lack of an absolute relationship for RF-induced block of the "fast" or "slow" pathways to the site of RF application supports this notion. The relationship of ablation of "fast" and "slow" pathway to the site of delivery of RF in our first 300 cases of ablation for A-V nodal reentrant SVT is shown in Figure 13-56. We have seen three "slow" pathway blocks produced by lesions delivered at the apex of the triangle of Koch. Both had prior ablations at other institutions. No discrete anatomic pathways have ever been described. Nonspecific effects altering summation and inhibition of A-V nodal conduction as well as the anisotropy of the compact node and transitional cells are probable contributing factors to the successful ablation of A-V nodal tachycardia. The persistence of dual A-V nodal pathways in 40% of patients who remain free of clinical arrhythmias suggests an alteration in the functional capabilities of the circuit to perpetuate themselves, perhaps related to change in the size of the potential reentrant circuit (e.g., smaller) such that a greater (steeper) curvature is needed to turn around in the smaller space, which results in the failure of conduction.

I do not think the results of ablation provide any clue in helping to resolve the issue of whether or not some part of the atrium is required for A-V nodal reentry. Clearly, in the vast majority of, if not in all, cases, successful ablation is associated with a change in A-V nodal conduction of one form or another. In addition, successful ablation almost always is associated with the induction of junctional rhythms and not ectopic atrial rhythms. Most A-V nodal conduction curves following A-V nodal modification demonstrate an upward shift to the right of one or both pathways following successful ablation. Regardless of the site of ablation, dual A-V nodal pathways may still be present, conduction over the fast or slow pathway may be slower, yet no A-V nodal tachycardia results.

The overall success rate of modification of the A-V node to cure A-V nodal reentrant tachycardia can be expected to exceed 95%.[116,117] The success rates are similar whether ablation is aimed at the retrograde fast pathway or antegrade slow pathway, or whether this is anatomically guided (i.e., ablating superior or inferior in Koch triangle) or electrogram-guided. Whether energy is delivered during SVT or sinus rhythm does not appear to influence the results, although it is easier to maintain a stable catheter position in sinus rhythm. The major reason why ablation should be carried out in sinus rhythm and not during SVT is that an unstable catheter position may result in inadvertent A-V block. In summary, the delivery of RF energy to the posterior third of the triangle of Koch has a high efficacy rate of curing A-V nodal tachycardia. The exact mechanism by which this works is uncertain. While accelerated junctional rhythms appear to be necessary to achieve successful ablation, they are not necessarily sufficient. The ideal end points include loss of slow pathway conduction, a prolonged Wenckebach cycle, and persistence of intact antegrade and retrograde conduction. Persistence of dual pathways is seen in 40%. If dual pathways are present with single echo complexes, recurrent clinical A-V nodal reentry is rare. We accept an echo zone associated with dual pathways of 30 msec or less. If dual pathways or single echoes can be produced over a wide range of coupling intervals, we have found that the addition of isoproterenol and/or atropine often induces more sustained A-V nodal tachycardia. As such we usually give additional lesions until an echo zone of 30 msec or less or loss of slow pathway conduction is achieved. In all instances, prior to termination of the study, stimulation is repeated following isoproterenol and/or atropine. Absence of slow pathway conduction or a very narrow window of slow pathway conduction is associated with a recurrence rate of less than 2%.

The major complication of RF ablation to cure A-V nodal tachycardia is the development of heart block. The risk of heart block appears to be less than 1% and does not seem to be able to be improved upon no matter how careful the investigator. Congenital abnormalities are often associated with displacement of the A-V node, and a forme fruste of these congenital abnormalities (which may go undetected) may be related to inadvertent A-V block. In the absence of complete heart block, prolonged A-V conduction can be produced, which can lead to a pacemaker syndrome or exercise intolerance, should Wenckebach occur at fast rates. Fortunately these complications are extremely rare. Controversy exists as to how to deal with patients who have failed ablations. While some believe that prior slow pathway ablation indicates a high incidence of A-V block should fast pathway ablation be undertaken and vice versa, the data supporting this fear is at best limited. While in most instances repeated ablation in the similar region of a prior failed ablation is sufficient, occasionally one must deliver RF energy at the opposite region—either near the os of the CS or in the fast pathway region. We have not had any evidence of A-V block in the nearly dozen patients who have been referred to us for failed ablations elsewhere. It is, however, a generally held belief that repeated ablations for A-V nodal tachycardia are associated with a higher risk of A-V block, and patients should be made aware of this.

Cryoablation is used in some centers, particularly in pediatric electrophysiology, in an attempt to reduce the risk of inadvertent A-V block. Although the use of larger tip (6 mm) catheters has eliminated the concept of cryomapping, cryoablation certainly offers the security of perfect catheter stability during energy delivery. Recent comparative studies of cryoablation and RF have been rather uniform in the following conclusions: (1) the incidence of heart block with RF is quite low, but essentially not seen with cryoablation; (2) acute procedural success is high (96% to 100%) with both methods and recurrence is higher with cryoablation (9% to 15%).[63,164]

### Junctional Tachycardia

Junctional tachycardia, which has a focal, nonreentrant mechanism, is important to distinguish from A-V nodal tachycardia. Although traditionally it is associated with digitalis toxicity or in the early period following cardiac surgery, it also has a paroxysmal form and may cause significant symptoms. Various maneuvers have been proposed to distinguish these two arrhythmias. If an atrial extrastimulus is delivered during tachycardia when the His is refractory perturbs the timing of the next His, this confirms participation of the slow pathway, consistent with A-V nodal tachycardia. Alternatively, if an earlier extrastimulus advances the timing of the His immediately following without terminating the tachycardia, this indicates that the retrograde fast pathway is not required for the maintenance of the tachycardia, diagnosing junctional tachycardia.[165] Overdrive pacing during tachycardia has also been used for this purpose, observing the response upon cessation: atrial-His-His-atrial response in junctional tachycardia and an atrial-His-atrial response in A-V nodal tachycardia.[166] These maneuvers may also be helpful immediately following slow pathway ablation, to distinguish between recurrent

AVNRT and the frequent occurrence of nonsustained junctional rhythm following atrial stimulation, particularly during isoproterenol administration.

Ablation of junctional tachycardia can be successful, but is not as effective as for A-V nodal tachycardia and has a higher incidence of heart block. Most reports of ablation in this circumstance are in pediatric patients. The largest included 11 patients (including 5 adults), and ablation was successful without heart block in 9 patients. The strategy in this series was ablation at the site of earliest atrial activation in patients with V-A conduction, and empiric slow pathway ablation in the setting of V-A block.[167] Cryoablation has also been used in this application with reasonable success.[168]

## Surgical and Catheter Ablation Techniques to Manage other Atrial Arrhythmias

Atrial arrhythmias that have been ablated either surgically or through the delivery of energy have included atrial tachycardias, atrial flutter, and atrial fibrillation.[10–13] Catheter ablation has clearly become the treatment of choice for atrial tachycardia and atrial flutter, for which excellent results can be expected. Ablation for atrial fibrillation is widely performed using catheter and surgical techniques; the optimal indications for either strategy are still being determined.

## Ablation of Atrial Tachycardia

Atrial tachycardias that are incessant and due to abnormal automaticity or triggered activity are often drug refractory and as such are most often treated by ablation. Microreentrant atrial tachyarrhythmias are more easily managed with drugs so that ablation is not usually considered until there is a drug failure. Macroreentrant atrial tachycardias are more like atrial flutter and will be discussed in that subsection.

Incessant atrial tachycardias are an important cause of tachycardia-mediated cardiomyopathy. They are also difficult to treat with antiarrhythmic agents. These atrial tachycardias can occur from a wide variety of areas in the heart but seem to have the propensity for the crista terminalis, both atrial appendages, the coronary sinus, the regions of the mitral and tricuspid annulae, as well as the pulmonary veins. Why these structures are prone to develop these rhythms is unclear.[169–175]

Since the vast majority of incessant atrial tachycardias are focal in origin and due to abnormal automaticity or triggered activity, the goal of mapping is to find the earliest site of activation. It is important to recognize that sedation of these patients might terminate the tachycardia. If the tachycardias are not incessant, catecholamine infusion and/or use of theophylline or atropine (in the case of a catecholamine-mediated triggered activity) may be necessary to induce the arrhythmia. The first step in mapping atrial tachycardias is using the electrocardiogram to regionalize the source of the arrhythmia. P waves associated with tachycardias arising in the crista have a right-to-left orientation such that they are positive and broad in leads I and II and positive in the aVL. They are also biphasic in lead $V_1$. Tachycardias arising in the septum near the os of the CS have inverted P waves in the inferior leads with positive P waves in aVR and aVL. P waves in tachycardias arising in the left atrial appendage are positive in II, III, and aVF with III being more positive than lead II and positive in $V_1$. These are not too dissimilar from the left superior pulmonary vein P waves, which are positive in II, III, and aVF and upright in $V_1$. Those tachycardias arising from the right superior pulmonary veins are narrower with positive orientation in II, III, and aVF with II and III being similar and biphasic to slightly positive in lead $V_1$. They are isoelectric in lead I. In general, P waves associated with tachycardias arising near the septum are narrower than those arising on the right or left free wall. Once seen, the P wave is analyzed and the tachycardia origin regionalized. A systematic approach can then be planned. Most left atrial tachycardias are approached via a transseptal catheterization, which in many laboratories is performed under intracardiac ultrasound guidance. The fossa is at the level of the His bundle catheter and about 2 to 3 cm posterior to it. The amplitude of the voltage of electrograms at the fossa is somewhat lower than the surrounding tissue. The fossa ovalis may be stained with dye prior to its puncture to verify location, even if ultrasound is used. During left atrial procedures once the sheath is passed into the left atrium, heparinization is administered to maintain an ACT in excess of 250 to 300 seconds. Some operators prefer to heparinize prior to the transseptal puncture to avoid thrombus which can be introduced into the left atrium via the transseptal sheath. I have not observed any difference in outcomes.

A variety of mapping techniques have been utilized to localize focal tachycardia. These include:

1. A simple roving catheter using unipolar and bipolar signals to find the site with the earliest bipolar and unipolar signals. Unipolar signals can be filtered or unfiltered, but the unfiltered signals offer directional information. As stated earlier under mapping of bypass tracts, unipolar recordings from the tip and second pole are useful to assure that the distal pole is recording the earliest activity, since it is the pole through which RF energy is delivered. Low-amplitude early signals followed by a sharper discrete signal may represent an early component of a fragmented electrogram or a far field signal associated with a second, discrete local signal. This is most likely to happen in the superior posterior right atrium where a low-amplitude signal preceding a sharper higher-frequency signal may actually represent electrical activity generated from the right superior pulmonary vein. This can be suggested if unipolar electrograms are simultaneously recorded. In this instance the unipolar electrogram will demonstrate a sharp negative deflection which times with the later, high-frequency potential, signifying that the earlier potential is a far field signal (Fig. 13-57). Another clue that this might be the case is if left atrial activation recorded in the CS is earlier than a lateral recording from the right atrium. Coupled with the positive P wave in $V_1$, a right superior pulmonary vein focus should be suspected.
2. A second method involves the use of two roving catheters. These catheters are each moved in tandem so that the earliest electrogram is recorded.

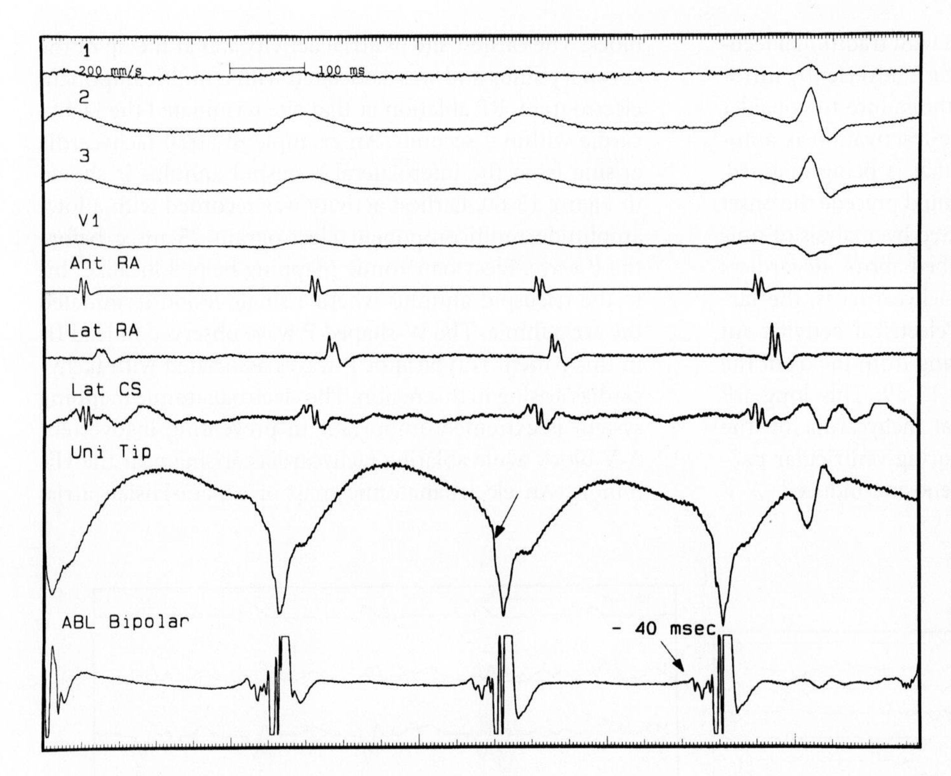


**FIGURE 13-57** *The role of unipolar recordings in mapping atrial tachycardia.* Atrial tachycardia with high-degree block is shown with reference electrograms from the anterior and lateral right atrium and the lateral coronary sinus. The ablation of bipolar electrogram is shown on the bottom. The recorded electrograms precede the P wave by 40 msec. The ablation catheter is located in the superior posterior right atrium. The electrogram is characterized by a low-amplitude, slower moving fragmented signal, followed by a high-frequency large amplitude signal. The unipolar recording from the tip shows that the intrinsicoid deflection corresponds to the later high-frequency deflection. The low-frequency deflection is not associated with local activation in the unipolar recording suggesting that it is a far-field electrogram. In this case the site of origin was the right superior pulmonary artery.

3. Simultaneous multisite data acquisition can often help rapidly regionalize and localize the tachycardia origin. This is most commonly done with a basket catheter from which multiple recordings[79] can demonstrate the site at which the tachycardia arises. More detailed mapping, however, is necessary to find the precise site to ablate. This is particularly useful if tachycardia episodes are short lived and/or cannot be reproducibly initiated by administration of catecholamines.
4. An important mapping technique involves pacing at sites of interest. If one is at the site of origin, pacing at this site should demonstrate a similar activation pattern to other sites being recorded in the right and left atrium as during the tachycardia.[174] As described in Chapter 8 this method suggests that focal activation of the atrium from the site designated to be the site of origin is indeed the site of origin. This form of pace mapping is sometimes referred to as electrogram mapping, but merely is a more precise form of pace mapping (Fig. 13-58).
5. In most laboratories, electroanatomic mapping is used for atrial tachycardia. The precision in mapping that this

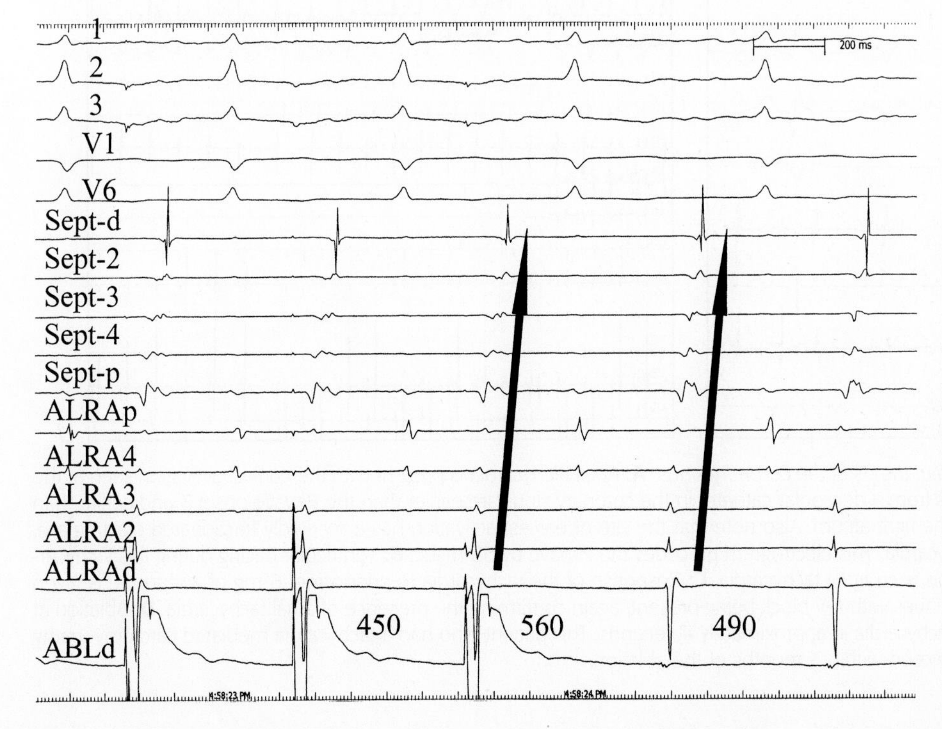


**FIGURE 13-58** Use of paced activation mapping to confirm focal atrial tachycardia is occurring at the site from which the earliest map site is recorded. Five surface ECGs and decapolar catheters from the septum and anterolateral right atrium are shown with electrograms from the ablation catheter. On the right-hand part of the panel, the activation sequence during the tachycardia is seen. Note the tachycardia has a cycle length of 490 msec and the low-amplitude signal recorded in the ablation catheter precedes a W-shaped P wave by 35 msec. Pacing at this site at 450 msec (first three electrograms in the tracing) demonstrates a P-wave morphology and atrial activation sequence identical to that of the tachycardia. This confirms that this site was indeed the focus of the atrial tachycardia. See text for discussion.

technique allows is much higher than with traditional techniques. One potential error that can be inadvertently introduced by this method, however, is the failure to consider additional sites when a site of earliest activation is automatically assigned in the chamber that is being mapped. Putative sites of earliest activation should precede the onset of the surface p wave, and can be vetted by analysis of unipolar recordings or pacing as described above. Regardless of where the site of origin of the tachycardia is, the target site usually shows fragmented electrical activity. An example of an atrial tachycardia arising from the os of the coronary sinus is shown in Figure 13-59. This long RP tachycardia was proven to be atrial tachycardia by the absence of retrograde conduction during ventricular pacing and persistence following adenosine-induced A-V block. The earliest site of atrial activity was at the lip of the coronary sinus and was associated with a multicomponent electrogram. RF ablation at that site terminated the tachycardia within 4 seconds. An example of atrial tachycardia arising from the inferolateral tricuspid annulus is shown in Figure 13-60. Earliest activity was recorded with a low-amplitude multicomponent electrogram 25 msec before the P wave. Electroanatomic mapping helped localize this to the tricuspid annulus where a single lesion terminated the arrhythmia. The W-shaped P wave observed in lead III in this patient is typical of P waves associated with tachycardias arising in this region. The electroanatomic mapping system is extremely important in preventing inadvertent A-V block while ablating tachycardias arising near the His bundle. An electroanatomic map of a para-Hisian atrial

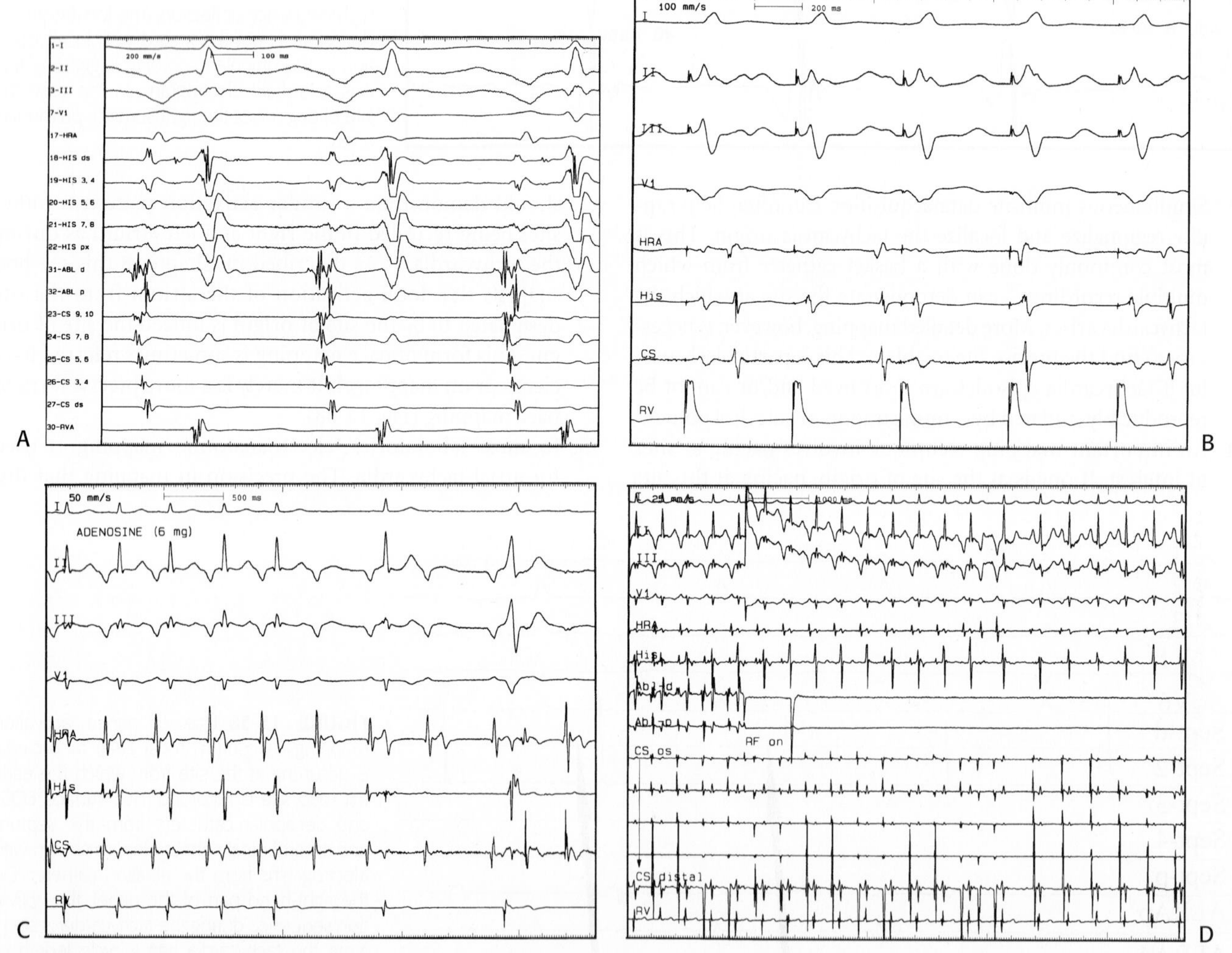


**FIGURE 13-59** *Ablation of atrial tachycardia at the os of the coronary sinus.* **A:** Atrial tachycardia is present with the earliest activation seen at the os of the coronary sinus. Note that recordings from a decapolar catheter in the coronary sinus are earlier than the P-wave onset 3 and earlier than recordings from the His bundle catheter in the right atrium. Also note that the site of earliest activation has a markedly fractionated electrogram, typical of sites of earliest activity in atrial tachycardia. This electrogram precedes the P wave by 55 msec. **B:** Ventricular pacing during this tachycardia shows V-A dissociation confirming that this is an atrial tachycardia. **C:** Response of the tachycardia to adenosine: 6 mg of adenosine is given and the tachycardia slows minimally but continues with A-V block being present, again confirming the presence of atrial tachycardia. **D:** Ablation at the site of earliest activation terminates the tachycardia in approximately 4 seconds. This patient who had a tachycardia mediated cardiomyopathy demonstrated normalization of ventricular function within 3 months of the ablation.

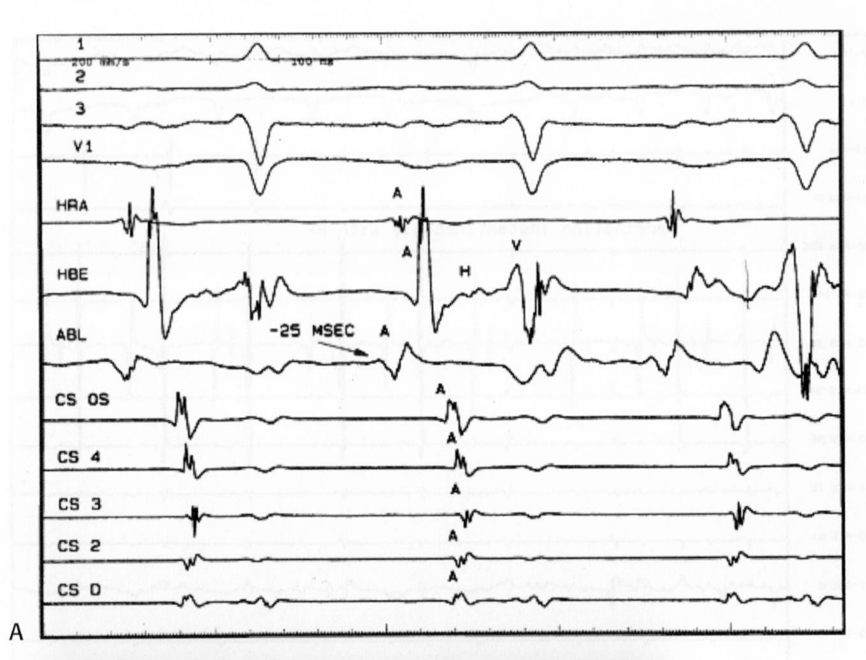


A

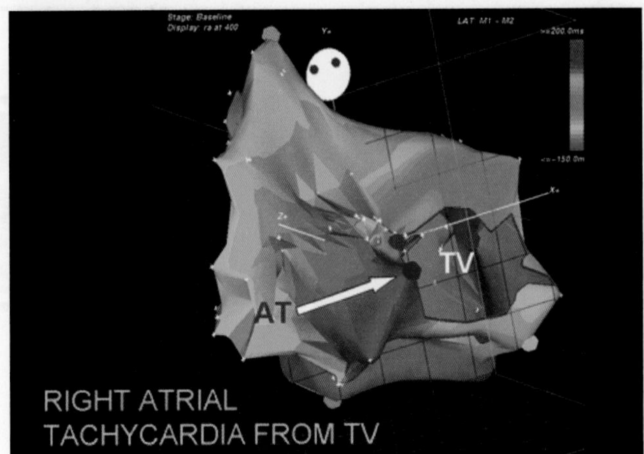


B

**FIGURE 13-60** *Role of electroanatomic mapping to guide ablation of focal tachycardia.* **A:** Atrial tachycardia is present. Note the morphology of the P wave has a W-like configuration. The earliest activation was shown to be recorded in the inferolateral right atrium at the tricuspid annulus. **B:** Electroanatomical mapping of the atrial tachycardia shown on top reveals earliest activation at the lateral tricuspid annulus. There is sequential spread to the rest of the atrium. Ablation at the earliest site (*red-brown dot*) at which the *white arrow* is pointed, was successful.

tachycardia is shown in Figure 13-61. The map clearly delineated the His bundle and allowed for the ablation to be accurately delivered 1 cm superior to the proximal His bundle recording site where nearly instantaneous termination of the arrhythmia occurred. Of note we have seen three cases of atrial tachycardia mapped to just above the His bundle catheter which actually arose and were ablated from the noncoronary cusp in the aorta (Fig. 13-62). An electroanatomic map of a right atrial tachycardia arising near a scar, just below the superior vena cava is shown in Figure 13-63 and an analog map of an atrial tachycardia from the superior crista is shown in Figure 13-64. A Carto map of a focal atrial tachycardia at the mitral annulus is shown in Figure 13-65. In Figure 13-66 electroanatomic mapping demonstrated a small reentrant circuit near the mitral annulus adjacent to the septum. This tachycardia would have been totally missed had only right atrial mapping been performed. As one can see on the isochronic map in the right atrium, earliest activity (red) occurs in the region of the apex of the triangle of Koch adjacent to the His bundle recording site (orange dots). Ablation at this site may have potentially produced heart block, but not cure the tachycardia that was shown to arise in the left atrium as a small reentrant circuit adjacent to the mitral annulus. Reentrant excitation is shown by arrows as the color spreads from red to orange to yellow to green to blue and then purple adjacent to the initial site of red at the mitral annulus. The burgundy color marks the site of adjacent early and late activity. RF energy adjacent to the mitral annulus on the septum terminated this arrhythmia.

The success rate for ablation of focal paroxysmal atrial tachycardia is highly variable and depends on the expertise of the investigator and the cause of the atrial arrhythmia. When atrial tachycardias are present incessantly the success rate approaches 90%, although there is a recurrence rate as high as 25%.[169–175] The early NASPE 1998 registry reports a success rate of 70% and a complication rate of 3%.[116] These success rates do not truly reflect the difficulty of atrial tachycardia ablation. Since these arrhythmias may not be reliably present

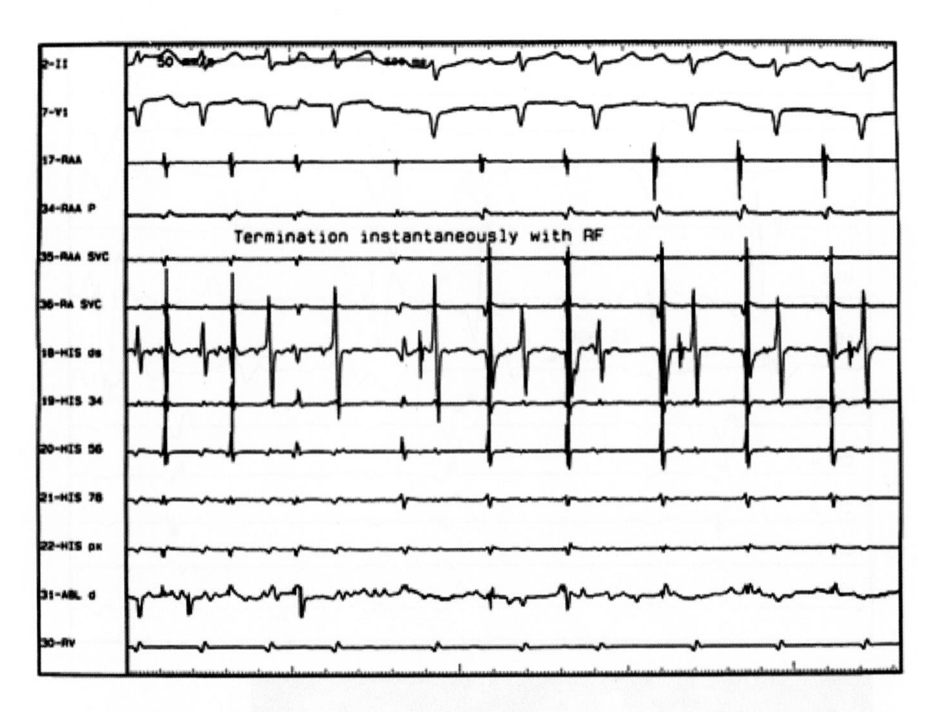


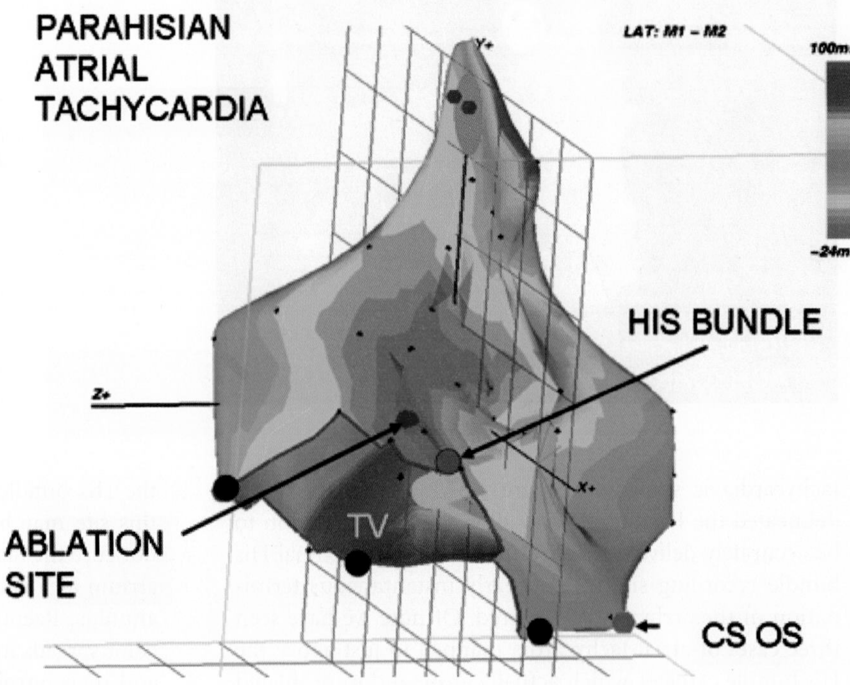


**FIGURE 13-61** *Use of electroanatomic mapping to prevent inadvertent heart block during ablation of an atrial tachycardia, just adjacent to the His bundle.* An electroanatomic map in a patient with atrial tachycardia occurring 5 mm superior to the His bundle is shown in the **bottom panel**. The site of earliest activation is denoted by the *brown dot.* The site of the His bundle is shown by *blue.* Three-msec isochrones are shown in this tracing. The catheter was able to be positioned above the His bundle safely and RF energy delivered at this site. Application of RF energy at this site immediately terminated the tachycardia (**top panel**).

at the time of the electrophysiology study, a true success rate on an intention to treat basis cannot be determined. Clearly it would be lower than the 90% or more success rate of persistent tachycardias. Thus, the mechanism of the focal arrhythmia also influences outcome.[176]

In patients in whom ablation fails and pharmacologic therapy cannot be appropriately applied, two potential therapeutic options are available. One is to ablate the A-V junction and implant a pacemaker. The other is to surgically resect or isolate the tachycardia. Success of surgery depends on being able to map the tachycardia at the time of surgery. In the absence of doing this, procedures such as a left atrial isolation can be performed if the tachycardia is localized to the specific atrium (Fig. 13-67). We operated on a patient with a tumor-related right atrial tachycardia that was mapped to the limbus of the fossa ovalis in the laboratory in the preablation era. This tachycardia could not be induced in the operating room, but mapping of isolated frequent APCs induced by catecholamines provided enough information to localize the rhythm and ablate it (Fig. 13-68). Tachycardias that cannot be ablated and that have been shown to arise in the left or right atrial appendage can be cured by surgical removal of the appendage. This is certainly a smaller procedure than isolation of the left atrium and could be performed through a minithoracotomy or thoracoscopy

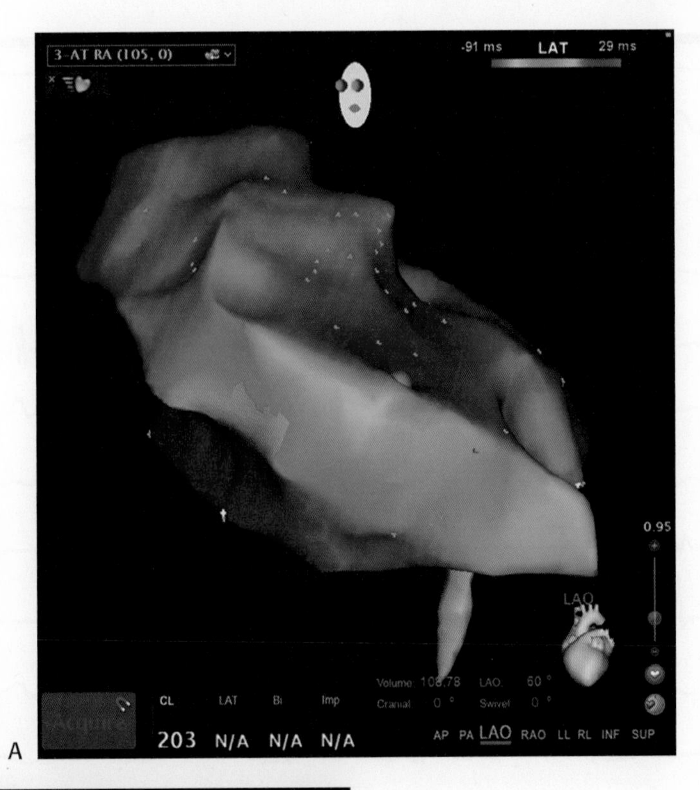


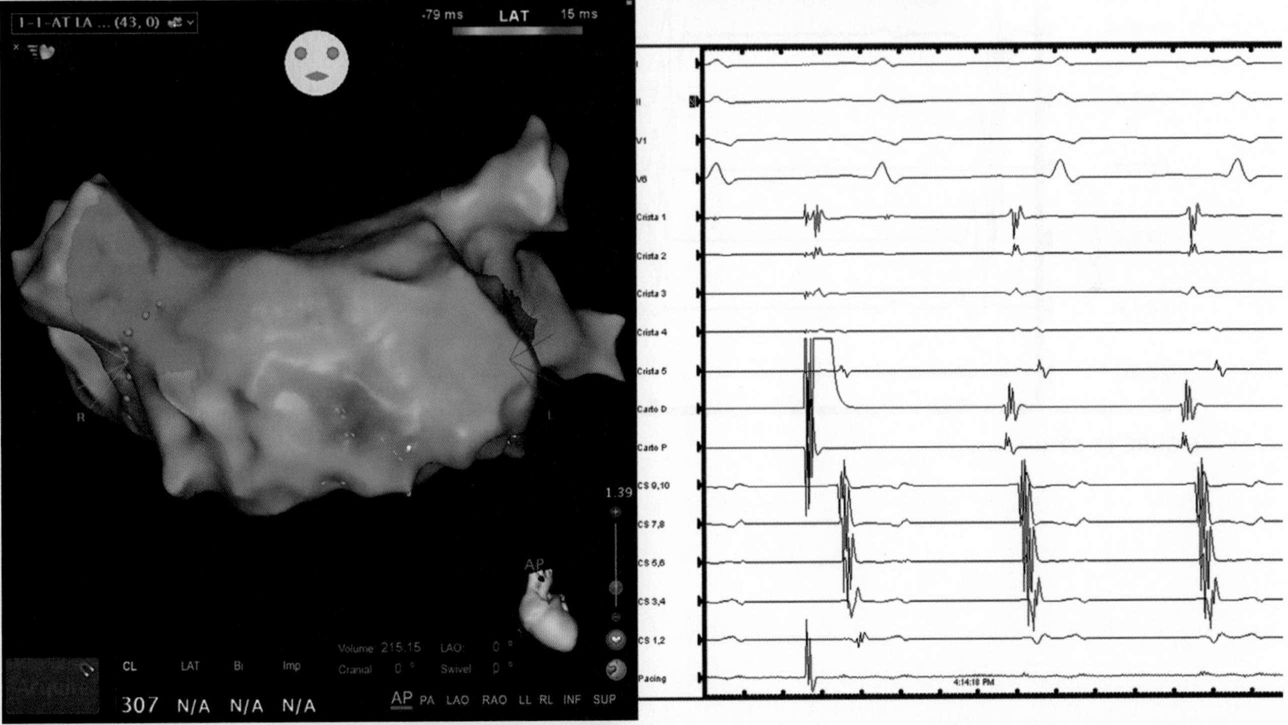


**FIGURE 13-62** *Ablation of a para-Hisian atrial tachycardia from the noncoronary sinus of Valsalva.* In **panel A**, an electroanatomic map of the right atrium during atrial tachycardia is shown. Note the broad area of earliest atrial activation just superior to the His bundle recording (denoted by the *yellow icon*); this sort of diffuse early activation is typical when mapping a chamber adjacent to the actual site of tachycardia origin. An activation map of the left atrium is shown in **panel B**. This registers a discreet early site, but pacing from this site causes subtle changes in the morphologies of the atrial electrograms compared to those recorded in tachycardia. Mapping of the noncoronary cusp (**panel C**) demonstrates a much earlier signal, and ablation at this site resulted in elimination of the atrial tachycardia without effecting A-V conduction.

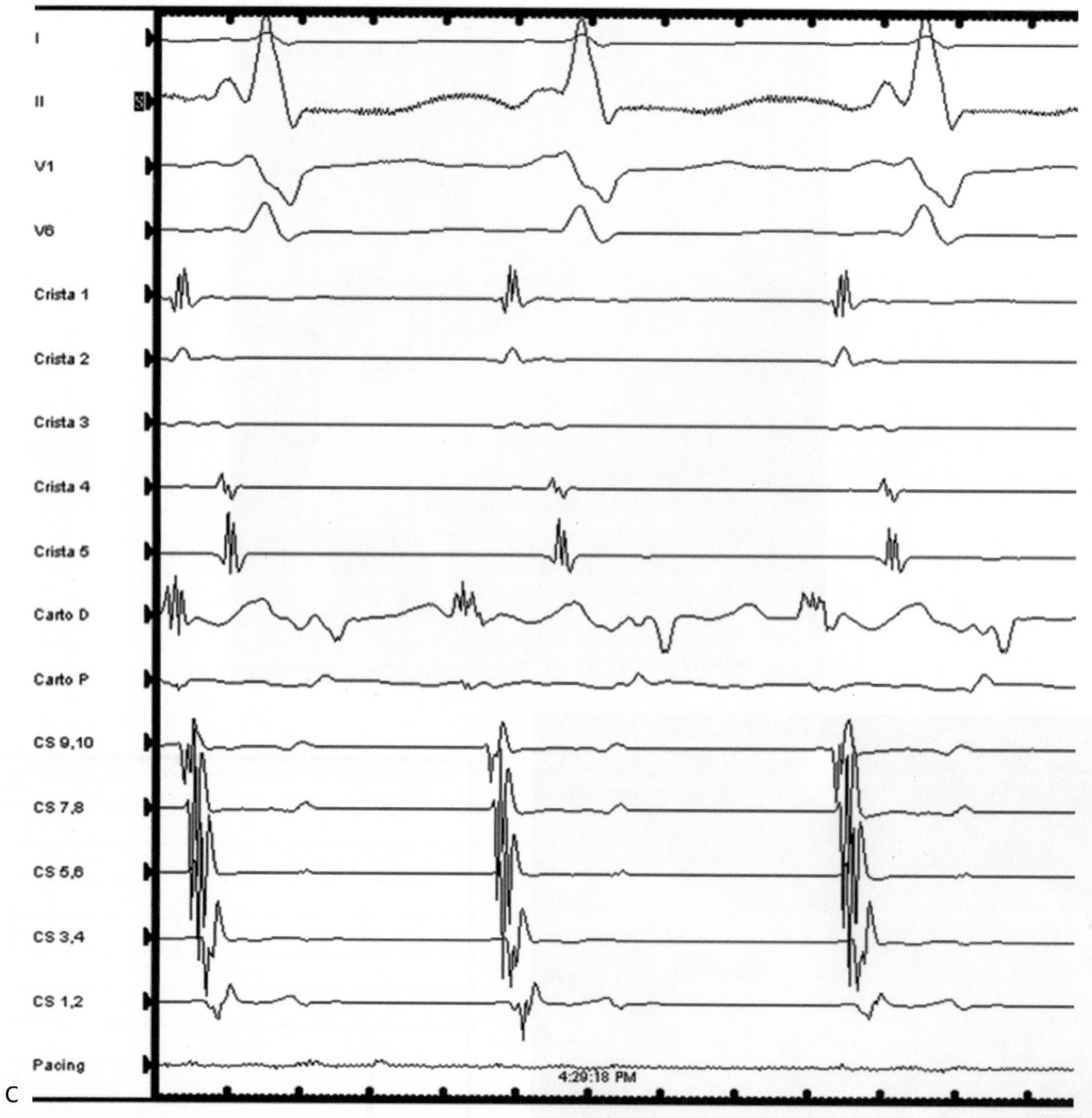


**FIGURE 13-62** *(Continued)*

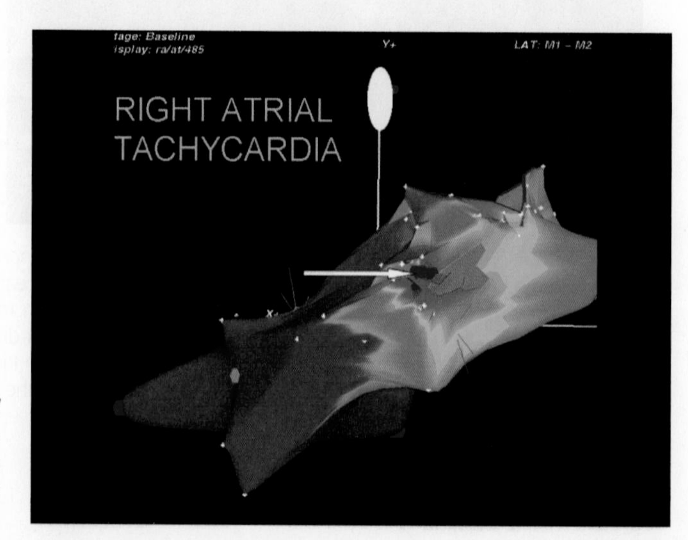


**FIGURE 13-63** *Scar-related atrial tachycardia from the superior and posterolateral right atrium.* Electroanatomic mapping of an atrial tachycardia is shown in this figure. Scar is shown in *gray* and *bright red* is the site of earliest atrial activation. The *red-brown dots* (*arrow*) are the site of successful ablation.

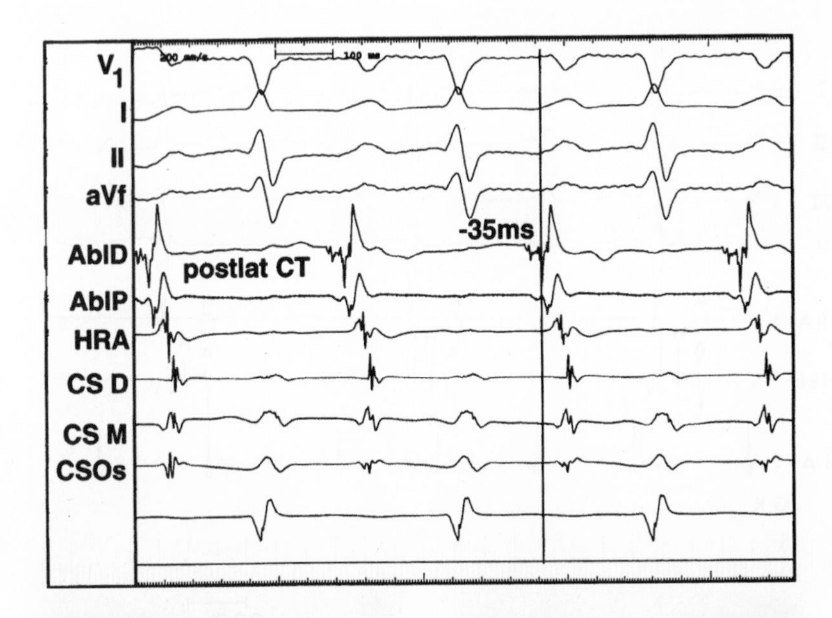


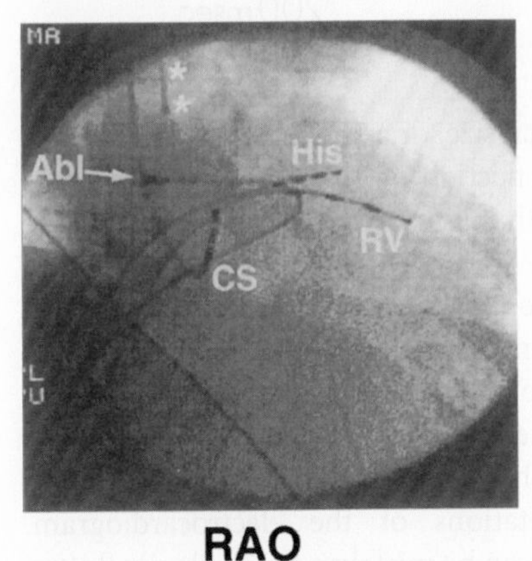


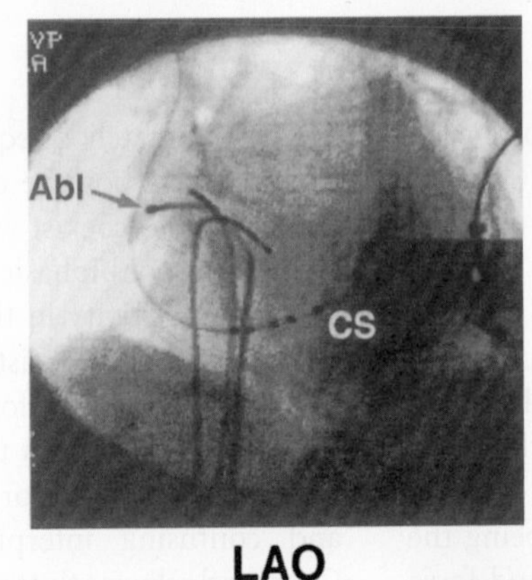


**FIGURE 13-64** Analog recordings and fluoroscopic images of catheter and ablation site shown in Figure 13-63. Analog records show fractionated earliest site 35 msec prior to the P wave. Fluoroscopic images of catheter position are shown on the bottom.

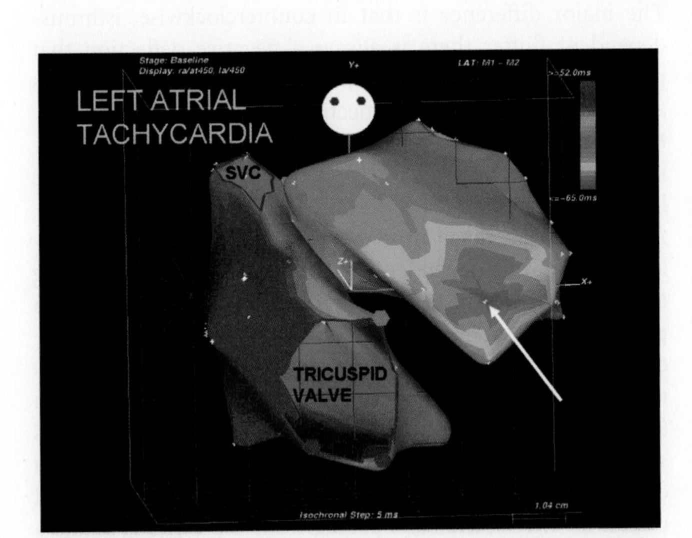


**FIGURE 13-65** *Electroanatomic map of focal atrial tachycardia just above the mitral annulus.* Electroanatomic mapping of an atrial tachycardia is shown with earliest activation in *red* and latest activation in *purple* at 5-msec isochronal steps. Note that the right atrium is late and it is activated in *blues and purples.* The earliest site of atrial activation (*white arrow*) is shown just superior to the mitral annulus in *red* and was a site at which a single RF application ablated the tachycardia.

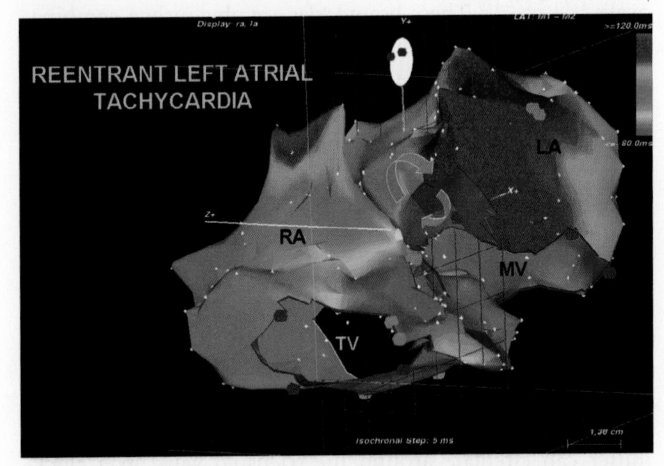


**FIGURE 13-66** *Electroanatomic mapping demonstrating small left atrial reentrant tachycardia.* The mapping of both the right and left atrium and 5-msec isochronal steps is shown in this figure. Earliest activation is seen in red, latest activation is seen in *purple.* The point at which earliest and latest activation meet is shown in *dark burgundy.* The *arrows* demonstrate reentrant excitation in this small area above the mitral annulus. A single lesion between the burgundy area and the mitral annulus terminated the tachycardia and prevented its reinitiation. If only right atrial activation were used, a focal tachycardia on the septum might have been suggested, leading to failed RF application and a potential for heart block.

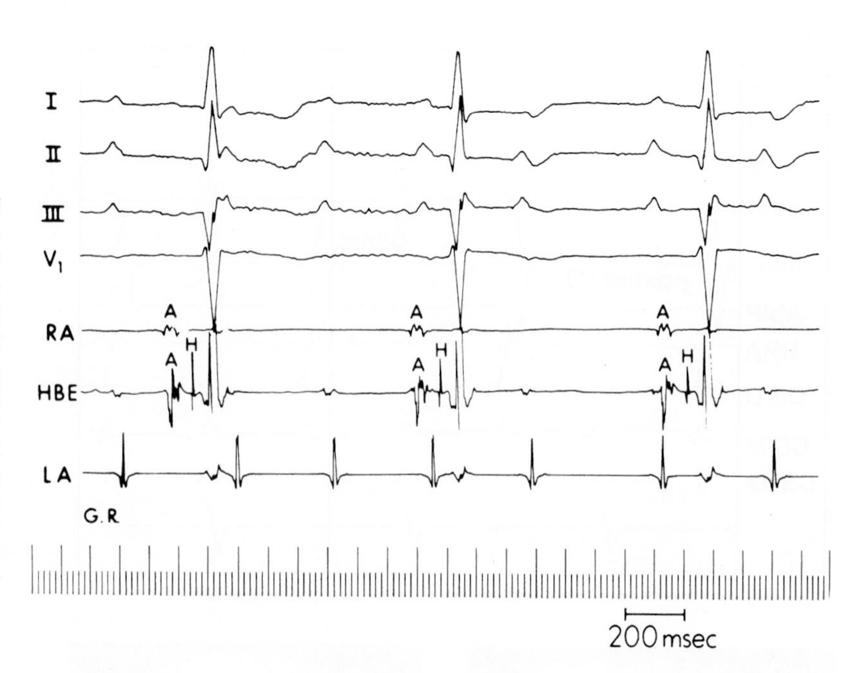


**FIGURE 13-67** *Isolation of atrium to manage atrial tachycardia.* Recordings, from the top down, are surface ECG leads I to III, $V_1$, bipolar catheter recordings of the right atrium (RA) and the His bundle, and a bipolar recording obtained by permanent electrodes sutured to the left atrial appendage (LA). The right and left atria are dissociated. Right atrial activity proceeds from the catheter positioned in the high RA to the atrial septum as recorded on the His bundle catheter, followed by conduction to the ventricle. An irregular left atrial tachycardia is present, which fails to propagate to either the right atrium or to the ventricles. (From Gallagher JJ, Cox JL, German LD, Kasell JH. Nonpharmacologic treatment of supraventricular tachycardia. In: Josephson MD, Wellens HJJ, eds. *Tachycardias: mechanisms, diagnosis, treatment*. Philadelphia, PA: Lea & Febiger, 1984:271.)

as long as the tachycardia has been mapped to the tip of the left atrial appendage.

## Ablation of Atrial Flutter and other Macroreentrant Atrial Arrhythmias

Typical atrial flutters are macroreentrant circuits involving the right atrium and may rotate in a clockwise or counterclockwise fashion.[169,170,175,177,178] The circuit has the tricuspid annulus as its anterior boundary with posterior boundaries being the coronary sinus inferior vena cava, crista terminalis, and fossa ovalis.[172,175,177–179] These boundaries are obviously a combination of anatomic structures and the functional consequences of propagation through those structures. Because typical flutters must proceed through an isthmus created by the tricuspid annulus, coronary sinus, and inferior vena cava, these flutters are now more appropriately termed "isthmus-dependent" flutter. Other macroreentrant circuits in either the right or left atrium are considered atypical flutters. The vast majority of clinically encountered atrial flutters are isthmus-dependent flutters; however, atypical flutters, which commonly complicate ablation therapy for atrial fibrillation, are certainly becoming increasingly frequent. Isthmus-dependent flutters frequently coexist with atrial fibrillation.

As described in detail in Chapter 9, isthmus-dependent flutter can circulate around the tricuspid valve in a clockwise or counterclockwise fashion (Fig. 13-69). Although typical electrocardiographic patterns have been described for isthmus-dependent flutter, these ECG characteristics are not always present. We have reviewed 200 consecutive cases of isthmus-dependent flutter in which the distal and/or proximal coronary sinus activation was recorded along with right atrial activation.[180] Counterclockwise flutter (the more common variety) may be characterized by pure negative deflections in the inferior leads, negative followed by positive deflections that are approximately of equal size, or a small negative deflection followed by a positive deflection of greater amplitude. These three varieties coexist with tall positive P waves, smaller positive P waves, or biphasic P waves in $V_1$, respectively. The degree to which positivity in the inferior leads is present appears to be related to the coexistence of heart disease and an enlarged left atrium. It is therefore apparent that propagation of atrial flutter to and through the left atrium is a major determinant of the flutter-wave morphology. This may lead to misleading and confusing interpretations of the electrocardiogram. Counterclockwise flutter can be mistaken for clockwise flutter, which generally has positive deflections in the inferior leads. The major difference is that in counterclockwise, isthmus-dependent flutter there is always a negative deflection that precedes the positive deflection. With clockwise flutter, there is a notching of the positive deflection in the middle of the flutter wave. Thus, despite the fact that isthmus-dependent flutter is a right atrial phenomenon, propagation to and through the left atrium determines its electrocardiographic appearance. As described in detail in Chapter 9, proof that one is dealing with isthmus-dependent flutter involves the use of pacing techniques to demonstrate the mechanism of the flutter. When pacing from components of the flutter circuit, the return cycle equals the flutter cycle length and the wavefront of activation is the same as that during flutter except for all amounts of fusion (caused by antidromic capture). Pacing from the isthmus shows no fusion of intra-atrial recordings because collision of wavefronts occurs within this slowly conducting, protected region of the circuit. Thus pacing from the isthmus shows a return cycle equal to the flutter cycle length, a paced atrial morphology equal to the flutter morphology, and a stimulus to coronary os electrogram equal to the spontaneous electrogram recorded by the pacing catheter and the coronary sinus electrogram during flutter. The response to entrainment from sites inside and outside the circuit is discussed in Chapter 9.

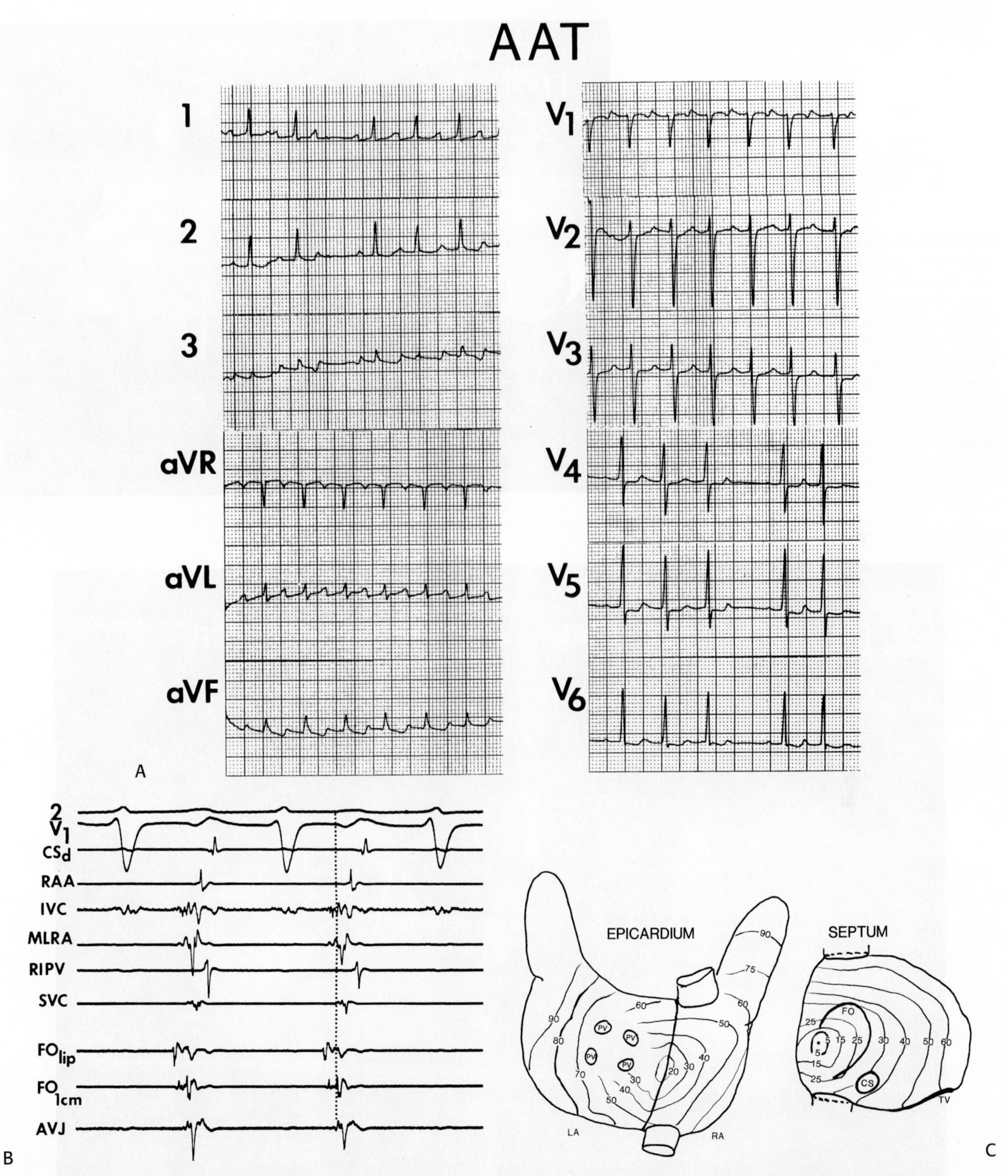


**FIGURE 13-68** *Surgical cure of right atrial tachycardia.* **A:** The 12-lead ECG of atrial tachycardia. **B:** Selective sites from the preoperative catheter map. **C:** Intraoperative epicardial and septal map. Earliest activity was from the posterior tip of the fossa ovalis (FO). AAT, automatic atrial tachycardia; MLRA, mid-lateral right atrium; RIPV, right inferior pulmonary vein.

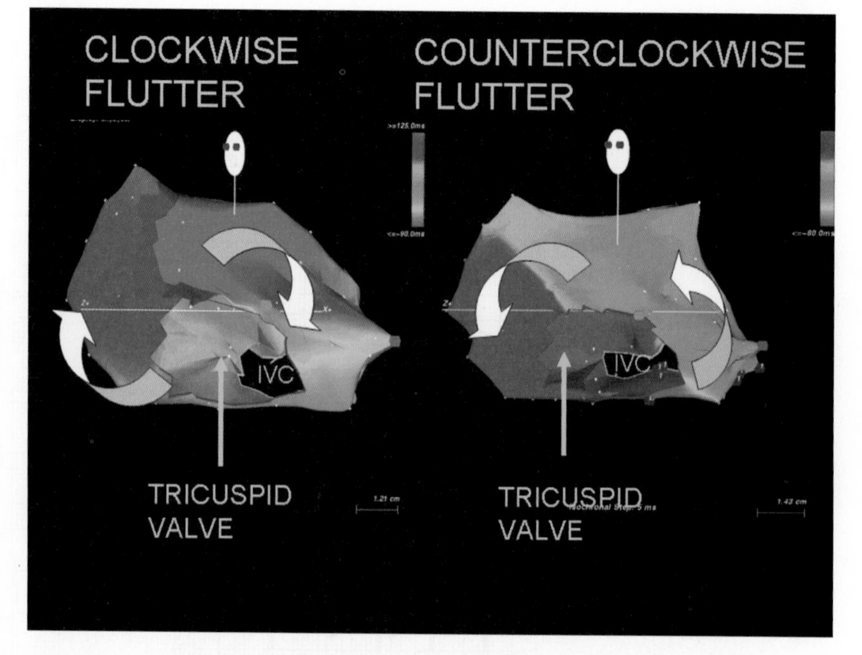


**FIGURE 13-69** *Electroanatomic mapping of isthmus-dependent flutter.* As described in Chapter 9, isthmus-dependent flutter can circulate around the tricuspid valve in a clockwise or counterclockwise direction as seen in the left anterior view. These two distinct patterns of activation are shown in the electroanatomic maps in this tracing. Activation proceeds from *red to orange to yellow to green* to a variety of *blues to purple.* The joining of the latest site with the earliest site is shown in *dark burgundy.* These activation maps are made in approximately 5-msec isochrones and clearly demonstrate the two types of rotation around the tricuspid annulus.

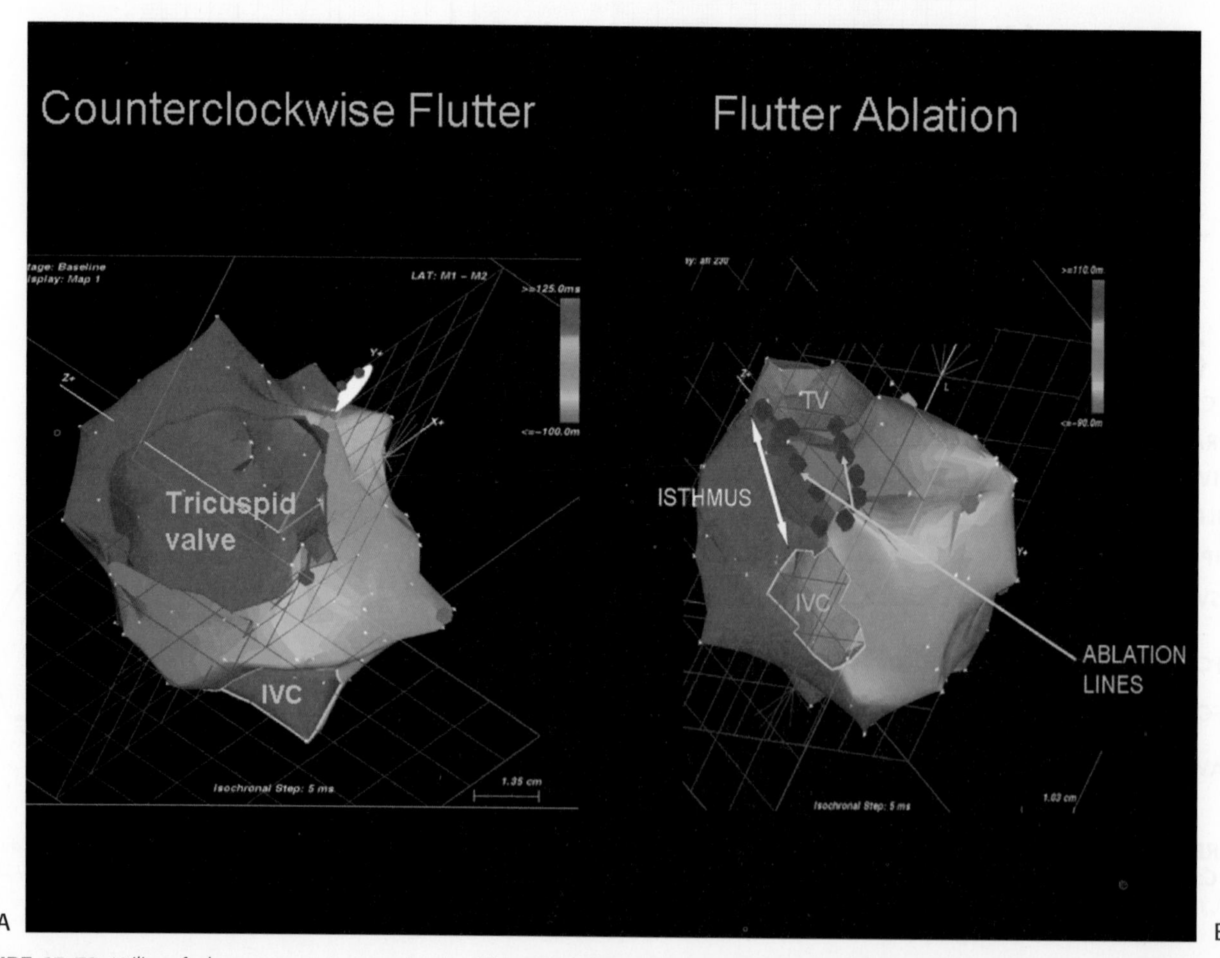


**FIGURE 13-70** *Utility of electroanatomic mapping in ablating atrial flutter.* **A:** Counterclockwise flutter is shown around the tricuspid valve. **B:** Using a posterior view, the isthmus between the tricuspid valve and inferior vena cava can be seen and linear lines of ablation can be drawn between the tricuspid valve and IVC. The *arrow* defines the isthmus that must be ablated. TV, tricuspid valve. IVC, inferior vena cava.

Electroanatomic mapping can be used in atrial flutter ablation (Fig. 13-70). Mapping systems allow one to rotate the heart to see the tricuspid-inferior vena cava isthmus and allows one to place RF lesions in a linear fashion between the tricuspid valve and inferior vena cava. We usually perform ablation during flutter. Invariably flutter is terminated during application of a critical lesion at the site of the ablation catheter (Fig. 13-71). Since termination of the flutter does not necessarily mean that the line is complete, continued ablation is performed during coronary sinus pacing. When true block has not been accomplished across the isthmus, pacing in the CS will demonstrate opposite wavefronts colliding in the lateral right atrium with one wavefront going clockwise through the unblocked isthmus and another wavefront going counterclockwise around the crista terminalis. This is what is seen prior to ablation (Fig. 13-72). When ablation of the tricuspid annulus is complete, clockwise propagation through the isthmus is not possible and the entire tricuspid annulus is activated in a counterclockwise direction (Fig. 13-72). This can be verified by the Carto system as demonstrated in Figure 13-73. Following the ablation, pacing at the coronary sinus os demonstrates block of the wavefront at the line of ablation in the isthmus with counterclockwise activation around the tricuspid annulus to block in that direction. To assure success, bidirectional block must also be shown.[175,181–183] In this instance, pacing from just lateral to the site of ablation will produce block toward the CS electrogram and activation of the tricuspid annulus only in a clockwise fashion in addition to block in the opposite direction as described above (Fig. 13-74). Electroanatomic mapping systems are also useful because they provide information about the voltage characteristics of the tissue involved in the isthmus. The lower the voltage the easier it is to achieve block in the tissue. Thus one might chose a path in the isthmus that is slightly longer through low-voltage tissue than a shorter route through high-voltage tissue, which represents a thicker atrial myocardium. Other appropriate endpoints of cavotricuspid isthmus ablation include widely split double potentials along the entire ablation line (isoelectric intervals of ≥110 msec),[184] absence of local atrial activity (electrograms <0.05 mV) along the ablation line or the reversal of unipolar electrogram polarity on two closely spaced electrodes, on either side of the ablation line during CS pacing.[185]

Some investigators prefer to ablate between the tricuspid annulus and the coronary sinus since it is the shortest path. This frequently fails, I believe, because the impulse can propagate through the Eustachian ridge (albeit slowly) to go around the IVC and produce a lower loop reentry. Analysis of Carto maps of atrial flutter frequently demonstrates simultaneous activation across the Eustachian ridge and around the IVC to produce a lower loop of reentrant excitation that meets the loop going counterclockwise around the tricuspid annulus in a figure-of-eight fashion (Fig. 13-75). This is also graphically shown using a basket catheter in Figure 13-76. Both the lower loop and upper loop can be simultaneously entrained. While the Eustachian ridge is believed to be a fixed obstacle that produces block because of the observation of double potentials that are often seen on either side of it, this may not in fact represent true block, but a very slowly propagating wavefront.[186] In fact, the ability to slowly conduct across the Eustachian ridge may be responsible for lower loop reentry that follows inadequate ablation of the isthmus because of placing ablation lines too medially, such that propagation across the Eustachian ridge is still possible. Ablation along the Eustachian ridge or between the tricuspid annulus and the

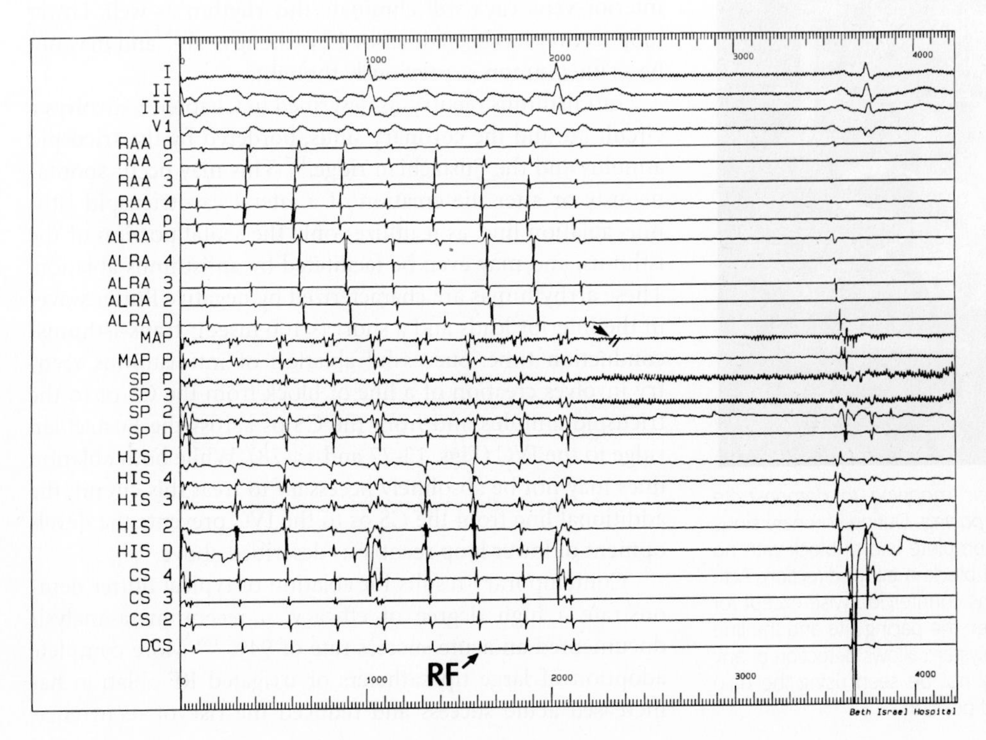


**FIGURE 13-71** *Termination of isthmus-dependent flutter during RF application.* Isthmus-dependent, counterclockwise flutter is shown on the left. Electrograms from the right atrial appendage (RAA), the anterolateral right atrium around the tricuspid annulus (LARA) with the distal (d) ALRA being misplaced at the lateral tricuspid annulus at the lateral border of the isthmus. Slow pathway proximal to distal. A decapolar catheter in the His bundle recording site and an octapolar catheter in the coronary sinus. During the formation of a linear lesion, atrial flutter terminates with block in the mapping/ablation catheter, which is positioned in the center of the isthmus.

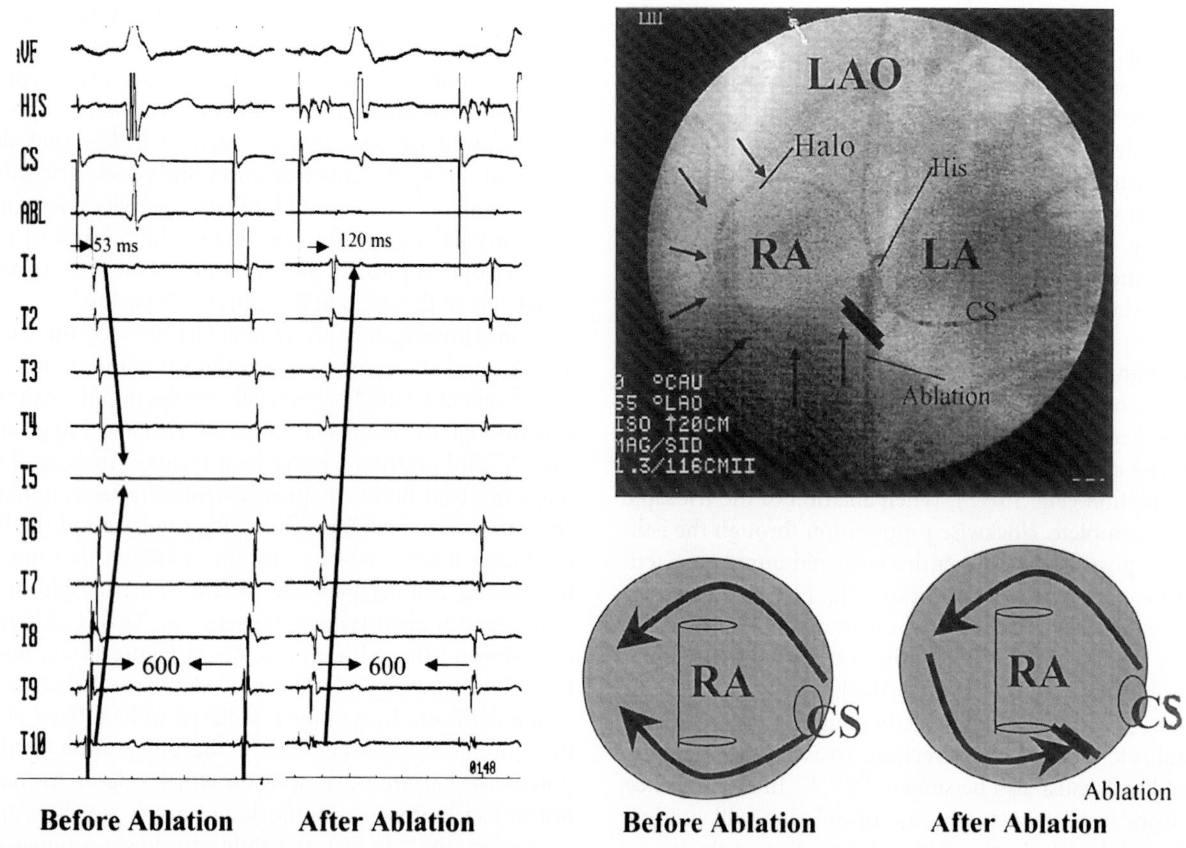


**FIGURE 13-72** *Demonstration of block across the isthmus using coronary sinus pacing.* In the top right is a fluoroscopic image showing a halo catheter positioned around the tricuspid annulus, the coronary sinus catheter, the His catheter, and the ablation catheter. Prior to and after ablation, the activation patterns around the tricuspid annulus using a halo catheter are shown on the left. Prior to ablation, pacing the coronary sinus demonstrates both superior and inferior wavefronts around the tricuspid annulus (**far left panel**). After ablation, a line of block appears to be created in the isthmus and activation of the tricuspid annulus only goes over the superior route (**middle panel**). This is schematically shown in the lower right-hand part of the figure.

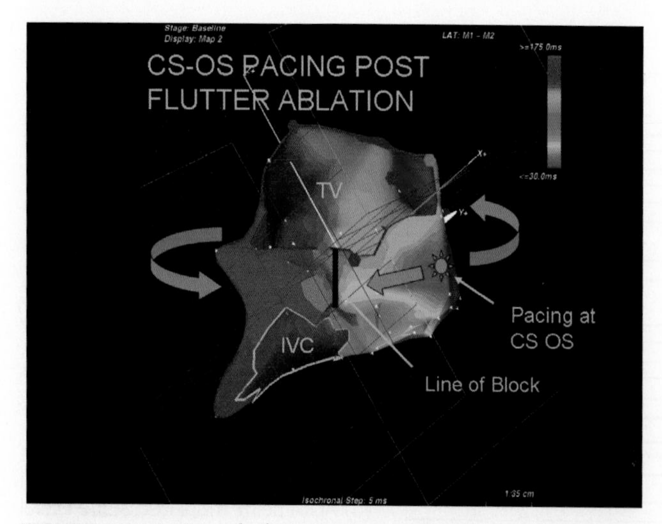


**FIGURE 13-73** *Use of electroanatomic mapping to demonstrate the line of block during coronary sinus pacing.* During coronary sinus pacing following ablation, one sees a complete line of block with no activation proceeding across that line of block in either direction. Activation of the entire tricuspid ring remains counterclockwise except for the small portion that is situated between the pacing site and the line of block. The electroanatomic mapping system allows detection of any breaks in the line of block, which may not be seen using the halo catheter or any single catheter in a fixed position.

inferior vena cava will eliminate this rhythm as well. Lower loop reentry has been described by Cheng et al.[187]and may not be as uncommon as previously thought.

Intraisthmus reentry, as described in Chapter 9, involves a circuit around the coronary sinus, bordered by the tricuspid annulus and the Eustachian ridge.[188] This may occur spontaneously or after the creation of a lateral cavotricuspid isthmus ablation line, as it utilizes only the septal portion of the isthmus, and may even be facilitated by an isthmus ablation. These arrhythmias are characterized by negative flutter waves in the inferior leads and a short (<100 msec) "trans-isthmus" conduction time. Successful ablation of intraisthmus reentry involves creation of a line of block from the CS os to the tricuspid annulus and from the CS os across the Eustachian ridge to the IVC (Figs. 13-77 and 13-78). While both ablation lines may not be absolutely necessary to treat this circuit, the additional line from the CS os to the IVC prevents the development of lower loop reentry as described above.

Contemporary results for ablation of typical flutter demonstrate a high degree of efficacy; a recent meta-analysis documented an acute success rate of 94%.[189] More complete adoption of large tip catheters or irrigated RF ablation has increased acute success and reduced the risk of recurrence.

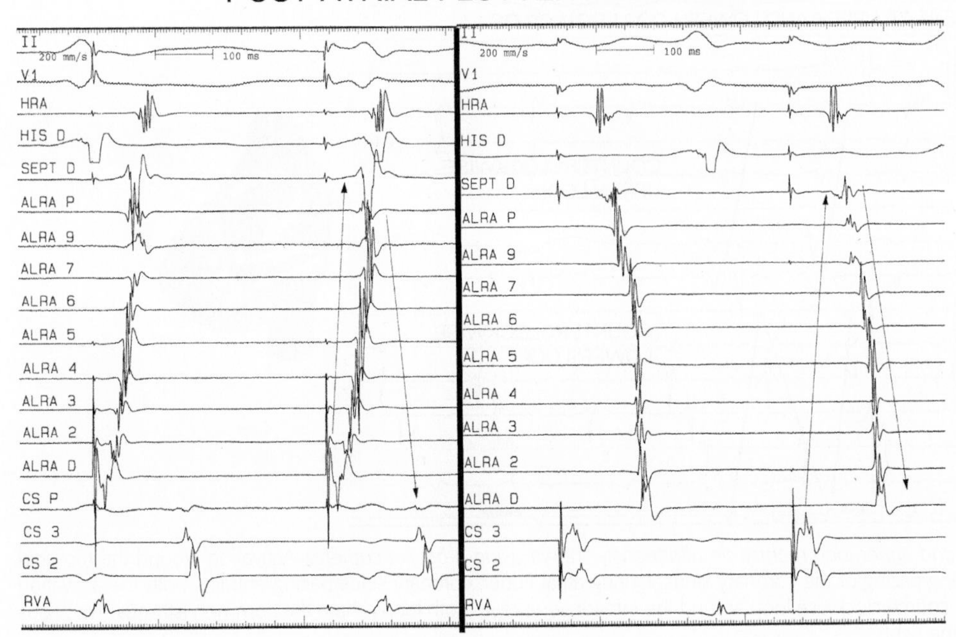


**FIGURE 13-74** *Demonstration of bidirectional block.* To assure success of flutter ablation bidirectional block should be demonstrated. This is necessary because occasionally one can demonstrate complete block in one direction but not in another. Pacing on either side of the To ablation line demonstrates that activation around the tricuspid annulus proceeds only in the direction away from the line. In the panel on the left, pacing in the lateral isthmus shows a clockwise activation around the tricuspid ring. Conversely, pacing the proximal coronary sinus demonstrates a clockwise pattern of activation around the tricuspid annulus.

One factor that can greatly complicate cavotricuspid isthmus ablation is abnormal anatomy, atrial pouches (which are more frequent in the medial isthmus) or thick pectinate ridges (more frequent in the lateral isthmus), or a prominent Eustachian ridge.[190] Although certainly not necessary for routine use, intracardiac echocardiography can be useful in difficult cases to visualize the underlying anatomy (Fig. 13-79).

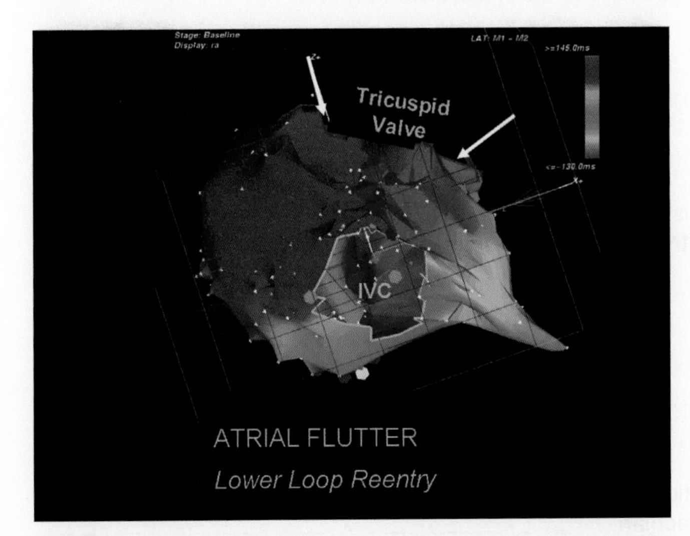


**FIGURE 13-75** *Demonstration of a lower loop of reentry using the electroanatomic mapping system.* Counterclockwise flutter is shown by analyzing the activation sequence around the tricuspid annulus. However, activation around the IVC, also demonstrates reentrant excitation. As in other electroanatomic maps, the earliest site of activation is arbitrarily shown in *red* with sequential activation to *orange, yellows, greens, blues, and purples.* A *dark burgundy line* demonstrates a line bordering the earliest and latest activation. Notice the densest isochrones appear in the tricuspid-inferior vena cava isthmus.

If bidirectional block can be demonstrated, the incidence of recurrent atrial flutter is less than 10%. In our laboratory it is 6%. Failure to demonstrate bidirectional block, however, is associated with a 20% recurrence rate of flutter. When recurrence occurs, noncontact mapping[67] or electroanatomic mapping has been very useful in defining the "leak" in the prior linear lesions. This facilitates sealing the leak and creating bidirectional block. Natale et al.[191] have demonstrated that a primary ablation approach to flutter is superior to pharmacologic approaches. Moreover, the incidence of subsequent atrial fibrillation (a common spontaneous accompaniment to atrial flutter) is less, in short-term follow-up (~1 year), than when pharmacologic therapy is used,[192] primarily in the absence of heart disease. The incidence of atrial fibrillation appearing after atrial flutter ablation in patients with normal hearts and atrial flutter as the only documented arrhythmia, is in the order of 10% at 1 year, whereas in the presence of organic heart disease, in particular hypertension, and heart failure, atrial fibrillation occurs in >80% in 3-year follow-up. Patients with concomitant atrial fibrillation can be recognized by ECG (atypical flutter patterns described above) or by echocardiographic enlarged left atria. This is not surprising since structural heart disease is a substrate for atrial fibrillation. In my opinion, patients who have flutter should undergo ablation as a primary procedure. In addition, in patients who have a history of flutter and fibrillation, the incidence of fibrillation episodes may be diminished by a flutter ablation. This suggests that flutter is involved in either the initiation and/or perpetuation of atrial fibrillation in a certain percentage of patients. This is another reason to consider flutter ablation in anyone who has this rhythm documented.

Left atrial flutters are more difficult to ablate, primarily because they are difficult to document. Electroanatomic mapping has been useful in this regard.[193] Many left atrial flutters

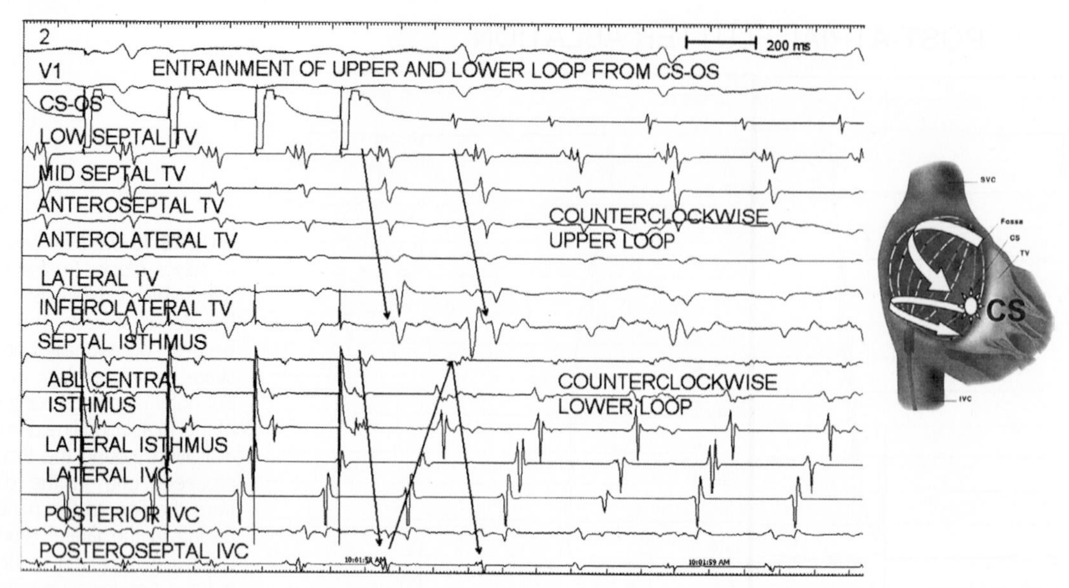


**FIGURE 13-76** *Demonstration of lower and upper loop reentry simultaneously shown using a basket catheter.* Activation around the tricuspid annulus (TV), and the IVC are shown during pacing of the coronary sinus. During atrial flutter, coronary sinus pacing entrains both the activation loop around the tricuspid annulus and the counterclockwise loop around the inferior vena cava. Both loops share the common isthmus. The loops are schematically shown in the figure on the right.

circulate around the mitral annulus with the pulmonary veins and fossa ovalis as posterior boundaries.[193] Scars from prior surgical procedures can provide obstacles that lead to atrial tachycardias with large excitable gaps. These are similar electrophysiologically to isthmus-dependent flutter. They can be caused by routine atriotomy incisions, postcardiac transplant, or following correction to congenital heart disease. Detailed mapping shows double potentials and low voltages in the area of incision. Electroanatomic mapping is invaluable in localizing "gaps" in the "scar" line through which the impulse can propagate and produce a macroreentrant circuit. Focal ablation at these gaps can cure the rhythm. An example is shown in Figure 13-80. The voltage map and double potentials define the "scar" region. Activation is possible where a small gap near the superior border of the "scar" (panel B) is. Ablation at this site cured the tachycardia. I believe these gaps are caused by the pressure of the "clamp" superior and/or inferior to the actual atriotomy scar.

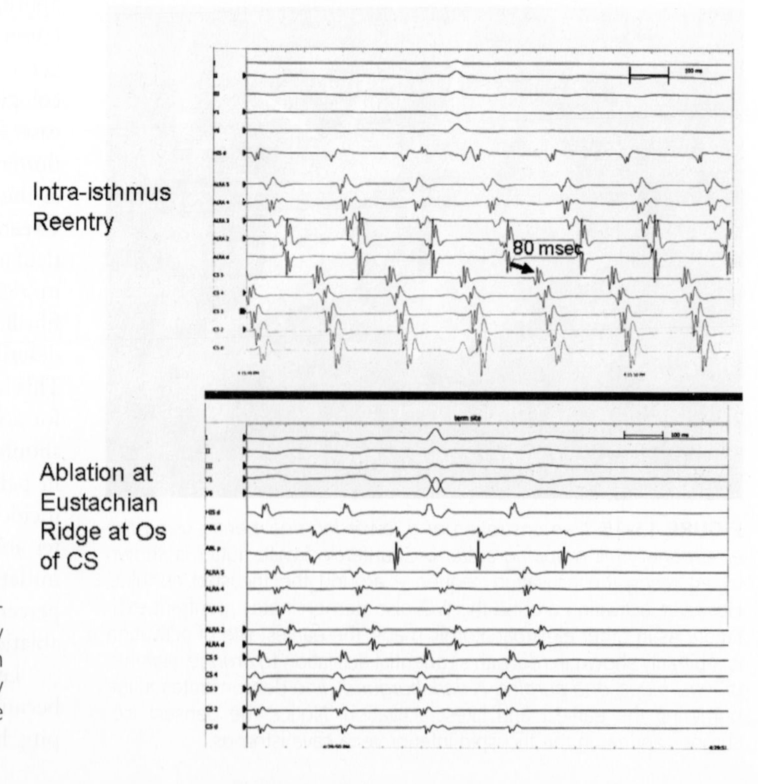


**FIGURE 13-77** *The requirement of ablation across the Eustachian ridge to treat intraisthmus reentry.* Intraisthmus reentry is shown on top with a typically short intraisthmus conduction time. Termination of the arrhythmia occurs with radiofrequency energy delivered along the coronary sinus os Eustachian ridge area. See text for explanation.

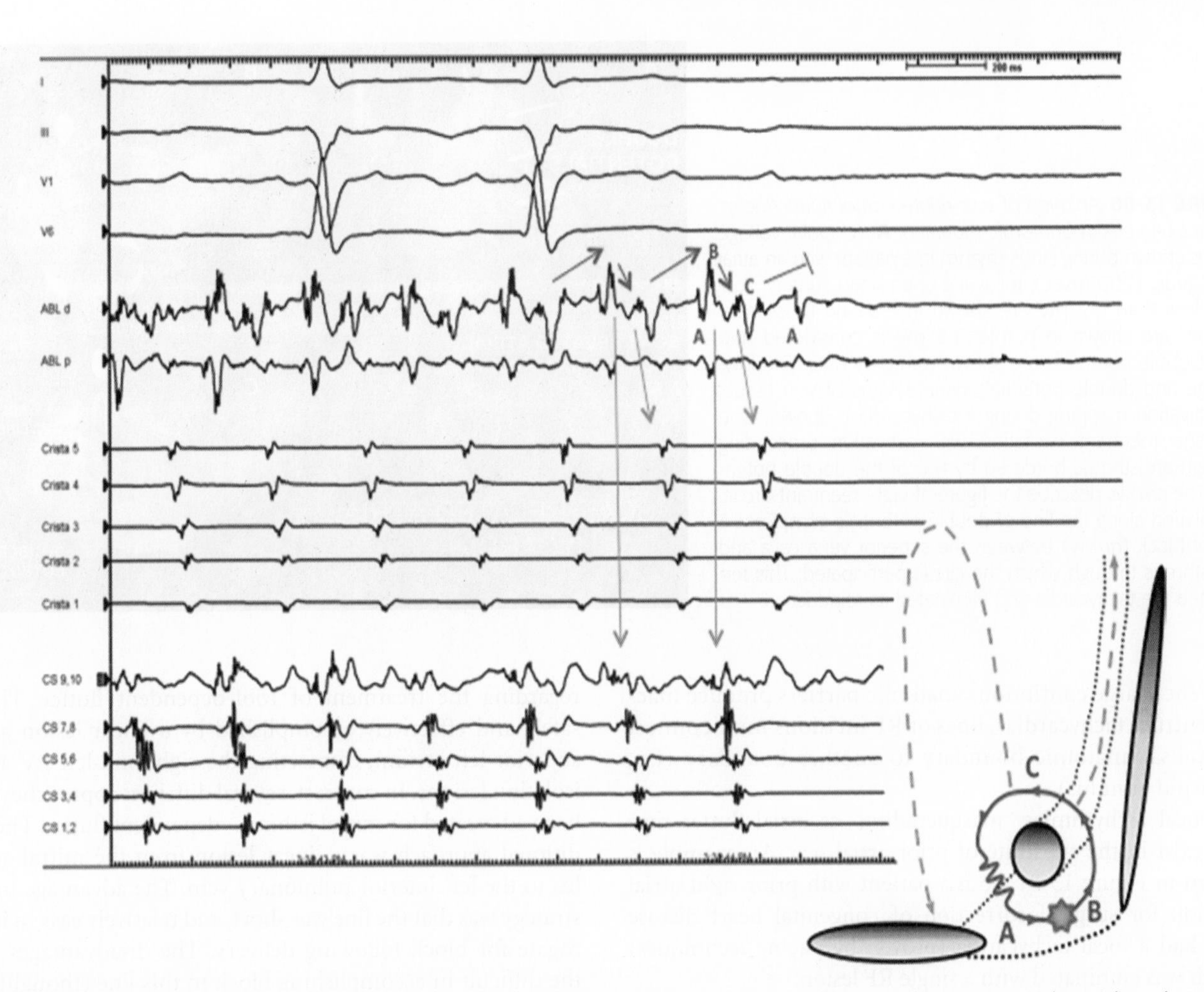


**FIGURE 13-78** Intraisthmus reentry. Four surface leads and intracardiac recordings from the ablation catheter, crista (right atrial) and coronary sinus decapolar catheters are shown during on-going tachycardia which is terminated by ablation between the coronary sinus and the IVC (denoted by the *star* on the schema). Note the extremely complex nature of the ABL catheter recording, which different components reflecting activation of different areas surrounding the coronary sinus, as explained in the schema (*inset*).

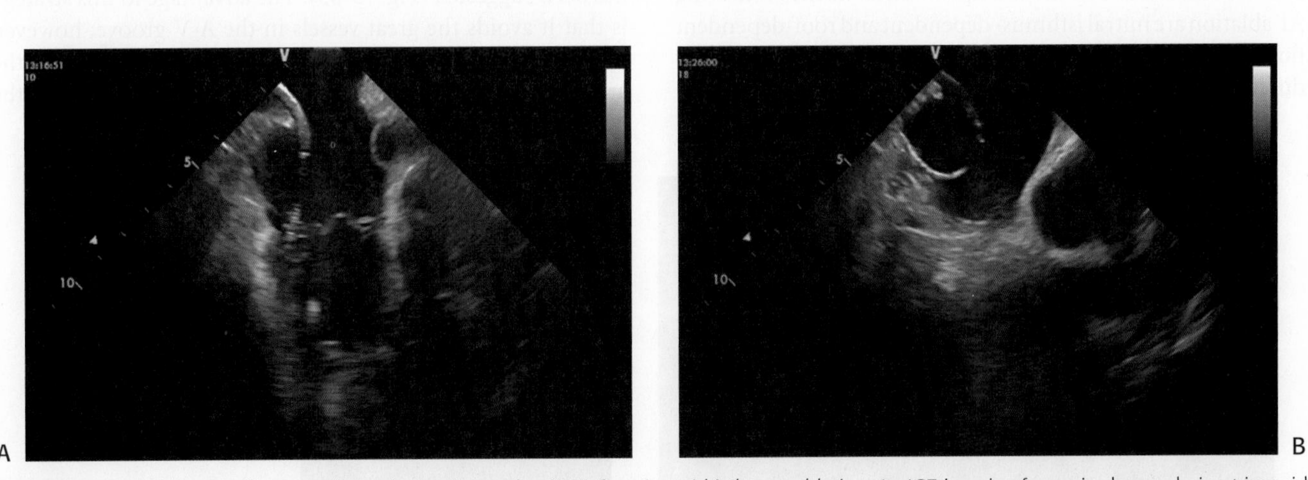


**FIGURE 13-79** *The use of intracardiac echocardiography (ICE) for tricuspid isthmus ablation.* An ICE imaging frame is shown during tricuspid isthmus ablation in a patient with a prominent *Eustachian* ridge (*arrow*). In **(A)**, the ablation catheter is positioned across the tricuspid valve (TV); simple pull back of the catheter would result in failure to contact the portion of isthmus close to the IVC because of "guarding" by the Eustachian ridge. ICE imaging allows recognition of this anatomic variant, and appropriate positioning of the ablation catheter **(B)**. (Courtesy of Luis Saenz, MD.)

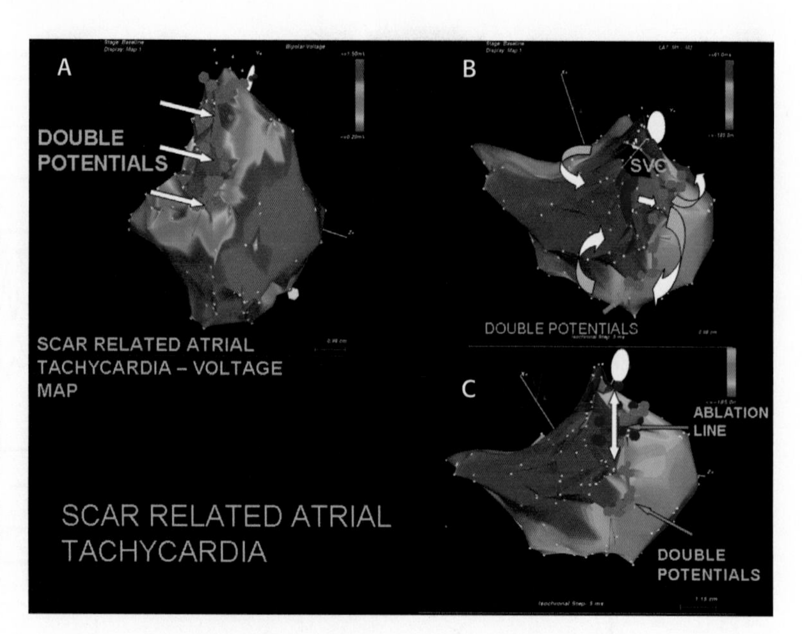


**FIGURE 13-80** *Ablation of scar-related atrial flutter/tachycardia using electroanatomic mapping.* **A:** A bipolar voltage map is shown during sinus rhythm in a patient with an atrial tachycardia (250 msec), following open heart surgery. Voltages less than 0.2 mV are shown in *red* and those over 1.5 mV are shown in purple. 1.5 mV is considered normal. Double potentials are shown with *gray dots.* The low-voltage and double potentials denote signs of scar tissue. **B:** Activation mapping during a tachycardia is shown. One can see reentrant excitation with activation proceeding through an isthmus bordered by two of the double potentials. The *arrows* describe the figure-of-eight reentrant circuit. **C:** Ablation along the line of double potentials completes a line of block (*arrow*) between the superior vena cava and the isthmus through which the circuit participated. This terminated the tachycardia and eliminated its reinduction.

When large continuous anatomic barriers produce macroreentrant tachycardias, lines of RF incisions must connect the causal anatomic boundary to another boundary (i.e., tricuspid annulus).

Focal arrhythmias "masquerading" as atrial flutter may also exist in the substrate of prior atrial scar. An example is shown in Figure 13-81 from a patient with prior right atrial incision for surgical correction of congenital heart disease who had a focal tachycardia (proven by pacing techniques) which was eliminated with a single RF lesion.

Atypical atrial flutters are also common after ablation of atrial fibrillation. In addition, as contemporary ablation strategies have focused on ablation more proximally within the atrium (antral ablation), the incidence of postprocedure flutters has increased. The most frequent atrial flutters following AF ablation are mitral isthmus–dependent and roof-dependent flutters. Importantly, these often coexist, sometimes at subtly different cycle lengths (Fig. 13-82). Little controversy exists regarding the treatment of roof-dependent flutter. This is safely and effectively accomplished by a linear lesion at the superior left atrium, connecting the right and left PV antral isolation lesions. In contrast, several different approaches have been advocated for mitral isthmus–dependent flutter. The traditional approach was a linear lesion from the mitral annulus to the left inferior pulmonary vein. The advantage to this strategy was that the line was short, and relatively easy to interrogate for block following delivery. The disadvantages were the difficult in accomplishing block in this line (thought secondary to cooling effects of the adjacent great cardiac vein), a substantial recurrence rate and possible damage to the left circumflex artery. More recently, an anterior line, connecting the anterior mitral annulus to the right superior pulmonary vein has been suggested (Fig. 13-83). The advantage to this strategy is that it avoids the great vessels in the A-V groove; however, it is a long linear lesion and has been reported to affect the arterial supply to the sinus node when it originates from the

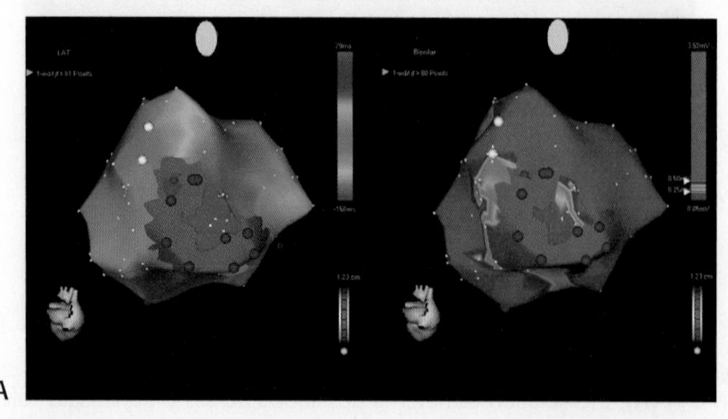


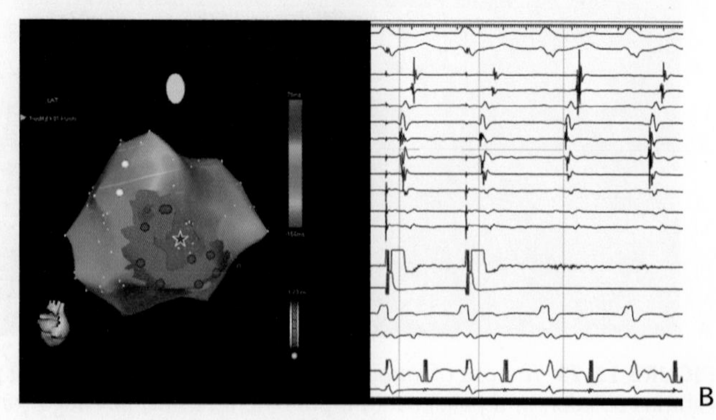


**FIGURE 13-81** *Ablation of a scar-related atrial tachycardia with a nonreentrant mechanism in a patient with remote atriotomy.* In **panel A**, electroanatomic maps of right atrial voltage and activation during atrial tachycardia are shown. The *gray* icons and surrounding *gray* color denote local bipolar electrogram voltage of <0.1 mV. In **panel B**, the ablation catheter is placed at the area denoted by the *blue star.* The electrogram recorded from this site was fractionated and low amplitude. Pacing at this site resulted in an intracardiac pace map match. Ablation at this site resulted in tachycardia termination and subsequent inability to reinduce.

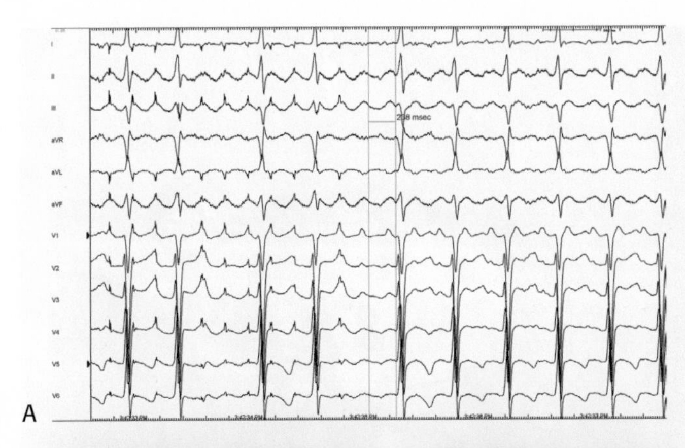


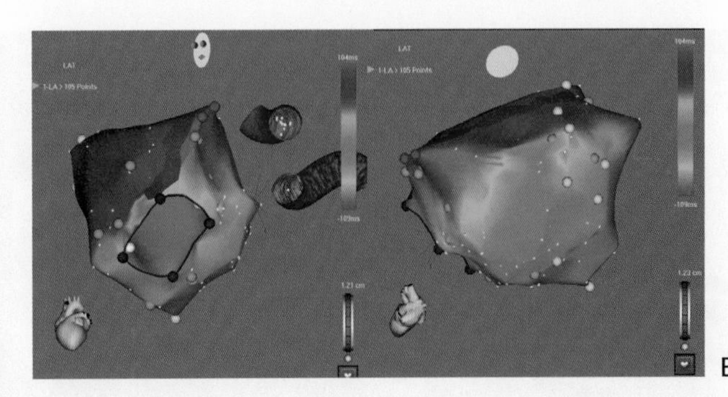


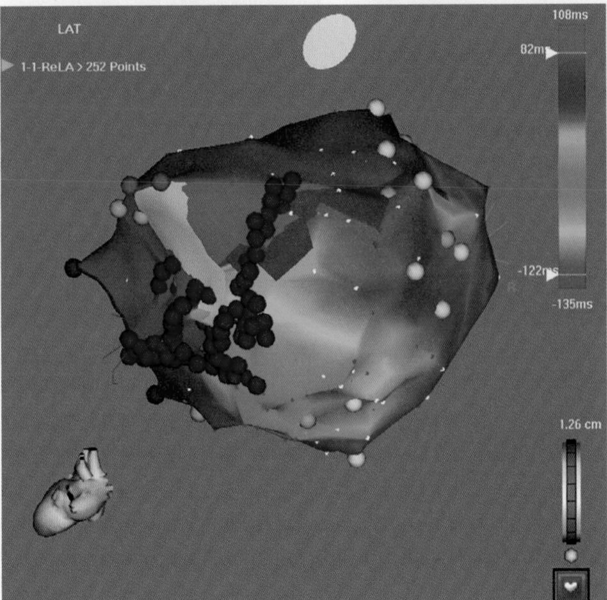


**FIGURE 13-82** *Coexisting mitral annular and roof dependent left atrial flutter in a patient with prior AF ablation.* In **A**, the 12 lead ECG is shown during atrial pacing and atrial flutter with a cycle length of 220 msec; note that overdrive pacing provides a clear demonstration of the P-wave morphology (p-wave onset denoted by the *red line*). In **B**, an electroanatomic activation map during atrial flutter is shown. Activation proceeds in a clockwise manner around the mitral annulus (**left**) and from top to bottom across the posterior wall (**right**); however, entrainment from the roof resulted in a long return cycle. After mitral isthmus ablation, a slightly different flutter continued, with a longer cycle length (240 msec). Activation mapping of the second flutter **(C)** demonstrated roof dependent flutter, which was ablated with a line from the left superior to the right superior pulmonary vein (roof line).

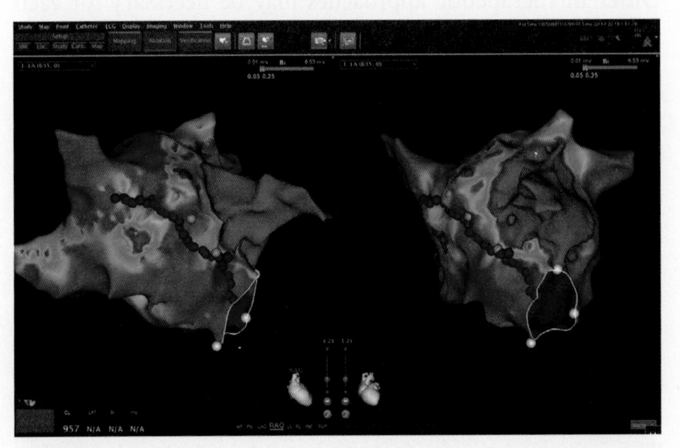

**FIGURE 13-83** *Anterior mitral annular line.* Right anterior and left anterior views of electroanatomic bipolar voltage maps of the left atrium in a patient with mitral annular flutter following ablation for atrial fibrillation. Note the very low voltages (which would be considered as scar by some investigators) at sites within the flutter circuit). A linear lesion connecting the anterior mitral annulus to the ostium of the right superior pulmonary vein (*red dots*) was constructed. Termination of the flutter occurred after approximately one-third of the line had been performed.

circumflex artery. As demonstrated by the Bordeaux group, incomplete linear lesions in the atrium can be proarrhythmic; this necessitates careful investigation of the line to assure that conduction block has been achieved (Fig. 13-84).[194,195]

## Ablative Techniques (Surgical and Catheter-Based) for Treatment of Atrial Fibrillation

Atrial fibrillation remains a therapeutic challenge. The goals of treatment of atrial fibrillation include rate control, prevention of atrial fibrillation and maintenance of sinus rhythm, and prevention of emboli. Prevention of emboli is primarily an anticoagulation issue; however, prevention of atrial fibrillation would be a better option. Pharmacologic therapy has neither been adequately able to provide rate control nor to prevent atrial fibrillation and maintain sinus rhythm, and is accompanied by significant side effects. As such, ablative techniques have been developed to deal with these issues. As stated earlier in the chapter, A-V nodal/junctional ablation provides the best method of rate control in patients who are

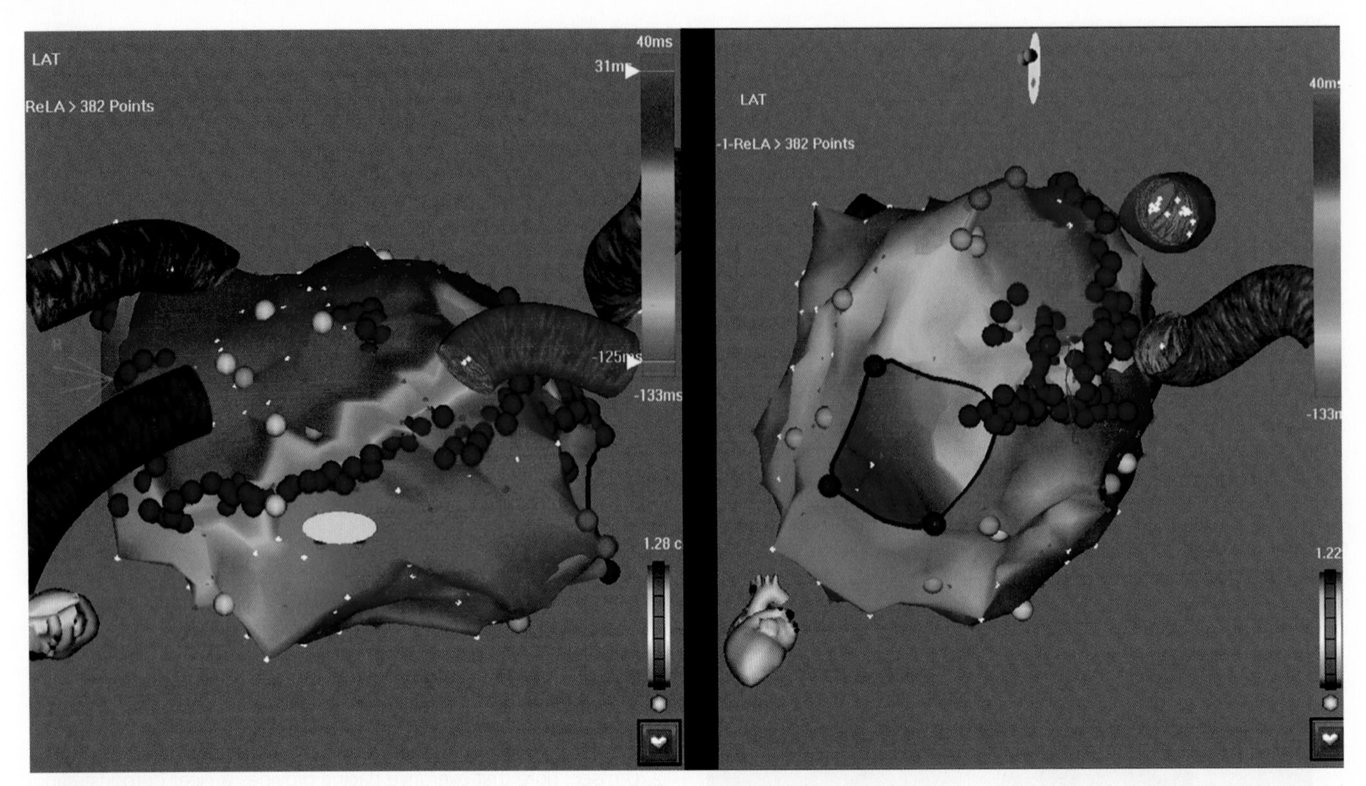


**FIGURE 13-84** *Verification of conduction block after linear lesion creation.* Electroanatomic activation mapping of the left atrium during left atrial appendage pacing shows conduction block across a roof line (**panel A**, superior projection) and a mitral annular line (posterior mitral annulus to left inferior pulmonary vein, panel B, LAO projection).

drug-refractory or intolerant of drugs. In fact, many patients prefer A-V junctional ablation with implantation of a pacemaker to combination pharmacotherapy. Ablation is carried out as described earlier in the chapter. The type of pacemaker implanted depends on the clinical situation. In patients with the Brady-Tachy syndrome, atrial-based pacing with mode switching is critical. Newer devices may also include preventative pacing, antitachycardia pacing, and defibrillation capabilities. The use of atrial-based pacing may actually decrease the incidence of atrial fibrillation, decrease cerebrovascular accidents, and improve heart failure. Although survival may not increase, patients experience marked improvement in the quality of life. Some of our happiest patients are those who have had "ablate and pace" therapy for atrial fibrillation. Nonetheless, recent data has suggested that this strategy may not optimally defend patients from risk. A randomized comparison of A-V junction ablation and biventricular pacing versus AF catheter ablation by Khan and coworkers demonstrated a superiority of the latter strategy, based on superior results in all metrics of a composite endpoint (ejection fraction, distance on the 6-minute walk test, and Minnesota Living with Heart Failure quality of life score) at 6 months.[196]

Prevention of atrial fibrillation is a much more complex issue, and is clearly more difficult to achieve. More uniformly successful treatment will ultimately require better understanding of the triggers and substrates responsible for initiating and maintaining atrial fibrillation. It is now obvious that atrial fibrillation is a heterogeneous group of disorders caused by a number of mechanisms, including (a) focal triggering mechanisms; (b) mother rotors, which gives off daughter wavelets leading to atrial fibrillation; and (c) random reentry as described in the multiple wavelet hypothesis. Different therapeutic approaches may be necessary for each mechanism. In addition, ablative procedures may also be used as part of so-called hybrid therapy; combinations of ablation and pharmacotherapy, ablation and pacing, and ablation and defibrillation (singly or in combination). Each of these will be described below.

Haissaguerre and his colleagues were the first to describe initiation of atrial fibrillation by repetitive foci originating in the pulmonary veins.[197–199] These investigators demonstrated that ectopic foci in the pulmonary veins could be recorded as sharp spikes preceding local left atrial activation that frequently triggered atrial tachycardia that degenerated into atrial fibrillation or initiated atrial fibrillation directly in the vein or ostial cuff. These observations have been substantiated by others.[200] The exact mechanism of triggering of these foci or the mechanism by which they specifically initiate atrial fibrillation has not yet been established. Catecholamines, stretch, and pressure may be the mechanisms of induction of such firing, but this does not necessarily explain their ability to initiate atrial fibrillation. In addition, we and other investigators have demonstrated that such firing could persist during stabilized atrial fibrillation, leading to the concept that such firing may also be a source of reinitiation or maintenance of atrial fibrillation. The typical patient in whom "focal atrial fibrillation" is the likely mechanism presents with multiple episodes of paroxysmal atrial fibrillation that are short lived and recur throughout the day. In some cases, these patients have prominent characteristics associated with autonomically modulated atrial fibrillation. In between episodes, multiple atrial premature depolarizations are seen that appear to arise primarily from a single focus, although it is difficult to document this definitively since such foci are only recorded on Holter monitors, which have only 1 to 3 ECG leads. In addition, early P waves often occur on T waves making their morphologic characteristics difficult to interpret. Although Haissaguerre and colleagues believe that nearly all cases of paroxysmal atrial fibrillation are manifestations of focal atrial fibrillation, the true incidence is probably significantly less. In many ways, focal atrial fibrillation may be the purest example "electrical" atrial fibrillation, in that it is not influenced by heart disease, aging, or other disorders that can add to the mechanistic complexity, particularly when atrial fibrillation becomes established. Examples of focal atrial fibrillation from Hassaiguerre's original description[197] are shown in Figure 13-85. Although the vast majority of focal triggers of atrial fibrillation appear to arise in the pulmonary veins (left and right superior pulmonary veins being most prominent), we and others have also recorded other sites of initiation of focal atrial fibrillation, including the coronary sinus, the atrial appendages, the superior vena cava, and the crista terminalis.[201–203] Of note, we have seen several young women in whom atrial fibrillation is initiated by A-V nodal reentry, the majority of which terminated with ablation at the os of the coronary sinus where atrial fibrillation appeared to initiate (see below). The coexistence of these two tachyarrhythmias has also been reported by others.[204] The high incidence of initiation in the pulmonary veins is believed to occur because of the thin cuff of muscular tissue that extends from the left atrium over the epicardial aspects of the pulmonary veins for a variable degree, sometimes as much as 3 cm. While near the ostia of the pulmonary veins this cuff is circumferential, as one moves more distally there is almost an unraveling such that one or more strands of muscular tissue coalesce to produce the proximal cuff. The anatomic complexity of these muscle fibers is shown in Figure 13-86. The variable coursing of these strands, and the poor coupling of cells in the musculature, lead to multicomponent electrograms within the pulmonary veins. What is special about cardiac myocytes in the pulmonary veins that makes them more likely to produce impulse formation is uncertain. Chen and colleagues[205] have studied isolated cardiac myocytes from the pulmonary veins of rabbits. The majority of myocytes had pacemaker activity and relatively long-action potential duration. These cells also demonstrated calcium-dependent slow inward currents and transient outward currents on depolarization, similar to those of nonpacemaker cells, but in addition they had a larger delayed rectifier. Whether human

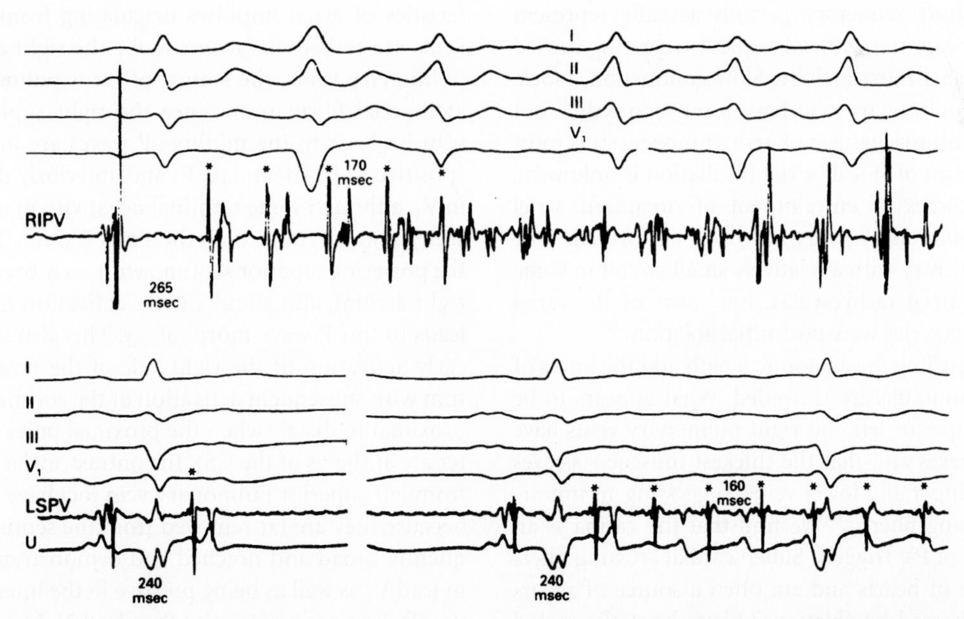


**FIGURE 13-85** *Initiation of focal atrial fibrillation from the pulmonary veins.* In the **top panel**, four surface ECG leads are shown with an electrogram obtained from the right inferior pulmonary vein. Note the double components of the electrogram from the right superior pulmonary vein. An atrial premature beat initiates atrial fibrillation. Note that the second spike noted in the pulmonary vein during sinus rhythms now becomes the initiating spike of the atrial tachyarrhythmia that induces atrial fibrillation. In the **bottom panel**, there is shown an electrogram from the left superior pulmonary vein. In the lower left panel, the sinus beat is associated with a low-amplitude left atrial potential followed by a higher-frequency component due to a potential from the pulmonary vein. An atrial premature beat follows, which is initiated from the pulmonary vein as shown by the spike proceeding the left atrial potential. In the right lower-hand panel, at another time, an atrial premature depolarization from the same pulmonary vein potential initiates a tachyarrhythmia that degenerates into atrial fibrillation. (From Haissaguerre M, Jais P, Shah DC, et al. Spontaneous initiation of atrial fibrillation by ectopic beats originating in the pulmonary veins. *N Engl J Med* 1998;339:659–666.)

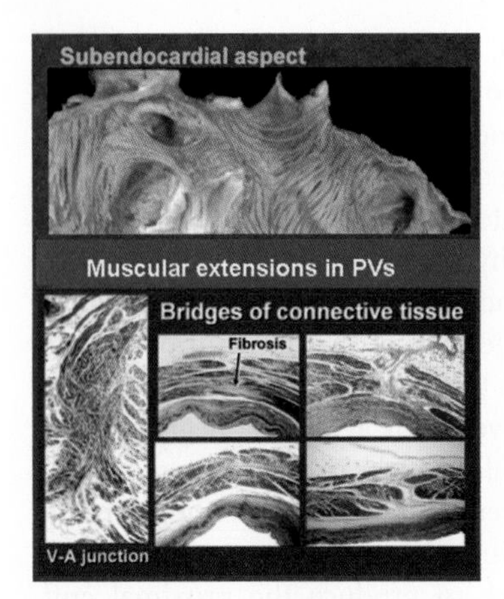
Subendocardial aspect
Muscular extensions in PVs
Bridges of connective tissue
Fibrosis
V-A junction
Changes in myocardial fibers orientation in the crucial posterior region of the LA-PV junction & the presence of structural discontinuities may confer abnormal conduction properties *that*
*set the scene* for:
Fragmented non-uniform anisotropic conduction and possibly microreentry

**FIGURE 13-86** Role of Atrial Structure on Arrhythmogenesis.

tissue is similar or whether these findings distinguish patients with and without the syndrome of focal AF is not well studied. The complex interdigitation of pulmonary vein muscle fibers and left atrial fibers and the variable angles and curvature produce an ideal pathophysiologic substrate for slow conduction and block due to nonuniform anisotropy and influence of curvature, leading to reentry. Studies in humans have also shown that the distal pulmonary veins have shorter refractory periods than the adjacent left atrium[200,206,207] have found that the refractory periods of pulmonary veins in patients with paroxysmal AF are significantly shorter than those in patients without AF (as short as 80 msec). Others have postulated that these apparent short refractory periods actually represent local nerve tissue capture, with subsequent triggering caused by gangionated plexi burst activity. Slow conduction, block, and reentry in a pulmonary vein have been reported,[207] but the frequency of this mechanism of arrhythmogenesis is most common mechanism of "focal" atrial fibrillation is unknown. No systematic studies of entrainment of organized atrial tachycardias in pulmonary veins has been performed. One study suggested reentry with a relatively small circuit in some pulmonary vein atrial tachycardias, but most of the atrial tachycardias in this series were postinitial ablation.[208]

More data regarding the anatomic length and thickness of pulmonary vein musculature is needed. What appears to be true is that the superior left and right pulmonary veins have longer muscle sleeves and that the thickest muscular sleeves are between the upper and lower veins, suggesting an important role of crossing fibers.[209] We find that the carina is an important source of PV triggers. Subepicardial crossing fibers are seen in ≈40% of hearts and are often a source of recurrences if not addressed by ablation. Others have also noted that recurrent PV triggers for AF are mapped to these carina areas, presumably because of this muscle thickness.[210] I personally do not believe we have identified any special characteristics of electrograms in pulmonary veins that distinguish patients with or without focal atrial fibrillation. I say this because virtually all patients with or without atrial fibrillation have similar looking pulmonary vein potentials. This is analogous to the situation in which "slow pathway potentials" were felt to be specific markers related to the physiology of A-V nodal tachycardia. Pulmonary vein potentials, analogous to "slow pathway potential," appear to be ubiquitous. More importantly, introduction of catheters into the pulmonary veins can lead to triggering within the pulmonary vein, providing targets for those investigators looking for targets. An example of this phenomenon from a patient who had no evidence of atrial fibrillation and who had her pulmonary veins mapped through a patent foramen ovale is shown in Figure 13-87. Multicomponent potentials were seen in all of her pulmonary veins and were most prominent in the left superior pulmonary vein. With the introduction of the catheter into the left superior pulmonary vein, a pulmonary vein rhythm appeared that demonstrates clear initiation of the rhythm from the distal pole of the ablation catheter. Thus, in order to prevent unnecessary pulmonary vein ablations and their attendant complications it is incumbent upon the investigator to demonstrate that ectopic impulse formation in the pulmonary veins occurs spontaneously. More work is necessary to more fully characterize the electrophysiology of the pulmonary veins and the adjacent left atrium in order to more accurately identify a specific arrhythmogenic substrate.

The two methods most commonly used to identify a pulmonary vein source of spontaneous impulse formations are use of the electrocardiogram and use of mapping catheters along the posterior septum or anterolateral right atrium with the proximal poles along the posterior-superior septum, and within the coronary sinus.[211] The ECG morphologic characteristics of atrial impulses originating from the pulmonary veins are rather characteristic for the right and left superior pulmonary veins, the source of most pulmonary vein initiated atrial fibrillation. Since the right superior pulmonary vein is closer to the midline, P waves are inferiorly directed (positive in II, III, and AVF) and anteriorly directed (positive in $V_1$, although some terminal negativity may occasionally be seen), and narrower than the sinus P wave. The proximity to the posterior superior septum, with early breakthrough to the right atrium, and simultaneous activation of the left atrium leads to this P-wave morphology. This also leads to relatively early activation of the right side of the posterior atrial septum with subsequent activation of the coronary sinus, usually proximal to distal (when the proximal poles of the CS catheter are at the os of the CS). In contrast, atrial impulses arising from left superior pulmonary vein foci have broader P waves because they are far removed from the septum. They are frequently broad and notched and demonstrate total positivity in lead $V_1$ as well as being positive in the inferior leads (lead 3 usually being more positive than lead 2). In contrast to activation associated with foci originating in the right superior pulmonary vein, the left superior vein foci produces activation of the coronary sinus earlier than the right atrial catheter, particularly when the coronary sinus catheter is positioned with its distal pole anteriorly. These two observations can provide evidence for a pulmonary vein origin for the spontaneous ectopy and initiation of atrial fibrillation, and justify

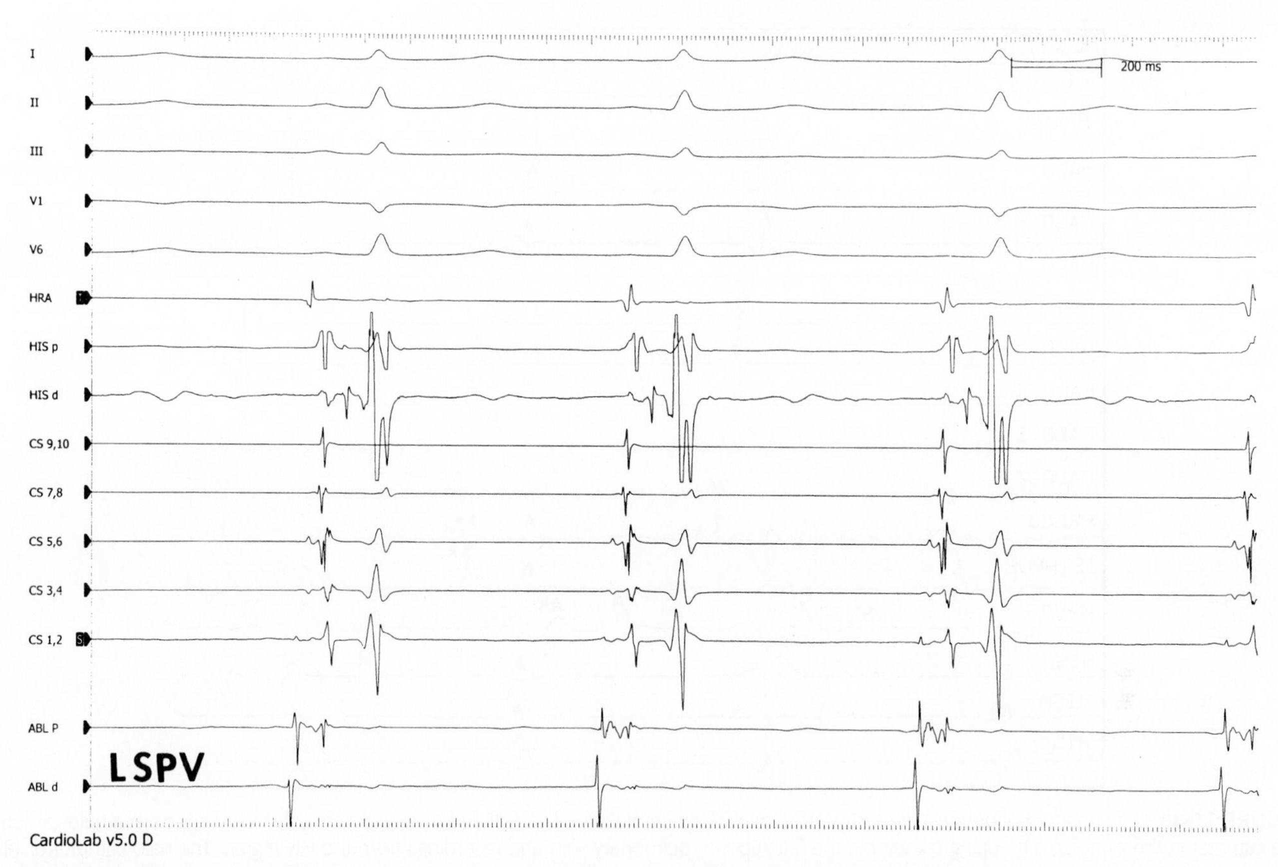


**FIGURE 13-87** *Mechanical initiation of pulmonary vein activity.* This tracing comes from a young person without any history of atrial fibrillation, but in whom a catheter was placed in the left superior pulmonary vein (LVSV). An ectopic atrial arrhythmia was initiated from that ablation/mapping catheter as demonstrated by earliest activation from the distal tip of the ablation catheter with subsequent activation to the proximal portion of the pulmonary vein associated with a layer left atrial component. Thus, initiation of atrial tachyarrhythmias from the pulmonary veins by mechanical induction of catheter introduction itself can produce misleading rhythms that should not be targeted for ablation. See text for discussion.

subsequent transseptal catheterization to further explore this mechanism of atrial fibrillation. Of note, negative P waves in lead 1 are never seen in left or right pulmonary vein foci, since the pulmonary veins are posterior in the chest. A negative P wave in lead 1 suggests a left atrial appendage or lateral mitral annulus origin. It is not unusual for there to be lack of such ectopy, however. Sedation is one of the major factors in inhibiting ectopic impulse formation. As such, I recommend that no sedative be given when one is attempting to demonstrate spontaneous atrial impulse formation. Moreover, it is most commonly necessary to add pharmacologic agents to facilitate impulse formation. Such agents include isoproterenol, epinephrine, theophyline, and adenosine. Because of the unreliability of seeing all potential sources of pulmonary vein foci, we do not rely on them for ablation of atrial fibrillation. We do, however, target focal pulmonary vein tachycardias (see below).

Once the appearance of pulmonary vein foci has been suggested, transseptal catheterization should be performed. Although some investigators use a single transseptal puncture followed by introduction of two guidewires and then reintroduction of two sheaths, I prefer two (or occasionally three) separate transseptal procedures. I believe the latter approach is associated with less femoral vein bleeding and local complications as well as a lower incidence of persistent atrial septal defect following a procedure. Intracardiac ultrasound or transesophageal echocardiography may also be employed to facilitate catheter positioning. Once the left atrium is entered the goals for the procedure are to identify vein and/or branch of the vein from which the impulse arises and localize either the earliest site of activation within that vein or branch, or the segment from which the earliest activation is recorded. Different techniques have been used to achieve these goals. The initial method used was point-by-point activation mapping in the pulmonary veins. This method is still useful, particularly using electroanatomic mapping, which allows one to tag the anatomic location of individual potentials. The initiation of atrial ectopic impulse formation in the pulmonary veins only after a catheter has been introduced into the pulmonary veins does not signify that the source of atrial fibrillation has been identified. The catheter should be withdrawn to assess whether or not this impulse formation exists spontaneously. This is in contrast to an ongoing atrial tachyarrhythmia in which a pulmonary vein is explored and early activation found (Fig. 13-88). One of the other clues that this rhythm was not flutter is simultaneous activation from high to low on the lateral right atrial free wall and on the septum. This is demonstrated in this

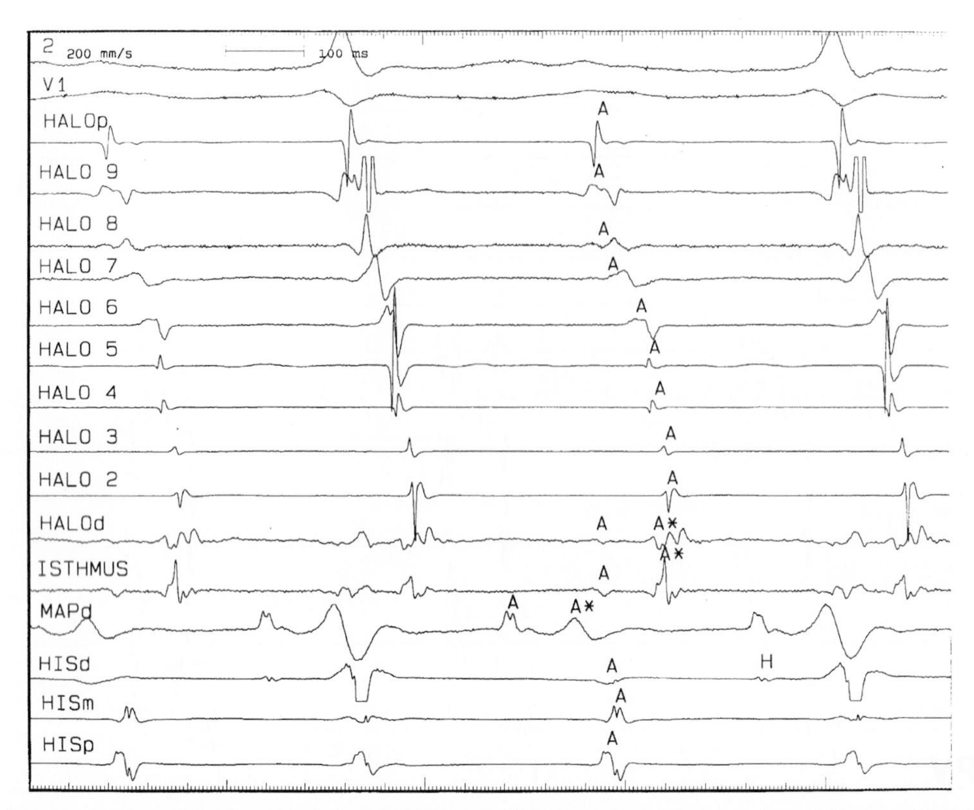


**FIGURE 13-88** *Left superior pulmonary vein tachycardia mimicking atrial flutter.* Leads II and $V_1$ are shown with recordings from a halo catheter, the catheter in the isthmus, a mapping catheter in the left superior pulmonary vein and recordings from the His region. The halo catheter distally records the lateral isthmus and proximally the superior septum. The tachycardia is present at approximately 310-msec cycle length. Activation of the lateral wall and the septum is high to low. The isthmus catheter is adjacent to the halo catheter distal, which was at the site of a prior ablation for proven isthmus-dependent flutter. The split electrograms are at the site of block produced by the prior linear lesion. The high–low sequence of activation proves that this is not clockwise flutter. The activation in the left superior pulmonary vein records a pulmonary vein potential of 130 msec prior to the P wave with a later left atrial potential (A*). Subsequent ablation of the pulmonary vein focus eliminated the need for antiarrhythmic therapy and the patient has been free of arrhythmia since.

figure in which there is simultaneous high-to-low activation along the lateral right atrial wall (halo 6 through halo 2) and the septum (halo 7 to 9 and the His bundle recording). Ablation of the focal tachycardia, which was initially performed in the pulmonary vein, is now done by targeting the exit site from the vein at the ostial cuff, or more commonly, by isolating the entire vein.

Occasionally, far field potentials can be recorded within pulmonary veins that confuse the issue. Because of this, some investigators suggest placing multipolar catheters in each pulmonary vein (primarily the superior pulmonary veins initially) to see the sequence of activation of impulse formation.[212] While this has advantages in allowing far field activity from one vein to be distinguished from local activity in another vein or the left atrial appendage, and facilitates diagnosing the earliest site, it also is associated with a high incidence of iatrogenic impulse formation from the catheters themselves. An example of an atrial premature complex, mapped to the pulmonary vein, initiating atrial fibrillation, and successful ablation of that site is shown in Figure 13-89. In panel A of this figure, a premature atrial complex is seen in the middle of the tracing, which is associated with early activation in the pulmonary vein associated with a local left atrial electrogram, suggesting the recording site is at the ostial cuff. Following the next sinus beat another atrial premature beat from this site initiates atrial fibrillation. Delivery of RF energy at that site in sinus rhythm initially produces an accelerated atrial rhythm followed by sinus rhythm, which is associated with local left atrial electrogram and loss of the pulmonary vein potential. Another example of an atrial tachyarrhythmia that was demonstrated to initiate atrial fibrillation at other times is shown in Figure 13-90. In the top panel the 12-lead ECG shows paroxysms of an atrial tachyarrhythmia that looks like either coarse atrial fibrillation or an atrial flutter-like rhythm. Intracardiac recordings guided by the Carto mapping system showed this earliest activity arose from the left superior pulmonary vein. The local electrogram in sinus rhythm at this site showed a complex electrogram with left atrial activity followed by a sharp spike representing activity from the pulmonary vein. Atrial tachyarrhythmia begins on the subsequent beats, which is associated with early activity first in the pulmonary vein potential with subsequent left atrial activity. This pulmonary vein activity precedes the P wave by 58 msec. RF ablation at this site terminated the arrhythmia almost immediately (see panel C). The patient has been free of arrhythmias on no medicines for 10 years. The Carto system was extremely useful in localizing the earliest site of activation

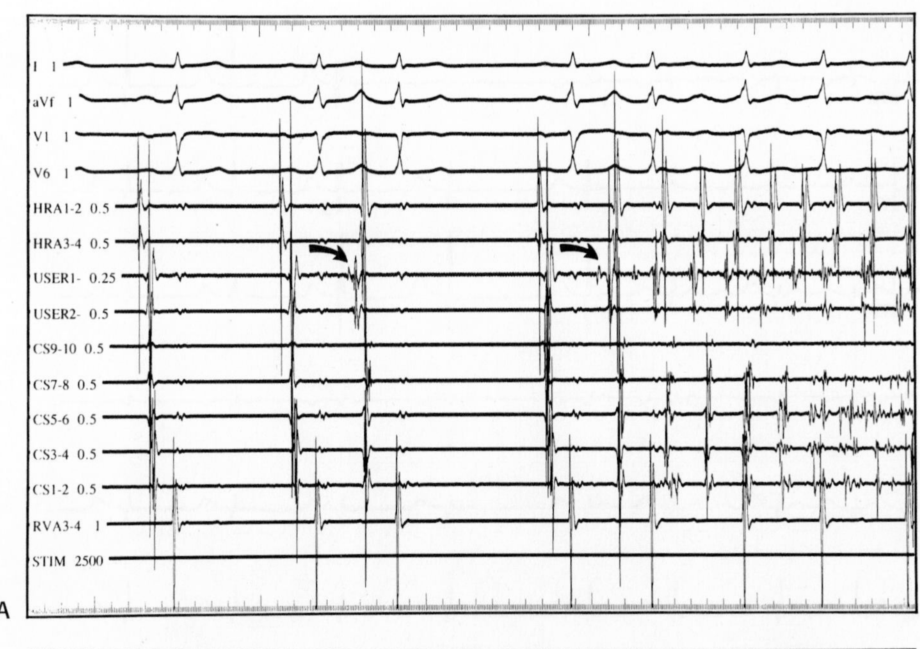


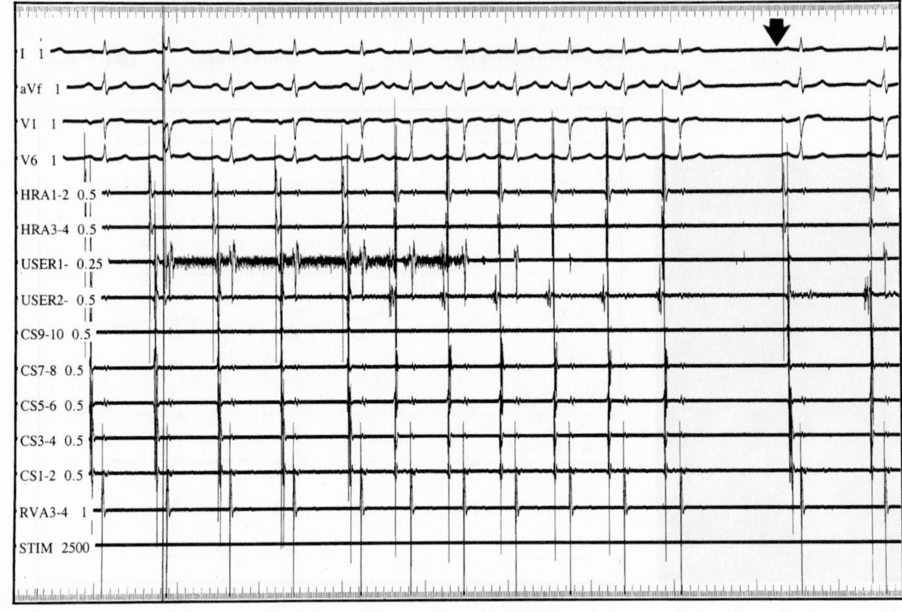


**FIGURE 13-89** *Mapping and ablation of pulmonary vein focus initiating atrial fibrillation.* **Panel A:** (**top**) The pulmonary vein APC (*curved arrow*) initiates an atrial tachyarrhythmia that degenerates to atrial fibrillation. **Panel B:** (**bottom**) Radiofrequency application at this site in sinus rhythm produces an accelerated rhythm from the pulmonary vein followed by sinus rhythm. The patient has had no further episodes of atrial tachyarrhythmia.

to the left superior pulmonary vein and anatomically tagging the earliest electrogram, at which site ablation was carried out. Although most ectopic impulse formations initiating atrial fibrillation appear to arise from the pulmonary veins, other sites may also be responsible as mentioned above. Figure 13-91 was recorded from a patient in whom initiation of atrial fibrillation by A-V nodal tachycardia began in the coronary sinus, 5 mm from the OS. RF ablation at that site terminated the atrial fibrillation, and sinus rhythm has been maintained thereafter for 36 months on no medicines.

Mapping and ablation of pulmonary vein foci is different from mapping atrial tachyarrhythmias, however. Mapping of pulmonary vein foci is limited by (a) ablation at sites that appear early but that are proximal to a more distal branching earlier site resulting in failure; (b) multiple foci are common (recurrences due to atrial ectopic formation in other pulmonary veins, antral sites proximal to the ablation, or at non-pulmonary vein related sites—perhaps only 65% arise *in* the pulmonary veins, 85% if antrum is included); (c) spontaneous or pharmacologically induced pulmonary vein foci are unreliable; (d) presence of atrial fibrillation prohibits identification of initiating foci; a high failure rate with most patients requiring 3 or 4 sessions; and (e) a high incidence of pulmonary vein stenosis. The latter complication is most frequently associated with the delivery of multiple lesions deep within the pulmonary veins at sites that are smaller than the ostial cuff. Pulmonary hypertension, pulmonary hemorrhage, hemoptysis, phrenic nerve paralysis, and strokes have all been reported.[213]

In order to improve the safety and efficacy of ablation of pulmonary vein triggers of atrial fibrillation, several techniques

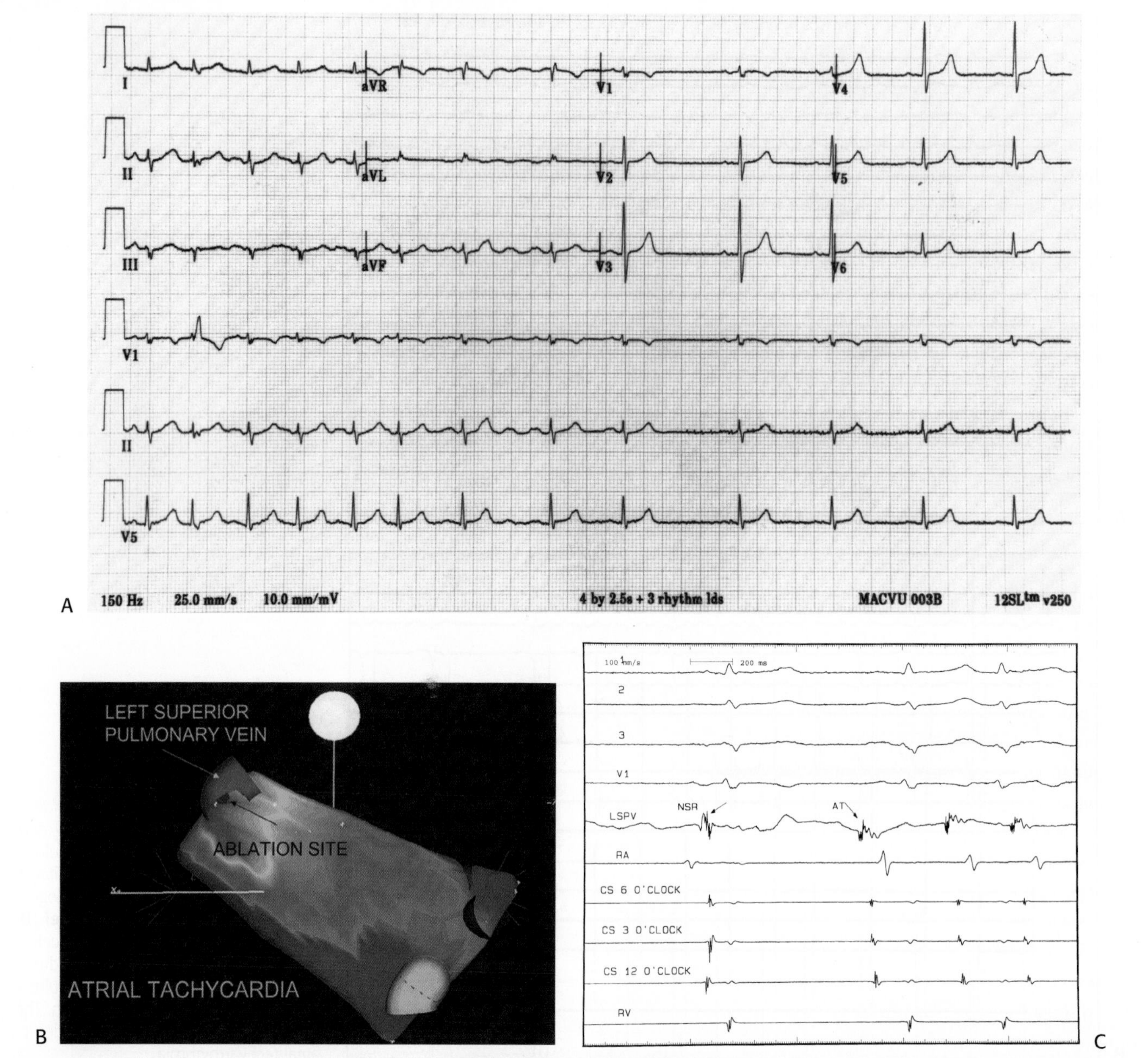


**FIGURE 13-90** *Ablation of atrial tachycardia radiating from the left superior pulmonary vein aided by electroanatomical mapping.* Paroxysmal atrial tachycardia at a cycle length of 250 msec is seen in the ECG in **panel A**. Analog records of sinus rhythm and the onset of atrial tachycardia are shown in **panel C**. Recordings shown are from the superior, lateral and inferior coronary sinus, the right atrium and the left superior pulmonary vein, along with four surface ECG leads. During sinus rhythm, the left superior pulmonary vein (LSPV) shows an initial slow component due to left atrial activation caused by a rapid, somewhat fractionated component (*arrow*) due to activation of the pulmonary vein. CS activation superiorly (12 o'clock) occurs prior to 3 o'clock and 6 o'clock recordings from the CS suggesting activation over Bachmann bundle. Atrial tachycardia then begins with reversal of the electrical signals in the left superior pulmonary vein with subsequent activation of the left atrium. This pulmonary vein focus was confirmed by electroanatomical mapping (**panel B**) to be just inside the left superior pulmonary vein. Ablation at this site immediately terminated the tachycardia and the patient has remained in sinus rhythm off of antiarrhythmic agents for 2 years.

have been developed. These include electrophysiologic map–guided isolation of the pulmonary veins, nonmap-guided approaches which include encircling the pulmonary veins with RF lesions (not documenting isolation), ablating areas of vagal or ganglionic innervation, and/or ablating fractionated electrograms. In none of the nonmap-guided approaches is pulmonary vein isolation attempted, and as such there is no real electrophysiologic endpoint. One cannot use termination of atrial fibrillation alone as and end point since it may occur spontaneously or additional mechanisms of initiation may still be present.

The technique of pulmonary vein isolation was developed by the group at Bordeaux[214] and further popularized by Chen and his colleagues from Taiwan. This technique employs the use of a mapping catheter that has a spiral curved tip on which 10 to 20 electrodes are placed. This is a mini-version of the halo

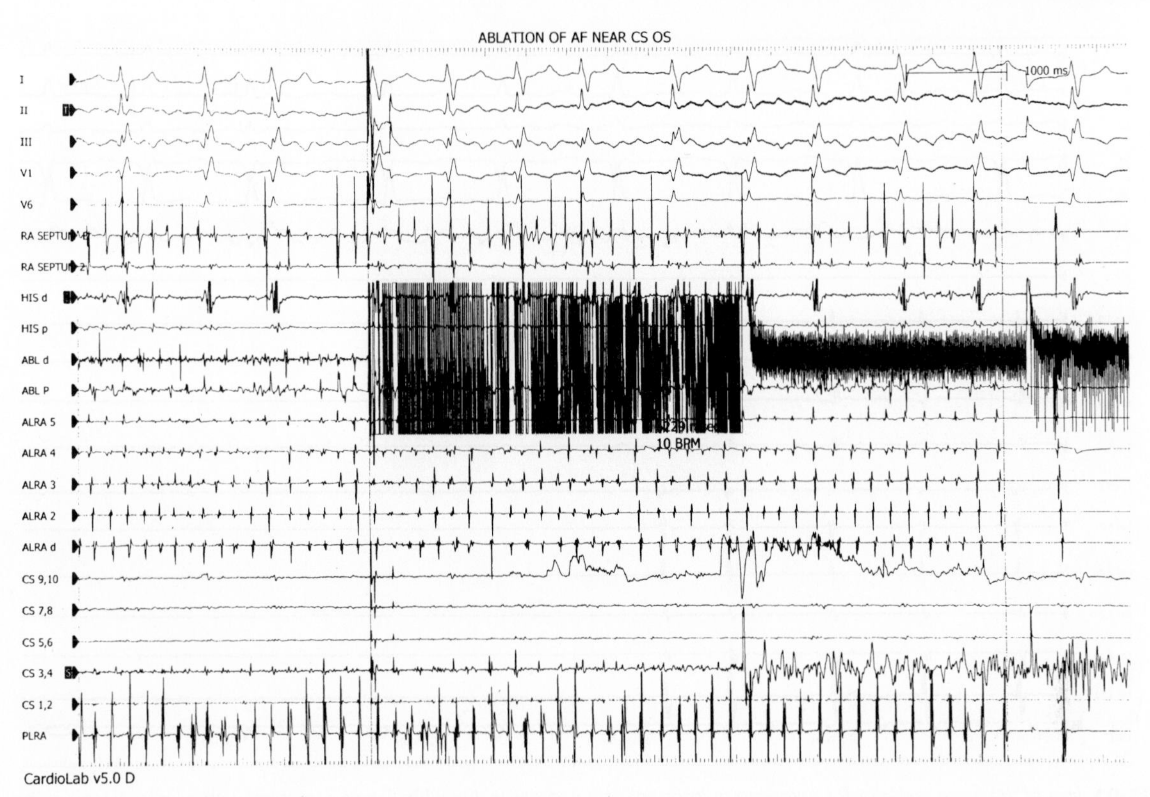


**FIGURE 13-91** *Termination of atrial fibrillation by ablation adjacent to the os of the coronary sinus.* Electrical signals from the septum, the His bundle area and ablation catheter adjacent to the coronary sinus ostium, the anterolateral right atrium, the coronary sinus and the posterolateral right atrium are shown. During A-V nodal tachycardia, atrial fibrillation began spontaneously with the initiating electrograms occurring just under the os of the CS at the site at which the ablation catheter was placed. Delivery of RF energy at this site terminated atrial fibrillation in approximately 5 seconds. Note the organization of electrograms from the septum, the anterolateral right atrium, and the coronary sinus prior to termination.

catheter used around the tricuspid ring for atrial flutter. The catheter is positioned at the ostium or just inside the ostium of the pulmonary vein and analysis of segmental activation is recorded. Although many investigators analyze bipolar pairs (i.e., 5 in a decapolar lasso), we use overlapping poles, yielding 10 to 20 bipolar pairs which maximize the areas of recording and subsequent stimulation (see below). An example is shown in Figure 13-92. It is important to make sure one records activity from the ostial cuff and to stay out of the tubular portion of the vein (Fig. 13-93). Some investigators have suggested the use unipolar recordings, but we have not found them of incremental value. RF catheters used for AF ablation include conventional 4-mm and 8-mm tip, and internally and externally irrigated tip catheters; externally irrigated RF catheters are most frequently used, bolstered by FDA approval for AF ablation. A cryoballoon catheter is also approved for pulmonary vein isolation (Fig. 13-6). At present, a laser balloon catheter manufactured by Cardiofocus, is in clinical trials (Fig. 13-5).

The best end point for pulmonary vein isolation is uncertain. Identifying pulmonary vein potentials, which may be fused with left atrial electrograms, is best accomplished by pacing the CS or adjacent left atrial sites (e.g., left atrial appendage) (Figs. 13-94 and 13-95). Left atrial–PV connections may be theoretically identified by the site of bipolar electrogram reversal or the use of unipolar electrograms. I do not think that targeting these individual sites is better than targeting "early" sites. Certainly, elimination of all pulmonary vein potentials is the end point that most investigators use. This may only require segmental ablation around the lasso. More often, circumferential lesions are placed. It is important that one demonstrates isolation of pulmonary vein potentials from the left atrium. This requires proximal positioning of the lasso at the ostium so that both left atrial and pulmonary vein potentials are recorded (Fig. 13-96). Failure to ablate at a proximal site may leave an ostial cuff of arrhythmogenic tissue but isolate the distal areas of the pulmonary vein. Other investigators have used small versions of the basket catheter placed within the pulmonary vein instead of the lasso to provide longitudinal and circumferential activation data. In my opinion this offers no advantage. Ouyang et al.[212,215] have suggested a double lasso technique by which lassos are simultaneously placed in ipsilateral pulmonary veins (Fig. 13-97). This technique theoretically provides a better visual approximation of large circumferential lesions that can be used to isolate the veins. I have not found this generally advantageous since the lassos are often placed more distal in the vein. As such the circumferential lesions are not that much different than ostial lesions placed using a single lasso. Review of the published data supports this contention, since with loss of pulmonary vein potentials, no left atrial potentials are recorded. I do find it useful when veins are small and you want landmarks to keep the ablation sites removed from the ostia.

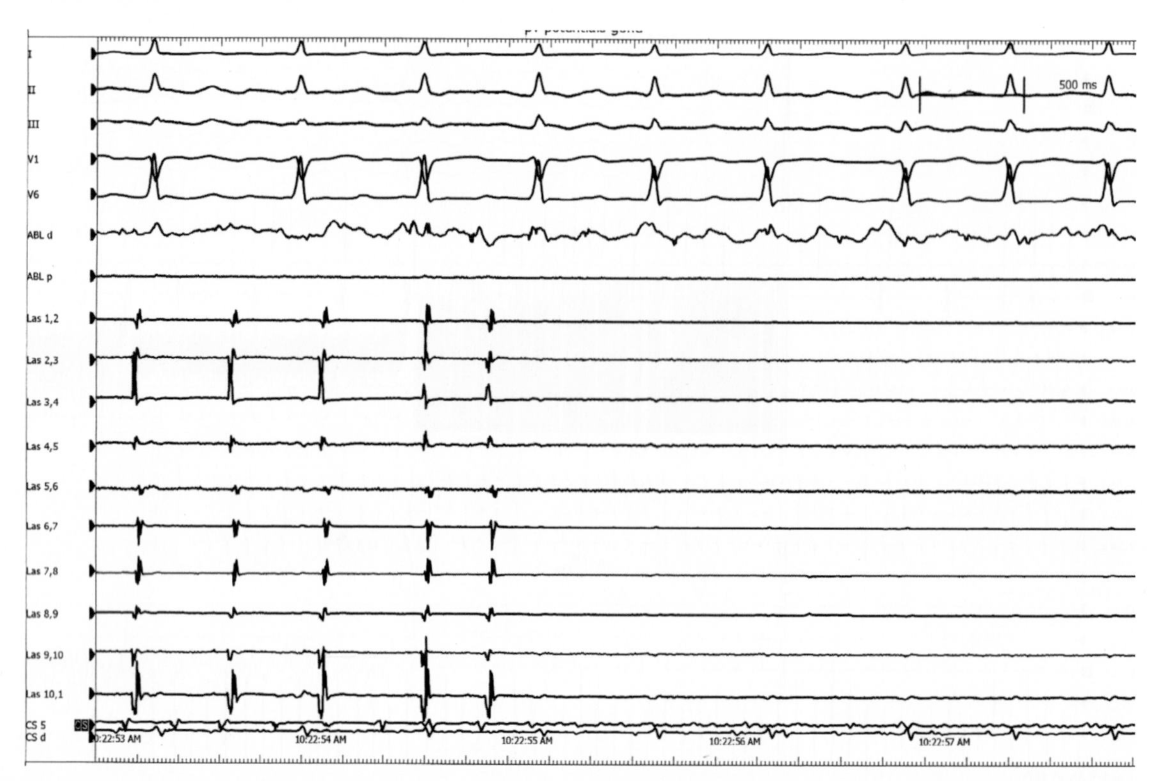


**FIGURE 13-92** *Use of the lasso catheter for detecting pulmonary vein potentials.* Atrial fibrillation is present with a lasso placed in the left superior pulmonary vein. Recordings from the ablation catheter, coronary sinus (bottom two recordings), and 10 bipolar pairs from the lasso. During radiofrequency application proximal to lasso poles 2, 3 there is abrupt loss of activity on the lasso. See text for discussion.

I do not rely on loss of pulmonary vein potentials as proof of isolation. At best this represents entrance block, since the recordings are done during sinus rhythm, coronary sinus pacing, or atrial fibrillation. I require the additional demonstration of exit block.[216,217] In ~30% of PVs that have lost local PV potentials, left atrial capture by pacing the lasso, typically in one to three bipolar pairs, typically in the same, but occasionally from different segments (Fig. 13-98). Ablation at sites of earliest left atrial capture eliminates this conduction, producing exit block (Fig. 13-99). One concern of using entrance block is ensuring against far field capture of adjacent the left or right atrial appendage when pacing within the PV. Simultaneous recordings from the appendage can help to distinguish appendage capture from pulmonary vein conduction. Using the ablation catheter to pace is often misleading since only a small area can be simulated, which is frequently missed by the

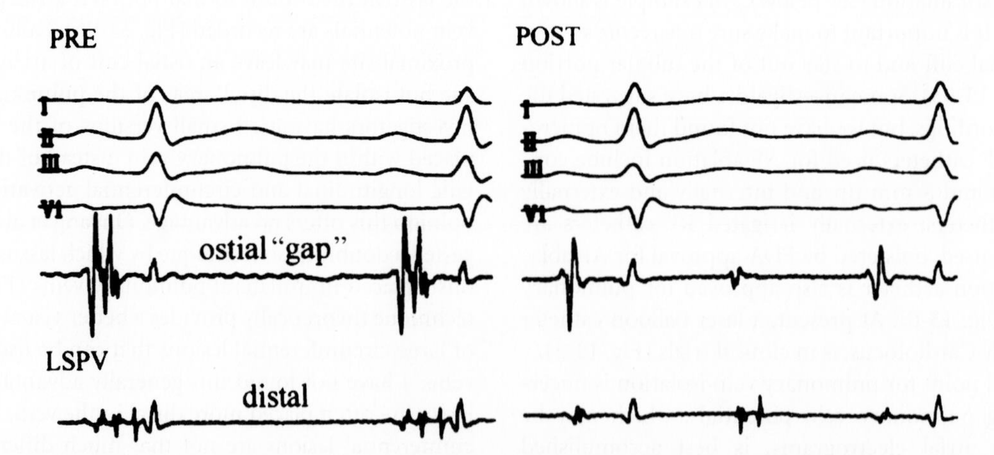


**FIGURE 13-93** *Isolation of pulmonary vein potentials by ostial segmental ablation.* Preablation during sinus rhythm, a local left atrial potential is associated with a complex pulmonary vein potential at the ostium and two discrete pulmonary vein potentials more distally. Postsegmental ablation, all that is seen during sinus rhythm is a local left atrial electrogram. The distal pulmonary vein potential can be seen as isolated from the left atrium. Ectopic impulse formation in the muscle sleeve of the vein generating this electrogram cannot lead to propagated responses. (Courtesy of Haissaguerre M, Shah DC, et al. Catheter ablation of chronic atrial fibrillation targeting the reinitiating triggers. *J Cardiovasc Electrophysiol* 2000;11:2–10.)

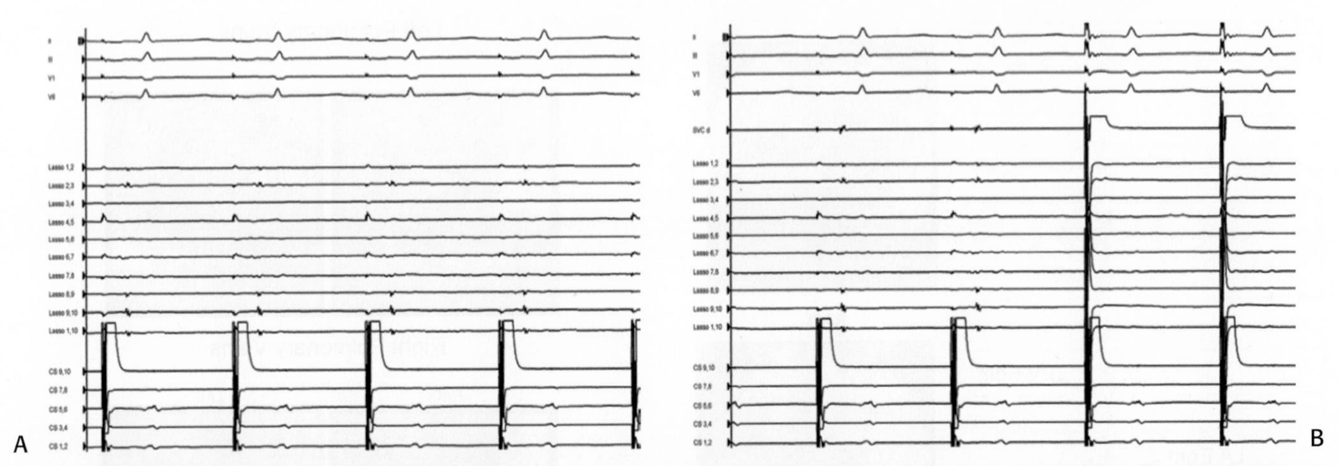

**FIGURE 13-94** *Pacing the SVC to diagnose right superior pulmonary vein far field electrograms.* Four surface ECG leads and intracardiac recordings from an RSPV circular catheter (Lasso) and the coronary sinus are shown. During CS pacing **(A)**, relatively sharp signals are observed on the Lasso at most recording sites. The ablation catheter is positioned in the SVC **(B)**, and records electrograms that are simultaneous in timing, and pacing from the SVC pulls in the Lasso electrograms; both of these observations strongly suggest that these signals are far field recordings from the adjacent right atrium/SVC.

ablation catheter. It is particularly encouraging and useful if one sees local capture of PV electrograms in the lasso which fail to activate the left atrium (Figs. 100 and 13-101). Induction of a PV tachycardia with exit block is also a good sign. Obviously the termination of atrial fibrillation on the ECG with continuation of atrial fibrillation or atrial flutter isolated to the PV is not only proof of concept but also an excellent endpoint (Figs. 13-102 and 13-103).

Many groups feel strongly that just as pulmonary vein foci are operative in the initiation AF initiation, non-PV foci participate in the same physiology and thus should be provoked, mapped, and ablated.[201,203,218] Typically these non-PV triggers are induced with high-dose isoproterenol (20 μg/min) following completion of PV isolation; in addition, this isoproterenol challenge may result in acute recovery of PV conduction.[219] Non-PV triggers are fairly common (as frequent as 10%), and appear to arise from sites that are common for paroxysmal atrial tachycardia in patients without atrial fibrillation, the crista terminalis, mitral and tricuspid annuli, the Eustachian ridge, and the superior vena cava (Fig. 13-104). Mapping of these evanescent triggers is typically difficult, as they often cause the prompt initiation of atrial fibrillation, just as is the case with pulmonary vein triggers. Use of reference catheters (i.e., multipolar catheters in the right atrium and coronary sinus) can be helpful to "triangulate" putative sites of origin (see discussion above),[211] but often multiple cardioversions and reinitiations are required for sufficient localization. This can lead to postablation pulmonary edema. I do not believe non-PV firing that does not initiate AF should be targeted. Larger randomized trials demonstrating improved outcome

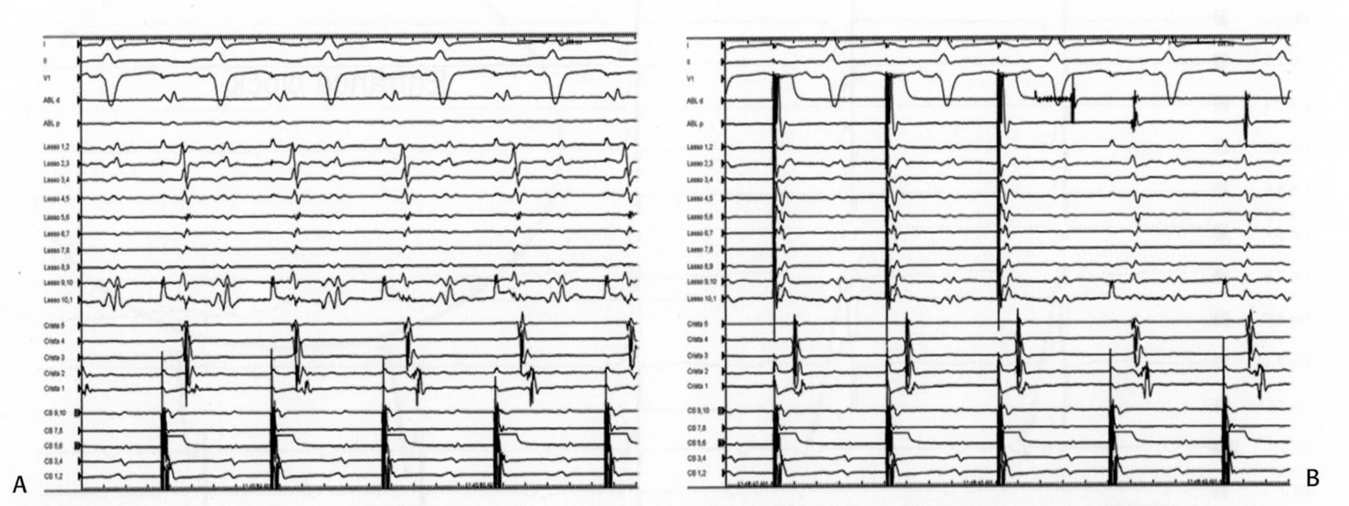

**FIGURE 13-95** *Pacing the left atrial appendage to diagnose left superior pulmonary vein far field electrograms.* In **A**, there are large signals recorded on the circular mapping catheter (Lasso) during CS pacing. The ablation catheter is placed within the left atrial appendage **(B)**. LAA pacing pulls in the Lasso electrograms, indicating that these are far field recordings from the adjacent LAA rather than persistent atrial to PV conduction.

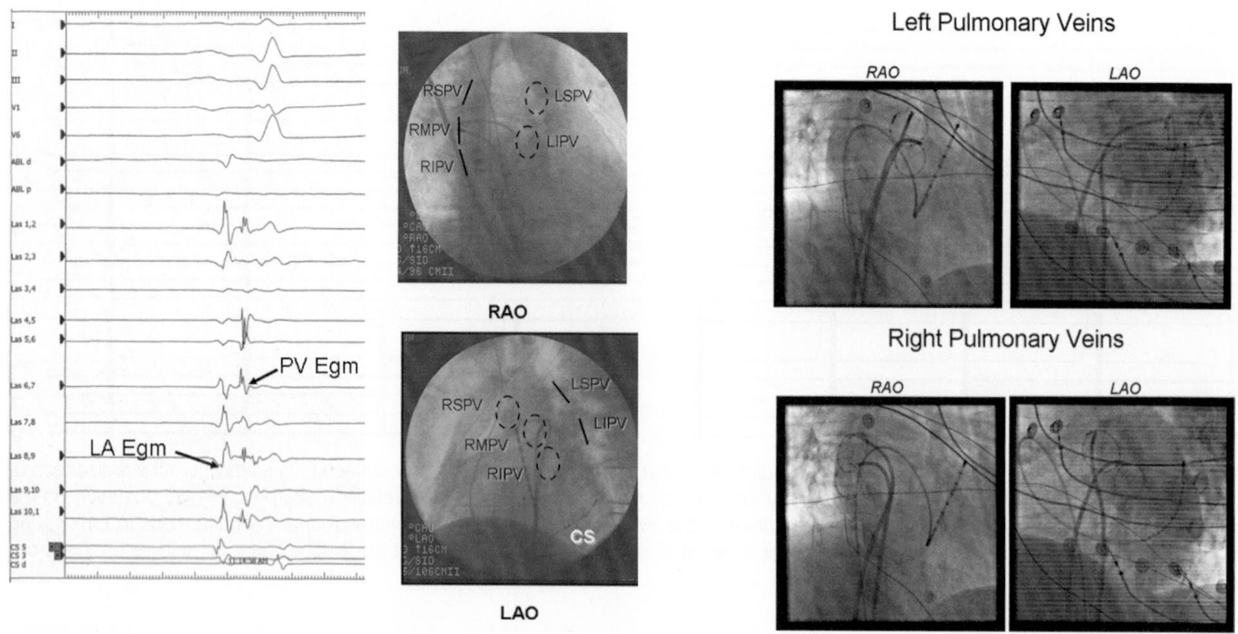


**FIGURE 13-96** *Good positioning of a circular mapping catheter within the pulmonary vein.* Analog recordings from a lasso positioned at the LA-left superior PV junction. This positioning is characterized by both left atrial and PV potentials on the same bipole. Schematic positions are shown on RAO and LAO fluoroscopic images to the right.

**FIGURE 13-97** *Double lasso technique for guiding pulmonary vein isolation.* Circular mapping catheters are positioned in the left (top) and right (bottom) pulmonary veins to guide circumferential ablation. See text.

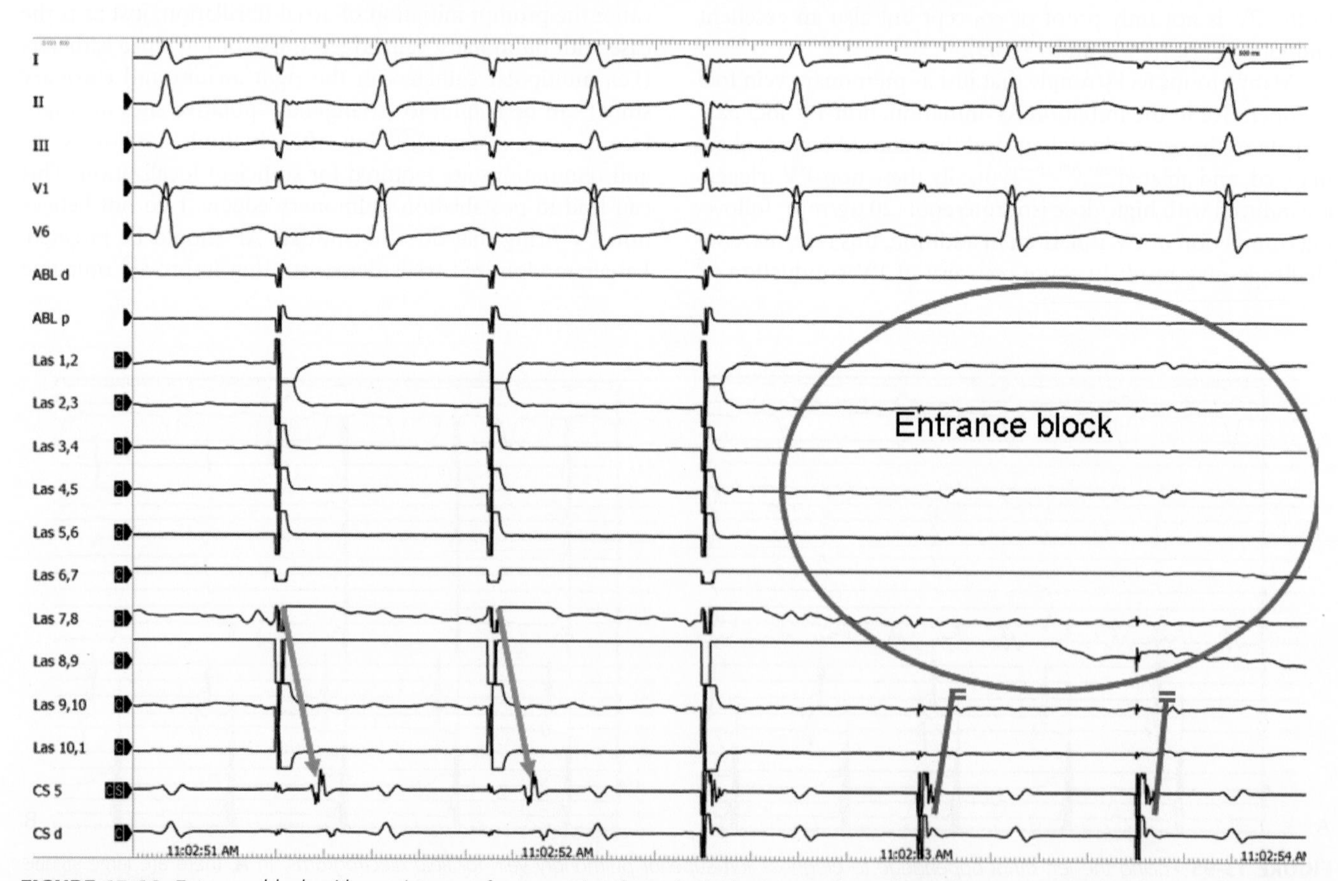


**FIGURE 13-98** *Entrance block with persistence of propagation from the pulmonary vein to the atrium.* Pacing from poles 7, 8 on the lasso produce left atrial capture (*green arrows*). Pacing the CS demonstrates entrance block (no PV potentials) at sites recorded by the lasso. See text for discussion.

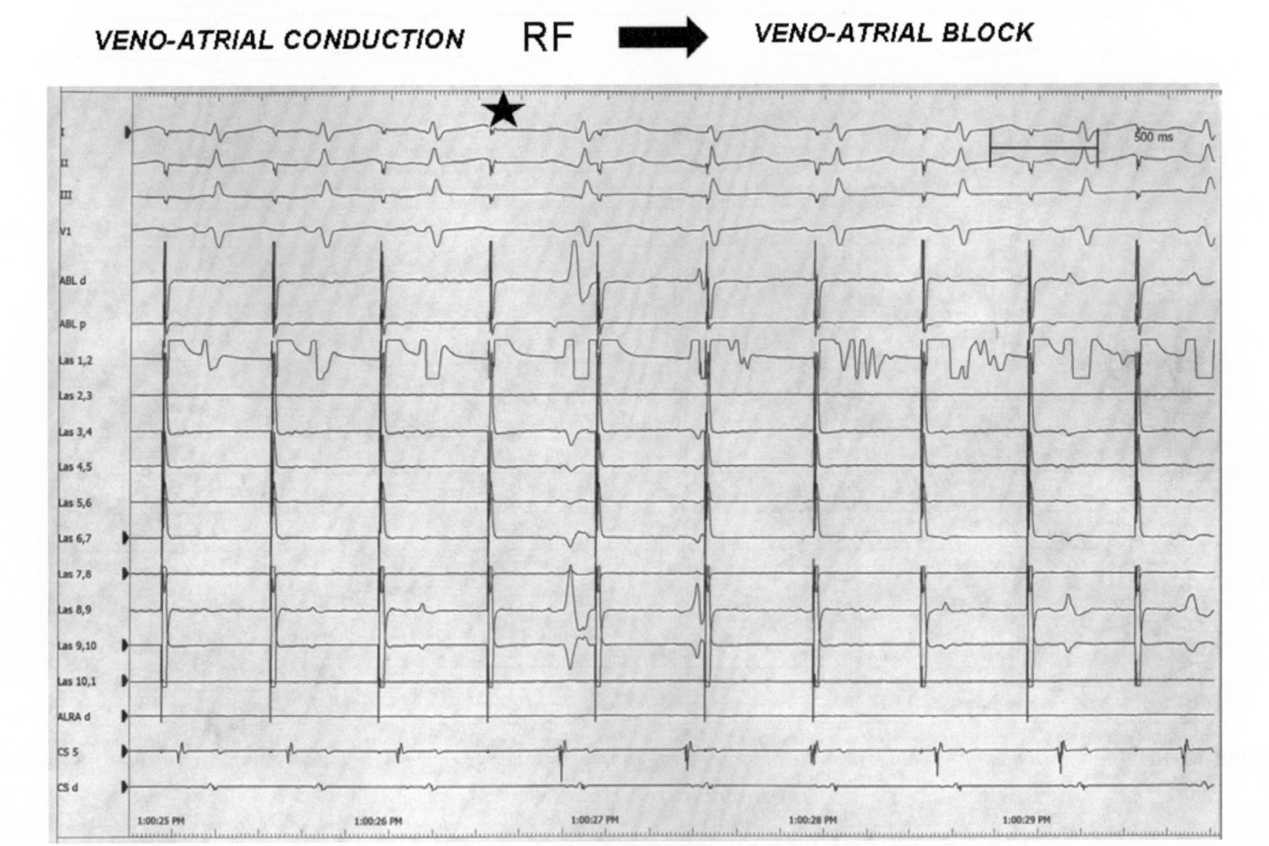


**FIGURE 13-99** *Achieving exit block during lasso pacing.* Pacing lasso poles 1,2 demonstrates venoatrial conduction. RF application at earliest left atrial activation produces venoatrial block.

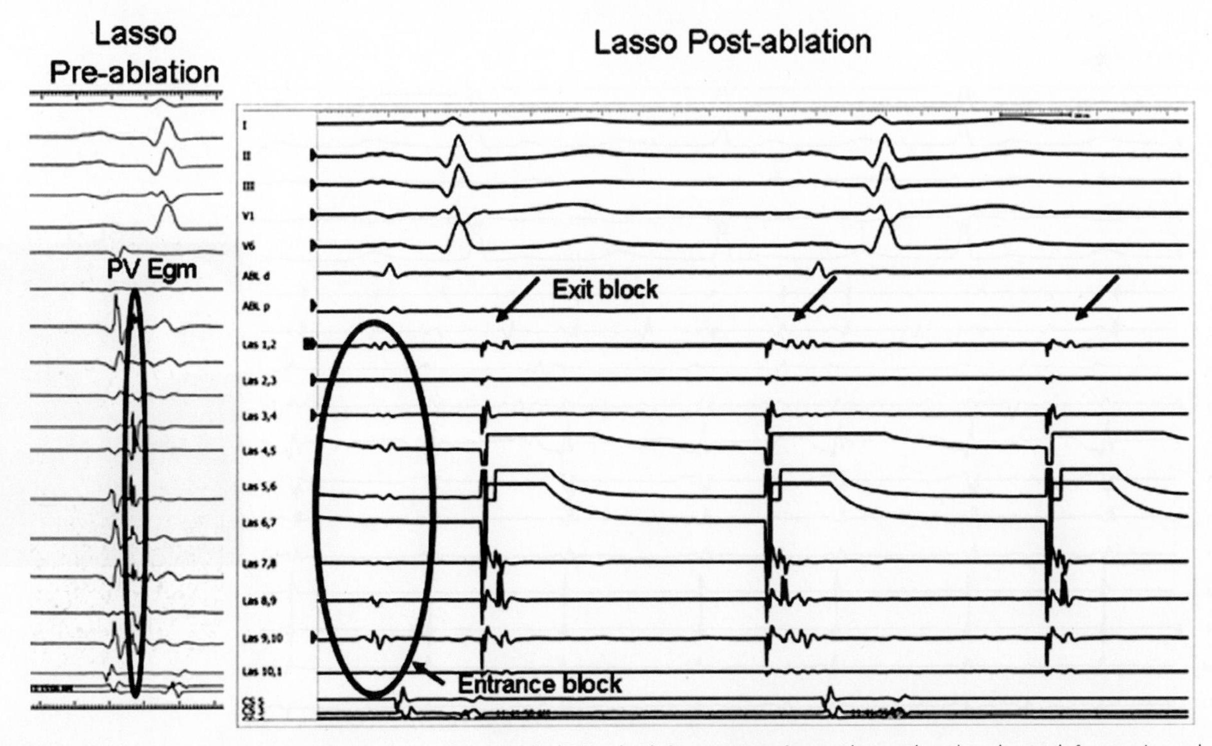


**FIGURE 13-100** *Demonstration of both entrance and exit block.* On the left are EGMs from a lasso placed at the LA-left superior pulmonary vein ostium. Both atrial and PV potentials are seen. Following ablation entrance block is shown by loss of PV potentials. Pacing lasso poles 6, 7 produces local capture of PV potentials which fail to conduct to the left atrium, identifying the presence of exit block. See text.

PV pacing 200 ms

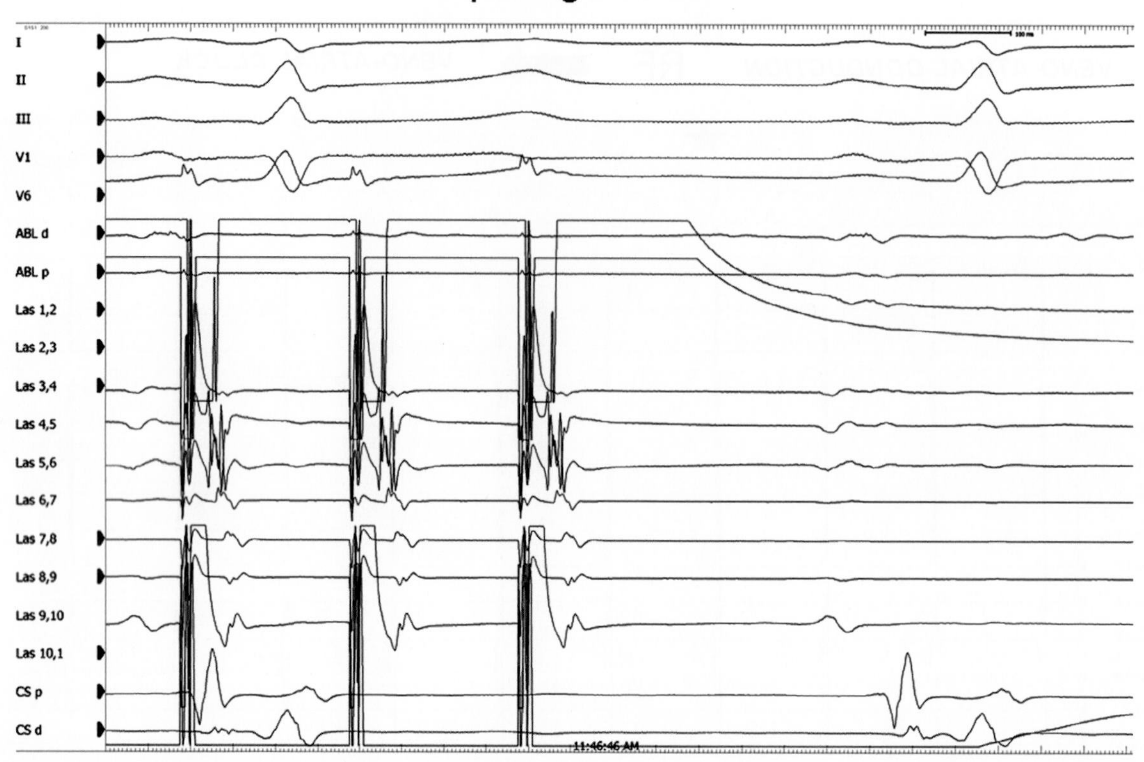


**FIGURE 13-101** *Demonstration of exit block from pulmonary vein.* Following ablation pacing poles 1, 2 at 200-msec captures PV EGMs but fails to depolarize the left atrium. See text.

*Veno-atrial block during AT in PV with 2 to 1 block in RSPV*

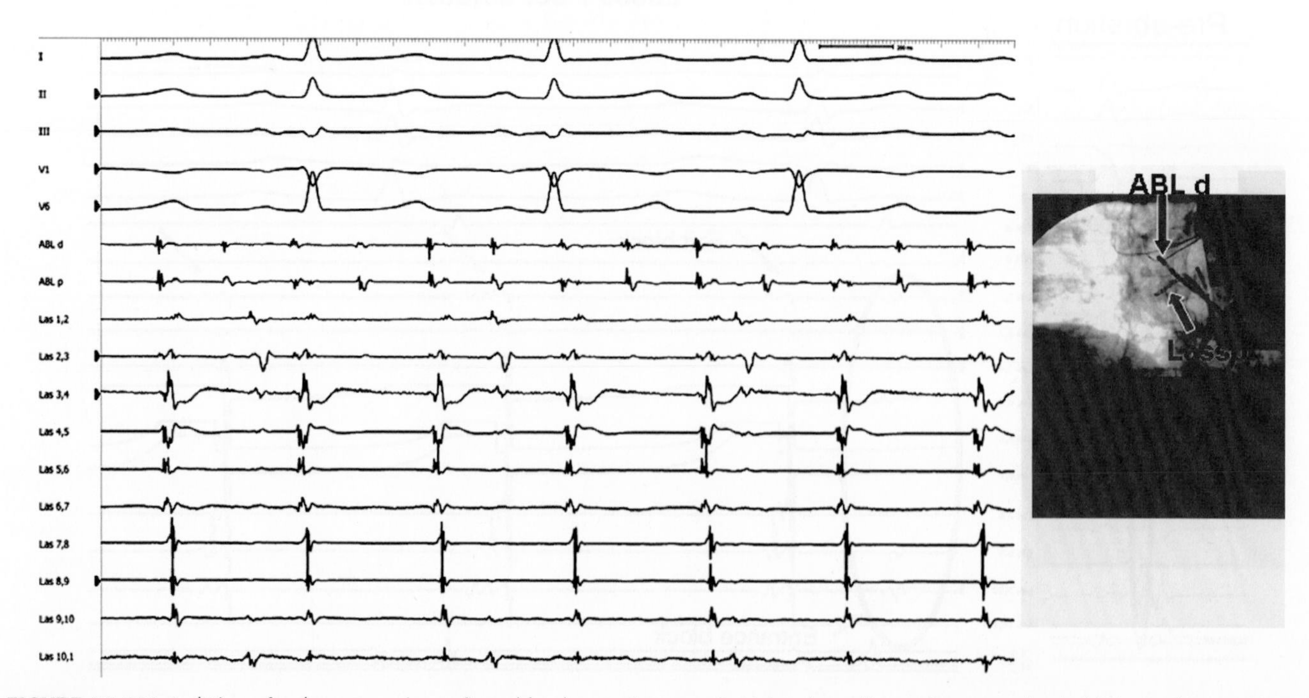


**FIGURE 13-102** Isolation of pulmonary vein confirmed by the persistence of atrial tachycardia on the more distal ablation catheter with 2 to 1 block to the lasso while the left atrium is in *sinus rhythm.*

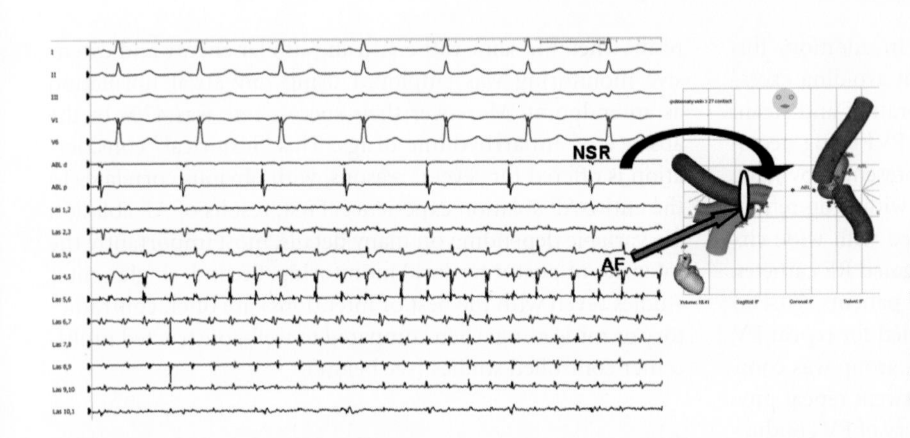


**FIGURE 13-103** *Isolation of atrial fibrillation to the right superior pulmonary vein.* During circumferential ablation around the right superior pulmonary vein during atrial fibrillation, sinus rhythm occurred, but atrial fibrillation persisted, trapped within the pulmonary vein. The ablation catheter in the left atrium shows sinus rhythm.

targeting non-PV triggers are needed before routinely recommending this time-consuming and potentially dangerous procedure.

The Achilles' heel of pulmonary vein isolation is recovery of conduction following apparently successful ablation. This is evident from multiple reports characterizing electrophysiologic findings during repeat procedures for recurrent AF. The underlying concept is that pulmonary vein isolation may well be sufficient (at least in some subtypes of AF) if it could be reliably achieved. The experience that launches this thought experiment comes from series of lung transplant surgery, in which "cut and sew" isolation of the pulmonary vein is performed to reimplant the graft. In these series, atrial fibrillation is essentially absent following the healing phase, although it is prevalent in patients with thoracic surgery in general.[220]

There have been two general schools of thought on increasing the long-term success of pulmonary vein isolation: (1) additional ablation of the posterior wall and (2) mechanical enhancements to improve the likelihood of initial lesion success. Natale and coworkers champion the former strategy, based on the idea that the entire posterior wall arises from the same tissue as the pulmonary veins in an embryologic sense.[221,222] In addition, posterior wall isolation provides a second level of defense for reconnection of the posterior aspects of the pulmonary vein antrum. The posterior wall has also been implicated in stretch-related changes in electrophysiology that may be important for the atrial remodeling that fosters atrial fibrillation. Walters and coworkers recently examined the role of acute stretch on atrial–pulmonary vein electrophysiology in an intraoperative mapping study. Left atrial stretch produced by acute volume expansion slowed conduction at the PV–atrial junction and increased the frequency of fractionated atrial electrograms.[223] Finally, elimination of the lesions that isolated the posterior wall had an important negative effect on outcome of surgical ablation of AF.[224]

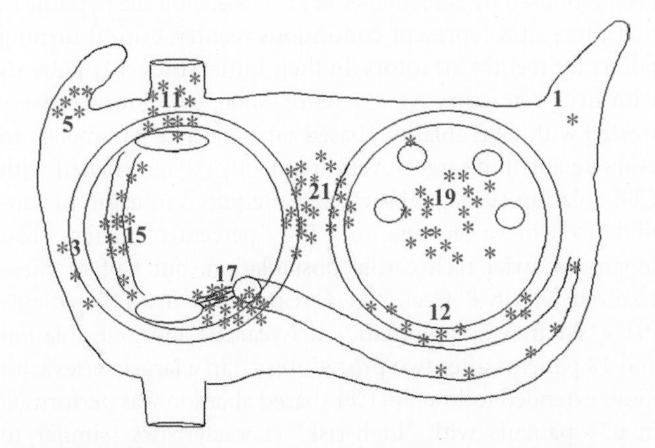


**FIGURE 13-104** *Schema of frequent sites for non-PV triggers.* In a series of 731 patients, a total of 137 non-PV triggers were found, with sites designated by *asterisks.* Frequent sites include the posterior left atrium (which would be encompassed by wide antral isolation in many cases), the left and right sides of the fossa ovalis, the Eustachian ridge and the superior vena cava.

There have been two important technologies that improve catheter stability and increase the likelihood for durable PV isolation. The first is the use of jet ventilation. Catheter stability is negatively affected by the movement of the heart caused by excursion of the diaphragm. This is a huge problem with conscious sedation and spontaneous breathing, but remains a problem with mechanical ventilation during general anesthesia. Hutchinson and coworkers presented a sequential study three groups of 100 consecutive patients referred for AF ablation. The three groups were stratified by exposure to improvements in technology, including image integration, steerable sheaths, and jet ventilation; none of these were used in the first group, image integration and steerable sheaths for the second and all three in the third. Although the patients were not matched, the characteristics of the group were "sicker" (more persistent AF, larger LA dimensions, higher body mass index) progressing from group 1 to 3. Single procedure freedom from recurrent AF at 12 months was 52%, 66%, and 74% in the three groups, respectively.[225] I have used apnea for ablation in unstable areas with the same results at Hutchinson et al. and none of the downsides of JET ventilation including hypercarbia and prolonged time to wake up. The second technology that offers improved effectiveness of lesions to produce PV isolation is catheters that provide real-time contact force sensors (ThermoCool SmartTouch, Biosense Webster; TactiCath, St. Jude Medical). Both catheters were used in clinical studies (TOCCATA, EFFICAS I and II, and Smart AF) to demonstrate the hypothesis that the feedback provided by this technology would reduce the frequency of (previously inadvertent) ineffective lesions, resulting in improved short-term arrhythmia free survival.[49,52,226] In addition, this technology should provide safer ablation, but avoiding excessive contact, reducing the incidence of perforation and steam pop. One recent challenge to the concept of PVI being necessary for successful AF ablation was recently presented by Jiang and coworkers.[227] In this study, 392 patients with drug refractory paroxysmal atrial fibrillation were treated with wide circumferential PV isolation using an open irrigated RF catheter, confirmed with entrance block. At 1 year, 276 patients (70.4%) were free from recurrence and 32 were enrolled for repeat PV mapping to assess PV–atrial conduction; this group was compared with a group of 43 patients who underwent repeat procedures for recurrent atrial fibrillation. Recovery of PV conduction was observed in 29 of 32 patients (including conduction in all four PVs in 10 patients). This was no different than the observed recovery of conduction in patients with AF recurrence (40 of 43 patients). The authors concluded that PV isolation may not be required for short-term control of atrial fibrillation. They hypothesized that this effect might be secondary to (1) elimination of triggers without isolation, (2) modification of the adjacent ganglionated plexi, which may affect the pathogenesis of AF (see below), or (3) inadvertent ablation of an AF rotor (see below). Of interest, similar observations have been reported in the past;[228,229] however, most felt these results were due to the relatively ineffective catheter technology available at that time, though irrigated ablation was used in some subjects in the Pratola study.

In reaction to the concept of PV isolation, and in large part because of the initial complications of pulmonary vein stenosis, several groups proposed initial hypotheses that could be roughly grouped under the concept of "substrate" ablation. If one were to view PV isolation strategies as preventing the initiation of AF, substrate ablation strategies are aimed at destroying the maintenance of AF. The initial substrate ablation method was reported by Pappone et al.[230] This method used electroanatomic mapping to provide circumferential lesions somewhat distant from the veins, which virtually eliminated the possibility of pulmonary vein stenosis, but without the intent of testing for isolation. Over time, various iterations of this concept were tested, eventually including ablation lesions even farther from the tubular portions of the PVs and typically including both of the ipsilateral PVs in the circumferential lesion set, with the addition of linear lesions superior-posterior wall of the left atrium as well as a "line" between the left inferior pulmonary vein and the mitral annulus.[231] Oral et al.[232] published a paper supporting this approach by comparing a Lasso-based approach using entrance block as an endpoint using a nonirrigated 4-mm tip catheter versus circumferential lesions and linear lesions using an 8-mm tip catheter at higher power with additional lesions delivered within the circles to abolish electrograms. Although the methodology of that study was challenged at the time (particularly because of the difference in catheter technology used in the two groups) it showed a slightly better outcome with the nonmap-guided approach using ***symptomatic*** atrial fibrillation as an endpoint. Karch et al.[233] demonstrated the opposite result when the same catheter using similar energy and extensive monitoring was employed using ***any*** atrial fibrillation as an endpoint. Moreover their success rate was 42% in the absence of antiarrhythmic drugs. This "historical" consideration is offered for several reasons, with obvious correlates to the entire AF ablation experience. First, results of AF ablation are variable depending on many details, most importantly the intensity of postprocedural monitoring. Second, single center studies (even with the best of intentions) are often contradictory or misleading when compared to well-constructed multicenter controlled studies (see below).

### Role of Linear Lesions to the Mitral Annulus and/or Across the Roof or Posterior Left Atrial Wall

Several investigators employ additional linear lesions to more closely mimic the Cox surgical Maze procedure (see below).[194,232,234,235] These are meant to prevent macroreentrant rhythms around the mitral annulus and around the pulmonary veins. Only Jais et al.[236] meticulously demonstrated block across these, and made the important points that (1) durable linear lesions (particularly mitral annular lines) are difficult to achieve and (2) gaps in the linear lesion (either related to recovery or unsuccessful initial procedures) are intensely proarrhythmic in terms of recurrent left atrial flutter. Substrate-based ablation including the use of linear lesions has been demonstrated to have a 15% to 30% incidence of left atrial flutter after ablation.[237] In some studies, these recurrent atrial arrhythmias were not counted in reports of AF free survival. I do not think that these linear lesions are necessary unless one documents a clinically relevant macroreentrant circuit. Moreover the potential collateral damage done by this additional ablation, including stroke, proarrhythmia, coronary occlusion, phrenic nerve paralysis, and esophageal fistulas, far exceeds the benefit.

Another non-PV map-guided approach is ablation of complex fractionated electrograms (CFE). This technique has been espoused by Nademanee et al.[238] based on the hypothesis that these sites represent continuous reentry, critical turning points for reentry, or rotors. In their initial study, 121 patients with drug refractory AF (57 paroxysmal, 64 "chronic") were treated with CFE ablation, based on subjective parameters to evaluate ablation targets. Very frequently AF terminated with CFE ablation (95%, although 28% required infusion of ibutilide to achieve termination). Fifty percent of patients had organized atrial tachycardia postablation, but half of these resolved within 8 weeks. At 1-year follow-up, 110 patients (91%) AF free (symptomatic) at 1 year; 92 after one ablation and 18 patients after two procedures.[238] In a larger series with more extended follow-up, CFE-based ablation was performed in 674 patients with "high-risk" characteristics (similar to AFFIRM patients). Monitoring for asymptomatic recurrence was very limited, but 81% of patients were free of symptomatic recurrence at a mean follow-up of 836 days.[239] However, other investigators were not able to reproduce these results.[240,241] Some effort was placed on mapping system–based algorithms

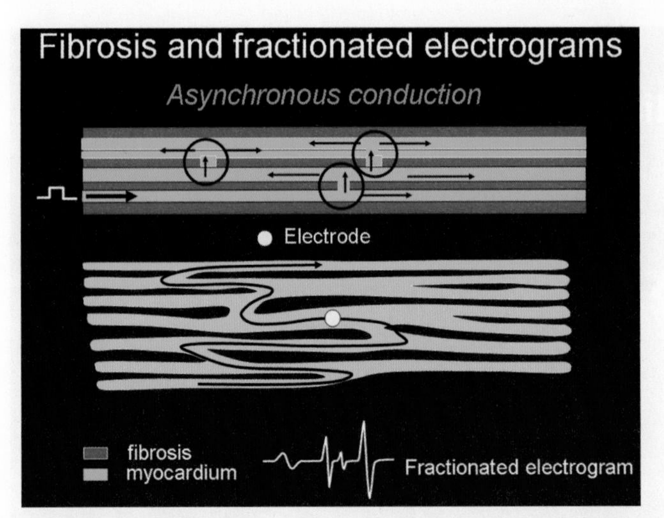


**FIGURE 13-105** *Mechanisms of fractionated electrograms.* Fractionated electrograms are the manifestation of asynchronous conduction. This is usually produced by fibrosis or altered gap junctions. They may also be recorded if the electrode records different simultaneous wavefronts. See text. (Courtesy of Dr. J de Bakker.)

Relationship of Fractionated Electrical Activity to Atrial Cycle Length

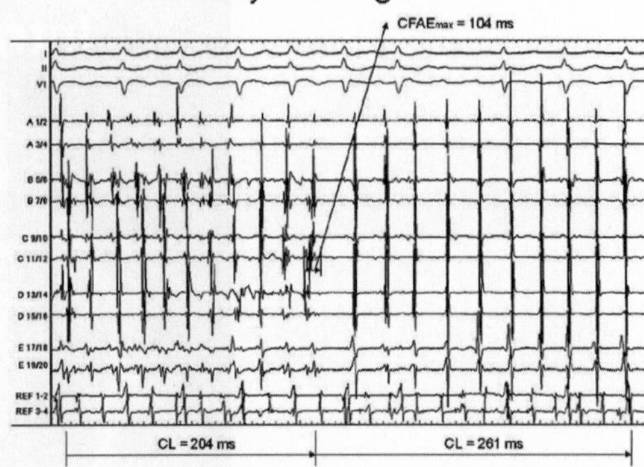


**FIGURE 13-106** *Effect of cycle length on development and disappearance of fractionated electrograms.* Recordings from a 20 pole flower electrode demonstrate fractionated signals appear at short cycle lengths and disappear at longer cycle lengths, suggesting they are a consequence of not a driver of the arrhythmia. (From Rostock T RM, Sanders P, Takahashi Y, et al. High-density activation mapping of fractionated electrograms in the atria of patients with paroxysmal atrial fibrillation. *Heart Rhythm* 2006;3(1):27–34, with permission.)

to make the determination of CFE more objective, but this did not seem to rescue the approach. Addition of CFE to PVI appeared to enhance success rates in persistent AF in several small single center studies and one multicenter study.[242]

Unfortunately there are little data to support the CFE hypothesis, and there are many problems with the underlying assumptions. There is no proof that such EGMs during AF represent any of the above. They may represent overlapping wavefronts of activation in a three-dimensional (3D) structure and/or nonuniform anisotropic conduction. Any form of asynchronous conduction results in fragmented electrograms (Fig. 13-105). Fractionated electrograms come and go, and are rate related; as such they cannot be required for maintenance of AF (Fig. 13-106).[243] A detailed study using monophasic action potential recording to determine the mechanism of CFE by Narayan and coworkers[244] demonstrated that the majority of CFEs were related to far field activation, AF acceleration or disorganization; only 8% of CFE recordings were considered consistent with "drivers." The endpoint of decreased EGM during AF or normalization of EGM on return to NSR is meaningless. The vast majority of such EGMs are around the PVs in areas frequently ablated during PV isolation; perhaps this is the mechanism. Finally, ablation of all fractionated electrograms will result in unnecessary ablation of the posterior wall of the LA, which is potentially dangerous. As such, I do not recommend this approach.

Pappone et al.[245] proposed potential mechanisms for the efficacy of substrate-based ablation:

- Exclusion of 23% of atrial volume
- Pulmonary vein isolation or change in conduction of triggers (affecting ability to induce AF)
- Elimination of anchor points for rotors or mother waves in the posterior venous atrium
- Ablation of the ligament of Marshall
- Autonomic denervation

All of these are conceptually possible, but the actual mechanism is not proven. The only consistent finding that has been documented is that pulmonary vein isolation has been shown to prevent AF. The extent of isolation required remains to be determined, but when patients have been restudied for recurrent AF, pulmonary vein reconnection is routinely observed regardless of whether segmental or circumferential isolation of individual veins or continuous circular lesions around ipsilateral veins is used.[194,214,215,228,246–249]

Moreover reisolation of the veins eliminates recurrences. As such I believe an electrophysiologic approach with well-defined endpoints should be the goal in the management of an electrophysiologic disorder. I believe MRI may offer the most accurate view of the pulmonary veins and this technology coupled with the Carto system, which is based on MRI, would be the ideal combination tool to accurately encircle the pulmonary veins. Other investigators rely on other forms of image integration (i.e., CT angiography), intracardiac echocardiography (Fig. 13-107) or "fast" electroanatomic mapping, using multielectrode catheters. In any case, it seems that increased experience has led to a better understanding of pulmonary vein antral anatomy, no matter the methodology. A figure demonstrating the use of ICE/multielectrode mapping reconstruction of the left atrium and wide circumferential PV ablation is shown in Figure 13-108.

I believe that pulmonary vein isolation, with demonstration of bidirectional block, should be the initial approach for all patients with paroxysmal atrial fibrillation. Even if one could do this, however, the number of cases in which atrial fibrillation would be "cured" is uncertain. Clearly however, there is a subpopulation of patients with paroxysmal atrial

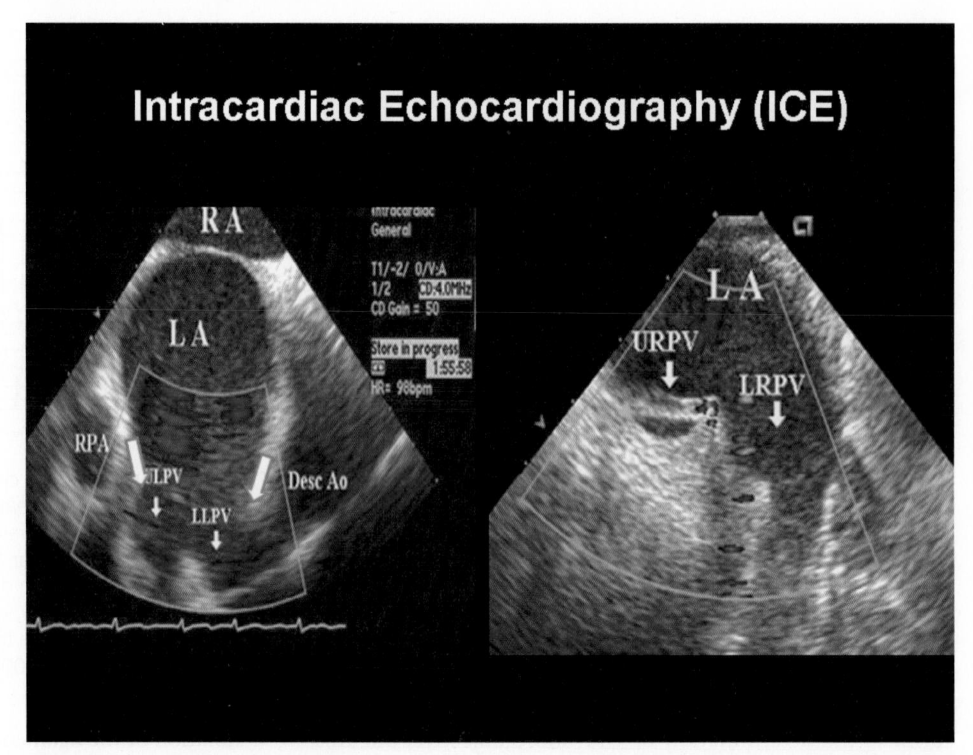


**FIGURE 13-107** *Use of intracardiac ultrasound (ICE) to define pulmonary vein ostia.* ICE demonstrates a common ostium of the left pulmonary veins even though they appeared as separate structures using other imaging modalities. The right pulmonary veins are shown on the right. ICE also allows assessment of pulmonary vein velocities and the presence of pericardial fluid.

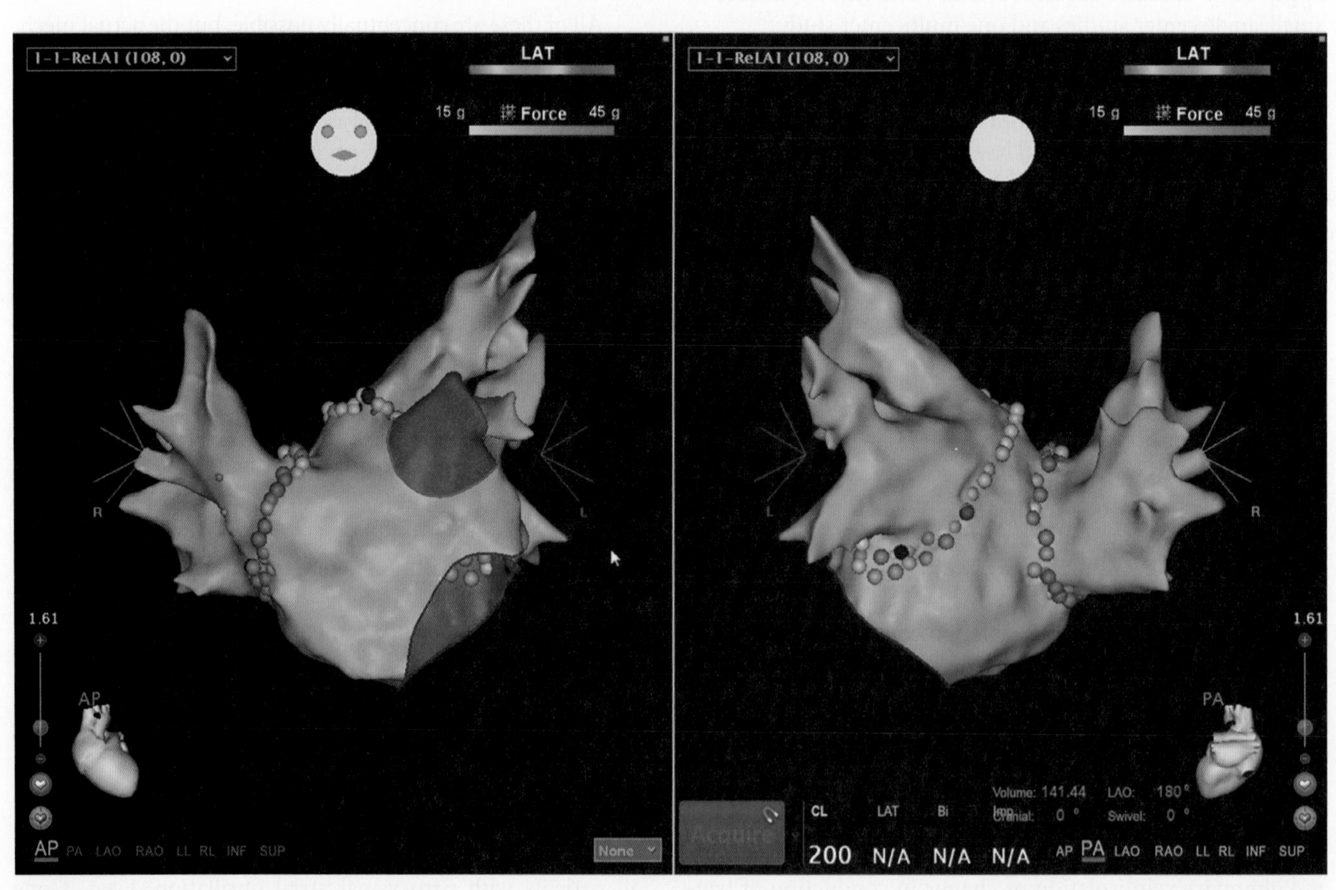


**FIGURE 13-108** *Multielectrode mapping to construct a shell of the left atrium.* AP and PA projections of a left atrial map which was performed with multielectrode mapping informed by reference to intracardiac echocardiography. The left atrial body is shown in *light green* and the left atrial appendage in *dark green.* Individual ablation lesions are shown as *pink–red icons* which are graded (10–45 grams) representations of contact force.

fibrillation in whom the pulmonary veins play a prominent role in the genesis of the arrhythmia and in whom isolation of the pulmonary veins or ablation of specific foci can "cure" their paroxysmal atrial fibrillation. Although a high efficacy rate of isolation of the pulmonary veins from the left atrial myocardium has been reported, I believe, the true success rate at preventing symptomatic or asymptomatic atrial fibrillation with such ablations is in the order of 50% to 75%, including those requiring drugs. There are several reasons recurrent AF following PVI: (a) impulse formation occurs in the proximal cuff of tissue that is left in connection to the left atrium; (b) other sites of impulse formation outside the isolated pulmonary veins are a source of atrial fibrillation triggers; (c) the mechanism of atrial fibrillation is neither focal nor related to the pulmonary veins; (d) incomplete isolation and/or reconnection of the pulmonary veins. How one defines success marked influences reported outcomes; that is, symptomatic versus asymptomatic AF, duration of AF, after recurrent procedures, etc. We consider >10 seconds of any AF a failure and extensively monitor our patients. We routinely use either a patient-triggered monitor for 2 weeks, transmitted three times daily without symptoms and with any symptoms or a continuous autotriggered monitor for 1 to 2 weeks. Monitoring is for the first 2 weeks postablation and at 1, 3, 6, 9, and 12 months following the ablation with continuous monitoring whenever possible. Our success rate with this type of monitored follow-up is ~75% at a mean of 15 months. Use of symptomatic AF as an endpoint underestimates recurrent AF by 15% to 25%, particularly in those patients with persistent AF or those on drugs. These findings have been corroborated by others.[250,251] The Hopkins group[251] found that 82% of the AF events that occurred were detected and transmitted by the CardioNet system, not by patients that is, they were asymptomatic and 60% of the events that patients triggered were non-AF events.

At present, consensus regarding pulmonary vein isolation compared to PVI "plus" seems to be established for the following points:[252]

1. Electrophysiologically documented pulmonary vein isolation is a necessary component, and the foundation of all AF ablation strategies.
2. Wide (antral) circumferential ablation is preferable to ostial ablation. This was tested in a randomized trial by Arentz and coworkers.[253] In this randomized study 110 patients with paroxysmal or persistent AF were treated with ostial (individual) PV ablation versus wide area circumferential ablation of ipsilateral PV pairs; open irrigated RF ablation and entrance block was confirmed in all patients. Wide circumferential ablation was associated with longer procedural and ablation times, but shorter fluoroscopy times; freedom from AF at 15 ± 4 months was 49% in the ostial and 67% in the circumferential ablation group. These results were confirmed in a review and meta-analysis by Proietti et al.[254] It is unclear whether wider circumferential ablation is more durable, or if this technique actually benefits from some of the mechanisms listed under substrate ablation, such as modification of the cardiac autonomic nervous system or interruption of AF rotors.
3. Additional substrate ablation is often advocated for persistent AF. This is in response to a sentinel paper by the Michigan group that largely influenced behavior for decades going forward, comparing the response of paroxysmal and persistent AF to segmental PVI using nonirrigated 4-mm tip RF catheters.[246] After 5 months of follow-up and no monitoring, 70% of paroxysmal patients were free of symptoms compared to 22% of those with persistent AF; the vast majority of recurrent events occurred in what would now be considered the blanking period. In addition, several studies employing sequential observational outcome data and meta-analysis of single center studies[255] appeared to favor additional ablation for persistent AF. Recently, however, Verma and colleagues presented the results of the STAR AF II trial.[256] This trial enrolled 589 patients with persistent atrial fibrillation randomized to pulmonary vein isolation (PVI; $n = 64$) versus PVI plus ablation by CFE (PVI + CFE; $n = 254$) versus PVI plus empiric linear ablation (PVI + lines; $n = 250$). Although surprising to many, the PVI alone group had slightly higher freedom from recurrent AF after single (59%, 48%, and 44% in the PVI, PVI + CFAE PVI + lines groups, respectively, $p = 0.15$) or repeat procedures; PVI alone was also associated with reduced procedural and fluoroscopy time and less major complications.
4. It is becoming increasingly clear that improved treatment of comorbidities (obesity, sleep apnea, hypertension) has an important effect on postablation AF recurrence. Several series have demonstrated that poorly treated hypertension or untreated severe sleep apnea almost completely eliminates the impact of catheter ablation.[257–259] The recent ARREST AF trial examined the effect of active risk factor management postablation in 149 patients with a BMI ≥27 kg/m$^2$ and ≥1 cardiac risk factor.[260] Sixty-one patients accepted this intervention, and 88 patients who did not served as a control group. There were no baseline differences between the two groups. Active risk factor management resulted in greater reductions in weight (−13.2 ± 5.4 kg vs. −1.5 ± 5.1 kg; $p < 0.002$) and improvements in glycemic control and serum lipid abnormalities. In addition, single and multiple ablation procedures (87% with risk factor management compared with 17.8% for the control group) arrhythmia free survival was significantly better in the intervention group, as was symptom score related to AF. This study discloses an important opportunity that is often under recognized by electrophysiologists, both to improve AF ablation success, and to provide better overall medical care to our patients.

Several ablation strategies that are not specifically focused on pulmonary vein isolation have continued to evolve in recent years: ablation of the gangionated plexi to modify the intrinsic cardiac nervous system, extensive ablation to terminate persistent AF, and ablation guided by the identification of rotors.

### Ablation/Modification of the Autonomic Nervous System for Control of AF

The role of the autonomic nervous system in the pathogenesis of AF has been investigated for decades.[261] More recently, beautiful collaborative anatomic and physiologic investigation have led to an improved understanding of the influence of the intrinsic cardiac autonomic nervous system.[262–266] High-intensity stimulation of the cervical vagus trunk or local cardiac ganglionated plexi causes AF in experimental models. The finding of sudden bradycardia (A-V block during AF or sinus pauses) during ablation around the pulmonary veins suggested that catheter ablation can effect ganglionated plexi, perhaps even promoting remodeling. This seems to mesh well with a general hypothesis that atrial fibrillation (at least in some patients) may be caused and/or maintained by hyperactivity of the cardiac autonomic nervous system. Attempts at directly ablating ganglionated plexi (extinguishing the "vagal" response to high-frequency stimulation) either with catheter or surgical ablation have not convincingly improved the outcome of catheter ablation (Fig. 13-109);[267] this observation does not negate the impact of autonomic nervous system physiology in the genesis of AF.

### Stepwise Ablation (Ablation to Termination of Persistent AF)

Stepwise ablation typically utilized in persistent and especially long lasting persistent AF is an attempt to sequentially target

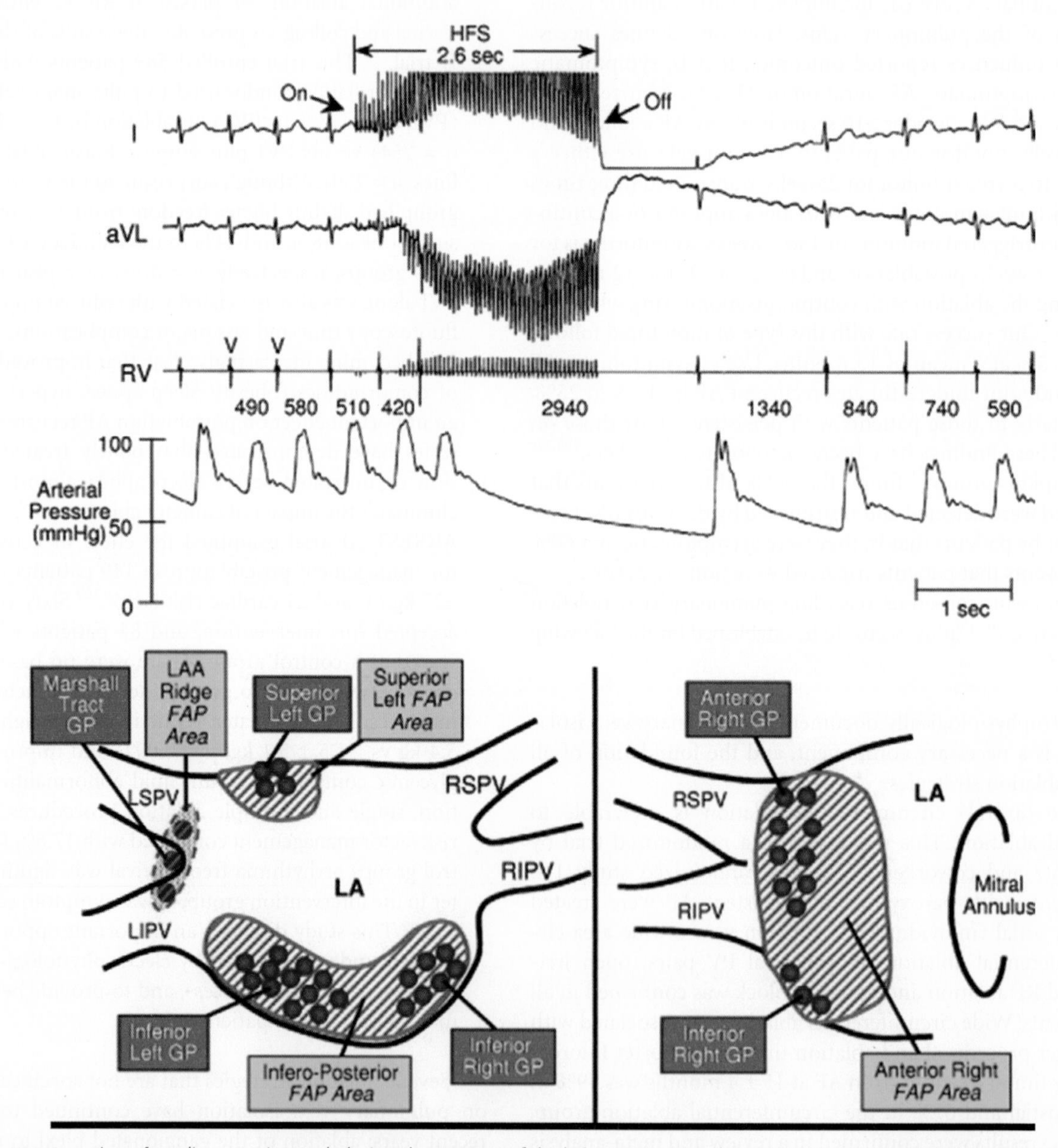


**FIGURE 13-109** *Location of cardiac gangionated plexi.* In the **top panel**, high-frequency stimulation (HFS) at a left atrial site produces a "vagal response" with prominent reduction in heart rate during ongoing atrial fibrillation, signifying stimulation of a plexus. Such stimulation mapping can reveal the location of the four major ganglionated plexi, here shown schematically (**bottom panel**) in the context of an electroanatomic map. (Adapted from Nagakawa H. *Heart Rhythm* 2009;6:S26–S34, with permission.)

anatomic areas that may be involved in the maintenance of atrial fibrillation.[268,269] At various stages in the stepwise approach, the prevailing AF cycle length progressively prolongs, and termination of AF (either to sinus rhythm or to an organized atrial tachycardia which can then be mapped and ablated.) is seen in approximately 80% of patients. The ablation strategy includes the following steps: pulmonary vein isolation, electrogram-guided ablation (continuous or fragmented electrograms, CFEs), linear lesions (mitral annulus, roof, cavotricuspid isthmus), right atrial CFE ablation, and mapping of organized rhythms that may result. In patients with successful AF termination, only 5% will have AF recurrence; however recurrent atrial tachycardias are seen in almost 50%.[270,271] In many ways, this represents the ultimate (nonsurgical) expression of substrate ablation, encompassing all possible mechanisms of AF maintenance (described above), but also admitting to all of the potential perils of extensive ablation, including proarrhythmia, procedural complications, and potential destruction of atrial mechanical function.

### *Focal Impulse and Rotor Modulation for Ablation of Atrial Fibrillation*

The biologic plausibility of spiral wave reentry has been convincingly demonstrated in model systems and experimental arrhythmias. Recent improvements in electrogram mapping and electrocardiographic imaging have reignited interest in the hypothesis that a focal source with resultant fibrillatory conduction could be responsible for the maintenance of AF in at least some patients. Narayan and colleagues devised a proprietary signal processing technique that can identify relatively stable focal arrhythmias and rotors that have the following characteristics (Fig. 13-110): (1) they are relatively stable over time, (2) they are multiple (mean 2.1 ± 1.0 rotors/

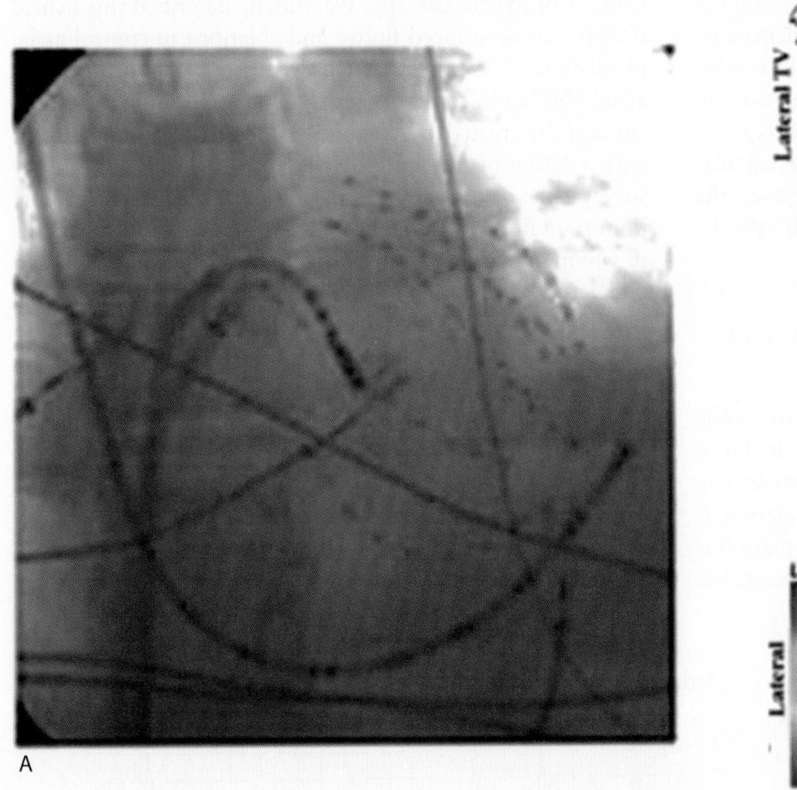


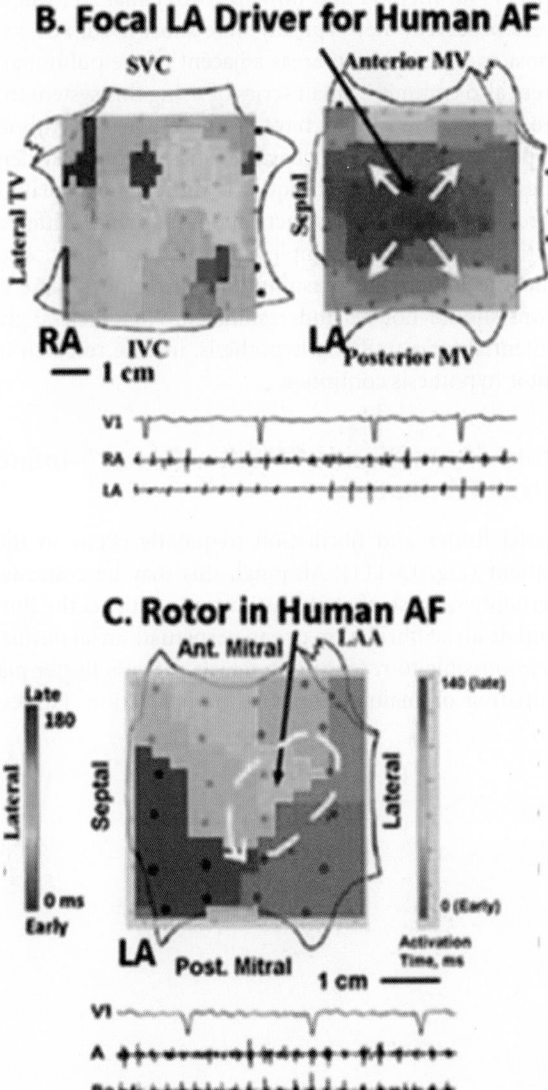


**FIGURE 13-110** *Focal impulse and rotor mapping (FIRM).* In **A**, the multielectrode "basket" catheter which is used in this strategy is shown deployed in the left atrium. In **B**, a color-coded phase map during AF is shown of the right and left atrium, demonstrating a focal left atrial driver; in **C**, a map of the left atrium is shown which demonstrates a rotor. (Courtesy of SM Narayan, MD.)

focal sources in the CONFIRM trial) (3) ablation at these sites results in AF termination and the subsequent inability to induce atrial fibrillation, and (4) they appear to be "conserved" in that repeat mapping in patients with recurrent AF reveals recurrence of the same focal drivers.[272] In the CONFIRM trial, 92 consecutive patients (70% persistent AF) were randomized 1:2 to focal impulse/rotor ablation (FIRM guided) + conventional ablation versus conventional ablation alone (FIRM blinded). After 1.2 ± 0.4 procedures and over a mean follow-up of 890 days, freedom from AF was greater in the FIRM treatment group (77.8% vs. 38.5%, $p < 0.001$).[273]

These results have been challenged on the basis of the results of another form of electrocardiographic imaging system, devised by Yoram Rudy.[274] This system uses inverse solution mathematics to merge cardiac CT anatomic data with epicardial biatrial activation mapping. In a study of 36 patients, multiple wavelet reentry was the most common mechanism (92%) and rotors were detected only rarely with this (15%) method and only in paroxysmal AF; when rotors were observed, they typically were short lived. Focal sources, most commonly from areas adjacent to the pulmonary veins were also common. Small series of using this system to visualize and localize sources have been presented.[275] Although the apparent differences in characteristics of rotors evidenced by these two imaging techniques is difficult to explain (endocardial/epicardial, phase/activation mapping, differences in patient subsets), the complexity of the mathematics required and the underlying presumptions to support these calculations should not be underestimated. Nonetheless, given the potential for a unifying hypothesis, intense research into the rotor hypothesis continues.

## Role of Ablation in "Mother Flutter"–Induced Atrial Fibrillation

Atrial flutter and fibrillation frequently occur in the same patient (Fig. 13-111). Although this may be coincidental, it certainly suggests that at least in some patients the flutter can initiate atrial fibrillation or can perpetuate atrial fibrillation. It is impossible to recognize in which patients flutter plays this initiating or maintaining role for fibrillation. However, the ease with which a flutter ablation can be accomplished suggests that such an ablation may be a reasonable approach to patients who have both flutter and fibrillation. Movsowitz et al.[192] showed a decrease in the incidence of atrial fibrillation over short-term follow-up in those patients who had a flutter ablation. They found a decrease in fibrillation of ~40% although these were short-term data in a small number of patients. In my experience atrial fibrillation is likely to recur in patients with structural heart disease the longer the follow-up. Anticoagulation should be maintained for all patients with a prior history of stroke and asymptomatic atrial fibrillation. However, under specific circumstances, that is, the absence of structural heart disease, age less than 65, no documented atrial fibrillation (asymptomatic or symptomatic) for >6 months following the procedure, or other risk factors for stroke, anticoagulation may be discontinued.

In the majority of cases the first episode of atrial flutter occurs after a patient has been placed on an antiarrhythmic agent with sodium channel blocking affects for atrial fibrillation. The common association of atrial flutter and fibrillation, as well as the frequent change of atrial fibrillation to atrial flutter by class I antiarrhythmic agents, led us to develop the concept of **hybrid therapy**. We initially described this hybrid therapy (drug-induced flutter and ablation) to control atrial fibrillation.[276] We investigated whether patients in whom atrial fibrillation could be converted to atrial flutter would be successfully treated by combining the antiarrhythmic agent with ablation of the flutter. Huang et al.[276] from our laboratory was the first to report application of this concept. Several important findings came out of that study. First, most patients in whom conversion from fibrillation to flutter occurred had either (a) paroxysmal atrial fibrillation with "coarse" atrial fibrillation or (b) fibrillation or flutter on different occasions. Second, all cases that look like flutter on the ECG are not isthmus-dependent flutter when studied by intracardiac mapping and program stimulation. Those patients with isthmus-dependent flutter proven at EP study and successful flutter ablations, as described earlier in the chapter, remained free from recurrences of atrial flutter or fibrillation as long as their antiarrhythmic therapy was maintained. Patient compliance and the development of CHF or angina, requiring cessation

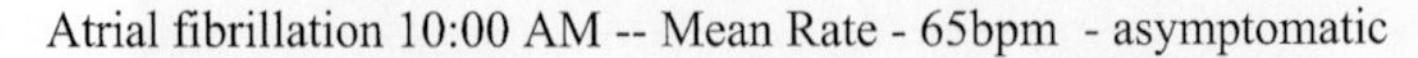

Atrial fibrillation 10:00 AM -- Mean Rate - 65bpm - asymptomatic


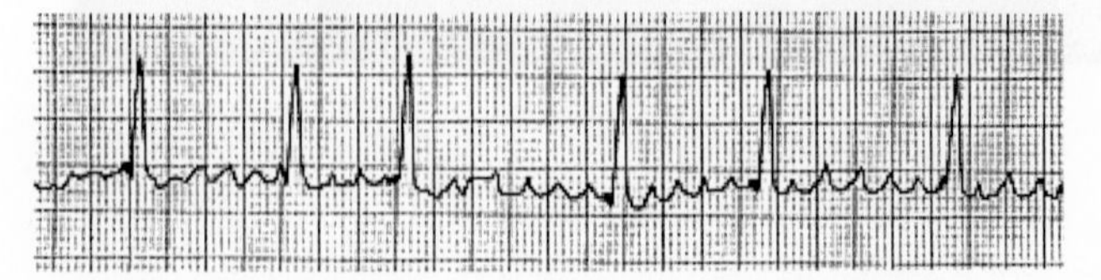


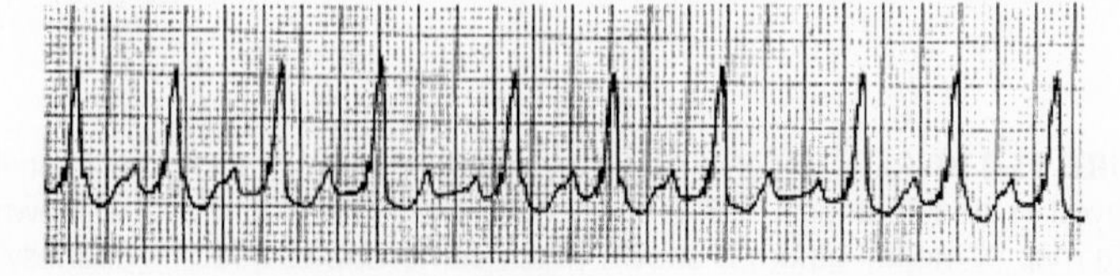

**FIGURE 13-111** Occurrence of atrial flutter and fibrillation in the same patient.

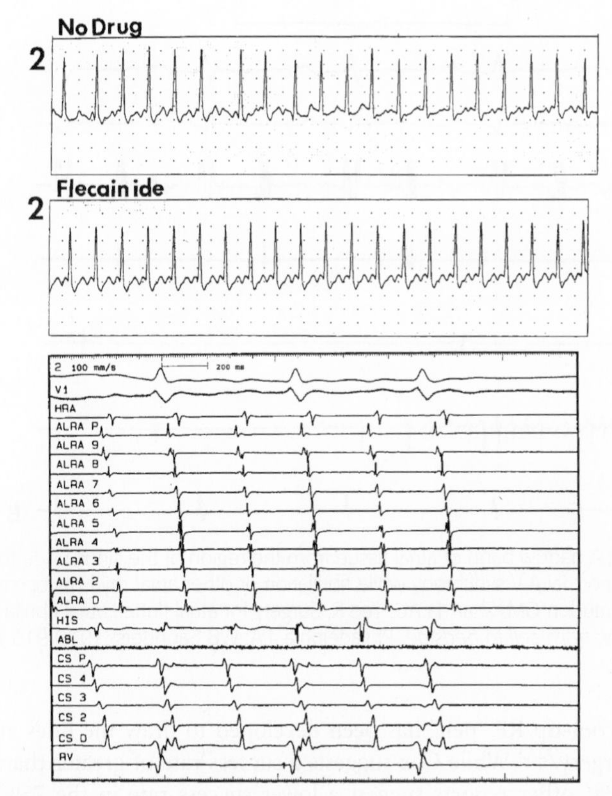


**FIGURE 13-112** *Hybrid therapy for atrial fibrillation.* The **top panel** shows 1 of 30 paroxysms of atrial fibrillation experienced daily by this young physician. Following the administration of flecainide (**second panel**) atrial flutter resulted. This was shown to be isthmus-dependent with classical atrial activation sequences (and entrainment characteristics) (**bottom panel**). Linear ablation to the isthmus terminated this flutter at the site of the ablation (**bottom panel**). Bidirectional block was confirmed and the patient has been free of arrhythmias while maintaining flecainide for 4 years. (From Huang DT, Monahan KH, Zimetbaum PJ, et al. Hybrid pharmacologic and ablative therapy—a novel and effective approach for the management of atrial fibrillation. *J Cardiovasc Electrophysiol* 1998;9:462–469.)

of Class 1C agents, are the most common limitations of the approach. An example of this combined therapy is shown in Figure 13-112. Nabar and colleagues[277] had similar findings in drug-induced flutter. The agents most commonly associated with the change from fibrillation to flutter are 1C agents and amiodarone. The 1A agents have also been associated with this, but their frequency of use has markedly diminished in the past decade. Other investigators have noted similar experiences.[191] We have noted that the ability to document atrial flutter degenerating to atrial fibrillation in a given patient may select out those patients most likely to benefit from this form of approach. An example of a patient with flutter-induced atrial fibrillation and completion of the flutter line that terminated the atrial fibrillation is shown in Figure 13-113. A larger series of patients needs to be evaluated to see how often flutter lesions can prevent atrial fibrillation and if we can better select those patients in whom this procedure might work. The major limiting features of this approach are failure of patient compliance, drug side effects, progressive disease process (e.g., CHF), or development of active CAD, prohibiting use of Class 1C agents. As suggested above, failure to document pure isthmus-dependent flutter, as practiced in many laboratories, is another feature precluding a successful outcome.

## Role of Ablation in "Multiple Wavelet" Atrial Fibrillation

Most cases of persistent and permanent atrial fibrillation are probably based on the mechanism of multiple wavelet reentry. We have also demonstrated this to be the case using intraoperative mapping techniques as described in Chapter 9. To date, the only technique that has been reproducibly shown to actually cure this type of atrial fibrillation is surgical ablation using the Maze procedure described by Cox et al.[11,12,71,74] or its variants.[72,73] While other surgical techniques have included left atrial isolation[10,70] or the creation of a corridor between the sinus node and the A-V node (Fig. 13-114), these atrial isolation procedures were, not surprisingly, unsuccessful in maintaining sinus rhythm. The development of the Maze by Dr. James Cox[11,12,71,74] provided the first cure of persistent atrial fibrillation. This procedure has undergone several iterations,

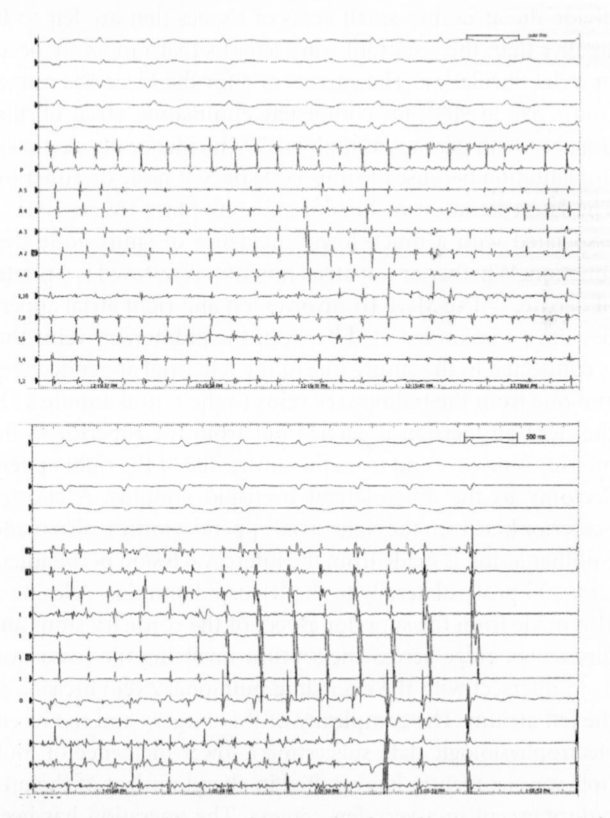

**FIGURE 13-113** *Ablation of tricuspid valve-inferior vena cava isthmus to terminate atrial fibrillation perpetuated by atrial flutter.* In the **top panel**, atrial flutter is present, which begins to change subtly as noted by a change in the relationship of the proximal coronary sinus electrogram with the other right atrial electrograms. Persistent atrial fibrillation subsequently developed as seen in the **bottom panel**. Radiofrequency ablation (after 45 minutes of atrial fibrillation) across the isthmus, when completed, terminates atrial fibrillation. The patient has had no episodes of flutter or fibrillation in 6 months off medicine.

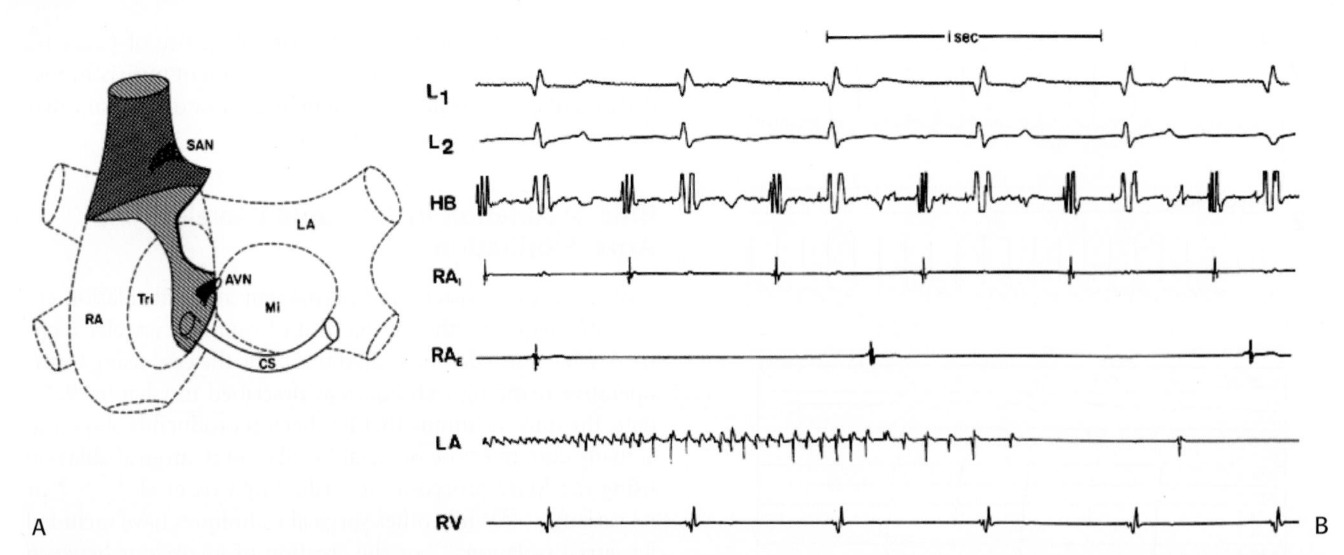


**FIGURE 13-114** *Corridor procedure for the prevention of atrial fibrillation.* **A:** A narrow band of atrial tissue from the region of the sinus node to the A-V junction is isolated from the remainder of the atria. **B:** This maintains normal A-V synchrony while fibrillation or other atrial rhythms occur elsewhere. Mi, mitral valve; SAN, sinoatrial node; Tri, tricuspid valve. (From Guiraudon GM, Sharma AD, Yee R. Surgery for atrial flutter, atrial fibrillation, and atrial tachycardia. In: Zipes DP, Jalife J, eds. *Cardiac electrophysiology: from cell to bedside*. Philadelphia, PA: WB Saunders, 1990:915.)

but they all involve a series of right and left atriotomies, which divide the atria into small areas of tissues that are felt to be smaller than the reentrant wave lengths that randomly occur in atrial fibrillation. The success rate for the Maze has ranged from 75% to 90%, for completely eliminating atrial fibrillation, but with perhaps as high as 25% incidence of pacemaker implantation because of sinus node or A-V node dysfunction. The latest iteration of the cut and sew Maze (Maze III)[71] is associated with a much lower incidence of sinus node dysfunction. Whether or not atrial function is restored is a matter of debate.[278] The Maze III involves left and right atrial appendectomy, a lesion inserted between the pulmonary veins that is connected to the suture line of the left atrial appendectomy and one from the pulmonary veins to the mitral annulus. On the right an incision is carried out from the superior to the inferior vena cave and from the suture line of the right appendectomy to the anterolateral tricuspid annulus. A shorter, posterior line from the right atrial appendectomy is also made. Another lesion is made from the intercaval lesion perpendicularly and posterolaterally to the tricuspid annulus. A lesion is also made from the superior aspect of the coronary sinus and Eustachian ridge across the septum involving the fossa ovalis to intersect with the encircling pulmonary vein incision in the left atrium. The complexity of this surgery and the recent electrophysiologic data suggesting a lower incidence of multiple wavelet reentry has resulted in abandonment of the procedure except in a very few centers. The operation has been modified to be employed in combination with mitral valve surgery.[279–282] Most of these other procedures have focused on encircling the pulmonary veins on the left side, bilateral appendage removal, and lines connecting the mitral annulus to the encircling lesion. A variety of other incisions have been employed in both the right and left atria, but they are more limited than the original Maze procedure. Most recently, a cool-tip RF "pen" has been developed to draw the lines at surgery.[72,73] While Cox suggests a success rate of greater than 90%, other reports suggest a lower success rate in the 75% range with size of the left atrium being the most important determinant for success. Reduction atrioplasty has also been incorporated into the procedure in order to eliminate excess tissue. The delayed left atrial activation and left atrial incisions make it difficult for me to believe that normal atrial transport is present. Moreover, even if the atria were to contract reasonably, the delayed and irregular atrial activation would unlikely lead to synchronous atrial contraction and appropriate filling of the left ventricle. A study[282] compared patients undergoing the Maze procedure with mitral valve repair with patients with preoperative atrial fibrillation who did not have a Maze procedure accompanying mitral valve repair. Although survival was no different at 2 years, there was a marked reduction in atrial fibrillation in the Maze-treated group who also had better outcome in terms of the combined end point of stroke or anticoagulation-related bleeding. This suggests that a variant of the Maze procedure could be safely employed as a concomitant procedure in patients undergoing mitral valve repair or other cardiac surgery in whom atrial fibrillation has been a problem. Whether the Maze procedure alone as an isolated procedure for treating atrial fibrillation has long-term better outcomes and quality of life than either some of the newer catheter-based procedures to "cure" atrial fibrillation (e.g., pulmonary vein isolation) or simply ablating the A-V junction and implanting a pacemaker is uncertain. Moreover little evidence is available to suggest surgical maze, or any procedure, can be expected to result in long-term sinus rhythm in patients with chronic (permanent) AF of greater than 5 to 7 years duration. At this point in time, permanent atrial fibrillation as an isolated clinical entity should be an unusual indication for Maze procedures.

Currently there is active surgical interest in performing "mini-mazes" which are left atrial RF or cryothermal pulmonary vein isolation procedures with additional "lines" made to recreate the incisions of the Maze III. Perhaps the most impressive of these experiences has been logged by the Washington University group. In a recent observational study, a comparison was made between results with the Cox Maze III and the minimally invasive Cox Maze IV in which lesions are delivered with bipolar RF (Atricure, West Chester, OH) and cryoablation. Follow-up of 100 patients with paroxysmal AF treated with the stand alone Cox Maze IV demonstrated 90% freedom from AF (84% freedom from AF off antiarrhythmic drugs) at 2 years.[283] Edgerton and coworkers, applied the Dallas lesion set which replicates the Maze III with RF ablation using thoracoscopic, beating heart surgery with linear lesions, LAA removal, and partial autonomic denervation in a group of 30 patients with persistent and/or long lasting persistent AF; at 6 months, 80% of patients were free of recurrence.[284] Minimally invasive surgical approaches using RF, microwave, or cryothermal energy sources are being pursued, but these are primarily pulmonary vein isolation procedures.

There remains interest in combining surgical and catheter ablation for AF, the so-called hybrid approach. The justification given for this approach for thoracoscopic procedures is that the endocardial catheter–based approach is necessary for ablation of atrial flutter, or adjuvant ablation within the coronary sinus or CFAE ablation (Fig. 13-115). Endocardial ablation is absolutely necessary for endoscopic transdiaphragmatic ablation using the nContact device. This procedure deploys a monopolar, unidirectional large electrode to the pericardial space using endoscopic techniques; ablation around the pulmonary veins is limited by the pericardial reflections; completion of PV isolation is performed with catheter ablation. Gehi and coworkers reported results in 101 mostly persistent AF patients. Freedom from AF at 12 months with antiarrhythmic therapy was 66% after a single ablation. However, there were two periprocedural deaths in this experience, one from atrioesophageal fistula, although the risk of this has subsequently been markedly reduced with improved surgical techniques.[285] A randomized trial in patients with persistent AF (catheter ablation vs. hybrid ablation using the nContact system) is presently enrolling patients.

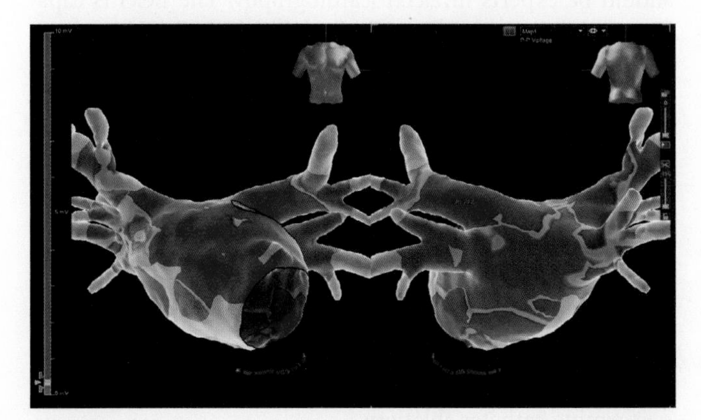

**FIGURE 13-115** *Effect of epicardial ablation (step 1 of hybrid procedure).* Sinus rhythm left atrial endocardial voltage maps (AP and PA projections) are shown from a patient with immediately following epicardial ablation using limited access from a subxyphoid approach. In this schema, bipolar voltage > 0.5 mV are "normal" (*violet*), with other colors (*blue to red*) representing lower voltages (0.5–0.2 mV) and <0.2 is designated by the gray color. The posterior wall is well ablated, as are many areas around the PV antra, limited by the pericardial reflections; these areas are approached by catheter ablation (step 2).

Catheter-based procedures involving linear lesions in the right and left atria have also been employed to treat persistent, or even permanent, atrial fibrillation.[242,255,268,270,286–288] Initial attempts to mimic the Maze procedure using catheters showed feasibility; however, the duration of the procedure and extremely high complication rate has led to its abandonment. Isolation of the superior vena cava and coronary sinus has been advocated in addition to pulmonary vein isolation in order to minimize the potential for development/maintenance of multiple wavelet reentry, as discussed above. Extensive substrate–based ablation, particularly stepwise ablation to AF termination is the most recent catheter-based iteration to attack this physiologic mechanism. As noted earlier, many investigators are targeting fractionated electrograms and "ganglia" as well. The problems with limited follow-up in single center studies in this context, especially in light of the STAR AF II trial,[256] was discussed above.

I occasionally will give lesions at the site of Bachmann bundle and/or the os of the coronary sinus in order to impair interatrial conduction. Total isolation of the coronary sinus from the left atrium has been suggested as part of an "individualized approach" to atrial fibrillation.[289] This is an area of active investigation, and with the development of better mapping and ablating tools, as well as better and more precise anatomic localization techniques (e.g., MRI), successful catheter-based therapy may be developed. Using primarily pulmonary vein isolation and caval-tricuspid lesions (if typical flutter is present) we have ~50% success rate with concomitant use of drugs in the majority of such patients.

In the future, linear right atrial lesions may decrease the number of wavelets and allow antitachycardia pacing to terminate the remaining arrhythmias or drugs to prevent them. In addition, if one could decrease the number of wavelets, the energy required for atrial defibrillation might be reduced to such an extent that it could be "painless." What lesion set will be necessary to achieve any of these end points has not been established. The lesions set may not be the same for all people. It is necessary to understand the pathophysiologic substrate of each patient. With aging and fibrosis, our ability to "cure" persistent or permanent atrial fibrillation diminishes, and use of these aggressive surgical and/or catheter-based tools will likely be less beneficial. As such our goal should be the prevention of chronic AF, when I believe ablation offers no benefit, since the multitude of ablation sites renders the left atrium nonfunctional. In this instance I doubt improvement over an "ablate and pace" strategy is possible.

## CONTROL OF VENTRICULAR ARRHYTHMIAS BY ABLATIVE TECHNIQUES

The possibility of surgical ablation of VT was realized when Couch[290] recognized the association of cardiac aneurysm with VT, which was subsequently cured by excision of the aneurysm. Although a variety of techniques including coronary bypass grafting, aneurysmectomy (with or without bypass grafting), ventriculotomy, and cryosurgery had been used in the late 1960s and early 1970s to treat "malignant ventricular arrhythmias," the exact efficacy of such procedures could not be established because (a) the surgical series usually dealt with poorly characterized arrhythmias (from isolated complex ectopy to ventricular fibrillation); (b) the clinical setting, coronary anatomy, and ventricular function were not uniformly characterized; (c) electrophysiologic studies and mapping were not performed; (d) there was no systematic pre- or postoperative evaluation of the success of surgical therapy; (e) there was obvious selective reporting of cases.

Our own limited experience using these early techniques to treat monomorphic VT was abysmal, with high operative mortality (primarily related to perioperative ventricular tachyarrhythmia recurrences) and a greater than 20% failure rate at 1 year. The development and refinement of catheter-based mapping techniques and programmed stimulation allowed the underlying mechanisms and pathophysiologic substrates of ventricular tachycardia to be established. As described in detail in Chapter 11, electrophysiologic studies allow demonstration of the mechanism of VT (reentrant vs. focal) and provide the ability to localize the arrhythmia by catheter mapping or intraoperative mapping in combination with stimulation techniques. The ability to localize the origin of focal VT, to define critical sites required for maintenance of macroreentrant VT, or characterize a pathophysiologic substrate for arrhythmias that are unstable and cannot be mapped has allowed further development of surgical and catheter-based procedures to destroy the site of origin, ablate the critical pathways associated with reentrant excitation, or isolate arrhythmogenic areas from the remainder of the heart, or render them incapable of developing arrhythmias. The ability to identify these sites in a 3D space allowed for precise localization of critical sites to enable catheter ablation to "cure" the arrhythmia. Although coronary artery disease remains the most common underlying etiology for recurrent sustained ventricular tachycardia, other pathophysiologic substrates exist (e.g., idiopathic dilated cardiomyopathy, right ventricular dysplasia—now called arrhythmogenic cardiomyopathy due to the recognition of left ventricular forms of this disease, postoperative tetralogy of Fallot, sarcoidosis, etc.). Uniform tachycardias may also be observed in normal hearts (see Chapter 11), a situation in which catheter-based therapy is now being widely applied as primary therapy. With the development of deflectible, easily steerable ablation catheters and new data acquisition systems allowing for either multisite simultaneous data acquisition (small or large basket catheters or the EnSite noncontact mapping probe system)[291–294] and the ability to precisely define points of data acquired in a 3D space (Carto, Navex, and Rhythmia electroanatomic mapping systems), catheter-based ablation of a variety of ventricular tachyarrhythmias has become widely accepted and frequently used in the management of ventricular arrhythmias. Catheter ablation of uniform VT has in fact supplanted cardiac surgery, which had been the only method to "cure" ventricular tachyarrhythmias associated with coronary artery disease or other structural entities. The decline of the surgical intervention for ventricular tachycardias has primarily resulted due to the widespread implementation of ICD therapy. This strategy offers a virtually negligible morbidity and mortality associated with implantation and high success rate in terminating ventricular tachyarrhythmias and preventing of sudden cardiac death. However, it should be remembered that an ICD is not a "cure." It requires recurrent arrhythmias to have any value. I believe the high mortality rate (10%–15%) noted in surgical series in the 1980s would be significantly less now due to better myocardial preservation techniques and additional methods to facilitate the surgical procedure itself. Thus, I believe surgical therapy for ventricular tachyarrhythmias, primarily associated with coronary artery disease, is underutilized today. Nevertheless, while the bulk of this section will deal with catheter-based ablative techniques, our surgical experience will also be described.

### Role of the ECG in Localization of Tachycardias

Before VT ablation is attempted, the investigator should have an idea of where the tachycardia might come from based purely on the ECG of the spontaneous or induced VT morphology. It is thus imperative that all people doing ablations should be experts in electrocardiography. The ECG is capable of regionalizing the arrhythmia to areas less than 15 to 20 $cm^2$, even in the most abnormal hearts. The ability to localize the origin of ventricular tachycardias by the surface ECG is greater in normal hearts than in abnormal hearts because of the absence of factors that can limit the accuracy of the ECG. These factors include fibrosis, infarction, metabolic abnormalities, prior surgery, aneurysms, and distortions of the chest wall that would otherwise alter the position of the heart relative to the chest wall. Notwithstanding these limitations, the ECG provides a "first best guess" as to where the tachycardia exit might be. This is critical because it limits the area to be mapped by the investigator. This reduces the time spent in performing catheter ablations.

The role of the ECG in localizing sites of origin of VT was described in detail in Chapter 11. There are some fairly simple general rules that should be applied. First, the presence of QS complexes in any lead suggests that the wavefront is moving away from that site, thus, providing a quick regionalization of where the tachycardia originates and/or exits. While this is a good rule of thumb in normal hearts, a dense infarct is an area of inexcitable tissue and may be associated with a QS even if

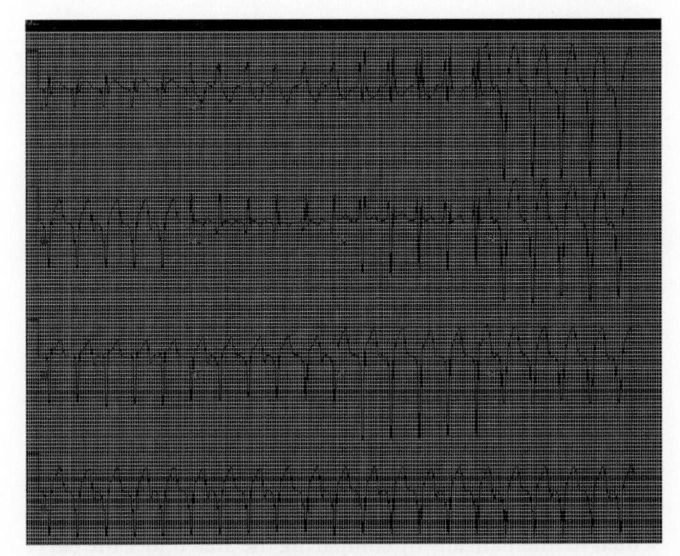

**FIGURE 13-116** *Use of the surface ECG during VT to regionalize exit site.* A 12-lead ECG is shown in a patient with hypertrophic cardiomyopathy with apical aneurysm. During VT, QRS complexes in leads I, aVF and $V_3$ to $V_6$ have q waves, signifying apical origin. See text for discussion.

the VT arises elsewhere. This can lead to confounding ECGs in patients with multiple infarctions. Nevertheless, QS complexes in the inferior leads suggest the tachycardia is coming from the inferior wall. Tachycardias that have Q waves in $V_{1-2}$ arise from the anterior septum, the mid-precordial leads ($V_3$–$V_4$) arise from the anterior wall, $V_{4-6}$ involve the apex (Fig. 13-116).

The vast majority of LBBB-type tachycardias in the setting of coronary disease arise on or adjacent to the LV septum. In the absence of coronary disease they can originate in the right ventricle (idiopathic right ventricular outflow tract [RVOT] tachycardia or right ventricular cardiomyopathy) but can arise in either the right ventricle or septum in other myopathic states. Ventricular tachycardias with an LBBB-type pattern arising in the left ventricular outflow tract (LVOT) can be distinguished from those arising in the RVOT by broader and taller r waves in $V_{1-2}$ and early transitions ($V_{2-3}$) as discussed in Chapter 11.[295–297] This is logical since the LVOT is posterior to the RVOT. On the other hand, VTs with RBBB morphologies virtually always arise in the left ventricle. The narrower the QRS complex, the more likely it is to arise near the septum and/or be associated with a normal heart. Idiopathic ventricular tachycardias which arise in the endocardium or midmyocardium usually have rapid initial forces. Those VTs that arise on the epicardium are characterized by wider QRS complexes and slurred upstrokes. The peak intrinsicoid deflection is typically >50% of the QRS in the precordial leads.[298] While this can be seen in endocardial VTs arising in dense scar, it is less common and the amplitude of the QRS is lower. Although **not** helpful in healed infarction, epicardial sites of origin can also be predicted when "focus leads" (lead I for the basal anterior or lateral walls, inferior leads for the inferior wall) have a qS morphology (Fig. 13-117).[299,300] The posterobasal areas (circumflex territory) are not seen by the standard precordial leads, so that monophasic slurred R waves in $V_{1-2}$ and aVR may be the only clues to that site of origin.

In general, the wider the VT QRS (in the absence of antiarrhythmic agents) the slower the intraventricular conduction. This situation typically takes place in the setting of a very scarred

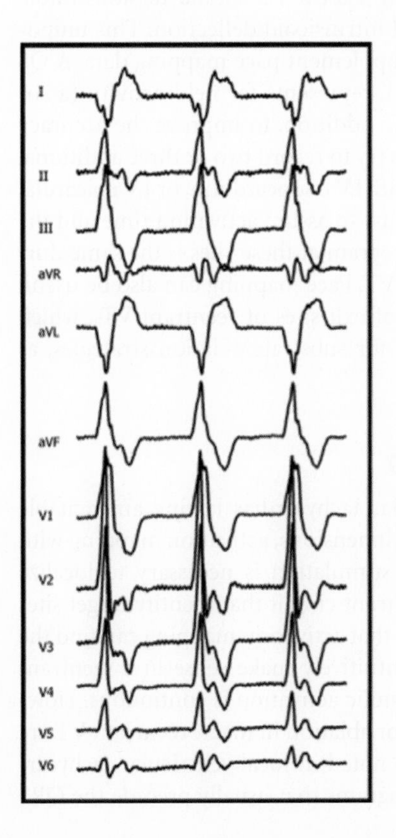


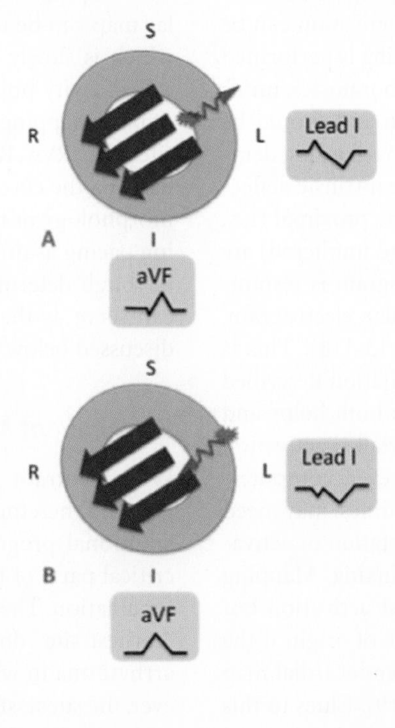


**FIGURE 13-117** *Use of the surface ECG to determine epicardial vs. endocardial exit site in basal lateral VT.* In the left panel, a 12-lead ECG during VT in a patient with nonischemic cardiomyopathy. There is a QS in lead I, and no initial q wave in the inferior leads. In the right panel, a schematic representation of activation from an endocardial (**top**) and epicardial exit site. From an endocardial site, there is a small initial vector (*blue arrow*) toward lead I (which results in an initial r wave) and away from aVF (which results in an initial q wave). From an endocardial site, this relationship is reversed. See text for discussion. (From Valles E. *Circ Arrhythm Electrophysiol* 2010;3:63–71, with permission.)

heart with VT arising from the free wall. It can also be seen in epicardial VTs. The administration of antiarrhythmic agents with sodium channel blocking capabilities and/or the presence of metabolic abnormalities (hyperkalemia, acidosis) can produce extremely wide QRSs in either supraventricular or ventricular tachycardias. Marked splintering of the QRS suggests the presence of scar, a clue to the underlying substrate of the VT. Characteristic ECG patterns of VTs arising at different locations in the left ventricle in stable coronary artery disease have been described by our laboratory and are reviewed in Chapter 11.

## Mapping Techniques for Ventricular Tachycardia

Several types of ventricular tachyarrhythmias lend themselves to catheter ablation. Direct ablation of a specific ventricular tachycardia requires that it must be present (inducible or spontaneous), uniform in morphology, and hemodynamically tolerated. The exact mechanism of the VT is less important in deciding whether VT is ablatable, but it does direct the mapping techniques used. There are four general strategies to select target sites for ablation: activation mapping, pace mapping, entrainment mapping, and substrate mapping. These have been described in Chapter 11 but are reviewed here.

### *Activation Mapping*

Activation mapping is most useful for tachycardias that are focal in origin—that is, either caused by abnormal automaticity, triggered activity, or theoretically, microreentry. It obviously requires detailed mapping during ongoing VT (which requires tolerated VT) or sequential mapping of frequent PVCs in the context of idiopathic VT. This strategy is easier to utilize in normal tissue as the local point of activation can be assigned precisely. Although activation mapping is performed using bipolar electrogram analysis in most laboratories, unfiltered and/or filtered unipolar recordings can and should be used as well. Sites of origin should have the tip recording demonstrating a QS potential with a rapid negative intrinsic deflection that is earlier than that recorded from the proximal (i.e., second pole). Unipolar recordings (filtered and unfiltered) are necessary to demonstrate that the tip electrogram is responsible for the earliest activation of the bipolar electrogram, which is also recorded simultaneously (Fig. 13-118). This is analogous to mapping techniques in pre-excitation described in Chapter 10. The use of mapping systems both helps and hinders this strategy. The ability to display detailed activation times in 3D is extraordinarily helpful; however, computer-based automatic assignment of activation times may need considerable editing. In addition, misinterpretation of activation maps can lead to "chamber-centric" thinking. Mapping a given chamber will always a site of earliest activation but this does not necessarily represent the VT site of origin if the incorrect chamber is being mapped, or if an endocardial map is performed for an epicardial VT (Fig. 13-119). Clues to this phenomenon include a broad area of similarly early sites, and the absence of a QS unipolar deflection, as described above. When there is reason for doubt, activation mapping should be supplemented by other data, such as pace mapping or entrainment mapping from the putative early site, or by mapping surrounding chambers prior to ablation attempts.

### *Pace Mapping*

Pace mapping is based on the hypothesis that replication of the tachycardia morphology by pacing at the tachycardia rate will identify the site from which the focal arrhythmia arises. The precision of pace mapping has been undermined by the concept of "12 of 12 match" which apparently means that the paced QRS morphology vaguely resembles the VT in each ECG lead. The point of this strategy in normal myocardium is to produce an exact match, even to the point of individual notches on each ECG lead (Fig. 13-120). This can be represented mathematically by comparing the area under the curve in each lead, and some mapping systems provide similar automatically derived comparative data.[301] Pace mapping can be reasonably accurate in patients with normal hearts, discrepancies can occur if the focus arises in diseased tissue. Increasing the strength of the stimulus can excite areas distant from the "point" of stimulation, even if unipolar pacing is used since the catheter tip is usually 4 or 5 mm long and high current may be required to pace diseased tissue. Nevertheless, this method provides reasonable "localizing" information.[302] We have noted similar pace maps over an area of 2 to 4 $cm^2$, as a result I try never to use pace mapping as the ***sole*** method of judging the site of origin of a focal rhythm because of these limitations. As discussed above, the unipolar signal recorded from the site of origin of a focal VT should demonstrate a QS complex with a rapid intrinsicoid deflection. This unipolar map can be used to supplement pace mapping data. A QS which is slowly inscribed, represents far field activity (a so-called cavity potential). In addition, to improve the accuracy of pace mapping, I always try to record two or three additional sites (i.e., RVA, RVOT, HBE, LV endocardium, or LV epicardial base via the coronary sinus) to assure activation time and the morphology of the electrogram at these sites is the same during pacing as during the VT. Pace mapping can also be useful in rough determination of exit sites of reentrant VTs, which can serve as the context for substrate ablation strategies, as discussed below.

### *Entrainment Mapping*

With reentrant ventricular tachycardias having an excitable gap, and therefore, finite dimensions, activation mapping with additional programmed stimulation is necessary to localize critical parts of that reentrant circuit that identify target sites for ablation. The concept that activation mapping can find the "earliest site" does not intuitively make sense in a reentrant arrhythmia in which diastolic activation is continuous. However, the successful sites for ablation in macroreentrant VT are in fact earlier than those noted in focal ventricular tachycardias. The diastolic electrograms that usually precede the QRS

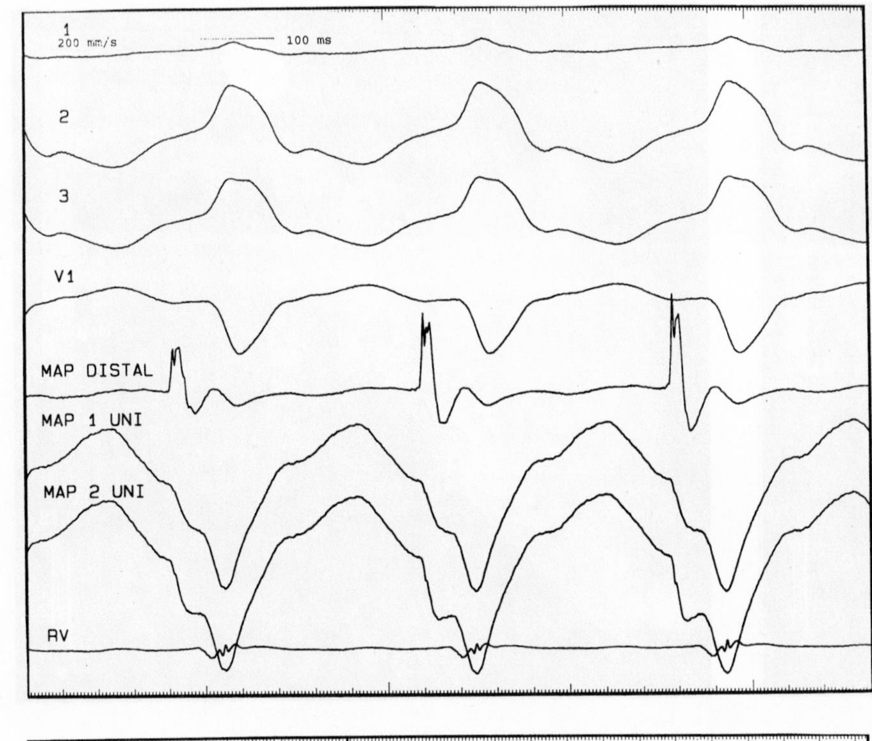


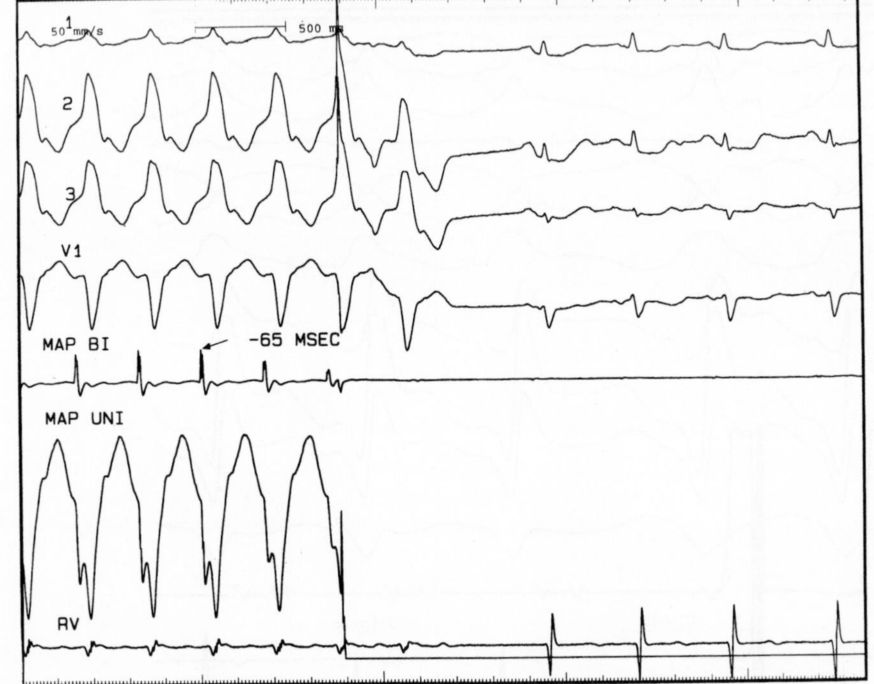


**FIGURE 13-118** *Bipolar and unipolar recordings in a patient with right ventricular outflow tract tachycardia.* **A:** ECG leads of ventricular tachycardia are shown simultaneously with the distal bipolar mapping catheter and unipolar recording from the distal and second pole of the ablation catheter. The distal mapping catheter records electrical activation 65 msec prior to the onset of the QRS. In addition, the tip electrode has the earliest unipolar deflection, which proceeds out of the second pole. **B:** Application of RF active site terminates the arrhythmia virtually instantaneously. There has been no recurrence in 2 years' follow-up.

by >50 msec must be verified as early and contributing to the subsequent QRS rather than late sites outside of the reentrant circuit that are activated passively. We have found that in some cases exit sites can be 100 msec or more prior to the QRS. Entrainment mapping supplements activation mapping during sustained, tolerated VT to precisely identify sites that are within the protected isthmus of the reentrant circuit and critical to the continuation of the tachycardia. As discussed above, pace mapping should not be used as a primary technique for determining critical sites for ablation for scar-related macroreentrant ventricular tachycardia. In macroreentrant ventricular tachycardia, the QRS begins once the impulse exits from the electrocardiographically silent diastolic pathway to excite the bulk of normal myocardium. Downer et al.,[303,304] using simultaneous multisite epicardial and endocardial recordings, have shown this can take place 50 msec before the onset of the QRS in patients with coronary disease since the impulse may still transverse abnormal tissue (and relatively "silent" in terms

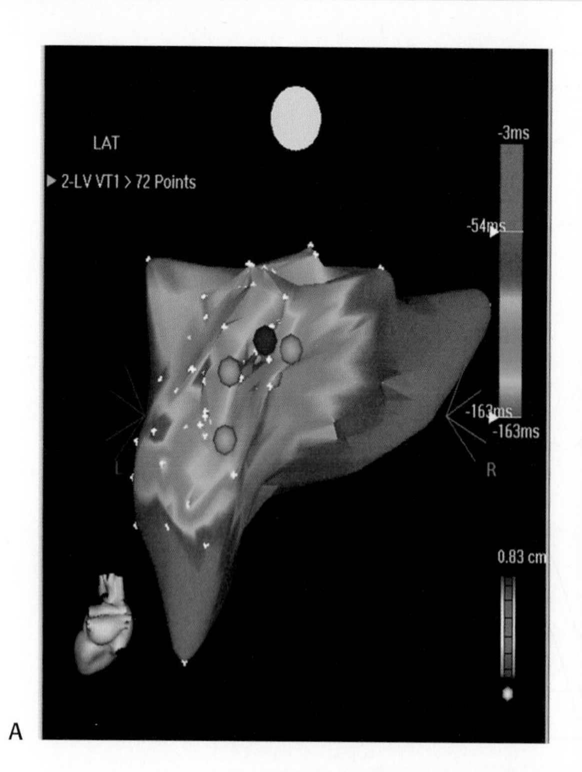


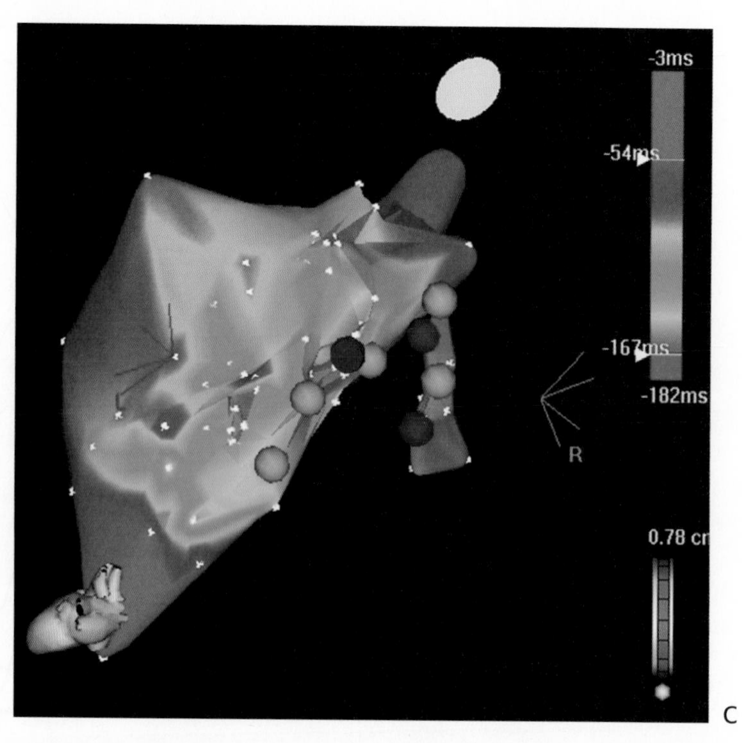


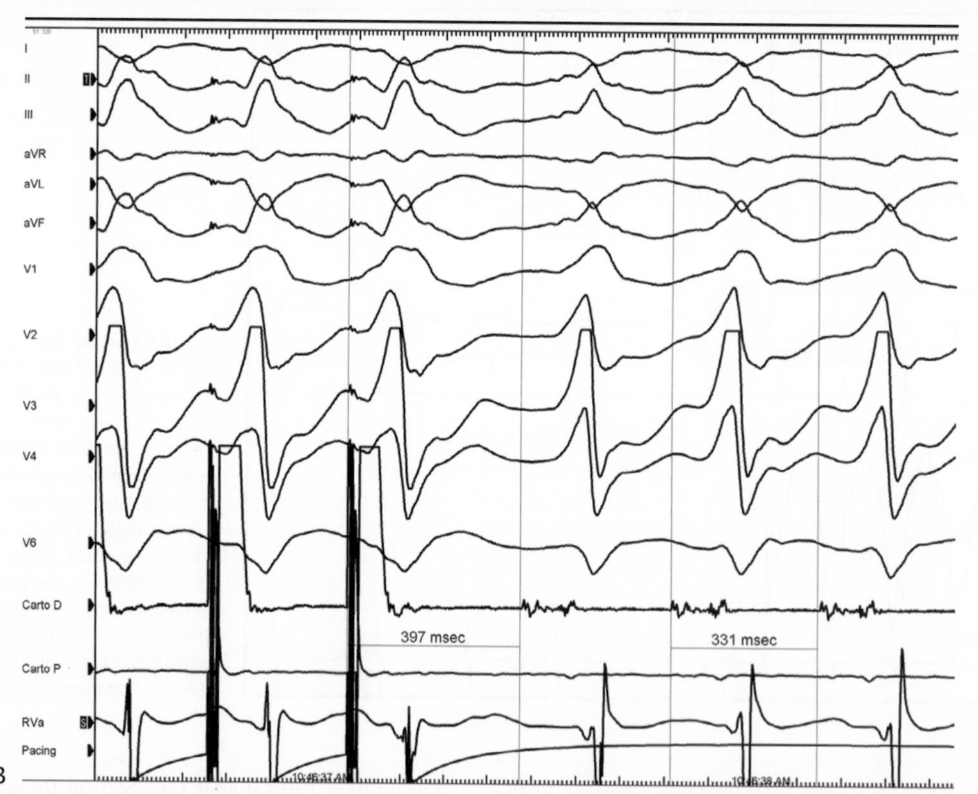


**FIGURE 13-119** *Activation and pace mapping findings in a chamber adjacent to VT origin.* In **A**, LV endocardial activation mapping during a right bundle, right inferior axis VT is shown. Note that there is a diffuse area of early activation. In **B**, overdrive pacing from an early endocardial site (the *blue dot* in **Panel A**) demonstrates fusion, and the return cycle is longer than the VT cycle length. Note also that the paced QRS has a small r wave in lead I (consistent with endocardial origin) that is missing in VT (suggesting epicardial origin). **C** shows a left lateral view of LV endocardial and coronary sinus activation mapping. Earlier activation is found in the adjacent CS, and successful ablation (*red dots*) was performed within.

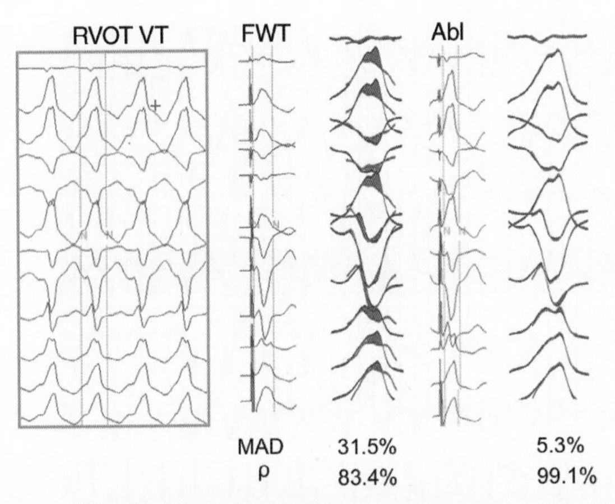


**FIGURE 13-120** *Use of the MAD score to objectify pace map results.* A 12-lead ECG during RV outflow tract VT is shown in the left panel. Pacing from a distant site, the RVOT free wall (**middle panel**) produces a poor match, which can be compared lead by lead for overlap (VT QRS in *blue,* pace map QRS in *red,* discordance in *gray*). The discordance can be quantified into the MAD score, which is high for this site. Pacing from the site of successful ablation (**right panel**) produces an excellent match, and a corresponding low MAD score. (From Gerstenfeld EP, Dixit S, Callans DJ, et al. Quantitative comparison of spontaneous and paced 12-lead electrocardiogram during right ventricular outflow tract ventricular tachycardia. *J Am Coll Cardiol* 2003;41:2046–2053, with permission.)

of its ability to contribute to the surface QRS) even after it exits the reentrant circuit to excite the myocardium. As stated above, we have seen sites recorded 100 msec prior to the QRS to be in scar defined by electroanatomic mapping as having voltage ≤0.5 mV(see below) but not in the critical central common pathway targeted for ablation (see subsequent sections). At best, a pace map that appears similar to the ventricular tachycardia would only identify the exit to the normal myocardium and may be distant from the critical points of reentrant circuit required for precise ablation. More importantly, however, is the fact that during sinus rhythm pacing from any specific site will lead to ventricular activation away from that site. Since the myocardium will be activated in a centrifugal fashion the resultant QRS almost invariably differs from that seen during ventricular tachycardia, in which the myocardium is activated orthodromically in one direction from that exit site. An example of this is shown in Figure 13-121. Ventricular tachycardia is shown in panel A. Pacing at the site within the central common pathway at which the tachycardia was subsequently successfully ablated results in a QRS that is distinctly different from the ventricular tachycardia. Pacing from a site 2 cm laterally, which was shown to be outside this central common pathway, produced an identical QRS to the ventricular tachycardia. Thus, relying on the most accurate pace map would have led to an inappropriate site for catheter ablation. For such macroreentrant arrhythmias, entrainment mapping must be used to identify sites critical to the reentrant circuit, that is, a central common pathway. This technique can also provide information about the size of that isthmus and its relationship to anatomy. Although multisite data acquisition systems that involve multiple contact recordings (large basket catheter)[291] or mathematically derived noncontact methodology (EnSite system)[292–294,305] can occasionally demonstrate the general path of diastolic activation, all components of the diastolic pathway portrayed by these techniques may not be in a protected isthmus or central common pathway. Therefore these technologies may not provide adequate targets for focal ablation, although they may suggest targets for a larger series of lesions producing a line of block. If one's goal is to terminate and eliminate a ventricular tachycardia with ablation at a single site, at this point in time entrainment mapping offers the only way to direct such ablation. The use of the small multipolar mapping catheters (PentArray by Biosense or Orion by Rhythmia) may allow one to more accurately record the critical diastolic pathway (see Fig. 11-213). The methodology of entrainment mapping that was described in Chapter 11 will be reviewed in subsequent paragraphs along with its use in defining targets for ablation.

Stevenson et al.[306] have devised a simplistic scheme to help understand the various sites inside and outside of a reentrant circuit, and, more specifically, the sites to target for ablation. These are shown in Figure 13-121. As shown here, and explained in detail in Chapter 11, the reentrant circuit involves a central common pathway that is the target for ablation, as well as pathways attached to the central isthmus that are dead ends. Inner loop pathways can serve as a potential component of a new reentrant circuit should the central common pathway be ablated. The purpose of mapping is to define the central common pathway (i.e., protected isthmus) as the target site for ablation. Much has been made of whether this is a zone of slow conduction. Conduction through this central pathway may be normal (as it usually is) or slow, but this is not important. Finding the protected isthmus is important, and success of ablation is independent of the speed of propagation of the impulse through that isthmus. The key characteristic of the protected isthmus is that the tachycardia circuit is confined within this area, allowing for the destruction of the circuit with limited ablation. The steps outlined in Chapter 11 include (a) finding the site of earliest activation closest to mid-diastole or continuous activity; (b) demonstrating that this diastolic electrogram bears a fixed relationship to the subsequent QRS despite spontaneous or pacing-induced oscillations by the tachycardia cycle length; (c) performing entrainment mapping to demonstrate an entrained morphology identical to the VT morphology, a stimulus to QRS approximately equal to the electrogram to QRS during the tachycardia (within 10 msec), and a postpacing interval equal to the ventricular tachycardia cycle length (within 10 msec) as long as the pacing is carried out at cycle lengths slightly shorter than the native tachycardia. If pacing is carried out too rapidly, delays in various components of the circuit may occur such that the postpacing interval and the stimulus to QRS may exceed the VT cycle length and electrogram to QRS during the tachycardia, respectively. Obviously, in order to accomplish activation mapping, the tachycardia must be present spontaneously or inducible.

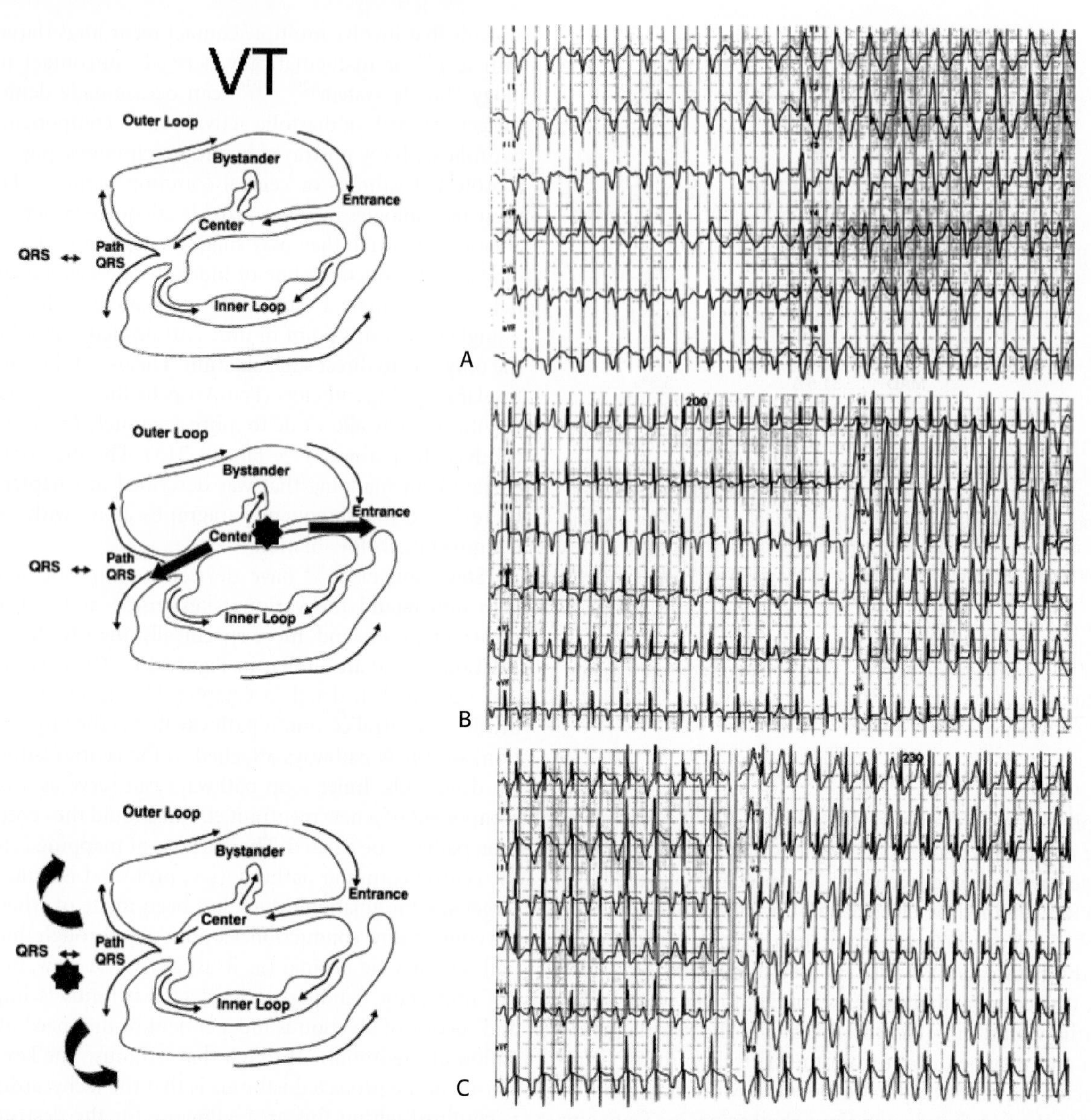


**FIGURE 13-121** *Failure of pace mapping to accurately locate isthmus of critical conduction during reentrant ventricular tachycardia associated with coronary artery disease.* **A:** (**top**) Shows the 12-lead of the ventricular tachycardia. **B:** (**middle**) Shows the pace map during sinus rhythm from the site ultimately shown to be in the center of the isthmus at which successful ablation was carried out. Note that this QRS does not resemble that of the native tachycardia. **C:** (**bottom**) Shows pace mapping from a site 2 cm lateral to the critical isthmus. Its morphology is identical to the tachycardia. These findings demonstrate the limitations of pace mapping. Dots in schema show pacing site relative to anatomic parts of the circuit. See text for discussion.

The initial step in entrainment mapping ventricular tachycardia is to identify the earliest presystolic electrogram closest to mid-diastole. In general we focus our mapping to areas that, based on the QRS, are likely to yield presystolic sites. These presystolic sites are sites that have exited from the central common pathway to produce a QRS. Thus, if the onset of the QRS represents the exit to the mass of myocardium, activity prior to that may be within the central common pathway or in scar tissue around it. Based on intraoperative mapping studies,[303,307] the time from the exit of the protected isthmus to the myocardium initiating the onset of the QRS may be as long as 50 msec. As noted earlier, we have seen sites that were presystolic by 100 msec be outside the isthmus and outside of the circuit. As such, we generally do not target sites that are less than 50 msec presystolic. The earliest sites closest to mid-diastole may appear as isolated mid-diastolic potentials, fragmented low-amplitude signals only within diastole, or most commonly, fragmented signals that extend from diastole to systole. As noted in Chapter 11, unfiltered unipolar signals are not very helpful in scar-related tachycardias because far field activity frequently dominates the signal. This is shown in Figure 13-122 in which the early presystolic site (site 3) on the midseptum is 55 msec prior to the QRS in the bipolar recording, but is associated with a much later unipolar recording. Note that site 1 to 2 is also presystolic but is not as early. Unipolar filtered recordings may be useful to assure that the tip electrode, which is the ablation

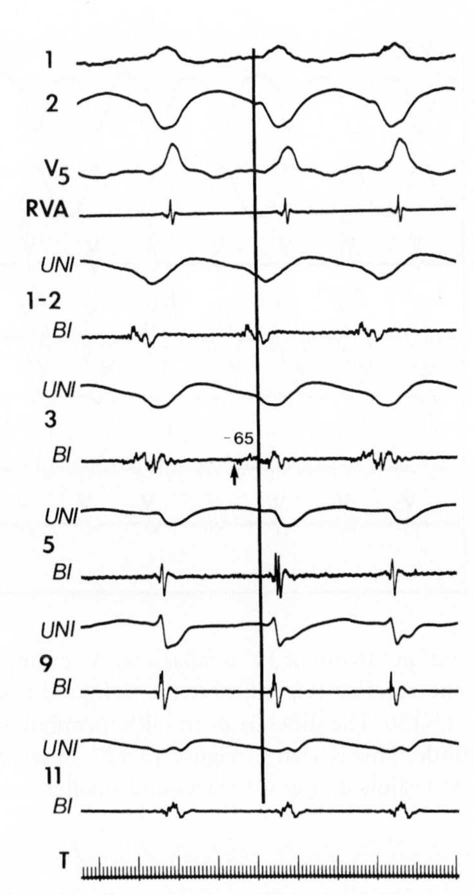


**FIGURE 13-122** *Map of ventricular tachycardia associated with coronary artery disease.* Unipolar and bipolar recordings from selected sites during VT with an RBBB left superior axis morphology. The earliest endocardial activity was 65 msec before the QRS at the midseptum (site 3). Unipolar signals are not useful in determining early sites, because electrical signals from the small number of fibers giving rise to diastolic activity are dominated by activation of more distant, larger muscle mass. See Chapter 11.

electrode, is responsible for the early component of the bipolar electrogram. Occasionally one can trace the diastolic pathway itself with careful mapping (see Fig. 11-221).Using the Carto system (Fig. 13-123) or the new Rhythmia system (see Figs. 11-213 and 13-124), one can actually record the entire reentrant circuit. Even more uncommon is the recording of continuous electrical activity throughout diastole (Fig. 13-125). As stressed in Chapter 11, "continuous" electrogram is significant only if one can demonstrate that it is not a passive electrogram whose duration equals a tachycardia cycle length, that it is required for initiation and maintenance of the tachycardia, and is localized.[308,309]

Since all diastolic signals may not necessarily be part of a reentrant circuit and may reflect late activation from unrelated, dead-end pathways, other methods must be used to demonstrate that these diastolic signals (particularly those that are isolated) are part of the circuit. As carefully outlined in Chapter 11 the demonstration that a mid-diastolic electrogram maintains its morphology and bears a constant relationship to the subsequent QRS during spontaneous or pacing-induced

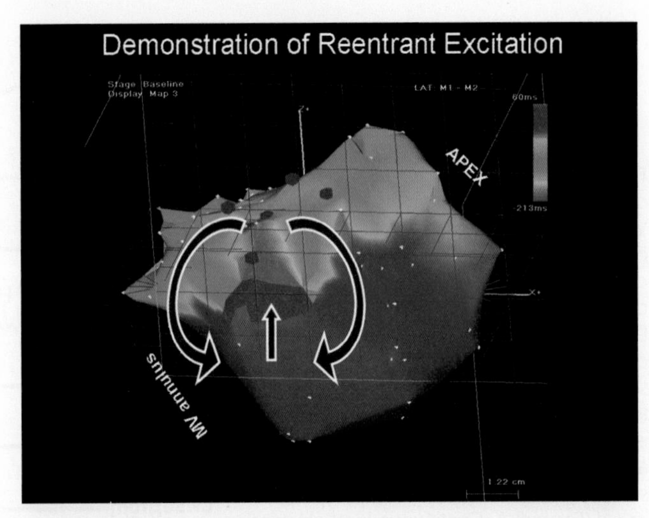


**FIGURE 13-123** *Demonstration of reentrant excitation using electroanatomic mapping.* Activation of the posterobasal septum during scar-related VT shows figure-of-eight reentrant excitation.

(i.e., pacing at sites distant from the circuit) changes in cycle length suggests that the electrogram is orthodromically activated during the tachycardia. If concealed entrainment can be shown at that site (see below) or a single extra stimulus can reset the circuit from that site with a morphology identical to the VT and with a return cycle length and stimulus to QRS equal to the VT cycle length and electrogram to QRS, respectively, the electrogram is not only in the circuit, but in the isthmus.

It is the response of overdrive pacing (entrainment) or single extrastimuli (resetting) that is most useful in demonstrating that an electrogram is not only in the reentrant circuit, but is within the central common pathway that is the

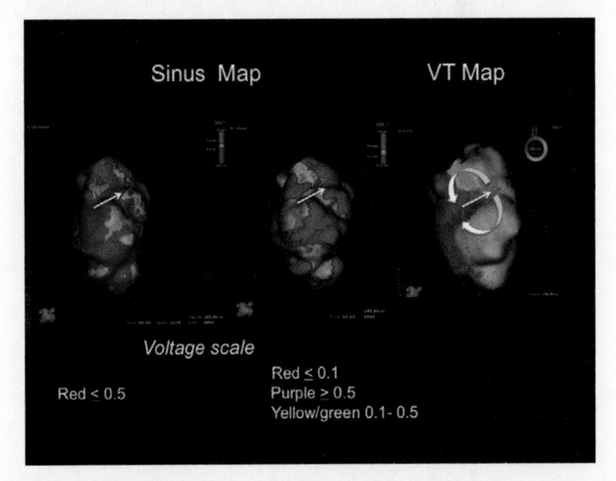


**FIGURE 13-124** *Relation of sinus rhythm mapping to activation mapping of VT.* Sinus rhythm maps in a porcine model of anterior infarction are shown in the left two panels. *Red* is dense scar, *purple* is normal. Different voltage settings are used. On the far left voltage <0.5 mV is shown in *red.* In the middle panel *red* is ≤0.1 mV is in *red; yellow/green* 0.1 to 0.5mV, and *purple* ≥0.5 mV. The *arrow* shows the same site using the different scales. Note that what appeared to be dense scar on the left is "viable" in the middle. Note the *arrow* shows a zone of viable area between two small areas of dense scar. On the far right is an activation map during VT which shows the isthmus in the same site as the *arrow.* See text for discussion.

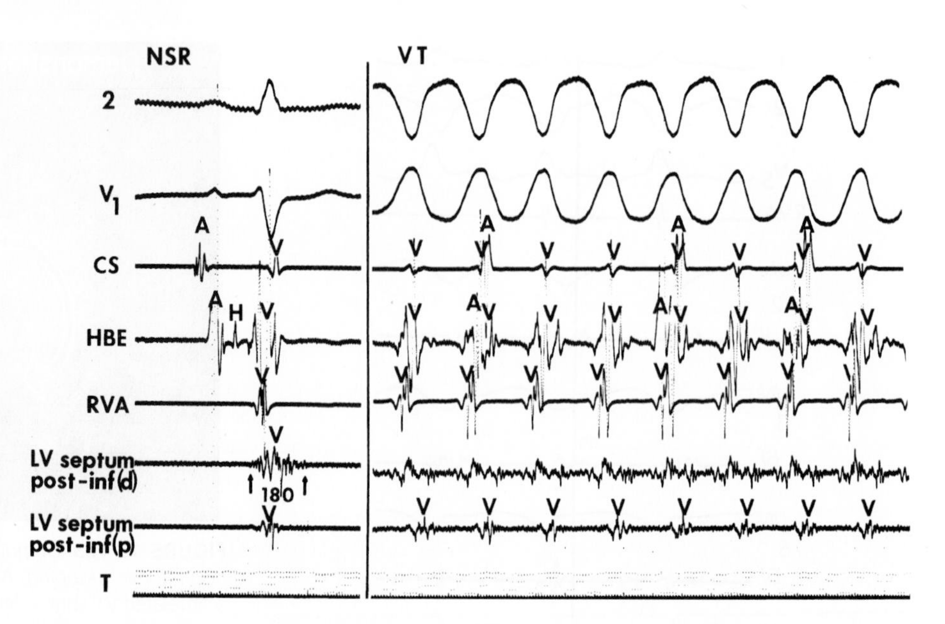


**FIGURE 13-125** *Local continuous electrical activity during ventricular tachycardia.* Ventricular tachycardia in a patient with coronary artery disease is shown. Proximal and distal bipolar recordings from a quadripolar catheter position on the septum are shown. During VT continuous fractionated activity is observed only in the distal recording. Note in sinus rhythm, the electrogram recorded from the bipolar pair that was continuous during VT is fractionated, of long duration (180 msec), and extends beyond the QRS. NSR, normal sinus rhythm. (From Josephson ME, Horowitz LN, Farshidi A. Continuous local electrical activity: A mechanism of recurrent ventricular tachycardia. *Circ* 1978;57:659.)

target of ablation. The first and simplest finding that would suggest one is within or adjacent to the isthmus is that the QRS during entrainment is identical to that of the ventricular tachycardia. Identical means 12 out of 12 leads that match the VT QRS, including amplitude and notches. The concept of a "pretty good" or "10 out of 12" is fallacious. An example of an entrainment map that is identical to the tachycardia is shown in Figure 13-126. The differences in QRS morphologies can be very subtle. This is seen in Figure 13-127, in which leads 2, 3, and AVF show deeper QS waves and smaller terminal R

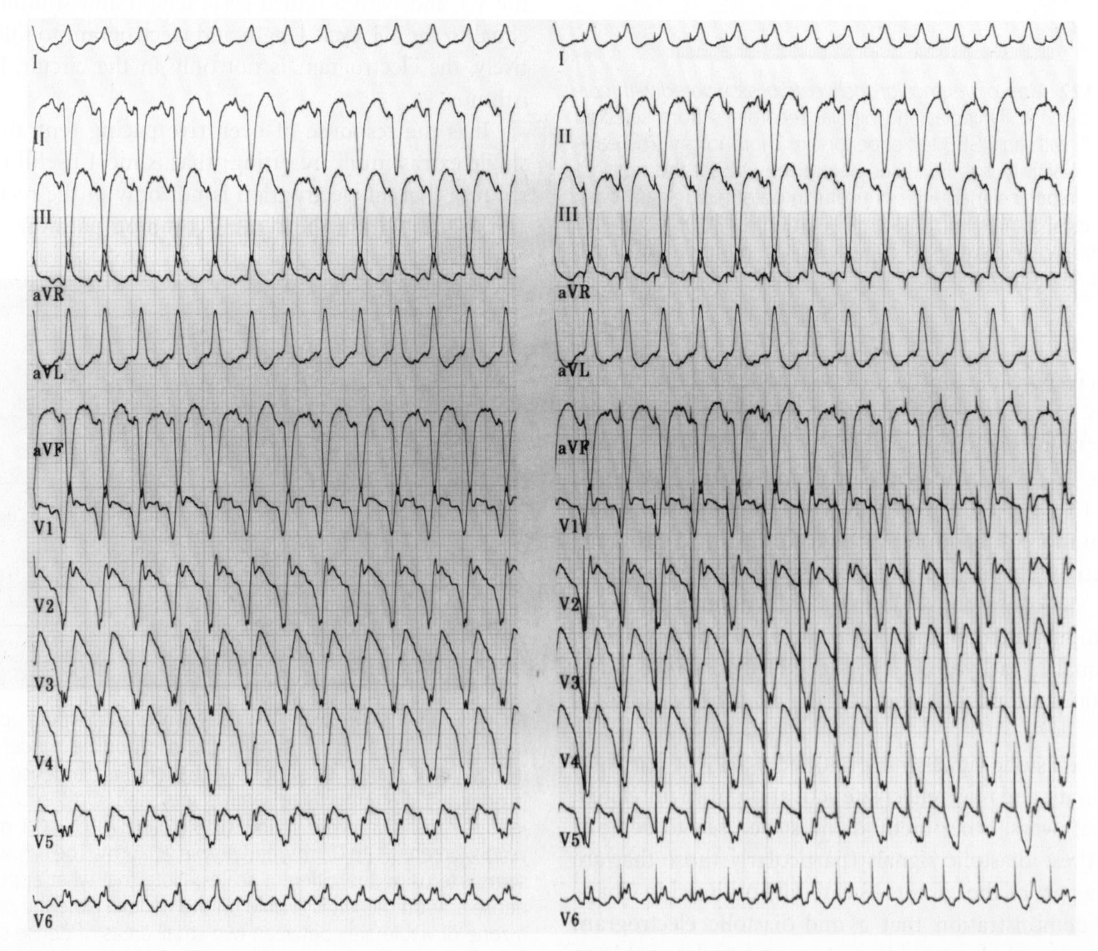


**FIGURE 13-126** *Example of exact entrainment map.* Ventricular tachycardia is shown on the left. Entrainment of that ventricular tachycardia is shown on the right. Note that the QRS morphology in all 12 leads is identical with comparable notching and amplitudes. See text for discussion.

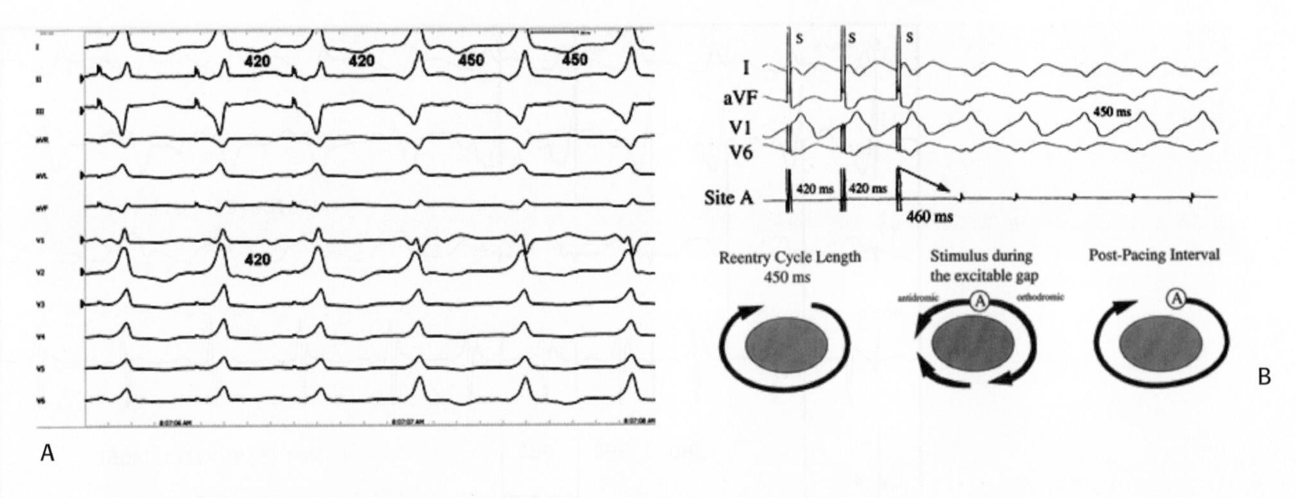


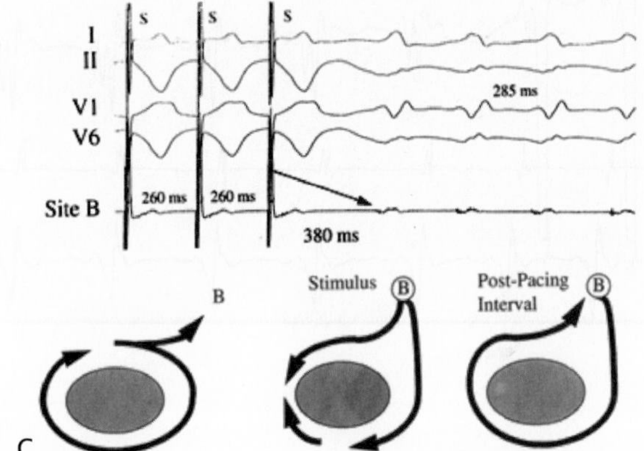


**FIGURE 13-127** *Response of VT to overdrive pacing on the left.* **A:** Ventricular pacing at a diastolic site. The QRS has a *similar* morphology but careful analysis showed subtle but distinct differences from that of the tachycardia. The stimulus to QRS exceeds 75% of the VT cycle length but the return cycle equals the VT cycle length suggesting the site is in the circuit but proximal to the entrance of the isthmus. **B:** Schematically shown is pacing from within the tachycardia circuit, but outside the central common pathway. This produces differences between the paced morphology and the tachycardia morphology but a return cycle approximating that of the VT cycle. The stimulus to QRS is short suggesting this is near the exit. **C:** When the pacing site is outside the reentrant circuit, not only will the paced morphology be markedly different than the tachycardia morphology, but the return cycle will exceed the tachycardia cycle length. See text for discussion.

waves than during VT. Subtle differences in QRS amplitude are important because this suggests one is near the exit site but not within the isthmus. If one is outside the central common pathway (or protected isthmus) but still within the reentrant circuit, entrainment will produce a QRS that is slightly different from the ventricular tachycardia (demonstrate fusion) but the return cycle will approximate the VT cycle length (Fig. 13-127). On the other hand, as shown in panel B of Figure 13-127, if the electrogram is outside the reentrant circuit, not only will the QRS differ from the ventricular tachycardia QRS, but the return cycle will be longer than the tachycardia cycle length. Another example of pacing outside the tachycardia circuit is shown in Figure 13-128. In this case, entrainment of ventricular tachycardia associated with an inferior wall infarction from the local left ventricular site produces a QRS that is slightly different than the native ventricular tachycardia QRS and has a return cycle that exceeds its ventricular tachycardia cycle length by 60 msec. The length of the central common pathway can be determined by the size of the zone from which concealed entrainment can be demonstrated (Fig. 13-129). We have found this isthmus to be 1 to 5 cm in length with an average of ~2.2 cm. It may actually be much shorter if higher-resolution mapping is done to define the barriers (fixed or anatomic) that form the isthmus (Fig. 13-130). Other investigators have found slightly longer isthmuses;[310–312] the reasons for this is unclear, but probably reflect location of VTs, extent of scar in individual patients, but most probably the inability to distinguish the end of a functional or anatomic barrier relative to the entrainment map.

The third criterion for identifying a central common pathway is the relationship of stimulus to QRS interval during overdrive pacing and the electrogram to QRS during spontaneous VT. If the electrogram is from a site in the central common pathway, the stimulus to QRS should equal the electrogram to QRS, the VT morphology will be the same as the paced morphology, and the return cycle will equal the tachycardia cycle. An example in which all three criteria are met is shown in Figure 13-131. On top the return cycle is identical to the tachycardia cycle and the stimulus to QRS equals the electrogram to QRS and the QRS is a match. In the bottom panel, once all three criteria are met, application of RF energy immediately terminates ventricular tachycardia. Another example of the use of these three criteria to identify the central common pathway is shown in Figure 13-132. In panel A, ventricular tachycardia with an RBBB superior axis is seen. The cycle length of 442 msec and the electrogram to QRS is 115 msec. Entrainment mapping shows a morphology equal to the tachycardia morphology, a return cycle equal to the tachycardia cycle, and a stimulus to QRS virtually identical to the electrogram to QRS. Application of RF energy at this site terminates the tachycardia in three and a half seconds

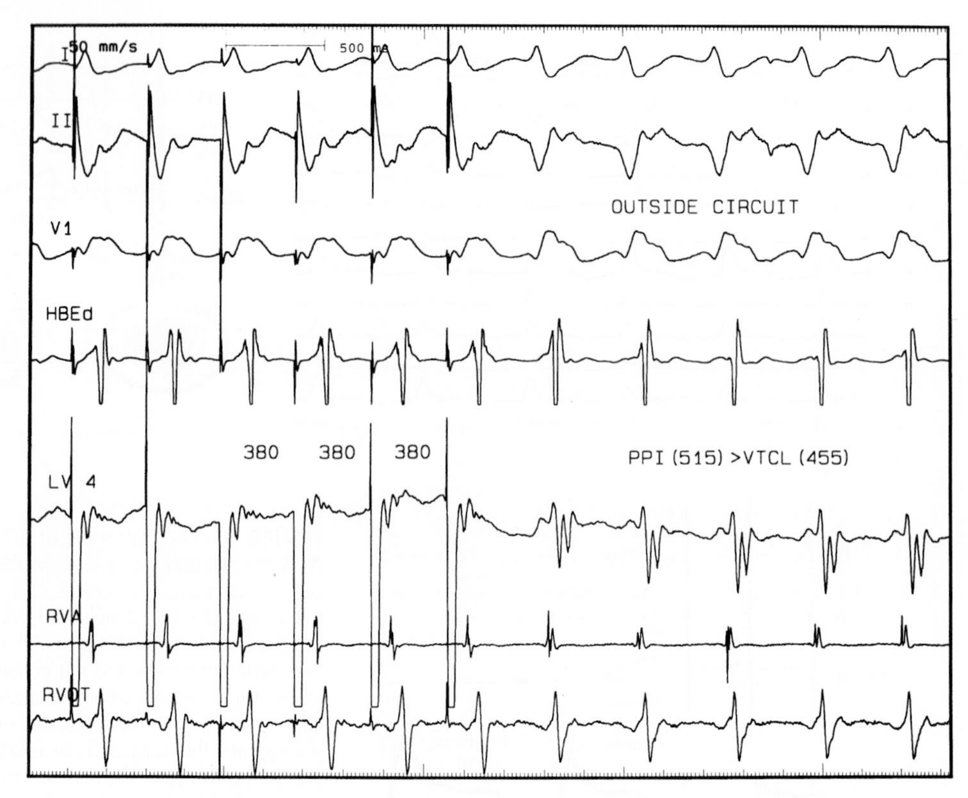


**FIGURE 13-128** *Analog recordings during overdrive pacing from a site outside the reentrant circuit.* Ventricular tachycardia is present in a patient with an inferior myocardial infarction. Pacing a site outside the tachycardia circuit produces a QRS that is distinctly different from the tachycardia. In addition, the post pacing interval exceeds the tachycardia cycle length by 60 msec.

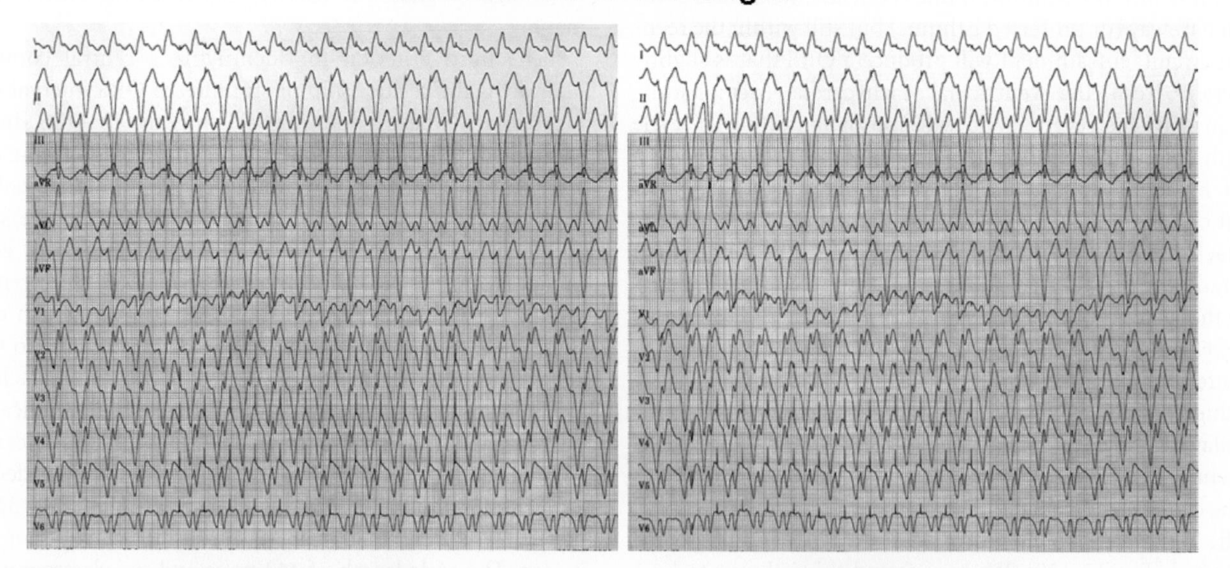


**FIGURE 13-129** Use of entrainment to assess length of protected isthmus. Ventricular tachycardia with an LBBB, left axis morphology is shown. Pacing at sites of diastolic activity produced exact entrainment maps with stimulus to QRS ranging from 90 to 220 msec over a 4.5-cm area. The 90-msec site is close to the exit, and the 160-msec site was felt to be mid-isthmus. See text for discussion.

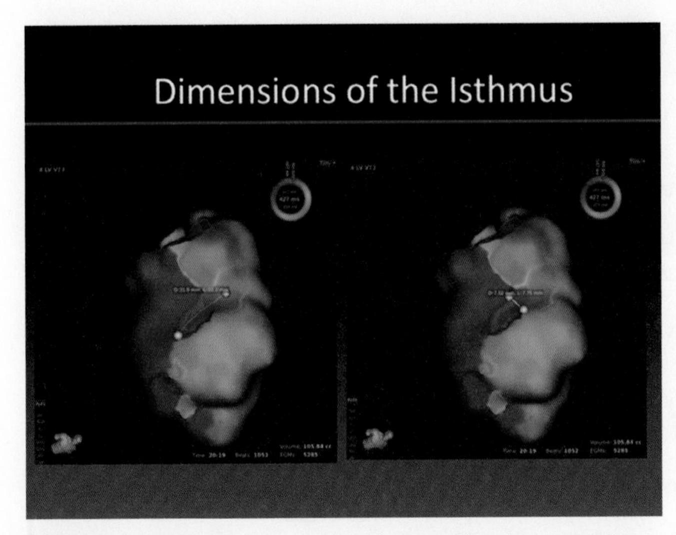


**FIGURE 13-130** *Activation mapping characterizing the VT circuit.* Two panels show activation mapping during VT. The length and width of the isthmus are shown by *yellow lines.*

(panel B).Two additional criteria for identifying a critical isthmus are:

1. Delay of the return cycle or termination of the VT during resetting in the absence of ventricular capture.[35]
2. Termination or delay of the VT with a stimulus that captures the local myocardium but fails to exit the circuit (nonpropagated stimulus) or a true subthreshold stimulus (a stimulus that fails to capture myocardium during sinus rhythm). The response to true subthreshold stimuli results from depolarizing tissue enough to make it inexcitable or partially excitable to the oncoming wavefront, but not enough to produce local capture. Both types of responses identify critical sites in the VT circuit and suggest a narrow isthmus.

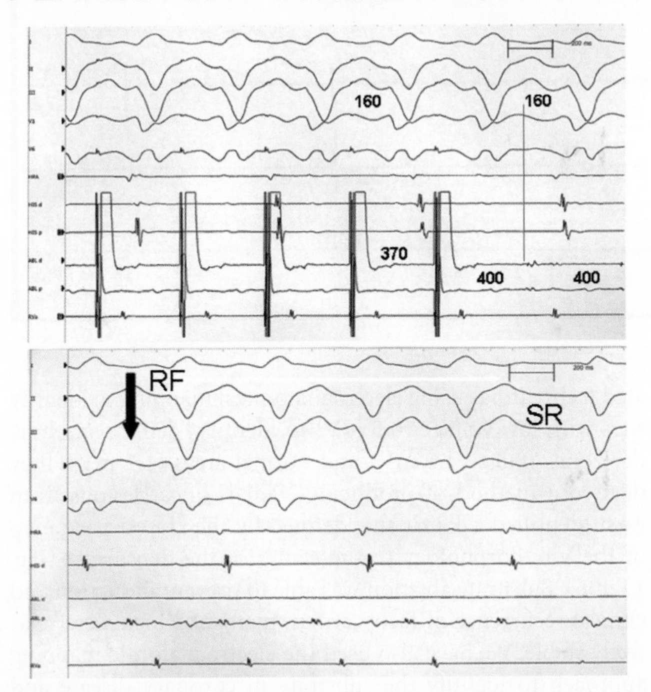


**FIGURE 13-131** *Ablation with perfect entrainment map.* This is the same patient as in Figure 13-129. Entrainment from the mid-isthmus is shown with stimulus-QRS, EGM-QRS (160 msec), a return cycle, VT cycle length (400 msec), and a perfect ECG match. Radiofrequency application at this site terminated the VT in 1.5 seconds.

The electrical anatomic mapping systems (Biosense, Navix and Rhythmia) allow one to define the size of the isthmus by identifying in 3D space all the sites from which concealed entrainment can be demonstrated. In Figure 13-133, areas of pace mapping during sinus rhythm (blue circles) produced QRS identical to VT with a stimulus to QRS from 20 to 190 msec over an area of 1.53 cm in length and 0.5 cm in width. A lesion placed near the exit (site of shortest stimulus-QRS) prevented induction of VT. This is the basis for use of substrate mapping to ablate VT (see ablation of untolerated VT below). The site at which termination occurs can be identified by assessing the effect on local electrograms. In Figure 13-134, RF energy terminates ventricular tachycardia after the diastolic signal and prior to the exit site. This confirms that the block occurred proximal to the exit site from the isthmus. We normally deliver RF energy for 2 minutes at the site at which the tachycardia is terminated and then test to see if the tachycardia is still inducible. If the tachycardia is not inducible no further lesions are given. Large isthmuses often require two to three lesions at adjacent sites usually within 1 $cm^2$. Occasionally, additional lesions are given at the same site if late potentials are seen at that site after termination of the VT. An example of such ablation is shown in Figure 13-135. In panel A, ventricular tachycardia is present and the target ablation site is shown with an isolated mid-diastolic potential preceding the QRS by 145 msec. Both the distal and second poles demonstrated this mid-diastolic potential, which was slightly earlier in the distal tip. RF energy delivered at this site immediately terminated the tachycardia. The sinus complexes that were recorded in the same electrograms demonstrated a late potential. An additional 2-minute application of RF energy was delivered at the same site, which resulted in loss of the late potential. Stimulation at that time revealed no inducible arrhythmia. The patient has been free of arrhythmias for many years on no medicines.

### *Substrate Mapping*

In the presence of ***unstable monomorphic and/or polymorphic*** ventricular tachycardias, detailed activation mapping and entrainment mapping are not possible. This is also true for transient arrhythmias. Multisite data acquisition systems as described above may provide useful information in such cases as to the earliest site of activation. However, these methodologies do not necessarily allow one to do a discrete ablative procedure. As such, ablation in these arrhythmias must be aimed at producing larger lesions to disrupt the potential circuit. These are indirect methods based on identification of the arrhythmogenic substrate in patients with structural heart

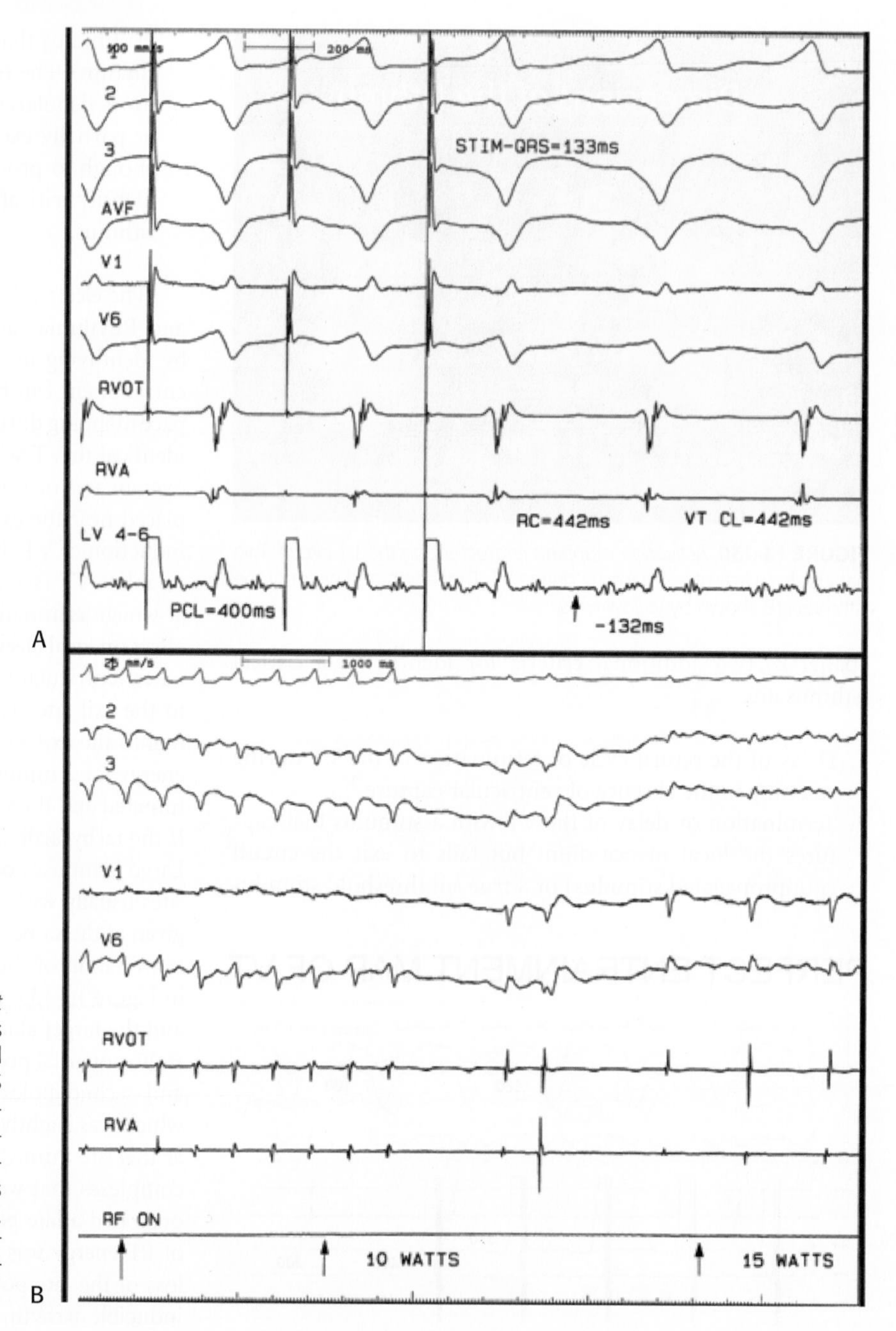


**FIGURE 13-132** *Effectiveness of all entrainment criteria to guide ablation.* **A:** Ventricular pacing is being carried out at a presumed site in the central common pathway. During entrainment the QRS approximates that of the tachycardia. The stimulus to QRS and return cycle also are nearly identical to the electrogram to QRS during a tachycardia and VT cycle length. **B:** RF application at this site terminates the tachycardia in 3.5 seconds. Following ablation, the tachycardia was no longer inducible. The patient has been free of ventricular tachycardia for over 10 years, off medications.

disease (Table 13-1). This substrate is defined by abnormal electrograms as defined by amplitude (voltage) and duration, particularly whether or not these electrograms are noted after the QRS (late potentials). These features of electrograms in coronary artery disease were described more than 20 years ago in our EP laboratory[313,314] and at the time of surgery.[315] At that time it was obvious that these abnormalities of electrograms extended far beyond the sites of exit of individual ventricular tachycardias. As such, abnormal electrograms were used for guiding surgical procedures in which these abnormal electrograms were encircled or removed in order to cure ventricular tachycardia.[316,317] This semidirected surgical procedure had a 50% to 85% success rate. Marchlinski et al.[318] were the first apply this concept to catheter ablation of poorly tolerated tachycardias using electroanatomical mapping to identify sites with low voltage (0.5 mV) to identify "dense scar," border zones (0.5 to 1.5 mV) and normal areas (1.5 mV), they devised a method of producing "radial" linear lesions from each identified VT exit site, defined by the closest pace map of the VT morphology to the center of the dense scar (Fig. 13-136). Substrate ablation was able to prevent induction and clinical recurrence of tachycardias, many of which were relatively stable. We have also used the electroanatomic mapping approach to identify the substrate in coronary disease and have shown that the site of successful ablation in the central, common pathway is located in infarcted tissue with late activation, low voltage, and often associated with late potentials (Fig. 13-137). If the poorly tolerated VTs are monomorphic,

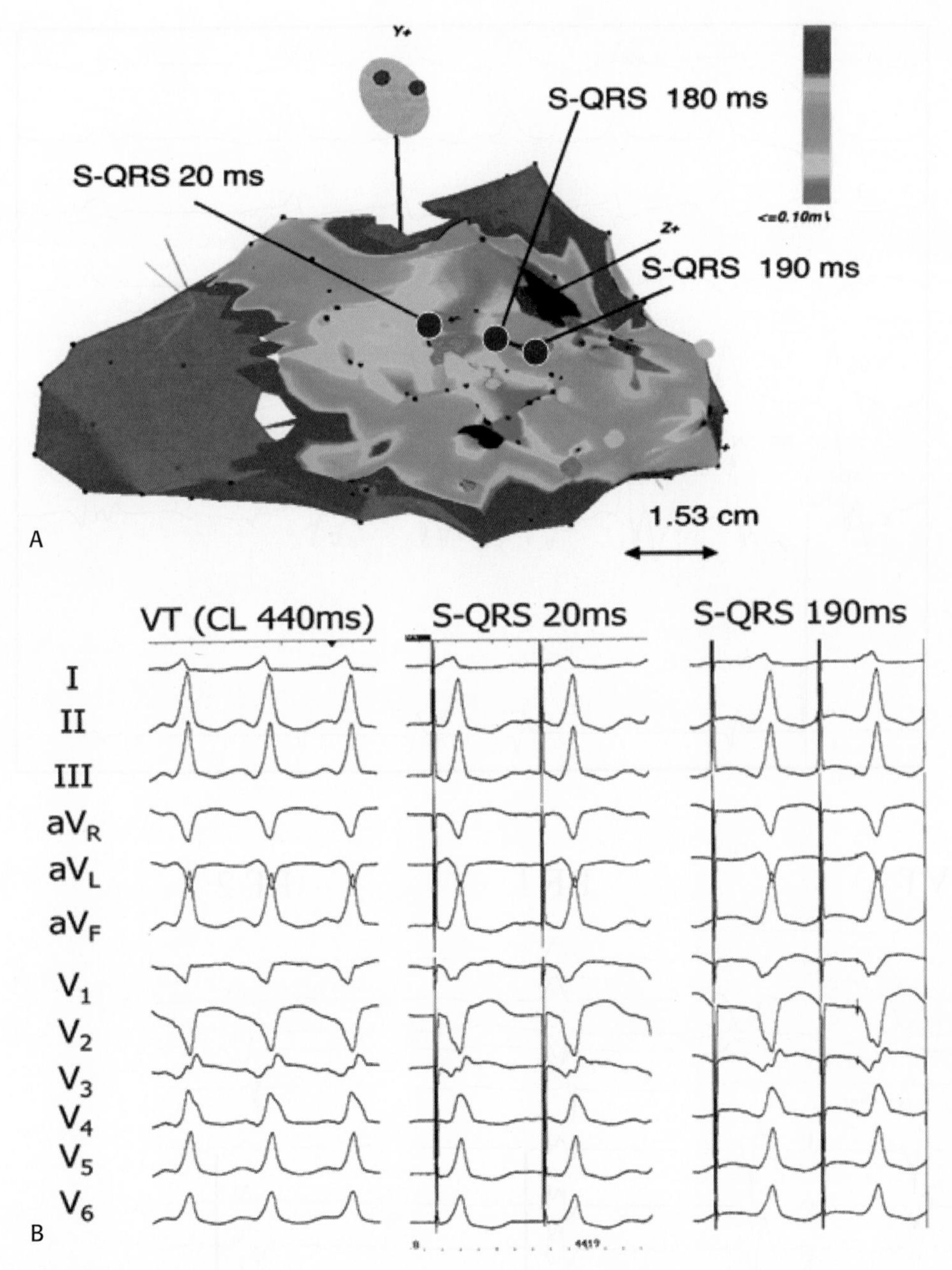


**FIGURE 13-133** *Pace mapping in scar to identify central isthmus.* Areas of pace mapping during sinus rhythm (*blue circles*) produced a QRS identical to VT with a stimulus to QRS ranging from 20 to 190 msec over an area of 1.53 cm in length and 0.5 cm in width. The scar is *red; black* being inexcitable tissue. Ablation across the exit of this channel prevented VT.

pace mapping can be used to identify an exit site from the scar and can identify the potential isthmus. Linear lesions **perpendicular** to the isthmus (i.e., tangent to the scar) can guide ablation of these tachycardias.

The concept of using voltage mapping to understand the morphology of ventricular scar and to plan ablation strategies is powerful. However, recent investigation suggests that there are significant limitations to this strategy which may explain, in part, the limited success rate of this technique. Although the voltage gradient in transmural infarction is very steep, repeated measures at the border of the infarct often are disparate, presumably related to the inherent inaccuracy of mapping with large tip catheters and differences in orientation; these errors would be expected to be magnified noninfarct related scar, in which the gradient is not always as steep. The promise of mapping with very small electrodes in this setting may enhance our knowledge of the interaction of infarct anatomy and VT circuit physiology (Fig. 13-124). At times, isolated late potentials (a certain signal of slow conduction) can be sufficiently high enough in amplitude to not "qualify" as scar in electroanatomic mapping. Finally, voltage maps constructed in different rhythms (sinus and RV pacing, sinus and VT) often have significant differences, confirming the fact that voltage is mainly a measure of underlying conduction velocity which is influenced by infarct anatomy, tissue contact, and the relationship of the wave front of activation to the bipolar recording electrodes (see Chapter 11) (Figs. 13-138 to 13-140). These limitations may be further magnified when unipolar voltage mapping techniques (see below) are employed.

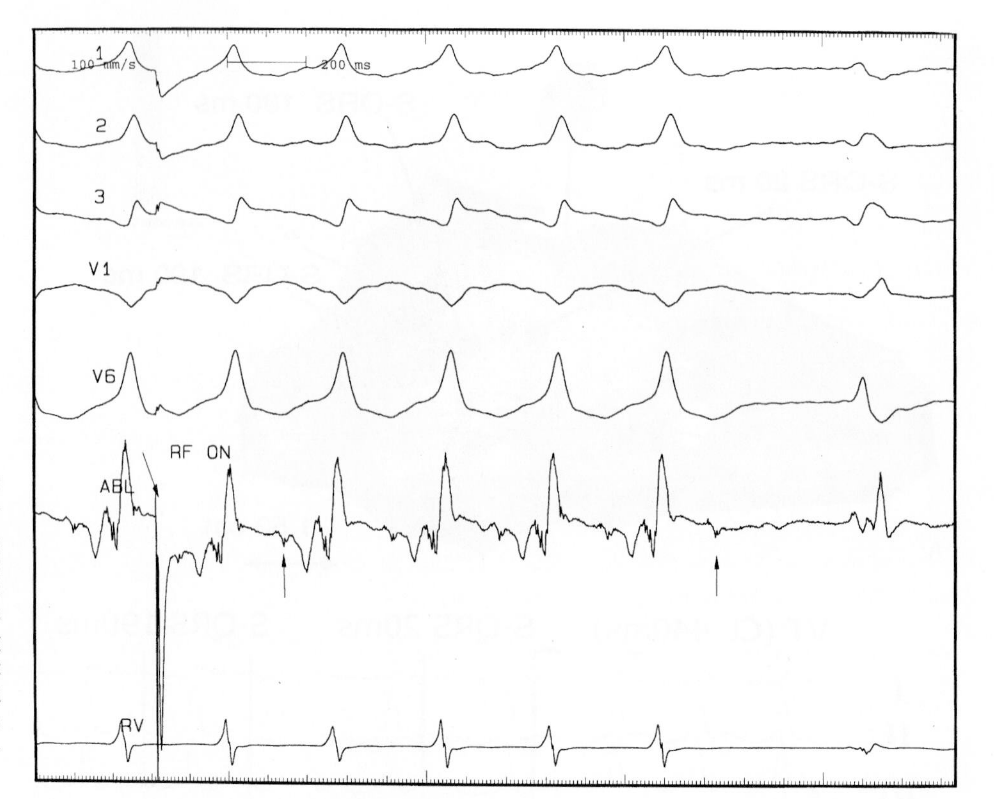


**FIGURE 13-134** *Site of block in the reentrant circuit deduced by RF application.* During ventricular tachycardia, mid-diastolic potential was observed (*small arrow*). This site demonstrated concealed entrainment. Ablation at this site terminated tachycardia by blocking between this diastolic site and a systolic electrogram. This suggested that block occurred between the central common pathway and the exit site of the tachycardia circuit. See text for discussion.

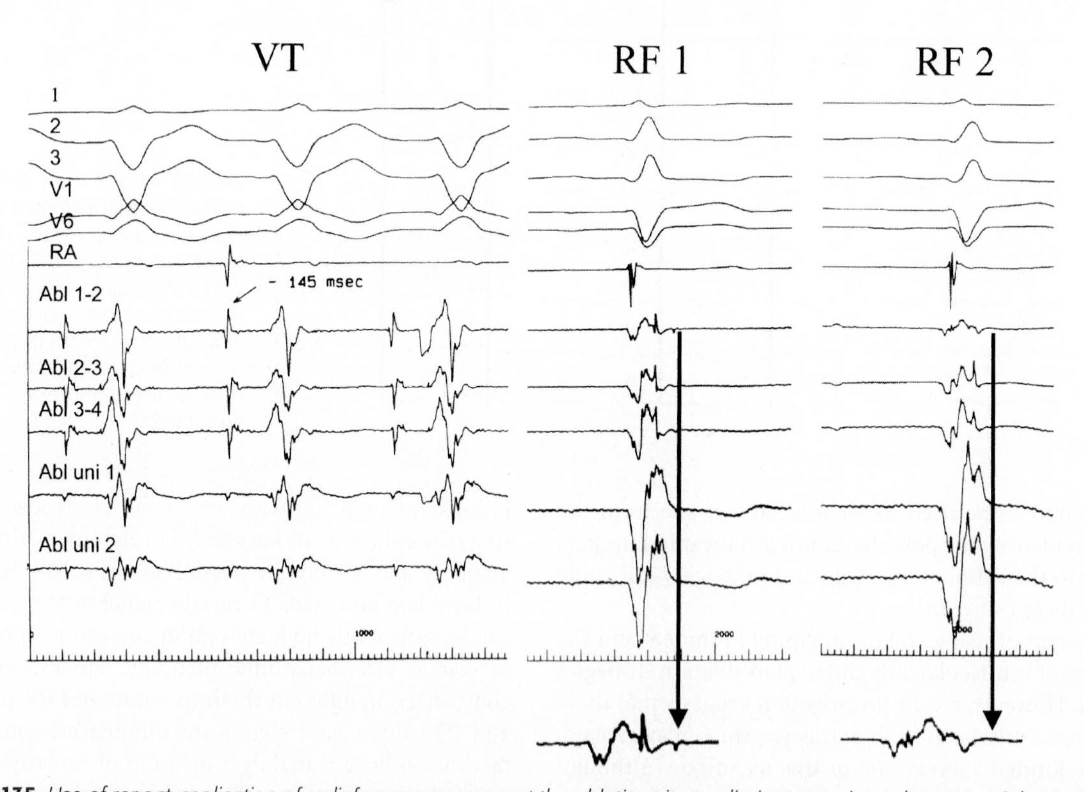


**FIGURE 13-135** *Use of repeat application of radiofrequency energy at the ablation site to eliminate persistent late potentials.* Ventricular tachycardia with a right bundle left superior axis is present. The site of earliest activation is shown in this panel. An isolated mid-diastolic electrogram was present 145 msec prior to the onset of the QRS and appeared in both the distal and second pole of the ablation catheter (**left panel**). Concealed entrainment criteria were met at this site. Delivery of RF energy at this site immediately terminated the tachycardia. After completion of 2 minutes of RF application, small late potentials were still observed in all bipolar recordings and in the distal unipolar recording (**middle panel**). An additional 1 minute of RF energy application was applied, which resulted in loss of the late potentials (**right panel**). No tachycardia was inducible at the end of the study. The patient has been free of recurrent VT in follow-up.

**TABLE 13-1 Methods of Substrate-Based Ablation for Ventricular Tachycardia**

- Define endocardial surface with detailed mapping and area of abnormal signals (>100 sites)
- Define areas with voltage ≥1.5 mV, <0.1 mV, and <0.5 mV, and all late potentials
- Induce VT
- If untolerated VT(s) induced, pace along 0.5–1.5 mV border to find site with best pace map and define area between that site and scar with similar pace maps and longer stimulus QRS
- Make linear lesion parallel to border to dense scar with or without a line perpendicular to the border into the dense scar
- Identify potential isthmuses by:
  - Changing voltage thresholds to 0.5–0.1 mV with 0.1 mV representing dense scar
  - Identifying sites of electrical inexcitability (i.e., no capture at 10 mA, 2 msec pulse width)
- Connect areas of dense scar or electrically inexcitable tissue with ablation line
- Eliminate all late potentials
- Encircle entire scar, if small

These initial strategies for substrate ablation were fairly successful, but limited in a way in their dependence on identification of specific morphologies of uniform VT. More often than not in the current era, patients with recurrent VT are treated with pre-existing ICDs, and the 12-lead ECG is unavailable. Programmed stimulation is used to reproduce VT morphologies to serve as the anchors for linear lesions. If a specific clinically relevant morphology is not inducible at

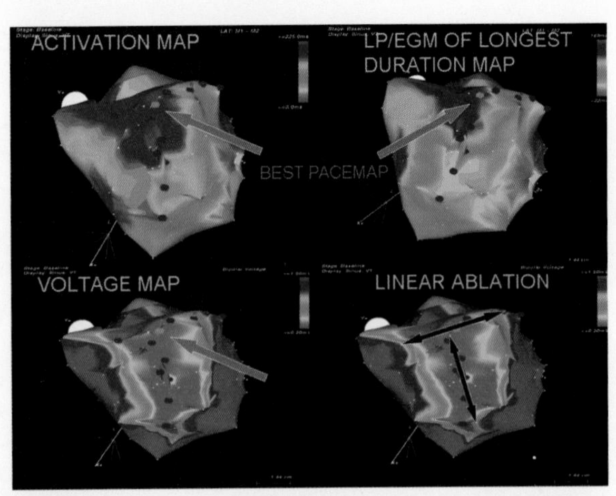


**FIGURE 13-137** *Use of activation map, late potential map and voltage map to guide linear ablations for untolerated ventricular tachycardia.* This patient had an inferoposterior infarction. All views are of the inferoposterior wall. On the top left is an activation map that showed latest activation in the midinferior wall. In the upper right is a late potential map in which the latest activation is also shown in *purple.* Again it coincides with the activation map. A voltage map was performed and shown in the lower left. *Red* indicates voltages less than 0.3 mV, the border zone is defined in *blue* between 1.25 and 1.5 mV, and normal tissue in *purple* exceeds 1.5 mV. Note that the whole inferior wall, which includes the late activation and late potential map site, is low voltage representing scar tissue. The *pink dot* represents the best pace map obtained in this patient. Note that it was between the border zone and the deepest part of the scar. A linear lesion was made from the border zone through the site of best pace map to the dense scar. A perpendicular lesion was also made through the dense scar. This patient has had no recurrent arrhythmias in follow-up.

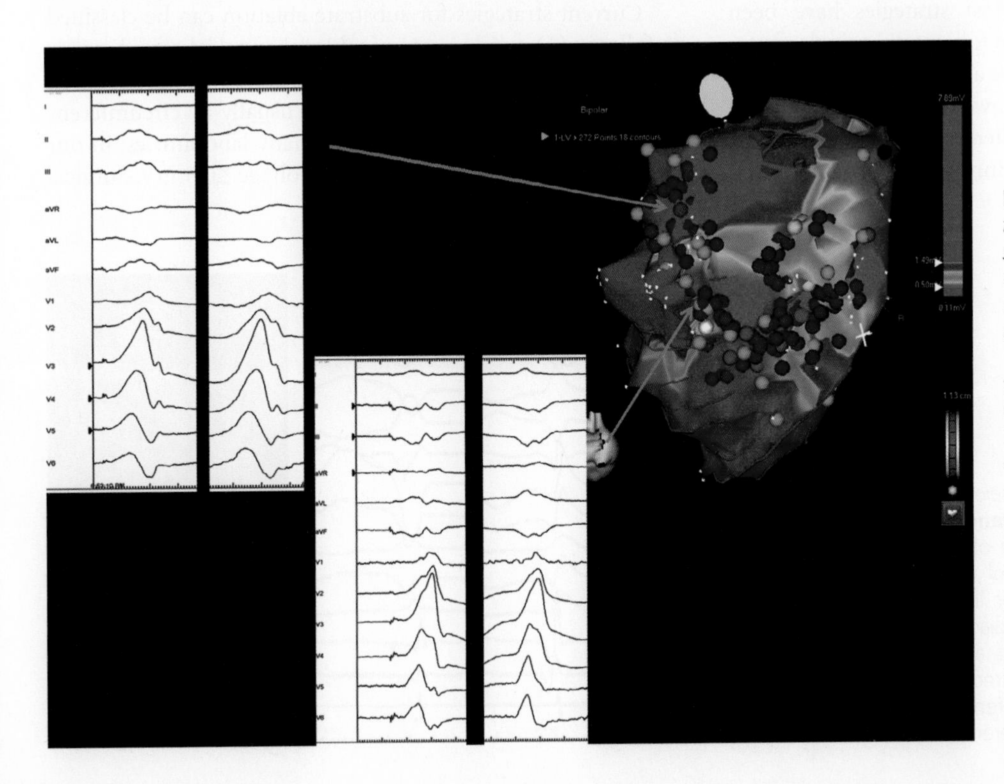

**FIGURE 13-136** *Substrate-based ablation with linear lesions positioned at presumed circuit exit sites.* Electroanatomic mapping is performed during sinus rhythm (near PA view), with bipolar voltage >1.5 mV denoted in *purple,* and < 0.5 mV in *red.* Two VT morphologies were induced in this patient with inferior infarction: VT1–RB iso I, cycle length 300 msec and VT2–RBLS, cycle length 440; neither were hemodynamically tolerated. Approximation of the circuit exit sites was performed with pace mapping at the edge of the voltage map abnormalities. Note that pace maps are not perfect matches, but approximate the VT QRS morphology. From that fulcrum point, linear lesions are constructed through the exit site to an anatomic barrier or the interior of the scar. See text for discussion.

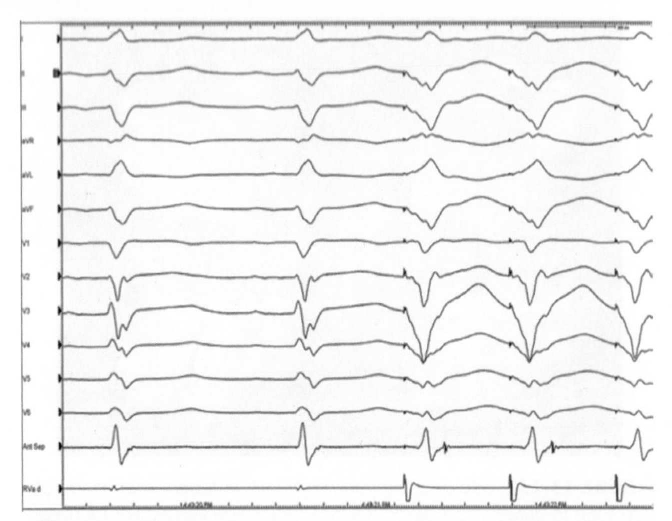

**FIGURE 13-138** *Alterations in bipolar electrogram with changes in rhythm.* Surface 12-lead ECG, and intracardiac recordings from a mapping catheter placed near and anterior septal infarct (Ant Sept) and RV apical catheter are shown. During sinus rhythm, the mapping catheter records a relatively high-voltage, bland electrogram. During RV pacing, a late potential is discovered.

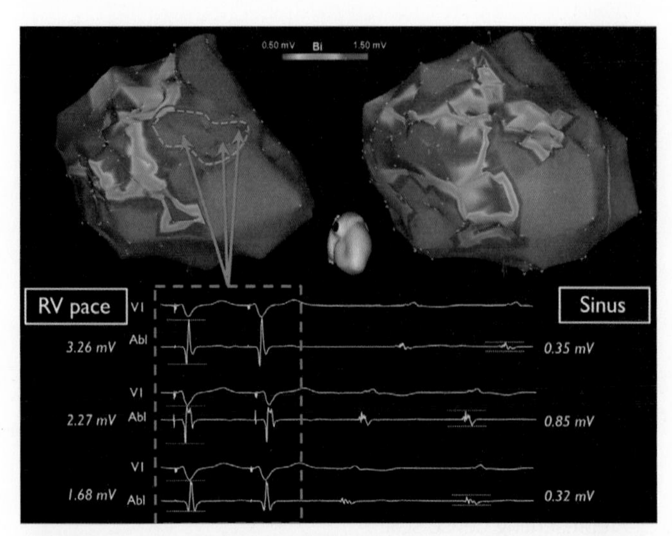


**FIGURE 13-140** *Alteration in voltage map with changes in rhythm.* Bipolar voltage mapping in a patient with anterior basal septal infarction during RV pacing (**right panel**) and sinus rhythm (**left panel**). Electroanatomical maps are shown at the top of each panel, and analog recordings from the mapping catheter at three septal sites at the bottom of each. Both the analog recordings and the voltage map are significantly different with the change in rhythm. (Courtesy of R. Tung, MD.)

that session, or, worse still, if no VT is inducible, these concepts cannot be successfully applied. In addition, although substrate ablation was based initially on surgery, the analogy fails; nonmapping-guided subendocardial resection (i.e., based on abnormal and fractionated EGMs and visible scar) theoretically removed all possible arrhythmia substrate, but was much less successful than surgery based on VT mapping. The concern about the limitations of programmed stimulation (both preablation in identifying all possible morphologies, as well as afterward for test of success) has led to more extensive, surrogate strategies. Most strategies have been evaluated with relatively short-term follow-up in single center observational studies. To date, there are no randomized comparisons of strategies. In general, however, the trend is toward more extensive ablation, albeit limited to the area of scar. This is certainly less elegant than entrainment mapping, and in a way the quantity of lesions is an expression of our frustration with localization techniques, the vagaries of permanent lesion formation in abnormal tissue and concerns about progression of the substrate with time. Although extensive ablation in truly densely scarred myocardium (i.e., >90% fibrosis) likely does not negatively affect function, when the extent of fibrosis is variable destruction of viable myocardium is possible. In addition each RF lesion does have a small but finite risk of thromboembolism.

Current strategies for substrate ablation can be classified as follows: (1) purely anatomic, (2) "channel" directed, or (3) late potential guided. The concept of purely anatomic ablation is typically viewed as scar exclusion, usually by circumferential ablation at the border zone in many laboratories; in our laboratory we isolate the area with voltage ≤0.5 mV. Surgical

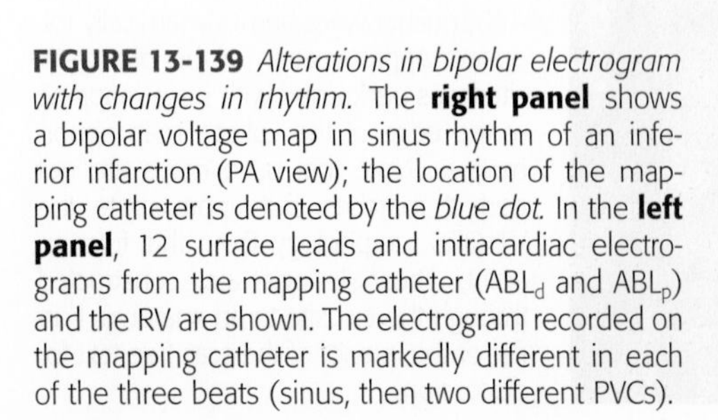

**FIGURE 13-139** *Alterations in bipolar electrogram with changes in rhythm.* The **right panel** shows a bipolar voltage map in sinus rhythm of an inferior infarction (PA view); the location of the mapping catheter is denoted by the *blue dot.* In the **left panel**, 12 surface leads and intracardiac electrograms from the mapping catheter ($ABL_d$ and $ABL_p$) and the RV are shown. The electrogram recorded on the mapping catheter is markedly different in each of the three beats (sinus, then two different PVCs).

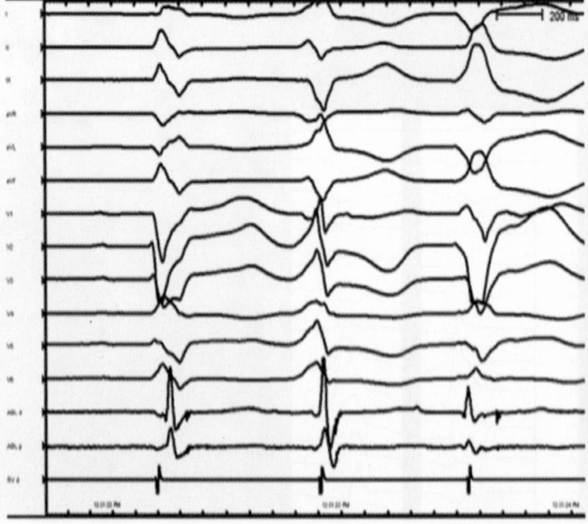

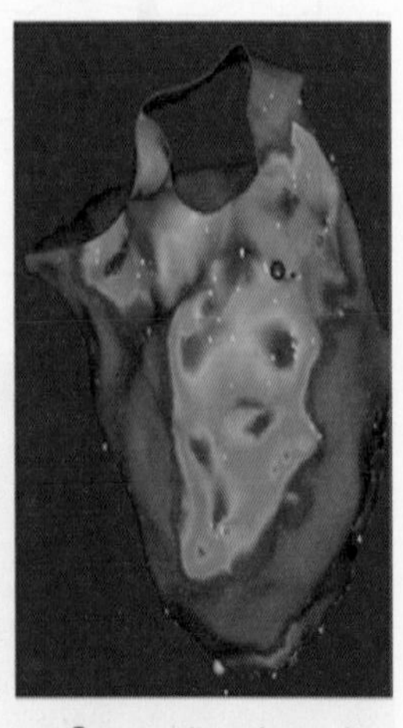

isolation in the border zones resulted in increased mortality because of necrosis of subjacent viable tissue. This would be exceptionally difficult (particularly given our documented trouble with durable ablation in the normal myocardium surrounding pulmonary veins!), and has not been subjected to even observational study. A conceptual variation of this idea is interrogating the "topography" of the scar using advanced imaging techniques, in an effort to determine areas that would be likely circuit sites.[319] An interesting extension of MR imaging merged with assumptions about fiber distribution and conduction velocity in normal and scarred myocardium is presently under investigation as a means to noninvasively localize presumptive VT circuits (Location of Ablation to Stop VT: A prospective study [LAST VT]).

Channel-based strategies conceptually interrogate the scar to find distinctive characteristics (voltage, conduction slowing) that may identify putative circuit locations. Two ideas from the Stevenson laboratory are examples of this general concept. The first described likely circuit locations between areas of inexcitable scar, extending the logical argument that this scar could not in itself support VT circuit conduction.[320] Another argued that areas within the scar that resulted in pace maps that approximated known VT morphologies, but with long stimulus to electrogram intervals were likely within VT circuits.[321] de Chillou and colleagues use "graded" pace mapping (using a matching algorithm) to identify the protected isthmus.[322] The best pace map match is at the exit, and the worst at the entrance to the isthmus (because of predominant antidromic capture). Another recent take on a similar idea focuses on pace map sites that produce more than a single morphology, supporting the idea that each exit morphology is from a distinct channel (Fig. 13-141).[323] Differential voltage mapping has been used to define areas within the scar with relatively preserved voltage, with the idea that these might serve as potential routes of preferential conduction as would be useful for VT circuits (Fig. 13-142).[311,324] A similar idea of preferential channels for conduction identified by isopotential mapping was demonstrated in a porcine model of infarction (Fig. 13-143).[325] A critique of channel identification was presented by Mountantonakis and coworkers, who found

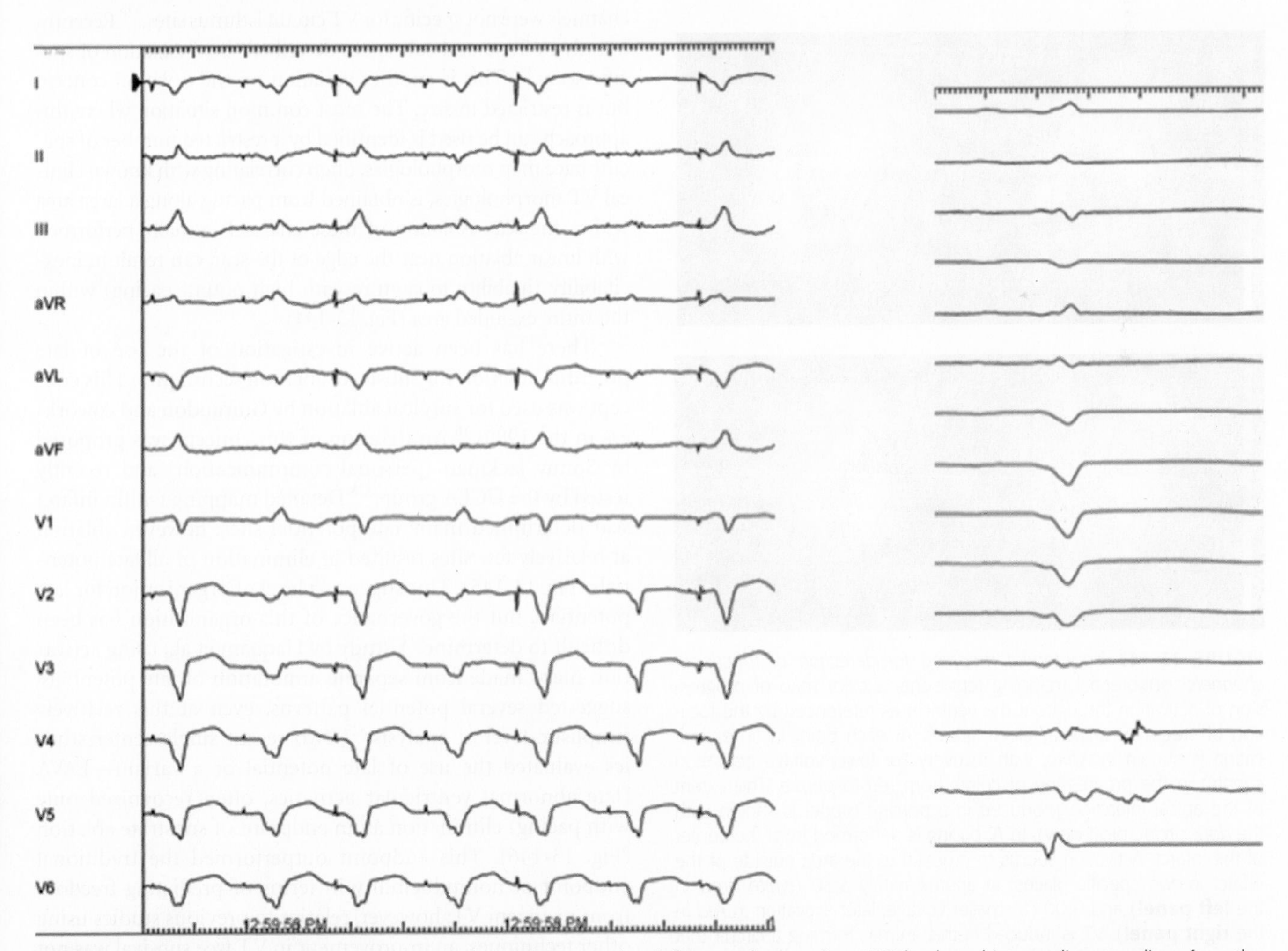


**FIGURE 13-141** *Multiple exit site morphologies during pacing.* In the **right panel**, 12 surface ECG leads and intracardiac recordings from the mapping/ablation RV catheters are shown. Note the dramatic isolated late potentials recorded on both bipoles of the ablation catheter. Pacing at this site (**left panel**) shows spontaneous variation between two different QRs morphologies, both of which matched inducible VTs. This suggests that this site is within a "crossroads" of two circuit channels. See text for discussion.

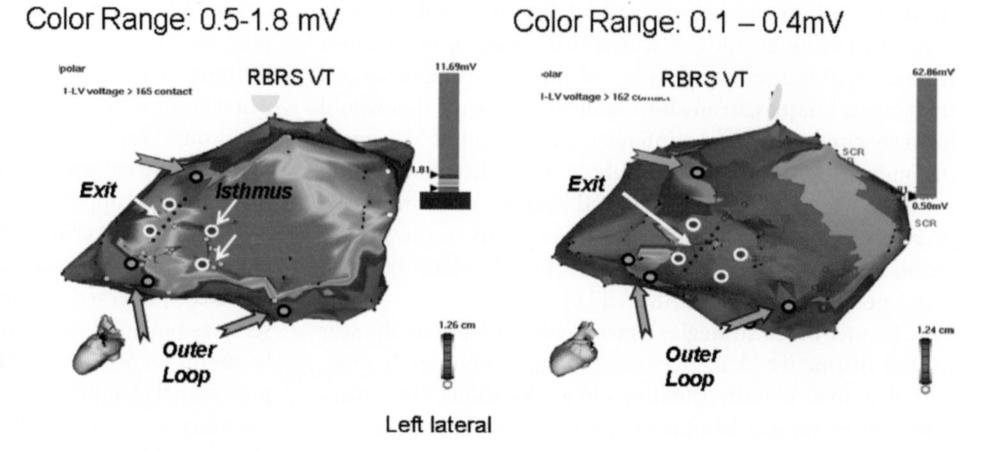


**FIGURE 13-142** *Identification of channels in scar by changing voltage scale.* The patient had VT from the posterolateral wall. A voltage map showed a large scar with voltage windows set at 0.5 to 1.8 mV. Entrainment suggested a viable isthmus within the assumed "dense" scar. Changing the voltage window to 0.1 to 0.4 mV identified relatively viable tissue bordered by true dense scar (*gray*). This correlated with the isthmus identified by entrainment. See text for discussion.

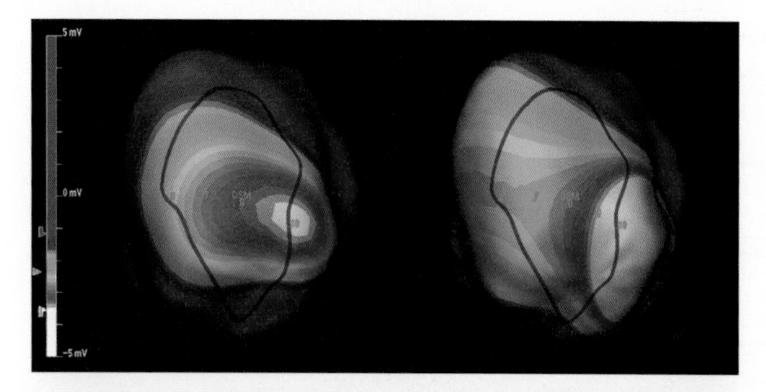

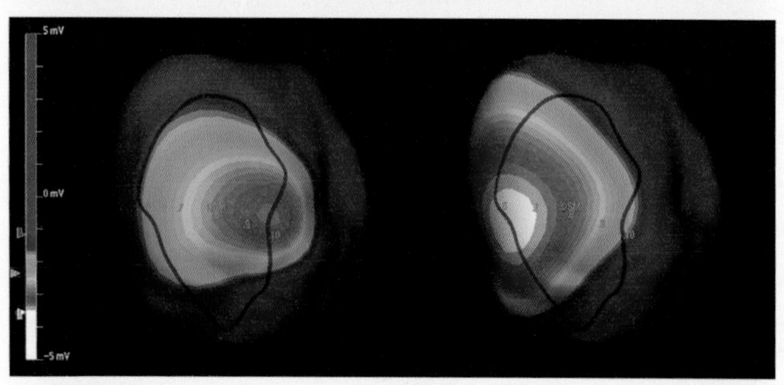

**FIGURE 13-143** *Isopotential mapping for detection of functional channels.* Isopotential mapping represents a color map of progression of activation throughout the ventricle as referenced by the location of steep qS unipolar electrograms. At each point in time, activation is shown in *white,* with recovery (or lower-voltage activation events) in the progression of colors from *red to purple.* The extent of the apical infarction produced in a porcine model is shown with the *dark circle* apical view). In **A**, pacing is performed from the center of the infarct. Activation seems to proceed to the area outside of the infarct in two specific places: at approximately 3:30 (*white area* in the **left panel**) and 9:00 (a smaller voltage, later activation in *red* in the **right panel**). VT is induced in this animal, forming a circuit that enters the scar at 3:30, and exits at 9:00. This suggests that functional channels, detected with pacing during sinus rhythm, may be important constructs for the VT circuit. (From Jacobson J. *Heart Rhythm* 2006;3:189–197, with permission).

channels were not specific for VT circuit isthmus sites.[326] Recently, a study by Tzou and colleagues described "box" isolation of specific scars.[327] This is another variation on the isolation concept but is restricted in size. The most common situation where this approach can be used is identified by a restricted number of specific pace map morphologies, often correlating with known clinical VT morphologies, is obtained from pacing along a large area within the scar. Ablation of these channels, usually performed with linear ablation near the edge of the scar, can result in inexcitability (inability to capture with high output pacing) within the entire excluded area (Fig. 13-144).

There has been active investigation of the use of late potential ablation for substrate ablation techniques. This concept was used for surgical ablation by Guiraudon and coworkers in the 1980s.[16] An iteration of this concept was proposed by Sonny Jackman (personal communication) and recently tested by the UCLA group.[328] Detailed mapping within infarct scar determined many late potential sites; however, ablation at relatively few sites resulted in elimination of all late potentials (Fig. 13-145). This suggests a level of organization for late potentials, but the governance of this organization has been difficult to determine. A study by Haqqani et al., using activation maps made from separate annotation of late potentials, suggested several potential patterns, even at this relatively simplistic level of analysis.[329] Two recent single center studies evaluated the use of late potential or a variant—LAVA (late abnormal ventricular activities, often recognized only with pacing) elimination as an endpoint of substrate ablation (Fig. 13-146). This endpoint outperformed the traditional endpoint of noninducibility in terms of predicting freedom from recurrent VT; however, relative to previous studies using other techniques, an improvement in VT free survival was not demonstrated using these endpoints.[330,331] Of great interest, the study by Jais and coworkers also established the possibility of endocardial ablation eliminating LAVA potentials on the

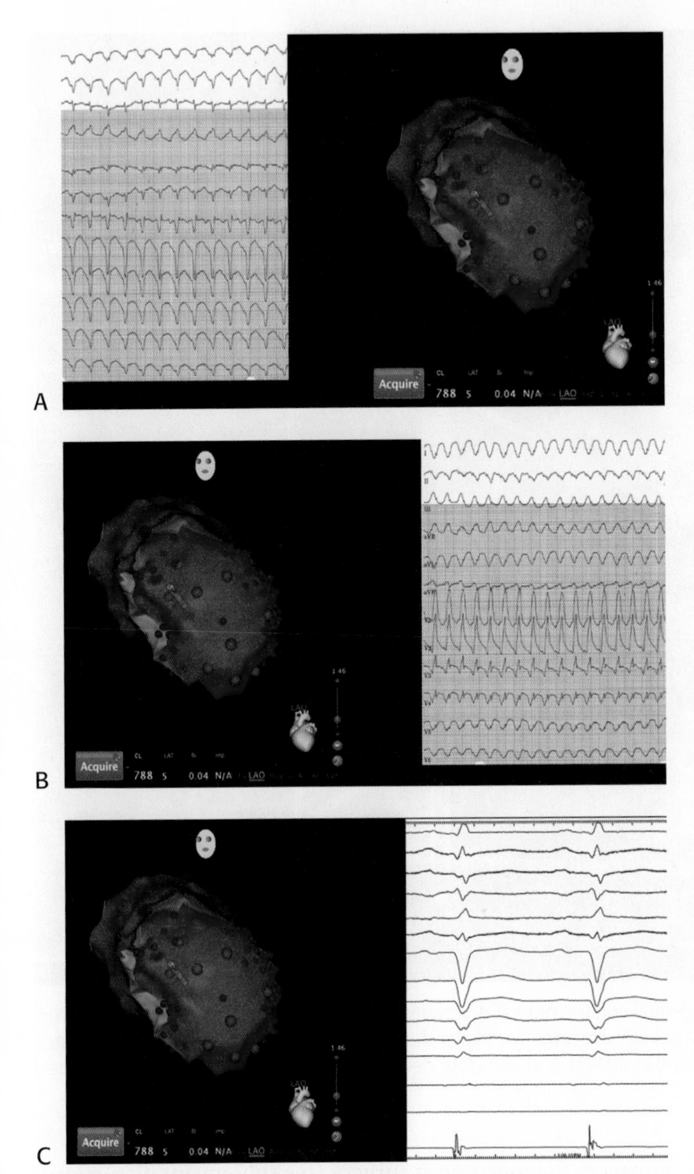


**FIGURE 13-144** *Box isolation.* In **A**, the **right panel** shows bipolar endocardial voltage mapping in a patient with extensive anterior infarction (RAO projection). Pacing from any site within the *yellow circle* (septal border of the infarct) produces an identical pace map (**left panel**) which matched the morphology of induced VT. **(B)** rotates the map to focus on the lateral infarct border, where pacing from sites within the *yellow circle* produced identical pace maps (**right panel**) for a different morphology of inducible VT. This suggests that the infarct is largely isolated from the healthy myocardium, except for specific channels that serve as exit sites during pacing within and during VT. Relatively limited ablation (**C**, *red dots*) resulted in inability to capture with high output pacing and inability to record electrograms within the infarct (**right panel**) as well as inability to reinduce either VT morphology.

epicardium. This suggests a transmural level of organization, at least in some patients. Finally, ablation of all late potential sites with individual ablation, often from both endocardial and epicardial surfaces, so-called scar homogenization, has been proposed.[332] Although in certain cases this requires delivery of a large number of ablation lesions, again the endpoint of late potential elimination is the guiding principle. The presence of late potentials is also affected be the wavefront of activation, which adds another limitation to this approach.

The presence of so many different strategies without any comparative data suggests we don't know how to identify the arrhythmogenic substrate. As such it makes recommendations about how to proceed quite difficult. When approaching substrate-based ablation, we often use a mixed approach, depending on the nature of the procedure. If a manageable number of VT morphologies are induced, morphology-specific ablation (anchored by identification of the exit site with pace mapping) is at least part of the procedure. If late potentials are plentiful, usually these would be attacked. If pacing within the scar from multiple sites suggests limited avenues of egress from the scar, limited isolation ("box isolation") ablation is a viable option.

Theoretically, noncontact mapping or large basket catheters would be expected to be effective in identification of target sites for ablation in poorly tolerated arrhythmias. This hypothesis has proven difficult to test even in observational studies. One limitation is the lack of associated software to accurately locate the scar tissue (voltage) or sites of late activation. Moreover, an additional catheter is needed to ablate through or around the scar tissue that is identified by these techniques. Animal studies have demonstrated a lack of correlation between substrate detected with noncontact mapping using the Ensite system and MRI. In a study of a porcine model of infarction with inducible untolerated ventricular tachycardia, the Carto electroanatomic map provides the most accurate correlation with the anatomic scar when compared to these other technologies.[333] Recent data from Anter et al. in our laboratory suggest an even tighter correlation using the Rhythmia mapping system.

Some groups have advocated the use of percutaneous hemodynamic support (Impella, Abiomed) to allow more detailed mapping during what would otherwise be poorly tolerated VT to allow precision ablation of the critical isthmus.[334–336] In general, series in which hemodynamic support is used have not conclusively demonstrated improved freedom from recurrent VT; however, there are clear cases that have been "rescued" by this technique after failed substrate ablation. It is also possible that hemodynamic support would VT ablation procedures safer, but this hypothesis has not been tested as yet in prospective studies.

## Additional Procedures after Failed Catheter Ablation

An important minority of patients continue to have clinically important recurrent ventricular tachycardia despite attempts at ablation. There has been a great deal of recent interest into various procedures that can serve to rescue these situations. Arrhythmia surgery (described in detail below) is one of these options. Anter and colleagues described a cohort of eight patients with nonischemic cardiomyopathy who had surgical cryoablation performed following unsuccessful catheter ablation.[337] The surgical ablation was not guided by mapping, except in the sense that energy was applied to sites of previous

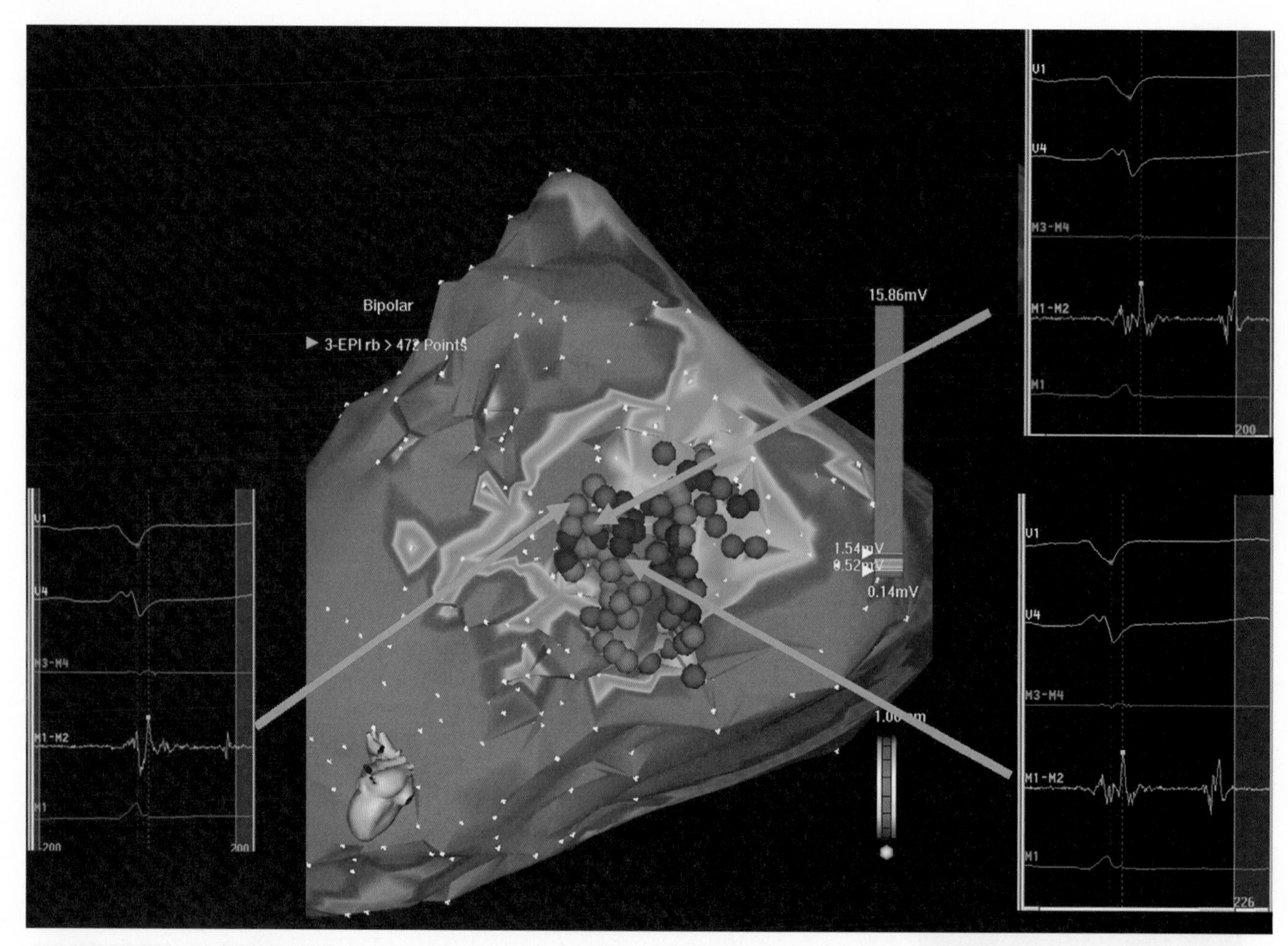


**FIGURE 13-145** *Late potential ablation.* An electroanatomic bipolar epicardial voltage map (PA view) is shown from a patient with nonischemic cardiomyopathy and recurrent VT. *Green icons* denote sites with fractionated electrograms (not late) during sinus rhythm; gray icons denote sites with isolated late potentials (electrograms from three such sites shown in the insets) and *red dots* denote ablation sites. After relatively limited ablation, all of the late and fractionated electrograms were eliminated.

catheter ablation lesions. The burden of VT as measured by appropriate ICD shocks was reduced from 6.6 in the preceding 3 months to 0.6 during the first 3 months following surgery. We have performed hybrid surgical and cryoablation in four nonischemic VT patients based on mapping and have been successful in all with a 3- to 5-year follow-up. Thus, mapping enhances the outcome at surgery (see subsequent discussion). There has been a resurgence in interest for transcoronary ethanol ablation (TCEA) for the treatment of refractory VT. Tokuda and coworkers presented results of this technique in 27 patients. Five patients had unsuitable coronary anatomy, and TCEA was not performed. Of the 22 patients that received

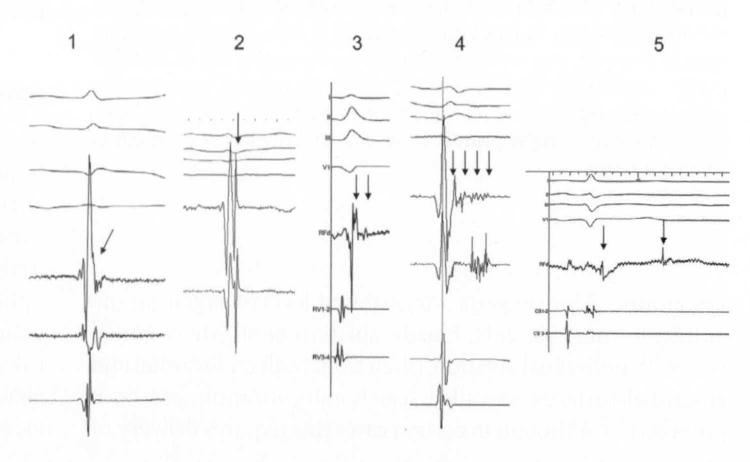


**FIGURE 13-146** *Characteristics of LAVA electrograms (arrows).* 1. The LAVA potential is fused with the terminal portion of the far-field ventricular signal. 2. The LAVA potential, a high-frequency, high-voltage component, occurs just after the far-field ventricular potential. 3. Two LAVAs occur in this electrogram, one within the QRS and one isolated, following the QRS. 4. Multiple LAVAs without isoelectric intervals. 5. Double-component LAVA signal, both following the QRS and one recorded very late after QRS offset. (From Jais P, Maury P, Khairy P, et al. Elimination of local abnormal ventricular activities: a new end point for substrate modification in patients with scar-related ventricular tachycardia. *Circulation* 2012;125:2184–2196, with permission).

TCEA, the targeted VT was no longer inducible in 18; however, freedom from VT was observed in only 36%, although an additional 27% had a reduction in arrhythmia burden.[338]

There is also considerable interest in the potential for neuraxial ablation for the treatment of refractory VT. Bourke and colleagues reported promising initial results in a critically ill population of 14 patients with refractory VT, often in the setting of VT storm, who were treated with thoracic epidural anesthesia and/or left stellate ganglionectomy.[339] These procedures resulted in a significant reduction in arrhythmia episodes in the majority of patients. Several small case studies of renal artery denervation have suggested a potential for benefit but there are no controlled trials to support this effort.

## Catheter Ablation of Ventricular Tachycardia Associated with Coronary Artery Disease

Coronary artery disease with prior myocardial infarction is the most common underlying substrate of sustained VT for which ablation is performed. These macroreentrant circuits involve both scar tissue and functional barriers through which the impulse circulates. In fact it is scar tissue separating viable myocytes that forms many of the circuitous and critical pathways in the reentrant circuits of such VTs. Different strategies of ablation should be employed for tolerated monomorphic VTs than for untolerated VTs. Although the relative incidence of tolerated versus untolerated VTs has been decreasing over the last decade due to early revascularization, if present, tolerated VTs should be ablated using an entrainment mapping strategy. If VT is hemodynamically stable, it allows for precise determination of critical sites for ablation. Since most patients with stable VT have significant myocardial dysfunction, limiting ablations to a small site by the mapping techniques described below, is safer for the patient, and, in my opinion, does not sacrifice survival benefit.

Which tachycardias require ablation is a matter of opinion. I prefer to target the spontaneous tachycardia or tachycardias originating in the same area at similar cycle lengths. I do not try to map and ablate all tachycardias that are induced. This is particularly true in patients who only present with stable tachycardias. These patients may have multiple, stable tachycardias, which may, depending on the investigator, be targets for ablation. However, the rapid untolerated tachycardias that may be induced in nearly 50% of such patients are not targeted for ablation in our laboratory. We have not found that such arrhythmias predict recurrences and sudden death due to these rapid arrhythmias.

We use the scheme as shown in Figure 13-147 as a basis for regionalizing the ventricular tachycardias associated with coronary artery disease, which by and large arise (or at least critical components of which arise) in the left ventricular endocardium. A small percentage of ventricular tachycardias associated with prior infarction with an LBBB QRS morphology may have the central common pathway identified on the right side of the septum. We have seen four such cases in which successful ablation was carried out from a site on

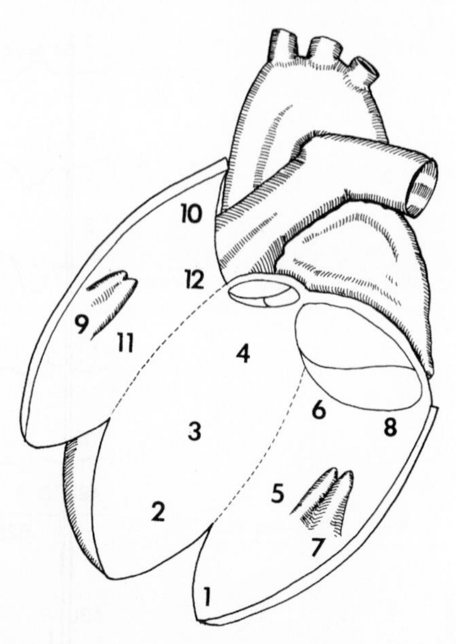


**FIGURE 13-147** Sites of endocardial catheter mapping in the left ventricle.

the right ventricular septum that demonstrated concealed entrainment. An example is shown in Figure 13-148 in a patient with an old inferior infarction. The patient had incessant VT and was in cardiogenic shock on a balloon pump. He had already had an ICD placed for prior cardiac arrest. No left ventricular site could be found that produced a paced QRS during entrainment that was identical to the VT QRS. Pacing on the right side of the septum produced a QRS identical to that of the tachycardia (panel A). The return cycle was slightly longer than the tachycardia cycle length (20 msec) because pacing was carried out at too rapid a rate (70 msec less that the VT cycle length). Nevertheless, the stimulus to QRS was equal to the electrogram to QRS suggesting that the delay was occurring at the entrance to the central common pathway due to antidromic penetration of the paced impulse. Not only did the stimulus to QRS equal the electrogram to QRS, but also the morphology of the stimulated electrogram was identical to the native electrogram. In addition, the right ventricular reference electrogram had both the same relationship to the stimulus as it did to the onset of the native electrogram. Because of these findings, RF energy was applied. At 1.8 seconds after the onset of delivery of RF energy the VT terminated and the patient's ICD pacing therapy took over control of the cardiac rhythm (panel B).

Occasionally, a macroreentrant circuit can be demonstrated with an impulse circulating around the edge of an aneurysm. This most often happens with inferior infarction in which the isthmus between the infarct and the annulus serves as the protected central common pathway of tachycardias that can go clockwise or counterclockwise. An example of a large inferoseptal aneurysm associated with ventricular tachycardia in which the earliest LV electrogram was recorded as an isolated diastolic potential just superior to the upper border of the aneurysm on the septum, 2 cm below the aortic valve

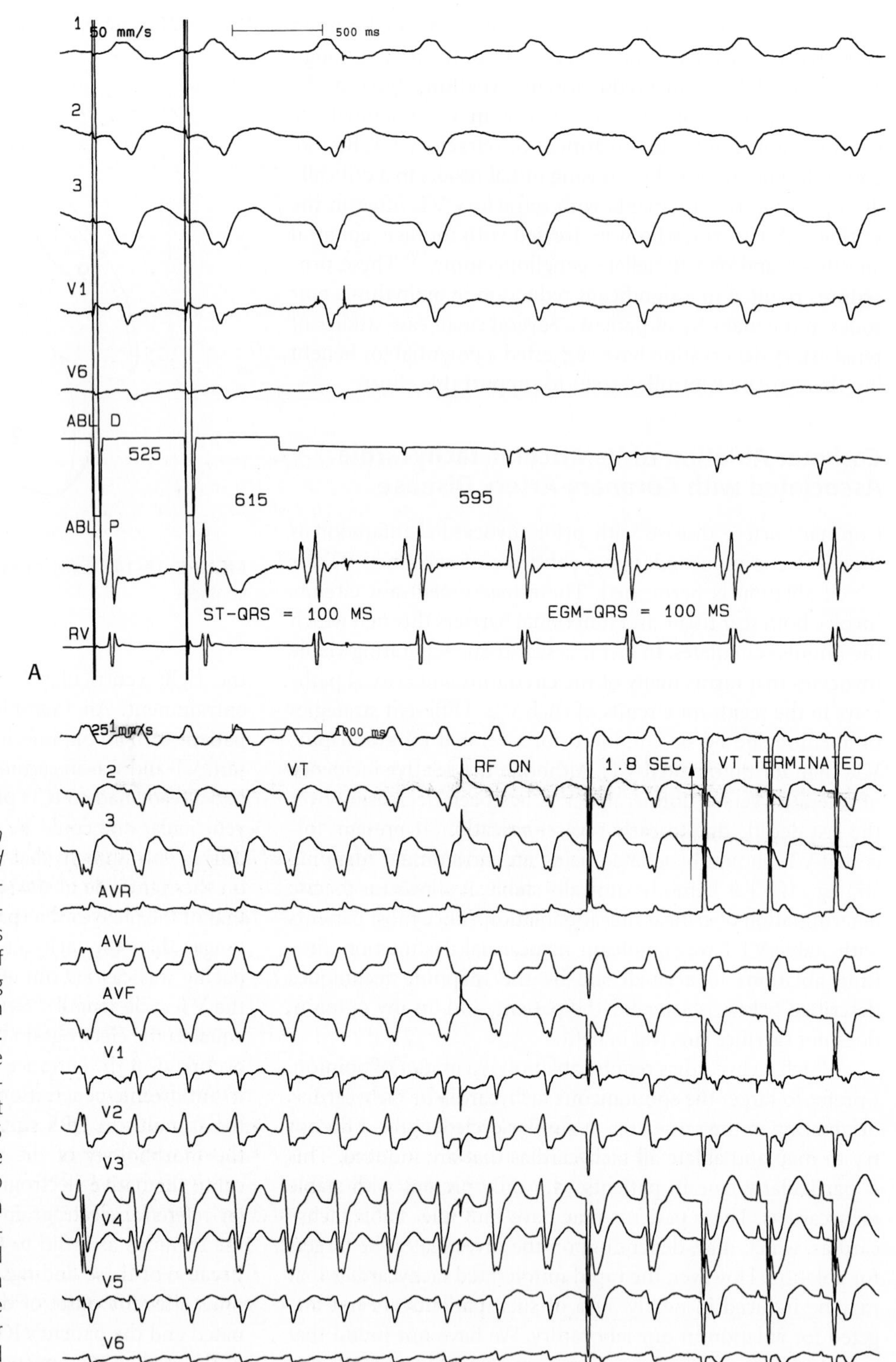


**FIGURE 13-148** *Role of entrainment in determining the need for a right-sided ablation in a patient with ventricular tachycardia associated with coronary artery disease.* **Panel A:** Ventricular tachycardia is present on the right at a cycle length of 595 msec with the earliest activation being recorded from the right ventricular septum 100 msec prior to the onset of the QRS. Pacing at this site at a rapid rate (cycle length 525 msec) does not alter the electrogram morphology, stimulus to QRS, but the return cycle is slightly prolonged to 615 msec as a result of the short-paced cycle length. The entrained QRS is identical to the tachycardia QRS. **Panel B:** Based on the excellent results of entrainment meeting all three criteria, RF energy was applied to this right ventricular septal site and in 1.8 seconds, VT was terminated. The patient's own ICD immediately took over ventricular pacing. The patient has not had recurrent VT in follow-up.

(Fig. 13-149). In addition, an equally early site was observed at the His bundle recording site. Entrainment mapping from the His bundle recording site produced a perfect entrainment map with the return cycle equal to the tachycardia cycle and a stimulus to QRS equal to the electrogram to QRS. Pacing from the earliest left ventricular site also produced a QRS identical to the VT QRS, with an identical return cycle to the tachycardia cycle length and an identical stimulus to QRS as the electrogram to QRS. Electroanatomic mapping delineated the large inferoseptal aneurysm and demonstrated a macroreentrant circuit around this giant aneurysm. A single lesion delivered just at the superior edge of the septal border of the aneurysm terminated the tachycardia and left A-V conduction intact. While reentrant excitation can occasionally be demonstrated using Carto, as stated above, stimulation as described above and in Chapter 11, is required to accurately define the

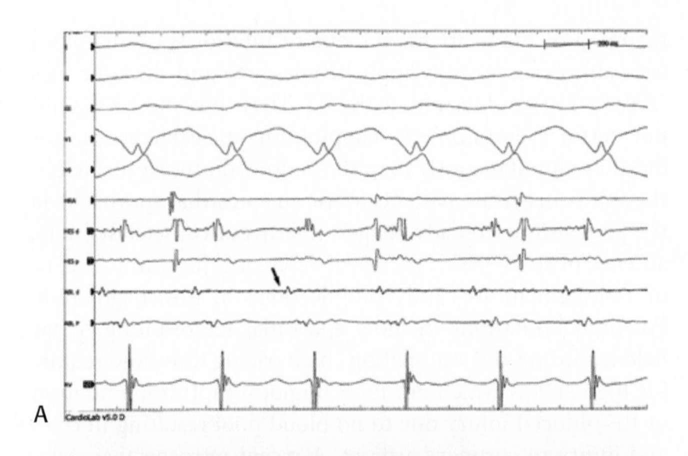


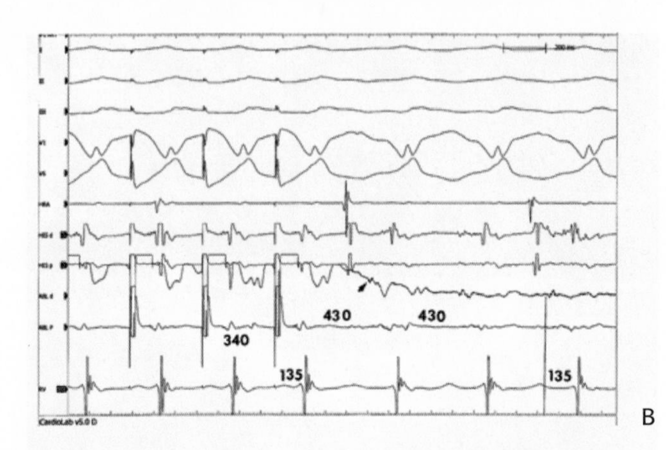


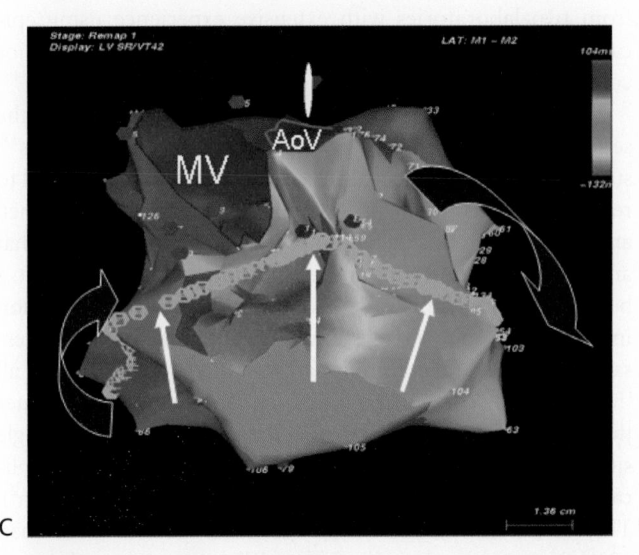


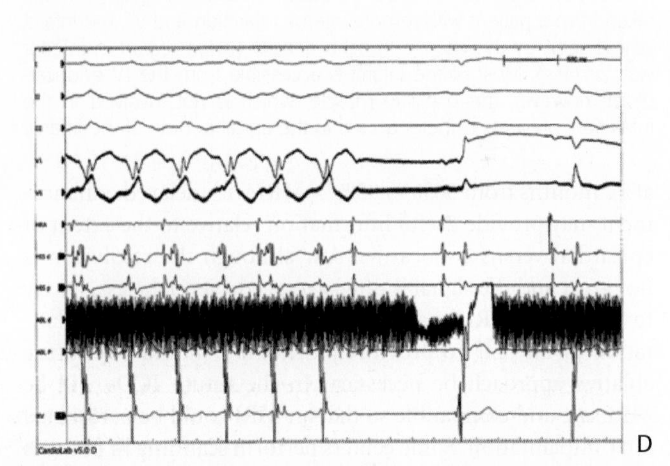


**FIGURE 13-149** *Macroreentrant ventricular tachycardia around the ventricular aneurysm.* **A:** A patient with a large ventricular aneurysm secondary to an old inferior infarction presented with incessant ventricular tachycardia. Mapping of the left ventricle showed the earliest site of activation to be a mid-diastolic potential 135 msec prior to the QRS located approximately 2 cm below the aortic valve and 1 cm medial to the mitral valve. Of note is that the ventricular electrogram in the His bundle recording site demonstrated equally early activity. The His bundle electrogram was recorded less than 4 mm away from the left ventricular diastolic potential. **B:** Entrainment mapping from the left ventricular site (as well as the His bundle site) produced an exact entrainment map. The paced QRS was identical to the VT QRS and the return cycle was identical to the tachycardia cycle. The stimulus to QRS was also identical to the electrogram at the onset of the QRS during the tachycardia. **C:** Electroanatomical mapping defined the borders of an aneurysm (*tan circles*) and demonstrated reentrant excitation around this aneurysm. **D:** Because all three criteria were met in the left ventricle as well as at the His bundle recording site, it was elected to ablate at the left ventricular site to prevent the possibility of heart block. RF energy delivered at this single site terminated tachycardia and made it noninducible. The patient has been free of arrhythmias off antiarrhythmic medications.

isthmus. The demonstration of an "early meets late" pattern does not necessarily define the critical isthmus for ablation. It may not be near the isthmus if an RV electrogram is used as the fiducial reference during mapping.

Recently there has been an increasing interest in the use of epicardial mapping. This has resulted from the observation at surgery that a subgroup of patients with blotchy infarctions and no aneurysms, usually on the inferior wall, have early activity noted on the epicardium.[307,340,341] Locations are suggested by a wide QRS, slurred initial forces of the QRS, QS complexes in leads directly overlying the area, inability to find a site earlier than 50 msec presystolic on the endocardium, failure to demonstrate concealed entrainment from the endocardium or requirement of very high stimulus strengths to achieve concealed entrainment. In some patients with inferior infarction, elements of the infarct scar are "protected" by the overlying posteromedial papillary muscle (Fig. 13-150). In such cases entrainment and ablation from the epicardium is possible (Fig. 13-151). This probably represents, at most, 5% to 10% of stable monomorphic VTs related to myocardial infarction. Several recent studies have addressed this issue. A retrospective analysis of a 444 patients with infarct-related VT demonstrated the use of epicardial approach was 6%; however, the authors pointed out that this might be an underestimate, as the enthusiasm for this technique was not high at the beginning of this series.[342] Tung and coworkers reported in a retrospective observational study that selective use of an epicardial approach improved the freedom from recurrent VT

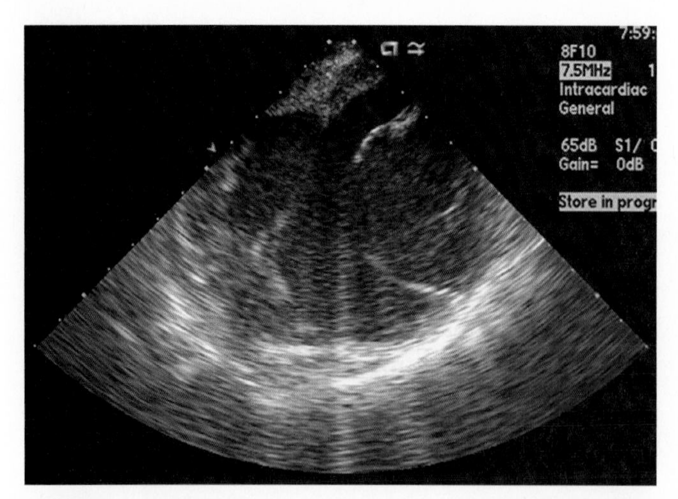


**FIGURE 13-150** *Relationship of inferior infarction and the posterior medial papillary muscle.* In this intracardiac echocardiographic image taken from a patient with remote inferior infarction and VT, the infarct scar is seen by the change in echo density (*white region* in inferior wall, *arrows*). Most of the infarct is accessible from the LV endocardium; however, the papillary muscle, which is not involved in the infarction, prevents catheter access to the apical portion of the infarct.

at 12 months from 56% to 85%[343] MRI with delayed enhancement may provide useful information relative to the extent of epicardial versus endocardial scar although the resolution is not great and the signal is often averaged. Nevertheless, we try to obtain an MRI in all patients before ablation or implantation of an ICD to provide information should any future ablative approach be necessary. In the future ICDs will be MRI safe and compatible so that an MRI could be performed after implantation. Some centers perform scanning in patients with ICDs; image degradation from the generator and leads can limit this approach. Improved filtering protocols are being developed to provide better imaging in this situation (Fig. 13-152).[344] Sosa et al.[345] were the first to use intrapericardial mapping of the heart for VT due to inferior wall infarction were able to successfully apply RF energy to mid-diastolic sites (Fig. 13-153) and terminate the VT. These investigators could not perform entrainment mapping for unclear reasons, nor did they simultaneously map the endocardium. Nevertheless, the ability in certain patients to use an epicardial approach via the pericardium has advantages in terms of catheter-stability, absence of stroke risk, absence of vascular injury, and absence of requirement for and complications of anticoagulation. Potential limitations include: epicardial fat resulting in far field recording and stimulation (high pacing threshold requiring high energy which produces nonlocal capture), limitation of RF-induced injury due to no blood pool resulting in char, and injury to coronary arteries. A recent retrospective series from two laboratories with extensive experience using epicardial access showed that these procedures had a 7% major complication rate related to epicardial access and ablation.[346]

The success rate of catheter ablation varies depending on the series and the endpoint.[306,347–358] Although some investigators[359] suggest that the postpacing interval is not important, they fail to recognize the requirement for multiple parameters to be met, and not just the postpacing interval. Others[353,360] suggest that any site with a long stimulus to QRS time is a useful target. I believe these individuals are also in error since any stimulation in a scar will lead to a long stimulus to QRS time but not necessarily in the central common pathway. In our experience, if all the criteria for concealed entrainment are met, there is greater than a 90% chance of terminating the tachycardia with a single site ablation.[354] This may mean using 2 to 4 minutes of RF applications at the same site, but it is at a single site (1 to 2 $cm^2$). The reinducibility rate of the targeted arrhythmia is less than 10%. Repeated local application of RF to cover the isthmus is performed to assure noninducibility. Failure is typically due to a deep intramural or epicardial location. At this point we would now try an epicardial approach for such patients. Moreover,

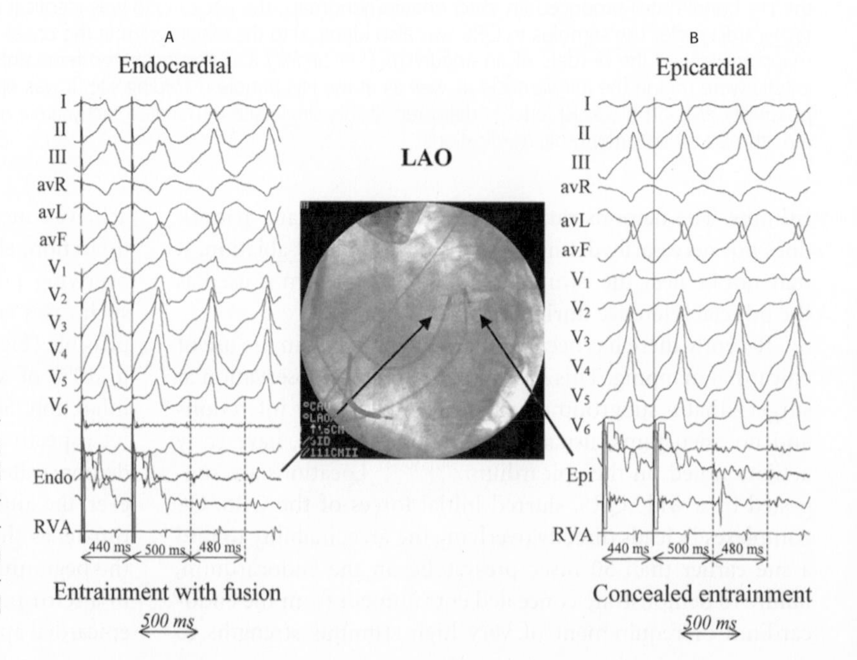


**FIGURE 13-151** *Endocardial and epicardial entrainment during an epicardial VT.* VT is present with an RBBB, right inferior axis. The earliest endocardial signal was 50 msec prior to the QRS. Pacing at this site produced a QRS slightly different than VT, with a reasonable return cycle, suggesting an outer loop. Pacing from the adjacent epicardium produced a perfect entrainment map. Ablation at this epicardial site terminated the VT. (Courtesy of Dr. Frank Marchlinski.)

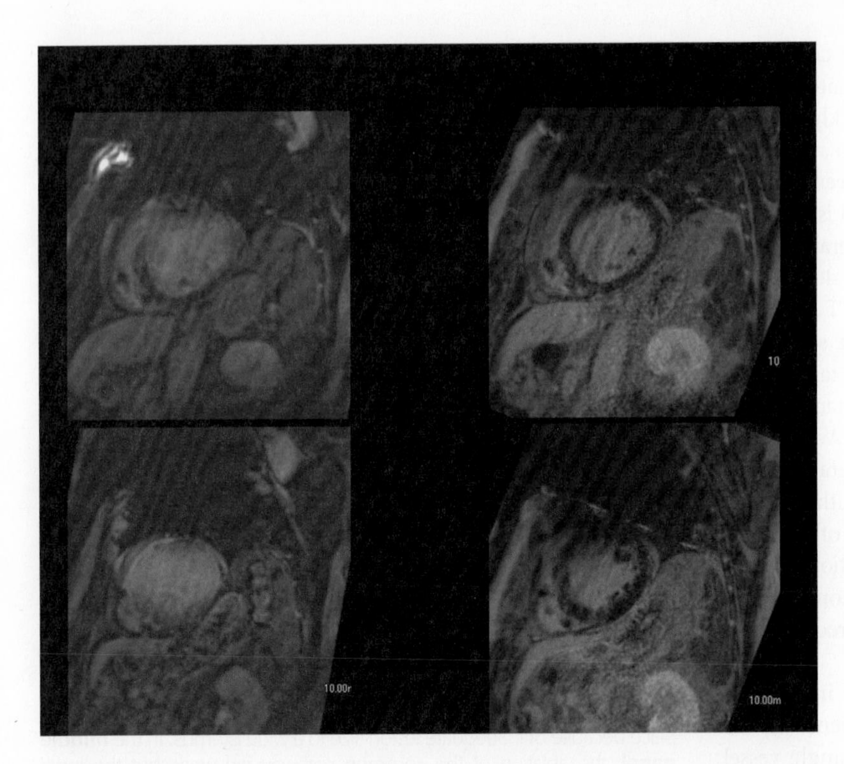

**FIGURE 13-152** *Improved filtering of ICD artifact during MR imaging.* Selected sections of cardiac MR late gadolinium enhancement images are shown in a patient with an implanted defibrillator, using traditional filtering (**left**) and improved filtering (**right**) protocols. The images on the right are much clearer than those on the left, although some image distortion related to the presence of the ICD can and the lead are still evident.

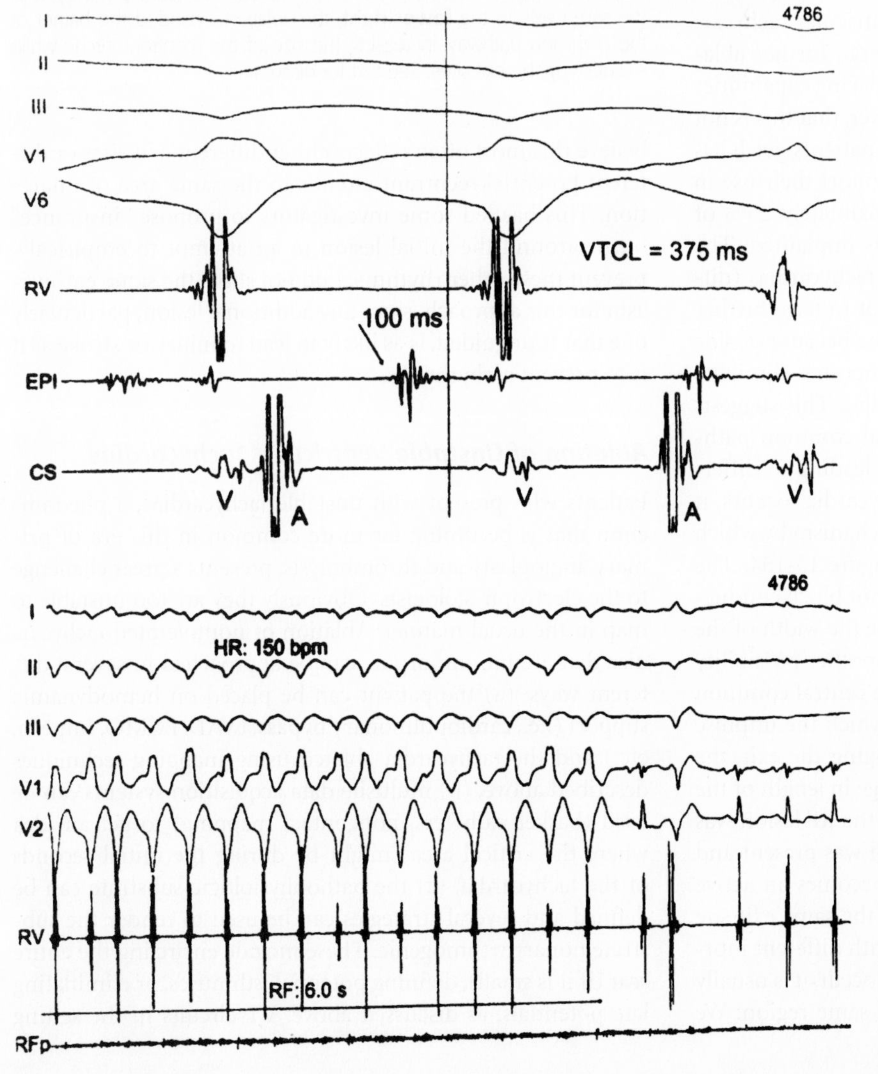


**FIGURE 13-153** *Use of intrapericardial mapping to locate an epicardial source of an arrhythmia.* Intrapericardial introduction of ablation catheter in a patient with ventricular tachycardia due to an old inferior infarction is shown. The epicardial flow detects a mid-diastolic potential 100 msec prior to the QRS. Application of radiofrequency energy at this site terminates the ventricular tachycardia in 6 seconds. See text for discussion. (From Sosa E, Scanavacco M, d'Avila A, et al. Nonsurgical transthoracic epicardial catheter ablation to treat recurrent ventricular tachycardia occurring late after myocardial infarction. *J Am Coll Cardiol* 2000;35(6):1442–1449.)

in analyzing the results of ablation when all three criteria are present, nearly 80% of the tachycardias are terminated within 10 seconds. The fact that termination occurs so quickly not only attests to the accuracy of those techniques, but also supports a subendocardial location for the critical sites in the reentrant circuit since the depths of penetration of an RF lesion is probably less than 2 mm at that short period of time. In general, the success rate appears to be 70% to 75% with a 25% to 40% recurrence rate.[306,345,347–358] Our recurrence rate of any VT is 25% in 2 years and 7% for the ablated VT. While there are some who suggest that all tachycardia morphologies should be targeted for ablation, I think it is reasonable to target tolerated tachycardias arising from a similar area as a clinical tachycardia. We have not found induced, rapid tachycardias that are untolerated to be clinically meaningful in patients who present only with tolerated tachycardias. If the patient is on drugs at the time of the ablation, one must maintain the drugs because the ablation actually should be considered a form of hybrid therapy in combination with the drug. In such cases stopping the drug will frequently be associated with recurrence.

Since the incidence of sudden death is so low in patients with tolerated tachycardias (see Chapter 11), I generally do not implant ICDs (particularly in patients with single vessel coronary disease without indications for primary prevention ICD therapy) unless there are recurrent ventricular tachycardias and the patient does not want to undergo further ablations and wishes to use the antitachycardia pacing capabilities to treat his arrhythmias. I would state; however, that this is not standard practice. The vast majority of the patients get ICDs despite the fact that there are *no* data to support their use in improving survival in such patients. Approximately 25% of our patients with stable VT have had ICDs implanted. The primary reason for these ICDs is recurrent tachycardias (different than the ablated VT) and the wish not to have further ablations or the necessity to stop amiodarone because of side effects. It is of interest that single lesions sometimes eliminate multiple morphologically distinct tachycardias. This suggests that several tachycardias can share a central common pathway with different exits from that pathway leading to different QRS morphologies. If the "clinical tachycardia" occurs, it is invariably at a longer cycle length. The mechanism by which this can occur is schematically shown in Figure 13-154. The RF lesion may in fact slow conduction and not block conduction in the central common pathway because the width of the pathway exceeds the size of the RF lesion. Another possibility is that the lesion increased the length of the central common pathway by increasing the barrier around which the impulse was circulated. If this occurs without changing the exit, the cycle length increase would be due to a change in length of the pathway. A third explanation would be that the RF lesion was actually successful, but an inner loop, which was present and not part of the primary reentrant circuit, becomes an active participant in a new longer circuit that has the same exit site as the original tachycardia. If tachycardias with different morphologies than the spontaneous tachycardia occur, it is usually one of the inducible tachycardias from the same region. We believe this most often reflects either different exit sites or different potential reentrant circuits in the same area of infarction. This has led some investigators to propose "insurance" burns around the initial lesion in an attempt to empirically prevent these other rhythms. I do not share the same enthusiasm for this approach, since any additional lesion, particularly one that is unguided, is as likely to lead to injury or stroke as it is to prevent arrhythmias.

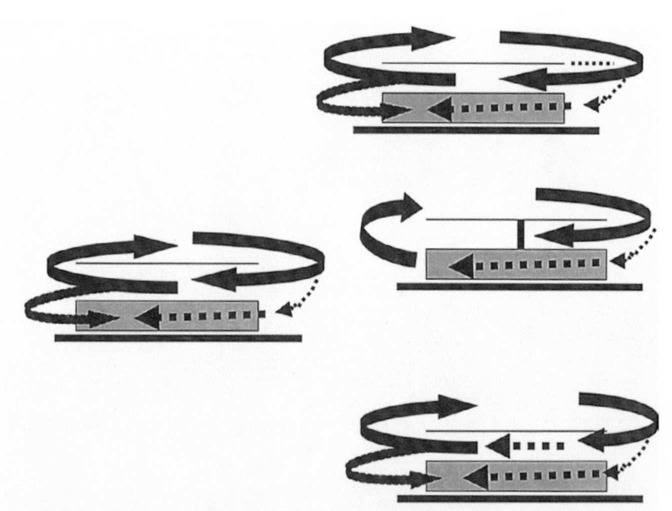

**FIGURE 13-154** *Potential mechanisms of recurrent ventricular tachycardia post-RF ablation with the same morphology as preablation.* On **top** is a proposed reentrant circuit with the main reentrant loop going through the right channel. An inner loop is shown on the left of the common pathway, shown in a stippled color. In the **lower panels** are three distinct mechanisms for the phenomenon of recurrence with the same morphology. In the lower left, failure to ablate the arrhythmia has taken place because of inadequate lesion size to a wide isthmus. In the **middle panel**, the ablation of the common pathway did work, but the inner loop now became active, producing a second reentrant pathway with the same exit. In the **lower right**, the ablation extended the barrier of the common pathway, increasing the size of the reentrant circuit while maintaining the exit sites. See text for discussion.

## Ablation of Unstable Ventricular Tachycardias

Patients who present with unstable tachycardias, a phenomenon that is becoming far more common in this era of primary angioplasty and thrombolysis, presents a great challenge to the electrophysiologists. Obviously they are too unstable to map in the usual manner. Ablation of nontolerated tachycardias that are monomorphic can be approached in several different ways: (a) the patient can be placed on hemodynamic support (i.e., cardiopulmonary bypass, LVAD, ECMO, Impella, etc.) and the tachycardia ablated using mapping techniques described above; (b) multisite data acquisition systems can be used (basket catheters, noncontact mapping) to get an idea where the critical areas might be during the initial seconds of the tachycardia; (c) the pathophysiologic substrate can be defined and several strategies can be used to render the substrate nonarrhythmogenic. These include encircling the entire scar (if it is small), defining potential isthmuses, or eliminating late potentials, as discussed above. VT circuits in the setting

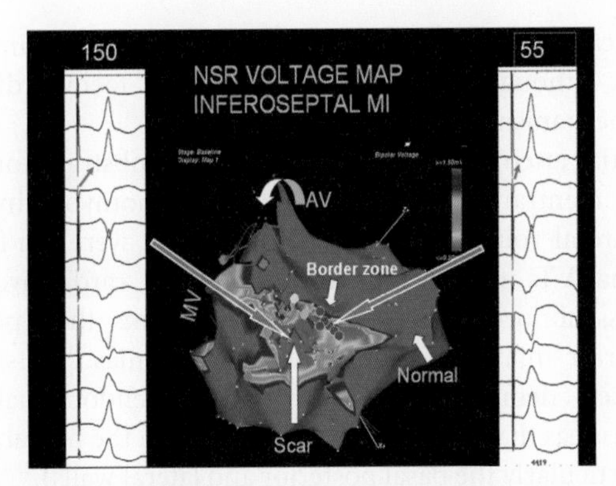


**FIGURE 13-155** *Method of substrate mapping.* A voltage map is performed during sinus rhythm (or ventricular pacing) to define normal (>1.5 mV), border zones (0.5–1.5 mV), and scar (<0.5 mV). Pacing at the border of the scar produces a QRS comparable to VT. Pacing progressively deeper in the scar while maintaining a similar QRS, but longer stimulus to QRS identifies a channel of conduction assumed to be the isthmus during VT. Ablation perpendicular to the exit, and, in some cases into the scar can prevent VT. *Dark reddish circles* are ablation sites. See text for discussion.

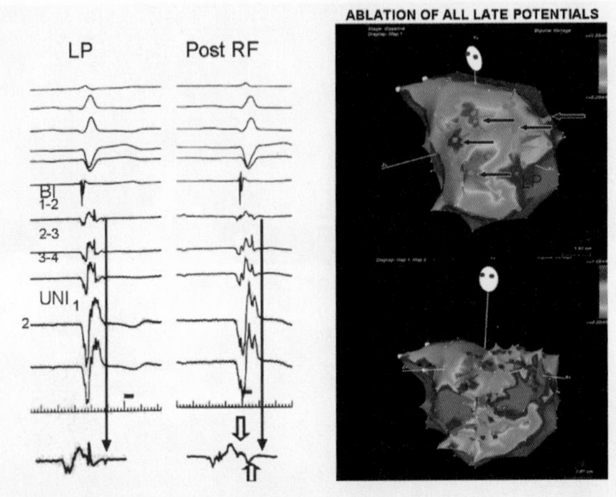


**FIGURE 13-156** *Targeting late potentials to ablate arrhythmogenic substrate.* The patient has a large apical infarction, but a poorly defined scar (Cato map on right). Late potentials were identified throughout the area (*blue circles and arrows*). RF application at sites of late potentials are delivered to eliminate them (*brown dots* bottom Carto map). Analog recordings of a site with late potentials seen in the distal bipolar pair (blowup bottom left) demonstrate loss of late potentials following RF application (*open arrows*).

of healed infarction often have apparent isthmus lengths of several centimeters (see discussion above), offering a sizeable opportunity for identification and interruption. Isthmuses may be defined in a number of ways. One method is to induce an untolerated monomorphic VT to obtain a 12-lead ECG. Pacing is then performed at the border zone (voltage 0.5 to 1.0 mV). At the site of best pace map, move into the scar and repeat pacing. A line of similar pace maps with an increasing stimulus to QRS defines a potential isthmus. A line of lesions is delivered perpendicular to the isthmus, tangential to the scar (Fig. 13-155).[361–363] Another method of defining an isthmus is to assess whether there are relatively preserved voltage areas within the 0.5-mV scar. This can be done by resetting the voltage limits to 0.3 to 0.5 mV as the upper limit and 0.1 mV as scar. Channels can be visualized and 0.1-mV scar can be connected with RF lesions closing the channel (Fig. 13-142). This method was first described by Arenal et al.[324] We chose the value of 0.1 mV to represent true dense scar based on our earlier work which demonstrated dense scar at surgery had endocardial amplitudes ≤0.1 mV. This has been confirmed by observations using MRI. Another method to assess dense scar bordering more viable tissue is to define it by electrical inexcitability.[320] These investigators noted that 0.5 mV was frequently excitable, and inexcitability was noted in the areas with voltage <0.1 mV. These methods are summarized in Table 13-1. One of the potential limitations of "voltage mapping" is that EGMs at sites of interest which have a small, isolated late potential but a rather large far field signal will be recorded as having "normal" voltage. This can be quite misleading and also can explain electrical inexcitability at sites which have reasonable voltage.[320] The use of isolated late potentials as target for ablation requires extensive and detailed mapping.[364] Such potentials may be recorded outside "scar," but this in many cases is a result of a large far field signal at the same site. Although late potentials are usually recorded during sinus rhythm, RV pacing usually allows more to be seen and may be preferable to recordings during sinus rhythm or atrial pacing. Ablation of all late potentials has been proposed by Jackman (personal communication) as the preferred approach in patients with large scars. It is, however, extremely time consuming to acquire the high-density maps required for this strategy I use this approach in the absence of inducible VTs, large scars, lack of ability to define channels (Fig. 13-156). High-density mapping with small electrodes (Biosense PentArray and Rhythmia Orion) facilitates the demonstration of isolated potentials within dense scar. Since multiple monomorphic as well as polymorphic tachycardias can be present combinations of ablative strategies are commonly used.

Linear lesions transverse (i.e., perpendicular) to the diastolic pathway may be all that is necessary to prevent arrhythmias. Currently there is a significant body of experience using the electrical anatomic mapping system to perform linear lesions through an identified substrate in patients with coronary disease. Marchlinski et al.[318] has used this technique to make linear lesions in patients receiving excessive shocks with ICDs. We also have used this system in patients with untolerated tachycardias. An example of a patient who had an untolerated tachycardia whose pace map (exit site) was in the midseptum and whose scar was inferoseptal is shown in Figure 13-157. Ablation perpendicular to the channel whose exit was defined by pace mapping along the scar border prevented VT. We completed a randomized controlled trial (SMASH-VT) comparing preventative substrate ablation guided by the Carto system versus standard therapy (ACE inhibitors and beta blockers) in 127 patients with coronary disease suffering from cardiac arrest.[357] The techniques described above were used in the ablation limb. All monomorphic tachycardias induced had pace maps to match to the 12-lead morphology of the tachycardia as closely

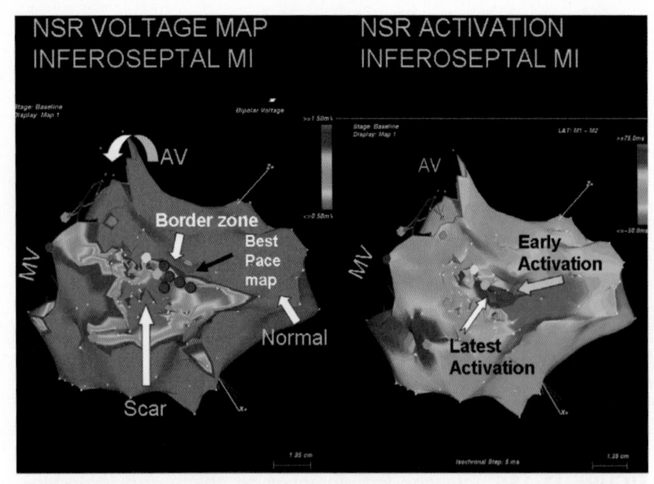


**FIGURE 13-157** *Substrate mapping for untolerated VT.* On the left a voltage map is shown in a patient with an inferoseptal MI. The best pace map was at the septal border. A linear lesion was made perpendicular to this site with an additional lesion just within the scar (*blue dots*). There has been no recurrence. Of note, the activation map at this site showed adjacent early and late activation, a theoretically (and in this case a reality) ideal substrate for reentry.

as possible. RF energy was delivered to construct a linear lesion through the site of the best pace map (exit site). An example of a patient in whom we evaluated delayed activation, late potentials, and voltage along with pace mapping is shown in Figure 13-156. If only polymorphic tachycardias or VF was induced, encirclement of the entire scar or ablation of all late potentials was performed. In a small number of patients connecting dense scar was employed. The results of the study showed a greater than 60% reduction of ICD shocks and total therapies that was highly significant and a trend an improved survival which was limited by patient numbers.

One remaining serious concern about extensive ablation techniques is thromboembolism. Open irrigation catheters have been proposed to be less thrombogenic,[365] but this has not been demonstrated in clinical situations. Cryoablation has not been used extensively in this application. Epicardial ablation does not promote thromboembolism, and may be helpful in this regard, but comes at the expense of introducing other potential complications.

## Role of Catheter Ablation in the Treatment of Ventricular Tachycardia Associated with Nonischemic Left Ventricular Tachycardia

Uniform monomorphic ventricular tachycardia can also complicate the course of nonischemic left ventricular tachycardia. This syndrome is a collection of different pathologies (idiopathic, sarcoidosis, myocarditis, etc.),[366] which all result in myocardial replacement fibrosis providing a qualitatively similar (but quantitatively much smaller) substrate for reentrant arrhythmias. The pathophysiology is not as well understood as healed infarction, due to the smaller experience both with applicable animal models and operative ablation experience in clinical situations. Scar-related reentry VT can occur in this setting, although bundle branch reentrant tachycardia and focal mechanisms are also observed.[367]

Initial attempts at understanding the substrate for scar-related reentrant VT in nonischemic cardiomyopathy used endocardial voltage mapping. Cassidy et al. were the first to note that VTs in patients with nonischemic cardiomyopathy had less abnormal endocardial electrograms than patients with prior infarction and similar arrhythmias.[314] Hsia and coworkers demonstrated relatively small endocardial low-voltage areas that consistently extended from the mitral annulus (particularly the basal posterior and lateral walls).[368] These areas of low voltage provided the substrate for ventricular tachycardia in nonischemic cardiomyopathy, analogous to the infarct tissue in ischemic cardiomyopathy. However, from the beginning, ablation of VT in this clinical setting was not as successful as in healed infarction. In general, perhaps because the degree of scarring is much smaller, VT in nonischemic cardiomyopathy tends to be more rapid, less well tolerated and more likely to require substrate ablation approaches. In addition, although different VT morphologies often share circuit elements in coronary disease VT, as discussed above, this does not appear to be the case in nonischemic cardiomyopathy. Although detailed mapping studies of the circuit in this setting are not available, it appears that the length of the critical isthmus in nonischemic cardiomyopathy is shorter.

In an early series of substrate ablation, the success rate in nonischemic cardiomyopathy was much less than that observed in coronary disease–related VT.[363] Soon thereafter, several points of evidence suggested that the endocardium may not be the only source for substrate in this condition. First, the work by Sosa and coworkers demonstrated the importance of epicardial mapping and ablation in Chagastic cardiomyopathy.[369] Second, there were individual patients with clear myocardial reentrant VT who had normal endocardial voltage maps. Finally, various investigators discovered the potential for epicardial sites of origin of other VTs, particularly in patients with previous failed endocardial ablations, either from the coronary venous system or from the epicardial surface.[298,370] Soejima and coworkers were the first to investigate the possibility of epicardial involvement in nonischemic cardiomyopathy, using percutaneous mapping in seven patients with failed endocardial ablation. In many, but not all of these patients, the extent of epicardial substrate was greater than endocardial.[371] Cano and coworkers provided a systematic experience of both endocardial and epicardial mapping in 22 patients with nonischemic cardiomyopathy referred for ablation. This population was "enriched" as 20 had prior failed endocardial ablation and the clinical VT morphology in the remaining 2 patients suggested epicardial exit.[372] Low-voltage areas were seen in 54% of endocardial and 82% epicardial maps and scar area was larger on the epicardial surface ($55.3 \pm 33.5$ cm$^2$ vs. $22.9 \pm 32.4$ cm$^2$) (Fig. 13-158). In addition to voltage abnormalities, epicardial electrograms were often wide (>80 msec duration), split and/or late; these abnormalities were only rarely observed in a reference population of

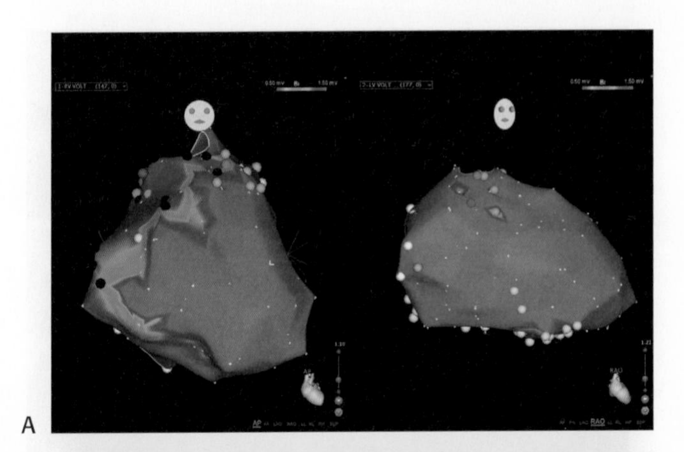


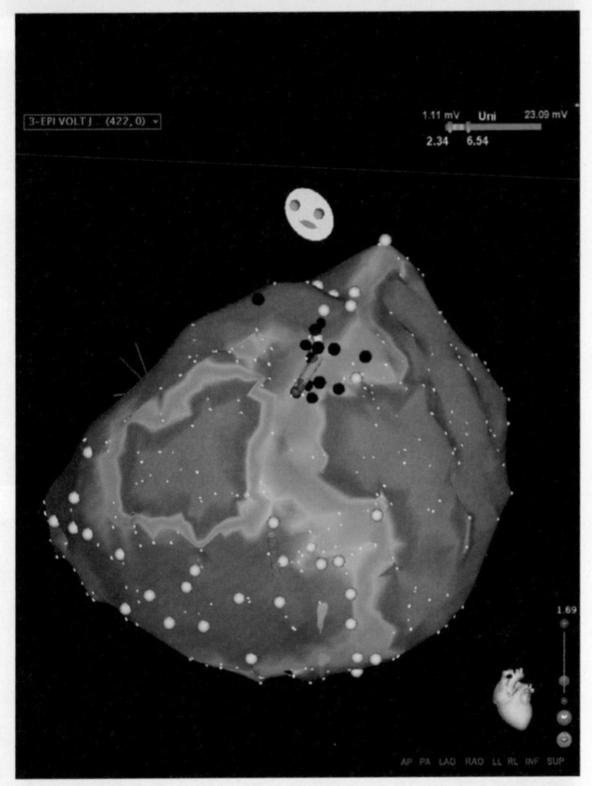


**FIGURE 13-158** *Epicardial substrate in nonischemic cardiomyopathy.* In **A**, RV and LV bipolar endocardial voltage maps are shown from a patient with nonischemic cardiomyopathy and recurrent VT; although there are some voltage abnormalities in the basal RV, they are fairly minimal. An epicardial bipolar voltage map is shown in **B**, demonstrating much more widespread RV and LV voltage abnormality. See text for discussion.

patients with epicardial mapping for idiopathic VT. At least one epicardial VT circuit was found in 18 patients, whereas only endocardial and/or intramural circuits were identified in 4. Over a mean follow-up of 18 ± 7 months, 71% of patients were free from recurrent VT, including 14 of 18 patients (78%) with epicardial VT.

These studies suggested that epicardial ablation, at least in selected patients would improve success rates. However, epicardial ablation introduces new considerations and additional risk. The presence of epicardial fat can have important impact on voltage mapping (low voltage recorded over normal tissue, particularly around the coronary arteries), and on energy delivery during ablation. As was shown by d'Avila and coworkers in experimental epicardial ablation, even a small layer of fat dramatically affects lesion depth during RF delivery.[373] This effect can be reduced with irrigated ablation. Most laboratories perform epicardial ablation under general anesthesia, because of the discomfort related to epicardial instrumentation and ablation. General anesthesia can negatively affect the ability to induce VT and may cause hypotension during previously tolerated arrhythmias because of vasodilation. The additional risks include RV perforation, damage to the epicardial coronary arteries and phrenic nerve palsy.[346]

Because of this risk/efficacy balance, we have used a provisional approach to the epicardium for patients with VT in the setting of nonischemic cardiomyopathy. Preprocedural MR imaging can demonstrate epicardial scar on delayed gadolinium images, but is not available in many programs in patients with pre-existing ICDs. Intraprocedural data that is compatible with epicardial circuits include the following: (1) A QRS morphology during VT with a qS in focus leads (typically lead I for the basal posterior lateral substrate in nonischemic cardiomyopathy; see discussion above). (2) Intracardiac echocardiographic (ICE) imaging that suggests epicardial substrate. In a small observational study, Bala and coworkers demonstrated that midmyocardial or epicardial abnormalities on ICE imaging (increased signal brightness) were correlated with areas of delayed gadolinium enhancement on MR imaging and epicardial bipolar voltage abnormalities during sinus rhythm mapping (Fig. 13-159).[374] (3) Endocardial unipolar voltage abnormalities that are significantly larger than bipolar.

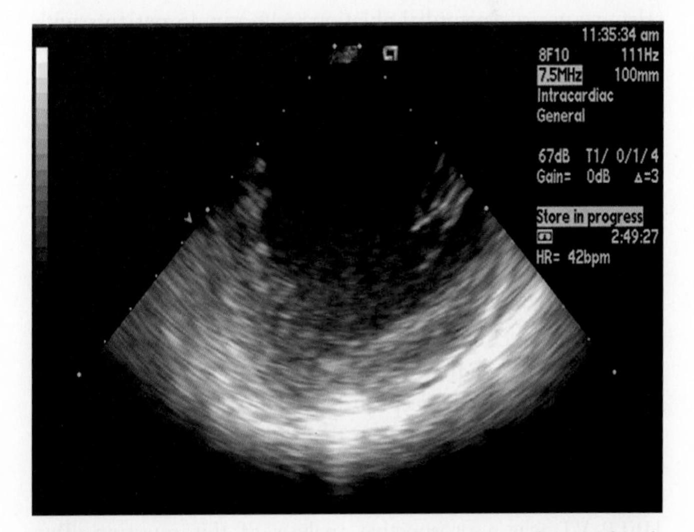


**FIGURE 13-159** *Use of intracardiac echocardiography to identify epicardial substrate.* A still frame echocardiographic image of the LV is shown from a patient with nonischemic cardiomyopathy and VT. Note the increased echodensity in the subepicardium (*arrows*) compared to the homogeneous density throughout the endocardium. In this patient, the endocardial voltage map was normal, and the epicardial voltage map abnormal, in a distribution that was predicted by the imaging. A mid-diastolic site was demonstrated during entrainment on the epicardium, and ablation there was successful.

Hutchinson et al. explored the utility of unipolar endocardial voltage mapping to predict epicardial scar.[375] In patients without heart disease undergoing endocardial and epicardial mapping for idiopathic VT, endocardial bipolar voltage, endocardial unipolar voltage (using a defined cutoff of 8.5 mV), and bipolar epicardial voltage were all normal. In 11 patients with nonischemic cardiomyopathy and VT who had normal endocardial bipolar voltage but abnormal endocardial unipolar voltage, the unipolar abnormalities correlated with abnormal epicardial bipolar voltage (Fig. 13-160). In addition, although endocardial unipolar voltage tended to over predict the size of epicardial bipolar abnormalities, some of this difference was secondary to midmyocardial scar, as demonstrated by MR imaging. The limitations of the use and interpretation of endocardial unipolar mapping are discussed in Chapter 11. (4) Inability to find abnormal endocardial potentials related to the circuit when VT is sufficiently well tolerated to map.

Even using a selective approach, the vast majority of VT ablation procedures in the setting of nonischemic cardiomyopathy involves epicardial ablation in our laboratory. However, the impact of epicardial ablation on success is still controversial. In certain circumstances, it has been demonstrated that endocardial ablation can eliminate epicardial late potentials, which may serve as arrhythmia substrate, provisionally providing a clear alternative to epicardial ablation.[331,376] A recent retrospective observational study from UCLA suggested that patients with nonischemic cardiomyopathy who had endocardial and epicardial ablation did not have improved outcome compared to those with endocardial ablation alone;[343] however, it may well be that patients who were offered epicardial ablation were not equivalent to those who were not. Piers and coworkers recently published an interesting study with selective use of epicardial ablation (64%) in 45 patients with nonischemic cardiomyopathy and VT.[377] These investigators found that although VT recurrence was frequent (53% at 25 ± 15 months), the VT burden was reduced by ≥ 75% in 79% of patients. Moreover, freedom from recurrence was influenced to a greater extent by acute efficacy, assessed by response to programmed stimulation, than by whether epicardial ablation was performed. Patients who were noninducible at the conclusion of the ablation procedure had low rates of recurrence (18%), but patients with partial success or failure (persistent induction of the targeted clinical VT) did less well (>70% recurrence). In summary, it seems that in a heterogeneous group of patients, the response to/need for epicardial ablation is heterogeneous.

In any case, it is fairly clear that independent of technique, results for ablation of VT in nonischemic cardiomyopathy are not as efficacious as in healed infarction. The recently published HELP VT was a prospective analysis of this question. Two hundred twenty-seven patients (63 with nonischemic cardiomyopathy, the remainder with coronary disease) were treated with catheter ablation. Although acute success was excellent (no VT inducible after ablation in 67 and 77% of nonischemic and ischemic heart disease groups, respectively) and not different between groups, freedom from VT in follow-up was much worse in the nonischemic group (40.5 vs. 57% at 1 year).[378]

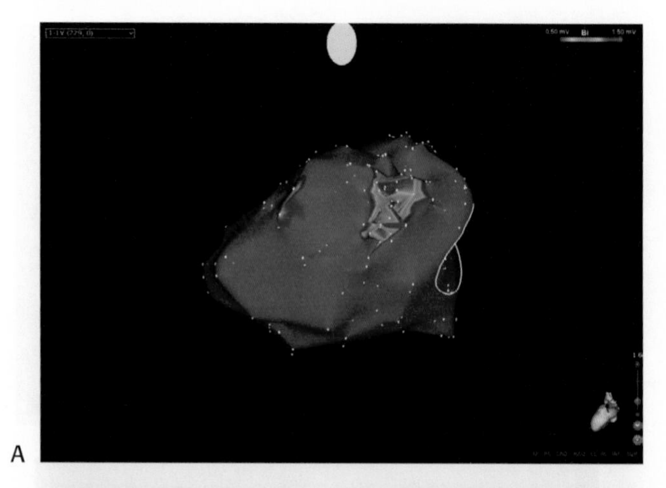
A

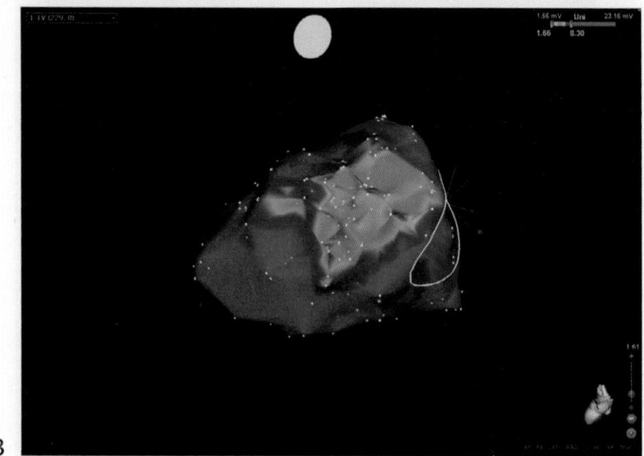
B

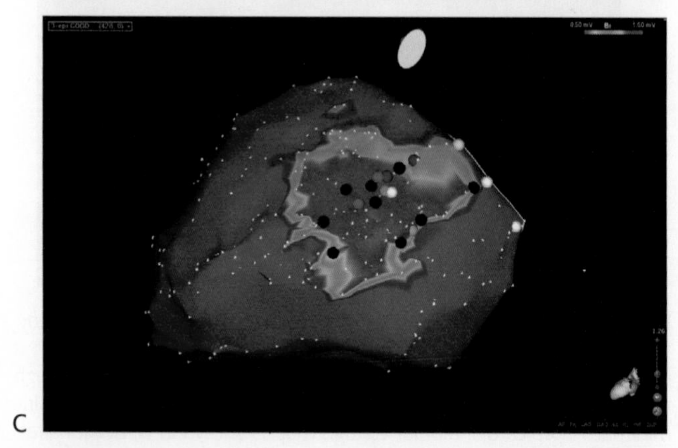
C

**FIGURE 13-160** *Use of unipolar mapping to predict epicardial bipolar voltage abnormalities.* Electroanatomic voltage maps (PA projection) recorded in a patient with cardiac sarcoid and ventricular tachycardia. **A** shows a small area of bipolar endocardial voltage abnormality; the endocardial unipolar voltage map demonstrates a larger abnormal area **(B)**, which correlates with a similar zone of bipolar voltage abnormality on the epicardium **(C)**, which served as the VT substrate in this patient.

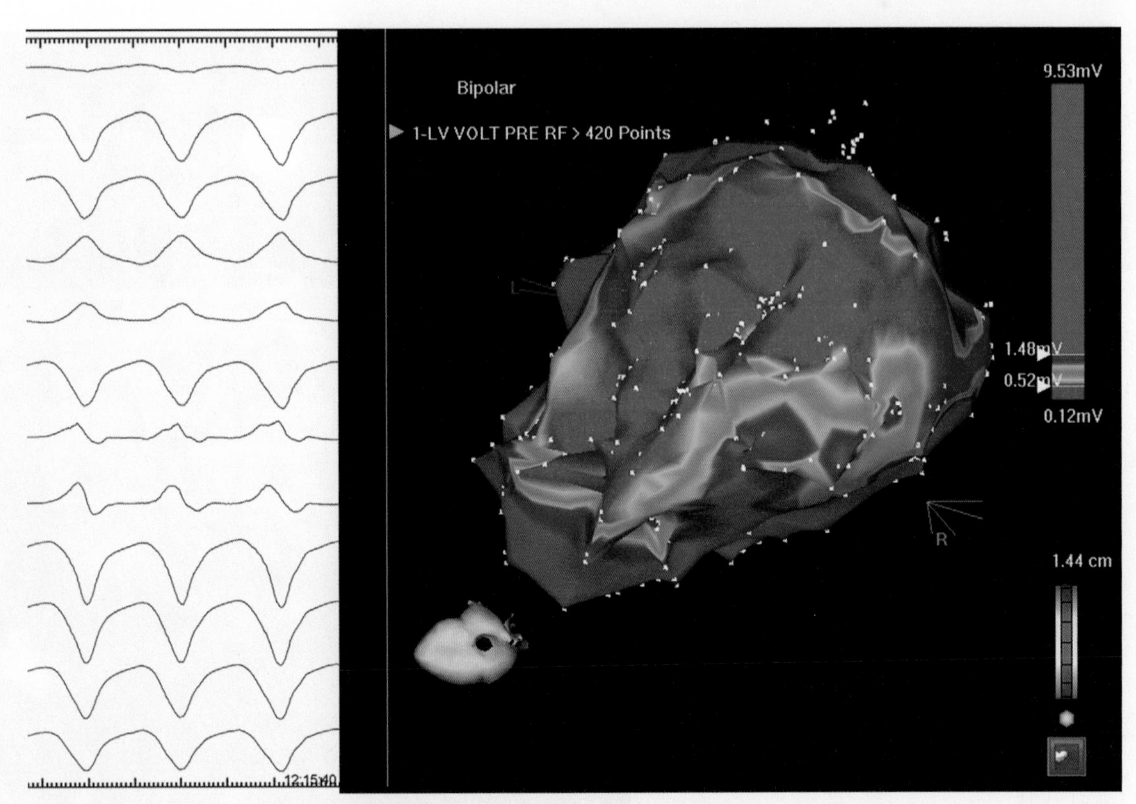


**FIGURE 13-161** *Apical extent of scar in nonischemic cardiomyopathy.* The **left panel** shows a 12-lead ECG of this patient's clinical VT; the QRS morphology is consistent with an apical site of origin. The corresponding LV endocardial bipolar voltage map (PA view) is shown in the **right panel**, which shows extensive voltage abnormalities, from the mitral annulus to the apex. Patients with apical scar in nonischemic cardiomyopathy have a poor prognosis.

Two groups of patients with nonischemic cardiomyopathy appear at particular risk for poor outcome. The pathophysiology in most forms of nonischemic cardiomyopathy (exceptions include sarcoid, myocarditis) involves predominantly basal involvement. From a group of 76 consecutive patients with nonischemic cardiomyopathy referred for VT ablation, Frankel and coworkers described 32 who had apical VTs judged by ECG morphology of LBBB with late transition (>V5), or RBBB morphology with early precordial transition (from positive to negative, <V3). These patients had larger endocardial/epicardial voltage abnormalities (extending farther from the mitral annulus), but importantly had worse transplant free survival than the remainder of the cohort (Fig. 13-161).[379] The second group of interest is patients with intraseptal substrate, either in an isolated form or in addition to the more frequent basal lateral substrate. Haqqani and coworkers were the first to describe the concept of isolated septal substrate in 31 patients (Fig. 13-162).[380] To the extent clinically possible, cardiac sarcoidosis was excluded in this cohort. Septal substrate was identified by RV/LV bipolar voltage mapping (and unipolar voltage mapping, particularly in eight patients with normal bipolar endocardial maps) and MR or CT imaging. Because of the potential for intramural VT circuits within the septum, the clinical response despite extensive ablation from both sides of the septum was not excellent; after a mean of 1.6 procedures per patient, recurrent VT was observed in 32% of patients over $20 \pm 28$ months. Heart block was present in eight patients prior to ablation, and was caused by extensive septal ablation in five. Oloriz and colleagues recently compared the results of ablation in patients with anteroseptal versus inferolateral scars in nonischemic cardiomyopathy. They found patients with septal scar had a higher rate of recurrent VT (74% vs. 25%) and required more frequent repeat procedures (59% vs. 7%).[381]

## Role of Catheter Ablation in the Treatment of Ventricular Tachycardia Associated with Right Ventricular Dysplasia

Right ventricular dysplasia is a primary cardiomyopathy characterized by fibrofatty replacement of the right ventricular free wall and in some patients the left ventricle as well. The disorder may be familial and several point gene mutations have been observed. Early in the disease, with little gross anatomic abnormalities, patients may present with nonsustained, catecholamine-triggered VT. Once fibrofatty replacement has been significant, patients present with sustained monomorphic tachycardias. Cardiac MRI is valuable in detecting fibrosis with delayed hyperenhancement and fat (less diagnostic). These arrhythmias are typically macroreentrant tachycardias, and as such, mapping and ablation follow the same guidelines as in coronary disease. Electrograms recorded in sinus rhythm in diseased areas are markedly fractionated and are of low amplitude

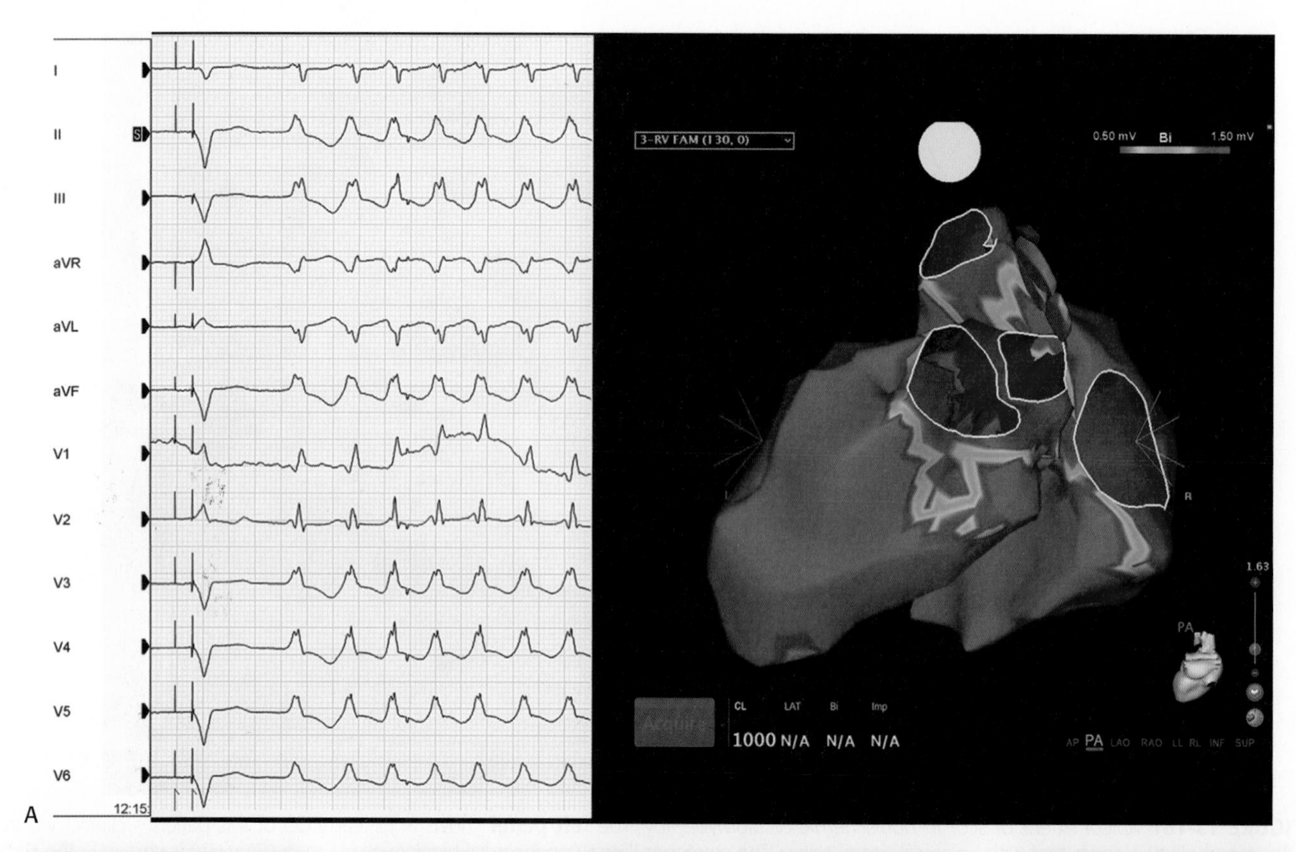


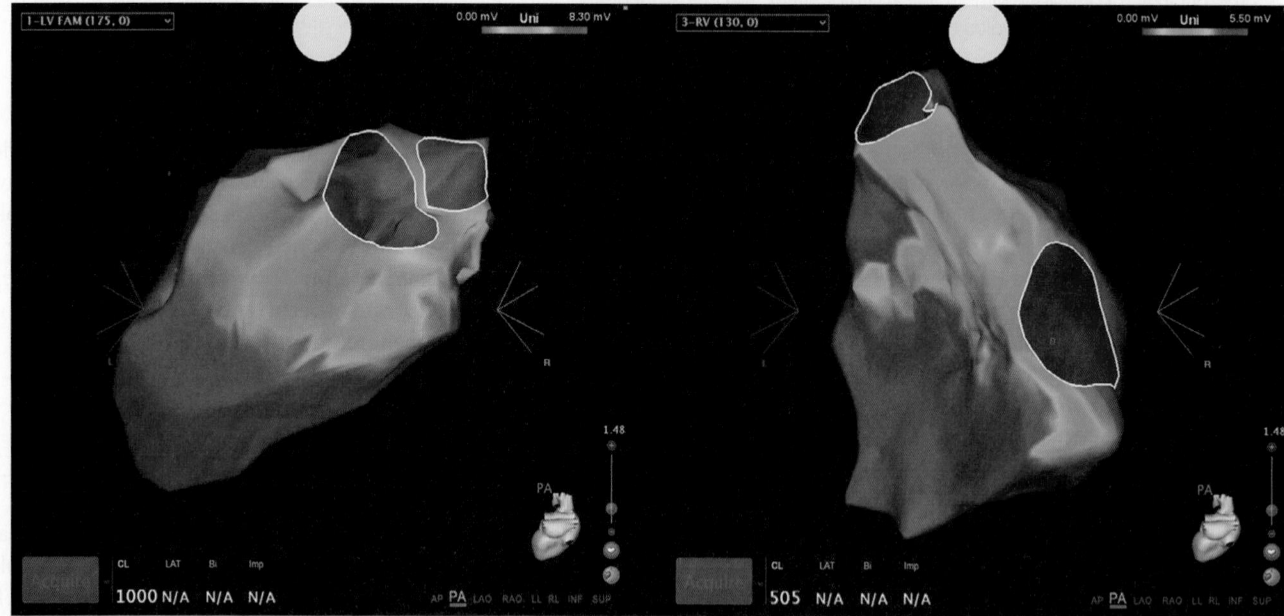


**FIGURE 13-162** *Septal substrate in nonischemic cardiomyopathy.* These figures are from a young patient with nonischemic cardiomyopathy, multiple morphologies of reentrant VT and heart block; there is no clinical evidence to support a diagnosis of cardiac sarcoid. In **Panel A**, the left figure shows a 12-lead ECG of one of his clinical VTs, a narrow right bundle, right inferior axis morphology; the right figure shows RV and LV endocardial bipolar voltage mapping which show possible small areas of basal scar. In **panel B**, unipolar voltage maps of the LV (**left**) and RV (**right**) show larger areas of scaring, which was confirmed by delayed gadolinium imaging.

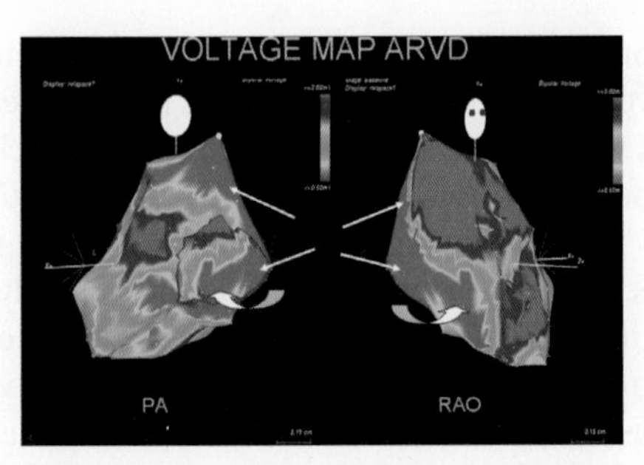


**FIGURE 13-163** *Voltage map of the right ventricle and arrhythmogenic right ventricular dysplasia.* PA and RAO views of a voltage map in a 35-year-old-man with arrhythmogenic right ventricular dysplasia. The *red areas* are all areas of abnormally low voltage consistent with fibrofatty replacement of the myocardium. *Purple areas* are normal. Note that the apex and basal free wall, as well as the posterior region around the outflow tract, show marked abnormalities of voltage. Right ventricular aneurysm and dyskinesis were present in all of these areas. The patient presented with multiple recurrent sustained ventricular tachycardia. See text for discussion.

(see Chapter 11). These patients have the most abnormal signal-averaged ECGs. The latest activation usually is at the base near the tricuspid annulus, but fragmented delayed activation can be obtained all over the free wall of the right ventricle. These diffuse abnormalities can be easily detected as low voltage along the free wall of the right ventricle (Fig. 13-163). For hemodynamically tolerated sustained monomorphic VT entrainment mapping should be carried out as in coronary disease.[382,383] If the entrainments mapping criteria described in Chapter 11 and earlier in this chapter are fulfilled, ablation is usually successful (Fig. 13-164). However, because of the diffuse disease, reentrant circuits may show a broad isthmus and good entrainment maps

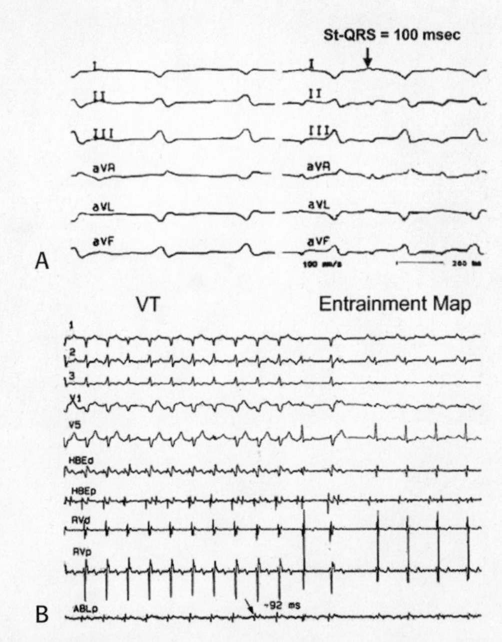


**FIGURE 13-164** *Ablation of ventricular tachycardia in arrhythmogenic right ventricular dysplasia guided by entrainment mapping.* In the **top panel (A)** an entrainment map from a site judged to be in the isthmus is shown. On the **bottom (B)**, application of radiofrequency energy at this site terminates VT. See text for discussion.

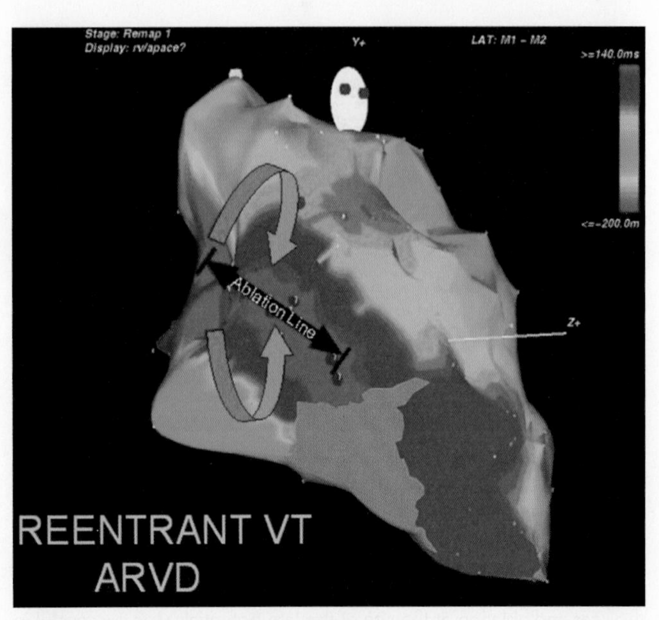


**FIGURE 13-165** *Requirement of a linear lesion to treat ventricular tachycardia in arrhythmogenic right ventricular dysplasia.* An electroanatomic map of a reentrant ventricular tachycardia and right ventricular dysplasia is shown. A broad reentrant wavefront was observed. As a consequence a linear line between the latest area of activation and the earliest area of activation was made. This terminated the tachycardia and prevented its recurrence.

can be seen over a very large area. This finding suggests single site ablation may not be effective and linear lesions over the isthmus or diastolic pathway are required (Fig. 13-165). Substrate mapping in such cases can be used to identify late potentials or voltage abnormalities that may guide therapy. Low voltage alone seems to be less useful in right ventricular dysplasias as a marker for ablation since it is so ubiquitous. However, use of variable voltage ranges (with its limitations, see discussion in Chapter 11) can often identify an apparent channel of viable muscle which is a useful target for ablation. Moreover, areas of late potentials may be distal to areas of low voltage, yet may be critical. In my experience these abnormalities are most common and severe at the inferolateral margin of the tricuspid valve extending to the adjacent free wall. As seen in Figure 13-166, ablation across an isthmus created by two scars in which late potentials were recorded was successful in preventing VT in a patient with right ventricular dysplasia. Note that the site of late potentials lies in between two areas of thin scar forming a narrow isthmus, while the low-voltage area is somewhat anterior to this and would not have provided a good site for ablation. We have successfully ablated tolerated monomorphic ventricular tachycardias in 25 patients with right ventricular dysplasia. In 17 of these, entrainment mapping was used to guide the ablation. In the remaining eight, due to extensive disease, substrate mapping was used in addition to entrainment mapping. While there remains some fear of perforation during ablation of patients with right ventricular dysplasia, we have not experienced any untoward effects. Fourteen of the patients who were ablated on antiarrhythmic drugs have maintained their antiarrhythmic therapy while 11 have stopped all medications. Only

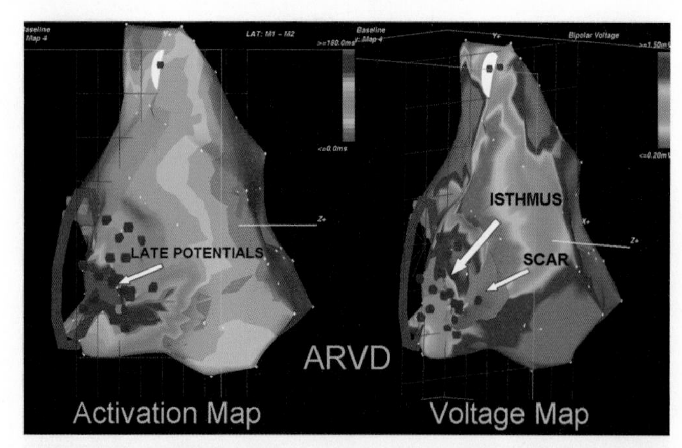


**FIGURE 13-166** *Use of late potentials and scar to guide ablation in right ventricular dysplasia.* An electroanatomic map of sinus rhythm is shown in a patient with right ventricular dysplasia. In the activation map, *gray areas* are scar, late potentials are denoted. The area of late potentials had relatively normal voltage. The voltage map demonstrates low amplitude superior to the scar and late potentials. Connection of the scar and ablation at the site of the late potentials was successful in preventing ventricular tachycardias. See text for discussion.

five patients have had an ICD implanted; one of whom also had hypertrophic obstructive cardiomyopathy. None of the patients have had a recurrence of the ablated VT. It must be stated that since right ventricular dysplasia may be a progressive disease, new ventricular tachycardias may occur. This happened in four of our patients, both of whom underwent a second ablation. As in coronary disease, the presentation of a tolerated monomorphic ventricular tachycardia predicts tolerated recurrences. Therefore, we do not routinely implant ICDs in such patients. While others have successfully ablated VT in patients with ARVD,[383–385] they routinely implant ICDs. I believe this is not only unnecessary in patients presenting with hemodynamically stable VT in terms of survival, the leads often cause or increase tricuspid regurgitation, which, may worsen right ventricular failure. For untolerated VTs a substrate approach is used.

Recent series from the Padua group have raised the important concept that even patients with a "secure" diagnosis of right ventricular dysplasia/cardiomyopathy by task force criteria may have other disease processes.[386,387] Selective RV biopsy guided by endocardial voltage mapping has demonstrated that some patients with presumed ARVC actually have sarcoidosis or myocarditis. This is not surprising because biopsies are generally taken from the septum and abnormalities at this site are not generally present in RV dysplasia.

Because the replacement fibrosis in this disease process begins at the epicardial surface and because of disappointing reports of endocardial ablation in ARVC,[388] some investigators have suggested an epicardial ablation approach. Garcia and colleagues reported the results of epicardial mapping and ablation in 13 patients with recurrent VT after endocardial ablation. Twenty-seven VTs were ablated from the epicardium sites that were adjacent to normal endocardial myocardium (77%) and/or endocardial sites where prior ablation was unsuccessful (85%) (Fig. 13-167).[389] Over a mean

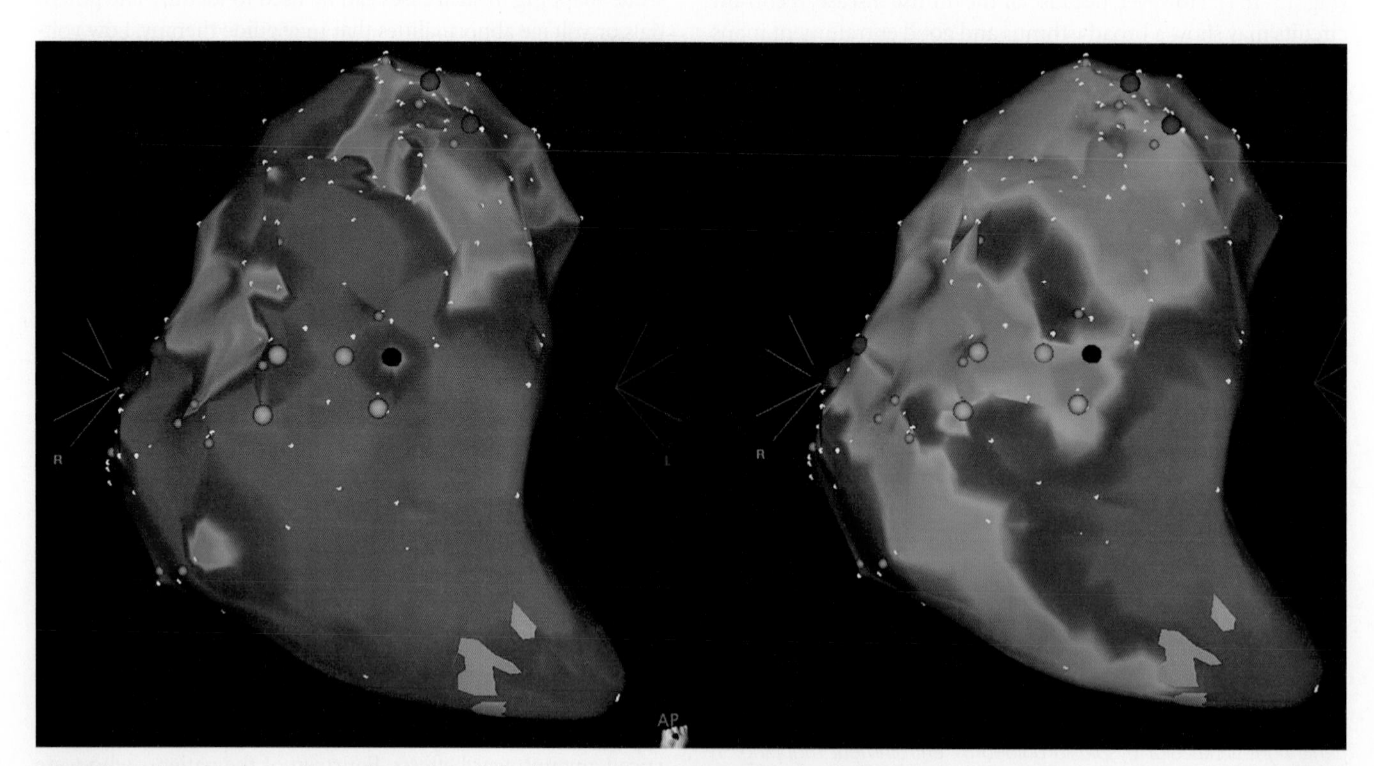


**FIGURE 13-167** *Bipolar and unipolar endocardial voltage mapping in ARVC.* Bipolar (**left**, voltage range 0.5 to 1.5 mV) and unipolar (**right**, voltage range 0.5 to 5.5 mV) are shown in a patient with ARVC and recurrent VT. The area of unipolar voltage abnormality exceeds that of bipolar, suggesting epicardial substrate > endocardial.

follow-up of 18 ± 13 months, 10 patients had no recurrent VT and 2 patients had only a single VT episode. Subsequent larger observational studies suggest an improved outcome in patients with a combined endo/epicardial ablation approach compared to endocardial alone.[385,390] In our experience, patients with ARVC typically have multiple VT morphologies, some which are best approached from the endocardium, some from the epicardium. Both approaches seem to be necessary in most patients.

## *The Role of Catheter Mapping and Ablation of Idiopathic Ventricular Tachycardias*

Idiopathic ventricular tachycardia can present as sustained monomorphic tachycardia, "bursts" of repetitive nonsustained tachycardia or isolated premature ventricular complexes. Although it can arise from any area of the heart, there are more frequent locations/syndromes, which are discussed below. In general, the prognosis of idiopathic VT is excellent, but there are exceptions. "Idiopathic VTs" can exist in patients with structural heart disease. Idiopathic VT can also be observed in patients with ion channel diseases, and may precipitate ventricular fibrillation in these patients.[391–393] Finally, very frequent premature complexes may cause cardiomyopathy, which is reversible with treatment of this arrhythmia.[394–396] Ablation of idiopathic VT is indicated for treatment of symptoms, in patients with suspected PVC-related cardiomyopathy, and when PVCs trigger episodes of ventricular fibrillation.

There are two main types of tachycardia mechanisms in patients without structural heart disease (the original definition of idiopathic ventricular tachycardias). The most common variety is due to triggered activity secondary to delayed afterdepolarizations, which are dependent on enhanced adenyl cyclase activity.[397–401] This is usually catecholamine-dependent but is also influenced by phosphodiesterase inhibitors and removal of inhibitors of adenyl cyclase activity (e.g., atropine blockade of negative influences of muscarinic stimulation). Enhancement of adenyl cyclase and cyclic AMP increases intracellular calcium influx by enhanced phosphorylation of the L-type calcium channel. This in turn leads to calcium release from the sarcoplasmic reticulum, enhanced sodium calcium exchange, and a transient inward current carried by sodium to produce the delayed afterdepolarizations. Conversely, termination can be facilitated by a variety of vagal maneuvers including carotid sinus pressure and Valsalva maneuver, administration of adenosine, calcium channel blockers, or sodium channel blockers. However, since these arrhythmias frequently arise in otherwise healthy patients, and since the treatment requires long-term therapy with beta blockers at reasonably high doses often with another agent, patients frequently opt for catheter ablation. These tachycardias usually arise in the RVOT, but are increasingly recognized in the LVOT (endocardial, epicardial, and supravalvular in the aortic cusps) as well. The LVOT VTs are more frequent in patients with structural heart disease, particularly

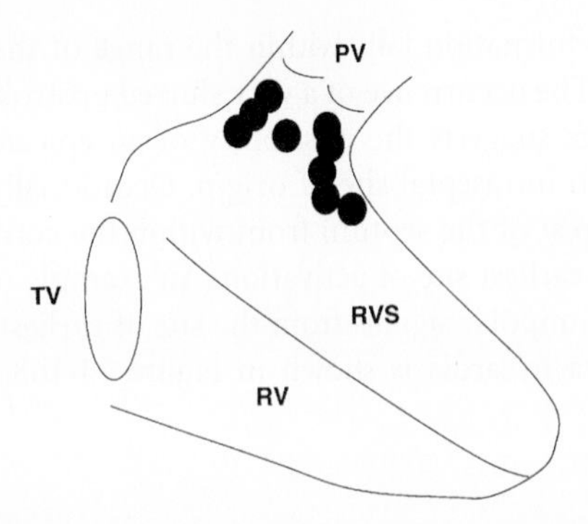


**FIGURE 13-168** *Schema of sites of origin of idiopathic right ventricular outflow tract tachycardia.* These tachycardias can occur anteriorly or basally in the right ventricular outflow tract. The site of earliest activation influences the morphology of the ventricular tachycardia. See text for discussion.

hypertension. Common RV sites seen in our laboratory are schematically shown in Figure 13-168. Finally triggered idiopathic VTs also arise in the Purkinje system, around the mitral annulus,[402] the epicardium adjacent to neurovascular bundles, or occasionally within prior scars.

Catecholamines are often necessary to facilitate a sustained arrhythmia, which can then be mapped. When arising at either the RVOT or LVOT these tachycardias usually have an LBBB and either right inferior or left inferior axis, depending on their location in the RVOT or LVOT. When they occur posterolateral to the LVOT (Aorto-mitral continuity and more lateral) or at other sites they have an RBBB morphology. Several ECG criteria can distinguish RV from LV origin, the most important of which are broader and taller R waves in $V_{1-2}$ and earlier transition in the precordial leads ($V_{2-3}$).[403] As described in Chapter 11, the closer the site of impulse formation is to the pulmonic valve, the more rightward and inferior the axis. The more posterior and inferior the site of impulse formation, the more leftward the axis. These morphologies serve as a guide to the initial site of activation mapping.[398] Those tachycardias arising around the mitral annulus have an RBBB and most often an inferior axis because of their frequent origin along the superior part of the annulus. The axis, however, can shift to the right and horizontal or even superior if the site of impulse formation is at the lateral or inferior aspects of the mitral annulus.[402]

Several approaches to mapping of these triggered tachycardias have been used. My own opinion is that a combination of mapping techniques is important. We use activation mapping using bipolar and unfiltered unipolar recordings. We also use pace mapping. The earliest bipolar recording in which the distal tip shows the earliest negative intrinsicoid deflection (QS deflection) is taken as the site of impulse formation. This is additionally confirmed by demonstrating an identical 12-lead match with a pace map. An identical pace map is useful because it is a focal tachycardia. Both methods are used because a QS unipolar recording and identical pace mapping can be demonstrated over a region of 1 to 1.5 cm, therefore, the more confirmatory information, the more likely the site of impulse formation falls within the range of the RF lesion produced. The occurrence of a very slurred upstroke and wide QS complex suggests the possibility of an epicardial site of origin or an intraseptal site of origin. Occasionally, mapping from the crest of the septum from within the coronary sinus reveals the earliest site of activation. An example of a bipolar signal and unipolar signals from the site of earliest activity in an RVOT tachycardia is shown in Figure 13-168. The distal mapping bipolar electrogram is 65 msec prior to the onset of the QRS. The associated unipolar electrograms demonstrate an earlier negative intrinsic deflection in the distal pole and the proximal pole. RF application at this site immediately terminates the tachycardia (panel B in Fig. 13-168). An example of an identical pace map in an RVOT tachycardia is shown in Figure 13-169. RF ablation at this site at which the earliest bipolar recording was 58 msec before the QS and was

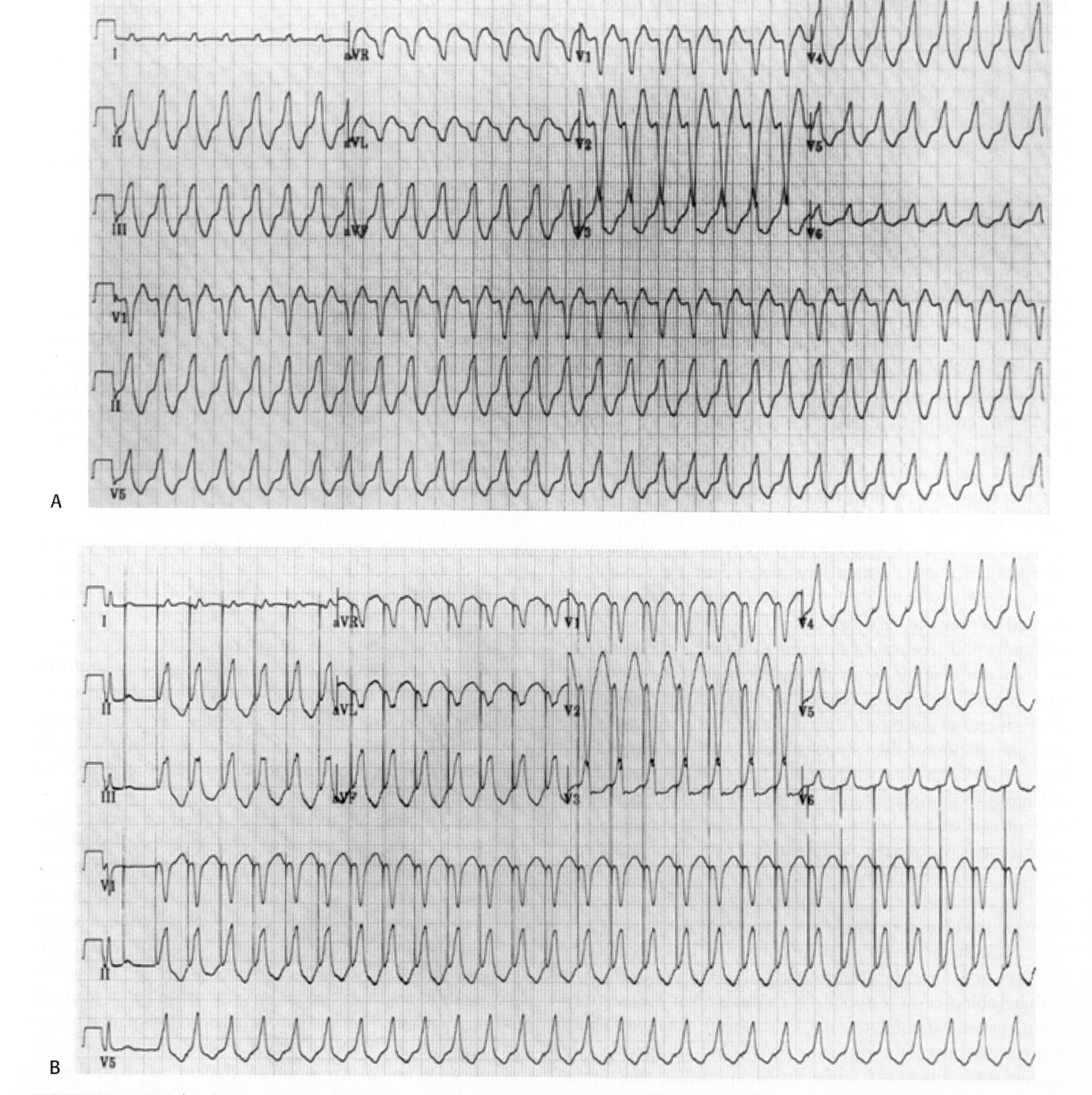


**FIGURE 13-169** *Role of pace mapping in localizing the site of origin in idiopathic RV outflow tract tachycardia.* **Panel A** shows ventricular tachycardia and **(B)** demonstrates an identical pace map from the earliest site of activation.

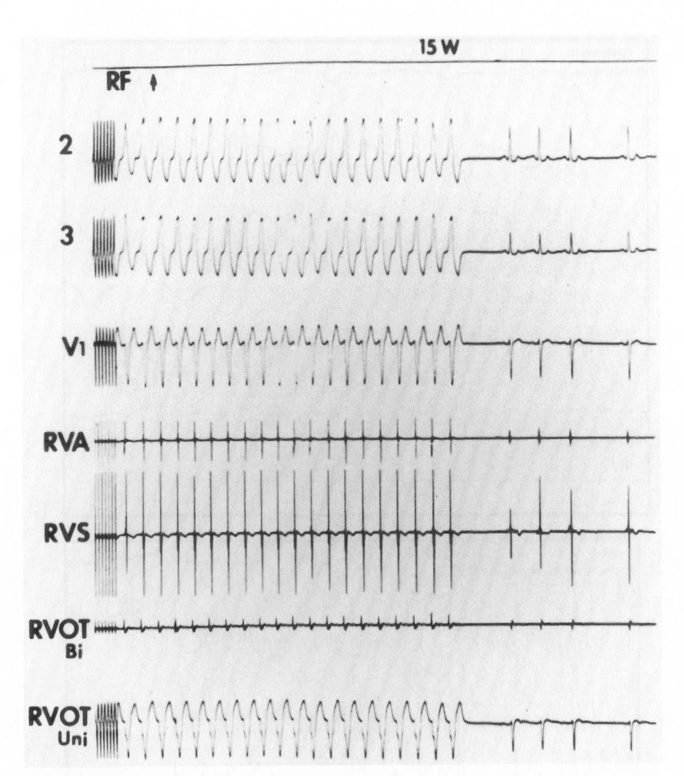


**FIGURE 13-170** *RF application of idiopathic RV outflow tract tachycardia.* This patient is the same as that described in Figure 13-169. Surface ECG leads along with additional right ventricular leads and bipolar and unipolar electrograms from the site of origin are displayed. Application of RF energy terminates the arrhythmia within 3 seconds. There has been no recurrence.

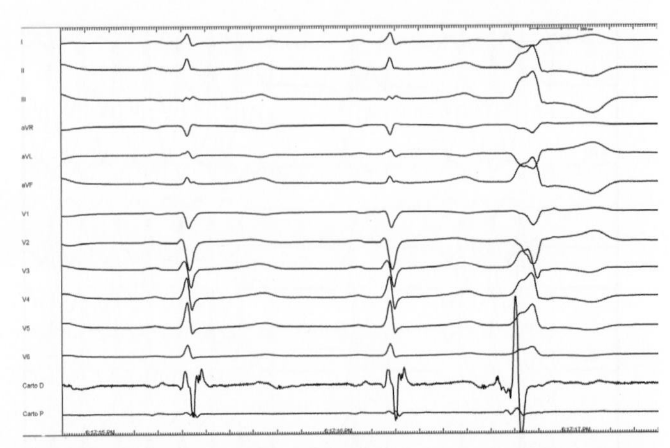

**FIGURE 13-171** *Activation mapping in sinus of Valsalva VT.* Surface 12-lead ECG and intracardiac recordings from the distal and proximal mapping catheter (Carto). During sinus rhythm, there is a sharp potential at the end of the far field ventricular electrogram (*red arrow*) which is later than the QRS offset. During a premature ventricular beat, this same signal becomes a prepotential. See text for discussion.

associated with a QS deflection in the unipolar recording, terminated the tachycardia in 3 seconds (Fig. 13-170). Epicardial mapping via the pericardium, coronary sinus, or retrograde aortic approach has demonstrated some sites of origin at the crest of the septum in or under the coronary cusps.[394,397,404]

As noted earlier, catecholamine-triggered ventricular tachycardia can also occur at the LVOT. These tachycardias behave similarly to those in the outflow tract and are often repetitive and made worse on exercise. The most typical locations are the right and left sinuses of Valsalva and the junction of the left and right coronary cusp. Activation mapping and pace mapping are carried out as described for the RVOT. However, there are two important differences when mapping in the sinuses of Valsalva. First, sites of successful ablation often have very early signals, which are thought to arise from relatively isolated muscle bundles (Fig. 13-171). In fact, there is very little myocardium associated with the cusps, and as mentioned above, most arrhythmias probably arise from the crest of the ventricular septum. Because of this, careful mapping of the entire surface of each sinus is required. Intracardiac echocardiography can be very helpful in this regard (Fig. 13-172). Second, although perfect pace maps can be obtained from the sinuses, often pacing at the site of successful ablation does not look anything like ventricular tachycardia; this is the case for the same reason described for the first point.

LVOT tachycardias may also arise near the mitral ring close to the coronary arteries and are often epicardial.[397,404] Attempted ablation from the distal-most coronary sinus or aortic cusp must be performed with caution in view of the potential damage of the adjacent coronary artery. Careful endocardial and epicardial mapping must be performed to decide where the ablation should be delivered. An example of an LVOT tachycardia that was found to be endocardial is shown in Figure 13-173 (panels A–D). Repetitive monomorphic tachycardia with the characteristic right bundle (with

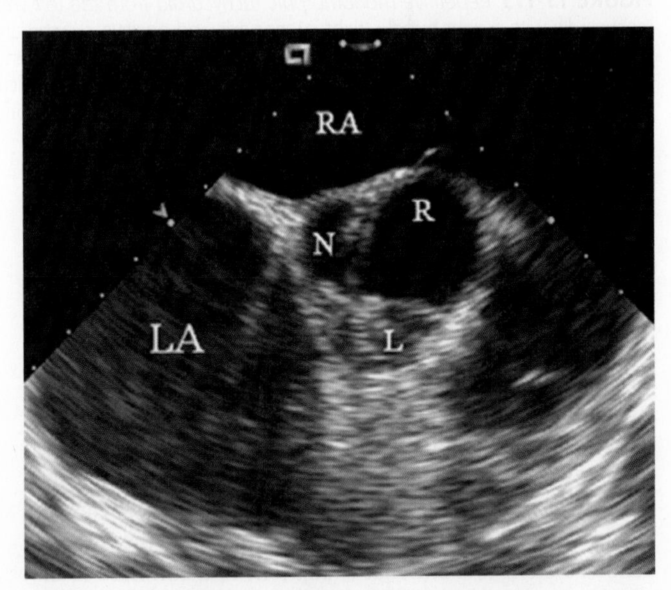


**FIGURE 13-172** *Use of intracardiac echocardiography to map the sinuses of Valsalva.* The image transducer is placed in the right atrium in this example, though this cross-sectional view of the aortic valve is often easier to obtain with the transducer in the RV outflow tract. A mapping catheter is seen with the left cusp (L). Imaging can assist in mapping the entire semilunar dimension of both the left and right cusps.

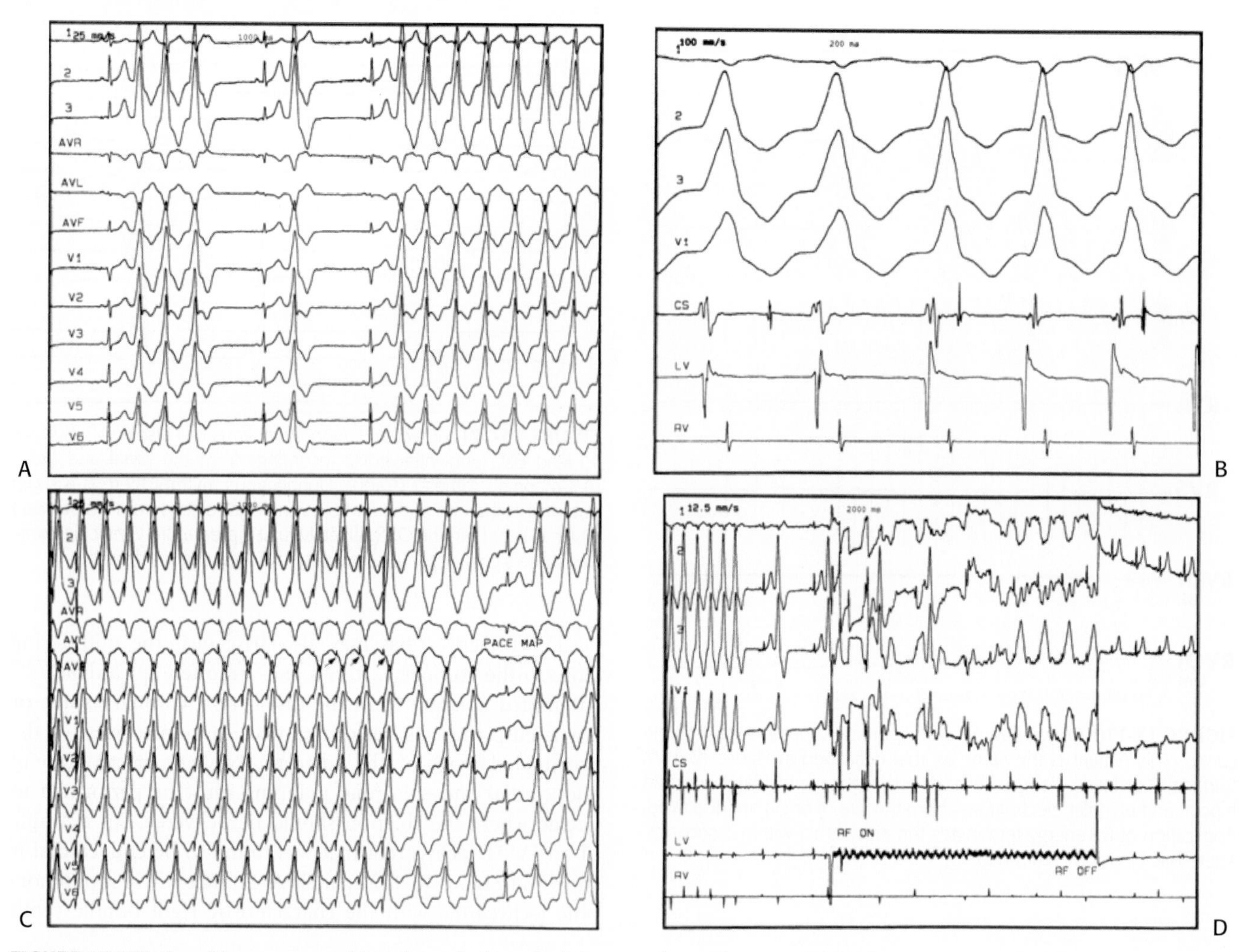


**FIGURE 13-173** *Repetitive monomorphic tachycardia from the left ventricular outflow tract.* **Panel A**. Shows repetitive bouts of monomorphic tachycardia with a right bundle, right inferior axis and positive concordance in the precordial leads. **Panel B**. Demonstrates the endocardial earliest site in the LV preceded the earliest site recorded in the coronary sinus. **Panel C**. Demonstrates that pace mapping from the endocardial site that replicates the tachycardia morphology. **Panel D**. Shows RF application at this site that eliminated all episodes of repetitive monomorphic tachycardia. The patient has been free of symptoms and tachycardia off antiarrhythmic agents.

positive concordance in the precordium), right inferior axis morphology is shown in panel A. The tachycardia had an earlier left ventricular endocardial bipolar electrogram than the simultaneously recorded epicardial left ventricular electrogram from the coronary sinus. Earliest activity was seen 35 msec before the QS. A pace map from that site revealed an identical QRS to the tachycardia (panel C) and ablation at that site eliminated all the tachycardia and sustained arrhythmias within seconds. The patient has been free of arrhythmias on no medications. Patients with organic heart disease, particularly hypertrophic ventricles, may also experience triggered rhythms. Occasionally, when VT is mapped from the coronary venous system to a site that is adjacent to a coronary artery, ablation from an "adjacent" location, such as the left coronary cusp or the endocardium can be successful.[405] This, again is an expression of the usual origin of such tachycardias from the crest of the septum or the epicardium of the ostium of the LVOT; various mapping locations can provide a vantage point to approach this source with ablation.

Focal tachycardias which also behave as triggered arrhythmias can arise from the papillary muscles, particularly the posterior medial papillary muscle. These tachycardias can be very difficult to map and ablate, given the confusing and intricate 3D structure, high degree of motility and rich distribution of the Purkinje network (which can facilitate multiple exits from the same site of origin). Considering the papillary muscle as a separate "chamber" on intracardiac echocardiography and/or 3D mapping system can be helpful (Fig. 13-174). VT can also arise from the myocardium close or subjacent to the papillary muscles. An example of a triggered rhythm originating from the lateral wall of the left ventricle adjacent to the papillary muscle in a patient with hypertensive cardiomyopathy is shown in Figure 13-175. The earliest endocardial electrogram is 78 msec before the QRS and is associated with a sharp negative intrinsic deflection. RF energy delivered at that site terminated the arrhythmia after 3 seconds. The patient has been free of arrhythmias and on no medications. The range of activation times at the earliest site of triggered rhythms ranges

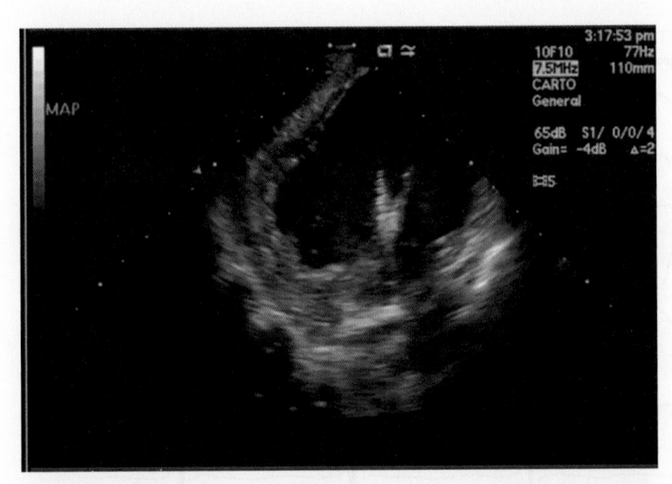


**FIGURE 13-174** *Use of three-dimensional ultrasound reconstruction to map papillary muscle VT.* This figure shows a 3D electroanatomic map constructed of individual 2D slices of LV intracardiac echo images (Biosense Webster, CARTO Sound). After reconstruction, the posterior medial papillary muscle was considered a separate "chamber" and activation mapping was performed in the context of that anatomy.

from 25 to 90 msec, the latter only occurring in the presence of organic heart disease.

A second variety of idiopathic ventricular tachycardia is that arising in the left ventricle, which is reentrant and verapamil-sensitive.[398,401,406–408] This tachycardia has a characteristic of an RBBB, left superior axis morphology or right superior axis morphology and has its earliest ventricular activation either at the level of the posterior third or apical third of the septum, respectively. These tachycardias characteristically have relatively narrow QRS complexes and rapid initial forces in the absence of antiarrhythmic drugs or associated, but unrelated, hypertrophy. These tachycardias, as described in Chapter 11, are reentrant in nature because:

1. They can be induced and terminated by programmed stimulation.
2. They exhibit an inverse relationship between the initiating coupling interval and the first complex of the tachycardia.
3. Entrainment and resetting with fusion are possible from multiple sites in the right ventricle and from the atrium as well.

Electrograms in sinus rhythm are normal although in some patients isolated diastolic potentials have been reported and identify a critical entrance to a zone of slow conduction (see below). In my experience, the tachycardias with a right bundle, left superior axis morphology are more reproducibly initiated and stable than those with right superior axis. There are multiple opinions as to what is the best methodology to use to guide ablation of these arrhythmias. Activation mapping has been used, but the guidelines for target have varied depending on the authors. Some authors recommend looking for the earliest Purkinje spike, which precedes the onset of ventricular activation as the target for ablation.[409] An example of sinus rhythm and a tachycardia demonstrating Purkinje potentials prior to the onset of the tachycardia is shown in Figure 13-176. Another example of such a Purkinje potential preceding the QRS associated with a QS unipolar recording is shown in Figure 13-177. Jackman's group[409] has popularized this method and has a superb success rate using this method. The number of ablations required, however, to successfully treat these arrhythmias using this method is unclear. Moreover, identifying the earliest Purkinje spike may be quite difficult since they are ubiquitous on the septum in the region of these arrhythmias. I don't personally believe that the Purkinje fiber is critical to successful ablation. An example of a patient in whom a Purkinje fiber was identified after the onset of the earliest bipolar and unipolar recording, yet in whom ablation was successful at that site, is shown in Figure 13-178. The earliest bipolar electrogram preceded the QS by only 25 msec with the Purkinje spike appearing 10 msec before the QRS (but after local LV activation). Nonetheless RF application delivered at this site, which was the earliest site of ventricular activation, eliminated the tachycardia in less than 300 msec.

Entrainment mapping has also been used successfully, but is extremely difficult to achieve. I have accomplished this in only two patients. Occasionally an exact entrainment map is possible, a fact I believe occurred because of a very small isthmus and/or reentrant circuit that is present in these patients. An example of an entrainment map is shown in Figure 13-179. In both patients in whom entrainment mapping was achieved, delivery of RF energy at that was immediately successful. Two groups have described the presence of late diastolic potentials in sinus rhythm as well as during the tachycardia that defined a potential entrance to the slowly conducting pathway in the circuit.[410,411] These investigators described diastolic potentials that follow the QRS by a fixed period of time and are associated with a changing relationship to the subsequent QRS, which is preceded by a Purkinje potential. I, too, have seen such potentials in a majority of our patients. The Purkinje potential associated with the diastolic potential is, however, never the earliest Purkinje potential recorded, and may not even be recorded (Fig. 13-180). Antegrade Purkinje conduction is suggested in Figure 13-180, panel C. The delay induced by pacing or associated with spontaneous oscillations occurs between the late diastolic potential and the Purkinje spike (Fig. 13-181). Ablation at these sites produced delay between the diastolic potential and Purkinje spike until the tachycardia is terminated at which time the diastolic potential remains as a late potential in sinus rhythm. An example of ablation of one of these VTs at a site with a diastolic potential, but no Purkinje potential is shown in Figure 13-182. The antegrade limb of the reentrant circuit (i.e., diastolic pathway) appears to be sensitive to verapamil (prior to the diastolic EGM), lidocaine and procainamide may also terminate the VT, but in the few cases reported this occurs between the diastolic potential and the Purkinje potential or the ventricular EGM.[410] The retrograde limb of the circuit is unclear. My concept of the circuit in this VT is described in Figure 13-183. Although most people believe the Purkinje system is involved, I do not for

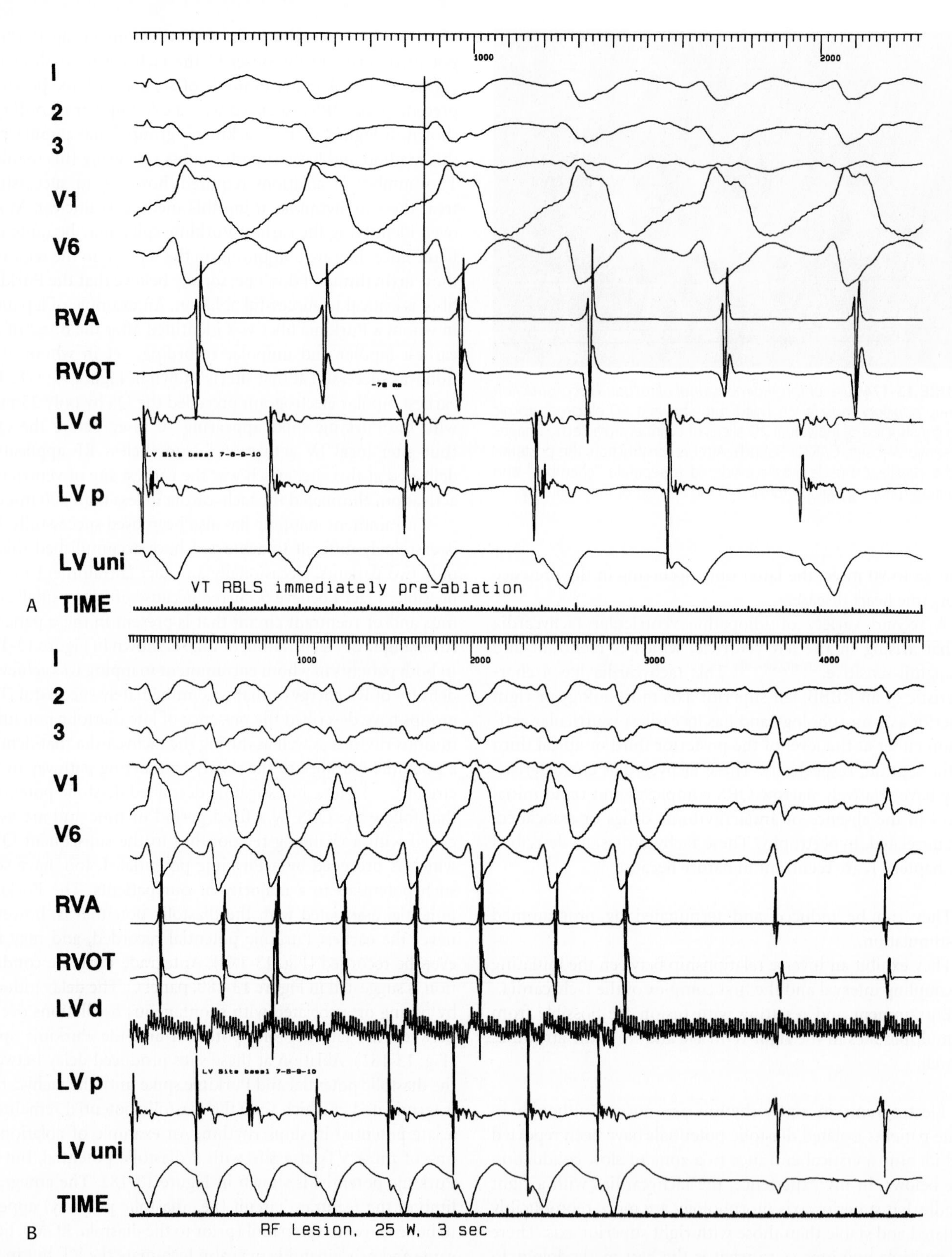


**FIGURE 13-175** *Ablation of ventricular tachycardia due to triggered activity in a patient with hypertensive cardiomyopathy.* **A:** VT with an RBBB pattern is shown. The earliest mapped site came from the posterolateral free wall (7-8-9-10) and was 78 msec before the QRS. Bipolar and unipolar (pole #2) electrograms recorded from this site are shown. **B:** Following delivery of RF energy (25 W) for 3 seconds, the VT slows, oscillates, and terminates. RF energy was delivered for a total of 45 seconds. The VT was no longer inducible.

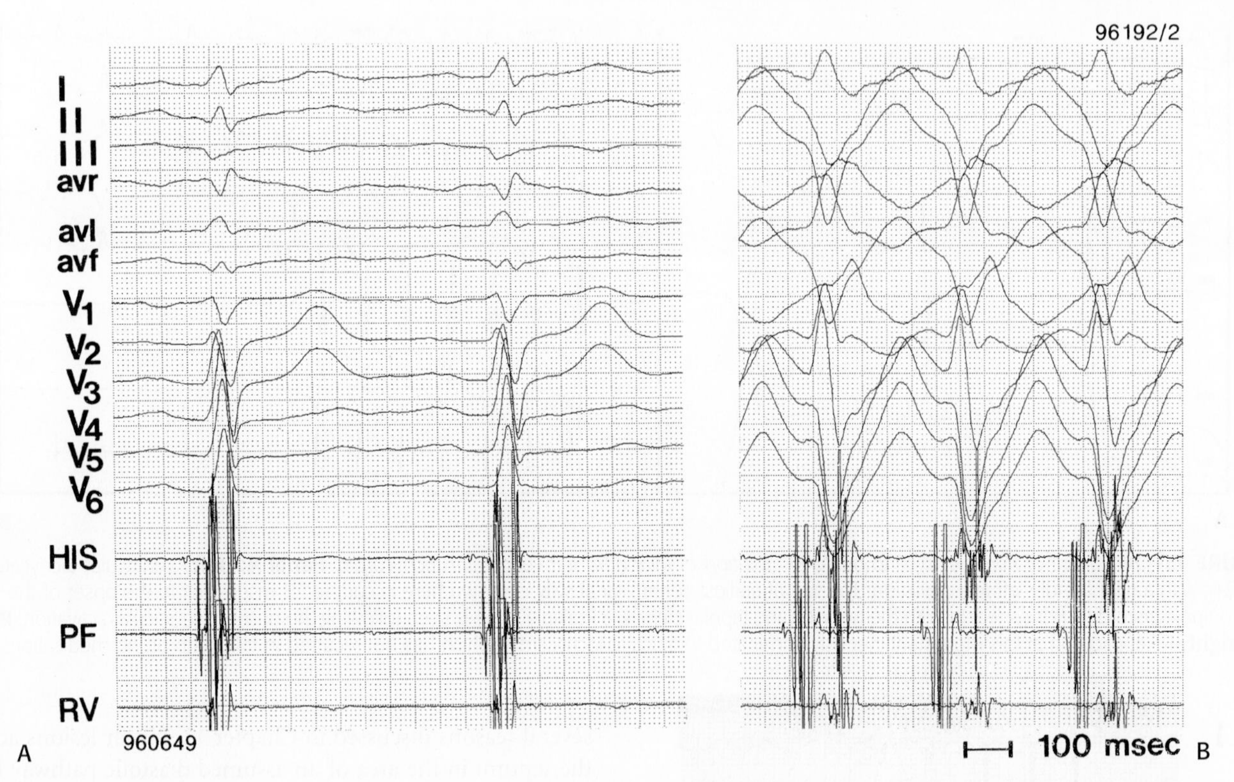


**FIGURE 13-176** *Purkinje potentials in idiopathic left ventricular tachycardia.* **Panel A:** Sinus rhythm is shown. A Purkinje fiber potential proceeds each QRS. **Panel B:** During the tachycardia, the site at which the Purkinje spike was recorded in sinus rhythm records a Purkinje spike proceeding the QRS. This site was targeted for RF ablation, which was successful.

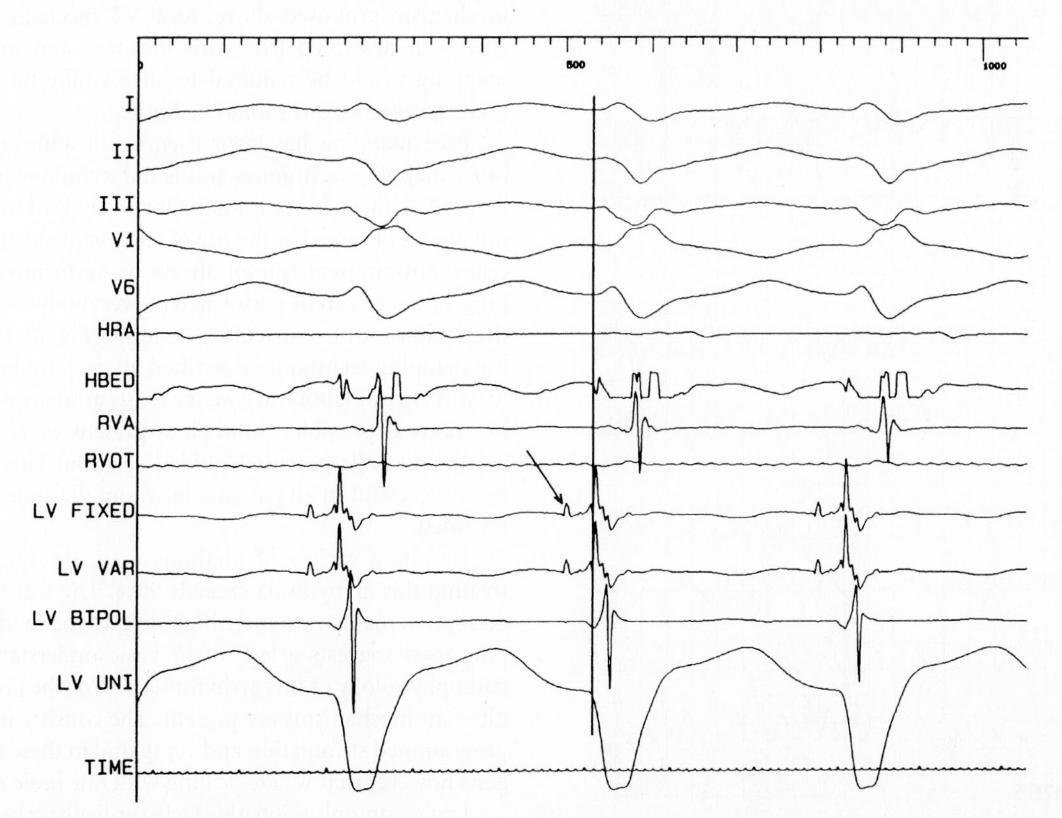


**FIGURE 13-177** *Purkinje potential associated with earliest site of ventricular activation.* Idiopathic left ventricular tachycardia is shown with bipolar and unipolar recordings. The earliest site of ventricular activation is shown. The unipolar recording shows a QS configuration and the bipolar recording proceeds the onset of the QRS by 25 msec. This in turn is preceded by a Purkinje spike by an additional 30 msec. This site was a successful site of RF ablation of this tachycardia.

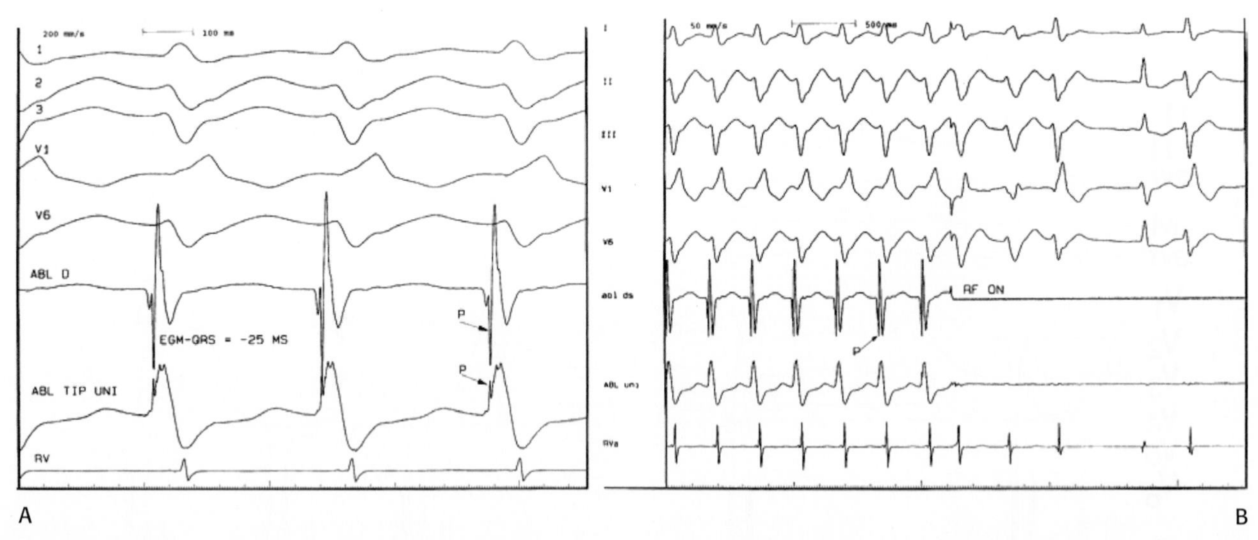

FIGURE 13-178 *Failure of Purkinje spike to guide RF ablation of idiopathic left ventricular tachycardia.* **Panel A:** (**left**) Ventricular tachycardia is present with a right bundle left axis deviation. The site of earliest ventricular activity is shown here occurring 25 msec prior to the onset of the QRS. The unipolar recording is inverted. In both the unipolar and bipolar signals, a Purkinje spike is seen following the onset of ventricular activation. **Panel B:** (**right**) RF application at this site instantaneously terminated ventricular tachycardia, which has not recurred in follow-up on no medications.

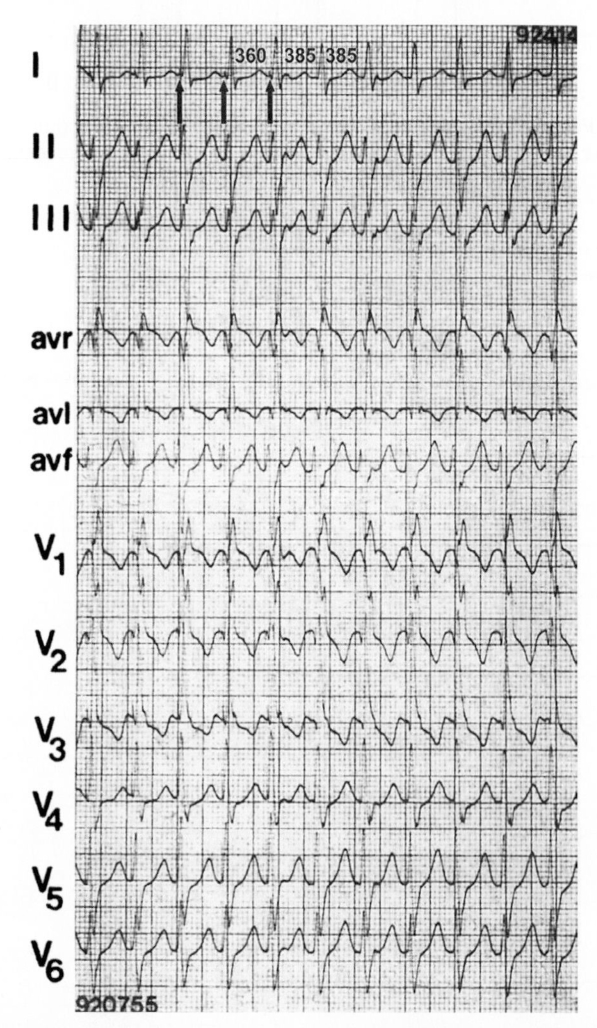

FIGURE 13-179 *Entrainment mapping of idiopathic left ventricular tachycardia.* A 12-lead ECG during entrainment (**left**) and resumption of VT (**right**) demonstrates an exact entrainment map and a return cycle identical to the VT cycle length.

several reasons discussed in Chapter 11. Linear lesions across the septum in the area of an assumed diastolic pathway have been proposed in patients in whom the VT cannot be induced particularly after catheter-induced trauma.[412] While this may be reasonable in patients in whom the VT has the reentrant mechanism proposed above, focal VT mechanisms are have also been described from this location, and more detailed mapping would be required to successfully target these. As such, empiric lesions should be limited.

Pace mapping has been used as an adjuvant to all the other mapping techniques and is the technique least likely to be used as the sole technique. Obviously Purkinje spikes are not always observed at the site of successful ablation and concealed entrainment cannot always be performed. Pace mapping, however, can be performed in everybody as can mapping the earliest site of ventricular activation (Fig. 13-184). Since all the mapping techniques described above have been reported to work, in our laboratory we try to use as many possible combinations as possible, although at present we always initially use the diastolic potential–guided ablation. This method has been successful in all patients in whom diastolic signals were recorded.

Despite a variety of methods used, the success rate for treating this arrhythmia exceeds 90%. The fact that the success rate remains extremely high despite the method of mapping used suggests a lack of or basic understanding of the pathophysiology of this arrhythmia and/or the possibility that different mechanisms are present. The consistent response to programmed stimulation and verapamil in these patients suggests however that we are dealing with one basic mechanism.

Less commonly idiopathic tachycardias have been described arising on or near the epicardium which are reentrant.[413] Whether these are truly idiopathic or represent sequelae of unrecognized myopericarditis is unclear. Epicardial mapping and

## DIASTOLIC POTENTIALS AND IDIOPATHIC LV VT

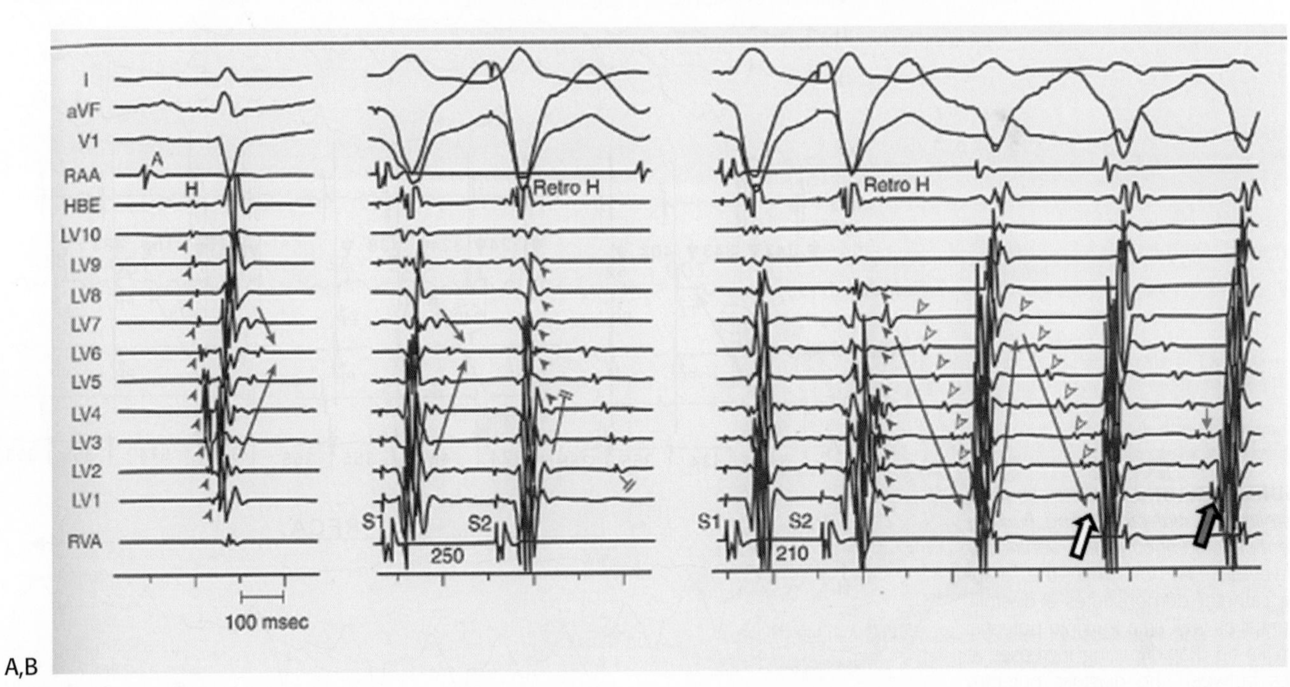


**FIGURE 13-180** *Relationship of diastolic potentials and idiopathic VT.* Electrograms from a decapolar catheter placed from superior basal to mid-inferior LV septum. During sinus rhythm sequential antegrade His–Purkinje activation is seen (*filled arrowheads* **Panel A**). Late poentials represent activation in two directions. With VPDs (**Panel B**), there is block in retrograde propagation of the late potential followed by prolonged antegrade activation. No VT is induced. Note apparent Purkinje potentials on EGMs from LV3 and LV4. With an earlier VPD, VT is induced. VT onset is the latest diastolic potential, which is associated with a later Purkinje potential. An earlier Purkinje potential is seen in LV3 which appears to conduct distally. See text.

entrainment mapping as described above in Chagas disease are utilized.

### Catheter Ablation of Miscellaneous Ventricular Tachycardias

Bundle branch reentrant ventricular tachycardias are macroreentrant ventricular arrhythmias using the right and left bundle branches in either an antegrade or a retrograde direction. These are described in detail in Chapter 11. While there is varied opinion about how frequently bundle branch reentrant ventricular tachycardias are responsible for spontaneously occurring events, it is clear that they can cause cardiac arrest in patients with prior conduction disturbances, particularly those with cardiomyopathy (idiopathic, hypertrophic, or "ischemic"). Patients with cardiomyopathy most frequently have bundle branch reentry using the right bundle antegradely and the left bundle retrogradely (Fig. 13-185). These patients almost always have a left-sided intraventricular conduction disturbance in sinus rhythm with a long H-V. In such patients, ablation of the right bundle branch can cure the arrhythmia.[414–416] The left bundle branch can also be a site of ablation and is equally as effective. Moreover, left bundle branch ablation is not fraught with the potential complication of heart block, because the bundle branch that has the greatest conduction delay in sinus rhythm is the bundle branch that is ablated. Nevertheless, because of ease of the approach, the right bundle branch is most frequently ablated. I do not generally ablate bundle branch reentrant VT unless it is the sole arrhythmia a patient has. This may be the case in patients with myotonic dystrophy or primary conduction disturbances, in which case a primary ablative approach is reasonable. However, in patients with cardiomyopathy, multiple VT types are commonly present; in such instances an ICD is placed, with or without the use of antiarrhythmic therapy. If recurrent shocks due to bundle branch reentry occur, ablation is a reasonable approach. Reversed bundle branch reentrant tachycardia, that is, with an RBBB configuration, is much rarer. As stated in Chapter 11, I have only seen one such patient who has had this as the sole arrhythmia. In that patient, ablation of the right bundle branch cured the tachycardia (see Chapter 11).

Another tachycardia that uses the His–Purkinje conduction system is intrafascicular reentry. This also is described in detail in Chapter 11. This disorder almost always occurs in patients with prior myocardial infarction and bifascicular block. Occasionally, it may occur in patients without infarction who have bifascicular block. In this instance the right bundle branch is permanently blocked in both directions. One of the fascicles that appears blocked is in fact slowly conducting. With the development of block in that one fascicle, a

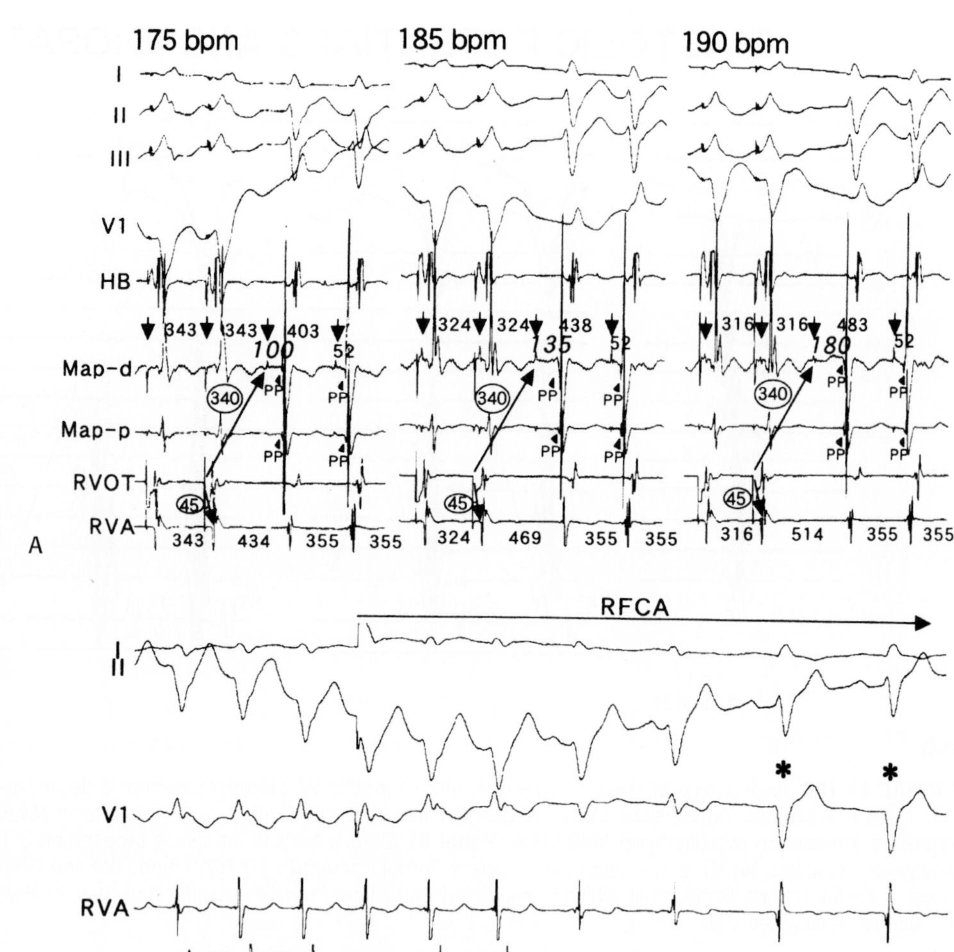


**FIGURE 13-181** *Demonstration of diastolic potential proceeding Purkinje potential in idiopathic left ventricular tachycardia.* **A:** On **top**, the mapping catheter demonstrates a diastolic potential as well as a Purkinje potential from its tip. Rapid pacing increases at times between the diastolic potential and the Purkinje potential. **B: (bottom)** RF energy at this site produced progressive prolongation between the diastolic potential and the Purkinje spike until failure of conduction occurred between the diastolic potential and the Purkinje spike terminating ventricular tachycardia. In the two sinus complexes that follow, the diastolic potential now appears as a late diastolic potential, while the Purkinje spike proceeds the QRS. See text for discussion. (From Tsuchiya T, Okumura K, Honda T, et al. Significance of late diastolic potential preceding Purkinje potential in Verapamil-sensitive idiopathic left ventricular tachycardia. *Circulation* 1999; 99:2408–2413.)

macroreentrant circuit is set up using the "primary conducting fascicle" antegradely and the antegradely blocked fascicle in the retrograde direction. Thus the tachycardia morphology is identical to that of the sinus rhythm since the sinus QRS complex is dominated by conduction only over the primary conducting fascicle as it is during intrafascicular reentry. This tachycardia is characterized by an H-V interval significantly shorter than that in sinus (usually 40 to 80 msec shorter). Activation of the conducting system goes from left bundle branch to the His bundle and then to the proximal right bundle branch. The reason for the shortened H-V is the fact that the H-V interval is determined by antegrade conduction from the turnaround site in the fascicle minus the retrograde conduction to the His bundle. Ablation of such tachycardias is not only difficult, but is virtually never curative since these patients typically have large infarctions and multiple arrhythmias. It is worth ablating them when these tachycardias become incessant, as they can.[417] In such instances, ablation of the fascicles may be difficult and ablation at the bifurcation of the left bundle is most easily accomplished. In such instances a pacemaker is virtually always necessary. Since in both bundle branch reentry and intrafascicular reentry, myocardial dysfunction is the dominant clinical problem, and other ventricular tachycardias are frequently present, an ICD with dual chamber pacing capability is the most important therapy.

Ventricular tachycardia can be a complication of surgery for tetralogy of Fallot. This usually takes the form of a macroreentrant circuit around the ventriculotomy incision at the outflow tract. Mapping of this tachycardia usually shows a complete reentrant circuit around the ventriculotomy scar in either a clockwise or counterclockwise direction (Fig. 13-186). The majority of such patients have tachycardias circulating in

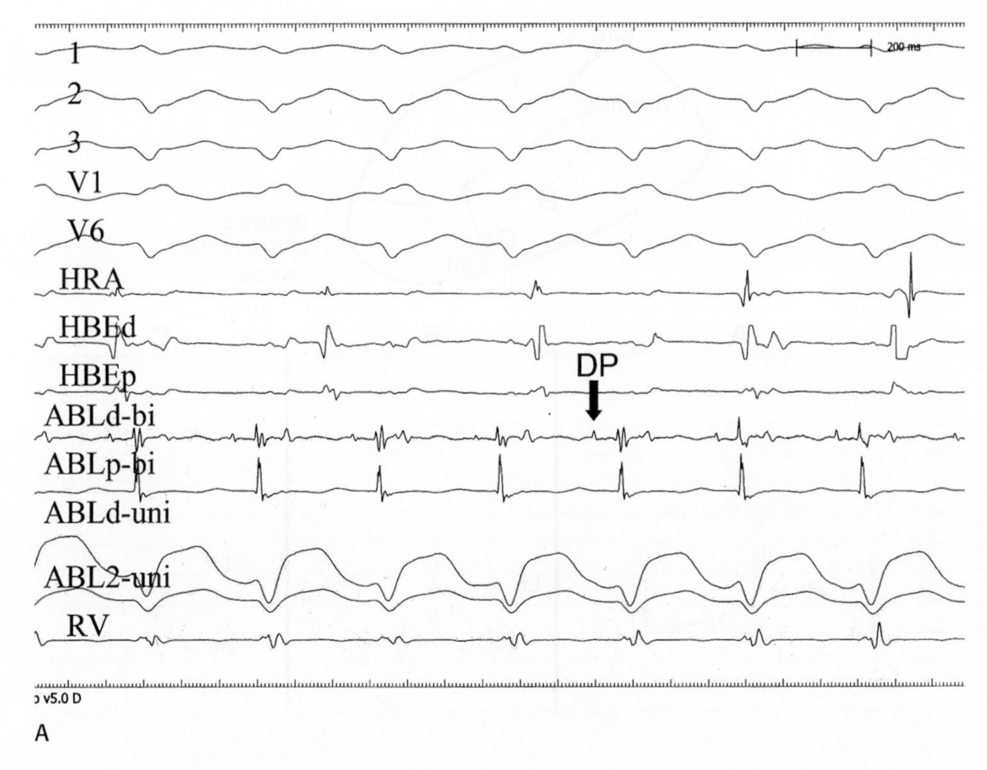


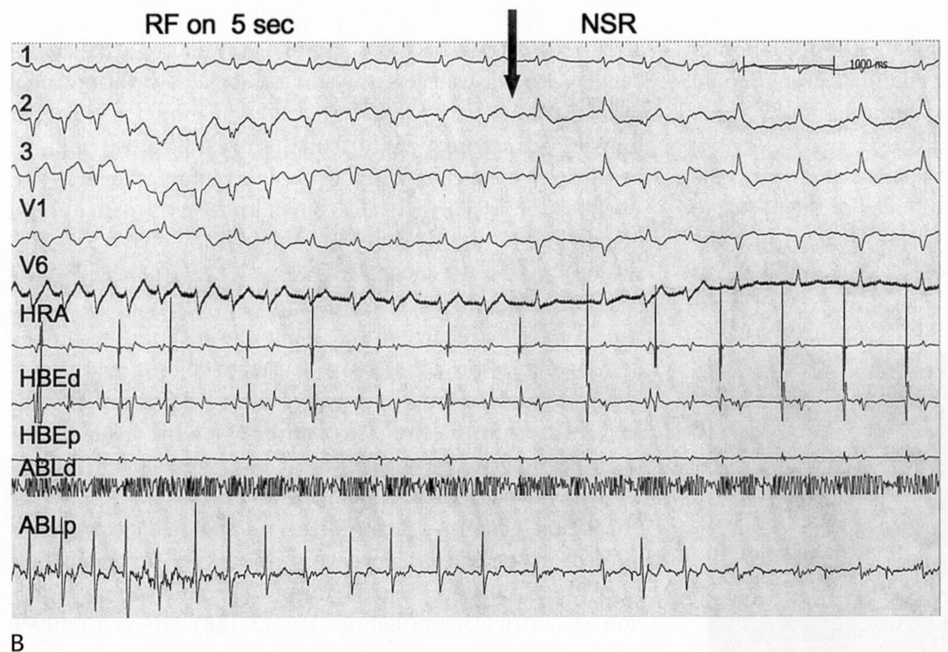


**FIGURE 13-182** *RF ablation of idiopathic left ventricular tachycardia guided by a diastolic potential in the absence of a Purkinje potential.* **A:** Ventricular tachycardia is seen. A diastolic potential is observed at a site that demonstrates neither a Purkinje potential nor the earliest ventricular activation. **B:** Application of RF energy at this site terminates the tachycardia. A late potential is seen after the sinus complexes. See text for discussion.

a clockwise fashion around the ventriculotomy or infundibulotomy usually and utilize the conotruncal isthmus.[418,419] The morphology of this tachycardia is dictated by the pattern of activation around the scar. Most commonly, an LBBB or RBBB and right inferior axis is seen during clockwise rotation around the scar. Less commonly, an LBBB left axis morphology is noted. In the past, this tachycardia was approached easily with cardiac surgery in which completion of the ventriculotomy scar to the pulmonary valve cured the tachycardia. One must make sure, however, that the tachycardia does not arise at a different site. Occasionally tachycardias arise in the region of the ventricular septal defect repair in which case an isthmus is present between the circling wavefront and the tricuspid annulus. Ablation of that isthmus with cryothermal application, RF application, or transection by scalpel can cure this arrhythmia. Detailed mapping and entrainment techniques are obviously necessary to discern the critical sites for ablation. Recently, electroanatomical mapping has allowed one to map and ablate such rhythms with RF catheter ablation (Fig. 13-186). The principals are the same. If one can demonstrate circus movement around the

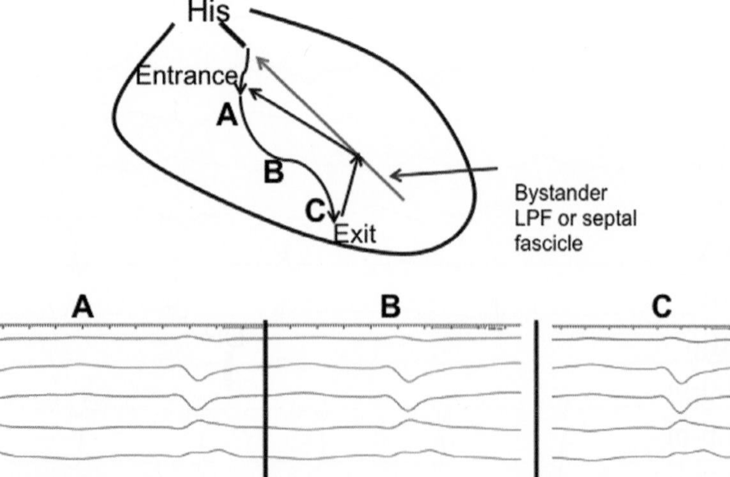


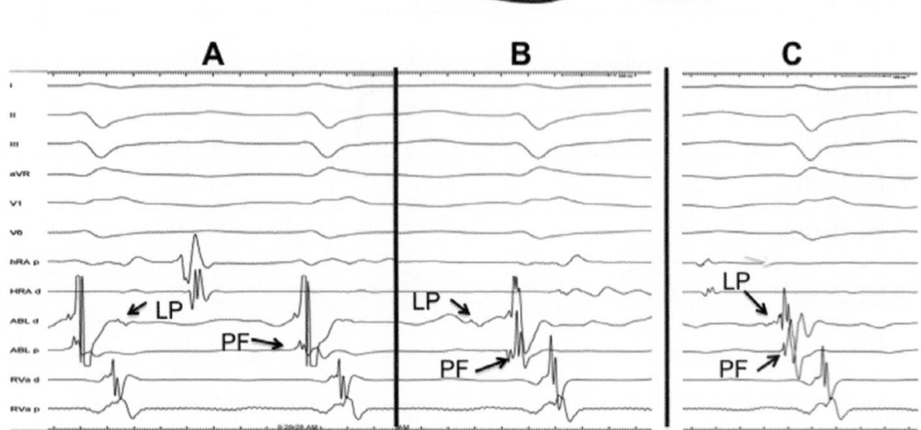


**FIGURE 13-183** *Reentrant circuit of Verapamil Sensitive VT.* On the top is a schema of the reentrant circuit. Antegrade conduction goes from high septum toward the inferior septum (**A**, **B**, **C**) over a decrementally conducting, verapamil-sensitive pathway. The retrograde limb which is not well characterized is attached to the distal Purkinje system (septal or posterior fascicle) which acts as a bystander. **Panels A, B, and C** below are recordings from the corresponding points in the schema. One can see a late potentials (LP) moving more distal. In **C** the LP is adjacent to the Purkinje fiber potential (PF). See text for discussion.

ventriculotomy scar, the VT can be cured by RF application to extend the scar to the pulmonary valve. Alternatively one could theoretically cure the VT by creating a linear lesion from the ventriculotomy scar to the tricuspid valve.

Another congenital anomaly that is associated with ventricular tachyarrhythmias is Ebstein anomaly of the tricuspid valve. In this disorder the tricuspid valve displaced into the ventricle creating an atrialized portion of the ventricle. This atrialized ventricle becomes part of a very dilated atrial chamber. As such, the wall gets thin and is associated with abnormal fractionated signals. We have recently encountered a patient in whom an automatic ventricular tachycardia arose from the atrialized ventricle just distal to the His bundle recording site. The location is schematically shown in the electroanatomical map in Figure 13-187, panel A. A single lesion delivered at this site terminated the tachycardia (Fig. 13-187, panel B). Ventricular tachyarrhythmias can occur in a variety of disorders, and if they are recurrent and stable the mapping technique described in prior sections can be used to ablate them.

A recent report by Nademanee describes epicardial catheter ablation in the Brugada syndrome for the treatment of recurrent ventricular fibrillation.[420] In nine patients with typical type I Brugada ECG patterns and recurrent ventricular fibrillation, ablation of low voltage, fractionated electrograms located on the epicardial aspect of the RVOT not only abolished the Brugada ECG pattern, but prevented acute induction of ventricular fibrillation (Fig. 13-188). No recurrent VF was noted in average 20 months' follow-up; all patients except one (who remained on amiodarone) were withdrawn from antiarrhythmic drugs.

**FIGURE 13-184** *Use of pace mapping and ventricular activation to guide ablation in idiopathic left ventricular tachycardia.* Pace mapping and activation mapping provide the only method of observing RF ablation in the absence of entrainment mapping.

## Intraoperative Mapping and Surgical Ablation of Ventricular Tachycardias

With the development and wide spread utilization of implantable defibrillator therapy, the practice of surgical ablation of ventricular arrhythmias has diminished considerably. The development of curative surgery for ventricular arrhythmias in healed infarction provided so much insight

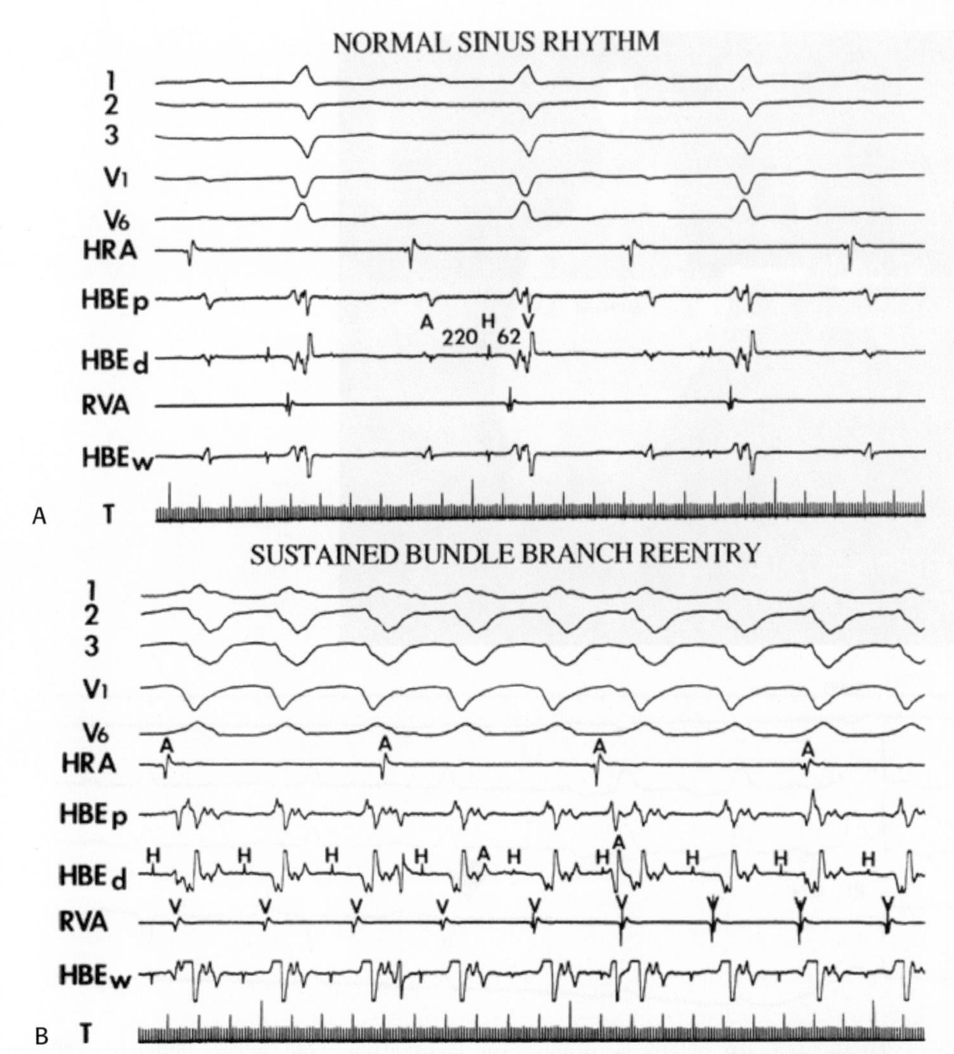


**FIGURE 13-185** *Ventricular tachycardia that is due to bundle branch reentry.* **A:** ECG in sinus rhythm of a patient with VT that is due to bundle branch reentry **(B)**. In sinus rhythm, there is a left-sided intraventricular conduction defect (IVCD) with a slightly prolonged H-V of 62 msec. **B:** VT that is due to bundle branch reentry is shown. Note that the H-V is similar to that in NSR. A-V dissociation is present. See Chapter 11 and text for discussion.

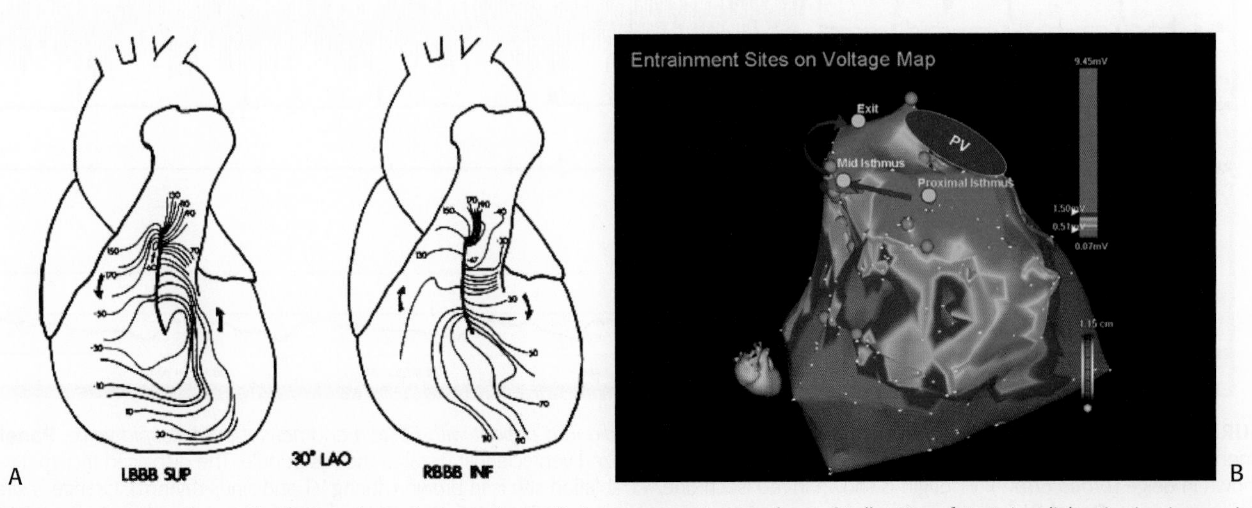


**FIGURE 13-186** *Mapping and ablation of ventricular tachycardia in postoperative tetralogy of Fallot.* **Panel A:** Epicardial activation in ventricular tachycardia following repair of tetralogy of Fallot. Two VTs are present, both showing continuous activity around the ventriculotomy scar. The LBBB superior axis is caused by a counterclockwise activation pattern, while the RBBB inferior axis is caused by a clockwise activation pattern. **Panel B:** Electroanatomic map of VT with a clockwise rotation around infundibulotomy scar. See text for discussion.

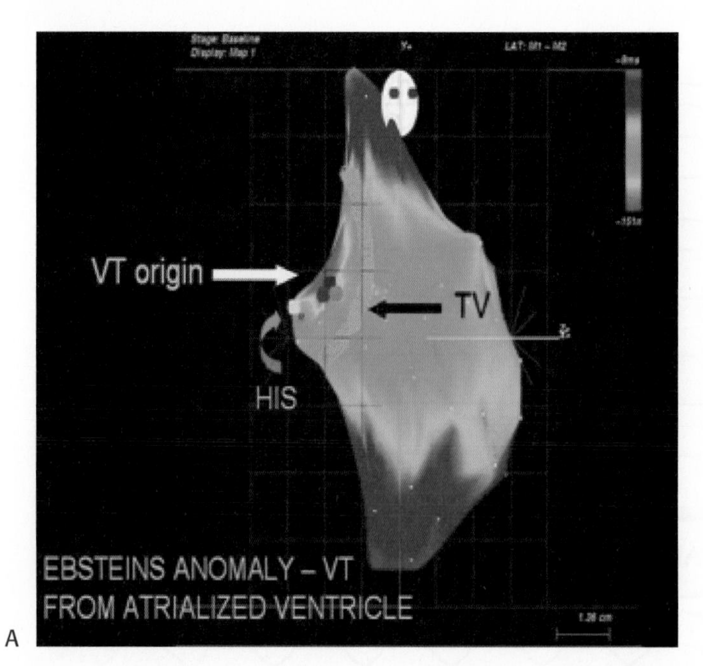


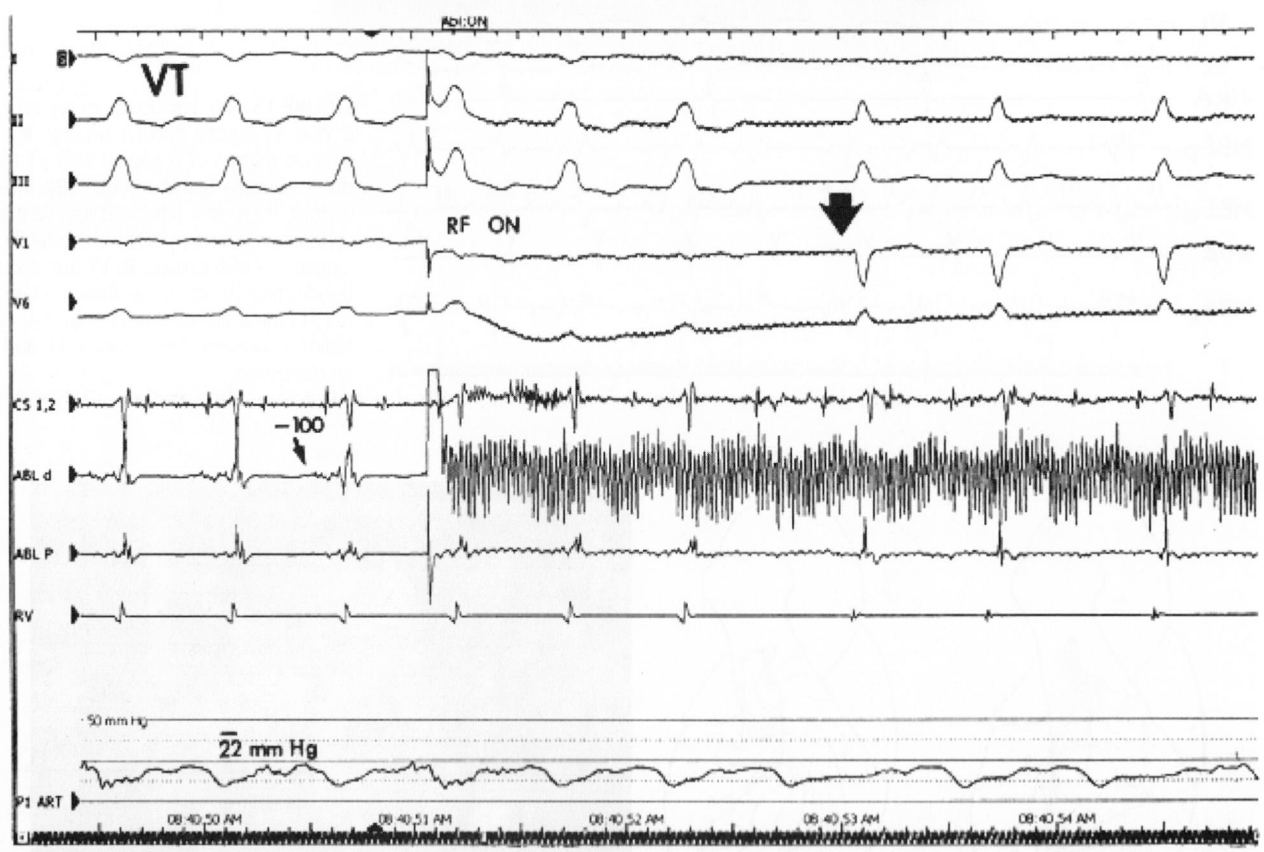


**FIGURE 13-187** *Mapping and ablation of incessant ventricular tachycardia in a patient with Ebstein anomaly of the tricuspid valve.* **Panel A:** Demonstrates an electroanatomic map of automatic VT arising in the atrialized ventricle just distal to the His bundle. The displaced tricuspid valve is shown in beige (*broad arrow*). VT origin is shown in *red* isochrone. VT ablation site is in brown (during VT and sinus rhythm). Orange is site of pressure recording. **Panel B:** Earliest site of activation was 100 msec presystolic and fractionated. RF application terminates VT in 1 second. Note atrial pressure wave at RV recording site (*orange dot* in **Panel A**).

Epicardial Mapping and Ablation in Brugada Syndrome

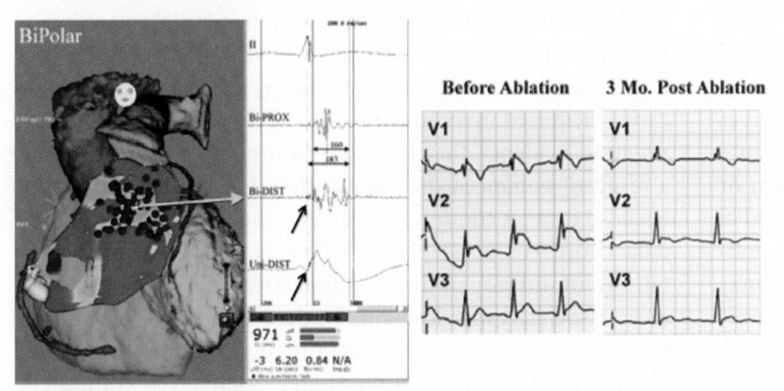


**FIGURE 13-188** *Epicardial ablation in the Brugada syndrome.* The **left panel** shows an electroanatomic voltage map (AP projection) during epicardial mapping of the RVOT in a patient with Brugada syndrome. At the point shown, a broad fractionated electrogram is shown. The surface ECG preprocedure and following ablation is shown in the **right panel**. Ablation of abnormal electrograms on the epicardium of the RVOT can normalize the Brugada ECG pattern. (Adapted from Nademanee K, Veerakul G, Chandanamattha P, et al. Prevention of ventricular fibrillation episodes in Brugada syndrome by catheter ablation over the anterior right ventricular outflow tract epicardium. *Circulation* 2011;123:1270–1279.)

into the pathophysiology of VT and the logic associated with mapping in abnormal myocardium that consideration of this experience continues to be of great value.

Despite the advances in catheter ablation of ventricular tachycardias, the successful ablation of arrhythmias is not uniform. In particular, in the setting of coronary artery disease, surgery offers a single procedure in which coronary revascularization, aneurysmectomy with ventricular remodeling, and cure of ventricular tachyarrhythmias can take place. At present ICDs are used in most institutions, primarily because of ease of implantation, low associated morbidity and mortality, with equal reimbursement as surgery. ICDs, however, do not cure the arrhythmia, or alter the state of vascular disease or myocardial function. Thus, particularly in coronary artery disease in which revascularization is necessary, antiarrhythmic surgery can play an important role. The marked decline in its use is not logical from a medical standpoint, but has been driven by the economics. Catheter mapping is an integral part of any surgical approach to ventricular tachycardia since it offers a greater opportunity to localize all potential tachycardia circuits in an individual patient, something that may not be possible in the operating room under general anesthesia. The role of the electrophysiologist is to select those patients who might benefit from a surgical procedure and localize the tachycardias accurately enough so that the surgeon can ablate the arrhythmogenic area without unnecessarily destroying tissue unrelated to the tachycardia. Obviously, the selection of patients in whom surgery is indicated depends not only on the presence of a drug-resistant tachycardia and the need for revascularization, but on the presence of a team of electrophysiologists and surgeons. The variability of results of surgery, as well as selection of operative candidates, is most dependent on the team of electrophysiologists and surgeons. While the majority of centers refuse to operate on patients with ejection fractions less than 25%, nearly 50% of our arrhythmia surgical patients had ejection fractions lower than 25%. In fact, 27% had ejection fractions less than 20%. In addition to skilled electrophysiologists and surgeons, the desire for a cure must be weighed against the morbidity and mortality of the operation and subsequent morbidity and mortality and success of implanting an ICD for tachycardia termination and defibrillation. In centers in which a team of surgeons and electrophysiologists do not have significant experience in arrhythmia surgery, ICDs are a reasonable approach. Nevertheless, I believe surgery is underutilized and should still be considered as an important option for patients with ventricular tachycardia (stable or unstable) caused by coronary artery disease who (a) require revascularization; (b) are undergoing aneurysmectomy and/or mitral valve placement for ventricular dysfunction associated with prior infarction; and (c) have recurrent VT, early after an infarction, and who need revascularization.[421] Surgery should also be considered in those patients with ventricular tachycardia following repair of tetralogy of Fallot in whom catheter ablation cannot be performed. Obviously, in patients with coronary artery disease, percutaneous revascularization and VT ablation is an alternative to surgical intervention and carries with it a lower mortality and morbidity. However, this approach does not address the marked ventricular dysfunction that is associated with aneurysms.

In all patients who are candidates for ventricular tachycardia surgery, an identifiable substrate for the VT should be present (i.e., either prior infarction or prior surgery). The substrate provides a rational basis for undertaking surgery, even in the absence of mapping, although this is less desirable. In such patients arrhythmia surgery may be directed at the electrophysiologic substrate either by direct visualization of the substrate (e.g., myocardial scar) or the presence of abnormal electrical signals that identify the substrate (sinus rhythm mapping showing fragmented electrograms). It is important to recognize that in the presence of such a substrate, tachycardias are almost always inducible and, if tolerated, are mappable in the electrophysiology laboratory and are certainly mappable in the operating room regardless of the hemodynamic status. In patients with an inducible sustained monomorphic tachycardia who presented with a cardiac arrest, revascularization alone is insufficient to prevent the arrhythmia. The ability to induce this arrhythmia implies the presence of a fixed substrate, and either percutaneous or operative revascularization has not been shown to alter this substrate.[4,340] While ICDs can improve survival, they certainly do not alter the frequency of such arrhythmic events. Revascularization should only be considered a primary therapy for cardiac arrest in patients with no inducible arrhythmias and multivessel disease, with a positive thallium test and ejection fractions greater than 40% without significant scar.

Once in the operating room, map-guided surgery provides the best results for sustained uniform tachycardias because (a) 15% of tachycardias arise outside regions of visible scar or abnormal electrograms; (b) in the setting of recent myocardial infarction, visible landmarks of the entire arrhythmogenic substrate are not distinct and well defined; (c) tachycardias may arise in deeper areas of the myocardium that would not normally be addressed by routine, nonmap-guided procedures. A variety of surgical procedures have been developed to manage VT. These involve resection, incision, cryoablation, laser photoablation/coagulation, or combinations of the above, of the arrhythmogenic tissue. All of these procedures may be map-guided, or either visually directed or electrogram-directed (sinus rhythm mapping) to remove or isolate the pathophysiologic substrate. Of the nonmap-guided procedures, extended subendocardial resection, encircling subendocardial ventriculotomy or cryoablation, an extended laser photocoagulation/vaporization, have been employed. DC ablation via a mapping balloon catheter has also been used. Details of these operative procedures have been reviewed elsewhere.[4,5,13–16] The relative merits of surgery versus other procedures have also been reviewed.[421–423]

## Intraoperative Mapping Techniques for Ventricular Tachycardia

Sequential point-by-point activation during a sustained tachycardia, using a hand-held stick or finger electrode, was the first mapping method used and is still useful. This technique obviously requires a stable monomorphic tachycardia for all designated mapping sites to be acquired. Simultaneous multisite data acquisition systems using either preformed plaques, epicardial sock electrodes, or endocavitary balloon electrodes are also available. Harris et al.[307] were the first to use simultaneous balloon endocardial and sock epicardial mapping to localize the tachycardia sites of origin. Most of these multisite data acquisition systems are computerized and allow acquisition of 64 to 256 simultaneous sites of activation. Many of these are commercially available, although several institutions have developed their own in-house systems. These computer techniques should be user-friendly and interactive. Obviously, these systems will allow assessment of nonsustained arrhythmias. Regardless of the ability to record multiple sites, several limitations still exist. These include (a) an unknown relevance of nonsustained or polymorphic arrhythmias to the spontaneous sustained arrhythmias that a patient has exhibited; (b) the inability for the computer to accurately analyze low-amplitude multicomponent signals, for which no good software program exists; (c) the inability of the computer to deal with intermittent signals; (d) the length of time it takes for the investigator to completely check and validate the computer-designated activation times. Moreover, while these tools offer exceptional power to further understand the arrhythmogenic mechanisms, reentrant pathways, and the physiology of initiation and termination of arrhythmias, it is uncertain whether they have added to the success of surgery. Although more data can be acquired in a shorter period of time, there is at present no good evidence that the surgical results have improved as a result of enhanced data acquisition. In part this may result because it takes too long to validate the computer-generated data (hours to days). As noted previously, additional limitations of intraoperative computerized mapping are those areas associated with low-amplitude multicomponent signals, which frequently exhibit intermittent conduction or block, phenomena that cannot be accurately analyzed by computers, and the ability to use the system because of failure to induce all arrhythmias observed preoperatively. As stated earlier, catheter mapping and identifying the areas of interest before entering the operating room offer the best opportunity to deal with these problems. As such, simplified techniques that are directed toward areas of interest have yielded a surgical efficacy comparable to or exceeding the results using computers costing several hundred thousands of dollars. Thus, the greater the expertise and understanding of the ventricular arrhythmias, the less equipment required to perform successful surgery. This in no way detracts from the importance of computer-assisted data acquisition. Such rapid data acquisition can shorten mapping time and allow exploration of both the epicardium and endocardium in more patients than when a computerized activation system is not available. Of note, most of the activation maps of human VT demonstrate a monoregional onset of activation with centrifugal spread from that site[307,340,424–426] although figure-of-eight reentry and continuous circular reentrant activation have also been recorded.[303,304,307,340,426] Nonetheless, in my opinion the most important use of the computer is to achieve a greater understanding of the mechanisms underlying the arrhythmias and to map the pathways of reentrant excitation. Ultimately this may allow further development of ablative techniques that can be applied without opening the heart. The virtual cessation of surgical approaches to treat ventricular tachyarrhythmias has prevented us from learning more about their mechanisms and subsequently limited our ability to further understand these arrhythmias. Since we have had the largest surgical series of patients with ventricular tachycardia, I will describe our results, which are primarily on the finger point roving mapping along with small plaques of 20 to 40 simultaneous electrodes and, when appropriate, we will relate these data to those obtained using computerized systems.

Most of the intraoperative mapping data that have been acquired have come from patients with VT associated with coronary artery disease. As such, the following paragraphs will specifically relate to data acquired in patients with coronary artery disease; those patients with tachycardia arising from other disorders will be briefly mentioned at the end of this section. The majority of patients with VT associated with coronary artery disease have large myocardial infarctions frequently

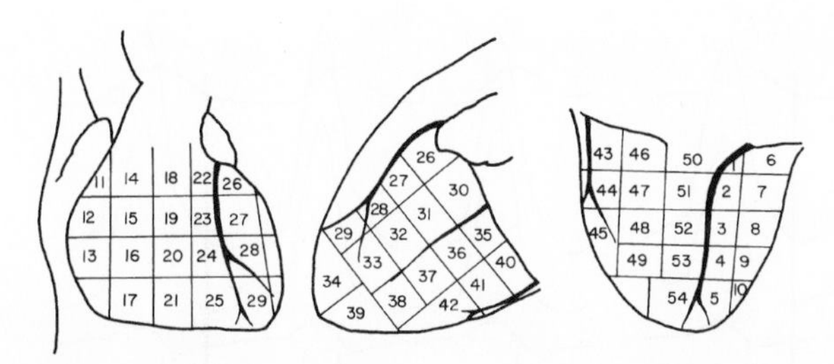

**FIGURE 13-189** *Epicardial mapping schema.* The heart is shown in the anterior, left lateral, and inferoposterior view. Fifty-four predetermined mapping sites are marked.

associated with left ventricular aneurysms. Depending on the patient population, aneurysms are present in nearly 85% of patients with VT associated with anterior apical infarctions and in 50% of patients with VT associated with inferior infarctions. Patient selection markedly influences the reported incidence of aneurysms and the ejection fractions in the surgical series. The differences in anatomy of patients operated on give rise to different results of activation mapping, because certain patterns of activation are more commonly associated with particular anatomies. Thus, patients with left ventricular aneurysms usually have subendocardial sites of origin, while those tachycardias associated with blotchy, nontransmural infarctions with aneurysms may have subendocardial, intramural, or subepicardial sites of origin (see subsequent paragraphs).

Endocardial and/or epicardial mapping may be performed sequentially by a hand-held probe or plaque or simultaneously by computerized multisite acquisition. When sequential mapping procedures are employed, a predetermined grid delineating sites to be mapped is used. An example of such a grid that we use for epicardial mapping is shown in Figure 13-189 in which electrograms from 54 epicardial segments are sampled. Our endocardial mapping system is shown in Figure 13-190. Following an anterior or inferior ventriculotomy into a scarred area, endocardial mapping is undertaken in a clockwise fashion using 12 sites at 1-cm increasing radii. With anterior infarction, noon is taken as that point that is closest to the junction of the free wall and apical septum following ventriculotomy or aneurysmectomy. With inferior infarction, the longitudinal incision is usually made from the apical to basal portion of the inferior scar; this incision is usually 1 to 3 cm in length. Noon is typically designated as the site midway between the apical and basal aspect of the incision on the septum. With computerized systems, an epicardial sock electrode is most commonly used, usually containing 56 to 128 electrodes, which are variably spaced depending on the heart size and the site of the electrodes (apical vs. basal). The larger the heart size, the wider the electrode distance, which limits the accuracy of the mapping data. Computerized endocardial mapping balloon systems with multiple electrodes have also been used.[303,304,307,425] In addition to sequential mapping, we also use relatively high-density plaques with 20 to 40 bipolar or unipolar electrodes recorded from either a 2.5 to 4 $cm^2$ plaque to better define activation in specific areas of interest suggested by the sequential map and/or prior catheter mapping.

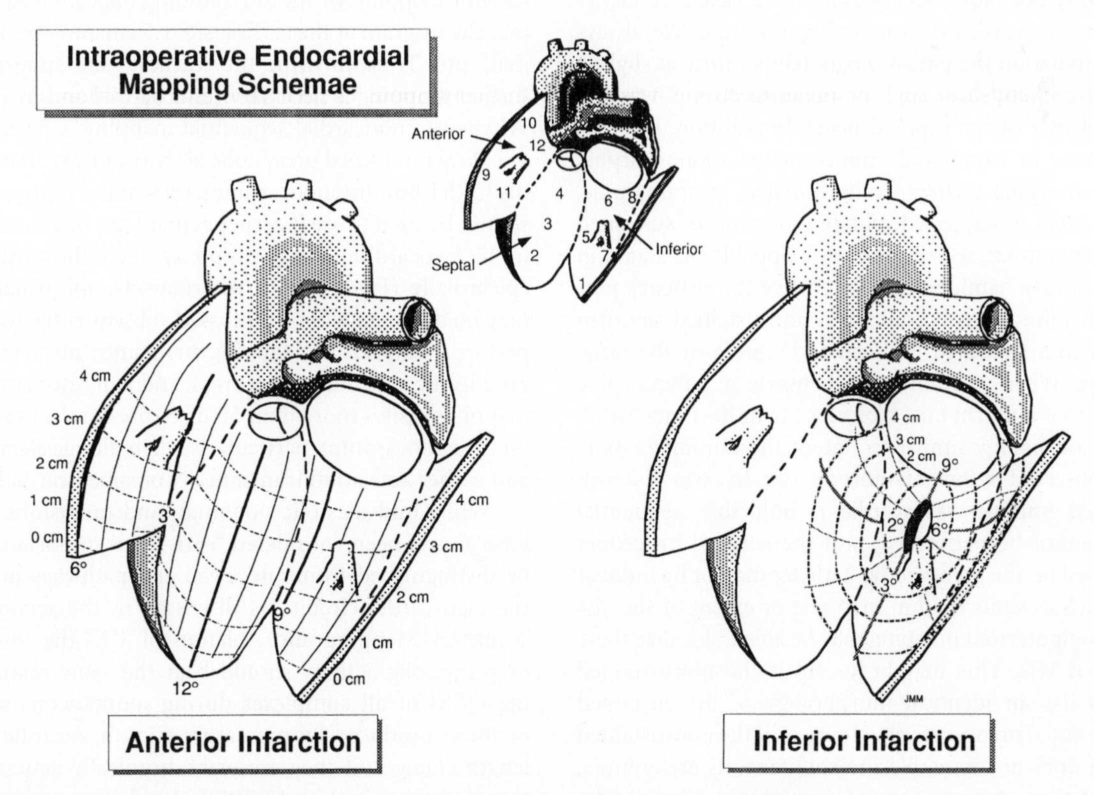


**FIGURE 13-190** *Intraoperative endocardial mapping schema.* A schema of the catheter mapping sites is shown on **top**. On the **bottom** the methods for endocardial sequential mapping of VT are shown for VTs arising in anterior and inferior.

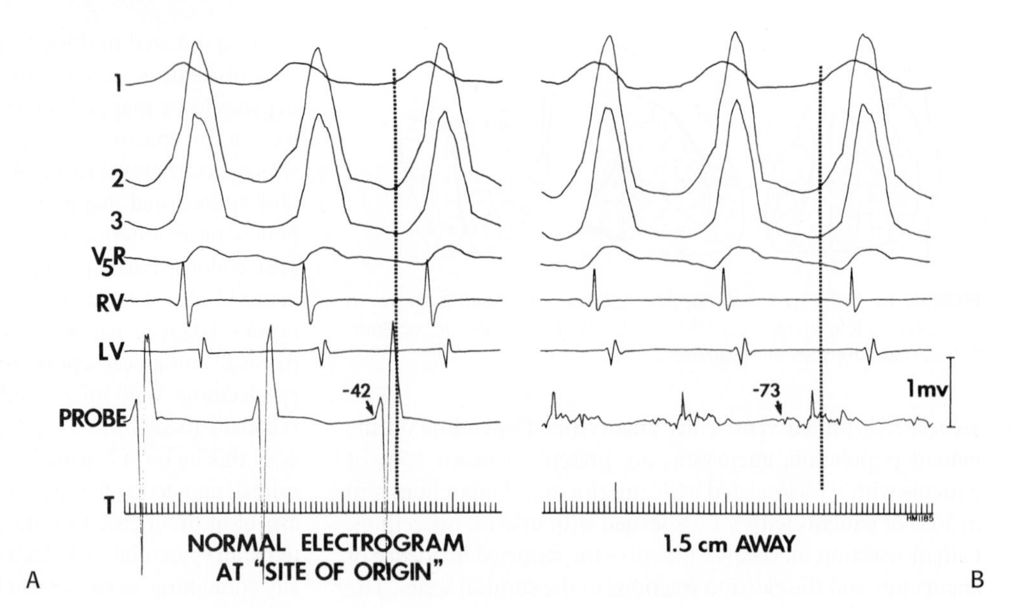


**FIGURE 13-191** *Qualitative characteristics of site of origin.* ECG leads are shown with RV and LV reference electrograms and an electrogram from a mapping probe. **A:** An early site with a normal electrogram is virtually never the earliest "site of origin." **B:** The "site of origin" is typically low amplitude and multicomponent. See text for discussion.

Obviously, to map VT, it must be present or inducible intraoperatively. While all morphologically distinct tachycardias that have been observed preoperatively may not be induced intraoperatively (hence, the need for preoperative catheter mapping), it is possible to induce at least one sustained uniform tachycardia in 90% to 95% of patients. Some investigators have found it difficult to induce sustained uniform tachycardias intraoperatively, which has led them to necessarily employ nonmapped-guided techniques. I believe one of the major reasons for inability to initiate a sustained tachycardia is that the exposed heart is hypothermic. We always attempt to maintain the patient's core temperature at slightly hyperthermic levels, since core temperature does not necessarily reflect that of the exposed heart. In addition, in occasional patients in whom only nonsustained monomorphic VT or polymorphic tachycardia is initiated, procainamide, initially in small doses, may facilitate induction of sustained uniform arrhythmias, which are then mappable. As stated in Chapter 11, procainamide does not change the patient's pattern of activation when it converts a nonsustained uniform tachycardia to a sustained uniform tachycardia of the same morphology. When procainamide converts a polymorphic tachycardia to a uniform one, typically, the uniform tachycardia has a morphology similar to one of the dominant morphologies observed in the polymorphic run. In cases in which no sustained uniform tachycardia is inducible, sequential mapping cannot be performed, and the surgical procedure must be based on the preoperative catheter map or by indirect methods such as sinus rhythm mapping or extent of the visible scar. Computerized mapping may be able to localize these nonsustained VTs. This may be useful if the nonsustained arrhythmia has an identical morphology to the sustained arrhythmia noted preoperatively. However, if the nonsustained tachycardia does not resemble the spontaneous arrhythmia, surgical ablation of nonsustained arrhythmia localized by the computer may have no clinical significance. Moreover, intraoperatively it is virtually impossible to state with certainty that any induced nonsustained VT has an identical morphology to the sustained arrhythmia observed spontaneously or induced preoperatively since 12-lead ECGs cannot be performed when the chest is opened.

If one uses sequential mapping, it is important to recognize that the earliest site recorded is virtually never a normal electrogram. This is shown in Figure 13-191, in which a normal-appearing electrogram was noted to be early (–42 msec). Careful mapping of the surrounding area showed an abnormal electrogram at the earliest site 1.5 cm away from the "normal" site. Thus, anytime the "earliest" site appears normal, further mapping is necessary (endocardial and/or epicardial). Whenever endocardial sequential mapping is performed and one does not record presystolic activity at least 50 msec before the QRS from the endocardium, intramural plunge electrodes should be used to see if earlier activity can be recorded deeper in the myocardium, on the opposite site of the septum or subepicardially (Fig. 13-192). Alternatively, epicardial mapping may be done. As will be discussed subsequently, we routinely perform endocardial mapping first, since most tachycardias arise in the subendocardial areas, and will resort to epicardial mapping if sites more than 50 msec presystolic are not found on the endocardium, particularly when plunge electrodes suggest earlier activation transmurally or subepicardially.

While mid-diastolic potentials and presystolic potentials have always been considered "early," it is important that they be distinguished from late, dead-end pathways unrelated to the tachycardia circuit. As discussed in the section entitled "Catheter Mapping and Ablation of VT," the mid-diastolic or presystolic activity should bear the same relationship to the QRSs of all complexes during spontaneous oscillations or those produced by premature stimuli, regardless of cycle length changes, if they are orthodromically activated by the reentrant circuit (Fig. 13-193). Overdrive pacing producing entrainment of the tachycardia can be used to distinguish early

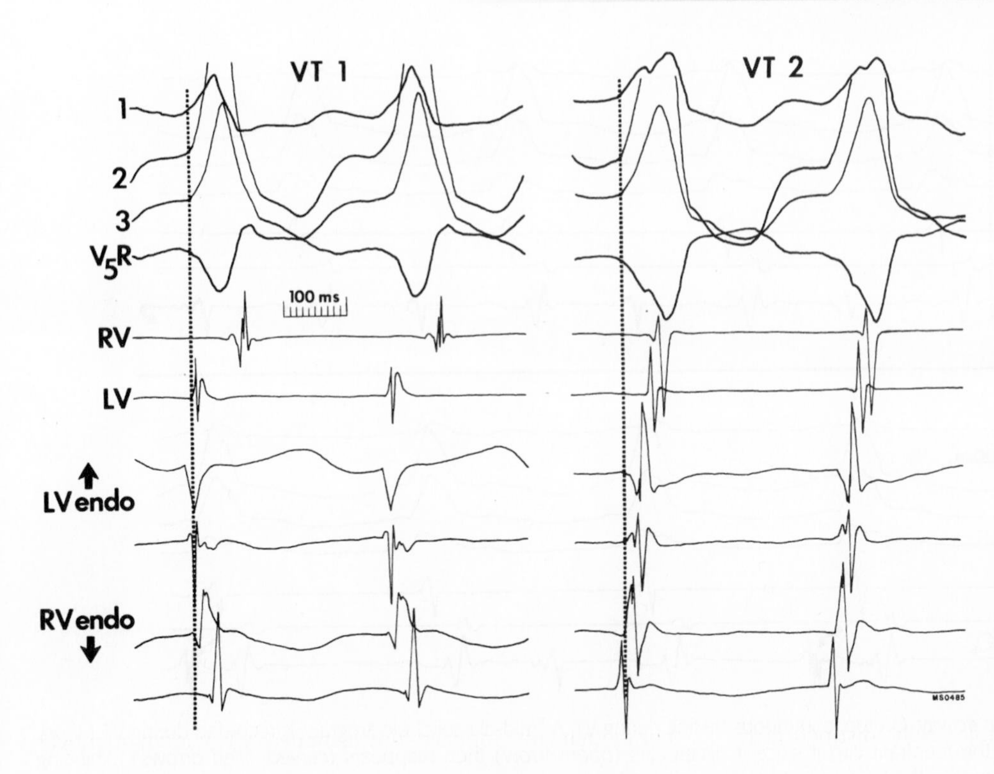


**FIGURE 13-192** *Use of intramural recordings.* An intramural plunge electrode records across the septum such that LV and RV endocardial sites are sampled. During VT1, LV endocardial activity precedes RV endocardial activity. During VT2, RV activity precedes LV activity.

from late sites, as described in Chapter 11. Fitzgerald et al.[427] have suggested that isolated mid-diastolic potentials are optimal sites for ablations. This is incorrect and misleading, since such electrograms may be totally unrelated to the tachycardia circuit. This is demonstrated in Figure 13-194, in which an isolated mid-diastolic potential is observed during VT in the top panel. In the bottom panel, this mid-diastolic potential occasionally disappeared without affecting the tachycardia. When it reappeared, it did so in a Wenckebach pattern, suggesting it was a recording from a dead-end pathway to which conduction delay and block was occurring, and was therefore unrelated to the tachycardia circuit. If one is not fortunate enough to observe such phenomena either spontaneously or following pacing, local pressure or transient cryoablation may yield similar results. As shown in Figure 13-195, focal pressure with the probe at a site which has early diastolic activity produces loss of that electrical signal while the tachycardia continues unaffected. Such local failure of conduction is very common and may occur in very circumscribed areas (Fig. 13-196). Miller et al.[428] have shown that such local failure of conduction occurs in 65% of VTs and in 86% of patients who have VT. Sites of conduction failure usually occur within 2.5 cm of a site of origin (exit site) of a tachycardia, suggesting that this phenomenon is one observed in arrhythmogenic tissue, but not

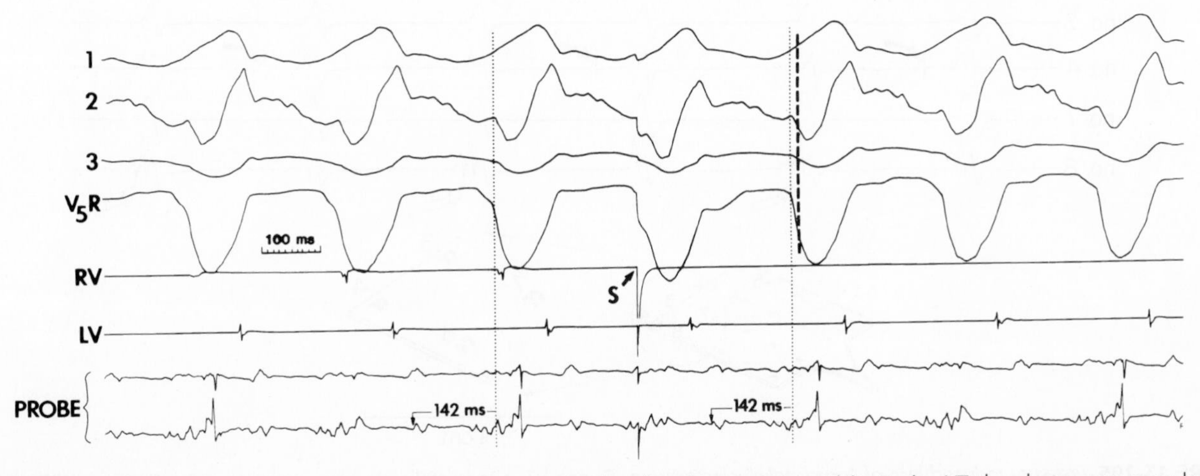


**FIGURE 13-193** *Use of resetting to demonstrate an electrogram is related to the reentrant activity.* During VT, the electrogram recorded with the probe has multiple components in early and late diastole. The early diastolic component is 142 msec before the QRS. To see if this is part of tissue in the orthodromic pathway and not an unrelated signal from a dead-end pathway, an RV extrastimulus is introduced which resets the VT. The *dark vertical dashed line* represents the time at which the QRS would have normally occurred. The electrogram maintains the same relationship to the reset complex as it did throughout the VT.

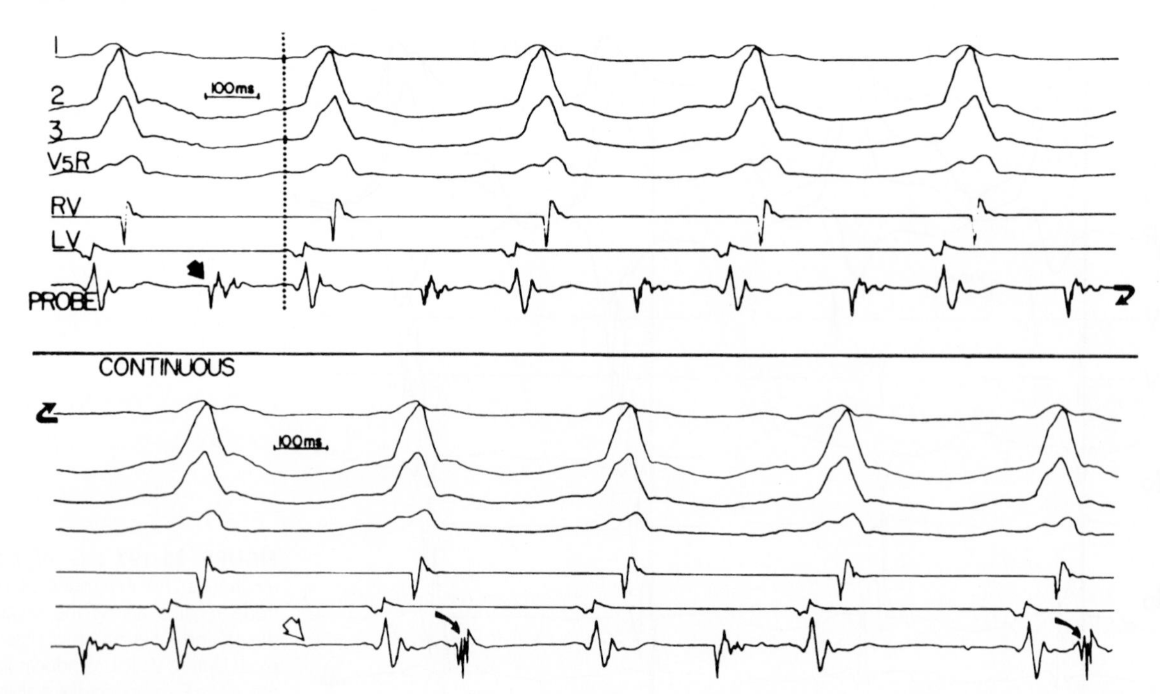


**FIGURE 13-194** *Transient mid-diastolic activity.* On top, continuous tracing during VT. A "mid-diastolic" electrogram is recorded during VT (*short, filled arrow*). This signal is not part of the reentrant circuit since it disappears (*open arrow*) then reappears (*curved, filled arrows*) exhibiting Wenckebach type block without any change in the VT. See text for discussion.

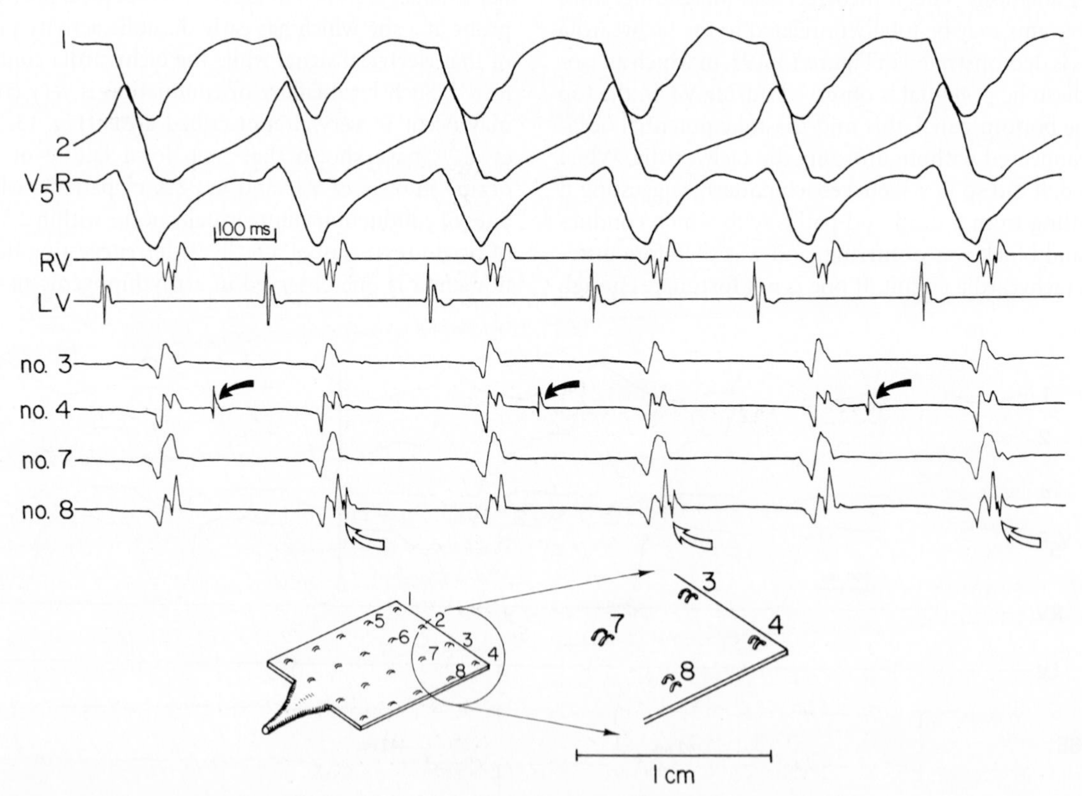


**FIGURE 13-195** *Pressure-induced loss of "presystolic" electrogram.* During VT, a presystolic electrogram is recorded. Pressure with the probe (*filled arrows*), abolishes the "presystolic" potential without affecting the tachycardia (*open arrow*). Note the "presystolic" potential reappears as mid-diastolic activity, which, of course, is unrelated to the VT. See text for explanation.

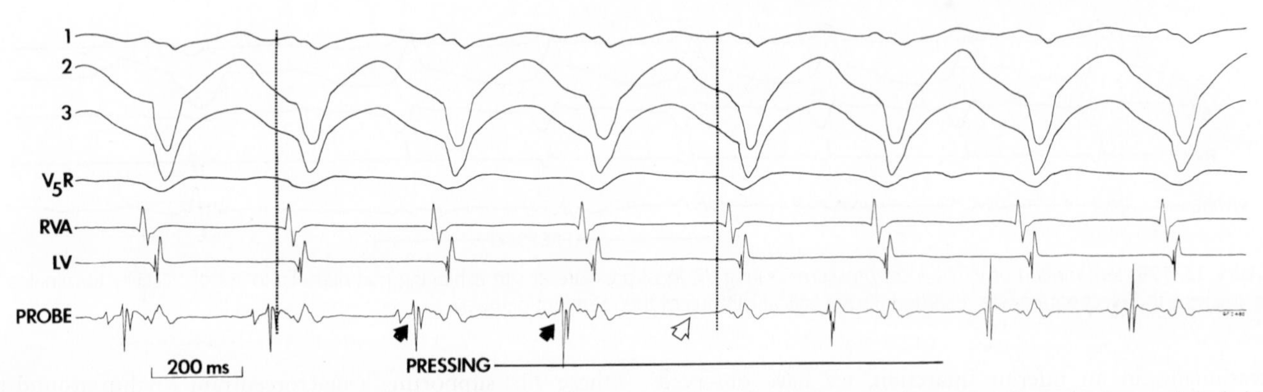


**FIGURE 13-196** *Demonstration of failure of conduction in a circumscribed area.* During VT, mapping was performed using a relatively high-density (20 bipolar pair) plaque. Selected recordings demonstrate 2:1 conduction to electrode 4 (*filled arrow*) and a 2:1 loss of an electrogram component at electrode 8. Adjacent sites 5 mm away show no conduction abnormalities. (From Miller JM, Vassallo JA, Hargrove WC, et al. Intermittent failure of local conduction during ventricular tachycardia. *Circulation* 1985;72:1286.)

necessarily at the exit site or in the isthmus of the tachycardia circuit. Computerized data acquisition might fail to recognize or misinterpret this phenomenon and may provide misleading information, since in many cases a perturbation such as stimulation or focal pressure is required to interpret the data accurately. Thus, reliance on computer analysis alone may be inadequate. One must have the ability to stimulate during the tachycardia and note responses before making a final determination of tachycardia site of origin. This is more likely to happen if electrophysiologists are actively involved in the mapping procedure and can immediately identify potential sites that require such perturbations to provide diagnostic information. In my opinion, this is less likely to happen when the computer analyzes three or four beats of VT, following which the physician must review 64 to 256 electrograms and then decide whether or not a perturbation should be performed.

Conversely, response to perturbations such as pressure or local cryothermia can demonstrate sites that are important. In Figure 13-197 focal pressure at specific mid-diastolic sites within 2 cm of each other slow the VT, but pressure elsewhere has no effect on the tachycardia, thus demonstrating the focal nature of pressure changes. In Figure 13-198, focal pressure terminates VT in the absence of any mechanically induced ventricular premature complexes. In an analogous manner, cryothermia or laser photocoagulation may produce similar effects. This is demonstrated in Figure 13-199, in which laser photocoagulation slows VT and then terminates it by producing block in the tachycardia circuit proximal to orthodromic activation of a mid-diastolic potential.[340]

The results of most series of intraoperative mapping of VT have demonstrated a focal origin, with centrifugal spread of electrical activity to the remainder of the heart; this has recently been termed monoregional spread.[307,310,424,425,429] In addition, continuous loop reentry (or circular reentry) has been observed, in which sequential activation throughout the cardiac cycle is observed.[303,304,340,341,429,430] These two types of activation patterns are schematically shown in Figure 13-200. Analog records of a complete reentrant circuit on the ventricular septum from a 3-$cm^2$ area are shown in Figure 13-201.

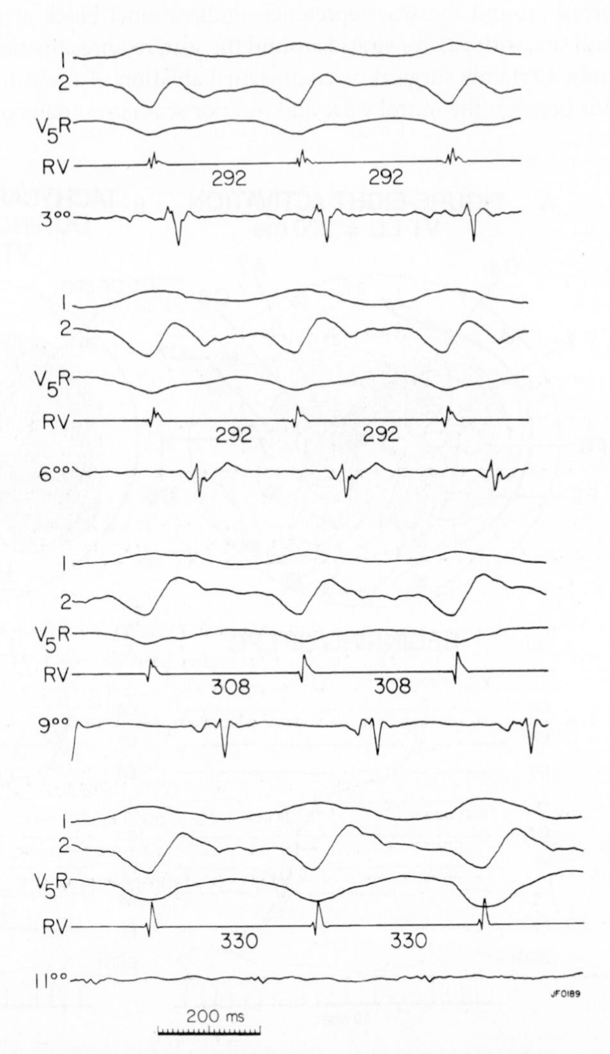


**FIGURE 13-197** *Slowing of VT by local pressure suggesting recording from the circuit.* During VT, focal pressure is delivered at 3, 6, 9, 11 o'clock; 2 cm (°°) from the edge of the ventriculotomy. Slowing was only produced over a 2 cm area from 9°° to 11°°. The absence of change in QRS suggests the mid-diastolic recorded at these sites was a critical part of the pathway.

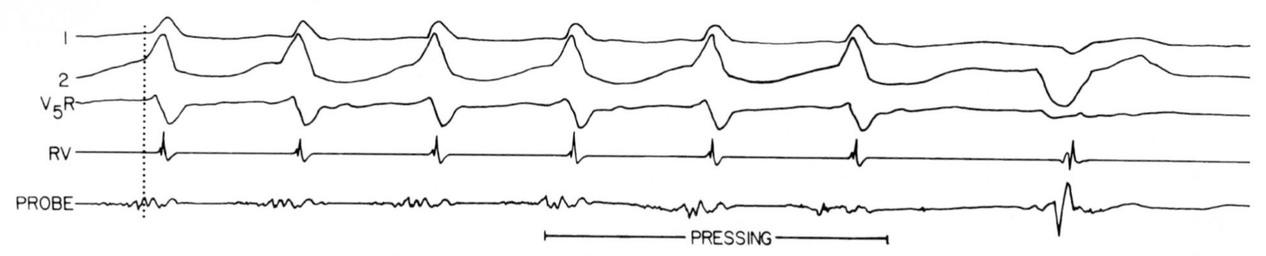


**FIGURE 13-198** *Termination of VT by local pressure.* During VT, local pressure at site exhibiting mid-diastolic to systolic activity terminates VT. This suggests the electrogram was recorded from a critical isthmus of the reentrant pathway.

Occasionally, in an inferior infarction, we have observed circumferential activation around the scar throughout the cardiac cycle in both a counterclockwise and a clockwise direction, producing two morphologically distinct VTs (Fig. 13-202). Of interest, all but one of our patients demonstrating circular activation around an inferior wall scar had an additional monoregional tachycardia. How often circular spread around the scar represents unidirectional block at a focal site, with passive spread around the scar, requires further study. Certainly surgical or cryothermal ablation of the isthmus between the mitral valve and inferior scar cures many of these VTs, supporting a macroreentrant rhythm around the scar. As can be seen in Figure 13-202, areas of slow conduction can appear during systole and/or during diastole and thus are not relegated to areas showing diastolic activity. This points out that there is no one specific "zone of slow conduction" but that many sites within and outside of a reentrant circuit may exhibit slow conduction. In a small percentage of patients, we have observed activation patterns meeting neither continuous nor centrifugal (monoregional) spread, primarily due to failure to record activity throughout the cardiac cycle. These undefined tachycardia patterns of endocardial activation

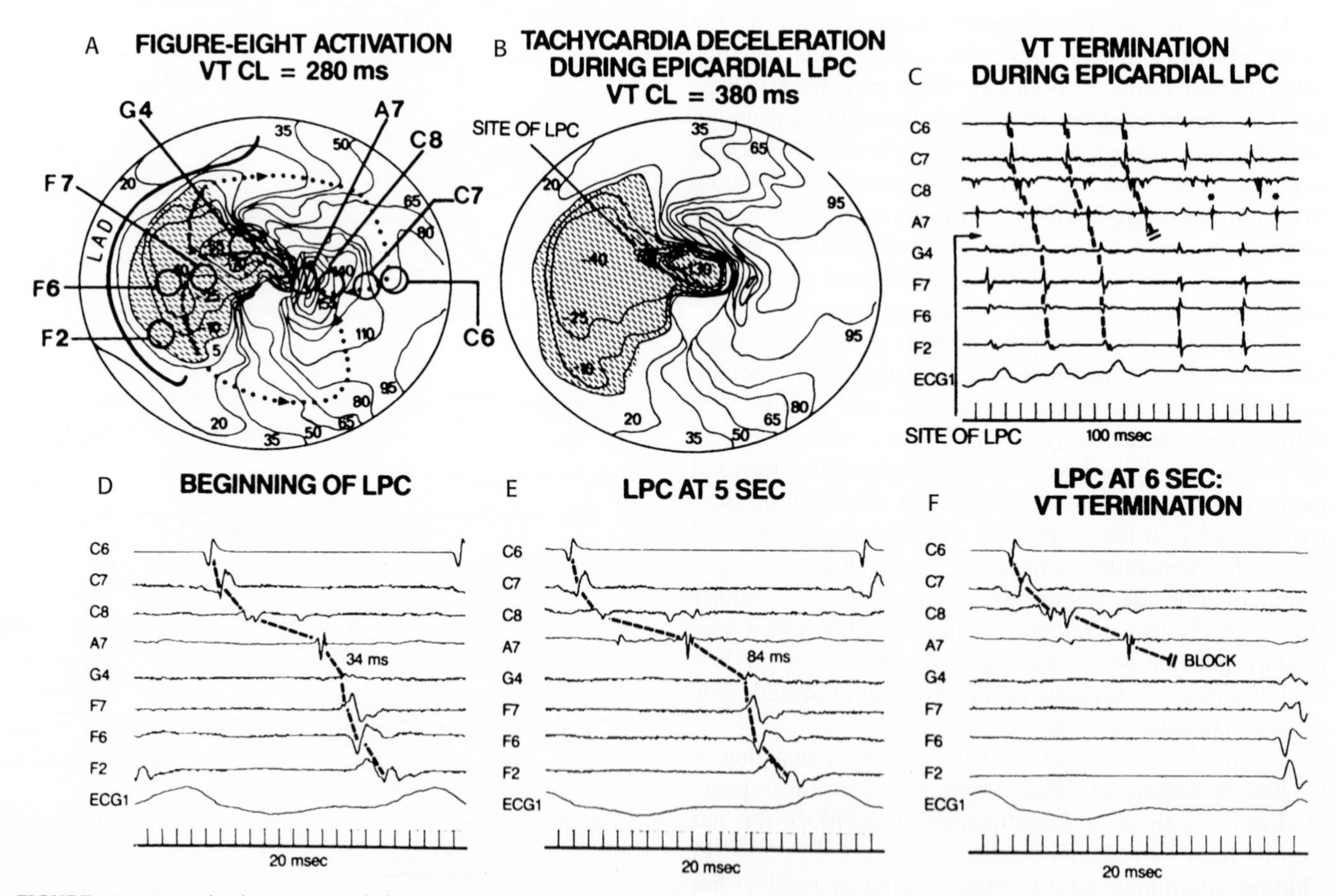


**FIGURE 13-199** *Activation maps and electrograms of deceleration and interruption of figure-of-eight reentry tachycardia using epicardial laser photocoagulation.* **A:** Global epicardial activation of a VT complex. Diastolic activity is marked by darkened area. **B:** Global epicardial activation of a VT complex after deceleration induced by laser photocoagulation (LPC). **C–F:** Epicardial electrograms spanning diastole during VT. LPC-induced deceleration and termination resulted from conduction delay and block between two sides of irradiated area. (From Littmann L, Svenson RH, Gallagher JJ, et al. Functional role of the epicardium in postinfarction ventricular tachycardia. Observations derived from computerized epicardial activation mapping, entrainment and epicardial laser photoablation. *Circulation* 1991;83:1577.)

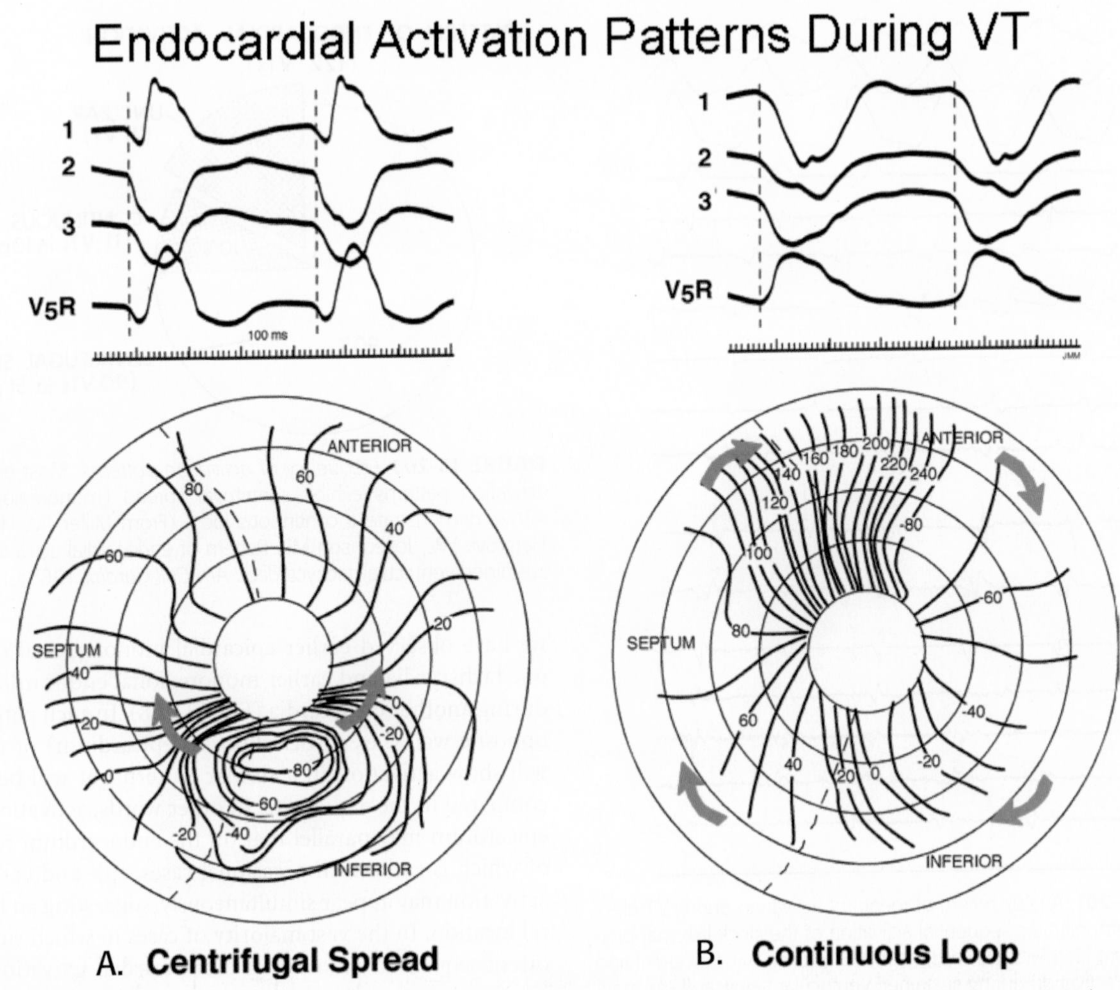


**FIGURE 13-200** *Centrifugal spread and continuous loop activation pattern.* Two VTs are shown. The VT on **left** shows a ventricular spread from a focal septal site (monoregional spread). On the **right**, VT shows a continuous wave of activation around a scar. (From Miller JM, Harken AH, Hargrove WC, Josephson ME. Pattern of endocardial activation during sustained ventricular tachycardia. *J Am Coll Cardiol* 1985;6:1260.)

may represent focal activation with an intramural loop or continuous activity within an intramural loop that is not detected from the subendocardium or the epicardium in these cases. In our experience of those tachycardias in which a clear pattern of activation could be determined, 90% had centrifugal spread (i.e., were monoregional), while others had circular or continuous loop activation patterns. As stated before, all but one of our patients who had "continuous loop" tachycardias also manifested tachycardias with monoregional spread (Fig. 13-203). The use of high-density mapping in areas of apparent monoregional spread has suggested reentry using a classic figure-of-eight model in some cases. While reentrant excitation can be observed in a two-dimensional (2D) planar dimension (Fig. 13-204), we and others have observed more complex types of activation sequences suggesting a 2D circuit that was not a simple figure-of-eight model (Fig. 13-205).[424,425]

The vast majority of published mapping data during VT associated with coronary artery disease suggests that the origin of the arrhythmia, or at least critical areas responsible for the arrhythmia, are either subendocardial (inner 2 to 5 mm) or intraseptal.[303,304,307,340,424–426] Subendocardial or septal "origins" of VT associated with coronary disease are reported in 85% to 97% of cases. Only 3% to 15% appear to be subepicardial in nature. The subendocardial "origin" may be disparate from the earliest epicardial breakthrough, even when tachycardias arise from the left ventricular free wall. These disparities may be marked, as shown in Figure 13-206, in which the earliest endocardial site of activation is 6 cm away from the earliest epicardial breakthrough. Such discrepancies arise as a result of variable patterns of slow activation through diseased tissue from the site of "origin" (exit site) toward viable myocardium, be it on the epicardium or intramural myocardium. In all cases in which tachycardias arise in the septum, by definition there is no correlation between epicardial activation and the origin of the tachycardia. In septal tachycardias, epicardial activation usually begins paraseptally; however, it may begin superiorly (anteriorly) or inferiorly, regardless of where on the septum the tachycardia originates. In our experience, in virtually all cases in which tachycardias arise in the septum, the earliest epicardial breakthrough occurs after the onset of the QRS, even if the earliest epicardial site is reasonably near the site of septal origin (Fig. 13-207).[429] In rare patients,

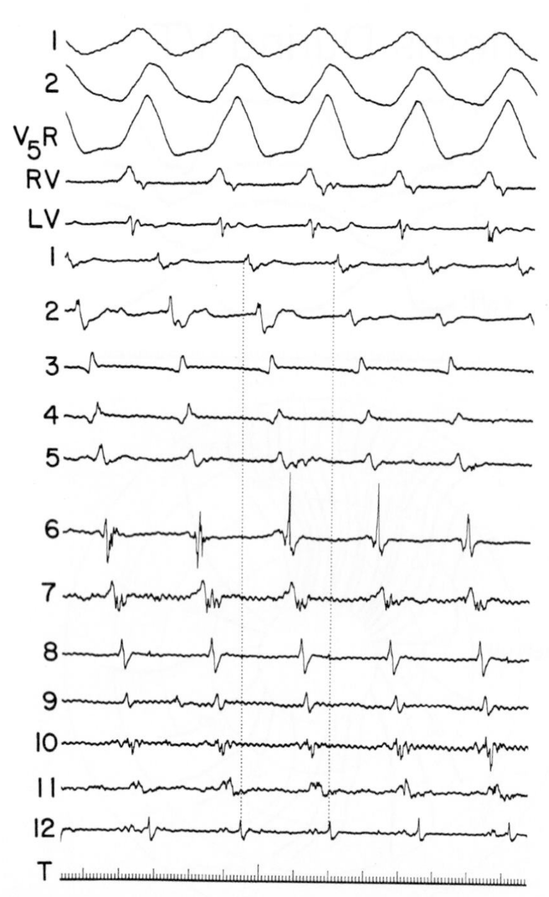


**FIGURE 13-201** Analog record of reentrant activation during VT electrograms demonstrates sequential activation of the clock-like mapping system. (From Horowitz LN, Josephson ME, Harken AH. Epicardial and endocardial activation during sustained ventricular tachycardia in man. *Circulation* 1980;61:1227.)

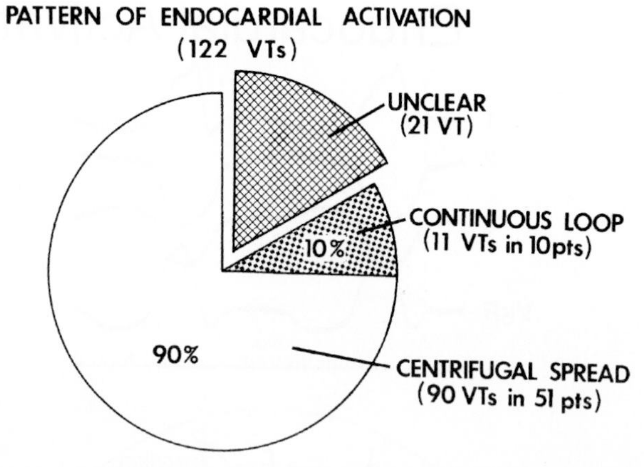


**FIGURE 13-203** *Frequency of activation patterns.* Most endocardial activation patterns exhibit centrifugal spread (monoregional); only ≈10% demonstrate a continuous loop. (From Miller JM, Harken AH, Hargrove WC, Josephson ME. Pattern of endocardial activation during sustained ventricular tachycardia. *J Am Coll Cardiol* 1985;6:1260.)

we have observed earlier epicardial monoregional spread in one tachycardia and earlier monoregional endocardial spread during another tachycardia (Fig. 13-208). In such patients, the opposite wall (i.e., myocardium or epicardium) of the heart will show activation in a similar pattern but will be delayed compared to the earlier site. In other words, activation on the epicardium may parallel that on the endocardium regardless of which is earliest. In occasional cases, epi- and endocardial activation may appear simultaneously, suggesting an intramural location. In the vast majority of cases in which simultaneous or sequential endocardial and epicardial activation during

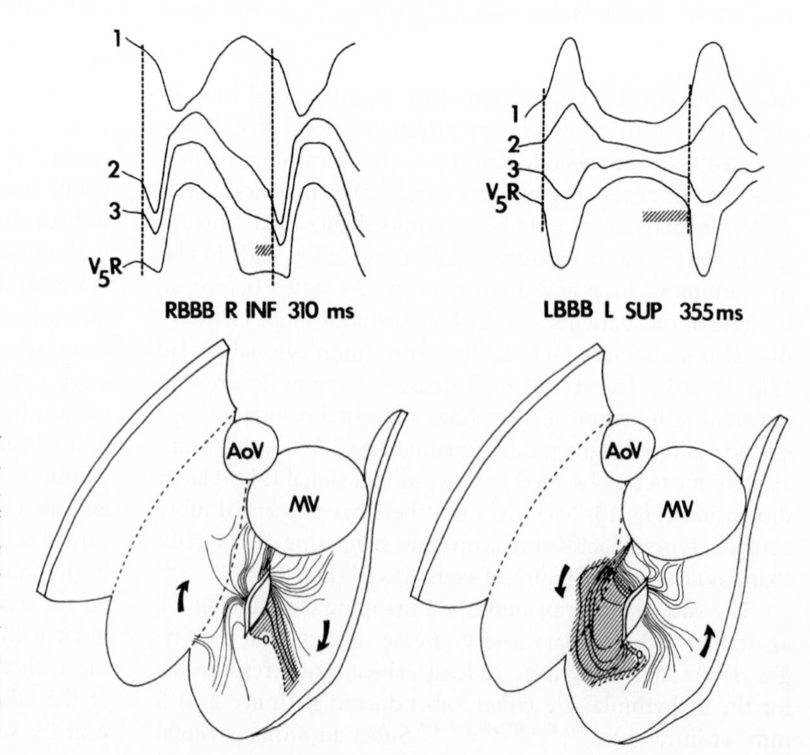


**FIGURE 13-202** *Circumferential spread around inferior ventriculotomy.* Two VTs from a patient with inferior infarction are shown. The RBBB VT demonstrates clockwise activation around the inferior ventriculotomy. Multiple areas of slow conduction are seen. The shaded areas denote the second half of diastole. The LBBB VT shows counterclockwise activation with multiple areas of slow conduction. The regions of slow conduction vary somewhat dependent on the clockwise or counterclockwise activation. (From Miller JM, Harken AH, Hargrove WC, Josephson ME. Pattern of endocardial activation during sustained ventricular tachycardia. *J Am Coll Cardiol* 1985;6:1260.)

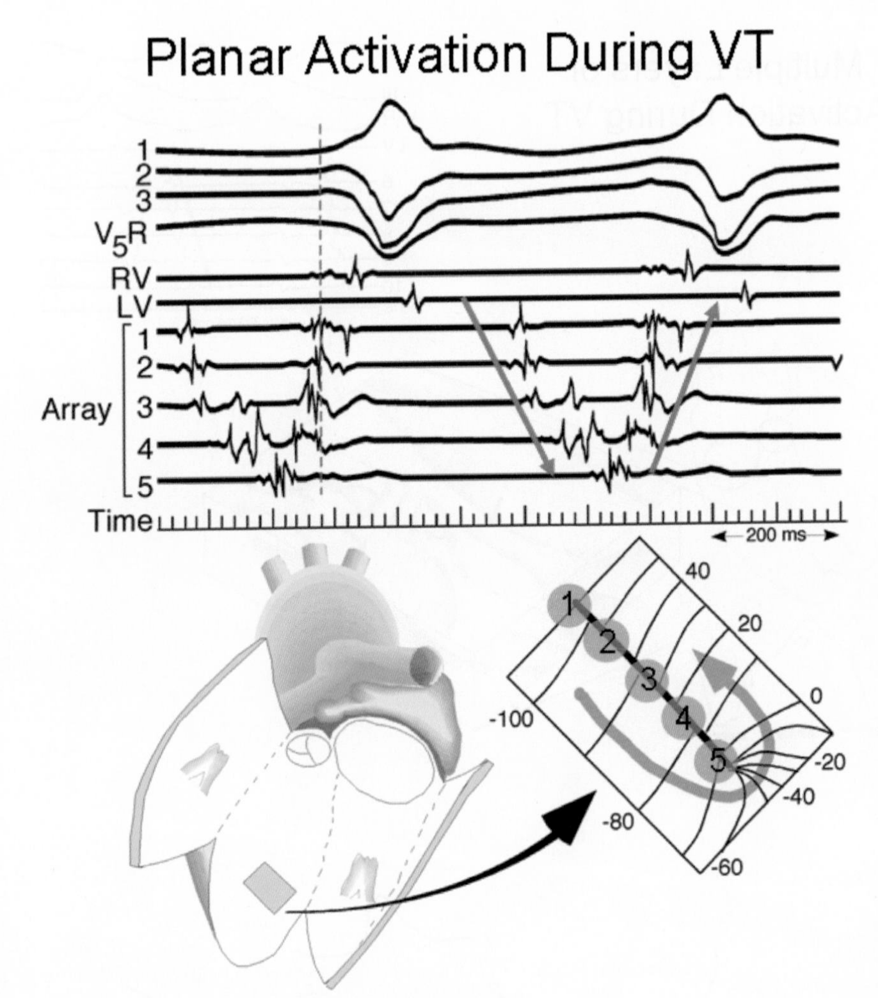


**FIGURE 13-204** *Reentrant excitation in a two-dimensional planar area.* VT with an LBBB, left axis is shown. A plaque on the septum shows sequential activation around poles 1 to 5.

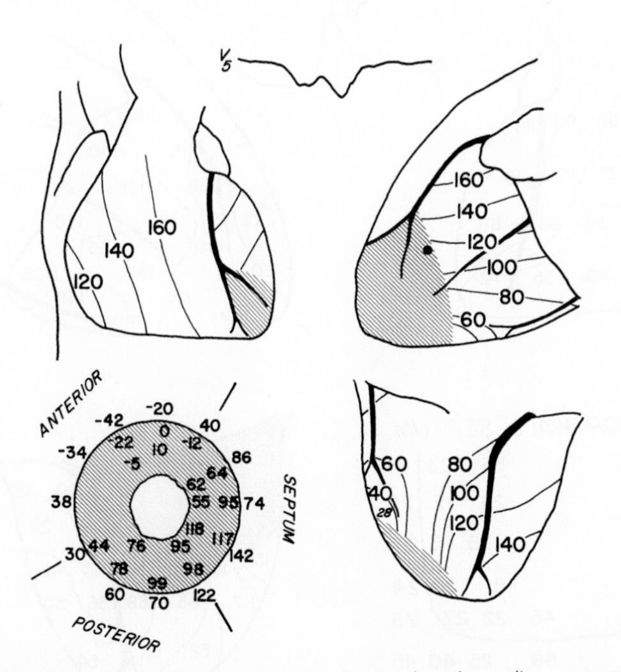


**FIGURE 13-205** *High-density map in focal tachycardia suggests superficial and deeper activation pattern.* A high-density plaque revealed a protected isthmus of activation at one level and slow conduction perpendicular to the isthmus at another level. Endocardial activation is in *red* and deeper activation in *blue.*

the same tachycardia has been obtained, earliest activation has been recorded from the endocardial electrodes.

Several investigators have observed that patients in whom earliest activation occurs on the epicardium do not have aneurysms and usually have inferior infarctions.[307,340,341] Thus, the relative incidence of early epicardial activation versus subendocardial activation in different surgical series may have to do with patient selection. It is still important to realize that Harris et al.,[307] who have the greatest experience in simultaneous intraoperative endocardial and epicardial mapping, have found the earliest activation on the endocardium in 92.5% of tachycardias mapped. Obviously, the site of earliest activation is important in directing the type of surgical procedure. If tachycardias were indeed found to be subepicardial in origin, then a ventriculotomy would not be necessary, and tachycardias could be cured with a "closed" approach using laser photocoagulation[55,56,340] or cryoablation. Even if such patients could also be cured via an endocardial approach, it seems reasonable, although not proven, that an epicardial approach should be associated with less morbidity and shorter recovery period. In the future, simultaneous multisite data acquisition will also include intramural electrical activation using relatively atraumatic electrodes made from very thin printed circuit boards. Such data may provide more

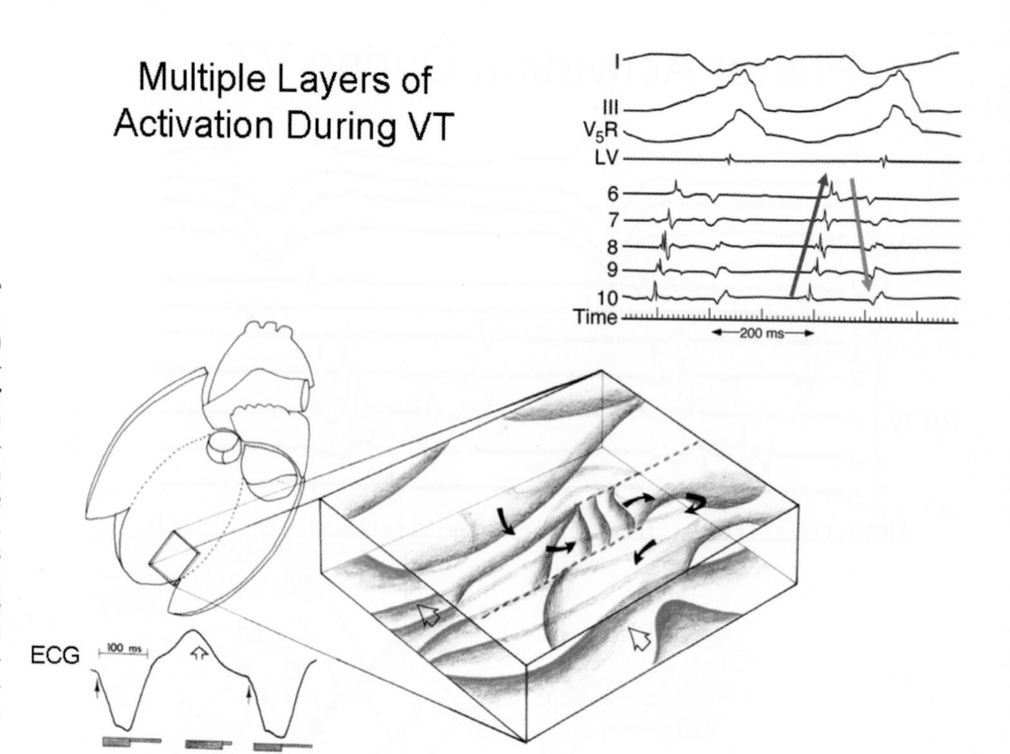


**FIGURE 13-206** *Markedly disparate epicardial and endocardial activation.* Epicardial activation in a patient with an apical infarction is shown in anterior (**upper left**), left lateral (**upper right**), and inferior (**lower right**) views. *Shaded areas* represent aneurysm. The earliest epicardial activation is 28 msec following the QRS at the inferoapical border of the aneurysm. The earliest endocardial activation is at the apical-superior free wall 2 cm, from the septum 42 msec before the QRS. (From Horowitz LN, Josephson ME, Harken AH. Epicardial and endocardial activation during sustained ventricular tachycardia in man. *Circulation* 1980;61:1227.)

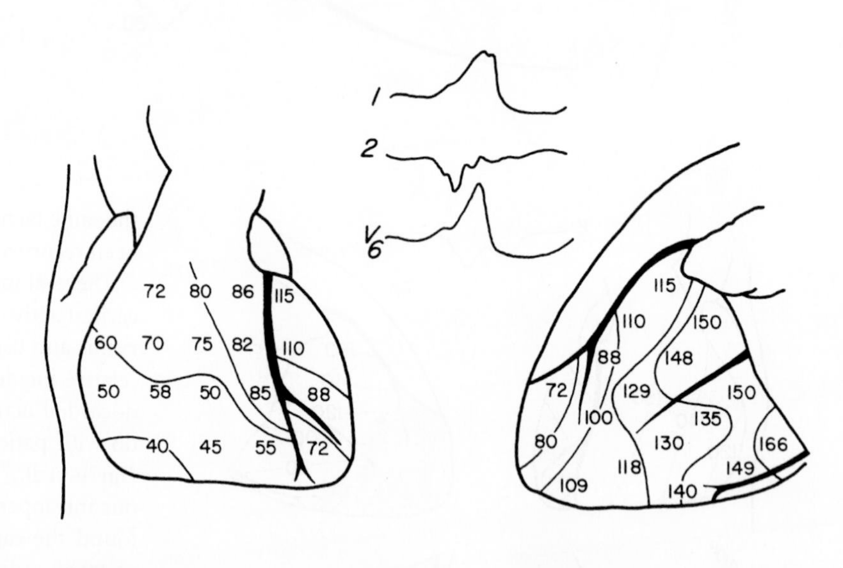


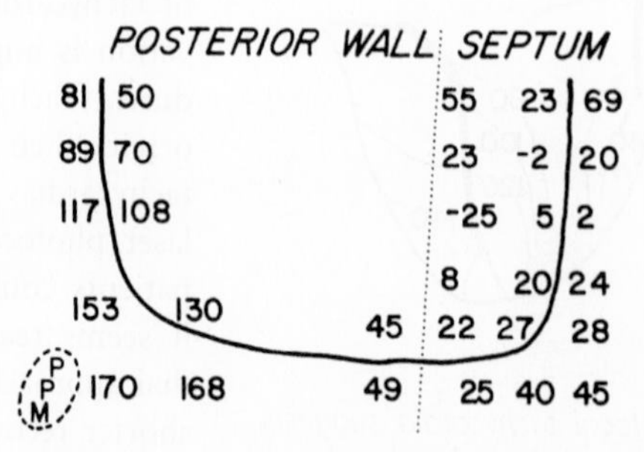


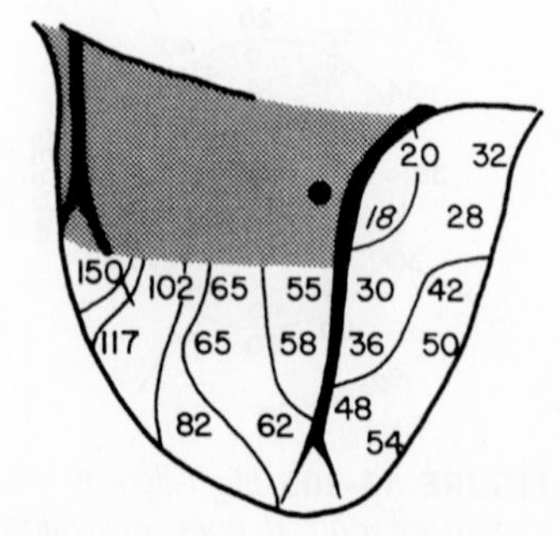


**FIGURE 13-207** *Epicardial and endocardial activation during VT arising on the basal septum.* Epicardial maps of VT are shown in the anterior, lateral, and inferior views (clockwise). The shaded area is the region of inferior scar. Epicardial breakthrough is at the paraseptal base of the RV, 18 msec after the onset of the QRS. Endocardial activation (**lower left**) shows earliest activation on the left side of the basal septum 25 msec before the onset of the QRS (*filled circle*, **lower right**). (From Horowitz LN, Josephson ME, Harken AH. Epicardial and endocardial activation during sustained ventricular tachycardia in man. *Circulation* 1980;61:1227.)

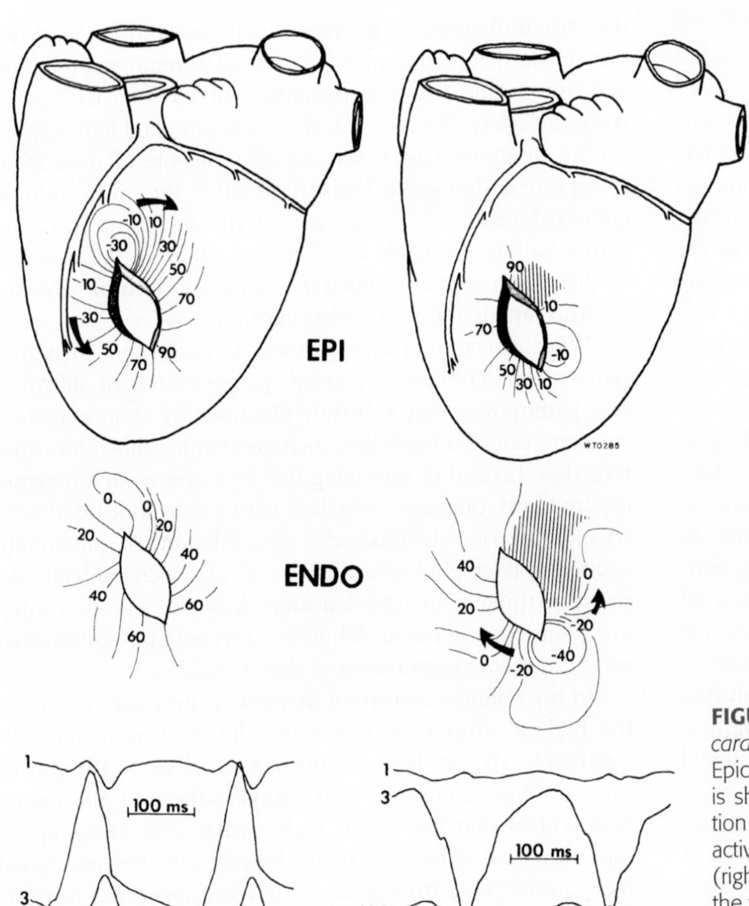


**FIGURE 13-208** *Epicardial and endocardial ventricular tachycardias.* Two VTs arose at the cut edge of a traumatic aneurysm. Epicardial (EPI) and endocardial (ENDO) activation during each VT is shown. The VT on the left (inferior axis) shows earliest activation at the epicardium with a centrifugal spread. The endocardial activation parallels epicardial activation. The VT with a superior axis (right) shows earliest activation to be focal from the inferior edge of the ventriculotomy on the endocardium. Epicardial spread parallels endocardial activation.

information about the routes of reentrant excitation during VT. Currently, I believe that the use of transmural needles to record such activity is too traumatic and, thus, has not added significantly useful clinical data to alter surgical approaches based on standard mapping techniques.

Other methods of activation may also be used in the future. Limitations of developing accurate isochronic maps are recognized,[431] and as a result two techniques have been developed that may have value. First is a vector approach in which moment-to-moment direction of activation can be plotted and can distinguish slow conduction from block. This has been used experimentally by Kadish et al.[432] in canine models of infarction. Another potential method is isopotential mapping in which DC recordings showing negative activity define a region from which activation occurs.[433] Such data provide information relative to monoregional spread toward which a surgical intervention could be targeted. This technique may be especially useful in septal tachycardias although it is limited by the resolution of the system such that very low-amplitude signals are missed.

If activation mapping of VT cannot be accomplished either in the catheterization laboratory or in the operating room, intraoperative mapping during sinus rhythm may be performed to define abnormal electrophysiologic sites analogously to that done in the catheterization laboratory.[434] Examples of normal, fractionated (and late) and split electrograms recorded using a bipolar signal with a 2-mm interelectrode distance are shown in Figure 13-209. Although epicardial and/or endocardial late potentials have been felt to present delayed activation and potential markers for sites of origin of tachycardia, we have

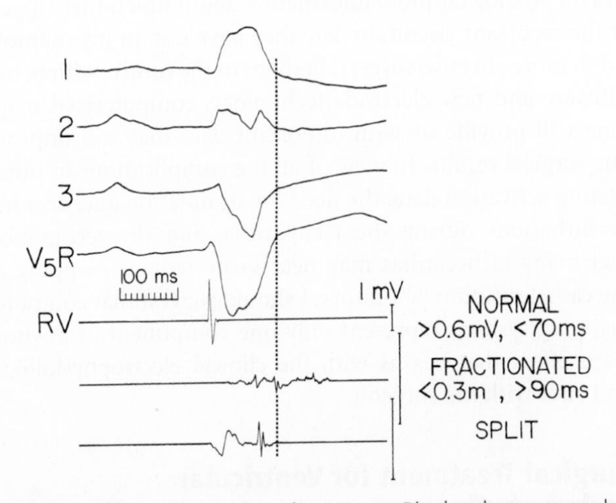


**FIGURE 13-209** *Sinus rhythm electrogram.* Bipolar electrograms during sinus rhythm recorded using electrodes with a 2-mm interelectrode distance. Normal electrograms are >0.6 mV and <70 msec in duration. Fractionated electrograms and split electrograms are also shown.

not found this to be the case in coronary artery disease.[313,434,435] We have found isolated epicardial late potentials to be rather uncommon in the setting of coronary artery disease (14%) and, even when present, not to be useful in localizing sites of origin of VT.[435] Certainly in all cases, instances of tachycardias that arise on the septum, epicardial late potentials have no significance regarding location of the tachycardia. Even when epicardial late potentials and VT arise on the free wall of the heart, there is still only a 50% chance that the epicardial late potential will be in a site within 2 cm of the origin of VT.[435] Fontaine et al.[316,436] have also found a low incidence of epicardial late potentials and a poor correlation of such potentials to VT origin in the setting of coronary artery disease. Such late potentials, however, may be important in the setting of cardiomyopathies. Preliminary data from our laboratory have shown a better correlation of epicardial later potentials, positive signal-averaged ECGs and inducible arrhythmias in patients with dilated cardiomyopathies.[437,438] Similarly, Fontaine and colleagues[439,440] have found a high incidence of epicardial late potentials in patients with arrhythmogenic right ventricular dysplasia, a phenomenon they call postexcitation. When intraoperative endocardial activation during sinus rhythm had been analyzed for fragmented electrograms and late potentials as markers for VTs, no correlation could be found.[434] Although the "site of origin" of VT may be associated with abnormal electrograms, split electrograms, late potentials, and broad electrograms are found more often at other sites. These are the same results that Cassidy et al.[313] found during catheter sinus rhythm mapping.

Thus, only activation mapping of VT is adequate to guide surgery. Endocardial catheter mapping and intraoperative mapping are necessary to provide the surgeon with the most information available to direct the surgery. In some instances, catheter-acquired mapping data may be the only data available. The good correlation of catheter and intraoperative mapping validate the use of catheter-acquired data.[441,442] Although complicated computerized mapping systems are available, and do provide far more information about functional aspects of the reentrant circuit, to date they have not, in my opinion, led to more effective surgery. Perhaps in the future, with better software and new electrode technology, computerized mapping will provide us with important data that will improve our surgical results. In view of all the complications in interpreting activation data, the need for stimulation and/or other perturbations during the tachycardia, and the recognition that many tachycardias may necessarily require mapping in the catheterization laboratory, I should suggest that computer mapping systems represent only one component of a whole team effort that begins with the clinical electrophysiologist and ends with the surgeon.

## Surgical Treatment for Ventricular Tachyarrhythmias

Once the site of origin of the tachycardia has been identified, a variety of surgical approaches may be undertaken to ablate the arrhythmogenic focus. We initially developed a localized subendocardial resection as the method of removing only the arrhythmogenic tissue in patients with VT associated with coronary artery disease.[15] Focal cryoablation and laser vaporization or photocoagulation are also capable of destroying specific arrhythmogenic tissue from either the epicardium or endocardium.[4,5,53–56,340] Map-guided ablation using an endocardial balloon electrode has also been reported.[443] The endocardial electrodes from which the earliest of "critical" sites are recorded are used for DC ablation of these areas.

When activation mapping cannot be performed, then procedures aimed to remove a visible pathophysiologic substrate or a pathophysiologic substrate identified by abnormal electrograms can be undertaken, such as extended subendocardial resection. Instead of removing this scar or area of abnormal electrograms, one may encircle it with a subendocardial ventriculotomy or subendocardial cryoablation, or potentially encircling laser photocoagulation, all of which probably do the same thing as an extended subendocardial resection without removing the tissue. All of the directed and nondirected procedures have been reviewed elsewhere.[4,5]

In my opinion, activation mapping is necessary to ensure the highest surgical success rate. This is demonstrated in Figure 13-210, which shows the variety of sites of origin of four sustained uniform VTs in a single patient. In this figure, it is evident that two of the tachycardias arise at the apical septum within visible scar tissue; however, the two additional tachycardias arise from areas of normal appearing myocardium and would not be cured by a visually guided or, in this

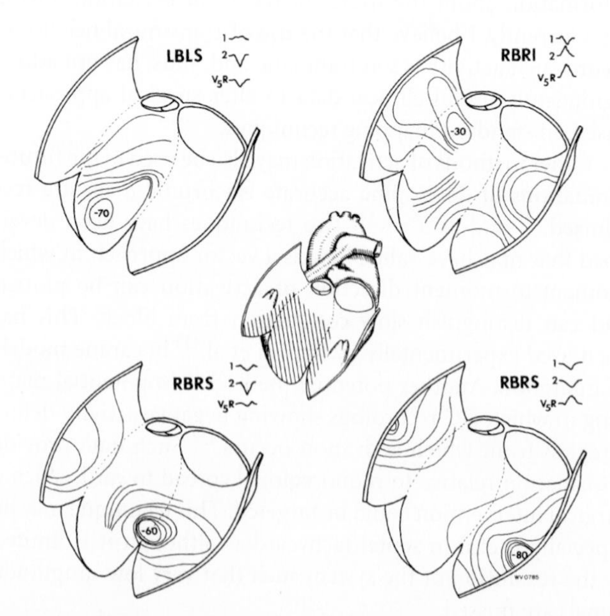


**FIGURE 13-210** *Requirement of mapping to guide therapy.* In the center is a schema of the opened LV with the *shaded area* representing visual scar. Four VTs were present in this patient. The two VTs on the **left** arose in the proximity to each other on the septum, within the area of visible scar. The remaining two VTs (**right**) arose outside the area of visible scar. See text for discussion.

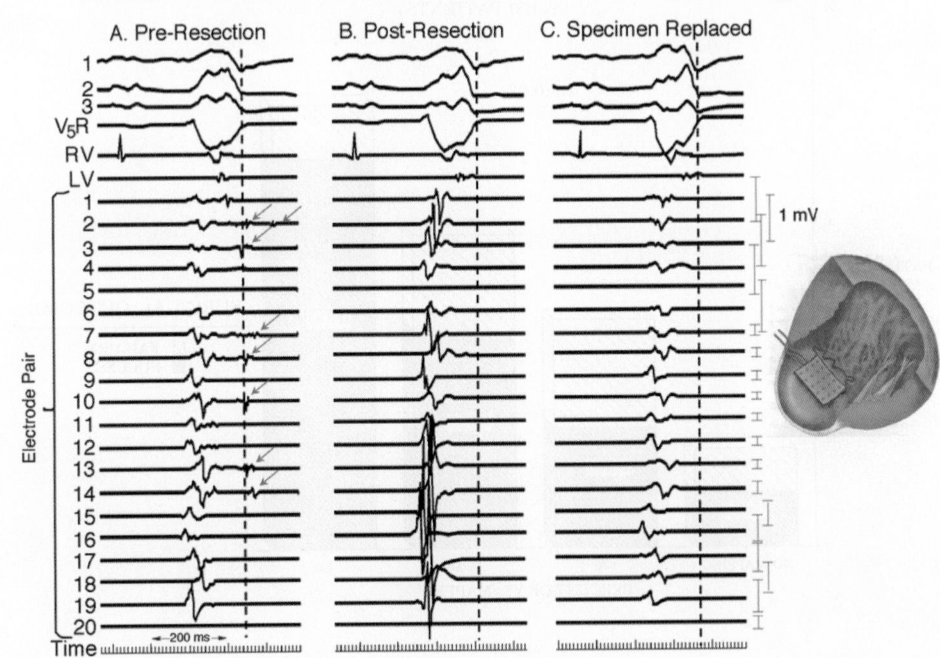


**FIGURE 13-211** *Influence of mapping on surgical outcome.* The effect of mapping on surgical outcome for 100 consecutive patients is shown in the bar graph. Failure was defined as inducible sustained VT postoperatively. Success was defined as no inducible arrhythmia. The greater the extent of mapping, the greater the likelihood of success. (Adapted from Miller JM, Gottlieb CD, Marchlinski FE, et al. Does ventricular tachycardia mapping influence the success of antiarrhythmic surgery? *J Am Coll Cardiol* 1988;11:112A.)

particular case, an electrogram-guided surgical procedure. Although one cannot compare surgical series, some of which use nonguided procedures, and some of which use mapping, in our own institution, we have been able to compare the results of nonmap-guided surgery with that guided by variable degrees of mapping.[444] In patients without adequate data, nonmap-guided therapy was used, and when mapping was performed, directed surgical therapy was used. I believe that visually guided extended subendocardial resection in our hands is the same as that in anyone else's hands, but surgery guided by mapping, as shown in Figure 13-211, increased the number of successfully treated tachycardias. Miller et al.[444] demonstrated in 100 consecutive cases that the greater the extent of mapping, the better the surgical outcome. In patients with 50% of all tachycardias mapped, there was only a 50% success rate, while if all the tachycardias were mapped, there was a nearly 90% success rate. Success was defined as noninducibility of any sustained arrhythmia postoperatively; and, in fact, there was 100% clinical success rate in this group of patients. Thus, in my opinion, an attempt at catheter and intraoperative mapping should always be made before any surgical procedure since the outcome can only be improved by such information. Failure to do so, by virtue of choice or inability to initiate arrhythmias, portends a poorer prognosis for the patient.

Miller et al.[445] have attempted to analyze the mechanism by which subendocardial resection is successful by recording over the mapped area of origin during sinus rhythm with a moderately high-density plaque. A subendocardial resection was then performed, and the plaque was replaced in the exact same position. As shown in Figure 13-212, before subendocardial resection, electrograms recorded from the area of origin of the tachycardia demonstrated either no activity or abnormal, fractionated electrograms, with 40% of the sites showing late potentials. Following subendocardial resection, electrograms recorded from the same area were larger in amplitude, narrower in duration, and there has been an eradication of late potentials. These changes, tabulated in Table 13-2, demonstrate that subendocardial resection results in a higher percentage of normal electrograms and eradication of split and late potentials.[445] These data suggest that subendocardial resection removes the critical areas of slow conduction that are required for reentry. Whether or not it removes the whole reentrant circuit is unknown, but certainly, absence of late potentials and normalization of the electrograms suggest improved conduction. How cryoablation or laser photocoagulation work is unclear, but both produce homogeneous lesions. One could imagine then that instead of removing areas of slow conduction, these two techniques homogeneously destroy these areas, leaving only those areas with better conduction, thereby preventing the recurrence of reentry.

We have used adjunctive cryoablation with subendocardial resection in one-third of our patients. This is particularly important when tachycardias are associated with inferior infarctions, to prevent surgical damage to the mitral valve or papillary muscles. Cryothermal ablation does not injure the mitral annulus and can be used to destroy arrhythmogenic tissue at the base of the papillary muscle without requiring removal of the papillary muscle, necessitating mitral valve replacement. Of note, we have never observed a tachycardia arising from the papillary muscle per se; when VTs arise in the region of the papillary muscle, the origin of the tachycardia is always at its base or in the subadjacent free wall myocardium. In addition, cryothermal ablation is used if endocardial activation does

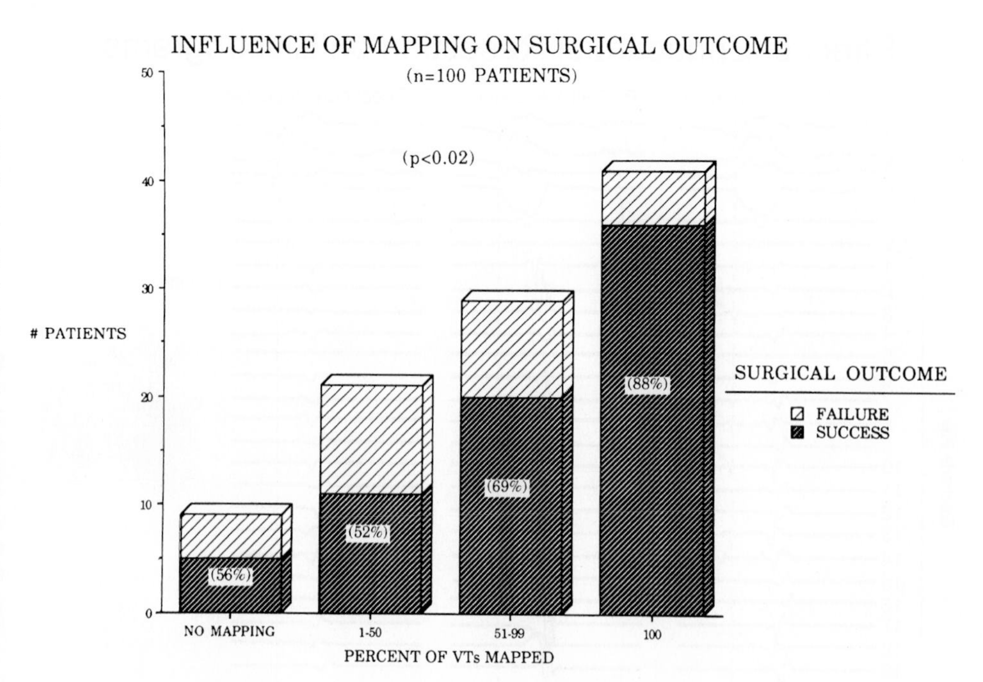


**FIGURE 13-212** *Mechanism of subendocardial resection.* Electrograms from the area from which VT arose are recorded in sinus rhythm using a plaque of 20 bipolar electrograms. Preoperatively, all electrograms are abnormal or fractionated, and many sites exhibit late potentials (*arrows*). Following subendocardial resection, recordings from the same area show "normalization" of electrograms and "amputation" of all late potentials. Placing the resected tissue over the cut endocardial surface makes the "normalized" electrograms look like the large far field components seen in **panel A**. This suggest the resected area acts as an insulator of signals from deeper layers. (Adapted from Miller JM, Vassallo JA, Rosenthal ME, et al. Endocardial late and split potentials: eradication by subendocardial resection. *Circulation* 1985;74:11.)

not show early activity and a transmural plunge shows earlier activation. These deeper layers are then cryoablated following standard subendocardial resection.

As stated earlier in this section, when tachycardias arise from an anterior infarction, our surgical approach is sequential resection in the warm, beating heart. This allows us to judge the success of the subendocardial resection and/or cryoablative lesion. Unfortunately, a sequential surgical procedure is not possible with inferior infarction, since it is virtually impossible to manipulate the heart with the inferior surgical approach without inducing ventricular fibrillation. Epicardial photocoagulation or cryoablation for those tachycardias that appear subepicardial is quite reasonable.

## Results of Surgery

The success of surgery depends on the definition of "success." It is also influenced by the type of patient who has undergone the surgical procedure as well as the electrophysiologists and surgeons involved in the procedures. Although a surgical registry has been established by Borggrefe,[317] the Hospital of the University of Pennsylvania supplied almost 50% of all the data in the registry. Our results provide a single institution's view of this electrophysiologic/surgical problem. As stated earlier in the chapter, nearly 50% of our patients had ejection fractions <25%, a number that is frequently used as a cutoff for surgical procedures at other institutions. As a consequence, nearly half of our patients would be or had been rejected at other institutions; in fact, most of our patients were referred to us from physicians at institutions with cardiothoracic surgical programs. We define our surgical results as following:

- Primary surgical success is defined by the absence of spontaneous or inducible arrhythmias on no antiarrhythmic agents following surgery.
- Clinical success is defined by the absence of spontaneous ventricular arrhythmias on or off antiarrhythmic drugs following discharge from the hospital.

**TABLE 13-2 Distribution of Electrogram Type Pre- and Postsubendocardial Resection**

| | Normal | Fractionated | Split | Other Abnormal | Late |
|---|---|---|---|---|---|
| Preresection | 8 (7%) | 28 (23%) | 13 (11%) | 71 (59%) | 38 (32%) |
| Postresection | 56 (55%) | 15 (12%) | 0 (0%) | 39 (33%) | 0 (0%) |

Subendocardial resection "normalizes" electrograms, decreases fractionated electrograms, and eliminates split and late potentials.

Data from Miller JM, Vassallo JA, Rosenthal ME, et al. Endocardial late and split potentials: eradication by subendocardial resection. *Circulation* 1985;74:11.

**TABLE 13-3 Effect of Experience on Outcome: Primary Success, Clinical Success, and Noninducibility**

| | First (%) | Second (%) | Third (%) | Fourth (%) |
|---|---|---|---|---|
| Primary success | 64 | 71 | 63 | 81 |
| Primary failure | 36 | 29 | 37 | 19 |
| Clinical success[a] | 82 | 94 | 91 | 94 |
| Clinical failure[a] | 18 | 6 | 9 | 6 |
| NI | 76 | 75 | 71 | 83 |
| I | 34 | 25 | 29 | 17 |

[a]$p = 0.05$.
I, inducibility; NI, noninducibility.
$p$ = NS.

- Inducible VT is defined by the initiation of any uniform VT regardless of whether or not it was observed before operation or intraoperatively regardless of cycle length of the induced rhythm.
- Noninducible VT is defined as failure to induce a sustained uniform VT; nonsustained VT or polymorphic tachycardia/VF is considered noninducible.
- Sudden cardiac death in this study was defined as an instantaneous death or death during sleep that was unmonitored or a monitored sudden death caused by a ventricular tachyarrhythmia. A monitored sudden death that was documented to be asystole was not considered an arrhythmogenic sudden cardiac death.

The two most important results are primarily surgical success and clinical success. As expected, we had a learning curve, and the results of both our primary and clinical success reflect this experience. If we divide our patients (who now number approximately 350) into the first, second, third, and fourth group of 100 patients, we observed an increase in primary success from nearly 64% to 81%, and our clinical success increased from 82% to 94% (Table 13-3). If we look at inducibility following surgery, of the first 100 patients, 76% had no inducible uniform VT, and in the last group that number is nearly 83%. If we look at the influence of inducibility on clinical success, we see that if the patient initially had no inducible arrhythmia, there was a 95% clinical success rate (5 years); but even if the patient initially had a postoperative inducible arrhythmia, there was a 76% success rate (Table 13-4). This is in part due to the fact that 40% of those patients who initially had inducible arrhythmias had those arrhythmias rendered noninducible by antiarrhythmic therapy before discharge. If we analyze those patients who had inducible VT initially and who then underwent drug studies, those patients whose tachycardias were rendered noninducible had an 88% success rate while still nearly 70% of patients whose tachycardias remained inducible had a good clinical outcome (Table 13-5). The fact that nearly 70% of patients who still have inducible arrhythmias on drugs at discharge nevertheless do well requires an explanation.

Miller et al.[446,447] analyzed our experience and demonstrated that induction of tachycardias that were comparable to those preoperatively—defined by identical morphology at a cycle length within 50 msec of preoperative arrhythmia—had a 50% recurrence rate. Conversely, if the postoperative tachycardias that were induced were polymorphic or had tachycardia cycle lengths 50 msec shorter than the preoperative tachycardia, only a 15% recurrence rate was observed (Fig. 13-213). In addition, tachycardias that were only inducible from the left ventricle had a lower incidence of recurrence. Of interest is the subgroup of patients in whom "never before seen" tachycardias were induced postoperatively. Most of these patients had used amiodarone preoperatively. All of these patients were readily controlled on antiarrhythmic agents afterward,

**TABLE 13-4 Inducibility of VT Postsubendocardial Resection and Clinical Outcome**

| | NI (%) | I (%) |
|---|---|---|
| Success | 95 | 76 |
| Failure | 5 | 24 |

VT, ventricular tachycardia.
$p = 0.0001$.

**TABLE 13-5 Inducibility of VT on Drugs Postsubendocardial Resection and Clinical Outcome**

| | NI (%) | I (%) |
|---|---|---|
| Success | 88 | 72 |
| Failure | 12 | 28 |

VT, ventricular tachycardia.
$p = 0.117$.

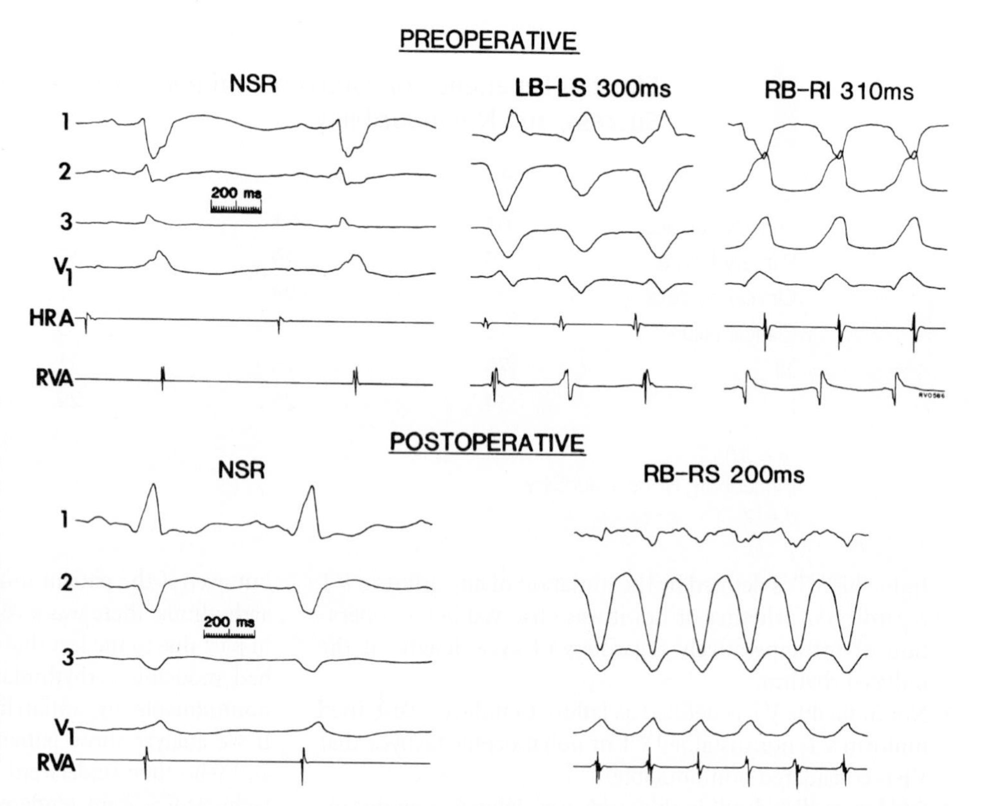


**FIGURE 13-213** *Effect of type of induced postoperative arrhythmia on outcome.* Patients with VT induced that are polymorphic or with a cycle length >50 msec shorter than control have a low incidence of recurrence. VTs of similar morphology and cycle length have a ≈50% recurrence rate. (From Miller JM, Hargrove WC, Josephson ME. Significance of "nonclinical" ventricular arrhythmias induced following surgery for ventricular tachyarrhythmias. In: Breithardt G, Borggrefe M, Zipes DP, eds. *Nonpharmacological therapy of tachyarrhythmias.* Mount Kisco, NY: Futura Publishing, 1987:133.)

suggesting that the reason for the new tachycardia was the absence of or a decrease of amiodarone effect. The apparent inability of amiodarone to suppress such tachycardias makes it doubtful that other antiarrhythmic agents would be effective.

Another method proposed to assess the postoperative outcome is use of the signal-averaged ECG. We have evaluated the role of the signal-averaged ECG in defining postoperative successes. Marcus et al.[448] demonstrated that if the low-amplitude late potential and/or prolonged QRS duration is normalized, noninducibility will be observed in the postoperative study, and an excellent outcome is to be expected. Unfortunately, only a minority of patients had such response. More often, the late potential and prolonged QRS duration remain, or may even be more prolonged, yet the clinical outcome is good. These data are not surprising, since our surgical approach is one of the limited resection of abnormal areas and not extended resection. As long as one leaves a significant amount of scar tissue and areas of normal activation, it is not surprising that the signal-averaged ECG would remain abnormal.

A subgroup of patients in whom surgery has been particularly gratifying are those patients with recurrent VT early after myocardial infarction. We [449] have demonstrated in a retrospective study of 87 patients that patients who had frequent (≥3) episodes of early postinfarction VT had significantly better survival when surgery was used than when medical therapy guided by electrophysiologic studies was used at our institution. Surgical therapy in fact was uniformly successful in patients with less than two episodes, but medical therapy was also more often successful. Thus, the difference in survival of medically and surgically treated patients did not meet statistical significance in this subgroup. Nonetheless, the high mortality both from arrhythmia and reinfarction, and heart failure in the group of patients with frequent episodes of recurrent VT, suggests that early operative intervention may be the therapy of choice (Fig. 13-214). I have reviewed our operative results in patients operated on for VT occurring less than 2 months following infarction versus those occurring more than 2 months after infarction. Two months was an arbitrary time limit, but in fact the mean time of VT was 3 weeks following infarction. The operative survival and results were at least as good as those procedures for tachycardias occurring later than 2 months after infarction (Tables 13-6 to 13-8). DiMarco et al.[450] demonstrated results similar to our previously reported data.[451]

Our overall surgical results show a 50% to 60% 5-year survival. The sudden death rate was less than our sudden death rate following implantable defibrillator, and we have observed approximately a 5% overall clinical recurrence of VT with a mean follow-up of 5.5 years. While these results seem good, more work is necessary to develop more precise surgical approaches to such patients.

## Ventricular Tachycardia Unassociated with Coronary Artery Disease

There are few systematic studies providing intraoperative mapping and surgical data for VT unassociated with coronary artery disease. Iwa et al.[452] and Guiraudon et al.[16] summarized their results in groups of patients with cardiomyopathies using ventriculotomies and cryothermal injury. How applicable these 10- to 20-year-old data are to present day patients is

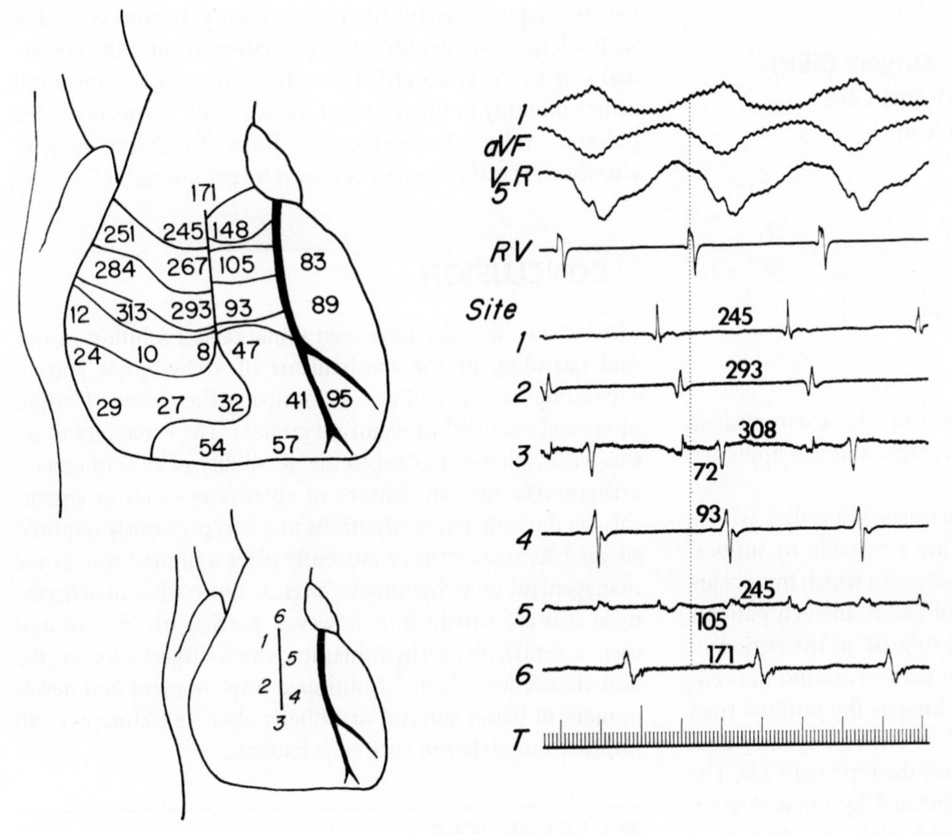


**FIGURE 13-214** *Effect of medical and surgical therapy on VT early postmyocardial infarction.* The effects of VT frequency and medical versus surgical therapy are shown. Regardless of frequency, arrhythmia-free survival was better with surgery than EPS-guided medical therapy. It is highly significant for frequent VT. (From Kleinman RB, Miller JM, Buxton AE, et al. Prognosis following sustained ventricular tachycardia occurring early after myocardial infarction. *Am J Cardiol* 1986;62:528.)

unclear. These approaches have virtually been abandoned for ICDs. We have not found management of sustained uniform VT in the setting of cardiomyopathy by drugs or surgery to improve longevity. Idiopathic left ventricular aneurysms are a cause of ventricular tachyarrhythmias that may be surgically ablated. Aizawa et al.[453] reported five such cases, and we have had two cases in which surgical approaches were successful. Recognition of this entity is important since surgery has a high success rate with relatively low risk.

Another group of patients in whom surgery has been employed for many years have been those with right ventricular dysplasia. Fontaine et al.[439,440] reported the use of ventriculotomy in such patients, but the procedure was not often successful. This led to the development of right ventricular isolation by Guiraudon et al.[454,455] The concept behind this procedure was that the arrhythmogenic right ventricle demonstrates little ventricular function and is unnecessary from a hemodynamic standpoint. Therefore, if the tachycardia remained in the free wall of the right ventricle, which is the normal site of origin of such tachycardias, isolation of that area from the rest of the myocardium would allow "normal" ventricular function despite the presence of the tachycardia. The technical procedure of disarticulation of the right ventricular free wall from the remainder of the ventricle is a difficult

**TABLE 13-6 Operative Mortality (SER) in Patients with Ventricular Tachycardia Early (<2 Mo) After Infarction**

| | VT <2 MO (%) | VT >2 MO (%) |
|---|---|---|
| Survival | 83 | 87 |
| Death | 17 | 13 |

SER, subendocardial resection.
$p = 0.36$.

**TABLE 13-7 Outcome of Surgery in Patients with VT Early (<2 Mo) or Later (>2 Mo) After Infarction**

| | VT <2 MO (%) | VT >2 MO (%) |
|---|---|---|
| Primary success | 71 | 67 |
| Early recurrence | 4 | 5 |
| Inducible | 21 | 22 |
| Late recurrence | 1 | 1 |
| Sudden death | 3 | 5 |

Primary surgical success was defined as noninducible, no clinical event.
Early recurrence was defined as an in-hospital event.
Late recurrence was defined as an event postdischarge.
$p$ = NS.

TABLE 13-8 Clinical Outcome of Surgery (SER) for VT Early (<2 Mo) and Late (>2 Mo) After Infarction

| | VT <2 MO (%) | VT >2 MO (%) |
|---|---|---|
| Success | 95 | 87 |
| Failure | 5 | 13 |

Clinical outcome refers to early and late events.
*p* = 0.06.

and time-consuming surgical task but can be accomplished. Surgical morbidity and mortality was high, and this approach has been abandoned.

Regardless of cause, any tachycardias associated with a known pathophysiologic substrate are amenable to surgical intervention. The most common situation in which this occurs is VT following repair of tetralogy of Fallot. In such patients the majority of tachycardias appear to arise in the region of the scar, often occurring in a circular pattern around the ventriculotomy or infundibulotomy as long as the outflow tract has not been replaced by a patch.[418] In this case reentry goes around the conotruncal septum above the repaired VSD. The morphology of the tachycardia is dictated by the activation wavefront (Fig. 13-187). Typically, left bundle or right bundle inferior axis tachycardias are associated with a clockwise activation pattern around the RVOT, whereas LBBB tachycardias, with superior axis, are associated with counterclockwise revolution around the RVOT. Tachycardias may also arise in the region of the ventricular septal defect repair. In cases in which circus movement around the scar is observed, continuation of the ventriculotomy to the pulmonary annulus will obliterate the narrow isthmus through which the uppermost part of the circulating wavefront must pass and terminate the arrhythmia. This area is invariably associated with very slow conduction manifested by tight isochrones during mapping or continuous activity during electrophysiologic study. Analog recordings from a left bundle, left axis deviation-type tachycardia in a patient with counterclockwise activation around the scar is shown in Figure 13-215. The surgical approach to VT in these

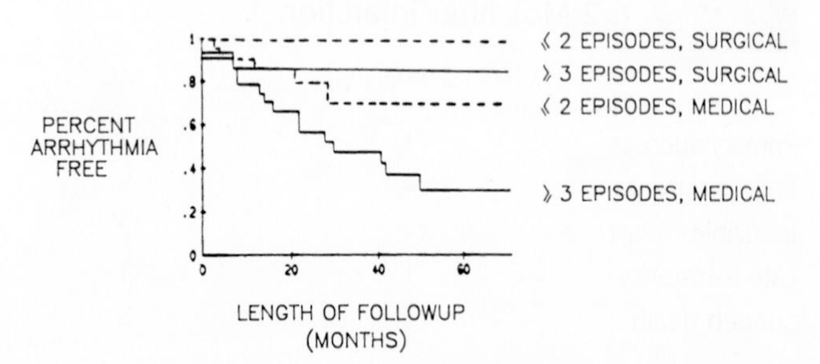


**FIGURE 13-215** *Analog recordings during epicardial mapping of ventricular tachycardia in a patient following repair of tetralogy of Fallot.* Electrograms suggest activation in a counterclockwise fashion around the ventriculotomy scar.

patients requires careful attention to ensure that one is dealing with a large macroreentrant circuit either around the epicardial scar or the endocardial scar. In both cases, a transmural ventriculotomy in the region of the scar with extension to the pulmonic valve will cure the arrhythmia. If tachycardias arise elsewhere, specific approaches must be employed.

## CONCLUSION

The last two decades have seen remarkable evolution in our understanding of the mechanisms of arrhythmias and in expanding our capabilities of localizing their sites of origin or critical sites within reentrant circuits. The capability to do this with catheters has led to the possibility of cure of certain arrhythmias through delivery of ablative energies or chemicals via the catheter, in situations that had previously required surgery. As such, surgery currently plays a limited role in the management of arrhythmias. Surgical approaches to arrhythmias still are worthwhile, however, particularly for AF and certain ventricular arrhythmias for which surgery remains the best chance for a "cure." Continued improvement and development of better surgical or catheter ablative techniques will improve our ability to cure such patients.

## REFERENCES


1. Cobb FR, Blumenschein SD, Sealy WC, et al. Successful surgical interruption of the bundle of kent in a patient with Wolff-Parkinson-White syndrome. *Circulation* 1968;38:1018–1029.
2. Sealy WC, Hattler BG Jr., Blumenschein SD, et al. Surgical treatment of Wolff-Parkinson-White syndrome. *Ann Thorac Surg* 1969;8:1–11.
3. Gallagher JJ. Surgical treatment of arrhythmias: current status and future directions.*Am J Cardiol* 1978;41:1035–1044.
4. Josephson ME, Harken AH. Surgical therapy of arrhythmias. *Cardiac Therapy* 1983:337.
5. Cox JL. Surgical management of cardiac arrhythmias. *Cardiac Pacing Electrophysiol* 1991:436.
6. Iwa T, Mitsui T, Misaki T, et al. Radical surgical cure of Wolff-Parkinson-White syndrome: the kanazawa experience. *J Thorac Cardiovasc Surg* 1986; 91:225–233.
7. Ferguson TB, Cox JL. Surgical treatment for the Wolff-Parkinson-White syndrome: the endocardial approach. *Cardiac Electrophysiol* 1990:697–907.
8. Guiraudon GM, Klein GJ, Gulamhusein S, et al. Surgical repair of Wolff-Parkinson-White syndrome: a new closed-heart technique. *Ann Thorac Surg* 1984;37:67–71.
9. Guiraudon GM, Klein GJ, Sharma AD, et al. Surgery for the Wolff-Parkinson-White syndrome: the epicardial approach. *Cardiac Electrophysiol* 1990:907.
10. Guiraudon GM, Sharma AD, Yee R. Surgery for atrial flutter, atrial fibrillation, and atrial tachycardia. *Cardiac Electrophysiol* 1990:915.
11. Cox JL, Schuessler RB, D'Agostino HJ Jr., et al. The surgical treatment of atrial fibrillation. Iii. Development of a definitive surgical procedure. *J Thorac Cardiovasc Surg* 1991;101:569–583.
12. Cox JL. The surgical treatment of atrial fibrillation. Iv. Surgical technique. *J Thorac Cardiovasc Surg* 1991;101:584–592.
13. Johnson DC, Boss DL, Uther JB. The surgical cure of atrioventricular junctional reentrant tachycardia. *Cardiac Electrophysiol* 1990:921.
14. Guiraudon G, Fontaine G, Frank R, et al. Encircling endocardial ventriculotomy: a new surgical treatment for life-threatening ventricular tachycardias resistant to medical treatment following myocardial infarction. *Ann Thorac Surg* 1978;26:438–444.
15. Josephson ME, Harken AH, Horowitz LN. Endocardial excision: a new surgical technique for the treatment of recurrent ventricular tachycardia. *Circulation* 1979;60:1430–1439.

16. Guiraudon G, Fontaine G, Frank R, et al. Surgical treatment of ventricular tachycardia guided by ventricular mapping in 23 patients without coronary artery disease. *Ann Thorac Surg* 1981;32:439–450.
17. Bogen DK, Derbyshire GJ, Marchlinski FE, et al. Is catheter ablation on target? *Am J Cardiol* 1987;60:1387–1392.
18. Bardy GH, Coltorti F, Stewart RB, et al. Catheter-mediated electrical ablation: the relation between current and pulse width on voltage breakdown and shock-wave generation. *Pacing Clin Electrophysiol* 1986;9: 1381–1383.
19. Levine JH, Merillat JC, Stern M, et al. The cellular electrophysiologic changes induced by ablation: comparison between argon laser photoablation and high-energy electrical ablation. *Circulation* 1987;76:217–225.
20. Haines DE, Watson DD, Verow AF. Electrode radius predicts lesion radius during radiofrequency energy heating. Validation of a proposed thermodynamic model. *Circ Res* 1990;67:124–129.
21. Haines DE. The biophysics of radiofrequency catheter ablation in the heart: the importance of temperature monitoring. *Pacing Clin Electrophysiol* 1993;16:586–591.
22. Langberg JJ, Gallagher M, Strickberger SA, et al. Temperature-guided radiofrequency catheter ablation with very large distal electrodes. *Circulation* 1993;88:245–249.
23. Panescu D, Whayne JG, Fleischman SD, et al. Three-dimensional finite element analysis of current density and temperature distributions during radio-frequency ablation. *IEEE Trans Biomed Eng* 1995;42:879–890.
24. Neven K, van Driel V, van Wessel H, et al. Safety and feasibility of closed chest epicardial catheter ablation using electroporation. *Circ Arrhythm Electrophysiol* 2014;7:913–919.
25. Neven K, van Driel V, van Wessel H, et al. Myocardial lesion size after epicardial electroporation catheter ablation after subxiphoid puncture. *Circ Arrhythm Electrophysiol* 2014;7:728–733.
26. van Driel VJ, Neven KG, van Wessel H, et al. Pulmonary vein stenosis after catheter ablation: electroporation versus radiofrequency. *Circ Arrhythm Electrophysiol* 2014;7:734–738.
27. Wittkampf FH, Nakagawa H. Rf catheter ablation: lessons on lesions. *Pacing Clin Electrophysiol* 2006;29:1285–1297.
28. Fontaine G, Volmer W, Nienaltowska E, et al. Approach to the physics of fulguration. *Ablation Cardiac Arrhythm* 1987.
29. Scheinman MM. Catheter ablation. Present role and projected impact on health care for patients with cardiac arrhythmias. *Circulation.* 1991; 83:1489–1498.
30. Jones JL, Lepeschkin E, Jones RE, et al. Response of cultured myocardial cells to countershock-type electric field stimulation. *Am J Physiol* 1978; 235:H214–H222.
31. Bardy GH, Ivey TD, Coltorti F, et al. Developments, complications and limitations of catheter-mediated electrical ablation of posterior accessory atrioventricular pathways. *Am J Cardiol* 1988;61:309–316.
32. Fisher JD, Brodman R, Kim SG, et al. Attempted nonsurgical electrical ablation of accessory pathways via the coronary sinus in the Wolff-Parkinson-White syndrome. *J Am Coll Cardiol* 1984;4:685–694.
33. Bockeria LA, Kupatadze NI, Saprigin DB, et al. Surgical treatment of the Wolff-Parkinson-White syndrome by epicardial electrical ablation. *Ann Thorac Surg* 1991;51:563–572.
34. Lemery R, Leung TK, Lavallee E, et al. In vitro and in vivo effects within the coronary sinus of nonarcing and arcing shocks using a new system of low-energy dc ablation. *Circulation* 1991;83:279–293.
35. Moore EN, Schafer W, Kadish A, et al. Electrophysiological studies on cardiac catheter ablation. *Pacing Clin Electrophysiol* 1989;12:150–158.
36. Kempf FC Jr., Falcone RA, Iozzo RV, et al. Anatomic and hemodynamic effects of catheter-delivered ablation energies in the ventricle. *Am J Cardiol* 1985;56:373–377.
37. Bardy GH, Coltorti F, Ivey TD, et al. Effect of damped sine-wave shocks on catheter dielectric strength. *Am J Cardiol* 1985;56:769–772.
38. du Pre BC, van Driel VJ, van Wessel H, et al. Minimal coronary artery damage by myocardial electroporation ablation. *Europace* 2013;15:144–149.
39. Huang SK, Graham AR, Lee MA, et al. Comparison of catheter ablation using radiofrequency versus direct current energy: biophysical, electrophysiologic and pathologic observations. *J Am Coll Cardiol* 1991; 18:1091–1097.
40. Huang SK, Graham AR, Bharati S, et al. Short- and long-term effects of transcatheter ablation of the coronary sinus by radiofrequency energy. *Circulation* 1988;78:416–427.
41. Langberg JJ, Lee MA, Chin MC, et al. Radiofrequency catheter ablation: the effect of electrode size on lesion volume in vivo. *Pacing Clin Electrophysiol* 1990;13:1242–1248.
42. Langberg JJ, Chin M, Schamp DJ, et al. Ablation of the atrioventricular junction with radiofrequency energy using a new electrode catheter. *Am J Cardiol* 1991;67:142–147.
43. Jackman WM, Wang XZ, Friday KJ, et al. Catheter ablation of atrioventricular junction using radiofrequency current in 17 patients. Comparison of standard and large-tip catheter electrodes. *Circulation* 1991;83:1562–1576.
44. Yokoyama K, Nakagawa H, Wittkampf FH, et al. Comparison of electrode cooling between internal and open irrigation in radiofrequency ablation lesion depth and incidence of thrombus and steam pop. *Circulation* 2006;113:11–19.
45. Haines DE, Stewart MT, Dahlberg S, et al. Microembolism and catheter ablation i: a comparison of irrigated radiofrequency and multielectrode-phased radiofrequency catheter ablation of pulmonary vein ostia. *Circulation Arrhythm Electrophysiol* 2013;6:16–22.
46. Verma A, Debruyne P, Nardi S, et al. Evaluation and reduction of asymptomatic cerebral embolism in ablation of atrial fibrillation, but high prevalence of chronic silent infarction: results of the evaluation of reduction of asymptomatic cerebral embolism trial. *Circulation Arrhythm Electrophysiol* 2013;6:835–842.
47. Herrera Siklody C, Deneke T, Hocini M, et al. Incidence of asymptomatic intracranial embolic events after pulmonary vein isolation: comparison of different atrial fibrillation ablation technologies in a multicenter study. *J Am Coll Cardiol* 2011;58:681–688.
48. Yokoyama K, Nakagawa H, Shah DC, et al. Novel contact force sensor incorporated in irrigated radiofrequency ablation catheter predicts lesion size and incidence of steam pop and thrombus. *Circulation Arrhythm Electrophysiol* 2008;1:354–362.
49. Reddy VY, Shah D, Kautzner J, et al. The relationship between contact force and clinical outcome during radiofrequency catheter ablation of atrial fibrillation in the toccata study. *Heart Rhythm* 2012;9:1789–1795.
50. Andrade JG, Monir G, Pollak SJ, et al. Pulmonary vein isolation using "contact force" ablation: the effect on dormant conduction and long-term freedom from recurrent atrial fibrillation-a prospective study. *Heart Rhythm* 2014;11:1919–1924.
51. Nakagawa H, Kautzner J, Natale A, et al. Locations of high contact force during left atrial mapping in atrial fibrillation patients: electrogram amplitude and impedance are poor predictors of electrode-tissue contact force for ablation of atrial fibrillation. *Circulation Arrhythm Electrophysiol* 2013;6:746–753.
52. Natale A, Reddy VY, Monir G, et al. Paroxysmal AF catheter ablation with a contact force sensing catheter: results of the prospective, multicenter smart-af trial. *J Am Coll Cardiol* 2014;64:647–656.
53. Saksena S. Laser ablation for tachyarrhythmia control: current status and future development. *Cardiac Arrhythm* 1987:803.
54. Selle JG, Svenson RH, Sealy WC, et al. Successful clinical laser ablation of ventricular tachycardia: a promising new therapeutic method. *Ann Thorac Surg* 1986;42:380–384.
55. Svenson RH, Gallagher JJ, Selle JG, et al. Neodymium:YAG laser photocoagulation: a successful new map-guided technique for the intraoperative ablation of ventricular tachycardia. *Circulation* 1987;76:1319–1328.
56. Svenson RH, Littmann L, Gallagher JJ, et al. Termination of ventricular tachycardia with epicardial laser photocoagulation: a clinical comparison with patients undergoing successful endocardial photocoagulation alone. *J Am Coll Cardiol* 1990;15:163–170.
57. Littmann L, Svenson RH, Tomcsanyi I, et al. Modification of atrioventricular node transmission properties by intraoperative neodymium-yag laser photocoagulation in dogs. *J Am Coll Cardiol* 1991;17:797–804.
58. Narula OS, Bharati S, Chan MC, et al. Microtransection of the his bundle with laser radiation through a pervenous catheter: correlation of histologic and electrophysiologic data. *Am J Cardiol* 1984;54:186–192.
59. Lee BI, Gottdiener JS, Fletcher RD, et al. Transcatheter ablation: comparison between laser photoablation and electrode shock ablation in the dog. *Circulation* 1985;71:579–586.
60. Schmidt B, Metzner A, Chun KR, et al. Feasibility of circumferential pulmonary vein isolation using a novel endoscopic ablation system. *Circ Arrhythm Electrophysiol* 2010;3:481–488.
61. Dukkipati SR, Kuck KH, Neuzil P, et al. Pulmonary vein isolation using a visually guided laser balloon catheter: the first 200-patient multicenter clinical experience. *Circulation Arrhythm Electrophysiol* 2013;6: 467–472.
62. Andrade JG, Khairy P, Dubuc M. Catheter cryoablation: biology and clinical uses. *Circ Arrhythm Electrophysiol* 2013;6:218–227.

63. Hanninen M, Yeung-Lai-Wah N, Massel D, et al. Cryoablation versus RF ablation for AVNRT: a meta-analysis and systematic review. *J Cardiovasc Electrophysiol* 2013;24:1354–1360.
64. Packer DL, Kowal RC, Wheelan KR, et al. Cryoballoon ablation of pulmonary veins for paroxysmal atrial fibrillation: first results of the North American Arctic Front (STOP AF) pivotal trial. *J Am Coll Cardiol* 2013;61:1713–1723.
65. Natale A, Pisano E, Shewchik J, et al. First human experience with pulmonary vein isolation using a through-the-balloon circumferential ultrasound ablation system for recurrent atrial fibrillation. *Circulation* 2000;102:1879–1882.
66. Neven K, Schmidt B, Metzner A, et al. Fatal end of a safety algorithm for pulmonary vein isolation with use of high-intensity focused ultrasound. *Circ Arrhythm Electrophysiol* 2010;3:260–265.
67. Ross DL, Johnson DC, Denniss AR, et al. Curative surgery for atrioventricular junctional ("AV nodal") reentrant tachycardia. *J Am Coll Cardiol* 1985;6:1383–1392.
68. Johnson DC, Nunn GR, Richards DA, et al. Surgical therapy for supraventricular tachycardia, a potentially curable disorder. *J Thorac Cardiovasc Surg* 1987;93:913–918.
69. Williams JM, Ungerleider RM, Lofland GK, et al. Left atrial isolation: new technique for the treatment of supraventricular arrhythmias. *J Thorac Cardiovasc Surg* 1980;80:373–380.
70. Leitch JW, Klein G, Yee R, et al. Sinus node-atrioventricular node isolation: long-term results with the "corridor" operation for atrial fibrillation. *J Am Coll Cardiol* 1991;17:970–975.
71. Cox JL, Boineau JP, Schuessler RB, et al. Modification of the maze procedure for atrial flutter and atrial fibrillation. I. Rationale and surgical results. *J Thorac Cardiovasc Surg* 1995;110:473–484.
72. Melo J, Adragao PR, Neves J, et al. Electrosurgical treatment of atrial fibrillation with a new intraoperative radiofrequency ablation catheter. *Thorac Cardiovasc Surg* 1999;47(Suppl 3):370–372.
73. Melo J, Adragao P, Neves J, et al. Endocardial and epicardial radiofrequency ablation in the treatment of atrial fibrillation with a new intra-operative device. *Eur J Cardiothorac Surg* 2000;18:182–186.
74. Cox JL, Schuessler RB, Lappas DG, et al. An 8 1/2-year clinical experience with surgery for atrial fibrillation. *Ann Surg* 1996;224:267–273; discussion 273–265.
75. Holman WL, Ikeshita M, Lease JG, et al. Elective prolongation of atrioventricular conduction by multiple discrete cryolesions: a new technique for the treatment of paroxysmal supraventricular tachycardia. *J Thorac Cardiovasc Surg* 1982;84:554–559.
76. Holman WL, Ikeshita M, Lease JG, et al. Alteration of antegrade atrioventricular conduction by cryoablation of peri-atrioventricular nodal tissue. Implications for the surgical treatment of atrioventricular nodal reentry tachycardia. *J Thorac Cardiovasc Surg* 1984;88:67–75.
77. Klein GJ, Guiraudon GM, Perkins DG, et al. Controlled cryothermal injury to the AV node: feasibility for av nodal modification. *Pacing Clin Electrophysiol* 1985;8:630–638.
78. Cox JL, Holman WL, Cain ME. Cryosurgical treatment of atrioventricular node reentrant tachycardia. *Circulation* 1987;76:1329–1336.
79. Wood DL, Hammill SC, Porter CB, et al. Cryosurgical modification of atrioventricular conduction for treatment of atrioventricular node reentrant tachycardia. *Mayo Clin Proc* 1988;63:988–992.
80. Gonzalez R, Scheinman M, Margaretten W, et al. Closed-chest electrode-catheter technique for his bundle ablation in dogs. *Am J Physiol* 1981; 241:H283–H287.
81. Scheinman MM, Morady F, Hess DS, et al. Catheter-induced ablation of the atrioventricular junction to control refractory supraventricular arrhythmias. *JAMA* 1982;248:851–855.
82. Gallagher JJ, Svenson RH, Kasell JH, et al. Catheter technique for closed-chest ablation of the atrioventricular conduction system. *N Engl J Med* 1982;306:194–200.
83. Gallagher JJ, Cox JL, German LD,Nonpharmacologic treatment of supraventricular tachycardia. *Tachycardias: Mechanisms, diagnosis, treatment.* 1984:271.
84. Jackman WM, Friday KJ, Scherlag BJ, et al. Direct endocardial recording from an accessory atrioventricular pathway: localization of the site of block, effect of antiarrhythmic drugs, and attempt at nonsurgical ablation. *Circulation* 1983;68:906–916.
85. Critelli G, Gallagher JJ, Perticone F, et al. Transvenous catheter ablation of the accessory atrioventricular pathway in the permanent form of junctional reciprocating tachycardia. *Am J Cardiol* 1985;55:1639–1641.
86. Haissaguerre M, Warin JF, Regaudie JJ, et al. [catheter ablation after the direct electrical recording of the bundle of kent. Apropos of 3 cases]. *Arch Mal Coeur Vaiss* 1986;79:1072–1079.
87. Ruder MA, Mead RH, Gaudiani V, et al. Transvenous catheter ablation of extranodal accessory pathways. *J Am Coll Cardiol* 1988;11:1245–1253.
88. Warin JF, Haissaguerre M, Lemetayer P, et al. Catheter ablation of accessory pathways with a direct approach. Results in 35 patients. *Circulation* 1988;78:800–815.
89. Haissaguerre M, Warin JF. Closed-chest ablation of left lateral atrioventricular accessory pathways. *Eur Heart J* 1989;10:602–610.
90. Morady F, Scheinman MM, Kou WH, et al. Long-term results of catheter ablation of a posteroseptal accessory atrioventricular connection in 48 patients. *Circulation* 1989;79:1160–1170.
91. Smith RT Jr., Gillette PC, Massumi A, et al. Transcatheter ablative techniques for treatment of the permanent form of junctional reciprocating tachycardia in young patients. *J Am Coll Cardiol* 1986;8:385–390.
92. Kuck KH, Schluter M, Geiger M, et al. Radiofrequency current catheter ablation of accessory atrioventricular pathways. *Lancet* 1991;337:1557–1561.
93. Haissaguerre M, Dartigues JF, Warin JF, et al. Electrogram patterns predictive of successful catheter ablation of accessory pathways. Value of unipolar recording mode. *Circulation* 1991;84:188–202.
94. Jackman WM, Wang XZ, Friday KJ, et al. Catheter ablation of accessory atrioventricular pathways (Wolff-Parkinson-White syndrome) by radiofrequency current. *N Engl J Med* 1991;324:1605–1611.
95. Warin JF, Haissaguerre M, D'Ivernois C, et al. Catheter ablation of accessory pathways: technique and results in 248 patients. *Pacing Clin Electrophysiol* 1990;13:1609–1614.
96. Haissaguerre M, Warin JF, Lemetayer P, et al. Closed-chest ablation of retrograde conduction in patients with atrioventricular nodal reentrant tachycardia. *N Engl J Med* 1989;320:426–433.
97. Calkins H, Sousa J, el-Atassi R, et al. Diagnosis and cure of the Wolff-Parkinson-White syndrome or paroxysmal supraventricular tachycardias during a single electrophysiologic test. *N Engl J Med.* 1991;324:1612–1618.
98. Epstein LM, Scheinman MM. Modification of the atrioventricular node. A new approach to the treatment of supraventricular tachycardias. *Cardiol Clin* 1990;8:567–574.
99. Haissaguerre M, Warin JF, D'Ivernois C, et al. Fulguration for av nodal tachycardia: results in 42 patients with a mean follow-up of 23 months. *Pacing Clin Electrophysiol.* 1990;13:2000–2007.
100. Lee MA, Morady F, Kadish A, et al. Catheter modification of the atrioventricular junction with radiofrequency energy for control of atrioventricular nodal reentry tachycardia. *Circulation* 1991;83:827–835.
101. Swartz JP, Cohen AI, Fletcher RD, et al. Right coronary epicardial mapping improves accessory pathway catheter ablation success [abstract]. *Circulation* 1989;80:111.
102. Cosio FG, Anderson RH, Kuck KH, et al. Living anatomy of the atrioventricular junctions. A guide to electrophysiologic mapping. A Consensus Statement from the Cardiac Nomenclature Study Group, Working Group of Arrhythmias, European Society of Cardiology, and the Task Force on Cardiac Nomenclature from NASPE. *Circulation* 1999;100: e31–e37.
103. Smeets J, Allessie M, Kirchlof CH, et al. High resolution mapping of ventriculo-atrial conduction over the accessory pathway in patients with the Wolff-Parkinson-White syndrome. *Eur Heart Abs. J* 1990;11:1.
104. Jackman WM, Friday KJ, Yeung-Lai-Wah JA, et al. New catheter technique for recording left free-wall accessory atrioventricular pathway activation. Identification of pathway fiber orientation. *Circulation* 1988; 78:598–611.
105. Niebauer MJ, Daoud E, Goyal R, et al. Assessment of pacing maneuvers used to validate anterograde accessory pathway potentials. *J Cardiovasc Electrophysiol.* 1995;6:350–356.
106. Jackman WM, Friday KJ, Fitzgerald DM, et al. Localization of left free-wall and posteroseptal accessory atrioventricular pathways by direct recording of accessory pathway activation. *Pacing Clin Electrophysiol* 1989;12: 204–214.
107. Jackman WM, Kuck KH, Friday KJ, et al. Catheter recordings of accessory atrioventricular pathway activation. *Cardiac Electrophysiol* 1990:491.
108. Joyner RW. Effects of the discrete pattern of electrical coupling on propagation through an electrical syncytium. *Circ Res* 1982;50:192–200.
109. Spach MS, Miller WT 3rd, Dolber PC, et al. The functional role of structural complexities in the propagation of depolarization in the atrium of the dog. Cardiac conduction disturbances due to discontinuities of effective axial resistivity. *Circ Res* 1982;50:175–191.

110. Spach MS, Miller WT 3rd, Geselowitz DB, et al. The discontinuous nature of propagation in normal canine cardiac muscle. Evidence for recurrent discontinuities of intracellular resistance that affect the membrane currents. *Circ Res* 1981;48:39–54.
111. Kuck KH, Friday KJ, Kunze KP, et al. Sites of conduction block in accessory atrioventricular pathways. Basis for concealed accessory pathways. *Circulation* 1990;82:407–417.
112. Kuck KH, Jackman WM, Friday KJ, et al. Sites of conduction block in accessory atrioventricular pathways. Basis for concealed accessory pathways. *Cardiac Electrophysiol* 1990:503.
113. Calkins H, Yong P, Miller JM, et al. Catheter ablation of accessory pathways, atrioventricular nodal reentrant tachycardia, and the atrioventricular junction: final results of a prospective, multicenter clinical trial. The atakr multicenter investigators group. *Circulation* 1999;99:262–270.
114. Kay GN, Epstein AE, Dailey SM, et al. Role of radiofrequency ablation in the management of supraventricular arrhythmias: experience in 760 consecutive patients. *J Cardiovasc Electrophysiol* 1993;4:371–389.
115. Morady F. Radio-frequency ablation as treatment for cardiac arrhythmias. *N Engl J Med* 1999;340:534–544.
116. Scheinman MM, Huang S. The 1998 NASPE prospective catheter ablation registry. *Pacing Clin Electrophysiol* 2000;23:1020–1028.
117. Morady F. Catheter ablation of supraventricular arrhythmias: state of the art. *J Cardiovasc Electrophysiol* 2004;15:124–239.
118. Hogenhuis W, Stevens SK, Wang P, et al. Cost-effectiveness of radiofrequency ablation compared with other strategies in Wolff-Parkinson-White syndrome. *Circulation* 1993;88:II437–II446.
119. Pappone C, Vicedomini G, Manguso F, et al. Risk of malignant arrhythmias in initially symptomatic patients with Wolff-Parkinson-White syndrome: results of a prospective long-term electrophysiological follow-up study. *Circulation* 2012;125:661–668.
120. Pappone C, Vicedomini G, Manguso F, et al. Wolff-Parkinson-White syndrome in the era of catheter ablation: insights from a registry study of 2169 patients. *Circulation* 2014;130:811–819.
121. Obeyesekere MN, Klein GJ. The asymptomatic Wolff-Parkinson-White patient: time to be more proactive? *Circulation* 2014;130:805–807.
122. Pediatric and Congenital Electrophysiology Society (PACES), Heart Rhythm Society (HRS), American College of Cardiology Foundation (ACCF), et al. PACES/HRS expert consensus statement on the management of the asymptomatic young patient with a Wolff-Parkinson-White (WPW, ventricular preexcitation) electrocardiographic pattern: developed in partnership between the Pediatric and Congenital Electrophysiology Society (PACES) and the Heart Rhythm Society (HRS). Endorsed by the governing bodies of PACES, HRS, the American College of Cardiology Foundation (ACCF), the American Heart Association (AHA), the American Academy of Pediatrics (AAP), and the Canadian Heart Rhythm Society (CHRS). *Heart Rhythm* 2012;9:1006–1024.
123. Manolis AS, Wang PJ, Estes NA 3rd. Radiofrequency ablation of left-sided accessory pathways: transaortic versus transseptal approach. *Am Heart J* 1994;128:896–902.
124. Swartz JF, Tracy CM, Fletcher RD. Radiofrequency endocardial catheter ablation of accessory atrioventricular pathway atrial insertion sites. *Circulation* 1993;87:487–499.
125. Farre J, Grande A, Martinell J, et al. Atrial unipolar waveform analysis during retrograde conduction over left-sided accessory atrioventricular pathways. *Cardiac Arrhythm* 1987:243.
126. Nakagawa H, Jackman WM. Catheter ablation of paroxysmal supraventricular tachycardia. *Circulation* 2007;116:2465–2478.
127. Otomo K, Gonzalez MD, Beckman KJ, et al. Reversing the direction of paced ventricular and atrial wavefronts reveals an oblique course in accessory av pathways and improves localization for catheter ablation. *Circulation* 2001;104:550–556.
128. Giorgberidze I, Saksena S, Krol RB, et al. Efficacy and safety of radiofrequency catheter ablation of left-sided accessory pathways through the coronary sinus. *Am J Cardiol* 1995;76:359–365.
129. Stavrakis S, Jackman WM, Nakagawa H, et al. Risk of coronary artery injury with radiofrequency ablation and cryoablation of epicardial posteroseptal accessory pathways within the coronary venous system. *Circ Arrhythm Electrophysiol* 2014;7:113–119.
130. Ticho BS, Saul JP, Hulse JE, et al. Variable location of accessory pathways associated with the permanent form of junctional reciprocating tachycardia and confirmation with radiofrequency ablation. *Am J Cardiol* 1992;70:1559–1564.
131. McClelland JH, Wang X, Beckman KJ, et al. Radiofrequency catheter ablation of right atriofascicular (mahaim) accessory pathways guided by accessory pathway activation potentials. *Circulation* 1994;89:2655–2666.
132. Hindricks G. The Multicentre European Radiofrequency Survey (MERFS): complications of radiofrequency catheter ablation of arrhythmias. The Multicentre European Radiofrequency Survey (MERFS) investigators of the Working Group on Arrhythmias of the European Society of Cardiology. *Euro Heart J* 1993;14:1644–1653.
133. Bohnen M, Stevenson WG, Tedrow UB, et al. Incidence and predictors of major complications from contemporary catheter ablation to treat cardiac arrhythmias. *Heart Rhythm* 2011;8:1661–1666.
134. Zhou L, Keane D, Reed G, et al. Thromboembolic complications of cardiac radiofrequency catheter ablation: a review of the reported incidence, pathogenesis and current research directions. *J Cardiovasc Electrophysiol* 1999;10:611–620.
135. Durrer D, Roos JP. Epicardial excitation of the ventricles in a patient with Wolff-Parkinson-White syndrome (type b). *Circulation* 1967;35:15–21.
136. Ferguson TH, Lesh MD, Haines DE. *Electrophysiology self assessment program [book 8]*. Bethesda, MD: American College of Cardiology and North American Society for Pacing and Electrophysiology, 1996..
137. Evans GT Jr., Scheinman MM, Scheinman MM, et al. The percutaneous cardiac mapping and ablation registry: final summary of results. *Pacing Clin Electrophysiol* 1988;11:1621–1626.
138. Evans GT, Huang WH. Car investigators. Comparison of direct current radiofrequency energy for catheter ablation of the atrioventricular junction: results of a prospective multicenter study [abstract]. *Circulation* 1990;82:719.
139. Evans GT, Huang WH. Car investigators. In-hospital mortality after direct current catheter ablation of the atrioventricular junction: a prospective international multicenter study [abstract]. *Circulation* 1990;82:691.
140. Twidale N, Sutton K, Bartlett L, et al. Effects on cardiac performance of atrioventricular node catheter ablation using radiofrequency current for drug-refractory atrial arrhythmias. *Pacing Clin Electrophysiol* 1993;16:1275–1284.
141. Brignole M, Gianfranchi L, Menozzi C, et al. Influence of atrioventricular junction radiofrequency ablation in patients with chronic atrial fibrillation and flutter on quality of life and cardiac performance. *Am J Cardiol* 1994;74:242–246.
142. Kay GN, Ellenbogen KA, Giudici M, et al. The ablate and pace trial: a prospective study of catheter ablation of the av conduction system and permanent pacemaker implantation for treatment of atrial fibrillation. Apt investigators. *J Interv Card Electrophysiol* 1998;2:121–135.
143. Feld GK, Fleck RP, Fujimura O, et al. Control of rapid ventricular response by radiofrequency catheter modification of the atrioventricular node in patients with medically refractory atrial fibrillation. *Circulation* 1994;90:2299–2307.
144. Morady F, Hasse C, Strickberger SA, et al. Long-term follow-up after radiofrequency modification of the atrioventricular node in patients with atrial fibrillation. *J Am Coll Cardiol* 1997;29:113–121.
145. Doshi RN, Daoud EG, Fellows C, et al. Left ventricular-based cardiac stimulation post av nodal ablation evaluation (the pave study). *J Cardiovasc Electrophysiol* 2005;16:1160–1165.
146. Orlov MV, Gardin JM, Slawsky M, et al. Biventricular pacing improves cardiac function and prevents further left atrial remodeling in patients with symptomatic atrial fibrillation after atrioventricular node ablation. *Am Heart J* 2010;159:264–270.
147. Ousdigian KT, Borek PP, Koehler JL, et al. The epidemic of inadequate biventricular pacing in patients with persistent or permanent atrial fibrillation and its association with mortality. *Circ Arrhythm Electrophysiol* 2014;7:370–376.
148. Jackman WM, Beckman KJ, McClelland JH, et al. Treatment of supraventricular tachycardia due to atrioventricular nodal reentry, by radiofrequency catheter ablation of slow-pathway conduction. *N Engl J Med* 1992;327:313–318.
149. Haissaguerre M, Gaita F, Fischer B, et al. Elimination of atrioventricular nodal reentrant tachycardia using discrete slow potentials to guide application of radiofrequency energy. *Circulation* 1992;85:2162–2175.
150. Niebauer MJ, Daoud E, Williamson B, et al. Atrial electrogram characteristics in patients with and without atrioventricular nodal reentrant tachycardia. *Circulation* 1995;92:77–81.
151. Jazayeri MR, Hempe SL, Sra JS, et al. Selective transcatheter ablation of the fast and slow pathways using radiofrequency energy in patients with atrioventricular nodal reentrant tachycardia. *Circulation* 1992;85:1318–1328.

152. Kay GN, Epstein AE, Dailey SM, et al. Selective radiofrequency ablation of the slow pathway for the treatment of atrioventricular nodal reentrant tachycardia. Evidence for involvement of perinodal myocardium within the reentrant circuit. *Circulation* 1992;85:1675–1688.
153. Langberg JJ, Leon A, Borganelli M, et al. A randomized, prospective comparison of anterior and posterior approaches to radiofrequency catheter ablation of atrioventricular nodal reentry tachycardia. *Circulation* 1993;87:1551–1556.
154. Roman CA, Wang X, Friday KJ, et al. Catheter technique with selective ablation of slow pathway and a-v nodal reentrant tachycardia [abstract]. *Pacing Clin Electrophysiol.* 1990;13:498.
155. Anselme F, Hook B, Monahan K, et al. Heterogeneity of retrograde fast-pathway conduction pattern in patients with atrioventricular nodal reentry tachycardia: observations by simultaneous multisite catheter mapping of Koch's triangle. *Circulation* 1996;93:960–968.
156. Loh P, de Bakker JM, Hocini M, et al. Reentrant pathway during ventricular echoes is confined to the atrioventricular node : high-resolution mapping and dissection of the triangle of koch in isolated, perfused canine hearts. *Circulation* 1999;100:1346–1353.
157. McGuire MA, Bourke JP, Robotin MC, et al. High resolution mapping of koch's triangle using sixty electrodes in humans with atrioventricular junctional (av nodal) reentrant tachycardia. *Circulation* 1993;88:2315–2328.
158. Boyle NG, Anselme F, Monahan K, et al. Origin of junctional rhythm during radiofrequency ablation of atrioventricular nodal reentrant tachycardia in patients without structural heart disease. *Am J Cardiol.* 1997; 80:575–580.
159. Chen J, Josephson ME. Recent advances in AVNRT: mechanisms and therapy.. *Cardiac Electrophysiol Rev* 2000;4:43–49.
160. Jais P, Haissaguerre M, Shah DC, et al. Successful radiofrequency ablation of a slow atrioventricular nodal pathway on the left posterior atrial septum. *Pacing Clin Electrophysiol* 1999;22:525–527.
161. Altemose GT, Scott LR, Miller JM. Atrioventricular nodal reentrant tachycardia requiring ablation on the mitral annulus. *J Cardiovasc Electrophysiol* 2000;11:1281–1284.
162. Sorbera C, Cohen M, Woolf P, et al. Atrioventricular nodal reentry tachycardia: slow pathway ablation using the transseptal approach. *Pacing Clin Electrophysiol* 2000;23:1343–1349.
163. Lockwood D, Otomo K, Wang Z, et al. Electrophysiologic characteristics of atrioventricular nodal reentrant tachycardia: implications for reentrant circuits. In: Zipes DP Jalife J, ed. *Cardiac electrophysiology: from cell to bedside.* 4th ed. Philadelphia, PA: Saunders, 2004:537–557.
164. Deisenhofer I, Zrenner B, Yin YH, et al. Cryoablation versus radiofrequency energy for the ablation of atrioventricular nodal reentrant tachycardia (the cyrano study): results from a large multicenter prospective randomized trial. *Circulation* 2010;122:2239–2245.
165. Padanilam BJ, Manfredi JA, Steinberg LA, et al. Differentiating junctional tachycardia and atrioventricular node re-entry tachycardia based on response to atrial extrastimulus pacing. *J Am Coll Cardiol* 2008;52: 1711–1717.
166. Fan R, Tardos JG, Almasry I, et al. Novel use of atrial overdrive pacing to rapidly differentiate junctional tachycardia from atrioventricular nodal reentrant tachycardia. *Heart Rhythm* 2011;8:840–844.
167. Hamdan M, Van Hare GF, Fisher W, et al. Selective catheter ablation of the tachycardia focus in patients with nonreentrant junctional tachycardia. *Am J Cardiol* 1996;78:1292–1297.
168. Collins KK, Van Hare GF, Kertesz NJ, et al. Pediatric nonpost-operative junctional ectopic tachycardia medical management and interventional therapies. *J Am Coll Cardiol* 2009;53:690–697.
169. Lesh MD, Van Hare GF, Epstein LM, et al. Radiofrequency catheter ablation of atrial arrhythmias. Results and mechanisms. *Circulation* 1994;89: 1074–1089.
170. Feld GK. Catheter ablation for the treatment of atrial tachycardia. *Prog Cardiovasc Dis* 1995;37:205–224.
171. Kalman JM, Olgin JE, Karch MR, et al. "Cristal tachycardias": origin of right atrial tachycardias from the crista terminalis identified by intracardiac echocardiography. *J Am Coll Cardiol* 1998;31:451–459.
172. Kalman JM, Olgin JE, Saxon LA, et al. Activation and entrainment mapping defines the tricuspid annulus as the anterior barrier in typical atrial flutter. *Circulation* 1996;94:398–406.
173. Kay GN, Chong F, Epstein AE, et al. Radiofrequency ablation for treatment of primary atrial tachycardias. *J Am Coll Cardiol* 1993;21:901–909.
174. Tracy CM, Swartz JF, Fletcher RD, et al. Radiofrequency catheter ablation of ectopic atrial tachycardia using paced activation sequence mapping. *J Am Coll Cardiol* 1993;21:910–917.
175. Lesh MD. Catheter ablation of atrial flutter and tachycardia. *Cardiac Electrophysiol* 1990:1009–1027.
176. Chen SA, Chiang CE, Yang CJ, et al. Radiofrequency catheter ablation of sustained intra-atrial reentrant tachycardia in adult patients. Identification of electrophysiological characteristics and endocardial mapping techniques. *Circulation* 1993;88:578–587.
177. Kalman JM, Olgin JE, Saxon LA, et al. Electrocardiographic and electrophysiologic characterization of atypical atrial flutter in man: use of activation and entrainment mapping and implications for catheter ablation. *J Cardiovasc Electrophysiol* 1997;8:121–144.
178. Cosio FG, Lopez-Gil M, Arribas F, et al. Mechanisms of induction of typical and reversed atrial flutter. *J Cardiovasc Electrophysiol* 1998;9:281–291.
179. Olgin JE, Kalman JM, Fitzpatrick AP, et al. Role of right atrial endocardial structures as barriers to conduction during human type I atrial flutter. Activation and entrainment mapping guided by intracardiac echocardiography. *Circulation* 1995;92:1839–1848.
180. Marine JE, Korley VJ, Obioha-Ngwu O, et al. Different patterns of interatrial conduction in clockwise and counterclockwise atrial flutter. *Circulation* 2001;104:1153–1157.
181. Poty H, Saoudi N, Nair M, et al. Radiofrequency catheter ablation of atrial flutter. Further insights into the various types of isthmus block: application to ablation during sinus rhythm. *Circulation* 1996;94:3204–3213.
182. Schwartzman D, Callans DJ, Gottlieb CD, et al. Conduction block in the inferior vena caval-tricuspid valve isthmus: association with outcome of radiofrequency ablation of type I atrial flutter. *J Am Coll Cardiol* 1996;28: 1519–1531.
183. Cosio FG, Arribas F, Lopez-Gil M, et al. Radiofrequency ablation of atrial flutter. *J Cardiovasc Electrophysiol* 1996;7:60–70.
184. Tada H, Oral H, Sticherling C, et al. Double potentials along the ablation line as a guide to radiofrequency ablation of typical atrial flutter. *J Am Coll Cardiol* 2001;38:750–755.
185. Villacastin J, Almendral J, Arenal A, et al. Usefulness of unipolar electrograms to detect isthmus block after radiofrequency ablation of typical atrial flutter. *Circulation* 2000;102:3080–3085.
186. Nakagawa H, Lazzara R, Khastgir T, et al. Role of the tricuspid annulus and the eustachian valve/ridge on atrial flutter. Relevance to catheter ablation of the septal isthmus and a new technique for rapid identification of ablation success. *Circulation* 1996;94:407–424.
187. Cheng J, Cabeen WR Jr., Scheinman MM. Right atrial flutter due to lower loop reentry: mechanism and anatomic substrates. *Circulation* 1999;99: 1700–1705.
188. Yang Y, Varma N, Keung EC, et al. Reentry within the cavotricuspid isthmus: an isthmus dependent circuit. *Pacing Clin Electrophysiol* 2005; 28:808–818.
189. Perez FJ, Schubert CM, Parvez B, et al. Long-term outcomes after catheter ablation of cavo-tricuspid isthmus dependent atrial flutter: a meta-analysis. *Circ Arrhythm Electrophysiol* 2009;2:393–401.
190. Asirvatham SJ. Correlative anatomy and electrophysiology for the interventional electrophysiologist: right atrial flutter. *J Cardiovasc Electrophysiol* 2009;20:113–122.
191. Natale A, Newby KH, Pisano E, et al. Prospective randomized comparison of antiarrhythmic therapy versus first-line radiofrequency ablation in patients with atrial flutter. *J Am Coll Cardiol* 2000;35:1898–1904.
192. Movsowitz C, Callans DJ, Schwartzman D, et al. The results of atrial flutter ablation in patients with and without a history of atrial fibrillation. *Am J Cardiol* 1996;78:93–96.
193. Jais P, Shah DC, Haissaguerre M, et al. Mapping and ablation of left atrial flutters. *Circulation* 2000;101:2928–2934.
194. Jais P, Hocini M, Hsu LF, et al. Technique and results of linear ablation at the mitral isthmus. *Circulation* 2004;110:2996–3002.
195. Shah AJ, Pascale P, Miyazaki S, et al. Prevalence and types of pitfall in the assessment of mitral isthmus linear conduction block. *Circ Arrhythm Electrophysiol* 2012;5:957–967.
196. Khan MN, Jais P, Cummings J, et al. Pulmonary-vein isolation for atrial fibrillation in patients with heart failure. *N Engl J Med* 2008;359:1778–1785.
197. Haissaguerre M, Jais P, Shah DC, et al. Spontaneous initiation of atrial fibrillation by ectopic beats originating in the pulmonary veins. *N Engl J Med* 1998;339:659–666.
198. Haissaguerre M, Jais P, Shah DC, et al. Catheter ablation of chronic atrial fibrillation targeting the reinitiating triggers. *J Cardiovasc Electrophysiol* 2000;11:2–10.
199. Jais P, Haissaguerre M, Shah DC, et al. A focal source of atrial fibrillation treated by discrete radiofrequency ablation. *Circulation* 1997;95:572–576.

200. Chen SA, Hsieh MH, Tai CT, et al. Initiation of atrial fibrillation by ectopic beats originating from the pulmonary veins: electrophysiological characteristics, pharmacological responses, and effects of radiofrequency ablation. *Circulation* 1999;100:1879–1886.
201. Lin WS, Tai CT, Hsieh MH, et al. Catheter ablation of paroxysmal atrial fibrillation initiated by non-pulmonary vein ectopy. *Circulation* 2003; 107:3176–3183.
202. Lee SH, Tai CT, Hsieh MH, et al. Predictors of non-pulmonary vein ectopic beats initiating paroxysmal atrial fibrillation: implication for catheter ablation. *J Am Coll Cardiol* 2005;46:1054–1059.
203. Elayi CS, Di Biase L, Bai R, et al. Administration of isoproterenol and adenosine to guide supplemental ablation after pulmonary vein antrum isolation. *J Cardiovasc Electrophysiol* 2013;24:1199–1206.
204. Sauer WH, Alonso C, Zado E, et al. Atrioventricular nodal reentrant tachycardia in patients referred for atrial fibrillation ablation: response to ablation that incorporates slow-pathway modification. *Circulation* 2006; 114:191–195.
205. Chen YJ, Chen SA, Chang MS, et al. Arrhythmogenic activity of cardiac muscle in pulmonary veins of the dog: implication for the genesis of atrial fibrillation. *Cardiovasc Res* 2000;48:265–273.
206. Jais P, Hocini M, Macle L, et al. Distinctive electrophysiological properties of pulmonary veins in patients with atrial fibrillation. *Circulation* 2002;106:2479–2485.
207. Kumagai K, Ogawa M, Noguchi H, et al. Electrophysiologic properties of pulmonary veins assessed using a multielectrode basket catheter. *J Am Coll Cardiol* 2004;43:2281–2289.
208. Gerstenfeld EP, Marchlinski FE. Mapping and ablation of left atrial tachycardias occurring after atrial fibrillation ablation. *Heart Rhythm* 2007;4:S65–S72.
209. Ho SY, Cabrera JA, Tran VH, et al. Architecture of the pulmonary veins: relevance to radiofrequency ablation. *Heart* 2001;86:265–270.
210. Valles E, Fan R, Roux JF, et al. Localization of atrial fibrillation triggers in patients undergoing pulmonary vein isolation: importance of the carina region. *J Am Coll Cardiol* 2008;52:1413–1420.
211. Ashar MS, Pennington J, Callans DJ, et al. Localization of arrhythmogenic triggers of atrial fibrillation. *J Cardiovasc Electrophysiol* 2000;11: 1300–1305.
212. Ouyang F, Bansch D, Ernst S, et al. Complete isolation of left atrium surrounding the pulmonary veins: new insights from the double-lasso technique in paroxysmal atrial fibrillation. *Circulation* 2004;110:2090–2096.
213. Saad EB, Marrouche NF, Saad CP, et al. Pulmonary vein stenosis after catheter ablation of atrial fibrillation: emergence of a new clinical syndrome. *Ann Intern Med* 2003;138:634–638.
214. Haissaguerre M, Shah DC, Jais P, et al. Electrophysiological breakthroughs from the left atrium to the pulmonary veins. *Circulation* 2000; 102:2463–2465.
215. Ouyang F, Antz M, Ernst S, et al. Recovered pulmonary vein conduction as a dominant factor for recurrent atrial tachyarrhythmias after complete circular isolation of the pulmonary veins: lessons from double lasso technique. *Circulation* 2005;111:127–135.
216. Essebag V, Baldessin F, Reynolds MR, et al. Non-inducibility post-pulmonary vein isolation achieving exit block predicts freedom from atrial fibrillation. *Eur Heart J* 2005;26:2550–2555.
217. Gerstenfeld EP, Dixit S, Callans D, et al. Utility of exit block for identifying electrical isolation of the pulmonary veins. *J Cardiovasc Electrophysiol* 2002;13:971–979.
218. Beldner SJ, Zado ES, Lin D, et al. Anatomic targets for nonpulmonary vein triggers: identification with intracardiac echo and magnetic mapping. *Heart Rhythm* 2004;1(Suppl):S237, abstract.
219. Sauer WH, McKernan ML, Lin D, et al. Clinical predictors and outcomes associated with acute return of pulmonary vein conduction during pulmonary vein isolation for treatment of atrial fibrillation. *Heart Rhythm* 2006;3:1024–1028.
220. Lee G, Wu H, Kalman JM, et al. Atrial fibrillation following lung transplantation: double but not single lung transplant is associated with long-term freedom from paroxysmal atrial fibrillation. *Eur Heart J* 2010;31: 2774–2782.
221. Marrouche NF, Dresing T, Cole C, et al. Circular mapping and ablation of the pulmonary vein for treatment of atrial fibrillation: impact of different catheter technologies. *J Am Coll Cardiol* 2002;40:464–474.
222. Khaykin Y, Skanes A, Champagne J, et al. A randomized controlled trial of the efficacy and safety of electroanatomic circumferential pulmonary vein ablation supplemented by ablation of complex fractionated atrial electrograms versus potential-guided pulmonary vein antrum isolation guided by intracardiac ultrasound. *Circ Arrhythm Electrophysiol* 2009;2:481–487.
223. Walters TE, Lee G, Spence S, et al. Acute atrial stretch results in conduction slowing and complex signals at the pulmonary vein to left atrial junction: insights into the mechanism of pulmonary vein arrhythmogenesis. *Circ Arrhythm Electrophysiol* 2014;7:1189–1197.
224. Voeller RK, Bailey MS, Zierer A, et al. Isolating the entire posterior left atrium improves surgical outcomes after the cox maze procedure. *J Thorac Cardiovasc Surg* 2008;135:870–877.
225. Hutchinson MD, Garcia FC, Mandel JE, et al. Efforts to enhance catheter stability improve atrial fibrillation ablation outcome. *Heart Rhythm* 2013;10:347–353.
226. Neuzil P, Reddy VY, Kautzner J, et al. Electrical reconnection after pulmonary vein isolation is contingent on contact force during initial treatment: results from the EFFICAS I study. *Circ Arrhythm Electrophysiol* 2013;6:327–333.
227. Jiang RH, Po SS, Tung R, et al. Incidence of pulmonary vein conduction recovery in patients without clinical recurrence after ablation of paroxysmal atrial fibrillation: mechanistic implications. *Heart Rhythm* 2014;11:969–976.
228. Cappato R, Negroni S, Pecora D, et al. Prospective assessment of late conduction recurrence across radiofrequency lesions producing electrical disconnection at the pulmonary vein ostium in patients with atrial fibrillation. *Circulation* 2003;108:1599–1604.
229. Pratola C, Baldo E, Notarstefano P, et al. Radiofrequency ablation of atrial fibrillation: is the persistence of all intraprocedural targets necessary for long-term maintenance of sinus rhythm? *Circulation* 2008;117: 136–143.
230. Pappone C, Rosanio S, Oreto G, et al. Circumferential radiofrequency ablation of pulmonary vein ostia: a new anatomic approach for curing atrial fibrillation. *Circulation* 2000;102:2619–2628.
231. Pappone C, Rosanio S, Augello G, et al. Mortality, morbidity, and quality of life after circumferential pulmonary vein ablation for atrial fibrillation: outcomes from a controlled nonrandomized long-term study. *J Am Coll Cardiol* 2003;42:185–197.
232. Oral H, Scharf C, Chugh A, et al. Catheter ablation for paroxysmal atrial fibrillation: segmental pulmonary vein ostial ablation versus left atrial ablation. *Circulation* 2003;108:2355–2360.
233. Karch MR, Zrenner B, Deisenhofer I, et al. Freedom from atrial tachyarrhythmias after catheter ablation of atrial fibrillation: a randomized comparison between 2 current ablation strategies. *Circulation* 2005;111: 2875–2880.
234. Pappone C, Manguso F, Vicedomini G, et al. Prevention of iatrogenic atrial tachycardia after ablation of atrial fibrillation: a prospective randomized study comparing circumferential pulmonary vein ablation with a modified approach. *Circulation* 2004;110:3036–3042.
235. Hocini M, Jais P, Sanders P, et al. Techniques, evaluation, and consequences of linear block at the left atrial roof in paroxysmal atrial fibrillation: a prospective randomized study. *Circulation* 2005;112: 3688–3696.
236. Jais P HM, Hsu LF, Sanders P, et al. Technique and results of linear ablation at the mitral isthmus. *Circulation* 2004;110(19):2996–3002.
237. Gerstenfeld EP, Callans DJ, Dixit S, et al. Mechanisms of organized left atrial tachycardias occurring after pulmonary vein isolation. *Circulation* 2004;110:1351–1357.
238. Nademanee K, McKenzie J, Kosar E, et al. A new approach for catheter ablation of atrial fibrillation: mapping of the electrophysiologic substrate. *J Am Coll Cardiol* 2004;43:2044–2053.
239. Nademanee K, Schwab MC, Kosar EM, et al. Clinical outcomes of catheter substrate ablation for high-risk patients with atrial fibrillation. *J Am Coll Cardiol* 2008;51:843–849.
240. Oral H, Chugh A, Good E, et al. Radiofrequency catheter ablation of chronic atrial fibrillation guided by complex electrograms. *Circulation* 2007;115:2606–2612.
241. Oral H, Chugh A, Good E, et al. Randomized evaluation of right atrial ablation after left atrial ablation of complex fractionated atrial electrograms for long-lasting persistent atrial fibrillation. *Circ Arrhythm Electrophysiol* 2008;1:6–13.
242. Elayi CS, Verma A, Di Biase L, et al. Ablation for longstanding permanent atrial fibrillation: results from a randomized study comparing three different strategies. *Heart Rhythm* 2008;5:1658–1664.
243. Rostock T, Rotter M, Sanders P, et al. High-density activation mapping of fractionated electrograms in the atria of patients with paroxysmal atrial fibrillation. *Heart Rhythm* 2006;3(1):27–34.

244. Narayan SM, Wright M, Derval N, et al. Classifying fractionated electrograms in human atrial fibrillation using monophasic action potentials and activation mapping: evidence for localized drivers, rate acceleration, and nonlocal signal etiologies. *Heart Rhythm* 2011;8:244–253.
245. Pappone C, Oreto G, Rosanio S, et al. Atrial electroanatomic remodeling after circumferential radiofrequency pulmonary vein ablation: efficacy of an anatomic approach in a large cohort of patients with atrial fibrillation. *Circulation* 2001;104:2539–2544.
246. Oral H, Knight BP, Tada H, et al. Pulmonary vein isolation for paroxysmal and persistent atrial fibrillation. *Circulation* 2002;105:1077–1081.
247. Lemola K, Hall B, Cheung P, et al. Mechanisms of recurrent atrial fibrillation after pulmonary vein isolation by segmental ostial ablation. *Heart Rhythm* 2004;1:197–202.
248. Nanthakumar K, Plumb VJ, Epstein AE, et al. Resumption of electrical conduction in previously isolated pulmonary veins: rationale for a different strategy? *Circulation* 2004;109:1226–1229.
249. Gerstenfeld EP, Callans DJ, Dixit S, et al. Incidence and location of focal atrial fibrillation triggers in patients undergoing repeat pulmonary vein isolation: implications for ablation strategies. *J Cardiovasc Electrophysiol* 2003;14:685–690.
250. Senatore G, Stabile G, Bertaglia E, et al. Role of transtelephonic electrocardiographic monitoring in detecting short-term arrhythmia recurrences after radiofrequency ablation in patients with atrial fibrillation. *J Am Coll Cardiol* 2005;45:873–876.
251. Vasamreddy CR, Dalal D, Dong J, et al. Symptomatic and asymptomatic atrial fibrillation in patients undergoing radiofrequency catheter ablation. *J Cardiovasc Electrophysiol* 2006;17:134–139.
252. Calkins H, Kuck KH, Cappato R, et al. 2012 HRS/EHRA/ECAS Expert Consensus Statement on Catheter and Surgical Ablation of Atrial Fibrillation: recommendations for patient selection, procedural techniques, patient management and follow-up, definitions, endpoints, and research trial design. *Europace* 2012;14:528–606.
253. Arentz T, Weber R, Burkle G, et al. Small or large isolation areas around the pulmonary veins for the treatment of atrial fibrillation? Results from a prospective randomized study. *Circulation* 2007;115:3057–3063.
254. Proietti R, Santangeli P, Di Biase L, et al. Comparative effectiveness of wide antral versus ostial pulmonary vein isolation: a systematic review and meta-analysis. *Circ Arrhythm Electrophysiol* 2014;7:39–45.
255. Brooks AG, Stiles MK, Laborderie J, et al. Outcomes of long-standing persistent atrial fibrillation ablation: a systematic review. *Heart Rhythm* 2010;7:835–846.
256. Verma A, Investigators SAIS. Optimal method and outcomes of catheter ablation of persistent af: the star af ii study. European cardiac society meetings, Barcelona. 2014.
257. Katritsis DG, Pokushalov E, Romanov A, et al. Autonomic denervation added to pulmonary vein isolation for paroxysmal atrial fibrillation: a randomized clinical trial. *J Am Coll Cardiol* 2013;62:2318–2325.
258. Mohanty S, Mohanty P, Di Biase L, et al. Long-term outcome of catheter ablation in atrial fibrillation patients with coexistent metabolic syndrome and obstructive sleep apnea: impact of repeat procedures versus lifestyle changes. *J Cardiovasc Electrophysiol* 2014;25:930–938.
259. Fein AS, Shvilkin A, Shah D, et al. Treatment of obstructive sleep apnea reduces the risk of atrial fibrillation recurrence after catheter ablation. *J Am Coll Cardiol* 2013;62:300–305.
260. Pathak RK, Middeldorp ME, Lau DH, et al. Aggressive risk factor reduction study for atrial fibrillation and implications for the outcome of ablation: the arrest-af cohort study. *J Am Coll Cardiol* 2014;64:2222–2231.
261. Coumel P, Attuel P, Lavallee J, et al. The atrial arrhythmia syndrome of vagal origin [in french]. *Arch Mal Coeur Vaiss* 1978;71:645–656.
262. Hou Y, Scherlag BJ, Lin J, et al. Ganglionated plexi modulate extrinsic cardiac autonomic nerve input: effects on sinus rate, atrioventricular conduction, refractoriness, and inducibility of atrial fibrillation. *J Am Coll Cardiol* 2007;50:61–68.
263. Lu Z, Scherlag BJ, Lin J, et al. Autonomic mechanism for initiation of rapid firing from atria and pulmonary veins: evidence by ablation of ganglionated plexi. *Cardiovasc Res* 2009;84:245–252.
264. Nakagawa H, Scherlag BJ, Patterson E, et al. Pathophysiologic basis of autonomic ganglionated plexus ablation in patients with atrial fibrillation. *Heart Rhythm* 2009;6:S26–34.
265. Patterson E, Po SS, Scherlag BJ, et al. Triggered firing in pulmonary veins initiated by in vitro autonomic nerve stimulation. *Heart Rhythm* 2005;2:624–631.
266. Po SS, Scherlag BJ, Yamanashi WS, et al. Experimental model for paroxysmal atrial fibrillation arising at the pulmonary vein-atrial junctions. *Heart Rhythm* 2006;2:201–208.
267. Pokushalov E, Romanov A, Katritsis DG, et al. Ganglionated plexus ablation vs linear ablation in patients undergoing pulmonary vein isolation for persistent/long-standing persistent atrial fibrillation: a randomized comparison. *Heart Rhythm* 2013;10:1280–1286.
268. Haissaguerre M, Hocini M, Sanders P, et al. Catheter ablation of long-lasting persistent atrial fibrillation: clinical outcome and mechanisms of subsequent arrhythmias. *J Cardiovasc Electrophysiol* 2005;16:1138–1147.
269. Haissaguerre M, Sanders P, Hocini M, et al. Catheter ablation of long-lasting persistent atrial fibrillation: critical structures for termination. *J Cardiovasc Electrophysiol* 2005;16:1125–1137.
270. O'Neill MD, Wright M, Knecht S, et al. Long-term follow-up of persistent atrial fibrillation ablation using termination as a procedural endpoint. *Eur Heart J* 2009;30:1105–1112.
271. Jais P, Matsuo S, Knecht S, et al. A deductive mapping strategy for atrial tachycardia following atrial fibrillation ablation: importance of localized reentry. *J Cardiovasc Electrophysiol* 2009;20:480–491.
272. Narayan SM, Krummen DE, Shivkumar K, et al. Treatment of atrial fibrillation by the ablation of localized sources: confirm (conventional ablation for atrial fibrillation with or without focal impulse and rotor modulation) trial. *J Am Coll Cardiol* 2012;60:628–636.
273. Narayan SM, Baykaner T, Clopton P, et al. Ablation of rotor and focal sources reduces late recurrence of atrial fibrillation compared with trigger ablation alone: extended follow-up of the confirm trial (conventional ablation for atrial fibrillation with or without focal impulse and rotor modulation). *J Am Coll Cardiol* 2014;63:1761–1768.
274. Cuculich PS, Wang Y, Lindsay BD, et al. Noninvasive characterization of epicardial activation in humans with diverse atrial fibrillation patterns. *Circulation* 2010;122:1364–1372.
275. Haissaguerre M, Hocini M, Shah AJ, et al. Noninvasive panoramic mapping of human atrial fibrillation mechanisms: a feasibility report. *J Cardiovasc Electrophysiol* 2013;24:711–717.
276. Huang DT, Monahan KM, Zimetbaum P, et al. Hybrid pharmacologic and ablative therapy: a novel and effective approach for the management of atrial fibrillation. *J Cardiovasc Electrophysiol* 1998;9:462–469.
277. Nabar A, Rodriguez LM, Timmermans C, et al. Effect of right atrial isthmus ablation on the occurrence of atrial fibrillation: observations in four patient groups having type I atrial flutter with or without associated atrial fibrillation. *Circulation* 1999;99:1441–1445.
278. Ueshima K, Hashimoto K, Chiba M, et al. Recovery of atrial function after combined treatment with surgical repair for organic heart disease and maze procedure for atrial fibrillation. *J Thorac Cardiovasc Surg* 1997; 113:214–215.
279. Chua YL, Schaff HV, Orszulak TA, et al. Outcome of mitral valve repair in patients with preoperative atrial fibrillation. Should the maze procedure be combined with mitral valvuloplasty? *J Thorac Cardiovasc Surg* 1994;107:408–415.
280. Handa N, Schaff HV, Morris JJ, et al. Outcome of valve repair and the cox maze procedure for mitral regurgitation and associated atrial fibrillation. *J Thorac Cardiovasc Surg* 1999;118:628–635.
281. Hindricks G, Mohr FW, Autschbach R, et al. Antiarrhythmic surgery for treatment of atrial fibrillation–new concepts. *Thorac Cardiovasc Surg* 1999;47(Suppl 3):365–369.
282. Kawaguchi AT, Kosakai Y, Sasako Y, et al. Risks and benefits of combined maze procedure for atrial fibrillation associated with organic heart disease. *J Am Coll Cardiol* 1996;28:985–990.
283. Weimar T, Schena S, Bailey MS, et al. The cox-maze procedure for lone atrial fibrillation: a single-center experience over 2 decades. *Circ Arrhythm Electrophysiol* 2012;5:8–14.
284. Edgerton JR, Jackman WM, Mahoney C, et al. Totally thorascopic surgical ablation of persistent af and long-standing persistent atrial fibrillation using the "dallas" lesion set. *Heart Rhythm* 2009;6:S64–S70.
285. Gehi AK, Mounsey JP, Pursell I, et al. Hybrid epicardial-endocardial ablation using a pericardioscopic technique for the treatment of atrial fibrillation. *Heart Rhythm* 2013;10:22–28.
286. Haissaguerre M, Jais P, Shah DC, et al. Right and left atrial radiofrequency catheter therapy of paroxysmal atrial fibrillation. *J Cardiovasc Electrophysiol* 1996;7:1132–1144.
287. Garg A, Finneran W, Mollerus M, et al. Right atrial compartmentalization using radiofrequency catheter ablation for management of patients with refractory atrial fibrillation. *J Cardiovasc Electrophysiol* 1999; 10:763–771.

288. Gaita F, Riccardi R, Calo L, et al. Atrial mapping and radiofrequency catheter ablation in patients with idiopathic atrial fibrillation. Electrophysiological findings and ablation results. *Circulation* 1998;97:2136–2145.
289. Oral H CA, Good E, Sankaran S, et al. A tailored approach to catheter ablation of paroxysmal atrial fibrillation. *Circulation* 2006;113(15):1824–1831.
290. Couch OA, Jr. Cardiac aneurysm with ventricular tachycardia and subsequent excision of aneurysm; case report. *Circulation* 1959;20:251–253.
291. Eldar M, Ohad DG, Goldberger JJ, et al. Transcutaneous multielectrode basket catheter for endocardial mapping and ablation of ventricular tachycardia in the pig. *Circulation* 1997;96:2430–2437.
292. Khoury DS, Taccardi B, Lux RL, et al. Reconstruction of endocardial potentials and activation sequences from intracavitary probe measurements. Localization of pacing sites and effects of myocardial structure. *Circulation* 1995;91:845–863.
293. Schilling RJ, Peters NS, Davies DW. Simultaneous endocardial mapping in the human left ventricle using a noncontact catheter: comparison of contact and reconstructed electrograms during sinus rhythm. *Circulation* 1998;98:887–898.
294. Schilling RJ, Peters NS, Davies DW. Feasibility of a noncontact catheter for endocardial mapping of human ventricular tachycardia. *Circulation* 1999;99:2543–2552.
295. Ouyang F, Fotuhi P, Ho SY, et al. Repetitive monomorphic ventricular tachycardia originating from the aortic sinus cusp: electrocardiographic characterization for guiding catheter ablation. *J Am Coll Cardiol* 2002;39:500–508.
296. Iwai S CD, Kim RJ, Markowitz SM, et al. Right and left ventricular outflow tract tachycardias: evidence for a common electrophysiologic mechanism. *J Cardiovasc Electrophysiol* 2006;17(10):1052–1058.
297. Hachiya H AK, Yamauchi Y, Harada T, et al. Electrocardiographic characteristics of left ventricular outflow tract tachycardia. *Pacing Clin Electrophysiol* 2000;23(11 Pt 2):1930–1934.
298. Daniels DV, Lu YY, Morton JB, et al. Idiopathic epicardial left ventricular tachycardia originating remote from the sinus of valsalva: electrophysiological characteristics, catheter ablation, and identification from the 12-lead electrocardiogram. *Circulation* 2006;113:1659–1666.
299. Bazan V, Gerstenfeld EP, Garcia FC, et al. Site-specific twelve-lead ECG features to identify an epicardial origin for left ventricular tachycardia in the absence of myocardial infarction. *Heart Rhythm* 2007;4:1403–1410.
300. Valles E, Bazan V, Marchlinski FE. Ecg criteria to identify epicardial ventricular tachycardia in nonischemic cardiomyopathy. *Circ Arrhythm Electrophysiol* 2010;3:63–71.
301. Gerstenfeld EP, Dixit S, Callans DJ, et al. Quantitative comparison of spontaneous and paced 12-lead electrocardiogram during right ventricular outflow tract ventricular tachycardia. *J Am Coll Cardiol* 2003;41: 2046–2053.
302. Azegami K, Wilber DJ, Arruda M, et al. Spatial resolution of pacemapping and activation mapping in patients with idiopathic right ventricular outflow tract tachycardia. *J Cardiovasc Electrophysiol* 2005;16(8): 823–829.
303. Downar E, Kimber S, Harris L, et al. Endocardial mapping of ventricular tachycardia in the intact human heart. Ii. Evidence for multiuse reentry in a functional sheet of surviving myocardium. *J Am Coll Cardiol* 1992;20:869–878.
304. Downar E, Saito J, et al. Endocardial mapping of ventricular tachycardia in the intact human ventricle. III. Evidence of multiuse reentry with spontaneous and induced block in portions of reentrant path complex. *J Am Coll Cardiol* 1995;25:1591–1600.
305. Segal OR, Chow AW, Markides V, et al. Long-term results after ablation of infarct- ventricular tachycardia. *Heart Rhythm* 2005;2:474–482.
306. Stevenson WG, Khan H, Sager P, et al. Identification of reentry circuit sites during catheter mapping and radiofrequency ablation of ventricular tachycardia late after myocardial infarction. *Circulation* 1993;88: 1647–1670.
307. Harris L, Downar E, Mickleborough L, et al. Activation sequence of ventricular tachycardia: endocardial and epicardial mapping studies in the human ventricle. *J Am Coll Cardiol* 1987;10:1040–1047.
308. Josephson ME, Horowitz LN, Farshidi A. Continuous local electrical activity. A mechanism of recurrent ventricular tachycardia. *Circulation* 1978;57:659–665.
309. Josephson ME, Wit AL. Fractionated electrical activity and continuous electrical activity: fact or artifact? *Circulation* 1984;70:529–532.
310. Miller JM, Harken AH, Hargrove WC, et al. Pattern of endocardial activation during sustained ventricular tachycardia. *J Am Coll Cardiol* 1985;6:1280–1287.
311. Hsia HH, Lin D, Sauer WH, et al. Anatomic characterization of endocardial substrate for hemodynamically stable reentrant ventricular tachycardia: identification of endocardial conducting channels. *Heart Rhythm* 2006;3:503–512.
312. de Chillou C, Lacroix D, Klug D, et al. Isthmus characteristics of reentrant ventricular tachycardia after myocardial infarction. *Circulation* 2002;105:726–731.
313. Cassidy DM, Vassallo JA, Buxton AE, et al. The value of catheter mapping during sinus rhythm to localize site of origin of ventricular tachycardia. *Circulation* 1984;69:1103–1110.
314. Cassidy DM, Vassallo JA, Miller JM, et al. Endocardial catheter mapping in patients in sinus rhythm: relationship to underlying heart disease and ventricular arrhythmias. *Circulation* 1986;73(4):645–652.
315. Kienzle MG, Miller J, Falcone RA, et al. Intraoperative endocardial mapping during sinus rhythm: relationship to site of origin of ventricular tachycardia. *Circulation* 1984;70(6):957–965.
316. Fontaine G, Guiraudon G, Frank R, et al. Intraoperative mapping and surgery for the prevention of lethal arrhythmias after myocardial infarction. *Ann N Y Acad Sci* 1982;382:396–410.
317. Borggrefe M, Podczek A, Ostermayer J, et al. Long-term results of electrophysiologically guided antitachycardia surgery in ventricular tachyarrhythmias. A report on 665 patients.*Nonpharmacological Therapy of Tachyarrhythmias*. 1987:109.
318. Marchlinski FE, Callans DJ, Gottlieb CD, et al. Linear ablation lesions for control of unmappable ventricular tachycardia in patients with ischemic and nonischemic cardiomyopathy. *Circulation* 2000;101:1288–1296.
319. Ciaccio EJ, Ashikaga H, Kaba RA, et al. Model of reentrant ventricular tachycardia based on infarct border zone geometry predicts reentrant circuit features as determined by activation mapping. *Heart Rhythm* 2007; 4:1034–1045.
320. Soejima K, Stevenson WG, Maisel WH, et al. Electrically unexcitable scar mapping based on pacing threshold for identification of the reentry circuit isthmus: feasibility for guiding ventricular tachycardia ablation. *Circulation* 2002;106:1678–1683.
321. Brunckhorst CB, Stevenson WG, Soejima K, et al. Relationship of slow conduction detected by pace-mapping to ventricular tachycardia reentry circuit sites after infarction. *J Am Coll Cardiol* 2003;41:802–809.
322. de Chillou C, Groben L, Magnin-Poull I, et al. Localizing the critical isthmus of postinfarct ventricular tachycardia: the value of pace-mapping during sinus rhythm. *Heart Rhythm* 2014;11:175–181.
323. Tung R, Mathuria N, Michowitz Y, et al. Functional pace-mapping responses for identification of targets for catheter ablation of scar-mediated ventricular tachycardia. *Circ Arrhythm Electrophysiol* 2012;5: 264–272.
324. Arenal A, del Castillo S, Gonzalez-Torrecilla E, et al. Tachycardia-related channel in the scar tissue in patients with sustained monomorphic ventricular tachycardias: influence of the voltage scar definition. *Circulation* 2004;110:2568–2574.
325. Jacobson JT, Afonso VX, Eisenman G, et al. Characterization of the infarct substrate and ventricular tachycardia circuits with noncontact unipolar mapping in a porcine model of myocardial infarction. *Heart Rhythm* 2006;3:189–197.
326. Mountantonakis SE, Park RE, Frankel DS, et al. Relationship between voltage map "channels" and the location of critical isthmus sites in patients with post-infarction cardiomyopathy and ventricular tachycardia. *J Am Coll Cardiol* 2013;61:2088–2095.
327. Tzou WS, Frankel DS, Hegeman T, et al. Core isolation of critical arrhythmia elements for treatment of multiple scar-based ventricular tachycardias. *Circ Arrhythm Electrophysiol* 2015: pii: CIRCEP.114.002310.
328. Tung R, Mathuria NS, Nagel R, et al. Impact of local ablation on interconnected channels within ventricular scar: mechanistic implications for substrate modification. *Circ Arrhythm Electrophysiol* 2013;6:1131–1138.
329. Haqqani HM, Tschabrunn CM, Betensky BP, et al. Layered activation of epicardial scar in arrhythmogenic right ventricular dysplasia: possible substrate for confined epicardial circuits. *Circ Arrhythm Electrophysiol* 2012;5:796–803.
330. Vergara P, Trevisi N, Ricco A, et al. Late potentials abolition as an additional technique for reduction of arrhythmia recurrence in scar related ventricular tachycardia ablation. *J Cardiovasc Electrophysiol* 2012;23: 621–627.
331. Jais P, Maury P, Khairy P, et al. Elimination of local abnormal ventricular activities: a new end point for substrate modification in patients with scar-related ventricular tachycardia. *Circulation* 2012;125:2184–2196.

332. Di Biase L, Santangeli P, Burkhardt DJ, et al. Endo-epicardial homogenization of the scar versus limited substrate ablation for the treatment of electrical storms in patients with ischemic cardiomyopathy. *J Am Coll Cardiol* 2012;60:132–141.
333. Wrobleski D, Houghtaling C, Josephson ME, et al. Use of electrogram characteristics during sinus rhythm to delineate the endocardial scar in a porcine model of healed myocardial infarction. *J Cardiovasc Electrophysiol* 2003;14(5):524–529.
334. Bunch TJ, Mahapatra S, Madhu Reddy Y, et al. The role of percutaneous left ventricular assist devices during ventricular tachycardia ablation. *Europace* 2012;14 (Suppl 2):ii26–ii32.
335. Reddy YM, Chinitz L, Mansour M, et al. Percutaneous left ventricular assist devices in ventricular tachycardia ablation: multicenter experience. *Circ Arrhythm Electrophysiol* 2014;7:244–250.
336. Miller MA, Dukkipati SR, Chinitz JS, et al. Percutaneous hemodynamic support with impella 2.5 during scar-related ventricular tachycardia ablation (permit 1). *Circ Arrhythm Electrophysiol* 2013;6:151–159.
337. Anter E, Hutchinson MD, Deo R, et al. Surgical ablation of refractory ventricular tachycardia in patients with nonischemic cardiomyopathy. *Circ Arrhythm Electrophysiol* 2011;4:494–500.
338. Tokuda M, Sobieszczyk P, Eisenhauer AC, et al. Transcoronary ethanol ablation for recurrent ventricular tachycardia after failed catheter ablation: an update. *Circ Arrhythm Electrophysiol* 2011;4:889–896.
339. Bourke T, Vaseghi M, Michowitz Y, et al. Neuraxial modulation for refractory ventricular arrhythmias: value of thoracic epidural anesthesia and surgical left cardiac sympathetic denervation. *Circulation* 2010; 121:2255–2262.
340. Littmann L, Svenson RH, Gallagher JJ, et al. Functional role of the epicardium in postinfarction ventricular tachycardia. Observations derived from computerized epicardial activation mapping, entrainment, and epicardial laser photoablation.*Circulation* 1991;83:1577–1591.
341. Kaltenbrunner W, Cardinal R, Dubuc M, et al. Epicardial and endocardial mapping of ventricular tachycardia in patients with myocardial infarction. Is the origin of the tachycardia always subendocardially localized? *Circulation* 1991;84:1058–1071.
342. Sarkozy A, Tokuda M, Tedrow UB, et al. Epicardial ablation of ventricular tachycardia in ischemic heart disease. *Circ Arrhythm Electrophysiol* 2013;6:1115–1122.
343. Tung R, Michowitz Y, Yu R, et al. Epicardial ablation of ventricular tachycardia: an institutional experience of safety and efficacy. *Heart Rhythm* 2013;10:490–498.
344. Rashid S, Rapacchi S, Vaseghi M, et al. Improved late gadolinium enhancement MR imaging for patients with implanted cardiac devices. *Radiology* 2014;270:269–274.
345. Sosa E, Scanavacca M, d'Avila A, Oliveira F, Ramires JA. Nonsurgical transthoracic epicardial catheter ablation to treat recurrent ventricular tachycardia occurring late after myocardial infarction. *J Am Coll Cardiol* 2000;35:1442–1449.
346. Sacher F, Roberts-Thomson K, Maury P, . Epicardial ventricular tachycardia ablation a multicenter safety study. *J Am Coll Cardiol* 2010;55: 2366–2372.
347. Morady F, Harvey M, Kalbfleisch SJ, et al. Radiofrequency catheter ablation of ventricular tachycardia in patients with coronary artery disease. *Circulation* 1993;87:363–372.
348. Kim YH, Sosa-Suarez G, Trouton TG, et al. Treatment of ventricular tachycardia by transcatheter radiofrequency ablation in patients with ischemic heart disease. *Circulation* 1994;89:1094–1102.
349. Gonska BD, Cao K, Schaumann A, et al. Catheter ablation of ventricular tachycardia in 136 patients with coronary artery disease: results and long-term follow-up. *J Am Coll Cardiol* 1994;24:1506–1514.
350. Rothman SA, Hsia HH, Cossu SF, et al. Radiofrequency catheter ablation of postinfarction ventricular tachycardia: long-term success and the significance of inducible nonclinical arrhythmias. *Circulation* 1997;96: 3499–3508.
351. Wilber DJ, Kopp DE, Glascock DN, et al. Catheter ablation of the mitral isthmus for ventricular tachycardia associated with inferior infarction. *Circulation* 1995;92:3481–3489.
352. Callans DJ, Zado E, Sarter BH, et al. Efficacy of radiofrequency catheter ablation for ventricular tachycardia in healed myocardial infarction. *Am J Cardiol* 1998;82:429–432.
353. Stevenson WG, Friedman PL, Kocovic D, et al. Radiofrequency catheter ablation of ventricular tachycardia after myocardial infarction. *Circulation* 1998;98:308–314.
354. El-Shalakany A, Hadjis T, Papageorgiou P, et al. Entrainment/mapping criteria for the prediction of termination of ventricular tachycardia by single radiofrequency lesion in patients with coronary artery disease. *Circulation* 1999;99:2283–2289.
355. Kuck KH, Schaumann A, Eckardt L, et al., VTACH study group. Catheter ablation of stable ventricular tachycardia before defibrillator implantation in patients with coronary heart disease (vtach): a multicentre randomised controlled trial. *Lancet* 2010;375:31–40.
356. Stevenson WG, Wilber DJ, Natale A, et al., Multicenter Thermocool VT Ablation Trial Investigators. Irrigated radiofrequency catheter ablation guided by electroanatomic mapping for recurrent ventricular tachycardia after myocardial infarction: the multicenter thermocool ventricular tachycardia ablation trial. *Circulation* 2008;118:2773–2782.
357. Reddy V, Reynolds M, Neuzl P. Prevention of implantable defibrillator therapy by prophylactic catheter ablation in post-myocardial infarction patients: results of the substrate mapping and ablation in sinus rhythm to halt ventricular tachycardia (smash VT) trial. *New Engl J Med* 2007;357:2657–2665.
358. Calkins H, Epstein A, Packer D, et al. Catheter ablation of ventricular tachycardia in patients with structural heart disease using cooled radiofrequency energy: results of a prospective multicenter study. Cooled RF multi center investigators group. *J Am Coll Cardiol* 2000;35:1905–1914.
359. Bogun F, Bahu M, Knight BP, et al. Comparison of effective and ineffective target sites that demonstrate concealed entrainment in patients with coronary artery disease undergoing radiofrequency ablation of ventricular tachycardia. *Circulation* 1997;95:183–190.
360. Harada T, Stevenson WG, Kocovic DZ, et al. Catheter ablation of ventricular tachycardia after myocardial infarction: relation of endocardial sinus rhythm late potentials to the reentry circuit. *J Am Coll Cardiol* 1997;30:1015–1023.
361. Oza S, Wilber DJ. Substrate-based endocardial ablation of postinfarction ventricular tachycardia. *Heart Rhythm.* 2006;3(5):607–609.
362. Hsia HH, Lin D, Sauer WH, et al. Anatomic characterization of endocardial substrate for hemodynamically stable reentrant ventricular tachycardia: identification of endocardial conducting channels. *Heart Rhythm.* 2006;3(5):503–512.
363. Marchlinski F GF, Siadatan A, Sauer W, et al. Ventricular tachycardia/ventricular fibrillation ablation in the setting of ischemic heart disease. *J Cardiovasc Electrophysiol.* 2005;16(Suppl 1):S59–S70.
364. Arenal A, Glez-Torrecilla E, Ortiz M, et al. Ablation of electrograms with an isolated, delayed component as treatment of unmappable monomorphic ventricular tachycardias in patients with structural heart disease. *J Am Coll Cardiol* 2003;41:81–92.
365. Demolin JM, Eick OJ, Munch K, et al. Soft thrombus formation in radiofrequency catheter ablation. *Pacing Clin Electrophysiol* 2002;25:1219–1222.
366. Tokuda M, Tedrow UB, Kojodjojo P, et al. Catheter ablation of ventricular tachycardia in nonischemic heart disease. *Circ Arrhythm Electrophysiol* 2012;5:992–1000.
367. Delacretaz E, Stevenson WG, Ellison KE, et al. Mapping and radiofrequency catheter ablation of the three types of sustained monomorphic ventricular tachycardia in nonischemic heart disease. *J Cardiovasc Electrophysiol* 2000;11:11–17.
368. Hsia HH, Callans DJ, Marchlinski FE. Characterization of endocardial electrophysiological substrate in patients with nonischemic cardiomyopathy and monomorphic ventricular tachycardia. *Circulation* 2003; 108:704–710.
369. d'Avila A, Splinter R, Svenson RH, et al. New perspectives on catheter-based ablation of ventricular tachycardia complicating Chagas' disease: experimental evidence of the efficacy of near infrared lasers for catheter ablation of chagas' VT. *J Interv Card Electrophysiol* 2002;7:23–38.
370. Schweikert RA, Saliba WI, Tomassoni G, et al. Percutaneous pericardial instrumentation for endo-epicardial mapping of previously failed ablations. *Circulation* 2003;108:1329–1335.
371. Soejima K, Stevenson WG, Sapp JL, et al. Endocardial and epicardial radiofrequency ablation of ventricular tachycardia associated with dilated cardiomyopathy: the importance of low-voltage scars. *J Am Coll Cardiol* 2004;43:1834–1842.
372. Cano O, Hutchinson M, Lin D, et al. Electroanatomic substrate and ablation outcome for suspected epicardial ventricular tachycardia in left ventricular nonischemic cardiomyopathy. *J Am Coll Cardiol* 2009;54: 799–808.
373. d'Avila A, Houghtaling C, Gutierrez P, et al. Catheter ablation of ventricular epicardial tissue: a comparison of standard and cooled-tip radiofrequency energy. *Circulation.* 2004;109:2363–2369.

374. Bala R, Ren JF, Hutchinson MD, et al. Assessing epicardial substrate using intracardiac echocardiography during VT ablation. *Circ Arrhythm Electrophysiol* 2011;4:667–673.
375. Hutchinson MD, Gerstenfeld EP, Desjardins B, et al. Endocardial unipolar voltage mapping to detect epicardial ventricular tachycardia substrate in patients with nonischemic left ventricular cardiomyopathy. *Circ Arrhythm Electrophysiol* 2011;4:49–55.
376. Komatsu Y, Daly M, Sacher F, et al. Endocardial ablation to eliminate epicardial arrhythmia substrate in scar-related ventricular tachycardia. *J Am Coll Cardiol* 2014;63:1416–1426.
377. Piers SR, Leong DP, van Huls van Taxis CF, et al. Outcome of ventricular tachycardia ablation in patients with nonischemic cardiomyopathy: the impact of noninducibility. *Circ Arrhythm Electrophysiol* 2013;6:513–521.
378. Dinov B, Fiedler L, Schonbauer R, et al. Outcomes in catheter ablation of ventricular tachycardia in dilated nonischemic cardiomyopathy compared with ischemic cardiomyopathy: results from the prospective heart centre of leipzig VT (help-VT) study. *Circulation* 2014;129:728–736.
379. Frankel DS, Tschabrunn CM, Cooper JM, et al. Apical ventricular tachycardia morphology in left ventricular nonischemic cardiomyopathy predicts poor transplant-free survival. *Heart Rhythm* 2013;10:621–626.
380. Haqqani HM, Tschabrunn CM, Tzou WS, et al. Isolated septal substrate for ventricular tachycardia in nonischemic dilated cardiomyopathy: incidence, characterization, and implications. *Heart Rhythm* 2011;8: 1169–1176.
381. Oloriz T, Silberbauer J, Maccabelli G, et al. Catheter ablation of ventricular arrhythmia in nonischemic cardiomyopathy: anteroseptal versus inferolateral scar sub-types. *Circ Arrhythm Electrophysiol* 2014;7:414–423.
382. Harada T, Aonuma K, Yamauchi Y, et al. Catheter ablation of ventricular tachycardia in patients with right ventricular dysplasia: identification of target sites by entrainment mapping techniques. *Pacing Clin Electrophysiol* 1998;21:2547–2550.
383. Ellison KE, Friedman PL, Ganz LI, et al. Entrainment mapping and radiofrequency catheter ablation of ventricular tachycardia in right ventricular dysplasia. *Journal of the American College of Cardiology.* 1998; 32:724–728.
384. Marchlinski FE, Zado E, Dixit S, et al. Electroanatomic substrate and outcome of catheter ablative therapy for ventricular tachycardia in setting of right ventricular cardiomyopathy. *Circulation* 2004;110(16):2293–2298.
385. Bai R, Di Biase L, Shivkumar K, et al. Ablation of ventricular arrhythmias in arrhythmogenic right ventricular dysplasia/cardiomyopathy: arrhythmia-free survival after endo-epicardial substrate based mapping and ablation. *Circ Arrhythm Electrophysiol* 2011;4:478–485.
386. Corrado D, Basso C, Leoni L, et al. Three-dimensional electroanatomic voltage mapping increases accuracy of diagnosing arrhythmogenic right ventricular cardiomyopathy/dysplasia. *Circulation* 2005;111:3042–3050.
387. Corrado D, Thiene G. Cardiac sarcoidosis mimicking arrhythmogenic right ventricular cardiomyopathy/dysplasia: the renaissance of endomyocardial biopsy? *J Cardiovasc Electrophysiol* 2009;20:477–479.
388. Dalal D, Jain R, Tandri H, et al. Long-term efficacy of catheter ablation of ventricular tachycardia in patients with arrhythmogenic right ventricular dysplasia/cardiomyopathy. *J Am Coll Cardiol* 2007;50:432–440.
389. Garcia FC, Bazan V, Zado ES, et al. Epicardial substrate and outcome with epicardial ablation of ventricular tachycardia in arrhythmogenic right ventricular cardiomyopathy/dysplasia. *Circulation* 2009;120:366–375.
390. Philips B, Madhavan S, James C, et al. Outcomes of catheter ablation of ventricular tachycardia in arrhythmogenic right ventricular dysplasia/cardiomyopathy. *Circ Arrhythm Electrophysiol* 2012;5:499–505.
391. Haissaguerre M, Shah DC, Jais P, et al. Role of purkinje conducting system in triggering of idiopathic ventricular fibrillation. *Lancet* 2002; 359:677–678.
392. Haissaguerre M, Shoda M, Jais P, et al. Mapping and ablation of idiopathic ventricular fibrillation. *Circulation* 2002;106:962–967.
393. Haissaguerre M, Extramiana F, Hocini M, et al. Mapping and ablation of ventricular fibrillation associated with long-QT and Brugada syndromes. *Circulation* 2003;108:925–928.
394. Yarlagadda RK, Iwai S, Stein KM, et al. Reversal of cardiomyopathy in patients with repetitive monomorphic ventricular ectopy originating from the right ventricular outflow tract. *Circulation* 2005;112:1092–1097.
395. Bogun F, Crawford T, Reich S, et al. Radiofrequency ablation of frequent, idiopathic premature ventricular complexes: comparison with a control group without intervention. *Heart Rhythm* 2007;4:863–867.
396. Baman TS, Lange DC, Ilg KJ, et al. Relationship between burden of premature ventricular complexes and left ventricular function. *Heart Rhythm* 2010;7:865–869.
397. Callans DJ, Menz V, Schwartzman D, et al. Repetitive monomorphic tachycardia from the left ventricular outflow tract: electrocardiographic patterns consistent with a left ventricular site of origin. *J Am Coll Cardiol* 1997;29:1023–1027.
398. Coggins DL, Lee RJ, Sweeney J, et al. Radiofrequency catheter ablation as a cure for idiopathic tachycardia of both left and right ventricular origin. *J Am Coll Cardiol* 1994;23:1333–1341.
399. Varma N, Josephson ME. Therapy of "idiopathic" ventricular tachycardia. *J Cardiovasc Electrophysiol* 1997;8:104–116.
400. Morady F, Kadish AH, DiCarlo L, et al. Long-term results of catheter ablation of idiopathic right ventricular tachycardia. *Circulation* 1990;82: 2093–2099.
401. Klein LS, Shih HT, Hackett FK, et al. Radiofrequency catheter ablation of ventricular tachycardia in patients without structural heart disease. *Circulation* 1992;85:1666–1674.
402. Dixit S, Gerstenfeld EP, Lin D, et al. Identification of distinct electrocardiographic patterns from the basal left ventricle: distinguishing medial and lateral sites of origin in patients with idiopathic ventricular tachycardia. *Heart Rhythm* 2005;2(5):485–491.
403. Betensky BP, Park RE, Marchlinski FE, et al. The v(2) transition ratio: a new electrocardiographic criterion for distinguishing left from right ventricular outflow tract tachycardia origin. *J Am Coll Cardiol* 2011;57: 2255–2262.
404. Kanagaratnam L, Tomassoni G, Schweikert R, et al. Ventricular tachycardias arising from the aortic sinus of valsalva: an under-recognized variant of left outflow tract ventricular tachycardia. *J Am Coll Cardiol* 2001;37: 1408–1414.
405. Jauregui Abularach ME, Campos B, Park KM, et al. Ablation of ventricular arrhythmias arising near the anterior epicardial veins from the left sinus of valsalva region: ecg features, anatomic distance, and outcome. *Heart Rhythm* 2012;9:865–873.
406. Klein GJ, Millman PJ, Yee R. Recurrent ventricular tachycardia responsive to verapamil. *Pacing Clin Electrophysiol* 1984;7:938–948.
407. Ohe T, Shimomura K, Aihara N, et al. Idiopathic sustained left ventricular tachycardia: clinical and electrophysiologic characteristics. *Circulation* 1988;77:560–568.
408. Lee KL, Lauer MR, Young C, et al. Spectrum of electrophysiologic and electropharmacologic characteristics of verapamil-sensitive ventricular tachycardia in patients without structural heart disease. *Am J Cardiol* 1996;77: 967–973.
409. Nakagawa H, Beckman KJ, McClelland JH, et al. Radiofrequency catheter ablation of idiopathic left ventricular tachycardia guided by a purkinje potential. *Circulation* 1993;88:2607–2617.
410. Tsuchiya T, Okumura K, Honda T, et al. Significance of late diastolic potential preceding purkinje potential in verapamil-sensitive idiopathic left ventricular tachycardia. *Circulation* 1999;99:2408–2413.
411. Sasano T, Satake S, Azegami K, et al. Diastolic potentials observed in idiopathic left ventricular tachycardia. *Jpn Circ J* 1999;63:917–923.
412. Lin D, Hsia HH, Gerstenfeld EP, et al. Idiopathic fascicular left ventricular tachycardia: linear ablation lesion strategy for noninducible or nonsustained tachycardia. *Heart Rhythm* 2005;2:934–939.
413. Ouyang F, Bänsch D, Schaumann A, et al. Catheter ablation of subeicardial ventricular tachycardia using electroanatomic mapping. *Herz.* 2003;28:591–597.
414. Tchou P, Jazayeri M, Denker S, et al. Transcatheter electrical ablation of right bundle branch. A method of treating macroreentrant ventricular tachycardia attributed to bundle branch reentry. *Circulation* 1988;78: 246–257.
415. Langberg JJ, Desai J, Dullet N, et al. Treatment of macroreentrant ventricular tachycardia with radiofrequency ablation of the right bundle branch. *Am J Cardiol* 1989;63:1010–1013.
416. Volkmann H, Kuhnert H, Dannberg G, et al. Bundle branch reentrant tachycardia treated by transvenous catheter ablation of the right bundle branch. *Pacing Clin Electrophysiol* 1989;12:258–261.
417. Crijns HJ, Smeets JL, Rodriguez LM, et al. Cure of interfascicular reentrant ventricular tachycardia by ablation of the anterior fascicle of the left bundle branch. *J Cardiovasc Electrophysiol* 1995;6:486–492.
418. Harken AH, Horowitz LN, Josephson ME. Surgical correction of recurrent sustained ventricular tachycardia following complete repair of tetralogy of Fallot. *J Thorac Cardiovasc Surg* 1980;80:779–781.
419. Gonska BD, Cao K, Raab J, et al. Radiofrequency catheter ablation of right ventricular tachycardia late after repair of congenital heart defects. *Circulation* 1996;94:1902–1908.

420. Nademanee K, Veerakul G, Chandanamattha P, et al. Prevention of ventricular fibrillation episodes in Brugada syndrome by catheter ablation over the anterior right ventricular outflow tract epicardium. *Circulation* 2011;123:1270–1279.
421. Krishnan SC, Josephson ME. Surgery for postinfarction ventricular tachycardia: is it obsolete? *Pacing Clin Electrophysiol* 2000;23:1295–1301.
422. Kelly P, Ruskin JN, Vlahakes GJ, et al. Surgical coronary revascularization in survivors of prehospital cardiac arrest: its effect on inducible ventricular arrhythmias and long-term survival. *J Am Coll Cardiol* 1990;15: 267–273.
423. Bocker D, Breithardt G, Block M, et al. Management of patients with ventricular tachyarrhythmias: does an optimal therapy exist? *Pacing Clin Electrophysiol* 1994;17:559–570.
424. de Bakker JM, van Capelle FJ, Janse MJ, et al. Reentry as a cause of ventricular tachycardia in patients with chronic ischemic heart disease: electrophysiologic and anatomic correlation. *Circulation* 1988;77:589–606.
425. de Bakker JM, Janse MJ, Van Capelle FJ, et al. Endocardial mapping by simultaneous recording of endocardial electrograms during cardiac surgery for ventricular aneurysm. *J Am Coll Cardiol* 1983;2:947–953.
426. Downar E, Harris L, Mickleborough LL, et al. Endocardial mapping of ventricular tachycardia in the intact human ventricle: evidence for reentrant mechanisms. *J Am Coll Cardiol* 1988;11:783–791.
427. Fitzgerald DM, Friday KJ, Wah JA, et al. Electrogram patterns predicting successful catheter ablation of ventricular tachycardia. *Circulation* 1988;77:806–814.
428. Miller JM, Vassallo JA, Hargrove WC, et al. Intermittent failure of local conduction during ventricular tachycardia. *Circulation* 1985;72:1286–1292.
429. Horowitz LN, Josephson ME, Harken AH. Epicardial and endocardial activation during sustained ventricular tachycardia in man. *Circulation* 1980;61:1227–1238.
430. Josephson ME, Marchlinski FE, Cassidy DM, et al. Sustained ventricular tachycardia in coronary artery disease-evidence for reentrant mechanism. *Cardiac Electrophysiology and Arrhythmias.* 1985:409.
431. Ideker RE, Smith WM, Blanchard SM, et al. The assumptions of isochronal cardiac mapping. *Pacing Clin Electrophysiol* 1989;12:456–478.
432. Kadish AH, Spear JF, Levine JH, et al. Vector mapping of myocardial activation. *Circulation* 1986;74:603–615.
433. Harada A, D'Agostino HJ, Jr., Schuessler RB, et al. Potential distribution mapping. New method for precise localization of intramural septal origin of ventricular tachycardia. *Circulation* 1988;78:III137–147.
434. Kienzle MG, Miller J, Falcone RA, et al. Intraoperative endocardial mapping during sinus rhythm: relationship to site of origin of ventricular tachycardia. *Circulation* 1984;70:957–965.
435. Josephson ME, Simson MB, Harken AH, et al. The incidence and clinical significance of epicardial late potentials in patients with recurrent sustained ventricular tachycardia and coronary artery disease. *Circulation* 1982;66:1199–1204.
436. Fontaine G, Guiraudon G, Frank R, et al. Stimulation studies in epicardial mapping of VT. Study of mechanisms and selection for surgery. *Reentrant Arrhythmias: Mechanisms and Treatment.* 1977.
437. Perlman RL, Poll D, Josephson ME, et al. Relationship of signal averaged ecg and late epicardial electrograms to inducible arrhythmias in patients with idiopathic dilated cardiomyopathy [abstract]. *Circulation* 1990;82:354.
438. Perlman RL, Miller J, Kindwall KE, et al. Abnormal epicardial and endocardial electrograms in patients with idiopathic dilated cardiomyopathy: relationship to arrhythmias [abstract]. *Circulation* 1990;82:708.
439. Guiraudon G, Fontaine G, Frank R, et al. Is the reentry concept a guide to the surgical treatment of chronic ventricular tachycardia? *Medical and Surgical Management of Tachyarrhythmias.* 1980:138.
440. Fontaine G, Guiraudon G, Frank R, et al. Correlation between late potentials in sinus rhythm and earliest activation during chronic vt. *Medical and Surgical Management of Tachyarrhythmias.* 1980:138.
441. Josephson ME, Horowitz LN, Spielman SR, et al. Comparison of endocardial catheter mapping with intraoperative mapping of ventricular tachycardia. *Circulation* 1980;61:395–404.
442. Josephson ME, Horowitz LN, Spielman SR, et al. Role of catheter mapping in the preoperative evaluation of ventricular tachycardia. *Am J Cardiol* 1982;49:207–220.
443. Downar E, Mickleborough L, Harris L, Parson I. Intraoperative electrical ablation of ventricular arrhythmias: a "closed heart" procedure. *J Am Coll Cardiol* 1987;10:1048–1059.
444. Miller JM, Gottlieb CD, Marchlinski FE, et al. Does ventricular tachycardia mapping influence the success of antiarrhythmic surgery? [abstract]. *J Am Coll Cardiol* 1988;11:112A.
445. Miller JM, Tyson GS, Hargrove WC, 3rd, et al. Effect of subendocardial resection on sinus rhythm endocardial electrogram abnormalities. *Circulation* 1995;91:2385–2391.
446. Miller JM, Hargrove WC, Marchlinski FE, et al. Electrophysiologic studies after surgery for ventricular tachycardia: what to treat? [abstract]. *Circulation* 1987;76:165.
447. Miller JM, Hargrove WC, Josephson ME. Significance of "non-clinical" ventricular arrhythmias induced following surgery for ventricular tachyarrhythmias. *Nonpharmacological Therapy of Tachyarrhythmias* 1987:133.
448. Marcus NH, Falcone RA, Harken AH, et al. Body surface late potentials: effects of endocardial resection in patients with ventricular tachycardia. *Circulation* 1984;70:632–637.
449. Kleiman RB, Miller JM, Buxton AE, et al. Prognosis following sustained ventricular tachycardia occurring early after myocardial infarction. *Am J Cardiol* 1988;62:528–533.
450. DiMarco JP, Lerman BB, Kron IL, et al. Sustained ventricular tachyarrhythmias within 2 months of acute myocardial infarction: results of medical and surgical therapy in patients resuscitated from the initial episode. *J Am Coll Cardiol* 1985;6:759–768.
451. Miller JM, Marchlinski FE, Harken AH, et al. Subendocardial resection for sustained ventricular tachycardia in the early period after acute myocardial infarction. *Am J Cardiol* 1985;55:980–984.
452. Iwa T, Misaki T, Mukai K, et al. Surgical management of non-ischemic ventricular tachycardia. *Cardiac Arrhythmias: Recent Progress in Investigation and Management* 1988:271.
453. Aizawa Y, Murata M, Satoh M, et al. Five cases of arrhythmogenic left ventricular aneurysm unrelated to coronary occlusion. *Jpn Circ J* 1986;50: 45–55.
454. Guiraudon GM, Klein GJ, Gulamhusein SS, et al. Total disconnection of the right ventricular free wall: surgical treatment of right ventricular tachycardia associated with right ventricular dysplasia. *Circulation* 1983;67: 463–470.
455. Jones DL, Guiraudon GM, Klein GJ. Total disconnection of the right ventricular free wall: physiological consequences in the dog. *Am Heart J* 1984;107:1169–1177.

# INDEX

Note: Page number followed by *f* and *t* indicates figure and table respectively.

## Q



## R